Pediatric Endocrinology

THIRD EDITION

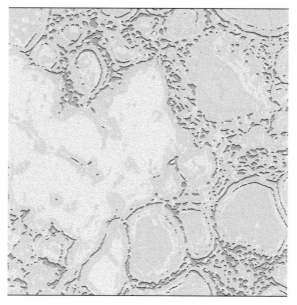

Mark A. Sperling, MD

Professor and Chair Emeritus

Department of Pediatrics

University of Pittsburgh School of Medicine

Division of Endocrinology, Metabolism, and Diabetes Mellitus

Children's Hospital of Pittsburgh

Pittsburgh, Pennsylvania

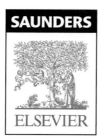

SAUNDERS

ELSEVIER

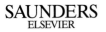

1600 John F. Kennedy Blvd.
Ste 1800
Philadelphia, PA 19103-2899

PEDIATRIC ENDOCRINOLOGY, THIRD EDITION   ISBN: 978-1-4160-4090-3

Copyright © 2008, 2002, 1996 by Saunders, an imprint of Elsevier Inc.

Notice

Knowledge and best practice in this field are constantly changing. As new research and experience broaden our knowledge, changes in practice, treatment and drug therapy may become necessary or appropriate. Readers are advised to check the most current information provided (i) on procedures featured or (ii) by the manufacturer of each product to be administered, to verify the recommended dose or formula, the method and duration of administration, and contraindications. It is the responsibility of the practitioner, relying on their own experience and knowledge of the patient, to make diagnoses, to determine dosages and the best treatment for each individual patient, and to take all appropriate safety precautions. To the fullest extent of the law, neither the Publisher nor the Editor assumes any liability for any injury and/or damage to persons or property arising out or related to any use of the material contained in this book.

The Publisher

Library of Congress Cataloging-in-Publication Data
Pediatric endocrinology / [edited by] Mark A. Sperling. — 3rd ed.
       p. ; cm.
       Includes bibliographical references and index.
       ISBN 978-1-4160-4090-3
    1. Pediatric endocrinology. I. Sperling, M.
       [DNLM: 1. Endocrine System Diseases. 2. Child. 3. Infant. WS 330
       P3712 2008]
       RJ418.P42 2008
       618.92'4—dc22

                                                            2007041424

Acquisitions Editor: Judith Fletcher
Developmental Editor: Colleen McGonigal
Project Manager: Bryan Hayward
Design Direction: Ellen Zanolle

Printed in the United States of America

Last digit is the print number: 9 8 7 6 5 4 3 2 1

To my parents, who gave and sustained my life; to my wife, Vera, "woman of valor";
and our children, Lisa and Steven, Jonathan and Shoshana, and grandchildren,
Jacob, Benjamin, Tzvi, Sydney, Rebecca, and Julian, who provide
meaning, joy, and continuity to our lives.

Foreword to the First Edition

The aim of the editor and contributors to this volume is to establish an effective bridge between the surging progress in biomedical science and the clinical practice of pediatric endocrinology. Half a century ago the biochemical elucidation of the structure and subsequent synthesis of steroid hormones provided the basis for a revolution in the diagnosis and treatment of a number of endocrine and nonendocrine disorders; that era was soon followed by a succession of fundamental discoveries: structure of peptide hormones, identification of releasing hormones from the brain, rapid and precise assay methods, and synthesis of peptide hormones by molecular biological techniques, to name but a few.

In no field has laboratory science been more effectively translated into clinical progress than in pediatric endocrinology. A glance at the roster of contributors to this volume may well provide insight into why; many who are responsible for the dramatic advances in the laboratory also pursue active clinical careers.

This volume includes many new sections that were not presented in previous texts devoted to clinical pediatric endocrinology. It will serve as a valuable reference for family physicians, internists, pediatricians, and other health professionals, covering as it does the gamut of information from basic molecular biology to practical considerations in the diagnosis and treatment of pediatric endocrine disorders.

Solomon A. Kaplan, MD

Preface

This third edition of *Pediatric Endocrinology* bears witness to the ongoing advances in this field, bringing together basic and clinical science and scientists for a deeper understanding of endocrine problems in infants and children, their diagnosis and their evidence-based treatment. No area of inquiry has been more impacted by the contribution of molecular biology, sophisticated imaging, and computer science to discover new knowledge, apply it, and manage it. There is not a single topic in this edition in which discoveries in the past five years have not occurred to provide new insights on old problems. To incorporate these comprehensive discoveries without significantly changing scope, size. and cost, it was necessary to realign some of the chapters. Hence, the chapters on "Organization and Integration of the Endocrine System" and "Imaging in Pediatric Endocrinology" have been reluctantly removed in this edition; the former is addressed in detail in more fundamental texts which approach endocrinology as the science of cell-to-cell communication via chemical messengers. In so doing, they blur previous concepts of hormones as chemical messengers produced in a single organ with specific effects on a limited number of other cell types. Instead, the newer understanding of endocrinology incorporates signal transduction cascades in various cell types in response to circulating messengers as diverse as cytokines into the family of "hormones."

The expanding horizons of sophisticated imaging could not be limited to a single chapter without compromising depth and quality; where relevant, appropriate references are provided in specific chapters, best exemplified by the use of 18-[F] L-DOPA positron emission tomography (PET) scanning to distinguish focal from diffuse hyperinsulinemia.

Taking the place of these realigned chapters is a new chapter on dyslipidemias and an expanded chapter on energy homeostasis and its disorders. These metabolic topics were deemed to be essential inclusions for this book, reflecting the importance of the epidemic of obesity and its consequences in pediatric populations throughout the developing and developed world, and the significant time commitment to management by pediatric endocrinologists. Likewise, management of dyslipidemias in children and adolescents is of increasing importance as data accumulate on the effectiveness and safety of lipid lowering agents in reversing intimal changes and delaying or preventing the consequences of atherosclerosis.

As in previous editions, the book is divided into seamless sections. First, there is an introductory section on molecular endocrinology and endocrine genetics, receptor transduction cascades, and the complexity of normal homeostasis as exemplified by the paradigm of bone mineral metabolism. Three chapters on endocrine disorders in newborns follow cover the topics of ambiguous genitalia, hypoglycemia, and abnormalities of thyroid function. These, together with calcium disorders, form the most common endocrine problems in the newborn nursery for which endocrine consultation is sought. A series of chapters on specific disorders in childhood follows, including thyroid, growth, posterior pituitary, diabetes mellitus, hypoglycemia, the adrenal cortex, pheochromocytoma and multiple endocrine neoplasias, puberty in the female, Turner syndrome, disorders of the testes, disorders of calcium and bone mineral metabolism, autoimmune polyglandular syndromes, disorders of energy balance, and lipid disorders in children and adolescents. Finally, the chapter on laboratory methods in pediatric endocrinology is included because of the importance of understanding the methodologies used in correct and appropriate interpretation of test results. Each chapter has a comprehensive bibliography, which, like all modern hard paper texts, may be somewhat out of date by the time of publication.

From an editor's point of view, it has been a pleasure to welcome new contributors from Europe and Israel to the list of recognized authorities in their respective fields; the text is enriched by their expertise and so too will be its readers.

For any oversight, omissions, or errors, we extend our apologies with request for indulgence and forgiveness from our readers. As always, we welcome your input to improve the value of this book.

Mark A. Sperling
Pittsburgh, Pennsylvania
Spring 2008

Acknowledgments

I gratefully acknowledge the contributions and support of each of the authors, who are my colleagues and friends. Our post-doctoral trainees, residents, and students provided constructive critique. Ms Kathy Wypychowski provided invaluable secretarial assistance. I thank Elsevier and their staff for their support; it has been a pleasure working with them to bring this third edition to print.

Contents

Contributors

John C. Achermann, MD
Wellcome Trust Senior Research Fellow in Clinical
   Science
Developmental Endocrinology Research Group
Clinical and Molecular Genetics Unit
UCL Institute of Child Health
University College
London, United Kingdom

Steven D. Chernausek, MD
Professor of Pediatrics
Department of Pediatrics
University of Oklahoma Health Sciences Center
Oklahoma City, Oklahoma

Pinchas Cohen, MD
Professor of Pediatrics
CMRI Edith Kinney Gaylord Chair
Director, CMRI Diabetes & Metabolic Research Center
UCLA School of Medicine
Director, Division of Endocrinology
Mattel Children's Hospital at UCLA
Los Angeles, California

David W. Cooke, MD
Associate Professor
Department of Pediatrics
Division of Pediatric Endocrinology
The Johns Hopkins University School of Medicine
Baltimore, Maryland

Sarah C. Couch, PhD, RD
Associate Professor
Department of Nutritional Sciences
University of Cincinnati
Cincinnati, Ohio

Steven Daniels, MD, PhD
Professor and Chairman
Department of Pediatrics
University of Colorado School of Medicine
The Children's Hospital
Denver, Colorado

Diva D. De León, MD
Assistant Professor of Pediatrics
Division of Endocrinology
Children's Hospital of Philadelphia
Philadelphia, Pennsylvania

Frank B. Diamond, Jr., MD
Professor of Pediatrics
University of South Florida College of Medicine
Tampa, Florida
All Children's Hospital
St. Petersburg, Florida

Charis Eng, MD, PhD
Sondra J. & Stephen R. Hardis Chair in Cancer Genomic
   Medicine
Chair and Director, Genomic Medicine Institute
Director, Center for Personalized Genetic Healthcare
Cleveland Clinic Foundation
Cleveland, Ohio

Delbert A. Fisher, MD
Professor Emeritus
Pediatrics and Medicine
David Geffen School of Medicine at UCLA
Los Angeles, California

Christa E. Flück, MD
Assistant Professor
Pediatric Endocrinology and Diabetology
University Children's Hospital Bern
Bern, Switzerland

Russel Grant, PhD
Director of Mass Spectrometry
LabCorp
Calabasas Hills, California

Annette Grueters, MD
Professor of Pediatrics and Endocrinology
Charite Children's Hospital
Humboldt University
Berlin, Germany

Michael J. Haller, MD
Assistant Professor of Pediatrics
Department of Pediatrics
University of Florida
Gainesville, Florida

Ieuan A. Hughes, MD, FRCP
Professor of Paediatrics
University of Cambridge School of Clinical Medicine
Department of Paediatrics
Addenbrooks Hospital
Cambridge, United Kingdom

Sharon J. Hyman, MD
Fellow, Pediatric Endocrinology and Diabetes
Mount Sinai School of Medicine
New York, New York

David R. Langdon, MD
Clinical Associate Professor of Pediatrics
University of Pennsylvania School of Medicine
Division of Endocrinology
The Children's Hospital of Philadelphia
Philadelphia, Pennsylvania

Peter A. Lee, MD, PhD
Professor, Department of Pediatrics
Penn State College of Medicine
Staff Attending Physician, Department of Pediatrics
MSHershey Medical Center
Hershey, Pennsylvania
Professor, Department of Pediatrics
Indiana University School of Medicine
Attending Physician, Department of Pediatrics
Riley Hospital for Children
Indianapolis, Indiana

Robert H. Lustig, MD
Professor of Clinical Pediatrics
Division of Endocrinology
Department of Pediatrics
University of California
San Francisco, California

Joseph A. Majzoub, MD
Chief, Division of Endocrinology
Children's Hospital Boston
Thomas Morgan Professor of Pediatrics
Professor of Medicine
Harvard Medical School
Boston, Massachusetts

Ram K. Menon, MD
Professor of Pediatrics
Professor of Molecular and Integrative Physiology
Director, Division of Endocrinology
Department of Pediatrics
University of Michigan Medical School
Ann Arbor, Michigan

Walter L. Miller, MD
Professor of Pediatrics
Chief of Endocrinology
University of California
San Francisco, California

Louis J. Muglia, MD, PhD
Alumni Endowed Professor of Pediatrics
Washington University Medical School
Director, Division of Pediatric Endocrinology and
    Diabetes
St. Louis Children's Hospital
St. Louis, Missouri

Sally Radovick, MD
Professor of Pediatrics
Director, Division of Pediatric Endocrinology
The Johns Hopkins University School of Medicine
Baltimore, Maryland

Robert Rapaport, MD
Emma Elizabeth Sullivan Professor
Director, Division of Pediatric Endocrinology and
    Diabetes
Mount Sinai School of Medicine
New York, New York

Alan M. Rice, MD
Assistant Professor and Division Director
Pediatric Endocrinology and Diabetes
University of Nevada School of Medicine
Las Vegas, Nevada

Scott A. Rivkees, MD
Professor and Associate Chair
Chief Section of Developmental Endocrinology and
    Biology
Department of Pediatrics
Yale University School of Medicine
New Haven, Connecticut

Allen W. Root, MD
Professor of Pediatrics
Department of Pediatrics
University of South Florida College of Medicine
Tampa, Florida
All Children's Hospital
St. Petersburg, Florida

Ron G. Rosenfeld, MD
Senior Vice-President for Medical Affairs
Lucile Packard Foundation for Children's Health
Palo Alto, California
Professor of Pediatrics
Stanford University
Stanford, California
Professor of Pediatrics
Oregon Health & Science University
Portland, Oregon

Robert L. Rosenfield, MD
Professor of Pediatrics and Medicine
The University of Chicago Pritzker School of Medicine
Section of Pediatric Endocrinology
Chicago, Illinois

Paul Saenger, MD
Professor of Pediatrics
Albert Einstein College of Medicine
Bronx, New York

Desmond A. Schatz, MD
Professor of Pediatrics
Department of Pediatrics
University of Florida
Gainesville, Florida

Mark A. Sperling, MD
Professor and Chair Emeritus
Department of Pediatrics
University of Pittsburgh School of Medicine
Division of Endocrinology, Metabolism, and Diabetes
    Mellitus
Children's Hospital of Pittsburgh
Pittsburgh, Pennsylvania

Charles A. Stanley, MD
Professor of Pediatrics
University of Pennsylvania School of Medicine
Director, Division of Endocrinology and Diabetes
Children's Hospital of Philadelphia
Philadelphia, Pennsylvania

Mark Stene, PhD
Director, Laboratory Operations
Quest Diagnostics
West Hills, California

Constantine A. Stratakis, MD, DSc
Chief, Section on Endocrinology and Genetics (SEGEN)
Director, Pediatric Endocrinology Training Program
DEB, NICHD, NIH
Bethesda, Maryland

William V. Tamborlane, MD
Professor of Pediatrics
Yale University School of Medicine
Director, Division of Endocrinology and Diabetes
Department of Pediatrics
New Haven, Connecticut

Massimo Trucco, MD
Hillman Professor of Pediatric Immunology
Head, Division of Immunogenetics
Children's Hospital of Pittsburgh
Rangos Research Center
University of Pittsburgh
Pittsburgh, Pennsylvania

Stuart A. Weinzimer, MD
Associate Professor of Pediatrics
Division of Pediatric Endocrinology and Diabetes
Yale Medical School
New Haven, Connecticut

Ram Weiss, MD
Assistant Professor of Pediatrics
Hadassah Hebrew University School of Medicine
Ein Kerem, Israel

William E. Winter, MD
Professor
Departments of Pediatrics and Pathology, Immunology,
    and Laboratory Medicine
University of Florida
Gainesville, Florida

Selma Feldman Witchel, MD
Associate Professor
Department of Pediatrics
University of Pittsburgh
Children's Hospital of Pittsburgh
Pittsburgh, Pennsylvania

Color Plates

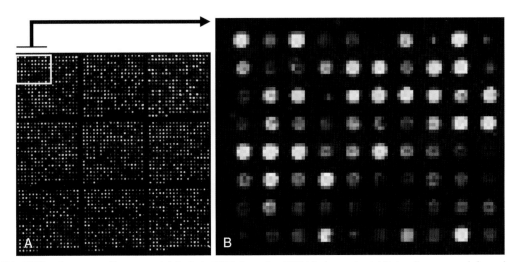

Figure 1-12. *(A)* cDNA microarray. Fluorescent labeled cDNA targets, ACTH-independent bilateral macronodular adrenal hyperplasia (Cy3), and ACTH-dependent hyperplasia (Cy5) were hybridized to glass slides containing genes involved in oncogenesis. Following laser activation of the fluorescent tags, fluorescent signals from each of the DNA "spots" are captured and subjected to analysis. *(B)* Magnified view of the microarray platform displaying the fluorescent signals: green (Cy3) and red (Cy5), with yellow representing overlap of these two colors. (see page 16.)

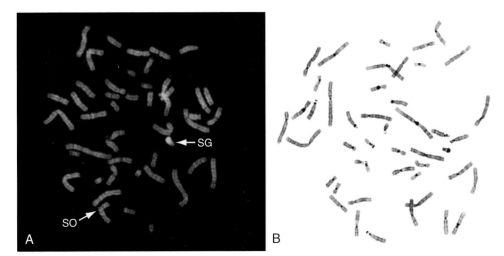

Figure 1-13. Human metaphase chromosomes. *(A)* After FISH using the chromosome-X–specific centromeric probe labeled with spectrum orange (SO) and chromosome-Y–specific heterochromatin labeled with spectrum green (SG). *(B)* With the inverted DAPI banding (similar to G-banding) allowing chromosomal identification. (see page 19.)

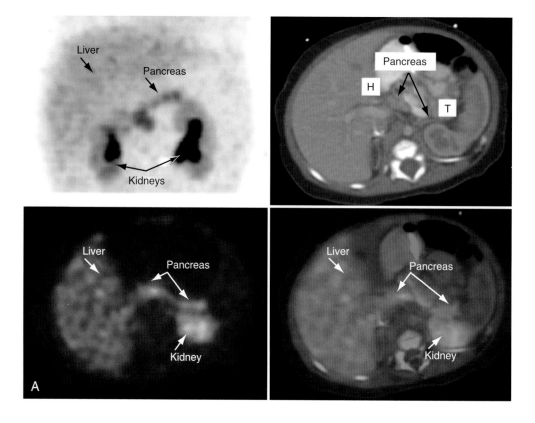

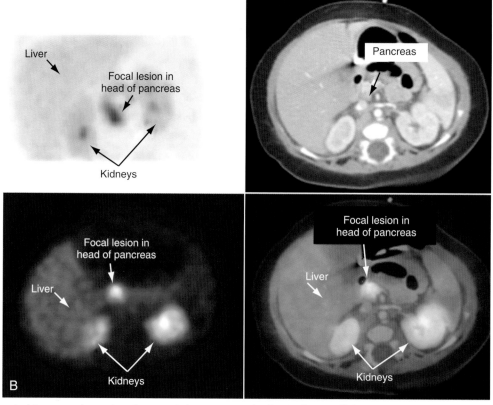

Figure 5-9. Computed tomography and positron emission tomography (CT/PET) using ^{18}Fluoro-L-Dopa. *(A)* Coregistration coronal view of a diffuse lesion and *(B)* focal lesion located in the head of the pancreas. L-DOPA uptake can be appreciated in the liver, in the kidneys, throughout the pancreas in the diffuse form *(A)* and in a focal area corresponding to the head of the pancreas *(B)*. [Used with permission from Hardy OT, Hernandez-Pampaloni M, Saffer J, et al. (2007). Diagnosis and localization of focal congenital hyperinsulinism by ^{18}F-fluorodopa PET scan. J Pediatr 150(2): 140-45.] (see pages 179-180)

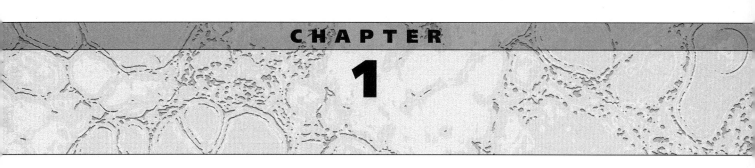

Molecular Endocrinology and Endocrine Genetics

Ram K. Menon, MD • Massimo Trucco, MD
• Constantine A. Stratakis, MD, DSc

Introduction

The study of the endocrine system has undergone a dramatic evolution in the last two decades, from the traditional physiologic studies that had dominated the field for many years to the discoveries of molecular endocrinology and endocrine genetics.[1,2] At the current time, the major impact of molecular medicine on the practice of pediatric endocrinology relates to diagnosis and genetic counseling for a wide variety of inherited endocrine disorders.

In contrast, the direct therapeutic application of this new knowledge is still in its infancy. This chapter is an introduction to basic principles of molecular biology, com-

mon laboratory techniques, and some examples of the recent advances made in clinical pediatric endocrinologic disorders—with an emphasis on endocrine genetics.

Basic Molecular Tools

ISOLATION AND DIGESTION OF DNA AND SOUTHERN BLOTTING

The human chromosome comprises a long double-stranded helical molecule of DNA associated with different nuclear proteins.[3,4] Because DNA forms the starting point of the synthesis of all protein molecules in the body, molecular techniques using DNA have proven crucial in the development of diagnostic tools for analyzing endocrine diseases. DNA can be isolated from any human tissue, including circulating white blood cells. About 200 micrograms of DNA can be obtained from 10 to 20 ml of whole blood, with the efficiency of DNA extraction being dependent on the technique used and the method of anticoagulation employed.

The extracted DNA can be stored almost indefinitely at an appropriate temperature. Furthermore, lymphocytes can be transformed with the Epstein-Barr virus to propagate indefinitely in cell culture as "immortal" cell lines—thus providing a renewable source of DNA. For performing molecular genetic studies, lymphoid lines are routinely the tissue of choice because a renewable source of DNA obviates the need to obtain further blood from the family. It should be noted that because the expression of many genes is tissue specific immortalized lymphoid cell lines cannot be used to analyze the abundance or composition of mRNA for a specific gene. Hence, studies involving mRNA necessitate the analysis of the tissue(s) expressing the gene—as outlined in the section on the analysis of RNA.

DNA is present in extremely large molecules. The smallest chromosome (chromosome 21) has about 50 million base pairs, and the entire haploid human genome is estimated to consist of 3 to 4 billion base pairs. This extreme size precludes the analysis of DNA in its native form in routine molecular biology techniques. The techniques for identification and analysis of DNA became feasible and readily accessible with the discovery of enzymes termed *restriction endonucleases*. These enzymes, originally isolated from bacteria, cut DNA into smaller sizes on the basis of specific recognition sites that vary from two to eight base pairs in length.[5,6]

The term *restriction* refers to the function of these enzymes in bacteria. A restriction endonuclease destroys foreign DNA (such as bacteriophage DNA) by cleaving the DNA at specific sites and thereby restricting the entry of foreign DNA in the bacterium. Several hundred restriction enzymes with different recognition sites are now commercially available. Because the recognition site for a given enzyme is fixed, the number and sizes of fragments generated for a particular DNA molecule remain consistent with the number of recognition sites and provide predictable patterns after separation by electrophoresis.

Analysis of the DNA fragments generated after digestion usually employs the technique of electrophoresis.[7] Electrophoresis exploits the property that the phosphate groups in the DNA molecule confer a negative charge to that molecule. Thus, when a mixture of DNA molecules of different sizes is electrophoresed through a sieve (routinely either agarose or acrylamide) the longer DNA molecules migrate more slowly relative to the shorter fragments. Following electrophoresis, the separated DNA molecules can be located by a variety of staining techniques—among which ethidium bromide staining is a commonly used method.

Although staining with ethidium bromide is a versatile technique, analysis of a few hundred base pairs of DNA in the region of interest is difficult when the DNA from all human chromosomes are cut and separated on the same gel. These limitations are circumvented by the technique of Southern blotting (named after its originator, Edward Southern) and the use of labeled radioactive (or, more commonly, nonradioactive) probes. Southern blotting involves digestion of DNA and separation by electrophoresis through agarose.[8] After electrophoresis, the DNA is transferred to a solid support (such as nitrocellulose or nylon membranes) that enables the pattern of separated DNA fragments to be replicated onto the membrane (Figure 1-1).

The DNA is then denatured (i.e., the two strands are physically separated) and fixed to the membrane, and the dried membrane is mixed with a solution containing the DNA probe. A DNA probe is a fragment of DNA that contains a nucleotide sequence specific for the gene or chromosomal region of interest. For purposes of detection, the DNA probe is labeled with an identifiable tag such as radioactive phosphorus (e.g., ^{32}P) or a chemiluminescent moiety. The latter has almost exclusively replaced radioactivity in recent years. The process of mixing the DNA probe with the denatured DNA fixed to the membrane is called hybridization, the principle being that there are only four nucleic acid bases in DNA [adenine (A), thymidine (T), guanine (G), and cytosine (C)] that always remain complementary on the two strands of DNA—A pairing with T, and G pairing with C.

Following hybridization, the membrane is washed to remove the unbound probe and exposed to an x-ray film either in a process called autoradiography to detect radioactive phosphorus or processed to detect the chemiluminescent tag. Only those fragments that are complementary and have bound to the probe containing the DNA of interest will be evident on the x-ray film, enabling analysis of the size and pattern of these fragments. As routinely performed, the technique of Southern analysis can detect a single-copy gene in as little as 5 μg of DNA (the DNA content of about 106 cells).

RESTRICTION FRAGMENT LENGTH POLYMORPHISM AND OTHER POLYMORPHIC DNA STUDIES

The number and size of DNA fragments resulting from the digestion of any particular region of DNA form a recognizable pattern. Small variations in a sequence between unrelated individuals may cause a restriction enzyme recognition site to be present or absent. This results in a variation in the number and size pattern of the DNA fragments produced by digestion with that particular enzyme. Thus, this region is said to be polymorphic for the particular enzyme tested [i.e., a restriction fragment length polymorphism (RFLP)] (Figure 1-2). The usefulness of RFLP is that it can be used as a molecular tag for tracing the inheritance of the maternal and paternal alleles.

Furthermore, the polymorphic region analyzed does not need to encode the genetic variation that is the cause of the disease being studied, but only to be located near the gene of interest. When a particular RFLP pattern can be shown to be associated with a disease, the likelihood of an offspring inheriting the disease can be determined from the offspring's RFLP pattern by comparing it with the RFLP

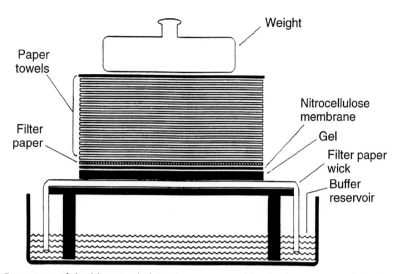

Figure 1-1. Southern blot. Fragments of double-stranded DNA are separated by size by agarose gel electrophoresis. To render the DNA single stranded (denatured), the agarose gel is soaked in an acidic solution. After neutralization of the acid, the gel is placed onto filter paper—the ends of which rest in a reservoir of concentrated salt buffer solution. A sheet of nitrocellulose membrane is placed on top of the gel and absorbent paper is stacked on top of the nitrocellulose membrane. The salt solution is drawn up through the gel by the capillary action of the filter paper wick and the absorbent paper towels. As the salt solution moves through the gel, it carries along with it the DNA fragments. Because nitrocellulose binds single-stranded DNA, the DNA fragments are deposited onto the nitrocellulose in the same pattern in which they existed in the agarose gel. The DNA fragments bound to the nitrocellulose are fixed to the membrane by heat or ultraviolet irradiation. The nitrocellulose membrane with the bound DNA can then be used for procedures such as hybridization to a labeled DNA probe. Techniques for transferring DNA to other bonding matrices, such as nylon, are similar. [Adapted from Turco E, Fritsch R, M. Trucco M (1990). Use of immunologic techniques in gene analysis. In RB Herberman, DW Mercer (eds.), *Immunodiagnosis of cancer*. New York: Marcel Dekker, 205.]

pattern of the affected or carrier parents. The major limitation of the RFLP technique is that its applicability for the analysis of any particular gene is dependent on the prior knowledge of the presence of convenient ("informative") polymorphic restriction sites that flank the gene of interest by at most a few kilobases. Because these criteria may not be fulfilled in any given case, the applicability of RFLP cannot be guaranteed for the analysis of a given gene.

In the early years of the molecular endocrinology era, the RFLP technique was the mainstay of experimental strategies employed for investigating the genetic basis of endocrine diseases. For example, RFLP-based genomic studies were used to identify mutations in the RET oncogene as the etiology of the multiple endocrine neoplasia type-2 syndrome. However, at present for routine disease mapping and whole genome and even gene-specific association studies the RFLP technique has been supplanted by more powerful and facile techniques such as microsatellite and single-nucleotide polymorphism studies (see material following). At present, RFLP analysis is only used within the context of a specific gene investigation.

POLYMERASE CHAIN REACTION

The polymerase chain reaction (PCR) is a technique that was developed in the late 1980s. It has indeed revolutionized molecular biology (Figure 1-3). PCR allows the selective logarithmic amplification of a desired fragment of DNA from a complex mixture of DNA that theoretically contains at least a single copy of the target fragment. In the typical application of this technique, some knowledge of the DNA sequences in the region to be amplified is

necessary so that a pair of specific short (approximately 18 to 25 bases in length) oligonucleotides ("primers") can be synthesized. The primers are synthesized in a manner such that they define the limits of the region to be amplified. The DNA template containing the segment to be amplified is heat denatured such that the strands are separated and then cooled to allow the primers to anneal to the respective complementary regions.

The enzyme Taq polymerase, a heat-stable enzyme originally isolated from the bacterium *Thermophilous aquaticus*, is then used to initiate synthesis (extension) of DNA. The DNA is repeatedly *denatured, annealed,* and *extended* in successive cycles in a machine called a thermocycler. This machine permits the process to be automated. In the usual assay, these repeated cycles of denaturing, annealing, and extension result in the synthesis of approximately 1 million copies of the target region in about 2 hours. To establish the veracity of the amplification process, the identity of the amplified DNA can be analyzed by electrophoresis, hybridization to RNA or DNA probes, or digestion with informative restriction enzyme(s) or can be subjected to direct DNA sequencing.

The relative simplicity combined with the power of this technique has resulted in widespread use of this procedure and has spawned a wide variety of variations and modifications that have been developed for specific applications.[9,10] From a practical point of view, the major drawback of PCR is the propensity to obtain cross-contamination of the target DNA. This drawback is the direct result of the extreme sensitivity of the method, which permits amplification from one molecule of the starting DNA template. Thus, unintended transfer of amplified sequences to items used in the

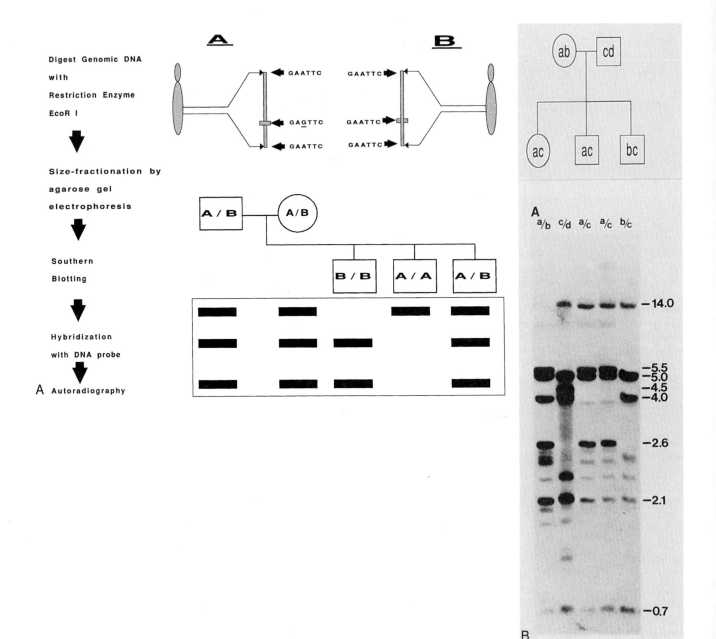

Figure 1-2. Restriction fragment length polymorphism. *(A)* Schematic illustration in which A and B represent two alleles that display a polymorphic site for the restriction enzyme EcoR I. EcoR I will cut DNA with the sequence GAATTC, and hence allele B will be cut by EcoR I at three sites to generate two fragments of DNA—whereas allele A will be cut by EcoR I only twice and not at the site (indicated by horizontal bar) where nucleotide G (underlined) replaces the nucleotide A present in allele B. Following digestion, the DNA is size fractionated by agarose gel electrophoresis and transferred to a membrane by Southern blot technique (see Figure 1-1 for details). The membrane is then hybridized with a labeled DNA probe that contains the entire sequence spanned by the three EcoR I sites. Autoradiography of the membrane will detect the size of the DNA fragments generated by the restriction enzyme digestion. In this particular illustration, both parents are heterozygous and possess both A and B alleles. Matching the pattern of the DNA bands of the offspring with that of the parents will establish the inheritance pattern of the alleles. For example, if allele A represents the abnormal allele for an autosomal recessive disease examination of the Southern blot will establish that (from left to right) the first offspring (B/B) is homozygous for the normal allele, the second offspring (A/A) homozygous for the abnormal allele, and the third offspring (A/B) a carrier. *(B)* RFLP analysis of the DQ-beta gene of the human lymphocyte antigen (HLA) locus. Genomic DNA from the members of the indicated pedigree was digested with restriction enzyme Pst I, size fractionated by agarose gel electrophoresis, and transferred to nitrocellulose membrane by Southern blot technique. The membrane was then hybridized with a cDNA probe specific for the DQ-beta gene, excess probe removed by washing at appropriate stringency, and analyzed by autoradiography. The sizes of the DNA fragments (in kilobases, kb) are indicated on the right. The pedigree chart indicates the polymorphic alleles (a, b, c, d), and the bands on the Southern blot corresponding to these alleles [a (5.5 kb), b (5.0 kb), c (14.0 kb), d (4.5 kb)] indicate the inheritance pattern of these alleles. [Adapted from Turco E, Fritsch R, Trucco M (1998). First domain encoding sequence mediates human class II beta-chain gene cross-hybridization. Immunogenetics 28:193.]

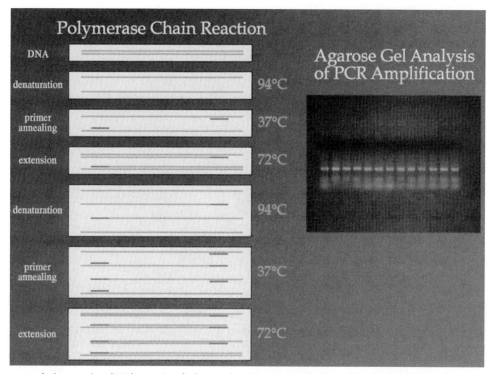

Figure 1-3. Polymerase chain reaction (PCR). A pair of oligonucleotide primers (solid red bars), complementary to sequences flanking a particular region of interest (shaded, stippled red bars), are used to guide DNA synthesis in opposite and overlapping directions. Repeated cycles of DNA denaturation, primer annealing, and DNA synthesis (primer extension) by DNA polymerase results in an exponential increase in the target DNA (i.e., the DNA sequence located between the two primers) such that this DNA segment can be amplified 1 x 106–107 times after 30 such cycles. The use of a thermostable DNA polymerase (i.e., Taq polymerase) allows for this procedure to be automated. Inset: The amplified DNA can be used for subsequent analysis (i.e., size fractionation by agarose gel electrophoresis). [Adapted from Trucco M (1992). To be or not to be ASP 57, that is the question. Diabetes Care 15:705.]

procedure will result in the amplification of DNA in samples that do not contain the target DNA sequence (i.e., a false positive result).

Cross-contamination should be suspected when amplification occurs in negative controls that did not contain the target template. One of the most common modes of cross-contamination is via aerosolization of the amplified DNA during routine laboratory procedures such as vortexing, pipetting, and manipulation of microcentrifuge tubes. Meticulous care to experimental technique, proper organization of the PCR workplace, and inclusion of appropriate controls are essential for the successful prevention of cross-contamination during PCR experiments.

In general, PCR applications are either directed toward the identification of a specific DNA sequence in a tissue or body fluid sample or are used for the production of relatively large amounts of DNA of a specific sequence—which is then used in further studies. Examples of the first type of application are very common in many fields of medicine; for example, in microbiology, wherein the PCR technique is used to detect the presence DNA sequences specific for viruses or bacteria in a biological sample. Prototypic examples of such an application in pediatric endocrinology include the use of PCR of the *SRY* gene for detection of Y chromosome material in patients with karyotypically defined Turner syndrome and for the rapid identification of chromosomal gender in cases of fetal or neonatal sexual ambiguity (Figure 1-4).[11]

Most PCR applications as research tools and for clinical use are directed toward the production of a target DNA or the complementary DNA of a target RNA sequence. The DNA that is made (amplified) is then analyzed by other techniques, such as RFLP analysis, allele-specific oligonucleotide hybridization, or DNA sequencing.

RNA ANALYSIS

The majority (>95%) of the chromosomal DNA represents non-coding sequences. These sequences harbor regulatory elements, serve as sites for alternate splicing, and are subject to methylation and other epigenetic changes that affect gene function. However, at present most disease-associated mutations in human genes have been identified in coding sequences. An alternative strategy for analyzing mutations in a given gene is to study its messenger RNA (mRNA), which is the product (via transcription) of the remaining 5% of chromosomal DNA that encodes for proteins. In addition, because the mRNA repertoire is cell and tissue specific the analysis of the mRNA sequences provides unique information about tissue-specific proteins produced in a particular organ or other tissue.

There are many techniques used in the analysis of mRNA, but one of the most commonly used methods is called Northern blotting (so named because it is based on the same principle as the Southern blot). In Northern

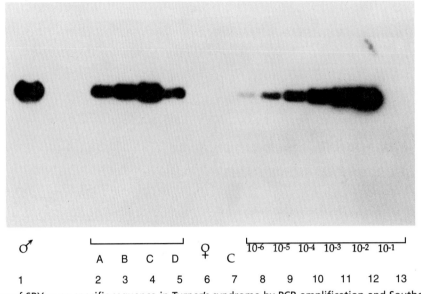

Figure 1-4. Detection of SRY-gene specific sequence in Turner's syndrome by PCR amplification and Southern blot. SRY-specific primers were used in PCR to amplify DNA from patients with 45X karyotype. The amplified DNA was size fractionated by agarose gel electrophoresis and transferred to membrane by Southern blotting. The membrane was then hybridized to labeled SRY-specific DNA and autoradiographed. From left to right: amplified male DNA (lane 1), amplified DNA from patients with 45X karyotype (lanes 2–5), amplified female DNA (lane 6), negative control with no DNA (lane 7), and serial dilution of male DNA (lanes 8–13). [Adapted from Kocova M, Siegel SF, Wenger SL, Lee PA, Trucco M (1993). Detection of Y chromosome sequence in Turner's Syndrome by Southern blot analysis of amplified DNA. Lancet 342:140.]

blotting, RNA is denatured by treating it with an agent such as formaldehyde to ensure that the RNA remains unfolded and in linear form.[12,13] The denatured RNA is then electrophoresed and transferred onto a solid support (such as nitrocellulose membrane) in a manner similar to that described for the Southern blot.[8] The membrane with the RNA molecules separated by size is probed with the gene-specific DNA probe labeled with an identifiable tag. As in the case of Southern blotting, the tag is either a radioactive label (e.g., ^{32}P) or more commonly a chemiluminescent moiety.

The nucleotide sequence of the DNA probe is complementary to the mRNA sequence of the gene and is hence called cDNA (complementary DNA). It is customary to use labeled cDNA (and not labeled mRNA) to probe Northern blots because DNA molecules are much more stable and easier to manipulate and propagate (usually in bacterial plasmids) than mRNA molecules. The Northern blot provides information regarding the amount (estimated by the intensity of the signal on autoradiography) and the size (estimated by the position of the signal on the gel in comparison to concurrently electrophoresed standards) of the specific mRNA.

Although the Northern blot technique represents a very versatile and straightforward method of analyzing mRNA, it has major drawbacks. Northern analysis is a relatively insensitive technique in terms of the concentration of mRNA that can be detected and in terms of the fine structure. Small changes in size or nucleotide composition of the mRNA being analyzed cannot be detected by this technique. Hence, for these types of specialized analyses newer methods [such as solution hybridization and reverse transcriptase-PCR (RT-PCR)] are employed.

Solution hybridization methods are based on the principle of hybridizing RNA in solution with either radioactively labeled DNA or RNA probes specific for the mRNA of interest. The main advantages of these methods are the enhanced sensitivity and the ability to yield information regarding the fine structure of the mRNA species being investigated. The enhanced sensitivity of these methods accrues from the fact that neither the mRNA being measured nor the probe being used are constrained by immobilization to a solid support, and hence do not require the additional steps of electrophoresis and transfer prior to hybridization (as in Northern blot analysis). In addition, the probe can be added in excess to drive the hybridization reaction to completion.

The two main types of solution hybridization use either single-stranded DNA (S1 nuclease protection assay) or RNA (ribonuclease protection assay) as the probe in the hybridization reaction. The greater sensitivity and the recent commercial availability of kits have propelled the popularity of the ribonuclease protection assay (RPA) as the solution hybridization method of choice for analysis of RNA (Figure 1-5). The first step in RPA is the synthesis of a radioactive single-stranded RNA probe. The RNA probe, which is complementary to the mRNA being analyzed, is synthesized by the RNA polymerase-directed transcription of a suitably engineered commercially available RNA expression vector. An excess of this synthesized RNA probe is then mixed with an aliquot of mRNA to be measured such that the RNA probe will hybridize to the complementary mRNA.

Separation of the hybridized from the free probe is achieved by exploiting the property of the enzyme RNase, which will only digest single-stranded RNA molecules.

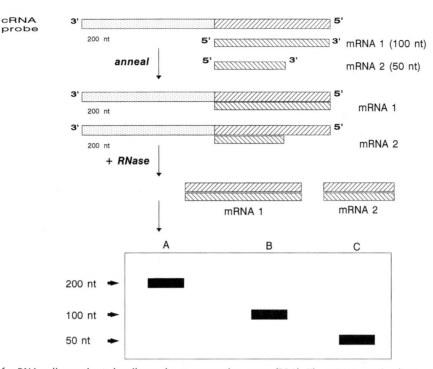

Figure 1-5. Detection of mRNA splice variants by ribonuclease protection assay (RPA). The mRNA species (100 and 50 nucleotides long) to be measured are represented by bars with cross hatches. A cRNA probe is synthesized with a region complementary to the mRNAs to be measured. This cRNA probe, which is internally labeled with ^{32}P is hybridized to the sample containing the target mRNAs. After hybridization, the unhybridized segments of the cRNA probe are digested with RNase enzyme. RNase enzyme will preferentially digest single-stranded RNA molecules and leave double-stranded RNA molecules intact. Hence, following RNase digestion RNase-resistant radioactivity will represent that segment(s) of the cRNA probe that was "protected" from RNase digestion by virtue of forming a double-stranded molecule with the target mRNA containing the complementary sequence. Following acrylamide gel electrophoresis, the RNase-resistant radioactivity is detected by autoradiography. Because the cRNA probe is always added in excess, the amount of the RNase-resistant radioactivity will be proportional to the concentration of the target mRNA. As depicted in the lower portion of the cartoon, the undigested probe (lane A) will electrophorese with a size distinct from the probe hybridized to mRNA 1 (lane B) or mRNA 2 (lane C).

Double-stranded RNA (such as that formed by the hybridization of the probe with the complementary RNA) is relatively resistant to digestion by RNase (such as RNase T1 or A). The RNase-resistant radioactive material is then size fractionated by electrophoresis and the double-stranded RNA molecules detected by autoradiography.

Because RNase is very discriminatory with respect to its ability to digest single-stranded RNA, while permitting double-stranded RNA to remain intact, even a single mismatch in the nucleotide sequence between the probe and the measured RNA will result in the probe RNA being digested at that point of mismatch (because the RNA will be single stranded at that point) and the appearance of additional radioactive bands after RNase digestion. Thus, this method is very useful for the detection and quantitation of internal splice variants wherein significant changes in one splice variant may be masked by the unchanged combined level of all mRNA variants analyzed by techniques such as Northern analysis. The major disadvantage of RPA is that it requires some prior knowledge of the RNA structure for the design of appropriate RNA probes.

One of the most sensitive methods for the detection and quantitation of mRNA currently available is the technique of quantitative RT-PCR (qRT-PCR).[9] This technique combines the unique function of the enzyme reverse tran-

scriptase with the power of PCR. qRT-PCR is exquisitely sensitive, permitting analysis of gene expression from very small amounts of RNA. Furthermore, this technique can be applied to a large number of samples and/or many genes (multiplex) in the same experiment. These two critical features endow this technique with a measure of flexibility unavailable in more traditional methods, such as Northern blot or solution hybridization analysis.

Whereas the detection of a specific mRNA by this technique is relatively straightforward, the precise quantitation of the mRNA in a given sample is more complicated. The first step in qRT-PCR analysis is the production of cDNA to the mRNA of interest. This is done by using the enzymes with RNA-dependent DNA polymerase activity that belong to the reverse transcriptase (RT) group of enzymes [e.g., Moloney murine leukemia virus (MMLV), avian myeloblastosis virus (AMV) reverse transcriptase, or an RNA-dependent DNA polymerase].

The RT enzyme, in the presence of an appropriate primer, will synthesize DNA complementary to RNA. The second step in the qRT-PCR analysis is the amplification of the target DNA, in this case the cDNA synthesized by the reverse transcriptase enzyme. The specificity of the amplification is determined by the specificity of the primer pair used for the PCR amplification. To establish the veracity of the amplification process, the identity of the amplified DNA can be analyzed by electrophoresis, hybridization to RNA or DNA probes, digestion with informative restriction enzyme(s), or subjection to direct DNA sequencing.

Whereas the detection of a specific mRNA by this technique is relatively straightforward, the precise quantitation of the mRNA in a given sample is more complicated. Because the production of DNA by PCR involves an exponential increase in the amount of DNA synthesized, relatively minor differences in any of the variables controlling the rate of amplification will cause a marked difference in the yield of the amplified DNA. In addition to the amount of template DNA, the variables that can affect the yield of the PCR include the concentration of the polymerase enzyme, magnesium, nucleotides (dNTPs), and primers. The specifics of the amplification procedure (including cycle length, cycle number, annealing, extension, and denaturing temperatures) also affect the yield of DNA.

Because of the multitude of variables involved, routine RT-PCR is unsuitable for performing a quantitative analysis of mRNA. To circumvent these pitfalls, alternative strategies have been developed. One technique for determining the concentration of a particular mRNA in a biological sample is a modification of the basic PCR technique called competitive RT-PCR.[9,14,15] This method is based on the co-amplification of a mutant DNA that can be amplified with the same pair of primers being used for the target DNA. The mutant DNA is engineered in such a way that it can be distinguished from the DNA of interest by size or by the inclusion of a restriction enzyme site unique to the mutant DNA.

The addition of equivalent amounts of this mutant DNA to all PCR reaction tubes serves as an internal control for the efficiency of the PCR process, and the yield of the mutant DNA in the various tubes can be used for the equalization of the yield of the DNA by PCR. It is important to ensure for accurate quantitation of the DNA of interest that the concentrations of the mutant and target template are nearly equivalent. Because the use of mutated DNA for normalization does not account for the variability in the efficiency of the reverse transcriptase enzyme, a variation of the original method has been developed.

In this modification, competitive mutated RNA transcribed from a suitably engineered RNA expression vector is substituted for the mutant DNA in the reaction prior to initiating the synthesis of the cDNA. Competitive RT-PCR can be used to detect changes of the order of two- to threefold of even very rare mRNA species. The major drawback of this method is the propensity to derive inaccurate results due to contamination of samples with the mRNA of interest. In theory, because the technique is based on PCR contamination by even one molecule of mRNA of interest can invalidate the results. Hence, scrupulous attention to laboratory technique and setup is essential for the successful application of this technique.

In general, there are two types of methods used for detection and quantitation of PCR products: the traditional "endpoint" measurements of products and the newer "real-time" techniques. Endpoint determinations (e.g., the competitive RT-PCR technique described previously) analyze the reaction after it is completed, whereas real-time determinations are made during the progression of the amplification process. Overall, the real-time approach is more accurate and is currently the preferred method. Advances in fluorescence detection technologies have made real-time measurement possible for routine use in the laboratory. One of the popular techniques that takes advantage of real-time measurements is the TaqMan (fluorescent 5'-nuclease) assay (Figure 1-6).[16,17]

The unique design of TaqMan probes, combined with the 5'-nuclease activity of the PCR enzyme (Taq polymerase), allows direct detection of PCR product by the release of fluorescent reporter during the PCR amplification by using specially designed machines (ABI Prism 5700/7700). The TaqMan probe consists of an oligonucleotide synthesized with a 5'-reporter dye (e.g., FAM; 6-carboxy-fluorescein) and a downstream 3'-quencher dye (e.g., TAMRA; 6-carboxy-tertamethyl-rhodamine). When the probe is intact, the proximity of the reporter dye to the quencher dye results in suppression of the reporter fluorescence primarily by Forster-type energy transfer. During PCR, forward and reverse primers hybridize to a specific sequence of the target DNA.

The TaqMan probe hybridizes to a target sequence within the PCR product. Because of its 5'- to 3'-nuclease activity, the Taq polymerase enzyme subsequently cleaves the TaqMan probe. The reporter dye and the quencher dye are separated by cleavage, resulting in increased laser-stimulated fluorescence of the reporter dye as a direct consequence of target amplification during PCR. This process occurs in every cycle and does not interfere with the exponential accumulation of product. Both primer and probe must hybridize to the target for amplification and cleavage to occur. The fluorescence signal is generated only if the target sequence for the probe is amplified during PCR.

Because of these stringent requirements, nonspecific amplification is not detected. Fluorescent detection takes place through fiber-optic lines positioned above optically nondistorting tube caps. Quantitative data are derived from a determination of the cycle at which the amplification product signal crosses a preset detection threshold. This cycle number is proportional to the amount of starting material, thus allowing for a measurement of the level of specific mRNA in the sample. An alternative machine (Light Cycler) also uses fluorogenic hydrolysis or fluorogenic hybridization probes for quantification in a manner similar to the ABI system.

Detection of Mutations in Genes

Changes in the structural organization of a gene that impact its function involve deletions, insertions, or transpositions of relatively large stretches of DNA—or more frequently single-base substitutions in functionally critical regions. The deletion or insertion of large stretches of DNA can usually be detected by Southern blotting and RFLP analysis. However, these analytic methods can be used for detecting point mutations only if the mutation

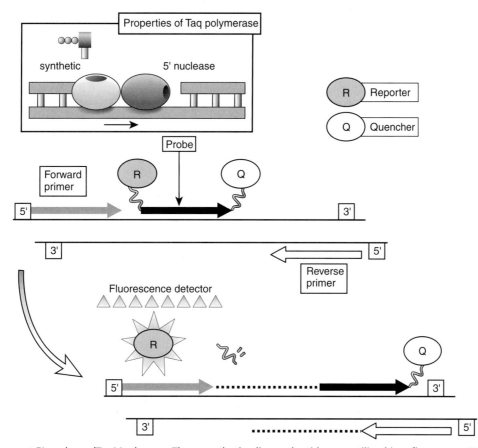

Figure 1-6. Fluorescent 5'-nuclease (TaqMan) assay. Three synthetic oligonucleotides are utilized in a fluorescent 5'-nuclease assay. Two oligonucleotides function as "forward" and "reverse" primers in a conventional PCR amplification protocol. The third oligonucleotide, termed the TaqMan probe, consists of an oligonucleotide synthesized with a 5'-reporter dye (e.g., FAM; 6-carboxy-fluorescein) and a downstream 3'-quencher dye (e.g., TAMRA; 6-carboxy-tertamethyl-rhodamine). When the probe is intact, the proximity of the reporter dye to the quencher dye results in suppression of the reporter fluorescence—primarily by Forster-type energy transfer. During PCR, forward and reverse primers hybridize to a specific sequence of the target DNA. The TaqMan probe hybridizes to a target sequence within the PCR product. Because of its 5'- to 3'-exonuclease activity, the Taq polymerase enzyme subsequently cleaves the TaqMan probe. The reporter dye and the quencher dye are separated by cleavage, resulting in increased fluorescence of the reporter dye as a direct consequence of target amplification during PCR. Both primers and probe must hybridize to the target for amplification and cleavage to occur. Hence, the fluorescence signal is generated only if the target sequence for the probe is amplified during PCR. Fluorescent detection takes place through fiber-optic lines positioned above the caps of the reaction wells. Inset: The two distinct functions of the enzyme Taq polymerase: the 5'-3' synthetic polymerase activity and the 5'-3' polymerase-dependent exonuclease activity.

involves the recognition site for a particular restriction enzyme such that the absence of a normally present restriction site or the appearance of a novel site unmasks the presence of the point mutation. More commonly, these techniques cannot be used for such an analysis—necessitating alternative procedures.

DIRECT METHODS

DNA sequencing is the current gold standard for obtaining unequivocal proof of a point mutation. However, DNA sequencing has its limitations and drawbacks. A clinically relevant problem is that current DNA sequencing methods do not reliably and consistently detect all mutations. For example, in many cases where the mutation affects only one allele (heterozygous) the heights of the peaks of the bases on the fluorescent readout corresponding to the wild-type and mutant allele are not always present in the predicted (1:1) ratio. This limits the

discerning power of "base-calling" computer protocols and results in inconsistent and/or erroneous assignment of DNA sequence to individual alleles.[18]

Because of this limitation, clinical laboratories routinely determine the DNA sequence of both alleles to provide independent confirmation of the absence/presence of a putative mutation. DNA sequencing can be labor intensive and expensive, although recent advances in pyrosequencing (see material following) have made it technically easier and cheaper.

Although the first DNA sequences were determined with a method that chemically cleaved the DNA at each of the four nucleotides,[19] the enzymatic or dideoxy method developed by Sanger et al. in 1977 is the one most commonly used for routine purposes (Figure 1-7).[20] This method uses the enzyme DNA polymerase to synthesize a complementary copy of the single-stranded DNA ("template") whose sequence is being determined. Single-stranded DNA can be obtained directly from viral

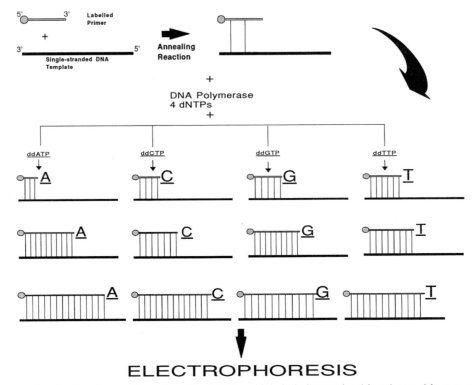

Figure 1-7. DNA sequencing by the dideoxy (Sanger) method. A 5′-end-labeled oligonucleotide primer with sequence complementarity to the DNA to be sequenced (DNA template) is annealed to a single strand of the template DNA. This primer is elongated by DNA synthesis initiated by the addition of the enzyme DNA polymerase in the presence of the four dNTPs (2′-deoxynucleoside triphosphates) and one of the ddNTPs (2′,3′-dideoxynucleoside triphosphates). Four such reaction tubes are assembled to use all four ddNTPs. The DNA polymerase enzyme will elongate the primer using the dNTPs and the individual ddNTP present in that particular tube. Because ddNTPs are devoid of 3′-hydroxyl group, no elongation of the chain is possible when such a residue is added to the chain. Thus, each reaction tube will contain prematurely terminated chains ending at the occurrence of the particular ddNTP present in the reaction tube. The concentrations of the dNTPs and the individual ddNTP present in the reaction tubes are adjusted so that the chain termination occurs at every occurrence of the ddNTP. Following the chain elongation-termination reaction, the DNA strands synthesized are size separated by acrylamide gel electrophoresis and the bands visualized by autoradiography.

or plasmid vectors that support the generation of single-stranded DNA or by partial denaturing of double-stranded DNA by treatment with alkali or heat.[21]

The enzyme DNA polymerase cannot initiate synthesis of a DNA chain de novo but can only extend a fragment of DNA. Hence, the second requirement for the dideoxy method of sequencing is the presence of a primer. A primer is a synthetic oligonucleotide 15 to 30 bases long, whose sequence is complementary to the sequence of the short corresponding segment of the single-stranded DNA template. The dideoxy method exploits the observation that DNA polymerase can use both 2′-deoxynucleoside triphosphate (dNTP) and 2′,3′-dideoxynucleoside triphosphates (ddNTPs) as substrates during elongation of the primer. Whereas DNA polymerase can use dNTP for continued synthesis of the complementary strand of DNA, the chain cannot elongate any further after addition of the first ddNTP because ddNTPs lack the crucial 3′-hydroxyl group.

To identify the nucleotide at the end of the chain, four reactions are carried out for each sequence analysis—with only one of the four possible ddNTPs included in any one reaction. The ratio of the ddNTP and dNTP in each reaction is adjusted so that these chain terminations occur at each of the positions in the template where the

nucleotide occurs. To enable detection by autoradiography, the newly synthesized DNA is labeled—usually by including in the reaction mixture radioactively labeled dATP (for the older manual methods) or, most commonly, currently fluorescent dye terminators in the reaction mixture (now in use in automated techniques). The separation of the newly synthesized DNA strands manually is done via high resolution denaturing polyacrylamide electrophoresis or with capillary electrophoresis in automatic sequencers.

Fluorescent detection methods have enabled automation and enhanced throughput. In capillary electrophoresis, DNA molecules are driven to migrate through a viscous polymer by a high electric field to be separated on the basis of charge and size. Although this technique is based on the same principle as identical to that used in slab gel electrophoresis, the separation is done in individual glass capillaries rather than gel slabs—facilitating loading of samples and other aspects of automation. Whereas manual methods allow the detection of about 300 nucleotide of sequence information with one set of sequencing reactions, automated methods using florescent dyes and laser technology can analyze 7,500 or more bases per reaction. To sequence larger stretches of DNA, it is necessary to divide the large piece of DNA into smaller fragments that can be individually sequenced. Alternatively, additional sequencing primers can be chosen near the end of the previous sequencing results—allowing the initiation point of new sequence data to be progressively moved along the larger DNA fragment.

One of the seminal technological advances in recent years has been the introduction of microarray-based methods for detection, and analysis of nucleic acids (see material following). For purposes of detection of mutations, the oligonucleotides fixed to the slide/membrane are complementary to all possible base substitutions or a subset of small deletions and insertions. Fluorescent labeled PCR probes derived from the patient and representing the genes to be tested are then hybridized to the microarrays. Following appropriate washing protocols, the retention of particular probes on the slide provide information regarding the presence/absence of a given mutation, deletion, or insertion.

There are limitations of microarray-based techniques. For example, similar to direct DNA sequencing methods microarray-based methods also suffer from the disadvantage of not being able to reliably or consistently detect heterozygous mutations. In addition, microarrays cannot be used to detect insertions of multiple nucleotides without exponentially increasing the number of oligonucleotides that must be immobilized on the glass slides.

The most exciting new technique in mutation identification is pyrosequencing. This is based on an enzymatic real-time monitoring of DNA synthesis by bioluminescence. This "read as you go" method uses nucleotide incorporation that leads to a detectable light signal from the pyrophosphate released when a nucleotide is introduced in the DNA strand.[22] The rapidity and reliability of this method far exceed other contemporary DNA sequencing techniques. However, the major limitation of this technique is that it can only be used to analyze short stretches of DNA sequence.

INDIRECT METHODS

Screening for mutations of the thousands of the sequence products provided by human genome analysis has proven to be a daunting task. Although the gold standard for identifying sequence alterations is direct sequencing, this method remains labor intensive and the least cost effective. Since the mid 1980s, the need for rapid, high-throughput, accurate, and economical mutation analysis systems has led to the development of several technologies as alternatives to analysis by direct sequencing that have allowed detection of single mutations in long stretches of DNA (200–600 bp). These techniques include restriction endonuclease digestion of PCR products (PCR-RFLP), denaturing gradient gel electrophoresis (DGGE), single-strand conformation polymorphism (SSCP), dideoxy fingerprinting (ddF), and heteroduplex mobility assay (HMA).

Most of these methods utilize PCR to amplify a region of the DNA, a physical or chemical treatment of amplified DNA (by restriction digestion or denaturation), separation of the amplicons by gel electrophoresis (by denaturing or nondenaturing), and visualization of the separated sequence strands (by autoradiography or fluorescence-based detection). Most recent modifications in some of these techniques allow simultaneous separation and detection of DNA fragments with the use of sophisticated equipment such HPLC and capillary electrophoresis.

Originally described in 1989, SSCP analysis has been a widely used method for the detection of mutations because of its simplicity and efficiency. In SSCP, DNA regions with potential mutations are first amplified by PCR in the presence of a radiolabeled dNTP (Figures 1-8 and 1-9). Single-stranded DNA fragments are then generated by denaturation of the PCR products and separated on a native polyacrylamide gel. As the denatured PCR product moves through the gel and away from the denaturant, it will regain a secondary structure that is sequence dependent. The electrophoretic migration of single-stranded DNA is a function of its secondary structure. Therefore, PCR products that contain substitution differences (as well as insertions and deletions) will have different mobility when compared with wild-type DNA.

Although SSCP is simple, rapid, and inexpensive, it also has some disadvantages. The major limitations of the technique are lack of sensitivity and the inability to provide information about the location of a mutation in a DNA fragment. Efficacy studies, in which the technique was evaluated against a known mutation, showed that the sensitivity of SSCP can be highly variable in identifying sequence alterations. This variability is seen not only between amplicons but within the same amplicon if examined under different conditions. Overall, SSCP detects previously identified sequence changes in as many as 90% and as little as 60% of the specimens—depending primarily on the sequence, the amplicon's size, and the location of the mutation.

To circumvent the disadvantages of SSCP, an alternative technique was proposed that became known as dideoxy-fingerprinting (ddF). ddF is essentially a hybrid of SSCP and dideoxy sequencing in which primer extension products are generated in the presence of one dideoxynucleotide and subjected to chemical denaturation and electrophoresis on a nondenaturing polyacrylamide gel to exploit differences in secondary structure of single-stranded conformers. The resulting electrophoretic pattern resembles sequencing gels in which the mobility of extension products is determined by both size and conformation. In ddF, single-base and other sequence changes may result in elimination of a normal band or appearance of an extra band (informative dideoxy component) and altered electrophoretic mobility of one or more sequence termination products (informative SSCP component). The intensity of bands may also be used for dosage analysis because detection of "half loss" would indicate heterozygous mutation.

There are three major advantages of ddF over conventional SSCP: the relative position of a mutation may be revealed due to addition or deletion of a dideoxy termination product; the sensitivity is increased because, unlike SSCP, there are multiple bands that exhibit altered mobility (making it unlikely that a mutation will be missed because the technique is based on the same extension principle as dideoxy sequencing, in which multiple DNA strands are generated that contain the sequence change); and it permits large PCR

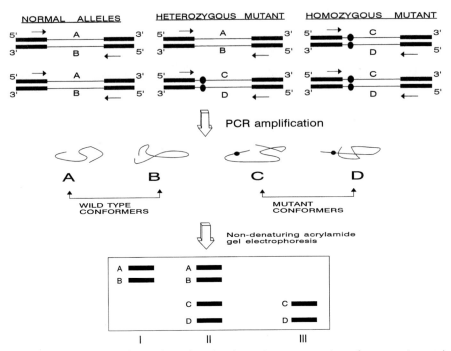

Figure 1-8. Single-stranded conformational polymorphism (SSCP). Schematic representation of an experiment designed to use SSCP to detect the presence of heterozygous and homozygous single–base-pair mutation (represented as a filled circle). The segment of DNA is amplified using PCR with flanking primers (represented by arrows). [32]P is incorporated into the newly synthesized DNA by end labeling the primers or by the addition of ^{32}P-dATP to the PCR reaction. Theoretically, four different types of conformers can be formed: A and B from the sense and anti-sense strand of the wild-type (normal) DNA, and C and D from the sense and anti-sense strands containing the single–base-pair mutation. Following PCR, the DNA is denatured and analyzed by nondenaturing gel electrophoresis. Lane I represents the wild-type conformers, lane II represents the wild-type and mutant conformers from an heterozygous patient, and lane III represents the presence of mutant conformers with the absence of wild-type conformers from a homozygous patient.

fragments to be generated only once and analyzed in smaller subfragments using different primers. The originally described ddF could screen the same size of DNA as SSCP (250-350 bp), but with a significantly higher level of detection.

In recent years, modifications of the original procedure have resulted in new and improved variants of ddF. Bidirectional ddF (bi-ddF), in which the dideoxy termination reaction is performed simultaneously with two opposing primers, has allowed larger fragments (~600 bp) to be screened with almost 100% sensitivity. RNA ddF (R-ddF), in which RNA is used as starting material, enables identification of mutations that result in splicing errors and allows screening of genes with large intronic regions. Denaturing fingerprinting (DnF), a modification of bi-ddF in which fingerprints are generated by performing denaturing gel electrophoresis on bidirectional "cycle-sequencing" reactions with each of two dideoxy terminators, has allowed screening of DNA regions with high GC content—avoiding the generation of "smearing" bands and thus increasing the sensitivity of the technique in identifying heterozygous mutations.

Further modifications have streamlined the previously cited procedures by adapting them to either automated fluorescent sequencers or capillary electrophoresis utilizing fluorescent dNTPs or primers (automated bi-ddf, capillary electrophoresis-ddf). Automated fingerprinting technology allows simultaneous analysis of a larger number of samples, higher reproducibility, faster data pro-

cessing, and the ability to analyze longer sequences from a single reaction.

DGGE is a method used to detect single-base pair substitutions (or small insertions or deletions) in genes.[23-25] Like SSCP, DGGE is also a PCR-based method and exploits the observation that when double-stranded DNA migrates through a polyacrylamide gel incorporating a gradient of chemical denaturing agents the mobility of the partially denatured ("melted") DNA molecule is extremely sensitive to its base composition. Thus, even single-base changes in the nucleotide composition of the DNA will result in altered mobility of the partially denatured DNA. G-C clamp is a modified DGGE procedure wherein the sensitivity of the procedure is enhanced by the incorporation of a G- and C-rich region at one end of the DNA.[24,26-28]

This manipulation is most readily done by modifying one of the primers used for the PCR. The addition of the G-C–rich region increases the melting point of the DNA fragment and makes it easier to detect changes in the nucleotide composition. Depending on the relative orientation of the chemical gradient and the electrical field during electrophoresis, DGGE could be parallel or perpendicular. The relative sensitivity of these two protocols has to be determined empirically for each application of this method. Denaturing high-performance liquid chromatography (DHPLC) is a related technique that detects a variation in the DNA sequence but uses HPLC instead of gel electrophoresis for separation of DNA

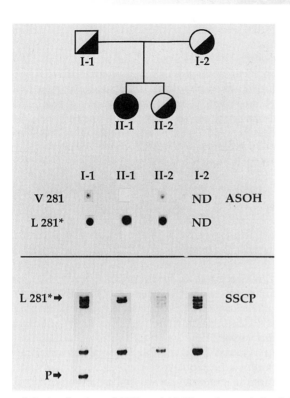

Figure 1-9. Application of SSCP and ASOH to the analysis of the 21-hydroxylase gene in congenital adrenal hyperplasia. Detection of a mutation of codon 281 from valine to leucine (V281L). Upper panel: Pedigree of a family with proband II-1, which was referred for evaluation of hirsutism and secondary amenorrhoea. Middle panel: ASOH results from both mutant and normal alleles at codon 281 show both the father and sister of the proband to be carriers of the V281L mutation, whereas the patient is homozygous. ASOH was not performed on the mother. The asterisk indicated the mutant allele (L281). Lower panel: SSCP analysis revealed that the two additional conformers, representing the L281 conformer, were detected at the top of the gel in this patient and her family. The greater intensity of the conformers in the proband compared to her family members and the disappearance of the normal V281 conformer (adjacent to the L281 conformers) are consistent with her being homozygous for this mutation. L281 indicates the mutant conformer. P indicates normal polymorphism. [Adapted from Siegel SF, Hoffman EP, Trucco M (1994). Molecular diagnosis of 21-hydroxylase deficiency: Detection of four mutations on a single gel. Biochem Med Metab Biol 51:66.]

fragments. The incorporation of HPLC allows for automation of this technique and significantly enhances throughput by this method.

Heteroduplex analysis is a variation of the SSCP method and is used to detect single-pair mismatches in double-stranded DNA.[29-31] When polymorphic PCR products are denatured and allowed to slowly cool to 37° C before being loaded onto a native gel, some of the polymorphic strands will reanneal to the slightly different complementary strand and form a double-stranded DNA molecule with a small number of mismatches (i.e., a heteroduplex). During electrophoresis, heteroduplexes migrate more slowly than homoduplexes and the resulting pattern can be visualized after autoradiography.

Although heteroduplex analysis would not detect abnormal sequences in a homozygous individual, it is pos-

sible to combine known DNAs with the DNA being tested to form the heteroduplexes and reveal the presence of the variant allele. Because of the technical similarity of the SSCP and heteroduplex analyses, the choice between the two methods can be dependent on which empirically performs best for each application. However, SSCP has the advantage of greater sensitivity because the definitive bands usually represent a major portion of the particular labeled molecule—whereas heteroduplex analysis must detect the fraction of labeled molecules that actually formed heteroduplexes.

Allele-specific oligonucleotide hybridization (ASOH) and reverse blot technique analyze DNA after amplification by PCR and detect sequence variations by the success or failure of hybridization of short oligonucleotide probes that either exactly match or mismatch the sequence being tested (Figure 1-10). The amplified target DNA is first denatured and applied to a nylon membrane in the form of a small dot. Once this target DNA is anchored to the membrane either by heating or by brief ultraviolet irradiation, the DNA is hybridized with a labeled (usually with ^{32}P) oligonucleotide that encompasses the variable nucleotides of the DNA sequence of interest. The membrane is then washed with a salt solution whereby the salt concentration and the temperature control the specificity ("stringency") of the procedure.

Following the wash, the probe remaining on the membrane is detected by autoradiography. When several nucleotide variations (i.e., alleles) are known to exist in the same target sequence, several identical membranes are prepared and each is hybridized with a different oligonucleotide probe complementary to one of the known sequence variations. Although the net result is similar to having actually sequenced the DNA region, the ASOH method is considerably less labor intensive and relatively less expensive than DNA sequencing. Hence, ASOH is one of the methods of choice for screening a large number of samples for a particular genetic variation.

The major disadvantage of this method is that it requires prior knowledge of the base changes involved in the mutation and the precise stringency parameters for hybridization and washing of the membrane. In effect, these limitations exclude the routine use of this method for the characterization of a new mutation but allow the use of this method for the rapid screening of large number of samples for a previously characterized mutation.

A variation of the original method to perform ASOH is called the reverse blot technique (Figure 1-10).[32] The difference when compared to ASOH is that the amplified target DNA is labeled and then hybridized to an anchored unlabeled probe. Because the length of the DNA molecules is an important factor facilitating binding to the membrane, a key to the design of this method was the development of a relatively simple means of synthesizing (using the PCR) a stretch of DNA that contained multiple copies (i.e., a polymer) of the relatively short allele-specific oligonucleotide probes.[33]

In practice, the amplified DNA is nonradioactively labeled by previously tagging the PCR primers with fluorescein or biotin. After hybridization of the denatured PCR product in the presence of a membrane containing

CONVENTIONAL DOT BLOT

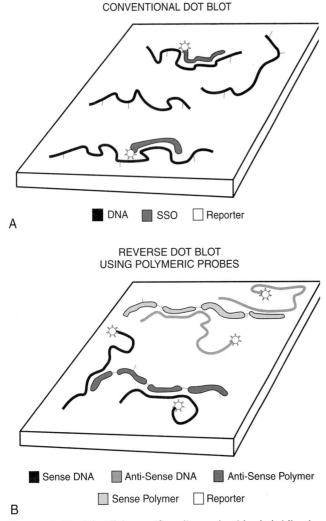

■ DNA ■ SSO □ Reporter

A

REVERSE DOT BLOT
USING POLYMERIC PROBES

■ Sense DNA ■ Anti-Sense DNA ■ Anti-Sense Polymer

□ Sense Polymer □ Reporter

B

Figure 1-10. (A) Allele-specific oligonucleotide hybridization (ASOH). The denatured (single-stranded) target DNA is anchored to a membrane, which is then treated (hybridized) with a solution of a short DNA segment of the gene of interest [sequence-specific oligonucleotide (SSO)]. The SSO is tagged with a reporter molecule, such as [32]P. Unbound probe DNA is removed by washing with buffer solutions. Appropriate stringency conditions of hybridization and washes limit the hybridization of the probe specifically to its complementary segment in the target DNA molecule. Depending on the manner in which the DNA is spotted onto the membrane, this procedure is referred to as a dot blot or a slot blot. (B) Reverse dot blot. In this variation of the conventional ASOH procedure, the DNA probes (sense and anti-sense polymer) tagged with the reporter molecule are fixed to a membrane and the denatured target DNA (sense and anti-sense DNA) is then hybridized to the immobilized probe. Similar to the ASOH procedure, appropriate stringency conditions of hybridization and washes limit the hybridization of target DNA to those that contain the complementary segment to the immobilized probe. The advantages of this method include the increased sensitivity derived from the ability to fix multiple copies (polymer) of the probe to the membrane and that both complementary strands of the probe sequence are present on the membrane. [Adapted from Trucco M (1992). To be or not to be ASP 57, that is the question. Diabetes Care 15:705.]

all of the relevant polymeric probes, and washing, the retained PCR products are revealed by detection via enzyme activity linked to fluorescein antibodies or to streptavidin. This method is especially useful for testing alleles that are highly polymorphic because a large number of probes and controls are easily tested using a single small membrane. Other advantages include the ability to use nonradioactive tracers, better reproducibility, and the potential for automation.

Certain classes of mutations are inherently difficult to detect using the traditional methods of detection outlined previously.[18] These types of mutations include promoter region, 3' untranslated region (UTR), or intronic region mutations affecting levels of transcript of mRNA or deletions of entire genes or of contiguous exons. Thus, if the genomic region examined is deleted from the mutant allele, PCR-based methods will be unable to detect this mutation because the PCR product obtained from the genomic DNA will be exclusively derived from the wild-type allele and thus appear to be normal. Promoter regions, 3'UTR, and intronic regions usually span genomic segments several orders larger than the coding exons and are thus not easily accessible for analysis with the methods outlined previously.

Different strategies need to be implemented for the analysis and detection of such mutations. Thus, deletions of one or more exons can be detected by quantitative hybridizations, quantitative PCR, Southern blotting, or fluorescence in situ hybridization—with the combined use of such methods enhancing the sensitivity of the testing protocol. A particularly promising and novel technique, termed *conversion*, exploits the principle that the diploid state of the human genome is converted to a haploid state that is then analyzed by one of the traditional methods.[34] The critical advantage of this manipulation is that heterozygous mutations are much easier to detect in the haploid state because of the absence of the normal wild-type sequence.

Positional Genetics in Endocrinology

THE PRINCIPLES OF POSITIONAL GENETICS

For the purpose of disease gene identification, the candidate gene approach relies on partial knowledge of the genetic basis of the disease under investigation. This process was successful in identifying disease genes whose function was obvious. For example, the genetic defects of most of the hereditary enzymatic disorders [including congenital adrenal hyperplasia (CAH) syndromes] became known in the late 1980s when the introduction of PCR made the tools of molecular biology widely available to the medical and genetic research community. However, at about the same time research on diseases without any obvious candidate genes [e.g., the multiple endocrine neoplasia (MEN) syndromes] and on diseases in which the screening of obvious candidate genes failed to reveal mutations was ongoing.

It was in these diseases that the application of "reverse genetics" (or more appropriately termed *positional cloning*)[35,36] yielded information regarding the genetic basis of

Linkage
analysis

Chromosomal
localization and mapping

Candidate gene screening
in the chromosomal locus;
contig construction (if needed)
and cloning of new genes

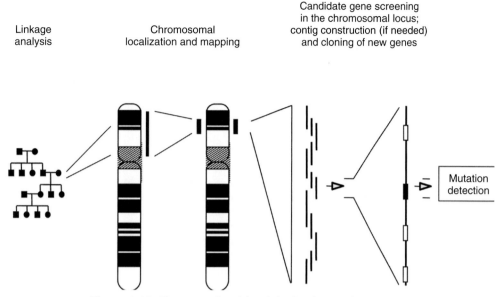

Mutation
detection

Figure 1-11. The steps of positional cloning (see text).

these disease states. Positional cloning is complemented by the Human Genome Project (HGP) and the Internet in making available in a fast and controlled manner information that would otherwise be inaccessible.[37] The process of positional genetics is outlined in Figure 1-11.

The first step is the collection of clinical information from families with affected members, the determination of the mode of inheritance of the defect (autosomal dominant or recessive, X-linked, complex inheritance), and the phenotyping of subjects (or tissues) following well-established criteria for the diagnosis of the disorder. If inheritance is not known, formal segregation analysis needs to be performed to determine the autosomal or X-linked (and the recessive or dominant) nature of the inheritance.[38] Once this determination is made and the penetrance of the disorder is known, appropriate linkage software may be used.[39] For more information on currently available computer software packages, the reader may check *http://darwin.case.edu* and other related links.

Linkage is examined with polymorphic markers that span the entire human genome.[36] Any marker that shows polymorphism and is known to lie close to or within a putative disease gene may be used. Genetic linkage can be defined as the tendency for alleles close together on the same chromosome to be transmitted together as an intact unit through meiosis. The strength of linkage can then be used as a unit of measurement to find out how close genetically different loci are to each other. This unit of map distance is an approximation of physical distance but is also highly dependent on other factors (e.g., the frequency of recombination is not the same in both genders, differing along the length of chromosomes and through the various chromosomes). The likelihood [logarithm of odds (LOD) score] method is widely used for linkage analysis.

Once a locus on a chromosome has been identified, narrowing of the region (this region is usually several thousands of base pairs in length) is accomplished by analyzing informative recombinations in the cohort of

patients and families available for study. The disease region may harbor already mapped genes. Online databases [Gen Bank, ENSEMBL at www.ensembl.org, and others, and especially for clinicians the Online Mendelian Inheritance in Man (OMIM)][40] may provide the necessary information. If a transcript is a reasonable candidate, mutation screening may identify the disease gene. If, however, these steps fail to identify the disease gene cloning of new sequences from the area may be needed.

This is usually done through the construction of a "contig," a contiguous array of human DNA clones covering the disease region. These DNA clones are maintained in large vectors such as bacterial artificial chromosomes (BACs). P1 and cosmid clones may also be used for coverage of the entire region or a subset of it. Contig construction may take a long time, depending on the genetic distance to be covered and the features of the genomic region. The identification of new genes and the construction of the contig are also called "chromosomal walking." The building blocks of this "walk" are the individual clones, which are linked by sequence-tagged sites (STSs) that are present in more than one clone—thus providing critical information that allows for the proper aligning of these clones.

Polymorphic markers (including those that were used for the linkage part of the process) are the most useful STSs because they provide a direct link between the genetic and the physical mapping data. Individual clones can be sequenced. Genes are identified in this process through their unique sequence features or through in vitro translation. The latter usually provides expressed sequence tags (ESTs), which can then be analyzed through software that is available online to determine the full gene structure and to identify redundancies (multiple ESTs or STSs of the same gene) and other errors.

Each of the newly identified genes may be screened for mutations, as long as the expression profile of the identified transcript matches the spectrum of the tissues affected by the disease under investigation. Although this is helpful for most diseases, for others the expression profile may even be misleading. Thus, the presence of a transcript in an affected tissue is not always necessary. Complete segregation of the disease with an identified mutation, functional proof, and/or mutations in two or more families with the same disease are usually required as supportive evidence that the cloned sequence is the disease gene.[41]

POSITIONAL CLONING OF ENDOCRINE GENES

A number of genes were identified by positional cloning in endocrinology in the 1990s. It is worth noting that endocrine tumor syndromes, despite their rarity and small overall impact on everyday clinical endocrine practice, are seminal examples of diseases whose molecular etiology was elucidated by positional cloning. Positional cloning played an essential role in unraveling the etiology of these syndromes because for most endocrine tumor syndromes there were no obvious candidate genes. Futhermore, positional cloning of genes responsible for familial tumor syndromes was greatly assisted by the use of neoplastic tissue for studies such as loss of heterozygosity (LOH), comparative genomic hybridization (CGH), and other fluoroscent in situ hybridization (FISH) applications.

These techniques narrow the genetically defined chromosomal regions and thus facilitate the identification of the responsible genes. LOH studies were critical to the identification of von-Hippel-Lindau disease (VHL-elongin),[42] MEN 1 (menin),[43] Cowden disease (PTEN),[44] Peutz-Jeghers syndrome (STK11/LKB1),[45,46] and Carney complex (PRKAR1A)[47] genes.

Expression Studies: Microarrays and SAGE

Advances in biotechnology, instrumentation, robotics, computer sciences, and the completion of genome sequencing initiatives for several organisms (including the human) have resulted in the development of novel and powerful techniques. A seminal example of such a technique is the development of the microarray technology. Microarrays contain thousands of oligonucleotides deposited or synthesized in situ on a solid support, typically a coated glass slide or a membrane. In this technique, a robotic device is used to print DNA sequences onto the solid support. The DNA probes immobilized on the microarray slide as spots can be cloned cDNA or gene fragments (ESTs) or oligonucleotides corresponding to known genes or putative open reading frames.

The arrays are hybridized with fluorescent targets prepared from RNA extracted from tissue/cells of interest. The RNA is labeled with fluorescent tags such as Cy3 and Cy5. The prototypic microarray experimental paradigm consists of comparing mRNA abundance in two different samples. One fluorescent target is prepared from control mRNA, and the second target labeled with a different fluorescent label is prepared from mRNA isolated from the treated cells or tissue under investigation. Both targets are mixed and hybridized to the microarray slide, resulting in target gene sequences hybridizing to their complementary sequences on the microarray slide. The microarray is then excited by laser and the fluorescent intensity of each spot is determined with the relative intensities of the two colored signals on individual spots being proportional to the number of specific mRNA transcripts in each sample (Figure 1-12). Analysis of the fluorescent intensity

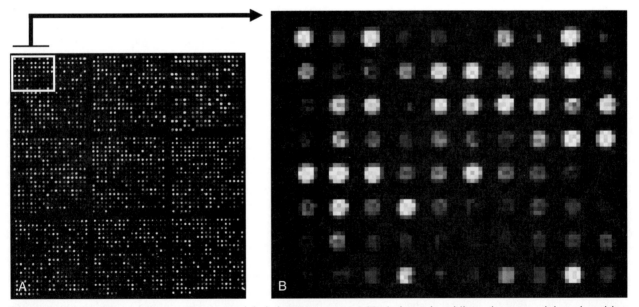

Figure 1-12. (A) cDNA microarray. Fluorescent labeled cDNA targets, ACTH-independent bilateral macronodular adrenal hyperplasia (Cy3), and ACTH-dependent hyperplasia (Cy5) were hybridized to glass slides containing genes involved in oncogenesis. Following laser activation of the fluorescent tags, fluorescent signals from each of the DNA "spots" are captured and subjected to analysis. (B) Magnified view of the microarray platform displaying the fluorescent signals: green (Cy3) and red (Cy5), with yellow representing overlap of these two colors. (See color plates.)

data yields an estimation of the relative expression levels of the genes in the sample and control sample. Microarrays enable individual investigators to perform large-scale analysis of model organisms and to customize arrays for special genome applications.

Most endocrine human genes participate in complex and highly interactive signaling pathways. They not only directly control a number of genes but modulate the functioning of a larger complement of genes by cross-talking with a multitude of signaling pathways. As noted elsewhere,[48] this is analogous to the Internet—the relevant genes being "nodes" or "hubs" in this Internet-like structure.[49] It was recently stated that "progress in dissecting signaling pathways has begun to lay out a circuitry that will likely mimic electronic integrated circuits in complexity and finesse, where transistors are replaced by proteins (e.g., kinases and phosphatases) and the electrons by phosphates and lipids."[50] Although this statement related to cancer research,[50] translational medicine today identifies these complex interactions to be ubiquitous[51]—making it no surprise that 30,000 to 40,000 genes (rather than the previously predicted 100,000 genes)[52] are sufficient to produce the human phenotype. It is not the number of genes that is critical but the regulation of expression of these genes and the number, quality, and temporospatial organization of interactions among their protein products.

An excellent example of an endocrine transcriptome is that recently presented by Roberts et al.:[53] the description of mitogen-activated protein kinase (MAPK) pathways during yeast pheromone response. Similar analytic strategies are currently being applied to investigations in a wide variety of fields of study, including that of endocrine tumors.[54] In this process (investigations by microarrays), simultaneous collection of information for hundreds of genes at a time (or the entire genome, depending on the type of the array used) have become the standard approach. An example from a recent study[55] is shown in Figure 1-12. Endocrine concepts and the reemergence of signaling as the chief means of understanding the complex interactions of genes may shape the new bioinformatics tools needed for the analysis of these data, and may direct the development of new drugs tailored to insights provided by these initiatives.[56,57]

Currently, in addition to the transcriptional profiling of any tissue performed by applying various types of microarrays there is the alternative technology of generating libraries of ESTs. An advanced expansion of EST libraries, especially in terms of high-throughput and transcript quantitation, is serial analysis of gene expression (SAGE). SAGE is based on generating, cloning, and sequencing concatenated short-sequence tags—each representing a single transcript derived from mRNA from target tissue.[58] Analysis of the transcriptional data gained by both methods is most commonly performed using clustering algorithms that group genes and samples on the basis of expression profiles, and statistical methods scoring the genes on the basis of their relevance to clinical manifestations.

The method of choice for global expression profiling depends on several factors, including technical, labor, price, time and effort involved, and most importantly the type of information sought. When comparing microarrays to EST libraries, an appreciable advantage of the latter is its inherent ability to identify transcripts without prior knowledge of the genes' coding sequences. This is the reason for its important potential for cloning and sequencing novel transcripts and genes. On the other hand, recent technical advances in the development of expression arrays, their abundance and commercial availability, and the relative speed with which analysis can be done are all factors that make arrays more useful in routine applications.

In addition, array content can now be readily customized to cover gene clusters and pathways of interest to the entire genome. Some studies examine series of tissue-specific transcripts and/or genes known to be involved in particular pathology. Others directly use arrays covering the entire genome. Another factor that needs to be considered prior to embarking on any high-throughput approach is whether individual or pooled samples will be investigated. Series of pooled samples reduce the price, the time spent, and the number of the experiments down to the most affordable. Investigating individual samples, however, is important for identifying unique expression ratios in a given type of tissue or cell.

A requirement of all high-throughput screening approaches is confirmation of findings (expression level of a given gene/sequence) by other independent methods. A select group of genes is tested. These genes are selected from the series of sequences that were analyzed either because they were found to have significant changes or due to their particular interest with regard to their expression in the studied tissue or their previously identified relationship to pathology or developmental stage. The confirmation process attempts to support the findings on three different levels: reliability of the high-throughput experiment (for this purpose, the same samples examined by the EST libraries or microarrays are used), trustfulness of the observations in general (to achieve this, larger number of samples are examined—assessment of which by high-throughput approaches is often unaffordable in terms of price and/or labor), and verification of expression changes at the protein level.[59]

A commonly used confirmatory technique is quantitative real-time reverse transcription PCR (qRT-PCR). For verification at the protein level, immunohistochemistry (IHC) and Western blot are the two most commonly chosen techniques. IHC is not quantitative but has the advantage of allowing for the observation of the exact localization of a signal within a cell (cytoplasmic versus nuclear) and the tissue (identifying histologically the tissue that is stained). Modern Western blot methods require a smaller amount of protein lysate than older techniques, and have the advantage of offering high-resolution quantitation of expression without the use of radioactivity.

Chromosome Analysis and Molecular Cytogenetics

Chromosomes represent the most condensed state in metamorphosis of the genome during a cell cycle. Condensation of the genetic material at metaphase stage is a crucial event that provides precise and equal segregation of chromosomes between the two newborn daughter cells during the next step, anaphase. This is followed by relaxation of the genetic content after cell division. This ability of the genome to transform from a molecular level (DNA) to materialistic submicroscopic stage (chromosome) provides a unique opportunity to visualize the genome of an individual cell of an organism. Different chromosomal abnormalities related to particular diseases or syndromes can be detected at this stage by karyotyping chromosomes.

Chromosomes can be individually recognized and classified by size or shape (ratio of the short/long arm) or by using differential staining techniques. In the past, identification of chromosomes was restricted to chromosome groups only. The introduction of chromosome banding technique revolutionized cytogenetic analysis.[60] The banding patterns are named by the following abbreviations: G (Giemsa), R (reverse), Q (Quinacrine), and DAPI (4'6'-diamino-2-phenylindole). The last two give a pattern similar to G-banding. Further development of high-resolution banding techniques[61] enabled the study of chromosomes at earlier stages of mitosis, prophase, and prometaphase. Chromosomes are longer and have enriched banding pattern at those stages, providing great details for identification of chromosomal aberrations.

OUTLINE OF METHODS

Preparation of quality chromosomes is an art. Many different methods for chromosome isolation have been developed in cytogenetics within the last half century. The main principle behind all methods is to arrest cells at metaphase by disruption of the cell spindle. Metaphase spindle is a structure composed of tubular fibers (formed in the cell) to which the chromosomes are attached by kinetochors (centrosomes). The spindle separates the chromosomes into the two daughter cells. The agent commonly used for spindle disruption is colcemid. The exposure time to colcemid varies depending on the proliferative activity of cells. Cells with a high proliferative index need a shorter time of exposure to a high concentration of colcemid (0.1–0.07 ug/ml for 10 to 20 minutes).

Slow-growing cells require longer exposure (1–4 hours or overnight with a lower concentration of 0.01–0.05 ug/ml). Prolonged exposure to colcemid or the use of high concentrations increases the proportion of chromosomes at late metaphase, resulting in shortening of the chromosomes. Conversely, a short exposure with a high concentration of colcemid reduces the total yield of metaphases. The optimum strikes a balance of these parameters. There are some additional modifications that allow for the enrichment of long (prometaphase) chromosomes by using agents that prevent DNA condensation, such as actinomycin D, ethidium bromide, or BrDU. Cell synchronization techniques can also significantly increase the total yield of metaphase chromosomes.

APPLICATIONS

Chromosomes are invaluable material for the evaluation of genome integrity and its preservation at the microscopic chromosomal level. The areas of application include prenatal diagnostics, genetic testing of multiple familial syndromes (including cancer), positional cloning of the genes,

and physical mapping (assignment of the genes to chromosomes and subchromosomal regions). The number and morphology of all 23 chromosome pairs in humans can be examined using G-banding differential staining of chromosomes obtained from a peripheral blood sample.

Abberations in the number of chromosomes or visible chromosomal alterations (such as translocations, deletions, and inversions involving extended regions) can be detected by this method. Recent advances such as spectral karyotyping (SKY) allow for better visualization of aneuploidy and translocations between different chromosomes.[62] Subtle rearrangements, such as submicroscopic deletions or cryptic translocations (an exchange of the small distal telomeric regions between the two nonhomologous chromosomes), can be visualized using specific probes in the fluorescent in situ hybridization (FISH) technique (Figure 1-13).[63]

FUTURE DEVELOPMENTS

Chromosome analysis will remain a powerful analytical tool in clinical and research fields for the foreseeable future. Possible strategies for improving existing methods include automation and linearization of the genetic content by increasing resolution to visualize at the level of the chromosome, chromatin, DNA, and gene. Another possible direction of development is functional analysis of the genome using constitutional chromosomes and labeled expressed sequences from particular tissues mapped directly to their original position on chromosomes (expression profiling).

Molecular Basis of Pediatrc Endocrinopathies

The past two decades haves witnessed the increasing application of recombinant DNA technology to the understanding of the pathogenesis of endocrinopathies. Although this new approach to endocrinologic disorders has resulted in the delineation of new syndromes, its major impact has been in facilitating the diagnosis of these disorders. Genetic counseling that includes anticipatory surveillance, as in multiple endocrine neoplasia (MEN) syndromes (see Chapter 13), is also one of the areas of clinical pediatric endocrinology experiencing major impact from this "new" knowledge. For example, it is becoming increasingly clear that phenotypically homogenous clinical syndromes may result from different genotypic abnormalities and that similar genetic abnormalities may have very different clinical manifestations.

In contrast, therapeutic implications of such knowledge are still limited. Hence, the earlier hopes of spectacular gains from gene therapy have not been realized and significant problems need to be addressed before gene therapy becomes a reality in routine patient care. However, targeted pharmacotherapy exploiting knowledge gained regarding molecular mechanisms and pathogenesis has been successfully employed in the treatment of some diseases (such as androgen insensitivity and thyroid cancer). The following section explores a couple of seminal examples of clinical endocrine disorders whose molecular

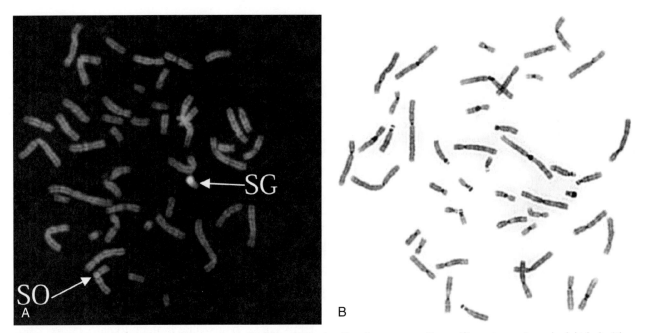

Figure 1-13. Human metaphase chromosomes. *(A)* After FISH using the chromosome-X–specific centromeric probe labeled with spectrum orange (SO) and chromosome-Y–specific heterochromatin labeled with spectrum green (SG). *(B)* With the inverted DAPI banding (similar to G-banding) allowing chromosomal identification. (See color plates.)

basis has been elucidated. Details of the specific disorders are elaborated in the respective chapters of this book.

DEFECTS IN PEPTIDE HORMONES

Genomic Deletions Causing Human Endocrine Disease

One of the early discoveries regarding the molecular basis of endocrinopathies was the absence of the gene coding for a particular peptide hormone. The entire gene could be missing, or only a part of the gene could be deleted. In either case, this resulted in the inability to synthesize a functional peptide so that the patient presents with clinical features indicative of deficiency of the hormone. A classic example of this type of endocrinopathy relevant to pediatric endocrinology is isolated growth hormone deficiency, type 1A (IGHD 1A).[64] In this syndrome the gene for human growth hormone-N (hGH-N) is deleted. Disease results when both alleles of hGH-N are absent (indicative of an autosomal recessive inheritance).

In the human, there are two hGH genes (hGH-N and hGH-V)—and both of them, along with the three placental lactogen (chorionic somatomammotropin) genes, are clustered along a 48-kilobase region of DNA. hGH-N is expressed in the pituitary gland and is the source of circulating growth hormone in the human, whereas hGH-V is expressed only in the placenta and its biologic function is not clear at this time. In autosomal recessive type 1A isolated growth hormone deficiency, although hGH-V is intact the absence of the active gene (hGH-N) results in deficiency of circulating growth hormone and the growth-hormone–deficient phenotype. In the original case description, the infants were of relatively normal size at birth but developed severe growth failure during the first year

of life. A distinctive feature of these infants was the propensity to develop antibodies against growth hormone in response to exogenously administered growth hormone. This feature, although common, is not invariably present in patients with IGHD 1A. The state-of-the-art method for screening for a hGH-N deletion is based on PCR amplification of the highly homologous regions of DNA on the long arm of chromosome 17 that flank the hGH-N gene.[65,66]

The presence of convenient restriction enzyme sites, such as SmaI, in the amplified DNA is exploited to ascertain the presence or absence of deletions in this region of the chromosome. Although this PCR-based approach is useful in most cases, it does not identify all cases with abnormalities in the hGH-N gene. In particular, more rigorous methods are required for the identification of the less common causes of IGHD-1A (such as point mutations). The study of the hGH-hPL gene cluster has also shed light on the function of prolactin because several studies have identified subjects with hPL deletions. These deletions do not result in overt clinical abnormalities, and specifically do not cause clinical effects in pregnant patients—suggesting that despite high levels of hPL found during pregnancy hPL serves no essential function in the human.[67]

Point Mutations

Peptide hormones act by binding to a specific receptor, which then results in the biologic actions attributed to that particular hormone. The binding of the peptide hormone to its receptor, classically described as the lock-and-key mechanism, is a very precise mechanism dependent on the complementary structures of the receptor and the site on the hormone involved in binding to the receptor. A change in the nucleotide sequence of the gene coding for a peptide hormone that results in altering an amino acid residue of the hormone can affect the function of the hormone if this change interferes with the hormone's ability to bind or activate the receptor.

Historically, point mutations resulting in aberrant protein production were well described with hemoglobin. This was possible because hemoglobin is present in abundant quantities in the blood, enabling purification and analysis of hemoglobin from patients suspected of having hemoglobinopathies. On the other hand, peptide hormones are present in infinitesimally lesser amounts in circulation—making their direct purification and analysis from blood a more daunting task. With the advent of recombinant DNA technology, it became feasible to clone and analyze the gene coding for the hormone directly without having to resort to purification of the protein from blood or tissue. This approach resulted in the identification of several clinical syndromes due to mutant hormones. One of the classic examples of this type of molecular pathology is non-insulin diabetes mellitus (NIDDM) due to mutant insulins.[68] A number of patients have been described with point mutations in the insulin gene.

In general, these patients present with hyperglycemia, hyperinsulinemia, and normal insulin sensitivity—a clinical picture that is attributed to the production of an abnormal insulin molecule with reduced biologic activity. Thus, Insulin Chicago is characterized by a single nucleotide change (TTC to TTG) that results in the substitution of a leucine for phenylalanine residue at position 25 of the B chain (Phe-B25-Leu). Similarly, the other two well-characterized point mutations are characterized by the change of a single amino acid residue and result in the formation of Insulin Wakayama (Val-A3-Leu) and Insulin Los Angeles (Phe-B24-Ser). These mutations are located within the putative receptor-binding region of the insulin molecule, and the insulin molecules transcribed from these mutant genes are characterized by low binding potency (<5% compared to normal) for the insulin receptor.

A separate class of mutations in the insulin gene gives rise to the syndrome of hyperproinsulinemia with or without clinically significant carbohydrate intolerance. Thus, two mutations described involve substitution of a histidine for an arginine at position 65 in one case and histidine at position 10 of the B chain changed to aspartic acid in the other. Although the original descriptions of these mutant insulins relied on the purification and analysis of the abnormal insulin molecule per se, the current availability of PCR-based methods to screen for these mutations has greatly simplified the laboratory diagnosis of this syndrome.

Another example of point mutations resulting in a phenotype that is especially relevant to pediatric endocrinologists is hypopituitarism secondary to abnormalities in transcription factors that orchestrate embryologic development of the anterior pituitary gland.[69,70] POU1F1 (also known as PIT1 or GHF-1) was the first transcription factor identified as playing a specific role in pituitary development. The POU1F1/PIT-1 gene encodes a 291–amino-acid Pit Oct Unc (POU) homeodomain DNA binding nuclear protein present in somatotrophs, lactotrophs, and thyrotrophs. POU1F1/PIT-1 is necessary for the

normal development of these pituitary cell types. The first indication that abnormalities in POU1F1/PIT-1 may result in a phenotypic change was derived from studies on strains of mice with genetic forms of dwarfism.

The Snell and Jackson strains of dwarf mice are characterized by a deficiency of growth hormone, prolactin, and TSH. In 1990, Li et al. reported that Snell phenotype was caused by a missense mutation and that the Jackson phenotype was caused by a rearrangement in the POU1F1/PIT-1 gene.[71] Since this landmark study, several recessive and dominant types of POU1F1/PIT-1 abnormality have been recognized in sporadic cases and in multiplex families with hypopituitarism.[72-74] POU1F1/PIT-1 activates growth hormone and prolactin gene expression, and can bind to and transactivate the TSH-B promoter. Accordingly, patients with POU1F1/PIT-1 mutations demonstrate growth hormone, prolactin, and variable TSH deficiencies.[72] The syndrome can be inherited in an autosomal dominant or recessive manner, but POU1F1/PIT-1 mutations are not a common cause of combined pituitary hormone deficiencies.

HESX1 is a paired-like homeodomain transcription factor expressed in the developing pituitary gland. Mutations in this gene leading to decreased activity have been found in two siblings with panhypopituitarism, absent septum pellucidum, optic nerve hypoplasia, and agenesis of the corpus callosum—implicating HESX1 in the mediation of forebrain development.[75,76] Another mutation in HESX1 was recently discovered in a patient with septo-optic dysplasia and isolated growth hormone deficiency.[77] Experimental evidence suggests that this particular mutation results in the production of an altered HESX1 protein with enhanced DNA binding activity that abrogates the transcriptional activity of PROP1, another transcription factor necessary for pituitary development.

PROP1 is thought to be involved in the differentiation of somatotropes, thyrotropes, lactotropes, and gonadotropes. Mutations in PROP1 leading to reduced DNA binding and transcriptional activity have been identified in patients with combined pituitary hormone deficiency. These patients have a deficiency of TSH, growth hormone, prolactin, LH, and FSH.[78] Patients with a demonstrated gonadotropin deficiency may present with failure to enter puberty spontaneously, whereas other patients do enter puberty but have subsequent loss of gonadotropin secretion. Although PROP1 is directly implicated in the differentiation of only four of the five anterior pituitary cell types, some patients have been described with ACTH deficiency. PROP1 mutations are believed to be relatively common (32%–50%) genetic causes of combined pituitary hormone deficiency.[79]

Rathke's pouch initially forms but fails to grow in LHX3-knockout mice.[80] Humans have been found to have mutations in the LHX3 gene (a LIM-type homeodomain protein), and demonstrate complete deficits of growth hormone, PRL, TSH, and gonadotropins in addition to a rigid cervical spine leading to limited head rotation. LHX4 is a related protein that (similar to LHX3) regulates proliferation and differentiation of pituitary lineages. A patient has been identified with a dominant mutation in this protein, demonstrating deficiencies of growth hormone, TSH, and ACTH; a small sella turcica; a hypoplastic anterior hypophysis; an ectopic posterior hypophysis; and a deformation of the cerebellar tonsil into a pointed configuration.[81]

Finally, Rieger syndrome is a condition with abnormal development of the anterior chamber of the eye, dental hypoplasia, and a protuberant umbilicus associated with growth hormone deficiency. All mutations in RIEG (Pitx2) found thus far have been heterozygous, with an autosomal dominant inheritance.[82]

DEFECTS IN PEPTIDE HORMONE RECEPTORS

Molecular defects resulting in phenotypic abnormalities in humans have been described in a variety of peptide hormone receptors, including growth hormone, LH, FSH, TSH, ACTH, and insulin. It is expected that this list will continue to expand in the future. Mutations in receptors for peptide hormone interfere in the actions of the hormone by altering the binding of the hormone, by altering the number of the receptors available for binding to the hormone, by interfering with the synthesis or intracellular processing of the receptor, or by disrupting the activation of the postreceptor signaling pathways.

In general, mutations in the receptor result in decreased actions of the cognate hormone. However, mutations involving G-protein–linked receptors are exceptions to this generalization and can result in a phenotype characterized by "over-activity" of the particular hormone system. Examples of these "gain-of-function" mutations include mutations in the LH receptor responsible for familial testotoxicosis[83] and mutations in the TSH receptor causing thyrotoxicosis[84] (see Chapter 2).

Insulin Receptor

Following the initial reports in 1988, a variety of mutations have been identified in the insulin receptor gene—with the majority of them being in patients with genetic syndromes associated with acanthosis nigricans and insulin resistance.[85] Patients with leprechaunism (a congenital syndrome characterized by extreme insulin resistance, fasting hypoglycemia, and intrauterine growth retardation) have two mutant alleles of the insulin receptor gene. Another syndrome associated with acanthosis nigricans and extreme insulin resistance, the Rabson-Mendenhall syndrome, has been linked to two different mutations within the insulin receptor gene existing in a compound heterozygous state.

The syndrome of type A insulin resistance is a heterogeneous collection of conditions defined by the presence of insulin resistance, acanthosis nigricans, and hyperandrogenism in the absence of lipoatrophy or obesity. Molecular analysis of the insulin receptor gene has revealed that several of these patients have mutations in one or both alleles of the insulin receptor gene. The initial expectation that mutations in the insulin receptor would provide the molecular basis for the common type of type 2 (NIDDM) diabetes mellitus has not been fulfilled. And, no alterations in the insulin receptor gene were identified in a study of Pima Indians—an ethnic group

with a greater than 50% incidence of type 2 diabetes mellitus. It is noteworthy, however, that recent studies have advanced the search for genetic variations that influence the propensity to develop type 2 diabetes mellitus.[86,87]

Positional-cloning–based analysis suggests that specific polymorphisms in the CAPN10 gene are associated with type 2 diabetes mellitus in the Finnish and Mexican-American (Pima Indian) populations. Whether these genetic variations in the CAPN10 gene, a chromosome 2 gene that encodes a widely expressed calpain-like cysteine protease, are causal factors for Type 2 diabetes mellitus or are merely co-segregating markers remains to be established. However, current studies have not excluded the possibility that polymorphisms in the insulin receptor gene may confer a genetic predisposition for the precipitation of the development of NIDDM by obesity and/or hypertension.

Growth Hormone Receptor

Genetic abnormalities in the growth hormone receptor result in the primary form of the syndrome of growth hormone insensitivity, also called Laron syndrome.[88] The human growth hormone receptor gene located on the proximal part of the short arm of chromosome 5 spans approximately 90 kilobases and includes nine exons (numbered 2 through 10) that encode the receptor protein and additional exons in the 5'UTR region of the gene. The growth hormone receptor protein contains an open reading frame of 638 amino acids that predicts a 246-amino-acid-long extracellular ligand-binding domain, a single membrane-spanning domain, and a cytoplasmic domain of 350 amino acids. In the human, the extracellular portion of the receptor exists in circulation as the growth-hormone–binding protein (GHBP).

Exon 2 encodes a signal sequence, exons 3 through 7 the extracellular GHB domain, exon 8 the transmembrane domain, and exons 9 and 10 the cytoplasmic domain and the 3'UTR region. The mutations that have been described in the growth hormone receptor gene include large deletions, nonsense mutations, splice mutations, and frameshift mutations.[89] The diagnosis of growth hormone insensitivity due to mutations in the growth hormone receptor gene is considered when patients demonstrate elevated growth hormone levels and low IGF-1 levels.

Because the GHBP is the cleaved extracellular portion of the growth hormone receptor, patients with mutations in the growth hormone receptor that results in decreased synthesis of the receptor protein can demonstrate low GHBP levels in circulation. However, mutations in the growth hormone receptor gene that selectively involve the transmembrane or intracellular domains may demonstrate normal or even enhanced circulating levels of GHBP. For example, a patient with a mutation that inhibits dimerization of the receptor had normal GHBP levels because the receptor had a normal GHB site.[90] Another set of affected individuals had a mutation of the transmembrane domain of the receptor, leading to a truncated growth hormone receptor product postulated to be more easily released from the cell membrane. In addition, elevated GHBP levels were noted.[91]

Recombinant DNA Technology and Therapy for Pediatric Endocrine Diseases

From a therapeutic point of view, recombinant DNA technology can be exploited to tailor pharmacotherapy according to the genotype of a patient (i.e., targeted pharmacotherapy), to manipulate genes within the human body (gene therapy), or to engineer prokaryotic or eukaryotic cells to produce proteins (such as hormones) that can then be administered for therapy or diagnosis. Whereas targeted pharmacotherapy and gene therapy are largely restricted to the research arena, the use of hormones produced by recombinant DNA technology is well established in clinical endocrinology. Historically, insulin was the first hormone synthesized by recombinant DNA technology to be approved for clinical use.[92,93] At present, a variety of recombinant hormones (including growth hormone, LH, FSH, TSH, PTH, and erythropoietin) are being used clinically or are in advanced stages of clinical trials.

On a theoretical basis, it should be possible to synthesize any protein hormone whose gene has been cloned and DNA sequence determined. Thus, recombinant DNA technology makes it possible to insert the gene coding for a particular protein hormone into a host cell such that the protein is produced by the host cell's protein synthesizing machinery. The synthesized protein is then separated from the rest of the host cell proteins to obtain the pure form of the hormone of interest. Both prokaryotic and eukaryotic cells can serve as the host cell for the production of proteins by this technology. Because post-translational modifications such as glycosylation may be essential for the optimal action of a protein hormone, the choice of the specific cell system utilized for the production of a particular protein hormone is critical. Prokaryotic cell systems such as *Escherichia coli* are suitable for the production of protein hormones that do not need post-translational modifications, such as growth hormone.[94]

Eukaryotic cell systems such as CHO (Chinese hamster ovary) cells, which are capable of post-translational modification of the protein, are useful for the production of hormones (such as TSH) that require glycosylation for optimal bioefficacy.[95] In addition, eukaryotic cells are capable of synthesizing proteins that undergo the appropriate folding—a step that is not carried out by prokaryotic cells. The advantages of the use of recombinant DNA for the production of these proteins include the possibility of a limitless supply of a highly pure form of a protein and the absence of the risk of contamination with biologic pathogens associated with extraction of proteins from human or animal tissue. In addition, this technology permits the development of hormone analogues and antagonists with much greater ease than conventional protein synthesis protocols.

The influence of genetic factors on the metabolism of various drugs is a well-established phenomenon, with the effect of various isozymes of cytochrome p450 on the circulating half-life of drugs such as anticonvulsants being a classic example of this interaction. Another example of the role of genotype on the choice of pharmacotherapy is the phenomenon of drug-induced hemolytic anemia in patients with G6PD deficiency. The recent genomic revolution has allowed for the exploitation of computational approaches to identifying polymorphisms of known genes encoding proteins with different functional characteristics. These single-nucleotide variations (also called single-nucleotide polymorphisms or SNPs) occur with varying frequencies in different ethnic populations and are the focus of intense scrutiny at this particular time.

The promise these SNPs hold out is that analysis of these SNPs for a given gene will allow the investigator to predict the response of the particular individual to a class of drugs or chemicals. This pharmacogenomic approach to clinical therapeutics has already been successful in demonstrating an association between specific polymorphisms in the beta-adrenergic receptor and response to beta-agonists in patients with bronchial asthma, and polymorphisms in hydroxytryptamine receptors and response to neuroleptic drugs. The widespread application of the tools of molecular biology to unravel the molecular basis of action of hormones has also yielded benefits by allowing for customization of pharmacotherapy of endocrine diseases and syndromes based on the specific individual genetic defect.

One such example is the report of directed pharmacologic therapy of an infant with ambiguous genitalia due to a mutation in the androgen receptor.[96] In this infant with an M807T mutation in the androgen receptor, in vitro functional studies had indicated that the mutant receptor exhibited loss of binding capacity for testosterone with retention of binding for dihydrotestosterone (DHT). Furthermore, this differential binding was also reflected in the better preservation of the transactivation potential of DHT compared to testosterone. These in vitro findings were exploited to treat the infant with DHT, resulting in restoration of male genital development. This case illustrates that in selected cases in vitro functional assays can help identify subsets of patients with ambiguous genitalia and androgen insensitivity who would respond to targeted androgen therapy. It can be anticipated that in the coming years more examples of such innovative therapeutic strategies and "customized" hormonal treatment protocols will become routinely implemented in the practice of clinical pediatric endocrinology.

Concluding Remarks

The application of recombinant DNA technology has resulted in a tremendous increase in our understanding of physiologic processes and pathologic conditions. The U.S. government sponsored Human Genome Project initiative launched in 1992 has catalyzed this revolution, which is currently being fueled by both public sector efforts and private sector entrepreneurship. The central goal of this initiative, which represents collaborative efforts among scientists in the United States and around the world, is to sequence the entire 3 to 4 billion base pairs of the human genome and to construct a detailed genetic and physical map of the entire human genome (i.e., each of the 24 different human chromosomes).

Such a map, along with advances in communication and computers, will allow a scientist to locate and isolate any human DNA sequence of interest. Recent achievements, such as the draft sequence of the human genome, are major milestones toward the fulfillment of this goal and have resulted in a paradigm shift in the way that novel genes are being discovered and in the analysis of the function of hormones and related proteins.[97] In the traditional paradigm, investigators seeking to discover new genes or to analyze the function of known proteins needed to devote a significant part of their time to conducting "bench research" in "wet laboratories." The new approach in this "post-genomic" era takes advantage of the unprecedented power of computational biology to "mine" nucleotide, protein sequence, and other related databases.

In the future, most researchers will deal with abstract models and data sets stored in computer databases. Hence, initial discoveries of novel genes or novel interactions between known proteins or intracellular signaling pathways could be made using the analytic power of computational software tools (functional genomics). These initial insights can then be verified and expanded upon by traditional benchtop methods. The advantages of this new paradigm are obvious, with computational approaches taking a significantly shorter time and with fewer demands on manpower. The new paradigm can also easily expand the scope of the search to include multiple molecules and organisms (phylogenetic profiling).

One of the key contemporaneous scientific developments that have enabled the efficient and widespread use of this new paradigm is the expansion of the Internet. The Internet has enabled the capture, storage, analysis, and dissemination of the enormous amounts of data generated by the Human Genome Project in a manner that is efficient, protects the privacy of individuals, and is easily accessible for legitimate use. Several public-domain web-accessible databases are currently serving as the major repositories for this information. GenBank is the major repository for sequence information and is currently supported by the National Institutes of Health. One of the main sources of the physical location, clinical features, inheritance patterns, and other related information of specific gene defects is the Online Mendelian Inheritance in Man (OMIM) operated by Johns Hopkins University in Baltimore, Maryland.

Johns Hopkins University also operates the online Genome Database (GDB), which allows scientists to identify polymorphisms and contacts for gene probes and other related research tools. The ever-expanding number of endocrine (and other) disorders that can be attributed to changes in the nucleotide sequence of specific genes has also increased the necessity for the availability of accurate, reliable, and timely genetic tests such as mutation detection. One source for such information is a collaborative website *(www.genetests.org)* that maintains an up-to-date catalog of commercially available and research-based tests for inherited disorders.

With the ubiquitous use of these powerful tools in laboratories around the world, genes are being cloned and genetic diseases being mapped at a very rapid pace. In all of this excitement, one still needs to keep in mind that whereas this "new" science has allowed for hitherto inaccessible areas of human biology to be probed and studied, a lot remains to be understood with respect to individual disease processes. Hence, at the present time we have only a rudimentary understanding of the correlations between phenotype and genotype in many of the common genetic diseases (such as congenital adrenal hyperplasia).

These lacunae in our knowledge dictate that clinicians should be cautious about basing therapeutic decisions solely on the basis of molecular and genetic studies. This is especially true in the area of prenatal diagnosis and termination of pregnancy based on genetic analysis. As we improve our understanding of the molecular and genetic basis of disease and translate this knowledge into gains at the bedside, it behooves us both as individuals and as a society to be cognizant of critical issues relating to privacy of health data and to remain vigilant against misuse by inappropriate disclosure of this powerful knowledge.

REFERENCES

1. Weintraub BD (1994). *Molecular endocrinology: Basic concepts and clinical correlations.* New York: Raven Press.
2. Shupnik M (2000). *Gene engineering in endocrinology, First edition.* Totowa, NJ: Humana Press.
3. Alberts B, Johnson A, Lewis J, Raff M, Roberts K, Walter P (2002). *Molecular biology of the cell.* New York: Garland Science.
4. Lodish H, Scott M, Matsudaira P, Darnell J, Zipursky L, Kaiser C, et al. (2003). *Molecular cell biology, Fifth edition.* New York: W. H. Freeman.
5. Roberts R (1989). Restriction enzymes and their isoschizomers. Nucl Acids Res 17:r347.
6. Nathans D, Smith H (1975). Restriction endonucleases in the analysis and restructuring of DNA molecules. Annu Rev Biochem 44:273–293.
7. Sambrook J, Russell D (2001). *Molecular cloning: A laboratory manual, Third edition.* Cold Spring Harbor, NY: Cold Spring Harbor Laboratory Press.
8. Southern E (1975). Detection of specific sequences among DNA fragments separated by gel electrophoresis. J Mol Biol 98:503–517.
9. Innis M, Gelfand D, Sninsky J (1999). *PCR applications: Protocols for functional genomics.* San Diego: Academic Press.
10. Innis M, Gelfand D, Sninsky J, White T (1990). *PCR protocols: A guide to methods and applications.* San Diego: Academic Press.
11. Kocova M, Siegel S, Wenger S, Lee P, Trucco M (1993). Detection of Y chromosome sequence in Turner's Syndrome by Southern blot analysis of amplified DNA. Lancet 342:140–143.
12. Lehrach H, Diamond D, Wozney J, Boedtker H (1977). RNA molecular weight determinations by gel electrophoresis under denaturing conditions. Biochemistry 16:4743–4751.
13. Thomas P (1980). Hybridization of denatured RNA and small DNA fragments transferred to nitrocellulose. Proc Natl Acad Sci USA 77:5201–5205.
14. Rudert W, Kocova M, Rao A, Trucco M (1994). Fine quantitation by competitive PCR of circulating donor cells in posttransplant chimeric recipients. Transplantation 58:964–965.
15. Gilliland G, Perrin S, Blanchard K, Bunn H (1990). Analysis of cytokine mRNA and DNA: Detection and quantitation by competitive polymerase chain reaction. Proc Natl Acad Sci USA 87:2725–2729.
16. Applied Biosystems (1997). *User Bulletin 2: ABI Prism 7700 Sequence Detection System, Relative Quantitation of Gene Expression.* Forest City, CA. Applied Biosystems.
17. Applied Biosystems (1998). *User Bulletin 5: ABI Prism 7700 Sequence Detection System, Multiplex PCR with Taqman Probes.* Forest City, CA. Applied Biosystems.
18. Yan H, Kinzler K, Vogelstein B (2000). Genetic testing: Present and future. Science 289:1890–1892.
19. Maxam A, Gilbert W (1980). Sequencing end-labeled DNA with base-specific chemical cleavages. Methods Enzymol 65:499–560.

20. Sanger F, Nicklen S, Coulson A (1977). DNA sequencing with chain-terminating inhibitors. Proc Natl Acad Sci USA 74:5463–5467.

21. Hattori M, Sakaki Y (1986). Dideoxy sequencing using denatured plasmid templates. Anal Biochem 152:232–238.

22. Ahmadian A, Ehn M, Hober S (2006). Pyrosequencing: History, biochemistry and future. Clin Chim Acta 363(1/2):83–94.

23. Myers R, Maniatis T, Lerman L (1985). Detection and localization of single base changes by denaturing gradient gel electrophoresis. In Wu R (ed.), *Methods in enzymology*. San Diego: Academic Press.

24. Abrams E, Murdaugh S, Lerman L (1990). Comprehensive detection of single base changes in human genomic DNA using denaturing gradient gel electrophoresis and a GC clamp. Genomics 7:463–475.

25. Gejman P, Weinstein L (1994). *Detection of mutations and polymorphisms of the Gs alpha subunit gene by denaturing gradient gel electrophoresis*. Orlando: Academic Press.

26. Myers R, Fischer S, Maniatis T, Lerman L (1985). Modification of the melting properties of duplex DNA by attachment of a GC-rich DNA sequence as determined by denaturing gradient gel electrophoresis. Nucl Acids Res 13:3111–3129.

27. Myers R, Fischer S, Lerman L, Maniatis T (1985). Nearly all single base substitutions in DNA fragments joined to a GC-clamp can be detected by denaturing gradient gel electrophoresis. Nucl Acids Res 13:3145.

28. Sheffield V, Cox D, Lerman L, Myers R (1989). Attachment of a 40-base pair G + C rich sequence (GC clamp) to genomic DNA fragments by the polymerase chain reaction results in improved detection of single-base changes. Proc Natl Acad Sci USA 86:232–236.

29. Nagamine C, Chan K, Lau Y-F (1989). A PCR artifact: Generation of heteroduplexes. Am J Hum Genet 45:337–339.

30. White M, Carvalho M, Derse D, O'Brien S, Dean M (1992). Detecting single base substitutions as heteroduplex polymorphisms. Genomics 12:301–306.

31. Keen J, Lester D, Inglehearn C, Curtis A, Bhattacharya S (1991). Rapid detection of single base mismatches as heteroduplexes on Hydrolink gels. Trends Genet 7:5.

32. Rudert W, Trucco M (1992). Rapid detection of sequence variations using polymers of specific oligonucleotides. Nucl Acids Res 20:1146.

33. Rudert W, Trucco M (1990). DNA polymers of protein binding sequences generated by PCR. Nucl Acids Res 18:6460.

34. Yan H, Papadopoulos N, Marra G, Perrera C, Jiricny J, Boland C, et al. (2000). Conversion of diploidy to haploidy. Nature 403:723–724.

35. Collins F (1992). Positional cloning: Let's not call it reverse anymore. Nature Genetics 1:3–6.

36. Collins F (1995). Positional cloning moves from perditional to traditional. Nature Genetics 9:347–350.

37. Borsani G, Ballabio A, Banfi S (1998). A practical guide to orient yourself in the labyrinth of genome databases. Hum Mol Genet 7:1641–1648.

38. Khoury M, Beaty T, Cohen B (1993). *Fundamentals of genetic epidemiology, First edition*. New York: Oxford University Press.

39. Terwilliger J, Ott J (1994). *Handbook of human genetic linkage*. Baltimore: The Johns Hopkins University Press.

40. Online Mendelian Inheritance in Man (OMIM) (2007). In National Library of Medicine: McKusick-Nathans Institute for Genetic Medicine, Johns Hopkins University (Baltimore, MD) and National Center for Biotechnology Information, National Library of Medicine (Bethesda, MD), Center for Medical Genetics, Johns Hopkins University and National Center for Biotechnology Information.

41. Bishop M (1997). Gene mapping and isolation: Access to databases. Methods Mol Biol 68:237–259.

42. Linehan W, Lerman M, Zbar B (1995). Identification of the von Hippel-Lindau (VHL) gene. JAMA 273:564–570.

43. Chandrasekharappa S, Guru S, Manickam P, Olufemi S, Collins F, Emmert-Buck M, et al. (1997). Positional cloning of the gene for multiple endocrine neoplasia-type 1. Science 276:404–407.

44. Liaw D, Marsh D, Li J, Dahia P, Wang S, Zheng Z, et al. (1997). Germline mutations of the PTEN gene in Cowden disease, an inherited breast and thyroid cancer syndrome. Nat Genet 16:64–67.

45. Hemminki A, Markie D, Tomlinson I, Avizienyte E, Roth S, Loukola A, et al. (1998). A serine/threonine kinase gene defective in Peutz-Jeghers syndrome. Nature 391:184–187.

46. Jenne D, Reimann H, Nezu J, Friedel W, Loff S, Jeschke R, et al. (1998). Peutz-Jeghers syndrome is caused by mutations in a novel serine threonine kinase. Nat Genet 18:38–43.

47. Kirschner L, Carney J, Pack S, Taymans S, Giatzakis C, Cho Y, et al. (2000). Mutations of the gene encoding the protein kinase A type I-alpha regulatory subunit in patients with the Carney complex. Nat Genet 26:89–92.

48. Vogelstein B (2000). Complexity in cancer. Nature 408:307–311.

49. Barabasi A, Oltvai Z (2004). Network biology: Understanding the cell's functional organization. Nat Rev Genet 5:101–113.

50. Hanahan D, Weinberg R (2000). The hallmarks of cancer. Cell 100:57–70.

51. Hillan K, Quirke P (2001). Preface to genomic pathology: A new frontier. J Pathol 195:1–2.

52. The Genome International Sequencing Consortium (2001). Initial sequencing and analysis of the human genome. Nature 409:860–921.

53. Roberts C, Nelson B, Marton M, Stoughton R, Meyer M, Bennett H, et al. (2000). Signaling and circuitry of multiple MAPK pathways revealed by a matrix of global gene expression profiles. Science 287:873–880.

54. Alizadeh A, Ross D, Perou C, van de Rijn M (2001). Towards a novel classification of human malignancies based on gene expression patterns. J Pathol 195:41–52.

55. Bourdeau I, Antonini S, Lacroix A, Kirschner L, Matyakhina L, Lorang D, et al. (2004). Gene array analysis of macronodular adrenal hyperplasia confirms clinical heterogeneity and identifies several candidate genes as molecular mediators. Oncogene 23:1575–1585.

56. Marton M, DeRisi J, Bennett H, Iyer V, Meyer M, Roberts C, et al. (1998). Drug target validation and identification of secondary drug target effects using DNA microarrays. Nat Med 4:1293–1301.

57. Khan J, Wei J, Ringner M, Saal L, Ladanyi M, Westermann F, et al. (2001). Classification and diagnostic prediction of cancers using gene expression profiling and artificial neural networks. Nat Med 7:673–679.

58. Dinel S, Bolduc C, Belleau P, Boivin A, Yoshioka M, Calvo E, et al. (2005). Reproducibility, bioinformatic analysis and power of the SAGE method to evaluate changes in transcriptome. Nucleic Acids Res 33:e26.

59. Velculescu VE, Madden S, Zhang L, Lash A, Yu J, Rago C, et al. (1999). Analysis of human transcriptomes. Nat Genet 23:387–388.

60. Caspersson T, Zech L, Johansson C (1970). Differential binding of alkylating fluorochromes in human chromosomes. Exp Cell Res 60:315–319.

61. Yunis J (1976). High resolution of human chromosomes. Science 191:1268–1270.

62. Schrock E, du Manoir S, Veldman T, Schoell B, Wienberg J, Ferguson-Smith M, et al. (1996). Multicolor spectral karyotyping of human chromosomes. Science 273(5274):494–497.

63. Cremer T, Lichter P, Borden J, Ward D, Manuelidis L (1988). Detection of chromosome aberrations in metaphase and interphase tumor cells by in situ hybridization using chromosome specific library probes. Hum Genet 80:235–246.

64. Phillips J, Hjelle B, Seeburg P, Zachmann M (1981). Molecular basis for familial isolated growth hormone deficiency. Proc Natl Acad Sci USA 78:6372–6375.

65. Vnencak-Jones C, Phillips J, De Fen W (1990). Use of polymerase chain reaction in detection of growth hormone gene deletions. J Clin Endocrinol Metab 70:1550–1553.

66. Kamijo T, Phillips J (1992). Detection of molecular heterogeneity in GH-1 gene deletions by analysis of polymerase chain reaction amplification products. J Clin Endocrinol Metab 74:786–789.

67. Hill D (1992). What is the role of growth hormone and related peptides in implantation and the development of the embryo and fetus. Horm Res 38:28–34.

68. Steiner D, Tager H, Chan S, Nanjo K, Sanke T, Rubenstein A (1990). Lessons learned from molecular biology of insulin-gene mutations Diabetes Care 13:600–609.

69. Rosenfeld M, Briata P, Dasen J, Gleiberman A, Kioussi C, Lin C, et al. (2000). Multistep signaling and transcriptional requirements for pituitary organogenesis in vivo. Recent Prog Horm Res 55:1–13; discussion 13–14.

70. Cushman L, Camper S (2001). Molecular basis of pituitary dysfunction in mouse and human. Mamm Genome 12:485–494.

71. Li S, Crenshaw E, Rawson E, Simmons D, Swanson L, Rosenfeld M (1990). Dwarf locus mutants lacking three pituitary cell types result from mutations in the POU-domain gene Pit-1. Nature 347:528–533.

72. Hendriks-Stegeman B, Augustijn K, Bakker B, Holthuizen P, van der Vliet P, Jansen M (2001). Combined pituitary hormone deficiency caused by compound heterozygosity for two novel mutations in the POU domain of the Pit1/POU1F1 gene. J Clin Endocrinol Metab 86:1545–1550.

73. Drouin J (2006). Molecular mechanisms of pituitary differentiation and regulation: Implications for hormone deficiencies and hormone resistance syndromes. Front Horm Res 35:74–87.

74. Quentien M, Barlier A, Franc J, Pellegrini I, Brue T, Enjalbert A (2006). Pituitary transcription factors: From congenital deficiencies to gene therapy. J Neuroendocrinol 18:633–642.

75. Dattani M, Martinez-Barbera J, Thomas P, Brickman J, Gupta R, Martensson I, et al. (1998). Mutations in the homeobox gene HESX1/Hesx1 associated with septo-optic dysplasia in human and mouse. Nat Genet 19:125–133.

76. Thomas P, Dattani M, Brickman J, McNay D, Warne G, Zacharin M, et al. (2001). Heterozygous HESX1 mutations associated with isolated congenital pituitary hypoplasia and septo-optic dysplasia. Hum Mol Genet 10:39–45.

77. Cohen R, Cohen L, Botero D, Yu C, Sagar A, Jurkiewicz M, et al. (2003). Enhanced repression by HESX1 as a cause of hypopituitarism and septooptic dysplasia. J Clin Endocrinol Metab 88:4832–4839.

78. Wu W, Cogan J, Pfaffle R, Dasen J, Frisch H, O'Connell S, et al. (1998). Mutations in PROP1 cause familial combined pituitary hormone deficiency. Nat Genet 18:147–149.

79. Deladoey J, Fluck C, Buyukgebiz A, Kuhlmann B, Eble A, Hindmarsh P, et al. (1999). "Hot spot" in the PROP1 gene responsible for combined pituitary hormone deficiency. J Clin Endocrinol Metab 84:1645–1650.

80. Zhao Y, Morales D, Hermesz E, Lee W, Pfaff S, Westphal H (2006). Reduced expression of the LIM-homeobox gene Lhx3 impairs growth and differentiation of Rathke's pouch and increases cell apoptosis during mouse pituitary development. Mech Dev 123:605–613.

81. Machinis K, Pantel J, Netchine I, Leger J, Camand O, Sobrier M, et al. (2001). Syndromic short stature in patients with a germline mutation in the LIM homeobox LHX4. Am J Hum Genet 69:961–968.

82. Sadeghi-Nejad A, Senior B (1974). Autosomal dominant transmission of isolated growth hormone deficiency in iris-dental dysplasia (Rieger's syndrome). J Pediatr 85:644–648.

83. Shenker A, Laue L, Kosugi S, Merendino J Jr., Minegishi T, Cutler G Jr. (1993). A constitutively activating mutation of the lutenizing hormone receptor in familial male precocious puberty. Nature 365:652–654.

84. Duprez L, Parma J, Van Sande J, Rodien P, Sabine C, Abramowicz M, et al. (1999). Pathology of the TSH receptor. J Pediatr Endocrinol Metab 12:295–302.

85. Taylor S, Arioglu E (1998). Syndromes associated with insulin resistance and acanthosis nigricans. J Basic Clin Physiol Pharmacol 9:419–439.

86. MT M (2005). Genetics of type 2 diabetes mellitus. Diabetes Res Clin Pract 68:S10–S21.

87. Mercado M, McLenithan J, Silver K, Shuldiner A (2002). Genetics of insulin resistance. Curr Diab Rep 2:83–95.

88. Laron Z, Pertzelan A, Mannheimer S (1966). Genetic pituitary dwarfism with high serum concentrations of growth hormone: A new inborn error of metabolism. Isr J Med Sci 4:883–894.

89. Rosenbloom A (1999). Growth hormone insensitivity: Physiologic and genetic basis, phenotype, and treatment. J Pediatr Endocrinol Metab 135:280–289.

90. Duquesnoy P, Sobrier M, Duriez B, Dastot F, Buchanan C, Savage M, et al. (1994). A single amino acid substitution in the exoplasmic domain of the human growth hormone (GH) receptor confers familial GH resistance (Laron syndrome) with positive GH-binding activity by abolishing receptor homodimerization. Embo J 13:1386–1395.

91. Woods K, Fraser N, Postel-Vinay M, Savage M, Clark A (1996). A homozygous splice site mutation affecting the intracellular domain of the growth hormone (GH) receptor resulting in Laron syndrome with elevated GH-binding protein. J Clin Endocrinol Metab 81:1686–1690.

92. Goeddel D, Kleid D, Bolivar F, Heyneker T, Yansura D, Crea R, et al. (1979). Expression in Escherichia coli of chemically synthesized genes for human insulin. Proc Natl Acad Sci USA 76:106–110.

93. Riggs A (1981). Bacterial production of human insulin. Diabetes Care 4:64–68.

94. Goeddel D, Heyneker H, Hozumi T, Arentzen R, Itakura K, Yansura D, et al. (1979). Direct expression in Escherichia coli of a DNA sequence coding for human growth hormone. Nature 281:544–548.

95. Gesundheit N, Weintraub B (1986). Mechanisms and regulation of TSH glycosylation. Adv Exp Med Biol 205:87–105.

96. Ong Y, Wong H, Adaikan G, Yong E (1999). Directed pharmacological therapy of ambiguous genitalia due to an androgen receptor gene mutation. Lancet 354:1444–1445.

97. Hsu S, Hsueh A (2000). Discovering new hormones, receptors, and signaling mediators in the genomic era. Mol Endocrinol 14:594–604.

Receptor Transduction of Hormone Action

ALAN M. RICE, MD • SCOTT A. RIVKEES, MD

Introduction

Hormones exert their actions by activating specific receptors. Activation of these receptors stimulates intracellular responses that influence cellular physiology and, at times, gene expression. The specificity of hormone action is thus determined by the affinity of hormones for different receptors, receptor distribution, and effector and genetic responses to ligand occupancy.

Over the past two decades, our understanding of hormone action has increased greatly—in part due to the cloning of many receptors that transduce hormone action. Four major receptor superfamilies have been identified that share common structural elements and/or effector systems. These families include the G-protein–coupled receptors (GPCRs), cytokine receptors, tyrosine kinase receptors (RTKs), and nuclear receptors (Table 2-1). This chapter reviews major features of these important receptor families. Mutations influencing receptor function leading to endocrine disorders are also highlighted.

G-Protein–Coupled Receptors

More than 1% of the genome of vertebrates encodes GPCRs.[1] Most of these GPCRs are odorant and pheromone receptors.[1] It is also important to note that most of the receptors that transduce the effects of hormones are GPCRs (Table 2-2).

The GPCR superfamily is divided into eight major classes.[1,2] These receptors contain an N-terminal extracellular domain that is frequently called the ectodomain or exodomain.[3] These receptors also contain seven putative transmembrane helixes (TM-I to TM-VII) connected by three intracellular (i1 through i3) and three extracellular

(e1 through e3) loops that are often collectively called the serpentine region (Figure 2-1).[3,4] The C-terminal intracellular region is usually referred to as the endodomain.[3]

GPCRs are activated by a wide variety of signals, including proteins, nucleotides, amino acid residues, Ca^{2+}, light, and odorants (Figure 2-1).[1] It is postulated that alteration of the conformation of transmembrane domains by ligand binding changes the conformation of intracellular loops, leading to activation of heterotrimeric guanosine nucleotide binding proteins (G proteins) (Figure 2-1).[5,6] When a GPCR is activated by a ligand, guanosine 5'-diphosphate (GDP) is converted to guanosine 5'-triphosphate (GTP)—which causes the heterotrimeric G protein to dissociate into active $G\alpha$-GTP and $G\beta\gamma$ subunits (Figure 2-1).[5-7] GTPase then converts GTP into GDP, which inactivates $G\alpha$ and increases affinity of $G\alpha$ for $G\beta\gamma$ leading to reformation of the inactive heterotrimeric G protein.[5-7] Active $G\alpha$ and $G\beta\gamma$ subunits can alter the activity of transmembrane channels, and the activity of intracellular effector enzymes that include phospholipase C, adenylyl cyclase, and kinases (Figure 2-1).[1,7]

Specificity in ligand binding is conferred by variations in the primary structures of the extracellular and intracellular domains.[1] Specificity of effector responses is conferred by the variations in the primary structure of intracellular domains and isoforms of the $G\alpha$ subunits of G proteins.[8,9] Some GPCRs couple predominantly with G proteins with $G\alpha_i$/$G\alpha_o$ subunits that act primarily to decrease adenylyl cyclase activity.[9-12] Other GPCRs couple predominantly with G proteins with $G\alpha_s$ subunits that act to increase adenylyl cyclase activity, or $G\alpha_q$/$G\alpha$[11,14,15,16] subunits that increase phospholipase C activity.[9,13,14]

Interestingly, data show that cytoskeletal proteins may module receptor–G-protein coupling. For example, the erythrocyte membrane cytoskeletal protein 4.1G can

TABLE 2-1
Major Types of Hormone Receptors

Receptor Class	Hormone Receptors
G-protein–coupled receptors	ACTH and other melanocortins, V2 vasopressin, LH, FSH, TSH, GnRH, TRH, GHRH, corticotropin releasing factor, somatostatin, glucagon, oxytocin, gastric inhibitory peptide, type 1 PTH, free fatty acid, GPR54, orexin, ghrelin, melanin-concentrating, calcitonin, glucagon-like peptide-1, and calcium-sensing receptors
Type I cytokine receptors	Growth hormone, prolactin, and leptin receptors
Receptor tyrosine kinases	Insulin, IGF-1, and fibroblast growth factor receptors
Nuclear receptors	Thyroid hormone, vitamin D3, PPARγ, HNF-4α, glucocorticoid, androgen, estrogen, mineralocorticoid, and DAX1 receptors

TABLE 2-2

G-Protein–Coupled Receptors and Clinical Conditions Associated with Receptor Mutations

Receptor	Germ Line Mutation	Endocrine Disorder
ACTH/melanocortin-2 receptor	Inactivating mutations (homozygous, compound heterozygous)	Familial glucocorticoid deficiency type 1
Melanocortin-4 receptor	Inactivating mutations (most heterozygous, some homozygous)	Obesity
V2 vasopressin receptor	Inactivating mutations (most X-linked recessive, rarely X-linked dominant)	X-linked nephrogenic diabetes insipidus
LH receptor	Inactivating mutations (homozygous, compound heterozygous)	Males: types I and II Leydig cell hypoplasia
		Females: asymptomatic or hypergonadotropic hypogonadism with primary amenorrhea
	Activating mutations (heterozygous)	Males: male limited precocious puberty
FSH receptor	Inactivating mutations (homozygous, compound heterozygous)	Females: autosomal recessive hypergonadotropic ovarian dysgenesis or milder hypergonadotropic hypogonadism
		Males: variable impairment of spermatogenesis
TSH receptor	Inactivating mutations (most homozygous or compound heterozygous, rarely heterozygous)	Resistance to TSH
	Activating mutations (heterozygous)	Autosomal-dominant inherited nonautoimmune hyperthyroidism/toxic adenomas
GnRH receptor	Inactivating mutations (homozygous or compound heterozygous)	Isolated hypogonadotropic hypogonadism
TRH receptor	Inactivating mutations (compound heterozygous)	Central hypothyroidism
GPR54	Inactivating mutations (homozygous, compound heterozygous)	Normosmic isolated hypogonadotropic hypogonadism
Ghrelin	Inactivating mutations (homozygous, possible heterozygous)	Short stature due to decreased growth hormone secretion
GHRH receptor	Inactivating mutations (homozygous/compound heterozygous)	Isolated growth hormone deficiency
Type 1 PTH receptor	Inactivating mutations (homozygous, heterozygous)	Blomstrand's chondrodysplasia if homozygous and rarely if heterozygous; enchondromatosis if heterozygous
	Activating mutations (heterozygous)	Jansen's metaphyseal chondrodysplasia
Calcium-sensing receptor	Inactivating mutations (heterozygous, homozygous)	Familial benign hypocalciuric hypercalcemia typical if heterozygous, neonatal severe hyperparathyroidism rarely if heterozygous, typical if homozygous
	Activating mutations (heterozygous)	Autosomal-dominant hypocalcemic hypocalciuria, Bartter syndrome type V

interfere with A1 adenosine receptor signal transduction.[15] 4.1G also influences mGlu1alpha-mediated cAMP accumulation, increases the ligand-binding ability of mGlu1alpha, and alters its cellular distribution.[16] 4.1G may also play a role in receptor-receptor dimerization.

Receptor agonist-independent and agonist-induced homo- and heterodimerization have increasingly been recognized as important determinants of GPCRs function.[17] For example, the GPCR somatostatin receptor 5 (SSTR5) primarily exist as monomers in the absence of an agonist. However, they form homodimers in the presence of an agonist.[18] Furthermore, it has been shown that SSTR5 can form heterodimers with type 2 dopamine receptors (DRD2)—another GPCR—in the presence of hsst2 agonist or dopamine.[19] Agonist-induced activation of SSTR5-DRD2 heterodimers in China hamster ovary (CHO)

cells expressing SSTR5 and DRD2 is increased when compared to agonist-induced activation of monomers and homodimers in CHO cells expressing only SSTR5 or DRD2.[19] Heterodimerization of receptors may also lead to inactivation of one of the receptors in the complex. For example, heterodimerization of somatostatin receptor 2A (sst2A) with somatostatin receptor 3 (SSTR3) appears to lead to inactivation of the heterodimerized SSTR3 without inactivating the heterodimerized SSTR2.[20]

GPCRs can form heterodimers with nonreceptor transmembrane proteins. Both the calcitonin receptor (CALCR) and the calcitonin receptor-like protein (CALCRL) can form heterodimers with three different receptor-activity–modifying proteins (RAMPs): RAMP1, RAMP2, and RAMP3.[21-23] Whereas CALCRs can be activated by ligand in the absence of heterodimerization with a RAMP, CALCRLs

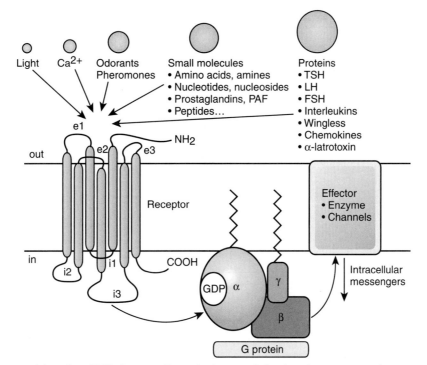

Figure 2-1. GPCR structure and function. GPCRs have an N-terminal extracellular domain, seven putative transmembrane domains separated by three extracellular loops (e1-e3) and three intracellular loops (i1-i3), and a C-terminal intracellular domain. Ligand binding results in the exchange of GTP for GDP, which induces dissociation of the G protein into a GTPα subunit and a βγ subunit. Then these subunits alter the activity of intracellular effector enzymes and transmembrane channels, resulting in the alteration of intracellular levels of second messengers that can include cAMP and calcium. [Adapted with permission from Bockaert J, Pin JP (1999). Molecular tinkering of G-protein–coupled receptors: An evolutionary success. Embo J 18:1724.]

are only activated by ligand if heterodimerized with a RAMP.[21,22] RAMPs alter the ligand specificity of the heterodimerized receptor.

CALCRs that are not in heterodimers with RAMPS are activated by calcitonin and thus constitute the classic CALCR.[21,22] However, CALCRs heterodimerized with RAMP1, RAMP2, and RAMP3 bind amylin and constitute amylin1, amylin2, and amylin3 receptors, respectively.[21,22] CALCRLs dimerized with RAMP1 bind calcitonin gene-related peptide and constitute the calcitonin gene-related peptide receptor.[21,22] CALCRLs dimerized with RAMP2 and RAMP3 bind adrenomedullin, and constitute adrenomedullin1 and adrenomedullin2 receptors, respectively.[21,22] RAMPS alter function of other GPCRs that transduce hormone action. The distribution and function of parathyroid hormone 1 and 2 receptors are altered by binding to RAMP2 and RAMP3, respectively.[24] The distribution and function of the glucagon receptor is altered by binding to RAMP2.[24]

Dimerization/heterodimerization may occur in the endoplasmic reticulum (ER) shortly after protein synthesis occurs.[25] The ER plays a role in determining whether or not a protein will be expressed elsewhere in the cell, thus protecting the cell from misfolded and (likely) mutant proteins.[25] The non-heterodimerized CALCRL is an orphan receptor because the CALCRLs cannot leave the ER for the cell membrane unless heterodimerized with RAMPs.[26]

Failure of the endoplasmic reticulum to export mutant GPCR homodimers and mutant GPCR wild-type GPCR heterodimers to the cell membrane has been unequivocally found to be the cause of two dominant negative endocrine conditions, and to occur without apparent clinical effect in a third endocrine condition. A dominant negative mutation is a heterozygous mutation that results in a phenotype that would only be expected in the presence of a homozygous mutation. Some V2 vasopressin receptor gene mutations that are known to cause nephrogenic diabetes insipidus encode mutant V2 vasopressin receptors that form dimers in the ER that cannot be exported to the cell membrane.[27]

These mutant receptors also interfere with cell surface expression of wild-type receptors by forming heterodimers with the wild-type receptors that cannot be exported from the ER to the cell membrane.[28] This finding explains why females heterozygous for these V2 vasopressin receptor gene mutations do not concentrate their urine with even high doses of desmopressin, a synthetic V2 vasopressin receptor agonist, in spite of being able to produce wild-type V2 vasopressin receptors.[29] A similar phenomenon explains dominant transmission of partial TSH receptor resistance in patients heterozygous for some inactivating TSH receptor mutations.[30] In these patients, mutant TSH receptors form oligomers with wild-type receptors and prevent export of wild-type receptors from the endoplasmic reticulum to the cell membrane.[30]

Similarly, misfolding and misrouting of some mutant gonadotropin-releasing hormone (GnRH) receptors in the endoplasmic reticulum (as well as oligomerization of these mutant GnRH receptors with wild-type GnRH receptors) decrease cell membrane expression of wild-type GnRH receptors.[31-33] This phenomenon, however, has not been found to have clinical implications in relatives of probands homozygous or compound heterozygous for mutations that cause isolated hypogonadotropic hypogonadism (IHH) because individuals heterozygous for these mutations demonstrate an intact GnRH-gonadotropin axis and do not have clinical signs of IHH. Thus, in these individuals enough wild-type GnRH receptors do not oligimerize with mutant GnRH receptors and are transported to the cell membrane to maintain sufficient normal GnRH-GnRH receptor interactions to avoid development of IHH.[32]

It has been recognized that many GPCRs (including lutenizing hormone, thyroid-stimulating hormone thyrotropin-releasing hormone, glucagon-like peptide-1, melanocortin, and cannabinoid receptors) activate G proteins in the absence of ligand binding.[34,35] Thus, these receptors are constitutively active and cellular G-protein activation increases linearly with increased cell surface expression of the receptors.[36] It has also been recognized that there are ligands (often called inverse agonists) that decrease the activity of these receptors.[37] Receptor ligands that neither increase nor decrease the activity of receptors are now frequently referred to as neutral antagonists.[35]

The term *antagonists* is applied to these ligands because they block activation and inactivation of receptors by agonists and inverse agonists, respectively.[35] The term *agonist* only refers to receptor ligands that increase receptor activity.[35] A scale has been formulated to express the continuity in receptor ligand function—from −1 (representing a full inverse agonist), to 0 (representing a neutral antagonist), to +1 (representing a full agonist).[35,37] It is possible that inverse agonists play a role in treating medical conditions caused by GPCR mutations that lead to increased constitutional activation of the receptor.[35]

Receptor desensitization and resensitization play a role in GPCR activity. During the past decade, mechanisms of GPCR desensitization and resensitization have been elucidated. Three processes for receptor desensitization have been described.[38,39] The first receptor desensitization process is rapid uncoupling of the G protein from GPCRs.[39] This process occurs within seconds to minutes after initiation of the process and occurs as a result of phosphorylation of GPCRs.[39] G-protein–receptor kinases (GRKs) have been increasingly recognized as playing a major role when this process involves homologous desensitization.[38]

Homologous or agonist-dependent desensitization occurs after agonist activation of the receptor that is desensitized.[39] GRK-mediated phosphorylation of serine and threonine residues in the third intracellular loop or the C-terminal intracellular domain leads to activation of β-arrestins, which in turn inactivate adenylyl cyclase (Figure 2-2).[38-41] Second-messenger–dependent protein kinases also contribute to receptor desensitization when

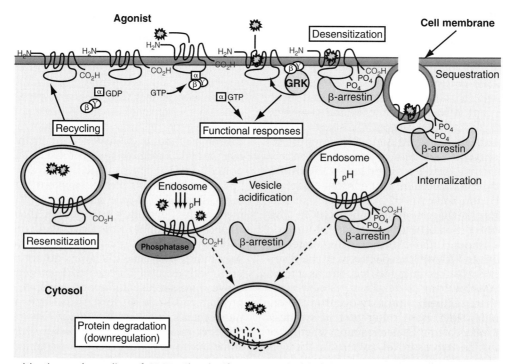

Figure 2-2. Desensitization and recycling of GPCRs. Shortly after an agonist binds a GPCR, G-protein–receptor kinases phosphorylation of serine and threonine residues in the third intracellular loop or the C-terminal intracellular domain leads to activation of β-arrestin. Activation of β-arrestin inactivates adenylyl cyclase and initiates sequestration of the GPCR in clathrin-coated vesicles. Dephosphorylation of the sequestered receptor and subsequent disassociation of the receptor from β-arrestin is followed by recycling of the GPCR to the cell membrane. Alternatively, once sequestered the GPCR can be destroyed in lysosomes. [Adapted with permission from Saunders C, Limbird LE (1999). Localization and trafficking of α2-adrenergic subtypes in cells and tissues. Pharmacol Ther 84:200.]

this process involves homologous desensitization, but also participate in receptor desensitization when desensitization involves heterologous desensitization. Heterologous or agonist-independent desensitization occurs as a result of activation of a different receptor from the one that is desensitized.[39]

The second receptor desensitization process is internalization/sequestration of GPCRs. This process is slower than receptor phosphorylation-induced uncoupling of the G protein from GPCRs and occurs within minutes to hours after initiation of the process. This process is reversible because the receptors can be recycled to the cell surface (Figure 2-2).[39] GRKs and β-arrestins play a role in initiating internalization/sequestration of β2-adrenergic, LH, FSH, TSH, TRH, vasopressin V2, angiotensin II type 1A, and other G-protein–coupled receptors in clathrin-coated vesicles (Figure 2-2).[38,42-49] Dephosphorylation of the sequestered receptor followed by disassociation of the receptor from β-arrestin is necessary for the receptor to be recycled to the cell membrane and resensitized (Figure 2-2).[14]

The third receptor desensitization process is down-regulation. With down-regulation the number of intracellular GPCRs decreases due to increased lysosomal degradation and decreased synthesis of the receptors due to alteration of transcriptional and post-transcriptional regulatory mechanisms (Figure 2-2).[50,51] Down-regulation is a slow process that occurs within several hours to days after initiation of the processes that lead to its development.[52]

One of the ways the Arg137His V2 vasopressin receptor mutation interferes with mutant receptor function and causes X-linked nephrogenic diabetes insipidus is by altering desensitization and recycling of the mutant receptor.[53] In vitro studies have revealed that the mutant receptor is constitutively phosphorylated. Thus, even in the absence of ligand binding the mutant receptor is bound by β-arrestin—which in turn leads to sequestration of the mutant receptor within clathrin-coated vesicles. Recycling of the mutant receptor back to the cell membrane requires the mutant receptor to be dephosphorylated and disassociated from β-arrestin. However, the mutant receptor remains constitutively phosphorylated while sequestered and thus cannot be disassociated from β-arrestin and recycled to the cell membrane—thereby reducing cell membrane expression of the mutant receptor.

Some investigators suggest that most GPCR-inactivating mutations can be classified by the effects of the mutations into one of five classes.[54] Class I inactivating mutations interfere with receptor biosynthesis. Class II inactivating mutations interfere with receptor trafficking to the cell surface. Class III inactivating mutations interfere with ligand binding. Class IV inactivating mutations impede receptor activation. Class V inactivating mutations do not cause discernible defects in receptor biosynthesis, trafficking, ligand binding, or activation but may cause medical disorders. There are also inactivating mutations that interfere with receptor function via multiple mechanisms and thus cannot be placed into one class.

Of the eight classes of GPCRs, only classes A, B, and C contain receptors for mammalian hormones (Figure 2-3).[2] Class A receptors contain the rhodopsin-like receptors

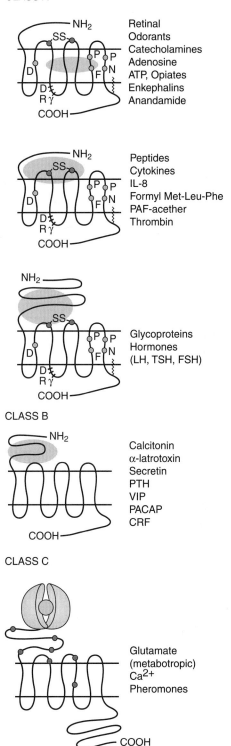

Figure 2-3. Examples of class A, B, and C GPCRs. The orange oval represents the ligand. These receptors can differ in amino acid sequence, in length of the N-terminal extracellular and C-terminal cytoplasmic domains, and in the receptor regions involved with ligand-receptor interactions. [Adapted with permission from Bockaert J, Pin JP (1999). Molecular tinkering of G protein-coupled receptors: An evolutionary success. Embo J 18:1725.]

and are divided into at least 15 groups.[2,55] Four of these groups contain receptors activated by hormones. These are the peptide receptor, hormone protein receptor, gonadotropin-releasing hormone (GnRH) receptor, and the thyrotropin-releasing hormone (TRH) and secretagogue receptor groups.[2]

The peptide receptor group includes the angiotensin, adrenocorticotropin hormone (ACTH)/melanocortin, oxytocin, somatostatin, and vasopressin receptors.[2] The hormone protein receptor group includes the receptors for glycoprotein hormones, including follicle-stimulating hormone (FSH), leutinizing hormone (LH), and thyrotropin (TSH) receptors.[2] These receptors have large extracellular N-terminal domains and ligand-binding sites that include the first and third extracellular loops (Figure 2-3).[1,2] There is also much similarity in amino acid sequence among these receptors (Figure 2-3).[1] The GnRH receptor group only contains the GnRH receptor.[2] The TRH and secretagogue receptor group includes the TRH receptor and the growth hormone secretagogue receptor.[2]

Class B GPCRs are structurally similar to members of the hormone protein receptor group (Figure 2-3).[1] However, unlike the glycoprotein hormone receptors class B GPCRs do not share similar amino acid sequences.[1] This family contains receptors for high-molecular-weight hormones, including calcitonin, glucagon, gastric inhibitory peptide, parathyroid hormone (PTH), and corticotrophin-releasing factor (CRF).[1,2,56]

Class C receptors have a very large extracellular domain with two lobes separated by a hinge region that closes on the ligand (Figure 2-3).[57] This region has also been called the "Venus's-flytrap" domain or module due to the trapping mechanism of the hinge region.[58] This family includes the calcium-sensing receptor (CASR).[1,2]

Class A Receptors That Transduce Hormone Action

THE PEPTIDE RECEPTOR GROUP

Adrenocorticotropin and Melanocortin-2 Receptors

It is important to note that a newly accepted name for the ACTH receptor is melanocortin-2 receptor (MC2R) because the ACTH receptor is one of five members of the melanocortin receptor family of GPCRs.[54] For the purpose of clarity, when discussing interactions between ACTH and its receptor the older name will be used for the remainder of this chapter. The ACTH receptor gene is located on the short arm of chromosome 18.[59] The ACTH receptor has a small extracellular and intracytoplasmic domain. Adrenocorticotropin-induced activation of ACTH receptor in the *zona fasciculata* and *zona reticularis* of the adrenal cortex stimulates $G\alpha_s$, resulting in increased intracellular cAMP levels that stimulate steroidogenesis by activating cAMP-dependent kinases.[60-62]

Hereditary isolated glucocorticoid deficiency, resistance to ACTH, and familial glucocorticoid deficiency (FGD) are

the same names for an autosomal recessive syndrome that consists of glucocorticoid deficiency accompanied by normal mineralocorticoid secretion. FGD has been classified further as FGD types 1 and 2 and the triple A syndrome.[63] Patients with FGD type 1 are homozygous or compound heterozygous for point mutations, resulting in ACTH receptors with abnormal function.[63-69] In contrast, patients with FGD type 2 have ACTH resistance that is not caused by ACTH receptor mutations.[62,63,70] Triple A (Allgrove syndrome) is an autosomal recessive syndrome characterized by ACTH-resistant adrenal insufficiency, achalasia, and alacrima—which is also not caused by ACTH receptor gene mutations.[63,67,71]

Patients with FGD type 1 usually present during infancy or early childhood with hypoglycemia.[66,72-76] Less commonly, patients may present with a severe infection, frequent minor infections, or childhood asthma that resolves with treatment with physiologic doses of glucocorticoids.[63,66,72] Hyperpigmentation may be seen as early as the first month of life, but usually becomes apparent after the fourth month of life.[64-66,72-74,77] Neonates may also suffer from jaundice.[66,74,76,78] Tall stature accompanied by an advanced bone age, in spite of normal age of onset of puberty, appears to be common in children with FGD type 1.[63,66,69,72,73,77] Patients with FGD type 2 have normal heights.[63,79]

At presentation, plasma cortisol, androstenedione, and dihydroepiandrosterone levels are low or low normal—and plasma ACTH levels are elevated.[63,66,72-76] When supine, patients with FGD type 1 have renin and aldosterone levels that are near normal.[63,73,75,76] Histologically, the *zona fasciculata* and *zona reticularis* are atrophied with FGD.[72] However, demonstrating the lack of an essential role for ACTH in the embryologic development and maintenance of the *zona glomerulosa,* adrenal cortices in patients with all types of FGD contains *zona glomerulosa* cells.[63,71-73,77,80]

Abnormalities in ACTH receptor expression may be seen in other conditions. Evidence suggests that the ACTH receptor-$G\alpha_s$-adenylyl cyclase-cAMP cascade maintains differentiation of adrenocortical cells, and that impairment of this cascade leads to dedifferentiation and increased proliferation of adrenocortical cells.[81,82] Adrenocortical carcinomas from some patients have been found to have a loss of heterozygosity (LOH) for the ACTH receptor gene, resulting markedly in decreased ACTH receptor mRNA expression.[82] Growth of the tumors with LOH for the ACTH receptor gene also may be more aggressive than the other tumors. An activating mutation of G_{i2} that constitutively suppresses adenylyl cyclase activity has also been found in adrenocortical tumors.[81] Thus, decreased ACTH receptor activity may be associated with tumorigenesis.

Interestingly, many patients with ACTH-independent macronodular adrenal hyperplasia (AIMAH)—a cause of ACTH-independent Cushing's syndrome—exhibit increased glucocorticoid levels in response to non-corticotropin hormones that do not normally induce glucocorticoid release.[83-88] These hormones include gastric inhibitory peptide, exogenous arginine and lysine vasopressin, lutenizing hormone, human chorionic gonadotropin, angiotensin II, catecholamines, leptin, and serotonin receptor agonists.[83-88] Increased expression of the receptors for these ligands in the abnormal adrenal glands has been implicated as a possible explanation for the abnormal induction of glucocorticoid release by these non-corticotropin ligands.[88] However, receptors for some of these ligands are expressed in normal adrenal glands.[88] Thus, the mechanism for this phenomenon remains to be fully elucidated.

Other Melanocortin Receptors

Murine studies reveal that melanocortin-3 receptor (MC3R), another of the five members of the melanocortin receptor family, regulates fat deposition.[54] The role of the MC3R in humans is less clear. Homozygosity for a pair of single-nucleotide polymorphisms of the MC3R gene that result in production of partially inactive MC3Rs was found to be associated with pediatric-onset obesity in Caucasian American and African American children.[89]

The melanocortin-4 receptor (MC4R) is another member of the melanocortin receptor family and plays a role in controlling appetite and weight.[90] The MC4R has baseline constitutive activity that can be inhibited by the inverse agonist agouti-related peptide (AgRP).[90,91] Activation of the MC4R by its natural agonist α-melanocyte stimulating hormone (α-MSH) produces anorexigenic effects.[90,92,93] Naturally occurring inactivating MC4R mutations have been identified in some individuals with hyperphagia, increased lean body mass, obesity, and hyperinsulinism due to insulin resistance and increased linear growth.[94-96]

Most of these obese individuals were heterozygous for the identified mutations, and an autosomal dominant mode of inheritance was identified in their blood relatives.[95,96] However, five obese children from a consanguineous kindred were found to be homozygous for an N62S missense mutation.[95] Family members heterozygous for the N62S mutation were noted to be nonobese. These MC4R mutations are thought to be the most common monogenic cause of human obesity. In one study, 5.8% of 500 probands with severe childhood obesity were found to be heterozygous or homozygous for MC4R mutations.[96] AgRP gene polymorphisms appear to be associated with anorexia nervosa.[97,98]

Very little is known about melanocortin-5 receptors (MC5Rs) in animals and humans. There is only weak evidence from a single linkage and association study of families in Quebec suggesting that MC5Rs may also play a role in regulating body weight and fat mass.[99]

Another member of the melanocortin receptor family, the melanocortin-1 receptor (MC1R), controls skin and hair pigmentation. Activation of MC1Rs in skin and hair follicle melanocytes with the pro-opiomelanocortin (POMC)-derived peptides α-melanocyte stimulating hormone (α-MSH) and ACTH leads to release of eumelanin, a brown-black pigment, from the melanocytes.[100,101] Inhibition of MC1R baseline constitutive activity by agouti protein leads to release of pheomelanin, a red-yellow pigment, from the melanocytes.[101]

Inactivating homozygous mutations of the POMC gene cause hypoadrenalism, red hair, fair skin, and early-onset obesity due to lack of ACTH production from the POMC precursor, lack of ACTH and α-MSH-induced melanocyte release of eumelanin resulting from activation of MC1Rs, and lack of α-MSH-induced anorectic effects resulting from activation of MC4Rs, respectively.[102] Heterozygosity for Arg236Gly and Tyr221Cys POMC gene mutations are associated with hyperphagia, early-onset obesity, and increased linear growth.[102,103] In one study, 5 out of 538 unrelated probands with severe early-onset obesity were found to be heterozygous for the Tyr221Cys POMC gene mutation.[103]

Vasopressin Receptors

Nephrogenic diabetes insipidus (NDI) occurs when the renal response to arginine vasopressin (AVP) is impaired. NDI is characterized by polydipsia and polyuria that is not responsive to vasopressin and vasopressin analogs.[104] X-linked NDI is caused by inactivating mutations of the V2 vasopressin receptor (AVPR2) gene located at Xq28.[105-108] An autosomal recessive variant of NDI is also caused by loss-of-function mutations in the gene for the aquaporin-2 AVP-sensitive water channel.[109,110]

More than 100 inactivating AVPR2 gene mutations have been identified that cause X-linked NDI.[104] Some of these mutations are complete gene deletions or mutations that cause abnormal mRNA splicing. Other mutations result in receptors with abnormal trafficking to the plasma membrane, ligand binding, or G_s activation.[104,111]

Gain-of-function mutations in the V2 vasopressin receptor have also been reported.[112] DNA sequencing of two patient's V2R gene identified missense mutations in both, with resultant changes in codon 137 from arginine to cysteine or leucine. These mutations resulted in constitutive activation of the receptor and a syndrome of inappropriate antidiuretic hormone secretion (SIADH)-like clinical picture, which was termed *nephrogenic syndrome of inappropriate antidiuresis.*[112]

THE HORMONE PROTEIN RECEPTOR GROUP

The glycoprotein hormones include TSH, FSH, LH, and HCG. These hormones are composed of similar α subunits that dimerize with hormone-specific β subunits. TSH, FSH, and LH bind to the extracellular N-terminal domain of the TSH, FSH, and LH receptors, respectively.[1,2,113,114] The effects of hCG are mediated by the LH receptor.[115]

Glycoprotein hormone receptors have a large (350–400 residues) extracellular N-terminal domain, also known as the ectodomain, that participates in ligand binding (Figure 2-3).[3,115] The ectodomain includes leucine-rich repeats that are highly conserved among the glycoprotein hormone receptors.[3,115] There is 39% to 46% similarity of the ectodomain and 68% to 72% similarity of the transmembrane or serpentine domain among the three glycoprotein hormone receptors.[3]

Activated glycoprotein hormone receptors increase G_s coupling to adenylyl cyclase, leading to increased intracellular cAMP levels and protein kinase A (PKA) activation.[115] Mutations leading to endocrine dysfunction have been reported for each of the glycoprotein hormone receptors.

LH Receptors

Both inactivating and activating mutations of the LH receptor have been found in humans.[115] The LH receptor gene is located in chromosome 2 p21 and consists of 11 exons.[116,117] Exon 1 encodes a peptide that directs the LH receptor to the plasma membrane.[115] Exons 2 through 10 encode the ectodomain.[115] The last exon encodes the transmembrane domains that are also known as the serpentine regions.[3,115,116] Single nonsense mutations, amino acid changes, and partial gene deletions have been found that lead to expression of LH receptors with decreased activity.[115] Single–amino-acid changes have also been found that lead to activation of G_s in the absence of ligand binding.[115]

Inactivating mutations of the LH receptor gene require homozygosity or compound heterozygosity to alter endocrine function because the presence of one normal receptor allele in the heterozygous state can compensate for the decreased function of a mutated allele.[115] In contrast, activating mutations of the LH receptor gene cause endocrine disorders in the heterozygous state.[115]

In the fetus, LH receptors are primarily activated by hCG.[115] Leydig cells begin to express LH receptors shortly after testicular differentiation at 8 weeks of gestation.[115] Thereafter, androgen production due to activation of these receptors by hCG plays an important role in the development of male genitalia and testicular descent.[115] Thus, male infants with inactivating mutations of the LH receptor may present with abnormally developed genitalia—including micropenis, cryptorchidism, and intersex..[115]

Males with mutations that completely inactivate the LH receptor may present with male pseudohermaphroditism accompanied by failure of fetal testicular Leydig cell differentiation. This phenotype, which is known as type I Leydig cell hypoplasia, includes female external genitalia with a blind-ending vagina, absence of Müllerian derivatives, and inguinal testes with absent or immature Leydig cells.[118-125] In addition, patients have elevated serum LH levels, normal serum FSH levels, and decreased serum testosterone levels that do not increase in response to HCG administration.[118-125] Mutations that lead to this phenotype include a nonsense mutation (Arg545Stop) that results in a receptor that is missing TM4-7, an Ala593Pro change, and a TM7 deletion (ΔLeu608, Val609) that decreases cell surface expression of the LH receptor.[123,124,126] These mutant receptors are unable to couple to G_s.[123,124,126]

Males with mutations that do not completely inactivate the LH receptor present with type II Leydig cell hypoplasia, which is characterized by a small phallus and decreased virilization.[122] A mutation that leads to this phenotype includes the insertion of a charged lysine at position 625 of TM7 in place of hydrophobic isoleucine that disrupts signal transduction.[127] Another mutation (Ser616Tyr, found in patients with mild Leydig cell hypoplasia) is associated with decreased cell surface expression of the LH receptor.[124,127] Other deletion and nonsense mutations have also been found to cause mild Leydig cell hypoplasia.[115]

Males with inactivating mutations of the LH receptor may also present with a phenotype intermediate in severity between type I and type II Leydig cell hypoplasia. A compound heterozygote patient with Ser616Tyr on one allele and an inactivating deletion (Δexon 8) on the other allele presented with Leydig cell hypoplasia, hypoplastic phallus, and hypospadias.[128] The Cys131Arg mutation has also been found in patients with Leydig cell hypoplasia, small phallus, and hypospadias.[129] This mutation is located in the leucine-rich repeat segment of the LH receptor extracellular domain and interferes with high-affinity ligand binding.[129]

Deletion of exon 10 of the LH receptor gene results in an LH receptor that binds LH and HCG normally.[130] However, although there is normal intracellular signaling in response to binding of the mutant receptor by HCG there is impaired intracellular signaling in response to binding of the mutant receptor by LH.[130] Because HCG is the main in utero LH receptor-activating hormone, and second-messenger response of the mutant receptors to HCG is not impaired, it is not surprising that a male patient found to be homozygous for the mutation was born with normal male genitalia.[54,130] Pubertal progression and later gonadal function, however, are dependent on LH activation of the LH receptor.[54,130]

Because deletion of exon 10 of the LH receptor gene results in a mutant LH receptor with diminished intracellular signaling in response to LH, it is also not surprising that the patient homozygous for this mutation was found to have delayed pubertal development, small testes, and hypergonadotropic hypogonadism when evaluated at the age of 18 years.[130] Prolonged HCG therapy resulted in normalization of testicular testosterone production, increased testicular size, and the appearance of spermatozoa in semen.[130]

Males with mutations that constitutively activate LH receptors present with male-limited precocious puberty (MLPP), also known as testotoxicosis—which may be familial or sporadic.[125,131,132] Boys with this condition present with GnRH-independent precocious puberty before the age of 4 years when the Asp578Gly is present, and as early as the first year of life when the Asp578Tyr mutation is present.[115,133-135] Patients with this condition may have an enlarged phallus at birth.[133]

During the first five years of life, patients with MLPP have very low LH and FSH levels and testosterone levels in pubertal ranges.[136] During adolescence and adult life, testosterone levels do not increase above age-appropriate concentrations and gonadotropin levels normalize.[115,136-138] Thus, adolescents and adults with MLPP do not usually manifest signs of androgen excess (such as hirsutism or severe acne).[115,136] Most mutations that cause MLPP are located in TM6 and i3, regions that participate in receptor-G protein coupling.[115] Somatic activating mutations cause sporadic Leydig cell adenomas.[90]

In contrast to males, the LH receptor is not known to play an important role in females until puberty. During puberty, activation of LH receptors on ovarian theca cells leads to the production of androgens that are converted to estrogens by aromatase in granulose cells.[115] LH, along with FSH, also plays a role in inducing the differentiation of follicles into Graaffian follicles and triggers ovulation and release of the oocyte.[115]

Females with inactivating mutations of the LH receptor may be asymptomatic or present with primary amenorrhea.[115] Females with complete inactivating LH receptor mutations may present with primary amenorrhea, inability to ovulate, and decreased estrogen and progesterone levels accompanied by elevated LH and FSH levels.[124,139] Affected individuals may have signs of low estrogen levels, including a hypoplastic uterus, a thin-walled vagina, decreased vaginal secretions, and decreased bone mass.[124,139]

FSH Receptors

Inactivating and activating FSH receptor mutations have also been described.[140] However, FSH receptor mutations are considerably less common than LH receptor mutations.[140] The FSH receptor gene is located in chromosome 2 p21 and contains 10 exons.[141] The last exon of the FSH receptor gene encodes the transmembrane and intracellular domains.[142]

FSH is required in females for normal follicle maturation and the regulation of estrogen production by ovarian granulosa cells.[140,143,144] FSH is required in pubertal males for Sertoli cell proliferation, testicular growth, and the maintenance of spermatogenesis.[140,145]

The first inactivating mutation of the FSH receptor was found in Finnish females with autosomal recessive inherited hypergonadotropic ovarian dysgenesis (ODG). ODG is characterized by primary amenorrhea, infertility, and streak or hypoplastic ovaries in the presence of a 46XX karyotype and elevated gonadotropin levels.[146] Twenty-two out of 75 Finnish patients with ODG were found to be homozygous for a C566T point mutation in exon 7 of the FSH receptor gene.[147] This mutation leads to the production of an FSH receptor with an Ala189Val substitution in an area of the extracellular ligand-binding domain that is thought to play a role in turnover of the receptor or in directing the receptor to the plasma membrane.[147] The mutated receptor demonstrates normal ligand-binding affinity but has decreased binding capacity and impaired signal transduction in transfected MSC-1 cells.[147] Males homozygous for this mutation have variable impairment of spermatogenesis and low to low-normal testicular volume but are not azoospermic and can be fertile.[148] The C556T point mutation is uncommon outside Finland, where the carrier frequency is 0.96%.[149]

Compound heterozygosity for mutations that cause partial loss of FSH receptor function may cause endocrine dysfunction in women.[150,151] Women may present with infertility, secondary amenorrhea, osteoporosis, and a history of delayed onset of puberty accompanied by elevated LH and FSH, low-normal plasma estradiol, low plasma inhibin B levels, slightly enlarged ovaries with immature follicles, and a small uterus.[150] This may be caused by FSH receptor gene mutations that result in an Ile160Thr mutation in the extracellular domain that impairs cell surface expression, and an Arg573Cys mutation in e3 that interferes with signal transduction.[150] Other women present with primary amenorrhea, and very elevated gonadotropin, low plasma estradiol and inhibin B levels, normal-size ovaries with immature follicles, and a normal-size uterus.[151] This condition is associated with an Asp224Val substitution in the extracellular domain leading to impaired cells surface expression, and a Leu601Val substitution in e3 impairing signal transduction.[151]

An activating mutation of the FSH receptor has also been described. Surprisingly, a hypophysectomized male was found to be fertile and to have serum testosterone levels above 4.9 nmol/l and normal testis volume in spite of undetectable gonadotropin levels.[152] This patient was found to be heterozygote for an A1700G mutation in exon 10 of the FSH receptor gene that resulted in an Asp567Gly substitution in an area of the third intracytoplasmatic loop that is highly conserved among FSH, LH, and TSH receptors.[152-154] The same substitution in corresponding areas of the LH and TSH receptors results in constitutively active receptors, and is found in MLPP and thyroid adenomas, respectively.[152-154]

TSH Receptors

The TSH receptor gene is located on chromosome 14 and contains 10 exons, with the first nine exons encoding the large extracellular domain and the tenth exon coding the remainder of the receptor.[155-158] At low extracellular TSH concentrations, TSH receptor activation leads to stimulation of $G\alpha_s$—which activates adenylyl cyclase, resulting in increased intracellular cAMP levels.[159,160] At higher extracellular TSH concentrations, activation of the TSH receptor also stimulates the G_q and G_{11} proteins—activating phospholipase C and resulting in the production of diacylglycerol and inositol phosphate.[160]

TSH receptors differ from the other glycoprotein hormone receptors in that they exist in two equally active forms.[161,162] These are the single-chain and two-subunit forms of the TSH receptor (Figure 2-4). The single-chain form of the TSH receptor is made up of three contiguous subunits: the A subunit, C peptide, and B subunit.[162-164] The A subunit begins at the N-terminal of the extracellular domain and contains most of the extracellular domain.[162-164] The C peptide is connected to the C-terminal of the A subunit and continues the extracellular domain.[162-164] The C peptide contains a 50-amino-acid sequence that is only found in TSH receptors.[162-164] The B subunit is connected to the C-terminal of the C peptide and contains the TMs and the C-terminal cytoplasmic portion of the receptor.[162-164] The two-subunit form of the receptor is missing the C-peptide, which is cleaved from the protein during intracellular processing and consists of the A and B subunits attached by disulfide bonds.[165-168] It is surprising that both receptor forms are activated equally by TSH because the C-peptide and nearby regions of the A and B subunits participate in signal transduction.[161-163,169,170]

Spontaneous single-allele mutations of the TSH receptor gene leading to replacement of Ser-281 (near the C-terminal of the A subunit, with Ile, Thr, or Asn) result in a constitutively active TSH receptor that may cause intrauterine or congenital hyperthyroidism, or toxic adenomas.[164,171-173] Activating somatic mutations that cause toxic adenomas have also been found in different transmembrane domains of the TSH receptor.[174-181] More specifically, clusters of mutations are located in the i3 and TM6 regions—found to be involved with signal transduction in all glycoprotein hormone receptors.[174-176,178-180]

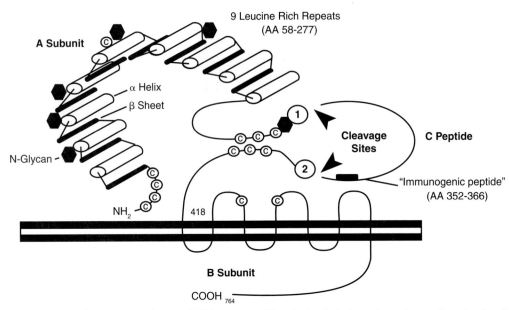

Figure 2-4. The TSH receptor. There are two forms of TSH receptors. The single-chain form is made up of an A subunit, C peptide, and B subunit. Post-translational cleavage of the C peptide from the single chain form results in the two-subunit form. This form consists of the A subunit joined to the B subunit by disulfide bonds between the C-terminal cysteine residues of the A subunit and the N-terminal cysteine residues of the B subunit. [Reproduced with permission from Rapoport B, Chazenbalk GD, Jaume JC, McLachlan SM (1998). The thyrotropin (TSH) receptor: Interaction with TSH and autoantibodies. Endocr Rev 19:676. Copyright 1998, The Endocrine Society.]

The prevalence of activating mutations of the TSH receptor in toxic adenomas has been estimated to range from 2.5% in Japan to 86% in Brazil.[177,178,180,182-185]

Activating somatic mutations of the TSH receptor have also been found in multinodular goiters.[186] Interestingly, different activating mutations have been found in separate nodules in the same individual.[186] Some well-differentiated thyroid carcinomas have activating mutations of the TSH receptor.[187-189] Activating mutations of the Gαs gene have also been found in toxic adenomas and differentiated thyroid carcinomas.[81,190,191] Activating germ line mutations of the TSH receptor can cause sporadic or autosomal dominant inherited nonautoimmune hyperthyroidism that presents in utero, during infancy, or during childhood.[173,192-200] These mutations have been found in the N-terminal extracellular and transmembrane domains.[173,192-200]

Patients with one allele producing constitutively active TSH receptors and one normal allele may present with hyperthyroidism.[162] In contrast, homozygosity or compound heterozygosity for mutations resulting in TSH receptors with reduced function is required to cause clinically apparent thyroid disease.[162] Most known loss-of-function TSH receptor mutations are located in the N-terminal extracellular domain.[201] A spontaneous Asp410Asn substitution, near the carboxy-terminus of the C peptide, results in a TSH receptor with normal ligand binding affinity and impaired Gαs-mediated signal transduction.[202] Patients homozygous for this type of mutation present with compensated hypothyroidism.[202]

Patients homozygous or compound heterozygous for loss-of-function mutations of the TSH receptor present with the syndrome of resistance to TSH (RTSH). Loss-of-function mutations of the TSH receptor that cause RTSH have been identified in the N-terminal extracellular domain, TM4, i2, e1, and e3.[203] Clinical severity of RTSH may range from a euthyroid state accompanied by elevated TSH levels (fully compensated RTSH), to mild hypothyroidism unaccompanied by a goiter (partially compensated hypothyroidism), to congenital thyroid hypoplasia accompanied by profound hypothyroidism (uncompensated RTSH).[62,202,204-208] In patients with uncompensated RTSH, a small bilobar thyroid gland is located at the normal site.[62] Because the sodium-iodide symporter is TSH dependent,[131] iodine and (99m) Pertechnetate uptakes are diminished or absent in patients with RTSH.[62,209] Some families have been found to have an autosomal-dominant form of RTSH that is not caused by a mutation of the TSH receptor.[210,211]

HCG and TSH Receptors During Pregnancy

Due to its structural similarity with TSH, HCG can activate the TSH receptor.[212] During pregnancy, HCG activation of TSH receptors leads to elevation in thyroid hormones seen after the ninth week of gestation—and decreases in TSH levels between the ninth and twelfth weeks of gestation.[213] This phenomenon does not usually result in maternal hyperthyroidism (gestational thyrotoxicosis).[213,214] However, when HCG levels are abnormally elevated due to a molar pregnancy or choriocarcinoma hyperthyroidism may occur.[215-219]

A mother and daughter were identified with recurrent gestational hyperthyroidism and normal serum HCG levels.[220] These individuals were found to be heterozygous for a point mutation in the TSH receptor gene, resulting in a Lys183Arg substitution in the extracellular domain of the receptor. It is believed that this substitution increases activation of the receptor by HCG, causing gestational hyperthyroidism.

HCG and FSH Receptors During Pregnancy

Promiscuous activation of wild-type FSH receptors by excessively elevated HCG and TSH levels during pregnancy, and promiscuous activation of mutated FSH receptors by normal levels of HCG and TSH during pregnancy, have been found to cause spontaneous ovarian hyperstimulation syndrome.[221-224] Ovarian hyperstimulation syndrome may occur spontaneously or iatrogenically as a result of ovarian stimulation treatment. The ovaries enlarge as multiple ovarian cysts form in association with the extravascular fluid shifts thought to result from increased mesothelial capillary permeability.

The extravascular fluid shifts may cause life-threatening pleural and/or pericardial effusions, and/or ascites.[225] Surprisingly, the heterozygous promiscuity-inducing FSH receptor gene mutations alter the serpentine domain rather than the ectodomain.[221-224] This finding reveals that transmembrane domain plays a role in conferring FSH receptor specificity. Interestingly, these mutations also cause the FSH receptor to be constitutively active.[3]

THE GONADOTROPIN-RELEASING HORMONE RECEPTOR GROUP

Gonadotropin-Releasing Hormone Receptors

The GnRH receptor gene is located on 4q13 and includes three exons.[226,227] Unlike glycoprotein hormone receptors, GnRH receptors lack an intracellular C-terminal domain.[228,229] The GnRH receptor also differs from most endocrine GPCRs in that its actions are mediated by G_q/G_{11} stimulation of phospholipase C activity.[230] Phospholipase C cleaves phosphatidylinositol-4,5-diphosphate (PIP2) to inositol 1,4,5-triphosphate (IP3) and diacylglycerol, leading to increased protein kinase C (PKC) activity.[231,232]

Some patients with IHH (idiopathic) have been found to be homozygous or compound heterozygous for loss-of-function mutations in the gene for the GnRH receptor.[233-235] Unlike patients with Kallman's syndrome, they have a normal sense of smell.[233-235] GnRH receptor mutations that cause IHH result in decreased binding of GnRH and/or impaired GnRH receptor signal transduction, or decreased cell GnRH receptor cell membrane expression due to misrouting of GnRH receptor oligomers from the endoplasmic reticulum.[32,33,233-235]

Female patients with mutations that partially compromise GnRH receptor function may present with primary amenorrhea and infertility associated with a normal or small uterus and small ovaries with immature follicles.[233,236] Males with the same mutations may present with incomplete hypogonadotropic hypogonadism (characterized by a delayed and incomplete puberty) or with complete hypogonadotropic hypogonadism, characterized by absent puberty.[233,236]

Some patients with IHH due to mutated GnRH receptors have partial or normal gonadotropin responses to exogenous GnRH.[233,234] However, decreased amplitude in the pulsatile LH secretion can be observed in these patients.[233] Females with a partial or normal gonadotropin response to exogenous GnRH are more likely than nonresponders to become fertile in response to pulsatile exogenous GnRH.[233,237]

THE THYROTROPIN-RELEASING HORMONE AND SECRETAGOGUE RECEPTOR GROUP

Thyrotropin-Releasing Hormone Receptors

Like the GnRH receptor, TRH receptor activation leads to increased phospholipase C activity.[238] To date, only inactivating mutations that cause endocrine dysfunction have been reported for the TRH receptor. One patient has been identified with central hypothyroidism due to mutated TRH receptors.[239] He presented during the ninth year of life with short stature (−2.6 SD) accompanied by a delayed bone age (−4.1 SD), low plasma thyroxine level, and normal plasma TSH level. Exogenous TRH did not induce an increase in plasma TSH and prolactin levels. He was found to be compound heterozygous for TRH receptor gene mutations, resulting in receptors with decreased binding.

OTHER CLASS A RECEPTORS THAT TRANSDUCE HORMONE ACTION

Free Fatty Acid Receptor 1

At the time of discovery of a new GPCR, the ligand for the newly discovered receptor is often unknown. Thus, until a specific ligand is discovered these GPCRs are known as orphan receptors. According to the Human Genome Organization (HUGO) Gene Nomenclature Committee, these G-protein–coupled orphan receptors should be named alphanumerically GPR followed by a number until their ligand is known. Once a specific ligand is identified, a more specific name is given the receptor.

The ligands for GPR40 were unknown when the receptor was first discovered. The HUGO Gene Nomenclature Committee changed the name of the receptor to free fatty acid receptor 1 (FFAR1) when the ligands were identified as medium- and long-chain fatty acids. With rare exceptions that are clearly identified, HUGO Gene Nomenclature Committee recommendations are followed in this chapter (see *http://www.gene.ucl.ac.uk/nomenclature/index.html* for more information on receptor nomenclature).

FFAR1 is one of several GRCRs for lipid mediators. Lipid mediators are intercellular lipid messengers that include sphingosine 1-phosphate, sphingosylphosphorylcholine, dioleoyphosphatidic acid, lysophosphatidic acid, eicosatetraenoic acid, bile acids, and free fatty acids.[55] FFAR1 is activated by medium- and long-chain fatty acids, whereas FFAR2 (formerly known as GPR43) and FFAR3 (formerly known as GPR 41) are activated by shorter-chain fatty acids.[55] There is now evidence that FFAR1 activation by medium- and long-chain fatty acids has endocrine implication. FFAR1 is expressed in human pancreatic β-islet cells.[240]

Fatty-acid–induced stimulation of FFAR1 in β-islet cells leads to activation of the $G\alpha_q$-phospholipase C second-messenger pathway, which in turn leads to release of calcium from the endoplasmic reticulum that augments insulin-mediated increases in intracellular calcium concentrations due to glucose-induced activation of voltage-gated calcium channels.[241-244] Because an increased intracellular calcium concentration induces insulin release, FFAR1-mediated augmentation of glucose-mediated increases in the intracellular calcium concentration leads to amplification of glucose-stimulated insulin release.[241-244]

Wild-type mice placed on an 8-week high-fat diet develop glucose intolerance, insulin resistance, hypertriglyceridemia, and hepatic steatosis—whereas FFAR1 knockout mice on the same diet do not develop these conditions.[245] The clinical relevance for humans is yet unclear. However, an Arg211His polymorphism in the FFAR1 gene may explain some of the variation in insulin secretory capacity found in Japanese men. Arg/Arg homozygotes had lower serum insulin levels, homeostasis model of insulin resistance, and homeostasis model of beta-cell function than His/His homozygotes.[246]

GPR54

Separate groups of investigators from France and the United States simultaneously found homozygous inactivating GPR54 mutations that cause IHH in consanguineous French and Saudi Arabian kindreds, respectively.[247-249] The United States group also found an African American patient with IHH due to compound heterozygous inactivating GPR54 mutations.[248] Since then, a patient with a Jamaican father and a Turkish-Cypriot mother, and with cryptorchidism and micropenis at birth and undetectable LH and FSH levels at 2 months of age, was found to have compound heterozygous GPR54 mutations.[250]

Unlike patients with Kallmann syndrome, these patients' sense of smell is intact. Furthermore, in contrast to patients with isolated hypogonadotropic hypogonadism due to GnRH mutations patients with IHH due to GPR54 mutations also exhibit increases in gonadotropin levels in response to exogenous GnRH. Thus, inactivating homozygous and compound heterozygous GPR54 mutations are a rare cause of normosmic IHH.[249,250]

Ligands for GPR54 derive from a single precursor protein, kisspeptin-1.[251,252] The longest derivative protein that acts as a ligand for GPR54 is metastin, which is named metastin because metastin is a metastasis suppressor gene in melanoma cells.[251] Metastin consists of kisspeptin-1 69-121.[251,252] However, shorter C-terminal peptides derived from kisspeptin-1 bind and activate GPR54.[251] Administration of metastin to adult male volunteers increases LH, FSH, and testosterone levels.[253] Recent animal research suggests that metasin and GPR54 play a role in the timing of onset of puberty, in modulating sex steroid feedback on GnRH release from the hypothalamus, and in the timing of onset of puberty.[249]

Orexin Receptors

Orexins act on orexin receptors, located predominantly in the hypothalamus, to control food intake and play a role in the regulation of sleep/wakefulness.[254-256] There are two types of orexin receptors, the orexin-1 and the orexin 2 receptors.[256] There are also two types of orexins, orexin A and orexin B, formed from the precursor peptide preproorexin.[256] Orexins are also known as hypocretins, and orexin A is synonymous with hypocretin-1 and orexin B with hypocretin-2.[255,256] Orexin A acts on orexin-1 and orexin-2 receptors, whereas orexin B only acts on orexin-2 receptors.[254,257,258]

Like most class A GPCRs, orexin receptors couple with $G_{q/11}$ and G_i/G_o to activate phospholipase C and inactivate adenylyl cyclase, respectively.[256,259-261] Surprisingly, however, recent evidence suggests that orexin receptors also couple with G_s—which increases adenylyl cyclase activity.[261] Orexins increase food intake and duration of wakefulness.[254,255,262] Orexin A and activation of the orexin-1 receptor have greater orexigenic effects than orexin B and activation of the orexin-2 receptor.[263] The orexin-2 receptor mediates the arousal effect of orexins.[263] Most patients with idiopathic narcolepsy have diminished levels of orexins in cerebral spinal fluid and lack orexin-containing neurons.[255,264-267]

Ghrelin Receptors

Another class A receptor that transduces hormone action is the ghrelin receptor. The receptor is also known as the growth hormone secretagogue receptor type 1a because the receptor is also activated by a family of synthetic growth hormone secretagogues.[90,263] Ghrelin is a product of post-translational modification of the ghrelin gene product proghrelin.[268] Ghrelin is mainly produced in the stomach.[269,270] Ghrelin activation of ghrelin receptors located in the hypothalamus and pituitary somatotrophs results in growth hormone secretion.[271] The ghrelin receptor also has an orexigenic role.

Plasma ghrelin levels are elevated just prior to eating, and decrease rapidly after eating.[272,273] In addition, intravenous administration of ghrelin to humans increases appetite and food intake.[274] Plasma ghrelin levels are elevated in individuals with Prader Willi syndrome.[275] Thus, hyperphagia in patients with Prader Willi syndrome may be due at least in part to overactivation of ghrelin receptors by ghrelin. Screening of 184 extremely obese children and adolescents for mutations of the ghrelin receptor gene failed to identify a single mutation likely to cause obesity.[276]

Short individuals in two unrelated Moroccan kindreds were found to have a C to A transversion at position 611 in the first exon of the ghrelin receptor gene.[277] This transversion results in replacement of the apolar and neutral amino acid alanine at position 204 of the receptor by the polar and charged amino acid glutamate. This mutation interferes with normal constitutive activity of the receptor, and decreases cell membrane expression of the receptor. Receptor activation by ghrelin, however, is preserved. Two-thirds of individuals in the kindreds heterozygous for the mutation had height greater than or equal to 2 standard deviations below the mean. One heterozygous individual's height was 3.7 standard deviations below the mean. Prior to onset of growth hormone therapy, the only individual in the kindreds homozygous for the mutation had a height 3.7 standard deviations below the mean. Whereas the patient homozygous for the mutation became overweight during puberty, the weight of the patients heterozygous for the mutation varied from underweight to overweight.

Another product of post-translational modification of proghrelin, obestatin, appears to play a role in controlling appetite and weight.[268] Activation of the obestatin receptor, previously known as GPR39, in rats results in decreased food intake and weight.

Melanin-Concentrating Hormone Receptors

Formerly known as SLC-1 or GPR24, the type 1 melanin-concentrating hormone (MCH) receptor (MCHR1)—and the more recently discovered type 2 MCH receptor (MCHR2), formerly known as SLT or GPR145—may play a role in regulating feeding and energy metabolism in humans.[278-281] When activated by MCH, MCHR1 couples with $G_{q/11}$ and $G_{i/o}$ to increase phospholipase C activity and inhibit adenylyl cyclase activity, respectively.[278,279,282] When activated by MCH, MCHR2 couples with $G_{q/11}$ to increase phospholipase C activity.[280,281]

Studies in rodents reveal that MCH is an orexigenic hormone, and treatment of rodents with MCHR1 antagonists decreases food intake, weight, and body fat.[278,283,284] Little is known about the role of MCHR2 in animals, and both receptors in humans. Analysis of the MCHR1 gene in more than 4,000 obese German, Danish, French, and American children and adolescents revealed several single-nucleotide polymorphisms and gene variations in the German children and adolescents that may be associated with obesity.[285] Another study of 106 American subjects with early-onset obesity failed to definitively identify MCHR1 and MCHR2 mutations as a cause of obesity.[286]

Class B Receptors That Transduce Hormone Action

GROWTH-HORMONE–RELEASING HORMONE RECEPTOR

The growth-hormone–releasing (GHRH) receptor gene is located at 7p14.[287] GHRH receptors interact with G_s to stimulate adenylyl cyclase, resulting in increased intracellular cAMP levels that lead to somatotroph proliferation and growth hormone secretion.[288] Thus, it is not surprising that activating mutations in $G\alpha_s$ leading to constitutive activation of adenylyl cyclase have been found in some growth-hormone–secreting pituitary adenomas in humans.[289]

Some patients with isolated growth hormone deficiency have been found to be homozygous or compound heterozygous for inactivating mutations in the GHRH receptor gene.[288] The same mutation was found in three apparently unrelated consanguineous kindreds from India, Pakistan, and Sri Lanka.[287,290,291] A different mutation has been identified in a Brazilian kindred.[288] Both mutations result in the production of markedly truncated proteins with no receptor activity.[288,291] In another family, two sibling with isolated growth hormone deficiency were found to be compound heterozygous for inactivating GHRH receptor gene mutations.[292]

Individuals in these kindreds homozygous or compound heterozygous for inactivating GHRH receptor gene mutations experienced severe postnatal growth failure that resulted in proportionate short stature.[287,288,291,292] Males have high-pitched voices and moderately delayed puberty.[287,288,291] Unlike infants with complete growth hormone deficiency, they do not have frontal bossing, microphallus, or hypoglycemia.[287,291,292] Their bone age was delayed with respect to chronologic age but advanced with respect to height age.[291] Some patients were found to have pituitary hypoplasia.[287,291] Growth velocity increased with exogenous growth hormone therapy.[287,288,291,292]

GASTRIC INHIBITORY POLYPEPTIDE RECEPTORS

The gastric inhibitory peptide receptor (GIPR) gene is located on the long arm of chromosome 19.[293] Two functional isoforms exist in humans due to alternate splicing.[294] GIPR activation induces $G\alpha_s$ activation of adenylyl cyclase.[294-296] Gastric inhibitory polypeptide (GIP) is also known as glucose-dependent insulinotropic polypeptide and is released by K cells in the small intestine in response to food. GIP has numerous physiologic actions, including stimulation of glucagon, somatostatin, and insulin release by pancreatic islet cells.[297,298] GIP does not normally induce cortisol release from adrenocortical cells.[299,300]

Circulating cortisol levels in patients with food-dependent or GIP-dependent Cushing's syndrome rise abnormally in response to food intake.[83,84] These patients may have adrenal adenomas or nodular bilateral adrenal hyperplasia that overexpress GIPRs that abnormally stimulate cortisol secretion when activated.[299,301] Thus, in these patients postprandial GIP release leads to activation of these abnormally expressed and functioning adrenal GIPRs—resulting in excessive adrenal cortisol secretion.[299,300]

PARATHYROID HORMONE AND PARATHYROID-HORMONE–RELATED PEPTIDE RECEPTORS

Two types of PTH receptors have been identified. The type 1 PTH receptor (PTHR1) is activated by PTH and parathyroid-hormone–related peptide (PTHrP) and mediates PTH effects in bone and kidney.[302] In spite of 51% homology to the PTHR1, the type 2 PTH receptor (PTHR2) is only activated by PTH.[302-305] The PTHR2 is expressed in the brain and pancreas and its function is largely unknown.[302,303]

The PTHR1 has a large amino-terminal extracellular domain containing six conserved cysteine residues.[302] Ligand binding induces the PTHR1 to interact with G_s and G_q proteins, leading to activation of the adenylyl cyclase/protein kinase A and phospholipase C/protein kinase C second-messenger pathways, respectively.[306-311] Interestingly, mutations in i2 interfere with coupling of the PTHR1 to G_q without interfering with coupling to G_s—whereas mutations in i3 disrupt coupling of the receptor to both G proteins.[312,313]

Loss-of-function PTHR1 gene mutations cause Blomstrand's chondrodysplasia.[302] This lethal disorder is characterized by accelerated chondrocyte differentiation, resulting in short-limbed dwarfism, mandibular hypoplasia, lack of breast and nipple development, and severely impacted teeth.[302,314] One patient with this rare condition was found to be homozygous for a point mutation that resulted in a Pro132Leu substitution in the N-terminal domain that interferes with ligand binding.[315,316] Another patient was found to be homozygous for a frame-shift mutation that results in a truncated receptor lacking TM5-7, and contiguous intracellular and extracellular domains.[317]

A third patient was found to have a maternally inherited mutation that altered splicing of maternal mRNA, resulting in a PTHR1 with a deletion of residues 373 through 383 in TM5 (which also interferes with ligand binding).[318] In spite of heterozygosity for the mutation, the patient was unable to produce normal PTHR1s because for unknown reasons the paternal allele, was not expressed.[318] Heterozygosity for an Arg150Cys PTHR1 gene mutation was found in two out of six patients with enchondromatosis.[319] Enchondromatosis is an autosomal-dominant condition characterized by benign cartilage tumors and increased risk for the development of osteosarcomas.[14]

Some cases of Jansen's metaphyseal chondrodysplasia have been found to be caused by constitutively activating mutations of the PTHR1 gene.[320-322] This autosomal-dominant disorder is characterized by short-limbed dwarfism due to impaired terminal chondrocyte differentiation and delayed mineralization accompanied by hypercalcemia.[320,321] Interestingly, constitutive activation appears to result predominantly in excessive $G\alpha_s$ activity because adenylyl cyclase activity is increased and PLC activity is unchanged in COS-7 cells expressing mutated receptors.[320-322]

OTHER CLASS B RECEPTORS THAT TRANSDUCE HORMONE ACTION

Other class B receptors that transduce hormone action include glucagon-like peptide-1, glucagon, calcitonin, and corticotrophin-releasing factor receptors.[323] Class B receptors usually couple with heterotrimeric G_s proteins, leading to activation of adenylyl cyclase—which in turn leads to elevated intracellular cAMP levels.[323,324] (See Chapter 10 for discussion of the role of GLP1 in promoting insulin secretion and the use of GLP1 analogues or inhibitors of GLP1 breakdown in therapy.)

Class C Receptors That Transduce Hormone Action

CALCIUM-SENSING RECEPTORS

The calcium-sensing receptor (CaSR) is located on the long arm of chromosome 3 (3q21.1).[325] The CaSR has a large amino-terminal domain that contains nine potential glycosylation sites.[326] Binding of ionized calcium to the CaSR leads to activation of phospholipase C, presumably via activation of a G_q protein.[326,327]

The CaSR is an integral component of a feedback system that utilizes parathyroid hormone and renal tubular calcium reabsorption to keep the serum concentrations of ionized calcium in a narrow physiologic range.[328] Increased extracellular ionized calcium concentrations activate CaSRs in parathyroid chief and renal tubular epithelial cells, leading to decreased PTH release and renal tubular calcium reabsorption.[326,329] When ionized calcium concentrations fall, CaSR activation decreases—leading to increased PTH release and renal tubular calcium reabsorption.[326,329]

Recent evidence suggests that the CaSR also binds another cation, magnesium, and thus may play a role in magnesium homeostasis by altering reabsorption of magnesium in the thick ascending limb of Henle in the kidneys.[330,331] It is probable that increased peritubular levels of magnesium activate renal CaSRs, leading to inhibition of reabsorption of magnesium from the thick ascending limb of Henle—which in turn leads to increased renal excretion of magnesium.[330,331]

Autosomal-dominant familial benign hypocalciuric hypercalcaemia (FBH) and neonatal severe hyperparathyroidism (NSHPT) are caused by loss-of-function mutations of the CaSR gene.[332,333] Most of these mutations are located in the N-terminal extracellular domain.[334,335] With few exceptions, individuals heterozygous for loss-of-function mutations have FBH—whereas individuals homozygous for such mutations have NSHPT.[336,337] Therefore, children of consanguineous FBH parents are at risk for NSHPT.[334,338,339] Occasionally, infants with NSHPT are heterozygous for CaSR gene mutations.[340]

Decreased CaSR function impedes calcium ion suppression of PTH release and renal tubular calcium reabsorption.[333] Thus, FBH is characterized by mild hypercalcemia that is accompanied by inappropriately normal or elevated serum PTH levels and by relatively low urinary calcium excretion.[336,341,342] Individuals with FBH may also have hypermagnesemia as a result of decreased peritubular inhibition of magnesium reabsorption from the thick ascending loops of the kidneys by the CaSR.[331] There are three type of FBH: FBH type 1 (FBH1), FBH type 2 (FBH2), FBH type 3 (FBH3).[343]

FBH1 is due to heterozygous loss-of-function mutations of the CaSR gene on 3q21.1.[343] Two other chromosome loci have been identified in patients with FBH without CaSR gene mutations. FBH2 has been mapped to 19p13.3 and is biochemically and clinically similar to FBH1.[343,344] FBH3, which is also known as the Oklahoma variant (FBH$_{OK}$), has been mapped to 19q13.[343,345] Adults with FBH3 have hypophosphatemia, elevated serum PTH levels, and osteomalacia in addition to the clinical and biochemical findings found in individuals with FBH1 and FBH2.[343,346] NSHPT is characterized by severe hypercalcemia accompanied by elevated circulating PTH levels, undermineralization of bone, rib cage deformity, and multiple long-bone and rib fractures.[336]

Activating mutations of the CaSR gene may cause autosomal-dominant hypocalcemic hypercalciuria (ADHH), also known as autosomal dominant hypocalcemia, as increased CaSR function leads to increased calcium ion suppression of PTH release and suppression of renal tubular calcium reabsorption.[327,343,347-351] ADHH is characterized by hypocalcemia and hypomagnesemia accompanied by inappropriately normal or increased urinary calcium excretion and inappropriately normal or low serum PTH levels.[327,349-351] Patients with ADHH may be asymptomatic or may present with tetany, muscle cramps, or seizures during infancy or childhood.[349-352] Similar to inactivating mutations, most activating mutations are located in the N-terminal extracellular domain.[347,349,350,352] Treatment of patients with ADHH with vitamin D or its metabolites is contraindicated because treatment with these vitamins results in worsening hypercalciuria and nephrolithiasis, in nephrocalcinosis, and in renal impairment.[349,350]

Bartter syndrome type V, like other types of Bartter syndrome, is characterized by hypokalemic metabolic alkalosis and by hyperaldosteronism due to elevated renin levels.[353,354] Patients with Bartter syndrome type V, unlike patients with other types of Bartter syndrome, may also have symptomatic hypocalcemia and are at risk for developing nephrocalcinosis due to hypercalciuria.[353,354] Evidence from in vitro functional expression studies suggests that patients with mild or moderate heterozygous gain-of-function mutations of the CaSR develop ADHH, whereas those with severe heterozygous gain-of-function mutations of the CaSR develop Bartter syndrome type V.[353-355]

Some single–amino-acid polymorphisms of the CaSR gene appear to be predictive of whole-blood ionized and serum total calcium levels, and may increase risk for bone and mineral metabolism disorders in individuals with other genetic and environmental risk factors for these disorders.[356-358] Individuals heterozygous or homozygous for a Gln1011Glu CaSR gene polymorphism tend to have higher calcium levels than individuals with the polymorphism.[358,359] The 15.4% of 387 healthy young Canadian women with at least one CaSR gene allele with an Ala986Ser polymorphism were found to have higher total calcium levels than the remainder of the women without the polymorphism.[357]

Another study of 377 unrelated healthy Italian adult males and females found that 24% of study subjects were heterozygous or homozygous for the Ala986Ser polymorphism, and confirmed the finding that individuals without the polymorphism have lower whole-blood ionized calcium levels than individuals with the polymorphism.[358] The Ala986Ser polymorphism has also been associated with Paget disease and primary hyperparathyroidism.[359-361] Individuals with a less common Arg990Gly polymorphism tend to have lower whole-blood ionized calcium levels than individuals without the polymorphism.[358] The Arg-990Gly polymorphism has been found to be associated with hypercalciuria and nephrolithiasis.[361,362]

Auto-antibodies against the CaSR that interfere with binding of calcium to the receptor may cause autoimmune hypocalciuric hypercalcemia.[363] These patients have the clinical and biochemical features of patients with FBH.[363] Conversely, auto-antibodies that activate the CaSR cause autoimmune-acquired hypoparathyroidism.[364] Both conditions may occur in association with other autoimmune conditions (such as autoimmune thyroiditis), with celiac disease in patients with autoimmune hypocalciuric hypercalcemia, and with autoimmune thyroiditis and autoimmune polyglandular syndrome types 1 and 2 in patients with autoimmune-acquired hypoparathyroidism.[363-365]

Auto-antibodies that activate the CaSR were found in approximately one-third of individuals with acquired hypoparathyroidism.[365]

G-Protein Gene Disorders

Inactivating and activating mutations of the GNAS1 gene that encodes $G\alpha_s$ cause endocrine disorders.

INACTIVATING MUTATIONS OF THE GNAS1 GENE

Pseudohypoparathyroidism type Ia (PHP-Ia; Albright hereditary osteodystrophy) and pseudopseudohypoparathyroidism (PPHP) are caused by heterozygous inactivating mutations of the GNAS1 gene that encodes $G\alpha_s$.[366-370] PHP-Ia is characterized by hypocalcemia, hyperphosphatemia, elevated circulating PTH levels, short stature, obesity, mental retardation, brachycephaly, short fingers, and short fourth and fifth metacarpals.[366-369] Some patients may also have a small phallus, reflecting the same defect in LH receptor transduction. FSH and TSH also may be affected. PPHP is characterized by the same somatic features as PHP-Ia in the absence of resistance to PTH.[366,367,370] Interestingly, patients who inherit these mutations from their mothers have PHP-Ia and patients who inherit these mutations from their fathers have PPHP.[366-370]

It is now known that in the renal proximal tubules $G\alpha_s$ can only be encoded from the maternally inherited GNAS1 allele, whereas elsewhere in the body $G\alpha_s$ can be encoded from either the maternally or paternally inherited GNAS1 allele.[371] Thus, patients with maternally inherited inactivating GNAS1 gene mutations are not able to express $G\alpha_s$ in the proximal tubules and have PHP-Ia.[371] Patients with paternally inherited inactivating GNAS1 gene mutations have wild-type maternally inherited GNAS1 alleles and thus have normal $G\alpha_s$ expression in the proximal renal tubules and have PPHP.[371]

Pseudohypoparathyroidism type Ib (PHP-Ib) is characterized by resistance to parathyroid hormone in the absence of the somatic features of PHP-Ia. It was thought that PHP-Ib is caused by inactivating mutations in the PTHR1 gene.[372] However, no deleterious PTHR1 gene mutations have been found in patients with PHP-Ib.[373,374]

Instead of PTHR1 gene mutations, defective imprinting is now thought to play a role in causing PHP-Ib. In most tissues, $G\alpha_s$ is encoded by both GNAS1 alleles.[371] However, in the renal proximal tubules $G\alpha_s$ is only encoded by the maternal GNAS1 allele.[371] The exon 1A region of the GNAS1 gene contains a region that is imprinted in the oocyte by methylation of the DNA.[371,375] This region is not imprinted in most PHP-Ib patients.[375] Thus, failure to maternally imprint the maternally inherited GNAS1 allele is now thought to play a role in causing most cases of PHP-Ib.[368,375] $G\alpha_s$ cannot be expressed in the renal proximal tubules of these patients due to lack of a maternal GNAS1 allele. The PHP-Ib syndrome is also limited to renal resistance to PTH rather than (as in Albright's hereditary osteodystrophy) having other clinical manifestations because $G\alpha_s$ expression in nonrenal tissues does not require a maternally imprinted GNAS1 allele.[376] One patient with PHP-Ib was found to have paternal uniparental isodisomy for chromosome 20, which contains the GNAS1 gene.[377] Thus, the patient was found to have two paternally inherited GNAS1 alleles. Thus, lack of a maternally imprinted GNAS1 allele also appears to have played a role in causing this patient's PHP-Ib.

ACTIVATING MUTATIONS OF THE GNAS1 GENE

When a GPCR is activated by a ligand, GDP is converted to GTP—which causes the heterotrimeric G protein to dissociate into active $G\alpha$-GTP and $G\beta\gamma$ subunits.[5-7] GTPase then converts GTP into GDP, which inactivates $G\alpha$ and increases affinity of $G\alpha$ for $G\beta\gamma$—leading to reformation of the inactive heterotrimeric G protein.[5-7] Arg^{201} and Gln^{227} of $G\alpha_s$ are critical to GTPase activity.[376] GNAS1 mutations that result in substitutions of these amino acid residues by amino acid residues that disrupt GTPase activity prolong the active state of $G\alpha_s$.[376] Somatic mutations of these residues that disrupt GTPase activity are present in approximately 40% of growth-hormone–secreting and some ACTH-secreting and nonsecreting pituitary tumors; in some parathyroid, thyroid, and adrenal tumors; and in some intramuscular myxomas.[81,378,379]

More widespread mosaic Arg^{201} $G\alpha_s$ mutations that decrease GTPase activity cause fibrous dysplasia or (when tissue distribution of the mutation is very widespread) McCune Albright syndrome, which is characterized by the triad of café au lait spots, polyostic fibrous dysplasia, and gonadotropin-independent precocious puberty.[380,381] Patients with McCune Albright syndrome may also have excessive growth hormone production, hyperthyroidism, and Cushing's syndrome—as well as associated nodularity of the pituitary and the thyroid and adrenal glands due to overactive $G\alpha_s$ subunits in GHRH, TSH, and ACTH receptors, respectively.[381,382] Hypophosphatemia, which is not uncommon in patients with McCune Albright syndrome, appears to be due in yet unknown ways to fibrous dysplasia. Patients with McCune Albright syndrome may also have nonendocrine problems such as hepatobiliary abnormalities, cardiomyopathy, and sudden death due to overactive $G\alpha_s$ subunits in nonendocrine GPCRs.[382]

Cytokine Receptors

Cytokines are molecules produced by one cell that act on another cell.[383] Thus, the term can apply not only to molecules with immunologic functions but to hormones. Therefore, growth hormone, prolactin, and leptin are classified as type I cytokines.[384] These and other type I cytokines, (including ILs 2–9, 11–13, and 15; erythropoietin; thrombopoietin; and granulocyte-colony–stimulating factor) are characterized by a four α-helical bundle structure and signaling via type I cytokine receptors.[384] Type II cytokines include the interferons and IL-10 and do not include hormones.[384]

Type I cytokines are divided into long-chain and short-chain cytokines.[384] Prolactin, leptin, and growth hormone belong to the long-chain subclass of type I cytokines because their helixes are 25 amino acids in length.[384] The short-chain type I cytokines, including IL-2 and stem cell factor, have helixes of approximately 15 amino acids in length.[384]

STRUCTURE AND FUNCTION OF TYPE I CYTOKINE RECEPTORS

All type I cytokine receptors have four conserved cysteine residues, fibronectin type II modules, a Trp-Ser-X-Trp-Ser motif in the extracellular domain, and a praline-rich Box 1/Box 2 region in the cytoplasmic domain.[384,385] With the exception of stem cell factor, type I cytokine receptors do not contain catalytic domains such as kinases.[384]

Type I cytokine receptors for long-chain type I cytokines require homodimerization for activation.[384,386] First, the ligand binds a monomeric receptor.[384,386] Then, the ligand interacts with a second receptor to induce receptor dimerization and activation.[384,386] Activated receptors then stimulate members of the Janus family of tyrosine kinases (Jak kinases) to phosphorylate tyrosine residues in itself and the cytoplasmic region of the receptors.[384,387] Signal transducers and activators of transcription (STATs) then dock on the phosphorylated cytoplasmic receptor domains or Jak kinases via an SH2 domain and are tyrosine phophorylated.[384] The phosphorylated STATs then dissociate from the receptors or Jak kinases, form homo- or heterodimers, and translocate to the nucleus.[384,388,389] In the nucleus, the STAT dimers bind and alter the activity of regulatory regions of target DNA.[384,388,390]

There are four Jak kinases.[388,391] Jak3 is only expressed in lymphohematopoietic cells, whereas Jak1, Jak2, and Tyk2 are expressed in every cell.[384,392,393] There are seven STATs (Stat1, Stat2, Stat3, Stat4, Stat5a, Stat5b, and Stat6), which have different SH2 domain sequences that confer different receptor specificities.[384,387-389]

CYTOKINE RECEPTORS THAT TRANSDUCE HORMONE ACTION

The actions of growth hormone, prolactin, and leptin are mediated via specific type I cytokine receptors.[384] Mutations of the growth hormone receptor (GHR) and the leptin receptor have been found that are associated with endocrine disorders (Table 2-3).

Growth Hormone Receptors

The GHR gene is located on the short arm of chromosome 5 (5p13.1-p12), and 9 of the 13 exons of the gene encode the receptor.[394-397] A secretion signal sequence is encoded by exon 2, the N-terminal extracellular ligand binding domain is encoded by exons 3 through 7, the single transmembrane domain is encoded by exon 9, and the C-terminal cytoplasmic domain is encoded by exons 9 and 10.[394-397] Growth hormone binding protein (GHBP) is the product of proteolytic cleavage of the extracellular domain of the GHR from the rest of the receptor.[398] Approximately 50% of circulating growth hormone is bound to GHBP.[398]

TABLE 2-3

Cytokine Receptors and Clinical Conditions Associated with Receptor Mutations

Receptor	Germ Line Mutation	Endocrine Disorder
Growth hormone receptor	Some inactivating (heterozygous)	Partial growth hormone insensitivity with mild to moderate growth failure
	Inactivating (homozygous, compound heterozygous)	Growth hormone insensitivity/ Laron syndrome with moderate to severe postnatal growth failure
Leptin receptor	Inactivating (homozygous)	Obesity and hypogonadotropic hypogonadism

Growth-hormone–induced receptor dimerization stimulates Jak2, resulting in tyrosyl phosphorylation of Stat1, Stat3, and Stat5.[399-403] Then the STATs translocate to the nucleus, where they regulate growth-hormone–responsive genes.[400-403] In particular, growth hormone indirectly controls growth by regulating production of insulin-like growth factor-1 (IGF-1)—which has direct effects on cell proliferation and hypertrophy.[404] Jak2 also activates the mitogen activated protein (MAP) kinase and insulin receptor substrate pathways.[405-407] However, the extent to which these pathways contribute to growth hormone action is as yet unknown.[397]

Patients are considered to have growth hormone insensitivity (GHI) if they do not exhibit appropriate growth and metabolic responses to physiologic levels of growth hormone.[398] The phenotype of GHI is variable and ranges from isolated moderate postnatal growth failure to severe postnatal growth failure accompanied by the classic features of Laron syndrome in Ecuadorean patients with GHR deficiency.[398,408-411] Features of GHR deficiency include frontal temporal hairline recession, prominent forehead, decreased vertical dimension of face, hypoplastic nasal bridge, shallow orbits, blue sclera, small phallus prior to puberty, crowded permanent teeth, absent third molars, small hands and feet, hypoplastic fingernails, hypomuscularity, delayed age of onset for walking, high-pitched voice, increased total and low-density lipoprotein cholesterol, and fasting hypoglycemia.[398,411] All patients with GHI have normal or elevated circulating growth hormone levels, markedly decreased circulating IGF-1 levels, and a delayed bone age.[398]

Patients homozygous or compound heterozygous for deletion of exons 5 and 6—or homozygous or compound heterozygous for numerous nonsense, missense, frame-shift, and splice-point mutations throughout the GHR gene—have been found to have GHI characterized by severe postnatal growth failure and usually low or absent circulating GHBP levels.[398,412,413] Patients homozygous or compound heterozygous for the Arg274Thr or the Gly223Gly splice mutations that result in a truncated receptor that cannot be anchored to the plasma membrane (or that result in the Asp152His missense mutation that interferes with GHR dimerization) have normal circulating GHBP levels.[398]

Patients heterozygous for mutations that alter the GHR have dimerization complexes that consist of two wild-type receptors (a wild-type receptor and a mutant receptor) and two mutant receptors. Thus, heterozygosity for

loss-of-function GHR gene mutations may have a dominant negative effect because the wild-type receptor/ mutant receptor dimers may not be able to function normally. As expected from this phenomenon, some patients with moderate to severe growth failure have been found to be heterozygous for loss-of-function point or splice mutations of the GHR gene that alter the cytoplasmic or extracellular domains.[398,414-417]

Some patients with severe short stature and GHI do not have GHR mutations. Rather, they have defects in GHR-mediated intracellular signaling—including impaired STAT activation.[418]

Leptin Receptors

The leptin receptor [LEPR (also known as Ob-R)] gene is located at 1p31. There are five isoforms of LEPR due to alternative splicing of the LEPR gene transcript (Figure 2-5).[419] Only the Ob-Rb isoform contains both the Jak kinase binding and STAT motifs necessary to maximally transduce the effects of leptin.[419] The Ob-Ra, Ob-Rc, and Ob-Rd isoforms contain intact extracellular and transmembrane but are missing the STAT motif from their cytoplasmic domains.[419] The Ob-Re isoform is missing the transmembrane and cytoplasmic domains.[419] Thus, the Ob-Rb isoform is thought to be the main isoform involved in mediating the effects of leptin.[419]

Three sisters from a consanguineous kindred were found to be homozygous for a splice mutation in the LEPR gene that resulted in expression of an 831 amino acid protein (Ob-Rhd) that lacks transmembrane and cytoplasmic domains.[420] They had been hyperphagic and morbidly obese since birth.[420] They were found to have elevated circulating leptin levels, decreased TSH and GH secretion, and failure of pubertal development due to hypogonadotropic hypogonadism.[420] Heterozygous carriers of the mutation are not morbidly obese and do not have delayed or absent puberty.[420]

More recently, in studies of 300 obese subjects 3% had nonsense or missense LEPR mutations. Individuals with mutations had hyperphagia, severe obesity, altered immune function, and delayed puberty due to hypogonadotropic hypogonadism. Importantly, circulating leptin levels were within the range predicted by the elevated fat mass, and clinical features were less severe than those of subjects with congenital leptin deficiency.[421]

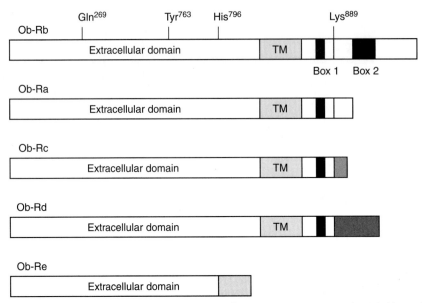

Figure 2-5. Leptin receptor isoforms. There are five leptin receptor isoforms. Box 1 represents the Jak kinase binding motif, and box 2 represents the STAT motif. The Ob-Rb isoform is the only isoform that contains Jak kinase binding and STAT motifs, and is thus thought to be the main isoform involved in mediating the effects of leptin. The Ob-Ra, Ob-Rc, and Ob-Rd isoforms are missing the STAT motif. The Ob-Re isoform is missing the transmembrane (TM) and cytoplasmic domains. [Reproduced with permission from Chen D, Garg A (1999). Monogenic disorders of obesity and body fat distribution. J Lipid Res 40:1737.]

Receptor Tyrosine Kinases

The receptor tyrosine kinase (RTK) superfamily consists of 15 receptor tyrosine kinase families (Figure 2-6).[422] With one exception, these families consist of receptors with one membrane-spanning domain (Figure 2-6).[422] The single-membrane–spanning receptors typically contain an N-terminal extracellular portion, a transmembrane helix, a juxtamembrane region, a tyrosine kinase (TK) domain, and a C-terminal region (Figure 2-6).[422] These receptors require dimerization to be maximally activated.[422-424] Receptors belonging to insulin RTK family differ from other RTKs, as they contain two membrane-spanning polypeptide chains linked by disulfide bonds to two intervening extracellular peptide chains and thus do not dimerize (Figure 2-6).[421]

Activation of RTKs leads to phosphorylation of tyrosine residues in the activation loop (A-loop) in the TK domain(s), resulting in activation of the TK(s).[421,425] Activation of the TK(s), in turn, induces the transfer of phosphate from adenosine triphosphate (ATP) to tyrosine residues in the cytosolic portion of the receptor and in cytosolic proteins that serve as docking sites for second messengers.[421]

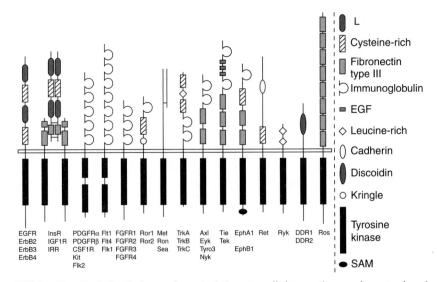

Figure 2-6. The fifteen RTK families. Each family has a characteristic extracellular portion, and a cytoplasmic portion that contains a tyrosine kinase domain. [Reproduced with permission from Hubbard SR (1999). Structural analysis of receptor tyrosine kinases. Prog Biophys Mol Biol 71:344.]

There is a growing body of evidence suggesting that members of the receptor tyrosine kinase superfamily can directly and indirectly interact with heterotrimeric G proteins. The insulin, insulin-like growth factor-1, and insulin-like growth factor-2 receptors appear to directly interact with $G_{i/o}$ and $G_{q/11}$, $G_{i/o}$, and G_i, respectively.[426] The fibroblast growth factor receptors appear to directly and indirectly interact with G_s.[426] Congenital alteration of function of receptors in the insulin and the fibroblast growth factor RTK families leads to endocrine disorders (Table 2-4).

INSULIN RECEPTOR TYROSINE KINASE FAMILY

The insulin RTK family includes the insulin receptor (INSR) and the insulin-like growth factor-1 receptor (IGF1R).[423] These receptors are heterotetramers consisting of two α and β subunits in a αββα configuration (Figure 2-7).[427-429] The cysteine-rich extracellular α subunits are linked by disulfide bonds, and each α subunit is linked to a plasma membrane-spanning and cytosolic β subunit by disulfide bonds.[429,430] Each β subunit contains a TK domain and a C-terminal region that contain tyrosine residues.[421]

Both insulin and insulin-like growth factor-1 (IGF-1) can bind INSRs and IGF1Rs. However, insulin has greater affinity for the INSR and IGF-1 has greater affinity for the IGF1R. Ligand binding alters the conformation of the receptor, resulting in *trans*-autophosphorylation of the C-terminal tyrosine residues on one β subunit by the TK on the other β subunit.[431,432] The phosphorylated tyrosine residues create motifs that can be bound by Src homology 2 (SH2)-domain-containing proteins, including Shc, Grb-2, SHP2, nck, phosphatidylinositol-3-kinase (PI3K), and Crk.[433-437] The receptor TK also phosphorylate tyrosine residues in insulin receptor substrate proteins (IRS), including IRS-1 and IRS-2, that bind INSRs and IGF1Rs.[437-440] When phosphorylated, these tyrosine residues create motifs that are bound by SH2-domain-containing proteins.[433,434,436,437,440] Thus, insulin receptor substrates can serve as docking proteins—allowing SH2-domain-containing proteins to indirectly interact with INSRs and IGF1Rs when stearic constraints do not permit direct interactions between the proteins and the

receptors.[433,434,437] Ultimately, IRSs, SH2-domain-containing proteins, and other proteins (including mSOS) interact to activate the Ras/Raf/MAPKK/MAPK and PI3K/protein kinase B (PKB) cascades (Figure 2-7).[436,437,440]

Activation of the Ras/Raf/ MAPKK/MAPK cascade increases mitogenesis and proliferation, and activation of the PI3K/PKB cascade increases glucose uptake and glycogen synthesis.[429,441-446] Evidence suggests that IGF1 has a greater effect on cell growth than on glucose metabolism because activation of the IGF1R stimulates the Ras/MAPK cascade more than INSR activation.[429,445] Conversely, it appears that insulin has a greater effect on glucose metabolism because INSR activation stimulates the PI3K/PKB cascade more than IGF1R activation.[429,446]

The Insulin Receptor

The INSR gene is located on 19p and contains 22 exons.[447] αβ half-receptor precursors are derived from proteolysis of a single proreceptor comprised of α and β subunits in tandem and disulfide linkage of these subunits.[437,447,448] These αβ half-receptor precursors then join to form a single αββα heterotetrameric insulin receptor.[448] Interestingly, αβ half-receptor precursors encoded by one allele may combine with αβ half-receptor precursors encoded by the other allele to form a single insulin receptor.[449] This phenomenon explains how heterozygote mutations resulting in impaired β subunit tyrosine kinase activity can have a dominant negative effect because activation of the INSR requires trans-autophosphorylation of one β subunit by the other β subunit.[449]

Patients with "type A syndrome" have acanthosis nigricans and severe inherited insulin resistance in the absence of INSR autoantibodies.[450-452] Patients with this syndrome tend to be lean and develop glucose intolerance.[452,453] Females with this syndrome also exhibit signs of ovarian hyperandrogenism, including hirsutism, severe acne, oligomenorrhea, and infertility.[450-452]

Patients with "type B syndrome" present during adulthood with acanthosis nigricans, ovarian hyperandrogenism, and severe insulin resistance in association with signs of autoimmune disease—including alopecia areata, vitiligo, primary biliary cirrhosis, arthritis, and nephritis.[450-452,454] Surprisingly, these patients may present with fasting

TABLE 2-4

Receptor Tyrosine Kinases and Clinical Conditions Associated with Receptor Mutations

Receptor	Germ Line Mutation	Endocrine Disorder
Insulin receptor	Inactivating (heterozygous)	Some cases of type A syndrome
	Inactivating (homozygous, compound heterozygous)	Rabson Mendenhall, Donohue (leprechaunism), and some cases of type A syndromes
IGF-1 receptor	Gene deletion (heterozygous)	Pre- and postnatal growth failure
FGFR1	Inactivating mutation (heterozygous)	Kallmann syndrome, missing teeth, cleft palate
FGFR3	Activating mutations (heterozygous)	Achondroplasia, severe achondroplasia with developmental delay and acanthosis nigricans, thanatophoric dysplasia types I and II, and platyspondylic lethal skeletal dysplasias (San Diego types)

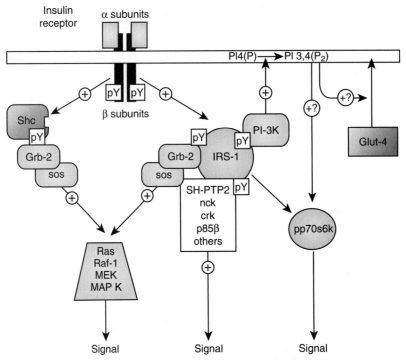

Figure 2-7. Insulin receptor signaling. IRS proteins, SH2-domain–containing proteins (including Grb-2 and Shc), and other proteins (including SOS) interact to activate the Ras/Raf-1/MAP K cascade and PI-3K/PKB cascades, and other enzymes—including SH-PTP2 (SHP2) and p70(s6k). [Adapted with permission from White MF (1997). The insulin signaling system and the IRS proteins. Diabetologia 40:S10.]

hypoglycemia that may or may not be accompanied by postprandial hyperglycemia.[450-452,454] Hodgkin's disease and ataxia-telangiectasia are also associated with this syndrome.[452] Patients with type B syndrome are distinguished from patients with type A syndrome by the presence of anti-INSR antibodies in the plasma that block insulin binding.[450-452,454]

The term *HAIR-AN* (hyperandrogenism, insulin resistance, and acanthosis nigricans) has also been used to describe women with features of types A and B syndromes in association with obesity.[452] However, this term is imprecise because many women who have been labeled as having HAIR-AN may actually have type A or B syndrome or severe polycystic ovary syndrome.[452]

Patients with Rabson-Mendenhall syndrome present during childhood with severe insulin resistance.[455-457] Although patients with this disorder may present initially with fasting hypoglycemia, eventually they develop severe diabetes ketoacidosis that is refractory to insulin therapy.[457] Patients with this condition also have acanthosis nigricans, accelerated linear growth, dystrophic nails, premature and dysplastic dentition, coarse facial features, and pineal hyperplasia.[453,455-457]

Patients with leprechaunism or Donohue syndrome are also severely insulin resistant.[458,459] Patients present during infancy with severe intrauterine and postnatal growth retardation, lipoatrophy, and acanthosis nigricans.[456,458] They also have dysmorphic features that include globular eyes, micrognathia, and large ears.[456,458] Affected male infants commonly have penile enlargement, whereas affected female infants often have clitoromegaly and hirsutism.[456,458] In spite of hyperinsulinemia associated with glucose intolerance or diabetes

mellitus, the major glucose metabolism problem for these patients is fasting hypoglycemia.[456,458] Unlike patients with Rabson-Mendenhall syndrome, patients with leprechaunism do not present with diabetic ketoacidosis.[457] Many patients with this condition do not survive past the first year of life.[456,458]

Mutations in the INSR have been found in 10% to 15% of patients with type A syndrome, and in all patients with Rabson-Mendenhall syndrome and leprechaunism.[452,459,460] These mutations are divided into five classes.[452,453,461] Class I mutations are frame-shift or nonsense mutations that prematurely terminate translation and thus interfere with INSR synthesis. Class II mutations interfere with post-translational processing and intracellular trafficking of the INSR. Class III mutations decrease insulin binding to the INSR. Class IV mutations are point mutations usually located on the intracellular region of the β subunit that decrease INSR TK activity. Class V mutations increase INSR degradation by increasing insulin-induced endocytosis and degradation of the receptors.

Patients with Rabson-Mendenhall syndrome and leprechaunism are homozygous or compound heterozygous for these mutations.[452,462-466] Some patients with type A syndrome have been found to be heterozygous for dominant negative β-subunit mutations that reduces TK activity by 75%.[461,466-471] Other patients with type A syndrome have been found to be homozygous or compound heterozygous for α-subunit mutations that interfere with receptor trafficking to the plasma membrane, β-subunit mutations that interfere with TK activity, or mutations that interfere with proreceptor cleavage into α and β subunits. Still other patients have been found to have decreased INSR mRNA levels that may be due to a loss-of-function mutation in the INSR gene promoter.[453,472-476] Interestingly, one patient with leprechaunism with parents with type A syndrome has been described.[466] The proband was found to be homozygous for an INSR mutation that decreases TK activity, and the parents were found to be heterozygous for the mutation.[466]

The Insulin-Like Growth Factor-1 Receptor

The growth-promoting effects of IGF-1 are mediated by IGR1Rs. IGF1R αβ subunits are encoded by a single gene.[448] Like the insulin receptor, an αβ half-receptor precursor is produced that then joins with a half-receptor precursor that may be encoded from the other allele to form a complete heterotetrameric IGF1R.[448] The IGF1R has 100-fold less affinity for insulin than for IGF1.[477]

Patients who are heterozygous for a ring chromosome 15, resulting in deletion of the IGF1R gene, present with intrauterine growth retardation and postnatal growth failure accompanied by delayed bone age, mental retardation, cardiac abnormalities, cryptorchidism, and dysmorphic features that include microcephaly, triangular face, frontal bossing, hypertelorism, and brachydactyly.[478,479] Similarly, IUGR and postnatal growth failure are commonly found in patients heterozygous for deletion of distal 15q that results in deletion of the IGF1R gene. Patients with deletion of distal 15q often have microcephaly, triangular facies, hypertelorism, high-arched palate, micrognathia, cystic kidneys, and lung hypoplasia or dysplasia.[477,480-482] However, the ring chromosome and deleted area of distal 15q may also be missing other genes—and it is unknown to what extent absence of the IGF1R gene contributes to the phenotype found in these patients.[477,479]

It has been suggested African Efe Pygmies are short due to resistance to IGF1.[477] T-cell lines established from Efe Pygmies have decreased IGF1R gene expression, cell surface expression, receptor autophosphorylation, and intracellular signaling when compared with T-cell lines established from American controls.[477] However, no IGF1R gene mutation has been identified in Efe Pygmies that can account for these findings.[477]

In addition to defective INSR function, some patients with leprechaunism and Rabson-Mendenhall syndrome are resistant to the glucose lowering or growth promotion of IGF1 and have abnormal IGF1R function—resulting in decreased ligand binding or altered intracellular signaling.[477,483-487] No deleterious IGF1R gene mutation has been identified in patients with these syndromes, and many patients with leprechaunism and Rabson-Mendenhall syndrome have normally functioning IGF1Rs and no evidence of IGF1 resistance.[477,488]

The Fibroblast Growth Factor Receptor Family

There are four members of the fibroblast growth factor receptor (FGFR) tyrosine kinase family.[421] These are FGFR1, FGFR2, FGFR3, and FGFR4. These receptors consist of a single polypeptide chain that contains an N-terminal extracellular region, a transmembrane region, and a cytosolic region (Figure 2-6).[421] The extracellular region contains three immunoglobulin-like domains: IgI, IgII, and IgIII (Figure 2-6).[489] The cytosolic region contains a TK domain split into two segments (TK1 and TK2) by an intervening amino acid segment.[489]

At least 13 types of fibroblast growth factors (FGFs) have been identified.[489] As monomers, FGFs can only bind a single FGFR—forming an inactive 1:1 complex.[423] FGFR activation by dimerization occurs when two or more FGF molecules in 1:1 complexes are linked by heparan sulfate proteoglycans.[423]

Activation of FGFRs increases receptor TK activity.[489] Increased TK activity leads to autophosphorylation of a tyrosine residue in the C-terminal region, resulting in a binding site for the SH2 domain of phospholipase Cγ (PLCγ).[490,491] Once PLCγ is bound to this site, it is phosphorylated and activated.[490,491] In chondrocytes, activation of FGFR3 also induces activation of STAT1.[492]

FIBROBLAST GROWTH FACTOR RECEPTOR 1

In 2003, inactivating FGFR1 gene mutations were identified as a cause of autosomal-dominant Kallmann syndrome (KS).[493] Individuals with KS have anosmia and isolated hypogonadotropic hypogonadism.[494,495] The FGFR1, which is located on 8p12, plays a role in olfactory and GnRH neuronal migration from the nasal placode to the olfactory bulb and in the subsequent migration of the GnRH neurons to the hypothalamus.[493] Prior to identification of these FGFR1 gene mutations, X-linked KS was found to be caused by inactivating KAL1 gene mutations.[494,496,497] The KAL1 gene is located on the X chromosome and encodes anosmin-1.[494,496,497] Anosmin-1 is a ligand for the FGFR1 receptor.[498] Like FGFR1s, anosmin-1 plays a role in olfactory and GnRH neuronal migration to the nasal placode, and in the subsequent migration of GnRH neurons to the hypothalamus.[494,498,499]

There is a high penetrance for anosmia and signs of hypogonadotropic hypogonadism, (including lack of puberty, microphallus, and cryptorchidism) in the 10% of KS patients with X-linked KS due to KAL1 gene mutations.[494] Female carriers of KAL1 gene mutations do not have anosmia or isolated hypogonadotropic hypogonadism.[494] In contrast to patients with KS due to KAL1 gene mutations, the approximately 10% of KS patients with FGFR1 gene mutations (even within the same kindred) exhibit variable phenotypes ranging from anosmia and complete hypogonadotropic hypogonadism (characterized by cryptorchidism and microphallus in males and absent pubertal development in both genders) to anosmia and/or delayed puberty.[493,500,501]

It has also been noted that in most kindreds with FGFR1 gene mutations females present with more mild KS phenotypes than males.[493,501] Female carriers may even be asymptomatic.[493,501] Because the KAL1 gene is located on the X chromosome, females may produce more anosmin-1 than males.[493] Thus, a possible explanation for milder KS phenotypes in females with FGFR1 gene mutations may be that the increased anosmin-1 levels in females may lead to increased anosmin-1–induced activation of the mutant FGFR1s that may partially compensate for the mutation.[493] Interestingly, missing teeth and cleft palate are not an uncommon finding in individuals with KS due to FGFR1 gene mutations, whereas unilateral renal agenesis and bilateral synkinesia are associated with KS due to KAL1 gene mutations.[500]

FIBROBLAST GROWTH FACTOR RECEPTOR 3

In addition to variants of Kallmann syndrome, FGFR mutations cause many conditions—including Pfeiffer syndrome (activating mutations of FGFR1 and FGFR2), Crouzon syndrome (FGFR2 mutations), Crouzon syndrome with acanthosis nigricans (an FGFR3 mutation), Apert syndrome (FGFR2 mutations), and craniosynostosis (FGFR3 mutations).[489] Several autosomal-dominant short-limb dwarfism syndromes—including achondroplasia, severe achondroplasia with developmental delay and acanthosis nigricans (SADDAN), hypochondroplasia, and three types of platyspondylic lethal skeletal dysplasias (PLSD) [thanatophoric dysplasia I (TDI), thanatophoric dysplasia II (TDII), and San Diego types (PLSD-SD)]—are often caused by heterozygous constitutively activating FGFR3 gene mutations.[502-505]

Individuals with achondroplasia have activating mutations in the transmembrane domain of FGFR3, with the Gly380Asn found in >95% of achondroplastic patients.[503,506-508] Forty to 70% of individuals with hypochondroplasia have an activating Asn540Lys mutation in the TK1 domain.[503,509-512] All individuals with TDII have an activating Lys650Glu mutation in the activating loop of the TK2 domain, and >90% of individuals with TDI and PLSD-SD have FGFR3 mutations.[503,505] Patients with SADDAN have an activating mutation in the same codon as patients with TDII.[513] Instead of the Lys650Glu mutation associated with TDII, patients with SADDAN have a Lys650Met mutation.[513] However, unlike patients with TDII patients with SADDAN do not have craniosynostosis and a cloverleaf skull—and often survive past childhood.[513]

The FGFR3 gene is primarily expressed in endochondral growth plates of long bones, brain, and skin pre- and postnatally.[514,515] Constitutional activation of FGFR3s in chondrocytes leads to growth arrest and apoptosis.[492,516,517] In addition, constitutive activation of FGFR3s is also postulated to alter neuronal migration because patients with SADDAN, TDI, and TDII have neurologic abnormalities that may include developmental delay, paucity of white matter, polymicrogyria, dysplastic temporal cortex, dysplasia of nuclei, and neuronal heterotopia.[513,518-520] Furthermore, constitutive activation of FGFRs in skin fibroblasts and keratinocytes is thought to cause the acanthosis nigricans seen in patients with SADDAN and Crouzon syndrome with acanthosis nigricans.[521] However, it is not yet known why some activating FGFR3 mutations effect the skeletal system, central nervous system, and the skin whereas other activating FGFR3 mutations only effect the skeletal system.[513]

Nuclear Receptors

Using a phylogenetic tree based on the evolution of two highly conserved nuclear receptor domains (the DNA-binding C domain and the ligand-binding E domain, V), Laudet divided nuclear receptors into six related subfamilies and a subfamily. Subfamily 0 contains receptors, such as the embryonic gonad (EGON) and DAX1 receptors, that do not have a conserved C or the E domain (Figure 2-8).[522,523] Subfamily 1 includes the peroxisome proliferator-activated retinoic acid, thyroid hormone, and vitamin D3 receptors. Subfamily 2 includes the hepatocyte nuclear factor-4α (HNF-4α) and retinoid X receptors (RXRs). Subfamily 3 contains the steroid receptors.

Subfamilies 4 and 5 contain the NGFIB and the FTZ-F1 orphan receptors, respectively. Subfamily 6 consists of the GCNF1 orphan receptor. Recent evidence suggests that subfamily 3 (which includes the glucocorticoid, androgen, progesterone, and mineralocorticoid receptors) rapidly evolved from a common steroid receptor gene about 500 million years ago.[524]

GENERAL STRUCTURE OF THE NUCLEAR RECEPTORS

Nuclear receptors are made up of four domains: A/B, C, D, and E (Figure 2-9).[522] Supporting the notion that nuclear receptor subfamilies are derived from a common ancestral orphan receptor, the C and E domains are highly conserved among the subfamilies.[522] Mutation of several nuclear receptors are associated with endocrine disorders (Table 2-5).

The A/B domain is located at the N-terminal and contains the activation function 1 (AF-1)/τ 1 domain.[525] The AF-1/τ 1 domain regulates gene transcription by interacting with proteins (such as the Ada and TFIID complexes) that induce transcription.[526,527] This transactivation function of the AF-1/τ 1 domain is not dependent on binding of the nuclear hormone receptor to its ligand and is not specific in its choice of DNA target sequences.[522,528-530] Thus, specificity of action of the nuclear hormone receptor is determined by the function of other nuclear hormone receptor domains.

The C domain has characteristics that help to confer specificity of action on each nuclear hormone receptor. This domain consists of two zinc-finger motifs responsible for the DNA-binding activity of the receptor and the selection of dimerization partners.[531,532] Each zinc-finger module consists of a zinc ion surrounded by the sulfurs of four cysteine residues, resulting in a tertiary structure containing helixes.[531,532] The P-box lies near the cysteines of the first zinc finger and contains the three to four amino acids responsible for specificity of binding to response elements.[532,533] The D-box consists of a loop of five amino acids attached to the first two cysteines of the second zinc finger that provides the interface for nuclear receptor dimerization.[532]

The D "hinge" domain contains nuclear localization signals and contributes to the function of the adjacent C and E domains.[522] Thus, the N-terminal portion of the domain contributes to DNA binding and heterodimerization and

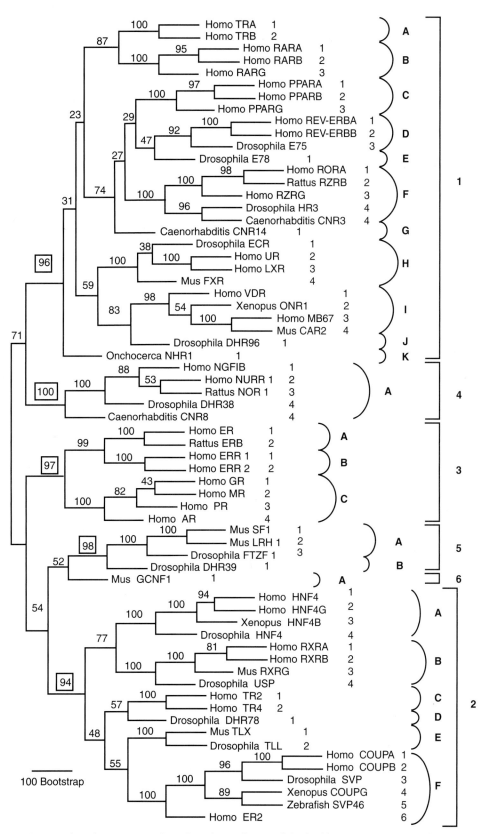

Figure 2-8. Phylogenetic tree of nuclear receptors based on the evolution of the highly conserved C and E domains. Numbers at the right side of the figure represent subfamilies, and capital letters represent groups of more closely related receptors. The small numbers to the right of the receptor names are used in combination with the subfamily letters and group letters in a proposed nuclear receptor nomenclature. This nomenclature proposes that nuclear receptors should be named NR, followed by subfamily number, group letter, and individual receptor number. Thus, the mineralocorticoid receptor is named NR3C2 and the PPARγ receptor is named NR1C3 according to this nomenclature. Numbers to the left of the receptor names represent bootstrap values. Values that define subfamilies with more than one member are boxed. [Reproduced with permission from the Nuclear Receptors Nomenclature Committee (1999). A unified nomenclature system for the nuclear receptor subfamily. Cell 97:161.]

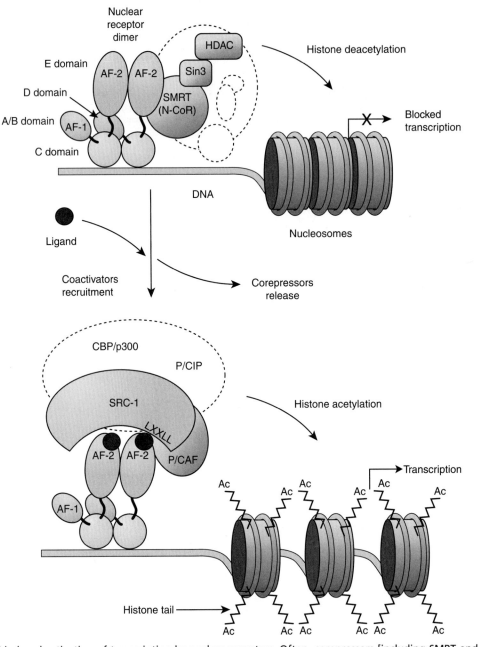

Figure 2-9. Ligand-induced activation of transcription by nuclear receptors. Often, corepressors [including SMRT and nuclear receptor copressor (N-CoR)] bind a nuclear receptor that is not bound by its ligand. These corepressors then associate with Sin3, which in turn associates with a histone deacetylases (HDAC). Then, HDAC represses transcription by deacetylating histone tails—resulting in compaction of the nucleosomes into structures that are inaccessible to transcription factors. Ligand binding induces structural changes in the E domain that result in release of the corepressor/Sin3/HDAC complexes from the receptor, and binding of coactivator complexes that may include steroid receptor coactivator 1 (SRC-1), p300/cAMP responsive element binding protein (CBP), p300/CBP-associated factor (P/CAF), or p300/CBP cointegrator-associated protein (pCIP) to the LXXLL motif of the AF2-AD. Then, the coactivator complexes induce transcription by acetylating (Ac) the histone tails—resulting in decompaction of the nucleosomes into structures that are accessible to transcription factors. Dashed lines are used to represent coactivator and corepressor complexes because their composition in vivo is yet unknown. [Adapted with permission from Robyr D, Wolffe AP, Wahli W (2000). Nuclear hormone receptor coregulators in action: Diversity for shared tasks. Mol Endocrinol 14:339. Copyright 2000, The Endocrine Society.]

the C-terminal portion contributes to ligand binding.[533-536] The nuclear localization signal plays a particularly important role in the function of glucocorticoids and mineralocorticoid receptors because these receptors bind their ligand in the cytoplasm and must then localize to the nucleus to alter gene transcription.[525]

The E domain is known as the ligand-binding domain (LBD) or the hormone-binding domain. In addition to ligand binding, the E domain has effects on dimerization and transactivation.[522] The LBD consists of 11 to 12 α helixes (named H1 through H12) and contains a ligand-binding pocket that is made up of portions of some of

TABLE 2-5

Nuclear Receptors and Clinical Conditions Associated with Receptor Mutations

Receptor	Germ Line Mutation	Endocrine Disorder
Thyroid hormone receptor β (TRβ)	Inactivating mutations (heterozygous and homozygous)	Generalized resistance to thyroid hormones
Vitamin D3 receptor	Inactivating mutations (homozygous)	Vitamin D3 resistance
PPARγ2	Inactivating mutations (heterozygous)	Obesity or early-onset type II diabetes mellitus
HNF-4	Inactivating mutations (heterozygous)	Maturity-onset diabetes of the young (MODY) type I
Glucocorticoid receptor	Inactivating mutations (heterozygous)	Glucocorticoid resistance
Androgen receptor	Inactivating mutations (X-linked recessive)	Androgen insensitivity syndrome, Kennedy's disease
Estrogen receptor α (ERα)	Inactivating mutations (homozygous)	Tall stature and incomplete epiphyseal fusion
Mineralocorticoid receptor	Inactivating mutations (heterozygous, homozygous) Activating mutations (homozygous)	Pseudohypoaldosteronism type I Syndrome of apparent mineralocorticoid excess
DAX1	Inactivating mutations (X-linked recessive)	X-linked adrenal hypoplasia congenita

the different helixes.[537-540] For example, the thyroid receptor (TR) LBD has a ligand-binding cavity that includes components from H2, H7, H8, H11, and H12.[540] The contribution of different parts of LBD to the ligand-binding pocket accounts for the finding that mutation of single–amino-acid molecules in different helixes of the LBD can interfere with ligand binding.[525]

Unlike the AF-1/τ 1 transcriptional activating factor, the E domain activation factor 2 (AF2-AD) requires ligand binding to function (Figure 2-9).[538-545] Often, when the receptor is not bound by its ligand corepressor complexes simultaneously bind the LBD and transcriptional machinery consisting of protein complexes that place transcription factors on nucleosome binding sites (Figure 2-9).[538-545] The corepressor complexes then suppress gene transcription by using histone deacetylases to compact the nucleosomes into inaccessible structures (Figure 2-9).[546-549] Ligand binding induces structural rearrangements in the E-domain that lead to release of these corepressor complexes from the transcriptional machinery and the LBD, and exposure of the transcriptional machinery and the LXXLL motif of the AF2-AD to coactivator complexes (Figure 2-9).[538-545] These coactivator complexes have histone acetyltransferase activity that acts to relax nucleosome structures, enabling transcription factors to access nucleosome binding sites (Figure 2-9).[550]

Most nuclear receptors are capable of binding their hormone response element and repress transcription when they are not bound by their ligand.[551] However, in the absence of ligand steroid receptors are bound to a complex of heat-shock proteins instead of their response element and do not appear to repress transcription.[552]

Agonists and antagonists have different effects upon the interaction between the ligand binding pocket and AF2-AD. For example, when 17β-estradiol binds to the estrogen receptor the position of the AF2-AD containing H12 is altered so that coactivators can access the LBD-binding coactivator binding site.[537] However, when the estrogen antagonist raloxifene binds at the same site the coactivator binding site on H12 remains blocked by other portions of H12.[537]

Although some of the nuclear receptors are fully active when bound as monomers to DNA, the hormone receptors in the nuclear receptor superfamily are most active when bound as homodimers or heterodimers (Figure 2-9).[522] RXRs, hepatocyte nuclear factor 4, and the steroid receptors can bind DNA as homodimers or heterodimers.[522,553,554] The α isoform of the estrogen receptor (ESR1) is particularly promiscuous, and is able heterodimerize with HNF4-α and retinoic acid receptors, the β isoform of the estrogen receptor (ESR2), RXR and the thyroid receptors.[553,554] As a homodimer, RXR binds the dINSRect repeat 1 (DR1).[555] It can also join the thyroid, vitamin D3, and peroxisome proliferator-activated receptors to form heterodimers.[522,556-558]

Interestingly, it has also been suggested that some steroid hormones also act on transmembrane receptors—and these interactions may be responsible for the acute cellular effects of steroids.[559] Progesterone has been shown to interact with the G-protein–coupled uterine oxytocin, nicotinic acetylcholine, GABA$_A$, NMDA, and sperm cell membrane progesterone receptors.[560-565] Cell membrane estrogen and glucocorticoids receptors have also been identified.[566-569]

Subfamily 1 Nuclear Receptors: Thyroid Hormone, Vitamin D3, and Peroxisome Proliferator-Activated Receptors

THYROID HORMONE RECEPTORS

The two thyroid hormone receptor (THR) isoforms—thyroid hormone receptor α (THRA) and thyroid hormone receptor β (THRB)—are encoded by different c-erbA genes on chromosomes 17 and 3, respectively.[536,570] THRs that are not occupied by the thyroid hormone triiodothyronine (T3) exist as homodimers or heterodimers with RXRs that are attached to DNA thyroid hormone response elements in association with corepressor proteins.[571] Thyroid hormone binding induces the release of the corepressors from the THR.[571] A coactivator, steroid receptor coactivator-1 (SRC-1), is then able to attach to the THR—enabling activation of transcription.[571]

Generalized resistance to thyroid hormones (GRTH) is due to mutations in the THRB gene.[570,572,573] Patients with this syndrome have impaired receptor response to triiodothyronine (T3).[570] They have elevated T3 and thyroxine (T4) levels with normal TSH levels.[570,572,573] The clinical manifestations are variable but may include goiter, attention deficit disorder, hearing defects, learning disabilities, poor weight gain, mental retardation, and delayed boned age.[570,572,573]

Mutations have been found in the D and E domains of THRBs of GRTH patients.[570,574,575] Thus, these mutations alter ligand binding or transactivation.[570,575,576] However, most mutant THRBs retain the ability to repress transactivation of target genes through interactions with corepressors.[575,576] Some of the GRTH mutant receptors continue to associate with corepressors and are unable to bind the coactivator SRC-1 even when bound by T3.[576,577] Thus, mutant THRBs have a dominant negative effect in the heterozygote state because they are able to interfere with the function of wild-type receptors by repressing transcription of target DNA.[570,575,576]

Patients who are homozygous for deleterious mutations of THRB demonstrate more severe clinical abnormalities than patients who are heterozygous for the mutations. One such patient with a deletion of both THRB alleles presented with deaf mutism, dysmorphic features, and stippled epiphyses.[578] This condition is inherited in an autosomal recessive mode because the mutant allele is missing the THRB gene and is therefore unable to produce a THRB with corepressor function.[578] Another patient homozygous for a THRB mutant ("kindred S receptor") with an amino acid deletion in the ligand-binding domain presented with mental retardation, very delayed bone age, and very elevated T3 and T4 levels.[574,579] Heterozygous carriers of the kindred S receptor mutation have milder clinical manifestations of GRTH because this mutant THRB retains corepressor activity and thus has dominant negative effects.[574,579,580]

VITAMIN D3 RECEPTOR

Severe rickets, hypocalcemia, secondary hyperparathyroidism, and increased 1,25-dihydroxyvitamin D3 (D3) levels occur in patients with the autosomal recessive syndrome of "vitamin D3 resistance."[581] These patients have defective vitamin D3 receptors (VDRs). Mutations causing this syndrome have been found in the zinc fingers of the DNA-binding domain (C domain), leading to decreased or abolished receptor binding to regulatory elements of target genes.[582] Causative mutations have also been found that lead to the production of receptors that have decreased or abolished ability to bind D3 and heterodimerize with retinoid X receptors (RXRs), which are required for the VDR to maximally transactivate target genes.[582,583]

Less severe mutations in the VDR are associated with decreased gastrointestinal calcium absorption and bone mineral density, even during childhood, and an increased risk for osteoporosis and fractures.[584-589] However, it has not been possible to replicate these findings in some ethnic groups.[590-594] Thus, other factors (such as estrogen receptor genotype, dietary calcium, and age) probably contribute to the effects of VDR polymorphisms on bone mineral metabolism.[587,589,595,596]

VDR polymorphisms have been associated with pre- and postnatal growth failure. Absence of VDR alleles digested by BSMI in the presence of homozygosity for estrogen receptor alleles digested by PVU II estrogen receptor polymorphism is associated with decreased pre- and postnatal linear growth.[597] In addition, girls homozygous for VDR alleles digested by TaqI have been found to be shorter than girls who do not have the polymorphism.[598]

Other important associations have been found with VDR polymorphisms. Homozygous polymorphisms have been reported to be associated with primary hyperparathyroidism.[599] In addition, the presence of VDR alleles digested by TaqI is associated with increased risk for the development of early-onset periodontal disease.[600] Conversely, absence of such alleles has been associated with familial calcium nephrolithiasis.[601] Absence of alleles digested by BSMI may be a risk factor for the development of sarcoidosis.[602] However, the presence of these alleles is associated with hypercalciuria and nephrolithiasis and increased risk in women for the development of metastatic breast cancer.[603,604] Absence of alleles digested by ApaI may be a risk factor for the development of psoriasis.[605] VDR polymorphisms have also been associated with increased susceptibility to tuberculosis, leprosy, and other infections.[606-609]

PPARγ

The orphan nuclear receptor PPARγ2 has a role in regulating adipocyte differentiation and metabolism. This orphan receptor, as the term indicates, does not have a known ligand. Recent evidence suggests that mutations in the gene encoding PPARγ2 may cause obesity. A missense mutation leading to a Pro115Gln substitution near a site of serine phosphorylation at position 114 that suppresses transcriptional activation in PPARγ2 was found in some morbidly obese patients.[610] The Pro115Gln substitution interferes with phosphorylation of the serine at position 114, leading to increased transcriptional activation by PPARγ—which in turn leads to increased adipocyte differentiation and triglyceride accumulation.[610]

Two other mutations in the PPARγ2 gene have been identified that cause severe insulin resistance, early-onset type 2 diabetes mellitus, and hypertension by the end of the third decade of life.[611] These mutations lead to amino acid substitutions that disturb the orientation of H12 in the E domain leading to decreased ligand-dependent transactivation by AF-2/AD and coactivator recruitment.[611] In addition, these mutant receptors interfere with wild-type receptor function in a dominant-negative manner by continuously suppressing target gene transcription.[611]

Subfamily 2 Nuclear Receptors: Hepatocyte Nuclear Factor and Retinoid X Receptors

This subfamily includes the HNF receptors and the RXR. RXRs form heterodimers with other nuclear receptors (including the estrogen, vitamin D, and thyroid hormone receptors) and with PPARγ (RXRs are discussed elsewhere in this chapter).

HNF

Alteration of another orphan nuclear receptor, HNF-4α, also causes an endocrine disorder. Mutations of the HNF-4α gene on chromosome 20 that alter the ligand-binding domain (E domain) or the DNA-binding domain (C domain) have been found in patients with maturity-onset diabetes of the young type I (MODY1).[612-615] Patients with MODY usually develop diabetes mellitus by the end of the third decade of life. They have a defect in glucose-mediated stimulation of insulin secretion.[613,616]

Carriers of a glycine-to-serine substitution in codon 115 in the DNA-binding domain (C domain) appear to be at increased risk for developing low-insulin diabetes mellitus.[617] Hepatocyte nuclear factors 3 (HNF-3α, -3β, and -3γ) are also regulators of the early-onset type 2 diabetes genes HNF-1 α, HNF-4 α, and IPF-1/PDX-1—which are associated with MODY types 3, 1, and 4, respectively.[618-621]

Subfamily 3 Nuclear Receptors: The Steroid Receptors and Glucocorticoid, Androgen, Estrogen, and Mineralocorticoid Receptors

GLUCOCORTICOID RECEPTORS

Glucocorticoid resistance is clinically characterized by the presence of elevated plasma cortisol and ACTH levels, accompanied by the effects of hyperaldosteronism and hyperandrogenism in the absence of striae and central fat deposition.[536,622,623] Excess adrenal steroids are made in an attempt to make sufficient cortisol to overcome glucocorticoid resistance. Thus, patients with this disorder may also suffer from hypokalemia, hypertension, fatigue, severe acne, hirsutism, irregular menses, and infertility.[622,623] Boys may present with isosexual precocity.[624]

A single Ile 559 to Asp 559 mutation in the DNA-binding domain is responsible for many cases of glucocorticoid resistance.[625] This mutation has a dominant negative effect in that it is able to inhibit the function of the wild-type allele in the heterozygote state.[625] Thus, glucocorticoid resistance is often an autosomal-dominant familial disease. Glucocorticoid resistance can also be caused by a mutation in the nuclear localization signal consensus that interferes with hormone-induced nuclear translocation of the glucocorticoid receptor.[626] According to the HUGO Gene Nomenclature Committee, the glucocorticoid receptor is also known as the nuclear receptor subfamily 3, group C, member 1 (NR3C1). However, the HUGO Gene Nomenclature Committee also acknowledges the alias GR for the glucocorticoid receptor. GR will be used as the abbreviation for glucocorticoid receptor for the remainder of this chapter.

ACTH-secreting pituitary macroadenomas can also be caused by a frame-shift mutation in the GR gene that interferes with signal transduction.[625] Patients with this mutation manifest the symptoms of glucocorticoid resistance. The tumor develops as a result of impaired negative feedback regulation by glucocorticoids of the hypothalamic-pituitary axis.

ANDROGEN RECEPTORS

The human androgen receptor (AR) gene is located on the X chromosome. Known disorders characterized by AR dysfunction due to AR gene mutations are only expressed in patients with a 46 XY karyotype.[627] Thus, these disorders are either transmitted by X-linked recessive inheritance or are due to sporadic mutations.

Numerous mutations of the AR gene have been found to cause androgen insensitivity syndrome (AIS; testicular feminization). The phenotype of this syndrome can vary in severity from partial undervirilization to complete AIS characterized by intraabdominal testes, absence of mullerian structures, absence of androgen-induced body hair such as pubic and axillary hair, and a female appearance.[627-629] Incomplete AIS refers to individuals with ambiguous external genitalia with an enlarged clitoris or microphallus and patients with Reifenstein syndrome.[628] Reifenstein syndrome is characterized by severe hypospadias with scrotal development and severe gynecomastia.[628]

The phenotypic heterogeneity of AIS is due to the wide variety of locations for the mutations causing AIS. Functional consequences of each mutation causing AIS relate to the function of the domain in which the mutation is located. However, the degree of impairment of mutated receptor function in in vitro studies does not always correlate with the phenotypic severity of the syndrome.[630]

Mutations in exons that code for the AR hormone-binding domain decrease hormone-binding affinity.[631] However, these mutations do not abolish the hormone-binding capability of the receptor.[631] Thus, patients with these mutations usually present with the incomplete AIS or occasionally with complete AIS.[631-634] Patients with mutations in the hormone-binding domain do not appear to respond to treatment with high doses of testosterone.[631] Mutations in the DNA-binding domain lead to failure of target gene regulation. Thus, patients with these mutations usually manifest the complete AIS.[635,636]

Complete AIS is also caused by a point mutation that results in a premature termination condition, leading to transcription beginning downstream of the termination signal and the AF1/tau1 domain.[637] Numerous other mutations have been described that cause truncation or deletion of the AR and complete AIS.[638-641] Two patients with ambiguous genitalia and partial virilization were found to be mosaic for mutant ARs.[642,643]

Some patients with Reifenstein syndrome have been found to have a mutation in the DNA-binding domain that abolishes receptor dimerization.[644] Other patients have been found to have a mutation in a different area of the DNA-binding domain that does not effect receptor dimerization, or to have mutations in the hormone-binding domain in the E domain.[645-648] The Ala596Thr mutation in the D-box area of the DNA-binding domain has been associated with an increased risk of breast cancer.[649]

AIS is also a feature of Kennedy's disease, which is an X-linked recessive condition causing spinal and muscular atrophy.[632] This condition is caused by extension of a poly-CAG segment in the AR gene exon that codes for the N-terminus of the AR, leading to an increased number of glutamine residues in the A/B domain.[650,651] ARs with a polyQ region increased to 48 glutamine residues accumulate abnormally in transfected cells due to misfolding and aberrant proteolytic processing.[652] Because polyQ extension does not completely abolish of transactivation, patients with Kennedy's disease exhibit a mild partial AIS phenotype consisting of normal virilization accompanied by testicular atrophy, gynecomastia, and infertility.

ESTROGEN RECEPTORS

Two major full-length estrogen receptor isoforms have been identified in mammals. Estrogen receptor α (ESR1) was discovered first and mediates most of the known actions of estrogens.[536] ESR1 is expressed primarily in the uterus, ovaries, testes, epididymis, adrenal cortices, and kidneys.[653] Estrogen receptor β (ESR2) was discovered in 1996.[654] ESR1 and ESR2 share 95% and 50% homology in the DBD and LBD, respectively.[655] There is little homology in the N-terminal between the two isoforms.[655] ESR2 is expressed primarily in the uterus, ovaries, testes, prostate, bladder, lung, and brain.[653] Although ESR2 has a high affinity for estrogens, it has less transactivating ability than ESR1 and has not yet been found to be involved in any pathologic condition.[536,656,657]

There is evidence supporting the existence of other functional estrogen receptors.[658] Some of these putative estrogen receptors localize to the cell membrane instead of or in addition to the nucleus. A 46-kDa amino terminal truncated product of ESR1, named ER46, localizes to the cell membrane and mediates estrogen actions that are initiated at the cell membrane.[659] Another of these putative estrogen receptors has been named ER-X and is postulated to be a G-protein–coupled receptor that localizes to the cell membrane.[660] Another putative receptor is the aptly named heterodimeric putative estrogen receptor (pER), which has been found on the cell and nuclear membranes.[661] The pER acts as a serine phosphatase.[661] Five other estrogen-binding proteins have also been identified, and at least three of them localize to the cell membrane.[662-665]

It had been thought that androgens are the main hormones responsible for closing the epiphyses during puberty. In 1994, however, it was shown from extensive studies of a 28-year-old man with incomplete epiphyseal closure and continued linear growth (in spite of otherwise normal pubertal development) that the estrogen receptor mediates epiphyseal closure.[666] He was found to have a homozygous C-to-T point mutation of codon 157 of the second exon in the ESR1 gene, introducing a premature termination signal. Expression of this gene leads to the production of a nonfunctional ESR1 lacking both the DNA- and hormone-binding domains. He was also found to have increased estradiol levels, impaired glucose tolerance with hyperinsulinemia, and decreased bone density.

Further strengthening the association between ESR1 and epiphyseal closure is the observation that women with ESR1-positive breast cancer and a mutation in the B domain (B' allele) of ESR1 have an increased incidence of spontaneous abortion and tall stature.[667] These associations were not found in female carriers of the allele without breast cancer or with ESR1-negative breast cancer. Thus, a second (as yet undiscovered) mutation is likely to play a role in the development of tall stature and spontaneous abortions in female carriers with ESR1-positive breast cancer.

MINERALOCORTICOID RECEPTORS

Mineralocorticoid resistance is also known as pseudohypoaldosteronism (PHA). Both sporadic and familial cases with either autosomal-dominant or -recessive cases have been reported.[668-672] Clinical presentation of patients with PHA ranges from asymptomatic salt wasting; to growth failure; to chronic failure to thrive, lethargy, and emesis; to life-threatening dehydration accompanied by severe salt wasting.[669-671,673-675] Patients with the severe forms of PHA typically present within a year of birth and may even present in utero with polyhydramnios due to polyuria.[676] Biochemically, the condition is characterized by urinary salt wasting, hyponatremia, elevated plasma potassium, aldosterone, and renin activity and urinary aldosterone metabolism that are unresponsive to the mineralocorticoid treatment.[677-679]

Two forms of PHA are recognized. PHA type I consists of classical PHA (due to renal tubular mineralocorticoid resistance) and PHA type II with kidney, intestine, salivary and/or sweat gland mineralocorticoid resistance.[680] Unlike PHA type I, PHA type II is not due to defective mineralocorticoid function. Rather, it is due to increased chloride reabsorption by the renal tubule. Patients with these conditions present with hyperkalemia that only responds to treatment with non-chloride ions, such as bicarbonate or sulfate, which increase delivery of sodium to the distal tubule.[681]

A transient form of mineralocorticoid resistance probably due to abnormal maturation of aldosterone receptor function also exists.[682] This variant of PHA is known as the syndrome of early-childhood hyperkalemia. Children with this disorder present with failure to thrive or linear growth failure accompanied by hyperkalemia and metabolic acidosis. This condition resolves spontaneously by the second half of the first decade of life.

The cause of PHA type I is not well understood. The HUGO Nomenclature Committee refers to the mineralocorticoid receptor as the nuclear receptor subfamily 3, group C, member 2 (NR3C2) but accepts the alias MR for the mineralocorticoid receptor. MR will be used in the remainder of this chapter. MRs from patients with PHA type I exhibit decreased or absent binding to aldosterone.[683] Mutations have been identified in the genes for MR in patients with PHA type I.[684] However, these mutations are not thought to be solely responsible for causing this condition because they have also been found in individuals without PHA.[684] Altered MR transcription does not appear to cause PHA type I because MR mRNA levels are not decreased in patients with this condition.[683] Thus, it has been hypothesized that PHA type I may be due to a defective post-receptor event that may involve cofactors involved in ligand binding.[677,684]

An interesting syndrome involving overactivation of the MRs is the syndrome of apparent mineralocorticoid excess. Patients with this autosomal-recessive condition can exhibit pre- and postnatal growth failure, hypervolemic hypertension, medullary nephrocalcinosis, and hypokalemic metabolic alkalosis accompanied by hyporeninemic hypoaldosteronism.[685-688] Patients with this syndrome may also be asymptomatic and exhibit only biochemical abnormalities.[689] Patients with this syndrome also have increased serum and urinary cortisol-to-cortisone ratios.[688] This syndrome is caused by mutations in the 11 β-hydroxysteroid dehydrogenase type 2 (11 β-HSD2) genes that reduce the activity of the enzyme.[687,688,690-692] 11 β-HSD2 converts the active glucocorticoid cortisol to inactive cortisone. Thus, decreased activity of 11 β-HSD2 increases cortisol levels in MR-containing tissues, leading to increased binding and activation of MRs by cortisol.[687,688]

Subfamily 0 Nuclear Receptors: DAX1

Subfamily 0 nuclear receptors include DAX1.[523] DAX1 plays a role in the regulation of steroid, mullerian-inhibiting substance, and gonadotropin production.

DAX1

The dosage-sensitive sex-reversal adrenal hypoplasia congenital critical region on the X chromosome gene 1 (DAX1) is an orphan nuclear receptor because its ligand has not yet been identified.[693] It has homologies in the E domain to other orphan receptors, including RXRs.[694] However, DAX1 has an unusual DNA-binding C domain that contains a tract of amino acid repeats instead of zinc finger motifs.[694] DAX1 inhibits steroidogenic factor 1 (SF-1)-mediated transcription. SF-1 is another orphan nuclear receptor that regulates transcription of adrenal and gonadal steroid hydroxylases, mullerian-inhibiting substance, and gonadotropin genes.[695,696]

DAX1 gene mutations have been identified that cause X-linked adrenal hypoplasia congenita.[694] Patients with this condition have congenital adrenal insufficiency and are therefore deficient in glucocorticoid, mineralocorticoid, and androgen production.[694,697] Gonadotropin deficiency and azoospermia also occur in these patients.[697,698] Female carriers may have delayed puberty.[698] All mutations that have been found to cause X-linked congenital adrenal hypoplasia are either located in or prevent transcription of the area of the E domain that inhibits SF-1-mediated transcription.[693,699-701] Thus, DAX1 mutations may cause X-linked congenital adrenal hypoplasia by altering SF-1 regulation of gonado- and adrenogenesis.[699] DAX1 deletion may also occur in the setting of the contiguous gene deletion syndrome, resulting in complex glycerol kinase deficiency (cGKD) if individuals have deletions extending from the GK gene into the Duchene muscular dystrophy (DMD) gene and/or involving a significant extension telomeric from DAX1.[702]

Summary

Understanding of receptors that transduce or influence hormone action has increased dramatically during the past decade. As molecular biology techniques improve, it is expected that knowledge of receptor action will continue to increase at a rapid pace. It is likely that subtle defects in receptor function (such as regulatory or promoter region mutations that increase or decrease receptor gene expression, or mutations in second messenger proteins) will be found that cause endocrine disorders. It is also likely that new receptors will be discovered that transduce or influence hormone action and that endocrine roles will be found for receptors that were not previously thought to mediate or alter hormone action.

REFERENCES

1. Bockaert J, Pin JP (1999). Molecular tinkering of G protein-coupled receptors: An evolutionary success. The EMBO Journal 18:1723–1729.
2. Horn F, Weare J, Beukers MW, Horsch S, Bairoch A, Chen W, et al. (1998). GPCRDB: An information system for G protein-coupled receptors. Nucleic Acids Res 26:275–279.
3. Vassart G, Pardo L, Costagliola S (2004). A molecular dissection of the glycoprotein hormone receptors. Trends in Biochemical Sciences 29:119–126.
4. Baldwin JM (1993). The probable arrangement of the helices in G protein-coupled receptors. The EMBO Journal 12:1693–1703.
5. Spengler D, Waeber C, Pantaloni C, Holsboer F, Bockaert J, Seeburg PH, et al. (1993). Differential signal transduction by five splice variants of the PACAP receptor. Nature 365:170–175.
6. Wess J (1997). G-protein-coupled receptors: Molecular mechanisms involved in receptor activation and selectivity of G-protein recognition. Faseb J 11:346–354.
7. Daaka Y, Luttrell LM, Ahn S, Della Rocca GJ, Ferguson SS, Caron MG, et al. (1998). Essential role for G protein-coupled receptor endocytosis in the activation of mitogen-activated protein kinase. J Biol Chem 273:685–688.
8. Eason MG, Liggett SB (1995). Identification of a Gs coupling domain in the amino terminus of the third intracellular loop of the alpha 2A-adrenergic receptor: Evidence for distinct structural determinants that confer Gs versus Gi coupling. J Biol Chem 270:24753–24760.

9. Fields TA, Casey PJ (1997). Signaling functions and biochemical properties of pertussis toxin-resistant G-proteins. Biochem J 321:561–571.

10. Limbird LE (1988). Receptors linked to inhibition of adenylate cyclase: Additional signaling mechanisms. Faseb J 2:2686–2695.

11. Rivkees SA, Barbhaiya H, AP IJ (1999). Identification of the adenine binding site of the human A1 adenosine receptor. J Biol Chem 274:3617–3621.

12. Reppert SM, Weaver DR, Stehle JH, Rivkees SA (1991). Molecular cloning and characterization of a rat A1-adenosine receptor that is widely expressed in brain and spinal cord. Mol Endocrinol 5:1037–1048.

13. Levitzki A, Marbach I, Bar-Sinai A (1993). The signal transduction between beta-receptors and adenylyl cyclase. Life Sciences 52:2093–2100.

14. Thompson MD, Burnham WM, Cole DE (2005). The G protein-coupled receptors: Pharmacogenetics and disease. Critical Reviews in Clinical Laboratory Sciences 42:311–392.

15. Lu D, Yan H, Othman T, Turner CP, Woolf T, Rivkees SA (2004). Cytoskeletal protein 4.1G binds to the third intracellular loop of the A1 adenosine receptor and inhibits receptor action. Biochem J 377:51–59.

16. Lu D, Yan H, Othman T, Rivkees SA (2004). Cytoskeletal protein 4.1G is a binding partner of the metabotropic glutamate receptor subtype 1 alpha. J Neurosci Res 78:49–55.

17. Csaba Z, Dournaud P (2001). Cellular biology of somatostatin receptors. Neuropeptides 35:1–23.

18. Rocheville M, Lange DC, Kumar U, Sasi R, Patel RC, Patel YC (2000). Subtypes of the somatostatin receptor assemble as functional homo- and heterodimers. J Biol Chem 275:7862–7869.

19. Rocheville M, Lange DC, Kumar U, Patel SC, Patel RC, Patel YC (2000). Receptors for dopamine and somatostatin: Formation of hetero-oligomers with enhanced functional activity. Science 288:154–157.

20. Pfeiffer M, Koch T, Schroder H, Klutzny M, Kirscht S, Kreienkamp HJ, et al. (2001). Homo- and heterodimerization of somatostatin receptor subtypes: Inactivation of sst(3) receptor function by heterodimerization with sst(2A). J Biol Chem 276:14027–14036.

21. Born W, Fischer JA, Muff R (2002). Receptors for calcitonin gene-related peptide, adrenomedullin, and amylin: The contributions of novel receptor-activity-modifying proteins. Receptors & Channels 8:201–209.

22. Born W, Muff R, Fischer JA (2002). Functional interaction of G protein-coupled receptors of the adrenomedullin peptide family with accessory receptor-activity-modifying proteins (RAMP). Microscopy Research and Technique 57:14–22.

23. Lerner UH (2006). Deletions of genes encoding calcitonin/alpha-CGRP, amylin and calcitonin receptor have given new and unexpected insights into the function of calcitonin receptors and calcitonin receptor-like receptors in bone. Journal of Musculoskeletal & Neuronal Interactions 6:87–95.

24. Christopoulos A, Christopoulos G, Morfis M, Udawela M, Laburthe M, Couvineau A, et al. (2003). Novel receptor partners and function of receptor activity-modifying proteins. J Biol Chem 278:3293–3297.

25. Angers S, Salahpour A, Bouvier M (2002). Dimerization: An emerging concept for G protein-coupled receptor ontogeny and function. Annu Rev Pharmacol Toxicol 42:409–435.

26. McLatchie LM, Fraser NJ, Main ML, Wise A, Brown J, Thompson N, et al. (1998). RAMPs regulate the transport and ligand specificity of the calcitonin-receptor-like receptor. Nature 393:333–339.

27. Morello JP, Salahpour A, Petaja-Repo UE, Laperriere A, Lonergan M, Arthus MF, et al. (2001). Association of calnexin with wild type and mutant AVPR2 that causes nephrogenic diabetes insipidus. Biochemistry 40:6766–6775.

28. Zhu X, Wess J (1998). Truncated V2 vasopressin receptors as negative regulators of wild-type V2 receptor function. Biochemistry 37:15773–15784.

29. Oksche A, Rosenthal W (1998). The molecular basis of nephrogenic diabetes insipidus. Journal of Molecular Medicine (Berlin, Germany) 76:326–337.

30. Calebiro D, de Filippis T, Lucchi S, Covino C, Panigone S, Beck-Peccoz P, et al. (2005). Intracellular entrapment of wild-type TSH receptor by oligomerization with mutants linked to dominant TSH resistance. Human Molecular Genetics 14:2991–3002.

31. Ulloa-Aguirre A, Janovick JA, Leanos-Miranda A, Conn PM (2004). Misrouted cell surface GnRH receptors as a disease aetiology for congenital isolated hypogonadotrophic hypogonadism. Human Reproduction Update 10:177–192.

32. Leanos-Miranda A, Ulloa-Aguirre A, Ji TH, Janovick JA, Conn PM (2003). Dominant-negative action of disease-causing gonadotropin-releasing hormone receptor (GnRHR) mutants: A trait that potentially coevolved with decreased plasma membrane expression of GnRHR in humans. The Journal of Clinical Endocrinology and Metabolism 88:3360–3367.

33. Brothers SP, Cornea A, Janovick JA, Conn PM (2004). Human loss-of-function gonadotropin-releasing hormone receptor mutants retain wild-type receptors in the endoplasmic reticulum: Molecular basis of the dominant-negative effect. Mol Endocrinol 18:1787–1797.

34. Seifert R, Wenzel-Seifert K (2002). Constitutive activity of G-protein-coupled receptors: cause of disease and common property of wild-type receptors. Naunyn-Schmiedeberg's Archives of Pharmacology 366:381–416.

35. Milligan G (2003). Constitutive activity and inverse agonists of G protein-coupled receptors: A current perspective. Mol Pharmacol 64:1271–1276.

36. Tiberi M, Caron MG (1994). High agonist-independent activity is a distinguishing feature of the dopamine D1B receptor subtype. J Biol Chem 269:27925–27931.

37. Milligan G, Bond RA, Lee M (1995). Inverse agonism: Pharmacological curiosity or potential therapeutic strategy? Trends in Pharmacological Sciences 16:10–13.

38. Ferguson SS (2001). Evolving concepts in G protein-coupled receptor endocytosis: The role in receptor desensitization and signaling. Pharmacological Reviews 53:1–24.

39. Mason D, Hassan A, Chacko S, Thompson P (2002). Acute and chronic regulation of pituitary receptors for vasopressin and corticotropin releasing hormone. Archives of Physiology and Biochemistry 110:74–89.

40. Lohse MJ, Benovic JL, Codina J, Caron MG, Lefkowitz RJ (1990). Beta-arrestin: A protein that regulates beta-adrenergic receptor function. Science 248:1547–1550.

41. Mukherjee S, Palczewski K, Gurevich V, Benovic JL, Banga JP, Hunzicker-Dunn M (1999). A direct role for arrestins in desensitization of the luteinizing hormone/choriogonadotropin receptor in porcine ovarian follicular membranes. Proceedings of the National Academy of Sciences of the United States of America 96:493–498.

42. Bouvier M, Hausdorff WP, De Blasi A, O'Dowd BF, Kobilka BK, Caron MG, et al. (1988). Removal of phosphorylation sites from the beta 2-adrenergic receptor delays onset of agonist-promoted desensitization. Nature 333:370–373.

43. Hunzicker-Dunn M, Gurevich VV, Casanova JE, Mukherjee S (2002). ARF6: A newly appreciated player in G protein-coupled receptor desensitization. FEBS Letters 521:3–8.

44. Troispoux C, Guillou F, Elalouf JM, Firsov D, Iacovelli L, De Blasi A, et al. (1999). Involvement of G protein-coupled receptor kinases and arrestins in desensitization to follicle-stimulating hormone action. Mol Endocrinol 13:1599–1614.

45. Lazari MF, Liu X, Nakamura K, Benovic JL, Ascoli M (1999). Role of G protein-coupled receptor kinases on the agonist-induced phosphorylation and internalization of the follitropin receptor. Mol Endocrinol 13:866–878.

46. Nakamura K, Lazari MF, Li S, Korgaonkar C, Ascoli M (1999). Role of the rate of internalization of the agonist-receptor complex on the agonist-induced down-regulation of the lutropin/choriogonadotropin receptor. Mol Endocrinol 13:1295–1304.

47. Nakamura K, Liu X, Ascoli M (2000). Seven non-contiguous intracellular residues of the lutropin/choriogonadotropin receptor dictate the rate of agonist-induced internalization and its sensitivity to non-visual arrestins. J Biol Chem 275:241–247.

48. Frenzel R, Voigt C, Paschke R (2006). The human thyrotropin receptor is predominantly internalized by beta-arrestin 2. Endocrinology 147:3114–3122.

49. Oakley RH, Laporte SA, Holt JA, Caron MG, Barak LS (2000). Differential affinities of visual arrestin, beta arrestin1, and beta arrestin2 for G protein-coupled receptors delineate two major classes of receptors. J Biol Chem 275:17201–17210.

50. Lohse MJ (1993). Molecular mechanisms of membrane receptor desensitization. Biochimica et Biophysica Acta 1179:171–188.

51. Morris AJ, Malbon CC (1999). Physiological regulation of G protein-linked signaling. Physiological Reviews 79:1373–1430.

52. Scearce-Levie K, Lieberman MD, Elliott HH, Conklin BR (2005). Engineered G protein coupled receptors reveal independent regulation of internalization, desensitization and acute signaling. BMC Biology [electronic resource] 3:3.

53. Barak LS, Oakley RH, Laporte SA, Caron MG (2001). Constitutive arrestin-mediated desensitization of a human vasopressin receptor mutant associated with nephrogenic diabetes insipidus. Proceedings of the National Academy of Sciences of the United States of America 98:93–98.

54. Tao YX (2006). Inactivating mutations of G protein-coupled receptors and diseases: structure-function insights and therapeutic implications. Pharmacology & Therapeutics 111:949–973.

55. Im DS (2004). Discovery of new G protein-coupled receptors for lipid mediators. Journal of Lipid Research 45:410–418.

56. Krasnoperov VG, Bittner MA, Beavis R, Kuang Y, Salnikow KV, Chepurny OG, et al. (1997). Alpha-latrotoxin stimulates exocytosis by the interaction with a neuronal G-protein-coupled receptor. Neuron 18:925–937.

57. O'Hara PJ, Sheppard PO, Thogersen H, Venezia D, Haldeman BA, McGrane V, et al. (1993). The ligand-binding domain in metabotropic glutamate receptors is related to bacterial periplasmic binding proteins. Neuron 11:41–52.

58. Silve C, Petrel C, Leroy C, Bruel H, Mallet E, Rognan D, et al. (2005). Delineating a Ca2+ binding pocket within the venus flytrap module of the human calcium-sensing receptor. J Biol Chem 280:37917–37923.

59. Magenis RE, Smith L, Nadeau JH, Johnson KR, Mountjoy KG, Cone RD (1994). Mapping of the ACTH, MSH, and neural (MC3 and MC4) melanocortin receptors in the mouse and human. Mamm Genome 5:503–508.

60. Mesiano S, Jaffe RB (1997). Developmental and functional biology of the primate fetal adrenal cortex. Endocrine Reviews 18:378–403.

61. Miller WL (1988). Molecular biology of steroid hormone synthesis. Endocrine Reviews 9:295–318.

62. Tiosano D, Pannain S, Vassart G, Parma J, Gershoni-Baruch R, Mandel H, et al. (1999). The hypothyroidism in an inbred kindred with congenital thyroid hormone and glucocorticoid deficiency is due to a mutation producing a truncated thyrotropin receptor. Thyroid 9:887–894.

63. Clark AJ, Weber A (1998). Adrenocorticotropin insensitivity syndromes. Endocrine Reviews 19:828–843.

64. Clark AJ, McLoughlin L, Grossman A (1993). Familial glucocorticoid deficiency associated with point mutation in the adrenocorticotropin receptor. Lancet 341:461–462.

65. Tsigos C, Arai K, Hung W, Chrousos GP (1993). Hereditary isolated glucocorticoid deficiency is associated with abnormalities of the adrenocorticotropin receptor gene. The Journal of Clinical Investigation 92:2458–2461.

66. Weber A, Toppari J, Harvey RD, Klann RC, Shaw NJ, Ricker AT, et al. (1995). Adrenocorticotropin receptor gene mutations in familial glucocorticoid deficiency: relationships with clinical features in four families. The Journal of Clinical Endocrinology and Metabolism 80:65–71.

67. Tsigos C, Arai K, Latronico AC, DiGeorge AM, Rapaport R, Chrousos GP (1995). A novel mutation of the adrenocorticotropin receptor (ACTH-R) gene in a family with the syndrome of isolated glucocorticoid deficiency, but no ACTH-R abnormalities in two families with the triple A syndrome. The Journal of Clinical Endocrinology and Metabolism 80:2186–2189.

68. Naville D, Barjhoux L, Jaillard C, Faury D, Despert F, Esteva B, et al. (1996). Demonstration by transfection studies that mutations in the adrenocorticotropin receptor gene are one cause of the hereditary syndrome of glucocorticoid deficiency. The Journal of Clinical Endocrinology and Metabolism 81:1442–1448.

69. Slavotinek AM, Hurst JA, Dunger D, Wilkie AO (1998). ACTH receptor mutation in a girl with familial glucocorticoid deficiency. Clin Genet 53:57–62.

70. Weber A, Clark AJ (1994). Mutations of the ACTH receptor gene are only one cause of familial glucocorticoid deficiency. Human Molecular Genetics 3:585–588.

71. Allgrove J, Clayden GS, Grant DB, Macaulay JC (1978). Familial glucocorticoid deficiency with achalasia of the cardia and deficient tear production. Lancet 1:1284–1286.

72. Shepard TH, Landing BH, Mason DG (1959). Familial Addison's disease. Am J Dis Child 97:154–162.

73. Migeon CJ, Kenny EM, Kowarski A, Snipes CA, Spaulding JS, Finkelstein JW, et al. (1968). The syndrome of congenital adrenocortical unresponsiveness to ACTH: Report of six cases. Pediatr Res 2:501–513.

74. Monteleone JA, Monteleone PL (1970). Hereditary adrenocortical unresponsiveness to ACTH—another case. Pediatrics 46:321–322.

75. Spark RF, Etzkorn JR (1977). Absent aldosterone response to ACTH in familial glucocorticoid deficiency. The New England Journal of Medicine 297:917–920.

76. Davidai G, Kahana L, Hochberg Z (1984). Glomerulosa failure in congenital adrenocortical unresponsiveness to ACTH. Clinical Endocrinology 20:515–520.

77. Kelch RP, Kaplan SL, Biglieri EG, Daniels GH, Epstein CJ, Grumbach MM (1972). Hereditary adrenocortical unresponsiveness to adrenocorticotropic hormone. The Journal of Pediatrics 81:726–736.

78. Lacy DE, Nathavitharana KA, Tarlow MJ (1993). Neonatal hepatitis and congenital insensitivity to adrenocorticotropin (ACTH). J Pediatr Gastroenterol Nutr 17:438–440.

79. Clark AJ, Cammas FM, Watt A, Kapas S, Weber A (1997). Familial glucocorticoid deficiency: One syndrome, but more than one gene. Journal of Molecular Medicine (Berlin, Germany) 75:394–399.

80. Petrykowski W, Burmeister P, Bohm N (1975). Familiar glucocorticoid insufficiency. Klin Padiatr 187:198–215.

81. Lyons J, Landis CA, Harsh G, Vallar L, Grunewald K, Feichtinger H, et al. (1990). Two G protein oncogenes in human endocrine tumors. Science 249:655–659.

82. Reincke M, Mora P, Beuschlein F, Arlt W, Chrousos GP, Allolio B (1997). Deletion of the adrenocorticotropin receptor gene in human adrenocortical tumors: Implications for tumorigenesis. The Journal of Clinical Endocrinology and Metabolism 82:3054–3058.

83. Lacroix A, Bolte E, Tremblay J, Dupre J, Poitras P, Fournier H, et al. (1992). Gastric inhibitory polypeptide-dependent cortisol hypersecretion: A new cause of Cushing's syndrome. The New England Journal of Medicine 327:974–980.

84. Reznik Y, Allali-Zerah V, Chayvialle JA, Leroyer R, Leymarie P, Travert G (1992). Food-dependent Cushing's syndrome mediated by aberrant adrenal sensitivity to gastric inhibitory polypeptide. The New England Journal of Medicine 327:981–986.

85. Lacroix A, N'Diaye N, Mircescu H, Hamet P, Tremblay J (1998). Abnormal expression and function of hormone receptors in adrenal Cushing's syndrome. Endocrine Research 24:835–843.

86. Arnaldi G, Gasc JM, de Keyzer Y, Raffin-Sanson ML, Perraudin V, Kuhn JM, et al. (1998). Variable expression of the V1 vasopressin receptor modulates the phenotypic response of steroid-secreting adrenocortical tumors. The Journal of Clinical Endocrinology and Metabolism 83:2029–2035.

87. Daidoh H, Morita H, Hanafusa J, Mune T, Murase H, Sato M, (1998). In vivo and in vitro effects of AVP and V1a receptor antagonist on Cushing's syndrome due to ACTH-independent bilateral macronodular adrenocortical hyperplasia. Clinical Endocrinology 49:403–409.

88. Bourdeau I, Stratakis CA (2002). Cyclic AMP-dependent signaling aberrations in macronodular adrenal disease. Annals of the New York Academy of Sciences 968:240–255.

89. Feng N, Young SF, Aguilera G, Puricelli E, Adler-Wailes DC, Sebring NG, (2005). Co-occurrence of two partially inactivating polymorphisms of MC3R is associated with pediatric-onset obesity. Diabetes 54:2663–2667.

90. Smit MJ, Vischer HF, Bakker RA, Jongejan A, Timmerman H, Pardo L, et al. (2006). Pharmacogenomic and structural analysis of constitutive G protein-coupled receptor activity. Annu Rev Pharmacol Toxicol [volume/pages].

91. Siegrist W, Drozdz R, Cotti R, Willard DH, Wilkison WO, Eberle AN (1997). Interactions of alpha-melanotropin and agouti on B16 melanoma cells: Evidence for inverse agonism of agouti. Journal of Receptor and Signal Transduction Research 17:75–98.

92. Vergoni AV, Bertolini A, Wikberg JE, Schioth HB (1999). Selective melanocortin MC4 receptor blockage reduces immobilization stress-induced anorexia in rats. European Journal of Pharmacology 369:11–15.

93. Vergoni AV, Bertolini A, Guidetti G, Karefilakis V, Filaferro M, Wikberg JE, et al. (2000). Chronic melanocortin 4 receptor blockage causes obesity without influencing sexual behavior in male rats. The Journal of Endocrinology 166:419–426.

94. Yeo GS, Farooqi IS, Aminian S, Halsall DJ, Stanhope RG, O'Rahilly S (1998). A frameshift mutation in MC4R associated with dominantly inherited human obesity. Nature Genetics 20:111–112.

95. Farooqi IS, Yeo GS, Keogh JM, Aminian S, Jebb SA, Butler G, et al. (2000). Dominant and recessive inheritance of morbid obesity associated with melanocortin 4 receptor deficiency. The Journal of Clinical Investigation 106:271–279.

96. Farooqi IS, Keogh JM, Yeo GS, Lank EJ, Cheetham T, O'Rahilly S (2003). Clinical spectrum of obesity and mutations in the melanocortin 4 receptor gene. The New England Journal of Medicine 348:1085–1095.

97. Vink T, Hinney A, van Elburg AA, van Goozen SH, Sandkuijl LA, Sinke RJ, et al. (2001). Association between an agouti-related protein gene polymorphism and anorexia nervosa. Molecular Psychiatry 6:325–328.

98. Adan RA, Vink T (2001). Drug target discovery by pharmacogenetics: Mutations in the melanocortin system and eating disorders. Eur Neuropsychopharmacol 11:483–490.

99. Chagnon YC, Chen WJ, Perusse L, Chagnon M, Nadeau A, Wilkison WO, et al. (1997). Linkage and association studies between the melanocortin receptors 4 and 5 genes and obesity-related phenotypes in the Quebec Family Study. Molecular Medicine (Cambridge, Mass.) 3:663–673.

100. Wakamatsu K, Graham A, Cook D, Thody AJ (1997). Characterisation of ACTH peptides in human skin and their activation of the melanocortin-1 receptor. Pigment Cell Research 10:288–297.

101. Graham A, Wakamatsu K, Hunt G, Ito S, Thody AJ (1997). Agouti protein inhibits the production of eumelanin and phaeomelanin in the presence and absence of alpha-melanocyte stimulating hormone. Pigment Cell Research 10:298–303.

102. Challis BG, Pritchard LE, Creemers JW, Delplanque J, Keogh JM, Luan J, et al. (2002). A missense mutation disrupting a dibasic prohormone processing site in pro-opiomelanocortin (POMC) increases susceptibility to early-onset obesity through a novel molecular mechanism. Human Molecular Genetics 11:1997–2004.

103. Lee YS, Challis BG, Thompson DA, Yeo GS, Keogh JM, Madonna ME, et al. (2006). A POMC variant implicates beta-melanocyte-stimulating hormone in the control of human energy balance. Cell Metabolism 3:135–140.

104. Pasel K, Schulz A, Timmermann K, Linnemann K, Hoeltzenbein M, Jaaskelainen J, et al. (2000). Functional characterization of the molecular defects causing nephrogenic diabetes insipidus in eight families. The Journal of Clinical Endocrinology and Metabolism 85:1703–1710.

105. Bichet DG, Hendy GN, Lonergan M, Arthus MF, Ligier S, Pausova Z, et al. (1992). X-linked nephrogenic diabetes insipidus: from the ship Hopewell to RFLP studies. American Journal of Human Genetics 51:1089–1102.

106. Rosenthal W, Seibold A, Antaramian A, Lonergan M, Arthus MF, Hendy GN, et al. (1992). Molecular identification of the gene responsible for congenital nephrogenic diabetes insipidus. Nature 359:233–235.

107. Lolait SJ, O'Carroll AM, McBride OW, Konig M, Morel A, Brownstein MJ (1992). Cloning and characterization of a vasopressin V2 receptor and possible link to nephrogenic diabetes insipidus. Nature 357:336–339.

108. Knoers N, van den Ouweland A, Dreesen J, Verdijk M, Monnens LA, van Oost BA (1993). Nephrogenic diabetes insipidus: identification of the genetic defect. Pediatr Nephrol 7:685–688.

109. Deen PM, Verdijk MA, Knoers NV, Wieringa B, Monnens LA, van Os CH, et al. (1994). Requirement of human renal water channel aquaporin-2 for vasopressin-dependent concentration of urine. Science 264:92–95.

110. van Lieburg AF, Verdijk MA, Knoers VV, van Essen AJ, Proesmans W, Mallmann R, et al. (1994). Patients with autosomal nephrogenic diabetes insipidus homozygous for mutations in the aquaporin 2 water-channel gene. American Journal of Human Genetics 55:648–652.

111. Ala Y, Morin D, Mouillac B, Sabatier N, Vargas R, Cotte N, et al. (1998). Functional studies of twelve mutant V2 vasopressin receptors related to nephrogenic diabetes insipidus: Molecular basis of a mild clinical phenotype. J Am Soc Nephrol 9:1861–1872.

112. Feldman BJ, Rosenthal SM, Vargas GA, Fenwick RG, Huang EA, Matsuda-Abedini M, et al. (2005). Nephrogenic syndrome of inappropriate antidiuresis. N Engl J Med 352:1884–1890.

113. Ben-Menahem D, Hyde R, Pixley M, Berger P, Boime I (1999). Synthesis of multi-subunit domain gonadotropin complexes: A model for alpha/beta heterodimer formation. Biochemistry 38:15070–15077.

114. Lustbader JW, Lobel L, Wu H, Elliott MM (1998). Structural and molecular studies of human chorionic gonadotropin and its receptor. Recent Progress in Hormone Research 53:395–424.

115. Themmen AP, Martens JW, Brunner HG (1998). Activating and inactivating mutations in LH receptors. Molecular and Cellular Endocrinology 145:137–142.

116. Tsai-Morris CH, Buczko E, Wang W, Xie XZ, Dufau ML (1991). Structural organization of the rat luteinizing hormone (LH) receptor gene. J Biol Chem 266:11355–11359.

117. Minegishi T, Nakamura K, Takakura Y, Miyamoto K, Hasegawa Y, Ibuki Y, et al. (1990). Cloning and sequencing of human LH/hCG receptor cDNA. Biochemical and Biophysical Research Communications 172:1049–1054.

118. Schwartz M, Imperato-McGinley J, Peterson RE, Cooper G, Morris PL, MacGillivray M, et al. (1981). Male pseudohermaphroditism secondary to an abnormality in Leydig cell differentiation. The Journal of Clinical Endocrinology and Metabolism 53:123–127.

119. Toledo SP, Arnhold IJ, Luthold W, Russo EM, Saldanha PH (1985). Leydig cell hypoplasia determining familial hypergonadotropic hypogonadism. Prog Clin Biol Res 200:311–314.

120. el-Awady MK, Temtamy SA, Salam MA, Gad YZ (1987). Familial Leydig cell hypoplasia as a cause of male pseudohermaphroditism. Hum Hered 37:36–40.

121. Martinez-Mora J, Saez JM, Toran N, Isnard R, Perez-Iribarne MM, Egozcue J, Audi L (1991). Male pseudohermaphroditism due to Leydig cell agenesia and absence of testicular LH receptors. Clinical Endocrinology 34:485–491.

122. Toledo SP (1992). Leydig cell hypoplasia leading to two different phenotypes: male pseudohermaphroditism and primary hypogonadism. Clinical Endocrinology 36:521–522.

123. Kremer H, Kraaij R, Toledo SP, Post M, Fridman JB, Hayashida CY, et al. (1995). Male pseudohermaphroditism due to a homozygous missense mutation of the luteinizing hormone receptor gene. Nature Genetics 9:160–164.

124. Latronico AC, Anasti J, Arnhold IJ, Rapaport R, Mendonca BB, Bloise W, et al. (1996). Brief report: Testicular and ovarian resistance to luteinizing hormone caused by inactivating mutations of the luteinizing hormone-receptor gene. The New England Journal of Medicine 334:507–512.

125. Chan WY (1998). Molecular genetic, biochemical, and clinical implications of gonadotropin receptor mutations. Molecular Genetics and Metabolism 63:75–84.

126. Latronico AC, Chai Y, Arnhold IJ, Liu X, Mendonca BB, Segaloff DL (1998). A homozygous microdeletion in helix 7 of the luteinizing hormone receptor associated with familial testicular and ovarian resistance is due to both decreased cell surface expression and impaired effector activation by the cell surface receptor. Mol Endocrinol 12:442–450.

127. Martens JW, Verhoef-Post M, Abelin N, Ezabella M, Toledo SP, Brunner HG, et al. (1998). A homozygous mutation in the luteinizing hormone receptor causes partial Leydig cell hypoplasia: Correlation between receptor activity and phenotype. Mol Endocrinol 12:775–784.

128. Laue LL, Wu SM, Kudo M, Bourdony CJ, Cutler GB Jr., Hsueh AJ, et al. (1996). Compound heterozygous mutations of the luteinizing hormone receptor gene in Leydig cell hypoplasia. Mol Endocrinol 10:987–997.

129. Misrahi M, Meduri G, Pissard S, Bouvattier C, Beau I, Loosfelt H, et al. (1997). Comparison of immunocytochemical and molecular features with the phenotype in a case of incomplete male pseudohermaphroditism associated with a mutation of the luteinizing hormone receptor. The Journal of Clinical Endocrinology and Metabolism 82:2159–2165.

130. Gromoll J, Eiholzer U, Nieschlag E, Simoni M (2000). Male hypogonadism caused by homozygous deletion of exon 10 of the luteinizing hormone (LH) receptor: Differential action of human chorionic gonadotropin and LH. The Journal of Clinical Endocrinology and Metabolism 85:2281–2286.

131. Schedewie HK, Reiter EO, Beitins IZ, Seyed S, Wooten VD, Jimenez JF, et al. (1981). Testicular leydig cell hyperplasia as a cause of familial sexual precocity. The Journal of Clinical Endocrinology and Metabolism 52:271–278.

132. Rosenthal SM, Grumbach MM, Kaplan SL (1983). Gonadotropin-independent familial sexual precocity with premature Leydig and germinal cell maturation (familial testotoxicosis): Effects of a potent luteinizing hormone-releasing factor agonist and medroxyprogesterone acetate therapy in four cases. The Journal of Clinical Endocrinology and Metabolism 57:571–579.

133. Gondos B, Egli CA, Rosenthal SM, Grumbach MM (1985). Testicular changes in gonadotropin-independent familial male sexual precocity: Familial testotoxicosis. Arch Pathol Lab Med 109:990–995.

134. Egli CA, Rosenthal SM, Grumbach MM, Montalvo JM, Gondos B (1985). Pituitary gonadotropin-independent male-limited autosomal dominant sexual precocity in nine generations: familial testotoxicosis. The Journal of Pediatrics 106:33–40.

135. Kremer H, Mariman E, Otten BJ, Moll GW Jr., Stoelinga GB, Wit JM, et al. (1993). Cosegregation of missense mutations of the luteinizing hormone receptor gene with familial male-limited precocious puberty. Human Molecular Genetics 2:1779–1783.

136. Rosenthal IM, Refetoff S, Rich B, Barnes RB, Sunthornthepvarakul T, Parma J, et al. (1996). Response to challenge with gonadotropin-releasing hormone agonist in a mother and her two sons with a constitutively activating mutation of the luteinizing hormone receptor: A clinical research center study. The Journal of Clinical Endocrinology and Metabolism 81:3802–3806.

137. Oerter KE, Uriarte MM, Rose SR, Barnes KM, Cutler GB Jr. (1990). Gonadotropin secretory dynamics during puberty in normal girls and boys. The Journal of Clinical Endocrinology and Metabolism 71:1251–1258.

138. Latronico AC, Abell AN, Arnhold IJ, Liu X, Lins TS, Brito VN, et al. (1998). A unique constitutively activating mutation in third transmembrane helix of luteinizing hormone receptor causes sporadic male gonadotropin-independent precocious puberty. The Journal of Clinical Endocrinology and Metabolism 83:2435–2440.

139. Toledo SP, Brunner HG, Kraaij R, Post M, Dahia PL, Hayashida CY, et al. (1996). An inactivating mutation of the luteinizing hormone receptor causes amenorrhea in a 46,XX female. The Journal of Clinical Endocrinology and Metabolism 81:3850–3854.

140. Tapanainen JS, Vaskivuo T, Aittomaki K, Huhtaniemi IT (1998). Inactivating FSH receptor mutations and gonadal dysfunction. Molecular and Cellular Endocrinology 145:129–135.

141. Minegishi T, Nakamura K, Takakura Y, Ibuki Y, Igarashi M, Minegish T (1991). Cloning and sequencing of human FSH receptor cDNA. Biochemical and Biophysical Research Communications 175:1125–1130.

142. Heckert LL, Daley IJ, Griswold MD (1992). Structural organization of the follicle-stimulating hormone receptor gene. Mol Endocrinol 6:70–80.

143. Jones GS, Acosta AA, Garcia JE, Bernardus RE, Rosenwaks Z (1985). The effect of follicle-stimulating hormone without additional luteinizing hormone on follicular stimulation and oocyte development in normal ovulatory women. Fertil Steril 43:696–702.

144. Durham CR, Zhu H, Masters BS, Simpson ER, Mendelson CR (1985). Regulation of aromatase activity of rat granulosa cells: Induction of synthesis of NADPH-cytochrome P-450 reductase by FSH and dibutyryl cyclic AMP. Molecular and Cellular Endocrinology 40:211–219.

145. Knobil E (1980). The neuroendocrine control of the menstrual cycle. Recent Progress in Hormone Research 36:53–88.

146. Aittomaki K, Herva R, Stenman UH, Juntunen K, Ylostalo P, Hovatta O, et al. (1996). Clinical features of primary ovarian failure caused by a point mutation in the follicle-stimulating hormone receptor gene. The Journal of Clinical Endocrinology and Metabolism 81:3722–3726.

147. Aittomaki K, Lucena JL, Pakarinen P, Sistonen P, Tapanainen J, Gromoll J, et al. (1995). Mutation in the follicle-stimulating hormone receptor gene causes hereditary hypergonadotropic ovarian failure. Cell 82:959–968.

148. Tapanainen JS, Aittomaki K, Min J, Vaskivuo T, Huhtaniemi IT (1997). Men homozygous for an inactivating mutation of the follicle-stimulating hormone (FSH) receptor gene present variable suppression of spermatogenesis and fertility. Nature Genetics 15:205–206.

149. Jiang M, Aittomaki K, Nilsson C, Pakarinen P, Iitia A, Torresani T, et al. (1998). The frequency of an inactivating point mutation (566C-->T) of the human follicle-stimulating hormone receptor gene in four populations using allele-specific hybridization and time-resolved fluorometry. The Journal of Clinical Endocrinology and Metabolism 83:4338–4343.

150. Beau I, Touraine P, Meduri G, Gougeon A, Desroches A, Matuchansky C, et al. (1998). A novel phenotype related to partial loss of function mutations of the follicle stimulating hormone receptor. The Journal of Clinical Investigation 102:1352–1359.

151. Touraine P, Beau I, Gougeon A, Meduri G, Desroches A, Pichard C, et al. (1999). New natural inactivating mutations of the follicle-stimulating hormone receptor: Correlations between receptor function and phenotype. Mol Endocrinol 13:1844–1854.

152. Gromoll J, Simoni M, Nieschlag E (1996). An activating mutation of the follicle-stimulating hormone receptor autonomously sustains spermatogenesis in a hypophysectomized man. The Journal of Clinical Endocrinology and Metabolism 81:1367–1370.

153. Laue L, Chan WY, Hsueh AJ, Kudo M, Hsu SY, Wu SM, et al. (1995). Genetic heterogeneity of constitutively activating mutations of the human luteinizing hormone receptor in familial male-limited precocious puberty. Proceedings of the National Academy of Sciences of the United States of America 92:1906–1910.

154. Tonacchera M, Van Sande J, Parma J, Duprez L, Cetani F, Costagliola S, et al. (1996). TSH receptor and disease. Clinical Endocrinology 44:621–633.

155. Libert F, Lefort A, Gerard C, Parmentier M, Perret J, Ludgate M, et al. (1989). Cloning, sequencing and expression of the human thyrotropin (TSH) receptor: Evidence for binding of autoantibodies. Biochemical and Biophysical Research Communications 165:1250–1255.

156. Nagayama Y, Kaufman KD, Seto P, Rapoport B (1989). Molecular cloning, sequence and functional expression of the cDNA for the human thyrotropin receptor. Biochemical and Biophysical Research Communications 165:1184–1190.

157. Misrahi M, Loosfelt H, Atger M, Sar S, Guiochon-Mantel A, Milgrom E (1990). Cloning, sequencing and expression of human TSH receptor. Biochemical and Biophysical Research Communications 166:394–403.

158. Gross B, Misrahi M, Sar S, Milgrom E (1991). Composite structure of the human thyrotropin receptor gene. Biochemical and Biophysical Research Communications 177:679–687.

159. Dumont JE, Lamy F, Roger P, Maenhaut C (1992). Physiological and pathological regulation of thyroid cell proliferation and differentiation by thyrotropin and other factors. Physiological Reviews 72:667–697.

160. Allgeier A, Offermanns S, Van Sande J, Spicher K, Schultz G, Dumont JE (1994). The human thyrotropin receptor activates G-proteins Gs and Gq/11. J Biol Chem 269:13733–13735.

161. Russo D, Chazenbalk GD, Nagayama Y, Wadsworth HL, Seto P, Rapoport B (1991). A new structural model for the thyrotropin (TSH) receptor, as determined by covalent cross-linking of TSH to the recombinant receptor in intact cells: Evidence for a single polypeptide chain. Mol Endocrinol 5:1607–1612.

162. Rapoport B, Chazenbalk GD, Jaume JC, McLachlan SM (1998). The thyrotropin (TSH) receptor: interaction with TSH and autoantibodies. Endocrine Reviews 19:673–716.

163. Chazenbalk GD, Tanaka K, McLachlan SM, Rapoport B (1999). On the functional importance of thyrotropin receptor intramolecular cleavage. Endocrinology 140:4516–4520.

164. Tanaka K, Chazenbalk GD, McLachlan SM, Rapoport B (1999). Thyrotropin receptor cleavage at site 1 involves two discontinuous segments at each end of the unique 50-amino acid insertion. J Biol Chem 274:2093–2096.

165. Kajita Y, Rickards CR, Buckland PR, Howells RD, Rees Smith B (1985). Analysis of thyrotropin receptors by photoaffinity labelling: Orientation of receptor subunits in the cell membrane. Biochem J 227:413–420.

166. Loosfelt H, Pichon C, Jolivet A, Misrahi M, Caillou B, Jamous M, et al. (1992). Two-subunit structure of the human thyrotropin receptor. Proceedings of the National Academy of Sciences of the United States of America 89:3765–3769.

167. Misrahi M, Ghinea N, Sar S, Saunier B, Jolivet A, Loosfelt H, et al. (1994). Processing of the precursors of the human thyroid-stimulating hormone receptor in various eukaryotic cells (human thyrocytes, transfected L cells and baculovirus-infected insect cells). European Journal of Biochemistry / FEBS 222:711–719.

168. Tanaka K, Chazenbalk GD, McLachlan SM, Rapoport B (1999). Subunit structure of thyrotropin receptors expressed on the cell surface. J Biol Chem 274:33979–33984.

169. Nagayama Y, Wadsworth HL, Chazenbalk GD, Russo D, Seto P, Rapoport B (1991). Thyrotropin-luteinizing hormone/chorionic gonadotropin receptor extracellular domain chimeras as probes for thyrotropin receptor function. Proceedings of the National Academy of Sciences of the United States of America 88:902–905.

170. Nagayama Y, Rapoport B (1992). Role of the carboxyl-terminal half of the extracellular domain of the human thyrotropin receptor in signal transduction. Endocrinology 131:548–552.

171. Kopp P, Muirhead S, Jourdain N, Gu WX, Jameson JL, Rodd C (1997). Congenital hyperthyroidism caused by a solitary toxic

adenoma harboring a novel somatic mutation (serine281—>isoleucine) in the extracellular domain of the thyrotropin receptor. The Journal of Clinical Investigation 100:1634–1639.

172. Duprez L, Parma J, Costagliola S, Hermans J, Van Sande J, Dumont JE, et al. (1997). Constitutive activation of the TSH receptor by spontaneous mutations affecting the N-terminal extracellular domain. FEBS Letters 409:469–474.

173. Gruters A, Schoneberg T, Biebermann H, Krude H, Krohn HP, Dralle H, et al. (1998). Severe congenital hyperthyroidism caused by a germ-line neo mutation in the extracellular portion of the thyrotropin receptor. The Journal of Clinical Endocrinology and Metabolism 83:1431–1436.

174. Parma J, Duprez L, Van Sande J, Cochaux P, Gervy C, Mockel J, et al. (1993). Somatic mutations in the thyrotropin receptor gene cause hyperfunctioning thyroid adenomas. Nature 365:649–651.

175. Porcellini A, Ciullo I, Laviola L, Amabile G, Fenzi G, Avvedimento VE (1994). Novel mutations of thyrotropin receptor gene in thyroid hyperfunctioning adenomas: Rapid identification by fine needle aspiration biopsy. The Journal of Clinical Endocrinology and Metabolism 79:657–661.

176. Paschke R, Tonacchera M, Van Sande J, Parma J, Vassart G (1994). Identification and functional characterization of two new somatic mutations causing constitutive activation of the thyrotropin receptor in hyperfunctioning autonomous adenomas of the thyroid. The Journal of Clinical Endocrinology and Metabolism 79:1785–1789.

177. Russo D, Arturi F, Wicker R, Chazenbalk GD, Schlumberger M, DuVillard JA, et al. (1995). Genetic alterations in thyroid hyperfunctioning adenomas. The Journal of Clinical Endocrinology and Metabolism 80:1347–1351.

178. Russo D, Arturi F, Suarez HG, Schlumberger M, Du Villard JA, Crocetti U, et al. (1996). Thyrotropin receptor gene alterations in thyroid hyperfunctioning adenomas. The Journal of Clinical Endocrinology and Metabolism 81:1548–1551.

179. Parma J, Duprez L, Van Sande J, Hermans J, Rocmans P, Van Vliet G, et al. (1997). Diversity and prevalence of somatic mutations in the thyrotropin receptor and Gs alpha genes as a cause of toxic thyroid adenomas. The Journal of Clinical Endocrinology and Metabolism 82:2695–2701.

180. Fuhrer D, Holzapfel HP, Wonerow P, Scherbaum WA, Paschke R (1997). Somatic mutations in the thyrotropin receptor gene and not in the Gs alpha protein gene in 31 toxic thyroid nodules. The Journal of Clinical Endocrinology and Metabolism 82:3885–3891.

181. Krohn K, Fuhrer D, Holzapfel HP, Paschke R (1998). Clonal origin of toxic thyroid nodules with constitutively activating thyrotropin receptor mutations. The Journal of Clinical Endocrinology and Metabolism 83:130–134.

182. Parma J, Van Sande J, Swillens S, Tonacchera M, Dumont J, Vassart G (1995). Somatic mutations causing constitutive activity of the thyrotropin receptor are the major cause of hyperfunctioning thyroid adenomas: Identification of additional mutations activating both the cyclic adenosine 3',5'-monophosphate and inositol phosphate-Ca2+ cascades. Mol Endocrinol 9:725–733.

183. Paschke R, Ludgate M (1997). The thyrotropin receptor in thyroid diseases. The New England Journal of Medicine 337:1675–1681.

184. Takeshita A, Nagayama Y, Yokoyama N, Ishikawa N, Ito K, Yamashita T, et al. (1995). Rarity of oncogenic mutations in the thyrotropin receptor of autonomously functioning thyroid nodules in Japan. The Journal of Clinical Endocrinology and Metabolism 80:2607–2611.

185. Nogueira CR, Kopp P, Arseven OK, Santos CL, Jameson JL, Medeiros-Neto G (1999). Thyrotropin receptor mutations in hyperfunctioning thyroid adenomas from Brazil. Thyroid 9:1063–1068.

186. Holzapfel HP, Fuhrer D, Wonerow P, Weinland G, Scherbaum WA, Paschke R (1997). Identification of constitutively activating somatic thyrotropin receptor mutations in a subset of toxic multinodular goiters. The Journal of Clinical Endocrinology and Metabolism 82:4229–4233.

187. Russo D, Arturi F, Schlumberger M, Caillou B, Monier R, Filetti S, Suarez HG (1995). Activating mutations of the TSH receptor in differentiated thyroid carcinomas. Oncogene 11:1907–1911.

188. Spambalg D, Sharifi N, Elisei R, Gross JL, Medeiros-Neto G, Fagin JA (1996). Structural studies of the thyrotropin receptor and Gs alpha in human thyroid cancers: Low prevalence of mutations predicts infrequent involvement in malignant transformation. The Journal of Clinical Endocrinology and Metabolism 81:3898–3901.

189. Russo D, Tumino S, Arturi F, Vigneri P, Grasso G, Pontecorvi A, et al. (1997). Detection of an activating mutation of the thyrotropin receptor in a case of an autonomously hyperfunctioning thyroid insular carcinoma. The Journal of Clinical Endocrinology and Metabolism 82:735–738.

190. O'Sullivan C, Barton CM, Staddon SL, Brown CL, Lemoine NR (1991). Activating point mutations of the gsp oncogene in human thyroid adenomas. Mol Carcinog 4:345–349.

191. Suarez HG, du Villard JA, Caillou B, Schlumberger M, Parmentier C, Monier R (1991). gsp mutations in human thyroid tumours. Oncogene 6:677–679.

192. Duprez L, Parma J, Van Sande J, Allgeier A, Leclere J, Schvartz C, et al. (1994). Germline mutations in the thyrotropin receptor gene cause non-autoimmune autosomal dominant hyperthyroidism. Nature Genetics 7:396–401.

193. Fuhrer D, Wonerow P, Willgerodt H, Paschke R (1997). Identification of a new thyrotropin receptor germline mutation (Leu629Phe) in a family with neonatal onset of autosomal dominant nonautoimmune hyperthyroidism. The Journal of Clinical Endocrinology and Metabolism 82:4234–4238.

194. Tonacchera M, Van Sande J, Cetani F, Swillens S, Schvartz C, Winiszewski P, et al. (1996). Functional characteristics of three new germline mutations of the thyrotropin receptor gene causing autosomal dominant toxic thyroid hyperplasia. The Journal of Clinical Endocrinology and Metabolism 81:547–554.

195. Schwab KO, Sohlemann P, Gerlich M, Broecker M, Petrykowski W, Holzapfel HP, et al. (1996). Mutations of the TSH receptor as cause of congenital hyperthyroidism. Exp Clin Endocrinol Diabetes 104:124–128.

196. Kopp P, van Sande J, Parma J, Duprez L, Gerber H, Joss E, et al. (1995). Brief report: congenital hyperthyroidism caused by a mutation in the thyrotropin-receptor gene. The New England Journal of Medicine 332:150–154.

197. de Roux N, Polak M, Couet J, Leger J, Czernichow P, Milgrom E, et al. (1996). A neomutation of the thyroid-stimulating hormone receptor in a severe neonatal hyperthyroidism. The Journal of Clinical Endocrinology and Metabolism 81:2023–2026.

198. Holzapfel HP, Wonerow P, von Petrykowski W, Henschen M, Scherbaum WA, Paschke R (1997). Sporadic congenital hyperthyroidism due to a spontaneous germline mutation in the thyrotropin receptor gene. The Journal of Clinical Endocrinology and Metabolism 82:3879–3884.

199. Schwab KO, Gerlich M, Broecker M, Sohlemann P, Derwahl M, Lohse MJ (1997). Constitutively active germline mutation of the thyrotropin receptor gene as a cause of congenital hyperthyroidism. The Journal of Pediatrics 131:899–904.

200. Esapa CT, Duprez L, Ludgate M, Mustafa MS, Kendall-Taylor P, Vassart G, et al. (1999). A novel thyrotropin receptor mutation in an infant with severe thyrotoxicosis. Thyroid 9:1005–1010.

201. Costagliola S, Sunthorntepvarakul T, Migeotte I, Van Sande J, Kajava AM, Refetoff S, et al. (1999). Structure-function relationships of two loss-of-function mutations of the thyrotropin receptor gene. Thyroid 9:995–1000.

202. de Roux N, Misrahi M, Brauner R, Houang M, Carel JC, Granier M, et al. (1996). Four families with loss of function mutations of the thyrotropin receptor. The Journal of Clinical Endocrinology and Metabolism 81:4229–4235.

203. Tonacchera M, Agretti P, Pinchera A, Rosellini V, Perri A, Collecchi P, et al. (2000). Congenital hypothyroidism with impaired thyroid response to thyrotropin (TSH) and absent circulating thyroglobulin: Evidence for a new inactivating mutation of the TSH receptor gene. The Journal of Clinical Endocrinology and Metabolism 85:1001–1008.

204. Sunthornthepvarakui T, Gottschalk ME, Hayashi Y, Refetoff S (1995). Brief report: resistance to thyrotropin caused by mutations in the thyrotropin-receptor gene. The New England Journal of Medicine 332:155–160.

205. Clifton-Bligh RJ, Gregory JW, Ludgate M, John R, Persani L, Asteria C, et al. (1997). Two novel mutations in the thyrotropin (TSH) receptor gene in a child with resistance to TSH. The Journal of Clinical Endocrinology and Metabolism 82:1094–1100.

206. Biebermann H, Schoneberg T, Krude H, Schultz G, Gudermann T, Gruters A (1997). Mutations of the human thyrotropin receptor gene causing thyroid hypoplasia and persistent congenital hypothyroidism. The Journal of Clinical Endocrinology and Metabolism 82:3471–3480.

207. Abramowicz MJ, Duprez L, Parma J, Vassart G, Heinrichs C (1997). Familial congenital hypothyroidism due to inactivating mutation of the thyrotropin receptor causing profound hypoplasia of the thyroid gland. The Journal of Clinical Investigation 99:3018–3024.

208. Gagne N, Parma J, Deal C, Vassart G, Van Vliet G (1998). Apparent congenital athyreosis contrasting with normal plasma thyroglobulin levels and associated with inactivating mutations in the thyrotropin receptor gene: are athyreosis and ectopic thyroid distinct entities? The Journal of Clinical Endocrinology and Metabolism 83:1771–1775.

209. Saito T, Endo T, Kawaguchi A, Ikeda M, Nakazato M, Kogai T, et al. (1997). Increased expression of the Na+/I- symporter in cultured human thyroid cells exposed to thyrotropin and in Graves' thyroid tissue. The Journal of Clinical Endocrinology and Metabolism 82:3331–3336.

210. Mimouni M, Mimouni-Bloch A, Schachter J, Shohat M (1996). Familial hypothyroidism with autosomal dominant inheritance. Arch Dis Child 75:245–246.

211. Xie J, Pannain S, Pohlenz J, Weiss RE, Moltz K, Morlot M, et al. (1997). Resistance to thyrotropin (TSH) in three families is not associated with mutations in the TSH receptor or TSH. The Journal of Clinical Endocrinology and Metabolism 82:3933–3940.

212. Grossmann M, Weintraub BD, Szkudlinski MW (1997). Novel insights into the molecular mechanisms of human thyrotropin action: structural, physiological, and therapeutic implications for the glycoprotein hormone family. Endocrine Reviews 18:476–501.

213. Harada A, Hershman JM, Reed AW, Braunstein GD, Dignam WJ, Derzko C, et al. (1979). Comparison of thyroid stimulators and thyroid hormone concentrations in the sera of pregnant women. The Journal of Clinical Endocrinology and Metabolism 48:793–797.

214. Hershman JM (1999). Human chorionic gonadotropin and the thyroid: hyperemesis gravidarum and trophoblastic tumors. Thyroid 9:653–657.

215. Karp PJ, Hershman JM, Richmond S, Goldstein DP, Selenkow HA (1973). Thyrotoxicosis from molar thyrotropin. Arch Intern Med 132:432–436.

216. Kenimer JG, Hershman JM, Higgins HP (1975). The thyrotropin in hydatidiform moles is human chorionic gonadotropin. The Journal of Clinical Endocrinology and Metabolism 40:482–491.

217. Higgins HP, Hershman JM, Kenimer JG, Patillo RA, Bayley TA, Walfish P (1975). The thyrotoxicosis of hydatidiform mole. Ann Intern Med 83:307–311.

218. Nagataki S, Mizuno M, Sakamoto S, Irie M, Shizume K (1977). Thyroid function in molar pregnancy. The Journal of Clinical Endocrinology and Metabolism 44:254–263.

219. Anderson NR, Lokich JJ, McDermott WV Jr., Trey C, Falchuk KR (1979). Gestational choriocarcinoma and thyrotoxicosis. Cancer 44:304–306.

220. Rodien P, Bremont C, Sanson ML, Parma J, Van Sande J, Costagliola S, et al. (1998). Familial gestational hyperthyroidism caused by a mutant thyrotropin receptor hypersensitive to human chorionic gonadotropin. The New England Journal of Medicine 339:1823–1826.

221. Vasseur C, Rodien P, Beau I, Desroches A, Gerard C, de Poncheville L, et al. (2003). A chorionic gonadotropin-sensitive mutation in the follicle-stimulating hormone receptor as a cause of familial gestational spontaneous ovarian hyperstimulation syndrome. The New England Journal of Medicine 349:753–759.

222. Smits G, Olatunbosun O, Delbaere A, Pierson R, Vassart G, Costagliola S (2003). Ovarian hyperstimulation syndrome due to a mutation in the follicle-stimulating hormone receptor. The New England Journal of Medicine 349:760–766.

223. Montanelli L, Delbaere A, Di Carlo C, Nappi C, Smits G, Vassart G, et al. (2004). A mutation in the follicle-stimulating hormone receptor as a cause of familial spontaneous ovarian hyperstimulation syndrome. The Journal of Clinical Endocrinology and Metabolism 89:1255–1258.

224. De Leener A, Montanelli L, Van Durme J, Chae H, Smits G, Vassart G, et al. (2006). Presence and absence of follicle-stimulating hormone receptor mutations provide some insights into spontaneous ovarian hyperstimulation syndrome physiopathology. The Journal of Clinical Endocrinology and Metabolism 91:555–562.

225. Delbaere A, Smits G, De Leener A, Costagliola S, Vassart G (2005). Understanding ovarian hyperstimulation syndrome. Endocrine 26:285–290.

226. Fan NC, Jeung EB, Peng C, Olofsson JI, Krisinger J, Leung PC (1994). The human gonadotropin-releasing hormone (GnRH) receptor gene: cloning, genomic organization and chromosomal assignment. Molecular and Cellular Endocrinology 103:R1–R6.

227. Kottler ML, Lorenzo F, Bergametti F, Commercon P, Souchier C, Counis R (1995). Subregional mapping of the human gonadotropin-releasing hormone receptor (GnRH-R) gene to 4q between the markers D4S392 and D4S409. Hum Genet 96:477–480.

228. Kakar SS, Musgrove LC, Devor DC, Sellers JC, Neill JD (1992). Cloning, sequencing, and expression of human gonadotropin releasing hormone (GnRH) receptor. Biochemical and Biophysical Research Communications 189:289–295.

229. Chi L, Zhou W, Prikhozhan A, Flanagan C, Davidson JS, Golembo M, et al. (1993). Cloning and characterization of the human GnRH receptor. Molecular and Cellular Endocrinology 91:R1–R6.

230. Stojilkovic SS, Reinhart J, Catt KJ (1994). Gonadotropin-releasing hormone receptors: structure and signal transduction pathways. Endocrine Reviews 15:462–499.

231. Hokin LE (1985). Receptors and phosphoinositide-generated second messengers. Annu Rev Biochem 54:205–235.

232. Berridge MJ (1987). Inositol trisphosphate and diacylglycerol: two interacting second messengers. Annu Rev Biochem 56:159–193.

233. de Roux N, Young J, Misrahi M, Genet R, Chanson P, Schaison G, et al. (1997). A family with hypogonadotropic hypogonadism and mutations in the gonadotropin-releasing hormone receptor. The New England Journal of Medicine 337:1597–1602.

234. Seminara SB, Hayes FJ, Crowley WF Jr. (1998). Gonadotropin-releasing hormone deficiency in the human (idiopathic hypogonadotropic hypogonadism and Kallmann's syndrome): Pathophysiological and genetic considerations. Endocrine Reviews 19:521–539.

235. Pralong FP, Gomez F, Castillo E, Cotecchia S, Abuin L, Aubert ML, et al. (1999). Complete hypogonadotropic hypogonadism associated with a novel inactivating mutation of the gonadotropin-releasing hormone receptor. The Journal of Clinical Endocrinology and Metabolism 84:3811–3816.

236. de Roux N, Young J, Brailly-Tabard S, Misrahi M, Milgrom E, Schaison G (1999). The same molecular defects of the gonadotropin-releasing hormone receptor determine a variable degree of hypogonadism in affected kindred. The Journal of Clinical Endocrinology and Metabolism 84:567–572.

237. Seminara SB, Beranova M, Oliveira LM, Martin KA, Crowley WF Jr., Hall JE (2000). Successful use of pulsatile gonadotropin-releasing hormone (GnRH) for ovulation induction and pregnancy in a patient with GnRH receptor mutations. The Journal of Clinical Endocrinology and Metabolism 85:556–562.

238. Gershengorn MC (1989). Mechanism of signal transduction by TRH. Annals of the New York Academy of Sciences 553:191–196.

239. Collu R, Tang J, Castagne J, Lagace G, Masson N, Huot C, et al. (1997). A novel mechanism for isolated central hypothyroidism: Inactivating mutations in the thyrotropin-releasing hormone receptor gene. The Journal of Clinical Endocrinology and Metabolism 82:1561–1565.

240. Tomita T, Masuzaki H, Iwakura H, Fujikura J, Noguchi M, Tanaka T, et al. (2006). Expression of the gene for a membrane-bound fatty acid receptor in the pancreas and islet cell tumours in humans: Evidence for GPR40 expression in pancreatic beta cells and implications for insulin secretion. Diabetologia 49:962–968.

241. Itoh Y, Kawamata Y, Harada M, Kobayashi M, Fujii R, Fukusumi S, et al. (2003). Free fatty acids regulate insulin secretion from pancreatic beta cells through GPR40. Nature 422:173–176.

242. Fujiwara K, Maekawa F, Yada T (2005). Oleic acid interacts with GPR40 to induce Ca2+ signaling in rat islet beta-cells: mediation by PLC and L-type Ca2+ channel and link to insulin release. American Journal of Physiology 289:E670–677.

243. Shapiro H, Shachar S, Sekler I, Hershfinkel M, Walker MD (2005). Role of GPR40 in fatty acid action on the beta cell line INS-1E. Biochemical and Biophysical Research Communications 335:97–104.

244. Itoh Y, Hinuma S (2005). GPR40, a free fatty acid receptor on pancreatic beta cells, regulates insulin secretion. Hepatol Res 33:171–173.

245. Steneberg P, Rubins N, Bartoov-Shifman R, Walker MD, Edlund H (2005). The FFA receptor GPR40 links hyperinsulinemia, hepatic

steatosis, and impaired glucose homeostasis in mouse. Cell Metabolism 1:245–258.

246. Ogawa T, Hirose H, Miyashita K, Saito I, Saruta T (2005). GPR40 gene Arg211His polymorphism may contribute to the variation of insulin secretory capacity in Japanese men. Metabolism: Clinical and Experimental 54:296–299.

247. de Roux N, Genin E, Carel JC, Matsuda F, Chaussain JL, Milgrom E (2003). Hypogonadotropic hypogonadism due to loss of function of the KiSS1-derived peptide receptor GPR54. Proceedings of the National Academy of Sciences of the United States of America 100:10972–10976.

248. Seminara SB, Messager S, Chatzidaki EE, Thresher RR, Acierno JS Jr., Shagoury JK, et al. (2003). The GPR54 gene as a regulator of puberty. The New England Journal of Medicine 349:1614–1627.

249. Seminara SB (2005). Metastin and its G protein-coupled receptor, GPR54: Critical pathway modulating GnRH secretion. Frontiers in Neuroendocrinology 26:131–138.

250. Semple RK, Achermann JC, Ellery J, Farooqi IS, Karet FE, Stanhope RG, et al. (2005). Two novel missense mutations in g protein-coupled receptor 54 in a patient with hypogonadotropic hypogonadism. The Journal of Clinical Endocrinology and Metabolism 90:1849–1855.

251. Kotani M, Detheux M, Vandenbogaerde A, Communi D, Vanderwinden JM, Le Poul E, et al. (2001). The metastasis suppressor gene KiSS-1 encodes kisspeptins, the natural ligands of the orphan G protein-coupled receptor GPR54. J Biol Chem 276:34631–34636.

252. Ohtaki T, Shintani Y, Honda S, Matsumoto H, Hori A, Kanehashi K, et al. (2001). Metastasis suppressor gene KiSS-1 encodes peptide ligand of a G-protein-coupled receptor. Nature 411:613–617.

253. Dhillo WS, Chaudhri OB, Patterson M, Thompson EL, Murphy KG, Badman MK, et al. (2005). Kisspeptin-54 stimulates the hypothalamic-pituitary gonadal axis in human males. The Journal of Clinical Endocrinology and Metabolism 90:6609–6615.

254. Sakurai T, Amemiya A, Ishii M, Matsuzaki I, Chemelli RM, Tanaka H, et al. (1998). Orexins and orexin receptors: A family of hypothalamic neuropeptides and G protein-coupled receptors that regulate feeding behavior. Cell 92:573–585.

255. Sutcliffe JG, de Lecea L (2000). The hypocretins: excitatory neuromodulatory peptides for multiple homeostatic systems, including sleep and feeding. Journal of Neuroscience Research 62:161–168.

256. Spinazzi R, Andreis PG, Rossi GP, Nussdorfer GG (2006). Orexins in the regulation of the hypothalamic-pituitary-adrenal axis. Pharmacological Reviews 58:46–57.

257. de Lecea L, Kilduff TS, Peyron C, Gao X, Foye PE, Danielson PE, et al. (1998). The hypocretins: hypothalamus-specific peptides with neuroexcitatory activity. Proceedings of the National Academy of Sciences of the United States of America 95:322–327.

258. Ammoun S, Holmqvist T, Shariatmadari R, Oonk HB, Detheux M, Parmentier M, et al. (2003). Distinct recognition of OX1 and OX2 receptors by orexin peptides. The Journal of Pharmacology and Experimental Therapeutics 305:507–514.

259. Smart D, Jerman JC, Brough SJ, Rushton SL, Murdock PR, Jewitt F, et al. (1999). Characterization of recombinant human orexin receptor pharmacology in a Chinese hamster ovary cell-line using FLIPR. British Journal of Pharmacology 128:1–3.

260. Kane JK, Tanaka H, Parker SL, Yanagisawa M, Li MD (2000). Sensitivity of orexin-A binding to phospholipase C inhibitors, neuropeptide Y, and secretin. Biochemical and Biophysical Research Communications 272:959–965.

261. Holmqvist T, Johansson L, Ostman M, Ammoun S, Akerman KE, Kukkonen JP (2005). OX1 orexin receptors couple to adenylyl cyclase regulation via multiple mechanisms. J Biol Chem 280:6570–6579.

262. Sakurai T (1999). Orexins and orexin receptors: Implication in feeding behavior. Regulatory Peptides 85:25–30.

263. Xu YL, Jackson VR, Civelli O (2004). Orphan G protein-coupled receptors and obesity. European Journal of Pharmacology 500:243–253.

264. Nishino S, Ripley B, Overeem S, Lammers GJ, Mignot E (2000). Hypocretin (orexin) deficiency in human narcolepsy. Lancet 355:39–40.

265. Peyron C, Faraco J, Rogers W, Ripley B, Overeem S, Charnay Y, et al. (2000). A mutation in a case of early onset narcolepsy and a generalized absence of hypocretin peptides in human narcoleptic brains. Nature Medicine 6:991–997.

266. Nishino S, Ripley B, Overeem S, Nevsimalova S, Lammers GJ, Vankova J, et al. (2001). Low cerebrospinal fluid hypocretin (Orexin) and altered energy homeostasis in human narcolepsy. Annals of Neurology 50:381–388.

267. Sutcliffe JG, de Lecea L (2002). The hypocretins: Setting the arousal threshold. Nature Reviews 3:339–349.

268. Zhang JV, Ren PG, Avsian-Kretchmer O, Luo CW, Rauch R, Klein C, et al. (2005). Obestatin, a peptide encoded by the ghrelin gene, opposes ghrelin's effects on food intake. Science 310:996–999.

269. Kojima M, Hosoda H, Date Y, Nakazato M, Matsuo H, Kangawa K (1999). Ghrelin is a growth-hormone-releasing acylated peptide from stomach. Nature 402:656–660.

270. Date Y, Kojima M, Hosoda H, Sawaguchi A, Mondal MS, Suganuma T, et al. (2000). Ghrelin, a novel growth hormone-releasing acylated peptide, is synthesized in a distinct endocrine cell type in the gastrointestinal tracts of rats and humans. Endocrinology 141:4255–4261.

271. Davenport AP, Bonner TI, Foord SM, Harmar AJ, Neubig RR, Pin JP, et al. (2005). International Union of Pharmacology. LVI: Ghrelin receptor nomenclature, distribution, and function. Pharmacological Reviews 57:541–546.

272. Cummings DE, Purnell JQ, Frayo RS, Schmidova K, Wisse BE, Weigle DS (2001). A preprandial rise in plasma ghrelin levels suggests a role in meal initiation in humans. Diabetes 50:1714–1719.

273. Tschop M, Wawarta R, Riepl RL, Friedrich S, Bidlingmaier M, Landgraf R, et al. (2001). Post-prandial decrease of circulating human ghrelin levels. Journal of Endocrinological Investigation 24:RC19–RC21.

274. Wren AM, Seal LJ, Cohen MA, Brynes AE, Frost GS, Murphy KG, et al. (2001). Ghrelin enhances appetite and increases food intake in humans. The Journal of Clinical Endocrinology and Metabolism 86:5992.

275. Cummings DE, Clement K, Purnell JQ, Vaisse C, Foster KE, Frayo RS, et al. (2002). Elevated plasma ghrelin levels in Prader Willi syndrome. Nature Medicine 8:643–644.

276. Wang HJ, Geller F, Dempfle A, Schauble N, Friedel S, Lichtner P, et al. (2004). Ghrelin receptor gene: identification of several sequence variants in extremely obese children and adolescents, healthy normal-weight and underweight students, and children with short normal stature. The Journal of Clinical Endocrinology and Metabolism 89:157–162.

277. Pantel J, Legendre M, Cabrol S, Hilal L, Hajaji Y, Morisset S, et al. (2006). Loss of constitutive activity of the growth hormone secretagogue receptor in familial short stature. The Journal of Clinical Investigation 116:760–768.

278. Chambers J, Ames RS, Bergsma D, Muir A, Fitzgerald LR, Hervieu G, et al. (1999). Melanin-concentrating hormone is the cognate ligand for the orphan G-protein-coupled receptor SLC-1. Nature 400:261–265.

279. Saito Y, Nothacker HP, Wang Z, Lin SH, Leslie F, Civelli O (1999). Molecular characterization of the melanin-concentrating-hormone receptor. Nature 400:265–269.

280. Hill J, Duckworth M, Murdock P, Rennie G, Sabido-David C, Ames RS, et al. (2001). Molecular cloning and functional characterization of MCH2, a novel human MCH receptor. J Biol Chem 276:20125–20129.

281. Wang S, Behan K, O'Neill K, Weig B, Fried S, Laz T, et al. (2001). Identification and pharmacological characterization of a novel human melanin-concentrating hormone receptor, mch-r2. J Biol Chem 276:34664–34670.

282. Hawes BE, Kil E, Green B, O'Neill K, Fried S, Graziano MP (2000). The melanin-concentrating hormone receptor couples to multiple G proteins to activate diverse intracellular signaling pathways. Endocrinology 141:4524–4532.

283. Borowsky B, Durkin MM, Ogozalek K, Marzabadi MR, DeLeon J, Lagu B, et al. (2002). Antidepressant, anxiolytic and anorectic effects of a melanin-concentrating hormone-1 receptor antagonist. Nature Medicine 8:825–830.

284. Shearman LP, Camacho RE, Sloan Stribling D, Zhou D, Bednarek MA, Hreniuk DL, et al. (2003). Chronic MCH-1 receptor modulation alters appetite, body weight and adiposity in rats. European Journal of Pharmacology 475:37–47.

285. Wermter AK, Reichwald K, Buch T, Geller F, Platzer C, Huse K, et al. (2005). Mutation analysis of the MCHR1 gene in human obesity. European Journal of Endocrinology/European Federation of Endocrine Societies 152:851–862.

286. Gibson WT, Pissios P, Trombly DJ, Luan J, Keogh J, Wareham NJ, et al. (2004). Melanin-concentrating hormone receptor mutations and human obesity: Functional analysis. Obesity Research 12:743–749.

287. Maheshwari HG, Silverman BL, Dupuis J, Baumann G (1998). Phenotype and genetic analysis of a syndrome caused by an inactivating mutation in the growth hormone-releasing hormone receptor: Dwarfism of Sindh. The Journal of Clinical Endocrinology and Metabolism 83:4065–4074.

288. Salvatori R, Hayashida CY, Aguiar-Oliveira MH, Phillips JA III, Souza AH, Gondo RG, et al. (1999). Familial dwarfism due to a novel mutation of the growth hormone-releasing hormone receptor gene. The Journal of Clinical Endocrinology and Metabolism 84:917–923.

289. Vallar L, Spada A, Giannattasio G (1987). Altered Gs and adenylate cyclase activity in human GH-secreting pituitary adenomas. Nature 330:566–568.

290. Wajnrajch MP, Gertner JM, Harbison MD, Chua SC Jr., Leibel RL (1996). Nonsense mutation in the human growth hormone-releasing hormone receptor causes growth failure analogous to the little (lit) mouse. Nature Genetics 12:88–90.

291. Netchine I, Talon P, Dastot F, Vitaux F, Goossens M, Amselem S (1998). Extensive phenotypic analysis of a family with growth hormone (GH) deficiency caused by a mutation in the GH-releasing hormone receptor gene. The Journal of Clinical Endocrinology and Metabolism 83:432–436.

292. Salvatori R, Fan X, Phillips JA III, Prince M, Levine MA (2001). Isolated growth hormone (GH) deficiency due to compound heterozygosity for two new mutations in the GH-releasing hormone receptor gene. Clinical Endocrinology 54:681–687.

293. Yamada Y, Hayami T, Nakamura K, Kaisaki PJ, Someya Y, Wang CZ, et al. (1995). Human gastric inhibitory polypeptide receptor: Cloning of the gene (GIPR) and cDNA. Genomics 29:773–776.

294. Gremlich S, Porret A, Hani EH, Cherif D, Vionnet N, Froguel P, et al. (1995). Cloning, functional expression, and chromosomal localization of the human pancreatic islet glucose-dependent insulinotropic polypeptide receptor. Diabetes 44:1202–1208.

295. Wheeler MB, Gelling RW, McIntosh CH, Georgiou J, Brown JC, Pederson RA (1995). Functional expression of the rat pancreatic islet glucose-dependent insulinotropic polypeptide receptor: Ligand binding and intracellular signaling properties. Endocrinology 136:4629–4639.

296. Tseng CC, Zhang XY (1998). Role of regulator of G protein signaling in desensitization of the glucose-dependent insulinotropic peptide receptor. Endocrinology 139:4470–4475.

297. Beck B (1989). Gastric inhibitory polypeptide: A gut hormone with anabolic functions. Journal of Molecular Endocrinology 2:169–174.

298. Fehmann HC, Goke R, Goke B (1995). Cell and molecular biology of the incretin hormones glucagon-like peptide-I and glucose-dependent insulin releasing polypeptide. Endocrine Reviews 16:390–410.

299. N'Diaye N, Tremblay J, Hamet P, De Herder WW, Lacroix A (1998). Adrenocortical overexpression of gastric inhibitory polypeptide receptor underlies food-dependent Cushing's syndrome. The Journal of Clinical Endocrinology and Metabolism 83:2781–2785.

300. Lebrethon MC, Avallet O, Reznik Y, Archambeaud F, Combes J, Usdin TB, et al. (1998). Food-dependent Cushing's syndrome: Characterization and functional role of gastric inhibitory polypeptide receptor in the adrenals of three patients. The Journal of Clinical Endocrinology and Metabolism 83:4514–4519.

301. de Herder WW, Hofland LJ, Usdin TB, de Jong FH, Uitterlinden P, van Koetsveld P, et al. (1996). Food-dependent Cushing's syndrome resulting from abundant expression of gastric inhibitory polypeptide receptors in adrenal adenoma cells. The Journal of Clinical Endocrinology and Metabolism 81:3168–3172.

302. Mannstadt M, Juppner H, Gardella TJ (1999). Receptors for PTH and PTHrP: Their biological importance and functional properties. Am J Physiol 277:F665675.

303. Usdin TB, Gruber C, Bonner TI (1995). Identification and functional expression of a receptor selectively recognizing parathyroid hormone, the PTH2 receptor. J Biol Chem 270:15455–15458.

304. Behar V, Pines M, Nakamoto C, Greenberg Z, Bisello A, Stueckle SM, et al. (1996). The human PTH2 receptor: Binding and signal transduction properties of the stably expressed recombinant receptor. Endocrinology 137:2748–2757.

305. Turner PR, Mefford S, Bambino T, Nissenson RA (1998). Transmembrane residues together with the amino terminus limit the response of the parathyroid hormone (PTH) 2 receptor to PTH-related peptide. J Biol Chem 273:3830–3837.

306. Abou-Samra AB, Jueppner H, Westerberg D, Potts JT Jr., Segre GV (1989). Parathyroid hormone causes translocation of protein kinase-C from cytosol to membranes in rat osteosarcoma cells. Endocrinology 124:1107–1113.

307. Tamura T, Sakamoto H, Filburn CR (1989). Parathyroid hormone 1-34, but not 3-34 or 7-34, transiently translocates protein kinase C in cultured renal (OK) cells. Biochemical and Biophysical Research Communications 159:1352–1358.

308. Dunlay R, Hruska K (1990). PTH receptor coupling to phospholipase C is an alternate pathway of signal transduction in bone and kidney. Am J Physiol 258:F223–231.

309. Partridge NC, Bloch SR, Pearman AT (1994). Signal transduction pathways mediating parathyroid hormone regulation of osteoblastic gene expression. Journal of Cellular Biochemistry 55:321–327.

310. Offermanns S, Iida-Klein A, Segre GV, Simon MI (1996). G alpha q family members couple parathyroid hormone (PTH)/PTH-related peptide and calcitonin receptors to phospholipase C in COS-7 cells. Mol Endocrinol 10:566–574.

311. Schwindinger WF, Fredericks J, Watkins L, Robinson H, Bathon JM, Pines M, et al. (1998). Coupling of the PTH/PTHrP receptor to multiple G-proteins: Direct demonstration of receptor activation of Gs, Gq/11, and Gi(1) by [alpha- 32P]GTP-gamma-azidoanilide photoaffinity labeling. Endocrine 8:201–209.

312. Iida-Klein A, Guo J, Takemura M, Drake MT, Potts JT Jr., Abou-Samra A, et al. (1997). Mutations in the second cytoplasmic loop of the rat parathyroid hormone (PTH)/PTH-related protein receptor result in selective loss of PTH-stimulated phospholipase C activity. J Biol Chem 272:6882–6889.

313. Huang Z, Chen Y, Pratt S, Chen TH, Bambino T, Nissenson RA, et al. (1996). The N-terminal region of the third intracellular loop of the parathyroid hormone (PTH)/PTH-related peptide receptor is critical for coupling to cAMP and inositol phosphate/Ca2+ signal transduction pathways. J Biol Chem 271:33382–33389.

314. Wysolmerski JJ, Cormier S, Philbrick WM, Dann P, Zhang JP, Roume J, et al. (2001). Absence of functional type 1 parathyroid hormone (PTH)/PTH-related protein receptors in humans is associated with abnormal breast development and tooth impaction. The Journal of Clinical Endocrinology and Metabolism 86:1788–1794.

315. Karaplis AC, He B, Nguyen MT, Young ID, Semeraro D, Ozawa H, et al. (1998). Inactivating mutation in the human parathyroid hormone receptor type 1 gene in Blomstrand chondrodysplasia. Endocrinology 139:5255–5258.

316. Zhang P, Jobert AS, Couvineau A, Silve C (1998). A homozygous inactivating mutation in the parathyroid hormone/parathyroid hormone-related peptide receptor causing Blomstrand chondrodysplasia. The Journal of Clinical Endocrinology and Metabolism 83:3365–3368.

317. Karperien M, van der Harten HJ, van Schooten R, Farih-Sips H, den Hollander NS, Kneppers SL, et al. (1999). A frame-shift mutation in the type I parathyroid hormone (PTH)/PTH-related peptide receptor causing Blomstrand lethal osteochondrodysplasia. The Journal of Clinical Endocrinology and Metabolism 84:3713–3720.

318. Jobert AS, Zhang P, Couvineau A, Bonaventure J, Roume J, Le Merrer M, et al. (1998). Absence of functional receptors for parathyroid hormone and parathyroid hormone-related peptide in Blomstrand chondrodysplasia. The Journal of Clinical Investigation 102:34–40.

319. Hopyan S, Gokgoz N, Poon R, Gensure RC, Yu C, Cole WG, et al. (2002). A mutant PTH/PTHrP type I receptor in enchondromatosis. Nature Genetics 30:306–310.

320. Schipani E, Kruse K, Juppner H (1995). A constitutively active mutant PTH-PTHrP receptor in Jansen-type metaphyseal chondrodysplasia. Science 268:98–100.

321. Schipani E, Langman CB, Parfitt AM, Jensen GS, Kikuchi S, Kooh SW, et al. (1996). Constitutively activated receptors for parathyroid hormone and parathyroid hormone-related peptide in Jansen's metaphyseal chondrodysplasia. The New England Journal of Medicine 335:708–714.

322. Schipani E, Langman C, Hunzelman J, Le Merrer M, Loke KY, Dillon MJ, et al. (1999). A novel parathyroid hormone (PTH)/PTH-related peptide receptor mutation in Jansen's metaphyseal chondrodysplasia. The Journal of Clinical Endocrinology and Metabolism 84:3052–3057.

323. Holz GG, Chepurny OG (2003). Glucagon-like peptide-1 synthetic analogs: New therapeutic agents for use in the treatment of diabetes mellitus. Current Medicinal Chemistry 10:2471–2483.

324. Holz GG, Leech CA, Habener JF (2000). Insulinotropic toxins as molecular probes for analysis of glucagon-like peptide-1 receptor-mediated signal transduction in pancreatic beta-cells. Biochimie 82:915–926.

325. Janicic N, Soliman E, Pausova Z, Seldin MF, Riviere M, Szpirer J, et al. (1995). Mapping of the calcium-sensing receptor gene (CASR) to human chromosome 3q13.3-21 by fluorescence in situ hybridization, and localization to rat chromosome 11 and mouse chromosome 16. Mamm Genome 6:798–801.

326. Brown EM, Gamba G, Riccardi D, Lombardi M, Butters R, Kifor O, et al. (1993). Cloning and characterization of an extracellular Ca(2+)-sensing receptor from bovine parathyroid. Nature 366:575–580.

327. Mancilla EE, De Luca F, Baron J (1998). Activating mutations of the Ca2+-sensing receptor. Molecular Genetics and Metabolism 64:198–204.

328. Brown EM, Pollak M, Chou YH, Seidman CE, Seidman JG, Hebert SC (1995). The cloning of extracellular Ca(2+)-sensing receptors from parathyroid and kidney: molecular mechanisms of extracellular Ca(2+)-sensing. J Nutr 125:1965S–1970S.

329. Brown EM, Hebert SC (1995). A cloned Ca(2+)-sensing receptor: a mediator of direct effects of extracellular Ca2+ on renal function? J Am Soc Nephrol 6:1530–1540.

330. Hebert SC, Brown EM, Harris HW (1997). Role of the Ca(2+)-sensing receptor in divalent mineral ion homeostasis. The Journal of Experimental Biology 200:295–302.

331. Chattopadhyay N (2000). Biochemistry, physiology and pathophysiology of the extracellular calcium-sensing receptor. The International Journal of Biochemistry & Cell Biology 32:789–804.

332. Thakker RV (1998). Disorders of the calcium-sensing receptor. Biochimica et Biophysica Acta 1448:166–170.

333. Pearce S, Steinmann B (1999). Casting new light on the clinical spectrum of neonatal severe hyperparathyroidism. Clinical Endocrinology 50:691–693.

334. Chou YH, Pollak MR, Brandi ML, Toss G, Arnqvist H, Atkinson AB, et al. (1995). Mutations in the human Ca(2+)-sensing-receptor gene that cause familial hypocalciuric hypercalcemia. American Journal of Human Genetics 56:1075–1079.

335. Health H III, Odelberg S, Jackson CE, Teh BT, Hayward N, Larsson C, et al. (1996). Clustered inactivating mutations and benign polymorphisms of the calcium receptor gene in familial benign hypocalciuric hypercalcemia suggest receptor functional domains. The Journal of Clinical Endocrinology and Metabolism 81:1312–1317.

336. Marx SJ, Attie MF, Spiegel AM, Levine MA, Lasker RD, Fox M (1982). An association between neonatal severe primary hyperparathyroidism and familial hypocalciuric hypercalcemia in three kindreds. The New England Journal of Medicine 306:257–264.

337. Marx SJ, Fraser D, Rapoport A (1985). Familial hypocalciuric hypercalcemia: Mild expression of the gene in heterozygotes and severe expression in homozygotes. The American Journal of Medicine 78:15–22.

338. Pollak MR, Brown EM, Chou YH, Hebert SC, Marx SJ, Steinmann B, et al. (1993). Mutations in the human Ca(2+)-sensing receptor gene cause familial hypocalciuric hypercalcemia and neonatal severe hyperparathyroidism. Cell 75:1297–1303.

339. Janicic N, Pausova Z, Cole DE, Hendy GN (1995). Insertion of an Alu sequence in the Ca(2+)-sensing receptor gene in familial hypocalciuric hypercalcemia and neonatal severe hyperparathyroidism. American Journal of Human Genetics 56:880–886.

340. Pearce SH, Trump D, Wooding C, Besser GM, Chew SL, Grant DB, et al. (1995). Calcium-sensing receptor mutations in familial benign hypercalcemia and neonatal hyperparathyroidism. The Journal of Clinical Investigation 96:2683–2692.

341. Marx SJ, Attie MF, Levine MA, Spiegel AM, Downs RW Jr., Lasker RD (1981). The hypocalciuric or benign variant of familial hypercalcemia: Clinical and biochemical features in fifteen kindreds. Medicine (Baltimore) 60:397–412.

342. Marx SJ, Spiegel AM, Levine MA, Rizzoli RE, Lasker RD, Santora AC, et al. (1982). Familial hypocalciuric hypercalcemia: The relation to primary parathyroid hyperplasia. The New England Journal of Medicine 307:416–426.

343. Thakker RV (2004). Diseases associated with the extracellular calcium-sensing receptor. Cell Calcium 35:275–282.

344. Heath H III, Jackson CE, Otterud B, Leppert MF (1993). Genetic linkage analysis in familial benign (hypocalciuric) hypercalcemia: Evidence for locus heterogeneity. American Journal of Human Genetics 53:193–200.

345. Lloyd SE, Pannett AA, Dixon PH, Whyte MP, Thakker RV (1999). Localization of familial benign hypercalcemia, Oklahoma variant (FBHOk), to chromosome 19q13. American Journal of Human Genetics 64:189–195.

346. McMurtry CT, Schranck FW, Walkenhorst DA, Murphy WA, Kocher DB, Teitelbaum SL, et al. (1992). Significant developmental elevation in serum parathyroid hormone levels in a large kindred with familial benign (hypocalciuric) hypercalcemia. The American Journal of Medicine 93:247–258.

347. Pollak MR, Brown EM, Estep HL, McLaine PN, Kifor O, Park J, et al. (1994). Autosomal dominant hypocalcaemia caused by a Ca(2+)-sensing receptor gene mutation. Nature Genetics 8:303–307.

348. Finegold DN, Armitage MM, Galiani M, Matise TC, Pandian MR, Perry YM, et al. (1994). Preliminary localization of a gene for autosomal dominant hypoparathyroidism to chromosome 3q13. Pediatr Res 36:414–417.

349. Baron J, Winer KK, Yanovski JA, Cunningham AW, Laue L, Zimmerman D, et al. (1996). Mutations in the Ca(2+)-sensing receptor gene cause autosomal dominant and sporadic hypoparathyroidism. Human Molecular Genetics 5:601–606.

350. Pearce SH, Williamson C, Kifor O, Bai M, Coulthard MG, Davies M, et al. (1996). A familial syndrome of hypocalcemia with hypercalciuria due to mutations in the calcium-sensing receptor. The New England Journal of Medicine 335:1115–1122.

351. De Luca F, Ray K, Mancilla EE, Fan GF, Winer KK, Gore P, et al. (1997). Sporadic hypoparathyroidism caused by de Novo gain-of-function mutations of the Ca(2+)-sensing receptor. The Journal of Clinical Endocrinology and Metabolism 82:2710–2715.

352. Pearce S (1999). Extracellular "calcistat" in health and disease. Lancet 353:83–84.

353. Vargas-Poussou R, Huang C, Hulin P, Houillier P, Jeunemaitre X, Paillard M, et al. (2002). Functional characterization of a calcium-sensing receptor mutation in severe autosomal dominant hypocalcemia with a Bartter-like syndrome. J Am Soc Nephrol 13:2259–2266.

354. Watanabe S, Fukumoto S, Chang H, Takeuchi Y, Hasegawa Y, Okazaki R, et al. (2002). Association between activating mutations of calcium-sensing receptor and Bartter's syndrome. Lancet 360:692–694.

355. Hebert SC (2003). Bartter syndrome. Current Opinion in Nephrology and Hypertension 12:527–532.

356. Cole DE, Peltekova VD, Rubin LA, Hawker GA, Vieth R, Liew CC, et al. (1999). A986S polymorphism of the calcium-sensing receptor and circulating calcium concentrations. Lancet 353:112–115.

357. Cole DE, Vieth R, Trang HM, Wong BY, Hendy GN, Rubin LA (2001). Association between total serum calcium and the A986S polymorphism of the calcium-sensing receptor gene. Molecular Genetics and Metabolism 72:168–174.

358. Scillitani A, Guarnieri V, De Geronimo S, Muscarella LA, Battista C, D'Agruma L, et al. (2004). Blood ionized calcium is associated with clustered polymorphisms in the carboxyl-terminal tail of the calcium-sensing receptor. The Journal of Clinical Endocrinology and Metabolism 89:5634–5638.

359. Miedlich S, Lamesch P, Mueller A, Paschke R (2001). Frequency of the calcium-sensing receptor variant A986S in patients with primary hyperparathyroidism. European Journal of Endocrinology/European Federation of Endocrine Societies 145:421–427.

360. Donath J, Speer G, Poor G, Gergely P, Jr., Tabak A, Lakatos P (2004). Vitamin D receptor, oestrogen receptor-alpha and calcium-sensing receptor genotypes, bone mineral density and biochemical markers in Paget's disease of bone. Rheumatology (Oxford, England) 43:692–695.

361. Scillitani A, Guarnieri V, Battista C, De Geronimo S, Muscarella LA, Chiodini I, et al. (2006). Primary hyperparathyroidism and the presence of kidney stones are associated with different haplotypes of the calcium-sensing receptor. The Journal of Clinical Endocrinology and Metabolism [volume/pages].

362. Vezzoli G, Tanini A, Ferrucci L, Soldati L, Bianchin C, Franceschelli F, et al. (2002). Influence of calcium-sensing receptor gene on urinary

calcium excretion in stone-forming patients. J Am Soc Nephrol 13:2517–2523.

363. Kifor O, Moore FD Jr., Delaney M, Garber J, Hendy GN, Butters R, et al. (2003). A syndrome of hypocalciuric hypercalcemia caused by autoantibodies directed at the calcium-sensing receptor. The Journal of Clinical Endocrinology and Metabolism 88:60–72.

364. Li Y, Song YH, Rais N, Connor E, Schatz D, Muir A, et al. (1996). Autoantibodies to the extracellular domain of the calcium sensing receptor in patients with acquired hypoparathyroidism. The Journal of Clinical Investigation 97:910–914.

365. Mayer A, Ploix C, Orgiazzi J, Desbos A, Moreira A, Vidal H, et al. (2004). Calcium-sensing receptor autoantibodies are relevant markers of acquired hypoparathyroidism. The Journal of Clinical Endocrinology and Metabolism 89:4484–4488.

366. Hayward BE, Kamiya M, Strain L, Moran V, Campbell R, Hayashizaki Y, et al. (1998). The human GNAS1 gene is imprinted and encodes distinct paternally and biallelically expressed G proteins. Proceedings of the National Academy of Sciences of the United States of America 95:10038–10043.

367. Hayward BE, Moran V, Strain L, Bonthron DT (1998). Bidirectional imprinting of a single gene: GNAS1 encodes maternally, paternally, and biallelically derived proteins. Proceedings of the National Academy of Sciences of the United States of America 95:15475–15480.

368. Juppner H, Schipani E, Bastepe M, Cole DE, Lawson ML, Mannstadt M, et al. (1998). The gene responsible for pseudohypoparathyroidism type Ib is paternally imprinted and maps in four unrelated kindreds to chromosome 20q13.3. Proceedings of the National Academy of Sciences of the United States of America 95:11798–11803.

369. Nakamoto JM, Sandstrom AT, Brickman AS, Christenson RA, Van Dop C (1998). Pseudohypoparathyroidism type Ia from maternal but not paternal transmission of a Gsalpha gene mutation. American Journal of Medical Genetics 77:261–267.

370. Wilson LC, Oude Luttikhuis ME, Clayton PT, Fraser WD, Trembath RC (1994). Parental origin of Gs alpha gene mutations in Albright's hereditary osteodystrophy. Journal of Medical Genetics 31:835–839.

371. Weinstein LS, Yu S, Warner DR, Liu J (2001). Endocrine manifestations of stimulatory G protein alpha-subunit mutations and the role of genomic imprinting. Endocrine Reviews 22:675–705.

372. Silve C, Santora A, Breslau N, Moses A, Spiegel A (1986). Selective resistance to parathyroid hormone in cultured skin fibroblasts from patients with pseudohypoparathyroidism type Ib. The Journal of Clinical Endocrinology and Metabolism 62:640–644.

373. Fukumoto S, Suzawa M, Kikuchi T, Matsumoto T, Kato S, Fujita T (1998). Cloning and characterization of kidney-specific promoter of human PTH/PTHrP receptor gene: Absence of mutation in patients with pseudohypoparathyroidism type Ib. Molecular and Cellular Endocrinology 141:41–47.

374. Bettoun JD, Minagawa M, Kwan MY, Lee HS, Yasuda T, Hendy GN, et al. (1997). Cloning and characterization of the promoter regions of the human parathyroid hormone (PTH)/PTH-related peptide receptor gene: Analysis of deoxyribonucleic acid from normal subjects and patients with pseudohypoparathyroidism type 1b. The Journal of Clinical Endocrinology and Metabolism 82:1031–1040.

375. Liu J, Litman D, Rosenberg MJ, Yu S, Biesecker LG, Weinstein LS (2000). A GNAS1 imprinting defect in pseudohypoparathyroidism type IB. The Journal of Clinical Investigation 106:1167–1174.

376. Spiegel AM, Weinstein LS (2004). Inherited diseases involving g proteins and g protein-coupled receptors. Annual Review of Medicine 55:27–39.

377. Bastepe M, Lane AH, Juppner H (2001). Paternal uniparental isodisomy of chromosome 20q—and the resulting changes in GNAS1 methylation—as a plausible cause of pseudohypoparathyroidism. American Journal of Human Genetics 68:1283–1289.

378. Williamson EA, Ince PG, Harrison D, Kendall-Taylor P, Harris PE (1995). G-protein mutations in human pituitary adrenocorticotrophic hormone-secreting adenomas. Eur J Clin Invest 25:128–131.

379. Okamoto S, Hisaoka M, Ushijima M, Nakahara S, Toyoshima S, Hashimoto H (2000). Activating Gs(alpha) mutation in intramuscular myxomas with and without fibrous dysplasia of bone. Virchows Arch 437:133–137.

380. Shenker A, Weinstein LS, Sweet DE, Spiegel AM (1994). An activating Gs alpha mutation is present in fibrous dysplasia of bone in the McCune-Albright syndrome. The Journal of Clinical Endocrinology and Metabolism 79:750–755.

381. Weinstein LS, Shenker A, Gejman PV, Merino MJ, Friedman E, Spiegel AM (1991). Activating mutations of the stimulatory G protein in the McCune-Albright syndrome. The New England Journal of Medicine 325:1688–1695.

382. Shenker A, Weinstein LS, Moran A, Pescovitz OH, Charest NJ, Boney CM, et al. (1993). Severe endocrine and nonendocrine manifestations of the McCune-Albright syndrome associated with activating mutations of stimulatory G protein GS. The Journal of Pediatrics 123:509–518.

383. Cohen S, Bigazzi PE, Yoshida T (1974). Commentary. Similarities of T cell function in cell-mediated immunity and antibody production. Cell Immunol 12:150–159.

384. Leonard WJ, Lin J-X (2000). Cytokine receptor signaling pathways. J of Allergy and Clin Immunol 105:877–888.

385. Davies DR, Wlodawer A (1995). Cytokines and their receptor complexes. Faseb J 9:50–56.

386. de Vos AM, Ultsch M, Kossiakoff AA (1992). Human growth hormone and extracellular domain of its receptor: Crystal structure of the complex. Science 255:306–312.

387. Greenlund AC, Morales MO, Viviano BL, Yan H, Krolewski J, Schreiber RD (1995). Stat recruitment by tyrosine-phosphorylated cytokine receptors: an ordered reversible affinity-driven process. Immunity 2:677–687.

388. Darnell JE Jr., Kerr IM, Stark GR (1994). Jak-STAT pathways and transcriptional activation in response to IFNs and other extracellular signaling proteins. Science 264:1415–1421.

389. Horvath CM, Darnell JE (1997). The state of the STATs: Recent developments in the study of signal transduction to the nucleus. Curr Opin Cell Biol 9:233–239.

390. Darnell JE Jr. (1997). STATs and gene regulation. Science 277:1630–1635.

391. Leonard WJ, O'Shea JJ (1998). Jaks and STATs: biological implications. Annu Rev Immunol 16:293–322.

392. Witthuhn BA, Silvennoinen O, Miura O, Lai KS, Cwik C, Liu ET, Ihle JN (1994). Involvement of the Jak-3 Janus kinase in signalling by interleukins 2 and 4 in lymphoid and myeloid cells. Nature 370:153–157.

393. Johnston JA, Kawamura M, Kirken RA, Chen YQ, Blake TB, Shibuya K, et al. (1994). Phosphorylation and activation of the Jak-3 Janus kinase in response to interleukin-2. Nature 370:151–153.

394. Leung DW, Spencer SA, Cachianes G, Hammonds RG, Collins C, Henzel WJ, et al. (1987). Growth hormone receptor and serum binding protein: purification, cloning and expression. Nature 330:537–543.

395. Kelly PA, Ali S, Rozakis M, Goujon L, Nagano M, Pellegrini I, et al. (1993). The growth hormone/prolactin receptor family. Recent Progress in Hormone Research 48:123–164.

396. Rosenfeld RG, Rosenbloom AL, Guevara-Aguirre J (1994). Growth hormone (GH) insensitivity due to primary GH receptor deficiency. Endocrine Reviews 15:369–390.

397. Campbell GS (1997). Growth-hormone signal transduction. The Journal of Pediatrics 131:S42–44.

398. Rosenbloom AL (1999). Growth hormone insensitivity: Physiologic and genetic basis, phenotype, and treatment. The Journal of Pediatrics 135:280–289.

399. Argetsinger LS, Campbell GS, Yang X, Witthuhn BA, Silvennoinen O, Ihle JN, et al. (1993). Identification of JAK2 as a growth hormone receptor-associated tyrosine kinase. Cell 74:237–244.

400. Meyer DJ, Campbell GS, Cochran BH, Argetsinger LS, Larner AC, Finbloom DS, et al. (1994). Growth hormone induces a DNA binding factor related to the interferon-stimulated 91-kDa transcription factor. J Biol Chem 269:4701–4704.

401. Wood TJ, Sliva D, Lobie PE, Pircher TJ, Gouilleux F, Wakao H, et al. (1995). Mediation of growth hormone-dependent transcriptional activation by mammary gland factor/Stat 5. J Biol Chem 270:9448–9453.

402. Smit LS, Meyer DJ, Billestrup N, Norstedt G, Schwartz J, Carter-Su C (1996). The role of the growth hormone (GH) receptor and JAK1 and JAK2 kinases in the activation of Stats 1, 3, and 5 by GH. Mol Endocrinol 10:519–533.

403. Hansen LH, Wang X, Kopchick JJ, Bouchelouche P, Nielsen JH, Galsgaard ED, et al. (1996). Identification of tyrosine residues in

the intracellular domain of the growth hormone receptor required for transcriptional signaling and Stat5 activation. J Biol Chem 271:12669–12673.

404. Rajaram S, Baylink DJ, Mohan S (1997). Insulin-like growth factor-binding proteins in serum and other biological fluids: Regulation and functions. Endocrine Reviews 18:801–831.

405. VanderKuur J, Allevato G, Billestrup N, Norstedt G, Carter-Su C (1995). Growth hormone-promoted tyrosyl phosphorylation of SHC proteins and SHC association with Grb2. J Biol Chem 270:7587–7593.

406. Argetsinger LS, Hsu GW, Myers MG Jr., Billestrup N, White MF, Carter-Su C (1995). Growth hormone, interferon-gamma, and leukemia inhibitory factor promoted tyrosyl phosphorylation of insulin receptor substrate-1. J Biol Chem 270:14685–14692.

407. Argetsinger LS, Norstedt G, Billestrup N, White MF, Carter-Su C (1996). Growth hormone, interferon-gamma, and leukemia inhibitory factor utilize insulin receptor substrate-2 in intracellular signaling. J Biol Chem 271:29415–29421.

408. Laron Z, Pertzelan A, Mannheimer S (1966). Genetic pituitary dwarfism with high serum concentration of growth hormone: A new inborn error of metabolism? Isr J Med Sci 2:152–155.

409. Laron Z, Pertzelan A, Karp M (1968). Pituitary dwarfism with high serum levels of growth hormone. Isr J Med Sci 4:883–894.

410. Laron Z (1974). The syndrome of familial dwarfism and high plasma immunoreactive human growth hormone. Birth Defects Orig Artic Ser 10:231–238.

411. Rosenbloom AL, Guevara-Aguirre J, Rosenfeld RG, Francke U (1999). Growth hormone receptor deficiency in Ecuador. The Journal of Clinical Endocrinology and Metabolism 84:4436–4443.

412. Wojcik J, Berg MA, Esposito N, Geffner ME, Sakati N, Reiter EO, et al. (1998). Four contiguous amino acid substitutions, identified in patients with Laron syndrome, differently affect the binding affinity and intracellular trafficking of the growth hormone receptor. The Journal of Clinical Endocrinology and Metabolism 83:4481–4489.

413. Walker JL, Crock PA, Behncken SN, Rowlinson SW, Nicholson LM, Boulton TJ, et al. (1998). A novel mutation affecting the interdomain link region of the growth hormone receptor in a Vietnamese girl, and response to long-term treatment with recombinant human insulin-like growth factor-I and luteinizing hormone-releasing hormone analogue. The Journal of Clinical Endocrinology and Metabolism 83:2554–2561.

414. Goddard AD, Covello R, Luoh SM, Clackson T, Attie KM, Gesundheit N, et al. (1995). Mutations of the growth hormone receptor in children with idiopathic short stature. The Growth Hormone Insensitivity Study Group. The New England Journal of Medicine 333:1093–1098.

415. Goddard AD, Dowd P, Chernausek S, Geffner M, Gertner J, Hintz R, et al. (1997). Partial growth-hormone insensitivity: The role of growth-hormone receptor mutations in idiopathic short stature. The Journal of Pediatrics 131:S51–55.

416. Ayling RM, Ross R, Towner P, Von Laue S, Finidori J, Moutoussamy S, et al. (1997). A dominant-negative mutation of the growth hormone receptor causes familial short stature. Nature Genetics 16:13–14.

417. Iida K, Takahashi Y, Kaji H, Nose O, Okimura Y, Abe H, et al. (1998). Growth hormone (GH) insensitivity syndrome with high serum GH-binding protein levels caused by a heterozygous splice site mutation of the GH receptor gene producing a lack of intracellular domain. The Journal of Clinical Endocrinology and Metabolism 83:531–537.

418. Freeth JS, Silva CM, Whatmore AJ, Clayton PE (1998). Activation of the signal transducers and activators of transcription signaling pathway by growth hormone (GH) in skin fibroblasts from normal and GH binding protein-positive Laron Syndrome children. Endocrinology 139:20–28.

419. Chen D, Garg A (1999). Monogenic disorders of obesity and body fat distribution. Journal of Lipid Research 40:1735–1746.

420. Clement K, Vaisse C, Lahlou N, Cabrol S, Pelloux V, Cassuto D, et al. (1998). A mutation in the human leptin receptor gene causes obesity and pituitary dysfunction. Nature 392:398–401.

421. Farooqi IS, Wangensteen T, Collins S, Kimber W, Matarese G, Keogh JM, et al. (2007). Clinical and molecular genetic spectrum of congenital deficiency of the leptin receptor. N Engl J Med 356:237–247.

422. Hubbard SR (1999). Structural analysis of receptor tyrosine kinases. Prog Biophys Mol Biol 71:343–358.

423. Spivak-Kroizman T, Lemmon MA, Dikic I, Ladbury JE, Pinchasi D, Huang J, et al. (1994). Heparin-induced oligomerization of FGF molecules is responsible for FGF receptor dimerization, activation, and cell proliferation. Cell 79:1015–1024.

424. Heldin CH (1995). Dimerization of cell surface receptors in signal transduction. Cell 80:213–223.

425. Pawson T (1995). Protein modules and signalling networks. Nature 373:573–580.

426. Patel TB (2004). Single transmembrane spanning heterotrimeric g protein-coupled receptors and their signaling cascades. Pharmacological Reviews 56:371–385.

427. Ebina Y, Ellis L, Jarnagin K, Edery M, Graf L, Clauser E, et al. (1985). The human insulin receptor cDNA: The structural basis for hormone-activated transmembrane signalling. Cell 40:747–758.

428. Ullrich A, Gray A, Tam AW, Yang-Feng T, Tsubokawa M, Collins C, et al. (1986). Insulin-like growth factor I receptor primary structure: Comparison with insulin receptor suggests structural determinants that define functional specificity. The EMBO Journal 5:2503–2512.

429. Urso B, Cope DL, Kalloo-Hosein HE, Hayward AC, Whitehead JP, O'Rahilly S, et al. (1999). Differences in signaling properties of the cytoplasmic domains of the insulin receptor and insulin-like growth factor receptor in 3T3-L1 adipocytes. J Biol Chem 274:30864–30873.

430. Garrett TP, McKern NM, Lou M, Frenkel MJ, Bentley JD, Lovrecz GO, et al. (1998). Crystal structure of the first three domains of the type-1 insulin-like growth factor receptor. Nature 394:395–399.

431. Treadway JL, Morrison BD, Soos MA, Siddle K, Olefsky J, Ullrich A, et al. (1991). Transdominant inhibition of tyrosine kinase activity in mutant insulin/insulin-like growth factor I hybrid receptors. Proceedings of the National Academy of Sciences of the United States of America 88:214–218.

432. Frattali AL, Treadway JL, Pessin JE (1992). Transmembrane signaling by the human insulin receptor kinase: Relationship between intramolecular beta subunit trans- and cis-autophosphorylation and substrate kinase activation. J Biol Chem 267:19521–19528.

433. Lee CH, Li W, Nishimura R, Zhou M, Batzer AG, Myers MG Jr., et al. (1993). Nck associates with the SH2 domain-docking protein IRS-1 in insulin-stimulated cells. Proceedings of the National Academy of Sciences of the United States of America 90:11713–11717.

434. Skolnik EY, Batzer A, Li N, Lee CH, Lowenstein E, Mohammadi M, et al. (1993). The function of GRB2 in linking the insulin receptor to Ras signaling pathways. Science 260:1953–1955.

435. Myers MG Jr., Grammer TC, Wang LM, Sun XJ, Pierce JH, Blenis J, et al. (1994). Insulin receptor substrate-1 mediates phosphatidylinositol 3'-kinase and p70S6k signaling during insulin, insulin-like growth factor-1, and interleukin-4 stimulation. J Biol Chem 269:28783–28789.

436. Myers MG Jr., Wang LM, Sun XJ, Zhang Y, Yenush L, Schlessinger J, et al. (1994). Role of IRS-1-GRB-2 complexes in insulin signaling. Molecular and Cellular Biology 14:3577–3587.

437. White MF (1997). The insulin signalling system and the IRS proteins. Diabetologia 40 Suppl 2:S2–17.

438. Gustafson TA, He W, Craparo A, Schaub CD, O'Neill TJ (1995). Phosphotyrosine-dependent interaction of SHC and insulin receptor substrate 1 with the NPEY motif of the insulin receptor via a novel non-SH2 domain. Molecular and Cellular Biology 15:2500–2508.

439. Craparo A, O'Neill TJ, Gustafson TA (1995). Non-SH2 domains within insulin receptor substrate-1 and SHC mediate their phosphotyrosine-dependent interaction with the NPEY motif of the insulin-like growth factor I receptor. J Biol Chem 270:15639–15643.

440. White MF, Yenush L (1998). The IRS-signaling system: A network of docking proteins that mediate insulin and cytokine action. Curr Top Microbiol Immunol 228:179–208.

441. Denton RM, Tavare JM (1995). Does mitogen-activated-protein kinase have a role in insulin action? The cases for and against. European Journal of Biochemistry/FEBS 227:597–611.

442. Hara K, Yonezawa K, Sakaue H, Ando A, Kotani K, Kitamura T, et al. (1994). 1-Phosphatidylinositol 3-kinase activity is required for insulin-stimulated glucose transport but not for RAS activation in CHO cells. Proceedings of the National Academy of Sciences of the United States of America 91:7415–7419.

443. Clarke JF, Young PW, Yonezawa K, Kasuga M, Holman GD (1994). Inhibition of the translocation of GLUT1 and GLUT4 in 3T3-L1

cells by the phosphatidylinositol 3-kinase inhibitor, wortmannin. Biochem J 300:631–635.

444. Okada T, Kawano Y, Sakakibara T, Hazeki O, Ui M (1994). Essential role of phosphatidylinositol 3-kinase in insulin-induced glucose transport and antilipolysis in rat adipocytes. Studies with a selective inhibitor wortmannin. J Biol Chem 269:3568–3573.

445. Lammers R, Gray A, Schlessinger J, Ullrich A (1989). Differential signalling potential of insulin- and IGF-1-receptor cytoplasmic domains. The EMBO Journal 8:1369–1375.

446. Kalloo-Hosein HE, Whitehead JP, Soos M, Tavare JM, Siddle K, O'Rahilly S (1997). Differential signaling to glycogen synthesis by the intracellular domain of the insulin versus the insulin-like growth factor-1 receptor: Evidence from studies of TrkC-chimeras. J Biol Chem 272:24325–24332.

447. Seino S, Seino M, Bell GI (1990). Human insulin-receptor gene. Diabetes 39:129–133.

448. Frattali AL, Treadway JL, Pessin JE (1992). Insulin/IGF-1 hybrid receptors: implications for the dominant-negative phenotype in syndromes of insulin resistance. Journal of Cellular Biochemistry 48:43–50.

449. Treadway JL, Frattali AL, Pessin JE (1992). Intramolecular subunit interactions between insulin and insulin-like growth factor 1 alpha beta half-receptors induced by ligand and Mn/MgATP binding. Biochemistry 31:11801–11805.

450. Kahn CR, Flier JS, Bar RS, Archer JA, Gorden P, Martin MM, et al. (1976). The syndromes of insulin resistance and acanthosis nigricans: Insulin-receptor disorders in man. The New England Journal of Medicine 294:739–745.

451. Moller DE, Flier JS (1991). Insulin resistance: Mechanisms, syndromes, and implications. The New England Journal of Medicine 325:938–948.

452. Tritos NA, Mantzoros CS (1998). Clinical review 97: Syndromes of severe insulin resistance. The Journal of Clinical Endocrinology and Metabolism 83:3025–3030.

453. Hunter SJ, Garvey WT (1998). Insulin action and insulin resistance: diseases involving defects in insulin receptors, signal transduction, and the glucose transport effector system. The American Journal of Medicine 105:331–345.

454. Taylor SI, Grunberger G, Marcus-Samuels B, Underhill LH, Dons RF, Ryan J, et al. (1982). Hypoglycemia associated with antibodies to the insulin receptor. The New England Journal of Medicine 307:1422–1426.

455. Mendenhall E (1950). Tumor of the pineal gland with high insulin resistance. J Indiana State Med Assoc 43:32–36.

456. Mantzoros CS, Flier JS (1995). Insulin resistance: The clinical spectrum. Adv Endocrinol Metab 6:193–232.

457. Longo N, Wang Y, Pasquali M (1999). Progressive decline in insulin levels in Rabson-Mendenhall syndrome. The Journal of Clinical Endocrinology and Metabolism 84:2623–2629.

458. Donohue W, Uchida I (1954). Leprechaunism: A euphemism for a rare familial disorder. The Journal of Pediatrics 45:505–519.

459. Whitehead JP, Soos MA, Jackson R, Tasic V, Kocova M, O'Rahilly S (1998). Multiple molecular mechanisms of insulin receptor dysfunction in a patient with Donohue syndrome. Diabetes 47:1362–1364.

460. Whitehead JP, Humphreys P, Krook A, Jackson R, Hayward A, Lewis H, et al. (1998). Molecular scanning of the insulin receptor substrate 1 gene in subjects with severe insulin resistance: Detection and functional analysis of a naturally occurring mutation in a YMXM motif. Diabetes 47:837–839.

461. Taylor S, Wertheimer E, Hone J, et al. (1994). Mutations in the insulin receptor gene in patients with genetic syndromes of extreme insulin resistance. In Draznin B, LeRoith D (eds.), *Molecular biology of diabetes*. Philadelphia: Humana Press 1–23.

462. Kadowaki T, Bevins CL, Cama A, Ojamaa K, Marcus-Samuels B, Kadowaki H, et al. (1988). Two mutant alleles of the insulin receptor gene in a patient with extreme insulin resistance. Science 240:787–790.

463. Krook A, Brueton L, O'Rahilly S (1993). Homozygous nonsense mutation in the insulin receptor gene in infant with leprechaunism. Lancet 342:277–278.

464. Wertheimer E, Lu SP, Backeljauw PF, Davenport ML, Taylor SI (1993). Homozygous deletion of the human insulin receptor gene results in leprechaunism. Nature Genetics 5:71–73.

465. Psiachou H, Mitton S, Alaghband-Zadeh J, Hone J, Taylor SI, Sinclair L (1993). Leprechaunism and homozygous nonsense mutation in the insulin receptor gene. Lancet 342:924.

466. Takahashi Y, Kadowaki H, Momomura K, Fukushima Y, Orban T, Okai T, et al. (1997). A homozygous kinase-defective mutation in the insulin receptor gene in a patient with leprechaunism. Diabetologia 40:412–420.

467. Moller DE, Flier JS (1988). Detection of an alteration in the insulin-receptor gene in a patient with insulin resistance, acanthosis nigricans, and the polycystic ovary syndrome (type A insulin resistance). The New England Journal of Medicine 319:1526–1529.

468. Odawara M, Kadowaki T, Yamamoto R, Shibasaki Y, Tobe K, Accili D, et al. (1989). Human diabetes associated with a mutation in the tyrosine kinase domain of the insulin receptor. Science 245:66–68.

469. Taira M, Hashimoto N, Shimada F, Suzuki Y, Kanatsuka A, Nakamura F, et al. (1989). Human diabetes associated with a deletion of the tyrosine kinase domain of the insulin receptor. Science 245:63–66.

470. Cama A, de la Luz Sierra M, Ottini L, Kadowaki T, Gorden P, Imperato-McGinley J, et al. (1991). A mutation in the tyrosine kinase domain of the insulin receptor associated with insulin resistance in an obese woman. The Journal of Clinical Endocrinology and Metabolism 73:894–901.

471. Moller DE, Cohen O, Yamaguchi Y, Assiz R, Grigorescu F, Eberle A, et al. (1994). Prevalence of mutations in the insulin receptor gene in subjects with features of the type A syndrome of insulin resistance. Diabetes 43:247–255.

472. Yoshimasa Y, Seino S, Whittaker J, Kakehi T, Kosaki A, Kuzuya H, et al. (1988). Insulin-resistant diabetes due to a point mutation that prevents insulin proreceptor processing. Science 240:784–787.

473. Accili D, Frapier C, Mosthaf L, McKeon C, Elbein SC, Permutt MA, et al. (1989). A mutation in the insulin receptor gene that impairs transport of the receptor to the plasma membrane and causes insulin-resistant diabetes. The EMBO Journal 8:2509–2517.

474. Kadowaki T, Kadowaki H, Rechler MM, Serrano-Rios M, Roth J, Gorden P, et al. (1990). Five mutant alleles of the insulin receptor gene in patients with genetic forms of insulin resistance. The Journal of Clinical Investigation 86:254–264.

475. Kusari J, Takata Y, Hatada E, Freidenberg G, Kolterman O, Olefsky JM (1991). Insulin resistance and diabetes due to different mutations in the tyrosine kinase domain of both insulin receptor gene alleles. J Biol Chem 266:5260–5267.

476. O'Rahilly S, Moller DE (1992). Mutant insulin receptors in syndromes of insulin resistance. Clinical Endocrinology 36:121–132.

477. Jain S, Golde DW, Bailey R, Geffner ME (1998). Insulin-like growth factor-I resistance. Endocrine Reviews 19:625–646.

478. Butler MG, Fogo AB, Fuchs DA, Collins FS, Dev VG, Phillips JAD (1988). Two patients with ring chromosome 15 syndrome. American Journal of Medical Genetics 29:149–154.

479. de Lacerda L, Carvalho JA, Stannard B, Werner H, Boguszewski MC, Sandrini R, et al. (1999). In vitro and in vivo responses to short-term recombinant human insulin-like growth factor-1 (IGF-I) in a severely growth-retarded girl with ring chromosome 15 and deletion of a single allele for the type 1 IGF receptor gene. Clinical Endocrinology 51:541–550.

480. Pasquali F, Zuffardi O, Severi F, Colombo A, Burgio GR (1973). Tandem translocation 15-13. Ann Genet 16:47–50.

481. Kristoffersson U, Heim S, Mandahl N, Sundkvist L, Szelest J, Hagerstrand I (1987). Monosomy and trisomy of 15q24-- --qter in a family with a translocation t(6;15)(p25;q24). Clin Genet 32:169–171.

482. Roback EW, Barakat AJ, Dev VG, Mbikay M, Chretien M, Butler MG (1991). An infant with deletion of the distal long arm of chromosome 15 (q26.1-- --qter) and loss of insulin-like growth factor 1 receptor gene. American Journal of Medical Genetics 38:74–79.

483. Rechler MM (1982). Leprechaunism and related syndromes with primary insulin resistance: Heterogeneity of molecular defects. Prog Clin Biol Res 97:245–281.

484. Kaplowitz PB, D'Ercole AJ (1982). Fibroblasts from a patient with leprechaunism are resistant to insulin, epidermal growth factor, and somatomedin C. The Journal of Clinical Endocrinology and Metabolism 55:741–748.

485. Backeljauw PF, Alves C, Eidson M, Cleveland W, Underwood LE, Davenport ML (1994). Effect of intravenous insulin-like growth factor I in two patients with leprechaunism. Pediatr Res 36:749–754.

486. Longo N, Singh R, Griffin LD, Langley SD, Parks JS, Elsas LJ (1994). Impaired growth in Rabson-Mendenhall syndrome: Lack of effect

of growth hormone and insulin-like growth factor-I. The Journal of Clinical Endocrinology and Metabolism 79:799–805.

487. Desbois-Mouthon C, Danan C, Amselem S, Blivet-Van Eggelpoel MJ, Sert-Langeron C, et al. (1996). Severe resistance to insulin and insulin-like growth factor-I in cells from a patient with leprechaunism as a result of two mutations in the tyrosine kinase domain of the insulin receptor. Metabolism: Clinical and Experimental 45:1493–1500.

488. Kuzuya H, Matsuura N, Sakamoto M, Makino H, Sakamoto Y, Kadowaki T, et al. (1993). Trial of insulinlike growth factor I therapy for patients with extreme insulin resistance syndromes. Diabetes 42:696–705.

489. Burke D, Wilkes D, Blundell TL, Malcolm S (1998). Fibroblast growth factor receptors: lessons from the genes. Trends in Biochemical Sciences 23:59–62.

490. Mohammadi M, Dionne CA, Li W, Li N, Spivak T, Honegger AM, et al. (1992). Point mutation in FGF receptor eliminates phosphatidylinositol hydrolysis without affecting mitogenesis. Nature 358:681–684.

491. Peters KG, Marie J, Wilson E, Ives HE, Escobedo J, Del Rosario M, et al. (1992). Point mutation of an FGF receptor abolishes phosphatidylinositol turnover and Ca2+ flux but not mitogenesis. Nature 358:678–681.

492. Su WC, Kitagawa M, Xue N, Xie B, Garofalo S, Cho J, et al. (1997). Activation of Stat1 by mutant fibroblast growth-factor receptor in thanatophoric dysplasia type II dwarfism. Nature 386:288–292.

493. Dode C, Levilliers J, Dupont JM, De Paepe A, Le Du N, Soussi-Yanicostas N, et al. (2003). Loss-of-function mutations in FGFR1 cause autosomal dominant Kallmann syndrome. Nature Genetics 33:463–465.

494. Oliveira LM, Seminara SB, Beranova M, Hayes FJ, Valkenburgh SB, Schipani E, et al. (2001). The importance of autosomal genes in Kallmann syndrome: genotype-phenotype correlations and neuroendocrine characteristics. The Journal of Clinical Endocrinology and Metabolism 86:1532–1538.

495. Pitteloud N, Hayes FJ, Boepple PA, DeCruz S, Seminara SB, MacLaughlin DT, et al. (2002). The role of prior pubertal development, biochemical markers of testicular maturation, and genetics in elucidating the phenotypic heterogeneity of idiopathic hypogonadotropic hypogonadism. The Journal of Clinical Endocrinology and Metabolism 87:152–160.

496. Franco B, Guioli S, Pragliola A, Incerti B, Bardoni B, Tonlorenzi R, et al. (1991). A gene deleted in Kallmann's syndrome shares homology with neural cell adhesion and axonal path-finding molecules. Nature 353:529–536.

497. Legouis R, Hardelin JP, Levilliers J, Claverie JM, Compain S, Wunderle V, et al. (1991). The candidate gene for the X-linked Kallmann syndrome encodes a protein related to adhesion molecules. Cell 67:423–435.

498. Gonzalez-Martinez D, Kim SH, Hu Y, Guimond S, Schofield J, Winyard P, et al. (2004). Anosmin-1 modulates fibroblast growth factor receptor 1 signaling in human gonadotropin-releasing hormone olfactory neuroblasts through a heparan sulfate-dependent mechanism. J Neurosci 24:10384–10392.

499. Bick DP, Schorderet DF, Price PA, Campbell L, Huff RW, Shapiro LJ, et al. (1992). Prenatal diagnosis and investigation of a fetus with chondrodysplasia punctata, ichthyosis, and Kallmann syndrome due to an Xp deletion. Prenatal Diagnosis 12:19–29.

500. Albuisson J, Pecheux C, Carel JC, Lacombe D, Leheup B, Lapuzina P, et al. (2005). Kallmann syndrome: 14 novel mutations in KAL1 and FGFR1 (KAL2). Human Mutation 25:98–99.

501. Pitteloud N, Meysing A, Quinton R, Acierno JS Jr., Dwyer AA, Plummer L, et al. (2006). Mutations in fibroblast growth factor receptor 1 cause Kallmann syndrome with a wide spectrum of reproductive phenotypes. Molecular and Cellular Endocrinology 254/255:60–69.

502. Bonaventure J, Rousseau F, Legeai-Mallet L, Le Merrer M, Munnich A, Maroteaux P (1996). Common mutations in the gene encoding fibroblast growth factor receptor 3 account for achondroplasia, hypochondroplasia and thanatophoric dysplasia. Acta Paediatr Suppl 417:33–38.

503. Bonaventure J, Rousseau F, Legeai-Mallet L, Le Merrer M, Munnich A, Maroteaux P (1996). Common mutations in the fibroblast growth factor receptor 3 (FGFR 3) gene account for achondroplasia, hypochondroplasia, and thanatophoric dwarfism. American Journal of Medical Genetics 63:148–154.

504. Brodie SG, Kitoh H, Lipson M, Sifry-Platt M, Wilcox WR (1998). Thanatophoric dysplasia type I with syndactyly. American Journal of Medical Genetics 80:260–262.

505. Brodie SG, Kitoh H, Lachman RS, Nolasco LM, Mekikian PB, Wilcox WR (1999). Platyspondylic lethal skeletal dysplasia, San Diego type, is caused by FGFR3 mutations. American Journal of Medical Genetics 84:476–480.

506. Shiang R, Thompson LM, Zhu YZ, Church DM, Fielder TJ, Bocian M, et al. (1994). Mutations in the transmembrane domain of FGFR3 cause the most common genetic form of dwarfism, achondroplasia. Cell 78:335–342.

507. Bellus GA, Hefferon TW, Ortiz de Luna RI, Hecht JT, Horton WA, Machado M, et al. (1995). Achondroplasia is defined by recurrent G380R mutations of FGFR3. American Journal of Human Genetics 56:368–373.

508. Ezquieta Zubicaray B, Iguacel AO, Varela Junquera JM, Jariego Fente CM, Gonzalez Gancedo P, (1999). [Gly380Arg and Asn-540Lys mutations of fibroblast growth factor receptor 3 in achondroplasia and hypochondroplasia in the Spanish population]. Med Clin (Barc) 112:290–293.

509. Bellus GA, McIntosh I, Smith EA, Aylsworth AS, Kaitila I, Horton WA, et al. (1995). A recurrent mutation in the tyrosine kinase domain of fibroblast growth factor receptor 3 causes hypochondroplasia. Nature Genetics 10:357–359.

510. Prinos P, Costa T, Sommer A, Kilpatrick MW, Tsipouras P (1995). A common FGFR3 gene mutation in hypochondroplasia. Human Molecular Genetics 4:2097–2101.

511. Ramaswami U, Rumsby G, Hindmarsh PC, Brook CG (1998). Genotype and phenotype in hypochondroplasia. The Journal of Pediatrics 133:99–102.

512. Fofanova OV, Takamura N, Kinoshita E, Meerson EM, Iljina VK, Nechvolodova OL, et al. (1998). A missense mutation of C1659 in the fibroblast growth factor receptor 3 gene in Russian patients with hypochondroplasia. Endocr J 45:791–795.

513. Bellus GA, Bamshad MJ, Przylepa KA, Dorst J, Lee RR, Hurko O, et al. (1999). Severe achondroplasia with developmental delay and acanthosis nigricans (SADDAN): Phenotypic analysis of a new skeletal dysplasia caused by a Lys650Met mutation in fibroblast growth factor receptor 3. American Journal of Medical Genetics 85:53–65.

514. Peters K, Ornitz D, Werner S, Williams L (1993). Unique expression pattern of the FGF receptor 3 gene during mouse organogenesis. Dev Biol 155:423–430.

515. Werner S, Weinberg W, Liao X, Peters KG, Blessing M, Yuspa SH, et al. (1993). Targeted expression of a dominant-negative FGF receptor mutant in the epidermis of transgenic mice reveals a role of FGF in keratinocyte organization and differentiation. The EMBO Journal 12:2635–2643.

516. Naski MC, Colvin JS, Coffin JD, Ornitz DM (1998). Repression of hedgehog signaling and BMP4 expression in growth plate cartilage by fibroblast growth factor receptor 3. Development 125:4977–4988.

517. Legeai-Mallet L, Benoist-Lasselin C, Delezoide AL, Munnich A, Bonaventure J (1998). Fibroblast growth factor receptor 3 mutations promote apoptosis but do not alter chondrocyte proliferation in thanatophoric dysplasia. J Biol Chem 273:13007–13014.

518. Wongmongkolrit T, Bush M, Roessmann U (1983). Neuropathological findings in thanatophoric dysplasia. Arch Pathol Lab Med 107:132–135.

519. Ho KL, Chang CH, Yang SS, Chason JL (1984). Neuropathologic findings in thanatophoric dysplasia. Acta Neuropathol 63:218–228.

520. Shigematsu H, Takashima S, Otani K, Ieshima A (1985). Neuropathological and Golgi study on a case of thanatophotoric dysplasia. Brain Dev 7:628–632.

521. Cruz PD, Jr., Hud JA Jr. (1992). Excess insulin binding to insulin-like growth factor receptors: Proposed mechanism for acanthosis nigricans. J Invest Dermatol 98:82S–85S.

522. Laudet V (1997). Evolution of the nuclear receptor superfamily: early diversification from an ancestral orphan receptor. Journal of Molecular Endocrinology 19:207–226.

523. Laudet V, Auwerx J, Gustafsson J-A, Wahli W for the Nuclear Receptors Nomenclature Committee (1999). A unified nomenclature system for the nuclear receptor superfamily. Cell 97:161–163.

524. Baker ME (1997). Steroid receptor phylogeny and vertebrate origins. Molecular and Cellular Endocrinology 135:101–107.

525. Kumar R, Thompson EB (1999). The structure of the nuclear hormone receptors. Steroids 64:310–319.

526. Ford J, McEwan IJ, Wright AP, Gustafsson JA (1997). Involvement of the transcription factor IID protein complex in gene activation by the N-terminal transactivation domain of the glucocorticoid receptor in vitro. Mol Endocrinol 11:1467–1475.

527. Henriksson A, Almlof T, Ford J, McEwan IJ, Gustafsson JA, Wright AP (1997). Role of the Ada adaptor complex in gene activation by the glucocorticoid receptor. Molecular and Cellular Biology 17:3065–3073.

528. Hollenberg SM, Evans RM (1988). Multiple and cooperative transactivation domains of the human glucocorticoid receptor. Cell 55:899–906.

529. Bocquel MT, Kumar V, Stricker C, Chambon P, Gronemeyer H (1989). The contribution of the N- and C-terminal regions of steroid receptors to activation of transcription is both receptor and cell-specific. Nucleic Acids Res 17:2581–2595.

530. Tasset D, Tora L, Fromental C, Scheer E, Chambon P (1990). Distinct classes of transcriptional activating domains function by different mechanisms. Cell 62:1177–1187.

531. Freedman LP, Luisi BF, Korszun ZR, Basavappa R, Sigler PB, Yamamoto KR (1988). The function and structure of the metal coordination sites within the glucocorticoid receptor DNA binding domain. Nature 334:543–546.

532. Luisi BF, Xu WX, Otwinowski Z, Freedman LP, Yamamoto KR, Sigler PB (1991). Crystallographic analysis of the interaction of the glucocorticoid receptor with DNA. Nature 352:497–505.

533. Lee MS, Kliewer SA, Provencal J, Wright PE, Evans RM (1993). Structure of the retinoid X receptor alpha DNA binding domain: a helix required for homodimeric DNA binding. Science 260:1117–1121.

534. Wilson TE, Paulsen RE, Padgett KA, Milbrandt J (1992). Participation of non-zinc finger residues in DNA binding by two nuclear orphan receptors. Science 256:107–110.

535. Laudet V, Adelmant G (1995). Nuclear receptors: Lonesome orphans. Curr Biol 5:124–127.

536. Tenbaum S, Baniahmad A (1997). Nuclear receptors: structure, function and involvement in disease. The international Journal of Biochemistry & Cell Biology 29:1325–1341.

537. Brzozowski AM, Pike AC, Dauter Z, Hubbard RE, Bonn T, Engstrom O, et al. (1997). Molecular basis of agonism and antagonism in the oestrogen receptor. Nature 389:753–758.

538. Bourguet W, Ruff M, Chambon P, Gronemeyer H, Moras D (1995). Crystal structure of the ligand-binding domain of the human nuclear receptor RXR-alpha. Nature 375:377–382.

539. Renaud JP, Rochel N, Ruff M, Vivat V, Chambon P, Gronemeyer H, et al. (1995). Crystal structure of the RAR-gamma ligand-binding domain bound to all-trans retinoic acid. Nature 378:681–689.

540. Wagner RL, Apriletti JW, McGrath ME, West BL, Baxter JD, Fletterick RJ (1995). A structural role for hormone in the thyroid hormone receptor. Nature 378:690–697.

541. Danielian PS, White R, Lees JA, Parker MG (1992). Identification of a conserved region required for hormone dependent transcriptional activation by steroid hormone receptors. The EMBO Journal 11:1025–1033.

542. Barettino D, Vivanco Ruiz MM, Stunnenberg HG (1994). Characterization of the ligand-dependent transactivation domain of thyroid hormone receptor. The EMBO Journal 13:3039–3049.

543. Durand B, Saunders M, Gaudon C, Roy B, Losson R, Chambon P (1994). Activation function 2 (AF-2) of retinoic acid receptor and 9-cis retinoic acid receptor: Presence of a conserved autonomous constitutive activating domain and influence of the nature of the response element on AF-2 activity. The EMBO Journal 13:5370–5382.

544. Schwabe JW (1996). Transcriptional control: How nuclear receptors get turned on. Curr Biol 6:372–374.

545. Wurtz JM, Bourguet W, Renaud JP, Vivat V, Chambon P, Moras D, et al. (1996). A canonical structure for the ligand-binding domain of nuclear receptors. Nat Struct Biol 3:87–94.

546. Chen H, Lin RJ, Schiltz RL, Chakravarti D, Nash A, Nagy L, et al. (1997). Nuclear receptor coactivator ACTR is a novel histone acetyltransferase and forms a multimeric activation complex with P/CAF and CBP/p300. Cell 90:569–580.

547. Nagy L, Kao HY, Chakravarti D, Lin RJ, Hassig CA, Ayer DE, et al. (1997). Nuclear receptor repression mediated by a complex containing SMRT, mSin3A, and histone deacetylase. Cell 89:373–380.

548. Alland L, Muhle R, Hou H Jr., Potes J, Chin L, Schreiber-Agus N, et al. (1997). Role for N-CoR and histone deacetylase in Sin3-mediated transcriptional repression. Nature 387:49–55.

549. Heinzel T, Lavinsky RM, Mullen TM, Soderstrom M, Laherty CD, Torchia J, et al. (1997). A complex containing N-CoR, mSin3 and histone deacetylase mediates transcriptional repression. Nature 387:43–48.

550. Grunstein M (1997). Histone acetylation in chromatin structure and transcription. Nature 389:349–352.

551. Jenster G (1998). Coactivators and corepressors as mediators of nuclear receptor function: An update. Molecular and Cellular Endocrinology 143:1–7.

552. Smith DF, Toft DO (1993). Steroid receptors and their associated proteins. Mol Endocrinol 7:4–11.

553. Lee SK, Choi HS, Song MR, Lee MO, Lee JW (1998). Estrogen receptor, a common interaction partner for a subset of nuclear receptors. Mol Endocrinol 12:1184–1192.

554. Barrett TJ, Spelsberg TC (1998). Steroid receptors at the nexus of transcriptional regulation. J Cell Biochem Suppl 31:185–193.

555. Zhang XK, Lehmann J, Hoffmann B, Dawson MI, Cameron J, Graupner G, et al. (1992). Homodimer formation of retinoid X receptor induced by 9-cis retinoic acid. Nature 358:587–591.

556. Hermann T, Hoffmann B, Zhang XK, Tran P, Pfahl M (1992). Heterodimeric receptor complexes determine 3,5,3'-triiodothyronine and retinoid signaling specificities. Mol Endocrinol 6:1153–1162.

557. Zhang XK, Hoffmann B, Tran PB, Graupner G, Pfahl M (1992). Retinoid X receptor is an auxiliary protein for thyroid hormone and retinoic acid receptors. Nature 355:441–446.

558. Chen ZP, Shemshedini L, Durand B, Noy N, Chambon P, Gronemeyer H (1994). Pure and functionally homogeneous recombinant retinoid X receptor. J Biol Chem 269:25770–25776.

559. Watson CS, Gametchu B (1999). Membrane-initiated steroid actions and the proteins that mediate them. Proc Soc Exp Biol Med 220:9–19.

560. Chen HC, Farese RV (1999). Steroid hormones: Interactions with membrane-bound receptors. Curr Biol 9:R478–481.

561. Baldi E, Luconi M, Bonaccorsi L, Forti G (1998). Nongenomic effects of progesterone on spermatozoa: Mechanisms of signal transduction and clinical implications. Front Biosci 3:D1051–1059.

562. Bergeron R, de Montigny C, Debonnel G (1996). Potentiation of neuronal NMDA response induced by dehydroepiandrosterone and its suppression by progesterone: Effects mediated via sigma receptors. J Neurosci 16:1193–1202.

563. Ke L, Lukas RJ (1996). Effects of steroid exposure on ligand binding and functional activities of diverse nicotinic acetylcholine receptor subtypes. Journal of Neurochemistry 67:1100–1112.

564. Maitra R, Reynolds JN (1999). Subunit dependent modulation of GABAA receptor function by neuroactive steroids. Brain Research 819:75–82.

565. Grazzini E, Guillon G, Mouillac B, Zingg HH (1998). Inhibition of oxytocin receptor function by direct binding of progesterone. Nature 392:509–512.

566. Pietras RJ, Szego CM (1977). Specific binding sites for oestrogen at the outer surfaces of isolated endometrial cells. Nature 265:69–72.

567. Berthois Y, Pourreau-Schneider N, Gandilhon P, Mittre H, Tubiana N, Martin PM (1986). Estradiol membrane binding sites on human breast cancer cell lines: Use of a fluorescent estradiol conjugate to demonstrate plasma membrane binding systems. J Steroid Biochem 25:963–972.

568. Gametchu B, Watson CS, Pasko D (1991). Size and steroid-binding characterization of membrane-associated glucocorticoid receptor in S-49 lymphoma cells. Steroids 56:402–410.

569. Nenci I, Marchetti E, Marzola A, Fabris G (1981). Affinity cytochemistry visualizes specific estrogen binding sites on the plasma membrane of breast cancer cells. J Steroid Biochem 14:1139–1146.

570. Refetoff S (1994). Resistance to thyroid hormone: An historical overview. Thyroid 4:345–349.

571. Apriletti JW, Ribeiro RC, Wagner RL, Feng W, Webb P, Kushner PJ, et al. (1998). Molecular and structural biology of thyroid hormone receptors. Clin Exp Pharmacol Physiol Suppl 25:S2–11.

572. Usala SJ, Bale AE, Gesundheit N, Weinberger C, Lash RW, Wondisford FE, et al. (1988). Tight linkage between the syndrome of generalized thyroid hormone resistance and the human c-erbA beta gene. Mol Endocrinol 2:1217–1220.

573. Refetoff S, Weiss RE, Usala SJ (1993). The syndromes of resistance to thyroid hormone. Endocrine Reviews 14:348–399.

574. Usala SJ, Menke JB, Watson TL, Wondisford FE, Weintraub BD, Berard J, et al. (1991). A homozygous deletion in the c-erbA beta thyroid hormone receptor gene in a patient with generalized thyroid hormone resistance: Isolation and characterization of the mutant receptor. Mol Endocrinol 5:327–335.

575. Piedrafita FJ, Ortiz MA, Pfahl M (1995). Thyroid hormone receptor-beta mutants associated with generalized resistance to thyroid hormone show defects in their ligand-sensitive repression function. Mol Endocrinol 9:1533–1548.

576. Yoh SM, Chatterjee VK, Privalsky ML (1997). Thyroid hormone resistance syndrome manifests as an aberrant interaction between mutant T3 receptors and transcriptional corepressors. Mol Endocrinol 11:470–480.

577. Liu Y, Takeshita A, Misiti S, Chin WW, Yen PM (1998). Lack of coactivator interaction can be a mechanism for dominant negative activity by mutant thyroid hormone receptors. Endocrinology 139:4197–4204.

578. Takeda K, Sakurai A, DeGroot LJ, Refetoff S (1992). Recessive inheritance of thyroid hormone resistance caused by complete deletion of the protein-coding region of the thyroid hormone receptor-beta gene. The Journal of Clinical Endocrinology and Metabolism 74:49–55.

579. Ono S, Schwartz ID, Mueller OT, Root AW, Usala SJ, Bercu BB (1991). Homozygosity for a dominant negative thyroid hormone receptor gene responsible for generalized resistance to thyroid hormone. The Journal of Clinical Endocrinology and Metabolism 73:990–994.

580. Sakurai A, Miyamoto T, Refetoff S, DeGroot LJ (1990). Dominant negative transcriptional regulation by a mutant thyroid hormone receptor-beta in a family with generalized resistance to thyroid hormone. Mol Endocrinol 4:1988–1994.

581. Hughes MR, Malloy PJ, Kieback DG, Kesterson RA, Pike JW, Feldman D, et al. (1988). Point mutations in the human vitamin D receptor gene associated with hypocalcemic rickets. Science 242:1702–1705.

582. Whitfield GK, Selznick SH, Haussler CA, Hsieh JC, Galligan MA, Jurutka PW, et al. (1996). Vitamin D receptors from patients with resistance to 1,25-dihydroxyvitamin D3: point mutations confer reduced transactivation in response to ligand and impaired interaction with the retinoid X receptor heterodimeric partner. Mol Endocrinol 10:1617–1631.

583. Kristjansson K, Rut AR, Hewison M, O'Riordan JL, Hughes MR (1993). Two mutations in the hormone binding domain of the vitamin D receptor cause tissue resistance to 1,25 dihydroxyvitamin D3. The Journal of Clinical Investigation 92:12–16.

584. Ames SK, Ellis KJ, Gunn SK, Copeland KC, Abrams SA (1999). Vitamin D receptor gene Fok1 polymorphism predicts calcium absorption and bone mineral density in children. J Bone Miner Res 14:740–746.

585. Gennari L, Becherini L, Masi L, Gonnelli S, Cepollaro C, Martini S, et al. (1997). Vitamin D receptor genotypes and intestinal calcium absorption in postmenopausal women. Calcified Tissue International 61:460–463.

586. Ferrari S, Rizzoli R, Chevalley T, Slosman D, Eisman JA, Bonjour JP (1995). Vitamin-D-receptor-gene polymorphisms and change in lumbar-spine bone mineral density. Lancet 345:423–424.

587. Feskanich D, Hunter DJ, Willett WC, Hankinson SE, Hollis BW, Hough HL, et al. (1998). Vitamin D receptor genotype and the risk of bone fractures in women. Epidemiology 9:535–539.

588. Gennari L, Becherini L, Mansani R, Masi L, Falchetti A, Morelli A, et al. (1999). FokI polymorphism at translation initiation site of the vitamin D receptor gene predicts bone mineral density and vertebral fractures in postmenopausal Italian women. J Bone Miner Res 14:1379–1386.

589. Gong G, Stern HS, Cheng SC, Fong N, Mordeson J, Deng HW, et al. (1999). The association of bone mineral density with vitamin D receptor gene polymorphisms. Osteoporos Int 9:55–64.

590. Eccleshall TR, Garnero P, Gross C, Delmas PD, Feldman D (1998). Lack of correlation between start codon polymorphism of the vitamin D receptor gene and bone mineral density in premenopausal French women: The OFELY study. J Bone Miner Res 13:31–35.

591. Cheng WC, Tsai KS (1999). The vitamin D receptor start codon polymorphism (Fok1) and bone mineral density in premenopausal women in Taiwan. Osteoporos Int 9:545–549.

592. Deng HW, Li J, Li JL, Johnson M, Gong G, Recker RR (1999). Association of VDR and estrogen receptor genotypes with bone mass in postmenopausal Caucasian women: Different conclusions with different analyses and the implications. Osteoporos Int 9:499–507.

593. Gross C, Krishnan AV, Malloy PJ, Eccleshall TR, Zhao XY, Feldman D (1998). The vitamin D receptor gene start codon polymorphism: A functional analysis of FokI variants. J Bone Miner Res 13:1691–1699.

594. Hansen TS, Abrahamsen B, Henriksen FL, Hermann AP, Jensen LB, Horder M, et al. (1998). Vitamin D receptor alleles do not predict bone mineral density or bone loss in Danish perimenopausal women. Bone 22:571–575.

595. Ferrari SL, Rizzoli R, Slosman DO, Bonjour JP (1998). Do dietary calcium and age explain the controversy surrounding the relationship between bone mineral density and vitamin D receptor gene polymorphisms? J Bone Miner Res 13:363–370.

596. Gennari L, Becherini L, Masi L, Mansani R, Gonnelli S, Cepollaro C, et al. (1998). Vitamin D and estrogen receptor allelic variants in Italian postmenopausal women: Evidence of multiple gene contribution to bone mineral density. The Journal of Clinical Endocrinology and Metabolism 83:939–944.

597. Suarez F, Rossignol C, Garabedian M (1998). Interactive effect of estradiol and vitamin D receptor gene polymorphisms as a possible determinant of growth in male and female infants. The Journal of Clinical Endocrinology and Metabolism 83:3563–3568.

598. Tao C, Yu T, Garnett S, Briody J, Knight J, Woodhead H, et al. (1998). Vitamin D receptor alleles predict growth and bone density in girls. Arch Dis Child 79:488–493; discussion 493–484.

599. Carling T, Ridefelt P, Hellman P, Juhlin C, Lundgren E, Akerstrom G, et al. (1998). Vitamin D receptor gene polymorphism and parathyroid calcium sensor protein (CAS/gp330) expression in primary hyperparathyroidism. World J Surg 22:700–706; discussion 706–707.

600. Hennig BJ, Parkhill JM, Chapple IL, Heasman PA, Taylor JJ (1999). Association of a vitamin D receptor gene polymorphism with localized early-onset periodontal diseases. J Periodontol 70:1032–1038.

601. Jackman SV, Kibel AS, Ovuworie CA, Moore RG, Kavoussi LR, Jarrett TW (1999). Familial calcium stone disease: TaqI polymorphism and the vitamin D receptor. J Endourol 13:313–316.

602. Niimi T, Tomita H, Sato S, Kawaguchi H, Akita K, Maeda H, et al. (1999). Vitamin D receptor gene polymorphism in patients with sarcoidosis. Am J Respir Crit Care Med 160:1107–1109.

603. Ruggiero M, Pacini S, Amato M, Aterini S, Chiarugi V (1999). Association between vitamin D receptor gene polymorphism and nephrolithiasis. Miner Electrolyte Metab 25:185–190.

604. Ruggiero M, Pacini S, Aterini S, Fallai C, Ruggiero C, Pacini P (1998). Vitamin D receptor gene polymorphism is associated with metastatic breast cancer. Oncol Res 10:43–46.

605. Park BS, Park JS, Lee DY, Youn JI, Kim IG (1999). Vitamin D receptor polymorphism is associated with psoriasis. J Invest Dermatol 112:113–116.

606. Roy S, Frodsham A, Saha B, Hazra SK, Mascie-Taylor CG, Hill AV (1999). Association of vitamin D receptor genotype with leprosy type. J Infect Dis 179:187–191.

607. Hill AV (1998). The immunogenetics of human infectious diseases. Annu Rev Immunol 16:593–617.

608. Roth DE, Soto G, Arenas F, Bautista CT, Ortiz J, Rodriguez R, et al. (2004). Association between vitamin D receptor gene polymorphisms and response to treatment of pulmonary tuberculosis. J Infect Dis 190:920–927.

609. Saito M, Eiraku N, Usuku K, Nobuhara Y, Matsumoto W, Kodama D, et al. (2005). ApaI polymorphism of vitamin D receptor gene is associated with susceptibility to HTLV-1-associated myelopathy/tropical spastic paraparesis in HTLV-1 infected individuals. J Neurol Sci 232:29–35.

610. Ristow M, Muller-Wieland D, Pfeiffer A, Krone W, Kahn CR (1998). Obesity associated with a mutation in a genetic regulator of adipocyte differentiation. The New England Journal of Medicine 3392:953–959.

611. Barroso I, Gurnell M, Crowley VE, Agostini M, Schwabe JW, Soos MA, et al. (1999). Dominant negative mutations in human

PPARgamma associated with severe insulin resistance, diabetes mellitus and hypertension. Nature 402:880–883.

612. Sladek FM, Dallas-Yang Q, Nepomuceno L (1998). MODY1 mutation Q268X in hepatocyte nuclear factor 4alpha allows for dimerization in solution but causes abnormal subcellular localization. Diabetes 47:985–990.

613. Lindner T, Gragnoli C, Furuta H, Cockburn BN, Petzold C, Rietzsch H, et al. (1997). Hepatic function in a family with a nonsense mutation (R154X) in the hepatocyte nuclear factor-4alpha/MODY1 gene. The Journal of Clinical Investigation 100:1400–1405.

614. Furuta H, Iwasaki N, Oda N, Hinokio Y, Horikawa Y, Yamagata K, et al. (1997). Organization and partial sequence of the hepatocyte nuclear factor-4 alpha/MODY1 gene and identification of a missense mutation, R127W, in a Japanese family with MODY. Diabetes 46:1652–1657.

615. Bulman MP, Dronsfield MJ, Frayling T, Appleton M, Bain SC, Ellard S, et al. (1997). A missense mutation in the hepatocyte nuclear factor 4 alpha gene in a UK pedigree with maturity-onset diabetes of the young. Diabetologia 40:859–862.

616. Yamagata K, Furuta H, Oda N, Kaisaki PJ, Menzel S, Cox NJ, et al. (1996). Mutations in the hepatocyte nuclear factor-4alpha gene in maturity-onset diabetes of the young (MODY1). Nature 384:458–460.

617. Malecki MT, Yang Y, Antonellis A, Curtis S, Warram JH, Krolewski AS (1999). Identification of new mutations in the hepatocyte nuclear factor 4alpha gene among families with early onset Type 2 diabetes mellitus. Diabet Med 16:193–200.

618. Fajans SS, Bell GI (2006). Phenotypic heterogeneity between different mutations of MODY subtypes and within MODY pedigrees. Diabetologia 49:1106–1108.

619. Fajans SS, Bell GI, Polonsky KS (2001). Molecular mechanisms and clinical pathophysiology of maturity-onset diabetes of the young. N Engl J Med 345:971–980.

620. Malecki MT, Klupa T (2005). Type 2 diabetes mellitus: From genes to disease. Pharmacol Rep 57:20–32.

621. Shih DQ, Stoffel M (2002). Molecular etiologies of MODY and other early-onset forms of diabetes. Curr Diab Rep 2:125–134.

622. Lamberts SW, Koper JW, Biemond P, den Holder FH, de Jong FH (1992). Cortisol receptor resistance: The variability of its clinical presentation and response to treatment. The Journal of Clinical Endocrinology and Metabolism 74:313–321.

623. Werner S, Thoren M, Gustafsson JA, Bronnegard M (1992). Glucocorticoid receptor abnormalities in fibroblasts from patients with idiopathic resistance to dexamethasone diagnosed when evaluated for adrenocortical disorders. The Journal of Clinical Endocrinology and Metabolism 75:1005–1009.

624. Malchoff CD, Javier EC, Malchoff DM, Martin T, Rogol A, Brandon D, et al. (1990). Primary cortisol resistance presenting as isosexual precocity. The Journal of Clinical Endocrinology and Metabolism 70:503–507.

625. Karl M, Lamberts SW, Koper JW, Katz DA, Huizenga NE, Kino T, et al. (1996). Cushing's disease preceded by generalized glucocorticoid resistance: Clinical consequences of a novel, dominant-negative glucocorticoid receptor mutation. Proc Assoc Am Physicians 108:296–307.

626. Malchoff DM, Brufsky A, Reardon G, McDermott P, Javier EC, Bergh CH, et al. (1993). A mutation of the glucocorticoid receptor in primary cortisol resistance. The Journal of Clinical Investigation 91:1918–1925.

627. McPhaul MJ, Marcelli M, Tilley WD, Griffin JE, Wilson JD (1991). Androgen resistance caused by mutations in the androgen receptor gene. Faseb J 5:2910–2915.

628. Jirasek JE (1971). Androgen-insensitive male pseudohermaphroditism. Birth Defects Orig Artic Ser 7:179–184.

629. Lubahn DB, Brown TR, Simental JA, Higgs HN, Migeon CJ, Wilson EM, et al. (1989). Sequence of the intron/exon junctions of the coding region of the human androgen receptor gene and identification of a point mutation in a family with complete androgen insensitivity. Proceedings of the National Academy of Sciences of the United States of America 86:9534–9538.

630. Bevan CL, Hughes IA, Patterson MN (1997). Wide variation in androgen receptor dysfunction in complete androgen insensitivity syndrome. The Journal of Steroid Biochemistry and Molecular Biology 61:19–26.

631. Tincello DG, Saunders PT, Hodgins MB, Simpson NB, Edwards CR, Hargreaves TB, et al. (1997). Correlation of clinical, endocrine and molecular abnormalities with in vivo responses to high-dose testosterone in patients with partial androgen insensitivity syndrome. Clinical Endocrinology 46:497–506.

632. MacLean HE, Warne GL, Zajac JD (1995). Defects of androgen receptor function: From sex reversal to motor neurone disease. Molecular and Cellular Endocrinology 112:133–141.

633. Peterziel H, Culig Z, Stober J, Hobisch A, Radmayr C, Bartsch G, et al. (1995). Mutant androgen receptors in prostatic tumors distinguish between amino-acid-sequence requirements for transactivation and ligand binding. International Journal of Cancer 63:544–550.

634. Brown TR, Lubahn DB, Wilson EM, French FS, Migeon CJ, Corden JL (1990). Functional characterization of naturally occurring mutant androgen receptors from subjects with complete androgen insensitivity. Mol Endocrinol 4:1759–1772.

635. McPhaul MJ, Marcelli M, Zoppi S, Griffin JE, Wilson JD (1993). Genetic basis of endocrine disease. 4. The spectrum of mutations in the androgen receptor gene that causes androgen resistance. The Journal of Clinical Endocrinology and Metabolism 76:17–23.

636. Marcelli M, Zoppi S, Grino PB, Griffin JE, Wilson JD, McPhaul MJ (1991). A mutation in the DNA-binding domain of the androgen receptor gene causes complete testicular feminization in a patient with receptor-positive androgen resistance. The Journal of Clinical Investigation 87:1123–1126.

637. Zoppi S, Wilson CM, Harbison MD, Griffin JE, Wilson JD, McPhaul MJ, et al. (1993). Complete testicular feminization caused by an amino-terminal truncation of the androgen receptor with downstream initiation. The Journal of Clinical Investigation 91:1105–1112.

638. Marcelli M, Tilley WD, Wilson CM, Griffin JE, Wilson JD, McPhaul MJ (1990). Definition of the human androgen receptor gene structure permits the identification of mutations that cause androgen resistance: premature termination of the receptor protein at amino acid residue 588 causes complete androgen resistance. Mol Endocrinol 4:1105–1116.

639. Trifiro M, Gottlieb B, Pinsky L, Kaufman M, Prior L, Belsham DD, et al. (1991). The 56/58 kDa androgen-binding protein in male genital skin fibroblasts with a deleted androgen receptor gene. Molecular and Cellular Endocrinology 75:37–47.

640. Quigley CA, Friedman KJ, Johnson A, Lafreniere RG, Silverman LM, Lubahn DB, et al. (1992). Complete deletion of the androgen receptor gene: definition of the null phenotype of the androgen insensitivity syndrome and determination of carrier status. The Journal of Clinical Endocrinology and Metabolism 74:927–933.

641. Ris-Stalpers C, Kuiper GG, Faber PW, Schweikert HU, van Rooij HC, Zegers ND, et al. (1990). Aberrant splicing of androgen receptor mRNA results in synthesis of a nonfunctional receptor protein in a patient with androgen insensitivity. Proceedings of the National Academy of Sciences of the United States of America 87:7866–7870.

642. Holterhus PM, Wiebel J, Sinnecker GH, Bruggenwirth HT, Sippell WG, Brinkmann AO, et al. (1999). Clinical and molecular spectrum of somatic mosaicism in androgen insensitivity syndrome. Pediatr Res 46:684–690.

643. Holterhus PM, Bruggenwirth HT, Hiort O, Kleinkauf-Houcken A, Kruse K, Sinnecker GH, et al. (1997). Mosaicism due to a somatic mutation of the androgen receptor gene determines phenotype in androgen insensitivity syndrome. The Journal of Clinical Endocrinology and Metabolism 82:3584–3589.

644. Gast A, Neuschmid-Kaspar F, Klocker H, Cato AC (1995). A single amino acid exchange abolishes dimerization of the androgen receptor and causes Reifenstein syndrome. Molecular and Cellular Endocrinology 111:93–98.

645. Kaspar F, Klocker H, Denninger A, Cato AC (1993). A mutant androgen receptor from patients with Reifenstein syndrome: identification of the function of a conserved alanine residue in the D box of steroid receptors. Molecular and Cellular Biology 13:7850–7858.

646. Klocker H, Kaspar F, Eberle J, Uberreiter S, Radmayr C, Bartsch G (1992). Point mutation in the DNA binding domain of the androgen receptor in two families with Reifenstein syndrome. American Journal of Human Genetics 50:1318–1327.

647. Nakao R, Yanase T, Sakai Y, Haji M, Nawata H (1993). A single amino acid substitution (gly743 —> val) in the steroid-binding domain of the human androgen receptor leads to Reifenstein

syndrome. The Journal of Clinical Endocrinology and Metabolism 77:103–107.

648. McPhaul MJ, Marcelli M, Zoppi S, Wilson CM, Griffin JE, Wilson JD (1992). Mutations in the ligand-binding domain of the androgen receptor gene cluster in two regions of the gene. The Journal of Clinical Investigation 90:2097–2101.

649. Wooster R, Mangion J, Eeles R, Smith S, Dowsett M, Averill D, et al. (1992). A germline mutation in the androgen receptor gene in two brothers with breast cancer and Reifenstein syndrome. Nature Genetics 2:132–134.

650. MacLean HE, Warne GL, Zajac JD (1996). Spinal and bulbar muscular atrophy: Androgen receptor dysfunction caused by a trinucleotide repeat expansion. J Neurol Sci 135:149–157.

651. Chamberlain NL, Driver ED, Miesfeld RL (1994). The length and location of CAG trinucleotide repeats in the androgen receptor N-terminal domain affect transactivation function. Nucleic Acids Res 22:3181–3186.

652. Stenoien DL, Cummings CJ, Adams HP, Mancini MG, Patel K, DeMartino GN, et al. (1999). Polyglutamine-expanded androgen receptors form aggregates that sequester heat shock proteins, proteasome components and SRC-1, and are suppressed by the HDJ-2 chaperone. Human Molecular Genetics 8:731–741.

653. Kuiper GG, Carlsson B, Grandien K, Enmark E, Haggblad J, Nilsson S, et al. (1997). Comparison of the ligand binding specificity and transcript tissue distribution of estrogen receptors alpha and beta. Endocrinology 138:863–870.

654. Mosselman S, Polman J, Dijkema R (1996). ER beta: identification and characterization of a novel human estrogen receptor. FEBS Letters 392:49–53.

655. Kuiper GG, Enmark E, Pelto-Huikko M, Nilsson S, Gustafsson JA (1996). Cloning of a novel receptor expressed in rat prostate and ovary. Proceedings of the National Academy of Sciences of the United States of America 93:5925–5930.

656. McInerney EM, Tsai MJ, O'Malley BW, Katzenellenbogen BS (1996). Analysis of estrogen receptor transcriptional enhancement by a nuclear hormone receptor coactivator. Proceedings of the National Academy of Sciences of the United States of America 93:10069–10073.

657. Pettersson K, Grandien K, Kuiper GG, Gustafsson JA (1997). Mouse estrogen receptor beta forms estrogen response element-binding heterodimers with estrogen receptor alpha. Mol Endocrinol 11:1486–1496.

658. Toran-Allerand CD (2004). Minireview: A plethora of estrogen receptors in the brain: where will it end? Endocrinology 145:1069–1074.

659. Li L, Haynes MP, Bender JR (2003). Plasma membrane localization and function of the estrogen receptor alpha variant (ER46) in human endothelial cells. Proceedings of the National Academy of Sciences of the United States of America 100:4807–4812.

660. Toran-Allerand CD, Guan X, MacLusky NJ, Horvath TL, Diano S, Singh M, et al. (2002). ER-X: a novel, plasma membrane-associated, putative estrogen receptor that is regulated during development and after ischemic brain injury. J Neurosci 22:8391–8401.

661. Rao BR (1998). Isolation and characterization of an estrogen binding protein which may integrate the plethora of estrogenic actions in non-reproductive organs. The Journal of Steroid Biochemistry and Molecular Biology 65:3–41.

662. Asaithambi A, Mukherjee S, Thakur MK (1997). Expression of 112-kDa estrogen receptor in mouse brain cortex and its autoregulation with age. Biochemical and Biophysical Research Communications 231:683–685.

663. Ramirez VD, Kipp JL, Joe I (2001). Estradiol, in the CNS, targets several physiologically relevant membrane-associated proteins. Brain Res Brain Res Rev 37:141–152.

664. Joe I, Ramirez VD (2001). Binding of estrogen and progesterone-BSA conjugates to glyceraldehyde-3-phosphate dehydrogenase (GAPDH) and the effects of the free steroids on GAPDH enzyme activity: physiological implications. Steroids 66:529–538.

665. Zheng J, Ramirez VD (1999). Purification and identification of an estrogen binding protein from rat brain: Oligomycin sensitivity-conferring protein (OSCP), a subunit of mitochondrial F0F1-ATP synthase/ATPase. The Journal of Steroid Biochemistry and Molecular Biology 68:65–75.

666. Smith EP, Boyd J, Frank GR, Takahashi H, Cohen RM, Specker B, et al. (1994). Estrogen resistance caused by a mutation in the estrogen-receptor gene in a man. The New England Journal of Medicine 331:1056–1061.

667. Lehrer S, Rabin J, Stone J, Berkowitz GS (1994). Association of an estrogen receptor variant with increased height in women. Hormone and Metabolic Research 26:486–488.

668. Kuhnle U, Nielsen MD, Tietze HU, Schroeter CH, Schlamp D, Bosson D, et al. (1990). Pseudohypoaldosteronism in eight families: Different forms of inheritance are evidence for various genetic defects. The Journal of Clinical Endocrinology and Metabolism 70:638–641.

669. Chitayat D, Spirer Z, Ayalon D, Golander A (1985). Pseudohypoaldosteronism in a female infant and her family: Diversity of clinical expression and mode of inheritance. Acta Paediatr Scand 74:619–622.

670. Hanukoglu A, Fried D, Gotlieb A (1978). Inheritance of pseudohypoaldosteronism. Lancet 1:1359.

671. Limal JM, Rappaport R, Dechaux M, Morin C (1978). Familial dominant pseudohypoaldosteronism. Lancet 1:51.

672. Bonnici F (1977). Autosomal recessive transmission of familial pseudohypoaldosteronism. Arch Fr Pediatr 34:915–916.

673. Rosler A (1984). The natural history of salt-wasting disorders of adrenal and renal origin. The Journal of Clinical Endocrinology and Metabolism 59:689–700.

674. Shigetomi S, Ojima M, Ueno S, Tosaki H, Kohno H, Fukuchi S (1986). Two adult familial cases of selective hypoaldosteronism due to insufficiency of conversion of corticosterone to aldosterone. Endocrinol Jpn 33:787–794.

675. Keszler M, Sivasubramanian KN (1983). Pseudohypoaldosteronism. Am J Dis Child 137:738–740.

676. Abramson O, Zmora E, Mazor M, Shinwell ES (1992). Pseudohypoaldosteronism in a preterm infant: Intrauterine presentation as hydramnios. The Journal of Pediatrics 120:129–132.

677. Kuhnle U, Keller U, Armanini D, Funder J, Krozowski Z (1994). Immunofluorescence of mineralocorticoid receptors in peripheral lymphocytes: Presence of receptor-like activity in patients with the autosomal dominant form of pseudohypoaldosteronism, and its absence in the recessive form. The Journal of Steroid Biochemistry and Molecular Biology 51:267–273.

678. Arai K, Chrousos GP (1995). Syndromes of glucocorticoid and mineralocorticoid resistance. Steroids 60:173–179.

679. Oberfield SE, Levine LS, Carey RM, Bejar R, New MI (1979). Pseudohypoaldosteronism: Multiple target organ unresponsiveness to mineralocorticoid hormones. The Journal of Clinical Endocrinology and Metabolism 48:228–234.

680. Hanukoglu A (1991). Type I pseudohypoaldosteronism includes two clinically and genetically distinct entities with either renal or multiple target organ defects. The Journal of Clinical Endocrinology and Metabolism 73:936–944.

681. Schambelan M, Sebastian A, Rector FC Jr. (1981). Mineralocorticoid-resistant renal hyperkalemia without salt wasting (type II pseudohypoaldosteronism): Role of increased renal chloride reabsorption. Kidney Int 19:716–727.

682. McSherry E (1981). Renal tubular acidosis in childhood. Kidney Int 20:799–809.

683. Komesaroff PA, Verity K, Fuller PJ (1994). Pseudohypoaldosteronism: Molecular characterization of the mineralocorticoid receptor. The Journal of Clinical Endocrinology and Metabolism 79:27–31.

684. Arai K, Tsigos C, Suzuki Y, Irony I, Karl M, Listwak S, Chrousos GP (1994). Physiological and molecular aspects of mineralocorticoid receptor action in pseudohypoaldosteronism: a responsiveness test and therapy. The Journal of Clinical Endocrinology and Metabolism 79:1019–1023.

685. New MI, Stoner E, DiMartino-Nardi J (1986). Apparent mineralocorticoid excess causing hypertension and hypokalemia in children. Clin Exp Hypertens [A] 8:751–772.

686. Muller-Berghaus J, Homoki J, Michalk DV, Querfeld U (1996). Diagnosis and treatment of a child with the syndrome of apparent mineralocorticoid excess type 1. Acta Paediatr 85:111–113.

687. Dave-Sharma S, Wilson RC, Harbison MD, Newfield R, Azar MR, Krozowski ZS, et al. (1998). Examination of genotype and phenotype relationships in 14 patients with apparent mineralocorticoid excess. The Journal of Clinical Endocrinology and Metabolism 83:2244–2254.

688. Morineau G, Marc JM, Boudi A, Galons H, Gourmelen M, Corvol P, et al. (1999). Genetic, biochemical, and clinical studies of

patients with A328V or R213C mutations in 11betaHSD2 causing apparent mineralocorticoid excess. Hypertension 34:435–441.

689. Ugrasbul F, Wiens T, Rubinstein P, New MI, Wilson RC (1999). Prevalence of mild apparent mineralocorticoid excess in Mennonites. The Journal of Clinical Endocrinology and Metabolism 84:4735–4738.

690. Monder C, Shackleton CH, Bradlow HL, New MI, Stoner E, Iohan F, et al. (1986). The syndrome of apparent mineralocorticoid excess: Its association with 11 beta-dehydrogenase and 5 beta-reductase deficiency and some consequences for corticosteroid metabolism. The Journal of Clinical Endocrinology and Metabolism 63:550–557.

691. Mune T, Rogerson FM, Nikkila H, Agarwal AK, White PC (1995). Human hypertension caused by mutations in the kidney isozyme of 11 beta-hydroxysteroid dehydrogenase. Nature Genetics 10:394–399.

692. Wilson RC, Harbison MD, Krozowski ZS, Funder JW, Shackleton CH, Hanauske-Abel HM, et al. (1995). Several homozygous mutations in the gene for 11 beta-hydroxysteroid dehydrogenase type 2 in patients with apparent mineralocorticoid excess. The Journal of Clinical Endocrinology and Metabolism 80:3145–3150.

693. Bassett JH, O'Halloran DJ, Williams GR, Beardwell CG, Shalet SM, Thakker RV (1999). Novel DAX1 mutations in X-linked adrenal hypoplasia congenita and hypogonadotrophic hypogonadism. Clinical Endocrinology 50:69–75.

694. Zanaria E, Muscatelli F, Bardoni B, Strom TM, Guioli S, Guo W, et al. (1994). An unusual member of the nuclear hormone receptor superfamily responsible for X-linked adrenal hypoplasia congenita. Nature 372:635–641.

695. Lynch JP, Lala DS, Peluso JJ, Luo W, Parker KL, White BA (1993). Steroidogenic factor 1, an orphan nuclear receptor, regulates the expression of the rat aromatase gene in gonadal tissues. Mol Endocrinol 7:776–786.

696. Ito M, Yu RN, Jameson JL (1998). Steroidogenic factor-1 contains a carboxy-terminal transcriptional activation domain that interacts with steroid receptor coactivator-1. Mol Endocrinol 12:290–301.

697. Muscatelli F, Strom TM, Walker AP, Zanaria E, Recan D, Meindl A, et al. (1994). Mutations in the DAX-1 gene give rise to both X-linked adrenal hypoplasia congenita and hypogonadotropic hypogonadism. Nature 372:672–676.

698. Seminara SB, Achermann JC, Genel M, Jameson JL, Crowley WF Jr. (1999). X-linked adrenal hypoplasia congenita: A mutation in DAX1 expands the phenotypic spectrum in males and females. The Journal of Clinical Endocrinology and Metabolism 84:4501–4509.

699. Ito M, Yu R, Jameson JL (1997). DAX-1 inhibits SF-1-mediated transactivation via a carboxy-terminal domain that is deleted in adrenal hypoplasia congenita. Molecular and Cellular Biology 17:1476–1483.

700. Zhang YH, Guo W, Wagner RL, Huang BL, McCabe L, Vilain E, et al. (1998). DAX1 mutations map to putative structural domains in a deduced three-dimensional model. American Journal of Human Genetics 62:855–864.

701. Hamaguchi K, Arikawa M, Yasunaga S, Kakuma T, Fukagawa K, Yanase T, et al. (1998). Novel mutation of the DAX1 gene in a patient with X-linked adrenal hypoplasia congenita and hypogonadotropic hypogonadism. American Journal of Medical Genetics 76:62–66.

702. Zhang YH, Huang BL, Niakan KK, McCabe LL, McCabe ER, Dipple KM (2004). IL1RAPL1 is associated with mental retardation in patients with complex glycerol kinase deficiency who have deletions extending telomeric of DAX1. Hum Mutat 24:273.

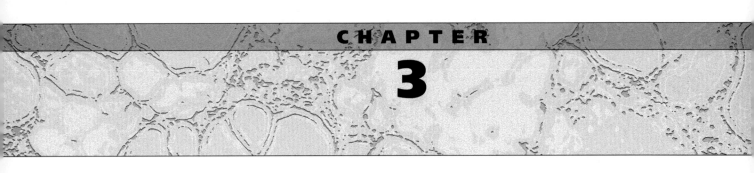

Disorders of Bone Mineral Metabolism: Normal Homeostasis

ALLEN W. ROOT, MD

Introduction

Calcium (Ca), phosphorus [as phosphate (HPO_4^{2-}) because this substance does not exist in the free state in living tissues], and magnesium (Mg) are elements essential to the structural integrity of the body and to the function of each of its cells[1] (Table 3-1). This chapter examines the genetic and physiologic mechanisms that regulate normal mineral homeostasis and bone development, composition, and strength from the prenatal period through adolescence. Table 3-2 lists some of the many genes that direct these processes. Figure 3-1 schematically depicts the factors that regulate serum concentrations of calcium and phosphate.

Calcium

Calcium is an essential component of the mineral portion of bone and is necessary for the function of each of the body's cells. Together, calcium and phosphate form the hydroxyapatite crystal $[Ca_{10}(PO_4)_{10}(OH)_2]$ of bone. Hydroxyapatite accounts for 65% of bone weight and provides its mechanical and weight-bearing strength.

Hydroxyapatite also serves as a reservoir for calcium that may be quickly needed for homeostatic and functional purposes. Although 99% of total body calcium is present in the slowly exchangeable deeply deposited skeletal crystal, it is the rapidly exchangeable 1% of body calcium in recently accumulated surface bone and in vascular, extracellular, and intracellular (soft tissues) spaces with which it is in equilibrium that modulates intercellular communication and intracellular signal transduction; neural transmission; cell-to-cell adhesion; clotting; striated, smooth, and cardiac muscular contraction; cardiac rhythmicity; enzyme action; synthesis and secretion of endocrine and exocrine factors; and cellular proliferation.[2]

Approximately 50% of total serum calcium is bound to albumin and globulin; 5% is complexed/chelated to citrate, phosphate, lactate, bicarbonate, and sulfate; and 45% is present as biologically active and closely regulated ionized Ca^{2+}_e. Serum total and ionized calcium concentrations are related to levels of albumin, creatinine, parathyroid hormone (PTH), phosphate, and serum pH. Approximately 75% of the variability in total serum calcium concentrations is accounted for by genetic factors.[3] The measured Ca^{2+}_e level is dependent on the serum pH (normal adult range

TABLE 3-1

Abbreviations

$1,25(OH)_2D_3$	1,25-Dihydroxyvitamin D_3 (calcitriol)	MAPK	Mitogen activated protein kinase
$24R,25(OH)_2D_3$	24,25-Dihydroxyvitamin D_3	MARRS	Membrane-associated rapid response steroid binding protein (see TBP-2)
$25OHD_3$	25-Hydroxyvitamin D_3 (calcidiol)	M-CSF	Macrophage colony stimulating factor
aa	Amino acid	MEPE	Matrix extracellular phosphoglycoprotein
ADHR	Autosomal-dominant hypophosphatemic rickets	Mg^{2+}	Magnesium
AF	Activating function	MMP	Matrix metalloproteinase
AMP	Adenosine monophosphate	Na^+	Sodium
ATP	Adenosine triphosphate	NFκB	Nuclear factor-κB
ATPase	Adenosine triphosphatase	NPT2	Sodium/phosphate transporter 2, kidney
BMAD	Bone mineral apparent density ~ volumetric BMD	NTx	Amino terminal cross-link telopeptide of collagen type I
BMC	Bone mineral content	OMIM	Online Mendelian Inheritance in Man
BMD	Bone mineral density	OPG	Osteoprotegerin
BMP	Bone morphogenetic protein	P3H1	Prolyl 3-hydroxylase-1
BRU	Bone remodeling unit	PHEX	Phosphate-regulating endopeptidase on the X chromosome
BTT	Bone transmission time	PICP	Carboxyl terminal propeptide of collagen type I
Ca^{2+}_e	Calcium (ionized, extracellular)		
Ca^{2+}_i	Calcium (ionized, intracellular)	PIIINP	Amino terminal propeptide of collagen type III
CaSR	Calcium-sensing receptor	PKA	Protein kinase A
Cl^-	Chloride	PLC	Phospholipase C
DAG	1,2-Diacylglycerol	PO_4	Phosphate (HPO_4^{2-})
DBP	Vitamin D binding protein	PTG	Parathyroid gland
DEXA	Dual energy x-ray absorptiometry	PTH	Parathyroid hormone
DNA	Deoxyribonucleic acid	PTHrP	PTH-related protein
Dpd	Deoxypyridinoline	PTHR1	PTH/PTHrP receptor (PTH/PTHrP-R)
ECF	Extracellular fluid	Pyr	Pyridinoline
ER	Estrogen receptor	QCT	Quantitative computed tomography
FGF	Fibroblast growth factor	QUS	Quantitative ultrasonography
FGFR	Fibroblast growth factor receptor	RANK	Receptor activator of NFκB
FRP4	Frizzled related protein-4	RANKL	RANK ligand
GABA	Gamma (γ) amino butyric acid	RNA	Ribonucleic acid
GDNF	Glial cell line-derived neurotrophic factor	RXR	Retinoic acid X receptor
$G_{i\alpha}$	Alpha subunit of inhibitory GTP-binding protein	SOS	Speed of sound
		SOX	SRY-Box
$G_{s\alpha}$	Alpha subunit of stimulatory GTP-binding protein	STAT	Signal transduction and transcription
		TALH	Thick ascending loop of Henle
$G_{q\alpha}$	Alpha subunit of another stimulatory GTP-binding protein	TBP-2	Thioredoxin binding protein-2 (see MARRS)
		TGF	Transforming growth factor
GH	Growth hormone	TIP	Tuberoinfundibular protein (hypothalamic)
GPCR	G-protein–coupled receptor	TLIMP	TBP-2-like inducible membrane protein
GMP	Guanosine monophosphate		
GTP	Guanosine triphosphate	TNF	Tumor necrosis factor
H^+	Hydrogen ion, proton	TNSALP	Tissue nonspecific alkaline phosphatase
		TR	Thyroid (hormone) receptor
ICTP	Carboxyl terminal cross-link telopeptide of collagen type I	TRAF	TNF receptor associated factor(s)
		TRANCE	TNF-related activation induced cytokine
IGF	Insulin-like growth factor (somatomedin)	TRAP	Tartrate-resistant acid phosphatase
Ihh	Indian hedgehog	TRP	Transient receptor potential (channel)
IL	Interleukin	VDR	Vitamin D receptor
IP_3	Inositol-1,4,5-trisphosphate	VDRE	Vitamin D response element
K^+	Potassium	VEGF	Vascular endothelial growth factor
LRP	Low-density lipoprotein receptor-related protein	XHR	X-linked hypophosphatemic rickets

a. A = adenine, C = cytidine, G = guanine, T = thymidne.

TABLE 3-2

Human Genes Involved in Mineral Homeostasis and Bone Metabolism

Protein	Gene	Chromosome	OMIM[a]
Aggrecan 1	AGC1	15q26.1	155760
Alkaline phosphatase	ALPL	1p36.1-p34	171760
Axis inhibitor 1	AXIN1	16p13.3	603816
β1-Catenin	CTNNB1	3p22-p21.3	116806
Bone morphogenetic protein-2	BMP2	20p12	112261
Bone morphogenetic protein-4	BMP4	14q22-q23	112262
Bone morphogenetic protein-7	BMP7	20	112267
BMP Receptor 1A	BMPR1A	10q22.3	601299
BMP Receptor 2	BMPR2	2q33	600799
C-type natriuretic protein	NPPC	2q24-qter	600296
Calbindin 3 (9 kDa)	CABP1	Xp	302020
Calcitonin	CALCA	11p15.2-p15.1	114130
Calcitonin receptor	CALCR	7q21.3	114131
Calcium-ATPase-channel	ATP2B1	12q21-q23	108731
Calcium release-activated calcium modulator 1	CRACM1	12q24	610277
Calcium sensing receptor	CASR	3q13.3-q21	601199
Calcium transport protein-5	TRPV5	7q35	606679
Calcium transport protein-1	TRPV6	7q33-q34	606680
Calcium channel, L-type, subunit α_1	CACNA1C	12p13.3	114205
Calmodulin 1	CALM1	14q24-q31	114180
Cartilage-associated protein	CRTAP	3p22	605497
β-Catenin	CTNNB1	3p22-p21.3	116806
Cathepsin K	CTSK	3q	603959
Chloride channel 5	CLCN5	Xp11.22	300008
Collagen type I(α1)	COL1A1	17q21.31-q24	120150
Collagen type I(α2)	COL1A2	7q22.1	120160
Collagen type II(α1)	COL2A1	12q13.11-q13.2	120140
Collagen type III(α1)	COL3A1	2q31	120180
Collagen type IV(α1)	COL4A1	13q34	120130
Collagen type IX(α1)	COL9A1	6q13	120210
Collagen type X(α1)	COL10A1	6q21-q22.3	120110
Collagen type XI(α1)	COL11A1	1p21	120280
Cyclophilin B	PIPB	15	123841
Cytochrome P450, III A, 4	CYP3A4	7q22.1	124010
Dikkopf	DKK1	10q11.2	605189
Disheveled 1	DVL1	1p36	601365
Distal-less 5	DLX5	7q22	600028
Fibroblast growth factor-1	FGF1 (acidic)	5q31	131220
Fibroblast growth factor-2	FGF2 (basic)	4q25-q27	176943
Fibroblast growth factor-5	FGF5	4q21	165190
Fibroblast growth factor-7	FGF7	15q15-q21.1	148180
Fibroblast growth factor-23	FGF23	12p13.3	605380
Fibroblast growth factor receptor-1	FGFR1	8p11.2-p11.1	136350
Fibroblast growth factor receptor-2	FGFR2	10q25.3-q26	176943
Fibroblast growth factor receptor-3	FGFR3	4p16.3	134934
Fibroblast growth factor receptor-4	FGFR4	5q35→qter	134935
Frizzled receptor	FZD1	7q21	603408
Frizzled related protein-4	FRP4	7p14-p13	606570
Glial cell missing 2 (PTG)	GCM2	6p24.2	603716
Guanine nucleotide binding protein, alpha stimulating	GNAS1	20q13.2	139320
Hairless	HR	8p21.1	602302
Heterogeneous nuclear ribonucleoprotein D	HNRPD	4q21.1-q21.2	601324
Indian hedgehog	IHH	2q33-q35	600726
Inositol trisphosphate receptor	ITPR1	3p26-p25	147265
Integrin αv	ITGAV	2q31	193210
Integrin β3	ITGB3	17q21.32	173470
Insulin-like growth factor I	IGF1	12q22-q24.1	147440
Insulin-like growth factor 1 receptor	IGF1R	15p25-q26	147370
Klotho	KL	13q12	604824

TABLE 3-2

Human Genes Involved in Mineral Homeostasis and Bone Metabolism (Continued)

Protein	Gene	Chromosome	OMIM[a]
Low density lipoprotein receptor-related protein 5	LRP5	11q13.4	603506
Low density lipoprotein receptor-related protein 6	LRP6	12p13.3-p11.2	603507
Macrophage-colony stimulating factor	CSF1	1p21-p13	120420
M-CSF receptor	CSF 1R	5q33.2-q33.3	164770
Matrix extracellular phosphoglycoprotein	MEPE	4q21.1	605912
Matrix GLA-protein	MGP	12p13.1-p13.2	154870
Mitochondrial RNA-processing endoribonuclease	RMRP	9p21-p12	157660
Naturetic peptide precursor C	NPPC	2q24-qter	600296
Naturetic peptide receptor B	NPR2	9p21-p12	108961
Nuclear factor-κB, Subunit 1	NFκB1	4q23-q24	164011
Nuclear factor-κB, Inhibitor	NFKB1A	14q13	164008
Osteocalcin	BGLAP	1q25-q31	112260
Osteonectin	SPARC	5q31.3-q32	182120
Osteopontin	SPP1	4q21-q25	166490
Osteoprotegerin	TNFRSF11B	8q24	602643
Osterix	SP7	12q13.13	606633
Paracellin-1 (Claudin 16)	CLDN16	3q27	603959
Parathyroid hormone	PTH	11p15.3-p15.1	168450
Peroxisome proliferator-activated receptor γ	PPARG	3p25	601487
PTH related protein	PTHLH	12p12.2-p11.2	168470
PTH (PTH/PTHrP) receptor 1	PTHR1	3p22-p21.1	168468
PTH receptor 2	PTHR2	2q33	601469
Patched 1	PTCH1	9q22.3	601309
Phosphate-regulating gene with homologies to endopeptidases on the X chromosome	PHEX	Xp22.1	307800
Pregnane X receptor	NR1I2	3q13-q21	603065
Prolyl 3-hydroxylase 1	LEPRE1	1p34	610339
Receptor activator of NF-κB (RANK)	TNFRSF11A	18q22.1	603499
RANK-Ligand	TNFSF11	13q14	602642
Retinoid X receptor α	RXRA	9q34.3	180245
Runt-related transcription factor 2	RUNX2	6p21	600211
Sclerostin	SOST	17q12-q21	605740
Sirtuin 1	SIRT1	10	604479
Smoothened	SMOH	7q31-q32	601500
Sodium calcium exchanger	SLC8A1	2p23-p22	182305
Sodium phosphate cotransporter Solute carrier family 34, member 1	SLC34A1	5q35	182309
Sodium phosphate cotransporter Solute carrier family 34, member 2	SLC34A2	4p15.3 1-p15.2	604217
Sodium phosphate cotransporter Solute carrier family 34, member 3	SLC34A3	9q34	609826
SRY-box 9	SOX9	17q24.3-q25.1	608160
T-cell factor/ lymphoid enhancement factor	LEF1	4q23-q25	153245
Transmembrane protein 142A	TMEM142A		610277
25-Hydroxylase	CYP2R1	11p15.2	608713
25OHD-1α hydroxylase	CYP27B1	12q13.1-q13.3	609506
25OHD-24 hydroxylase	CYP24A1	20q13.3-q13.3	126065
Tuberoinfundular peptide 39	TIP39	19q13.33	608386
Vascular endothelial growth factor	VEGF	6p12	192240
Vitamin D binding protein	GC	4q12	139200
Vitamin D receptor	VDR	12q12-q14	601769
Voltage-gated calcium channel α$_1$	CACNA1C	12p13.3	114205
Wingless 1	WNT1	12q12-q13	164820
Wingless 9A	WNT9A	1q42	602863

Source: *www3.ncbi.nlm.nih.gov/htbin-post/Omim.*
a. OMIM = Online Mendelian Inheritance in Man.

Phosphatonin–FGF23

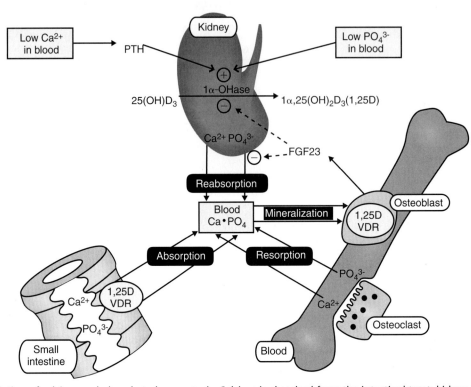

Figure 3-1. Regulation of calcium and phosphate homeostasis. Calcium is absorbed from the intestinal tract, kidney tubule, and bone in response to calcitriol [1,25(OH)$_2$D$_3$] and parathyroid hormone (PTH). Calcitonin inhibits resorption of calcium from bone. The Ca^{2+}-sensing receptor modulates the activity of the parathyroid glands and the renal tubules. Hypocalcemia and hypophosphatemia enhance renal tubular generation of calcitriol and absorption of intestinal phosphate. PTH inhibits renal tubular reabsorption of phosphate. Fibroblast growth factor-23 (FGF23), a phosphatonin secreted by osteoblasts, inhibits renal tubular reabsorption of phosphate and synthesis of calcitriol. [Reproduced with permission from Kolek OI, et al. (2005). 1α,25-Dihydroxyvitamin D$_3$ upregulates FGF23 gene expression in bone: The final link in a renal-gastrointestinal-skeletal axis that controls phosphate transport. Am J Physiol Gastrointest Liver Physiol 289:G1036–G1042.]

1.15-1.35 mmol/L at pH 7.4). An increase in alkalinity (higher pH) raises calcium binding to albumin, thus decreasing Ca$^{2+}_e$—whereas acidic changes (lower pH) decrease binding and thus increase Ca$^{2+}_e$. The relationship between pH and Ca$^{2+}_e$ is best described by an inversely S-shaped third-degree function.[4]

The serum concentration of Ca$^{2+}_e$ is maintained within narrow limits by an integrated system involving the plasma membrane Ca$^{2+}_e$ sensing receptor (CaSR), PTH and its receptor [PTH and PTH-related protein (PTHrP)-R], the thyroidal parafollicular C-cell product calcitonin and its receptor, and the vitamin D hormone system acting upon the intestinal tract, bone, and kidney[5] (Figure 3-1). With increase in serum Ca$^{2+}_e$ concentration, the CaSR on the chief cell of the parathyroid gland (PTG) is activated, which depresses PTH secretion instantly—whereas the CaSR in the distal renal tubule is activated, decreasing reabsorption of calcium filtered through the glomerulus and increasing urinary calcium excretion. When the serum Ca$^{2+}_e$ concentration falls, signaling through the CaSR also declines—thereby increasing PTH secretion and renal tubular reabsorption of filtered calcium, activating osteoclastic bone reabsorption, and somewhat later increasing synthesis of 1,25 dihydroxyvitamin D$_3$ (calcitriol) and intestinal absorption of ingested calcium.[1]

The intracellular concentration of cytosolic free Ca$^{2+}_i$ is 10,000-fold less than that in serum and extracellular fluid, a gradient maintained by extrusion of the cation through energy-dependent sodium-calcium exchangers.[2] Within the cell, Ca$^{2+}_i$ is primarily (99%) within mitochondria, associated with the endoplasmic reticulum, or bound to the inner plasma membrane—from which sites it can be released by chemical signals [e.g., inositol-1,4,5-trisphosphate (IP$_3$)]. IP$_3$ acts upon IP$_3$ receptors (encoded by ITPR1; see Table 3-2 for gene locus and OMIM site) located in the membrane of the endoplasmic reticulum to effect rapid egress of Ca^{2+} from storage and thereby quickly increase Ca$^{2+}_i$ levels.[6]

Ca$^{2+}_i$ serves as a second-messenger signal transducer that controls many cellular activities, including cell movement, secretion of synthesized products, transcription, and cell division and growth. Ca^{2+} enters the cell through transmembrane protein "pores," such as voltage-gated calcium channels that "open" in response to depolarization of the plasma membrane—permitting rapid influx of Ca^{2+} into the cell cytoplasm and leading to further depolarization of the membrane and activation of cell function.[7,8] These channels are widely distributed in the plasma membranes of all cells (e.g., neurons; cardiac, skeletal, and smooth muscle; endocrine glands; gastric mucosa; white blood cells; and platelets) and in cytoplasmic organelles such as mitochondria and the endoplasmic reticulum. They may be activated by high or low electrical voltage. The skeletal muscle high-voltage–activated calcium channel consists of five subunits: α_1, α_2, β, γ, and δ. The voltage-sensing pore-forming Ca^{2+}-binding α_1 subunit has four repeated domains, each with six transmembrane-spanning regions (or helixes) and intracytoplasmic amino and carboxyl terminals. Transmembrane helix 4 serves as the voltage sensor. The α_1 subunit also has a sequence of amino acids between transmembrane helixes 5 and 6 that is partially inserted into the membrane to serve as a "selectivity filter."[8]

The assembly, intracellular movement, interaction with other proteins, activation, and kinetic properties of the α_1 subunit are modified by the extracellular glycosylated α_2 subunit, the β subunit (a cytoplasmic globular protein), a small membrane-spanning δ subunit that is disulfide linked to form dimeric $\alpha_2\delta$, and a second transmembrane subunit γ.[7-9] (The subunit structure of the low-voltage–activated voltage-gated calcium channels is as yet unknown.) The voltage-gated calcium channels are currently designated in accord with their cloned specific α_1 subunits and have been termed Cav 1.1, Cav 1.2 (CACNA1C), and Cav 1.3 to Cav 3.3. Formerly, they were designated in accord with the high- or low-voltage strength required for activation and for their sensitivity to specific inhibitors (e.g., L, N, P, Q, R, and T subtypes).[7,8,10,11]

The high-voltage–dependent L-type calcium channels (Cav 1.1 through Cav 1.4) are present in skeletal, cardiac, and vascular smooth muscle; endocrine cells; neurons; and fibroblasts. L-type calcium channels are activated by the guanine triphosphate (GTP)-binding α_q subunit of G_q proteins through stimulation of phospholipase C (PLC), leading to phosphorylation of the channel protein. L-type calcium channels modulate the growth and proliferation of fibroblasts and smooth muscle cells, the synthesis of extracellular matrix collagen proteins, and the activation of specific transcription factors.[9]

In addition to traversing rapidly across the cell's plasma membrane through voltage-gated channels, Ca^{2+} enters the cytosol but at a markedly slower rate through bifunctional membrane-associated IP_3 receptors that also serve as calcium channels.[6,12] Encoded by ITPR1, the tetrameric IP_3 receptor has six transmembrane domains and a pore-forming loop between the fifth and sixth transmembrane segments. Whereas many IP_3 receptors/channels are expressed in the endoplasmic reticulum, only one to two such channels are expressed in the plasma membrane of each cell. A third site of Ca^{2+} entry into the cytosol is through a plasma membrane protein important to "store-operated" Ca^{2+} entry termed CRACM1 [or TMEM142A (transmembrane protein 142A) or ORAI1].[6]

Store-operated Ca^{2+} entry is triggered after Ca^{2+} release from storage sites has depleted intracellular stores of Ca^{2+}_i and is mediated by CRACM1, a protein with four transmembrane-spanning domains. Multiple copies of CRACM1 are expressed in each cell, permitting large amounts of Ca^{2+} to cross the plasma membrane through this route.[13] Loss-of-function mutations in ORAI1 have been identified in patients with severe combined immune deficiency.[14] Ca^{2+} is translocated not only through

specific Ca^{2+} channels but through paracellular transport channels.[15] Ca^{2+}_i is extruded from cell cytoplasm by calcium and energy-dependent adenosine triphosphate (ATP)-driven calcium pumps and in exchange for sodium (Na^+) through H^+-ATPase and Na^+-Ca^{2+} exchangers.[1,2]

There are many intracellular calcium-binding proteins (e.g., calcium-binding proteins 1 and 4, calbindin, sorcin, calmodulin, and so forth). Calmodulin 1 (CALM1) is a widely distributed 149-aa protein with an amino terminal "lobe" linked to a carboxyl terminal lobe that can assume more than 30 three-dimensional conformations. It is a member of a large family of calcium-modulated proteins.[8] Each lobe has two calcium-binding motifs. Calcium binding exposes hydrophobic "pockets" that allow calmodulin to bind to and regulate the activity of target proteins. While bound to a target protein, calmodulin can assume any of an exceedingly large number of conformations. This versatility enables calmodulin to act as a calcium sensor for many different proteins subserving distinct processes within a single cell, including the voltage-gated calcium channels and calcium/calmodulin-dependent protein kinases.

Gastrointestinal absorption of calcium is primarily an active and saturable process (stimulated by calcitriol) that regulates the availability of transmembrane calcium "pumps" and channels on the luminal and basolateral surface membranes of duodenal and jejunal enterocytes.[1] The ileum and colon are also able to absorb calcium when dietary intake is low or demand increases. Calcitriol acting through the vitamin D receptor (VDR) increases duodenal expression of calcium transport protein-1 (epithelial calcium channel 2 encoded by TRPV6-transient receptor potential-vanilloid 6), a luminal calcium channel with six transmembrane domains and intracytoplasmic amino and carboxyl terminals that form a homotetramer or heterotetramer combined with TRPV5. [There are six subfamilies of the transient receptor potential (TRP) family of ion channels, many of which are permeable to calcium.[16]]

After entering the enterocyte, calcium traverses its interior within the cytosol or within a lysosomal vesical bound to calbindin$_{9kd}$. After fusion of the vesicle with the basolateral plasma membrane, Ca^{2+} is extruded. Ca^{2+} is also released into the circulation through a basolateral Na^+-Ca^{2+} exchanger (SLC8A1) or a Ca^{2+}-Mg^{2+}-dependent ATPase calcium channel (ATPB21). When present in high amounts, luminal calcium may also be absorbed by diffusion along paracellular channels. PTH indirectly increases intestinal calcium absorption by enhancing renal 25-hydroxyvitamin D-1α hydroxylase activity and calcitriol synthesis. Growth hormone (GH) and estrogens also increase intestinal absorption of calcium. Glucocorticoids and thyroid hormone inhibit this process.

Intestinal calcium absorption is increased during adolescence, pregnancy, and lactation—and is depressed in patients with nutritional or functional vitamin D deficiency, chronic renal disease, and hypoparathyroidism. Calcium is excreted into the intestinal tract in the ileum and in pancreatic and biliary secretions. The amount of calcium ingested influences the net amount of calcium absorbed. The lower the calcium intake the greater the efficiency of its absorption. In the adult, when the dietary calcium intake is <200 mg/day fecal calcium excretion exceeds intake. Thus, active absorption of calcium cannot compensate for very low intake. As dietary calcium increases from 200 to 1,000 mg/day, active calcium absorption increases but at a progressively decreasing rate.

When dietary calcium exceeds 1,000 mg/day, active calcium absorption remains relatively constant at 300 mg/day but passive absorption of calcium through paracellular channels continues to increase.[1] Thus, hypercalcemia may result from dietary calcium excess (as in the milk-alkali syndrome). The availability of calcium for bone mineralization and cellular function is determined by its intake, absorption, excretion, and turnover. Intestinal calcium absorption is influenced by vitamin D status, its food source (the bioavailability of calcium in cow milk formulas is 38%, that in human breast milk is 58%; leafy green vegetables are also a good source of dietary calcium), the form of the calcium salt in supplements, and the presence in food of inhibitors of calcium absorption such as phytates, oxalates, or phosphates (e.g., cola beverages).[17]

It is currently recommended that infants (including those who are breast fed), children, and adolescents receive a minimum of 200 IU (5.0 μg) of cholecalciferol (vitamin D$_3$) daily, but this amount may be too low (vide infra).[18,19] Low calcium intake appears to be associated with increased fracture rate in children and adolescents, and therefore adequate dietary intake of calcium during infancy, childhood, and particularly adolescence has been considered necessary to attain a peak bone mass that may lessen the risk of fracture and the later development of osteopenia.[20]

In an effort to ensure optimal mineralization of the developing skeleton, age-related dietary intakes of elemental calcium for infants, children, and adolescents have been recommended (Table 3-3).[20] However, critical review of these recommendations suggests that after basal levels of calcium intake have been achieved (>500 mg/day in children and adolescents) increased calcium intake in dairy foods or supplements has only transient effects on indices of bone mineralization and no documented positive long-term effects on fracture rate or

future risk of osteoporosis.[17] Nevertheless, adherence to these guidelines has been strongly advocated by the American Academy of Pediatrics.[20] In addition to dietary intake of calcium and vitamin D status, the most significant modifiable determinant of bone mineralization is weight-bearing physical activity (vide infra).[21]

Calcium is primarily excreted by the kidney. Ultrafiltrable serum calcium (both Ca$^{2+}_e$ and that complexed or chelated) crosses the renal glomerular membrane. Ninety-eight percent of filtered calcium is reabsorbed by the renal tubule [70% in the proximal renal tubule primarily by a paracellular mechanism, 20% in the thick ascending loop of Henle (TALH) by the paracellular route through generation of a lumen-positive voltage differential by a sodium-potassium-chloride (Na$^+$K$^+$-2Cl$^-$) transporter, and 8% in the distal convoluted tubule by active transcellular transport regulated by PTH and calcitriol].[1,22] In the TALH, calcium and magnesium are reabsorbed through voltage-driven paracellular channels (in part through paracellin-1, a tight-junction protein channel instrumental in renal reabsorption of filtered calcium and magnesium).

Cells of the TALH also express the CaSR on their basolateral membrane. When activated by peritubular Ca^{2+}, this G-protein–coupled receptor (GPCR) decreases renal tubular reabsorption of calcium through the paracellular channels by inhibiting activity of the Na$^+$-K$^+$-2Cl$^-$ transporter and lowering lumen-positive voltage. In active transcellular calcium reabsorption, Ca^{2+} crosses the luminal or apical surface of the renal distal convoluted tubular cell from the tubular lumen through calcium transport protein-5 (renal epithelial calcium channel 1 encoded by TRPV5)—whose expression is increased by calcitriol, estradiol, and a low-calcium diet. The multifunctional β-glucuronidase transmembrane protein klotho (KL) is able to de-glycosylate TRPV5, thereby trapping it in the renal tubular cell membrane and prolonging its activity.[23]

PTH increases calcium reabsorption in the distal tubule by increasing chloride efflux from the basolateral membrane of the distal renal tubular cell, thus increasing the transmembrane voltage gradient.[2] Calcium exits the basolateral serosal surface of the renal tubular cell against a chemical gradient in exchange for Na$^+$ through the Na$^+$-Ca^{2+} exchanger with the aid of Mg^{2+}-dependent Ca^{2+}-ATPase. Increased glomerular filtration and/or decreased renal tubular reabsorption increase renal excretion of calcium, phosphate, and magnesium. Urinary excretion of calcium is augmented by increased dietary intake, hypercalcemia of diverse pathophysiology (with the exception of that associated with familial hypocalciuric hypercalcemia), expansion of extracellular volume, metabolic acidosis, and loop diuretics (furosemide) (Table 3-4).[1] PTH and PTHrP increase renal tubular reabsorption of Ca^{2+}, whereas glucocorticoids, mineralocorticoids, and Ca^{2+} itself suppress its reabsorption.

In utero, fetal serum calcium concentrations are quite high (12-13 mg/dL), because calcium is transported across the placenta against a chemical gradient—likely under the influence of placentally synthesized calcitriol. The high calcium levels in umbilical cord blood (12 mg/dL) decline rapidly postnatally to a nadir of 9 mg/dL between 24 and 48 hours of age, increase to approximately 10 mg/dL, stabilize, and then decline marginally

TABLE 3-3

Recommended Dietary Calcium Intake in Infants, Children, and Adolescents

Age (Years)	Dietary Intake (mg/day)	
	NAS	NIH
0-0.5	210	400
0.5-1	270	600
1-3	500	800
4-8	800	
4-5		800
6-10		1,000
9-18	1,300	
11-18		1,350

From American Academy of Pediatrics (1999). Calcium requirements of infants, children, and adolescents. Pediatrics 104:1152–1157.
NAS = National Academy of Science (1997 data), NIH = National Institutes of Health (1994 data).

TABLE 3-4

Factors Affecting Renal Excretion of Calcium, Phosphate, and Magnesium in Normal Subjects (Sites of Action)

	Calcium	Phosphate	Magnesium
Glomerular Filtration			
Increased	Hypercalcemia	Hyperphosphatemia Mild hypocalcemia	Hypermagnesemia
Decreased	Hypocalcemia Renal insufficiency	Hypophosphatemia Renal insufficiency Moderate hypercalcemia	Hypomagnesemia Renal insufficiency
Renal Tubular Reabsorption			
Increased	ECF volume depletion Hypocalcemia Phosphate administration Thiazide diuretics Metabolic alkalosis PTH PTHrP Calcitriol	ECF volume depletion Hypercalcemia Phosphate deprivation Chronic metabolic alkalosis	ECF volume depletion Hypocalcemia Hypomagnesemia PTH Metabolic alkalosis
Decreased	ECF volume expansion Hypercalcemia Phosphate deprivation Metabolic acidosis Loop diuretics Cyclosporin A	PTH/PTHrP Hypocalcemia Phosphate excess Metabolic alkalosis Thiazide diuretics FGF23 Calcitriol	ECF volume expansion Hypercalcemia Phosphate depletion Hypermagnesemia Loop diuretics Cyclosporin A Cisplantin Ethanol

Adapted from Favus MJ, Bushinsky DA, Lemann J Jr. (2006). Regulation of calcium, magnesium, and phosphate metabollism. In Favus MJ (ed.), *Primer on the metabolic bone diseases and disorders of mineral metabolism, Sixth edition.* Washington, D.C.: American Society for Bone and Mineral Research 76–83.
ECF = extracellular fluid.

over the next 18 months. In children and adolescents, serum calcium levels are slightly higher than in adults (8.5–10.5 mg/dL). In preterm infants or full-term ill infants, hypocalcemia is often present because the PTH secretory response to hypocalcemia is blunted and calcitonin secretion exaggerated and prolonged.

CALCIUM-SENSING RECEPTOR

Plasma Ca^{2+}_e concentrations are detected by the CaSR, a 1,079-aa cell membrane protein with seven transmembrane domains whose extracellular domain binds Ca^{2+}, Mg^{2+}, and specific aromatic amino acids.[24] Through its binding of Ca^{2+}_e, the CaSR finely regulates the concentration of this anion by modulating the secretion of PTH and the renal tubular reabsorption of calcium. The CaSR is encoded by *CASR* and is a member of the C family of GPCRs with extremely long extracellular domains (500- to 600-aa residues) and homologies with receptors that bind glutamate, γ-amino butyric acid, and pheromones.[25,26] The very long extracellular domain is heavily glycosylated, a post-translational modification essential to efficient movement of the receptor to the cell surface. This domain forms "pockets" into which the ligand binds.

Interestingly, this GPCR is biologically active in the dimeric form linked by cysteine residue numbers 129 and 131.[24] Homodimerization of the CaSR takes place in the endoplasmic reticulum after core N-linked glycosylation.

Homodimeric CaSR is then packaged within the Golgi apparatus, where it is further glycosylated and then transported to the cell membrane.[27] The CaSR is expressed on the plasma membrane of parathyroid chief cells, at the apical or basolateral membranes of most renal tubular cells (particularly the TALH and the collecting ducts), on the cell membranes of the parafollicular (C) cells of the thyroid, in cartilage, and in bone, lungs, adrenals, breast, intestines, skin, lens, placental cytotrophoblasts, and nervous tissue.[26,28]

The serum Ca^{2+}_e concentration is related to polymorphic variants of the CaSR. Seventy percent of individuals are homozygous for alanine at aa position 986 within the intracellular domain, 3% are homozygous for serine, and the remainder are heterozygous for the two aa. In heterozygous Arg986Ser and homozygous Ser986 subjects, Ca^{2+}_e concentrations are significantly higher than in those homozygous for Ala986.[29,30] In addition, there are cellular Ca^{2+} sensors unrelated structurally to the CaSR or to subtypes of the CaSR itself.[26] The CaSR also serves as a magnesium sensor and perhaps as a moderator of nutrient availability. By binding to the CaSR, aromatic L-amino acids appear to "sensitize" the receptor to a given level of Ca^{2+}_e.[24] The CaSR also modulates renal tubular reabsorption of magnesium, decreasing its reabsorption when serum cation values rise.

Although in the kidney the CaSR is expressed in greatest abundance in the basolateral (plasma) membranes of the medullary and cortical TALH, it is also found in glomerular cells and other segments of the renal tubule.[26] There too, increasing peritubular concentrations of Ca^{2+}_e and Mg^{2+}_e inhibit renal tubular reabsorption of filtered Ca^{2+}. Acting through the CaSR, rising serum Ca^{2+}_e concentrations stimulate release of calcitonin from thyroid C cells. The CaSR is expressed throughout the (rat) intestinal tract, where it may modulate the changes in intestinal motility that accompany low (increased) and high (depressed) serum Ca^{2+}_e values. Cell membrane CaSRs are present in (mouse, rat, bovine) articular and hypertrophic chondrocytes of the epiphyseal growth plate and to a lesser extent in proliferating and maturing chondrocytes.[31]

Osteoblasts, osteocytes, and osteoclasts also express the CaSR—and agonist (Ca^{2+}, neomycin, gadolinium) activation of the CaSR stimulates intracellular signal transduction.[31] The CaSR may mediate recruitment of osteoblast precursor cells to sites of high Ca^{2+} levels, the residue of local osteoclast activity, thus linking the bone-remodeling processes of resorption and formation.[20] In vitro Ca^{2+} inhibits bone reabsorptive activity of (rabbit) osteoclasts by causing the osteoclast to decrease secretion of acid and catabolic enzymes and to withdraw from the site of bone resorption.[32]

Through its intracellular carboxyl terminal, the CaSR is linked to G proteins that couple the ligand-receptor message to intracellular signal transduction pathways.[24,26,33,34] After binding of Ca^{2+} to the extracellular domain of the CaSR, $G_{\alpha q/11}$ dissociates from its $\beta\gamma$ subunit complex and activates membrane-bound PLC-β1. In turn, this enzyme hydrolyzes membrane-bound phosphatidylinositol 4,5-bisphosphate to diacylglycerol and IP_3—the latter leading to increased cytosolic concentrations of Ca^{2+}_i. Activation of the CaSR also stimulates activity of phospholipases A_2 and D and mitogen-activated protein kinases (MAPK) but inhibits that of adenylyl cyclase, the latter through stimulation of adenylate-cyclase–inhibitory $G_{\alpha i}$ activity.[24] Within the PTG, increases in plasma Ca^{2+}_e and consequently cytosolic Ca^{2+}_i concentrations suppress expression, synthesis, and secretion of PTH and inhibit proliferation of chief cells.

Decline in Ca^{2+}_e leads to increased PTH secretion, thus enabling the CaSR to exercise minute-to-minute control over the release of PTH and hence of the Ca^{2+}_e. In the kidney, binding of Ca^{2+}_e to the CaSR decreases not only transcellular transport of filtered Ca^{2+} but its paracellular transport in the TALH.[28] Inactivating mutations in CASR result in familial hypocalciuric hypercalcemia, whereas gain-of-function mutations in this gene are associated with autosomal-dominant hypoparathyroidism ("familial hypercalciuric hypocalcemia").[24]

The Ca^{2+}/CaSR complex inhibits antidiuretic hormone-induced renal tubular permeability to water by decreasing the number of apical water channels in the inner medullary collecting ducts, thus leading to polyuria. The CaSR also binds Mg^{2+} and regulates its urinary excretion in a manner similar to that of Ca^{2+}. The CaSR is widely expressed throughout the gastrointestinal tract, where it may regulate secretion of gastrin and gastric acid, intestinal motility, and nutrient absorption.[35] Expression of

the CaSR in the brain suggests a mechanism whereby Ca^{2+} may influence neural function locally by modulating neurotransmitter and neuroreceptor function (such as the metabotropic glutamate receptor, which also recognizes Ca^{2+}).

Calcimimetics are agonistic drugs that activate the CaSR. Calcilytics are antagonists of the CaSR.[35] As noted, the CaSR binds not only Ca^{2+}_e but Mg^{2+}_e, selected L-amino acids, and some antibiotics. The latter are designated type I calcimimetics. Synthetic compounds that bind to the transmembrane domains of the CaSR and increase the sensitivity of the CaSR to ambient Ca^{2+}_e are designated type II calcimimetics. The most widely employed of the calcimimetics is cinacalcet [N-[1-(R)-(-)-(1-naphthyl)ethyl]-3-[3-(trifluoromethyl)phenyl]-1-aminopropane hydrochloride], which has been effective in decreasing secretion of PTH in patients with primary or secondary hyperparathyroidism.[36] Calcilytics decrease the sensitivity of the CaSR to Ca^{2+}_e and thus increase the secretion of PTH and depress renal tubular reabsorption of Ca^{2+}. These compounds remain investigational at present but might in the future be useful for the treatment of some forms of metabolic bone disease.

Phosphate

Eighty-five percent of body phosphate is deposited in bone as hydroxyapatite. The remainder is intracellular (in the cytosol or mitochondria in the form of inorganic phosphate esters or salts, membrane phospholipids, and phosphorylated metabolic intermediate compounds) or in interstitial fluid or serum (0.1%), where it circulates as free orthophosphate anions HPO_4^{2-} and $H_2PO_4^-$ (55%), bound to proteins (10%), or complexed to calcium, magnesium, or sodium (35%).[1,22] At pH 7.4, serum HPO_4^{2-} and $H_2PO_4^-$ are present in a molar ratio of 4:1. In alkalotic states, the ratio increases—and with acidosis it declines. (At pH 7.4, 1 mmol/L of orthophosphate = 1.8 mEq/L = 3.1 mg/dL.) Intracellularly, cytosolic free phosphate concentrations approximate those in serum (i.e., 3–6 mg/dL). Phosphate is an integral and absolutely essential component of cellular and intracellular membrane phospholipids, ribonucleic (RNA) and deoxyribonucleic (DNA) acids, energy-generating ATP, and intracellular signal transduction systems.[2,37]

The serum phosphate concentration is regulated by intake, intestinal absorption, excretion, and renal tubular reabsorptive mechanisms and fluctuates with age, gender, growth rate, diet, and serum calcium levels.[1,38] Inasmuch as phosphate is found in all cells and foods, dietary deficiency is unusual. Dietary phosphate is absorbed across the intestinal brush border as HPO_4^{2-} in direct proportion to its intake, principally in the duodenum and jejunum. It is absorbed by both passive paracellular diffusion related to the luminal concentration of this anion and by an active transcellular mechanism stimulated by calcitriol.

The latter is an energy-requiring transport process with sodium through a Na^+-HPO_4^{2-} cotransporter protein (SLC34A2, solute carrier family 34, member 2) maintained by a calcitriol-dependent Na^+, K^+-ATPase. Phosphate is also secreted into the intestinal tract. When dietary phosphate intake falls below 310 mg/day in the adult, net phosphate absorption is negative. At low phosphate intakes, absorption is active in the duodenum, jejunum, and distal ileum—whereas at high intakes 60% to 80% of ingested phosphate is absorbed primarily by diffusion. Phosphate absorption can be impaired by its intraluminal precipitation as an aluminum or calcium salt and by intestinal malabsorption disorders.

Phosphate is filtered in the renal glomerulus and reabsorbed in the proximal (85%) and distal convoluted tubules. It is actively transported across the luminal membrane against an electrochemical gradient through specific Na^+-HPO_4^{2-} cotransporter proteins with the aid of Na^+, K^+-ATPase.[1,22] Expression of the renal Na^+-HPO_4^{2-} cotransporter protein (SLC34A1) is regulated by serum phosphate levels (hypophosphatemia increases expression), PTH, PTHrP, and fibroblast growth factor (FGF)-23. Phosphate exits the renal tubular cell with sodium through cation exchange for potassium. The maximal tubular reabsorption of phosphate approximates the filtered load.

Tubular phosphate reabsorption is increased by low phosphate intake and hypophosphatemia (due to decrease in filtered load), hypercalcemia (by decrease in the glomerular filtration rate), depletion of extracellular fluid volume, and metabolic alkalosis (Table 3-4). Renal tubular reabsorption of phosphate is depressed by high phosphate intake and by PTH- and PTHrP-mediated down-regulation of SLC34A1. Calcitriol, glucocorticoids, and thiazide diuretics decrease renal tubular reabsorption of phosphate. Phosphate is deposited in bone as hydroxyapatite dependent on local levels of calcium, phosphate, and alkaline phosphatase activity and is reabsorbed by osteoclasts whose activity is stimulated by PTH, calcitriol, and other osteoclast-activating factors. Serum concentrations of phosphate are highest in infancy and early childhood (4–7 mg/dL) and then decline during mid-childhood and adolescence to adult values (2.5–4.5 mg/dL).

PHOSPHATONINS

Renal tubular reabsorption of phosphate is regulated by several substances collectively termed *phosphatonins* (Figure 3-1). Phosphaturic agents have been identified in the serum of normal subjects and in patients with X-linked hypophosphatemic rickets (XHR), which is due to loss-of-function mutations in the membrane-bound 749-aa endopeptidase encoded by *PHEX* (phosphate-regulating gene with homologies to endopeptidases located on the X chromosome). They have also been identified in patients with autosomal-dominant hypophosphatemic rickets (ADHR-OMIM 193100), due to activating mutations in *FGF23*, and in patients with tumor-induced osteomalacia in which increased production of FGF23 and other phosphaturic agents has been identified.[38,39]

By inhibition of phosphate transport in the kidney, phosphatonins lead to hyperphosphaturia and hypophosphatemia. They also inhibit activity of 25-hydroxyvitamin D-1α hydroxylase, resulting in decreased synthesis and thus inappropriately normal or low serum concentrations of calcitriol and in impaired intestinal absorption of phosphate.[40] Among the best characterized of the phosphato-

nins is FGF23, generated as a 251-aa with a 24-aa signal sequence that is post-translationally glycosylated. It is expressed primarily by osteoblasts and osteocytes and to a lesser extent by the brain, thyroid, PTG, thymus, cardiac/skeletal muscle, liver, and intestines. In osteoblasts, expression of FGF23 is enhanced by calcitriol acting through the VDR and modified by a chondrocyte-derived secreted factor yet to be characterized.[41,42]

FGF23 induces renal phosphate wasting by down-regulating expression of *SLC34A1*, the Na^+-HPO_4^{2-} cotransporter expressed in the apical or luminal membrane of the proximal renal tubule. It also down-regulates expression of a related renal tubular Na^+-HPO_4^{2-} cotransporter encoded by *SLC34A3*, and of 25-hydroxyvitamin D-1α hydroxylase encoded by *CYP27B1*. FGF23 acts through binding to the c isoform of tyrosine kinase FGF receptors (FGFR) 1, 2, and 3. The genes encoding the FGFRs consist of 19 exons that may be alternatively spliced to include or to exclude exon 8 or exon 9 (encoding the third extracellular immunoglobulin-like domain of the FGF receptor, which helps to specify the ligand bound by the receptor). When exon 8 is included in the mRNA transcript, the b isoform of the FGFR is formed. When exon 9 is included in the transcript, the c isoform is produced. Although it is likely that FGF23 binds to multiple FGFR c isoforms, the multifunctional protein klotho has been reported to convert FGFR1(IIIc) into a specific FGF23 receptor in renal tissue.[38,43] Highly sulfated glycosaminoglycans facilitate ligand-receptor interaction.

FGF23 is measurable in normal adult sera with a mean concentration of 29 pg/mL that does not correlate with age or gender. Its concentration is inversely related to that of phosphate, and values rise when dietary phosphate increases and decline with phosphate restriction.[38] Serum values of FGF23 are increased in patients with XHR, ADHR, tumor-induced osteomalacia, and fibrous dysplasia associated with hypophosphatemia. In patients with ADHR, gain-of-function mutations (e.g., Arg179Trp) in *FGF23* result in resistance to degradation of the protein that is normally cleaved between Arg179 and Ser180. In subjects with tumor-induced osteomalacia, the production of FGF23 is greatly increased.

Serum FGF23 concentrations are also elevated in the Hyp mouse model of XHR. FGF23 may be a substrate for PHEX enzymatic activity, but it is unclear if it is the endogenous substrate for this enzyme.[40,44] In the Hyp mouse, biallelic "knockout" of Fgf23 reverses the hypophosphatemia and relative calcitriol deficiency—suggesting that FGF23 is of fundamental pathogenic importance in XHR. In familial tumoral calcinosis (OMIM 211900), loss-of-function mutations in FGF23 lead to accelerated intracellular degradation of FGF23 that prevents secretion of intact protein—resulting in decreased renal excretion of phosphate, in hyperphosphatemia, in relatively increased calcitriol levels, and in diffuse ectopic calcification.[38,45]

Tumors associated with hypophosphatemic osteomalacia also express *FRP4* (frizzled related protein-4), *MEPE* (matrix extracellular phosphoglycoprotein), and *FGF7*—all of which have phosphaturic properties.[38,46] FRP4 is a secreted 346-aa glycosylated protein that shares the structure of the extracellular domain of transmembrane frizzled receptors. The natural ligands of frizzled receptors are Wnt proteins, and their coreceptors are the cell surface low-density lipoprotein receptor-related proteins (LRP-5/6). These heterotrimeric complexes stabilize intracellular β-catenin and the attendant signal transduction systems and are essential for bone formation (vide infra).

Secreted FRP4 serves as a "decoy" receptor competing with the frizzled receptor for binding to Wnt, thus inhibiting the function of this receptor. FRP4 is expressed in bone cells and in large amounts by tumors with associated osteomalacia. In normal adults, the mean serum FRP4 concentration is 34 ng/mL. FRP4 inhibits sodium-dependent renal tubular phosphate reabsorption by inhibition of Wnt signaling, leading to hypophosphatemia. It also reduces expression of the gene encoding 25-hydroxyvitamin D_3-1α.hydroxylase.[40] MEPE is primarily expressed by osteoblasts, osteocytes, and odontoblasts—as well as by tumors associated with hypophosphatemic osteomalacia. It encodes a 525-aa 58-kDa protein, a member of the short-integrin-binding ligand-interacting glycoprotein family that also includes osteopontin. MEPE modulates osteoblast and osteoclast function and may both inhibit and support bone mineralization.[38] Although MEPE is able to inhibit sodium-dependent renal tubular phosphate reabsorption, its role in phosphate metabolism may be more complex inasmuch as knockout of MEPE in mice results in increased bone mass without altering serum phosphate or calcitriol values.[47] MEPE is associated with and may serve as a substrate for PHEX on the osteoblast surface.[44]

Magnesium

Magnesium is the fourth most abundant of the body cations. Two-thirds of body Mg is found in bone (primarily on the surface of the hydroxyapatite crystal, where 50% is freely exchangeable), one-third is intracellular, and 1% is in the ECF compartment.[1,2] In blood, magnesium (1.7-2.4 mg/dL = 0.7-1.0 mmol/L) is partially bound to proteins (30%), complexed to phosphate and other anions (15%), and found as free Mg^{2+}_e (55%). As with Ca^{2+}_e, Mg^{2+}_e levels rise as pH falls (increased acidity).[22]

Intracellularly, magnesium (0.5 mmol/L) is bound to ATP and other molecules. Ten percent is in the ionic form, and 50% within mitochondria. Mg^{2+}_e is a cofactor in many enzymatic reactions, including those that consume or produce ATP. Mg^{2+}_e alters free radicals and influences nitric oxide synthase activity, cyclic guanosine monophosphate generation, endothelin production, and immune function. Mg^{2+}_e decreases membrane excitability in nerve and muscle cells and blocks the excitatory N-methyl D-aspartate receptor. It is a necessary cofactor for the regulation of neuromuscular excitability, nerve conduction, enzyme activity, oxidative metabolism by mitochondria, glycolysis, phosphorylation, transcription, and translation. It is essential to the secretion (but not the synthesis) of PTH by the parathyroid chief cell.

Net intestinal magnesium absorption is directly related to dietary intake and independent of calcitriol.[1] Magnesium is passively absorbed primarily by diffusion through paracellular channels in proportion to the intestinal luminal concentration of this cation. In addition, there is a small component of active transcellular magnesium absorption. Magnesium is also excreted into the intestinal tract, where its absorption may be impaired by high phosphate intake, significant intestinal disease, or chronic laxative abuse.

Seventy percent of serum magnesium is ultrafiltrable and passes through the renal glomerular membrane. Ninety-five percent is reabsorbed: 15% in the proximal convoluted and straight tubules, 70% in the cortical TALH, and 10% in the distal convoluted tubule.[1,22] In the TALH, Mg^{2+} reabsorption occurs through a paracellular pathway that is impermeable to water.[48] Mg^{2+} is conducted from the lumen of the TALH to the interstitial space and vasculature by paracellin-1 (CLDN16, also termed claudin 16), a 305-aa tight-junction protein whose encoding gene is expressed only in the renal cortical TALH and distal convoluted tubule. Paracellin-1 has four transmembrane domains with intracellular carboxyl and amino terminals and is a member of the claudin family of proteins that bridge intercellular gaps within the tight junctions.[15,48]

Paracellin-1 is also utilized for Ca^{2+} reabsorption in the TALH. Loss-of-function mutations of CLDN16 lead to familial autosomal-recessive renal hypomagnesemia because of renal wastage of magnesium in association with hypercalciuria and renal calcification (OMIM 248250).[48,49] In the distal convoluted tubule, Mg^{2+} reabsorption is related to activity of a Na^+-Cl^- cotransporter and perhaps to paracellin-1. PTH increases magnesium reabsorption in the renal TALH and distal convoluted tubule, perhaps by regulating paracellin-1. On the other hand, hypermagnesemia and hypercalcemia (acting through the CaSR) decrease renal tubular magnesium reabsorption—as do expansion of extracellular fluid volume, metabolic alkalosis, phosphate depletion, loop diuretics, aminoglycoside antibiotics, and impaired renal function (Table 3-4).[1]

Alkaline Phosphatase

The gene (ALPL) encoding tissue-nonspecific alkaline phosphatase (TNSALP) is expressed in bone (synthesized and secreted by the osteoblast), liver, kidney, and skin fibroblast. ALPL is a 507-aa protein that by alternative processing during transcription and translation permits the osteoblast to synthesize and secrete a reasonably specific bone form. Although TNSALP circulates as a homodimer, in tissue it is a homotetrameric ectoenzyme (ectophosphatase) located on the cell surface anchored through its carboxyl terminal to cell membrane phosphatidylinositol-glycan. In bone, alkaline phosphatase binds to collagen type I and prepares skeletal matrix for mineralization, hydrolyzes organic phosphates (thus increasing the local concentration of phosphate to a value that exceeds the calcium X phosphate product, encouraging deposition of calcium phosphate as hydroxyapatite), transports inorganic phosphate and Ca^{2+} into the cell, and inactivates pyrophosphate and other inhibitors of mineralization by removing their phosphate moieties.

Among the endogenous substrates for TSNALP are phosphoethanolamine and pyridoxal-5'-phosphate. The hepatic form of TNSALP is formed by alternative splicing of exon 1 of *ALPL*. Hepatic alkaline phosphatase converts pyridoxal-5'-phosphate to pyridoxal, a compound essential for normal synthesis of neural γ-amino butyric acid (GABA)—an inhibitory neurotransmitter. Without pyridoxal-5'-phosphate, central nervous system levels of GABA are low and seizures may occur.[50] Loss-of-function mutations in ALPL lead to infantile, childhood, and adult forms of hypophosphatasia. Three genes encoding tissue-specific intestinal, placental, and germ cell alkaline phosphatase isoenzymes are clustered at chromosome 2q34-q37.

Parathyroid Hormone and Parathyroid-Hormone–Related Protein

PARATHYROID HORMONE

PTH is secreted by the chief cells of four paired PTGs that are derived from the endoderm of the dorsal segments of the third (paired inferior glands) and fourth (paired superior glands) pharyngeal pouches. Occasionally, there may be a fifth PTG embedded within the substance of the thyroid gland or in the mediastinum.[24] The thymus is formed by the endoderm of the third pharyngeal pouch and calcitonin-synthesizing parafollicular (C) cells of the thyroid by that of the fourth pharyngeal pouch. The mRNA of PTH has also been demonstrated in rodent thymus and hypothalamus.[51]

A critical factor for the development of the PTGs is the nuclear DNA binding transcription factor encoded by *Gcm2* (glial cell missing, drosophila, homolog of, 2). Although essential to neural glial cell development in insects, GCM is not expressed in mammalian brain but is expressed primarily in the rodent placenta and thymus *(Gcm1)* and in the PTG *(Gcm2)*. The pharyngeal pouch expression of *Gcm2* is maintained by a number of homeobox and transcription factors, including those encoded by Hoxa3, Pax1, Pax9, and Eya1. The human homolog of *Gcm2 (Gcm2* or *GCMB)* is expressed in the PTG and in intrathymic PTH-secreting adenomas but not by normal human thymus.[52] Intragenic deletion or missense mutations of *Gcm2* have been identified in subjects with familial autosomal-recessive hypoparathyroidism (Table 3-5).

Chief cells synthesize, store, and secrete PTH—a hormone that increases serum concentrations of calcium, lowers phosphate values, and exerts both anabolic and catabolic effects on bone [primarily in response to ambient Ca^{2+}_e concentrations that either enhance (when low) or repress (when high) transcription of *PTH* and secretion of PTH and regulate the rate of chief cell proliferation, responses mediated by the CaSR]. Calcimimetic drugs have inhibitory effects on PTH secretion. Higher phosphate values enhance transcription of *PTH*, secretion of PTH, and chief cell replication. 1α,25-dihydroxyvitamin D_3 (calcitriol) and its synthetic analogues inhibit transcription of *PTH*, secretion of PTH, and proliferation of chief cells.[24] In response to acute hypocalcemia, PTH stored in secretory vesicles is rapidly released. When hypocalcemia is prolonged, the secretion of PTH[1-84] is augmented by a decrease in its intracellular degradation and an increase in transcription of *PTH*. When hypocalcemia is extended, it is augmented by an increase in chief cell number.

The three exons of *PTH* encode the prepro-PTH sequence of 115 aa. The amino terminal 25-aa signal sequence (encoded by exon 2) is removed by furin, a prohormone convertase, as it leaves the endoplasmic reticulum [forming pro-PTH (90 aa)]. It is then further processed in the Golgi apparatus by furin to mature human PTH (84 aa). PTH is stored in secretory vesicles and granules. The stability, translation, and intracellular translocation of PTH mRNA are regulated by binding of cytosolic proteins to the 3'-untranslated region of PTH mRNA. These proteins include a member of the dynein complex that also binds to microtubules within the parathyroid chief cell and to HNRPD (heterogeneous nuclear ribnucleoprotein D or AUF1), which directs mRNA into the proteasomal pathway of degradation.[53]

TABLE 3-5

Parathyroid Hormone–Related Protein: Sites of Expression and Proposed Actions

Site	Action
Mesenchyma	
Periarticular cells	PTH-rP depresses the rate of differentiation of late-proliferating chondrocytes to hypertrophic chondrocytes, thus permitting increased proliferation and delay of ossification.
Bone	Enhances or depresses bone resorption.
Smooth muscle Vascular system Myometrium Urinary bladder	Relaxation.
Cardiac muscle	Positive chronotropic and inotropic effects.
Skeletal muscle	
Epithelia	
Skin	Perhaps regulates proliferation of keratinocytes.
Breast	Induces ductal branching, secreted into milk, and drives mobilization of calcium from maternal bone for transfer to nursing infant.
Teeth	Stimulates resorption of overlying bone enabling eruption.
Endocrine system	
Parathyroid glands	Stimulates transport of calcium.
Pancreatic islets	Stored and co-secreted with insulin.
Placenta	Enhances calcium transport.
Central nervous system	Neuroprotective by antagonizing excessive calcium-related excitotoxicity.

Compiled and adapted from Broadus AE, Nissenson RA (2006). Parathyroid hormone-related protein. In Favus MJ (ed.), *Primer on the metabolic bone diseases and disorders of mineral metabolism, Sixth edition*. Washington, D.C.: American Society for Bone and Mineral Research 99-106.

The full biologic activity of PTH[1-84] is found in its first 34-amino-acid sequence, and all of its renal effects are localized within the segment PTH[1-31]. Amino acid numbers 1 and 2 (serine-valine) comprise an activation sequence essential to the bioactivity of the amino terminal portion of PTH[1-84]. The PTGs secrete intact PTH[1-84], a phosphorylated form of PTH[1-84], and carboxyl terminal PTH fragments of varying length but do not secrete amino terminal fragments of PTH[1-84].[54,55] Intraglandular PTH[1-84] is degraded by cathepsins B and H (proteases colocalized with PTH[1-84] in secretory granules). PTH degradation represents an important mechanism regulating the release of bioactive PTH[1-84] and is accelerated when the Ca^{2+}_e concentration is elevated.

The half-life of circulating PTH[1-84] is approximately 2 minutes. It is rapidly metabolized by the liver and excreted by the kidney. In the hepatic Kupffer cells, PTH[1-84] is cleaved usually after either aa 33 or aa 36 to carboxyl terminal PTH peptides with half-lives of approximately 15 to 20 minutes. In the kidney, intact and carboxyl terminal fragments of PTH are filtered by the glomerulus, reabsorbed by the renal tubule, and then degraded to small fragments. Megalin (a multifunctional receptor expressed in coated pits on the luminal/apical surface, endocytic vacuoles, and lysosomes of proximal renal tubular cells; in the PTG; and in other epithelial structures) specifically recognizes intact PTH[1-84] and amino terminal fragments of PTH and mediates the renal tubular endocytosis of intact PTH[1-84] that has been filtered through the glomerulus.[28]

The classic functions of PTH[1-84] as well as its shorter peptide derivatives PTH[1-34] and PTH[1-31] upon regulation of calcium and phosphate homeostasis are carried out through the seven-transmembrane G-protein–coupled PTH/PTHrP receptor in the renal tubule and osteoblast. Thus, with equal potency PTH[1-84], PTH[1-34], and PTH[1-31] increase urinary excretion of phosphate by inhibiting its renal tubular reabsorption, the renal tubular and osteoclastic reabsorption of calcium thereby raising serum calcium concentrations common and the renal synthesis of calcitriol by enhancing expression of *CYP27B1* (encoding 25-hydroxyvitamin D_3-1α hydroxylase), thereby augmenting intestinal absorption of calcium. Mediated by the $G_{s\alpha}$ subunit of the G-protein and adenylyl cyclase, these actions involve generation of cyclic adenosine monophosphate (AMP) and signaling through protein kinase A (PKA). Whereas the first two residues of PTH[1-84] (serine-valine) are essential to activation of adenylyl cyclase, residues 15 through 34 are needed for high-affinity binding to its receptor. In addition to cyclic AMP, PTH[1-84] activates other signal transduction pathways in skeletal and kidney cells—including those involving PLC and cytosolic Ca^{2+} flux, PKC, and MAPK.[55]

As noted, multiple species of carboxyl terminal peptides derived from PTH[1-84] circulate. They are secreted directly by the PTG or returned to the circulation after metabolism of intact PTH[1-84] by hepatic Kupffer cells.[55] Indeed, carboxyl terminal fragments of PTH[1-84] are secreted in greater abundance from the PTG than is intact PTH[1-84], and the proportion of carboxyl terminal fragments secreted increases as the ambient Ca^{2+} concentration rises. Many of the circulating carboxyl terminal fragments of PTH are generated by hepatic uptake and degradation of PTH[1-84].

Amino terminal fragments generated by hepatic degradation of PTH[1-84] are degraded further within the liver and do not recirculate. PTH[1-84] and the carboxyl terminal fragments of PTH are filtered by the kidneys, and the carboxyl terminal fragments are reabsorbed by the renal tubules and further degraded intracellularly. The kidneys are not a major source of circulating carboxyl terminal fragments of PTH. Among the carboxyl terminal fragments of PTH found in circulation are PTH[7-84], [24-84], [34-84], [37-84], [41-84], [43-84]. They are extracted by the kidneys, muscle, and bone. The presence of as yet structurally uncharacterized receptors for these carboxyl terminal peptides of PTH[1-84] has been demonstrated by their biologic actions.

In addition to their classic effects on mineral homeostasis, several nonclassic actions of PTH[1-84] have been identified—including rapid and direct stimulation of intestinal calcium absorption independent of its effects on vitamin D metabolism, stimulation of hepatic gluconeogenesis, acute natriuresis and calciuresis, and enhancement of neutrophil movement *in vitro*.[55] Inasmuch as many of these nonclassic biologic effects of intact PTH are not replicated by the amino terminal fragment PTH[1-34], it has been suggested that they may be related to the carboxyl terminal portion of the protein.

Indeed, specific effects of carboxyl terminal PTH fragments have been observed [e.g., PTH[7-84] lowers serum calcium levels in parathyroidectomized rats (maintained eucalcemic by diet) and antagonizes PTH[1-84]-stimulated increase in calcium concentrations, urinary phosphate excretion, and bone turnover.[55] PTH[7-84] directly lowers the rate of bone resorption and suppresses the bone resorbing effects of PTH[1-34], calcitriol, prostaglandin E_2, and interleukin (IL)-11. PTH[7-84] also antagonizes osteoclastogenesis. On the other hand, PTH[39-84] and PTH[53-84] augment the biologic effects of PTH[1-34]. PTH[7-84] does not bind to the PTH/PTHrP receptor, nor does it inhibit PTH[1-84]-mediated increase in cyclic AMP generation—implying that PTH[7-84] acts through a unique receptor.

Because there are multiple circulating forms of PTH, its immunologic measurement is dependent on the specificity of the antibody or antibodies employed in the assay. When a polyclonal PTH radioimmunoassay is utilized, intact and carboxyl terminal fragments of PTH are usually measured. Use of dual monoclonal antibodies and immunometric assays has improved the specificity of immunologic assays. Nevertheless, most assays detect intact and selected fragments of PTH and are consequently rather poor predictors of bone turnover—particularly in patients with chronic renal insufficiency.[56] The comparability of PTH assays from different commercial sources is limited.[57] Employing a two-site immunochemiluminescent assay, serum PTH concentrations average approximately 11 to 13 pg/mL and range between 2.3 and 24.5 pg/mL in children and adolescents 2 to 16 years of age. Values do not vary with age but are a bit higher in girls than in boys.[58]

The synthesis and secretion of PTH[1-84] and its various fragments are modulated for the most part by the serum Ca^{2+}_e concentration acting through the CaSR expressed on the plasma membrane of the parathyroid chief cell. Because a change in serum Ca^{2+}_e concentration sensed by the parathyroid chief cell CaSR is quickly reflected in changes in cytosolic Ca^{2+}_i levels, the release of PTH is regulated on a minute-to-minute basis. Rapidly declining and steady-state low serum concentrations of Ca^{2+}_e increase PTH secretion by accelerating its release from storage sites in secretory granules. Hypocalcemia also raises PTG levels of PTH mRNA by increasing the transcription rate of *PTH* and enhancing the stability of PTH mRNA by its post-transcriptional binding to cytosolic proteins.[2,24] Hypercalcemia slightly deceases PTH transcription and cellular levels of PTH mRNA. The serum Ca^{2+}_e concentration also determines the form of PTH released by the PTG. During hypocalcemia, PTH^{1-84} is the predominant form secreted. In hypercalcemic states, carboxyl terminal fragments of PTH are released.

Low serum phosphate concentrations exert an independent and direct inhibitory effect on the transcription of *PTH*, post-transcriptional PTH mRNA stability, PTH secretion, and proliferation of parathyroid chief cells. Hyperphosphatemia enhances PTH secretion.[24] Prolonged hyperphosphatemia may contribute to the PTG hyperplasia frequently encountered in patients with chronic renal disease. Calcitriol directly inhibits *PTH* transcription acting through the VDR and a vitamin D response element (VDRE) in the 5'-untranslated region of *PTH*. Calcitriol also controls expression of *CASR* and of *VDR* and decreases proliferation of parathyroid cells. However, chronic hypocalcemia overcomes the suppressive effects of calcitriol on *PTH* transcription by decreasing VDR number in the PTG.[2] Hypomagnesemia and hypermagnesemia inhibit release but not synthesis of PTH. Other agents that increase PTH release include β-adrenergic agonists, dopamine, prostaglandin E, potassium (by decreasing cytosolic Ca^{2+}_i levels within the parathyroid chief cell), prolactin, lithium (by "resetting" the set point for PTH release), glucocorticoids, estrogens, and progestins. Prostaglandin $F_{2\alpha}$, α-adrenergic agonists, and fluoride suppress PTH release by increasing Ca^{2+}_i values.

PTH regulates the serum concentration of Ca^{2+}_e directly by stimulating its reabsorption in the distal renal tubule and from the skeleton, and indirectly by augmenting the intestinal absorption of calcium by increasing the synthesis of calcitriol. In bone, PTH enhances osteoclast activity indirectly by acting on and through the osteoblast.

When administered intermittently, PTH^{1-84} and amino terminal PTH^{1-34} exert anabolic effects upon skeletal mass. They augment bone formation by increasing osteoblast number by accelerating their differentiation from progenitor cells and from inactive bone-lining cells and by reducing their rate of death.[24] The anabolic effect of PTH may be mediated further by release of matrix-embedded growth factors and by local generation of insulin-like growth factor I (IGF-I). PTH stimulates calcitriol synthesis by increasing renal tubular expression of *CYP27B1,* the gene encoding 25-hydroxyvitamin D_3-1α-hydroxylase (the enzyme that catalyzes the synthesis of calcitriol from calcidiol). PTH depresses proximal and distal renal tubular reabsorption of phosphate by decreasing expression of *SLC34A1,* a Na^+-HPO_4 cotransporter protein, thus increasing the urinary excretion of this anion.

PARATHYROID HORMONE–RELATED PROTEIN

PTH and PTHrP have evolved from a common ancestor. They share 8 of their first 13 amino acids (the site of the activating domain for PTHR1), but their structures diverge thereafter. Both peptides bind with equal affinity to a common PTH/PTHrP receptor (PTHR1), but their receptor binding domains are distinct. PTHrP was initially identified as a primary mediator of hypercalcemia of malignancy. However, PTHrP is normally synthesized in many fetal and adult tissues (cartilage, bone, smooth, cardiac and skeletal muscle, skin, breast, intestines, PTGs, pancreatic islets, pituitary, placenta, and central nervous system) and plays a crucial role in chondrocyte differentiation and maturation, formation of the mammary gland and eruption of teeth, epidermal and hair follicle growth, and other developmental events.[59,60]

Whereas PTH acts as an endocrine hormone on tissues distant from the PTG, PTHrP is synthesized locally and acts primarily as a paracrine or juxtacrine (and perhaps intracrine) messenger. (A nuclear localization sequence is present in the latter half of the PTHrP molecule.[59]) Although the secretion of PTH is regulated by ambient calcium levels and fluctuates rapidly, the production of PTHrP is constitutive and is controlled at the point of expression of its encoding gene. The six exons of the gene encoding PTHrP (*PTHLH*) are transcribed and translated into 108-, 139-, 141-, and 173-aa isoforms employing coding sequences from exon 4 alone or from exons 4 and 5 or 6.[24] In addition, amino and carboxyl terminal and mid-region products of *PTHLH* are also formed by post-translational processing. The predominant isoform of PTHrP is the 141-aa sequence. In specific tissues, $PTHrP^{1-139}$ is cleaved by prohormone convertases to smaller peptides ($PTHrP^{1-36, \ 37-94, \ 107-139}$) that may act as paracrine factors or be secreted into the circulation. PTHrP secreted by fetal PTGs and a mid-region fragment of $PTHrP^{37-94}$ synthesized by the placenta increase placental calcium transport. $PTH^{107-139}$ inhibits bone resorption (and has been termed osteostatin).[60]

Serum concentrations of PTHrP are low except when it is secreted by tumors, leading to humoral hypercalcemia of cancer. There are high concentrations of PTHrP in breast milk. Although the effects of $PTHrP^{1-36}$ on calcium, phosphate, and vitamin D metabolism are similar to those of PTH, the major roles of this and other segments of PTHrP in many developmental processes (including those of breast, teeth, cartilage, and endochondral bone) distinguish PTHrP from PTH. In the cartilaginous growth plate, proximal periarticular proliferative chondrocytes synthesize PTHrP in response to Indian hedgehog (Ihh), a protein secreted by chondrocytes in their late proliferative and early prehypertrophic phases (Figure 3-2).

PTHrP then diffuses into and through the growth plate and signals prehypertrophic chondrocytes through PTHR1 to slow their rate of differentiation to hypertrophic

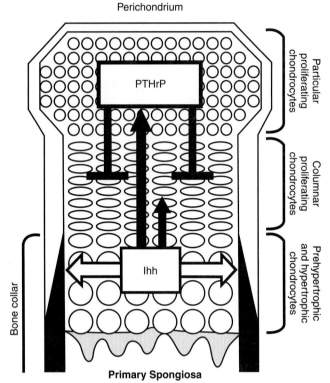

Figure 3-2. The epiphyseal cartilage growth plate consists of zones of proliferating, transitional, and hypertrophic chondrocytes. Indian hedgehog is synthesized by prehypertrophic chondrocytes. Receptors for parathyroid-hormone–related protein are expressed by proliferating and transitional chondrocytes. Indian hedgehog stimulates secretion of parathyroid-hormone–related protein from periarticular cells, and this in turn blocks further differentiation and maturation of late proliferating chondrocytes to hypertrophic chondrocytes—thus prolonging the period of cartilage growth. [Reproduced with permission by the American Society for Bone and Mineral Research from Broadus A (2006). Parathyroid hormone-related protein. In Favus M (ed.), *Primer on the metabolic bone diseases and disorders of mineral metabolism, Sixth edition.* Washington, D.C.: American Society for Bone and Mineral Research 99–106.]

chondrocytes, thus prolonging the stage of proliferation and delaying ossification.[59,60] Biallelic loss of PTHrP in knockout mice is lethal due to bony malformations. In these mice (*Pthlh*[-/-]), there is a decrease in the number of resting and proliferating chondrocytes, disruption of the columnar organization of the growth plate, premature acceleration of chondrocyte maturation and apoptosis, and inappropriate ossification resulting in a dwarfing phenotype (a domed and foreshortened cranium, short limbs, small thorax) similar to that of Blomstrand chondrodysplasia (a disorder associated with loss-of-function mutations of PTHR1).[61] Most of these mice die at birth.

Mice in which expression of Pthlh has been maintained only in chondrocytes survive, but display small stature, cranial chondrodystrophy, and failure of tooth eruption.[60] In the heterozygous state (*Pthlh*[+/-]), mouse fetal development is normal but by 3 months of age the trabeculae of the long bones are osteopenic. A similar bone phenotype is noted when loss of *Pthlh* expression

is confined to osteoblasts.[59] For comparison, in mice in which *Pth* has been "knocked out" there is decreased mineralization of cartilage matrix, expression of vascular endothelial growth factor (VEGF) and neovascularization, osteoblast number, and trabecular bone volume.[62] Thus, PTH and PTHrP are necessary to normal fetal endochondral bone development. PTHrP has also been identified in the nucleus of chondrocytes and other cells, where it may regulate cell proliferation and act as a survival factor.[59,63] Cortical thickness of long bones is increased in *Pth*- and *Pthlh*-null mouse models, indicating that the regulation of endochondral and periosteal osteoblast function differs.

The placental transport of calcium is dependent on PTHrP produced by the placenta itself because the maternal-fetal calcium gradient is lost in its absence and may be restored by administration of a mid-molecular fragment.[59] PTH and PTHrP are required for normal mineral homeostasis *in utero*. In mice that lack PTGs, fetal serum calcium and magnesium concentrations are low and phosphate levels are elevated. To a lesser extent, similar changes occur with loss of expression of *Pthlh*.[64] PTH does not regulate placental calcium transfer, whereas PTHrP is essential to this process. During lactation, mammary expression of *PTHLH* and secretion of PTHrP increases—whereas production of estrogens declines, permitting unopposed PTHrP-induced mobilization of maternal skeletal calcium necessary for the breast-fed infant but substantially decreasing maternal bone mineral content (a process reversed when lactation ceases).[65,66]

PARATHYROID HORMONE AND PARATHYROID-HORMONE–RELATED PROTEIN RECEPTORS

PTH and PTHrP utilize a common receptor (PTHR1), through which most of the "classic" physiologic functions of these peptides are exerted. PTHR1 is a 585-aa protein that shares its structure with that of the B family of GPCRs (calcitonin, GH-releasing hormone, secretin, glucagon, vasoactive intestinal polypeptide, corticotropin-releasing hormone) that are characterized by long extracellular amino terminal domains (~100-aa residues) with multiple cysteine residues forming disulfide bridges.[25] As a result of alternative mRNA splicing, there are several isoforms of the PTH/PTHrP receptor. PTHR1 recognizes the amino terminal sequences of PTH[1-84] and PTHrP as essential to activation (aa 1–9) and binding (aa 15–34).[2,55]

The amino terminal extracellular domain of PTHR1 contains six conserved cysteine residues that form three disulfide bonds; clustered near the first transmembrane domain are four glycosylated asparagine residues. PTH[15-34] binds to the extracellular domain and loops of the transmembrane domains of PTHR1, whereas the amino terminal of PTH[1-84] interacts with the transmembrane domains and their connecting extra- and intracellular loops (termed the J or juxtamembrane domain) to activate G_s- and G_q-proteins and their respective signal transduction pathways.[67]

PTHR1 is expressed in renal tubular cells and osteoblasts, skin, breast, heart, and pancreas, among other tissues—the latter sites reflecting the paracrine targets of PTHrP. It is coupled primarily through G_s-protein to adenylyl cyclase, cyclic AMP, and PKA—the initiating steps in intracellular transduction of the PTH signal. PTHR1 also activates G_q-proteins, thereby stimulating PLC activity and leading to hydrolysis of membrane phosphatidylinositol 1,4,5-trisphosphate to IP_3 and diacylglycerol, activation of PKC, release of Ca^{2+} from intracellular storage sites, and stimulation of the MAPK signal transduction pathway. PTH and calcitriol decrease expression of *PTHR1*.

Targeted loss of *PTHR1* is accompanied by impaired proliferation of chondrocytes and acceleration of chondrocyte maturation and calcification, an outcome mimicked by targeted loss of $G_{s\alpha}$ in chondrocytes.[55,59] Constitutively activating mutations of PTHR1 leads to hypercalcemia and Jansen metaphyseal chondrodysplasia, whereas inactivating mutations results in hypocalcemia and Blomstrand chondrodysplasia. The abnormalities of chondrocyte maturation seen experimentally with inactivating mutations of *Pthr1* are mimicked to an extent by loss of PTHrP function as well. Loss of PTH results in aberrant formation of primary spongiosa of long bone and in defective mineralization.[62]

After activation of the G-protein is complete, PTHR1 is phosphorylated by a GPCR kinase. It then associates with β-arrestin proteins and undergoes endocytosis. By an alternate pathway, carboxyl terminal PTH peptides may also promote endocytosis of PTHR1.[55] Once internalized, PTHR1 may be degraded, recycled to the cell membrane, or directed to the nucleus by importins-α_1 and -β where it is found in the nucleoplasm.[68] The role of nuclear PTHR1 in relaying the many biologic effects of PTH and PTHrP is unknown at present, but one can speculate that it might interact with DNA directly to regulate gene transcription.

A second PTH receptor *(PTHR2)* is selectively activated by PTH but does not recognize PTHrP. PTH specificity is determined by Ile^5 and Trp^{23} in native PTH, sites that affect activation and binding, respectively.[55] *PTHR2* encodes a 539-aa GPCR with 70% homology to PTHR1 that activates adenylyl cyclase. It is expressed predominantly in brain, testis, placenta, and pancreas, but not in bone or kidney. Its physiologic role is uncertain.[69] In response to PTH^{1-84}, PTHR2 enhances both cyclic AMP generation and Ca^{2+} mobilization. However, the naturally occurring endogenous ligand for PTHR2 is not PTH but is likely to be the 39-aa PTH-related hypothalamic tuberoinfundibular peptide (TIP39). This protein is also expressed in the testis and various central nervous system regions. TIP39, PTH, and PTHrP may have evolved from a common ancestral protein. A third PTH receptor that recognizes amino terminal sequences of PTH has been identified in zebra fish and is termed the type-3 zPTH receptor (zPTHR3). Rat PTH binds to this receptor and activates adenylyl cyclase.[55] This species also expresses a PTHR1-like protein. A human homolog for zPTHR3 has not been identified to date. Specific receptors recognizing the amino terminal sequences of PTHrP have been found in brain and skin. PTHrP stimulates release of arginine vasopressin from the supraoptic nucleus *in vitro*.[55]

Although as yet not specifically characterized, receptors for carboxyl terminal fragments of PTH^{1-84} have been identified as renal and bone cell binding sites for PTH^{1-84} from which intact hormone can be only partially displaced by PTH^{1-34} but can be further displaced by PTH^{53-84} and PTH^{69-84}.[55] In addition, in osteocytes, osteoblasts, and chondrocytes from which the PTH/PTHrP receptor has been knocked out and to which intact PTH^{1-84} but not PTH^{1-34} binds, labeled PTH^{1-84} can be displaced by carboxyl terminal $PTH^{19-84,\ 28-84,}$ $^{39-84}$ fragments. Important determinants for binding of PTH to the carboxyl terminal selective receptor(s) appear to be aa 24 through 27 (Leu-Arg-Lys-Lys) and aa 53 and 54 (Lys-Lys).

Furthermore, carboxyl terminal fragments of PTH exert biologic effects in intact and *PTHR1*-null cells—such as regulation of alkaline phosphatase activity in osteosarcoma cells and osteoblasts (but not generation of collagen type I), stimulation of Ca^{2+} uptake by osteosarcoma cells and chondrocytes, and cell survival *in vitro*. Thus, the physiologic actions of PTH likely reflect the integrated sum of the individual functions of the intact hormone and its carboxyl terminal fragments. Because carboxyl terminal fragments of PTHrP are not recognized by the membrane sites that bind carboxyl terminal fragments of PTH, a means of specifying cellular response to these closely related proteins potentially exists.

Calcitonin

Calcitonin is a 32-aa peptide that in mammals is secreted by the neural-crest–derived parafollicular (C) cells of the thyroid gland. It inhibits osteoclastic bone resorption, thus lowering blood calcium concentrations.[70] It is encoded by a six-exon gene *(CALCA)* that by alternative transcription and translation can form two products: a 141-aa protein from which calcitonin (exons 1-4) and katacalcin (a 21-aa hypocalcemic peptide adjacent to the carboxyl terminus of calcitonin) are derived and a 128-amino-acid protein from which is gleaned the 37-aa calcitonin-gene-related peptide-α (exons 1-3, 5, 6)—a vasodilator and neurotransmitter that also interacts with the calcitonin receptor. Calcitonin is also expressed by cells in the adenohypophysis and brain, and by neuroendocrine cells in the lung and elsewhere.

Calcitonin is produced in abundance by medullary carcinoma of the thyroid, and at times by other neuroendocrine tumors. The calcitonins of multiple species share similar structures, including five of the first seven amino terminal aa, a disulfide bridge between aa 1 and aa 7, glycine at aa residue 28, and a proline amide residue at carboxyl terminal aa 32. In the interior of the peptide, species other than human have several basic amino acids that make them more stable and easily recognized by the human calcitonin receptor and thus more biologically potent (e.g., therapeutically useful salmon calcitonin).

Calcitonin secretion is stimulated primarily by increasing serum concentrations of Ca^{2+}_e transduced by the CaSR expressed on the plasma membrane of the parafollicular cell.[2] Members of the gastrin-cholecystokinin intestinal peptide hormone family (gastrin, glucagon, pancreozymin) are also potent calcitonin secretagogues.[70]

Calcium, pentagastrin, and glucagon are effective stimuli employed to assess calcitonin secretion clinically. Somatostatin, calcitriol, and chromogranin A[1-40] inhibit (and chromogranin A[403-428] stimulates) calcitonin secretion. Calcitonin secretion falls as the ambient Ca^{2+}_e concentration declines.

The half-life of calcitonin is brief. It is metabolized primarily by the kidney but also by liver, bone, and thyroid gland. Serum levels of calcitonin are high in the fetus and newborn, fall rapidly after birth as serum Ca^{2+}_e values decline, and then fall more slowly (until three years of age)—remaining relatively constant thereafter (<12 pg/mL). After 10 years of age, serum concentrations of calcitonin are higher in males than in females. The physiologic role of calcitonin is unclear because serum calcium concentrations are normal in patients with both decreased (primary congenital or acquired hypothyroidism) and increased (medullary carcinoma of the thyroid) secretion of this peptide. However, disposal of a calcium load is slower in the calcitonin-deficient subject. Immunoassayable concentrations of calcitonin are increased in patients with medullary carcinoma of the thyroid, chronic renal insufficiency, and pycnodysostosis.[70] Individual commercial immunoassays for calcitonin may detect differing epitopes, have altered intra-assay dynamics, and provide inconsistent measurements.[71]

The biologic effects of calcitonin are mediated through its 490-aa GPCR encoded by *CALCR*, a member of the B family of GPCRs. Intracellular signaling of the CALCR is transduced through the adenylyl cyclase-cyclic AMP-PKA signal transduction pathway. Alternative splicing of *CALCR* results in two isoforms of the calcitonin receptor, one of which has an additional 16-aa inserted into its first intracellular loop between transdomains I and II. Accessory proteins that modulate function of the calcitonin receptor have also been described.[70] The calcitonin receptor is expressed in osteoclasts. When exposed to calcitonin, the osteoclast shrinks and bone resorbing activity declines quickly. Thus, calcitonin lowers serum calcium and phosphate levels—particularly in patients with hypercalcemia.

Polymorphic variants of *CALCR* have been related to variations in bone mineral density (BMD). In subjects heterozygous at aa 463 (Pro/Leu) in the third intracellular domain, BMD is greater than in individuals who are homozygous for either amino acid.[72] However, for the most part there has been little evidence that calcitonin plays a major role in mineral and skeletal homeostasis. In lactating women, serum levels of calcitonin rise and calcitonin is excreted in breast milk. Women who are breastfeeding their infants lose 5% to 10% of their trabecular bone mineral during 6 months of lactation. This is recouped rapidly when lactation ceases—much more quickly than when bone mass is lost because of other problems (e.g., glucocorticoid excess, bed rest).

Experimentally, in the female mouse in which the gene encoding calcitonin has been eliminated loss of calcitonin has no effect on maternal bone mineralization during pregnancy or on the rate of skeletal remineralization after weaning of pups. However, 21 days of lactation are associated with much more marked demineralization of the spine of the nursing mother without calcitonin than in the wt female—a response that is reversible by the administration of exogenous calcitonin during the interval of lactation.[73] Thus, in mammals calcitonin may be essential to the protection of maternal skeletal mass during lactation.

Vitamin D

Cholecalciferol (vitamin D_3) is synthesized in skin from cholesterol through 7-dehydrocholesterol. It is also present in oily fish such as salmon and mackerel. Ergocalciferol (vitamin D_2) is a plant and yeast sterol[74] (Figure 3-3). Vitamin D_2 differs from vitamin D_3 by the presence of a double bond between carbons 22 and 23 and a methyl group on carbon 24 in vitamin D_2. Both forms of vitamin D undergo similar chemical modifications to bioactive metabolites. However, physiologically vitamin D_2 is 3- to 10-fold less biologically effective in man than is vitamin D_3 because its product (25-hydroxyvitamin D_2) is cleared much more rapidly from serum than is 25-hydroxyvitamin D_3.[75] In skin, provitamin D_3 7-dehydrocholesterol is transformed to previtamin D_3 and then isomerized to vitamin D_3 by exposure to ultraviolet B-photon radiation (290–315 nm) and heat (37° C).[74,76]

The latitude, season of the year, and time of day influence the rate of synthesis of vitamin D_3 stimulated by exposure to sunlight. In higher latitudes, the path through which ultraviolet B photons from the sun travel is longer and fewer reach the target. Exposure of the back of a white adult to intense summer sun (mid July) for 10 to 12 minutes in the northeastern United States generates ~10,000 to 20,000 IU of vitamin D_3 over the next 24-hour interval.[19] (For black persons, 30 to 120 minutes of exposure to sunlight may be required for comparable effects.) Sun-screening agents and aging also decrease the cutaneous formation of cholecalciferol in response to sunlight.

Orally ingested vitamin D is packaged into chylomicrons and absorbed into the intestinal lymphatic system. It then enters the circulation and is transported to the liver by vitamin-D–binding protein (DBP), a polymorphic variant of the serum α2-globulin termed Gc (group-specific component) encoded by *GC*. In the liver, vitamin D is hydroxylated to 25-hydroxyvitamin D (25OHD; calcidiol is 25OHD$_3$) by vitamin D-25 hydroxylase—a 501-aa class I mitochondrial cytochrome P450 enzyme encoded by *CYP2R1*. In addition, there are other hepatic 25-hydroxylases that carry out this reaction (CYP27A1, CYP2J3).[74] Calcidiol exerts only a minimal inhibitory effect on its production. Thus, serum concentrations of 25OHD reflect body stores of vitamin D.

There are substantial data indicating that because of decreased exposure to sunlight and marginal dietary intake of vitamin D_3 body stores of this vitamin are deficient or insufficient in many North American subjects.[19] In addition, currently established normal values for serum concentrations of 25-hydroxyvitamin D (25OHD, 10–55 ng/mL) have likely been derived from populations that are not completely vitamin D sufficient. In populations

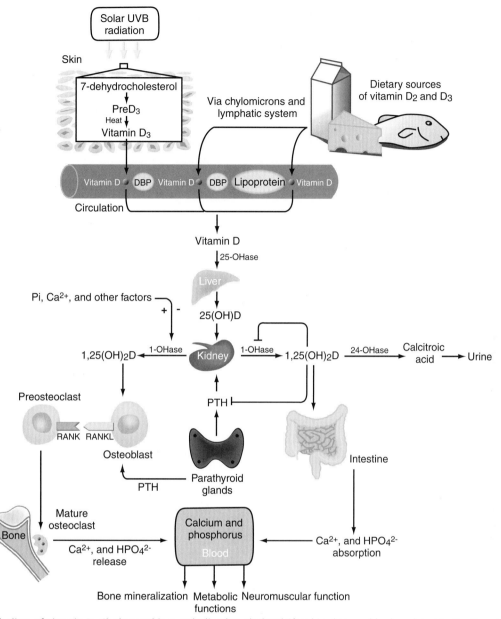

Figure 3-3. Metabolism of vitamin D. Cholesterol is metabolized to cholecalciferol in skin, and hydroxylated in the liver to calcidiol and in the kidney to calcitriol. Factors that regulate these processes are depicted (see text). [Reproduced with permission from Holick MF (2006). Resurrection of vitamin D deficiency and rickets. J Clin Invest 116:2062-2072.]

living in sun-rich environments, the lower normal concentration of serum 25OHD is 32 ng/mL—with a range to 100 ng/mL. Physiologic data such as the relationship between serum concentrations of 25OHD and those of PTH, intestinal absorption of calcium, and optimal bone mineralization support the concept that a serum 25OHD level of 32 ng/mL is the minimum normal value in humans and that 25OHD concentrations between 10 and 30 should be considered insufficient.

Although the current officially recommended minimal supplemental dose of vitamin D for breast and formula-fed infants and older children and adolescents is 200 IU/day, it is likely that 400 IU/day (10 μg) is more appropriate. It has been suggested that children, adolescents,

adults, and pregnant and nursing women should receive 400 to 600 IU (10-15 μg) of supplemental vitamin D daily. Some data suggest that the daily required amount of supplemental vitamin D may be closer to 2,000 IU/day (50 μg), and even more in pregnant and lactating women.[19,76,77]

Bound to DBP, calcidiol is transported to cells in the proximal convoluted and straight renal tubules. There it is further hydroxylated to the biologically active metabolite 1,25-dihydroxyvitamin D_3 [$1,25(OH)_2D_3$ or calcitriol] by the cytochrome P450 mitochondrial monooxygenase 25OHD-1α-hydroxylase encoded by *CYP27B1*.[78,79] *CYP27B1* has nine exons that encode a 508-aa protein with a mitochondrial signal sequence at its amino terminal and ferredoxin- and heme-binding sites within its structure. As a class I mitochondrial cytochrome P450 enzyme, 25OHD-1α-hydroxylase requires for catalytic activity electrons from NADPH that are ferried to the enzyme protein by the electron transport proteins ferredoxin and ferredoxin reductase.[80]

Although *CYP27B1* is expressed primarily in renal proximal convoluted and straight tubular cells, it may also be expressed by keratinocytes and hair follicles, osteoblasts, placental decidual and trophoblastic cells, the gastrointestinal and central nervous systems, testes, breast, and pancreatic islets. In monocytes and macrophages, expression of *CYP27B1* may be induced by inflammatory cytokines such as interferon-γ.[81] In the kidney, expression of *CYP27B1* in the proximal convoluted tubules is stimulated by PTH through cyclic AMP and in the straight tubules by calcitonin by a pathway independent of cyclic AMP. In addition, activity of 25OHD-1α-hydroxylase is increased by hypocalcemia and hypophosphatemia, PTHrP, 24R,25(OH)$_2$D$_3$, GH, insulin-like growth factor-I (IGF-I), and prolactin.[82]

Increased serum and tissue levels of Ca^{2+} and phosphate directly suppress expression of *CYP27B1* and thus depress 25OHD-1α-hydroxylase activity. Calcitriol exerts an indirect inhibitory effect upon renal *CYP27B1* expression and thus upon its own synthesis by inhibition of PTH synthesis in the PTG.[76] In activated monocytes, calcitriol actually enhances transcription of *CYP27B1*.[81] FGF23 depresses 25OHD-1α-hydroxylase activity, whereas calcitriol up-regulates FGF23 expression—effectively establishing an auto-control system for these compounds.[41] Inactivating mutations of *CYP27B1* result in vitamin-D–dependent rickets type I or 1α-hydroxylase deficiency (OMIM 264700), a disorder associated with hypocalcemia, hypophosphatemia, secondary hyperparathyroidism, severe rickets, and often alopecia.

Calcitriol is inactivated in bone, intestine, liver, and kidney by glucuronidation, sulfation, multisite (carbons 23, 24, and 26) hydroxylation, and lactone formation to water-soluble compounds (such as calcitroic acid) excreted in urine and bile.[76] In the kidney, 25OHD and 1,25(OH)$_2$D are converted to 24R,25(OH)$_2$D and 1,24R,25(OH)$_3$D, respectively, by 25OHD-24 hydroxylase encoded by *CYP24A1*—the first in a series of degradative hydroxylations. The expression of this gene is up-regulated by hypercalcemia, hyperphosphatemia, and calcitriol and is suppressed by hypocalcemia and PTH. Cleavage of the side chain between carbons 23 and 24 [which have been hydroxylated by hepatic cytochrome P450-3A (*CYP3A4*)-dependent enzymes] generates water-soluble calcitroic acid.[74]

Many drugs (e.g., phenobarbital, phenytoin, carbamazepine, rifampicin) that are known to impair bone mineralization by inactivating calcitriol do so by increasing its state of hydroxylation by binding to and activating the nuclear pregnane X receptor (*NR1I2*), which in turn increases expression of *CYP3A4*.[83] Calcitriol may also induce expression of hydroxylases that utilize cytochrome P450-3A, thereby enhancing its own hydroxylation and degradation.[84] Bound to DBP, calcidiol is filtered through the glomerular membrane and reabsorbed

by cells in the proximal renal tubule by the multifunctional receptor megalin (gp330)—expressed in coated pits on the luminal/apical surface, endocytic vacuoles, and lysosomes of proximal tubular cells.[28]

After uptake, the megalin-calcidiol complex enters the lysosome—where calcidiol is released, enters the cytosol, and is metabolized to calcitriol in mitochondria. The bulk of circulating calcitriol is bound to DBP, but it is its free fraction that is biologically active. Approximately 0.04% of calcidiol and 0.4% of calcitriol are present in free form in serum. Normal ranges of calcitriol concentrations are 8 to 72 pg/mL for neonates, 15 to 90 pg/mL for infants and children, and 21 to 65 pg/mL for adults.

Once calcitriol is synthesized, its three-dimensional configuration is flexible rather than fixed—enabling it to exert both genomic and nongenomic (rapid-response) actions.[85] The nuclear VDR serves as a transactivating transcription factor after binding to its ligand, calcitriol. The VDR is also associated with caveolae of the cell plasma membrane, flask-shaped invaginations of the membrane composed to a large extent of sphingolipids and cholesterol.[85,86] Through binding to the nuclear VDR, calcitriol regulates the expression of many genes involved in mineral and bone metabolism. These effects take place over hours to days as the processes of transcription, translation, and post-translational modifications to the encoded protein(s) occur in multiple cytosolic compartments.

Calcitriol also generates rapid responses evident within seconds to minutes after its contact with the cell. Examples of rapid cellular responses to calcitriol include immediate intestinal absorption of calcium (transcaltachia), opening of voltage-gated calcium and chloride channels in osteoblasts, endothelial cell migration, and pancreatic β cell secretion of insulin.[85] The three-dimensional flexibility of calcitriol structure is enabled by rotation of side chain carbon pairs 17-20, 20-22, 22-23, 23-24, and 24-25; by rotation of the carbon 6-7 bond around the B ring, and by A-ring chair-chair interconversion with formation of either an α- or β-configuration of the cyclohexane-like A ring (Figure 3-4). Rotation about the carbon 6-7 bond of the B ring allows calcitriol to assume an extended 6-s configuration or a 6-s-*cis* conformation. It is the trans form of calcitriol that is employed by the VDR for its genomic responses and the *cis* form for its rapid actions. For binding to DBP, calcitriol assumes yet another shape.[85]

Calcitriol primarily regulates intestinal and renal absorption of calcium and phosphate by enhancing expression of genes encoding calcium transporters and channels [e.g., calbindin-D$_{28K}$, calbindin-D$_{9K}$, TRPV5 (expressed primarily in the kidney) and TRPV6 (expressed predominantly in the intestinal tract)]. Calcitriol also promotes endochondral bone formation and increases length of the long bones by amplifying epiphyseal volume, proliferation, and differentiation of chondrocytes and mineralization of cartilage matrix.[87]

Furthermore, this sterol increases trabecular and cortical bone formation by augmenting osteoblast number and function—including alkaline phosphatase activity, osteocalcin synthesis, and type I collagen formation—and by

Vitamin D: Trans and CIS Configurations

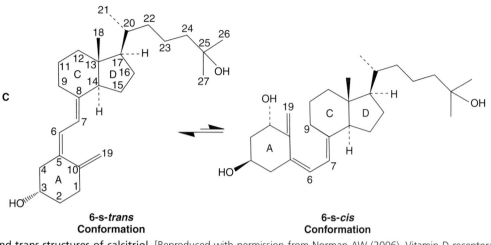

Figure 3-4. Cis and trans structures of calcitriol. [Reproduced with permission from Norman AW (2006). Vitamin D receptor: New assignments for an already busy receptor. Endocrinology 147:5542-5548.]

repressing bone resorption by osteoclasts. It does so by a direct cellular effect independent of endogenous PTH, evidenced by its activity in the mouse in which both *CYP27B1* and *Pth* have been knocked out.[87] Calcitriol directly suppresses transcription of *PTH* in the PTG, acting through the VDR. Vitamin D is also important for normal muscle development and is an integral component of the system requisite for achievement of optimal skeletal integrity and strength.[88]

Mediated by the VDR, calcitriol stimulates the absorption or reabsorption of calcium in the intestines, bone, and kidney. In the duodenum and proximal small intestine, calcitriol increases the efficiency of calcium uptake from the intestinal lumen by increasing the number of epithelial calcium transport channels (TRPV6) in enterocytes, its movement through the cytoplasm, and its transfer across the basal lateral membrane into the circulation—in part by the induction of calbindin$_{9k}$ (a calcium-binding protein), alkaline phosphatase, Ca-ATPase, calmodulin, and other proteins.[74] Calcitriol also increases jejunal and ileal absorption of phosphate through a transcellular mechanism utilizing the type II Na$^+$-HPO$_4^{2-}$ cotransporter protein (NPT2, encoded by *SLC34A1*) expressed on the luminal surface of the enterocyte.

When vitamin D stores are replete, 40% of dietary calcium and 80% of dietary phosphate may be absorbed. Even greater efficiency of mineral absorption is realized during growth spurts, pregnancy, and lactation. A major task of calcitriol is to maintain calcium and phosphate concentrations in blood at levels sufficient to sustain mineralization of osteoid-collagen-containing bone matrix synthesized by osteoblasts. Paradoxically, in states of calcium deficiency calcitriol acts indirectly within bone to stimulate monocytic stem cell differentiation into osteoclasts by stimulating osteoblast/stromal cell synthesis of osteoclast-activating factors such as the ligand for the receptor activator of nuclear factor κB (RANKL).

During periods of calcium deficiency, calcitriol is also able to promote bone resorption through osteoblast production of osteopontin—a bone matrix noncollagenous protein to which osteoclast cell surface integrin receptors bind.[89] Calcitriol stimulates osteoblasts to produce osteocalcin, bone-specific alkaline phosphatase, osteoprotegerin, osteonectin, and various cytokines.[74]

In addition to the classic effects of calcitriol upon mineral and skeletal metabolism, vitamin D and synthetically constructed ligands of the VDR have many non-calcemic actions.[90] Among the several synthetic vitamin D$_3$ analogues are alfacalcidiol [1α-(OH)D$_3$], calcipotriol [1α,25-(OH)$_2$-24-cyclopropyl-D$_3$], maxacalcitrol [1α,25-(OH)$_2$-22-oxa-D$_3$], and talcitol [1α,24R-(OH)$_2$D$_3$]. These vitamin D analogues have been engineered to retain the non-calcemic actions of the parent compound and reduce calcemic properties. Calcitriol and vitamin D$_3$ analogues exert many immunomodulatory effects.

In animal models of autoimmune diseases such as systemic lupus erythematosis, multiple sclerosis, type I diabetes mellitus, and inflammatory bowel disease, these agents inhibit T-lymphocyte differentiation into Th1 [IL-2, tumor necrosis factor (TNF)-α, and interferon-γ secreting] cells and thereby modify disease induction, course, and severity. Calcitriol and analogues also exert differentiating and antiproliferative effects on a variety of cells. Thus, calcitriol induces differentiation of promyelocytes into monocytes and macrophages.

These agents enhance differentiation of keratinocytes, and when administered orally or topically to patients with psoriasis vulgaris effectively ameliorate the disease. They are particularly effective when coadministered with a topical glucocorticoid. *In vitro*, calcitriol and its analogues inhibit growth of prostate, breast, and colon cancer cell lines—and clinical trials of these agents in patients with these neoplasms appear promising. Calcitriol and several of its analogues have been employed successfully in the treatment of osteoporosis, secondary hyperparathyroidism, and arthritis.[90] Calcitriol also enhances secretion of insulin and down-regulates activity of the renin-angiotensin system.[74]

VITAMIN D RECEPTOR

Calcitriol acts primarily by binding to the VDR, a 427-aa protein encoded by 11-exon *VDR*.[91] Because of two potential start site codons for transcription of VDR in exon 2, there is a second isoform of VDR with 424 aa. At its 5' end, the VDR has three noncoding exons (1A, 1B, 1C)—followed by exons 2 through 9, which encode the active protein [enabling transcription of three unique mRNA isoforms, depending on the splicing pattern of exons 1B and 1C (Figure 3-5A)].

As a member of the steroid/thyroid/vitamin-D receptor gene superfamily of nuclear-transcription–activating factors, the VDR has five domains: a short amino terminal segment of 24 aa (domains A/B) that houses a ligand-independent transactivation function termed activation function-*1* (AF-1), a DNA-binding domain (C) with two zinc fingers (exons 2 and 3), a "hinge" region (D), and a long carboxyl terminal ligand-binding domain (E) (exons 7, 8, 9). Structurally, the E domain consists of 12 α-helixes (H1–H12) and has two ligand-dependent transactivating regions (E1 between aa 232 and 272 and AF2 between aa 416 and 424) that recruit transcriptional cofactors when the VDR is activated by binding to calcitriol.[91]

Among the stimulants to the transcription of VDR are calcitonin, retinoic acid, estrogen, the transcription factor SP1, and β-catenin. In part, estrogens increase expression of VDR through binding to estrogen receptors present in the caveolae of the cell membrane and then through activation of the MAPK signal transduction pathway.[92] The *VDR* is expressed in the intestinal tract, distal renal tubule, osteoblast, keratinocyte, hair follicle, fibroblast, smooth and cardiac muscle, lung, bladder, thyroid, parathyroid, pancreas, adrenal cortex and medulla, pituitary, placenta, uterus, ovary, testis, prostate, activated T and B lymphocytes, macrophages, monocytes, spleen, thymus and tonsil, brain, spinal cord, and sensory ganglia.

Allelic polymorphisms (random variations in gene composition not known to affect structure or function) of VDR have been related to bone mineralization and linear growth (Figure 3-5B). These gene variants have been identified by examining restriction fragment length

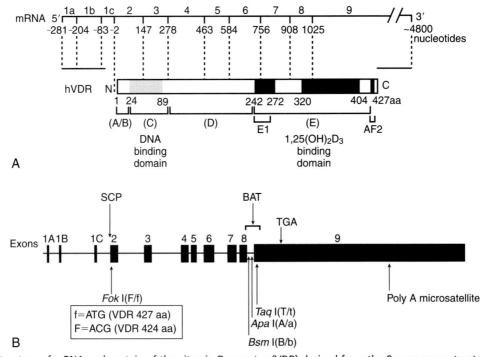

Figure 3-5. *(A)* Structure of mRNA and protein of the vitamin D receptor (VDR) derived from the 9-exon gene structure of VDR. The five domains of the VDR are depicted. Exons 2 and 3 encode the DNA-binding domain, and exons 7 through 9 encode the ligand-binding domain. Sites E1 and AF2 are subregions within the E domain that serve transactivating functions. Regions of homology shared with other members of the nuclear receptor steroid/thyroid hormone/vitamin-D superfamily are indicated by the gray and black areas. *(B)* Polymorphic variants of VDR. By convention, uppercase letters denote the absence (and lowercase letters the presence) of a polymorphic restriction site. The site of the start codon polymorphism (SCP) is depicted above the gene structure. It generates a FokI polymorphism and generates vitamin D receptor proteins of different lengths. The site of the BAT polymorphism is indicated above intron 10/exon 9. The BsmI, ApaI, and TaqI restriction sites are placed below the VDR gene structure. These polymorphic variants do not change the amino acid structure of the VDR. In exon 9, there is a poly A microsatellite of variable length. [Reproduced with permission from Malloy PJ, et al. (1999). The vitamin D receptor and the syndrome of hereditary 1,25-dihydroxyvitamin D-resistant rickets. Endocrine Reviews 20:156–188.]

polymorphisms (DNA fragments of varying lengths) defined by endonuclease digestion of *VDR* DNA by BsmI (B), TaqI (T), FokI (F), and ApaI (A). For example, in *VDR* there are BsmI cut sites in the 3' region and in exon 10. By convention, BB indicates absence of a BsmI cut site on both alleles, bb the presence of the cut site on both alleles, and Bb the heterozygous state.[91,93]

The BB *VDR* genotype has been variably associated with lower BMD in postmenopausal women and adult men, whereas the aa, bb, and TT genotypes have been linked to higher BMD in prepubertal girls.[94] Polymorphic variants of the *VDR* have also been associated with differences in intestinal calcium absorption (subjects with the bb genotype on a low-calcium diet absorb ingested calcium to a greater extent than do those with the BB pattern), in birth length (BB neonatal males are shorter than Bb and bb male infants), in growth in infancy (at 2 years of age BB girls are longer and heavier than bb girls, BB boys weigh less than bb boys although of similar length, and at 1 year of age tt infant females are heavier than TT or Tt subjects), in pubertal growth (boys with the BB genotype are smaller than their Bb and bb peers through puberty), and in adult stature (the adult stature of subjects with the bT haplotype is on average 1.6 cm greater than that of individuals with other haplotypes).[95,96] Polymorphic variants of *VDR* have also been linked to development of hyperparathyroidism and parathyroid tumors. The mechanism(s) by which polymorphic variants might exert these effects (or even if the associations are meaningful) is unclear. However, it has been suggested that the polymorphisms may influence the expression of the *VDR* or its function.

Whereas most members of the superfamily of nuclear-receptor–transactivating factors pair as homodimers to bind to their specific hormone response elements in the 5'-untranslated region of the target gene, the calcitriol-VDR complex teams through its E (ligand-binding) domain with its obligate partner [unliganded retinoid X receptor α *(RXRA)*] to form a heterodimer that then binds to a VDRE. The endogenous ligand for RXRα is 9-cis-retinoic acid. When unliganded, the bulk of the VDR is cytoplasmic. Binding of calcitriol to the VDR leads to heterodimerization with RXRα and translocation of the tripartite complex to the nucleus. However, the unliganded VDR can also be guided to its target gene within the nucleus by a multi-protein chromatin-remodeling complex termed WINAC (where it remains inactive until bound by calcitriol).[97]

The generic VDRE, located in the 5' upstream promoter region of the target gene, is composed of two directly repeated hexanucleotide sequences (5'-AG-G/T-TCA-3') separated by three base pairs (bp). RXRα binds to the 5' half of the VDRE, and the VDR to its 3' segment. After binding to the VDRE, the calcitriol-VDR-RXR complex recruits coactivating or corepressing comodulating proteins (e.g., SRC/p160 family, TRIP/SUG1, CPB/p300, TIF1, NcooR-1RIP13) into the promoter site and the general transcription apparatus of the target gene (TF-IIA, -B, TAF family).[90,91] Gene activation by the VDR complex is initiated by recruitment of a histone acetyltransferase complex to the promoter segment of the gene that destabilizes the region and leads to unwinding of DNA, thereby granting

access to basal transcription factors and RNA polymerase II that bring about RNA modeling of the target gene.

In addition to positive and negative regulation of target gene expression through binding to the VDRE, the VDR complex may also affect transcription by modifying the effect of other transcription factors.[90] Corepressors cause chromatin to compact, thereby silencing gene expression. Genes whose expression is regulated by the VDR are listed in Figure 3-6. Calcitriol acting through the VDR stimulates transcription or genes encoding calcium transport proteins (TRPV5/6), bone matrix proteins (osteopontin, osteocalcin), bone reabsorption factors (RANKL), and 25OHD-24-hydroxylase—and represses those that encode PTH and PTHrP. The calcitriol-VDR complex represses expression of multiple cytokines (IL-2, interferon-γ, granulocyte macrophage-colony stimulating factor) by negatively interacting with transcription factors that enhance their transcription (e.g., NF-κB).

Although the VDR is necessary for the actions of calcitriol in the intestines, kidney, bone, skin, and elsewhere, its loss does not interfere with embryogenesis and fetal development in humans with loss-of-function mutations in *Vdr* and vitamin D resistance or in mice in which *Vdr* has been knocked out. Newborn mice homozygous for targeted deletion of the second zinc finger (exon 3) and resultant truncation of the *Vdr* survive fetal life, appear normal at birth, and grow well for the first 24 days of life.[98] However, after weaning their rates of weight gain and linear growth and serum Ca^{2+}_e and phosphate levels decline and serum PTH concentrations and PTG weights increase.

In *Vdr*[-/-] mice as young as 15 days of age, osteoid surface is increased, bone mineralization decreased, and epiphyseal plate cartilage formation disorganized—with irregular columns of chondrocytes, increased matrix, and excessive vascularity relative to wt-type or heterozygous (*Vdr*[+/-]) mice.[69,99] In mice in which both *Vdr* and *Rxra* have been knocked out, development of the cartilage growth plate is even more disrupted than in *Vdr*[-/-] pups.[100] In addition, hair loss begins at 4 weeks of age and is complete by 4 months of age in homozygous *Vdr*[-/-] animals and is due to a defect in the growth cycle of hair follicles, a phenocopy of the generalized alopecia associated with loss of hairless *(HR)*, a transcriptional corepressor that interacts with the *VDR*.[90] (Vitamin D deficiency alone does not interfere with hair growth.)

At approximately 8 weeks of age, *Vdr*[-/-] mice are a bit smaller than their wt counterparts and have lower calcium concentrations and cortical bone density and thickness—although trabecular bone density is similar in *Vdr*[-/-] and wt animals.[101] *Vdr*[-/-] mice usually succumb between 4 and 6 months of age. However, maintenance of normal serum concentrations of calcium and phosphate by the feeding of high calcium-phosphate diets to *Vdr*[-/-] pups beginning at 16 days of age prevents the development of all of the skeletal abnormalities—suggesting that the main physiologic effects of calcitriol and the VDR are upon the intestinal absorption of calcium and phosphate and the maintenance of normal serum concentrations of these ions.[99] In pregnant *Vdr*[-/-] 8-week-old mice, fetal (*Vdr*[+/-]) epiphyseal cartilage is histologically abnormal and skeleton

Genes Regulated by Calcitriol/VDR

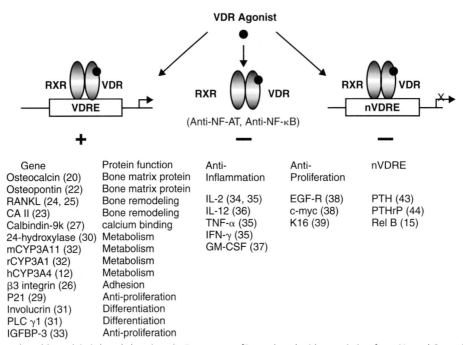

Gene	Protein function	Anti-Inflammation	Anti-Proliferation	nVDRE
Osteocalcin (20)	Bone matrix protein			
Osteopontin (22)	Bone matrix protein			
RANKL (24, 25)	Bone remodeling	IL-2 (34, 35)	EGF-R (38)	PTH (43)
CA II (23)	Bone remodeling	IL-12 (36)	c-myc (38)	PTHrP (44)
Calbindin-9k (27)	calcium binding	TNF-α (35)	K16 (39)	Rel B (15)
24-hydroxylase (30)	Metabolism	IFN-γ (35)		
mCYP3A11 (32)	Metabolism	GM-CSF (37)		
rCYP3A1 (32)	Metabolism			
hCYP3A4 (12)	Metabolism			
β3 integrin (26)	Adhesion			
P21 (29)	Anti-proliferation			
Involucrin (31)	Differentiation			
PLC γ1 (31)	Differentiation			
IGFBP-3 (33)	Anti-proliferation			

Figure 3-6. Genes regulated by calcitriol and the vitamin D receptor. [Reproduced with permission from Nagpal S, et al. (2005). Noncalcemic actions of vitamin D receptor ligands. Endocrine Reviews 26:662-687.]

mineralization subnormal. Both defects can be reversed by increasing maternal dietary calcium and phosphate intake.[101] Thus, absorption of intestinal calcium by non vitamin-D–dependent mechanisms can bypass the absorptive defect caused by loss of the VDR and by inference the deficiency of vitamin D itself.

As previously discussed, in addition to acting through the nuclear VDR to regulate gene expression calcitriol also has rapid nongenomic effects mediated through plasma membrane caveolae-associated VDRs (Figure 3-7).[85] The classic ligand-binding domain of the VDR recognizes the 6-s-*trans* configuration of calcitriol, whereas the 6-s-*cis* shape of the VDR mediates the nongenomic actions of calcitriol. An alternative VDR ligand binding domain that overlaps with the classic domain and accommodates the 6-s-*cis* conformation of calcitriol has been tentatively identified.[85] The mechanism(s) by which the 6-s-*trans* and 6-s-*cis* forms of calcitriol recognize the genomic or nongenomic "pockets" of the VDR has not been established at this writing.

In vitro, calcitriol induces expression of several membrane-associated rapid-response steroid-binding (MARRS) proteins such as the multifunctional thioredoxin-interacting protein-2 (TXNIP) and its homologue TXNIP-like inducible membrane protein, both of which are situated on the interior of the cell plasma membrane.[102-104] After binding of calcitriol to the plasma membrane-associated VDR, its signal is transmitted by several classical intracellular signal transduction systems—including adenylyl cyclase induction of cyclic AMP and PKA; PLC- and PLD-mediated increase in phosphoinositide turnover resulting in generation of 1,2-diacylglycerol and IP$_3$ that increase the permeability of

Ca^{2+} channels and release Ca^{2+} from cytosolic storage sites; G$_q$ protein through PLC-β1 activation and intracellular redistribution of PKC isoforms (α, β, δ); and Jun-activated kinase and the MAPK pathway.[102]

Within minutes after exposure of a vitamin-D–responsive tissue (e.g., intestine, chondrocyte, osteoblast) to calcitriol, there is increase in the intracellular concentration of Ca^{2+}$_i$ (transcaltachia) and activation of PLC, PKC, and MAPK.[85] In osteoblasts from *VDR$^{-/-}$* mice and in fibroblasts from patients with inactivating mutations of *VDR*, the rapid actions of calcitriol are lost—as is the association of the VDR with caveolae (evidence of the importance of the VDR to membrane-initiated responses to calcitriol).[102] The plasma membrane caveolae-associated VDR may link to G$_{sα}$ and thence to a calcium channel, to adenylyl cyclase, to PLC, or to caveolin—a protein that interacts with the nonreceptor tyrosine kinase Src and in turn with PLC or the kinase h-Ras.[102,105]

The physiologic role(s) of the rapid actions of vitamin D are not certain. In chondrocytes, there is MARRS-dependent enhancement of calcium flux, PKC activity, and matrix vesicle mineralization.[106] Vitamin-D3–mediated activation of TLIMP suppresses cell proliferation, perhaps in part by antagonizing the effects of IGF-I by increasing synthesis of IGF-binding protein-3.[104,107] The rapid effects of vitamin D may optimize its genomic effects by phosphorylation of proteins required by the VDR transcriptional complex. As expected, membrane-related phenomena are often better mimicked by analogs of calcitriol that are in the *cis* conformation than by calcitriol itself. A membrane-binding protein for 24,25(OH)$_2$D$_3$ has also been reported.[108]

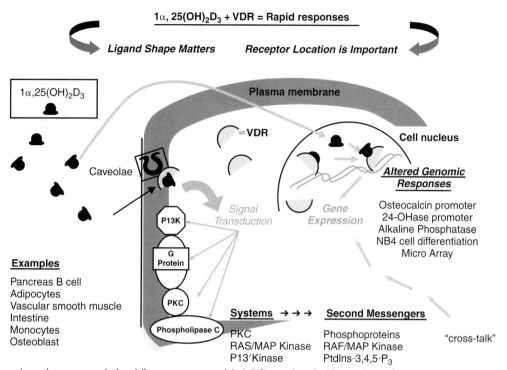

Figure 3-7. Genomic and nongenomic (rapid) responses to calcitriol. [Reproduced with permission from Norman AW (2006). Vitamin D receptor: New assignments for an already busy receptor. Endocrinology 147:5542-5548.]

Skeleton: Cartilage and Bone

The skeleton is the framework of the body. It consists of cartilage and bone—specialized forms of connective tissue that provide mechanical support for muscle/tendon insertion that enables movement, protective shielding for soft-tissue organs, repository for bone marrow, and reserve source of calcium, phosphate, and other metabolically important ions.[109,110] There are two primary bone shapes: flat bones (e.g., cranium, scapula, pelvis) and long bones (e.g., humerus, femur).[111] Flat bones develop by membranous bone formation, whereas long bones develop by endochondral and membranous bone formation.

The external surface of bone is enveloped by periosteum (containing blood vessels, nerve terminals, osteoblasts, and osteoclasts), whereas the interior of bone next to marrow is lined by endosteum. Long bones consist of a hollow shaft (diaphysis), distal to which are the metaphyses, cartilaginous growth plates, and epiphyses. The diaphysis consists of cortical bone and the metaphysis/epiphysis of trabecular bone surrounded by cortical bone. Eighty percent of the adult skeleton is dense cortical bone whose primary function is to provide mechanical strength. Twenty percent is cancellous bone, a network of trabeculae with a large surface area and increased turnover of bone constituents.

Bone matrix or osteoid is the component of bone that is composed of collagenous (collagen types I and III) and noncollagenous proteins (e.g., osteocalcin, osteopontin) secreted by osteoblasts—upon which the mineral phase of bone is deposited. Modeling of bone is the process that takes place during growth in which the shape and size of the bone are determined. Remodeling of bone is a continual process in which formed bone is periodically reabsorbed and replaced by new bone. Remodeling occurs in both the growing child and the adult. Osteoprogenitor pluripotent stromal mesenchymal stem cells provide a continuous supply of bone-forming osteoblasts, the network of osteocytes embedded throughout bone that monitor bone integrity and strength and bone-surface-lining cells. Osteoclasts derived from hematopoietic precursor cells mediate bone resorption.

Chondroblasts, osteoblasts, adipocytes, myoblasts, and fibroblasts are derived from a common mesenchymal cell (Figure 3-8).[112] Bone morphogenetic proteins (BMPs) are members of the transforming growth factor-β (TGFβ) superfamily that direct the transformation of a pluripotent mesenchymal cell into the pathway leading to formation of chondrocytes and osteoblasts. BMP-2, -4, and -7 are among the factors important for this differentiation process, although there is substantial redundancy in the system and other BMPs participate also. The BMPs act through designated cell membrane threonine/serine kinase receptors (e.g., BMPRIA, BMPR2). Depending on the interaction of the BMP receptors involved, intracellular signaling is transduced by the SMAD (mothers against decapentaplegic homolog) and/or MAPK pathways and induces synthesis of specific transcription factors that further the differentiation process.[113,114]

During early embryogenesis, bone is formed by condensation of mesenchymal cells in genetically determined patterns of position, arrangement, size, and shape.[115] Individual mesenchymal cells then differentiate either into chondrocytes that secrete a matrix of collagen

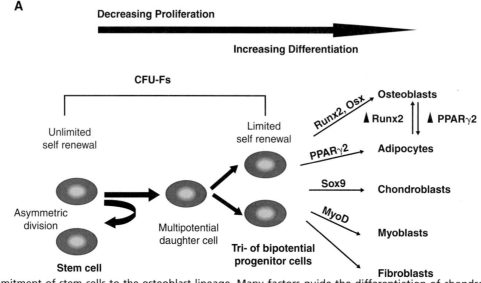

Figure 3-8. Commitment of stem cells to the osteoblast lineage. Many factors guide the differentiation of chondroblasts, osteoblasts, myoblasts, fibroblasts, and adipocytes from a common mesenchymal stem cell (see text). Bone morphogenetic proteins are involved in the earliest steps, leading to the differentiation of the common mesenchymal precursor cell. RUNX2 is necessary for the initial differentiation of the common progenitor cell of chondrocytes and osteoblasts and for further delineation of osteoblasts in association with osterix. PPARγ2 (peroxisome proliferator-activated receptor γ2) stimulates the differentiation of adipocytes. Osteoblasts and adipocytes may be interconverted, depending on the active transcription factor. MyoD is a muscle-specific transcription factor necessary for the development of myoblasts. [Reproduced with permission from Aubin JE, et al. (2006). Bone formation: Maturation and functional activities of osteoblast lineage cells. In Favus MJ (ed.), *Primer on the metabolic bone diseases and disorders of mineral metabolism, Sixth edition.* Washington, D.C.: American Society for Bone and Mineral Research 20–29.]

type II in the anlagen of endochondral bones or directly into osteoblasts in precursor regions of intramembranous bone, where they secrete a matrix rich in collagen type I. Differentiation of the pluripotent mesenchymal cell into an osteoblast is under the guidance of the canonical Wnt signaling pathway.[116] (The name Wnt is derived from combining and contracting the *Drosophila* gene *Wingless* with the corresponding mouse gene *Int.*)

Binding of secreted Wnt cytokines, a family of lipid-modified signaling glycoproteins with 350 to 400 aa and a conserved sequence of 22 cysteine residues (e.g., Wnt1, Wnt9A), to GPCR frizzled receptors (FZD1) and to the LRP 5/6 coreceptors also situated on the mesenchymal stem cell's plasma membrane leads to intracellular accumulation of β-catenin *(CTNNB1).*[117] Frizzled receptors act through the Gα$_q$-protein and PLC signal transduction pathway. LRP 5/6 *(LRP5, LRP6)* are long-chain proteins with a single transmembrane domain whose function is to prevent degradation of cytoplasmic β-catenin through the ubiquitination-proteasomal pathway. When a Wnt ligand binds to its frizzled receptor, the intracellular protein disheveled-1 *(DVL1)* is phosphorylated and inhibits glycogen-synthase-kinase-3-mediated phosphorylation of β-catenin—which slows its rate of degradation and releases it from binding to axin *(AXIN1),* another intracellular protein.

The intracellular domain of LRP5 then binds axin, permitting further increase in cytoplasmic levels of β-catenin.[118] In designated mesenchymal cells, increased levels of β-catenin acting as a transcriptional cofactor with T-cell factor/lymphoid enhancement factor *(LEF1)*

stimulates expression of runt-related transcription factor 2 *(RUNX2,* also termed core-binding factor alpha subunit 1 or CBFA1). The product of *RUNX2* is itself a transcription factor that stimulates production of osterix (encoded by *SP7).* RUNX2 and osterix, a 431-aa protein, are essential for differentiation of mesenchymal cells into osteoblasts and for the synthesis of osteocalcin and collagen type I(α1) by osteoblasts.[116]

Osteocalcin *(BGLAP)* plays an important role in normal mineralization of bone matrix. Other gene targets of RUNX2 include those encoding BMP4, FGFR1, Dickkopf, Wnt10a, and Wnt10b.[119] Thus, RUNX2 is not only central to initiation of osteoblastogenesis but to its maintenance. Wnt signaling also increases production of osteoprotegerin, a protein that inhibits osteoclastogenesis—thereby further increasing bone mass vide infra. When intracellular stores of β-catenin are depleted, mesenchymal cells differentiate as chondrocytes rather than osteoblasts.[120] Through changes in its state of phosphorylation, β-catenin also affects cell-to-cell adhesion and cell migration.[117]

The Wnt signaling pathway is opposed by inhibitors of LRP5 function [including secreted frizzled-related proteins, Dickkopf, and sclerostin *(SOST)*] that ensure orderly and normal bone mineralization. The axin-binding function of LRP5 is inhibited by binding of its extracellular domain to Dickkopf. Osteocytes are derived from osteoblasts after they have been embedded within mature bone. They form an interconnected network of long-cell processes within canaliculi that link deep osteocytes with newly formed osteocytes and with surface-lining cells.[118] Osteocytes detect mechanical strain by movement of fluid within these channels and respond by secreting growth factors and sclerostin. Because sclerostin inhibits Wnt signaling by binding to the extracellular domain of LRP5, when new bone formation is needed the secretion of sclerostin declines.

Cortical or compact bone is present in the cranium, scapula, mandible, ilium, and shafts of the long bones and has periosteal and endosteal surfaces—both of which are lined with layers of osteogenic cells. Cancellous (trabecular or spongy) bone is located in the vertebrae, basal skull, pelvis, and ends of the long bones. Because only 15% to 25% of trabecular bone volume is calcified (compared to 80%-90% of cortical bone volume) and thus has a far greater surface area, trabecular bone is metabolically quite active. It has a high turnover rate, making it more vulnerable to disorders that affect bone mineralization.

In flat bones (skull, ilium, mandible), intramembranous ossification begins with the local condensation of mesenchymal cells that then differentiate directly into preosteoblasts and osteoblasts and initiate the formation of irregularly calcified (woven) bone that is then replaced by mature lamellar bone.[109] Membranous bones grow by apposition, a process supported by development of new blood vessels induced by VEGF (a protein that also enhances bone formation).[121] The periosteum is a fibrous network in which osteoblasts synthesize peripheral compact bone. Cortical bone reinforces bone strength and complements and extends that provided by trabecular and endosteal bone. Tendons and ligaments insert and are fixed into cortical bone.

Chondrocyte differentiation and cartilage formation occur in mesenchymal regions in which activity of the canonical Wnt signaling pathway and the expression of VEGF are low but not totally absent. This results in increased expression of SOX9 and related SOX family members, transcription factors that direct differentiation of mesenchymal cells into chondrocytes that are characterized by synthesis and secretion of collagen types II, IX, and XI. The expression of SOX9 is stimulated by FGF signaling through the MAPK pathway. SOX9 is a 509-aa protein with an SRY homology domain that is also expressed in the testis, where it is responsible for differentiation of Sertoli cells.

Inactivating mutations of SOX9 lead to campomelic dysplasia and sex reversal in males (OMIM 114290). Target genes of SOX9 include those that encode collagen type II(α1) and aggrecan, a chondroitin sulfate proteoglycan core protein. A mutation in the gene encoding aggrecan leads to an autosomal-dominant form of spondyloepiphyseal dysplasia associated with premature degenerative arthropathy (OMIM 608361). SOX9 is expressed not only in chondrocytes in the resting phase but in those in the proliferative phase but not in chondrocytes in the hypertrophic phase of maturation.[114]

The pattern of endochondral bone development is directed by factors that are independent of bone formation (e.g., in transgenic mice in which Runx2 is inactivated, the cartilage "skeleton" forms normally but is not ossified).[116] [In humans, heterozygous inactivating mutations in RUNX2 result in cleidocranial dysplasia (OMIM 119600), manifested by growth retardation, hypoplasia of the clavicle and pelvis, delayed closure of cranial sutures, and defective tooth eruption.] Vertebrae evolve from the condensation and segmentation of paraxial mesoderm into somites under the direction and control of multiple genes, including Notch1, Sonic hedgehog, and Pax1 and Notch ligands encoded by DLL3 and JAG1.[116]

The appearance of limb buds, proliferating mesenchymal cells that grow out from the lateral body wall and are capped by an apical ectodermal ridge, heralds development of the cartilage anlagen of the long bones—a process of segmentation directed by homeobox genes (HOXA13, HOXD13), Sonic hedgehog, WNT7a, GLI3, TGFβ, FGF4, FGFR1, FGFR2, BMP2, BMP4, BMP6, BMP7, LMX1B, PITX1, TBX4, TBX5, TWIST, and other signaling, receptor, and transcription-regulating factors involved in differentiation, paracellular communication, and cell-to-cell interaction.[116,122,123] Mitochondrial RNA-processing endoribonuclease encoded by RMRP is a ribonucleoprotein essential to assembly of ribosomes and cyclin-dependent cell cycle activity as well as chondrocyte proliferation and differentiation.

Inactivating mutations of RMRP result in anauxetic dysplasia (OMIM 607095), a spondylometaepiphyseal dysplasia characterized by intrauterine and postnatal growth retardation (with adult stature <85 cm).[124] Histologically, the growth plates of these patients are depleted of chondrocytes. Different mutations of RMRP result in varying clinical manifestations [e.g., cartilage hair hypoplasia (OMIM 250250) and metaphyseal dysplasia without hypotrichosis (OMIM 250460)].

In bones of cartilaginous origin (long bones, vertebrae), mesenchymal stem cells differentiate initially into prechondrocytes and chondrocytes that secrete collagen type II into a matrix in which chondrocytes are embedded as the cartilage mold enlarges. In the center of the mold, chondrocyte proliferation ceases. The chondrocytes hypertrophy and begin to synthesize collagen type X and VEGF.[114] Blood vessels from the perichondrium together with cartilage-resorbing cells (chondroclasts) and osteoblasts and osteoclasts invade the hypertrophic region, destroy and reabsorb cartilage matrix and apoptotic chondrocytes, and deposit the primary spongiosa of bone that is later replaced by mature bone—a process dependent on normal function of the VDR.[42]

At the ends of the long bones, the cartilaginous epiphyseal growth plate develops—separating the epiphysis (a secondary ossification center at the end of a long bone) from the central metaphysis and diaphysis. Orderly columnar proliferation of chondrocytes in isogenous groups permits longitudinal growth of the long bone. Differentiation of resting chondrocytes from the reserve (resting, germinal, or stem cell) zone of the cartilage growth plate into the proliferating zone is initiated by BMP-6 and GH. Locally synthesized IGF-I induced by GH increases proliferation of chondrocytes (Figure 3-9).[125,126] The perichondrium contributes chondrocytes to the growth plate and supports its appositional growth. Sequentially, proliferating chondrocytes evolve into prehypertrophic chondrocytes and then into hypertrophic chondrocytes that secrete collagen type X into the matrix in which they are

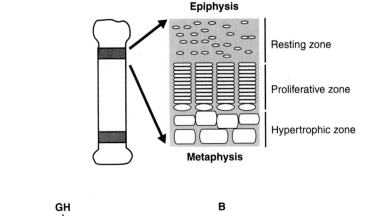

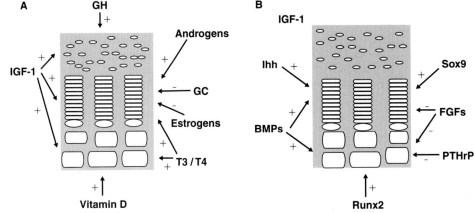

Figure 3-9. Hormones and growth factors affecting differentiation and proliferation of the cartilage growth plate. [Reproduced with permission from De Luca F (2006). Impaired growth plate chondrogenesis in children with chronic illness. Pediatr Res 59:625-629.]

embedded—thus contributing to interstitial growth of cartilage.

Central to the maturational development of chondrocytes are PTHrP and Indian hedgehog (Ihh). The latter is a 45-kDa protein synthesized by prehypertrophic and early hypertrophic chondrocytes whose expression is increased by BMP-6. Ihh acts through its receptor Patched 1 *(PTCH1)* and coreceptor Smoothened *(SMOH)* to stimulate transcription of genes that are essential to chondrocyte proliferation and maturation. Ihh directly stimulates chondrocytes in the reserve zone to differentiate into proliferating chondrocytes, thus increasing the number of proliferative chondrocytes and lengthening the cartilage growth plate.[127] It promotes cell division and growth by increasing expression of cyclins D and E, Wnts, and IGF-I. Ihh also regulates the generation of PTHrP by perichondrial cells on the articular surface, periarticular chondrocytes at the ends of the long bones, and most abundantly by early proliferative chondrocytes.[59,114]

PTHrP (through PTHR1) decreases the rate of differentiation of proliferating chondrocytes to prehypertrophic chondrocytes, thus antagonizing the effect of BMP-6. It prolongs the stage of chondrocyte proliferation by preventing premature hypertrophic differentiation and delays the generation of Ihh in a negative feedback loop.[127] PTHrP also enhances phosphorylation of SOX9 in prehypertrophic chondrocytes in the cartilage growth plate and thereby enhances its transcriptional activity. SOX9 contrib-

utes to the decelerating effect of PTHrP on the rate of differentiation of prehypertrophic to hypertrophic chondrocytes while maintaining the rate of chondrocyte proliferation and therefore continued elongation of the growth plate and long bone.[60,128] Thus, Ihh and PTHrP interact to determine the height of the growth plate and the length of the long bone. In mice in which *Ihh, Pthlh* (the gene encoding PTHrP), or *Pthr1* has been eliminated (knocked out), chondrocyte proliferation is decreased and there is accelerated differentiation into terminal hypertrophic chondrocytes and rapid replacement of cartilage by mineralized bone.[129]

In humans, inactivating mutations of *PTHR1* result in rapid chondrocyte maturation and Blomstrand chondrodystrophy (OMIM 215045)—whereas activating mutations in *PTHR1* lead to impaired chondrocyte maturation and Jansen metaphyseal chondrodysplasia (OMIM 156400). FGFs have dual effects upon chondrocyte proliferation and maturation. In part they enhance proliferation by increasing expression of *SOX9* and decreasing that of *Ihh*.[114] On the other hand, FGF18 inhibits chondrocyte proliferation and antagonizes the effects of BMPs acting through its cell surface tyrosine kinase receptor (FGFR3).[114,116]

Furthermore, spontaneous activating mutations of FGFR3 decrease the rate of chondrocyte proliferation and disturb their organization and are associated with achondroplasia and other chondrodysplasias. In hypertrophic chondrocytes, the expression of *Runx2* and *Vegf* is enhanced—contributing to the invasion from the perichondrium into hypertrophic cartilage of blood vessels, cartilage resorbing cells, and osteoblast precursor cells.[116] Ihh also enhances osteoblast differentiation in perichondrium. Subsequently, a primary ossification center is formed—and cartilage is replaced by trabecular bone and marrow (endochondral bone formation).

Stromal mesenchymal stems cells differentiate not only into osteoblasts [through Wnt signaling of Runx2, Dlx5 (another gene capable of stimulating osteoblastogenesis), and osterix] but into chondroblasts (through Sox9), adipocytes [through peroxisome proliferator-activated receptor γ2 (PPARγ2)], myoblasts, and fibroblasts (Figure 3-8). Committed osteoblasts and adipocytes appear to be able to re-differentiate one into the other cell type, depending on whether the expression of *Runx2* or Pparg is paramount. This process is directed by Wnt10b, which enhances expression of *Runx2, Dlx5,* and *Sp7* while suppressing that of *Pparg*.[112]

The nuclear NAD-dependent protein deacetylase encoded by Sirt1 also inhibits the adipocyte-differentiating effects of PPARγ2 by docking corepressors to this transcription factor, thereby diverting mesenchymal stem cells into the osteoblastogenic pathway.[130] BMP-2, -4, and -7 induce osteoblastogenesis acting through their heterodimeric cell surface receptors and transduce their intracellular signals through receptor-regulated SMADs 1, 5, and 8 (which heterodimerize with DNA-binding SMAD 4 to induce expression of *Runx2, Dlx5,* and *Sp7*).[131,132]

Osteoblasts have a life span of 3 months. They secrete type I collagen and many noncollagenous proteins that form osteoid into which calcium and phosphate are deposited as hydroxyapatite. In mature osteoblasts, Runx2, Dlx5, and osterix promote the synthesis of osteoblast-restricted proteins—including collagen type I(α1) and noncollagenous matrix proteins such as bone-specific alkaline phosphatase, osteocalcin, fibronectin, osteonectin, and osteopontin. Several factors (including TGFβ, platelet-derived growth factor, FGF, and IGF) enhance the proliferation and further differentiation of committed osteoblast precursors, but they cannot initiate this process.

Osteoblasts are heterogeneous and express diverse genes independent of the stage of the cell cycle and extent of differentiation. An early marker of the osteoblast is expression of bone alkaline phosphatase.[112] The heterogeneity of osteoblasts may relate to the variety of bone architectures and microenvironments. Actively bone-forming osteoblasts have an enlarged nucleus, plentiful Golgi apparatus, and abundant endoplasmic reticulum. When the rate of bone formation is low, osteoblasts are small and quiescent and incorporated into the endosteum separating bone mineral from marrow or into the undersurface of the periosteum.

Once differentiated, mature osteoblasts secrete collagenous and noncollagenous proteins—including collagen type I, bone-specific alkaline phosphatase, and calcium and phosphate binding proteins (osteocalcin, osteopontin, and osteonectin)—thus making bone matrix competent for mineralization. They also secrete many other proteoglycans and glycoproteins.[133] Osteocalcin, osteonectin, and various phosphoproteins account for approximately 10% of the noncollagenous proteins of bone matrix.[110] Osteoblasts control mineralization of matrix by regulating local concentrations of phosphate through synthesis of cell-membrane–bound alkaline phosphatase and by reducing levels of inhibitors of bone formation such as pyrophosphates.

Calcium and phosphate precipitate in bone matrix as hydroxyapatite crystals. After completing matrix synthesis and local bone formation, mature osteoblasts are embedded in bone as osteocytes (the most abundant cell in bone). Osteocytes are interconnected with each other and with surface osteoblasts by extension of plasma membranes through narrow canaliculi. They function as sensors of bone strength and mechanical integrity and act to identify sites of bone damage requiring repair (i.e., remodeling).[112] Osteocytes synthesize osteocalcin and sclerostin but not alkaline phosphatase. Osteocytes may live for several decades in quiescent bone but ultimately die.

Receptors for PTH[1-84] (PTHR1) and calcitriol (VDR) are expressed by osteoblasts.[134] PTH stimulates growth of osteoblast progenitor cells and inhibits apoptosis of osteoblasts and osteocytes, thereby enhancing bone formation and accounting for its therapeutic usefulness in treatment of osteopenic states. However, PTH[1-84] also promotes bone resorption via osteoblast production of an osteoclast-activating factor that increases osteoclastogenesis. In osteoblasts, carboxyl terminal fragments of PTH affect generation of alkaline phosphatase, procollagen I, and apoptosis—some of which effects may be opposite those of PTH[1-84]. There is a high density of binding sites for carboxyl fragments of PTH on osteocyte membranes, suggesting that these sequences may play a role in the mechano-sensory activity of the osteocyte network.[55]

Calcitriol increases synthesis of several noncollagenous matrix proteins, including osteocalcin. Glucocorticoids increase differentiation of osteoprogenitor cells but also accelerate apoptosis of osteoblasts and osteocytes.[112] Estrogens stimulate osteoblast proliferation and synthesis of collagen type I and inhibit apoptosis of osteoblasts and osteocytes. They enhance osteoclast apoptosis. Estrogens stimulate trabecular and endosteal bone growth and are thought to exert a biphasic effect on periosteal bone growth. Thus, in prepubertal boys and girls low amounts of estrogens enhance periosteal bone growth—whereas in pubertal and adult subjects estrogens oppose this process. Estrogens also accelerate growth plate fusion and inhibit bone resorption. Androgens primarily promote mineralization by conversion to estrogens, as evidenced by the osteopenia noted in adult males with aromatase deficiency or loss-of-function mutations in estrogen receptor (ER)α.[135] However, androgens also have a direct effect on bone mineralization because acting through the androgen receptor they increase periosteal bone growth during puberty in both males and females. However, the stronger bones of men compared to women reflect not increased volumetric bone mineral density but rather increased bone size due to greatly expanded periosteal bone width.[136]

Increased periosteal bone width in males is due in part to the androgen-induced effect of increased muscle mass, strain, and mechanical loading on bones. Nevertheless, estrogens too are necessary for normal periosteal bone growth because despite normal testosterone secretion the aromatase-deficient male has decreased periosteal bone width—a situation that can be reversed by administration of estrogen acting through ERα. A portion of the anabolic effects of estrogens on bone mineralization may be mediated through their stimulation of the GH/IGF-I axis. GH enhances proliferation and differentiation of osteoblast precursors, whereas IGF-I increases osteoblast function and trabecular and cortical bone volume and protects osteoblasts and osteocytes from apoptosis.[112]

IGF-I also mediates (some of) the stimulatory effects of PTH on osteoblast function.[137] The endogenous GH secretagogue ghrelin promotes proliferation and differentiation of osteoblasts and bone mineralization in vivo.[138] Leptin secreted by adipocytes or osteoblasts acting locally in bone exerts anabolic effects and promotes bone formation, whereas centrally active (hypothalamic ventromedial nucleus) leptin both impairs and promotes bone formation.[110]

In addition to their pivotal role in bone formation, osteoblasts and stromal cells regulate bone resorption by controlling the differentiation, maturation, and function of osteoclasts (Figure 3-10). They do so by expressing RANKL (an osteoclast activator) and a decoy acceptor protein for RANKL that inhibits osteoclastogenesis [osteoprotegerin (OPG)] in response to PTH, calcitriol, interleukins, and other cytokines (e.g., TNFα) and in response to prostaglandins. RANKL [also termed osteoprotegerin-ligand (OPGL)] is a member of the TNF ligand superfamily and is encoded by *TNFSF11*. It is expressed on the surface of (and its extracellular domain secreted by) bone marrow stromal cells and osteoblasts. RANKL binds to RANK expressed on the surface of primitive osteoclast progenitor cells, where it induces their further differentiation and activation (Figure 3-11).[139,140] (Transcription factors important in the very early commitment of the mesenchymal stem cell to the osteoclast lineage are those encoded by *PU.1, c-Fos,* and *MI.*[141])

RANKL is a 317-aa protein composed of cytoplasmic (48 aa), transmembrane (21 aa), and extracellular (248 aa) domains—with the binding site for RANK extending between aa 137 and aa 158. In the promoter region of TNFSF11 is a response element for RUNX2, the osteoblast-differentiating transcription factor. TNF-related activation-induced cytokine (TRANCE) is the soluble extracellular domain of RANKL released by a specific metalloprotease.

RANKL is also expressed in skeletal and lymphoid tissue, striated and cardiac muscle, lung, intestines, placenta, thyroid, pre-chondroblast mesenchymal cells, and hypertrophic chondrocytes. In addition to furthering osteoclast differentiation, RANKL enhances function of the mature osteoclast and inhibits its apoptosis. RANKL stimulates transcription of osteoclast-specific proteins such as tartrate-resistant acid phosphatase (TRAP), cathepsin K, β₃-integrin, and the calcitonin receptor. It also stimulates development of calcium resorption lacunae and pits. In

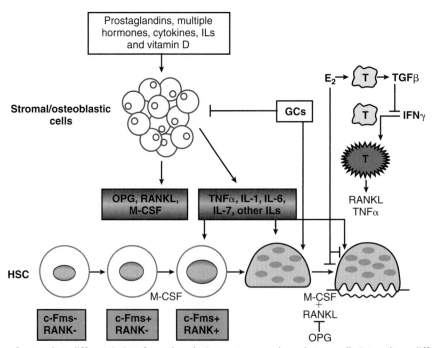

Osteoclastogenesis

Figure 3-10. Regulation of osteoclast differentiation from the pluripotent mesenchymal stem cell. Osteoclasts differentiate from precursor cells of monocyte/macrophage lineage in response to osteoblast/stromal cell secretion of macrophage-colony–stimulating factor (M-CSF) stimulated by parathyroid hormone (PTH) and other osteoclast-activating cell factors acting through its receptor (c-Fms) and stromal cell/osteoblast derived ligand for the receptor for activation of nuclear factor κB (RANKL). [Reproduced with permission from Ross FP (2006). Osteoclast biology and bone resorption. In Favus MJ (ed.), *Primer on the metabolic bone diseases and disorders of mineral metabolism, Sixth edition.* Washington, D.C.: American Society for Bone and Mineral Research 30-35.]

Effect of RANKL and OPG on osteoclast differentiation

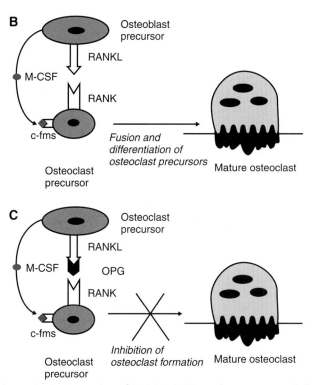

Figure 3-11. Interaction of RANK, RANKL, and osteoprotegerin in osteoclastogenesis. Osteoprotegerin serves as a pseudoreceptor for RANKL, thus preventing its association with RANK and thereby inhibiting osteoclastogenesis. [Reproduced with permission from Rogers A, Eastell R (2005). Circulating osteoprotegerin and receptor activator for nuclear factor kB ligand: Clinical utility in metabolic bone disease assessment. J Clin Endocrinol Metab 90:6323-6331.]

RANKL knockout mice, loss of osteoclasts leads to osteopetrosis. Because RANKL also affects differentiation and function of the immune system, these animals have thymic hypoplasia and lymph node agenesis. BMPs too stimulate osteoclast formation and function.[142]

OPG is a member of the TNF receptor superfamily and is synthesized and secreted by the stromal cell/osteoblast. It acts as a "decoy" receptor by binding to RANKL, thus inhibiting the interaction of RANKL and RANK and thereby osteoclastogenesis.[134,139] The 5 exon gene (*TNFRSF11B*) encoding human OPG is expressed also in the lung, liver, heart, kidney, intestinal cells, brain, thyroid, lymphocytes, and monocytes. Human OPG is synthesized as a 401-aa propeptide. After cleavage of the 21-aa signal peptide, the mature protein of 380 aa contains four cysteine-rich amino terminal domains and two carboxyl terminal "death" domains. It is glycosylated and released into the paracellular space as a disulfide-linked homodimer.

The synthesis of OPG is enhanced by IL-1α and -1β, TNFα, TNFβ, BMP-2, TGFβ, and estrogen—and is antagonized by calcitriol, glucocorticoids, and prostaglandin E_2. Through binding of RANKL, OPG inhibits the osteoclast-activating and bone-absorbing effects of calcitriol, PTH, and the interleukins. Overexpression of OPG in transgenic mice leads to osteopetrosis, whereas its knockout is associated with loss of cortical and trabecular bone and osteoporosis, multiple fractures, and hypercalcemia. The latter model is the experimental counterpart of juvenile Paget disease.[143,144]

In response to macrophage colony-stimulating factor (M-CSF) secreted by both mature osteoblasts and bone marrow stromal cells that acts through its receptor c-Fms expressed on the membrane of preosteoclasts, osteoclast progenitor cells further proliferate and differentiate.[134,140,141] Also expressed on the plasma membrane of the preosteoclast is transmembrane RANK (*TNFRSF11A*), a member of the TNF receptor superfamily. It is a 616-aa protein with a signal peptide (28 aa), cytoplasmic domain (383 aa), transmembrane domain (21 aa), and extracellular domain (184 aa) that is expressed in osteoclasts, fibroblasts, and B and T lymphocytes (Figure 3-11).

By cell-to-cell interaction, RANK on the surface of the prefusion osteoclast binds to RANKL expressed on the membrane of the osteoblast and/or stromal cell (or secreted by a monocyte) to induce osteoclast fusion and activation, leading to bone resorption. After binding of its ligand, RANK signals [through TNF receptor-associated factors (TRAFs)] a family of intracellular adaptor proteins that bind to the intracellular domain of RANK and activates several intracellular signaling cascades—including the classical pathway of nuclear factor κB (NFκB) activation, JNK-AP1, c-src-PI3K-AKT/PKB, and Ca^{2+}-calmodulin-calcineurin.[140]

In turn, there is enhanced generation of c-Fos, c-Jun, NFAT1c, and NFκB—transcription factors essential for osteoclast formation and function. Synthesis of interferon-β is also increased. This cytokine limits expression of c-Fos and consequently osteoclast differentiation, thus establishing an autoregulatory system for osteoclast production.[145] Osteopetrosis develops in transgenic mice in whom RANK is overexpressed or in whom NF-κB or TRAF-6 has been knocked out. In TRAF-6-depleted mice, osteoclasts develop normally but are not activated and do not form ruffled borders (structures essential to osteolysis).

NFκB subunit 1 (*NFKB1*) is a component of a widely expressed "master" transcription factor complex essential for cell differentiation, growth, and function within the hematopoietic and immune systems and the key regulatory element in osteoclastogenesis. The NFκB complex is composed of five subunits: NKκB1, NFκB2, RELA, RELB, and c-REL.[146] The subunits form homodimers or heterodimers with one another (e.g., NFκB1/RELA and NFκB2/RELB), which are trapped in the cytoplasm bound to specific inhibitors of NFκBs or IκBs (e.g., *NFKB1A*). After cell stimulation, phosphorylation of serine residues on IκB proteins targets them for ubiquitination and proteasomal destruction—thereby freeing the NFκB dimer and allowing it to enter the nucleus and activate target genes.

Within the nucleus there are DNA-binding motifs for NFκB (e.g., 5'-GGGA/GNNC/TC/TCC-3') that control the transcription of several hundred genes involved in cell replication and apoptosis, including the interleukins, TNFs, VEGF, and colony-stimulating factors. The intricate relationship between osteoblasts and osteoclasts provides the pathway(s) through which bone formation and bone resorption are linked. Thus, BMP and other factors induce osteoblast differentiation and production of RUNX2—leading to synthesis of RANKL that binds to RANK of the osteoclast precursor and enhances further differentiation and function of mature osteoclasts.[132] The effects of modifying agents and of disease processes on bone formation and bone resorption are mediated to a large extent by their influence on the RANKL-RANK-OPG system. Particularly at the level of the osteoblast/stromal cell production of RANKL and OPG may these effects be exerted, with the relative proportion of the two products being synthesized (or their ratio) regulating osteoclastogenesis and bone resorption.[139]

Mature osteoclasts are short-lived (approximately 2 weeks) bone-reabsorbing multi-nucleated giant cells. When attached to bone, the inferior surface of the osteoclast forms the ruffled border—a series of villus projections that bind to underlying bone at the site of bone resorption, creating an isolated microenvironment between the inferior surface of the cell membrane and the outer bone surface (Figure 3-12).[140,141] These villus structures anchor to the bone surface through interaction of dimeric αvβ3 integrins expressed on the osteoclast cell membrane and matrix-embedded osteopontin and other components that contain the amino acid sequence Arg-Gly-Asp (RGD).

Beneath this shield and into the isolated sealed zone the osteoclast pumps acid (H⁺ or protons) generated from carbon dioxide by carbonic anhydrase II and trans-

ported via an electrogenic proton pump and chloride ions transmitted through a chloride channel to form a highly acidic (pH 4.5) milieu that dissolves hydroxyapatite, the mineral phase of bone. The osteoclast also pumps lysosomal proteolytic enzymes [such as the cysteine proteases cathepsins K, B, and L and matrix metalloproteinases (MMP) such as MMP-9 a collagenase] that digest osteoid, the protein matrix of bone. Mutations in the genes controlling carbonic anhydrase II or the chloride channel result in osteopetrosis, whereas mutations in the gene encoding cathepsin K lead to pycnodysostosis (OMIM 265800).

The heterodimeric αvβ3 integrin (vitronectin receptor) consists of two transmembrane proteins (αv integrin, β3 integrin) with extra- and intracellular domains that attach the osteoclast to bone surface. They are crucial to normal osteoclast function. The integrins also transmit signals between the interior and exterior of the osteoclast. After the osteoclast contacts bone, it functionally polarizes into two realms. The inferior portion of the osteoclast above the ruffled membrane transports protons, chloride ions, and enzymes from the interior of the cell into the subcellular space and reabsorbs the products degraded by these agents. The superior portion of the osteoclast processes and excretes the reabsorbed materials. The absorptive lacuna is surrounded and isolated by a "sealing zone," whereas the osteoclast is encircled by an actin ring.[140] In the β3 integrin knockout mouse, the ruffled membrane is abnormal and osteoclast function impaired. Osteoclasts withdraw from the sites of bone resorption in response to the high local concentration of Ca²⁺.[32]

PTH[1-84], PTHrP, calcitriol, thyroid hormone, IL-1β, -3,-6, and -11, TNFα, prostaglandin E₂, and glucocorticoids stimulate expression of RANKL and M-CSF and depress that of OPG and hence favor osteoclast development and bone resorption. Calcitonin, estrogen, interferon-γ, IL-4, -10, and -18, TGFβ, glucocorticoids, and bisphosphonates antagonize these processes.[140] Estrogen maintains and augments bone mass by inhibiting its dissolution by suppressing T-cell production of osteoclast-activating cytokines such as IL-1, -6, and TNF and by suppressing expression of RANKL and increasing that of TGFβ.

Glucocorticoids decrease bone mineralization by depressing osteoblast differentiation, function, and life span and by prolonging the life span of osteoclasts. Receptors for calcitonin and to a limited extent for PTH are expressed by osteoclasts. Calcitonin antagonizes formation and activity of osteoclasts and accelerates their death. Interestingly, carboxyl terminal fragments of PTH[1-84] can inhibit osteoclast formation and function and antagonize the osteoclast-stimulating effects of PTH[1-84], calcitriol, prostaglandins, and interleukins.[55] Thus, they may exert a protective effect upon the skeleton and perhaps work in concert with intact PTH[1-84].

Bone modeling is accomplished by the independent action of osteoblasts and osteoclasts and is not dependent on prior bone resorption.[111] On the other hand, during bone remodeling (the process during which the strength, structure, and function of bone are renewed) bone resorption and deposition are sequentially linked. Bone remodeling is accomplished within the bone remodeling unit (BRU) of designated osteoclasts and osteoblasts. It is

Osteoclast Function

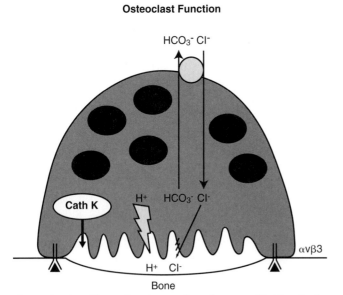

Figure 3-12. Differentiated osteoclasts form a ruffled border by adhering to bone surface through αvβ3 integrin receptors. A sub-osteoclast lacuna is formed by the dissolution of bone mineral and the resorption of organic bone matrix by osteoclast secreted acid and cathepsin K, respectively. Subsequently, osteoblasts are attracted to this pit (perhaps by the high local Ca²⁺ concentration) as new bone is formed in the continuing process of bone remodeling. [Reproduced with permission from Ross FP (2006). Osteoclast biology and bone resorption. In Favus MJ (ed.), *Primer on the metabolic bone diseases and disorders of mineral metabolism, Sixth edition.* Washington, D.C.: American Society for Bone and Mineral Research 30-35.]

a continuous process in which old cancellous and cortical bone is reabsorbed and replaced by new bone and takes place in the growing as well as the mature skeleton. The BRU is 1 to 2 mm in length, 0.2 to 0.4 mm in width, led by osteoclasts, and trailed by osteoblasts. In the adult skeleton, the life span of the BRU is 6 to 9 months—and 10% of the skeleton is turned over each year.

The site selected for remodeling may be random or may be targeted by osteocytes sensing a mechanical or stress defect. Bone remodeling occurs in four stages. Stage 1 is activation, in which osteoclast precursor cells target a resting bone surface, evolve into osteoclasts, convert the area into a BRU composed of a sub-osteocytic bone resorption compartment, and initiate stage 2. Stage 2 is bone resorption, during which the mineral phase of bone is solublized by acid and the protein component degraded by proteases. When complete, the osteoclast dies. This phase is followed by stage 3, reversal—in which monocytes, osteocytes, and osteoblasts perhaps attracted to the BRU through their detection of the high Ca^{2+} concentrations in the resorption lacunae or by growth factors (IGF-I and -II, TGFβ, BMP) released from the matrix or secreted by osteoclasts enter the area of reabsorbed bone and initiate the fourth stage. Stage 4 is renewed bone formation, in which osteoid is secreted, increase local concentrations of calcium and phosphate to levels that exceed their solubility, and are degraded pyrophosphates and proteoglycans that inhibit mineralization. The majority of osteoblasts and osteoclasts in the BRU are eliminated by programmed cell death (apoptosis), whereas some osteoblasts develop into osteocytes.[132]

Organic matrix proteins comprise 35% of bone, and type I collagen makes up 90% of these proteins.[133] Type I collagen is composed of a coiled triple helix of two polypeptide chains of collagen type I(α1) and one of (α2) that are cross-linked intramolecularly by disulfide bonds and intermolecularly at the amino (N) and carboxyl (C) telopeptides by pyridinium compounds that permit bundling of collagen molecules into fibrils and fibers (Figure 3-13).[147,148] Glycine occupies every third aa position in the collagen α peptides and permits the chains to coil. Proline, hydroxyproline, and hydroxylysine are also incorporated in large quantities. Proline is hydroxylated to 4-hydroxyproline and 3-hydroxyproline by prolyl 4-hydroxylase and prolyl 3-hydroxylase-1 (P3H1), respectively. Lysine is hydroxylated by lysyl hydroxylase and some hydroxylysine residues further glycosylated.

P3H1 (also termed leprecan, *LEPRE1*) specifically hydroxylates the proline residue at codon 986 in bone collagen type I(α1), a reaction that requires interaction of P3H1 with cartilage-associated protein *(CRTAP)* and cyclophilin B *(PIPB)*. CRTAP is expressed in the proliferative zone of developing cartilage and at the chondroosseous junction. Cyclophilin B is a peptidyl-prolyl cis-trans isomerase. That post-translational modifications of collagen type I(α1) are essential to normal bone formation is evidenced by the association of inactivating mutations of *CRTAP* with osteogenesis imperfecta types IIB (OMIM 610854) and VII (OMIM 610682) and of *LEPRE1* with osteogenesis imperfecta type VII.[149-151]

Amino and carboxyl terminal extensions of the propeptides of collagen are removed by proteolysis during formation of the mature collagen molecule and are partially secreted into extracellular space and serum. Pyridinoline (Pyr, hydroxylysyl-pyridinoline) and deoxypyridinoline (Dpd, lysyl-pyridinoline) form nonreducible pyridinium cross-links between mature collagen fibers, thus making them insoluble (Figure 3-14). Type I collagen predominates in bone but is also present in ligaments, tendons, fascia, and skin. Type II cartilage is composed of three procollagen type II(α1) chains and is primarily deposited in cartilage. Type III collagen [three procollagen type III(α1) chains] is present in bone, tendons, arteries, and intestine, and type IV [three procollagen type IV(α1)] cartilage is a component of cell basement membranes.

Type I Collagen

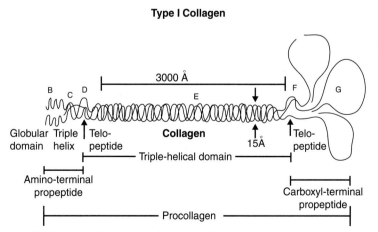

Figure 3-13. Type I collagen is a coiled triple helix of two polypeptide chains of collagen α1(I) and one of α2(I) that are cross-linked intramolecularly by disulfide bonds and intermolecularly at the amino and carboxyl telopeptides by pyridinium compounds. In the process of collagen formation, carboxyl and amino terminal propeptides are removed. [Reproduced with permission from Byers PH (1995). Disorders of collagen biosynthesis and structure. In Scriver CR, Beaudet AL, Sly WS, Vale D (eds.),,*The metabolic and molecular bases of inherited disease, Seventh edition.* New York: McGraw-Hill 4029-4077.]

Crossed-Linked Telopeptides

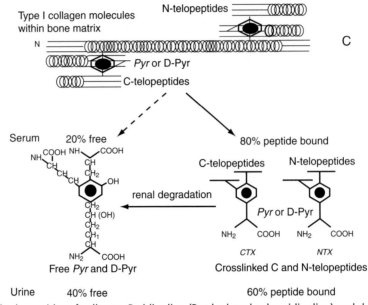

Figure 3-14. Pyridinium and telopeptides of collagen. Pyridinoline (Pyr, hydroxylysyl-pyridinoline) and deoxypyridinoline (D-Pyr or Dpd, lysyl-pyridinoline) form nonreducible pyridinium cross-links between mature collagen fibers, rendering them insoluble. Amino (N-) and carboxyl (C-) terminal extensions (NTx, CTx) of the propeptides of collagen are proteolytically removed during formation of mature collagen and secreted into extracellular space and serum. [Reproduced with permission from Garnero P, Delmas PD (1998). Biochemical markers of bone turnover: Applications for osteoporosis. Endocrinol Metab Clin NA 27:303-323.]

Measurement of serum concentrations of the procollagen I extension peptides such as the C-terminal extension of procollagen type I (PICP) and the N-terminal extension of procollagen type III (PIIINP) provides information about bone and collagen formation (as does determination of the osteoblast products, osteocalcin and bone-specific alkaline phosphatase). Degradation of mature bone matrix by osteoclasts catabolizes type I collagen and releases Pyr, Dpd, and the N- and C-telopeptides [NTx; ICTP (CTx) = amino or carboxyl terminal cross-link telopeptide of type I collagen, respectively]. The urinary excretion of hydroxyproline, hydroxylysine, Pyr, Dpd, and NTx reflects catabolism of collagen type I and bone resorption.

Serum/urine levels of markers of bone formation and resorption are higher in the fetus than mother[152] (Table 3-6). Fetal umbilical cord plasma PICP concentrations are highest in mid-gestation and decline in the last trimester to term values. After birth, PICP values fall in preterm neonates during the first 3 days of life and then increase steadily to peak values at 36 weeks postconceptual age. PICP levels in cord plasma are higher in males than females and correlate with gestational age and birth weight.[153] Urine levels of NTx at 2 days of age are higher in preterm than term neonates. Markers of bone turnover increase during the first 3 weeks of life in preterm infants.[154]

Values of bone formation and resorption markers are highest in infants and decline during childhood and adolescence to adult levels[155-160] (Tables 3-7A and B). In the normally menstruating young adult female, urine Pyr and Dpd levels fall during the first half of the cycle and increase during the second half. Serum concentrations of PICP have the reverse pattern. These data suggest that the fluctuations in estrogen secretion during the menstrual cycle alter the dynamics of bone formation and resorption.[161] Osteoprotegerin and RANKL are also measurable in serum, but their utility in children and adolescents has yet to be assessed.[139]

The adult skeleton is composed of mineral (50%-70%), organic matrix (20%-40%), water (5%-10%), and lipids (<3%). Ten percent to 15% of bone matrix is composed of noncollagenous peptides secreted by the osteoblast, including proteoglycans (chondroitin sulfate, heparan sulfate), glycoproteins, growth-stimulating proteins (BMP, TGFβ, IGF-I, and IGF-II), cell attachment peptides (integrin ligands such as osteopontin, osteonectin, fibronectin), and γ-carboxylated proteins or proteins derived from serum (e.g., albumin).[133] Macromolecular proteoglycans are composed of glycosaminoglycans (acidic polysaccharide side chain) linked to a core protein and are important to normal synthesis of collagen and bone development.

Osteonectin is a phosphorylated 35- for 45-kDa glycoprotein that binds Ca^{2+} and is necessary for growth and survival of osteoblasts and osteoclasts and for normal mineralization of matrix. Alkaline phosphatase is an 80-kDa glycoprotein essential to bone mineralization. Osteopontin (also termed *bone sialoprotein* or *secreted phosphoprotein 1*) is an 85-kDa sulfated and phosphorylated glycoprotein that contains the aa sequence [Arg-Gly-Asp (RGD)] necessary for linkage to integrins and hence for attachment of osteoclasts to bone. It also binds Ca^{2+} and hydroxyapatite and may play a role in the initiation of bone matrix mineralization. Osteopontin is secreted by osteoblasts in response to calcitriol. Osteocalcin is a 49-aa γ-carboxylic acid-containing 6-kDa peptide that likely

TABLE 3-6

Markers of Bone Formation and Resorption in Mothers and Neonates

	Maternal	Full-term Cord	24-29 wk Cord M	24-29 wk Cord F	29WK	30-34 wk Cord M	30-34 wk Cord F
Bone Formation							
Osteocalcin	19.6[1]	3.3[1]			14.1[2]		
ng/mL ±SD	2.6	0.3			9.4		
Bone Alkaline	273[1]	69[1]					
Phosphatase ± IU/L	11	12					
		M / F					
		822 (475-1420) / 824[3] (246-1450)	1950 (402-3372)	1103 (400-1808)		1392 (473-2939)	673[3] (128-2277)
PICP µg/L							
Bone Resorption							
ICT	2.7[1]	4.6[1]					
µg/L	±0.2	0.1					
Urine Pyridinoline							
Total		623 ± 235[2]			645 ± 227[2]		
Free		217 ± 92			248 ± 96		
Deoxypyridinoline							
Total		101 ± 41			106 ± 43		
Free		33 ± 14			34 ± 14		
N-Telopeptide (nmolBCE/mmol Creatinine)		1302 ± 790			3008 ± 1185		

1. Yamaga A, et al. (1999). Comparison of bone metabolic markers between maternal and cord blood. Horm Res 51:277–279.
2. Naylor KE, et al. (1999). Bone turnover in premature infants. Pediatr Res 45:363–366.
3. Seibold-Weiger K, et al. (2000). Plasma concentrations of the carboxyterminal propeptide of type I procollagen (PICP) in preterm neonates from birth to term. Pediatr Res 48:104-108.

regulates osteoclast activity and the interface between bone resorption and formation, whose synthesis is dependent on vitamin K activation of γ-carboxylases.

Calcium and phosphate deposit in extracellular matrix around the osteoblast. Type I collagen and osteopontin are important for the nucleation of hydroxyapatite and the determination of bone structure.[162] In the first phase of bone formation, hypertrophic chondrocytes and/or osteoblasts initiate bone crystal formation by generating 100 nm subsurface matrix vesicles containing among other components calcium, phosphate, alkaline phosphatase, calbindin-D_{9K}, carbonic anhydrase, pyrophosphatases, osteocalcin, and osteopontin. These vesicles are extruded from the osteoblast and attach to adjacent bone matrix—in cartilage to collagen types II and X and in bone to collagen type I. Ca^{2+} and $H_2PO_4^{2-}$ enter the vesicle through ion channels and possibly first form rudimentary crystals of calcium phosphate that enlarge, attain the structure of hydroxyapatite, and penetrate the vesicle wall. In the matrix, these crystals enlarge further and deposit about collagen type I.

Mineralization of bone is partially dependent on the extent of phosphorylation of osteopontin. When 40% of the phosphorylation sites of osteopontin are phosphorylated, bone mineralization is inhibited. When 95% of its sites are phosphorylated, hydroxyapatite formation is promoted—a process further enhanced by a complex of osteopontin and osteocalcin.[133,163] Osteocalcin is also synthesized by osteoblasts in response to calcitriol acting through the VDR/RXR heterodimer. Inhibition of calcification is an active process as well. In addition to osteopontin, matrix GLA protein (an 84-aa vitamin K-dependent peptide containing γ-carboxylated glutamate that is related to but distinct from osteocalcin and encoded by *MGP*) has great affinity for Ca^{2+} and inhibits precipitation of calcium and phosphate. *MGP* is expressed in arteries and chondrocytes but not in osteoblasts. In patients with biallelic loss-of-function nonsense mutations in *MGP* (Keutel syndrome, OMIM 245150), there is extensive calcification of cartilage and its experimental deletion in mice leads to calcification of both cartilage and arteries and early demise.[162]

Bone strength is determined by its size (height, width, depth), mineral mass, macro- and microarchitecture, and material properties (e.g., elasticity) of collagen that in turn are regulated not only by endocrine hormones and paracrine growth factors but by mechanical forces exerted upon the skeleton by the environment (gravity) and by the muscular system.[164,165] Bone mass and strength are determined by the loads placed on bone by biomechanical

TABLE 3-7A

Normal Values of Markers of Bone Deposition and Resorption in Male Children and Adolescents

Bone Formation

Bone-specific alkaline phosphatase[1,7] (µg/L)

CA	1	2	5	10	12	14	16	18
	103	62	74	88	90	102	96	62
	(89-114)	(52-72)	(62-86)	(74-102)	(74-106)	(82-122)	(78-114)	(38-86)

	P1*	P2	P3	P4	P5	
CA	10.5	12.1	13.2	13.8	15.1	
	41.3	54.0	59.8	53.6	33.3	
SD ±	19.2	27.2	33.1	25.1	36.7	

	P1*	P1*	P2	P3	P4	P5
CA	3-6	6-12				
Osteocalcin[2] (µg/L)	74	56	43	41	50	50
	(49-93)	(29-88)	(28-45)	(23-56)	(31-67)	(43-55)
PICP[2,3] (µg/L)		372	380	398	561	536
	(193-716)	(264-556)	(244-650)	(384-1,066)	(312-692)	
PIIINP[2] (µg/L)		593	704	920	882	
	(435-941)	(223-1,000)	(428-1,000)	(720-1,000)		

Bone Resorption,

	P1*	P1*	P2	P3	P4	P5
CA	3-6	6-12				
ICTP[2,3] (µg/L)		9.3	13.6	15.8	23.5	22.6
	(5.1-17)	(10.7-30.3)	(11.6-30.2)	(14.1-35.4)	(18.4-25.0)	

CA	2-10	11-17	Adults
Dpd[4]	40-120	2-118	6-26
Pyr[4]	150-400	17-410	23-65

(nmol/mmol creatinine/2 hours)

CA	4	6	8	10
Dpd[5]	20	20	14	17
	(17-24)	(15-22)	(12-16)	(13-19)
Pyr[5]	69	68	58	57
	(59-85)	(53-77)	(46-63)	(46-67)

(median - nmol/mmol creatinine - first morning void)

	P1*	P2	P3	P4	P5
Dpd[7]	258.8	313.0	273.1	245.1	141.9
SD ±	68.4	106.1	73.0	94.3	83.3
Pyr[7]	70.3	78.2	71.0	61.8	40.4
SD ±	21.9	29.3	22.1	25.8	32.3

(mean - nmol/mmol creatinine/2 hours)

CA	<1	5	10	15	>20
NTx[6]	1988	640	425	376	71
	(507-4942)	(189-1056)	(150-773)	(133-1146)	(43-154)

(nmol BCE**/mmol creatinine/2 hours)

CA = chronologic age (years).

Data presented as mean or median (range or SD).

* Pubertal stage.

** Bone collagen equivalent units.

1. Tobiume H, et al. (1997). Serum bone alkaline phosphatase isoenzyme levels in normal children and children with growth hormone (GH) deficiency: A potential marker for bone formation and response to GH therapy. J Clin Endocrinol Metab 82:2056-2061.

2. Sorva R, et al. (1997). Serum markers of collagen metabolism and serum osteocalcin in relation to pubertal development in 57 boys at 14 years of age. Pediatr Res 42:528-532.

3. Crofton PM, Wade JC, Taylor MRH, Holland CV (1997). Serum concentrations of carboxyl-terminal propeptide of type I procollagen, amino-terminal propeptide of type III procollagen, cross-linked carboxy-terminal telopeptide of type I collagen, and their interrelationships in school children. Clin Chem 43:1577-1581.

4. Nichols Institute/Quest #432-04/93.

5. Hussain SM, et al. (1999). Urinary excretion of pyridinium crosslinks in healthy 4-10 year olds. Arch Dis Child 80:370-373.

6. Bollen A-M, Eyre DR (1994). Bone resorption rates in children monitored by the urinary assay of collagen type I cross-linked peptides. Bone 15:31-34.

7. Mora S, et al. (1999). Biochemical markers of bone turnover and the volume and the density of bone in children at different stages of sexual development. J Bone Miner Res 14:1664-1671.

TABLE 3-7B

Normal Values of Markers of Bone Deposition and Resorption in Female Children and Adolescents

Bone Deposition

CA	1	2	5	10	12	14	16
Bone-specific alkaline phosphatase[1,7] (µg/L)							
	84	78	70	78	96	49	30
	(70-98)	(66-90)	(58-82)	(62-94)	(84-108)	(33-67)	(22-38)

	P1*	P2	P3	P4	P5		
CA	9.8	11.8	12.2	12.9	14.2		
	47.4	49.8	40.4	38.3	41.3		
SD ±	22.7	26.8	15.8	32.0	27.2		

	P1*	P1*	P2	P3-P4	P5	Adult
CA	3-6	6-12				
Osteocalcin	69	44	88	62	35	22
(µg/L)	(33-88)	(24-70)	(50-134)	(33-86)	(11-77)	(12-38)

	P1*	P2	P3	P4	P5
PICP[2]	374	408	442	401	203
(µg/L)	(242-406)	(258-558)	(307-577)	(190-612)	(100-306)

Bone Resorption

CA	4-8	9-13	14-15	16-18
ICTP[3]	9.2	12.0	7.4	5.0
(µg/dL)	(5.7-14.9)	(7.2-20)	(4.1-13.3)	(2.9-8.5)

CA	2-10	11-17	Adults
Dpd[4]	40-120	2-118	6-26
Pyr[4]	150-400	17-410	23-65
(nmol/mmol creatinine/2 hours)			

CA	4	6	8	10
Dpd[5]	21	19	17	14
	(17-25)	(14-21)	(13-18)	(13-18)
Pyr[5]	77	67	61	50
	(64-85)	(58-78)	(50-67)	(46-71)
(median - nmol/mmol creatinine - first morning void)				

	P1*	P2	P3	P4	P5
Dpd[7]	247.1	337.7	250.0	213.2	124.0
SD ±	249.5	120.4	96.7	91.1	43.3
Pyr[7]	69.8	97.6	68.5	59.8	33.8
SD ±	75.8	45.6	31.1	29.0	19.1
(mean - nmol/mmol creatinine/2 hours)					

CA	<1	1	5	10	15	>20
NTx[6]	2218	1207	728	515	217	67
	(872-45,702)	(477-2,752)	(335-1,615)	(116-12,410)	(107-653)	(13-137)
(nmol BCE/mmol creatinine)						

1. Tobiume H, et al. (1997). Serum bone alkaline phosphatase isoenzyme levels in normal children and children with growth hormone (GH) deficiency: A potential marker for bone formation and response to GH therapy. J Clin Endocrinol Metab 82:2056-2061.
2. Hertel NT, et al. (1993). Serum concentrations of type I and III procollagen propeptides in healthy children and girls with central precocious puberty during treatment with gonadotropin-releasing hormone analog and cyproterone acetate. J Clin Endocrinol Metab 76:924-927.
3. Crofton PM, et al. (1997). Serum concentrations of carboxyl-terminal propeptide of type I procollagen, amino-terminal propeptide of type III procollagen, cross-linked carboxy-terminal telopeptide of type I collagen, and their interrelationships in school children. Clin Chem 43:1577-1581.
4. Nichols Institute/Quest #432-04/93.
5. Hussain SM, et al. (1999). Urinary excretion of pyridinium crosslinks in healthy 4-10 year olds. Arch Dis Child 80:370-373.
6. Bollen A-M, Eyre DR (1994). Bone resorption rates in children monitored by the urinary assay of collagen type I cross-linked peptides. Bone 15:31-34.
7. Mora S, et al. (1999). Biochemical markers of bone turnover and the volume and the density of bone in children at different stages of sexual development. J Bone Miner Res 14:1664-1671.

forces exerted by muscles (the "mechanostat" model).[166] In this model, bone tissue monitors the stresses and strains (deformations) that are the result of mechanical forces placed upon it.[167]

In part, mechanical forces are recognized by osteocytes, whose rate of apoptosis declines in response to these dynamic changes. In addition, stromal cells modify their expression of RANKL—and thus the process of osteoclastogenesis. Deformation of the osteoblast cell membrane induced by mechanical forces (e.g., stretch, gravity, vibration) generates signals that are transmitted through alterations in configuration of its cytoskeleton that act upon cytoplasmic organelles and within the nucleus itself, increasing expression of transcription factors such *c-Fos* and *c-Myc*.

In response to mechanical stress, multiple growth factors likely generated by the osteoblast itself (FGF, IGF-I, TGFβ) act in an autocrine/paracrine manner upon their tyrosine kinase receptors expressed in the cell membrane of the osteoblast to activate phosphoinositide 3-kinase, PKB, and the MAPK signal transduction system. Prostaglandins activate G-protein–coupled receptors, adenylyl cyclase, PKA, and the cyclic AMP responsive transcription factor. PLC generation leads to increase in cytosolic Ca^{2+}_i and osteoblast function, as does influx of Ca^{2+} through L-type calcium channels in the cell membrane.[168]

One of the target genes affected by mechanical stimulation is *Runx2,* whose product is essential to osteoblast differentiation and expression and synthesis of osteoblast-related proteins such as collagen type I, bone-specific alkaline phosphatase, osteopontin, and collagenase-3.[169] Repetitive bone strain (an applied deforming force that might be compressive, lengthening, or angulating) leads to enhanced quantity and quality of bone (bone strength). It is this property that enables various exercises to increase bone mineralization at all ages and states of mobility.

The mechanisms that lead to increased bone mass are inactivated by decreased weight bearing, such as immobilization or decreased gravity (e.g., space flight), and lead to bone loss ("disuse osteoporosis"). Although bone strength is in part dependent on bone mass, it is the size of the bone that primarily determines its strength.[170] Clinically, this is illustrated by the increased rate of fractures in children with osteopetrosis ("marble bone disease") despite extremely dense bones with thick cortices and trabeculae.

Skeletal accretion of calcium begins early in fetal life and progresses through childhood and puberty. The skeleton accumulates 25 to 30 grams of calcium *in utero* and accrues 1,300 grams by adulthood.[171] The average total body bone mineral content (BMC) of the adult male is 2,800 g, and that of the adult female 2,200 g. Approximately 60% of total adult bone calcium is acquired during adolescence (26% in the two years prior to and after the peak velocity of BMC accrual) (Figure 3-15). Thirty-two percent of the mean BMC of the adult female lumbar spine (60 g) is deposited during this interval.[172]

It is recommended that the adolescent ingest 1,300 to 1,600 mg of elemental calcium daily in order to absorb and retain the 220 mg per day of calcium needed to achieve optimal adult bone mineral mass. Although calcium supplementation has been reported to increase radial and femoral BMC in children, extensive review of the effects of calcium supplementation in approximately 3,000 children and adolescents (3–18 years of age) did not support this conclusion. Nor did supplementation decrease fracture rate.[173,174]

As evidenced by the close concordance of bone mineral status between mothers and daughters, identical and fraternal twins and siblings, 60 to 80% of the peak or maximum adult bone mass is determined by genetic factors.[175] There are numerous candidate genes through which this parental relationship might be exercised, including those encoding the vitamin D, calcium-sensing, estrogen, low-density lipoprotein-related, leptin and β-adrenergic receptors, cytokines (e.g., IL-6, TGFβ) and growth factors (BMPs, IGF-I), and bone matrix proteins such as type I collagen and osteocalcin—emphasizing the fact that the regulation of bone mineralization is genetically complex and heterogeneous.[176]

In addition to intrafamilial factors, race, sex, body size, and composition are important genetic determinants of bone calcium content. In black males and female youths, there is higher whole-body, lumbar spine, total hip, and femoral neck BMD and bone mineral apparent density (BMAD) than in white, Asian, or Hispanic youth.[177] Asian female children and adolescents have lower whole-body and femoral neck BMD than do white and Hispanic subjects. Hispanic males have lower lumbar spine BMD than do white and Asian youth. Radial and femoral neck (peripheral) and vertebral (axial) BMDs correlate with sex, age, height, weight, body mass index, pubertal and postpubertal hormonal status, calcium intake, and exercise in children, adolescents, and adults.[178,179]

In young women, only 16% to 21% of peak vertebral and femoral bone mass can be accounted for by weight, height, physical activity as an adolescent, and the VDR genotype—emphasizing once more the essential role of multiple genetic factors in this process. Adult peak bone mass is inversely related to the risk of osteopenia and osteoporosis in later adulthood. In adults, a 10% increase in BMD reduces the risk of femoral neck fracture by 50%. Thus, it is essential that bone mass be maximized during childhood and adolescence.[180]

The effects of diminished physical activity on bone growth and strength are dramatically illustrated by those children with neurologic insults that prevent normal motion (Erb paresis, hemiplegia, spinal cord insults) and thus restrain limb growth.[166] During prolonged bed rest, the BMC of the peripheral skeleton substantially declines—whereas that of the cranium increases. Thirty minutes of programed exercise thrice weekly increases BMC of the femoral neck and lumbar spine in prepubertal boys and girls.[181,182] High-impact weight-bearing exercises (ballet, tennis, volleyball, gymnastics, soccer, rugby) increase mass of weight-bearing bones, particularly in children and adolescents.[172,183,184]

Exercise does so in part by augmenting periosteal bone acquisition and increasing the cortical thickness of long bones, particularly of the legs at their most distal extremes closest to the ground where weight bearing is maximal. Active boys and girls accrue more bone mineral than do relatively inactive youth at similar intakes of calcium (1,150 mg/day). At peak BMC velocity (Figure 3-15), the annual gain and total accumulation

Total Body Bone Mineral Content–Accrual Rate

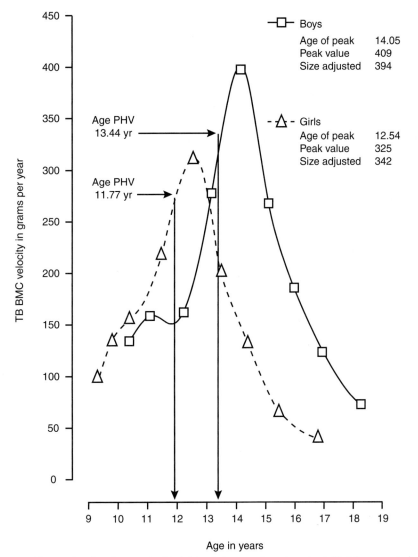

Figure 3-15. During adolescence, the peak rate of accrual of total body bone mineral content (BMC) occurs in boys and girls 0.7 years after attainment of peak height velocity (PHV). [Reproduced with permission from Bailey DA, et al. (1999). A six-year longitudinal study of the relationship of physical activity to bone mineral accrual in growing children: The University of Saskatchewan bone mineral accrual study. J Bone Miner Res 14:1672-1679.]

(over 2 years) of total body bone mineral in active boys and girls are 80 g/year and 120 g/yr (respectively) greater than in inactive adolescents. One year after peak BMC velocity, the total body, femoral neck, and lumbar spine BMCs are 9% to 17% greater in active than in relatively inactive subjects.

EFFECTS OF HORMONES AND GROWTH FACTORS ON THE SKELETON

Systemic hormones and growth factors (GH, IGF-I, PTH, leptin, thyroid and sex hormones, glucocorticoids) have substantial effects on chondrocyte proliferation, matura-tion, and function.[185] GH increases the synthesis of BMPs, directly enhances differentiation of prechondrocytes, supports proliferation of chondrocytes in the reserve or resting zone, and increases expression of *IGF1*. IGF-I then ensures the clonal expansion of committed chon-drocytes.[126] *In utero,* both IGF-I and IGF-II are essential for normal fetal growth as denoted by the *in utero* growth retardation experienced by the fetus with a loss-of-function mutation in *IGF1, IGF2,* or *IGFR1.*[185,186]

GH and IGF-I receptors are expressed in chondrocytes in the reserve, proliferative, and hypertrophic zones—whereas IGF-I and IGF-II are expressed predominantly in proliferating chondrocytes.[187] GH mediates chondrocyte proliferation and maturation and IGF-I synthesis through the Janus kinase-2 signal transduction and transcription 5b (JAK2-STAT5b) signal transduction system.[188] IGF-I coordinates chondrocyte proliferation and inhibits their apoptosis. It modulates their differentiation and maturation and their synthesis of matrix heparan sulfate proteoglycan, a matrix component necessary for efficient signaling of FGFs and their receptors.[126,186]

IGF-I also influences the interaction of Ihh and PTHrP. IGF-binding proteins (IGFBP) 1 through 6 are synthesized by growth plate chondrocytes, where they regulate levels of bioactive IGF-I as well as exert direct stimulatory/inhibitory effects on chondrocyte proliferation (depending on the stage of chondrocyte differentiation).[126,189] Neither GH nor IGF-I is necessary for patterning of the skeleton, however. Systemic loss of GH secretion or IGF-I production or inactivation of the IGF-I receptor greatly impairs linear growth of long bones postnatally. Selective loss of hepatic IGF-I production lowers total circulating levels of IGF-I to 25% of normal but does not adversely affect growth in transgenic mice, indicating that it is IGF-I synthesized by the cartilage growth plate that affects chondrocyte division by a paracrine mechanism.[190]

In patients with inactivating mutations of the GH receptor or deletion of the gene encoding IGF-I, administration of IGF-I enhances linear growth—indicating that this growth factor is able to stimulate cartilage proliferation without the initial differentiating effect of GH but does so to a lesser extent than does GH in the GH deficient subject. Thus, sufficient numbers of differentiated prechondrocytes are necessary for optimal IGF-I effect.[191] The GH secretagogue ghrelin is also synthesized and secreted by chondrocytes and affects their intracellular metabolism, but its physiologic significance in this region is unknown at present.[192]

Through expression of the GH receptor by osteoblasts, GH stimulates their differentiation, proliferation, and function—enhancing synthesis and secretion of osteocalcin, bone-specific alkaline phosphatase, and type I collagen. GH also increases expression of IGF-I by the osteoblast, as do estrogen, PTH, cortisol, calcitriol, and other factors. IGF-I is essential for GH-induced osteoblast proliferation *in vitro*. It also decreases expression of the GH receptor, whereas estrogen stimulates its expression.[193] In response to GH, IGFBP-3 and IGFBP-5 are synthesized by (rat) osteoblasts. IGFBP-4 expression is decreased by GH in rat and human osteoblasts.

The IGFBPs may augment or restrict activity of IGF-I and IGF-II. Thus, IGFBP-5 binds to bone cells, matrix, and hydroxyapatite and enhances the actions of IGF-I on bone. Expression of the GH receptor by the osteoblast is up-regulated by IGFBP inhibition of IGF-I activity. Acting through the osteoblast, GH increases osteoclast proliferation and activity. Human osteoclasts express receptors for IGF-I, which also enhances osteoclast formation and activation.

In children with GH deficiency and adults with childhood-onset or adult-onset GH deficiency, BMC and areal and volumetric BMDs are decreased—and increase when GH is administered.[193,194] Administration of GH to the GH-deficient subject is followed by increase in serum and urine levels of markers of bone formation and resorption (osteocalcin, bone-specific alkaline phosphatase, PICP, PIIINP, ICTP, Pyr, Dpd, and NTx), with maximal values achieved 3 to 6 months after beginning treatment. There is a biphasic response of bone mass during GH treatment. For approximately the first 6 months of GH administration, BMD declines as bone resorption exceeds formation. Thereafter, BMD increases steadily to positive values over the next 6 to 12 months.[193]

In subjects with GH receptor deficiency or IGF-I gene deletion, BMC and BMD are decreased relative to control subjects but volumetric BMD is not—suggesting that bone size but not bone mineral acquisition is impaired by isolated IGF-I deficiency.[195,196] Nevertheless, administration of IGF-I to subjects with deletion of *IGF1* enhances osteoblast function as documented by increased serum concentrations of osteocalcin and bone-specific alkaline phosphatase, BMC, and areal and volumetric BMDs.[196] In acromegalic patients, there is increased bone turnover—and variably increased lumbar spine and femoral neck BMD and iliac crest cortical and trabecular bone mass.[193]

Thyroid hormone receptors (TRα, TRβ) are expressed in the reserve and proliferative zones of the growth cartilage. Triiodothyronine, acting primarily through TRα, enables the differentiation of resting chondrocytes and their entrance into the proliferative phase. However, there thyroid hormone inhibits further chondrocyte proliferation and promotes differentiation to terminal hypertrophic chondrocytes and secretion of collagen type X.[126] They do so in part by disrupting the reciprocal interaction of Ihh and PTHrP, thereby accelerating chondrocyte maturation (effects mediated by FGFR3 and the STAT signaling pathway), and by down-regulation of IGF-I expression in chondrocytes.[126,197]

Thyroid hormone is essential also for invasion of the growth plate's hypertrophic zone by blood vessels and induction of metaphyseal trabecular bone formation. Thyroid hormones are necessary for fusion of the epiphyseal cartilage plate, although fusion may occur in the absence of thyroid hormone through the action of sex hormones. Through osteoblast-expressed receptors for thyroid hormone, triiodothyronine increases osteoblast production of osteocalcin, bone-specific alkaline phosphatase, and IGF-I. Thyroid hormones increase the rate of bone remodeling by expanding the number of osteoclasts and sites of bone resorption and the amount of bone resorptive surface. Urinary calcium excretion is increased by thyroid hormones. In excess, thyroid hormones can lead to net bone loss.

Estrogen and androgens promote chondrocyte maturation.[185] Although many of the effects of androgens are mediated by their conversion to estrogens, nuclear androgen receptors are expressed by chondrocytes and non-aromatizable androgens stimulate chondrocyte proliferation and long bone growth. Estrogens acting through ERα and ERβ expressed in chondrocytes exert dual effects on long bone growth—stimulatory at low levels and inhibitory at high values. Estrogens decrease chondrocyte proliferation and accelerate differentiation and senescence. Complete maturation and fusion of the growth plate are mediated solely by estrogens, as evidenced by the failure of growth plate fusion in young adult males with inactivating mutations of the genes encoding aromatase (the enzyme that converts androgens to estrogens) or ERα despite adult levels of testosterone.

Chondrocytes may also be capable of synthesizing estrogens from androgens because aromatase activity has been found in growth plate chondrocytes.[185] This observation suggests that locally produced (as well as systemic) estrogens may contribute to chondrocyte maturation and growth plate fusion. Sex hormones play major roles in the accretion of bone mineral in both females and males because the bulk of adult bone calcium stores are deposited during puberty, when the peak rate of accrual of total body BMC occurs in boys and girls 0.7 years after attainment of peak height velocity (PHV) and 0.4 to 0.5 years after peak accrual of lean body mass (a surrogate measurement of muscle mass)[172,198] (Figure 3-15).

After controlling for size, total body mass, and femoral neck peak, BMC velocity and BMC accrual over 2 years around the PHV are greater in males than in females. There is no gender effect on accrual of BMC of the lumbar spine, however. Both androgens (in part by conversion to estrogen) and estrogens markedly influence rates of bone formation and resorption, although it is the effect of estrogen that predominates—as evidenced by the marked osteopenia of adult males with androgen sufficiency but estrogen deficiency related to loss-of-function mutations in the genes encoding aromatase and ERα, by the beneficial effects of estrogen but not of testosterone on BMD in males with aromatase deficiency, by the very close association of BMD and serum levels of bioavailable estrogen in elderly men, and by the significant correlation in adult men treated with testosterone between changes in BMD and increases in serum concentrations of estradiol but not of testosterone.[132,199]

Nevertheless, the osteopenia of adult (46XY) females with complete androgen insensitivity due to loss-of-function mutations of the X-linked androgen receptor despite elevated serum testosterone and (endogenous or exogenous) estradiol concentrations and the fragile bone structure of the (Tfm) mouse counterpart of this disorder indicates that androgens, too, increase bone mineralization.[200] Furthermore, non-aromatizable dihydrotestosterone has a direct anabolic effect on bone because it stimulates the proliferation and maturation of osteoblasts, increases the production of procollagen I(α1), and prevents bone loss in orchidectomized rats.[201]

Estrogens have a biphasic effect on chondrocyte proliferation—increasing it at low doses and reducing it at higher doses. By accelerating their rate of maturation and apoptosis, estrogens lead to epiphyseal fusion.[199] Both males and females with systemic aromatase deficiency have delayed bone age, absent adolescent growth spurt, and marked osteopenia. Males are tall and eunuchoid, whereas females are short and hyperandrogenic (cliteromegaly, hirsutism). Administration of low doses of estrogens results in bone maturation in both genders. Estrogens increase bone mass primarily by suppressing bone resorption. They do so through inhibition of osteoclastogenesis and down-regulating osteoblast production of osteoclast-activating factors such as IL-6 (and its receptor), TNFα, and M-CSF; increasing production of osteoprotegerin; and accelerating apoptosis of mature osteoclasts.[132]

Estrogens also prolong the life span of osteoblasts and osteocytes. During adolescence, in the female not only does the rate of bone deposition increase but that of bone resorption declines.[202] Serum levels of IGF-I are positively correlated with lumbar spine BMD and metacarpal length and cortical thickness in early and mid-pubertal females. There is maturation-related increase in BMC and areal and volumetric BMD, and in metacarpal length, width, and cortical thickness—due in part to decline in width of the marrow cavity. These data suggest that the pubertal increase in production of GH and IGF-I (attributable specifically to increased estrogen synthesis in females) mediates longitudinal and periosteal skeletal growth and mineral acquisition during puberty. Estrogen may decrease endosteal bone resorption through inhibition of IL-6 generation—both systems contributing to increase in cortical bone mass.

Estrogens likely account for part of the pubertal growth spurt of girls and boys, acting both indirectly (by increasing the secretion of GH and the systemic and local production of IGF-I) and directly on the chondrocyte. Other gonadal hormones also influence bone quality.[203] Experimentally, inhibin A (a member of the TGFβ superfamily) increases total body BMD and bone volume and tibial biomechanical strength in transgenic mice through enhancement of osteoblast differentiation and function.[204]

The nuclear glucocorticoid receptor is expressed in chondrocytes in the proliferative and hypertrophic zones. Cortisol exerts an inhibitory effect on chondrocyte proliferation and maturation and hastens the death of hypertrophic chondrocytes.[126] Glucocorticoids act in part by depressing expression of the genes encoding the GH receptor, IGF-I, and IGF1R in growth plate chondrocytes and by regulating synthesis of IGFBPs and thereby indirectly function of IGF-I. However, glucocorticoids also increase expression of SOX9 and the earliest phase of chondrocyte differentiation. Glucocorticoids suppress osteoblastogenesis and accelerate the rate of apoptosis of osteoblasts and osteocytes, in part by suppressing expression of BMP-2 and RUNX2.[132] Secondarily, glucocorticoids decrease osteoclastogenesis but delay osteoclast death. In excess, glucocorticoids decrease trabecular bone and osteoid volumes and the rate of bone formation—contributing to bone weakness and collapse.

Transcripts of C-type natriuretic peptide (NPPC) and its receptor (NPR2) are expressed by chondrocytes. These peptides stimulate the growth of proliferative and hypertrophic chondrocytes, stimulate osteoblast function, and induce endochondral ossification.[205] Plasma concentrations of the amino terminal pro-C-type natriuretic peptide are positively related to growth velocity in normal children and adolescents.[206] Biallelic loss-of-function mutations in NPR2 have been identified in patients with acromesomelic dysplasia [Maroteaux type (OMIM 602875)].[207] In this disorder, there is shortening and deformation of the forearms, forelegs, and vertebrae—resulting in severely compromised adult stature.

After genetic influences, the factor to which bone mass is most closely related is weight. Although obese children, adolescents, and adults may have greater BMC and BMD than do slimmer subjects, it is primarily lean body mass (i.e., muscle) to which bone mass is related in these subjects.[208] Because osteoblasts and adipocytes arise from a common mesenchymal stem cell and can be interconverted, it is not surprising that the fat cell synthesizes and secretes a number of adipokines that exert effects on bone accumulation. Among these products is leptin, a 16-kDa protein that enhances osteoblast differentiation and maturation (but not proliferation) and inhibits adipocyte differentiation in human bone marrow stromal cells *in vitro*.[209] However, leptin concentrations are not correlated with whole-body BMD in either obese or nonobese late prepubertal or early pubertal subjects.[210]

Furthermore, in mice with loss-of-function mutations in leptin or its receptor bone mass is increased before onset of obesity due to increased osteoblast activity in the presence of normal osteoclast function. Bone mass can be reduced in these and wt animals by intracerebroventricular infusion of leptin, indicating that leptin can act centrally to inhibit bone formation.[211] Central infusion of leptin also decreases bone formation in sheep.[212] These and other data demonstrate that in addition to peripheral modulating factors there is central (hypothalamic) regulation of bone remodeling that is thought to be exerted through the sympathetic nervous system.[213] Adiponectin, another fat cell product, stimulates osteoclastogenesis by inducing osteoblast expression of RANKL and inhibiting that of osteoprotegerin.[214]

ASSESSMENT OF BONE MASS AND STRENGTH

Bone mass is determined by the three-dimensional size (volume) of the bone, its mineral content, and its material properties such as elasticity. Bone mineralization may be assessed by bone biopsy and histomorphometric analysis of bone formation and resorption.[215-217] Undecalcified transiliac biopsies permit limited assessment of bone modeling (changes in bone size, shape, mass), but detailed analysis of remodeling (bone renewal) as the iliac crest biopsy is primarily composed of trabecular bone with a limited amount of cortical bone. Although in children bone biopsies are usually reserved for research studies or for the evaluation of disorders of bone formation/mineralization not readily understood by noninvasive procedures (e.g., osteogenesis imperfecta, fibrous dysplasia), they have substantial clinical utility when applied appropriately by experienced personnel.[216]

During bone modeling, osteoblasts and osteoclasts are active on opposite bone surfaces across from one another. Thus, the bone surface may change position, size, or mass during the modeling process. Usually, modeling is associated with gain in bone mass because the rate of osteoblastic deposition of bone is more rapid than is that of osteoclastic resorption. During bone remodeling, osteoclastic resorption of bone is followed by osteoblastic replacement of the reabsorbed bone at the same surface with a net change of zero in bone mineral at the remodeling site under normal circumstances.

Histomorphometry enables quantitation of structural parameters of bone size and amount (cortical width, tra-

becular number, and thickness), static bone formation (thickness and surface of osteoid or unmineralized bone matrix, osteoblast surface), dynamic bone formation after labeling with a fluorochrome such as tetracycline (mineral apposition and bone formation rates), and static resorption (osteoclast number and appearance and extent of eroded surfaces). Iliac trabecular thickness but not trabecular number increases substantially between 2 and 20 years of age, whereas remodeling activity peaks in young children, declines, and then increases again during puberty.[215]

Noninvasive methods of assessment of skeletal mineralization include bone x-rays (of limited value), radiographic absorptiometry or photodensitometry, single-photon or single–x-ray absorptiometry, dual-photon or dual-energy x-ray absorptiometry (DEXA), spinal and peripheral quantitative computed tomography (pQCT), quantitative ultrasonography (QUS), quantitative magnetic resonance, and magnetic resonance microscopy.[170] DEXA has become the most frequently employed method of quantifying axial and peripheral bone mass and bone area (as well as body composition) because of its relatively low radiation dosage (5–10 μSv), ease of use and applicability for infants, rapidity (4 minutes for total body scan), accuracy, precision, and reproducibility under controlled circumstances.[170,218]

The ratios of attenuation of x-rays of two energies (70 kV, 140 kV) traversing the same pathway through the patient reflect the "density" and mass of the tissue through which the x-rays have crossed. Computer analysis of these captured energies then reconstructs the boundaries, density, and mass of the tissue. Two methods of imaging geometry have been employed in DEXA instruments: the earlier pencil beam DEXA instruments utilized a pinhole collimator linked to a single detector, whereas the newer fan beam DEXA units apply a slit collimator coupled with a multidetector array.[219]

Fan beam DEXA has the advantages of more rapid scan acquisition and improved resolution, making it especially useful for small children and infants.[220] Because of variability between instruments and analytical software programs (infant, pediatric, adult) employed for DEXA, the report of the DEXA scan should include not only the recorded data but the type of DEXA instrument and the software version employed for analysis. Because relatively low BMDs in children make it more difficult to distinguish clearly bone edges, specific infant and pediatric software must be used to address this problem.[221]

DEXA is employed to quantify bone mass and bone area in the axial (head, spine) and appendicular (limbs) skeleton. DEXA assesses a two-dimensional image, and therefore does not measure "true" BMD (the mass within a volume of uniform composition). DEXA measures the area(l) or surface mass of mineral within a region of bone of nonuniform composition (cortex, trabeculae, osteoid, marrow). It is expressed as g/cm^2.[222] Because DEXA does not take into account the depth of a bone, it underestimates BMD in small children and overestimates it in large subjects.[223]

In children and adolescents, bone size/volume increases with growth and maturation—and the larger the three-dimensional structure of bone the greater the recorded areal BMD [even though the actual or volumetric (v) BMD may not change substantially].[222] Therefore, calculated or "apparent" (v) BMDs (BMAD) (g/cm³) data have been generated in an attempt to correct this problem. Volumetric BMD increases as the cortex thickens, the number and width of trabeculae per unit volume rises, and the amount of hydroxyapatite per unit of trabecular volume accrues. Although during childhood and adolescence areal BMD of the femoral shaft increases with age, its vBMD remains relatively constant.[224]

On the other hand, vBMD of the lumbar spine increases in late puberty and early adulthood because of increasing thickness of trabeculae that is not gender specific but is greater in blacks than in whites after puberty.[222,225] Cross-sectional areas of cortical and trabecular bone increase with age, with males achieving greater increase in periosteal apposition than females during puberty. Cortical cross-sectional area is similar in white and black subjects.[226] Included in measurement of whole-body areal BMD is the head. This structure characteristically has twice the areal BMD of that of the rest of the skeleton and may comprise as much as 20% to 50% of the total BMD in children. Whole-body areal BMD correlates better with body height when the head BMD is excluded.[227,228]

Whole- or total body BMC and BMD, lumbar spine BMC and BMD, and femoral BMD are the most commonly measured indices of bone mass in childhood by DEXA and are reported as gm/cm². Data are often reported as a Z score, the number of standard deviations about the mean of peers matched for chronologic age and gender. (In adults, the DEXA T score is commonly reported. The T score is the number of standard deviations about the mean of maximal or peak bone mass recorded in healthy young adults aged 20 to 29 years. The T score should not be utilized in children and adolescents.)

In neonates and infants, it is recommended that whole-body BMC be the primary measurement when assessing bone mineralization.[229] In neonates with appropriate weight for gestational age (AGA), whole-body BMC by pencil-beam DEXA doubles between 32 and 40 weeks and increases 3.5-fold between birth weights of 1,000 and 4,000 grams. Neonates small for gestational age (SGA) have lower whole-body BMC than do AGA neonates of comparable gestational age, but they are similar to those of AGA infants with the same birth weights (Table 3-8).[230,231] In young adults (16-19 years) born prematurely with birth weights <1.5 kg, total body BMC is less than that of subjects born at term with normal birth weights but appropriate for their smaller stature.[232]

Utilizing fan-beam DEXA (QDR 4500A, Hologic Inc, Bedford, MA), whole-body BMC of 73 full-term neonates (birth weights 2,720 to 3,982 g) of both genders and of multiple ethnicities has been reported as 89.3 ± 14.1 (SD) grams with BMD of 0.240 ± 0.022 g/cm².[220] Areal BMD of the lumbar spine (L2-L4) is low in prematurely born infants but "catches up" to that of full-term infants by

TABLE 3-8

Whole-Body Bone Mineral Content (BMC g) and Density (g/cm²) by Pencil Beam Dual-Energy X-ray Absorptiometry in Prematurely Born and Full-term Appropriate- or Small-for-Gestational-Age Infants (AGA, SGA)

GA	BMC				BMD	
	AGA	SD	SGA	SD		AGA
32-33	21.9	(9.7)[1]				
34-35	32.0)	(11.3				
36-37	39.4	(15.9)	24.9	(7.4)		
38-39	45.5	(18.4)	27.0	(11.1)		
Birth Weight		**Range**				**Range**
1001-1500	22.9	(21.7-24.1)[2]			0.146	(0.141-0.150)
1501-2000	31.8	(30.9-32.8)			0.162	(0.158-0.165)
2001-2500	42.2	(41.7-43.2)			0.178	(0.175-0.181)
2501-3000	54.6	(53.9-55.3)			0.199	(0.196-0.202)
3001-3500	66.9	(66.0-67.9)			0.220	(0.217-0.224)
3501-4000	77.6	(76.3-78.8)			0.234	(0.229-0.238)
Postnatal Age						
9-90	103	(10)[3]			0.238	(0.022)
91-150	137	(20)			0.259	(0.024)
150-270	196	(27)			0.302	(0.018)
271-390	253	(41)			0.335	(0.029)

GA = gestational age (weeks), birth weight (g), postnatal age (days) (95% range).

1. Lapillone A, et al. (1997). Body composition in appropriate and in small for gestational age infants. Acta Paediatr 86:196–200.
2. Koo WWK, et al. (1996). Dual-energy x-ray absorptiometry studies of bone mineral status in newborn infants. J Bone Miner Res 11:1997-1002.
3. Koo WWK, et al. (1998). Postnatal development of bone mineral status during infancy. J Am Coll Nutr 17:65-70.

2 years of age.[233] Particular attention to detail must be exercised when assessing bone mineralization in very small subjects by DEXA because even apparently minor changes (position on the scanning table, prone or supine posture, number of blankets overlaid or wrapped around the subject, administration of a bolus of intravenous fluid prior to scanning, presence of a radiographic contrast agent) may affect measurement of BMC and BMD.[234,235] It is important to reemphasize that infant software be employed for data analysis of DEXA measurements in small subjects because adult and pediatric software underestimate bone area and BMC but overestimate BMD in this group.[234]

Whole-body (or total body) BMC is the more accurate and reliable of the measurements provided by DEXA compared to regional measurements, particularly in growing children and adolescents.[228] Whole-body BMC increases three- to fourfold between 6 and 17 years of age[177,236-238] (Tables 3-9A and B). Whole-body BMC is greater in adult males than in females because of the larger size of male bones. The gender difference in whole-body BMC appears after 15 years of age. Lumbar vertebral BMD approximately doubles between 3 and 15 years of age in boys (0.454 to 0.885 g/cm²) and girls (0.444 to 0.960 g/cm²); lumbar spine BMD increases rapidly between birth and 5 years in both sexes (between 13 and 15 years in boys, and between 12 and 14 years in girls)[236,238-240] (Table 3-9B and Table 3-10).

BMD of the femoral neck increases 1.5-fold during puberty. In females, the rate of maximal increase in whole-body BMC occurs in the year of menarche and follows the year of peak height velocity (Figure 3-15).[172,241] Peak BMC and BMD are reached at 18 to 20 years in both sexes, although there may be slight accrual of additional bone mass in the third decade of life. In girls with menarche

---

TABLE 3-9A

Whole-Body Bone Mineral Content (BMC g) and Areal(a) Bone Mineral Density (BMD g/cm²) by Pencil Beam Dual-Energy X-ray Absorptiometry in Children and Adolescents

CA	Males			Females	
	BMC[1]	aBMD[2]		BMC	aBMD
4-5		0.781 (0.05)			0.795 (0.02)
6-7	674 (149)	0.843 (0.03)		669 (152)	0.828 (0.06)
8-9	909 (187)	0.870 (0.04)		896 (185)	0.860 (0.05)
10-11	1186 (224)	0.894 (0.05)		1203 (223)	0.863 (0.07)
12-13	1540 (226)	0.961 (0.07)		1622 (267)	0.974 (0.09)
14-15	1965 (308)	1.030 (0.09)		2043 (294)	1.081 (0.07)
16-17	2395 (336)	1.133 (0.11)		2183 (268)	1.143 (0.09)
18-20		1.202 (0.11)			1.159 (0.07)
23-26[3]	2599 (511)	1.128 (0.11)		2308 (383)	1.088 (0.08)

CA = chronologic age (years).
Mean (SD).
1. Molgaard C, et al. (1997). Whole body bone mineral content in healthy children and adolescents. Arch Dis Child 76:9–15.
2. Boot AM, et al. (1997). Bone mineral density in children and adolescents: relation to puberty, calcium intake, and physical activity. J Clin Endocrinol Metab 82:57-62.
3. Bachrach LK, et al. (1999). Bone mineral acquisition in healthy Asian, Hispanic, black, and Caucasian youth: A longitudinal study. J Clin Endocrinol Metab 84:4702-4712.

TABLE 3-9B

Bone Mineral Density (g/cm²) by Fan-Beam Dual-Energy X-ray Absorptiometry in White Children in the United States (Hologic QDR 4500 Analyzed with Software Version 12.1) (mean ± SD)

CA	Males			Females		
	Whole Body	AP Spine	Total Hip	Whole Body	AP Spine	Total Hip
3	0.582 (0.039)	0.454 (0.047)	—	0.561 (0.039)	0.444 (0.046)	—
5	0.655 (0.046)	0.492 (0.052)	0.572 (0.062)	0.637 (0.046)	0.490 (0.054)	0.553 (0.061)
7	0.717 (0.052)	0.530 (0.058)	0.652 (0.070)	0.698 (0.053)	0.538 (0.062)	0.602 (0.069)
9	0.791 (0.060)	0.578 (0.066)	0.720 (0.080)	0.768 (0.060)	0.597 (0.075)	0.669 (0.081)
11	0.866 (0.068)	0.648 (0.084)	0.786 (0.092)	0.856 (0.068)	0.697 (0.099)	0.764 (0.097)
13	0.945 (0.077)	0.750 (0.112)	0.872 (0.110)	0.959 (0.073)	0.853 (0.116)	0.869 (0.110)
15	1.041 (0.089)	0.885 (0.125)	0.973 (0.129)	1.041 (0.075)	0.960 (0.111)	0.938 (0.112)
17	1.133 (0.101)	0.995 (0.123)	1.064 (0.143)	1.084 (0.075)	1.003 (0.107)	0.970 (0.110)
19	1.205 (0.111)	1.067 (0.120)	1.139 (0.152)	1.107 (0.074)	1.017 (0.105)	0.986 (0.108)

Zemel BS, et al. (2004). Reference data for whole body, lumbar spine and proximal femur for American children relative to age, gender and body size. J Bone Miner Res 19:(1):S231.

TABLE 3-10

Lumbar Spine Bone Mineral Content (BMC, L2–L4, g), Areal (aBMD - g/cm²), and Volumetric (vBMD-g/cm³) Bone Mineral Densities and Femoral Neck Areal Bone Mineral Density by Pencil Beam Dual-Energy X-ray Absorptiometry in Children and Adolescents

CA	Lumbar Spine			Femoral Neck[3]
	BMC[1]	aBMD[1,2]	vBMD[2]	
Males				
1	3.76 (1.54)	0.380 (0.06)		
3	9.37 (1.91)	0.565 (0.07)		
5	14.5 (1.72)	0.625 (0.06)	0.261 (0.03)	
7	19.4 (3.42)	0.720 (0.06)	0.282 (0.04)	
9	22.2 (2.17)	0.755 (0.08)	0.288 (0.03)	0.824
11	23.7 (2.22)	0.791 (0.07)	0.282 (0.03)	0.965 (0.072)
13	31.1 (8.04)	0.868 (0.13)	0.280 (0.03)	0.910 (0.119)
15	44.5 (13.1)	1.058 (0.10)	0.312 (0.03)	1.169 (0.132)
17	54.2 (9.46)	1.204 (0.11)	0.347 (0.04)	1.044 (0.096)
19	68.7 (4.81)	1.238 (0.10)	0.355 (0.03)	1.258 (0.109)
21	69.0 (5.25)	1.220 (0.12)		
23-26[4]		1.037 (0.15)		0.916 (0.136)
Females				
1	4.61 (1.24)	0.380 (0.06)		
3	9.91 (1.58)	0.565 (0.07)		
5	13.4 (1.40)	0.674 (0.07)	0.288 (0.02)	
7	16.4 (2.05)	0.710 (0.03)	0.290 (0.03)	
9	22.2 (3.65)	0.745 (0.08)	0.296 (0.04)	0.692 (0.079)
11	26.2 (4.10)	0.887 (0.14)	0.313 (0.03)	0.810 (0.061)
13	39.1 (6.98)	1.024 (0.15)	0.345 (0.04)	0.924 (0.101)
15	39.2 (6.47)	1.239 (0.12)	0.396 (0.04)	1.056 (0.207)
17	46.1 (5.1)	1.214 (0.11)	0.390 (0.03)	0.981 (0.122)
19	46.0 (5.95)	1.246 (0.15)	0.397 (0.05)	0.962 (0.072)
21	47.5 (6.59)	1.200 (0.12)		
23-26[4]		1.074 (0.12)		0.873 (0.114)

Pubertal Stage	Whole-Body BMD[2]	Lumbar Spine BMD[2]
Males		
I	0.86 (0.06)	0.69 (0.09)
II	0.94 (0.07)	0.82 (0.10)
III	1.02 (0.10)	0.91 (0.15)
IV	1.11 (0.12)	1.08 (0.17)
V	1.15 (0.09)	1.15 (0.09)
Females		
I	0.84 (0.05)	0.71 (0.08)
II	0.93 (0.05)	0.83 (0.07)
III	0.97 (0.08)	0.96 (0.15)
IV	1.08 (0.09)	1.14 (0.15)
V	1.15 (0.08)	1.22 (0.14)

CA = chronologic age.
Mean (SD).

1. del Rio L, et al. (1994). Bone mineral density of the lumbar spine in white Mediterranean Spanish children and adolescents: Changes related to age, sex, and puberty. Pediatr Res 35:362-366.
2. Boot AM, et al. (1997). Bone mineral density in children and adolescents: relation to puberty, calcium intake, and physical activity. J Clin Endocrinol Metab 82:57-62.
3. Kroger H, et al. (1993). Development of bone mass and bone density of the spine and femoral neck: A prospective study of 65 children and adolescents. Bone Mineral 23:171-182.
4. Bachrach LK, et al. (1999). Bone mineral acquisition in healthy Asian, Hispanic, black, and Caucasian youth: A longitudinal study. J Clin Endocrinol Metab 84:4702-4712.

before 12 years, there is greater peak BMD (at age 18-19 years) than in females with menarche after 14 years.[242] Similarly, in adult males with a history of delayed puberty there is lower lumbar spine BMD than in those with pubertal onset at 11 to 12 years.[243] A major drawback to the use of DEXA for determination of bone mineralization in children is the reliance of reference data on chronologic age independent of body size. Thus, a short child may appear to have decreased bone mineralization relative to chronologic age but a satisfactory value relative to height age.

Accordingly, assessment of bone mass relative to height is essential (Figure 3-16). DEXA measurements of bone mineralization are also affected by the composition of soft tissues that surround the axial skeleton. Thus, variations in fat about the bone may significantly influence the recorded DEXA measurements—limiting the use of DEXA in extremely thin or obese children.[244] Generally, BMC, areal BMD, and/or BMAD below −2 SDs for age and gender are considered abnormally low. However, DEXA measurements must always be interpreted in relationship to the patient's clinical findings.[223]

QCT measures volumetric BMD of both trabecular and cortical bone at any site but has been commonly applied to the lumbar spine.[225] However, the radiation dose delivered to the spine by this method is high (~30 μSv). During childhood, lumbar spine vBMD measured by QCT is simi-lar in black and white youth. During puberty, black males and females gain twice the vBMD recorded in whites (with no gender difference). In peripheral (p)QCT, bone mineralization is quantified in distal and/or proximal radial, femoral, or tibial sites (regions of cortical and trabecular bone). The delivered radiation dose (10 μSv) is low.

Peripheral QCT may be examined in the radius two-thirds of the distance between its proximal and distal ends and distally at a point that is 4% of forearm length, with a reference line being drawn through the most distal aspect of the cartilage growth plate when it is open or through the middle of the ulnar border of the articular cartilage when the growth plate is closed.[245-247] pQCT permits measurement of total and cortical bone area, cortical thickness, BMC (mg/mm), cortical and trabecular vBMD, periosteal and endosteal circumferences, and marrow area. Proximal and distal radial bone pQCT data between 6 and 40 years of age and pubertal stages I through V are recorded in Table 3-11.

Interestingly, at all ages total cross-sectional and cortical areas, cortical thickness, BMC, and BMD are greater in males than in females. As mirrored by the proximal radius, pQCT documents the prolonged period of periosteal expansion in males that ultimately accounts for their larger bone size. Widespread application of pQCT awaits standardization of protocols for data acquisition and

Bone Area–Bone Mineral Content Total Body

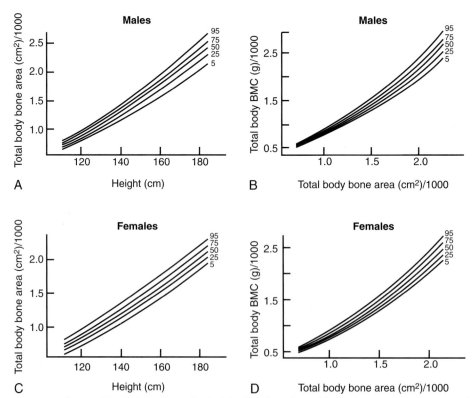

Figure 3-16. Reference curves for total body bone area for height (A, C) and total body bone mineral content (BMC) for bone area (B, D) in white male and female children and adolescents 6 to 17 years of age employing fan-beam dual-energy X-ray absorptiometry. [Reproduced with permission from Ward KA, et al. (2007). UK reference data for the Hologic QDR Discovery dual-energy x-ray absorptiometry scanner in healthy children and young adults aged 6-17 years. Arch Dis Child 92:53-59.]

TABLE 3-11A

Peripheral Quantitative Computed Tomography Non-dominant Proximal Radius (Mean ± SD)

Age	Total[1]	Cortical[1]	Cortical[2] Area	BMC[3] Area	vBMD[4] Thickness
Male					
6-7	73 (13)	37 (8)	1.45 (0.31)	52 (8)	579 (70)
8-9	86 (14)	47 (6)	1.71 (0.21)	61 (6)	601 (57)
10-11	98 (16)	52 (8)	1.78 (0.26)	68 (9)	596 (68)
12-13	108 (19)	57 (8)	1.85 (0.28)	73 (9)	589 (82)
14-15	123 (21)	72 (16)	2.27 (0.46)	91 (17)	645 (92)
16-17	128 (20)	83 (13)	2.63 (0.35)	105 (16)	720 (66)
18-23	151 (22)	95 (14)	2.75 (0.41)	121 (16)	719 (82)
Adult	158 (27)	97 (12)	2.74 (0.44)	125 (15)	711 (102)
Pubertal Stage					
I	87 (18)	45 (10)	1.64 (0.32)	61 (11)	593 (70)
II	108 (19)	57 (8)	1.88 (0.31)	74 (9)	597 (79)
III	114 (11)	59 (8)	1.84 (0.35)	75 (8)	574 (80)
IV	118 (19)	70 (13)	2.22 (0.32)	87 (16)	640 (66)
V	141 (23)	88 (17)	2.61 (0.47)	111 (19)	700 (90)
Female					
6-7	78 (12)	31 (8)	1.15 (0.39)	47 (6)	517 (84)
8-9	78 (13)	43 (8)	1.68 (0.35)	57 (9)	615 (90)
10-11	92(18)	51 (11)	1.84 (0.40)	65 (12)	619 (89)
12-13	100 (18)	61 (16)	2.14 (0.51)	77 (19)	662 (97)
14-15	109 (18)	70 (9)	2.38 (0.35)	89 (11)	722 (88)
16-17	114 (15)	73 (10)	2.42 (0.31)	94 (12)	717 (66)
18-23	111 (16)	71 (10)	2.42 (0.34)	93 (12)	749 (78)
Adult	117 (20)	75 (9)	2.48 (0.34)	99 (11)	763 (86)
Pubertal Stage					
I	81 (15)	40 (10)	1.50 (0.43)	55 (10)	577 (93)
II	90 (15)	50 (12)	1.81 (0.39)	65 (14)	607 (102)
III	89 (14)	53 (7)	1.98 (0.30)	68 (10)	648 (72)
IV	102 (17)	66 (8)	2.33 (0.34)	82 (9)	713 (85)
V	113 (16)	74 (11)	2.49 (0.34)	95 (13)	739 (75)

[1]mm^2 [2]mm [3]mg/mm [4]mg/cm^3

Neu CM, et al. (2001). Modeling of cross-sectional bone size, mass and geometry at the proximal radius: A study of normal bone development using peripheral quantitative computed tomography. Osteoporos Int 12:538-547.

analysis and larger reference databases. By direct comparison of bone mass data gathered by DEXA and tibial metaphyseal pQCT examinations in the same subjects (6-21 years), it has been observed that DEXA whole-body bone area and BMC for height correlate well with pQCT-derived cross-sectional area for tibial length.[248]

Although BMD values of the lumbar spine acquired by DEXA and QCT are reasonably well related, osteopenia is "identified" in children far more often by DEXA than by QCT because DEXA measurements do not account for body height and bone size.[244] Clearly, pQCT would appear to be the preferred method for quantitation of bone mineralization in children at this time.

Quantitative ultrasonography (QUS) measures the speed of a longitudinal sound (SOS) wave as it is propagated along a bone.[170] The rate of movement of sound through bone is dependent on its microstructural and macrostructural characteristics, mineral density, and elasticity—and is thought to be a measure of bone strength. It is an attractive method for assessment of bone because it does not utilize radiation, is low in cost, and the equipment is portable. Transmitter and receiver ultrasound transducers placed on either side of the examination site (os calcis, patella, tibia, radius, phalange) quantitate transmission velocity or signal attenuation and convert these observations to SOS. In a study of 1,085 children and adolescents, SOS increased steeply at the tibia and radius during the first 5 years of life, more slowly between 6 and 11 years of age, and then again more rapidly during pubertal development.[249]

In 3,044 healthy subjects ages 2 to 21 years, phalangeal QUS SOS and bone transmission time (BTT) increased over time and with advancing adolescent development—and were related to gender, age, height, and weight.[250] However, the overlap of QUS data between various ages makes interpretation of a single SOS measurement problematic. Serial assessment may be useful. Thus, in a cohort of 29 preterm infants tibial SOS values declined over time in neonates whose gestational ages were less than 29 weeks—suggesting progressive loss of bone strength in this population

TABLE 3-11B

Peripheral Quantitative Computed Tomography Non-dominant Distal Radius (Mean ± SD)

Age	vBMD-tot[1]	vBMD-Trab[1]	vBMD-cort[1]	CSA[2]
Males				
6-7	306 (34)	206 (32)	388 (42)	174 (31)
8-9	294 (34)	189 (34)	380 (41)	211 (31)
10-11	290 (33)	194 (32)	368 (41)	245 (37)
12-13	292 (38)	201 (36)	366 (47)	289 (47)
14-15	293 (35)	201 (33)	369 (47)	351 (70)
16-17	349 (56)	217 (30)	458 (86)	358 (49)
18-23	401 (60)	220 (42)	549 (83)	377 (64)
Adults	438 (56)	224 (46)	594 (81)	374 (45)
Pubertal Stage				
I	299 (32)	198 (31)	381 (41)	212 (47)
II	288 (40)	186 (31)	372 (52)	269 (43)
III	286 (33)	197 (36)	359 (37)	293 (44)
IV	296 (42)	210 (35)	367 (50)	334 (65)
V	361 (72)	215 (40)	481 (109)	377 (59)
Females				
6-7	290 (36)	191 (31)	370 (45)	164 (30)
8-9	283 (22)	186 (23)	362 (32)	185 (25)
10-11	281 (36)	191 (36)	355 (44)	237 (39)
12-13	295 (39)	197 (32)	376 (54)	260 (55)
14-15	303 (37)	179 (25)	407 (53)	297 (32)
16-17	350 (57)	186 (26)	483 (95)	300 (45)
18-23	371 (50)	195 (35)	516 (74)	295 (42)
Adults	395 (46)	182 (34)	569 (69)	281 (37)
Pubertal Stage				
I	284 (30)	187 (29)	363 (39)	188 (38)
II	277 (34)	190 (34)	348 (37)	239 (57)
III	288 (44)	204 (44)	356 (50)	250 (47)
IV	291 (43)	197 (32)	375 (56)	282 (30)
V	347 (54)	190 (28)	476 (87)	295 (43)

[1]mg/cm^3 [2]mm^2

Neu CM, et al. (2001). Bone densities and bone size at the distal radius in healthy children and adolescents: a study using peripheral quantitative computed tomography. Bone 28:227-232.

Rauch F, Schonau E (2005). Peripheral quantitative computed tomography of the distal radius in young subjects: New reference data and interpretation of results. J Musculoskelet Neuronal Interact 5:119-126

consistent with the development of osteopenia of prematurity.[251] Although there is marginal correlation between vBMD determined by pQCT and SOS measurements in children and adolescents, QUS may complement but is unlikely to replace assessment of mineralization by radiographic methods at this time.[252,253] Magnetic resonance imaging of the skeleton is being examined as a method of assessment of bone geometry and strength.[254]

Concluding Remarks

Calcium, phosphate, and magnesium are vital to normal moment-to-moment function of all cells, and calcium and phosphate compose the mineral phase of the skeleton.

This structure is essential to protection of body organs and to movement, and as a warehouse for these minerals. To an extent, the complex genetic and physiologic mechanisms that require vitamin D, PTH, and PTHrP to regulate calcium, phosphate, magnesium, and skeletal homeostasis have been deciphered—thereby permitting application of this information to the management of patients with derangements in this system (as detailed in an accompanying chapter).

In regard to this chapter, two manuscripts of interest have been published. The physiology and genetic regulation of bone formation and resorption have been reviewed in detail.[258] The most current data on whole-body and regional bone mineral content and density in North American children and adolescents analyzed by age, gender, and race have been presented[259] (Figure 3-17).

Bone Mineral Content Age, Gender, Race

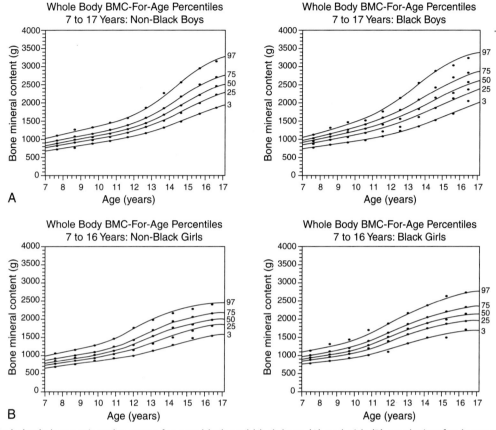

Figure 3-17. Whole-body bone mineral content for non-black and black boys (A) and girls (B) employing fan-beam dual-energy x-ray absorptiometry. [Reproduced with permission from Kalkwarf HJ, Zemel BS, Gilsanz V, et al. (2007). The bone mineral density in childhood study: Bone mineral content and density according to age, sex, and race. J Clin Endocrinol Metab 92:2087-2099.]

REFERENCES

1. Favus MJ, Bushinsky DA, Lemann J Jr. (2006). Regulation of calcium, magnesium, and phosphate metabolism. In Favus MJ (ed.), *Primer on the metabolic bone diseases and disorders of mineral metabolism, Sixth edition*. Washington D.C.:American Society for Bone and Mineral Research 76–83.
2. Bringhurst R, Demay MB, Kronenberg HM (2003). Hormones and disorders of mineral metabolism. In Larsen PR, Kronenberg HM, Melmed S, Polonsky KS (eds), *Williams textbook of endocrinology, Tenth edition*. Philadelphia: Saunders 1303–1371.
3. Williams PD, Puddey IB, Martin NG, Beilin LJ (1992). Plasma cytosolic free calcium concentration, total plasma calcium concentration and blood pressure in human twins: A genetic analysis. Clin Sci 82:493–504.
4. Dewitte K, Stockl D, Thienpont LM (1999). pH dependency of serum ionised calcium. Lancet 354:1793–1794.
5. Bushinsky DA, Monk RD (1998). Calcium. Lancet 352:306–311.
6. Gill DL, Spassova MA, Soboloff J (2006). Calcium entry signals: Trickles and torrents. Science 313:183–184.
7. Davila HM (1999). Molecular and functional diversity of voltage-gated calcium channels. Ann NY Acad Sci 868:102–117.
8. Halling DB, Aracena-Parks P, Hamilton SL (2005). Regulation of voltage-gated Ca²⁺ channels by calmodulin. Sci STKE 2005, re15.
9. Abernethy DR, Schwartz JB (1999). Calcium-antagonist drugs. N Engl J Med 341:1447–1457.
10. Burgess DL, Noebels JL (1999). Voltage-dependent calcium channel mutations in neurological disease. Ann NY Acad Sci 868:199–212.

11. Stea A, Dubel SJ, Snutch TP (1999). α1B N-type calcium channel isoforms with distinct biophysical properties. Ann NY Acad Sci 868:118–130.
12. Dellis O, Dedos SG, Tovey SC, et al. (2006). Ca²⁺ entry through plasma membrane IP₃ receptors. Science 313:229–233.
13. Vig M, Peinelt C, Beck A, et al. (2006). CRACM1 is a plasma membrane protein essential for store-operated Ca²⁺ entry. Science 312:1220–1223.
14. Feske S, Gwack Y, Prakriya M, et al. (2006). A mutation in Orai1 causes immune deficiency by abrogating CRAC channel function. Nature 441:179–185.
15. Wong V, Goodenough DA (1999). Paracellular channels! Science 285:62.
16. Nillus B, Voeta T, Peters J (2005). TRP channels in disease. Sci STKE 2005, re8.
17. Lanou AJ, Berkow SE, Barnard ND (2005). Calcium, dairy products, and bone health in children and young adults: A reevaluation of the evidence. Pediatrics 115:736–743.
18. Gartner LM, Greer FR (2003). Prevention of rickets and vitamin D deficiency: New guidelines for Vitamin D intake. Pediatrics 111:908–910.
19. Hollis BW (2005). Circulating 25-hydroxyvitamin D levels indicative of vitamin D sufficiency: Implications for establishing a new effective dietary intake recommendation for vitamin D. J Nutr 135:317–322.
20. Greer FR, Krebs NF (2006). Optimizing bone health and calcium intakes of infants, children, and adolescents. Pediatrics 117:578–585.
21. Greer FR (2005). Bone health: It's more than calcium intake. Pediatrics 115:792–794.

22. Bushinsky DA (1999). Calcium, magnesium, and phosphorus: Renal handling and urinary excretion. In Favus M (ed.), *Primer on the metabolic bone diseases and disorders of mineral metabolism, Fourth edition.* Philadelphia: Lippincott Williams & Wilkins 67–74.

23. Chang Q, Hoefs S, van der Kempt AW, et al. (2005). The beta glucuronidase klotho hydrolyzes and activates the TRPV5 channel. Science 310:490–493.

24. Brown EM, Juppner H (2006). Parathyroid hormone: Synthesis, secretion, and action. In Favus MJ (ed.), *Primer on the metabolic bone diseases and disorders of mineral metabolism, Sixth edition.* Washington, D.C.: American Society for Bone and Mineral Research 90–99.

25. Gether U (2000). Uncovering molecular mechanisms involved in activation of G protein-coupled receptors. Endocrine Reviews 21:90–113.

26. Yamaguchi T, Chattopadhyay N, Brown EM (2000). G protein-coupled extracellular Ca^{2+} (Ca^{2+}_o)-sensing receptor (CaR): Roles in cell signaling and control of diverse cellular functions. In O'Malley BW (ed.), *Hormones and signaling.* New York: Academic Press 209–253.

27. Pidasheva S, Grant M, Canaff L, et al. (2006). Calcium-sensing receptor dimerizes in the endoplasmic reticulum: Biochemical and biophysical characterization of the CASR mutants retained intracellularly. Hum Molec Genet 15:2200–2209.

28. Friedman PA (1999). Calcium transport in the kidney. Curr Opin Nephrol Hypertension 8:589–595.

29. Cole DEC, Peltekova VD, Rubin LA, et al. (1999). A986S polymorphism of the calcium-sensing receptor and circulating calcium concentrations. Lancet 353:112–115.

30. Scillitani A, Guarnieri V, de Geronimo S, et al. (2004). Blood ionized calcium is associated with clustered polymorphisms in the carboxyl-terminal tail of the calcium-sensing receptor. J Clin Endocrinol Metab 89:5634–5638.

31. Chang W, Tu C, Chen T-H, Komuves L, et al. (1999). Expression and signal transduction of calcium-sensing receptors in cartilage and bone. Endocrinology 140:5883–5893.

32. Zaidi M, Adebanjo OA (2000). Calcium handling by the osteoclast. The Endocrinologist 10:155–163.

33. Chattopadhyayl N, Yamaguchi T, Brown EM (1998). Ca^{2+} receptor from brain to gut: Common stimulus, diverse actions. Trends Endocrinol Metab 9:354–359.

34. De Luca F, Baron J (1998). The Ca^{2+}-sensing receptor: Molecular biology and clinical importance. Curr Opin Pediatr 10:435–440.

35. Steddon SJ, Cunningham J (2005). Calcimimetics and calcilytics: Fooling the calcium receptor. Lancet 365:2237–2239.

36. Dong BJ (2005). Cinacalcet: An oral calcimimetic agent for the management of hyperparathyroidism. Clin Therapeutics 27:1725–1751.

37. Weisinger JR, Bellorin-Font E (1998). Magnesium and phosphorus. Lancet 352:391–396.

38. White KE, Larsson TE, Econs MJ (2006). The roles of specific genes implicated as circulating factors in normal and disordered phosphate homeostasis: Frizzled related protein-4, matric extracellular phosphoglycoprotein, and fibroblast growth factor 23. Endocrine Reviews 27:221–241.

39. Drezner MK (2000). PHEX gene and hypophosphatemia. Kid Internat 57:9–18.

40. Jan de Beur SM (2006). Tumor-induced osteomalacia. In Favus MJ (ed.), *Primer on the metabolic bone diseases and disorders of mineral metabolism, Sixth edition.* Washington, D.C.: American Society for Bone and Mineral Research 345–351.

41. Kolek OI, Hines ER, Jones MD, et al. (2005). 1α,25-Dihydroxyvitamin D_3 upregulates FGF23 gene expression in bone: The final link in a renal-gastrointestinal-skeletal axis that controls phosphate transport. Am J Physiol Gastrointest Liver Physiol 289:G1036–G1042

42. Masuyama R, Stockmans I, Torrekens S, et al. (2006). Vitamin D receptor in chondrocytes promotes osteoclastogenesis and regulates FGF23 production in osteoblasts. J Clin Invest 116:3150–3159.

43. Yu X, Ibrahimi OA, Goetz R, et al. (2005). Analysis of the biochemical mechanisms for the endocrine actions of fibroblast growth factor-23. Endocrinology 146:4647–4656.

44. Campos M, Couture C, Hirata, IY, et al. (2003). Human recombinant PHEX has a strict S1' specificity for acidic residues and cleaves peptides derived from FGF23 and MEPE. Biochem J 373:271–279.

45. Benet-Pages A, Orlik P, Strom TM, Lorenz-Depiereux B (2005). An FGF23 missense mutation causes familial tumor calcinosis with hyperphosphatemia. Hum Molec Genet 14:385–390.

46. Carpenter TO, Ellis TK, Insogna RL, et al. (2004). Fibroblast growth factor 7: An inhibitor of phosphate transport derived from oncogenic osteomalacia-causing tumors. J Clin Endocrinol Metab 90:1012–1020.

47. Gowen LC, Petersen DN, Mansolf AL, et al. (2003). Targeted disruption of the osteoblast/osteocyte factor 45 gene (OF45) results in increased bone formation and bone mass. J Biol Chem 278:1998–2007.

48. Simon DB, Lu Y, Choate KA, et al. (1999). Paracellin-1, a renal tight junction protein required for paracellular Mg^{2+} resorption. Science 285:103–106.

49. Kausalya RJ, Amasheh S, Gunzel D, et al. (2006). Disease associated mutations affect intracellular traffic and paracellular Mg^{2+} transport function of Claudin16. J Clin Invest 116:878–891.

50. Whyte MP (1994). Hypophosphatasia and the role of alkaline phosphatase. Endocrine Reviews 15:439–461.

51. Gunther T, Chen Z-F, Kim J, et al. (2000). Genetic ablation of parathyroid glands reveals another source of parathyroid hormone. Nature 406:199–203.

52. Maret A, Bordeaux I, Ding C, et al. (2004). Expression of GCM by intra thymic parathyroid hormone-secreting adenomas indicates their parathyroid cell origin. J Clin Endocrinol Metab 89:8–12.

53. Epstein E, Sela-Brown A, Ringel I, et al. (2000). Dynein light chain binding to a 3'-untranslated sequence mediates parathyroid hormone mRNA association with microtubules. J Clin Invest 105:505–512.

54. D'Amour P, Brossard J, Rousseau L, et al. (2005). Structure of non-(1-84) PTH fragments secreted by parathyroid glands in primary and secondary hyperparathyroidism. Kidney Int 68:998–1007.

55. Murray TM, Rao LG, Divieti P, Bringhurst PR (2005). Parathyroid hormone secretion and action: Evidence for discrete receptors for the carboxyl-terminal region and related biological actions of carboxyl-terminal ligands. Endocrine Reviews 26:78–113.

56. Salusky IB, Juppner H (2004). New PTH assays and renal osteodystrophy. Pediatr Nephrol 19:709–713.

57. Cantor T, Yang Z, Caraiani N, Ilamathi E (2006). Lack of comparability of intact parathyroid hormone measurements among commercial assays for end-stage renal disease patients: Implication for treatment decisions. Clin Chem 52:1771–1776.

58. Vietri MT, Sessa M, Pilla P, et al. (2006). Serum osteocalcin and parathyroid hormone in healthy children assessed with two new automated assays. J Pediatr Endocrinol Metab 19:1413–1419.

59. Broadus AE, Nissenson RA (2006). Parathyroid hormone-related protein. In Favus MJ (ed.), *Primer on the metabolic bone diseases and disorders of mineral metabolism, Sixth edition.* Washington, D.C.: American Society for Bone and Mineral Research 99–106.

60. Strewler GJ (2000). The physiology of parathyroid hormone-related protein. New Engl J Med 342:177–185.

61. Nissenson RA (1998). Editorial: Parathyroid hormone (PTH)/PTHrP receptor mutations in human chondrodysplasia. Endocrinology 139:4753–4755.

62. Miao D, He B, Karaplis AC, Goltzman D (2002). Parathyroid hormone is essential for normal fetal bone formation. J Clin Invest 109:1173–1182.

63. Henderson JE, Amizuka N, Warshawsky H, et al. (1995). Nuclear localization of parathyroid hormone-related peptide enhances survival of chondrocytes under conditions that promote apoptotic death. Mol Cell Biol 15:4064–4075.

64. Kovacs CS, Chafe LL, Fudge NJ, et al. (2001). PTH regulates fetal blood calcium and skeletal mineralization independently of PTHrP. Endocrinology 142:4983–4993.

65. Buhimschi CS (2004). Endocrinology of lactation. Obstet Gynecol Clin North Am 31:963–979.

66. Sowers MF, Hollis BW, Shapiro B, et al. (1996). Elevated parathyroid hormone-related peptide associated with lactation and bone density loss. J Am Med Assn 276:549–554.

67. Iida-Klein A, Guo J, Takemura M, et al. (1997). Mutations in the second cytoplasmic loop of the rat parathyroid hormone (PTH)/PTH-related protein receptor results in selective loss of PTH-stimulated PLC activity. J Biol Chem 272:6882–6889.

68. Pickard BW, Hodsman AB, Fraher LJ, Watson PH (2006). Type 1 parathyroid hormone receptor (PTH1R) nuclear trafficking: Association of PTH1R with importin $_{α1}$ and $_β$. Endocrinology 147:3326–3332.

69. Usdin TB, Gruber C, Bonner TI (1996). Identification and functional expression of a receptor selectively recognizing parathyroid hormone: The PTH2 receptor. J Biol Chem 270:15455–15458.

70. Deftos LJ (2006). Calcitonin. In Favus MJ (ed.), *Primer on the metabolic bone diseases and disorders of mineral metabolism, Sixth edition*. Washington, D.C.: American Society for Bone and Mineral Research 115–117.

71. Leboeuf R, Langlois F, Martin M, et al. (2006). "Hook effect" in calcitonin immunoradiometric assay in patients with metastatic medullary thyroid carcinoma: Case report and review of the literature. J Clin Endocrinol Metab 91:361–364.

72. Taboulet J, Frenkian M, Frendo JL, et al. (1998). Calcitonin receptor polymorphism is associated with a decreased fracture risk in postmenopausal women. Hum Molec Genet 7:2129–2133.

73. Woodrow JP, Sharpe CJ, Fudge NJ, et al. (2006). Calcitonin plays a critical role in regulating skeletal mineral metabolism during lactation. Endocrinology 147:4010–4021.

74. Holick MF, Garabedian M (2006). Vitamin D photobiology, metabolism, mechanism of action, and clinical application. In Favus MJ (ed.), *Primer on the metabolic bone diseases and disorders of mineral metabolism, Sixth edition*. Washington, D.C.: American Society for Bone and Mineral Research 106–114.

75. Armas LAG, Hollis BW, Heaney RP (2004). Vitamin D_2 is much less effective than vitamin D_3 in humans. J Clin Endocrinol Metab 89:5387–5391.

76. Holick MF (2006). Resurrection of vitamin D deficiency and rickets. J Clin Invest 116:2062–2072.

77. Hollis BW, Wagner CL (2006). Nutritional vitamin D status during pregnancy: Reasons for concern. CMAJ 174:1287–1290.

78. Fu GK, Lin D, Zhang MYH, et al. (1997). Cloning of human 25-hydroxyvitamin D-1_-hydroxylase and mutations causing vitamin D-dependent rickets type 1. Molec Endocrinol 11:1961–1970.

79. Monkawa T, Yoshida T, Wakino S, et al. (1997). Molecular cloning of cDNA and genomic DNA for human 25-hydroxyvitamin D_3 1α-hydroxylase. Biochem Biophys Res Comm 239:527–533.

80. Wang JT, Lin C-J, Burridge SM, et al. (1998). Genetics of vitamin D 1α-hydroxylase deficiency in 17 families. Am J Hum Genet 63:1694–1702.

81. Overbaugh L, Stoffels K, Waer M, et al. (2006). Immune regulation of 25-hydroxyvitamin D-1α-hydroxylase in human monocytic THP1 cells: Mechanisms of interferon-α-mediated induction. J Clin Endocrinol Metab 91:3566–3574.

82. Murayama A, Takeyama K, Kitanaka S, et al. (1999). Positive and negative regulations of the renal 25-hydroxyvitamin D3 1 alpha-hydroxylase gene by parathyroid hormone, calcitonin, and 1 alpha,25(OH)2D3 in intact animals. Endocrinology 140:2224–2231.

83. Zhou C, Assem M, Tay JC, et al. (2006). Steroid and xenobiotic receptor and vitamin D receptor crosstalk mediates CYP24 expression and drug-induced osteomalacia. J Clin Invest 116:1703–1712.

84. Makishima M, Lu TT, Xie W, et al. (2002). Vitamin D receptor as an intestinal bile acid sensor. Science 296:1313–1316.

85. Norman AW (2006). Vitamin D receptor: New assignments for an already busy receptor. Endocrinology 147:5542–5548.

86. Root AW, Rogol AD (2005). Organization and function of the endocrine system. In Kappy M, Allen D, Geffner M (eds.), *Principles and practice of pediatric endocrinology*. Springfield, IL: Charles Thomas 3–76.

87. Xue Y, Karaplis AC, Hendry GN, et al. (2006). Exogenous 1,25-dihydroxyvitamin D_3 exerts a skeletal anabolic effect and improves mineral ion homeostasis in mice that are homozygous for both the 1α-hydroxylase and parathyroid hormone null alleles. Endocrinology 147:4801–4810.

88. Demay M (2003). Muscle: A nontraditional 1,25-dihydroxyvitamin D target tissue exhibiting classic hormone-dependent vitamin D receptor actions. Endocrinology 144:5135–5137.

89. Haussler MR, Haussler CA, Jurutka PW, et al. (1997). The vitamin D hormone and its nuclear receptor: molecular actions and disease states. J Endocrinol 154:S57–S73.

90. Nagpal S, Na S, Rathnachalam R (2005). Noncalcemic actions of vitamin D receptor ligands. Endocrine Reviews 26:662–687.

91. Malloy PJ, Pike JW, Feldman D (1999). The vitamin D receptor and the syndrome of hereditary 1,25-dihydroxyvitamin D-resistant rickets. Endocrine Reviews 20:156–188.

92. Gilad LA, Bresler T, Gnainsky J, et al. (2005). Regulation of vitamin D receptor expression via estrogen-induced activation of the ERK 1/2 signaling pathway in colon and breast cancer cells. J Endocrinol 185:577–592.

93. Wood RJ, Fleet JC (1998). The genetics of osteoporosis: Vitamin D receptor polymorphisms. Ann Rev Nutr 18:233–258.

94. Tao C, Yu T, Garnett S, et al. (1998). Vitamin D receptor alleles predict growth and bone density in girls. Arch Dis Child 79:488–494.

95. Lorentzon M, Lorentzon R, Nordstrom P (2000). Vitamin D receptor gene polymorphism is associated with birth height, growth to adolescence, and adult stature in healthy Caucasian men: A cross-sectional and longitudinal study. J Clin Endocrinol Metab 85:1666–1671.

96. Xiong D-H, Xu FH, Liu P-Y, et al. (2005). Vitamin D receptor gene polymorphisms are linked to and associated with adult height. J Med Genet 42:228–234.

97. Kitagawa H, Fujiki R, Yoshimura K, et al. (2003). The chromatin-remodel complex WINAC targets a nuclear receptor to promoters and is impaired in Williams syndrome. Cell 113:905–917.

98. Li YC, Pirro AE, Amling M, et al. (1997). Targeted ablation of the vitamin D receptor: An animal model of vitamin D-dependent rickets type II with alopecia. Proc Natl Acad Sci USA 94:9831–9835.

99. Amling M, Priemel M, Holzmann T, et al. (1999). Rescue of skeletal phenotype of vitamin D receptor-ablated mice in the setting of normal mineral ion homeostasis: Formal histomorphometric and biomechanical analyses. Endocrinology 140:4982–4987.

100. Yagishita N, Yamamoto Y, Yoshizawa T, et al. (2001). Aberrant growth plate development in VDR/RXR double null mutant mice. Endocrinology 142:5332–5341.

101. Rummens K, Van Cromphaut SJ, Carmeliet G, et al. (2003). Pregnancy in mice lacking the vitamin D receptor: Normal maternal skeletal response, but fetal hypomineralization rescued by maternal calcium supplementation. Pediatr Res 54:466–473.

102. Fleet JC (2004). Rapid, membrane-initiated actions of 1,25 dihydroxyvitamin D: What are they and what do they mean? J Nutrition 134:3215–3218.

103. Norman AW, Mizwicki MT, Norman DP (2004). Steroid-hormone rapid actions, membrane receptors and a conformational ensemble model. Nat Rev Drug Discov 3:21–41.

104. Oka S-I, Masutani H, Liu W, et al. (2006). Thioredoxin-binding protein-2-like inducible membrane protein is a novel vitamin D3 and peroxisome proliferator-activated receptor (PPAR) gamma ligand target protein that regulates PPAR gamma signaling. Endocrinology 147:733–743.

105. Huhtakangas JA, Olivera CJ, Bishop JE, et al. (2004). The vitamin D receptor is present in caveolae-enriched plasma membranes and binds 1α,25(OH)$_2$-vitamin D_3 in vivo and in vitro. Mol Endocrinol 18:2660–2671.

106. Boyan BD, Schwartz Z (2004). Rapid vitamin D dependent PKC signaling shares features with estrogen-dependent PKC signaling in cartilage and bone. Steroids 69:591–597.

107. Peng L, Malloy PJ, Feldman D (2004). Identification of a functional vitamin D response element in the human insulin-like growth factor binding protein-3 promoter. Mol Endocrinol 18:1109–1119.

108. Pedrozo HA, Schwartz Z, Rimes S, et al. (1999). Physiological importance of the 1,25(OH)2D3 membrane receptor and evidence for a membrane receptor specific for 24,25(O)2D3. J Bone Miner Res 14:856–857.

109. Baron R (1999). Anatomy and ultrastructure of bone. In Favus M (ed.), *Primer on the metabolic bone diseases and disorders of mineral metabolism, Fourth edition*. Philadelphia: Lippincott Williams & Wilkins 3–10.

110. Cohen MM Jr. (2006). The new bone biology: Pathologic, molecular, and clinical studies. Am J Med Genet 140A:2646–2706.

111. Dempster DW (2006). Anatomy and function of the adult skeleton. In Favus MJ (ed.), *Primer on the metabolic bone diseases and disorders of mineral metabolism, Sixth edition*. Washington, D.C.: American Society for Bone and Mineral Research 7–11.

112. Aubin JE, Lian JB, Stein GB (2006). Bone formation: Maturation and functional activities of osteoblast lineage cells. In Favus MJ (ed.), *Primer on the metabolic bone diseases and disorders of mineral metabolism, Sixth edition*. Washington, D.C.: American Society for Bone and Mineral Research 20–29.

113. Kaplan FS, Fiori J, Serrano de la Pena L, et al. (2006). Dysregulation of the BMP-4 signaling pathway in fibrodysplasia ossificans progressiva. Ann NY Acad Sci 1068:54–65.

114. Kronenberg HM (2003). Developmental regulation of the growth plate. Nature 423:332–336.

115. Karsenty G (2003). The complexities of skeletal biology. Nature 423:316–318.

116. Olsen BR (2006). Bone embryology. In Favus MJ (ed.), *Primer on the metabolic bone diseases and disorders of mineral metabolism, Sixth edition.* Washington, D.C.: American Society for Bone and Mineral Research 2–6.

117. Nelson WJ, Nusse R (2004). Convergence of Wnt, β-catenin, and cadherin pathways. Science 303:1483–1487.

118. Ott SM (2005). Sclerostin and Wnt signaling: The pathway to bone strength. J Clin Endocrinol Metab 90:6741–6743.

119. James MJ, Jarvinen E, Wang X-P, Thesleff I (2006). Different roles of Runx2 during early neural crest-derived bone and tooth development. J Bone Miner Res 21:1034–1044.

120. Hill TP, Spater D, Taketo MM, et al. (2005). Canonical Wnt/beta-catenin signaling prevents osteoblasts from differentiating into chondrocytes. Dev Cell 8:727–738.

121. Zelzer E, Olsen BR (2005). Multiple roles of vascular endothelial growth factor (VEGF) in skeletal development, growth, and repair. Curr Topics Dev Biol 65:169–187.

122. Bamshad M, Watkins WS, Dixon, ME, et al. (1999). Reconstructing the history of human limb development: Lessons from birth defects. Pediatr Res 45:291–299.

123. Marglies EH, Innis JW (2000). Building arms or legs with molecular models. Pediatr Res 47:2–3.

124. Thiel CT, Horn D, Zabel B, et al. (2005). Severely incapacitating mutations in patients with extreme short stature identify RNA-processing endoribonuclease *RMRP* as an essential cell growth regulator. Am J Hum Genet 77:795–806.

125. De Luca F (2006). Impaired growth plate chondrogenesis in children with chronic illness. Pediatr Res 59:625–629.

126. Robson H, Siebler T, Shalet SM, Williams GR (2003). Interactions between GH, IGF-I, glucocorticoids, and thyroid hormones during skeletal growth. Pediatr Res 52:137–147.

127. Kobayashi T, Soegiarto DW, Yang Y, et al. (2005). Indian hedgehog stimulates periarticular chondrocyte differentiation to regulate growth plate length independently of PTHrP. J Clin Invest 115:1734–1742.

128. Huang W, Chung U, Kronenberg HM, de Crombrugghe B (2001). The chondrogenic transcription factor Sox9 is a target of signaling by the parathyroid hormone-related peptide in the growth plate of endochondral bones. Proc Nat Acad Sci 98:160–165.

129. Lanske B, Karalis AC, Lee K, et al. (1996). PTH/PTHrP receptor in early development and Indian hedgehog-regulated bone growth. Science 273:663–666.

130. Backesjo C-M, Li Y, Lindgren U, Haldosen L-A (2006). Activation of Sirt1 decreases adipocyte formation during osteoblast differentiation of mesenchymal stem cells. J Bone Miner Res 21:993–1002.

131. Ducy P, Schinke T, Karsenty G (2000). The osteoblast: A sophisticated fibroblast under central surveillance. Science 289:1501–1504.

132. Manolagas SC (2000). Birth and death of bone cells: Basic regulatory mechanisms and implications for the pathogenesis and treatment of osteoporosis. Endocrine Reviews 21:115–137.

133. Robey PG, Boskey AL (2006). Extracellular matrix and biomineralization of bone. In Favus MJ (ed.), *Primer on the metabolic bone diseases and disorders of mineral metabolism, Sixth edition.* Washington, D.C.: American Society for Bone and Mineral Research 12–19.

134. Suda T, Takahashi N, Udagawa N, et al. (1999). Modulation of osteoclast differentiation and function by the new members of the tumor necrosis factor receptor and ligand families. Endocrine Reviews 20:345–357.

135. Bilezikian JP (2006). What's good for the goose's skeleton is good for the gander's skeleton. J Clin Endocrinol Metab 91:1223–1225.

136. Vanderschueren D, Venken K, Ophoff J, et al. (2006). Sex steroids and the periosteum: Reconsidering the roles of androgens and estrogens in periosteal expansion. J Clin Endocrinol Metab 91:378–382.

137. Bickle DB, Sakata T, Leary C, et al. (2002). Insulin-like growth factor I is required for the anabolic actions of parathyroid hormone on mouse bone. J Bone Miner Res 17:1570–1578.

138. Fukushima N, Hanada R, Teranishi H, et al. (2004). Ghrelin directly regulates bone formation. J Bone Miner Res 20:790–798.

139. Rogers A, Eastell R (2005). Circulating osteoprotegerin and receptor activator for nuclear factor κB ligand: Clinical utility in metabolic bone disease assessment. J Clin Endocrinol Metab 90:6323–6331.

140. Ross FP (2006). Osteoclast biology and bone resorption. In Favus MJ (ed.), *Primer on the metabolic bone diseases and disorders of mineral metabolism, Sixth edition.* Washington, D.C.: American Society for Bone and Mineral Research 30–35.

141. Teitelbaum SL (2000). Bone resorption by osteoclasts. Science 289:1504–1508.

142. Okamoto M, Murai J, Yoshikawa H, Tsumaloi N (2006). Bone morphogenetic proteins in bone stimulate osteoclasts and osteoblasts during bone development. J Bone Miner Res 21:1022–1033.

143. Hofbauer LC, Khosla S, Dunstan CR, et al. (2000). The roles of osteoprotegerin and osteoprotegerin ligand in the paracrine regulation of bone resorption. J Bone Min Res 15:2–12.

144. Whyte MP, Obrecht SE, Finnegan PM, et al. (2002). Osteoprotegerin deficiency and juvenile Paget's disease. N Engl J Med 347:175–184.

145. Takayangi H, Kim S, Matsuo K, et al. (2002). RANKL maintains bone homeostasis through c-Fos-dependent induction of interferon-B. Nature 416:744–749.

146. Karin M (2006). Nuclear factor-κB in cancer development and progression. Nature 441:431–436.

147. Byers PH (1995). Disorders of collagen biosynthesis and structure. In Scriver CR, Beaudet AL, Sly WS, Vale D (eds.), *The metabolic and molecular bases of inherited disease, Seventh edition.* New York: McGraw-Hill 4029–4077.

148. Garnero P, Delmas PD (1998). Biochemical markers of bone turnover: Applications for osteoporosis. Endocrinol Metab Clin NA 27:303–323.

149. Barnes AM, Chang W, Morello R, et al. (2006). Deficiency of cartilage-associated protein in lethal osteogenesis imperfecta. N Engl J Med 355:2757–2764.

150. Cabral WA, Chang W, Barnes AM, et al. (2007). Prolyl 3-hydroxylase 1 deficiency causes a recessive metabolic bone disorder resembling lethal/severe osteogenesis imperfecta. Nature Genet 39:359–365.

151. Morello R, Bertin TK, Chen Y, et al. (2006). CRTAP is required for prolyl 3-hydroxylation and mutations cause recessive osteogenesis imperfecta. Cell 127:291–304.

152. Yamaga A, Taga M, Hashimoto S, Ota C. (1999). Comparison of bone metabolic markers between maternal and cord blood. Horm Res 51:277–279.

153. Seibold-Weiger K, Wollmann HA, Ranke MB, Speer CP (2000). Plasma concentrations of the carboxyterminal propeptide of type I procollagen (PICP) in preterm neonates from birth to term. Pediatr Res 48:104–108.

154. Naylor KE, Eastell R, Shattuck KE, et al. (1999). Bone turnover in premature infants. Pediatr Res 45:363–366.

155. Bollen A-M, Eyre DR (1994). Bone resorption rates in children monitored by the urinary assay of collagen type I cross-linked peptides. Bone 15:31–34.

156. Crofton PM, Wade JC, Taylor MRH, Holland CV (1997). Serum concentrations of carboxyl-terminal propeptide of type I procollagen, amino-terminal propeptide of type III procollagen, cross-linked carboxy-terminal telopeptide of type I collagen, and their interrelationships in school children. Clin Chem 43:1577–1581.

157. Hussain SM, Mughal Z, Williams G, et al. (1999). Urinary excretion of pyridinium crosslinks in healthy 4-10 year olds. Arch Dis Child 80:370–373.

158. Mora S, Pitukcheewanont P, Kaufman FR, et al. (1999). Biochemical markers of bone turnover and the volume and the density of bone in children at different stages of sexual development. J Bone Miner Res 14:1664–1671.

159. Sorva R, Anttila R, Siimes MA, et al. (1997). Serum markers of collagen metabolism and serum osteocalcin in relation to pubertal development in 57 boys at 14 years of age. Pediatr Res 42:528–532.

160. Tobiume H, Kanzaki S, Hida S, et al. (1997). Serum bone alkaline phosphatase isoenzyme levels in normal children and children with growth hormone (GH) deficiency: A potential marker for bone formation and response to GH therapy. J Clin Endocrinol Metab 82:2056–2061.

161. Zittermann A, Scwarz I, Scheld K, et al. (2000). Physiologic fluctuations of serum estradiol levels influence biochemical markers of bone resorption in young women. J Clin Endocrinol Metab 85:95–101.

162. Schinke T, McKee MD, Karsenty G (1999). Extracellular matrix calcification: Where is the action? Nature Genet 21:150–151.

163. Gericke A, Qin C, Spevak L, et al. (2005). Importance of phosphorylation for osteopontin regulation of biomineralization. Calc Tiss Int. 77:45–54.

164. Chavassieux P, Seeman E, Delmas PD (2007). Insights into material and structural basis of bone fragility from diseases associated with fractures: How determinants of the biomechanical

properties of bone are compromised by disease. Endocrine Reviews 28:151–164.

165. Rubin C, Rubin J (2006). Biomechanics and mechanobiology of bone. In Favus MJ (ed.), Primer on the metabolic Bone Diseases and Disorders of Mineral Metabolism, 6th ed, American Society for Bone and Mineral Research, Washington, D.C., 2006, p 36–42.

166. Frost HM, Schonau E (2000). The "muscle-bone unit" in children and adolescents: A 2000 overview. J Pediatr Endocrinol Metab 13:571–590.

167. Rauch F (2006). Material matters: a mechanostat-based perspective on bone development in osteogenesis imperfecta and hypophosphatemic rickets. J Musculoskelet Neuronal Interact 6:142–146.

168. Hughes-Fulford M (2004). Signal transduction and mechanical stress. Sci STKE 2004, re12.

169. Salingcarnboriboon R, Tsuji K, Komori T, et al. (2006). Runx2 is a target of mechanical unloading to alter osteoblastic activity and bone formation in vivo. Endocrinology 147:2296–2305.

170. Specker L, Schonau E (2005). Quantitative bone analysis in children: Current methods and recommendations. J Pediatr 146:726–731.

171. Rigo J, De Curtis M, Pieltain C, et al. (2000). Bone mineral metabolism in the micropremie. Clin Perinatol 27:147–170.

172. Bailey DA, McKay HA, Mirwald RL, et al. (1999). A six-year longitudinal study of the relationship of physical activity to bone mineral accrual in growing children: The University of Saskatchewan bone mineral accrual study. J Bone Miner Res 14:1672–1679.

173. Bonjour J-P, Carrie A-L, Ferrari S, et al. (1997). Calcium-enriched foods and bone mass growth in prepubertal girls: A randomized, double-blind, placebo-controlled trial. J Clin Invest 99:1287–1294.

174. Winzenberg TM, Shaw K, Fryer J, Jones G (2006). Effects of calcium supplementation on bone density in healthy children: meta-analysis of randomised controlled trials. BMJ 333:775–778.

175. Greenfield EM, Goldberg VM (1997). Genetic determination of bone density. Lancet 350:1263–1254.

176. Liu Y-J, Shen H, Xiao P, et al. (2005). Molecular genetic studies of gene identification for osteoporosis, A 2004 update. J Bone Miner Res 21:1511–1535.

177. Bachrach LK, Hastie T, Wang M-C, et al. (1999). Bone mineral acquisition in healthy Asian, Hispanic, black, and Caucasian youth: A longitudinal study. J Clin Endocrinol Metab 84:4702–4712.

178. Rubin K, Schirduan V, Gendreau P, et al. (1993). Predictors of axial and peripheral bone mineral density in healthy children and adolescents, with special attention to the role of puberty. J Pediatr 123:863–870.

179. Rubin LA, Hawker GA, Peltekova V, et al. (1999). Determinants of peak bone mass: Clinical and genetic analyses in a young female Canadian cohort. J Bone Miner Res 14:633–643.

180. Weaver CM, Peacock M, Johnston CC Jr. (1999). Adolescent nutrition in the prevention of postmenopausal osteoporosis. J Clin Endocrinol Metab 84:1839–1843.

181. Bradney M, Pearce G, Sullivan C, et al. (1998). Moderate exercise during growth in prepubertal boys: Changes in bone mass, size volumetric density and bone strength: A controlled prospective study. J Bone Miner Res 13:1814–1821.

182. Morris FL, Naughton GA, Gibbs JL, et al. (1997). Prospective 10-month exercise intervention in premenarchal girls: positive effects on bone and lean mass. J Bone Miner Res 12:1453–1462.

183. Lehtonen-M, Mottonen T, Irjala K, et al. (2000). A 1-year prospective study on the relationship between physical activity, markers of bone metabolism, and bone acquisition in peripubertal girls. J Clin Endocrinol Metab 85:3726–3732.

184. Morel J, Combe B, Francisco J, Bernard J (2001). Bone mineral density of 704 amateur sportsman involved in different physical activities. Osteoporosis Int 12:152–157.

185. Van der Eerden BCJ, Karperien M, Wit J (2003). Systemic and local regulation of the growth plate. Endocrine Reviews 24:782–801.

186. Wang Y, Nishida S, Sakata T, et al. (2006). Insulin-like growth factor-I is essential for embryonic bone development. Endocrinology 147:4753–4761.

187. Cruickshank J, Grossman DI, Peng RK, et al. (2005). Spatial distribution of growth hormone receptor, insulin-like growth factor-1 receptor and apoptotic chondrocytes during growth plate development. J Endocrinol 184:543–553.

188. Rosenfeld R (2006). Molecular mechanisms of IGF-I deficiency. Horm Res 65(1):15–20.

189. Cohen P (2006). Overview of the IGF-I system. Horm Res 65(1):3–8.

190. Yakar S, Liu J-L, Stannard B, et al. (1999). Normal growth and development in the absence of hepatic insulin-like growth factor-I. Proc Natl Acad Sci 96:7324–7329.

191. Savage MO, Attie KM, David A, et al. (2006). Endocrine assessment, molecular characterization and treatment of growth hormone insensitivity. Nature Clin Prac Endocrin Metab 2:395–407.

192. Caminos JE, Gualillo O, Lago F, et al. (2005). The endogenous growth hormone secretagogue (ghrelin) is synthesized and secreted by chondrocytes. Endocrinology 146:1285–1292.

193. Ohlsson C, Bengtsson B-A, Isaksson OGP, et al. (1998). Growth hormone and bone. Endocrine Reviews 19:55–79.

194. Baroncelli GI, Bertelloni S, Ceccarelli C, Saggese G (1998). Measurement of volumetric bone mineral density accurately determines degree of lumbar undermineralization in children with growth hormone deficiency. J Clin Endocrinol Metab 83:3150–3154.

195. Bachrach LK, Marcus R, Ott SM, et al. (1998). Bone mineral histomorphometry and body composition in adults with growth hormone receptor deficiency. J Bone Miner Res 13:415–421.

196. Woods KA, Camacho-Huber C, Bergman RN, et al. (2000). Effects of insulin-like growth factor I (IGF-I) therapy on body composition and insulin resistance in IGF-I gene deletion. J Clin Endocrinol Metab 85:1407–1411.

197. Barnard JC, Williams AJ, Rabier B, et al. (2005). Thyroid hormones regulate fibroblast growth factor receptor signaling during chondrogenesis. Endocrinology 146:5568–5580.

198. Rauch F, Bailey DA, Baxter-Jones A, et al. (2004). The "muscle-bone unit" during the pubertal growth spurt. Bone 34:771–775.

199. Couse JF, Korach KS (1999). Estrogen receptor null mice: What have we learned and where will they lead us? Endocrine Reviews 20:358–417.

200. Marcus R, Leary C, Schneider DL, et al. (2000). The contribution of testosterone to skeletal development and maintenance: Lessons from the androgen insensitivity syndrome. J Clin Endocrinol Metab 85:1032–1037.

201. Vanderschueren D, Bouillon R (1995). Androgens and bone. Calcif Tissue Int 56:341–346.

202. Libanati C, Baylink DJ, Lois-Wenzel E, et al. (1999). Studies on potential mediators of skeletal changes occurring during puberty in girls. J Clin Endocrinol Metab 84:2807–2814.

203. Martin TJ, Gaddy D (2006). Bone loss goes beyond estrogen. Nature Med 12:612–613.

204. Perrien DS, Akel NS, Edwards PK, et al (2007). Inhibin A is an endocrine stimulator of bone mass and strength. Endocrinology 148:1654–1665.

205. Potter LR, Abbey-Hosch A, Dickey DM (2006). Natriuretic peptides, their receptors, and cyclic guanosine monophosphate-dependent signaling functions. Endocrine Reviews 27:47–72.

206. Prickett TMCR, Lynne AM, Barrell GK, et al. (2005). Amino-terminal proCNP: A putative marker of cartilage activity in post natal growth. Pediatr Res 58:334–340.

207. Bartels CF, Bukulmez H, Padayatti P, et al. (2004). Mutations in the transmembrane natriuretic peptide receptor NPR-B impair skeletal growth and cause acromesomelic dysplasia, type Maoteaux. Am J Hum Genet 75:27–34.

208. Janicka A, Wren TAL, Sanchez MM, et al. (2007). Fat mass is not beneficial to bone in adolescents and young adults. J Clin Endocrinol Metab 92:143–147.

209. Thomas T, Gori F, Khosla S, et al. (1999). Leptin acts on human marrow stromal cells to enhance differentiation to osteoblasts and to inhibit differentiation to adipocytes. Endocrinology 140:1630–1638.

210. Klein KO, Larmore KA, de Lancey E, et al. (1998). Effect of obesity on estradiol level, and its relationship to leptin, bone maturation, and bone mineral density in children. J Clin Endocrinol Metab 83:3469–3475.

211. Ducy P, Amling M, Takeda S, et al. (2000). Leptin inhibits bone formation through a hypothalamic relay: A central control of bone mass. Cell 100:197–207.

212. Pogoda P, Egermann M, Schnell JC, et al. (2006). Leptin inhibits bone formation not only in rodents but also in sheep. J Bone Miner Res 21:1591–1599.

213. Baldock PA, Allison S, McDonald MM, et al. (2006). Hypothalamic regulation of cortical bone mass: Opposing activity of Y2 receptor and leptin pathways. J Bone Miner Res 21:1600–1607.

214. Luo X-H, Guo L-J, Xie H, et al. (2006). Adiponectin stimulates RANKL and inhibits OPG expression in human osteoblasts through the MAPK signaling pathway. J Bone Miner Res 21:1648–1656.

215. Glorieux FH, Travers R, Taylor A, et al. (2000). Normative data for iliac bone histomorphometry in growing children. Bone 26:103–109.

216. Rauch F (2006). Watching bones at work: What we can see from bone biopsies. Pediatr Nephrol 21:457–462.

217. Recker RR, Barger-Lux MJ (2006). Bone biopsy and histomorphometry in clinical practice. In Favus MJ (ed.), *Primer on the metabolic bone diseases and disorders of mineral metabolism, Sixth edition*. Washington, D.C.: American Society for Bone and Mineral Research 161–169.

218. Bachrach LK (2005). Osteoporosis and measurement of bone mass in children and adolescents. Endocrinol Metab Clin N Am 34:521–535.

219. Koo WWK, Hammami M, Hockman EM (2004). Validation of bone mass and body composition measurements in small subjects with pencil beam dual energy x-ray absorptiometry. J Am Coll Nutr 23:79–84.

220. Hammami M, Koo WW, Hockman EM (2003). Body composition of neonates from fan beam dual energy x-ray absorptiometry measurement. J Parenteral Enteral Nutr 27:423–426.

221. Leonard MB, Propert KJ, Zemel BS, et al. (1999). Discrepancies in pediatric bone mineral density reference data: Potential for misdiagnosis of osteopenia. J Pediatr 135:182–188.

222. Seeman E (1998). Growth in bone mass and size: Are racial and gender differences in bone mineral density more apparent than real? J Clin Endocrinol Metab 83:1414–1419.

223. Ward KA, Ashby RL, Roberts SA, et al. (2007). UK reference data for the Hologic QDR Discovery dual-energy x ray absorptiometry scanner in healthy children and young adults aged 6-17 years. Arch Dis Child 92:53–59.

224. Lu PW, Cowell CT, Lloyd-Jones SA, et al. (1996). Volumetric bone mineral density in normal subjects aged 5-27 years. J Clin Endocrinol Metab 81:1586–1590.

225. Gilsanz V, Skaggs DL, Kovanlikaya A, et al. (1998). Differential effects of race on the axial and appendicular skeletons of children. J Clin Endocrinol Metab 83:1420–1427.

226. Miller PD, Leonard MB (2006). Clinical use of bone mass measurements in children and adults for the assessment and management of osteoporosis. In Favus MJ (ed.), *Primer on the metabolic bone diseases and disorders of mineral metabolism, Sixth edition*. Washington, D.C.: American Society for Bone and Mineral Research 150–161.

227. Brismar TB, Lindgren A-C, Ringertz H, et al. (1998). Total bone mineral measurements in children with Prader-Willi syndrome: The influence of the skull's bone mineral content per area (BMA) and of height. Pediatr Radiol 28:38–42.

228. Maynard LM, Guo SS, Chumlea WC, et al. (1998). Total-body and regional bone mineral content and areal bone mineral density in children aged 8-18 y; the Fels Longitudinal Study. Am J Clin Nutr 68:1111–1117.

229. Koo WWK (2000). Body composition measurements during infancy. NY Acad Sci 904:383–392.

230. Koo WWK, Walters J, Bush AJ, et al. (1996). Dual-energy x-ray absorptiometry studies of bone mineral status in newborn infants. J Bone Miner Res 11:997–1002.

231. Lapillone A, Braillon P, Claris O, et al. (1997). Body composition in appropriate and in small for gestational age infants. Acta Paediatr 86:196–200.

232. Weiler HA, Yuen CK, Seshia MM (2002). Growth and bone mineralization of young adults weighing less than 1500 grams at birth. Early Hum Devel 67:101–112.

233. Yeste D, Aslmar J, Clemente M, et al. (2004). Areal bone mineral density of the lumbar spine in 80 premature newborns. A prospective and longitudinal study. J Pediatr Endocrinol Metab 17:959–966.

234. Hammami M, Koo WW, Hockman EM (2004). Technical considerations for fan-beam dual-energy x-ray absorptiometry body composition studies in pediatric studies. J Parenteral Enteral Nutr 28:328–333.

235. Koo WW, Hockman EM, Hammami M (2004). Dual energy X-ray absorptiometry measurements in small subjects: conditions affecting clinical measurements. J Am Coll Nutr 23:212–219.

236. Boot AM, de Ridder MA, Pols HA, et al. (1997). Bone mineral density in children and adolescents: relation to puberty, calcium intake, and physical activity. J Clin Endocrinol Metab 82:57–62.

237. Molgaard C, Thomsen BL, Prentice A, et al. (1997). Whole body bone mineral content in healthy children and adolescents. Arch Dis Child 76:9–15.

238. Zemel BS, Leonard MB, Kalkwarf HJ, et al. (2004). Reference data for whole body, lumbar spine and proximal femur for American children relative to age, gender and body size. J Bone Miner Res 19(1):S231.

239. del Rio L, Carrascosa A, Pons F, et al. (1994). Bone mineral density of the lumbar spine in white Mediterranean Spanish children and adolescents: Changes related to age, sex, and puberty. Pediatr Res 35:362–366.

240. Kroger H, Kotaniemi A, Kroger L, Alhava E (1993). Development of bone mass and bone density of the spine and femoral neck: A prospective study of 65 children and adolescents. Bone Mineral 23:171–182.

241. McKay HA, Bailey DA, Mirwald RL, et al. (1998). Peak bone mineral accrual and age at menarche in adolescent girls: A 6-year longitudinal study. J Pediatr 133:682–687.

242. Takahashi Y, Minamitani K, Kobayashi Y, et al. (1996). Spinal and femoral bone mass accumulation during normal adolescence: Comparison with female patients with sexual precocity and with hypogonadism. J Clin Endocrinol Metab 81:1248–1253.

243. Finkelstein JS, Neer RM, Biller BMK, et al. (1992). Osteopenia in men with a history of delayed puberty. N Engl J Med 326:600–604.

244. Wren TALH, Liu X, Pitukcheewanont P, Gilsanz V (2005). Bone densitometry in pediatric patients: Discrepancies in the diagnosis of osteoporosis by DXA and CT. J Pediatr 146:776–779.

245. Neu CM, Rauch F, Manz F, Schonau E (2001). Modeling of cross-sectional bone size, mass and geometry at the proximal radius: A study of normal bone development using peripheral quantitative computed tomography. Osteoporos Int 12:538–547.

246. Neu CM, Manz F, Rauch F, et al. (2001). Bone densities and bone size at the distal radius in healthy children and adolescents: A study using peripheral quantitative computed tomography. Bone 28:227–232.

247. Rauch F, Schonau E (2005). Peripheral quantitative computed tomography of the distal radius in young subjects: New reference data and interpretation of results. J Musculoskelet Neuronal Interact 5:119–126.

248. Leonard MB, Shults J, Justine E, et al. (2004). Interpretation of whole body dual energy X-ray absorptiometry measures in children: Comparison with peripheral quantitative computed tomography. Bone 34:1044–1052.

249. Zadik Z, Price D, Diamond G (2003). Pediatric reference curves for multi-site quantitative ultrasound and its modulators. Osteoporos Int 14:857–862.

250. Baroncelli GI, Federico G, Vignolo M, et al. (2006). Cross-sectional reference data for phalangeal quantitative ultrasound from early childhood to young-adulthood according to gender, age, skeletal growth, and pubertal development. Bone 39:159–173.

251. Ashmeade T, Pereda L, Chen, Carver JD (2007). Longitudinal measurements of bone status in preterm infants. J Pediatr Endocrinol Metab 20:415–424.

252. Fielding KT, Nix DA, Bachrach LK (2003). Comparison of calcaneus ultrasound and dual x-ray absorptiometry in children at risk of osteopenia. J Clin Densit 6:7–15.

253. Fricke O, Tutlewski B, Schwahn B, Schoenau E (2005). Speed of sound: Relation to geometric characteristics of bone in children, adolescents, and adults. J Pediatr 146:764–768.

254. Loud KJ, Gordon CM (2006). Adolescent bone health. Arch Pediatr Adolesc Med 160:1026–1032.

255. American Academy of Pediatrics (1999). Calcium requirements of infants, children, and adolescents. Pediatrics 104:1152–1157.

256. Hertel NT, Stoltenberg M, Juul A, et al. (1993). Serum concentrations of Type I and III procollagen propeptides in healthy children and girls with central precocious puberty during treatment with gonadotropin-releasing hormone analog and cyproterone acetate. J Clin Endocrinol Metab 76:924–927.

257. Koo WWK, Bush AJ, Walters J, Carlson SE (1998). Postnatal development of bone mineral status during infancy. J Am Coll Nutr 17:65–70.

258. Zaidi M (2007). Skeletal remodeling in health and disease. Nature Med 13:791–801.

259. Kalkwarf HJ, Zemel BS, Gilsanz V, et al. (2007). The bone mineral density in childhood study: Bone mineral content and density according to age, sex, and race. J Clin Endocrinol Metab 92:2087–2099.

CHAPTER 4

Ambiguous Genitalia

SELMA FELDMAN WITCHEL, MD • PETER A. LEE, MD, PhD

Introduction

Under the auspices of the Lawson Wilkins Pediatric Endocrine Society (USA) and the European Society for Pediatric Endocrinology, an international consensus statement was formulated that recommended a revised classification of the medical terminology used for disorders of sex development to avoid confusing and derogatory terms.[1] This descriptive classification attempts to be sensitive to concerns of parents and flexible enough to incorporate novel molecular genetic information. The updated classification system integrates molecular genetic considerations into the nomenclature for "disorders of sexual differentiation (DSD)."[1]

Terms such as *pseudohermaphrodite, intersex,* and *gender labeling* in the diagnosis should be avoided.[2] To accommodate all DSD, the classification system is broad and includes some conditions that do not present with obvious abnormalities of genital development (Table 4-1). The DSD categories are sex chromosome DSDs such as 45,X/46,XY (formerly mixed gonadal dysgenesis) and ovotesticular DSD (formerly true hermaphroditism); 46,XY

DSDs such as disorders of testicular development, disorders of androgen synthesis and action (replacing and expanding the former category of male pseudohermaphroditism), and XY sex reversal; and 46,XX DSDs such as masculinization of the XX individual (replacing female pseudohermaphrodite) and XX sex reversal. Because of the complexities of chromosomal and gonadal development, some diagnoses can be included in more than one of the three major categories. Nevertheless, despite many recent advances the specific cause of genital ambiguity cannot always be identified—particularly among those with a 46,XY karyotype.

TABLE 4-1

Summary of Disorders Associated with Ambiguous Genitalia

Sex Chromosome DSD
- 45,X Turner syndrome
- 45,X/46,XY gonadal dysgenesis
- 46,XX/46,XY gonadal dysgenesis

46,XY DSD (Disorders of Testicular Differentiation)
- Denys-Drash syndrome (WT1 mutations)
- Frasier syndrome (WT1 mutations)
- XX gonadal dysgenesis
- XY gonadal dysgenesis
  - SRY positive
  - SRY negative
- Ovotesticular DSD
- Campomelic dwarfism (SOX9 mutations)
- Dosage sensitive sex reversal (duplications of DAX1)
- Desert hedgehog (DHH) mutations
- Monosomy distal chromosome 9p
- Xq28 deletion
- Vanishing testes
- ATR-X syndrome
- ARX
- Persistent Mullerian duct syndrome

46,XY (Disorders of Androgen Synthesis or Action)
- Steroidogenic factor-1 (SF-1 mutations)
- Leydig cell hypoplasia (LHR mutations)
- Smith-Lemli-Opitz syndrome (DHCR7)
- 3β-hydroxysteroid dehydrogenase deficiency (HSD3B2)
- 17α-hydroxylase/17,20-lyase deficiency (CYP17)
- Lipoid adrenal hyperplasia (StAR)
- 17β-hydroxysteroid dehydrogenase deficiency (HSD17B3)
- 5α-reductase deficiency (SRD5A2)
- Androgen insensitivity (AR)
- Hypogonadotropic hypogonadism
- P450 oxidoreductase deficiency (POR)

46XX, DSD
- 21-hydroxylase deficiency (CYP21)
- 11β-hydroxylase deficiency (CYP11B1)
- Placental aromatase deficiency (CYP19)
- Maternal hyperandrogenism
- XX males
- Ovotesticular DSD

Other
- IMAGe syndrome
- Environmental endocrine disrupters
- VACTERL syndrome
- MURCs syndrome
- Cloacal extrophy
- Aphallia

Ambiguous Genitalia: Talking with the Parents

For parents, the birth of a child is a long-anticipated, much desired, and exciting event. However, today the scenario has largely changed. In the past, the typical first question or statement after a child's birth related to the sex of the child: Is it a boy or a girl? Now, with the increased frequency of prenatal ultrasound examinations parents have usually been told the sex of their child and often have selected names for their son or daughter. Thus, when confronted with a newborn with genital ambiguity the issues occur in a different context. This immediately necessitates full disclosure, which allows parents to be actively involved in the medical decision-making process. The parents need to be quickly equipped to deal emotionally with these issues for themselves and to enable them to appropriately interact with their infant, family members, friends, and colleagues.

Initially, the parents need to hear that there has been a problem in the complex system that directs genital development—which makes it impossible to tell the sex of their child simply by examining the external genitalia. It is important to acknowledge that such development is not a consequence of anything that they, as parents, did or did not do. Despite openness and full disclosure, the parents may harbor guilt and negative feelings. Cultural attitudes, preexisting expectations, and family support systems influence the parents' responses to their child. The medical team needs to promote an open and caring network to provide support for the parents.

The initial treatment goal is to determine if there is an underlying or associated life-threatening condition that requires specific urgent treatment. If the child's gender remains unclear, information needs to be obtained to assist the parents in determining the most appropriate sex of rearing. Usually, this can be accomplished within a matter of hours or days. In more complex instances, the diagnostic process may take longer. In situations in which it is impossible to identify the specific etiology, the general DSD category provides a basis for decision making.

These considerations include the extent of external and internal reproductive system development, evidence of gonadal functionality (potential hormone secretion and fertility), and hormone responsiveness. In some instances, these factors are more relevant than the karyotype. When consensus has been reached regarding a diagnostic category, available outcome information for that diagnosis should be reviewed. Knowledge of the specific etiology, including details of the diagnosis, enables planning therapeutic interventions and genetic counseling for future pregnancies.

The first interview with the parents should set a positive and optimistic tone to promote parental bonding with their infant. Indeed, the emotional tone of this initial interaction is usually more meaningful than the factual information provided and is recalled by parents for many years. Respect for the family and individual perspectives together with a willingness to repeat or defer detailed explanations are crucial. In the midst of the emotional distress associated with the uncertainty of their infant's gender, parents cannot be expected to assimilate the vast amount of information that eventually needs to be shared.

Factual explanations regarding the process of sexual differentiation with a focus on their infant's situation should be initially outlined. Detailed explanations and discussion can be repeated multiple times as the child ages. The use of simple sketches and provision of pictures and diagrams can be helpful to explain the embryology of genital development to the parents. The primary goal at this point is to provide the parents with a basic understanding that the internal and external genital structures for both boys and girls develop from the same primordial tissues. It may be helpful to explain that there are not exclusively male and female hormones, but rather the environments in which male and female fetuses develop are characterized by differing relative amounts of these hormones. Thus, incomplete male or female development represents the consequences of the prenatal hormonal environment. Too much or too little androgen effect is reflected in the degree of prenatal virilization.

During this initial dialogue, showing the parents the specific physical findings of their infant is often beneficial. This can alleviate apprehension, increase their comfort to look at their infant's genitalia, and promote the goal of fostering their perception of their child as a human having the needs of any other infant. This approach allows for information to be presented in a manner that will minimize anxiety and better equip parents to participate in the decision-making process. Before parents can provide the best support for their infant, they must each personally reach a resolution with a commitment to a positive perspective concerning this situation. Discussion of many concerns (particularly those related to gender identity, pubertal development, sexual orientation, sexual function, and fertility) may be helpful. The intent is that honest discussions will engender positive feelings that enhance positive interactions and enable the parents to promote their child's self-esteem.

Unless the gender assignment is clear at this point, delay in naming the infant, announcing the baby's birth, and registering the birth can be recommended until more information becomes available. The message should be clear that there will be an appropriate sex of rearing for their child and that it is the parents' privilege and responsibility to participate in the process leading to a gender assignment. Until sex of rearing is established, it is best to refer to the infant as "your baby" or "your child." Terms such as *he*, *she*, and *it* should be avoided.

Sex Determination

Sex determination is the binary switch that launches the developmental destiny of the embryonic gonads to become testes or ovaries. Sexual differentiation refers to the process through which male or female phenotype develops. The gonads, internal genital ducts, and external genital structures all develop from bipotential embryologic tissues. Each cell in the developing gonad has the potential to differentiate into either a testicular or ovarian cell. However, "the fate decisions in individual cells are highly coordinated such that cells of discordant fate are rarely seen."[3] Thus, differentiation as male or female depends on regulated orchestration of the expression and interaction of specific genes and gene products.

Through Alfred Jost's experiments with fetal rabbits in the 1940s and 1950s, the requirements for a testis and testosterone for male sexual differentiation were established.[4] Chromosomal composition of the embryo, XX or XY, determines gonadal sex. The genetic locus primarily responsible for this binary switch, the sex-determining region on the Y *(SRY)* gene on the Y chromosome, was identified through studies of patients with disorders of sexual differentiation. Analysis of transgenic mice confirmed the essential role of SRY and provided further molecular understanding of testicular differentiation.[5,6]

Whereas the karyotype (46,XY or 46,XX) of the primordial gonad determines whether it differentiates into a testis or ovary, respectively, local factors (such as hormones secreted by the developing gonads or tissue-specific transcription factors) influence the ensuing differentiation of the internal and external genital structures.[7] Divergence from the normal sequence of events leads to disorders of sexual differentiation that can manifest as abnormal gonadal differentiation, inconsistent internal genital differentiation, or ambiguity of the external genitalia. Although genital ambiguity is usually not considered to be a medical emergency, it is highly distressing to the parents and extended family. Hence, prompt referral and evaluation by a team with expertise in disorders of sexual differentiation is beneficial. Information regarding our current knowledge of sexual differentiation is presented, followed by a discussion of the various causes and treatment for ambiguous genital development.

Development of the Reproductive System

UROGENITAL DIFFERENTIATION

In humans, at 4 to 6 weeks of gestation the urogenital ridges develop as an outgrowth of coelomic epithelium (mesothelium).[8] The gonads, adrenal cortex, kidney, and reproductive tract derive from the urogenital ridge (Figure 4-1). Physical contact with the mesonephros appears to be important for

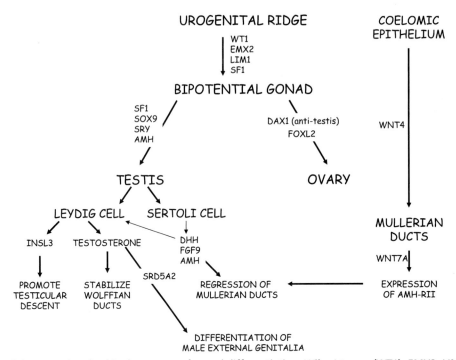

Figure 4-1. Cartoon of the genes involved in the process of sexual differentiation. Wilms' tumor (WT1), EMX2, LIM1, and steroidogenic factor-1 (SF1) play roles in differentiation of gonad from urogenital ridge. Genes involved in testicular differentiation include SF-1, SOX9, sex-determining region on Y (SRY), and anti-Mullerian hormone (AMH). The dosage-sensitive sex-adrenal hypoplasia congenital critical region on X (DAX1) appears to function as an anti-testis factor. Wnt4 promotes development of the Mullerian ducts, whereas Wnt7a promotes expression of the receptor for AMH (AMH-RII). Sertoli cells secrete AMH, which [acting through its cognate receptor (AMH-RII)] promotes regression of the Mullerian ducts. Leydig cells secrete testosterone and insulin-like hormone-3 (INSL3). Testosterone stabilizes the Wolffian ducts and is converted to DHT by 5α-reductase in target tissues to promote differentiation of the prostate and development of male external genitalia. INSL3 is involved in transabdominal testicular descent.

subsequent gonadal differentiation.[9] Due to their origin as part of the developing urogenital system, ovaries and testes are initially located high in the abdomen near the kidneys. One of the earliest morphologic changes is increased proliferation and size of developing 46,XY gonads.

TESTICULAR DIFFERENTIATION

The SRY protein is a nuclear high-mobility group (HMG) domain protein expressed in pre-Sertoli cells, where it triggers a molecular switch to induce Sertoli cell differentiation and initiate the process of male sexual differentiation. The HMG domain of the SRY protein binds to the minor DNA groove, where it functions as a transcription factor by bending DNA to presumably permit other proteins access to regulatory regions and to promote assembly of nucleoprotein transcription complexes.[10] A threshold SRY level must be achieved at a critical time to establish male sexual differentiation. Otherwise, the ovarian differentiation pathway is activated.[11] Yet, the factor(s) upregulating SRY expression remains elusive.

SRY expression is independent of the presence of germ cells. In addition to SRY, sequential expression of several other genes is required for normal male sexual differentiation. These genes include SRY-related HMG box-containing-9 (SOX9), anti-Mullerian hormone (AMH), dosage-sensitive sex reversal adrenal hypoplasia congenita critical region on X (DAX1), steroidogenic factor-1 (SF1), Wilms' tumor 1(WT1), GATA-binding-4 (GATA4), desert hedgehog (DHH), patched (PTC), wingless-related MMTV integration site 4 (WNT4), and WNT7a.

Using immunohistochemistry, SF1 and SOX9 proteins can be detected in human embryonic gonadal tissue at 6 to 7 weeks of gestation. At this time, SOX9 expression becomes limited to nuclei of Sertoli cells in a 46,XY fetus but remains cytosolic in a 46,XX fetus. SF1 and SOX9 protein expression precede that of AMH. Only after AMH protein expression and onset of overt testicular differentiation do Wilms' tumor (WT1) and GATA-4 protein expression increase in the fetal testis.[12] GATA4 belongs to a family of zinc finger transcription factors known as GATA-binding proteins because they bind to a consensus sequence in the promoter and enhancer regions of target genes.

Testicular differentiation occurs earlier than ovarian development. The testis consists of five cell types: supporting or Sertoli cells, endothelial cells, peritubular myoid cells, steroid-secreting Leydig cells, and germ cells. The first evidence of testicular differentiation is the appearance of primitive Sertoli cells at 6 to 7 weeks gestation in the human fetal testis. Cells, mostly endothelial cells, migrate from the mesonephros and interact with the pre-Sertoli cells to promote development of the testicular cords.[13] The testicular cords are precursors of the seminiferous tubules that will contain Sertoli and germ cells. In addition to the migration of mesonephric cells, testes show an increased rate of cell proliferation.[14]

SOX9 induces expression of prostaglandin D synthase (Pgds), an enzyme involved in prostaglandin synthesis.[15] In a positive feedback loop, developing Sertoli cells secrete prostaglandin D2—which binds to its cognate receptor to upregulate SOX9 expression and recruit additional Sertoli cells.[16,17] Phenotype-genotype studies of humans and mice demonstrate that SOX9 expression is a crucial step, downstream of SRY, in testis development. Fibroblast growth factor 9 (FGF9) is another signaling molecule important for testis development. In the mouse, the absence of FGF9 expression is associated with a premature decline in SOX9 expression—leading to arrested Sertoli cell differentiation, upregulation of Wnt4 expression, and male-to-female sex reversal of germ cells.[18]

Vascular development in the gonad is sexually dimorphic with the endothelial cells in the developing testis, forming a characteristic pattern consisting of a prominent coelomic vessel on the antimesonephric surface with branches between the testis cords.[19] This blood vessel is absent in the ovary. The signaling molecule, WNT4 suppresses formation of this coelomic vessel without affecting the development of its side branches.

Peritubular myoid cells are testis-specific smooth-muscle-like cells important to structural integrity and development of the testis cords. Factors relevant to peritubular myoid cell differentiation include desert hedgehog (DHH), which is secreted by Sertoli cells and its receptor Patched (Ptch1)—which is expressed on peritubular myoid cells.[20,21] The peritubular myoid cells surround the Sertoli cells, separating them from the Leydig cells—which are then sequestered in the interstitium.

Leydig cell differentiation depends on paracrine signals, including platelet-derived growth factor receptor-alpha [(PDGFR-α), DHH, PTCH1, and Aristaless-related homeobox (ARX)]. SF1 is expressed in Leydig cells to promote steroidogenic enzyme genes expression. The number of fetal Leydig cells reflects gonadotropin stimulation because the number is decreased in anencephalic male fetuses and increased in 46,XY fetuses, with elevated gonadotropin concentrations secondary to complete androgen insensitivity.[22] Differentiation of adult Leydig cells occurs postnatally.[23]

OVARIAN DIFFERENTIATION

Although ovarian differentiation has been considered the default pathway that occurs in the absence of SRY gene expression, accumulating evidence indicates that specific genes influence ovarian differentiation. Genes involved in cell cycle regulation were found to be overexpressed in developing XX gonads. Persistent DAX1 expression appears to play a role in ovarian differentiation. Other genes identified in developing ovaries include follistatin (Fst), Iroquois-3 (Irx3), Wnt4, and bone morphogenic protein-2 (Bmp2).[24]

The functions of Wnt4 include suppression of the androgen-secreting interstitial cells, inhibition of coelomic vascularization, and support of Mullerian derivatives—suggesting that it plays a major role in ovarian differentiation. Another gene postulated to influence ovarian differentiation is Forkhead L2 (FOXL2), a forkhead transcription factor.[23]

GERM CELL DIFFERENTIATION

Despite the requirement for germ cells in the postnatal ovary to maintain its structure, germ cells are not required for the initial development of ovaries or testes.[3] Primordial germ cells migrate from their origin in the hindgut to the developing gonadal ridges. Factors important for germ cell migration and colonization of the genital ridges include fragilis proteins 1 and 3 (IFITM1 and IFITM3) and stromal-cell–derived factor 1 (SDF1, also known as CXCL12) and its receptor CXCR4.[25,26]

The local environment directs the fate of the primordial germ cells.[3] Germ cell differentiation into a sperm or an egg is closely linked to the cell cycle decision between mitosis and meiosis.[27] In a human XX gonad, the germ cell meiosis begins at 10 to 11 weeks of gestation. This process appears to depend on retinoic acid, which is derived from mesonephric cells. Retinoic acid induces meiosis in an anterior-to-posterior wave and upregulates Stra8 (stimulated by retinoic acid gene 8) expression.[28]

In mice, Stra8 is necessary to premeiotic DNA replication. Thus, premeiotic DNA replication and the ensuing meiotic prophase are sexually dimorphic regulated steps of terminal differentiation characteristic of germ cells resident in the embryonic ovary.[29] After the first meiotic division, the primary oocyte becomes associated with granulosa cell precursors to constitute the primary follicle. In humans, primordial follicles are evident at 20 weeks of gestation. From a peak of 6.8 million oocytes at approximately 5 months of gestation, approximately 2 million are present at birth due to follicular atresia.[30] Accelerated follicular atresia contributes to the degeneration observed in streak gonads in X monosomy.

The developing somatic cells in the testis actively inhibit meiosis through expression of CYP26B1, a cytochrome P450 enzyme that degrades retinoic acid.[28,31] The germ cells in the testis enter a state of mitotic arrest. It has been suggested that fetal germ cells are programmed to enter meiosis and initiate oogenesis unless this process is inhibited.[32]

Maternal and paternal alleles are differentially imprinted such that monoallelic expression of specific genes occurs. During this process of imprinting, mature oocytes and sperm are differentially marked reflecting "parent-of-origin"–specific methylation patterns. In the primordial immature germ cells, inherited imprints are erased shortly after the germ cells enter the gonadal ridge. Sexually dimorphic methylation imprinting is subsequently reestablished in male and female gametes. This process occurs late in fetal development in the male and postnatally in female germ cells.[33,34] The importance of this imprinting process has been elucidated through study of parent-of-origin–dependent gene disorders such as Beckwith-Wiedemann, Prader-Willi, and Angelman syndromes and neonatal diabetes mellitus.

DIFFERENTIATION OF INTERNAL GENITAL STRUCTURES

The Wolffian duct originates as the excretory duct of the mesonephros and develops into the epididymis, vas deferens, ejaculatory duct, and seminal vesicle. The epididymis consists of four functional portions: initial segment, caput, corpus, and cauda. Sperm mature in the caput and corpus, whereas the cauda is primarily for storage. The Mullerian or paramesonephric duct originates as an invagination of the coelomic epithelium and develops into the Fallopian tubes, uterus, and upper third of the vagina.

In the male fetus, the Sertoli cells secrete anti-Mullerian hormone (AMH), also known as Mullerian inhibitory hormone (MIH). In human 46,XY fetuses, AMH expression can be detected by 7 weeks of gestation, is not dependent on the presence of germ cells within the testis, and promotes regression of the Mullerian ducts.[35] AMH, a member of the transforming growth factor-β (TGF-β) family, undergoes proteolytic cleavage to become biologically active. AMH binds to its receptor, AMH-RII, on the surface of the Mullerian duct mesenchymal cells to induce increased matrix metalloproteinase 2 expression.[36,37] The net result is degeneration and loss of basement membrane integrity of the epithelial and mesenchymal Mullerian cells, leading to regression of the Mullerian ducts.[38]

AMH expression is highly regulated because inappropriate expression in a 46,XX fetus would lead to uterine agenesis. In the 46,XX fetus with absence of both AMH and testosterone, the Mullerian duct derivatives persist and the Wolffian ducts regress. When a female fetus is inappropriately exposed to AMH (as in freemartin cattle), Mullerian duct regression and ovarian masculinization occur.[39,40]

The fetal hypothalamic-pituitary-gonadal (HPG) axis is active by mid-gestation, with peak fetal testosterone concentrations occurring at approximately 15 to 16 weeks of gestation. Prior to this time, placental hCG stimulates testosterone production by the fetal Leydig cells. Secretion of testosterone by the fetal Leydig cells stabilizes the Wolffian ducts in 46,XY fetuses. Region-specific signaling molecules such as bone morphogenic proteins (BMPs), homeobox genes (HOXA10 and HOXA11), growth differentiation factor 7 (GDF7), relaxin, an orphan G-protein–coupled receptor (LGR4), platelet-derived growth factor A (PDGFA), and its cognate receptor (PDGFRA) influence the development of the epididymis and seminal vesicle.[19]

The prostate, a male accessory sex gland, contributes to seminal fluid plasma and develops from the urogenital sinus. After the initial testosterone-dependent induction of prostate differentiation, subsequent development involves epithelial-mesenchymal interactions that lead to cell differentiation and branching morphogenesis. The requisite signaling molecules FGFs, sonic hedgehog (SHH), BMPs, HOXA13, and HOXD13 are similar to those required for external genital differentiation.[41,42]

DIFFERENTIATION OF EXTERNAL GENITAL STRUCTURES

The genital tubercle, urethral folds, and labioscrotal swellings give rise to the external genitalia. Under the influence of circulating androgens that are converted to dihydrotestosterone in the target tissues, the urethral folds fuse to form the corpus spongiosum and penile urethra, the genital tubercle develops into the corpora cavernosa of the penis, and the labioscrotal folds fuse to form the scrotum.

In the normal 46,XY human fetus, a cylindrical 2-mm phallus with genital swellings has developed by 9 weeks of gestation. By 12 to 14 weeks of gestation, the urethral folds have fused to form the cavernous urethra and corpus spongiosum. By 14 weeks, the external genitalia are clearly masculine apart from testicular location. The high incidence of hypospadias in humans suggests that urethral fusion is a delicate and finely regulated process.

In the 46,XX fetus, in the absence of androgens the urethral folds and labioscrotal swellings do not fuse and develop into the labia minora and labia majora, respectively. The genital tubercle forms the clitoris, and canalization of the vaginal plate creates the lower portion of the vagina.[43] By 11 weeks of gestation, the clitoris is prominent and the lateral boundaries of the urogenital sulcus have separated. Minimal clitoral growth, well-defined labia majora, hypoplastic labia minora, and separate vaginal and urethral perineal openings are present by 20 weeks of gestation.

By 33 days postconception, the human fetal adrenal cortex is distinct from the developing gonad. Due to its role as the source of DHEAS for placental estrogen biosynthesis, the fetal adrenal cortex grows rapidly. By 50 to 52 days postconception, expression of several steroidogenic enzymes, steroidogenic acute regulatory protein (StAR), 11β-hydroxylase (CYP11B1), 17α-hydroxylase/17,20-lyase (CYP17), and 21-hydroxylase (CYP21) in the fetal adrenal cortex have been demonstrated immunohistochemically.[44] Recent data indicate that transitory cortisol biosynthesis peaks at 8 to 9 weeks gestation.[44] This early cortisol biosynthesis coincides with transient adrenal expression of both nerve growth factor IB-like (NGFI-B) and 3β-hydroxysteroid dehydrogenase-2 (HSD3B2).[44] Concommitantly, ACTH can be detected in the anterior pituitary—suggesting the presence of negative feedback inhibition during the first trimester.[44] During the time male sexual differentiation begins, this negative feedback inhibition may serve to prevent virilization of female fetuses to ensure normal female sexual differentiation.[44,45]

SEXUAL DIFFERENTIATION OF THE BRAIN

Clinical investigations suggest that the brain is sexually dimorphic and that testosterone is a masculinizing hormone in human. Males with aromatase deficiency manifest male psychosexual behavior and gender identity. Alternatively, 46,XY individuals with complete androgen insensitivity syndrome (CAIS) develop female gender identity.[46,47] Preliminary data implicate genetic differences, independent of sex steroid exposure, as the molecular basis for some aspects of sexual dimorphism of the brain.[48] Postmortem histologic examination demonstrated that women have more synapses in the neocortex, whereas men have more neurons in this region.[49,50]

Lessons Learned from Transgenic Models

Sexual differentiation is a complex process in which precise spatiotemporal coordination and regulation of gene expression are crucial to achieve full reproductive capability.[51] Despite greater knowledge of the molecular details of sexual differentiation, the precise sequence of biologic events and all component factors remain to be elucidated. Investigation of normal and transgenic mice confirmed the crucial role of the sex-determining region on Y (SRY) gene in male differentiation when XX mice carrying only a 14-kb fragment of the Y chromosome showed a male phenotype.[52] In some instances, sex-reversal phenotypes have been fortuitous observations. Although investigation of transgenic mouse models has provided much information about sexual differentiation (Table 4-2), the mouse and human phenotypes may differ. For example, humans with a 45,X karyotype develop gonadal dysgenesis associated with infertility—whereas XO mice are fertile.

The following brief discussion of the spatiotemporal expression of specific genes and phenotypes of transgenic mice reviews the current understanding of sexual differentiation. Abnormal gonadal development has been described in mice homozygous for targeted deletions of genes involved in urogenital differentiation (such as Wt1, Sf1, Emx2, M33, and Lim1). In mice, these genes are expressed earlier in gestation than Sry, which is expressed transiently at 10.5 to 11 days postcoitum (d.p.c.).[53] For example, Wt1 is expressed throughout the intermediate mesoderm at 9 d.p.c. Subsequently, Wt1 is expressed in the developing gonad. The phenotype of Wt1 knockout mice includes embryonic lethality, failure of gonadal and kidney development, and abnormal development of the mesothelium, heart ,and lungs.[54] Unlike humans, as discussed later, heterozygous Wt1 mutations in mice are not associated with kidney tumors or genito-urinary anomalies.

Steroidogenic factor 1 (Sf1), also known as NR5A1, is an orphan nuclear hormone receptor that functions as a transcription factor. In mice, Sf1 is expressed from the earliest stages of gonadogenesis at 9 d.p.c. and regulates expression of steroidogenic enzyme genes in gonads and adrenals. At the onset of testicular differentiation, Sf1 expression becomes sexually dimorphic with increased expression in fetal testis and decreased expression in fetal ovaries.[55] The pathologic findings in mice homozygous for targeted deletion of Sf1 include absence of gonads, adrenal glands, and ventromedial hypothalamus—with decreased number of gonadotropes in the anterior pituitary.[56] Sf1 knockout mice have female internal and external genitalia irrespective of genetic sex and die shortly after birth secondary to adrenal insufficiency.[57] Pituitary-specific Sf1 knockout mice manifest hypogonadotropic hypogonadism, confirming the essential role of Sf1 in pituitary function.[58]

The protein encoded by the Sox9 gene contains a DNA-binding HMG domain and plays a major role in testicular differentiation. Following the onset of testicular differentiation, Sox9 expression increases in the testis and decreases in the ovary by 11.5 d.p.c. Ectopic expression of Sox9 in XX mice leads to testicular differentiation.[59] Mice with homozygous targeted deletion of the Sox9 gene die during mid-gestation.[60] Sox9 also plays a major role in chondrocyte differentiation and cartilage formation.[61]

Homozygous deletion of Emx2, a homeodomain transcription factor, results in an embryonic lethal phenotype associated with absence of kidneys, ureters, gonads—and in Wolffian and Mullerian duct derivatives.[62,63] As Wt1 expression is initially normal in the metanephric blastema of Emx2 knockout mice, Emx2 is likely downstream of Wt1. Interestingly, adrenal gland development is normal in Emx2 knockout mice. Lim1, also known as Lhx1, encodes a homeobox protein—which is important in the differentiation of intermediate mesoderm and the urogenital system.[64] Homozygous deletion of Lim1 is associated with absence of kidneys and gonads and with anterior head structures.[65]

Dax1 is first expressed in the genital ridge at 10.5 to 11 d.p.c. With differentiation of the testicular cords, Dax1 expression becomes sexually dimorphic—with decreased expression in the fetal testis. It continues to be expressed in the fetal ovary, where it appears to inhibit gonadal steroidogenesis.[66] Dax1 may interfere with steroidogenesis by inhibiting StAR expression and/or Sf1-mediated transactivation.[67,68] Dax1 functions as an adaptor molecule to recruit the nuclear receptor corepressor N-CoR to the Sf1 promoter, thus interfering with transactivation.[69,70] Rather than functioning to promote ovarian differentiation, it appears that Dax1 acts as an anti-testis factor. In male mice with targeted disruptions of the Dax1 gene, abnormalities of testicular germinal epithelium and male infertility develop despite normal testicular appearance at birth.[71] Female mice homozygous for targeted Dax1 mutation showed normal adult reproductive function.[72] Testicular development is delayed in XY mice carrying extra copies of mouse Dax1, but sex reversal is not observed unless the mouse also carries weak alleles of the SRY gene.[72]

At 11.5 days, Fgf9 is expressed in gonads of both sexes. By day 12.5, Fgf9 is detected only in testes. Mice homozygous for Fgf9-targeted deletions show male-to-female sex reversal with disruption of testis differentiation.[73] Loss of Fgf9 does not interfere with Sry expression, but prevents persistence of Sox9 expression in the developing testis. As discussed previously, Fgf9 inhibits Wnt4 expression.[18]

At 11.5 to 12.5 d.p.c, in both sexes Mullerian ducts arise from coelomic epithelium in the mesonephric region under the influence of Wnt4.[74] Male mice with homozygous targeted deletions of Wnt4 show normal testicular and Wolffian duct development, but Mullerian ducts never develop. The phenotype of female mice with homozygous deletions of Wnt4 includes absence of Mullerian duct derivatives, retention of Wolffian duct derivatives, and decreased oocyte development. In addition, the large coelomic blood vessel (typical of testicular differentiation) develops in the ovaries of female mice homozygous for targeted deletion of Wnt4.[75] Wnt4 appears to be involved in differentiation of Mullerian ducts, repression of endothelial migration from the mesonephros into the gonad, impeding migration of adrenal cells into the developing gonad, and maintenance of oocyte development.

Persistence of Mullerian duct derivatives and infertility were noted in male mice homozygous for targeted deletion of Wnt7a. One consequence of Wnt7a deletions is absence of Mullerian hormone receptor (AMH-RII) expression by Mullerian ducts. In females, although Mullerian duct derivatives develop they are abnormal—with loss of uterine glands, reduction in uterine stroma, and deficient coiling and elongation of the Mullerian duct. Thus, Wnt7a appears

TABLE 4-2

Consequences of Loss-of-Function Mutations in Genes Associated with DSD

Gene	Human Locus	Human Phenotype	Mouse Phenotype
WT1	11p13	Denys-Drash and Frasier syndrome	Homozygous: embryonic lethal with absence of kidney and gonads.
SRY	Yp11.3	46,XY Gonadal dysgenesis	"Knock-in" female-to-male sex reversal.
SOX9	17q24-25	Campomelic dysplasia and gonadal dysgenesis	Overexpression in XX mice results in female-to-male sex reversal. Heterozygous null associated with perinatal death, cleft palate, and skeletal abnormalities.
DHH	12q13.1	Gonadal dysgenesis	Abnormal peripheral nerves, infertility due to impaired spermatogenesis in males.
ATRX/XH2	Xq13.3	α-thalassemia, mental retardation, genital abnormalities, short stature	Phenotype of null is embryonic lethal. Overexpression associated with growth retardation, neural tube defects, and embryonic death.
ARX	Xp22.13	Lissencephaly, absence of the corpus callosum, microcephaly	Males have abnormal CNS development and abnormal testicular differentiation.
SF1/NR5A1	9q33	46,XY sex reversal with or without adrenal insufficiency	Absent adrenal glands, absent gonads, abnormal pituitary differentiation.
EMX2	10q26.1	Schizencephaly	Absence of kidneys, ureters, gonads, and genital tracts.
FGF9	13q11-q12	??	Male-to-female sex reversal, lung hypoplasia.
WNT4	1p35	46,XX, Uterine agenesis 46,XY, Male-to-female sex reversal	Males are normal. Females manifest female-to-male sex reversal.
WNT7A	3p25	Limb malformation syndromes	Persistent Mullerian duct derivatives in males. Abnormal Mullerian duct differentiation in females.
DAX1/NROB1	Xp21.3	Adrenal hypoplasia congenita; duplication associated with male-to-female sex reversal	Male infertility.
GATA4	8p23.2-p22	Congenital heart disease	Embryonic lethal, heart defects.
FOXL2	3q23	Blepharophimosis/ptosis/epicanthus inversus syndrome	Small, absence of eyelids, craniofacial anomalies, female infertility.
LHGCR	2p21	Leydig cell hypoplasia	NA.
DHCR7	11q12-q13	Smith-Lemli-Opitz syndrome	IUGR, cleft palate, neurologic abnormalities.
StAR	8p11.2	Congenital lipoid adrenal hyperplasia	All with female external genitalia. Neonatal death due to adrenal insufficiency.
CYP11A1	15q23-q24	Male-to-female sex reversal, adrenal insufficiency	Male-to-female sex reversal. Neonatal death due to adrenal insufficiency.
CYP19A1	15q21.1	Aromatase deficiency	Immature infertile female. Males are initially fertile, but develop disrupted spermatogenesis.
POR	7q11.2	Antley-Bixler syndrome	Embryonic lethal.
AMH	19p13.3-p13.2	Persistent Mullerian duct syndrome	Male has persistent Mullerian duct derivatives and infertility.
AMH-RII	12q13	Persistent Mullerian duct syndrome	Male has persistent Mullerian duct derivatives and infertility.
INSL3	19p13.2	Associated with cryptorchidism	Cryptorchidism in males. Overexpression in females associated with development of gubernaculum and aberrant ovarian location.
LGR8	13q13.1	Associated with cryptorchidism	Cryptorchidism.

to function as an epithelial-to-mesenchymal signal important in the sexually dimorphic differentiation of Mullerian duct derivatives. [76]

The phenotype associated with targeted disruption of c-kit ligand, a receptor tyrosine kinase also known as Steel factor, is complete lack of germ cells in the gonads.[77] Affected animals are sterile, but show normal sexual differentiation.[78] Both male and female mice homozygous for targeted deletion of the Stra8 gene show no overt phenotype apart from infertility.[29]

Mullerian inhibitory hormone (Amh) is first expressed at 12 d.p.c. Although direct control of Amh expression by the Sry gene product originally appeared to be an attractive hypothesis,[79] subsequent investigations have refuted this theory.[80] Rather, transcriptional regulation of Amh appears to involve both protein-protein and protein-DNA interactions—with Sf1 and Sox9 being two of the proteins involved.[81-83] Amh action is mediated by a heteromeric-signaling complex consisting of type I and type II serine/threonine kinase receptors. The Amh type II receptor binds Amh and recruits a type I receptor. SF1 appears to regulate expression of the Amh type II receptor (Amh-rIII) gene.[84] The phenotypes of the Amh and Amh-rII knockout mice are identical. In XY mice, both male and female internal genital structures are found. Male mice are infertile because the retained uterus blocks passage of sperm through the vas deferens.

The phenotype of male mice with targeted deletion of desert hedgehog (Dhh) includes infertility and impaired spermatogenesis.[85] These mice also showed abnormal peripheral nerves with extensive minifascicles within the endoneurium.[86] During development, expression of Dhh is limited to Sertoli cells and Schwann cells in peripheral nerves.[87] In mice, other key molecules in the development of male external genital structures include sonic hedgehog (Shh), fibroblast growth factors, Wnts, Bmps, Hoxa13, and Hoxad13. Specifically, Shh increases expression of Bmp4, Hoxa13, Hoxd13, and Ptc expression.[19] Expression of 5α-reductase in the genital tubercle mesenchyme occurs. Male mice homozygous for targeted deletions of the insulin-like hormone-3 (Insl3), Hoxa10, or leucine-rich repeat-containing Lgr8 genes show bilateral cryptorchidism.[88-91]

Investigations involving normal and transgenic mice have provided much information about the genes and gene products involved in sexual differentiation. Nevertheless, differences do exist between rodents and humans. Thoughtful examination of patients with disorders affecting sexual differentiation has elucidated many of the factors involved in human sexual differentiation.

Disorders of Gonadal Differentiation

WILMS' TUMOR GENE

The Wilms' tumor suppressor (WT1) gene, located at chromosome 11p13, plays an important role in both kidney and gonadal differentiation.[92] Although Wilms' tumor and genitourinary abnormalities can be associated with heterozygous WT1 deletions, only 6% to 15% of sporadic Wilms' tumors are associated with WT1 mutations.[93] Heterozygous deletions at chromosome 11p13 can be part of a contiguous gene deletion syndrome known as WAGR syndrome (Wilms' tumor, aniridia, genito-urinary anomalies, gonadoblastoma, and mental retardation).

Denys-Drash syndrome (characterized by genito-urinary anomalies, Wilms' tumor, and nephropathy) is due to mutations in the WT1 gene. Typically, the nephropathy begins during the first few years of life, manifests with proteinuria, and results in end-stage renal failure due to focal or diffuse mesangial sclerosis.[94-97] Among affected 46,XY individuals, the external genitalia can range from ambiguous to normal female. Affected 46,XX individuals show normal female external genital development. Internal genital differentiation varies because persistence of Wolffian and/or Mullerian structures is inconsistent. Typically, the gonads are dysgenetic in 46,XY individuals. The heterozygous missense mutations associated with Denys-Drash syndrome are believed to act in a dominant negative fashion.[98]

The features of Frasier syndrome include gonadal dysgenesis, progressive glomerulopathy, and an increased risk for gonadoblastoma. Wilms' tumor is extremely rare in Frasier syndrome.[99] The typical renal lesion is focal glomerular sclerosis. The majority of cases are associated with a specific point mutation in intron 9 of WT1.

In the fetal kidney, WT1 induces the mesenchymal-epithelial transition—leading to nephron formation.[100] Depending on cellular context, WT1 can function as a transcriptional activator, a transcriptional repressor, or tumor suppressor. The carboxyl terminal domain of the WT1 protein contains four zinc fingers that serve as the nucleic acid binding domain. Downstream target genes include WNT4 and AMHRII.[101] Through alternative splicing, multiple translation start sites, and post-translational RNA editing, multiple isoforms can be derived from this one gene. Distinct isoforms may have unique functions.

Alternative splicing between the third and fourth zinc fingers generates two isoforms differing by the presence or absence of three amino acids [lysine, threonine, and serine (KTS)]. Subnuclear localization studies have shown that the –KTS form colocalizes predominantly with transcription factors, whereas the +KTS form colocalizes mainly with splicing factors.[102] The ratio of the +KTS/–KTS isoforms appears to be tightly regulated. The mutation associated with Frasier syndrome alters splicing patterns, leading to decreased amounts of the +KTS isoform.

WNT4 GENE

WNT4 is a secreted molecule that binds to members of the frizzled family of receptors, resulting in transcriptional regulation of target genes. WNT4 increases follistatin expression, which inhibits formation of the coelomic vessel (anti-testis action) and supports ovarian germ cell survival (pro-ovarian action).[103] Duplication of the WNT4 gene, located at chromosome 1p31-1p35, has been associated with 46,XY male-to-female sex reversal. One such patient presented with ambiguous external genitalia accompanied by severe hypospadias, fibrous gonads, remnants of both Mullerian and Wolffian structures, cleft lip, microcephaly, and intrauterine growth retardation.[104] Loss of function WNT 4 mutations have been detected in two women with primary amenorrhea secondary to Mullerian duct abnormalities and androgen excess.[105,106] The phenotypes of these patients support the hypothesis that WNT4 plays a role in ovarian differentiation.

46,XY DISORDERS OF SEXUAL DIFFERENTIATION (GONADAL DYSGENESIS)

Phenotype/genotype studies of 46,XY sex-reversed patients played a major role in the localization of the Y chromosome gene responsible for the initial signal-promoting testicular differentiation. Subsequently, this gene was identified to be the sex-determining region on Y (SRY) gene located at Yp11.3 near the pseudoautosomal region on Yp. Identification of mutations in SRY in 46,XY females confirmed the vital role of SRY in testicular differentiation.

SRY is a gene with a single exon that codes for a 204-amino-acid protein and that contains an HMG DNA-binding domain flanked by nuclear localization signals (NLS). The majority of sex-reversing SRY mutations are located in the HMG/NLS domain and affect DNA-binding affinity, DNA bending ability, or nuclear localization.[107] Yet, only 15% to 20% of cases of 46,XY DSD due to gonadal dysgenesis can be attributed to SRY mutations.[108] Paternal mosaicism for SRY mutations in which different cells carry different SRY genes has been described.[109,110] More puzzling are the pedigrees in which fathers and unaffected brothers carry the identical mutant SRY allele as the propositus.[111,112] These paradoxical findings implicate involvement of other genes, gene-gene interactions, and gene-environment interactions in the process of sexual differentiation.

Individuals with sex chromosome DSDs due to partial or mixed gonadal dysgenesis usually present with asymmetric genital ambiguity (Figure 4-2). Somatic features of Turner syndrome such as short stature, webbed neck, cubitus valgus, and gonadal failure may be present. Multiple cell lines, including a monosomic X cell line, may be detected. The most common karyotype is 45,X/46,XY. However, there is much phenotypic heterogeneity associated with 45,X/46,XY karyotype in that internal and external genital differentiation ranges from normal male to ambiguous to female.[113,114] Whereas the typical histologic features consist of poorly developed seminiferous tubules surrounded by wavy ovarian stroma, gonadal differentiation can range from normal testis to streak gonads. At the time of puberty, virilization can occur.

Individuals with sex chromosome DSDs due to gonadal dysgenesis have an increased risk of developing gonadal tumors such as gonadoblastoma or dysgerminoma because a dysgenetic gonad carrying a Y chromosome has an increased risk for neoplastic changes.[115,116] Although gonadal tumors typically do not develop until the second decade of life, they can occur earlier.[117]

SOX9

Heterozygous loss of function mutations in the SOX9 gene are associated with autosomal-dominant campomelic dwarfism and male-to-female sex reversal.[118,119] Features of campomelic dwarfism include congenital bowing of long bones, hypoplastic scapulae, 11 pairs of ribs, clubfeet, micrognathia, and cleft palate. SOX9 mutations do not cause sex reversal in the absence of skeletal malformations.[120] Although the severity of the bone malformations varies, most affected individuals die shortly after birth due to respiratory failure. Approximately 75% of affected 46,XY fetuses show sex reversal, with external genital differentiation ranging from ambiguous to female. Gonadal dysgenesis and persistence of Mullerian duct derivatives are typical. Phenotypic heterogeneity with

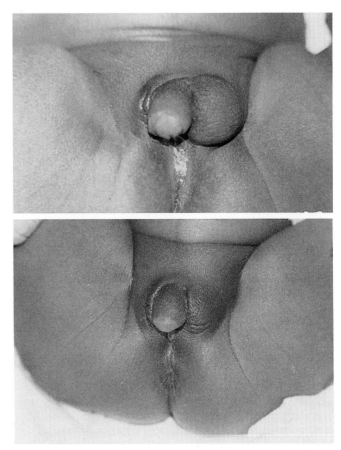

Figure 4-2. Genital ambiguity with asymmetry in patient with 46, XY disorder of sexual differentiation (mixed gonadal dysgenesis).

differing phenotypes (ovotesticular DSD or true hermaphroditism and complete sex reversal) in affected siblings has been described.[121]

SOX9 is a member of the SRY-related HMG domain gene family located at chromosome 17q24.3-17q25.1.[122] It is a 508-amino-acid protein containing an 80-amino-acid HMG domain involved in DNA binding and bending; a 41-amino-acid proline, glutamine, and alanine motif; and a C-terminal transactivation domain. Mutations in SOX9 can affect DNA-binding affinity, DNA bending ability, nuclear import, transactivation, and nuclear export.[123] An interstitial deletion of SOX9 in an affected patient provides the strongest evidence to date that haploinsufficiency is the mechanism responsible for the effects of SOX9.[124] Somatic cell mosaicism, de novo germ-line mutations, and mitotic gene conversion events have been described.[125]

DAX1

DAX1 is an orphan nuclear receptor that lacks a typical zinc finger DNA-binding domain. The gene (NROB1) coding for DAX1 is located on the short arm of the X chromosome and consists of two exons. Duplication of the DAX1 locus is associated with male-to-female sex reversal.[126] External genital differentiation ranges from female to ambiguous. Descriptions of internal genitalia include presence of Mullerian and Wolffian structures. Gonads are typically described as streaks. A submicroscopic interstitial duplication of the DAX1 gene was discovered during thorough evaluation of two sisters. The older sister had presented with primary amenorrhea, female external genitalia, 46,XY karyotype, and gonadal dysgenesis.[127]

Loss-of-function mutations are associated with X-linked adrenal hypoplasia congenita (AHC). In this disorder, development of the fetal adrenal cortex is normal. However, the adult or definitive adrenal cortex fails to develop—leading to postnatal adrenal insufficiency. Although the symptoms of adrenal insufficiency generally manifest in infancy or early childhood, phenotypic heterogeneity in severity and age at presentation occurs.[128] Unilateral or bilateral cryptorchidism can also occur.[129] At the age of expected puberty, hypogonadotropic hypogonadism due to hypothalamic and pituitary dysfunction may occur among affected males.[130] Delayed puberty has been recognized in heterozygous females.[131] One female homozygous for DAX1 mutations has been reported. Her phenotype was hypogonadotropic hypogonadism.[132] As part of a contiguous gene deletion syndrome, X-linked AHC can be associated with glycerol kinase deficiency, Duchenne muscular dystrophy, ornithine transcarbamylase deficiency, and mental retardation.[133]

DAX1/NROB1 is expressed throughout the HPG axis. The DAX1 protein functions as a transcriptional repressor of many genes, including SF1 and some steroidogenic enzyme genes. Nonsense mutations have been identified throughout the gene. Missense mutations account for 20% of mutations associated with AHC. These mutations tend to cluster in the carboxyl terminal of the protein corresponding to the putative ligand-binding domain and impair the transcriptional repression activity of the protein.[134,135] One missense point mutation, located in the hinge region of the protein, was identified in an 8-year-old girl with clinical and laboratory features indicative of adrenal insufficiency. Additional studies showed that this mutation hindered nuclear localization of the protein. Curiously, the hemizygous father and heterozygous younger sister of the proband did not manifest the AHC phenotype.[136]

Recently, an alternatively spliced form of DAX1 (DAX1A) has been identified and found to have a more ubiquitous expression pattern than DAX1. DAX1A is expressed in adrenals, gonads, and pancreas.[137,138] The deduced protein sequence of DAX1A contains 400 amino acids, compared with 470 amino acids for DAX1. Another member of the NROB family is small heterodimer partner (SHP). Among its actions, SHP influences expression of cholesterol, bile acid, and glucose homeostasis.[139] The protein domain structures of DAX1, DAX1A, and SHP lack the canonical DNA-binding domain, AF-1 modulator domain, and the hinge region—which are characteristics of nuclear hormone receptors. All three proteins can form homodimers or heterodimers with one other, as well as with other nuclear receptors. As transcriptional repressors, DAX1 and SHP repress gene transcription by direct protein-protein interactions with target genes and recruit additional corepressor proteins such as nuclear receptor corepressor

Alien.[140] DAX1, DAX1A, and SHP may have novel and complex interactions.[141]

DESERT HEDGEHOG

One patient with 46,XY DSD associated with a dysgenetic gonad was found to be homozygous for a single nucleotide substitution at the initiation codon, ATG→ACG, of the DHH gene. This variation was predicted to abolish initiation of translation at the normal start site. This patient's phenotype consisted of female external genitalia, polyneuropathy, a testis on one side, and a streak gonad on the other side. Histologic analysis of the sural nerve revealed extensive formation of minifascicles within the endoneurium.[142] Mutations in the DHH gene have been reported in several additional 46,XY patients with either complete or mixed gonadal dysgenesis.[143,144] The DHH gene is located on chromosome 12q12→q13.1 and encodes a protein consisting of 396 amino acids.[145]

CHROMOSOME 9p MONOSOMY

Monosomy for distal chromosome 9p has been reported in male-to-female sex reversal. External genitalia have been described as ambiguous or female. Differentiation of internal genitalia is highly variable, with the presence of Mullerian and Wolffian remnants being reported.[146] Description of the gonads has ranged from streak gonads to hypoplastic testes. In addition to sex reversal, clinical features include mental retardation, low-set ears, trigonocephaly, wide nasal bridge, and single palmar creases.[147,148] Neither the size of the deletion nor parental origin influences the degree of sex reversal.[149-151] Two genes related to double-sex (dsx) and mab-3 regulators of sexual differentiation in *Drosophila melanogaster* (DMRT1 and DMRT2)[152] have been mapped to 9p24. It has been suggested that these human genes, DMRT1 and DMRT2, play roles in testis differentiation.[153]

Although, to date no, mutations have been detected in either gene,[154] a submicroscopic deletion at 9p24.3 was identified in two 46,XY sex-reversed sisters. This deletion was also present in their fertile mother.[155] This small deletion (less than 700 kilobases) mapped 5' of both DMRT1 and DMRT2, but within 30 kilobases of DMRT1. Thus, the deletion could include a previously unidentified upstream exon or regulatory sequence(s) of DMRT1. Because karyotypes for most 9p deletion patients with sex reversal have been 46,XY, DMRT1 may be involved in testicular differentiation. Investigation of sexual differentiation in other species shows higher DMRT1 expression in testis compared to ovaries, whereas DMRT2 is not expressed in adult testis or in developing gonadal ridges.[156,157] Sexually dimorphic expression of DMRT1 was found in 6- and 7-week-old human fetuses, with expression limited to male fetuses.[158]

Xq28 DELETION

Sex reversal and myotubular myopathy are associated with interstitial deletions at Xq28. One family has been described in which there were two affected 46,XY infants in whom MTM1 and F18 (now known as CXorf6) genes were deleted.[159,160] Three nonsense mutations in CXorf6 were identified in three Japanese males with hypospadias.[161]

ATR-X SYNDROME

ATR-X (α-thalassemia, mental retardation, X-linked protein) syndrome is an X-linked disorder characterized by mild alpha-thalassemia, severe mental retardation, and genital abnormalities. The urogenital anomalies consist of ambiguous genitalia, cryptorchidism, hypoplastic scrotum, hypospadias, shawl scrotum, and small penis.[162,163] Other typical features include short stature, microcephaly, seizures, talipes equinovarus, and gastrointestinal problems. Facies are described as coarse, with midface hypoplasia, short nose, and widely spaced incisors.

The hemoglobin H inclusions can be demonstrated on brilliant cresyl blue stained peripheral blood smears.[164] The typical presence of Wolffian duct and absence of Mullerian duct structures indicates at least partial Sertoli and Leydig cell function. Histologic studies of testes suggest aberrant Leydig cell development.[165]

The molecular basis of this entity is mutations in the ATRX (also known as XH2 or XHP) gene located at Xq13.3.[166,167] The ATRX gene product is a member of the SWI/SNF DNA helicase family and contains functional domains involved in protein-protein and protein-DNA interactions. Based on in vitro evidence and its functional domains, the protein appears to play a role in chromatin remodeling.[168,169] Phenotype-genotype correlations are inconsistent. Urogenital anomalies are associated with mutations that truncate the protein and with mutations located in the plant homeodomain-like domain.[170] Skewed X-inactivation is typical of carrier females. Greater than 75% of cases are inherited from carrier mothers.[171] Carpenter-Waziri, Juber-Marsidi, and Smith-Fineman-Myers syndromes and X-linked mental retardation with spastic paraplegia are also associated with mutations in the ATRX gene.[172]

VANISHING TESTES

The terms *testicular regression syndrome* and *vanishing testes* are used to describe testicular absence in boys with undescended testes. In some instances, this situation is associated with ambiguous genitalia and under-virilization—which presumably represents regression of testicular tissue occurring between 8 and 14 weeks of gestation. Physical findings reflect duration of testicular function. At operation, a rudimentary spermatic cord and nubbin of testicular tissue may be identified. Histologic examination of the testicular nubbins often reveals hemosiderin-laden macrophages and dystrophic calcification. It has been suggested that an antenatal vascular accident associated with antenatal testicular torsion is a cause of testicular regression.[173] Although usually sporadic, familial testicular regression has been described.[174]

MULTIPLE CONGENITAL ANOMALIES

In affected 46,XY infants, the IMAGe syndrome is characterized by intrauterine growth retardation, metaphyseal dysplasia, adrenal hypoplasia, cryptorchidism, and micropenis in the absence of DAX1 or NR5A1/SF1 mutations.[175] The Pallister-Hall syndrome is associated with micropenis, hypospadias, hypothalamic hamartoma, postaxial polydactyly, and imperforate anus.[176] Features of the autosomal dominant Robinow syndrome include small penis, cryptorchidism, bulging forehead, hypertelorism, depressed nasal bridge, short stature, short limbs, and hemivertebrae.[177] Genital ambiguity in affected 46,XY individuals in association with X-linked lissencephaly, absence of the corpus callosum, and hypothalamic dysfunction (including temperature instability) has been described. This constellation of features has been associated with mutations in the ARX gene.[178-180]

OVOTESTICULAR DISORDER OF SEXUAL DIFFERENTIATION (TRUE HERMAPHRODITISM)

Ovotesticular DSD is defined as presence of ovarian tissue with follicles and testicular tissue with seminiferous tubules in the same individual. Although an ovotestis is the most commonly identified gonad, there can be an ovary on one side and a testis on the other. In most ovotestes, ovarian and testicular tissue show distinct separation in an end-to-end arrangement. Karyotypes are usually 46,XX. Mosaic karyotypes (46,XX/46,XY and 46,XX/47,XXY) have been described.[181] In some instances, Y chromosomal material such as the SRY gene can be detected by PCR amplification. However, ovotesticular DSD in the absence of Y chromosomal material has been reported.[182] In one patient in whom the peripheral blood karyotype was 46,XX, molecular genetic analysis showed a deletion of the promoter region of the SRY gene in the testicular tissue of an ovotestis.[183]

Several pedigrees in which both XX males and XX true hermaphrodites coexist have been described.[184,185] These families likely represent incomplete penetrance of mutations of genes involved in sexual differentiation.[186] Although most patients present in infancy or childhood, two phenotypic males who presented with bilateral gynecomastia have been reported.[187,188] Outcome regarding fertility has been disappointing. In a series of 33 patients followed longitudinally, germ cells identified in the testicular tissue during infancy degenerated—resulting in azoospermia. Although normal menstrual cycles have been reported in a few females, no pregnancies were documented in one series.[182] However, pregnancies have been reported in some females with ovotesticular DSD.[189-191]

46,XX TESTICULAR DISORDER OF SEXUAL DIFFERENTIATION

The frequency of the XX male syndrome is approximately 1 in 25,000 males.[192] The majority of 46,XX males are found to carry the SRY gene, have normal male genitalia, and often present with infertility.[193] In most instances, the SRY gene is located on an X chromosome due to illegitimate recombination between the X and Y chromosomes. An incidental finding was reported for a 61-year-old man with a history of small testes and azoospermia. His karyotype showed 46,XX, with the insertion of the SRY gene on the terminal end of chromosome 16q.[194] Rare instances of 46,XX males with absence of the SRY gene have been described.[195]

FOXL2

Mutations in the FOXL2 gene have been associated with the autosomal dominant blepharophimosis ptosis epicanthus inversus syndrome (BPES). The phenotype of BPES type 1 involves premature ovarian failure and malformations of the eyelid [which consist of small palpebral fissures (blepharophimosis)], ptosis, epicanthus inversus, and a broad nasal bridge.[196] FOXL2 is a forkhead transcription factor. Curiously, in goats mutations in this locus are responsible for the autosomal dominant phenotype characterized by the absence of horns in male and female goats (polledness). It is also associated with XX female-to-male sex reversal in a recessive manner.[197]

Disorders of Androgen Synthesis

Genital ambiguity can be a manifestation of alterations in sex steroid biosynthesis, which most commonly are secondary to mutations in a steroidogenic enzyme gene.

During fetal life, steroidogenic enzymes are expressed in placenta, testis, and adrenal (Figure 4-2). The fetal testis secretes testosterone that is converted to dihydrotestosterone in target tissues such as the prostate and external genitalia. Inborn errors of testosterone biosynthesis can lead to ambiguous genitalia in 46,XY fetuses. Specific proteins necessary to testosterone biosynthesis include SF1, LH receptor, steroidogenic acute regulatory peptide (StAR), 17α-hydroxylase/17,20-lyase, 3β-hydroxysteroid dehydrogenase type 2, 17β-hydroxysteroid dehydrogenase type 3, P450-oxidoreductase, and 5α-reductase type 2 (Figure 4-3). Inborn errors of glucocorticoid biosynthesis are often associated with the virilizing congenital adrenal hyperplasias.

The fetal adrenal cortex is derived from coelomic epithelium and consists of two major zones: the fetal zone and the adult zone. Because the human placenta does not express 17α-hydroxylase/17,20-lyase, it cannot directly convert progesterone to estrogens. The fetal zone is primarily responsible for DHEA synthesis, which is then sulfated to provide substrate for placental estrogen biosynthesis (Figure 4-3). The adult zone, which after birth differentiates into the three zones of the adult adrenal cortex, is primarily responsible for cortisol biosynthesis. By 10 weeks of gestation, the adrenal is secreting DHEAS and the hypothalamic-pituitary-adrenal axis is functional.

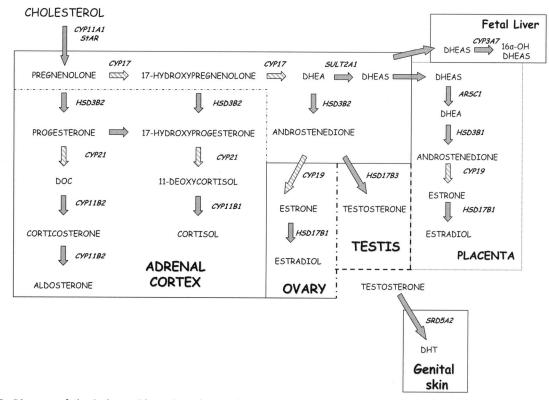

Figure 4-3. Diagram of classical steroidogenic pathways. Substrates, products, and genes involved in adrenal, ovarian, testicular, and placental steroidogenesis are indicated. Genes are 17α-hydroxylase/17,20-lyase (CYP17), 3β-hydroxysteroid dehydrogenase (HSD3B2), 21-hydroxylase (CYP21), 11β-hydroxylase (CYP11B1), aldosterone synthase (CYP11B2), aromatase (CYP19), 17β-hydroxysteroid dehydrogenase type 1 (HSD17B1), 17β-hydroxysteroid dehydrogenase type 3 (HSD17B3), 5α-reductase type 2 (SRD5A2), sulfotransferase (SULT2A1), and steroid sulfatase/arylsulfatase C (ARSC1). CYP3A7 is a cytochrome P450 enzyme expressed in fetal liver, where it catalyzes the 16α-hydroxylation of estrone (E1) and DHEA. Its expression decreases postnatally. Steroidogenic enzymes that utilize P450 oxidoreductase, a flavoprotein encoded by POR, to transfer electrons are indicated by hatched arrows.

SF1/NR5A1 GENE

The SF1/NR5A1 gene, located at chromosome 9q33, codes for a 461-amino-acid protein. One 46,XY patient heterozygous for an NR5A1/SF-1 mutation presented in the newborn period with adrenal insufficiency and was initially considered to have lipoid adrenal hyperplasia. The patient had female external genitalia, normal Mullerian structures, and streak gonads. Reevaluation prior to induction of puberty revealed normal gonadotropin response to GnRH stimulation. Functional studies showed that this mutation, G35E, fails to transactivate a known SF1 responsive reporter gene.[198]

A 46,XX female with adrenal insufficiency, adrenal hypoplasia, and an SF1/NR5A1 mutation showed normal ovarian morphology.[199] With identification of more patients heterozygous for missense mutations in the SF1/NR5A1 gene, it has become apparent that haploinsufficiency of SF1 can manifest a predominantly gonadal phenotype characterized by undervirilization of affected 46,XY fetuses without overt adrenal insufficiency.[200] Females heterozygous for missense mutations appear to lack an obvious phenotype.

LUTEINIZING HORMONE CHORIOGONADOTROPIN RECEPTOR GENE

Leydig cell hypoplasia is an autosomal recessive disorder characterized by failure of testicular Leydig cell differentiation secondary to inactivating LHCGR mutations and target cell resistance to LH.[201-203] The inability to respond to hCG or LH results in decreased Leydig cell testosterone biosynthesis. The phenotype of affected 46,XY infants ranges from undervirilization to female external genitalia. Affected individuals raised as females often seek medical attention for delayed breast development. Mullerian duct derivatives are absent because AMH is secreted by the unaffected Sertoli cells. Laboratory studies show elevated LH, low testosterone, and normal FSH concentrations. There is no significant testosterone response to hCG stimulation.

The LHCGR gene is mapped to chromosome 2p21.[204] The 674-amino-acid protein is a seven-transmembrane domain G-protein–coupled receptor. Specific mechanisms through which the loss-of-function mutations induce LH resistance include decreased receptor protein, decreased ligand binding, altered receptor trafficking, and impaired ability to activate G_s. Undervirilization with hypospadias, micropenis, and cryptorchidism has been described with incomplete loss-of-function missense mutations.[205] Genetic females, sisters of affected 46,XY individuals, who carry the identical mutations show normal female genital differentiation and normal pubertal development but have amenorrhea and infertility.[206,207] Genetic analysis may be helpful to distinguish LHCGR mutations from other disorders affecting testosterone biosynthesis (such as isolated 17,20-lyase deficiency).[208]

SMITH-LEMLI-OPITZ SYNDROME

Clinical features of this autosomal recessive disorder include multiple malformations, urogenital anomalies, mental retardation, failure to thrive, facial abnormalities, developmental delay, and behavioral abnormalities. The most common urogenital abnormalities include male-to-female sex reversal, hypospadias, and cryptorchidism. The facial abnormalities consist of a broad nose, upturned nares, micrognathia, short neck, and cleft palate.[209] Typical limb anomalies comprise short thumbs, syndactyly of the second and third toes, and post-axial polydactyly.

Several enzymes catalyze the conversion of lanosterol to cholesterol. Decreased activity of these enzymes leads to cholesterol deficiency. The enzyme, 7-dehydrocholesterol reductase, encoded by the 7-dehydrocholesterol reductase (DHCR7) gene catalyzes the last step in cholesterol biosynthesis. Smith-Lemli-Opitz (SLO) is due to mutations in the 7-dehydrocholesterol reductase (DHCR7) gene located at chromosome 11q12-q13.[210,211] Mutations in the DHCR7 gene are associated with elevated 7-dehydroxycholesterol concentrations. Demonstration of elevated 7-dehydroxycholesterol concentrations is required to confirm the diagnosis. To date, more than 80 mutations have been reported.[212]

As anticipated, mutations in this cholesterol biosynthetic pathway are associated with decreased cholesterol and accumulation of sterol intermediates proximal to the defective enzyme. Decreased cholesterol concentrations lead to decreased steroid concentrations because cholesterol serves as the precursor for glucocorticoid, mineralocorticoid, and sex steroid biosynthesis. In addition to its role as the precursor for steroid biosynthesis, cholesterol modification of sonic hedgehog protein (SHH) is necessary for normal signaling through its cognate receptor, Patched (PTCH), which contains a sterol sensing domain. In fibroblasts from patients with SLO, SHH signaling is impaired. Using transgenic mouse models, available data indicate that accumulation of sterol intermediates rather than cholesterol deficiency interferes with midline fusion of facial structures. These observations shed light on the molecular pathophysiology responsible for the cleft palate associated with SLO.[213,214]

Prenatal diagnosis can be performed by measurement of amniotic fluid DHCR7 concentrations.[215] Low plasma estriol and elevated 16α-hydroxy-estrogens concentrations are found in women pregnant with affected fetuses, presumably due to impaired fetal cholesterol production.[216] The incidence of biochemically confirmed SLO is estimated at 1/20,000 to 1/60,000 live births.[217] With the identification of the molecular basis for this disorder, a surprisingly high heterozygote carrier rate for DHCR7 mutations has been found. Because the prevalence of SLO at 16 weeks of gestation is comparable to the prevalence at birth, early fetal loss and/or reduced fertility of carrier couples may be occurring.[218]

CONGENITAL LIPOID ADRENAL HYPERPLASIA

This autosomal-recessive disorder is characterized by a severe defect in the conversion of cholesterol to pregnenolone, leading to impaired steroidogenesis of all adrenal and gonadal steroid hormones. Impaired testosterone biosynthesis in utero prevents male sexual differentiation. Hence, all affected fetuses (46,XY or 46,XX) have female external genitalia. Low or undetectable steroid hormone levels are consistent with this diagnosis. The hormone determinations to distinguish congenital lipoid adrenal hyperplasia from 3β-hydroxysteroid dehydrogenase deficiency should include 17-hydroxypregnenolone or pregnenolone. These hormones will be low in the former but elevated in the latter. Milder forms of this disorder with presentation beyond the newborn period have been described.[219]

Following cloning of the gene for steroidogenic acute regulatory protein (StAR), mutations in the StAR gene were identified among patients with congenital lipoid adrenal hyperplasia.[220-224] The StAR protein facilitates cholesterol transport across the mitochondria to P450scc.[225,226] In congenital lipoid adrenal hyperplasia, impaired cholesterol transport into mitochondria leads to accumulation of cholesterol esters and sterol auto-oxidation products. Ultimately, the lipid accumulation alters the cell cytostructure—provoking cell destruction and complete loss of StAR-dependent steroidogenesis.[227] Yet, the presence of low levels of StAR-independent steroidogenesis allows for preservation of Wolffian duct remnants in affected 46,XY fetuses and spontaneous pubertal mutation in affected 46,XX girls.[228,229]

SIDE CHAIN CLEAVAGE CYTOCHROME P450 ENZYME

The side chain cleavage enzyme (also known as cholesterol desmolase) is a cytochrome P450 enzyme encoded by the CYP11A1 gene mapped to chromosome 15q23-q24. This enzyme converts cholesterol to pregnenolone and is essential to steroidogenesis. Despite the crucial role of this enzyme for placental progesterone synthesis, rare fetuses with loss-of-function mutations on both alleles may be viable. Children affected with this autosomal-recessive disorder have female external genitalia irrespective of the karyotype and adrenal insufficiency. Postnatally, sizes of adrenals and gonads on ultrasound or magnetic resonance imaging have been variable but not enlarged. The absence of adrenal/gonadal tissue has been speculated to result from lipid accumulation similar to the cell destruction observed in patients with StAR mutations.[230-232]

VIRILIZING CONGENITAL ADRENAL HYPERPLASIAS

The virilizing congenital adrenal hyperplasias are a group of disorders due to mutations in the steroidogenic enzyme genes involved in cortisol biosynthesis. These genes are 3β-hydroxysteroid dehydrogenase type 2 (HSD3B2), 21-hydroxylase (CYP21), and 11β-hydroxylase (CYP11B1). The common pathophysiology is decreased negative feedback inhibition due to insufficient cortisol concentrations, but the specific manifestations and laboratory abnormalities vary depending on which enzyme gene is involved. Steroid intermediates proximal to the deficient enzyme accumulate.

Overall, relative cortisol deficiency leads to a diminution of negative feedback inhibition with subsequent increased ACTH secretion. The adrenal cortex responds by

proportionally increasing adrenal androgen production. Thus, the clinical signs and symptoms reflect androgen excess in addition to glucocorticoid and mineralocorticoid deficiencies. Indeed, the magnitude of glucocorticoid and mineralocorticoid deficiencies varies—generally in proportion to the severity of the enzyme deficiency.

The most common type of congenital adrenal hyperplasia (accounting for 90% to 95% of cases) is 21-hydroxylase deficiency due to mutations in the 21-hydroxylase (CYP21A2) gene located at chromosome 6p21.3 in the HLA class III region.[233-237] The reported incidence of 21-hydroxylase deficiency ranges from 1 in 5,000 to 1 in 15,000, with variation among ethnic/racial backgrounds.[238,239] Decreased 21-hydroxylase activity impairs conversion of 17-hydroxyprogesterone to 11-deoxycortisol in the zona fasciculata (the primary site of cortisol biosynthesis) and conversion of progesterone to deoxycorticosterone in the zona glomerulosa, the primary site of aldosterone biosynthesis.

In addition to the shunting of 17-OHP to androstenedione, DHEA, and DHEAS resulting in increased androgen concentrations in the affected female fetus, 17-OHP can be converted through an alternate route to DHT. This alternate route (the "backdoor pathway") involves 5α-reduction of 17-OHP to 5α-pregnane-17α-ol-3,20-dione, ultimately generating androstanediol—which is the substrate for 3α-reduction and conversion to DHT[240] (Figure 4-4). During fetal life, accumulation of 17-OHP due to mutations in CYP21A2, CYP11B2, or P450-oxidoreductase (POR) may increase flux through this "backdoor pathway"—leading to elevated DHT concentrations.[241]

Infant girls with classic salt-losing 21-hydroxylase deficiency usually present in the immediate neonatal period due to genital ambiguity (Figure 4-5). When the diagnosis is delayed, affected girls develop dehydration, hyponatremia, and hyperkalemia due to glucocorticoid and mineralocorticoid deficiencies. Among affected female infants, virilization of the external genitalia ranges from clitoromegaly to perineal hypospadias—with chordee to complete fusion of labiourethral and labioscrotal folds. The magnitude of external genital virilization may be so extensive that affected female infants appear to be males with bilateral undescended testes.[242,243] Unless identified by neonatal screening, infant boys typically present at 2 to 3 weeks of age with failure to thrive, poor feeding, lethargy, dehydration, hypotension, hyponatremia, and hyperkalemia. When the diagnosis is delayed or missed, congenital adrenal hyperplasia is potentially fatal. Newborn screening programs decrease the morbidity and mortality associated with acute adrenal insufficiency.

In affected infants, random 17-hydroxyprogesterone concentrations are usually elevated. Concentrations are greater than 5,000 ng/dL, and often much higher.[244] Androstenedione and progesterone concentrations are also typically elevated. In some instances, plasma renin activity (PRA) can be helpful to assess mineralocorticoid status. Measurement of 21-deoxycortisol is extremely helpful, but availability of this hormone assay is limited.[245,246] For female infants, a normal uterus is present and can be identified on ultrasound. Ovaries may be too small to be readily identified on ultrasound. Despite excessive antenatal androgen exposure, ovarian position is normal and internal Wolffian structures are not retained.

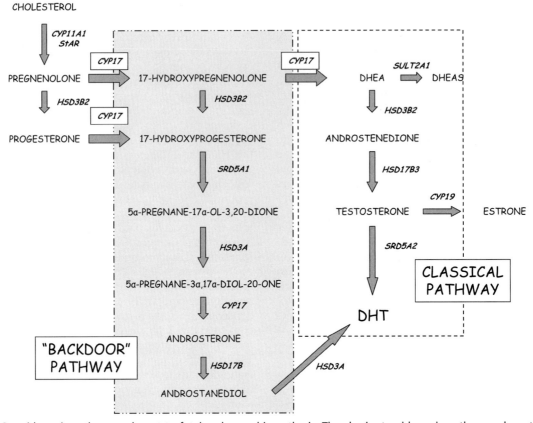

CHOLESTEROL

Figure 4-4. Steroidogenic pathways relevant to fetal androgen biosynthesis. The classic steroidogenic pathway relevant to the testis (light background) and the "backdoor pathway" (dark background) are indicated. Both pathways can generate DHT through the actions of target tissue enzymes capable of converting substrates, testosterone, and androstanediol into DHT. In the presence of elevated ACTH and 17-OHP concentrations due to CYP21, CYP11B1, or POR mutations, the backdoor pathway may contribute to the excessive androgen concentrations responsible for virilization of XX fetuses.

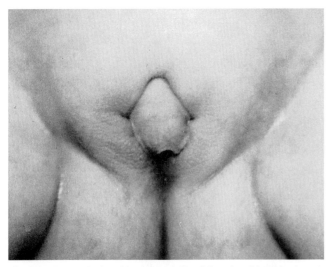

Figure 4-5. Genital ambiguity in virilized female with 21-hydroxylase deficiency. The labioscrotal folds are fused, and the clitoris is enlarged.

The spectrum of impaired 21-hydroxylase activity ranges from complete glucocorticoid and mineralocorticoid deficiencies to mild deficiencies manifested principally by compensatory excessive adrenal androgen secretion. Infants capable of adequate aldosterone synthesis do not usually manifest overt salt loss. Female infants capable of adequate aldosterone synthesis may still have sufficient androgen exposure in utero to virilize their external genitalia. In the absence of newborn screening programs, affected males capable of aldosterone biosynthesis may not be identified until they present with genital overgrowth or premature pubarche. Infants with the milder forms of congenital adrenal hyperplasia are generally not identified by most newborn screening programs.[247]

CYP21A2 is located approximately 30 kilobases from a highly homologous pseudogene, CYP21A1P. The tenascin-XB (TNXB) gene encoding an extracellular matrix protein is located on the DNA strand opposite CYP21A2.[248] At this time, more than 100 CYP21A2 mutations have been reported. However, only a few mutations account for the majority of affected alleles.[249,250] Most of the common mutations represent gene conversion events in which CYP21A2 has acquired deleterious CYP21A1P sequences. The frequency of specific mutations varies among ethnic groups.[251] Molecular genotyping can be a useful adjunct to newborn screening.[252,253] Caveats to bear in mind are that multiple mutations can occur on a single allele and that different CYP21A2 mutations can occur in one family.[254-256]

Congenital adrenal hyperplasia due to 11β-hydroxylase deficiency is characterized by glucocorticoid deficiency, excessive androgen secretion, and hypertension.

This enzyme is expressed in the zona fasciculate, where it converts 11-deoxycortisol to cortisol. This form of congenital adrenal hyperplasia is rare (3%–5% of cases) apart from the high incidence among Moroccan Jews, for whom the incidence approaches 1 in 6,000.[257] Despite the presence of the identical mutation, phenotypic heterogeneity for the magnitude of virilization and hypertension occurs even in a single family. Affected females may present with ambiguous genitalia. Typical laboratory findings are elevated serum concentrations of 11-deoxycortisol. Serum concentrations of 17-hydroxyprogesterone, androstenedione, and testosterone may be mildly elevated. PRA concentrations are low or suppressed. Although ACTH-stimulated hormone responses among heterozygotic carriers are usually normal, elevated 11-deoxycortisol and 11-deoxycorticosterone have been reported.[258,259]

Mutations in the 11β-hydroxylase (CYP11B1) gene have been identified in patients with 11β-hydroxylase deficiency.[260-262] The CYP11B1 gene is located at chromosome 8q22 in close proximity to a highly homologous gene CYP11B2, which codes for aldosterone synthase.[263] CYP11B1 is expressed in the zona fasciculate, whereas CYP11B2 is expressed primarily in the zona glomerulosa.[264]

3β-HYDROXYSTEROID DEHYDROGENASE DEFICIENCY

Congenital adrenal hyperplasia due to 3β-hydroxysteroid dehydrogenase type 2 deficiency leads to virilization of the external genitalia of 46,XX fetuses due to increased DHEA synthesis. Affected 46,XY fetuses have ambiguous genitalia characterized by undervirilization of the external genitalia secondary to testosterone deficiency. Despite decreased testosterone synthesis, affected 46,XY fetuses usually have intact Wolffian duct structures (including vas deferens). The NAD$^+$-dependent enzyme 3β-hydroxysteroid dehydrogenase/Δ^5-Δ^4-isomerase catalyzes the conversion of the Δ^5 steroid precursors, pregnenolone, 17-hydroxypregnenolone, and DHEA into the respective Δ^4-ketosteroids, progesterone, 17-hydroxyprogesterone, and androstenedione.[265]

Two isozymes encoded by two different highly homologous genes have been identified and mapped to chromosome 1p13.1.[266,267] The type 1 (HSD3B1) gene is expressed primarily in skin, placenta, prostate, and other peripheral tissues. The type 2 (HSD3B2) gene is the predominant form expressed in the adrenal cortex and gonads. Mutations in HSD3B2, but not HSD3B1, have been detected in patients with 3β-hydroxysteroid dehydrogenase deficiency congenital adrenal hyperplasia.[268-270] Acute adrenal insufficiency occurs in the newborn period when complete loss of function mutations impair biosynthesis of mineralocorticoids, glucocorticoids, and sex steroids. Typical presentations for the non–salt-losing forms include premature pubarche and (in 46,XY infants) perineal hypospadias.[271] Confirmatory laboratory findings include elevated pregnenolone, 17-hydroxypregnenolone, and DHEA concentrations with elevated ratios of Δ^5 to Δ^4 steroids. Because enzymatic activity of the type 1 isozyme is unimpaired, elevated 17-hydroxyprogesterone and androstenedione concentrations may be found.

17β-HYDROSTEROID DEHYDROGENASE DEFICIENCY

Saez and colleagues first described ambiguous genitalia in 46,XY fetuses due to 17β-hydroxysteroid dehydrogenase deficiency.[272] In this autosomal recessive disorder, external genitalia range from female with perineal hypospadias and a blind-ending vaginal pouch to ambiguous with labio-scrotal fusion to hypospadias. Testes are present and may be palpable in the labio-scrotal folds or incompletely descended. Despite the presence of female external genitalia, Wolffian structures are typically present. In The Netherlands, incidence was estimated to be 1:147,000.[273]

The 17β-hydroxysteroid dehydrogenase type 3 gene (HSD17B3) is located at chromosome 9q22 and is expressed in the testis, where it converts androstenedione to testosterone. Loss-of-function mutations result in testosterone deficiency and subsequent undervirilization of 46,XY fetuses.[274,275] When unrecognized, patients are usually considered to be female at birth. The clinical features are similar to those of 5α-reductase deficiency and androgen insensitivity. Phenotypic heterogeneity occurs.[276] Diagnostic laboratory features include increased basal and hCG-stimulated androstenedione to testosterone ratios.

At puberty, progressive virilization attributed to extra-testicular conversion of androstenedione to testosterone occurs.[277] With progressive virilization, affected individuals may choose to change gender identity from female to male. Increased conversion of androstendione to estrogen may cause gynecomastia. Appropriate male gender assignment can be made in infancy when the diagnosis is suspected and confirmed.[278] Affected females show no phenotype.[279,280]

5α-REDUCTASE DEFICIENCY

In this autosomal-recessive disorder, affected males have genital ambiguity characterized by differentiation of Wolffian structures, absence of Mullerian-derived structures, small phallus, urogenital sinus with perineal hypospadias, and blind vaginal pouch. At puberty, progressive virilization occurs with muscular development, voice change, and phallic enlargement. Facial hair tends to be scanty and the prostate is smaller than normal. Despite pronounced virilization at puberty, semen tends to be viscous and with low amount of ejaculate. The ducts to mature and transport sperm are inadequately developed, so that most affected men are unable to father children.

In one case report, intrauterine insemination with sperm from an affected male resulted in two pregnancies.[281] Deletions and mutations of the 5α-reductase type 2 gene (SRD5A2) have been identified in affected individuals.[282] The SRD5A2 gene is located at chromosome 2p23 and is expressed primarily in androgen target tissues. An isozyme (SRD5A1, located at chromosome 5p15) is expressed in skin and scalp. Clusters of individuals with SRD5A2 mutations have been described in regions of the Dominican Republic, Papua New Guinea, Turkey, and the Middle East.[283]

CYTOCHROME P450 OXIDOREDUCTASE DEFICIENCY

In 1985, a disorder with biochemical evidence suggesting decreased 17α-hydroxylase and 21-hydroxylase activity was initially reported.[284] Clinical features include genital ambiguity, craniosynostosis, midface hypoplasia, and radiohumeral synostosis. At birth, genital ambiguity occurs in both males and females. However, there is no progressive postnatal virilization. During pregnancy, some mothers develop signs associated with androgen excess such as acne, hirsutism, and clitoromegaly.[285] Typical laboratory findings include elevated 17-OHP, low sex steroid, and normal mineralocorticoid concentrations. Glucocorticoid deficiency can occur.

However, despite the apparent resemblance to combined steroidogenic enzyme deficiencies mutations were not identified in the CYP17A1 or CYP21A2 genes. Rather, this disorder is associated with mutations in the cytochrome P450 oxidoreductase (POR) gene. The POR gene codes for a protein involved in electron transfer from NADPH, which functions as a cofactor for steroidogenic and hepatic cytochrome P450 enzymes. The POR gene, mapped to chromosome 7q11-12, consists of 15 exons. Loss-of-function mutations appear to be scattered throughout the gene, without an apparent hot spot.

The skeletal malformations resemble those found in the Antley-Bixler syndrome, which is an autosomal dominant disorder associated with mutations in the fibroblast growth factor receptor 2 (FGFR2) gene. The molecular basis of the skeletal anomalies is unclear but may reflect impaired sterol biosynthesis.[286,287] Patients with Antley-Bixler syndrome due to FGFR2 mutations have normal steroidogenesis, whereas patients with POR mutations have abnormal steroidogenesis.[288]

The paradox in this disorder is the virilization of the female fetus and undervirilization of the male fetus. It has been suggested that the alternative backdoor pathway for androgen synthesis (Figure 4-4) occurs with conversion of 17-OHP to 5α-pregnane-3α,17α-diol-20-one through the sequential activity of 5α-reductase type 1 and 3α-hydroxysteroid dehydrogenase. Subsequently, 5α-pregnane-3α,17α-diol-20-one can be converted to androstenedione by the 17,20-lyase activity of CYP17A1.[289,290]

PLACENTAL AROMATOSE DEFICIENCY

Placental aromatase deficiency is a rare autosomal recessive disorder. During pregnancies with affected fetuses, progressive maternal virilization characterized by hirsutism, clitoral hypertrophy, acne, and frontal balding occurs. During pregnancy, testosterone, DHT, and androstenedione concentrations are elevated and estradiol, estrone, and estriol concentrations are low. In the postpartum period, some clinical features of androgen excess regress and the elevated androgen concentrations return to normal levels.

At birth, 46,XX infants are variably virilized with labioscrotal fusion, clitoromegaly, and perineal scrotal hypospadias.[291,292] Affected 46,XX individuals generally manifest delayed puberty characterized by minimal or absent breast development, primary amenorrhea, hypergonado-tropic hypogonadism, multi-cystic ovaries, and decreased bone mineral density.[293,294] At birth, affected 46,XY infants have normal internal and external genital development. Affected males have generally presented after puberty with tall stature, skeletal pain, delayed skeletal maturation, and infertility.[295] Investigation of aromatase-deficient men suggests that estrogen deficiency is associated with abdominal obesity, insulin resistance, dyslipidemia, and relative infertility.[296] Patients with less severe phenotypic features have been described.[297]

Aromatase is a cytochrome P450 enzyme that plays an important role in the biosynthesis of estrogens (C18 steroids) from androgens (C19 steroids). The aromatase gene, CYP19A1, maps to chromosome 15q21.2 and codes for a 503-amino-acid protein.[298] Inactivating mutations of CYP19A1 impair conversion of androgens to estrogens, leading to increased androgens.[299,300] In addition to its role in estrogen biosynthesis in adolescents and adults, aromatase located in the human placenta converts fetal adrenal androgens to estrogens and protects the mother from the potential virilizing effects of the fetal androgens. Tissue-specific aromatase expression is governed by several different promoters associated with alternative first exon usage.[301]

Maternal Hyperandrogenism

Maternal hyperandrogenism during gestation can be due to luteomas of pregnancy, androgen secreting tumors, and exposure to exogenous androgen. The excessive maternal androgen concentrations can cause virilization of the external genitalia of 46,XX fetuses. Organochlorinepesticides, polychlorinated biphenyls (PCBs), and alkylpolyethoxylates are considered to be "endocrine disruptors" because of their estrogenic and/or antiandrogenic properties. In addition, some pesticides can inhibit placental aromatase activity.[302] Genital ambiguity, described in three 46,XY infants born in heavily agricultural areas, was attributed to fetal exposure to endocrine disruptors (especially because no mutations were detected in the SRY or SRD5A2 genes).[303]

Prenatal treatment with diethylstilbesterol (DES), a nonsteroidal synthetic estrogen, is also associated with urogenital abnormalities of both male and female fetuses. Cryptorchidism has been noted in 46,XY fetuses.[304] It has been speculated that the frequency of cryptorchidism and poor semen quality is increasing because exposure to endocrine disruptors in the environment has increased.[305-308] One potential mechanism is that environmental hydroxylated PCB metabolites can bind to estrogen sulfotransferase, some with greater affinity than estradiol, leading to increased estrogen levels and cryptorchidism.[309]

Disorders of Androgen Action

During the process of sexual differentiation, androgen action is essential to retention of Wolffian duct derivatives, development of the prostate, and differentiation of male external genitalia. Complete androgen insensitivity

(CAIS) is characterized by female external genitalia, absence of Mullerian duct derivatives, sparse sexual hair, inguinal masses, spontaneous pubertal breast development due to aromatization of androgens to estrogens, and a 46,XY karyotype. Partial androgen insensitivity (PAIS) is characterized by clinical features suggestive of a partial biologic response to androgens.[310] Androgen insensitivity is an X-linked recessive disorder secondary to mutations in the androgen receptor (AR) gene, which is located near the centromere on Xq11-12.[311,312] Approximately 30% of cases represent de novo mutations. Somatic cell mosaicism can occur when the mutation arises in the post-zygotic stage and is associated with a lower recurrence risk.[313,314]

Clinical features of CAIS include inguinal or labial masses in an otherwise normal-appearing female infant or primary amenorrhea in an adolescent girl. Among patients with CAIS, Wolffian duct derivatives (e.g., vas deferens and epididymides) are absent because of deficient androgen action. Although rare exceptions have been described, Mullerian-derived structures are usually absent because Sertoli cell function is normal with in utero AMH secretion. It has been suggested that 1% to 2% of girls with bilateral inguinal herniae may have androgen insensitivity. The finding of a gonad within the hernia sac should prompt cytogenetic studies.[315] The expected LH surge in testosterone concentrations during the first few months of life may be absent in some infants with CAIS.[316]

Phenotypic features associated with PAIS include ambiguous genitalia with perineoscrotal hypospadias, microphallus, and bifid scrotum. Testicular position is variable, ranging from undescended to palpable in the scrotum. Infants with PAIS generally manifest the expected neonatal testosterone surge, suggesting that prenatal androgen responsiveness plays a role in imprinting of the HPG axis.[317] Features of mild androgen insensitivity (MAIS) include gynecomastia and infertility in otherwise normal males. Older chronological age at presentation is typical. In all instances, karyotype is 46,XY.

Typical laboratory findings are elevated LH and testosterone concentrations because testicular testosterone synthesis is unimpeded and there is loss of negative feedback inhibition of gonadotropins. LH is usually higher than FSH because testicular inhibin secretion is not impeded. FSH concentrations may be elevated or normal. Infants with PAIS may require dynamic endocrine tests to assess hCG-stimulated Leydig cell testosterone secretion and, more importantly, end-organ responsiveness to androgens. The risk for gonadal tumors is increased in the presence of a Y chromosome. Tumors associated with AIS include carcinoma-in-situ (CIS) and seminoma. In one series, only 2 of 44 subjects with CAIS had CIS. Both subjects were postpubertal.[318]

Androgen action is mediated by the androgen receptor, a member of the steroid/thyroid hormone family of hormone receptors. In common with other members of this receptor family, the androgen receptor is a ligand-dependent transcription factor with a characteristic modular structure. The major modules of the 110-kD protein include the amino-terminus transactivation (AF1), DNA-binding, and ligand-binding domains. Other features include a nuclear localization signal and another trans-activation domain (AF2) in the carboxy terminus ligand-binding domain. Although the androgen receptor is usually described as containing 910 amino acids, the actual number varies because of three polymorphic trinucleotide repeat regions [CAG, GGN (N = any nucleotide), and GCA] located in the amino terminal domain encoding polyglutamine, polyglycine, and polyproline repeat regions, respectively.[319,320]

The normal range for the polyglutamine repeat is 8 to 31, with an average length of 20 repeats. In vitro, AR transcriptional activity varies inversely with the number of repeats. Variation in the length of the CAG repeat, even within the normal range, appears to influence AR function—with long normal repeat lengths associated with infertility secondary to decreased spermatogenesis.[321,322] The role of CAG repeat length in male sexual differentiation is controversial at this time and awaits more data.[323] One possible mechanism is a cell-specific effect on transactivation.[324] The usual range for the polyglycine repeat is 10 to 30. The functional significance of the polyglycine repeat is unclear, but complete deletion reduces transactivation in vitro.[325] Reports regarding the role of CAG repeat length in females influencing ovarian hyperandrogenism, acne, and premature pubarche have been inconsistent.

Phosphorylation, acetylation, ubiquitylation, and sumoylation are post-translational modifications that influence AR transactivational function. The physiologic roles of these modifications remain to be established.[326,327] The DNA-binding domain (DBD) contains two zinc fingers that interact with DNA. X-ray crystallographic studies indicate that the three-dimensional structure of the ligand-binding domain (LBD) consists of 12 α-helixes that form the ligand-binding pocket. Kinetic and biochemical assays with molecular dynamic simulations of mutations identified in patients with CAIS indicate that the position of helix 12 is crucial to AR function.[328]

In the absence of ligand, the receptor is located primarily in the cytoplasm—where it is bound to chaperone proteins. Upon ligand binding, the conformation of the androgen receptor changes. The ligand-receptor complexes dimerize and move to the nucleus.[329] A key feature of androgen receptor dimerization is the intramolecular interaction between the N-terminal and C-terminal domains.[330] Binding of ligand stabilizes the androgen receptor and slows its degradation.[331] In the nucleus, the complex binds to androgen response elements (AREs) and alters target gene transcription. Nucleotide sequences of AREs in conjunction with specific AR amino acids confer greater specificity for transcriptional regulation of specific genes.[332]

Additional proteins (such as coactivators and other transcription factors) are involved in transcription. These other proteins presumably provide a physical bridge linking the basal transcription machinery, the ligand-receptor complex, and chromatin. Once the ligand dissociates from the receptor, the receptor dissociates from the DNA. The most important physiologic ligands are testosterone and dihydrotestosterone. The increased potency of dihydrotestosterone is attributed to the greater stability of the dihydrotestosterone-receptor complex compared to the testosterone-receptor complex.

Numerous AR mutations have been described in affected individuals. Complete loss-of-function mutations (such as deletions, insertions, and deletions associated with frame-shifts) and premature termination codons are typically associated with complete androgen insensitivity.[333] Partial loss-of-function mutations are typically missense mutations. Receptors with mutations in the DBD bind ligand normally but fail to transactivate target genes. Mutations in the LBD of the AR gene can be associated with decreased affinity for ligand, increased instability of the hormone-receptor complex, or increased susceptibility of the receptor to thermal denaturation.[334] In addition to hormone determinations, diagnostic evaluation may include DNA sequence analysis of the AR gene *(www. genetests.org and www.androgendb.mcgill.ca)*.

In general, the phenotype correlates with degree of impaired androgen action. However, clinical features can vary despite the presence of the identical mutation (even within the same family). Complete and partial androgen insensitivity associated with the same AR mutation can occur in siblings.[335] Different missense mutations at the same position can also be associated with differing phenotypes.[336,337] Factors potentially responsible for this phenotypic heterogeneity include individual variation in ligand concentration, variations within the AR or in other genes influencing androgen action and metabolism, variations in mRNA concentrations, and epigenetic phenomenon.[338]

In addition to androgen sensitivity, Kennedy's disease (also known as spinal and bulbar muscular dystrophy) is mapped to the androgen receptor locus. Kennedy's disease is a progressive neurodegenerative disorder with onset in the thirties or forties. This disorder is associated with excessive expansion of the CAG polyglutamine trinucleotide repeat region in exon 1 of the androgen receptor.[339] Repeat lengths greater than 35 are associated with spinal and bulbar muscular atrophy. In Kennedy's disease, aberrant degradation of misfolded AR generates insoluble aggregates—leading to cellular toxicity. In a mouse model, castration improved the neurologic phenotype—suggesting that the androgen-AR signaling pathway influences the phenotype of Kennedy's disease.[340] Mild symptoms of androgen insensitivity can be detected with slight decreases in AR mRNA and protein concentrations.[341]

Mullerian Duct Abnormalities

PERSISTENT MULLERIAN DUCT SYNDROME

The typical clinical features of PMDS include cryptorchidism, testicular ectopia associated with inguinal hernia, and hernia uteri inguinalis. Testicular differentiation is usually normal, but the male excretory ducts may be embedded in the Mullerian duct remnants or incompletely developed. Infertility may ensue secondary to cryptorchidism, intertwining of vas deferens and uterine wall, or lack of proper communication between the testes and excretory ducts. Testicular torsion is not uncommon because the testes may not be anchored properly to the bottom of the processus vaginalis.[342]

AMH is a member of the TGF-β family and signals through two different interacting membrane-bound serine/threonine receptors. The ligand, AMH, binds to the type II receptor—which leads to recruitment and phosphorylation of a type I receptor. The type II receptor is specific for AMH, whereas there are multiple subtypes of the type 1 receptors. Inheritance is autosomal recessive and associated with mutations in the AMH gene or in the Mullerian inhibitory hormone receptor (AMH-RII) gene.[343] AMH concentrations are low among patients with mutations in the AMH gene. Among patients with AMH-RII mutations, AMH concentrations are normal or elevated. The phenotypes of patients with AMH or AMH-RII mutations are comparable. Females who carry mutations on both AMH alleles appear to have normal fertility.

MULLERIAN DUCT ABNORMALITIES IN 46,XX INDIVIDUALS

Mayer-Rokitansky-Küster-Hauser syndrome refers to congenital absence of the vagina associated with uterine hypoplasia or aplasia. Primary amenorrhea is the typical presentation. Renal anomalies and skeletal malformations may be present. Unilateral renal agenesis was found in 29.8% of cases of Mullerian duct anomalies on magnetic resonance imaging (MRI).[344] The aggregation of Mullerian duct aplasia, renal aplasia, and cervico-thoracic somite dysplasia has been labeled MURCS syndrome.[345] Mullerian duct hypoplasia has been associated with facio-auriculo-vertebral anomalies such as Goldenhar syndrome.[346]

Transverse vaginal septa can occur sporadically or in association with other features, such as polydactyly in the McKusick-Kaufman syndrome.[347] Because of the high frequency associated anomalies, careful physical examination for skeletal malformations and renal sonography should be included in the diagnostic evaluation of women with abnormal development of the Mullerian duct system.[348]

Hypogonadotropic Hypogonadism

Hypogonadotropic hypogonadism may present with microphallus and/or cryptorchidism in male infants (see chapter 16). Genital ambiguity would not be anticipated because placental hCG secretion is unaffected. Decreased gonadotropin secretion presumably results in decreased testosterone secretion such that microphallus and cryptorchidism can occur.[349,350]

Kallmann syndrome is the eponym used for the X-linked recessive form of hypogonadotropic hypogonadism associated with anosmia due to failed migration of GnRH neurons from the olfactory placode into the forebrain along branches of the vomeronasal nerve.[351,352] Olfactory tract hypoplasia or aplasia has been found on MRI.[353] The molecular basis of this X-linked form is mutations in the Kallmann (KAL) gene (located at Xp22.3). This gene escapes X-inactivation, codes for a 680-amino-acid protein, and helps target GnRH neurons to the hypothalamus.[354,355]

Mutations in the GnRH receptor (GNRHR), fibroblast growth factor receptor 1 (FGFR1), and GPR54 genes are also associated with hypogonadotropic hypogonadism.[356-359] More recently, mutations in the genes coding for prokineticin receptor-2 (PROKR2) and its ligand [prokineticin-2 (PROK2)] have been associated with hypogonadotropic hypogonadism.[360]

Cryptorchidism

Cryptorchidism (undescended testes) is the most common disorder of sexual differentiation, affecting 3% of male infants. Because spontaneous descent often occurs during infancy, the prevalence decreases to 1% by 6 months of age.[361] Cryptorchidism has been associated with hypothalamic hypogonadism, aberrant testicular differentiation, impaired testosterone biosynthesis, androgen insensitivity, holoprosencephaly, abnormal AMH production or action, and abnormalities affecting INSL3/LGR8 function. Other associations include prune belly syndrome, bladder exotrophy, and renal anomalies. Cryptorchidism is also a feature of many syndromes (Table 4-3). Maternal diabetes mellitus, including gestational diabetes, may be a risk factor.[362]

During sexual differentiation, the gonads are positioned between two structures: the cranial suspensory ligament and the gubernaculum. Testicular descent is divided into two phases: intraabdominal and inguinoscrotal. Factors involved in gubernacular development during the intraabdominal phase include INSL3 and its receptor, LGR8. INSL3 is secreted by Leydig cells. Its receptor, LGR8, is a leucine-rich G-protein–coupled receptor expressed by the gubernaculum. By 13 or 14 weeks of gestation, the gubernaculum anchors the testis to the internal inguinal ring.[363] Androgen action during the intraabdominal phase appears to be limited to regression of the cranial suspensory ligament. In females, the cranial suspensory ligament persists as the suspensory ligament of the ovary. Testicular descent through the inguinal canal is usually accomplished by the end of seventh month of gestation, with completion of the inguinoscrotal phase by the end of week 35.[363]

Heterozygous missense INSL3 mutations have been identified in patients with cryptorchidism.[364] Mutations have also been identified in the LGR8 gene in males with cryptorchidism. Sequence variants have been identified in the HOXA10 gene in boys with cryptorchidism.[365] Typically, the testes of patients with androgen insensitivity have completed the intraabdominal phase but fail to undergo inguineoscrotal descent because this second phase is androgen dependent. However, the more complete the androgen insensitivity the greater likelihood of finding abdominal testes. Exposure of XX fetuses to androgen does not promote significant ovarian descent in humans, as evidenced by normal ovarian position in females with congenital adrenal hyperplasia.[366,367]

Cryptorchidism can be associated with decreased number of germ cells, impaired germ cell maturation, and decreased number of Leydig cells.[368] In some instances of unilateral cryptorchidism, abnormal histology is apparent

TABLE 4-3

Disorders Associated with Small Penis or Cryptorchidism

- Aarskog syndrome
- Börjeson-Forssman-Lehman syndrome
- Carnevale syndrome
- Cornelia de Lange syndrome
- Deletion 4p, 5p, 9p, 11q, 13q, 18q
- Duplication 3q, 10q, 15q
- Faciogenitopopliteal syndrome
- Goldenhar syndrome
- Holoprosencephaly
- Juberg-Marside syndrome
- Johanson-Blizzard syndrome
- Lenz-Majewski hyperostosis syndrome
- Lowe syndrome
- Malpeuch facial clefting syndrome
- McKusick-Kaufman syndrome
- Meckel-Gruber
- Miller-Dieker syndrome
- Multiple pterygium syndrome, Escobar variant
- Myotonic dystrophy
- Najjar-syndrome
- Noonan syndrome
- Pallister-Hall syndrome
- Pfeiffer
- Prader-Willi syndrome
- Robinow syndrome
- Rubinstein-Taybi syndrome
- Seckel syndrome
- Shprintzen-Goldbert
- Simpson-Golabi-Behmel, type 1
- Townes-Brocks syndrome
- Varadi-Papp syndrome
- VATER syndrome
- Weaver

in the contralateral normally descended testis.[369] However, it is unclear if these features represent consequences or causes of cryptorchidism.

Diagnosis

HISTORY

A detailed family history should be obtained. The family history should include ascertainment of unexplained infant deaths, consanguinity, and infertility. Infants with congenital adrenal hyperplasia may have died prior to diagnosis. Many DSDs are inherited as autosomal-recessive disorders. Infertility and gynecomastia may represent milder phenotypes for some DSDs. For X-linked disorders such as androgen insensitivity, there may be affected maternal family members (i.e., either amenorrheic or infertile aunts or partially virilized uncles). Pertinent questions include prenatal exposure to exogenous or endogenous androgens, estrogens, or potential endocrine disruptors. Maternal virilization during pregnancy should be queried.

PHYSICAL EXAMINATION

DSDs encompass a spectrum of physical findings. The specific physical findings range from micropenis, hypospadias, undescended testes, minimal clitoromegaly, and scrotalized labia to more extensive forms of genital ambiguity. Severe clitoromegaly with posterior labial fusion in an 46,XX patient may be difficult to distinguish from perineal hypospadias, undescended testes, and a bifid scrotum in an 46,XY individual. During the physical examination, attention should be focused on phallic size, symmetry of the external genitalia, presence and location of palpable gonads, and any additional anomalies.

The extent of virilization should be carefully documented, recording the configuration, stretched dorsal length, and diameter of the phallus (including the glans penis). The location of the urethral opening, degree of labiourethral fold fusion, and extent of labioscrotal fold fusion should also be noted. Labioscrotal folds fuse from posterior to anterior such that the appearance extends from posterior labial fusion, a partially fused hemiscrota, to completely fused scrotum with labiourethral fusion extending to a midline urethral opening. The position of the urethra should be noted, as well as whether one or two perineal openings are present.

Gonadal or adnexal structures may be identified upon careful palpation for content of the labioscrotal structures, scrotum or labia majora, inguinal region, and the lower abdomen. The groin area may be "milked" to maneuver the testis into the scrotum. The absence of palpable testes may indicate a genetic female with virilization, as occurs with adrenal hyperplasia or a genetic male with undescended or absent testes. Although structures palpated within the labioscrotal folds are usually testes, ovaries or even the uterine cervix can be found within the labioscrotal folds. Testes typically have a characteristic ovoid structure.

Symmetry or asymmetry of external genital differentiation may provide clues to the etiology of the genital ambiguity (Figure 4-6). Unilateral structures with asymmetry of other genital structures suggests ovotesticular or 45X/46,XY DSDs and is often associated with unilateral gonadal maldescent. Asymmetry implies differing local influences, which often reflect abnormalities in gonadal differentiation (Figures 4-6 and 4-7). Repeated examinations may be beneficial for diagnostic precision.

Penile length measurements extend from the tip of stretched penis from the pubic ramus. Normal length depends on gestational age, the lower limit (approximately −2.5 SD) at term being 2.0 cm. An isolated micropenis can be a consequence of decreased testosterone exposure in the second half of gestation due to Leydig cell failure, LH deficiency, androgen insensitivity syndrome, LHCGR mutations, or GH deficiency. A micropenis with hypospadias suggests more severe DSDs.

Clitoral length is usually less than 1.0 cm, although rare variations exist. Measurement of the clitoris requires a careful estimate of the proximal end and careful exclusion of overlying skin. The location of the urethral opening should be ascertained by visualization, witnessing the urinary stream, or with careful insertion of a firm catheter. If urination is observed, force, diameter, and direction

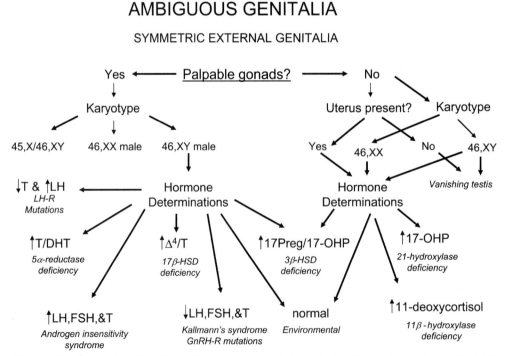

Figure 4-6. Algorithm for the approach to the child with symmetric genital ambiguity. The configuration of the labio-scrotal folds and presence/absence of palpable gonads is comparable on both sides. The presence or absence of palpable gonads directs the initial laboratory evaluation. Ultrasound examination to determine whether a uterus is present is helpful. For example, symmetric fusion of the labio-scrotal folds, nonpalpable gonads, and presence of a uterus provide strong circumstantial evidence for the diagnosis of a virilized female with congenital adrenal hyperplasia.

AMBIGUOUS GENITALIA

ASYMMETRIC EXTERNAL GENITALIA

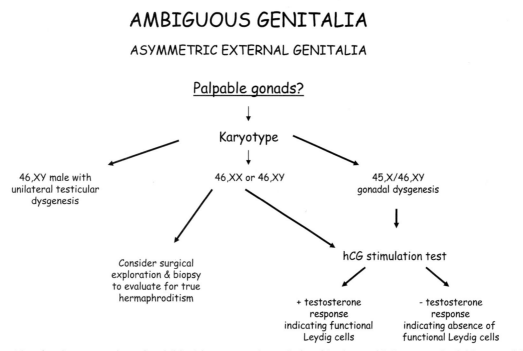

Figure 4-7. Algorithm for the approach to the child with asymmetric genital ambiguity. In this instance, the labio-scrotal folds may appear different or a gonad is palpable only on one side.

of the urinary stream should be noted. The position of the inserted catheter may also provide crucial initial information. If directed toward the anal opening and palpable under the perineal skin, the catheter is likely in a urogenital sinus—as occurs often with virilization of a 46,XX fetus secondary to 21-hydroxylase deficiency. However, a penile urethra is anticipated if the catheter is directed anteriorly and is nonpalpable.

The anogenital ratio is measured as the distance between the anus and the posterior fourchette divided by the distance between the anus and the base of the phallus. If the ratio is >0.5, this suggests a component of female differentiation and hence virilization with posterior labial fusion.[370] Because pelvic ultrasound is part of the initial laboratory assessment, a rectal examination may not be necessary. If present, a midline uterine cervix can often be palpated upon rectal exam.

The Prader scale is often used to classify the appearance of the external genitalia: (1) normal female genitalia with clitoromegaly, (2) partial labial fusion and clitoromegaly, (3) labioscrotal fusion so that there is a single opening from the urogenital sinus and clitoromegaly, (4) fusion of labioscrotal folds so that the single opening is at the base of the phallic structure, and (5) complete male virilization with penis-size phallus, complete labial fusion, and meatus on the glands. A recent description extends this traditional Prader classification to include urogenital sinus characteristics by defining the vaginal confluence in relation to the bladder neck and the meatus.[371]

In addition to the genital examination, the examination should include weight, length, and other features to ascertain whether findings are consistent with gestational age—particularly in the apparent female because the clitoris is more prominent in preterm infants in that there

is scant subcutaneous fat and clitoral growth is completed before the last trimester of fetal life.[372] A careful examination includes inspection for additional dysmorphic features because genital ambiguity may occur in association with other anomalies. These include midline facial defects, head size, and ear and digital anomalies. Infants with congenital adrenal hyperplasia may manifest hyperpigmentation of the genitalia and nipples due to adrenal insufficiency and ACTH hypersecretion.

LABORATORY STUDIES

Initial laboratory studies to assess genital ambiguity should include an abdominal/pelvic ultrasound and karyotype. The ultrasound will provide information regarding the presence or absence of a uterus. Information regarding the size and location of the gonads and adrenals may be obtained on ultrasound. When gonads are not palpable, the external genitalia are symmetrically ambiguous, and a uterus and possibly ovaries are present, the most likely diagnosis is a virilized 46,XX fetus with congenital adrenal hyperplasia. However, the possibility of markedly dysgenetic testes cannot be excluded. If the differential diagnosis based on the presentation includes congenital adrenal hyperplasia, the initial laboratory studies should include electrolytes, plasma renin activity, and serum 17-hydroxyprogesterone and cortisol levels.

The karyotype is essential to determine chromosomal sex even if prenatal chromosome testing was performed. In general, peripheral blood karyotypes are sufficient. However, the patient may be a mosaic with one or more additional cell lines restricted to gonadal tissue.[373] Other initial studies depend on the physical findings. If the external genitalia are symmetrically virilized to any degree in the absence of palpable gonads, particularly if a normal uterus is present, additional studies should be directed toward causes of virilization of a female infant. Because 21-hydroxylase deficiency is the most common cause of virilization and genital ambiguity in 46,XX infants, initial laboratory studies should include determination of 17-hydroxyprogesterone concentrations. If one or both gonads can be palpated, the intent of screening studies is to determine the adequacy of androgen synthesis and androgen action in a male infant. Determination of LH, FSH, and testosterone concentrations in infancy provides information regarding the function of the testes and the HPG axis (Table 4-4).

The pattern of steroid hormone concentrations provides evidence for specific defects in steroidogenesis (Table 4-4). The diagnosis of congenital adrenal hyperplasia due to 21-hydroxylase deficiency is confirmed by finding elevated 17-hydroxyprogesterone concentrations. Typically, 17-hydroxyprogesterone concentrations are greater than 10,000 ng/dL (300 nmol/L) in the affected neonate. For 11β-hydroxylase deficiency, 11-deoxycortisol and 17-hydroxyprogesterone concentrations are elevated. For 3β-hydroxysteroid dehydrogenase deficiency, pregnenolone, 17-hydroxypregnenolone, and DHEA concentrations are typically elevated. When salt-losing forms of congenital adrenal hyperplasia are included in the differential diagnosis, serum electrolytes and plasma renin activity should be monitored. Typically, hyponatremia and hyperkalemia are not present at birth and develop during the first week of life.

Newborn screening programs have been established in many states and countries to identify infants with classic congenital adrenal hyperplasia. Many screening programs measure whole-blood 17-hydroxyprogesterone concentrations eluted from a dried filter paper blood spot.[374] Whereas false negative 17-hydroxyprogesterone results are uncommon, slightly increased whole-blood 17-OHP concentrations are detected often enough (especially in preterm infants) to complicate clinical decision making regarding affected status and need to initiate glucocorticoid therapy. Etiologies of slightly increased 17-OHP concentrations include prematurity, cross-reacting steroids, sampling prior to 36 hours of age, heterozygosity for 21-hydroxylase deficiency, and late-onset congenital adrenal hyperplasia.

To avoid an excessive number of false positive screening results, the cutoff levels are typically selected to identify all infants with classic salt-losing or simple virilizing forms—often missing those infants with late-onset congenital adrenal hyperplasia. Improved specificity can be achieved by use of additional procedures such as organic extraction, chromatography, or GC/MS analysis. Prenatal or neonatal treatment with glucocorticoids can result in a false negative screening result.[375] If the differential diagnosis includes CAH, specific laboratory testing is warranted even if the newborn screen results are reported as negative for 21-hydroxylase deficiency.

For the milder forms of congenital adrenal hyperplasia, ACTH stimulation testing may be necessary to confirm the diagnosis. After a basal blood sample has been drawn, synthetic ACTH (0.25 mg) can be administered by intravenous bolus or intramuscular injection. A second blood sample to measure ACTH-stimulated hormone response can be obtained 30 or 60 minutes later. The milder forms of congenital adrenal hyperplasia generally do not affect external genital differentiation and are therefore not usually associated with genital ambiguity. Infants with late-onset congenital adrenal hyperplasia are generally not detected through newborn screening programs, presumably because the whole-blood 17-OHP concentrations determined from the newborn screening filter paper are lower than the values used as cutoffs.

In addition to the diagnostic evaluation for disorders of steroidogenesis, hormone measurements in the immediate neonatal period provide an index to the function of

TABLE 4-4
Normal Values (Mean and SD) for Full-Term and Preterm Infants from 2 Hours to 7 Days of Postnatal Life.

	2 Hours		24 Hours		4 Days		7 Days	
	PT	FT	PT	FT	PT	FT	PT	FT
Progesterone (ng/dl)								
Mean	3,900	5,730	679	1,250	56	88	53	50
SD	640	690	149	286	11	26	18	12
17-Hydroxyprogesterone								
Mean	713	886	286	94	214	79	237	124
SD	96	203	44	16	40	9	58	20
Cortisol (μg/dl)								
Mean	8.2	10.4	3.7	2.7	4.5	5.7	3.2	3.5
SD	2.5	2.6	0.9	1.2	1.4	1.7	1.0	1.6
Deoxycorticosterone (ng/dl)								
Mean	114	360	38	116	9	13	6	11
SD	13	65	7	38	2	7	2	7

PT = preterm (*n* = 8), FT = full-term (*n* = 12).

Data from Sippel et al. (1980). Plasma levels of aldosterone, corticosterone, 11-deoxycorticosterone, progesterone, 17-hydroxyprogesterone, cortisol, and cortisone during infancy and childhood. Pediatr Res 14:39; and from Doerr et al. (1988). Plasma mineralocorticoids, and progesterins in premature infants: Longitudinal study during the first week of life. Pediatr Res 23:525.

the HPG axis. Low testosterone and elevated gonadotropin concentrations in a 46,XY infant with ambiguous genitalia suggest inadequate testosterone biosynthesis. Elevated testosterone and gonadotropin concentrations in an infant with female external genitalia, bilateral labial masses, and 46,XY karyotype are consistent with the diagnosis of androgen insensitivity (Table 4-5).

Measurement of AMH may provide another assessment of testicular function because AMH concentrations reflect Sertoli cell function. AMH concentrations are sexually dimorphic, with high values in boys (20–80 ng/mL) during the first six years of life and low values in girls.[376] Thus, in the patient with nonpalpable gonads and absence of Mullerian structures AMH concentrations may help distinguish between anorchia and cryptorchidism.[377] In addition, AMH concentrations can be helpful in disorders of testicular dysgenesis or in virilized females to determine the presence of testicular tissue.[378] Inhibin B concentrations, lower in females than in males, provide another marker of Sertoli cell function.[379]

Assessment of the ability of a gonad to secrete testosterone may be helpful, especially for patients with evidence of testicular tissue by palpation or ultrasound and AMH levels indicating testicular tissue. This can be done by administering hCG and measuring hormone responses. To assess hormone responses, doses of 1,000 to 1,500 units can be injected subcutaneously either daily or every other day for one to five days—with blood sampling on the day after the last injection. Hormone determinations should include androstenedione, testosterone, and dihydrotestosterone.[380] Testosterone concentrations should more than double, and the T/DHT ratio should be <10:1. Intermittent injections can be given for up to three weeks to stimulate penile growth to demonstrate both testosterone secretion and target tissue responsiveness. Total dosage should not exceed 15,000 units of hCG.

Molecular genetic analyses have become increasingly available to determine and confirm the molecular basis of the genital ambiguity. Knowledge regarding the specific mutation enables more accurate genetic counseling for inherited disorders of sexual differentiation. The genetics laboratory can often perform fluorescent in situ hybridization (FISH), for the SRY gene, or other detailed chromosomal tests. For some DSDs, molecular genetic analysis of specific genes is available through commercial laboratories. Information regarding the particular details can be obtained from an NIH-funded web-based resource, Genetests *(http://www.genetests.com)*. In some instances, genetic testing is available through research laboratories.

Endoscopic studies can be used to locate the vaginal-urethral confluence in relation to the bladder neck and the single opening of the urogenital sinus. Using a cystoscope and catheter placement, these distances can be determined before or in conjunction with retrograde contrast studies performed to outline the urethra and to demonstrate (if present) the vagina, uterus, cervix, and uterine cavity. Such information is needed to plan for reconstructive surgery, to assess the risk of medical complications, and in certain instances to provide information to determine the sex of rearing. If such procedures are unhelpful, laparoscopy may be necessary to visualize and biopsy gonadal and internal genital structures. MRI may be helpful to define anatomic relationships.

Treatment

While awaiting results of the initial laboratory studies, attention is focused on the main decision: the gender of rearing. In the ideal situation, there is a specific DSD team comprised of a pediatric surgeon or pediatric urologist with expertise in urogenital reconstructive surgery, a behavioral science professional (psychologist, social worker, or psychiatrist), a pediatric endocrinologist, and a neonatalogist. Initially, the neonatalogist may facilitate coordination of care and communication with the parents. Long-term management needs to be delineated. In addition to the appointments necessary to the patient's medical, surgical, and psychological needs, additional sessions may benefit the parents to address their questions and concerns about their child.[381] These evaluations should be performed promptly and often necessitate transfer of the infant to a tertiary care facility.

The parents need to participate in discussions and decision making regarding the options for sex of rearing and possible surgical interventions. Honest, sensitive, and candid discussions with the parents can only benefit the child. As the child matures, honest explanations regarding the medical condition are essential. The child should progress from a silent partner to a full participating member in this decision-making process, with the child's wishes taking precedence where appropriate.

Once the diagnosis is confirmed as specifically as possible, therapy is instituted. When a specific diagnosis has been confirmed, decision making and therapy can be guided accordingly. Considerations for medical care

TABLE 4-5		
Normal Values (Ranges) From 2 to 12 Months by Sex		
	Male	**Female**
	(n = 14)	(n = 8)
Pregnenolone (ng/dl)	10 –137	18 – 87
17-Hydroxypregnenolone (ng/dl)	14 – 766	62 – 828
Progesterone (ng/dl)	5 – 80	5 – 53
17-Hydroxyprogesterone (ng/dl)	11 – 173	13 – 106
DHEA (ng/dl)	26 – 236	32 – 584
DHEAS (µg/dl)	2 – 38	4 – 111
Androstenedione (ng/dl)	6 – 54	12 – 78
Deoxycorticosterone (ng/dl)	7 – 57	7 – 52
Aldosterone (ng/dl)	2 – 129	6 – 71
11-Deoxycortisol (ng/dl)	10 – 200	10 – 156
Cortisol (µg/dl)	3 – 21	4 – 23
Testosterone (ng/dl)	0.6 – 501	0.3 – 8.1

Data from Lashansky et al. (1991). Normative data for adrenal steroidogenesis in a healthy pediatric population: Age- and sex-related changes after adrenocorticotropin stimulation. J Clin Endocrinol Metab 73:674; and from Lashansky et al. (1992). Normative data for the steroidogenic response of mineralocorticoids and their precursors to adrenocorticotropin in a healthy pediatric population. J Clin Endocrinol Metab 75:1491.

include sex of rearing, possible need for surgery and a timeline for planned surgery, plan for medical treatment, and timely and appropriate psychological counseling and support.

SEX OF REARING

Decisions regarding the appropriate sex of rearing are based on the specific pathophysiology, prognosis for spontaneous pubertal development, capacity for sexual activity and orgasm, and potential for fertility.[382] With the use of assisted techniques, the potential for fertility is more likely than in the past. Although current surgical techniques spare more of the neurovascular bundle of the phallus, surgery should be avoided except in those instances of severe ambiguity or markedly discordant genitalia to preserve sexual responsiveness.

In instances where a decision regarding sex of rearing is necessary, each child evaluated for genital ambiguity warrants careful consideration of the physical findings, laboratory information, and available outcome data. In most instances, children are raised in the gender consistent with the karyotype—acknowledging that there are rare exceptions of sex reversal. Limited longitudinal outcome studies are available regarding adult function and gender identity. Virtually all 46,XY CAIS patients identify themselves as female.

About a quarter of PAIS patients are dissatisfied with the gender assignment, regardless of whether they are raised as male or female. The majority of patients with 5α-reductase deficiency identify as male, whereas about half of those diagnosed with 17β-hydroxysteroid dehydrogenase self-reassign from female to male.[383,384] The majority of virilized 46,XX individuals with CAH identify as female. Of the few estrogen-deficient males identified, all are heterosexual and report normal libido and sexual function.[385] Thus, in spite of the accumulating evidence that androgen exposure to the CNS alters general and cognitive behavior much remains to be learned about the influences of nature and nurture on gender identity.[386]

Because the majority of 46,XX virilized females (primarily those with CAH) identify as female, this sex of rearing is usually recommended if the question arises in infancy. For virilized 46,XX patients with Prader stage 4 or 5 genitalia, the recent consensus conference felt that the outcome data was insufficient to support a sex of rearing as male despite the anecdotal data suggesting good adjustment when this has occurred with late diagnosis of CAH. For virilized females with CAH, the primary issue is not gender assignment but questions regarding genital surgery.

To date, more information and knowledge is available about physical sexual development than about psychosexual cognitive development. The primary factors, critical steps, and sequence of psychosexual development are unclear. Traditionally, psychosexual development has been viewed as having three components: gender identity, gender role, and sexual orientation. The development of gender identity begins as an infant with the self-recognition that one is a boy or girl. Gender role develops during childhood as a result of society's expectations concerning behavior and is influenced by prenatal hormonal exposure.

Gender roles are defined in part by the messages society relays concerning appropriate and inappropriate male and female behavior. Gender role may subsequently shift, depending on the individual's reaction to the expectations of society. How prenatal factors such as hormones and environmental exposures impact gender role has been difficult to ascertain. Sexual orientation may be apparent prior to puberty or not expressed until late in adult life, underlying the unknown influencing factors.

The effects of prenatal androgen exposure on gender identity are uncertain.[387,388] Prenatal androgen levels apparently influence gender-related behavior and cognitive function during childhood.[387] Yet, the impact on degrees of femininity and masculinity and cognitive function (spatial and verbal abilities) and handedness does not appear to persist into adult life.[389,390] Data obtained from some studies of the 46,XX CAH patient suggest that prenatal androgen exposure may be associated with reduced satisfaction with a female sex assignment.[391] Among virilized 46,XX individuals with CAH, an increased rate of homosexual orientation has been reported—primarily based on self-reported sexual imagery and sexual attraction, with reports of actual homosexual involvement being less well documented.[392-394]

Some females with classic CAH are more likely to question their female gender,[395] and the reported incidence of sex reassignment from female to male is greater than in the general population.[396] Among 46,XX CAH patients with gender self-reassignment, it was judged that factors contributing to this change were not genotype or phenotype but gender-atypical behavioral self-image and body image and development of erotic attraction to women.[397] Other studies concluded that psychological adjustment was comparable between females with CAH and their unaffected siblings.[398] In another study, gender identity of girls with CAH was comparable to the control group.[399] In these studies, the impact of environmental influences cannot be separated from the effects of prenatal hormonal exposures.

Female gender of rearing is appropriate for 46,XY individuals with complete androgen insensitivity because virilization and fertility are unattainable. The lack of androgen responsiveness limits androgen effect on the developing CNS of individuals with CAIS. Conversely, the decision regarding gender of rearing for individuals with partial androgen insensitivity may be problematic because the extent of androgen impact on CNS development and the androgen responsiveness of the genital development are uncertain. The clinical response to exogenous testosterone may benefit this decision-making process. Testosterone responsiveness may be ascertained by assessing penile growth following one or more intramuscular injections of 25-mg testosterone depot formulations.

Among individuals with DSD associated with gonadal dysgenesis, hCG-stimulated testosterone secretion and clinical response facilitates the decision regarding gender of rearing. The genital phenotype, ability of the Leydig cell to secrete testosterone, and extent of genital virilization in response to androgen stimulation are indicators regarding the potential for spontaneous pubertal development and need for hormone replacement therapy. Nevertheless, in gonadal dysgenesis the impact of prenatal androgen exposure on gender development processes is often indeterminate and cannot be reliably predicted from routine diagnostic studies in the newborn period.

Generally, with the exception of CAIS, 46,XY individuals with fetal androgen exposure manifested as partial genital masculinization should be raised as males unless there are extenuating individual circumstances. Caution, reflection, and dialog are appropriate before those with a 46,XY, karyotype are assigned female because fetal androgen exposure appears to impact strongly on self-concept as male despite compromised external genital development.

CONSIDERATIONS WITH REGARD TO SURGERY

For the virilized female patient with female sex of rearing, the extent of ambiguity in combination with the magnitude of clitoromegaly and posterior fusion must be carefully evaluated to determine whether genitoplasty, including clitoral reduction or clitoroplasty, should be considered. Another factor in the decision-making process is the location of the urethral outlet. If located high in the urogenital sinus, early surgery may be indicated to decrease the risk of recurrent urinary tract infections by providing a direct urinary outflow path. The current perspective is that girls with mild to moderate degrees of clitoromegaly do not need surgery because of the potential risk of compromising genital sensitivity.

One important point to share with parents of a virilized girl with CAH is that the stimulated genital tissues will regress after glucocorticoid therapy is begun. On one hand, the parents need to be informed that some (including patient advocacy) groups discourage genital surgery until the child is old enough to make her own decision. On the other hand, they must be empowered to make the choice with which they will be comfortable. This must be done with the understanding that their daughter may criticize them for this decision when she is older. Most parents of daughters with severe ambiguity still choose surgery.[400]

If there is agreement between the interdisciplinary medical team and the parents for surgery, the surgery is generally performed as soon as feasible. If surgery is anticipated, the operation should be described in a manner understandable to the parents. An experienced surgeon should discuss the options, risks, and benefits of surgery—including the innervation of the clitoris or penis and the surgical approach to be used to attempt to spare the neurovascular supply.[401,402] Although opinions vary as to whether surgery should be done in one or more stages and whether vaginal reconstruction should be attempted during infancy, the parents need to be informed that subsequent vaginoplasty is almost always required after puberty. Among patients who underwent vaginal reconstructive surgery during infancy, the frequency of postoperative vaginal stenosis has been reported to range from 0% to 77%.[403] Therapeutic goals for vaginal reconstruction surgery include adequate sexual function with minimal need for continual dilatation or lubrication.[404]

For the under-virilized male, decisions concerning genital surgery and when it occurs belong to the parents until the patient reaches adolescence and adulthood.

Most decide for surgery, except in the instances of minimal to moderate hypospadias. When discussing surgery with the parents, pertinent topics include common male concerns about the importance of being able to stand to urinate, adequacy of genital development, and capability of sexual activities. Because correction of hypospadias and chordee is generally performed in stages, this discussion also needs to cover the details of the surgical approach, the proposed schedule for follow-up visits, the likely number of surgical procedures, and the optimal age for each surgical stage. The surgeon should review the options, risks, and anticipated outcomes. If the precise location and differentiation status of the testes are unknown, the parents should be aware that exploration and biopsy may be performed.

Another consideration regarding the need for and timing of surgery is the relative risk for gonadal tumors. The aberrant fetal gonadal environment and subsequent anomalous germ cell differentiation is associated with the development of germ cell tumors. In general, CIS or gonadoblastoma are the most common germ cell tumors and precede the development of the more invasive neoplasms such as dysgerminoma, seminoma, and nonseminoma. The presence of Y chromosome material increases the propensity risk for gonadal tumors.[405] Increased and prolonged expression of immunohistochemical markers, OCT3/4 and testis-specific protein Y-encoded (TSPY), is common in CIS and gonadoblastoma.[406] In one series, TSPY was abundantly expressed in germ cells within dysgenetic testes and undifferentiated gonadal tissue—suggesting up-regulation when germ cells are located in an unfavorable environment.[406] It is hypothesized that the normal germ cell maturation process is interrupted, resulting in prolonged expression of OCT3/4, erased genomic imprinting, and subsequent immortalization of the cell.[407]

The reported prevalence of gonadoblastoma ranges from 15% to 30%, depending on age of the patient, gonadal histology, and diagnostic criteria used for CIS/gonadoblastoma. In one series of patients with Turner syndrome, 14/171 (8%) were positive for Y-chromosomal material. Among these 14 patients, the prevalence of gonadoblastoma was 33%.[408] A meta-analysis of 11 studies, all using PCR methodology, found that 5% of patients with Turner syndrome showed positive results for Y chromosome material.[407]

Frasier syndrome is also associated with gonadoblastoma. The prevalence of germ cell tumors is lower in androgen insensitivity and disorders of androgen biosynthesis. Nevertheless, limited sample size, ascertainment bias, inconsistent diagnostic criteria for malignant cells, and confusing terminology leave many questions to be answered. For example, which patients with DSD benefit from gonadal biopsy to assess risk for neoplasia? Another consideration is how many biopsies are necessary to be representative of the histology of the gonad. Laparoscopy and video-assisted gonadectomy are invaluable techniques when the risk for malignancy is high. Ultimately, the decision regarding gonadectomy involves consideration of the patient's phenotype (internal and external genital anatomy), karyotype, gender of rearing, psychosocial factors, and gonadal histology.

MEDICAL TREATMENT

With the exception of disorders affecting glucocorticoid and mineralocorticoid biosynthesis, most DSD conditions do not require specific medical therapy in infancy. At the time of expected puberty, patients with hypogonadism will need appropriate hormone replacement therapy. In general, hormone replacement therapy is initiated using low doses of the appropriate sex steroid hormone—with incremental increases designed to mirror spontaneous pubertal development. It is helpful to review with families the anticipated frequency of outpatient visits and how the adequacy of replacement therapy will be assessed.

For females, induction of puberty involves low-dose estrogen therapy—usually initiated between 10.5 to 12 years of age to avoid excessive acceleration of skeletal maturation. The initial estrogen dosage is usually the lowest available, such as 0.3 mg of conjugated estrogens every other day, 5 ug of ethinyl estradiol daily, or transdermal estrogen preparations (0.025 mg) weekly. Transdermal patches may be used only at night in an effort to mimic spontaneous puberty.[409] Matrix transdermal patches can also be cut into smaller pieces to provide a lower estrogen dosage. Based on clinical response and the patient's perception, the dose of estrogen can be increased in 6- to 12-month intervals such that complete replacement doses and development are achieved within 3 years.

Therapy involves the addition of a progestational agent after 12 months of estrogen therapy or when withdrawal bleeding occurs, whichever occurs sooner. Thereafter, cyclic estrogen-progesterone therapy should be used. Once full pubertal development has been reached, the estrogen dosage should be the minimum that will maintain normal menstrual flow and prevent calcium bone loss (equivalent to 0.625 conjugated estrogen or 20 ug ethinyl estradiol). Options for cyclic estrogen-progesterone therapy include low-dosage estrogen birth control pills or estrogen-progesten transdermal patches.

Another regimen involves a daily oral estrogen regimen or the transdermal form for 21 days—with the addition of progesterone, 5 to 10 mg of medroxyprogesterone acetate, or 200 to 400 mg of micronized progesterone daily added for 12 days (day 10 to day 21). This is followed by a week of no hormones. At this point, the replacement regimen may be extended so that less frequent withdrawal bleeding occurs. In the absence of a uterus, progesterone therapy becomes optional. Among patients with low circulating androgen levels, sexual hair growth and libido may be improved by administering small doses of DHEA or methyltestosterone. Gonadotropins hCG and/or hMG (human menopausal gonadotropin/recombinant FSH) are only used to stimulate ovulation or during assisted fertility attempts.

For males, testosterone hormone replacement typically begins at 12.5 to 14 years. In instances where the psychological impact is felt to be needed, therapy may be initiated one or two years earlier. If therapy is begun earlier to assure the patient concerning physical changes, the rate of skeletal maturation should be carefully monitored. Conversely, treatment may be delayed to allow for psychological or emotional maturity or catch-up growth. Testosterone therapy may be given by depot intramuscular injections or topically by a patch or gel. Depot testosterone (such as enanthate or cyprinate) is begun at a dosage 50 mg IM every four weeks, followed by increased dosing and frequency over about 3 years to a full replacement dosage of approximately 200 mg every 2 weeks. Availability of the gel in metered-dose pumps allows gradual increases of dosage from 1.25 g daily upward. Among those with differentiated testes and gonadotropin deficiency, assisted fertility techniques may involve intratesticular germ cell retrieval or hFSH/hLH stimulation.

For patients with CAH, carefully monitored hormone replacement therapy is essential. The goal of glucocorticoid therapy is suppression of excessive adrenal androgen secretion while maintaining normal growth and development. Typically, oral cortisol doses range from 8 to 20 mg/m^2/day. This range is based on provision of 1.5 to 2 times the daily cortisol production rate, 7 to 12 mg/m^2/day. Oral fludrocortisone (e.g., Florinef) is commonly used for mineralocorticoid replacement for patients with salt-losing CAH. Patients with simple virilizing CAH may benefit from mineralocorticoid replacement. The typical dose is 0.1 mg administered as a single daily dose. Neonates and infants may require higher fludrocortisone doses as well as salt supplementation because of relative mineralocorticoid resistance, higher aldosterone production rates, and relatively lower sodium intakes. Topics of discussion with parents include how to crush and administer tablets, what to do if doses are accidentally missed, and when to administer "stress" dosages.

For children with CAH, adequacy of replacement therapy is monitored by periodic reassessment of growth velocity, extent of virilization, and salt craving. Laboratory monitoring may include serum androgen and 17-OHP concentrations, skeletal maturation, and 24-hour urinary 17-ketosteroid excretion. Androstenedione concentrations are useful to assess adequacy of glucocorticoid replacement, whereas 17-hydroxyprogesterone concentrations are useful to assess for overtreatment. Determination of testosterone concentrations is helpful in girls and prepubertal boys. In pubertal and postpubertal girls, menstrual cyclicity is a sensitive indicator of hormone replacement therapy. Adequacy of mineralocorticoid replacement can be judged using plasma renin activity.

At times of physiological stress (such as fever greater than 101° F, persistent vomiting, significant trauma, and surgical procedures), the glucocorticoid dose should be increased. In general, two to three times the usual dose is sufficient to prevent adrenal insufficiency. Higher doses may be necessary for surgical procedures. All families should have at home and be able to administer injectable hydrocortisone (e.g., Solu-Cortef) intramuscularly in case of medical emergencies. Recommended intramuscular doses are 25 mg for infants, 50 mg for children less than 4 years of age, and 100 mg for all others.

During surgical procedures, additional hydrocortisone can be administered either as continuous intravenous infusion or intramuscular injection. Intravenous normal saline (0.9% NaCl) can be used if oral mineralocorticoid replacement is not tolerated by the patient. While receiving glucocorticoid replacement therapy (and occasionally in the newborn period), physiologically stressed individuals with

11β-hydroxylase deficiency may develop hyponatremia and hyperkalemia and benefit from mineralocorticoid therapy.

PSYCHOLOGICAL AND GENETIC COUNSELING AND SUPPORT

Longitudinal continuity of care and provision for support systems are essential because of the medical and psychological aspects of DSDs. If an experienced social worker, psychologist, or psychiatrist is available, careful assessment and counseling are valuable throughout childhood and adolescence. Although most such cases of 46,XY DSD do not require medical therapy during childhood, clinical visits with an endocrinologist are helpful intermittently to address the patient's and parents' concerns, update parents concerning new therapy and outcome data, and ensure that appropriate psychological support needs are being addressed. Some parents may find disorder-specific support groups (e.g., AIS, *www.aissg.org*; CAH, *www.caresfoundation.org*; Turner syndrome, *www.turnersyndrome.org*) to be helpful.

Many DSD conditions are inherited. The most common inheritance patterns are autosomal recessive or X-linked traits. Genetic counseling is indicated because parents are often interested to learn about recurrence risks. Because phenotypic heterogeneity occurs in some DSD disorders (i.e., partial androgen insensitivity), hormone determinations and genetic analyses (when available) for other family members may be beneficial.

Conclusions

Identification of genes involved in sexual differentiation has elucidated some of the molecular events responsible for normal and abnormal sexual differentiation. Knowledge of the genetic, hormonal, and environmental factors that influence sexual differentiation benefits the affected children, their parents, and their health care providers. This information enables better parental education regarding the etiology, natural history, and prognosis for their child. With understanding of factors that affect sexual differentiation, recurrence risks can be estimated. Despite the advances in characterizing the molecular basis of ambiguous genitalia, the most important consideration in the management of an infant with genital ambiguity remains the sensitivity and compassion demonstrated by health care professionals in their interactions with the family.

REFERENCES

1. Lee PA, Houk CP, Ahmed SF, Hughes IA, and the International Consensus Conference on Intersex Working Group (2006). Consensus statement on management of intersex disorders. Pediatrics 118: e488–500.
2. Vilain E, Achermann JC, Eugster EA, Harley VR, Morel Y, Wilson JD, et al. (2007). We used to call them hermaphrodites. Genetics in Medicine 9:65.
3. Kim Y, Capel B (2006). Balancing the bipotential gonad between alternative organ fates: A new perspective on an old problem. Dev Dynamics 235:2292.
4. Jost A (1947). Recherches sur la différenciation sexuelle de l'embryon del lapin. Arch Anat Microsc Morph Exp 36:271.
5. Sinclair AH, Berta P, Palmer MS, Hawkins JR, Griffiths BL, Smith MJ, et al. (1990). A gene from the human sex-determining region encodes a protein with homology to a conserved DNA-binding motif. Nature 346(6281):240.
6. Gubbay J, Collignon J, Koopman P, Capel B, Economou A, Munsterberg A, et al. (1990). A gene mapping to the sex-determining region of the mouse Y chromosome is a member of a novel family of embryonically expressed genes. Nature 346(6281):245.
7. Park SY, Jameson JL (1993). Transcriptional regulation of gonadal development and differentiation. Endocrinology 146:1035.
8. Wylie CC (1993). The biology of primordial germ cells. Eur Urol 23:62.
9. Parker KL, Schimmer BP (2006). Embryology and Genetics of the Mammalian Gonads and Ducts. In Knobil and Neill's Physiology of Reproduction, 3/e. St. Louis: Elsevier 313-336.
10. Capel B (1998). Sex in the 90s: SRY and the switch to the male pathway. Annu Rev Physiol 60:497.
11. Bullejos M, Koopman P (2005). Delayed Sry and Sox9 expression in developing mouse gonads underlies B6-Y(DOM) sex reversal. Dev Biol 278(2):473.
12. De Santa Barbara P, Moniot B, Poulat F, et al. (2000). Expression and subcellular localization of SF-1, SOX9, WT1, and AMH proteins during early human testicular development. Dev Dyn 217:293.
13. Capel B, Albrecht KH, Washburn LL, Eicher EM (1999). Migration of mesonephric cells into the mammalian gonad depends on Sry. Mech Dev 84:127.
14. Schmahl J, Eicher E, Washburn L, Capel B (2000). Sry induces cell proliferation in the mouse gonad. Development 127:65.
15. Wilhelm D, Hiramatsu R, Mizusaki H, Widjaja L, Combes AN, Kanai Y, et al. (2007). SOX9 regulates prostaglandin D synthase gene transcription in vivo to ensure testis development. Journal of Biological Chemistry 282:10553.
16. Wilhelm D, Martinson F, Bradford S, Wilson MJ, Combes AN, Beverdam A, et al. (2005). Sertoli cell differentiation is induced both cell-autonomously and through prostaglandin signaling during mammalian sex determination. Dev Biol 287:111.
17. Malki S, et al. (2005). Prostaglandin D2 induces nuclear. EMBO J 24:1798.
18. Kim Y, Kobayashi A, Sekido R, DiNapoli L, Brennan J, Chaboissier MC, et al. (2006). Fgf9 and Wnt4 act as antagonistic signals to regulate mammalian sex determination. PLoS Biol 4:1000.
19. Wilhelm D, Koopman P (2006). The makings of maleness: Towards an integrated view of male sexual development. Nature Review Genetics 7:620.
20. Jeanes A, Wilhelm D, Wilson MJ, Bowles J, McClive PJ, Sinclair AH, et al. (2005). Evaluation of candidate markers for the peritubular myoid cell lineage in the developing mouse testis. Reproduction 130:509.
21. Clark AM, Garland KK, Russell LD (2000). Desert hedgehog (Dhh) gene is required in the mouse testis for formation of adult-type Leydig cells and normal development of peritubular cells and seminiferous tubules. Biology of Reproduction 63:1825.
22. Zondek LH, Zondek T (1983). Ovarian hilar cells and testicular Leydig cells in anencephaly. Biol Neonate 43:211.
23. Wilhelm D, Palmer S, Koopman P (2007). Sex determination and gonadal development in mammals. Physiol Rev 87:1.
24. Nef S, Schaad O, Stallings NR, Cederroth CR, Pitetti JL, Schaer G, et al. (2005). Gene expression during sex determination reveals a robust female genetic program at the onset of ovarian development. Dev Biol 287:361.
25. Tanaka SS, Yamaguchi YL, Tsoi B, Lickert H, Tam PP (2005). IFITM/Mil/fragilis family proteins IFITM1 and IFITM3 play distinct roles in mouse primordial germ cell homing and repulsion. Dev Cell 9:745.
26. Molyneaux KA, Zinszner H, Kunwar PS, Schaible K, Stebler J, Sunshine MJ, et al. (2003). The chemokine SDF1/CXCL12 and its receptor CXCR4 regulate mouse germ cell migration and survival. Development 130:4279.
27. Kimble J, Page DC (2007). The mysteries of sexual identity. The germ cell's perspective. Science 316:400.
28. Bowles J, Knight D, Smith C, Wilhelm D, Richman J, Mamiya S, et al. (2006). Retinoid signaling determines germ cell fate in mice. Science 312:596.

29. Baltus AE, Menke DB, Hu YC, Goodheart ML, Carpenter AE, de Rooij DG, et al. (2006). In germ cells of mouse embryonic ovaries, the decision to enter meiosis precedes premeiotic DNA replication. Nature Genetics 38:1430.

30. Baker TG (1963). A quantitative and cytological study of germ cells in human ovaries. Proc R Soc Med Lond 158:417.

31. Koubova J, Menke DB, Zhou Q, Capel B, Griswold MD, Page DC (2006). Retinoic acid regulates sex-specific timing of meiotic initiation in mice. Proceeding of the National Academy of Science USA. 103:2474.

32. McLaren A, Southee D (1997). Entry of mouse embryonic germ cells into meiosis. Dev Biol 187;107.

33. Schaefer CB, Ooi SK, Bestor TH, Bourc'his D (2007). Epigenetic decisions in mammalian germ cells. Science 316:398.

34. Allegrucci C, Thurston A, Lucas E, Young L (2005). Epigenetics and the germline. Reproduction 129:137.

35. Münsterberg A, Lovell-Badge R (1991). Expression of the mouse anti-Müllerian hormone gene suggests a role in both male and female sexual differentiation. Development 113:613.

36. Roberts LM, Visser JA, Ingraham HA (2002). Involvement of a matrix metalloproteinase in MIS-induced cell death during urogenital development. Development 129:1487.

37. Zhan Y, Fujino A, MacLaughlin DT, Manganaro TF, Szotek PP, Arango NA, et al. (2006). Mullerian inhibiting substance regulates its receptor/SMAD signaling and causes mesenchymal transition of the coelomic epithelial cells early in Mullerian duct regression. Development 133:2359.

38. Catlin EA, MacLaughlin DT, Donahoe PK (1993). Müllerian inhibiting hormone substance: new perspectives and future directions. Microscopy Res Technique 25:121.

39. Vigier B, Watrin F, Magre S, et al. (1987). Purified bovine AMH induces a characteristic freemartin effect in fetal rat prospective ovaries exposed to it in vitro. Development 100:43.

40. Vigier B, Forest MG, Eychenne B, et al. (1989). Anti-Müllerian hormone produces endocrine sex-reversal of fetal ovaries. Proc Natl Acad Sci 86:3684.

41. Marker PC, Donjacour AA, Dahiya R, Cunha GR (2003). Hormonal, cellular, and molecular control of prostatic development. Dev Biol 253:156.

42. Zhang TJ, Hoffman BG, Ruiz de Algara T, Helgason CD (2006). SAGE reveals expression of Wnt signalling pathway members during mouse prostate development. Gene Expr Patterns 6:310.

43. Clarnette TD, Sugita Y, Hutson JM (1997). Genital anomalies in human and animal models reveal the mechanisms and hormones governing testicular descent. Br J Urol 79:99.

44. Goto M, Piper Hanley K, Marcos J, Wood PJ, Wright S, Postle AD, et al. (2006). In humans, early cortisol biosynthesis provides a mechanism to safeguard female sexual development. J Clin Invest 116:953.

45. White PC (2006). Ontogeny of adrenal steroid biosynthesis: why girls will be girls. J Clin Invest 116:872.

46. Grumbach MM, Auchus RJ (1999). Estrogen: Consequences and implications of human mutations in synthesis and action. J Clin Endocrinol Metab 84:4677.

47. Wilson JD (2001). Androgens, androgen receptors, and male gender role behavior. Horm Behav 40:358.

48. Arnold AP, Burgoyne PS (2004). Are XX and XY brain cells intrinsically different? Trends Endocrinol Metab 15:6.

49. de Courten-Myers GM (1999). The human cerebral cortex: Gender differences in structure and function, J Neuropathol Exp Neurol 58: 217.

50. Rabinowicz T, Dean DE, Petetot JM, de Courten-Myers GM (1999). Gender differences in the human cerebral cortex: more neurons in males: More processes in females. J Child Neurol 14:98.

51. Swain A, Lovell-Badge R (1999). Mammalian sex determination: A molecular drama. Genes Dev 13:755.

52. Koopman P, Gubbay J, Vivian N, et al. (1991). Male development of chromosomally female mice transgenic for Sry. Nature 351:117.

53. Hacker A, Capel B, Goodfellow P, et al. (1995). Expression of Sry, the mouse sex determining gene. Development 121:1603.

54. Kreidberg JA, Sariola H, Loring JM, et al. (1993). WT-1 is required for early kidney development. Cell 74:679.

55. Ikeda Y, Shen W-H, Ingraham HA, et al. (1994). Developmental expression of mouse steroidogenic factor-1, an essential regulator of the steroid hydroxylases. Mol Endocrinol 8:654.

56. Parker KL, Schimmer BP (1997). Steroidogenic factor 1: a key determinant of endocrine development and function. Endocr Rev 18:361.

57. Luo X, Ikeda Y, Schlosser DA, et al. (1995). Steroidogenic factor 1 is the essential transcript encoded by the mouse Ftz-F1 gene. Mol Endocrinol 9:1233.

58. Zhao L, Bakke M, Hanley NA, Majdic G, Stallings NR, Jeyasuria P, et al. (2004). Tissue-specific knockouts of steroidogenic factor 1. Mol Cell Endocrinol 215:89.

59. Vidal VP, Chaboissier MC, Rooij DG de, Schedl A (2001). Sox9 induces testis development in XX transgenic mice. Nat Genet 28:216.

60. Chaboissier MC, Kobayashi A, Vidal VIP, Lützkendorf S, Kant HJK van de, Wegner M, et al. (2004). Functional analysis of Sox8 and Sox9 during sex determination in the mouse. Development 131:1891.

61. Bi W, Deng JM, Zhang Z, et al. (1999). Sox9 is required for cartilage formation. Nat Genet 22:85.

62. Miyamoto N, Yoshida M, Kuratani S, et al. (1997). Defects of urogenital development in mice lacking Emx2. Development 124:1653.

63. Pellegrini M, Pantano S, Lucchini F, et al. (1997). Emx2 developmental expression in primorida of the reproductive and excretory systems. Anat Embryol 196:427.

64. Fujii T, Pichel JG, Taira M, et al. (1994). Expression patterns of the murine LIM class homeobox gene Lim1in the developing brain and excretory system. Developmental Dynamics 199:73.

65. Shawlot W, Behringer RR: Requirement for Lim1 in head-organizer function. Nature 374:425, 1995.

66. Swain A, Zanaria E, Hacker A, et al. (1996). Mouse Dax-1 expression is consistent with a role in sex determination as well as in adrenal and hypothalamus function. Nat Genet 12:404.

67. Ito M, Yu R, Jameson JL (1997). DAX-1 inhibits SF-1 mediated transactivation via a carboxy-terminal domain that is deleted in adrenal hypoplasia congenita. Mol Cell Biol 17:1476.

68. Zazopoulos E, Lalli E, Stocco DM, et al. (1997). DNA binding and transcriptional repression by DAX-1 blocks steroidogenesis. Nature 390:311.

69. Crawford PA, Dorn C, Sadovsky Y, et al. (1998). Nuclear receptor DAX-1 recruits nuclear receptor corepressor N-CoR to steroidogenic factor 1. Mol Cell Biol 18:2949.

70. Hanley NA, Rainey WE, Wilson DI, et al. (2001). Expression profiles of SF-1, DAX1, and CYP17 in the human fetal adrenal gland: Potential interactions in gene regulation. Mol Endocrinol 15:57.

71. Yu RN, Ito M, Saunders TL, et al. (1998). Role of Ahch in gonadal development and gametogenesis. Nat Genet 20:353.

72. Swain A, Narvaez V, Burgoyne P, Camerino G, Lovell-Badge R (1998). Dax1 antagonizes Sry action in mammalian sex determination. Nature 391:761.

73. DiNapoli L, Batchvarov J, Capel B (2006). FGF9 promotes survival of germ cells in the fetal testis. Development 133:1519.

74. Vainio S, Heikkila M, Kispert A, et al. (1999). Female development in mammals is regulated by Wnt-4 signalling. Nature 397:405.

75. Jeays-Ward K, Hoyle C, Brennan J, Dandonneau M, Alldus G, Capel B, et al. (2003). Endothelial and steroidogenic cell migration are regulated by WNT4 in the developing mammalian gonad. Development 130:3663.

76. Parr BA, McMahon AP (1998). Sexually dimorphic development of the mammalian reproductive tract requires Wnt-7a. Nature 395:707.

77. Besmer P, Manova K, Duttlinger R, Huang EJ, Packer A, Gyssler C, et al. (1993). The kit-ligand (steel factor) and its receptor c-kit/W: pleiotropic roles in gametogenesis and melanogenesis. Dev [volume]:125.

78. Brannan CI, Lyman SD, Williams DE, et al. (1991). Steel-Dickie mutation encodes a c-kit ligand lacking transmembrane and cytoplasmic domains. Proc Nat Acad Sci 88:4671.

79. Haqq CM, King CY, Ukiyama E, et al. (1994). Molecular basis of mammalian sexual determination: Activation of Müllerian inhibiting substance gene expression by SRY. Science 266:1494.

80. Shen WH, Moore CCD, Ikeda Y, et al. (1994). Nuclear receptor steroidogenic factor 1 regulates the Müllerian inhibiting substance gene: A link to the sex determination cascade. Cell 77:651.

81. de Santa Barbara P, Bonneaud N, Boizet B, et al. (1998). Direct interaction of SRY-related protein SOX9 and steroidogenic factor1 regulates transcription of the human anti-Müllerian hormone gene. Mol Cell Biol 18:6653.

82. Arango NA, Lovell-Badge R, Behringer RR (1999). Targeted mutagenesis of the endogenous mouse Mis gene promoter: In vivo definition of genetic pathways of vertebrate sexual development. Cell 99:409.

83. Kamachi Y, Uchikawa M, Kondoh H (2000). Pairing SOX off with partners in the regulation of embryonic development. Trends Genet 16:182.

84. de Santa Barbara P, Moniot B, Poulat F, et al. (1998). Steroidogenic factor-1 regulates transcription of the human anti-müllerian hormone receptor. J Biol Chem 273:29654.

85. Bitgood MJ, Shen L, McMahon AP (1996). Sertoli cell signaling by desert hedgehog regulates the male germline. Curr Biol 6:298.

86. Parmantier E, Lynn B, Lawson D, et al. (1999). Schwann cell-derived desert hedgehog controls the development of peripheral nerve sheath. Neuron 23:713.

87. Bitgood MJ, McMahon AP (1995). Hedgehog and Bmp genes are coexpressed at many diverse sites of cell-cell interaction in the mouse embryo. Dev Biol 172:126.

88. Zimmermann S, Steding G, Emmen JMA, et al. (1999). Targeted disruption of the Insl3 gene causes bilateral cryptorchidism. Mol Endocrinol 13:681.

89. Nef S, Parada L (1999). Cryptorchidism in mice mutant for Insl3. Nature Genetics 22:295.

90. Rijli FM, Matyas R, Pellegrini M, et al. (1995). Cryptorchidism and homeotic transformations of spinal nerves and vertebrae in Hoxa-10 mutant mice. Proc Natl Acad Sci 92:8185.

91. Gorlov IP, Kamat A, Bogatcheva NV, Jones E, Lamb DJ, Truong A, et al. (2002). Mutations of the GREAT gene cause cryptorchidism. Hum Mol Genet 11:2309.

92. Barbaux S, Niaudet P, Gubler M-C, et al. (1997). Donor splice-site mutations in WT1 are responsible for Frasier syndrome. Nature Genetics 17:467.

93. Varanasi R, Bardeesy N, Ghahremani M, et al. (1994). Fine structure analysis of the WT1 gene in sporadic Wilms tumors. Proc Natl Acad Sci 91:3554.

94. Denys P, Malvaux P, Berghe H van den, et al. (1967). Association d'un syndrome anatomo-pathologique de pseudohermaphroditisme masculin d'une tumeur de Wilms, d'une nephropathie-parenchymateuse et d'un mosaicisme XX/XY. Arch Fr Pediatr 24:729.

95. Drash A, Sherman F, Hartmann WH, et al. (1979). A syndrome of pseudohermaphroditism, Wilms' tumor, hypertension, and degenerative renal disease. J Pediatr 76:585.

96. Jadresic L, Leake J, Gordon I, et al. (1990). Clinicopathologic review of twelve children with nephropathy, Wilms' tumor, and genital abnormalities (Drash syndrome). J Pediatr 117:717.

97. Schmitt K, Zabel B, Tulzer G, et al. (1995). Nephropathy with Wilms tumour or gonadal dysgenesis: Incomplete Denys-Drash syndrome or separate diseases? European Journal of Pediatrics 154:577.

98. Bardeesy N, Zabel B, Schmitt K, et al. (1994). WT1 mutations associated with incomplete Denys-Drash syndrome define a domain predicted to behave in a dominant-negative fashion. Genomics 21:663.

99. Barbosa AS, Hadjuatgabasiou CG, Theodoridis C, et al. (1999). The same mutation affecting the splicing of WT1 gene is present on Frasier syndrome patients with or without Wilms' tumor. Hum Mutat 13:146.

100. Davies JA, Ladomery M, Hohenstein P, Michael L, Shafe A, Spraggon L, et al. (2004). Development of an siRNA-based method for repressing specific genes in renal organ culture and its use to show that the Wt1 tumour suppressor is required for nephron differentiation. Hum Mol Genet 13:235.

101. Klattig J, Sierig R, Kruspe D, Besenbeck B, Englert C (2007). The Wilms tumor protein Wt1 is an activator of the anti-Mullerian hormone receptor gene Amhr2. Mol Cell Biol 27:4355.

102. Larsson SH, Charlieu J-P, Miyagawa K, et al. (1995). Subnuclear localization of WT1 in splicing or transcription factor domains is regulated by alternative splicing. Cell 81:391.

103. Yao HH, Matzuk MM, Jorgez CJ, Menke DB, Page DC, Swain A, et al. (2004). Follistatin operates downstream of Wnt4 in mammalian ovary organogenesis. Dev Dyn 230:210.

104. Elejalde BR, Opitz JM, de Elejalde MM, Gilbert EF, Abellera M, Meisner L, et al. (1984). Tandem dup (1p) within the short arm of chromosome 1 in a child with ambiguous genitalia and multiple congenital anomalies. Am J Med Genet 17:723.

105. Biason-Lauber A, De Filippo G, Konrad D, Scarano G, Nazzaro A, Schoenle EJ (2007). WNT4 deficiency: A clinical phenotype distinct from the classic Mayer-Rokitansky-Kuster-Hauser syndrome, A case report. Hum Reprod 22:224.

106. Biason-Lauber A, Konrad D, Navratil F, Schoenle EJ (2004). A WNT4 mutation associated with Mullerian-duct regression and virilization in a 46,XX woman. N Engl J Med 351:792.

107. Fleming A., Vilain E (2004). The endless quest for sex determination genes. Clin Genet 67:15.

108. Harley VR, Clarkson MJ, Argentaro A (2003). The molecular action and regulation of the testis-determining factors, SRY (sex-determining region on the Y chromosome) and SOX9 [SRY-related high-mobility group (HMG) box 9]. Endocr Rev 24:466.

109. Schnitt-Ney M, Thiele H, Kaltwasser P, et al. (1995). Two novel SRY missense mutations reducing DNA binding identified in XY females and their mosaic father. Am J Hum Genet 56:862.

110. Hines RS, Tho SP, Zhang YY, et al. (1997). Paternal somatic and germ-line mosaicism for a sex-determining region on Y (SRY) missense mutation leading to recurrent 46,XY sex reversal. Fertil Steril 67:675.

111. Hawkins JR, Taylor A, Goodfellow PN, et al. (1992). Evidence for increased prevalence of SRY mutations in XY females with complete rather than partial gonadal dysgenesis. Am J Hum Genet 51:979.

112. Jager RJ, Harley VR, Pfeiffer RA, et al. (1992). A familial mutation in the testis-determining gene SRY shared by both sexes. Hum Genet 90:350.

113. Telvi L, Lebbar A, Del Pino O, et al. (1999). 45,X/46,XY mosaicism: Report of 27 cases. Pediatrics 104(2/1):304.

114. Mendez JP, Ulloa-Aguirre A, Kofman-Alfaro S, et al. (1993). Mixed gonadal dysgenesis: Clinical, cytogenetic, endocrinological, and histopathological findings in 16 patients. Am J Med Genet 46:263.

115. Lukusa T, Fryns JP, Kleczkowska A, et al. (1991). Role of gonadal dysgenesis in gonadoblastoma induction in 46, XY individuals. The Leuven experience in 46, XY pure gonadal dysgenesis and testicular feminization syndromes. Genet Couns 2:9.

116. Iezzoni JC, Von Kap-Herr C, Golden WL, et al. (1997). Gonadoblastomas in 45,X/46,XY mosaicism: Analysis of Y chromosome distribution by fluorescence in situ hybridization. Am J Clin Pathol 108:197.

117. Alikasifoglu A, Kandemir N, Caglar M, et al. (1996). Prepubertal gonadoblastoma in a 46,XY female patient with features of Turner syndrome. Eur J Pediatr 155:653.

118. Foster JW, Dominguez-Steglich MA, Guioli S, et al. (1994). Campomelic dysplasia and autosomal sex reversal caused by mutations in an SRY-related gene. Nature 372:525.

119. Wagner T, Wirth J, Meyer J, et al. (1994). Autosomal sex reversal and campomelic dwarfism are caused by mutations in and around the SRY-related gene SOX9. Cell 79:1111.

120. Meyer J, Sudbeck P, Held M, et al. (1997). Mutational analysis of the SOX9 gene in campomelic dysplasia and autosomal sex reversal: lack of genotype/phenotype correlations. Hum Molec Genet 6:91.

121. Cameron FJ, Hageman R M, Cooke-Yarborough C, et al. (1996). A novel germ line mutation in SOX9 causes familial campomelic dysplasia and sex reversal. Hum Molec Genet 5:1625.

122. Tommerup N, Schempp W, Meinecke P, et al. (1993). Assignment of an autosomal sex reversal locus (SRA1) and campomelic dysplasia (CMPD1) to 17q24.3-q25.1. Nature Genet 4:170.

123. Preiss S, Argentaro A, Clayton A, John A, Jans DA, Ogata T, et al. (2001). Compound effects of point mutations causing campomelic dysplasia/autosomal sex reversal upon SOX9 structure, nuclear transport, DNA binding, and transcriptional activation. J Biol Chem 276:27864.

124. Pfeifer D, Kist R, Dewar K, et al. (1999). Campomelic dysplasia translocation breakpoints are scattered over 1 Mb proximal to SOX9: evidence for an extended control region. Am J Hum Genet 65:111.

125. Pop R, Zaragoza MV, Gaudette M, Dohrmann U, Scherer G (2005). A homozygous nonsense mutation in SOX9 in the dominant disorder campomelic dysplasia: a case of mitotic gene conversion. Hum Genet 117:43.

126. Bardoni B, Zanaria E, Guioli S, et al. (1994). A dosage sensitive locus at chromosome Xp21 is involved in male to female sex reversal. Nature Genetics 7:497.

127. Barbaro M, Oscarson M, Schoumans J, Staaf J, Ivarsson SA, Wedell A (2007). Isolated 46,XY gonadal dysgenesis in two sisters caused by a Xp21.2 interstitial duplication containing the DAX1 gene. J Clin Endocrinol Metab [E-pub ahead of print].

128. Bernard P, Ludbrook L, Queipo G, Dinulos MB, Kletter GB, Zhang YH, et al. (2006). A familial missense mutation in the hinge region of DAX1 associated with late-onset AHC in a prepubertal female. Mol Genet Metab 88:272.

129. Peter M, Viemann M, Partsch C-J, et al. (1998). Congenital adrenal hyperplasia: Clinical spectrum, experience with hormonal diagnosis, and report on new point mutations of the DAX-1 gene. J Clin Endocrinol Metab 83:2666.

130. Habiby RL, Boepple P, Nachtigall L, et al. (1996). Adrenal hypoplasia congenita with hypogonadotropic hypogonadism. Evidence that DAX-1 mutations lead to combined hypothalamic and pituitary defects in gonadotropin production. J Clin Invest 98:1055.

131. Seminara SB, Achermann JC, Genel M, et al. (1999). X-linked adrenal hypoplasia congenita: a mutation in DAX1 expands the phenotypic spectrum in males and females. J Clin Endocrinol Metab 84:4501.

132. Merke DP, Tajima T, Baron J, et al. (1999). Brief report: Hypogonadotropic hypogonadism in a female caused by an X-linked recessive mutation in the DAX1 gene. N Engl J Med 340:1248.

133. Francke U, Harper JF, Darras BT, et al. (1987). Congenital adrenal hypoplasia, myopathy, and glycerol kinase deficiency: molecular genetic evidence for deletions. Am J Hum Genet 40:212.

134. Muscatelli F, Strom TM, Walker AP, et al. (1994). Mutations in the DAX-1 gene give rise to both X-linked adrenal hypoplasia congenital and hypogonadotropic hypogonadism. Nature 372:672.

135. Reutens AT, Achermann JC, Ito M, et al. (1999). Clinical and functional effects of mutations in the DAX-1 gene in patients with adrenal hypoplasia congenita. J Clin Endocrinol Metab 84:504.

136. Bernard P, Ludbrook L, Queipo G, Dinulos MB, Kletter GB, Zhang YH, et al. (2006). A familial missense mutation in the hinge region of DAX1 associated with late-onset AHC in a prepubertal female. Mol Genet Metab 88:272.

137. Ho J, Zhang YH, Huang BL, McCabe ER (2004). NR0B1A: An alternatively spliced form of NR0B1. Mol Genet Metab 83:330.

138. Hossain A, Li C, Saunders GF (2004). Generation of two distinct functional isoforms of dosage-sensitive sex reversal-adrenal hypoplasia congenita-critical region on the X chromosome gene 1 (DAX-1) by alternative splicing. Mol Endocrinol 18:1428.

139. Bavner A, Sanyal S, Gustafsson JA, Treuter E (2005). Transcriptional corepression by SHP: Molecular mechanisms and physiological consequences. Trends Endocrinol Metab 16:478.

140. Altincicek B, Tenbaum SP, Dressel U, Thormeyer D, Renkawitz R, Baniahmad A (2000). Interaction of the corepressor Alien with DAX-1 is abrogated by mutations of DAX-1 involved in adrenal hypoplasia congenita. J Biol Chem 275:7662.

141. Iyer AK, Zhang YH, McCabe ER (2006). Dosage-sensitive sex reversal adrenal hypoplasia congenita critical region on the X chromosome, gene 1 (DAX1) (NR0B1) and small heterodimer partner (SHP) (NR0B2) form homodimers individually, as well as DAX1-SHP heterodimers. Mol Endocrinol 20:2326.

142. Umehara F, Tate G, Itoh K, et al. (2000). A novel mutation of desert hedgehog in a patient with 46,XY partial gonadal dysgenesis accompanied by minifascicular neuropathy. Am J Hum Genet 67:1302.

143. Canto P, Vilchis F, Soderlund D, Reyes E, Mendez JP (2005). A heterozygous mutation in the desert hedgehog gene in patients with mixed gonadal dysgenesis. Mol Hum Reprod 11:833.

144. Canto P, Soderlund D, Reyes E, Mendez JP (2004). Mutations in the desert hedgehog (DHH) gene in patients with 46,XY complete pure gonadal dysgenesis. J Clin Endocrinol Metab 89:4480.

145. Tate G, Satoh H, Endo Y, Mitsuya T (2000). Assignment of desert hedgehog (DHH) to human chromosome bands 12q12- -q13.1 by in situ hybridization. Cytogenet Cell Genet 88:93.

146. Muroya K, Okuyama T, Goishi K, et al. (2000). Sex-determining gene(s) on distal 9p: Clinical and molecular studies in six cases. J Clin Endocrinol Metab 85:3094.

147. Hoo JJ, Fischer A, Fuhrmann W (1982). Familial tiny 9p/20p translocation: 9p24. The critical segment for monosomy 9p syndrome. Ann Genet 25:249.

148. Huret JL, Leonard C, Forestier B, et al. (1988). Eleven new cases of del(9p) and features from 80 cases. J Med Genet 25:741.

149. Bennett CP, Docherty Z, Robb SA, et al. (1993). Deletion 9p and sex reversal. J Med Genet 30:518.

150. Ogata T, Muroya K, Matsuo N, et al. (1997). Impaired male sex development in an infant with molecularly defined partial 9p monosomy: implication for a testis forming gene(s) on 9p. J Med Genet 34:331.

151. McDonald MT, Flejter W, Sheldon S, et al. (1997). XY sex reversal and gonadal dysgenesis due to 9p24 monosomy. Am J Med Genet 73:321.

152. Burtis KC, Baker BS (1989). Drosophila doublesex gene controls somatic sexual differentiation by producing alternatively spliced mRNAs encoding sex-specific polypeptides. Cell 56:997.

153. Raymond CS, Parker ED, Kettlewell JR, et al. (1999). A region of human chromosome 9p required for testis development contains two genes related to known sexual regulators. Hum Mol Genet 8:989.

154. Ottolenghi C, Veitia R, Barbieri M, et al. (2000). The human doublesex-related gene, DMRT2, is homologous to a gene involved in somitogeneis and encodes a potential bicistronic transcript. Genomics 64:179.

155. Calvari V, Bertini V, De Grandi A, et al. (2000). A new submicroscopic deletion that refines the 9p region for sex reversal. Genomics 65:203.

156. Smith CA, McClive PJ, Western PS, et al. (1999). Conservation of a sex-determining gene. Nature 402:601.

157. De Grandi A, Calvari V, Bertini V, et al. (2000). The expression pattern of a mouse doublesex-related gene is consistent with a role in gonadal differentiation. Mech Dev 90:323.

158. Moniot B, Berta P, Scherer G, et al. (2000). Male specific expression suggests role of DMRT1 in human sex determination. Mech Dev 91:323.

159. Bartsch O, Kress W, Wagner A, et al. (1999). The novel contiguous gene syndrome of myotubular myopathy (MTM1), male hypogenitalism and deletion in Xq28: Report of the first familial case. Cytogenet Cell Genet 85:310.

160. Laporte J, Kioschis P, Hu LJ, et al. (1997). Cloning and characterization of an alternatively spliced gene in proximal Xq28 deleted in two patients with intersexual genitalia and myotubular myopathy. Genomics 41:458.

161. Fukami M, Wada Y, Miyabayashi K, Nishino I, Hasegawa T, Nordenskjold A, et al. (2006). CXorf6 is a causative gene for hypospadias. Nature Genetics 38:1369.

162. Wilkie AOM, Zeitlin HC, Lindenbaum RH, et al. (1990). Clinical features and molecular analysis of the β-thalassemia/mental retardation syndromes. II. Cases without detectable abnormality of the β-globin complex. Am J Hum Genet 46:1127.

163. Reardon W, Gibbons RJ, Winter RM, et al. (1995). Male pseudohermaphroditism in sibs with the alpha-thalassemia/mental retardation (ATR-X) syndrome. Am J Med Genet 55:285.

164. McPherson EW, Clemens MM, Gibbons RJ, et al. (1995). X-linked alpha-thalassemia/mental retardation (ATR-X) syndrome: A new kindred with severe genital anomalies and mild hematologic expression. Am J Med Genet 55:302.

165. Tang P, Park DJ, Marshall Graves JA, Harley VR (2004). ATRX and sex differentiation. Trends Endocrinol Metab 15:339.

166. Gibbons RJ, Picketts DJ, Villard L, et al. (1995). Mutations in a putative global transcriptional regulator cause X-linked mental retardation with β-thalassemia (ATR-X syndrome). Cell 80:837.

167. Wada T, Kubota T, Fukushima Y, et al. (2000). Molecular genetic study of Japanese patients with X-linked alpha-thalassemia/mental retardation syndrome (ATR-X). Am J Med Genet 94:242.

168. Cardoso C, Timsit S, Villard L, et al. (1998). Specific interaction between the XNP/ATR-X gene product and the SET domain of the human EZH2 protein. Hum Mol Genet 7:679.

169. Gibbons RJ, McDowell TL, Raman S, et al (2000). Mutations in ATRX, encoding a SWI/SNF-like protein, cause diverse changes in the pattern of DNA methylation. Nat Genet 24:368.

170. Picketts DJ, Higgs DR, Bachoo S, et al. (1996). ATRX encodes a novel member of the SNF2 family of proteins: Mutations point to a common mechanism underlying the ATR-X syndrome. Hum Molec Genet 5:1899.

171. Badens C, Lacoste C, Philip N, Martini N, Courrier S, Giuliano F, et al. (2006). Mutations in PHD-like domain of the ATRX gene correlate with severe psychomotor impairment and severe

urogenital abnormalities in patients with ATRX syndrome. Clin Genet 70:57.

172. Gibbons RJ, Higgs DR (2000). Molecular-clinical spectrum of the ATR-X syndrome. Am J Med Genet 97:204.

173. Law H, Mushtaq I, Wingrove K, Malone M, Sebire NJ (2006). Histopathological features of testicular regression syndrome: Relation to patient age and implications for management. Fetal Pediatr Pathol 25:119.

174. Joss N, Briard ML (1980). Embryonic testicular regression syndrome: variable phenotypic expression in siblings. J Pediatr 97:200.

175. Vilain E, Le Merrer M, Lecointre C, et al. (1999). IMAGe, a new clinical association of intrauterine growth retardation, metaphyseal dysplasia, adrenal hypoplasia congenita, and genital anomalies. J Clin Endocrinol Metab 84:4335.

176. Topf KF, Kletter GB, Kelch RP, et al. (1993). Autosomal dominant transmission of the Pallister-Hall syndrome. J Pediatr 123:943.

177. Lee PA, Migeon CJ, Brown TR, et al. (1982). Robinow's syndrome: Partial primary hypogonadism in pubertal boys with persistence of micropenis. Am J Dis Child 136:327.

178. Dobyns WB, Berry-Kravis E, Havernick NJ, et al. (1999). X-linked lissencephaly with absent corpus callosum and ambiguous genitalia. Am J Med Genet. 86:331.

179. Ogata T, Matsuo N, Hiraoka N, et al. (2000). X-linked lissencephaly with ambiguous genitalia: Delineation of further case. Am J Med Genet 94:174.

180. Uyanik G, Aigner L, Martin P, Gross C, Neumann D, Marschner-Schafer H, et al. (2003). ARX mutations in X-linked lissencephaly with abnormal genitalia. Neurology 61:232.

181. Verkauskas G, Jaubert F, Lortat-Jacob S, Malan V, Thibaud E, Nihoul-Fekete C (2007). The long-term followup of 33 cases of true hermaphroditism: A 40-year experience with conservative gonadal surgery. J Urol 177:726.

182. Aleck KA, Argueso L, Stone J, et al. (1999). True hermaphroditism with partial duplication of chromosome 22 and without SRY. Am J Med Genet 85:2.

183. Jimenez AL, Kofman-Alfaro S, Berumen J, et al. (2000). Partially deleted SRY gene confined to testicular tissue in a 46,XX true hermaphrodite without SRY in leukocytic DNA. Am J Med Genet 93:417.

184. Kuhnle U, Schwarz HP, Lohrs U, et al. (1993). Familial true hermaphroditism: paternal and maternal transmission of true hermaphroditism (46,XX) and XX maleness in the absence of Y-chromosomal sequences. Hum Genet 92:571.

185. Ramos ES, Moreira-Filho CA, Vicente YA, et al. (1996). SRY-negative true hermaphrodites and an XX male in two generations of the same family. Hum Genet 97:596-598.

186. Sarafoglou K, Ostrer H (2000). Familial sex reversal: A review. J Clin Endocrinol Metab 85:483-493.

187. Alonso G, Pasqualini T, Busaniche J, Ruiz E, Chemes H (2007). True hermaphroditism in a phenotypic male without ambiguous genitalia: An unusual presentation at puberty. Horm Res 68:261.

188. Ouhilal S, Turco J, Nangia A, Stotland M, Manganiello PD (2005). True hermaphroditism presenting as bilateral gynecomastia in an adolescent phenotypic male. Fertil Steril 83:1041.

189 Talerman A, Verp MS, Senekjian E, Gilewski T, Vogelzang N (1990). True hermaphrodite with bilateral ovotestes, bilateral gonadoblastomas and dysgerminomas, 46,XX/46,XY karyotype, and a successful pregnancy. Cancer 66:2668.

190. Minowada S, Fukutani K, Hara M, Shinohara M, Kamioka J, Isurugi K, et al. (1984). Childbirth in true hermaphrodite. Eur Urol 10:414.

191. Starceski PJ, Sieber WK, Lee PA (1988). Fertility in true hermaphroditism. Adol Pediatr Gynecol 1:55.

192. de la Chapelle A, Hastbacka J, Korhonen T, Maenpaa J (1990). The etiology of XX sex reversal. Reprod Nutr Dev 1:39S.

193. Kadandale JS, Wachtel SS, Tunca Y, et al. (2000). Localization of SRY by primed in situ labeling in XX and XY sex reversal. Am J Med Genet 95:71.

194. Dauwerse JG, Hansson KB, Brouwers AA, Peters DJ, Breuning MH (2006). An XX male with the sex-determining region Y gene inserted in the long arm of chromosome 16. Fertil Steril 86:463.e1.

195. Rajender S, Rajani V, Gupta NJ, Chakravarty B, Singh L, Thangaraj K (2006). SRY-negative 46,XX male with normal genitals, complete masculinization and infertility. Mol Hum Reprod 12:341.

196. Uhlenhaut NH, Treier M (2006). Foxl2 function in ovarian development. Mol Genet Metab 88:225.

197. Vaiman D, Koutita O, Oustry A, Elsen JM, Manfredi E, Fellous M, et al. (1996). Genetic mapping of the autosomal region involved in XX sex-reversal and horn development in goats, Mamm. Genome 7:133–137.

198. Achermann JC, Ito M, Ito M, et al. (1999). A mutation in the gene encoding steroidogenic factor-1 causes XY sex reversal and adrenal failure in humans. (Letter) Nature Genet. 22:125.

199. Biason-Lauber A, Schoenle EJ (2000). Apparently normal ovarian differentiation in a prepubertal girl with transcriptionally inactive steroidogenic factor 1 (NR5A1/SF-1) and adrenocortical insufficiency. Am J Hum Genet 67:1563.

200. Lin L, Philibert P, Ferraz-de-Souza B, Kelberman D, Homfray T, Albanese A, et al. (2007). Heterozygous missense mutations in steroidogenic factor 1 (SF1/Ad4BP/NR5A1) are associated with 46,XY disorders of sex development with normal adrenal function. J Clin Endocrinol Metab 92:991.

201. Kremer H, Kraaij R, Toledo SPA, et al. (1995). Male pseudohermaphroditism due to a homozygous missense mutation of the luteinizing hormone receptor gene. Nat Genet 9:160.

202. Laue LL, Wu SM, Kudo M, et al. (1996). Compound heterozygous mutations of the luteinizing hormone receptor gene in Leydig cell hypoplasia. Mol Endocrinol 10:987.

203. Wu SM, Hallermeier KM, Laue L, et al. (1998). Inactivation of the luteinizing hormone/chorionic gonadotropin receptor by an insertional mutation in Leydig cell hypoplasia. Mol Endocrinol 12:1651.

204. Rousseau-Merck MF, Misrahi M, Atger M, et al. (1990). Localization of the human luteinizing hormone/chorion gonadotropin receptor gene (LHCGR) to chromosome 2p21. Cytogenet Cell Genet 54:77.

205. Misrahi M, Meduri G, Pissard S, et al. (1997). Comparison of immunocytochemical and molecular features with the phenotype in a case of incomplete male pseudohermaphroditism associated with a mutation of the luteinizing hormone receptor. J Clin Endocrinol Metab 82:2159.

206. Toldeo SPA, Brunner HG, Kraaij R, et al. (1996). An inactivation mutation of the luteinizing hormone receptor causes amenorrhea in a 46,XX female. J Clin Endocrinol Metab 81:3850.

207. Arnhold IJP, Latronico AC, Batista MC, et al. (1997). Ovarian resistance to luteinizing hormone: A novel cause of amenorrhea and infertility. Fertil Steril 67:394.

208. Richter-Unruh A, Korsch E, Hiort O, Holterhus PM, Themmen AP, Wudy SA (2005). Novel insertion frameshift mutation of the LH receptor gene: problematic clinical distinction of Leydig cell hypoplasia from enzyme defects primarily affecting testosterone biosynthesis. Eur J Endocrinol 152:255.

209. Dallaire L (1969). Syndrome of retardation with urogenital and skeletal anomalies (Smith-Lemli-Opitz syndrome): Clinical features and mode of inheritance. J Med Genet 6:113.

210. Moebius FF, Fitzky BU, Lee JN, et al. (1998). Molecular cloning and expression of the human delta7-sterol reductase. Proc Natl Acad Sci 95:1899.

211. Wassif CA, Maslen C, Kachilele-Linjewile S, et al. (1998). Mutations in the human sterol delta7-reductase gene at 11q12-13 cause Smith-Lemli-Opitz syndrome. Am J Hum Genet 63:55.

212. Witsch-Baumgartner M, Clayton P, Clusellas N, Haas D, Kelley RI, Krajewska-Walasek M, et al. (2005). Identification of 14 novel mutations in DHCR7 causing the Smith-Lemli-Opitz syndrome and delineation of the DHCR7 mutational spectra in Spain and Italy. Hum Mutat 25:412.

213. Engelking LJ, Evers BM, Richardson JA, Goldstein JL, Brown MS, Liang G (2006). Severe facial clefting in Insig-deficient mouse embryos caused by sterol accumulation and reversed by lovastatin. J Clin Invest 116:2356.

214. Porter FD (1995). Cholesterol precursors and facial clefting. J Clin Invest 116:2322.

215. Dallaire L, Mitchell G, Giguere R, et al. (1995). Prenatal diagnosis of Smith-Lemli-Opitz syndrome is possible by measurement of 7-dehydrocholesterol in amniotic fluid. Prenatal Diag 15:855.

216. Shackleton CHL, Roitman E, Kratz LE, et al. (1999). Equine type estrogens produced by a pregnant woman carrying a Smith-Lemli-Opitz fetus. J Clin Endocrinol Metab 84:1157.

217. Tint GS, Irons M, Elias ER, et al. (1994). Defective cholesterol biosynthesis associated with the Smith Lemli-Opitz syndrome. N Engl J Med 330:107.

218. Nowaczyk MJ, Waye JS, Douketis JD (2006). DHCR7 mutation carrier rates and prevalence of the RSH/Smith-Lemli-Opitz syndrome: Where are the patients? Am J Med Genet A 140:2057.

219. Baker BY, Lin L, Kim CJ, Raza J, Smith CP, Miller WL, et al. (2006). Nonclassic congenital lipoid adrenal hyperplasia: A new disorder of the steroidogenic acute regulatory protein with very late presentation and normal male genitalia. J Clin Endocrinol Metab 91:4781.

220. Lin D, Sugawara T, Strauss III JF, et al. (1995). Role of steroidogenic acute regulatory protein in adrenal and gonadal steroidogenesis. Science 267:1828.

221. Tee MK, Lin D, Sugawara T, et al. (1995). TβA transversion 11 bp from a splice acceptor site in the gene for steroidogenic acute regulatory protein causes congenital lipoid adrenal hyperplasia. Hum Mol Genet 4:2299.

222. Nakae J, Tajima T, Sugawara T, et al. (1997). Analysis of the steroidogenic acute regulatory protein (StAR) gene in Japanese patients with congenital lipoid adrenal hyperplasia. Hum Mol Genet 6:571.

223. Bose HS, Sato S, Aisenberg J, et al. (2000). Mutations in the steroidogenic acute regulatory protein (StAR) in six patients with congenital lipoid adrenal hyperplasia. J Clin Endocrinol Metab 85:3636.

224. Clark BJ, Wells J, King SR, et al. (1994). The purification, cloning, and expression of a novel luteinizing hormone-induced mitochondrial protein in MA-10 mouse Leydig tumor cells. Characterization of the steroidogenic acute regulatory protein (StAR). J Biol Chem 269:28314.

225. Kallen CB, Arakane F, Christenson LK, et al. (1998). Unveiling the mechanism of action and regulation of the steroidogenic acute regulatory protein. Mol Cell Endocrinol 145:39.

226. Miller WL (2007). StAR search: What we know about how the steroidogenic acute regulatory protein mediates mitochondrial cholesterol import. Mol Endocrinol 21:589.

227. Bose HS, Sugawara T, Strauss III JF, et al. (1996). The pathophysiology and genetics of congenital lipoid adrenal hyperplasia. N Engl J Med 335:1870.

228. Ogata T, Matsuo N, Saito M, et al. (1988). The testicular lesion and sexual differentiation in congenital lipoid adrenal hyperplasia. Helv Paediat Acta 43:531.

229. Bose HS, Pescovitz OH, Miller WL (1997). Spontaneous feminization in a 46,XX female patient with congenital lipoid adrenal hyperplasia caused by a homozygous frame shift mutation in the steroidogenic acute regulatory protein. J Clin Endocrinol Metab 82:1511.

230. Katsumata N, Ohtake M, Hojo T, Ogawa E, Hara T, Sato N, et al. (2002). Compound heterozygous mutations in the cholesterol side-chain cleavage enzyme gene (CYP11A) cause congenital adrenal insufficiency in humans. J Clin Endocrinol Metab 87:3808.

231. Hiort O, Holterhus PM, Werner R, Marschke C, Hoppe U, Partsch CJ, et al. (2005). Homozygous disruption of P450 side-chain cleavage (CYP11A1) is associated with prematurity, complete 46,XY sex reversal, and severe adrenal failure. J Clin Endocrinol Metab 90:538.

232. al Kandari H, Katsumata N, Alexander S, Rasoul MA (2006). Homozygous mutation of P450 side-chain cleavage enzyme gene (CYP11A1) in 46, XY patient with adrenal insufficiency, complete sex reversal, and agenesis of corpus callosum. J Clin Endocrinol Metab 91:2821.

233. Carroll MC, Campbell RD, Porter RR (1985). Mapping of steroid 21-hydroxylase genes adjacent to complement component C4 genes in HLA, the major histocompatibility complex in man. Proc Natl Acad Sci 82:521.

234. Higashi Y, Yoshioka H, Yamane M, et al. (1986). Complete nucleotide sequence of two steroid 21-hydroxylase genes tandemly arranged in human chromosome: a pseudogene and a genuine gene. Proc Natl Acad Sci 83:2841.

235. White PC, New MI, Dupont B (1986). Structure of human steroid 21-hydroxylase genes. Proc Natl Acad Sci 83:5111.

236. Rodrigues NR, Dunham I, Yu CY, et al. (1987). Molecular characterization of the HLA-lined steroid 21-hydroxylase B gene from an individual with congenital adrenal hyperplasia. EMBO J 6:1653.

237. Speiser PW, White PC (2003). Congenital adrenal hyperplasia. N Engl J Med 349:776.

238. Speiser PW, Dupont B, Rubinstein P, et al. (1985). High frequency of nonclassical steroid 21-hydroxylase deficiency. Am J Hum Genet 37:650.

239. Pang S, Clark A (1993). Congenital adrenal hyperplasia due to 21-hydroxylase deficiency: newborn screening and its relationship to the diagnosis and treatment of the disorder. Screening 2:105.

240. Auchus RJ (2004). The backdoor pathway to dihydrotestosterone. Trends Endocrinol Metab 15:432.

241. Hanley NA, Arlt W (2006). The human fetal adrenal cortex and the window of sexual differentiation. Trends Endocrinol Metab 17:391.

242. Prader A (1954). Der genitalbefund beim ppseudohermaphroditismus femininus der kengenitalen adrenogenitalen syndroms. Helv Paediatr Acta 9:231.

243. Grumbach MM, Ducharme JR (1960). The effects of androgens on fetal sexual development: Androgen-induced female pseudohermaphroditism. Fertil Steril 11:157.

244. Witchel SF, Nayak S, Suda-Hartman M, et al. (1997). Newborn screening for 21-hydroxylase deficiency: Results of CYP21 molecular genetic analysis. J Pediatr 131:328.

245. Gourmelen M, Gueux B, Pham HTM, et al. (1987). Detection of heterozygous carriers for 21-hydroxylase deficiency by plasma 21-deoxycortisol measurement. Acta Endocrinol 12:525.

246. Fiet J, Grueux B, Gourmelen M, et al. (1988). Comparison of basal and drenocorticotropin-stimulated plasma 21-deoxycortisol and 17-hydroxyprogesterone values as biological markers of late-onset adrenal hyperplasia. J Clin Endocrinol Metab 66:659.

247. Votava F, Torok D, Kovacs J, Moslinger D, Baumgartner-Parzer SM, et al. for the Middle European Society for Paediatric Endocrinology (2005). Congenital Adrenal Hyperplasia (MESPE-CAH) Study Group: Estimation of the false-negative rate in newborn screening for congenital adrenal hyperplasia. Eur J Endocrinol 152:869.

248. Bristow J, Tee MK, Gitelman SE, et al. (1993). Tenascin-X: a novel extracellular matrix protein encoded by the human XB gene overlapping P450c21B. J Cell Biol 122:265.

249. Wedell A, Thilén A, Ritzén EM, et al. (1994). Mutational spectrum of the steroid 21-hydroxylase gene in Sweden: Implications for genetic diagnosis and association with disease manifestation. J Clin Endocrinol Metab 78:1145.

250. Ferenczi A, Garami M, Kiss E, et al. (1999). Screening for mutations of 21-hydroxylase gene in Hungarian patients with congenital adrenal hyperplasia. J Clin Endocrinol Metab 84:2369.

251. Wilson RC, Nimkarn S, Dumic M, Obeid J, Azar M, Najmabadi H, et al. (2007). Ethnic-specific distribution of mutations in 716 patients with congenital adrenal hyperplasia owing to 21-hydroxylase deficiency. Mol Genet Metab 90:414.

252. Nordenström, Thilén A, Hagenfeldt L, et al. (1999). Genotyping is a valuable diagnostic complement to neonatal screening for congenital adrenal hyperplasia due to steroid 21-hydroxylase deficiency. J Clin Endocrinol Metab 84:1505.

253. Fitness J, Dixit N, Webster D, et al. (1999). Genotyping of CYP21, linked chromosome 6p markers, and a sex-specific gene in neonatal screening for congenital adrenal hyperplasia. J Clin Endocrinol Metab 84:960.

254. Wedell A, Chun X, Luthman H (1994). A steroid 21-hydroxylase allele concomitantly carrying four disease-causing mutations is not uncommon in the Swedish population. Hum Genet 93:204.

255. Witchel SF, Lee PA, Trucco M (1996). Who is a carrier? Detection of unsuspected mutations in 21-hydroxylase deficiency. Am J Med Genet 61:2.

256. Witchel SF, Smith R, Crivellaro CE, et al. (2000). CYP21 mutations in Brazilian patients with 21-hydroxylase deficiency. Hum Genet 106:414.

257. Rösler A, Lieberman E, Cohen T (1992). High frequency of congenital adrenal hyperplasia (classic 11β-hydroxylase deficiency) among Jews from Morocco. Am J Med Genet 42:827.

258. Rösler A, Cohen H (1995). Absence of steroid biosynthetic detects in heterozygote individuals for classic 11β-hydroxylase deficiency due to a R448H mutation in the CYP11B1 gene. J Clin Endocrinol Metab 80:3771.

259. Peter M, Sippell WG (1997). Evidence for endocrinological abnormalities in heterozygotes for adrenal 11β-hydroxylase deficiency of a family with the R448H mutation in the CYP11B1 gene. J Clin Endocrinol Metab 82:3506.

260. Merke DP, Tajima T, Chhabra A, et al. (1998). Novel CYP11B1 mutations in congenital adrenal hyperplasia due to steroid 11β-hydroxylase deficiency. J Clin Endocrinol Metab 83:270.

261. Curnow KM, Slutsker L, Vitek J, et al. (1993). Mutations in the CYP11B1 gene causing congenital adrenal hyperplasia and hypertension cluster in exons 6, 7, and 8. Proc Natl Acad Sci USA 90:4552.

262. White PC, Dupont J, New MI, et al. (1991). A mutation CYP11B1 (Arg448(His) associated with steroid 11-hydroxylase deficiency in Jews of Moroccan origin. J Clin Invest 87:1664.

263. Mornet E, Dupont J, Vitek A, et al. (1989). Characterization of two genes encoding human steroid 11β-hydroxylase(P-45011B). J Biol Chem 35:20961.

264. White PC (2001). Steroid 11 beta-hydroxylase deficiency and related disorders. Endocrinol Metab Clin North Am 30:61.

265. Simard J, Ricketts ML, Gingras S, Soucy P, Feltus FA, Melner MH (2005). Molecular biology of the 3beta-hydroxysteroid dehydrogenase/delta5-delta4 isomerase gene family. Endocr Rev 26:525.

266. Luu-The V, Lachance Y, Labrie C, et al. (1989). Full length cDNA structure and deduced amino acid sequence of human 3β-hydroxy-5-ene steroid dehydrogenase. Mol Endocrinol 3:1310.

267. Rhéaume E, Lachance Y, Zhao HF, et al. (1991). Structure and expression of a new cDNA encoding the almost exclusive 3β-hydroxysteroid dehydrogenase/(5-ene isomerase in human adrenals and gonads. Mol Endocrinol 5:1147.

268. Rhéaume E, Simard J, Morel Y, et al. (1992). Congenital adrenal hyperplasia due to point mutations in the type II 3β-hydroxysteroid dehydrogenase gene. Nat Genet 1:239.

269. Simard J, Rhéaume E, Sanchez R, et al. (1993). Molecular basis of congenital adrenal hyperplasia due to 3β-hydroxysteroid dehydrogenase deficiency. Mol Endocrinol 7:716.

270. Moisan AM, Ricketts ML, Tardy V, et al. (1999). New insight into the molecular basis of 3β-hydroxysteroid dehydrogenase deficiency: identification of eight mutations in the HSD3B2 gene in eleven patients from seven new families and comparison of the functional properties of twenty-five mutant enzymes. J Clin Endocrinol Metab 84:4410.

271. Gendrel D, Chaussain JL, Roger M, et al. (1979). Congenital adrenal hyperplasia due to blockade of 3β-hydroxysteroid dehydrogenase. Arch Fr Pédiatr 36:647.

272. Saez JM, De Peretti E, Morera AM, et al. (1971). Familial male pseudohermaphroditism with gynecomastia due to a testicular 17-ketosteroid reductase defect. I. Study in vivo. J Clin Endocr 32:604.

273. Boehmer ALM, Brinkmann AO, Sandkuijl LA, et al. (1999). 17β-hydroxysteroid dehydrogenase 3 deficiency: diagnosis, phenotypic variability, population genetics, and worldwide distribution of ancient and de novo mutations. J Clin Endocrinol Metab 84:4713.

274. Andersson S, Geissler WM, Wu L, et al. (1996). Molecular genetics and pathophysiology of 17-beta-hydroxysteroid dehydrogenase 3 deficiency. J Clin Endocr Metab 81:130.

275. Geissler WM, Davis DL, Wu L, et al. (1994). Male pseudohermaphroditism caused by mutations of testicular 17-beta-hydroxysteroid dehydrogenase 3. Nature Genet 7:34.

276. Lee YS, Kirk JM, Stanhope RG, Johnston DI, Harland S, Auchus RJ, et al. (2007). Phenotypic variability in 17beta-hydroxysteroid dehydrogenase-3 deficiency and diagnostic pitfalls. Clin Endocrinol (Oxford), [E-pub ahead of print].

277. Andersson S, Russell DW, Wilson JD (1996). 17β-hydroxysteroid dehydrogenase 3 deficiency. Trends Endocrinol Metab 7:121.

278. Gross DJ, Landau H, Kohn G, et al. (1986). Male pseudohermaphroditism due to 17β-hydroxysteroid dehydrogenase deficiency: Gender reassignment in early infancy. Acta Endocrinol 112:238.

279. Rösler A, Silverstein S, Abeliovich D (1996). A (R80Q) mutation in 17β-hydroxysteroid dehydrogenase type 3 gene among Arabs of Israel is associated with pseudohermaphroditism in males and normal asymptomatic females. J Clin Endocrinol Metab 81:1827.

280. Mendonça BB, Arnhold IJ, Bloise W, et al. (1999). 17β-hydroxysteroid dehydrogenase 3 deficiency in women. J Clin Endocrinol Metab 84:802.

281. Katz MD, Kligman I, Cai L-Q, et al. (1997). Paternity in intrauterine insemination with sperm from a man with 5-alpha-reductase-2 deficiency. New Eng J Med 336:994.

282. Andersson S, Berman DM, Jenkins EP, et al. (1991). Deletion of steroid 5-alpha-reductase gene in male pseudohermaphroditism. Nature 354:159.

283. Hochberg Z, Chayen R, Reiss N, et al. (1996). Clinical, biochemical, and genetic findings in a large pedigree of male and female patients with 5-alpha-reductase 2 deficiency. J Clin Endocr Metab 81:2821.

284. Peterson RE, Imperato-McGinley J, Gautier T, Shackleton C (1985). Male pseudohermaphroditism due to multiple defects in steroid biosynthetic microsomal mixed-function oxidases: A new variant of congenital adrenal hyperplasia. N Engl J Med 313:1182.

285. Shackleton C, Marcos J, Arlt W, Hauffa BP (2004). Prenatal diagnosis of P450 oxidoreductase deficiency (ORD): A disorder causing low pregnancy estriol, maternal and fetal virilization, and the Antley-Bixler syndrome phenotype. Am J Med Genet A 129:105.

286. Arlt W, Walker EA, Draper N, Ivison HE, Ride JP, Hammer F, et al. (2004). Congenital adrenal hyperplasia caused by mutant P450 oxidoreductase and human androgen synthesis: analytical study. Lancet 363:2128.

287. Fluck CE, Tajima T, Pandey AV, Arlt W, Okuhara K, Verge CF, et al. (2004). Mutant P450 oxidoreductase causes disordered steroidogenesis with and without Antley-Bixler syndrome. Nat Genet 36:228.

288. Huang N, Pandey AV, Agrawal V, Reardon W, Lapunzina PD, Mowat D, et al. (2005). Diversity and function of mutations in p450 oxidoreductase in patients with Antley-Bixler syndrome and disordered steroidogenesis. Am J Hum Genet 76:729.

289. Krone N, Dhir V, Ivison HE, Arlt W (2007). Congenital adrenal hyperplasia and P450 oxidoreductase deficiency. Clin Endocrinol (Oxford) 66:162.

290. Wilson JD, Auchus RJ, Leihy MW, Guryev OL, Estabrook RW, Osborn SM, et al. (2003). 5alpha-androstane-3alpha,17beta-diol is formed in tammar wallaby pouch young testes by a pathway involving 5alpha-pregnane-3alpha,17alpha-diol-20-one as a key intermediate. Endocrinology 144:575.

291. Shozu M, Akasofu K, Harada T, et al. (1991). A new cause of female pseudohermaphroditism: Placental aromatase deficiency. J Clin Endocrinol Metab 72:560.

292. Harada N, Ogawa H, Shozu M, et al. (1992). Genetic studies to characterize the origin of the mutation in placental aromatase deficiency. Am J Hum Genet 51:666.

293. Mullis PE, Yoshimura N, Kuhlmann B, et al. (1997). Aromatase deficiency in a female who is compound heterozygote for two new point mutations in the P450(arom) gene: Impact of estrogens on hypergonadotropic hypogonadism, multicystic ovaries, and bone densitometry in childhood. J Clin Endocr Metab 82:1739.

294. Ludwig M, Beck A, Wickert L, et al. (1998). Female pseudohermaphroditism associated with a novel homozygous G-to-A (V370-to-M) substitution in the P-450 aromatase gene. J Pediatr Endocrinol Metab 11:657.

295. Morishima A, Grumbach MM, Simpson ER, et al. (1995). Aromatase deficiency is male and female siblings caused by a novel mutation and the physiological role of estrogens. J Clin Endocrinol Metab 80:3689.

296. Jones ME, Boon WC, McInnes K, Maffei L, Carani C, Simpson ER (2007). Recognizing rare disorders: aromatase deficiency. Nat Clin Pract Endocrinol Metab 3:414.

297. Lin L, Ercan O, Raza J, Burren CP, Creighton SM, Auchus RJ, et al. (2007). Variable phenotypes associated with aromatase (CYP19) insufficiency in humans. J Clin Endocrinol Metab 92:982.

298. Chen S, Besman MJ, Sparkes RS, et al. (1988). Human aromatase: cDNA cloning, Southern blot analysis, and assignment of the gene to chromosome 15. DNA 7:27.

299. Lin L, Ercan O, Raza J, Burren CP, Creighton SM, Auchus RJ, et al. (2007). Variable phenotypes associated with aromatase (CYP19) insufficiency in humans. J Clin Endocrinol Metab 92:982.

300. Bulun SE (1996). Aromatase deficiency in women and men: would you have predicted the phenotypes? J Clin Endocr Metab 81:867.

301. Jones ME, Boon WC, Proietto J, Simpson ER (2006). Of mice and men: The evolving phenotype of aromatase deficiency. Trends Endocrinol Metab 17:55.

302. Vinggaard AM, Hnida C, Breinholt V, et al. (2000). Screening of selected pesticides for inhibition of CYP19 aromatase activity in vitro. Toxicol In Vitro 14:227.

303. Paris F, Jeandel C, Servant N, Sultan C (2006). Increased serum estrogenic bioactivity in three male newborns with ambiguous genitalia: A potential consequence of prenatal exposure to environmental endocrine disruptors. Environ Res 100:39.

304. Stillman RJ (1982). In vitro exposure to diethylstilbestrol: Adverse effects on the reproductive tract and reproductive performance in male and female offspring. Am J Obstet Gynecol 142:905.

305. Toppari J, Skakkebaek NE (1998). Sexual differentiation and environmental endocrine disrupters. Bailliere Clin Endocrinol Metab 12:143.

306. Ministry of Environment and Energy, Denmark (1995). Male reproductive health and environmental chemicals with estrogenic effects. Copenhagen: Danish Environmental Protection Agency, Miljoprojekt No 290.

307. Sharpe RM (1995). Another DDT connection. Nature 375:538.

308. Weidner IS, Moller H, Jensen TK, et al. (1998). Cryptorchidism and hypospadias in sons of gardeners and farmers. Environ Health Perspect 106:793.

309. Kester MHA, Bulduk S, Tibboel D, et al. (2000). Potent inhibition of estrogen sulfotransferase by hydroxylated PCB metabolites: a novel pathway explaining the estrogenic activity of PCBs. Endocrinol 141:1897.

310. Hughes IA, Deeb A (2006). Androgen resistance. Best Pract Res Clin Endocrinol Metab 20:577.

311. Migeon BR, Brown TR, Axelman J, et al. (1981). Studies of the locus for androgen receptor: Localization on the human X chromosome and evidence for homology with the Tfm locus in the mouse. Proc Natl Acad Sci USA 78:6339.

312. Brown CJ, Goss SJ, Lubahn DB, et al. (1989). Androgen receptor locus on the human X chromosome: Regional localization to Xq11-12 and description of a DNA polymorphism. Am J Hum Genet 44:264.

313. Hiort O, Sinnecker GH, Holterhus PM, Nitsche EM, Kruse K (1998). Inherited and de novo androgen receptor gene mutations: Investigation of single-case families. J Pediatr 132:939.

314. Kohler B, Lumbroso S, Leger J, Audran F, Grau ES, Kurtz F, et al. (2005). Androgen insensitivity syndrome: Somatic mosaicism of the androgen receptor in seven families and consequences for sex assignment and genetic counseling. J Clin Endocrinol Metab 90:106.

315. Deeb A, Hughes IA (2005). Inguinal hernia in female infants: A cue to check the sex chromosomes. BJU International 96:401.

316. Bouvattier C, Carel JC, Lecointre C, David A, Sultan C, Bertrand AM, et al. (2002). Postnatal changes of T, LH, and FSH in 46,XY infants with mutations in the AR gene. J Clin Endocrinol Metab 87:29.

317. Quigley CA (2002). The postnatal gonadotropin and sex steroid surge-insights from the androgen insensitivity syndrome. J Clin Endocrinol Metab 87:24.

318. Hannema SE, Scott IS, Rajpert-De Meyts E, Skakkebaek NE, Coleman N, Hughes IA (2006). Testicular development in the complete androgen insensitivity syndrome. J Pathol 208:518.

319. Brinkman AO, Faber PW, van Rooy HCJ, et al. (1989). The human androgen receptor: Domain structure, genomic organization and regulation of expression. J Steroid Biochem Molec Biol 34:307–310.

320. Lumbroso R, Beitel LK, Vasiliou DM, et al. (1997). Codon-usage variants in the polymorphic (GGN)n trinucleotide repeat of the human androgen receptor gene. Hum Genet 101:43.

321. Tut TG, Ghadessy FJ, Trifiro MA, et al. (1997). Long polyglutamine tracts in the androgen receptor are associated with reduced transactivation, impaired sperm production, and male infertility. J Clin Endocr Metab 82:3777.

322. Dowsing AT, Yong EL, Clark M, et al. (1999). Linkage between male infertility and trinucleotide repeat expansion in the androgen-receptor gene. Lancet 354:640.

323. Lim HN, Chen H, McBride S, et al. (2000). Longer polyglutamine tracts in the androgen receptor are associated with moderate to severe undermasculinized genitalia in XY males. Hum Molec Genet 9:829.

324. Beilin J, Ball EM, Favaloro JM, et al. (2000). Effect of the androgen receptor CAG repeat polymorphism on transcriptional activity: Specificity in prostate and non-prostate cell lines. J Mol Endocrinol 25:85–96.

325. Lee DK, Chang C (2003). Endocrine mechanisms of disease: Expression and degradation of androgen receptor, mechanism and clinical implication. J Clin Endocrinol Metab 88:4043.

326. Poukka H, Karvonen U, Janne OA, Palvimo JJ (2000). Covalent modification of the androgen receptor by small ubiquitin-like modifier 1 (SUMO-1). Proc Natl Acad Sci USA 97:14145.

327. Faus H, Haendler B (2006). Post-translational modifications of steroid receptors. Biomed Pharmacother 60:520.

328. Elhaji YA, Stoica I, Dennis S, Purisima EO, Trifiro MA (2006). Impaired helix 12 dynamics due to proline 892 substitutions in the androgen receptor are associated with complete androgen insensitivity. Hum Mol Genet 15:921.

329. Wong CI, Zhou ZX, Sar M, Wilson EM (1993). Steroid requirement for androgen receptor dimerization and DNA binding. Modulation by intramolecular interactions between the NH2-terminal and steroid binding domains. J Biol Chem 268:19004.

330. He B, Gampe RT Jr., Kole AJ, Hnat AT, Stanley TB, An G (2004). Structural basis for androgen receptor interdomain and coactivator interactions suggests a transition in nuclear receptor activation function dominance. Mol Cell 16:425.

331. Kemppainen JA, Lane MV, Sar M, et al. (1992). Androgen receptor phosphorylation, turnover, nuclear transport, and transcriptional activation. Specificity for steroids and antihormones. J Biol Chem 267:968.

332. Schoenmakers E, Verrijdt G, Peeters B, et al. (2000). Differences in DNA binding characteristics of the androgen and glucocorticoid receptors can determine hormone-specific responses. J Biol Chem 275:12290.

333. Quigley CA, Friedman KJ, Johnson A, et al. (1992). Complete deletion of the androgen receptor gene: Definition of the null phenotype of the androgen insensitivity syndrome and determination of carrier status. J Clin Endocr Metab 74:927.

334. McPhaul MJ, Griffin JE (1999). Male pseudohermaphroditism caused by mutations of the human androgen receptor. J Clin Endocrinol Metab 84:3435.

335. Rodien P, Mebarki F, Moszowicz I, et al. (1996). Different phenotypes in a family with androgen insensitivity caused by the same M708I point mutation in the androgen receptor gene. J Clin Endocrinol Metab 81:2994.

336. Elhaji YA, Wu JH, Gottlieb B, Beitel LK, Alvarado C, Batist G, (2004). An examination of how different mutations at arginine 855 of the androgen receptor result in different androgen insensitivity phenotypes. Mol Endocrinol 18:1876.

337. Kazemi-Esfarjani P, Beitel LK, Trifiro M, et al. (1993). Substitution of valine-865 by methionine or leucine in the human androgen receptor causes complete or partial androgen insensitivity, respectively with distinct androgen receptor phenotypes. Mol Endocrinol 7:37.

338. Holterhus P-M, Sinnecker GHG, Hiort O (2000). Phenotypic diversity and testosterone-induced normalization of mutant L712F androgen receptor function in a kindred with androgen insensitivity. J Clin Endocrinol Metab 85:3245.

339. La Spada AR, Wilson EM, Lubahn DB, et al. (1991). Androgen receptor gene mutations in X-linked spinal and bulbar muscular atrophy. Nature 352:77.

340. Katsuno M, Adachi H, Kume A, Li M, Nakagomi Y, Niwa H, et al. (2002). Testosterone reduction prevents phenotypic expression in a transgenic mouse model of spinal and bulbar muscular atrophy. Neuron 35:843.

341. Choong CS, Kemppainen JA, Zhou ZX, et al. (1996). Reduced androgen receptor gene expression with first exon CAG repeat expansion. Molec Endocr 10:1527.

342. Hutson JM, Davidson PM, Reece L, Baker ML, Zhou B (1994). Failure of gubernacular development in the persistent Mullerian duct syndrome allows herniation of the testes. Pediatr Surg Int 9:544.

343. Josso N, Belville C, di Clemente N, Picard JY (2005). AMH and AMH receptor defects in persistent Mullerian duct syndrome. Hum Reprod Update 11:351.

344. Li S, Qayyum A, Coakley FV, Hricak H (2000). Association of renal agenesis and mullerian duct anomalies. J Comput Assist Tomogr 24:829.

345. Duncan PA, Shapiro LR, Stangel JJ, et al. (1979). The MURCS association: Müllerian duct aplasia, renal duct aplasia, and cervicothoracic somite dysplasia. J Pediatr 95:399.

346. Wulfsberg EA, Grigsby TM (1990). Rokitansky sequence in association with the facio-auriculo-vertebral sequence: Part of a mesodermal malformation spectrum? Am J Med Genet 37:100.

347. Chityat D, Hahm SYE, Marion RW, et al. (1987). Further delineation of the McKusick-Kaufman hydrometrocolpospolydactyly syndrome. Am J Dis Child 141:1133.

348. Oppelt P, von Have M, Paulsen M, Strissel PL, Strick R, Brucker S, et al. (2007). Female genital malformations and their associated abnormalities. Fertil Steril 87:335.

349. Caron P, Chauvin S, Christin-Maitre S, et al. (1999). Resistance of hypogonadic patients with mutated GnRH receptor genes to pulsatile GnRH administration. J Clin Endocrinol Metab 84:990.

350. Semple RK, Achermann JC, Ellery J, Farooqi IS, Karet FE, Stanhope RG, et al. (2005). Two novel missense mutations in g protein-coupled receptor 54 in a patient with hypogonadotropic hypogonadism. J Clin Endocrinol Metab 90:1849.

351. Schwanzel-Fukuda M, Pfaff DW (1990). The migration of luteinizing hormone-releasing hormone (LHRH) neurons from the medial olfactory placode into the medial basal forebrain. Experientiat 46:956.

352. Schwanzel-Fukuda M, Bick D, Pfaff DW (1989). Luteinizing hormone releasing hormone (LHRH)-expressing cells do not migrate normally in an inherited hypogonadal (Kallmann) syndrome. Mol Brain Res 6:311.

353. Bick DP, Ballabio A (1993). Bringing Kallmann syndrome into focus. Am J Neuroradiol 14:852.

354. Franco B, Guioli S, Pragliola A, et al. (1991). A gene deleted in Kallmann's syndrome shares homology with neural cell adhesion and axonal path-finding molecules. Nature 353:529.

355. Maya-Nuñez G, Zenteno JC, Ulloa-Aguirre A, et al. (1998). A recurrent missense mutation in the KAL gene in patients with X-linked Kallmann's syndrome. J Clin Endocrinol Metab 83:1650.

356. De Roux N, Young J, Brailly-Tabard S, et al. (1999). The same molecular defects of the gonadotropin releasing hormone receptor determine a variable degree of hypogonadism in affected kindred. J Clin Endocrinol Metab 84:567.

357. de Roux N, Genin E, Carel JC, Matsuda F, Chaussain JL, Milgrom E (2003). Hypogonadotropic hypogonadism due to loss of function of the KiSS1-derived peptide receptor GPR54. Proc Natl Acad Sci USA 100:10972.

358. Seminara SB, Messager S, Chatzidaki EE, Thresher RR, Acierno JS Jr., Shagoury JK, et al. (2003). The GPR54 gene as a regulator of puberty. N Engl J Med 349:1614.

359. Dode C, Levilliers J, Dupont JM, De Paepe A, Le Du N, Soussi-Yanicostas N, et al. (2003). Loss-of-function mutations in FGFR1 cause autosomal dominant Kallmann syndrome. Nat Genet 33:463.

360. Dode C, Teixeira L, Levilliers J, Fouveaut C, Bouchard P, Kottler ML, et al. (2006). Kallmann syndrome: Mutations in the genes encoding prokineticin-2 and prokineticin receptor-2. PLoS Genet 2:e175.

361. Virtanen HE, Bjerknes R, Cortes D, Jorgensen N, Rajpert-De Meyts E, et al. (2007). Cryptorchidism: Classification, prevalence and long-term consequences. Acta Paediatr 96:611.

362. Virtanen HE, Tapanainen AE, Kaleva MM, Suomi AM, Main KM, Skakkebaek NE, et al. (2006). Mild gestational diabetes as a risk factor for congenital cryptorchidism. J Clin Endocrinol Metab 91:4862.

363. Virtanen HE, Cortes D, Rajpert-De Meyts E, Ritzen EM, Nordenskjold A, Skakkebaek NE, et al. (2007). Development and descent of the testis in relation to cryptorchidism. Acta Paediatr 96:622.

364. Tomboc M, Lee PA, Mitwally MF, et al. (2000). Insulin- like3/relaxin-like factor gene mutations are associated with cryptorchidism. J Clin Endocrinol Metab 85:4013.

365. Kolon TF, Wiener JS, Lewitton M, et al. (1999). Analysis of homeobox gene HOXA10 mutations in cryptorchidism. J Urol 161:275.

366. Scheffer IE, Hutson JM, Warne GL, et al. (1988). Extreme virilization in patients with congenital adrenal hyperplasia fails to induce descent of the ovary. Pediatr Surg Int 3:165.

367. Lee SMY, Hutson JM (1999). Effect of androgens on the cranial suspensory ligament and ovarian position. Anat Rec 255:306.

368. Cortes D, Thorup JM, Visfeldt J (2001). Cryptorchidism: Aspects of fertility and neoplasms. A study including data of 1,335 consecutive boys who underwent testicular biopsy simultaneously with surgery for cryptorchidism. Horm Res 55:21.

369. Huff DS, Fenig DM, Canning DA, Carr MG, Zderic SA, Snyder HM III (2001). Abnormal germ cell development in cryptorchidism. Horm Res 55:11.

370. Callegari C, Everett S, Ross M, Brasel JA (1987). Anogenital ratio: Measure of fetal virilization in premature and full-term newborn infants. J Pediatr 111:240.

371. Rink RC, Adams MC, Misseri R (2005). A new classification for genital amniguity and urogenital sinus anomalies. BJU Inter 95:638–642.

372. Riley WJ, Rosenbloom AL (1980). Clitoral size in infancy. J Pediatr 96:918.

373. Kocova M, Siegel SF, Wenger SL, et al. (1995). Detection of Y chromosome sequences in a 45X/46XXq- patient by Southern blot analysis of PCR-amplified DNA and fluorescent in situ hybridization (FISH). Am J Med Genet 55:483.

374. Torresani T, Grüters A, Scherz R, et al. (1994). Improving the efficacy of newborn screening for congenital adrenal hyperplasia by adjusting the cut-off level of 17β-hydroxyprogesterone to gestational age. Screening 3:77.

375. Van der Kamp HJ, Wit JM (2004). Neonatal screening for congenital adrenal hyperplasia. Eur J Endocrinol 151:U71.

376. Lee MM, Donahoe PK, Hasegawa T, et al. (1996). Mullerian inhibiting substance in humans: Normal levels from infancy to adulthood. J Clin Endocrinol Metab 81:571.

377. Guibourdenche J, Lucidarme N, Chevenne D, Rigal O, Nicolas M, Luton D, et al. (2003). Anti-Mullerian hormone levels in serum from human foetuses and children: Pattern and clinical interest. Mol Cell Endocrinol 211;55.

378. Rey RA, Belville C, Nihoul-Fekete C, et al. (1999). Evaluation of gonadal function in 107 intersex patients by means of serum anti-mullerian hormone measurement. J Clin Endocrinol Metab 84:627.

379. Bergada I, Milani C, Bedecarras P, Andreone L, Ropelato MG, Gottlieb S, et al. (2006). Time course of the serum gonadotropin surge, inhibins, and anti-Mullerian hormone in normal newborn males during the first month of life. J Clin Endocrinol Metab 91:4092.

380. Ng KL, Ahmed SF, Hughes IA (2000). Pituitary-gonadal axis in male undermasculinization. Arch Dis Child 82:54–58.

381. Jurgensen M, Hampel E, Hiort O, Thyen U (2006). "Any decision is better than none" decision-making about sex of rearing for siblings with 17beta-hydroxysteroid-dehydrogenase-3 deficiency. Arch Sex Behav 35:359.

382. Lerman SE, McAleer IM, Kaplan GW (2000). Sex assignment in cases of ambiguous genitalia and its outcome. Urol 55:8.

383. Imperato-McGinley J, Miller M, Wilson JD, Peterson RE, Shackleton C, Gajdusek DC (2001). A cluster of male pseudohermaphrodites with 5 alpha-reductase deficiency in Papua New Guinea. Clin Endocrinol (Oxford) 34:293.

384. Cohen-Kettenis PT (2005). Gender change in 46,XY persons with 5alpha-reductase-2 deficiency and 17beta-hydroxysteroid dehydrogenase-3 deficiency. Arch Sex Behav 34:399.

385. Carani C, Granata AR, Rochira V, Caffagni G, Aranda C, Antunez P, et al. (2005). Sex steroids and sexual desire in a man with a novel mutation of aromatase gene and hypogonadism. Psychoneuroendocrinology 30:413.

386. Glassberg KI (1999). Gender assignment and the pediatric urologist. J Urol 161:1308.

387. Meyer-Bahlburg HF, Dolezal C, Baker SW, Carlson AD, Obeid JS, New MI (2004). Prenatal androgenization affects gender-related behavior but not gender identity in 5-12-year old girls with congenital adrenal hyperplasia. Arch Sex Behav 33:97.

388. Berenbaum SA, Bailey JM (2003). Effects on gender identity of prenatal androgens and genital appearance: Evidence from girls with congenital adrenal hyperplasia. J Clin Endocrinol Metab 88:1102.

389. Long DN, Wisniewski AB, Migeon CJ (2004). Gender role across development in adult women with congenital adrenal hyperplasia due to 21-hydroxylase deficiency. J Pediatr Endocrinol Metab 17:1367.

390. Malouf MA, Migeon CJ, Carson KA, Petrucci L, Wisniewski AB (2006). Cognitive outcome in adult women affected by congenital adrenal hyperplasia due to 21-hydroxylase deficiency. Horm Res 65:142.

391. Hines M, Brook C, Conway GS (2004). Androgen and psychosexual development: Core gender identity, sexual orientation and recalled childhood gender role behavior in women and men with congenital adrenal hyperplasia (CAH). J Sex Res 41:75.

392. Dittmann RW, Kappes ME, Kappes MH (1992). Sexual behavior in adolescent and adult females with congenital adrenal hyperplasia. Psychoneuroendocrinology 17:153.

393. Zucker KJ, Bradley SJ, Oliver G, Blake J, Fleming S, Hood J (1996). Psychosexual development of women with congenital adrenal hyperplasia. Horm Behav 30:300.

394. Meyer-Bahlburg HF (2001). Gender and sexuality in classic congenital adrenal hyperplasia. Endocrinol Metab Clin North AM 30:155.

395. Wisniewski AB, Migeon CJ, Malouf MA, Geargart JP (2004). Psychosexual outcome in women affected by congenital adrenal hyperplasia due to 21-hydroxylase deficiency. J Urol 171:2497.

396. Meyer-Bahlberg HF, Dolezal C, Baker SW, Ehrhardt AA, New MI (2006). Gender development in women with congenital adrenal hyperplasia as a function of disorder severity. Arch Sex Behav 35: 667.

397. Meyer-Bahlburg HF, Gruen RS, New MI, Bell JJ, Morishima A, Shimshi M, et al. (1996). Gender change from female to male in classical congenital adrenal hyperplasia. Horm Behav 30:319.

398. Berenbaum SA, Korman Bryk K, Duck SC, Resnick SM (2004). Psychological adjustment in children and adults with congenital adrenal hyperplasia. J Pediatr 144:741.

399. Berenbaum SA, Bailey JM (2003). Effects on gender identity of prenatal androgens and genital appearance: Evidence from girls with congenital adrenal hyperplasia. J Clin Endocrinol Metab 88:1102.

400. Dayner JE, Lee PA, Houk CP (2004), Medical treatment of intersex: parental perspectives. J Urol 172:1762.

401. Baskin LS, Erol A, Li YW, Liu WH, Kurzrocl E, Cunha GR (1999). Anatomical studies of the human clitoris. J Urol 162:1015.

402. Akman Y, Lui W, Li YW, Baskin LS (2001). Penile anatomy under the pubic arch: Reconstructive implications. J Urol 166:225.

403. Creighton SM, Minto CL, Steele SJ (2001). Objective cosmetic and anatomical outcomes at adolescence of feminising surgery for ambiguous genitalia done in childhood. Lancet 358:124.

404. Gollu G, Yildiz RV, Bingol-Kologlu M, Yagmurlu A, Senyucel MF, Aktug T, et al. (2007). Ambiguous genitalia: an overview of 17 years' experience. J Pediatr Surg 42:840.

405. Fallat ME, Donahoe PK (2006). Intersex genetic anomalies with malignant potential. Curr Opin Pediatr 18:305.

406. Cools M, van Aerde K, Kersemaekers AM, Boter M, Drop SL, Wolffenbuttel KP, et al. (2005). Morphological and immunohisto-chemical differences between gonadal maturation delay and early germ cell neoplasia in patients with undervirilization syndromes. J Clin Endocrinol Metab 90:5295.

407. Cools M, Drop SL, Wolffenbuttel KP, Oosterhuis JW, Looijenga LH (2006). Germ cell tumors in the intersex gonad: Old paths, new directions, moving frontiers. Endocr Rev 27:468.

408. Mazzanti L, Cicognani A, Baldazzi L, Bergamaschi R, Scarano E, Strocchi S, et al. (2005). Gonadoblastoma in Turner syndrome and Y-chromosome-derived material. Am J Med Genet A 135:150.

409. Ankarberg-Lindgren C, Elfving M, Wikland KA, Norjavaara E (2001). Nocturnal application of transdermal estradiol patches produces levels of estradiol that mimic those seen at the onset of spontaneous puberty in girls. J Clin Endocrinol Metab 86:3039.

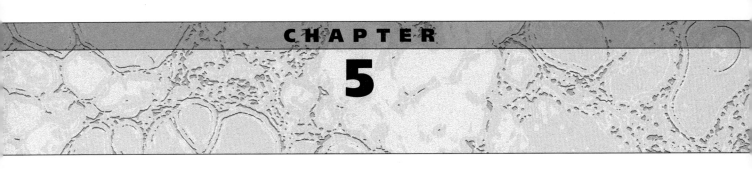

CHAPTER 5

Hypoglycemia in Neonates and Infants

DIVA D. DE LEÓN, MD • CHARLES A. STANELY, MD
• MARK A. SPERLING, MD

Introduction

One of the most important genetic and metabolic events that marks the transition from fetal to neonatal life is the adaptation from an environment that has a readily available and continuous source of glucose-maternal blood-to an environment in which glucose is provided in a limited and intermittent supply. The complex events involved in the maintenance of plasma glucose concentration must coordinate in their operation to avoid hypoglycemia and resultant damage to the central nervous system. A newborn or infant with hypoglycemia presents an urgent diagnostic and therapeutic challenge. The clinical features must be rapidly assessed and a plan of action developed based on the infant's age, maternal and parturition history, severity and persistence of hypoglycemic state, and all other relevant clinical clues.

PHYSIOLOGY OF PERINATAL GLUCOSE HOMEOSTASIS

A systematic approach to hypoglycemia in the newborn, infant, or child requires an appreciation of the central role of glucose in the body's fuel economy.[1] Glucose metabolism accounts for approximately half of basal daily energy needs. Glucose can be stored for energy in the form of glycogen and fat, and its carbon can be used for synthesis of protein and for structural components (such as cell membranes). The aerobic oxidation of glucose yields high energy by producing 38 mol of adenosine triphosphate (ATP) for each mole of glucose. Glucose is the principal metabolic fuel of the human brain.

All glucose extracted by the brain is oxidized, and thus cerebral glucose utilization parallels cerebral oxygen uptake. In infants of 5 weeks of age, cerebral glucose utilization already represents 71% to 93% of the adult level in most brain regions (ranging from 13 to 25 μmol/100g/min). At that age, the areas with highest metabolic rates for glucose are the sensorimotor cortex, thalamus, midbrain, brain stem, and cerebellar vermis. By 3 months, metabolic rates for glucose increase in the parietal, temporal, and occipital cortices, as well as in basal ganglia.

By 8 months, subsequent increases occur in the frontal cortex and various associative regions, concordant with the appearance of higher cortical and cognitive functions. Adult levels of cerebral glucose utilization (19 to 33 μmol/100g/min) are reached by 2 years of age, and continue to increase until 3 to 4 years of age—when they reach values ranging from 49 to 65 μmol/100g/min that are maintained to approximately 9 years of age. They then begin to decline, reaching adult levels by the end of the second decade.[2] Glucose uptake by the brain occurs by means of a carrier-mediated facilitated diffusion process that is glucose concentration dependent, as well as energy-, Na^+-, and insulin-independent.[3]

This process is mediated by facilitative glucose transporter (GLUT) proteins. The human genome contains 14 members of the GLUT family. Characterization of the different members has provided new insights into the regulation and significance of glucose transport and its disorders in various tissues[3-5] (Table 5-1). Several members of the GLUT family have been detected in the brain. GLUT1 is located at the blood-brain barrier,[6] and although some neurons express GLUT2 and GLUT4 the majority use GLUT3 as their primary transporter.[7]

Of major importance is the confirmation at a molecular level of biochemical evidence that glucose entry into brain cells and its subsequent metabolism are not dependent on insulin but rather are dependent on circulating arterial glucose concentration.[8] Therefore, a decrease in arterial glucose concentration or a defect in the glucose transport mechanism of the brain will result in intracerebral glucopenia and low cerebrospinal fluid glucose concentration (hypoglycorrhachia)—with attendant symptoms and signs of cerebral glucopenia as subsequently described.[8-10]

To prevent circulating arterial blood glucose from decreasing precipitously under normal physiologic conditions, and therefore to prevent impairment of vital function that depends on cerebral glucose metabolism, an elaborate defense mechanism has evolved.[1] This defense against hypoglycemia is integrated by the autonomic nervous system and by hormones that act synergistically to enhance glucose production through enzymatic modulation of glycogenolysis and gluconeogenesis while simultaneously limiting peripheral glucose use.[11,12] Thus, hypoglycemia is the result of a defect in one or several of the complex interactions that maintain a normal range of glucose concentration, preventing its fall to less than 70 mg/dL during fasting and its rise to more than 140 mg/dL during feeding.

These mechanisms are not fully developed in neonates, in whom there is an abrupt transition from intrauterine life (characterized by dependence on transplacental glucose supply) to extrauterine life (characterized ultimately by the autonomous ability to maintain precise glucose balance).[13] A neonate delivered prematurely whose enzymatic machinery mechanisms are not yet fully developed and expressed or one whose placental insufficiency resulted in intrauterine growth retardation with limited tissue nutrient deposits may be particularly vulnerable to hypoglycemia,[14] often with consequences to subsequent cerebral development or function.[15,16] Genetically determined defects in enzyme function or hormones are also relatively common,[17] and therefore hypoglycemia is an important cause of morbidity in the newborn period.[18] The key element in the transition to extrauterine life is separation from the placenta and the adaptations that follow.[13,19]

INTEGRATION OF GLUCOSE HOMEOSTASIS IN THE FETUS: SUBSTRATES, ENZYMES, HORMONES, AND RECEPTORS

Under normal nonstressed conditions, fetal glucose is derived entirely from the mother through placental transfer.[20,21] In humans, the evidence remains indirect in that infusion of stable nonradioactive glucose isotopes to steady-state-specific activity in the mother during labor yields an indistinguishable glucose specific activity in fetal arterial blood at birth.[22] This indicates that maternal and fetal glucose concentrations behave as a single pool, with no endogenous glucose production in the fetus.

TABLE 5-1

Characterization of Glucose Transporters

Subfamily	Name	Tissue Distribution	Glucose Transport Activity	Location of Human Gene	Regulation by Insulin
Class I	GLUT1	Erythrocytes, brain (blood-brain barrier), placenta	Erythrocyte:asymmetric carrier with exchange acceleration; $K_m\sim$5-30mmol/L (variable):Vmax (influx) < Vmax (efflux)	1p35-p31.3	Zero to minimal
	GLUT2	Liver, islet cells, kidney, small intestine	Low-affinity. Liver:simple, symmetric carrier; $K_m\sim$60mmol/L;intestine: asymmetric carrier: Vmax (efflux) < Vmax (influx)	3q26.1-q26.2	Zero to minimal
	GLUT3	Brain (neuronal), testis, placenta	High-affinity. Exchange $K_m\sim$10mmol/L	12p13.3	Zero
	GLUT4	Adipocytes, muscle	High-affinity. Adipocyte:simple, symmetric carrier; $K_m\sim$2-5mmol/L	17p13	Dependent on insulin
	GLUT14	Testis	?	12p13.31	?
Class II	GLUT5	Testis, small intestine, kidney	No glucose transport activity, fructose transporter	1p36.2	?
	GLUT7	Small intestine (enterocytes brush border membrane), colon, testis, prostate	High-affinity transport for glucose (K_m=0.3mM)	1p36.2	?
	GLUT9	Liver, kidney. Expressed at preimplantation stage in mouse	Proven glucose transport activity	4p16-p15.3	?
	GLUT11	Pancreas, kidney, placenta, heart, skeletal muscle	Low affinity for glucose (possible fructose transporter)	22q11.2	Mediates insulin-stimulated glucose uptake in embryos
Class III	GLUT6	Brain, spleen, leukocytes	Low affinity for glucose	9q34	?
	GLUT8	Testis, brain (neuronal), adipocytes, preimplantation embryos	High-affinity glucose transporter (possible multifunctional transporter)	9q33.3	?
	GLUT10	Liver, pancreas	Glucose transport activity with $K_m\sim$3mmol/L	20q13.1-q12	?
	GLUT12	Heart, prostate, breast cancer	Proven glucose transporter activity	6q23.2	?
	GLUT13 (HMIT)	Brain	No glucose transport activity, myo-inositol and related isomers transporter	12q12	?

There are important clinical consequences implicit in these findings. For example, acute hypoglycemia in a mother with diabetes will result in acute hypoglycemia in the fetus—with no ability to acutely compensate for the abrupt reduction in blood glucose supply.

The transfer of glucose across the placenta to the fetus occurs by facilitated diffusion along a concentration gradient. GLUT1 has been identified as the major isoform in the human placenta,[23] although other members of the family are expressed. Of note is the fact that the placental GLUTs are not regulated by insulin, suggesting that maternal glucose concentration and (more specifically) the maternal-fetal glucose gradient is the major determinant of placental glucose transfer independent of the maternal insulin concentration perfusing the placenta.[24,25]

Observations in infants with mutations of glucokinase, the glucose sensor of pancreatic beta cells, indicate that the physiologic "set point" for plasma glucose in the fetus is identical to that of older children and adults. Fetal glucose metabolism depends directly on simultaneous effects of fetal plasma glucose and insulin concentrations, which in experiments in near-term sheep have been shown to act additively to enhance fetal glucose utilization and oxidation to CO_2 according to saturation kinetics. The relative proportion of glucose oxidized in short-term studies does not change significantly over the physiologic range of fetal glucose utilization rates, indicating little effect of glucose or insulin on intracellular pathways of glucose metabolism.[26]

Although basal plasma concentrations of insulin and glucagon in the fetus are similar to those in the mother, their regulation differs. Acute hypoglycemia or hyperglycemia does not markedly affect fetal insulin or glucagon secretion. Long-term exposure to hyperglycemia is required to augment insulin secretion and promote glucagon suppression.[27,28] Conversely, chronic starvation of the mother will depress maternal and fetal glucose concentrations and cause diminished insulin but greater glucagon release in the fetus. This sluggishness of intrauterine pancreatic hormone secretion is in part related to immaturity of the cyclic adenosine monophosphate (AMP)-generating system, which occasionally extends into the newborn period.[28]

Studies in animals, principally in fetal sheep, indicate that a proportion of glucose used is oxidized and the remainder is used for tissue accretion.[29] Hyperinsulinemia in the fetus increases total glucose use, whereas the proportions used for oxidation and tissue accretion remain constant.[29] A large proportion of glucose use appears to be relatively independent of insulin and is markedly glucose concentration dependent.[30] Likewise, glucagon in physiologic doses does not increase fetal hepatic glucose output—and pharmacologic doses are required to demonstrate an effect.[31,32] In contrast to glucagon, at relatively physiologic concentrations catecholamines mobilize fetal glucose and free fatty acids by adrenergic mechanisms—reflecting the existence of functionally linked adrenergic receptors in fetal liver and adipose tissues.[33] In addition, in high doses catecholamines can exert appropriate modulation of fetal pancreatic hormone secretion by inhibiting insulin and stimulating glucagon release.[34,35]

CHANGES AT BIRTH

The acute interruption of maternal glucose transfer to the fetus at delivery imposes an immediate need to mobilize endogenous glucose. At least three related events facilitate this transition: changes in hormones, changes in their receptors, and changes in key enzyme activity. In all mammalian species, there is a threefold to fivefold abrupt increase in glucagon concentration within minutes to hours of birth.[19] Insulin, on the other hand, usually falls initially and remains in the basal range for several days without demonstrating the usual brisk response to physiologic stimuli such as glucose.

A dramatic surge in spontaneous catecholamine secretion is also characteristic of several mammalian species.[35] These changes in epinephrine, glucagon, and insulin may be interrelated because epinephrine is capable of stimulating glucagon and suppressing insulin release.[35] In addition, epinephrine can augment growth hormone secretion by α-adrenergic mechanisms—and growth hormone levels are considerably elevated at birth.

Acting synergistically, these hormonal changes at birth (characterized by high epinephrine, high glucagon, high growth hormone, and low insulin levels) would be expected to mobilize glucose through glycogenolysis and gluconeogenesis to activate lipolysis and promote ketogenesis.[1] This appears to be true because after birth in the human newborn the plasma glucose concentration declines, reaching a nadir by 1 hour of age and then rising spontaneously to plateau levels reached between 2 and 4 hours.[36] Liver glycogen stores become rapidly depleted within hours of birth, and gluconeogenesis from alanine (a major gluconeogenic amino acid) can account for approximately 10% of glucose turnover in the human newborn within several hours of age.[37] Free fatty acid concentrations also rise sharply in concert with the surges in glucagon and epinephrine and are followed later by an increase in ketone bodies. In this way, glucose can be spared for brain use—whereas free fatty acids and ketones provide alternative fuel sources for muscle and provide essential gluconeogenic cofactors such as acetyl-CoA and NADH from the hepatic fatty oxidation required to drive gluconeogenesis.[38]

In the early postnatal period, responses of the endocrine pancreas favor glucagon secretion at the relative expense of insulin secretion—perhaps because there is little need for acute insulin responses (AIRs) and so that blood glucose concentration can be protected. In the fetus, the high insulin receptor number tends to facilitate anabolic processes and growth while limiting gluconeogenesis—whereas a low glucagon receptor number (with incomplete functional linkage to cyclic AMP) further limits catabolic events in utero. In contrast, in the newborn there is a fall in insulin receptor number associated with a fall in insulin at a time when glucagon secretion rises abruptly and glucagon receptors become functional.

These coordinate changes serve to mobilize glucose and other fuel stores after the interruption of the maternal supply. The surge in epinephrine secretion and its coupling with appropriate receptors also augment glucose production and lipolysis. Key enzymes involved in glucose production change dramatically in the perinatal period. Thus, there is a rapid fall in glycogen synthase activity—whereas that of phosphorylase rises sharply after delivery.[14,39-41] The rate-limiting enzyme for gluconeogenesis, phosphoenolpyruvate carboxykinase (PEPCK), rises dramatically after birth—activated in part by the surge in glucagon and fall in insulin.[42] This framework is consistent with the insulin and with other hormonal and enzyme responses to acute hypoglycemia in the adult.[1] Failure of these changes to occur may lead to failure of extrauterine autonomy in newborn glucose metabolism.

HORMONAL AND METABOLIC SYSTEMS OF FASTING ADAPTATION

Hypoglycemia in neonates, infants, and children is essentially always a problem with fasting adaptation. Postprandial (reactive) hypoglycemia is exceedingly rare and is limited to a few unusual situations, such as postprandial hypoglycemia after Nissen fundoplication or hereditary fructose intolerance. Therefore, a consideration of the major hormonal and metabolic pathways that maintain fuel homeostasis during fasting provides an important framework for understanding the causes, diagnosis, and treatment of different forms of hypoglycemia.

The physiology of fasting homeostasis in infants is identical to that of adults, although the timing of adaptation is faster owing to the greater metabolic demands of infants and children. Table 5-2 outlines the sources of potential fasting fuels in an adult man with a metabolic rate of 1,800 kcal/day.[43] Note that hepatic glycogenolysis is sufficient to meet energy requirements for only a few hours. Beyond that time, glucose must be produced by hepatic gluconeogenesis from precursors such as amino acids, glycerol, and lactate recycled from glycolysis.

TABLE 5-2

Fuel Composition of Normal Adult

Fuel	Kg	Calories
Tissues		
Fat (adipose triglyceride)	15	141,000
Protein (mainly muscle)	6	24,000
Glycogen (muscle)	0.150	600
Glycogen (liver)	0.075	300
		165,900
Circulating Fuels		
Glucose (extracellular fluid)	0.020	80
Free fatty acids (plasma)	0.0003	3
Triglycerides (plasma)	0.003	30
		113

From Cahill GF (1970). Starvation in man. N Engl J Med 282:668.

The major source of gluconeogenic precursors is muscle protein. Although the pool of muscle protein is large, it is all required for body function and thus in contrast to stores of glycogen and fat there are no "reserves" of protein to draw on during fasting. To spare the use of essential protein during extended fasting, glucose consumption must be suppressed by switching on the mobilization and oxidation of fatty acids from adipose triglyceride stores.

Glucose homeostasis is very limited in children compared with adults, in part because of their smaller reserves of liver glycogen and muscle protein but also because of their relatively larger rates of glucose consumption due to their larger brain-to-body-mass ratio. For example, the fuel stores of a 10-kg infant are only 15% of those of an adult. However, the caloric needs are 60% of those of an adult and glucose turnover rates per kilogram are two- to threefold greater. Major organs (such as skeletal muscle) can readily oxidize free fatty acids, released from adipose tissue lipolysis, in place of glucose and thus limit the need for gluconeogenesis.

Brain cannot directly use free fatty acids, because they do not pass the blood-brain barrier. However, the brain can substitute glucose consumption with the ketones acetoacetate and β-hydroxybutyrate—which are released by the liver as the end product of hepatic fatty acid oxidation. Thus, as shown in Figure 5-1 the essential metabolic pathways of fasting adaptation are hepatic glycogenolysis, hepatic gluconeogenesis, adipose tissue lipolysis, and fatty acid oxidation and ketogenesis.[43] The key enzymatic steps in these pathways are shown in Figure 5-2. A defect in any one of these four pathways impairs fasting adaptation and can lead to fasting hypoglycemia.

The four metabolic systems of fasting adaptation (glycogenolysis, gluconeogenesis, lipolysis, and ketogenesis) are regulated by a fifth system: endocrine control. The most important hormone for control of fasting adaptation is insulin, which acts to inhibit all four of the metabolic systems (Table 5-3). These inhibitory effects of insulin are opposed by several counter-regulatory hormones, which as shown in Table 5-3 have overlapping effects on specific fasting metabolic pathways. Excessive secretion of insulin or deficiency of one or more counter-regulatory hormones can result in fasting hypoglycemia.

The operation of the metabolic and endocrine systems of fasting adaptation is evidenced by the changes in circulating levels of metabolic fuels and hormones during a fast. As shown in Figure 5-3, in young infants a 24-hour fast is accompanied by a gradual fall in glucose levels as hepatic glycogen stores are depleted, a progressive fall in

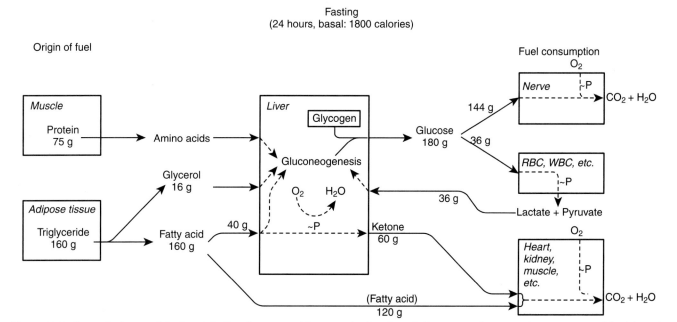

Figure 5-1. General scheme of fuel metabolism in a normal human who has fasted. Shown are the two primary sources of fuel (muscle and adipose tissue) and the three types of fuel consumers that use fatty acids and ketones: nerve, pure glycolyzers [e.g., red blood cells (RBCs) and white blood cells (WBCs), and the remainder of the body (e.g., heart, kidney, and skeletal muscle). ~P represents energy production. [From Cahill GF (1970). Starvation in man. N Engl J Med 282:668. Copyright © 1970 Massachusetts Medical Society. All rights reserved.]

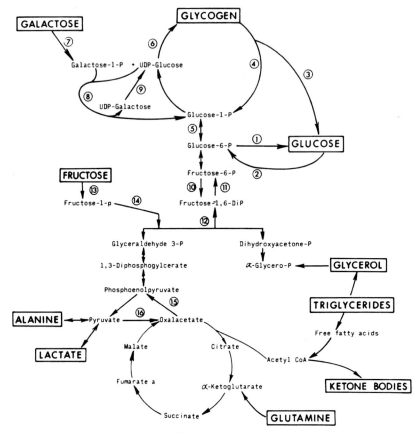

Figure 5-2. Key metabolic pathways of intermediary metabolism. Disruption of the elements of these pathways may be pathogenetic in the development of hypoglycemia. Not shown is the hormonal control of these pathways. Indicated are (1) glucose 6-phosphatase, (2) glucokinase, (3) amylo-1,6-glucosidase, (4) phosphorylase, (5) phosphoglucomutase, (6) glycogen synthetase, (7) galactokinase, (8) galactose 1-phosphate uridyl transferase, (9) uridine diphosphogalactose-4-epimerase, (10) phosphofructokinase, (11) fructose 1,6-diphosphatase, (12) fructose 1,6-diphosphate aldolase, (13) fructokinase, (14) fructose 1-phosphate aldolase, (15) phosphoenolpyruvate carboxykinase, and (16) pyruvate carboxylase. UDP is uridine diphosphate. [From Pagliara AS, et al. (1973). Hypoglycemia in infancy and childhood. J Pediatr 82(3): 365-79 and 82(4):558-77.]

TABLE 5-3

Hormonal Regulation of Fasting Metabolic Systems

Counter-Regulatory Hormone	Hepatic Glycogenolysis	Hapatic Gluconeogenesis	Adipose Tissue Lipolysis	Hepatic Ketogenesis
Insulin	Inhibits	Inhibits	Inhibits	Inhibits
Glucagon	Stimulates			Stimulates
Cortisol		Stimulates		
Growth Hormone			Stimulates	
Epinephrin	Stimulates	Stimulates	Stimulates	Stimulates

concentrations of gluconeogenic substrate (e.g., lactate, alanine) as they are used for hepatic gluconeogenesis, a brisk rise in free fatty acids as lipolysis is activated, and a dramatic rise in β-hydroxybutyrate (the major ketone) as hepatic ketogenesis is turned on.[1,44]

Levels of insulin diminish to less than 2 μU/mL, whereas there is a rise in the four major counter-regulatory hormones (catecholamines, glucagon, cortisol, and growth hormone) as the plasma glucose level falls. These hormonal changes

lead to a reversal of metabolic pathways from synthesis to breakdown in order to maintain glucose homeostasis. When insulin concentration is 2 μU/mL or greater at a time when blood glucose concentration is 50 mg/dL or less, there is a hyperinsulinemic state reflecting failure of the mechanisms that normally result in suppression of insulin secretion during fasting or hypoglycemia.[45-47]

Thus, a snapshot of the integrity of the metabolic and endocrine fasting systems can easily be obtained by

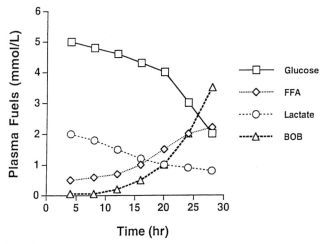

Figure 5-3. Changes in major metabolic fuels during fasting in a normal infant. Note that plasma glucose declines toward hypoglycemic values by 24 hours as hepatic glycogen reserves are depleted. The level of lactate, a representative gluconeogenic substrate, declines gradually during the fast. Late in fasting, levels of plasma free fatty acids (FFA) increase as lipolysis is activated—followed by an increase in β-hydroxybutyrate as rates of hepatic fatty acid oxidation and ketogenesis increase.

measuring the plasma levels of the major fuels and hormones at the end of a fast, when the blood glucose approaches hypoglycemic levels ("critical samples"). The use of these critical samples in diagnosing the cause of hypoglycemia is discussed at the end of the chapter.

The key hormone governing glycogen synthesis during and immediately after meals is insulin. Likewise, glycogen breakdown (and later, gluconeogenesis) depends on a low insulin concentration. The control of insulin secretion, its metabolic effects, and its mechanisms of action are detailed in Chapter 10. In this chapter, the following requires emphasis. The neural, hormonal, and metabolic changes (including the rise in blood glucose associated with feeding) lead to a rise in insulin. This rise in insulin serves to modulate the rise in blood glucose concentration and eventually to lower it through the activation of glycogen synthesis, enhancement of peripheral glucose uptake, and inhibition of gluconeogenesis. In addition, insulin stimulates lipid synthesis—simultaneously curtailing lipolysis and ketogenesis.

Table 5-3 summarizes the synergistic effects of the counter-regulatory hormones on key metabolic pathways and insulin action. There is a hierarchic redundancy in the interaction of these counter-regulatory hormones that provides a margin of safety ("fail-safe mechanism") if only one counter-regulatory hormone is impaired. Epinephrine and glucagon are quick acting, each signaling its effects by activation of cyclic AMP. Deficiencies of glucagon, as occurs in long-standing type I diabetes mellitus, can be largely compensated for by an intact autonomic nervous system with appropriate α- and β-adrenergic effects. Conversely, autonomic failure can be largely compensated for if glucagon secretion remains intact.[1]

Nevertheless, the defense against insulin-induced hypoglycemia is impaired by deficiency of glucagon or catecholamines—with hypoglycemia ensuing quite rapidly. Similarly, growth hormone deficiency can be compensated for in part by intact cortisol secretion (and vice versa). However, deficiency of either impairs the defense against insulin-induced hypoglycemia. Congenital

or acquired deficiencies in these hormones may result in hypoglycemia, which will occur when endogenous glucose production cannot be mobilized to meet energy needs in the postabsorptive state (i.e., 8 to 12 hours after meals or during fasting). Combined deficiency of several hormones, as occurs in hypopituitarism, may result in a hypoglycemia that is more severe or appears earlier during fasting than might occur with isolated hormone deficiency.

The intricate physiologic regulation that maintains glucose homeostasis provides a diagnostic framework with which to anticipate the phenotypes of infants with hypoglycemia of varying causes. The deficiency of substrates, an excess of insulin or a deficiency of hormones, and the absence, delay, deficiency, or missed timing of the development of activity of enzymes or transporters will affect the presentation of infantile hypoglycemia. Thus, this detailed presentation of the events leading to, involving, and after parturition allows rapid and specific diagnostic considerations to be entertained and to evolve to an appropriate treatment.

DEFINITION OF HYPOGLYCEMIA IN NEONATES AND INFANTS

The classic definition of symptomatic hypoglycemia is "Whipple's triad" (i.e., symptoms typical of hypoglycemia, a blood glucose value less than 50 mg/dL during symptoms, and relief of symptoms with treatment to raise the blood glucose level into the normal range). These three criteria were originally used for diagnosing insulinomas in adults but apply well to diagnosis of any form of hypoglycemia. In infants, children, and adults, the normal range for plasma glucose in the postabsorptive state equals plasma glucose levels between 70 and 100 mg/dL.

A plasma glucose level of 50 mg/dL is conventionally used for diagnosing hypoglycemia. Note that this value is a very conservative threshold, well below the threshold for hormonal and cognitive deficits to avoid overdiagnosing hypoglycemia. Falling glucose levels elicit a typical sequence of responses: plasma insulin levels decrease when plasma glucose falls to the range of 80 to 85 mg/dL; glucagon secretion increases when plasma glucose levels are in the range of 65 to 70 mg/dL; epinephrine, cortisol, and growth hormone responses are activated in the range of 65 to 70 mg/dL; acute symptoms may appear in the range of 50 to 55 mg/dL; and cognition is impaired when levels fall below 50 mg/dL.[1]

In some disorders, such as defects in ketogenesis, signs and symptoms may begin to appear during fasting at plasma glucose levels of 60 mg/dL. On the other hand, some patients (those with glucose 6-phosphatase deficiency) may have few symptoms of neuroglycopenia at plasma glucose levels as low as 20 to 30 mg/dL because their high plasma levels of lactate provide an alternative substrate for the brain. Thus, plasma glucose levels between 50 and 70 mg/dL should be regarded as suboptimal and below the goal for therapy for hypoglycemia.

Pediatric endocrinologists should be aware that there continues to be controversy about whether the previously cited standards for normal and abnormal plasma glucose levels should apply in the newborn period.[48,49] Because the risk for low blood glucose levels is high in neonates, especially in the first day after birth, it has been traditional to accept lower standards for hypoglycemia in newborns. The major rationale for this is statistical (i.e., low glucose is so frequent it must be "normal"). However, the authors do not recommend using lower standards for glucose in neonates. Instead, we use the same definition for hypoglycemia and the same targets for treatment of hypoglycemia in neonates as in older children. This is especially true for the diverse groups of neonates who have congenital hyperinsulinism (e.g., birth asphyxia, small for gestational age birth weight, maternal diabetes, genetic defects) because they lack alternative fuels, such as ketones, for brain metabolism when glucose levels are low.

There are a number of potential artifacts that can interfere with measuring glucose levels in neonates and infants (Table 5-4). Whole-blood glucose concentrations are 10% to 15% lower than plasma glucose levels because of lower erythrocyte versus plasma glucose concentrations. Blood samples that are not processed promptly can have erroneously low glucose levels, owing to glycolysis by red and white blood cells. At room temperature, the decline of whole-blood glucose can be 5 to 7 mg/dL/hr. The use of inhibitors, such as fluoride, in collection tubes avoids this problem.

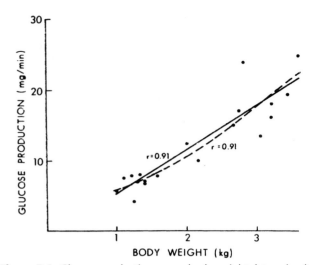

Figure 5-4. Glucose production versus body weight determined in 19 newborns with the use of stable isotopic techniques. These studies provide support for the calculated rates of glucose administration required to correct hypoglycemia. [From Bier DM, Leake RD, Haymond MW, et al. (1977). Measurement of "true" glucose production rates in infancy and childhood with 6,6-dideuteroglucose. Diabetes 26:1016.]

TABLE 5-4

Factors Affecting Measurement of Blood Glucose Concentration

- Whole-blood versus plasma glucose concentration (plasma is ~10%-15% higher)
- Duration between sample collection and sample measurement
- Presence or absence of glycolytic inhibitors in collection tubes
- Sample collection from indwelling lines without adequate flushing

Compiled from Sacks DB (1994). Carbohydrates. In Burtis CA, Ashwood ER (eds.), *Tietz textbook of clinical chemistry, Second edition.* Philadelphia: WB Saunders.

Hospital bedside glucose meters and similar home glucose meters are less precise than clinical laboratory methods and can be expected to have an error range of 10% to 15%. These methods are also prone to errors, such as outdated strips or short-sampling—most of which result in falsely low glucose values. For this reason, bedside monitors can be used for screening purposes—but any glucose value below 60 mg/dL should be verified in the clinical laboratory. Falsely low (or high) glucose values may occur with samples drawn from indwelling lines without adequate flushing of the saline (or glucose) infusate.

If a plasma glucose value below 50 mg/dL is verified, treatment should immediately be provided. Plasma glucose values below 60 mg/dL should be rechecked and treatment considered, if confirmed to be below 60 mg/dL. Symptomatic infants and neonates should be treated with intravenous dextrose (0.2 g/kg bolus, followed by infusion at 5 to 10 mg/kg/min). These rates approximate the normal hepatic glucose production rates in neonates and young infants (Figure 5-4). Asymptomatic neonates with plasma glucose levels below 50 mg/dL may be treated with oral glucose, but only if there is good reason to believe the problem is a transient one that will not recur. This applies essentially only to otherwise normal neonates during the first 12 to 24 hours after birth who have delayed feedings, such as with initiation of breastfeeding. Beyond the first day of life, all neonates with verified plasma glucose below 60 mg/dL should be suspected of having a hypoglycemic disorder.

CLINICAL SYMPTOMS AND SIGNS ASSOCIATED WITH HYPOGLYCEMIA

The clinical features of hypoglycemia in infants may be associated with both adrenergic and neuroglycopenic components (Table 5-5). Symptoms are often quite subtle,

TABLE 5-5

Symptoms of Spontaneous Hypoglycemia and Hypoglycemia in Infancy

Spontaneous Hypoglycemia		Hypoglycemia in Infancy
Symptoms Due in Part to Activation of Autonomic Nervous System Associated Epinephrin Release (Usually Associated with Rapid Decline in Blood Glucose Level)	Symptoms Due to Decreased Cerebral Glucose and Oxygen Use (Usually with Slow Decline in Blood Glucose Level and/or Severe Prolonged Hypoglycemia)	
Sweating	Headache	Cyanotic episodes
Shakiness, trembling	Visual disturbances	Apnea
Tachycardia	Lethargy, lassitude	"Respiratory distress"
Anxiety, nervousness	Restlessness, irritability	Refusal to feed
Weakness	Difficulty with speech and thinking, inability to	Brief myoclonic jerks
Hunger	concentrate	Wilting spells
Nausea, vomiting	Mental confusion	Nausea, vomiting
	Somnolence, stupor, prolonged sleep	Somnolence
	Loss of consciousness, coma	Subnormal temperature
	Hypothermia	Sweating
	Twitching, convulsions, "epilepsy"	
	Bizarre neurologic signs	
	Motor	
	Sensory	
	Loss of intellectual ability	
	Personality changes	
	Bizarre behavior	
	Outburst of tempor	
	Psychological disintegration	
	Manic behavior	
	Depression	
	Psychoses	
	Permanent mental of neurologic damage	

and a high index of clinical suspicion must be maintained. Therefore, any alteration in clinical status in a newborn that suggests a change in neurologic behavior, fall in temperature, change in feeding pattern, or presence of tremors must be considered a possible initial presentation of a hypoglycemic episode. Seizures must always be considered a possible manifestation of hypoglycemia.

Classification of Hypoglycemias

A logical approach to diagnosis and treatment must analyze a hypoglycemic event as a maladaptation to fasting. The classification scheme represented in Table 5-6 is based on this approach.

TRANSIENT NEONATAL HYPOGLYCEMIA

Developmental Immaturity of Fasting Adaptation

During the first day of life, normal infants are susceptible to hypoglycemia—especially if fasted after birth for any length of time. As shown in Figure 5-5, 10% of normal appropriate-for-gestational-age term neonates can develop plasma glucose values below 30 mg/dL when the first feeding is delayed for 6 hours after birth.[50] This high risk of hypoglycemia reflects immaturity of several of the fasting systems immediately after birth. As reported by Lubchenco and Bard, whereas plasma glucose levels fell below 50 mg/dL in one-third of term infants in the first 6 hours after delivery by the second day of life the frequency of glucose levels below 50 mg/dL was less than 0.5% and only occurred in small-for-gestational-age infants.[50] As these observations illustrate, the fasting systems mature very quickly after birth.

Studies in normal infants during the first postnatal fast indicate that their high susceptibility to hypoglycemia is associated with developmental lags in the capacity for both hepatic gluconeogenesis and ketogenesis.[51] This is consistent with studies in the guinea pig and rat, which show that hepatic phosphoenolpyruvate carboxykinase (one of the four gluconeogenic enzymes) as well as carnitine palmitoyl-transferase-1 (CPT-1) and β-hydroxy-β-methylglutaryl-CoA (HMG-CoA) synthase (the first and last steps in hepatic ketogenesis) are not expressed for up to 12 hours after birth[52-54] (Figure 5-6). The developmental lags in capacity for ketogenesis mean that during the first day of life, normal neonates lack the protection of generating alternative fuel for the brain during fasting

TABLE 5-6

Classification of Hypoglycemia in Infants and Children

Transient Neonatal Hypoglycemia

Developmental immaturity of fasting adaptation associated with inadequate substrate or immature enzyme function:

- Prematurity
- Normal newborn

Transient hyperinsulinism due to maternal factors:

- Maternal diabetes
- Intravenous glucose administration during labor and delivery
- Medications: oral hypoglycemics, terbutaline, propranolol

Prolonged Neonatal Hypoglycemia

Prolonged neonatal hyperinsulinism:

- Intrauterine growth retardation
- Prematurity
- Birth asphyxia
- Maternal toxemia/preeclampsia

Neonatal, Infantile, or Childhood Persistent Hypoglycemias

Hormonal Disorders

Hyperinsulinism

ATP-sensitive potassium channel congenital hyperinsulinism:

- Diffuse K_{ATP} channel HI
- Focal K_{ATP} channel HI
- Dominant K_{ATP} channel HI

Glutamate dehydrogenase congenital hyperinsulinism (hyperinsulinism/hyperammonemia syndrome):

- Glucokinase congenital hyperinsulinism
- Short-chain L-3-hydroxyacyl-CoA dehydrogenase congenital hyperinsulinism
- Congenital disorders of glycosylation
- Beckwith-Wiedemann syndrome
- Acquired islet adenoma
- Insulin administration (Munchausen by proxy)
- Oral sulfonylurea drugs

Counter-Regulatory Hormone Deficiency

- Panhypopituitarism
- Isolated growth hormone deficiency
- Adrenocorticotropic hormone deficiency
- Primary adrenal insufficiency
- Epinephrine deficiency

Glycogenolysis Disorders

- Amylo-1,6-glucosidase (debranching enzyme) deficiency (GSD 3)
- Liver phosphorylase deficiency (GSD 6)
- Phosphorylase kinase deficiency (GSD 9)
- Glycogen synthetase deficiency (GSD 0)

Gluconeogenesis Disorders

- Glucose 6-phosphatase deficiency (GSD 1a)
- Glucose 6-phosphate translocase deficiency (GSD 1b)
- Fructose 1,6-diphosphatase deficiency
- Pyruvate carboxylase deficiency

Lipolysis Disorders

- Propranolol

Fatty Acid Oxidation Disorders

- Carnitine transporter deficiency (primary carnitine deficiency)
- Carnitine palmitoyl-transferase 1 deficiency
- Carnitine translocase deficiency
- Carnitine palmitoyl-transferase 2 deficiency
- Very long-chain acyl-CoA dehydrogenase deficiency

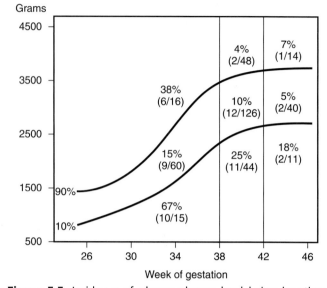

Figure 5-5. Incidence of plasma glucose level being less than 30 mg/dL before first feeding at 3 to 6 hours of age in newborns, classified by birth weight and gestational age. [From Lubchenko LO, Bard H (1971). Incidence of hypoglycemia in newborn infants by birth weight and gestational age. Pediatrics 47:831.]

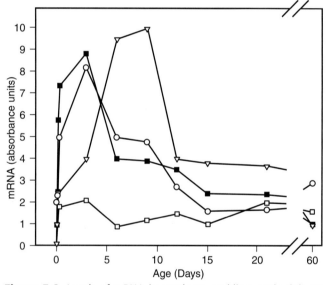

Figure 5-6. Levels of mRNA in newborn, suckling, and adult rat liver for phosphoenolpyruvate carboxykinase (triangles), mitochondrial β-hydroxy-β-methylglutaryl CoA synthase (circles), and carnitine palmitoyltransferase I (solid squares) and II (open squares). [From Hegardt FG (1999). Mitochondrial 3-hydroxy-3-methylglutaryl-CoA synthase: A control enzyme in ketogenesis. Biochem J 338:569.]

hypoglycemia. Fatty acids provided by the first feeding appear to play a key, possibly direct, role in activating transcription of these two important fatty acid oxidation and ketogenesis enzymes.[52,53]

In terms of fasting systems, the normal newborn is highly dependent on hepatic glycogen stores to maintain normoglycemia in the first 12 to 24 hours but rapidly acquires the full complement of fasting systems thereafter.

Normal term infants who are being breast fed unsuccessfully are at highest risk for hypoglycemia because of developmental immaturity of fasting adaptation and may require supplementation until milk production is adequate. Symptomatic hypoglycemia is rare in normal term infants who are fed early and is easily prevented by ensuring that feedings are given.

As shown in Figure 5-5, the risk of fasting hypoglycemia in the immediate postnatal period is considerably higher in preterm appropriate-for-gestational-age infants compared with normal full-term neonates. This increased risk may be explained by the fact that premature infants have the same developmental immaturity of ketogenesis and gluconeogenesis as term infants but lower glycogen reserves. In addition, hormonal responses are initially limited in preterm infants.[55] As discussed later in the chapter, the higher risk of fasting hypoglycemia on day 1 of life in infants who are large or small for gestational age most likely involves additional factors (especially hyperinsulinism).

Hypoglycemia in Normal Infants and Children (Ketotic Hypoglycemia)

The process of fasting adaptation is accelerated in infants and children compared with adults because of their relatively larger ratio of brain weight to body weight. Thus, normal infants may develop fasting hyperketonemia before 24 hours of fasting, whereas adults usually require more than 48 hours of fasting to reach the same point. For this reason, otherwise normal infants and children (as discussed in Chapter 11) are susceptible to fasting hypoglycemia during intercurrent illnesses (such as gastroenteritis)—which interfere with feeding. Beyond acute treatment of the hypoglycemia, these infants need no therapy. However, because of this increased susceptibility to hypoglycemia precautions to avoid prolonged fasting beyond 12 hours should be taken in children with ketotic hypoglycemia.

Early intervention with intravenous dextrose should be considered during intercurrent illnesses that might interrupt normal eating. Ketotic hypoglycemia has often been considered a specific diagnosis, but in most cases may simply represent normal infants who have accelerated fasting adaptation (e.g., smaller infants with less fuel reserve). A diagnosis of ketotic hypoglycemia should only be made after other conditions have been excluded (e.g., glycogen synthase deficiency, pituitary deficiency). Because the timing of hypoglycemia in patients with fatty acid oxidation disorders [such as medium-chain acyl-CoA dehydrogenase (MCAD) deficiency] is similar to that of ketotic hypoglycemia, specific measurements of plasma ketones are essential to diagnosis.

Transient Hyperinsulinism Due to Maternal Factors

Transient hyperinsulinism is a well-recognized complication in infants of diabetic mothers. Gestational diabetes affects approximately 2% of pregnant women, and approximately 1 in 1,000 pregnant women have insulin-dependent diabetes. At birth, infants born to these mothers may be large and plethoric—and their body stores of glycogen, protein, and fat are replete. Thus, in contrast to the transient hypoglycemia of the infant who is small for gestational age (whose body size and tissue nutrient content reflect diminished placental transfer) infants born to diabetic mothers are examples of nutrient surfeit and represent the opposite extreme of the spectrum. The classic clinical description of the effect of hyperinsulinism relates to the infant of the diabetic mother[56]:

> These infants are remarkable not only because like fetal versions of Shadrack, Meshack, and Abednego, they emerge at least alive from within the fiery metabolic furnace of diabetes mellitus, but because they resemble one another so closely they might well be related. They are plump, sleek, liberally coated with vernix caseosa, full-faced, and plethoric. The umbilical cord and placenta share in the gigantism. During their first 24 or more extrauterine hours, they lie on their backs, bloated and flushed, their legs flexed and abducted, their lightly closed hands on either side of the head, the abdomen prominent and their respiration sighing. They convey a distinct impression of having had such a surfeit of both food and fluid pressed upon them by an insistent hostess that they desire only peace so that they may recover from their excesses. On the second day their resentment of the slightest noise improves the analogy when their trembling anxiety seems to speak of intrauterine indiscretions of which we know nothing.

Hypoglycemia in infants of diabetic mothers is related chiefly to hyperinsulinemia and in part to diminished glucagon secretion. Hypertrophy and hyperplasia of their islets have been documented, as has their brisk, biphasic, and typically adult insulin response to glucose. This insulin response is absent in normal infants. Infants born to diabetic mothers also have a subnormal surge in plasma glucagon immediately after birth, subnormal glucagon secretion in response to stimuli, and (initially) excessive sympathetic activity that may lead to adrenomedullary exhaustion because urinary excretion of epinephrine is diminished. Thus, despite their abundance of tissue stores of available substrate the normal plasma hormonal pattern of low insulin, high glucagon, and catecholamines is reversed. Their endogenous glucose production is inhibited and glucose utilization is increased compared with that in normal infants, thus predisposing them to hypoglycemia.

Mothers whose diabetes has been well controlled during pregnancy in general have near-normal-sized infants who are less likely to develop neonatal hypoglycemia and other complications formerly considered typical of maternal diabetes. Nevertheless, treatment of infants born to mothers with diabetes commonly requires provision of intravenous glucose for a few days until the hyperinsulinemia abates. For these infants, glucose should be provided at a rate of 5 to 10 mg/kg/min. However, the appropriate dosage for each patient should be individually adjusted. During labor and delivery, maternal hyperglycemia should be avoided because it may result in fetal hyperglycemia—which predisposes to rebound hypoglycemia when the glucose supply is interrupted at birth. Other maternal factors that can result in transient neonatal hyperinsulinism include oral hypoglycemics (such as sulfonylureas) or other medications (terbutaline or propranolol).

By definition, transient hyperinsulinism as a cause of neonatal hypoglycemia in an infant of a diabetic mother should abate in 1 or 2 days. If the condition persists, organic hyperinsulinism must become a prominent consideration and the index of suspicion must remain high until it is ruled out. The potential risk of brain damage in an infant suffering from hyperinsulinism is high, placing this diagnosis in a critical position in the diagnostic evaluation of neonatal hypoglycemia.

PROLONGED NEONATAL HYPERINSULINISM: PERINATAL STRESSS-INDUCED HYPERINSULINISM

As shown in Figure 5-5, the risk of postnatal hypoglycemia is increased in neonates who are small for gestational age. Although this may sometimes be caused by poorer stores of glycogen, there is increasing evidence that prolonged hypoglycemia in some neonates exposed to perinatal stress such as birth asphyxia, maternal toxemia, prematurity, or intrauterine growth retardation or other peripartum stress is due to hyperinsulinism.[57-59] The estimated incidence of prolonged neonatal hyperinsulinism is 1:12,000 live births.[59]

The clinical presentation of perinatal stress-induced hyperinsulinism is characterized by high glucose utilization, and the response to fasting hypoglycemia shows an elevated plasma insulin level (although it may be normal in some), low β-hydroxybutyrate and free fatty acid levels, and a glycemic response to glucagon. Unlike the transient hyperinsulinism seen in the infant of the diabetic mother, perinatal stress-induced hyperinsulinism may persist for several days to several weeks. In a series of neonates diagnosed after 1 week of age, the median age of resolution was 6 months.[59] The mechanism responsible for the dysregulated insulin secretion is not known. AIR testing shows that in general the patterns of insulin response to secretagogues (calcium, tolbutamide, glucose, and leucine) in infants with prolonged neonatal hyperinsulinism resembled those of normal controls.[59] This suggests that the defect does not involve the ATP-dependent potassium (K_{ATP}) channel or glutamate dehydrogenase (GDH) sites.

Infants with prolonged neonatal hyperinsulinism usually respond very well to medical therapy with diazoxide.[57-59] Previously, it was common practice to use pharmacologic doses of glucocorticoids to treat such neonates with persistent hypoglycemia. Glucocorticoids are not effective in controlling hyperinsulinism, however. Their use as nonspecific therapy for neonatal hypoglycemia is not recommended.

Endocrine System Disorders

CONGENITAL HYPERINSULINISM

Congenital hyperinsulinism is the most common and most difficult to manage form of persistent hypoglycemia in neonates and infants.[60] Advances in defining the genetic basis of hyperinsulinism during the past decade have been rapid, and improvements in diagnosis and treatment can be expected to occur quickly in the future. As shown in Table 5-6, both recessive and dominantly expressed genetic forms of congenital hyperinsulinism have been described. In addition, a sporadic form of congenital hyperinsulinism associated with focal adenomatosis of the pancreas has been delineated. Unlike adults, insulinomas are not a cause of hyperinsulinism in infancy; these lesions and surreptitious insulin administration are discussed in Chapter 11.

Figure 5-7 outlines the major pathways regulating insulin release by pancreatic beta cells. Glucose-stimulated insulin secretion involves glucose uptake through the GLUT2 glucose transporter and phosphorylation by glucokinase (GK), leading to glucose oxidation and an increased ATP/ADP ratio that results in inhibition of a plasma membrane ATP-dependent potassium (K_{ATP}) channel. The β-cell K_{ATP} channel is a hetero-octameric complex consisting of two subunits: a K^+-selective pore-forming subunit (Kir6.2) and a regulatory subunit (SUR1). Four Kir6.2 subunits form the central pore, coupled to four SUR1 subunits. The K_{ATP} channel is inhibited by sulfonylurea drugs (used therapeutically to stimulate insulin secretion in type 2 diabetes) and activated by diazoxide (the main medical treatment for congenital hyperinsulinism).

In the unstimulated state, the ß-cell ATP-sensitive potassium channels are open—keeping a resting membrane potential of approximately –65 mV. Following the uptake and metabolism of glucose, an increase in the intracellular ATP/ADP ratio results in closure of ATP-sensitive potassium channels, depolarization of the cell membrane, and subsequent opening of voltage-dependent Ca^{2+} channels. The resulting increase in cytosolic Ca^{2+} concentration triggers release of stored insulin granules. Stimulation of insulin secretion by amino acids occurs through an allosteric activation of glutamate dehydrogenase (GDH) by leucine, which results in increased oxidation of glutamate—leading to increased ATP/ADP ratio, inhibition of K_{ATP}-channel activity, and membrane depolarization.

Genetic defects in these pathways associated with congenital hyperinsulinism include loss-of-function mutations of SUR1 (encoded by *ABCC8*) or Kir6.2 (encoded by *KCNJ11*) and gain-of-function mutations of glucokinase (encoded by *GCK*) or glutamate dehydrogenase (GDH; encoded by *GLUD1*).[60,61] Mutations of SUR1 and Kir6.2 are usually recessively expressed, however, a few dominantly expressed mutations of *ABCC8* and *KCNJ11* have been reported.[62-64] Mutations of *GCK* and *GLUD1* are dominantly expressed; sporadic, de novo mutations of the latter have been diagnosed more commonly than familial cases.[65] Loss-of-function mutations of *ABCC8* or *KCNJ1* transmitted from the paternal side have also been demonstrated to be responsible for congenital hyperinsulinism in infants with focal hyperinsulinism.[66] Recently, loss of function mutations in *HADHSC,* the gene encoding the mitochondrial enzyme short-chain L-3-hydroxyacyl-CoA (SCHAD),[67-69] was found to be associated with recessive congenital hyperinsulinism.

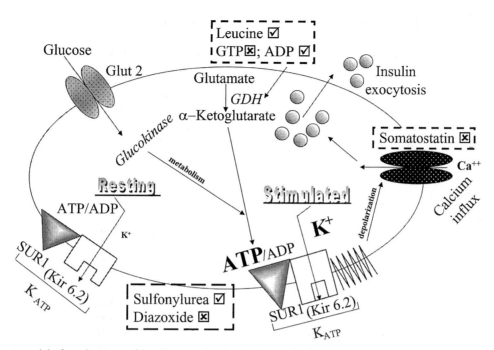

Figure 5-7. Current model of mechanisms of insulin secretion by the beta cell of the pancreas. Glucose transported into the beta cell by the insulin-independent glucose transporter GLUT2 undergoes phosphorylation by glucokinase and is then metabolized, resulting in an increase in the adenosine triphosphate/adenosine diphosphate (ATP/ADP) ratio. The increase in the ATP/ADP ratio closes the KATP channel and initiates the cascade of events characterized by increase in intracellular potassium concentration, membrane depolarization, calcium influx, and release of insulin from storage granules. Leucine stimulates insulin secretion by allosterically activating glutamate dehydrogenase (GDH) and by increasing the oxidation of glutamate, thereby increasing the ATP/ADP ratio and closure of the KATP channel. x = inhibition; (? = stimulation; and GTP = guanosine triphosphate. [From Sperling MA, Menon RK (1999). Hyperinsulinemic hypoglycemia of infancy. Endocrinol Metab Clin North Am 28:695.]

The clinical presentations of congenital hyperinsulinism vary with the severity of the disorder as well as the site of defect. The most severe cases have been associated with recessive or focal K_{ATP} channel defects and are often associated with macrosomia caused by fetal hyperinsulinemia. These infants may be confused with infants of diabetic mothers. They usually present with hypoglycemia in the first hours or days after birth. The hypoglycemia is difficult to control and often requires glucose infusion rates greater than 20 mg/kg/min. Less severe phenotypes of congenital hyperinsulinism are associated with defects of GDH, GK, SCHAD, and dominant K_{ATP} mutations. Episodes of hypoglycemia may not be recognized until 1 to 2 years of age or later.

It is often not easy to diagnose hyperinsulinism based solely on measurements of plasma insulin. This is because standard insulin assays are not sufficiently sensitive in the low range to distinguish a normal from an inadequately suppressed insulin concentration. Plasma insulin levels are rarely dramatically elevated in congenital hyperinsulinism; rather there is inadequate suppression of insulin at low plasma glucose concentrations. Therefore, the diagnosis of hyperinsulinism in infants is most frequently based on evidence of excessive insulin action at the time of hypoglycemia, such as inappropriate suppression of plasma β-hydroxybutyrate and free fatty acid levels and an inappropriate glycemic response to glucagon.

As shown in Table 5-7, at a plasma glucose level below 50 mg/dL, evidence of hyperinsulinism includes plasma

TABLE 5-7
Criteria for Diagnosing Hyperinsulinism Based on "Critical" Samples (Drawn at a Time of Fasting Hypoglycemia: Plasma Glucose <50 mg/dL)

1. Hyperinsulinemia (plasma insulin >2 mU/mL)*
2. Hypofattyacidemia (plasma FFA <1.5 mmol/L)
3. Hypoketonemia (plasma BOB <2.0 mmol/L)
4. Inappropriate glycemic response to glucagon, 1 mg IV (delta glucose >30 mg/dL)

*Depends on sensitivity of insulin assay.
BOB, β-hydroxybutyrate; FFA, free fatty acids.

insulin greater than 2 μU/mL; plasma β-hydroxybutyrate (BOB) less than 2.0 mmol/L; plasma free fatty acids (FFA) less than 1.5 mmol/L; and glycemic response to glucagon, 1 mg given intravenously, greater than 30 mg/ dL within 15 to 30 minutes.[70,71] Plasma concentrations of insulin-like growth factor binding protein-1 (IGFBP1) may be an additional indicator of insulin action on the liver.[72] Children with hyperinsulinism fail to show a rise in circulating IGFBP1 concentration during fasting, which is in contrast to normal subjects, who show a 10-fold increase during fasting.[72] In neonates, hypoglycemia due to hypopituitarism can mimic hyperinsulinism and may need to be formally excluded. Note that plasma levels of cortisol and growth hormone are frequently not elevated with

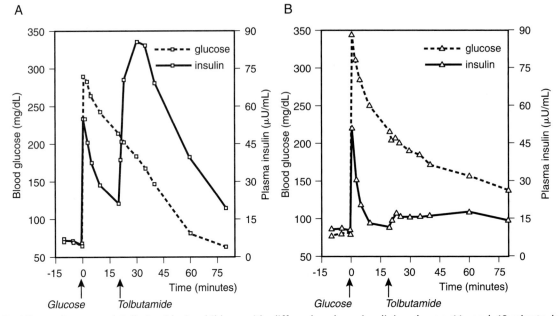

Figure 5-8. AIR to glucose and tolbutamide in children with diffuse k_{ATP} hyperinsulinism (mean 11- and 13-minute increments). *(A)* Normal adult control. *(B)* Patient with diffuse k_{ATP} hyperinsulinism. [From Grimberg A, Ferry RJ, Kelly A, et al. (2000). Dysregulation of insulin secretion in children with congenital hyperinsulinism due to sulfonylurea receptor mutations. Diabetes 50:322.]

hypoglycemia, hence the need for separate testing to rule out cortisol or growth hormone deficiency.

Additional tests for specific forms of congenital hyperinsulinism include plasma ammonia levels (GDH-HI), plasma acyl-carnitine profile (elevated 3-hydroxybutyryl-carnitine) and urine organic acids (3-hydroxyglutarate) (SCHAD-HI). Genetic testing is available for four of the five genes known to be associated with congenital hyperinsulinism through commercial laboratories *(ABCC8, KCNJ11, GLUD1, GCK)*. For research purposes, AIR tests have been useful in phenotypic characterization. Patients with K_{ATP}-HI display abnormal positive responses to calcium, abnormal negative response to the K_{ATP}-channel antagonist, tolbutamide, as well as impaired responses to glucose[73,74] (Figure 5-8). In contrast, infants with GDH-HI exhibit increased responses to leucine.[75]

K_{ATP}-Channel Hyperinsulinism

Recessive K_{ATP}-HI

Infants with this form of congenital hyperinsulinism frequently present as neonates who are large for gestational age with very severe hypoglycemia immediately after delivery. The genetic defects in these infants are loss of function of either the SUR1 or the Kir6.2 components of the ATP-sensitive potassium channel complex. These two genes are located on chromosome 11p, immediately adjacent to each other. More than 100 mutations of *ABCC8* and 20 mutations of *KCNJ11* have been found. Heterozygous carrier parents are normal. Common SUR1 founder mutations have been reported in Ashkenazi Jews and in Finland. The incidence of the severe hyperinsulinism phenotype seen with recessive K_{ATP}-HI has been estimated at 1 in 40,000 in Northern Europe and Finland, but it is as

high as 1 in 2,500 in Saudi Arabia—where the frequency of consanguinity is high.

As shown in Figure 5-7, because the mutations disrupt the K_{ATP} channel these patients are usually unresponsive to diazoxide treatment. Octreotide is helpful in short-term management. However, because of tachyphylaxis, octreotide is often not successful as the sole therapy for long-term management.[76] The use of calcium-channel blockers to decrease voltage-dependent calcium-channel activity has been proposed as an alternative medical therapy. A few reports of successful treatment with nifedipine are published,[77] but most centers have not had success with this drug.

Because of the lack of effective medical therapy, most infants with severe hypoglycemia due to K_{ATP}-HI require treatment with near-total (95% to 98%) pancreatectomy. Near-total pancreatectomy is associated with a high risk of later development of diabetes mellitus.[78] This most likely reflects not only the effects of pancreas resection but the fact that the loss of channel activity renders the beta cells unresponsive to hyperglycemia as well as to hypoglycemia.[73]

Histologically, in diffuse hyperinsulinism beta cells throughout the pancreas are functionally abnormal and have characteristic enlarged nuclei in about 2% to 5% of cells.[79] Previously, this form of hyperinsulinism was termed *nesidioblastosis*, although it is now recognized that islet neogenesis from ductal epithelium is a normal feature of early infancy.[80] The term *nesidioblastosis* should therefore be abandoned as a synonym for hyperinsulinism.

Focal K_{ATP}-HI (Focal Adenomatosis)

From 40% to 60% of the cases of K_{ATP}-HI (which require surgery) have focal disease.[81] Histologically, these lesions are small (usually less than 10 mm in diameter) and are characterized by the presence of confluent proliferation of endocrine cells (adenomatous hyperplasia). In contrast to true adenomas, the focal adenomatous hyperplasia includes exocrine acinar cells intermixed within the lesion. The morphology of islets away from the focal lesion is normal.[79]

Focal lesions arise by a "two-hit" mechanism of focal loss of heterozygosity for the maternal 11p15 region, leading to a somatic reduction to homozygosity (or hemizygosity) of a paternally inherited mutation of the *ABCC8* or *KCNJ11* gene. The 11p15 region, which carries the *ABCC8* and *KCNJ11* genes, contains several imprinted tumor suppressor genes (*H19* and *CDKN1C,* also known as p57kip2) that are only expressed on the maternal chromosome. Loss of these growth-suppressing genes may play an important permissive role in the clonal expansion of the lesion.[82]

Clinically, infants with focal lesions are indistinguishable from those with diffuse K_{ATP}-HI and nearly always require surgery. The focal lesions are potentially curable by surgery, whereas diffuse K_{ATP}-HI is not. Efforts to diagnose and localize focal lesions in infants with congenital

hyperinsulinism are therefore worthwhile. Interventional radiology studies, such as transhepatic portal venous insulin sampling[83] and selective pancreatic arterial calcium stimulation,[84] have only modest success and are technically difficult and highly invasive. Recently, position emission tomography (PET) scans with flurorine-18 L-3, 4-dihydroxyphenylalanine (¹⁸F-fluoro-L-DOPA) have been found to accurately discriminate focal from diffuse hyperinsulinism.[85-87] Pancreatic β-cells take up L-DOPA,[88] and DOPA decarboxylase is active in pancreatic islet cells.[89] In children with focal hyperinsulinism, there is local accumulation of ¹⁸F-fluoro-L-DOPA. Coregistration of PET and computed tomography (CT) images allows the anatomic localization of the lesion (Figure 5-9).

Dominant K_{ATP}-HI

A few cases of dominantly expressed mutations of *ABCC8* and one of *KCNJ11* have been reported.[62-64,90] The hypoglycemia in these patients is less severe than the recessive K_{ATP}-HI just described. Although birth weight in affected individuals is increased, the onset of

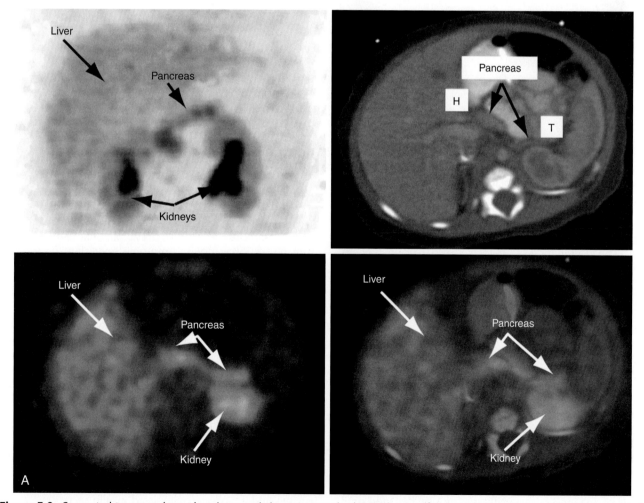

Figure 5-9. Computed tomography and positron emission tomography (CT/PET) using ¹⁸Fluoro-L-Dopa. *(A)* Coregistration coronal view of a diffuse lesion and *(B)* focal lesion located in the head of the pancreas. L-DOPA uptake can be appreciated in the liver, in the kidneys, throughout the pancreas in the diffuse form *(A)* and in a focal area corresponding to the head of the pancreas *(B)*. [Used with permission from Hardy OT, Hernandez-Pampaloni M, Saffer J, et al. (2007). Diagnosis and localization of focal congenital hyperinsulinism by ¹⁸F-fluorodopa PET scan. J Pediatr 150(2): 140-45.] (See color plates.)

Continued

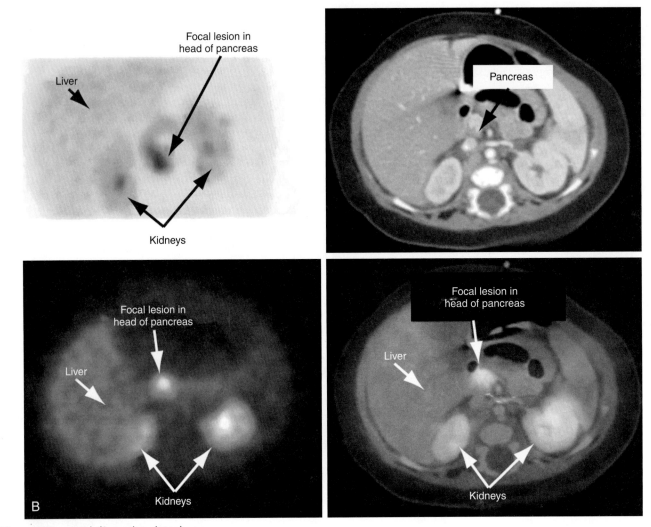

Figure 5-9. cont'd. (See color plates.)

hypoglycemic symptoms is often later in infancy or childhood. The dominant K_{ATP} defects retain responsiveness to diazoxide. These dominant K_{ATP} mutations presumably exert a dominant negative effect in the heteroctameric K_{ATP} channel complexes.

GDH-HI

Hyperinsulinism associated with gain-of-function mutations of *GLUD1* (encoding glutamate dehydrogenase, GDH) is also a dominant disorder.[65,91-94] Affected patients present with symptomatic hypoglycemia together with a characteristically persistent but asymptomatic elevation of plasma ammonia. This unusual hyperinsulinism/hyperammonemia (HI/HA) syndrome represents the second most common form of congenital hyperinsulinism after recessive K_{ATP}-HI. In GDH-HI, size at birth is normal. Episodes of symptomatic hypoglycemia are often not recognized until 1 to 2 years of age, and occasionally may not be detected until adulthood. Most cases are sporadic, owing to de novo mutations.

Familial cases showing autosomal-dominant patterns of inheritance comprise 20% of the identified probands.

Plasma ammonia levels in HI/HA patients usually range from 60 to 150 μmol/L. Ammonia levels are quite constant, and in contrast to urea cycle enzyme defects do not increase with protein feeding. The hyperammonemia does not appear to cause symptoms and does not require treatment.

GDH is a mitochondrial matrix enzyme that is a key regulator of amino acid and ammonia metabolism in pancreatic beta cells, liver, and brain. As shown in Figure 5-7, GDH functions in the beta cell pathway of leucine-stimulated insulin secretion. Leucine is an allosteric activator of the enzyme, causing increased oxidation of glutamate to α ketoglutarate and increased ATP production—which results in insulin release. The HI/HA mutations impair allosteric inhibition of GDH by high-energy phosphates (GTP and ATP), thus leading to excessive insulin release. Isolated islets from transgenic mice expressing a mutated human GDH exhibit normal glucose-stimulated insulin secretion but enhanced leucine- and amino-acid-stimulated insulin secretion.[95]

In the liver, increased GDH activity leads to hyperammonemia by overproduction of ammonia owing to increased glutamate oxidation and by depression of ammonia detoxification due to the depletion of tissue glutamate (because glutamate is the substrate for synthesis of N-acetylglutamate, a required allosteric activator of carbamoyl-phosphate synthetase, the rate-controlling step in ureagenesis). The consequences of increased GDH enzyme activity in the brain are less clear, but might explain the lack of hyperammonemic symptoms in affected individuals. The normal toxic effect of hyperammonemia is thought to be a consequence of increased levels of glutamate and glutamine in brain. Increased GDH activity in HI/HA patients may protect against this effect of hyperammonemia by depleting brain concentrations of glutamate.

Patients with GDH-HI have fasting hypoglycemia, which may be relatively mild. Patients may be able to fast for 8 to 12 hours before becoming hypoglycemic. However, these patients have dramatic protein-sensitive hypoglycemia—becoming severely hypoglycemic within 30 to 90 minutes of ingesting a protein meal[96] (Figure 5-10). Children with GDH-HI may present with an unusual pattern of absence seizure with EEG pattern of generalized epilepsy.[97] Patients with GDH-HI have been shown to have leucine-sensitive insulin secretion.[98] The diagnosis of GDH-HI can be suggested by the persistent mild elevation of plasma ammonia.

Unlike urea cycle enzyme defects, plasma amino acid and urinary amino acid levels are normal in GDH-HI. Plasma ammonia concentrations are not affected by protein feeding, fasting, or plasma glucose levels. GDH enzyme activity can be measured in cultured lymphoblasts to demonstrate impaired responsiveness to allosteric inhibition by GTP. Disease-causing missense mutations have been reported to occur in specific regions of the enzyme involved in GTP inhibition, including exons 6, 7, 10, 11, and 12. Diazoxide therapy, 5 to 10 mg/kg/day, is usually effective in controlling both fasting and protein-induced hypoglycemia in GDH-HI. Carbohydrate preloading may be helpful in avoiding the latter.

GK-HI

A less frequent form of congenital hyperinsulinism is due to activating mutations in *GCK* (encoding glucokinase). Glucokinase is a hexokinase that serves as the glucose sensor in pancreatic beta cells[99] (Figure 5-7). In GK-HI, activating mutations result in increased affinity of glucokinase for glucose, closure of K_{ATP} channels, and inappropriate insulin secretion. The beta cell glucose threshold for glucose-stimulated insulin secretion in children with GK-HI may be less than 2 mmol/L (38 mg/dL), whereas the normal glucose threshold is maintained close to 5 mmol/L (90 mg/dL). Five dominantly inherited mutations have been reported to date.[100] The age of onset and severity of symptoms vary markedly.[101-104] Some mutations seem to have a mild phenotype, with fasting hypoglycemia responsive to diazoxide. Others seem to lower the glucose threshold further and may be more difficult to treat.

SCHAD-HI HYPERINSULINISM

Recently, a mutation in *HADHSC* [the gene encoding the mitochondrial short-chain L-3-hydroxyacyl-CoA dehydrogenase (SCHAD)] was found to be associated with congenital HI.[67-69] SCHAD-HI is an autosomal-recessive disorder characterized by fasting hypoglycemia due to inappropriate insulin regulation. The biochemical hallmark, in addition to markers of increased insulin action, is increased levels of plasma 3-hydroxybutyryl-carnitine and increased levels of 3-hydroxyglutarate in urine.

In contrast to all other defects in fatty acid oxidation, children with SCHAD-HI have no signs of hepatic dysfunction or cardiomyopathy, or of affects on skeletal muscle. The clinical presentation of SCHAD-HI is heterogeneous, ranging from late onset of mild hypoglycemia to severe early onset of hypoglycemia in the neonatal period. Affected patients have been responsive to medical

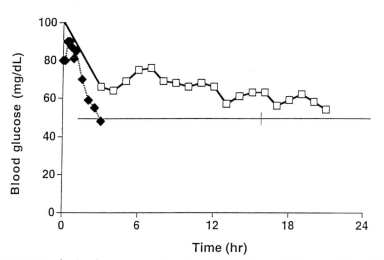

Figure 5-10 Blood glucose responses to fasting (open squares) and protein feeding (solid diamonds) in a 16-year-old girl with the hyperinsulinism/hyperammonemia syndrome caused by a dominantly expressed R269H regulatory mutation of glutamate dehydrogenase. [From Hsu BY, Kelly A, Thornton PS, et al. (2001). Protein-sensitive and fasting hypoglycemia in children with the hyperinsulinism/hyperammonemia syndrome. J Pediatr 138:383.]

therapy with diazoxide. The cause of dysregulated insulin secretion in SCHAD deficiency remains to be elucidated.

OTHER FORMS OF HYPERINSULINISM

Hyperinsulinism can be associated with complex syndromes such as Beckwith-Wiedemann syndrome (BWS) and the congenital disorders of glycosylation (CDG).

BWS is a clinically and genetically heterogenous disorder characterized by fetal overgrowth, hypoglycemia in up to 50% of patients, and a predisposition to childhood tumors. Among cases of BWS, 85% are sporadic and 15% are dominant. Genetic abnormalities in the imprinted region of chromosome 11 have been described in patients with BWS. These often lead to isodisomy for the paternal 11p, a region that is highly imprinted—including some maternally expressed growth-suppressing genes and the paternally expressed fetal growth-promoting *IGF2* gene. The hypoglycemia in BWS may be mild and transient, although in some cases it can be severe and persistent.[105] Some BWS patients respond to diazoxide, whereas others require partial pancreatectomy to control the hypoglycemia. At least two theories have been proposed to explain the hypoglycemia. One involves the insulin-like actions of IGFII. The second involves dysregulated insulin secretion due to loss of K_{ATP} channel genes on 11p.[106]

Hypoglycemia due to hyperinsulinism has been reported in patients with a few of the congenital disorders of glycosylation.[107-109] These inherited metabolic diseases result in hypoglycosylation of different extracellular glycoproteins. They usually affect multiple systems, such as the brain, liver, gastrointestinal system, and the skeleton.[110] Hypoglycosylation of the sulfonylurea receptor has been speculated to be the responsible mechanism for the dysregulated insulin secretion, but the mechanism of hyperinsulinism remains to be proven.

Other forms of hyperinsulinism include islet adenoma or carcinoma (both very rare in childhood), surreptitious insulin administration (Munchausen syndrome by proxy), and ingestion of insulin secretagogues such as sulfonylureas. The latter has occasionally been described in neonates as being caused by drug administration to the mother shortly before delivery. Exogenous insulin produces the usual features of hyperinsulinism (increased glucose use, suppression of lipolysis and ketogenesis, inappropriate glycemic response to glucagon). However, plasma levels of C-peptide are low—indicating suppression of endogenous insulin secretion. Surreptitious insulin administration can be suspected when plasma insulin concentrations at times of hypoglycemia are unusually high (100 μU/mL or greater). Note, however, that biosynthetic forms of insulin such as lispro insulin are not detectable by standard insulin assays.

Counter-Regulatory Hormone Deficiencies

Hypoglycemia associated with endocrine deficiency is usually caused by glucocorticoid or growth hormone deficiency. In patients with panhypopituitarism, isolated growth hormone deficiency, or a combination of ACTH deficiency and growth hormone deficiency the incidence of hypoglycemia is as high as 20%. In the newborn period, hypoglycemia may be the presenting feature of hypopituitarism. In males, a microphallus may provide a clue to a coexistent deficiency of gonadotropin[111,112] (Figure 5-11). Newborns with hypopituitarism may also have liver dysfunction resembling cholestatic liver disease, and some have midline malformations such as the syndrome of septo-optic dysplasia.[113]

Although older infants and children with pituitary deficiency present with ketotic hypoglycemia, in the neonatal period the hypoglycemia may mimic hyperinsulinism. These infants may represent a subset of perinatal stress-induced hyperinsulinism. However, their hypoglycemia is not responsive to diazoxide and only remits with replacement of deficient hormones (including thyroxine, as well as growth hormone and cortisol). When adrenal disease is severe (as in congenital adrenal hyperplasia caused by enzyme defects in cortisol synthesis, adrenal hemorrhage, or congenital absence or hypoplasia of the adrenals,[114,115]), disturbances in serum electrolytes with hyponatremia and hyperkalemia or ambiguous genitalia may provide diagnostic clues.

Abnormalities of the ACTH receptor or adrenal agenesis may also be phenotypically difficult to distinguish from cortisol deficiency of other causes, with the exception of the marked elevations of serum ACTH concentration noted if the ACTH receptor or adrenal gland is malfunctioning.[116] However, all states with ACTH elevations can be clinically suspected by virtue of the associated hyperpigmentation (see Chapter 12). These cases of isolated adrenal insufficiency very rarely cause

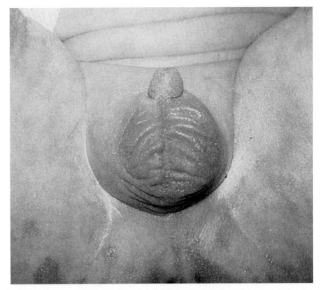

Figure 5-11. Micropenis and undescended testes in an infant with congenital hypopituitarism. The infant was hypoglycemic at 12 hours of age (glucose, 24 mg/dL). At 72 hours of age, he was jaundiced—and a liver biopsy demonstrated neonatal hepatitis. His endocrine evaluation was positive for hypothyroidism, low cortisol level, undetectable growth hormone level, and an elevated prolactin level (confirming hypothalamic hypopituitarism).

hypoglycemia in neonates, whereas in older infants and children treated congenital adrenal hyperplasia and isolated ACTH deficiency can cause profound stress-induced hypoglycemia.

The mechanism of hypoglycemia in growth hormone deficiency may be the result of decreased lipolysis. The mechanism of hypoglycemia with cortisol deficiency may be reduced liver glycogen reserves plus diminished gluconeogenesis, owing to a failure to supply endogenous gluconeogenic substrate in the form of amino acids from muscle proteolysis. Deficiency of either of these hormones can resemble the syndrome of ketotic hypoglycemia. Investigation of a child with hypoglycemia therefore requires exclusion of ACTH, cortisol, or growth hormone deficiency—and if diagnosed appropriate replacement with cortisol or growth hormone. Although glucagon deficiency[117,118] has been described, this disorder is exceedingly rare or nonexistent. Epinephrine deficiency is also rare, but must be a consideration in familial dysautonomia or in children treated with beta blockers.

Glycogen Storage Disorders

The glycogen storage disorders (GSDs) may present primarily as hepatic manifestations or muscular and cardiac manifestations. Hypoglycemia is a consistent feature of certain forms (e.g., glucose 6-phosphatase deficiency). Affected children may display a remarkable tolerance to their chronic hypoglycemia. Blood glucose values in the range of 20 to 50 mg/dL (1.1 to 2.7 mmol/L) are often not associated with the classic symptoms of hypoglycemia, possibly reflecting the use of ketones or lactic acid as alternative fuels by the central nervous system. These disorders are uncommon, but they present with distinct phenotypes and are important to diagnose correctly to avoid long-term sequelae.[119]

Glycogen is a globular structure with a variable molecular weight. It is found primarily in liver and muscle but is present in other cells. The arborized structure consists of straight-chain glucose residues attached through amylo-1,4 linkages, with branch points every 12 to 18 residues attached through a 1,6 linkage. Glycogen is synthesized from incorporation of sequential glucose-1-phosphate residues that have been converted to uridine diphosphoglucose and then incorporated by glycogen synthase. When the elongating glycogen chain consists of at least 11 residues, a branching enzyme transfers a chain of seven molecules to another chain by an α1-6 bound. Thus, glycogen synthase elongates the glycogen chain and the branching enzyme produces new branches—creating a molecule with a helical structure of 12 concentric tiers.

Glycogen degradation is the result of the activities of glycogen phosphorylase and a debranching enzyme. Glycogen phosphorylase catalyzes the rate-limiting step of glycogenolysis. It cleaves α1-4 linkages to remove glucose molecules from the glycogen chain as glucose-1-phosphate. The debranching enzyme has both transferase and glucosidase activity. When four glucose units remain before a branch point, the transferase activity of the debranching enzyme catalyzes the transfer of three glucose residues to an adjacent branch of the glycogen chain. Through a second enzymatic glucosidase component, the debranching enzyme next cleaves the α1-6 bond to release a free glucose moiety from the branch point. Glycogen phosphorylase is then able to continue removal of glucose residues from the glycogen chain.[120] This complex system offers many specific points of regulation and many sites for mutation.[121]

GLUCOSE 6-PHOSPHATASE DEFICIENCY (GSD TYPE I)

Glucose 6-phosphatase catalyzes the terminal steps of both hepatic gluconeogenesis and glycogenolysis. The phenotype of infants with type I GSD is characteristic, despite the fact that the glucose 6-phosphatase complex possesses a variety of sites for different mutations and several subtypes of GSD I have been described.[119] The most striking feature is the massive hepatomegaly that may fill the entire abdomen. Affected infants have profound elevations of plasma triglycerides, and their serum may be creamy.

Patients are often tachypneic secondary to respiratory compensation for their metabolic acidemia as a result of dramatic elevation in plasma lactate concentration. Although ketosis is often present, it is minimal compared to the dramatic lactic acidosis seen in untreated patients. Other consistent features are hyperuricemia to plasma concentrations that may precipitate gouty crises, hypophosphatemia, a bleeding diathesis secondary to impairment of platelet adhesiveness, and growth retardation.

Hypoglycemia may occur anytime these children are exposed to even brief periods of fasting. They are completely dependent on the provision of glucose from exogenous sources, with the exception of the small amount of free glucose—which is released as part of the process of debranching glycogen. Because less than 10% of glycogen consists of branch points, this mechanism provides little protection against hypoglycemia during fasting. Affected infants may be diagnosed soon after birth with hepatomegaly, and then hypoglycemia may be documented during the diagnostic evaluation. On the other hand, because lactate and ketones may provide adequate brain substrate to protect central nervous system function (and because in early infancy regular feedings are consistently provided) the diagnosis may be delayed for months until massive hepatomegaly brings the infant to medical attention.

Hepatomegaly, in the absence of splenomegaly or other signs of a generalized storage disorder, should suggest glycogen as the likely storage component causing liver enlargement. After infancy, affected patients may be seen walking with a waddling gait secondary to their prominent abdomen and muscle weakness—with blood glucose levels of less than 40 mg/dL and lactate levels of more than 8 to 10 mmol/L (apparently in total disregard of their hypoglycemia and with deep respirations reflecting their respiratory compensation for metabolic acidosis).

Glucose 6-phophatase is a multicomponent system consisting of a catalytic unit with its active site located on the luminal side of the endoplasmic reticulum, and transmembrane-spanning translocases that allow the entry of glucose 6-phophate to the catalytic subunit and the exit of Pi and glucose.[122] The gene for the catalytic unit has been cloned and located in a single copy on chromosome 17,[121] whereas the gene for the glucose 6-phosphate translocase is located on chromosome 11.[123] GSD type I is an autosomal-recessive disease. Molecular genetic evidence has unequivocally demonstrated that GSD type Ia[124] is caused by mutations in the catalytic unit, whereas mutations in glucose 6-phosphate translocase cause GSD type Ib.[123]

The clinical hallmark of patients with GSD type 1b is their susceptibility to infection as a consequence of neutropenia, mouth ulcers, and occasionally chronic enteritis (which is similar to Crohn disease).[119] Treatment with granulocyte-macrophage colony-stimulating factor to augment neutrophil production has been shown to ameliorate mouth ulcers and the enteritis.[125] Although two additional types have been reported [GSD type Ic[126] (presumably caused by a mutation in the putative Pi translocase) and GSD type Id[119] (due to a defect in the glucose translocase)], there is insufficient available evidence to sustain the existence of these defects.

Rapid onset of hypoglycemia is the hallmark of GSD type I, which occurs 2 to 3 hours after a meal immediately after intestinal absorption of carbohydrates is complete. Renal disease is a frequent complication of GSD type I (with an estimated prevalence of 30%).[127] Manifestations include proximal renal tubular dysfuntion (Fanconi-like syndrome), distal tubular acidification defect, and hypercalciuria. The widespread prevalence and serious prognosis of kidney involvement is manifested by severe glomerular hyperfiltration and microalbuminuria over time, systemic arterial hypertension, and consequently renal failure in a considerable number of patients.[128-130] The early implementation of treatment with angiotensin-converting enzyme inhibitors has been shown to delay the progression of renal damage.[127]

The pathologic findings include focal segmental glomerulosclerosis with interstitial fibrosis. The etiology of this renal involvement is unclear, but it seems to correlate negatively with metabolic control. It has been proposed that the dyslipidemia contributes to the kidney injury.[131] In addition to the characteristic hepatomegaly, the liver undergoes adenomatous changes. Ultrasound of older patients with glucose 6-phosphatase deficiency will frequently show multiple adenomas.[132,133] Reports of malignant degeneration of these lesions are noted.[134] Other complications of GSD I include osteopenia and growth retardation.

The goal of treatment of children with glucose-6-phosphate deficiency is to completely eliminate hypoglycemia and suppress secondary metabolic decompensation. Continuous nasogastric or intragastric feeding during the night or total parenteral nutrition has demonstrated either a reduction or an elimination of the metabolic and clinical findings through complete avoidance of hypoglycemia.[135] Oral uncooked cornstarch supplementation (1.6 g/kg per dose every 4 hours in infants and 1.7 to 2.5 g/kg per dose every 6 hours in older patients) has also been applied in treatment regimens.[136,137]

A typical regimen institutes daytime feedings every 3 to 4 hours that are calculated to provide adequate carbohydrate calories to suppress hepatic glucose output. Most of these calories consist of carbohydrates, primarily providing pure glucose as an energy source and avoiding disaccharides containing fructose or galactose. At night, the regimen consist of an intragastric infusion of glucose with or without protein designed to infuse at rates of about 125% calculated hepatic glucose output[138] for young infants. For older children, a regimen of uncooked cornstarch can be implemented.

Meticulous dietary control of blood glucose levels can lead to a significant clinical and metabolic improvement and prevention of complications. Adjunctive therapies should include careful monitoring of the uric acid level and treatment with allopurinol if the uric acid level remains elevated. With increasing awareness of the renal tubular dysfunction, treatment of the hyperfiltration state with an angiotensin-converting enzyme inhibitor should be initiated promptly.

AMYLO-1,6-GLUCOSIDASE DEFICIENCY (DEBRANCHER DEFICIENCY, GSD TYPE III)

The debraching enzyme, together with phosphorylase, is required for complete degradation of glycogen. The lack of activity of this enzyme results in incomplete breakdown of glycogen and glycogen accumulates. The human debranching enzyme gene is a large single-copy gene located on chromosome 1p21.[139] Debrancher deficiency GSD type III is an autosomal-recessive disease. The phenotype of debrancher deficiency, although similar, can be distinguished clinically from that of glucose 6-phosphatase deficiency (e.g., particularly in regard to lack of lactic academia and renal disease).

During infancy and childhood, hepatomegaly, hypoglycemia, hyperlipidemia, and short stature are the predominant features. The hepatomegaly may be quite marked in GSD type III. Although these individuals also share a propensity for developing hypoglycemia, it usually tends to be less severe. Moreover, these individuals have the capacity to undergo gluconeogenesis—whereas individuals with glucose 6-phosphatase deficiency lack this capacity. The general presentation of debrancher deficiency is hepatomegaly noted with growth retardation. Hypoglycemia is less often the presenting finding than in patients with glucose 6-phosphatase deficiency. The abnormality in liver function is less profound, and these individuals also may have muscle weakness and myotonia.

Approximately half of affected patients may have progressive skeletal muscle weakness and/or cardiomyopathy (type IIIa). In about 15% of patients, GSD III appears to involve only the liver (type IIIb). The patient's serum creatine kinase level can be used to determine muscle involvement. The debranching enzyme is active in leukocytes and erythrocytes, and thus these present easily accessible tissues for biochemical analysis.[140] Because of genetic heterogeneity in enzyme activity, leukocyte or erythrocyte enzyme testing has not been effective in determining the heterozygote state. Frequent feedings with high protein content have been successful in treatment of debrancher deficiency.[141,142]

GLYCOGEN PHOSPHORYLASE DEFICIENCY (GSD TYPE VI) AND PHOSPHORYLASE KINASE DEFICIENCY (GSD TYPE IX)

Glycogen storage disease due to reduction in liver phosphorylase activity is a heterogeneous group of disorders. Deficiency of phosphorylase kinase (GSD type IX) resulting in failure of hepatic phosphorylase activation is the most common of these disorders, whereas deficiency of liver glycogen phosphorylase (GSD type VI) is very rare. Phosphorylase kinase of liver and muscle is a complex enzyme consisting of four subunits (α, β, γ, and δ), of which the γ subunit is catalytically active.

Mutations in three different genes for PHK subunits can result in deficient activity of hepatic phosphorylase. X-linked GSD type IX caused by mutations in the gene encoding the liver isoform of the α subunit is the most common variant. Other less common variants of GSD type IX are autosomal recessive (affecting only liver) or are a form that affects both liver and muscle. GSD type VI is recessive and caused by mutations in liver glycogen phosphorylase.

The clinical phenotype is similar in GSD types VI and IX. Classically, the physical hallmark is hepatomegaly without splenomegaly. Although some patients have been reported with growth retardation and hypoglycemia, this tends to be the exception. The impaired glycogen breakdown in GSD types VI and IX leads to mild hypoglycemia after prolonged fasting. Unlike in GSD type I, blood levels of lactic acid and uric acid are normal. Mild elevation of triglycerides, cholesterol, and serum transaminase may be present. Muscular hypotonia can result in delayed motor development in patients with X-linked GSD type IX. Prolonged fasting should be avoided in these patients. A bedtime snack is usually sufficient to prevent hypoglycemia in the morning. Clinical and biochemical abnormalities gradually improve with age, and most adult patients are asymptomatic.

GLYCOGEN SYNTHASE DEFICIENCY (GSD TYPE 0)

Glycogen storage disease type 0 is caused by deficiency of the hepatic isoform of glycogen synthase.[143] Glycogen synthase catalyzes the formation of α-1,4 linkages that elongate chains of glucose molecules to form glycogen. Autosomal-recessive mutations in the *GYS2* gene located on chromosome 12p12.2 cause GSD 0.[144] In contrast to other forms of glycogenoses, in GSD type 0 there is marked decreased in liver glycogen content. GSD type 0 is the only GSD not associated with hepatomegaly. Children with GSD 0 are usually asymptomatic during early infancy, but experience fasting ketotic hypoglycemia when weaned from overnight feedings. They can be relatively asymptomatic because the increased plasma ketones are used as alternative brain fuel.

This condition mimics the syndrome of ketotic hypoglycemia and should be considered in the differential diagnosis. In addition to fasting hypoglycemia, deficiency of glycogen synthase results in postprandial hyperglycemia after ingestion of a carbohydrate-containing meal. After uptake by the liver, glucose is shunted into the glycolytic pathway—leading to postprandial hyperlactatemia and hyperlipidemia. Short stature and osteopenia are common in untreated children, but improve with appropriate metabolic control. The goal of treatment is to prevent hypoglycemia and to minimize metabolic acidosis. Dietary recommendations include a high-protein diet with complex carbohydrates. Uncooked cornstarch is used to prevent fasting ketotic hypoglycemia overnight.

DIAGNOSIS OF GLYCOGEN STORAGE DISORDERS

The diagnosis of glycogen storage disorders is based in grant part on the clinical presentation. The combination of clinical features, biochemical analysis, and mutation analysis allows for the specific types of GSD to be differentiated. Clinically, GSD type I can be easily differentiated by the severity of hypoglycemia (which occurs after a short period of fasting) and the association with lactic academia and hyperuricemia. As previously discussed, hypoglycemia is milder and usually happens after prolonged fasting in patients with other forms of GSD. Hepatomegaly is a common clinical feature in all the types except GSD type 0.

A fed glucagon stimulation testing with simultaneous assessment of blood glucose and lactate is also helpful in the diagnosis. In GSD type I, glucagon cause a rise in lactate levels (whereas blood glucose levels remain unchanged). Biochemical studies of leukocytes provide information on all glycogen storage diseases except glucose 6-phosphatase deficiency. The diagnosis of glucose 6-phosphatase deficiency may be made through enzymatic studies on liver biopsy tissue, but the availability of mutation analysis has made the need for liver biopsy obsolete. Mutation analysis is now available for GSD types Ia and Ib, as well as GSD type 0.

Disorders of Gluconeogenesis

GLUCOSE 6-PHOSPHATASE DEFICIENCY (GSD TYPE I)

Although this disorder is often classified among the glycogen storage diseases, it should be considered primarily a defect of gluconeogenesis.

FRUCTOSE 1,6-DIPHOSPHATASE DEFICIENCY

Fructose 1,6-diphosphatase is a key regulatory enzyme of gluconeogenesis. A deficiency of this enzyme results in a block of gluconeogenesis from all possible precursors below the level of fructose-1,6-diphosphate (i.e., fructose, glycerol, lactate, amino acids) (see Figure 5-2). Infusion of these gluconeogenic precursors results in lactic acidosis without a rise in glucose, and acute hypoglycemia may be provoked by inhibition of glycogenolysis. Normally, however, glycogenolysis remains intact and glucagon elicits a normal glycemic response in the fed but not in the fasted state. Hypoglycemia does not develop until fasted beyond glycogen reserves. In affected families, there may be a history of siblings with known hepatomegaly who died in infancy with unexplained metabolic acidosis.

Hepatomegaly in individuals with fructose 1,6-diphosphatase deficiency is due to lipid storage. The biochemical hallmark consists of lactic acidosis, ketosis, hyperlipidemia, and hyperuricemia. Their pathogenesis is related to the severity and duration of hypoglycemia and the resultant low levels of insulin and high levels of counter-regulatory hormones. Therapy in these infants consists of avoidance of fasting longer than 8 to 10 hours. A diet high in carbohydrates (56%, excluding fructose, which cannot be used), low in protein (12%), and normal in fat composition (32%) has permitted normal growth and development. Continuous nocturnal provision of calories through the intragastric infusion system described for type I glycogen storage disease is also applicable to children with fructose 1,6-diphosphatase deficiency. During intercurrent illnesses with vomiting, intravenous glucose infusion is necessary to prevent severe hypoglycemia and lactic acidemia.

PYRUVATE CARBOXYLASE DEFICIENCY

Pyruvate carboxylase is a mitochondrial enzyme that catalyzes conversion of pyruvate to oxalacetate, a key metabolite in gluconeogenesis. Clinical manifestations of pyruvate carboxylase deficiency include lactic acidosis and hypoglycemia. Other biochemical markers include elevated pyruvate and alanine.[145] In addition to lactic acidosis and hypoglycemia, a subgroup of patients develops hyperammonemia and elevation of plasma citrulline, lysine, and proline levels.

Mental retardation and seizures may be part of the presentation in some patients.[146] The severity of this condition varies from mild intermittent lactic acidosis without mental disability to severe, rapidly progressive, and often fatal disease. The diagnosis of pyruvate carboxylase deficiency is confirmed by measurement of enzyme activity in fibroblasts. Treatment is primarily symptomatic, with correction of the metabolic acidosis. Replacement of Krebs cycle intermediates (citrate, aspartate, or odd-chain fatty acid compounds) has been used, as well as supplementation with coenzymes of pyruvate dehydrogenase complex (thiamine and lipoic acid).[147,148]

PHOSPHOENOLPYRUVATE CARBOXYKINASE DEFICIENCY

This is a potential gluconeogenic disorder, and a few reported cases have been suggested to have a deficiency of this enzyme. None has been confirmed, however. Therefore, the existence of this defect remains uncertain.

Galactosemia

Galactose metabolism progresses through phosphorylation (galactose-1-P) and then through conjugation with uridine to form uridine diphosphate (UDP) galactose. UDP galactose may undergo epimerization to form UDP glucose (Figure 5-2). The clinical syndrome of galactosemia results from a deficiency of galactose 1-phosphate uridyl transferase. UDP galactose-4-epimerase deficiency may result in a similar syndrome, however.[149] Galactose 1-phosphate uridyl transferase is essential in infants consuming lactose as their primary carbohydrate source.

In infants with classic galactosemia, exposure to dietary galactose results in acute deterioration of multiple organ systems—including liver dysfunction, coagulopathy, poor feeding and weight loss, renal tubular dysfunction, cerebral edema, vitreous hemorrhage, neutropenia, and *Escherichia coli* sepsis.[150] Most state screening programs have included galactosemia in their newborn screening. The important clinical caveat is that hypoglycemia in an infant who has vomiting or diarrhea and jaundice (with or without hepatomegaly) should raise the diagnostic consideration of galactosemia. However, hypoglycemia is not a common feature unless severe hepatic failure has already developed.

A neonate with these findings and concomitant *Escherichia coli* sepsis should also be considered as possibly affected with galactosemia, because neonatal *E. coli* sepsis is increased in this disorder (often leading to death). The toxic accumulation of galactose 1-phosphate is proposed as a mechanism to explain the deleterious effects on certain tissues resulting in intellectual impairment, cataracts, hepatic dysfunction, renal tubular defects with Fanconi syndrome, and ovarian (but not testicular) failure. A galactose-restricted diet will effectively reverse many of the listed abnormalities and almost certainly will eliminate the likelihood of hypoglycemia. Long-term effects on mental function as well as on speech and ovarian function may persist despite appropriate dietary therapy, however.[151]

Hereditary Fructose Intolerance

Hereditary fructose intolerance (HFI) is an autosomal-recessive disorder caused by a deficiency in fructose-1-phosphate aldolase. This aldolase is the primary isoenzyme used during the incorporation of diet-derived fructose into the hepatic glycolytic and gluconeogenic pathways. HFI may be a diagnostic challenge. In the absence of fructose ingestion, patients are entirely normal. Ingestion or infusion of fructose, sucrose, and sorbitol results in the accumulation of fructose 1-phosphate in the liver and a depletion of intracellular phosphate and ATP pools. These metabolic disturbances result in decreased gluconeogenesis and glycogenolysis, which precipitate hypoglycemia.[152]

The severity of the clinical phenotype varies with the quantity of the dietary fructose exposure. Breast-fed or milk-based formula-fed infants are normal until fruits and juices are introduced into the diet. If a fructose- or sucrose-containing formula is fed during the neonatal period to an affected individual, the consequences may be lethal. Because many of the symptoms after fructose ingestion suggest gastrointestinal system disturbances, a soy or elemental formula containing sucrose may be tried—resulting in progressive deterioration of the infant. The worsening of symptoms and hypoglycemia with feedings should raise clinical suspicion. Biochemical confirmation of the diagnosis may be ascertained by enzyme assay of liver or small intestinal biopsy. Although intravenous fructose tolerance testing was used in the past, the risks to the patient and the availability of molecular diagnosis have made this method obsolete.

Symptoms after acute exposure to fructose include those of hypoglycemia, as well as nausea, abdominal pain, and vomiting. Chronic exposure results in failure to thrive and a clinical spectrum suggestive of chronic liver disease. Hypoglycemia may be missed in patients with HFI because the fall in blood glucose concentration may be transient.[153] Sorbitol ingestion causes biochemical abnormalities similar to fructose ingestion without fructosemia.[154] Treatment of this disorder involves strict dietary avoidance of fructose, sucrose, and sorbitol. This avoidance is often learned and self-imposed by patients if they reach 1 year of age.

Disorders of Fatty Acid Oxidation

At least 25 enzymes and transport proteins are involved in mitochondrial fatty acid metabolism, some of which have been recognized very recently. Defects in 22 of these have been shown to cause disease in humans, and although the first defects were identified 30 years ago most have been identified only in the past 15 years.[155] The inborn errors of metabolism associated with deficiencies of fatty acid oxidation (Figure 5-12) are inherited in autosomal-recessive fashion. All of these disorders may be provoked with fasting and exhibit life-threatening events with varying degrees of hypoglycemia associated with a relative deficiency in the generation of ketone bodies.[156] Disorders of fatty acid oxidation may be divided according to the site of the defect: defects of fatty acid and carnitine transport, β-oxidation defects, electron transport chain defects, and defects of ketone body synthesis and utilization.

The disorders of fatty acid oxidation share many clinical features and tend to be exacerbated with fasting because metabolism of fatty acids is maximal during fasting. Common events (such as immunization or intercurrent infections) will often decrease oral intake and result in symptoms and signs of a defect in fatty acid oxidation. The wide spectrum of clinical presentation includes hepatic, cardiac, and muscle manifestations.[157] The most important of these is the hepatic presentation characterized by acute life-threatening attacks of coma precipitated by fasting. This manifestation occurs in nearly all of the defects, and is more clearly exemplified by medium-chain acyl-coenzyme A dehydrogenase deficiency (MCAD).

Attacks are associated with hypoketotic hypoglycemia with little or no academia; elevation of serum urea, ammonia, and uric acid; liver function abnormalities; and hepatic steatosis. The risk of severe complications and

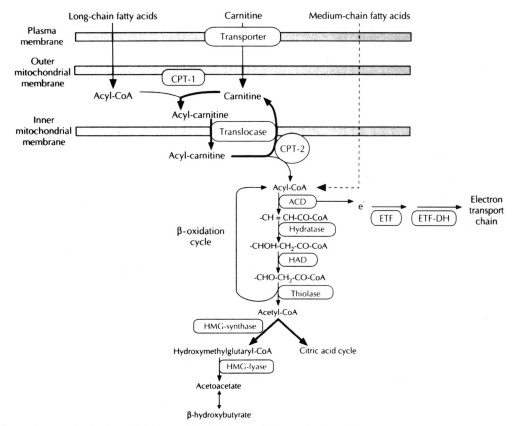

Figure 5-12. The pathways of mitochondrial fatty acid oxidation and ketone body synthesis. ACD = acyl-CoA dehydrogenase, CPT-1 and CPT-2 = carnitine palmitoyltransferase I and II, ETF 5 electron-transferring flavoprotein, ETF-DH = electron-transferring flavoprotein dehydrogenase, and HAD = hydroxyacyl-CoA dehydrogenase. [From Stanley CA, Hale DE (1994). Genetic disorders of mitochondrial fatty acid oxidation. Curr Opin Pediatr 6:476.]

death is very high unless appropriate treatment to reverse the catabolic state is implemented. The diagnosis of these cases may be confused with Reye's syndrome. Cardiac involvement frequently accompanies acute hepatic presentations, especially in defects affecting long-chain fatty acid oxidation.[158] The cardiac presentation can be acute or chronic, with dilated or hyperthrophic cardiomyopathy. This presentation can evolve to progressive heart failure at 2 to 3 years of age (or later in patients with muscle-kidney plasma membrane carnitine transporter defect).[159] The third manifestation of fatty acid oxidation disorders is acute or chronic muscle presentations.

The least severe cases can be seen in adults with the mild form of carnitine palmitoyl-transferase 2 deficiency who present with acute rhabdomyolysis and renal failure after strenuous exercise.[160] Some manifestations of fatty acid oxidation disorders, such as pigmentary retinopathy and peripheral neuropathy (which occur in long-chain 3-hydroxyacyl-CoA dehydrogenase deficiency), may be explained by toxic effects of fatty acid metabolites. Less common manifestations of fatty acid oxidation disorders involve congenital malformations[161] or the acute fatty liver of pregnancy or the HELLP (hemolysis, elevated liver enzymes, low platelets) syndrome in mothers heterozygous for long-chain 3-hydroxy-acyl-coenzyme A dehydrogenase deficiency (LCHAD) mutations.[162]

Because fatty acid oxidation is reduced with loss-of-function mutations in this pathway, a decreased ability to generate ketones during normal fasting and acute illness is common. Thus, these defects as a class are associated with hypoketotic hypoglycemia. Although hypoglycemia may be a prominent late feature of the severe mutations seen with MCAD, the phenotype of a defect of a fatty acid oxidation disorder may not manifest if a fasting state is avoided. A high index of suspicion for fatty acid oxidation defects is important because appropriate therapy may result in an interruption and prevention of these potentially life-threatening episodes.

The most commonly presenting deficiencies involve the mitochondrial acyl-CoA dehydrogenases with very long-, long-, medium-, and short-chain length specificities (VLCAD, LCAD, MCAD, and SCAD, respectively).[163] MCAD is the most frequent. Neonatal screening in Pennsylvania has shown an incidence of 1 in 9,000 live births.[164] Although there is significant heterogeneity in presentation of MCAD, the most frequent clinical presentation is one of intermittent hypoketotic hypoglycemia. Mild hyperammonemia and coma may be present with a Reye-like syndrome. A distinct association of the symptoms with fasting or substrate deprivation is consistent with this defect.

Affected patients have also been misdiagnosed with idiopathic sudden infant death syndrome.[165,166] Decreased plasma carnitine levels and an increase in the ratio of esterified to free carnitine is a frequently associated laboratory finding. VLCAD deficiency is commonly associated with cardiac and skeletal muscle myophaty, but hypoketotic hypoglycemia, hyperammonemia, and hepatocellular failure can also occur.[167] Although putative LCAD deficiency cases have been reported, all of the patients described before 1992 were subsequently proven to have VLCAD.[168] Hypoglycemia is not usual in SCAD deficiency.

Deficiencies of several steps of carnitine, acylcarnitine, and fatty acid transport into cells and mitochondria have been described.[169,170] A genetic defect of the plasma membrane carnitine transporter represents the only true entity of primary carnitine deficiency. Decreased carnitine accumulation in tissue and renal carnitine losses result in impairment of long-chain fatty acid metabolism, which can lead to severe hypoglycemia and dilated cardiomyophaty in infancy or childhood. This disorder (and no others) responds to carnitine supplementation. Liver carnitine palmitoyl transferase I (CPT I) deficiency is characterized by early-onset episodic hypoketotic hypoglycemia, sometimes with hyperammonemia and multiorgan system failure.

These patients can have elevated levels of plasma carnitine. Deficiency of the carnitine-acylcarnitine translocase presents with severe hypoketotic hypoglycemia, hyperammonemia, and cardiac arrhytmias in the neonatal period. Plasma carnitine levels are extremely low. Cardiomyopathy related to secondary carnitine deficiency may be present. CPT II deficiency is the most common of this group of disorders (with mostly muscle involvement), although a more severe variant similar to CPT I deficiency has also been reported.[171] The carnitine transporter defect may be effectively treated with oral carnitine supplementation, and a rapid reversal of the clinical syndrome (including cardiomyopathy) may be seen over weeks to months.[172,173]

Defects of other mitochondrial matrix enzymes involved in β-oxidation include deficiency of long-chain 3-hydroxy-acyl-coenzyme A dehydrogenase (LCHAD). LCHAD is one of the more severe fatty acid oxidation disorders, with a wide phenotypic spectra and diverse manifestations—including hypoglycemia, cardiomyopathy, skeletal myopathy, hepatocellular disease, pigmentary retinopathy, peripheral neuropathy, and sudden death. In the last decade, many patients with LCHAD deficiency have been reported who were born following pregnancies complicated with severe maternal liver disease (acute fatty liver of pregnancy and HELLP syndrome). Thus, a detailed prenatal history may be key to the diagnosis.[174] The vulnerability to maternal complications of pregnancy can also be seen in other fatty acid oxidation disorders.

Hypoketotic hypoglycemia can be part of the presentation in defects of ketone body production due to deficiency of 3-hydroxy 3-methylglutaryl-coenzyme A (HMG-CoA) lyase and HMG-CoA synthase deficiency. These two disorders can be differentiated by the large urinary excretion of 3-hydroxy-3-methylglutaric acid, which is pathognomonic for HMC-CoA lyase deficiency.

Evaluation of suspected errors in fatty acid oxidation should first include determination of the profile of plasma acyl-carnitines by mass spectrometry and measurement of plasma total, esterified, and free carnitine. Most, but not all, of the fatty acid oxidation disorders are associated with specific abnormalities of plasma acyl-carnitines—such as octanoyl-carnitine, which is diagnostically elevated in MCAD deficiency (Table 5-8). Determinations of urinary organic acids with assessment of the presence or absence of dicarboxylic aciduria are also very useful.

TABLE 5-8

Fatty Acid Oxidation Disorders with Distinguishing Metabolic Markers

Disorder	Plasma Acylcarnitines	Urinary Acylglycines	Urinary Organic Acids
VLCAD	Tetradecenoyl-		
MCAD	Octanoyl	Hexanoyl-	
		Suberyl-	
		Phenylpropionyl-	
SCAD	Butyryl-	Butyryl-	Ethylmalonic
LCHAD	3-Hydroxy-palmitoyl-		3-Hydroxydicarboxylic
	3-Hydroxy-oleoyl-		
	3-Hydroxy-linoleoyl-		
DER	Dodecadienoyl-		
ETF and ETF-DH	Butyryl-	Isovaleryl-	Ethylmalonic
	Isovaleryl-	Hexanoyl-	Glutaric
	Glutaryl-		Isovaleric
HMG-CoA lyase	Methylglutaryl-		3-Hydroxy-3-methyl-glutaric

DER, 2,4-dienoyl-coenzyme A reductase; ETF, electron-transferring flavoprotein; ETF-DH, ETF dehydrogenase; HMG-CoA, 3-hydroxy-3-methylglutaryl-coenzyme A; LCHAD, long-chain 3-hydroxyacyl-coenzyme A dehydrogenase; MCAD, medium-chain acyl-coenzyme A dehydrogenase; SCAD, short-chain acyl-coenzyme A dehydrogenase; VLCAD, very-long-chain acyl-coenzyme A dehydrogenase.

From Stanley CA (1990). Disorders of fatty acid oxidation. In Fernandes J, Bremer E, Saudubray J-M (eds.), *Inborn metabolic diseases: Diagnosis and treatment*. New York: Springer-Verlag 394-410.

Patients whose disorder cannot be identified by these tests may require further evaluations, including assays of fatty acid oxidation and specific enzyme assays in cultured skin fibroblasts or lymphoblasts. Since the early 1990s, the use of tandem mass espectometry has made newborn screening possible for most fatty acid oxidation disorders based on the acyl-carnitine profile in blood spots. Presymptomatic identification of these individuals can prevent catastrophic events such as sudden death. Direct DNA mutational analysis can be performed for many of these defects, which is particularly useful in MCAD and LCHAD deficiencies in which most cases are due to single common mutations.

The primary treatment of disorders of fatty acid oxidation is a devoted avoidance of fasting. For infants younger than 1 year old, 6 to 8 hours of fasting may be sufficient to precipitate an episode. On the other hand, as children become older they appear to be able to withstand periods of fasting of as long as 10 to 12 hours without decompensation. A high index of suspicion and rapid institution of intravenous glucose will often reverse an evolving episode. The presence of hypoglycemia is usually an event that occurs late in the evolution of an episode of metabolic decompensation. High-fat diets should be avoided, although normal amounts of dietary fats do not appear to be toxic. An adjunct approach may involve the use of cornstarch (as used for the treatment of type I glycogen storage disease) in doses of 1.5 to 2 g/kg. This may delay the adaptation from the fed to the fasted state. Riboflavin has been reported to be an adjunct in rare patients.[175] The use of carnitine has been advocated.[176] However, a systematic assessment of various treatment regimens in these defects has not been available.

The expansion of neonatal screening programs based on determination of blood acyl-carnitine profiles by mass spectrometry allows earlier identification of these disorders and allows preventive counseling to parents to significantly decrease the occurrence of life-threatening events in these syndromes. Some chemical agents (such as valproic acid, hypoglycin A, and atractyloside) mimic the fatty acid oxidation disorders outlined in Figure 5-12.[177] Valproic acid can block β-oxidation. Treatment of epilepsy with valproic acid has been associated with Reye-like syndromes, including hypoketotic hypoglycemia.[178] Some investigators have advocated treatment with carnitine for infants receiving valproic acid, but there is not universal agreement on this point.[178]

Jamaican vomiting sickness is caused by the toxin hypoglycin A, a component of the unripened ackee fruit (a Jamaican food staple). This chemical acts as an inhibitor of fatty acid oxidation and can produce a syndrome similar to that of a patient with MCAD deficiency with hypoketotic hypoglycemia.[179] Last, rare ingestions of plant atractyloside (such as found in the Mediterranean species *Atractylis gummifera*) have been associated with a syndrome of vomiting and hypoketotic hypoglycemia.[180] Atractyloside is an inhibitor of mitochondrial oxidative phosphorylation and prevents translocation of adenine nucleotides across the mitochondrial membrane.[181]

Drug-Induced Hypoglycemia

Drug-induced hypoglycemia is rare in neonates and young infants. The administration of medications to infants may represent the Munchausen by proxy syndrome. Rarely, it may represent a pharmaceutical dispensing error with substitution of an insulin secretogogue (e.g., glyburide) for another medication. Hypoglycemia can also occur as a side effect of therapy (i.e., beta-blockers). Toxic substances such as ethyl alcohol in various beverages or salicylates may be accidentally or deliberately used in detrimental ways in infants. As noted in the discussion of hyperinsulinism, injectable insulin is readily available—as are potent oral hypoglycemic agents. Occasionally, an infant will present with unexplained hypoglycemia and not fit readily into any diagnostic algorithm. In these rare instances, a careful history of drug or alcohol availability in the environment must be undertaken and pharmacy dispensing errors considered.

Defects of Glucose Transporters

GLUT1 DEFICIENCY

GLUT1 deficiency has now been diagnosed in a growing number of patients since the first reports in 1991.[9] The cloning of the human SLC2A1 (encoding *GLUT1*) gene confirmed the initial speculation involving a defect in glucose transport across the blood-brain barrier as the underlying mechanism for the classic presentation of infantile-onset epileptic encephalopathy associated with delayed neurologic development. The genetic inheritance of the condition behaves as an autosomal dominant trait, although spontaneous heterozygous mutation in the SLC2A1 gene can present sporadically in families.[182,183]

The phenotypic presentation is variable, from the classic presentation of developmental encephalopathy with seizures to nonclassic presentations with mental retardation, dysarthric speech, and intermittent ataxia without clinical seizures. It can also manifest as a movement disorder characterized by choreoathetosis and dystonia.[183] The biochemical hallmark is the finding of hypoglycorrhachia (low cerebrospinal fluid glucose concentration) despite normal plasma glucose concentrations. Treatment efforts have been based on providing alternative brain fuel sources by a ketogenic diet.[9,184] The ketogenic diet effectively controls the seizures and other paroxysmal activities, but is has less effect on the cognitive function.

GLUT2 DEFICIENCY

Fanconi-Bickel syndrome (characterized by hepatomegaly, glucose and galactose intolerance, and renal tubular dysfunction) is due to a recessive mutation of the GLUT2 plasma membrane transporter for glucose (encoded by *SLC2A2*).[185] GLUT2 is expressed in liver, renal tubular cells, enterocytes, and pancreatic beta cells. The clinical

TABLE 5-9

Differential Diagnosis of Hypoglycemia in Neonates and Infants

Disorder	Length of Fast (hr)	PLASMA FUELS AT END OF FAST (mmol/L)			
		Glucose	Lactate	Free Fatty Acids	β-Hydroxy-butyrate
Normal Infants	24-36	2.8	0.7-1.5	1.5-2.5	2.0-4.0
Endocrine System					
Hyperinsulinism	Varies	2.8	N	<1.5	<2.0
Cortisol deficiency	10-16	2.8	N	N	N
GH deficiency	10-16	2.8	N	N	N
Panhypopituitarism	10-16	2.8	N	N	N
Epinephrine deficiency (beta-blocker)	10-16	2.8	N	<1.5	<2.0
Glycogenolysis					
Debrancher deficiency (GSD3)	4-8	2.8	N	N	N
Phosphorylase deficiency (GSD6)	10-16	2.8	N	N	N
Phosphorylase kinase deficiency (GSD9)	10-16	2.8	N	N	N
Glycogen synthase deficiency (GSD0)	6-12	2.8	N	N	N
Gluconeogenesis					
Glucose 6-phosphatase deficiency (GSD1a and 1b)	2-4	2.8	4-8+	N	<2.0
Fructose 1,6-diphosphatase deficiency	8-12	2.8	4-8+	N	N
Pyruvate carboxylase deficiency	8-12	2.8	4-8+	N	N
Lypolysis					
Congenital lipodystrophy, familial dysautonomia, beta-blockers	10-16	2.8	N	<1.5	<2.0
Fatty Acid Oxidation	10-16	2.8	N	>2.5	<1.5
Carnitine transporter, CPT-1, Translocase, CPT-2, VLCAD, MCAD, SCAD, LCHAD, MADD, HMG-CoA synthase, HMG-CoA lyase deficiency					

For definitions of abbreviations, see Table 7-8 footnote.
GH, growth hormone; GSD, glycogen storage disease.

manifestations reflect impairment of glucose release from liver and of glucose reabsorption from renal tubular cells. Galactose clearance and conversion to glucose is delayed. Patients with GLUT2 deficiency usually present at an age of 3 to 10 months.

The typical clinical signs are hepatomegaly due to glycogen accumulation, a severe Fanconi-type renal tubulopathy with disproportionately severe glucosuria, glucose and galactose intolerance, rickets, and severely stunted growth.[186] These patients may present with a combination of fasting hypoglycemia and postprandial hyperglycemia. The therapeutic goal for patients with GLUT2 deficiency is to ameliorate the consequences of renal tubulopathy by replacing water, electrolytes, and alkali—and by providing phosphate and vitamin D supplementation. In terms of diet, an adequate caloric intake is recommended to compensate for renal and intestinal glucose loss—given as frequent feedings containing slowly absorbed carbohydrates (such as cornstarch) to avoid fasting hypoglycemia.

Systemic Disorders

Hypoglycemia may be a concomitant of severe systemic disease in neonates and infants. Neonatal sepsis is frequently complicated by hypoglycemia.[187] Malnourished infants, either deprived of caloric intake or suffering from malabsorption, may develop hypoglycemia as the malnutrition becomes severe.[188] Unique to newborns, hyperviscosity syndrome may be complicated by hypoglycemia. Up to 14% of infants with a hematocrit of more than 65% were noted to demonstrate hypoglycemia in one study.[189] A high index of suspicion for hypoglycemia should be maintained in any severely compromised neonate or infant.

Diagnosis

Treatment of hypoglycemia in neonates and infants requires making a specific diagnosis of the underlying cause. The diagnosis should be based on the combination of data obtained from the history, physical examination, laboratory findings, and (especially) the hormonal and fuel responses at the time of fasting hypoglycemia. Table 5-9 outlines the major distinguishing features of the various forms of hypoglycemic disorders in neonates and infants. As shown, the most important information required for diagnosis comes from tests on the blood and urine specimens obtained at a time of hypoglycemia (also known as the critical samples).

Important facts from the history include the duration of fasting that provoked hypoglycemia. Based on frequency,

PLASMA HORMONES AT END OF FAST

Insulin (mU/mL)	Cortisol (mg/dL)	Growth Hormone (ng/mL)	Glycemic Response to Glucagon (Mg/dl)	Physical Examination
<2	>20	>10	<30	
>1	N	N	>30	LGA
N	low	low	N	
N	N	low	N	Short stature
N	low	N	N	Short stature, midline facial malformation, optic hypoplasia, micropenis
N	N	N	N	
N	N	N	N	Hepatomegaly 4+
N	N	N	N	Hepatomegaly 2+
N	N	N	N	Hepatomegaly 2+
N	N	N	N	Hepatomegaly 1+
N	N	N	(↑ lactate)	Hepatomegaly 4+
N	N	N	N	Hepatomegaly 1+
N	N	N	N	
N	N	N	N	
N	N	N	N	Hepatomegaly 1+

hyperinsulinism should always be considered at the top of the list of differential diagnoses. Onset within a few hours of a meal would be consistent with hyperinsulinism or glucose 6-phosphatase deficiency, whereas onset after 10 to 12 hours would be consistent with a defect in fatty acid oxidation. Short stature would be consistent with pituitary deficiency, and this possibility would be supported by the presence of midline facial malformations, microphthalmia, or microphallus. Growth failure is also a prominent feature of glucose 6-phosphatase deficiency or debrancher deficiency glycogen storage disease. Both of these disorders are associated with massive hepatomegaly. Abnormal results of liver function tests (transaminases) and hyperammonemia, with or without elevated creatine kinase level, would suggest a possible fatty acid oxidation disorder.

Figure 5-13 outlines an algorithm for diagnosis of different forms of hypoglycemia based on readily available laboratory tests on the "critical" blood and urine samples. The first discriminant is a measure of acidemia at the time of hypoglycemia using the serum bicarbonate. If the acidemia is caused by elevations of the keto-acids β-hydroxybutyrate and acetoacetate), possibilities include a normal child fasted for too long (ketotic hypoglycemia), a defect in glycogenolysis (type 3 glycogen storage disease), or counter-regulatory hormone deficiency (e.g., hypopituitarism). If the acidemia is caused by an elevation of lactic acid, a block of gluconeogenesis should be suspected (e.g., glucose 6-phosphatase or fructose 1,6-diphosphatase deficiency or ethanol ingestion).

If there is no acidemia (i.e., absence of the normal elevation of ketones) but free fatty acid levels are high, a defect in fatty acid oxidation and ketogenesis can be suspected (e.g., MCAD deficiency). If ketones are not appropriately increased but the free fatty acid concentrations are also suppressed, hyperinsulinism can be suspected. In the neonatal period, the features of hyperinsulinism can be mimicked by congenital pituitary deficiency. Further tests can then be planned using the initial critical specimens to confirm the suspected diagnosis. These may include physiologic tests (such as the glucagon stimulation test at a time of hypoglycemia to confirm hyperinsulinism) or specialized laboratory tests (such as a plasma acyl-carnitine profile) to identify a defect in mitochondrial β-oxidation.

In some cases, a formal fasting test may be necessary to diagnose the cause of hypoglycemia. The goal of this test is to reproduce the setting in which hypoglycemia occurs in order to identify the underlying cause. The fasting test should be considered a method of testing a hypothesis that has already been developed, based on available clinical and laboratory data about the cause of the hypoglycemia. Thus, the test can be modified with additions or deletions to the basic protocol. This is important, because challenging an infant with fasting is not without risk—particularly if a genetic defect in fatty acid oxidation or adrenal insufficiency is present. Therefore, fasting or other diagnostic challenges should be done only in the hospital under carefully controlled settings with experienced physician and nursing staff readily available.

Infants younger than 1 year are usually fasted for up to 24 hours, whereas in older children the maximum fast is 36 hours. The fast is terminated when the plasma glucose

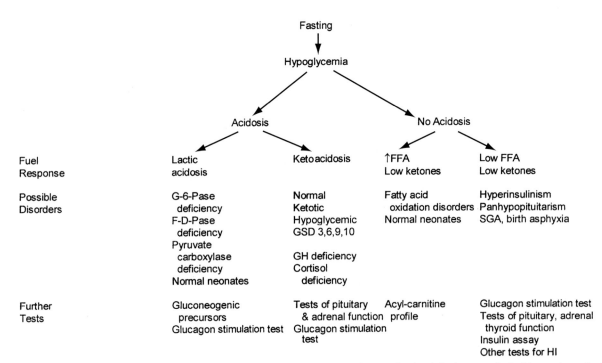

Figure 5-13 Algorithm for diagnosis of hypoglycemia based on "critical" blood tests obtained during a period of hypoglycemia. FFA = free fatty acids, GSD = glycogen storage disorder, HI = hyperinsulinism, and SGA = small for gestational age. [Modified from Stanley CA, Baker L (1978). Hypoglycemia. In Kaye R, Oski FA, Barness LA (eds.), *Core textbook of pediatrics*. Philadelphia: JB Lippincott 280-305.]

falls below 50 mg/dL, but may be ended sooner if plasma β-hydroxybutyrate rises to greater than 2.0 mmol/L or in the case of any adverse signs or symptoms. Periodic blood samples are obtained for analysis of major fuels and hormones and for appropriate ancillary tests (e.g., serum total carnitine, acyl-carnitine profile, liver transaminases, creatine phosphokinase, or urinary organic acids). If hyperinsulinism is suspected, the fasting test may be ended with glucagons (1 mg given intravenously) to evaluate the glycemic response.

Special note should be made that the most frequent cause of hypoglycemia in neonates, infants, and children (hyperinsulinism) often cannot be diagnosed based solely on the plasma insulin concentration. With very sensitive assays, serum insulin concentrations will be less than 1 to 2 μU/mL at times of hypoglycemia (i.e. below the sensitivity of most insulin assays). Therefore, the diagnosis must often be made based on evidence of inappropriate insulin effects: hypoketonemia, hypo-free fatty acidemia, and a positive glycemic response to glucagon.

Treatment

A rational therapeutic approach to the treatment of hypoglycemia relies on a systematic diagnostic evaluation. The key to effective treatment is diagnosis specific. The maintenance of euglycemia is critical to the preservation of central nervous system function. Even in the presence of an uncertain diagnosis, every effort must be used to maintain euglycemia until a diagnosis is made or hypoglycemia resolves. Intravenous glucose infusion remains the mainstay of emergency therapy. Glucose infusion rates may need to be increased as high as 15 to 25 mg/kg/min in infants with hyperinsulinism to maintain euglycemia. Hormones and drugs may be used as insulin antagonists or suppressants. In the case of congenital hyperinsulinism due to KATP mutations, surgery should be considered—especially in children with the focal form of the disease.

Conclusions

Since the early reports of neonatal hypoglycemia in the 1950s by McQuarrie[190] and Cornblath and colleagues,[191] our understanding of the pathogeneses and treatment of hypoglycemia in neonates and infants has progressed rapidly. The recent identification of the molecular causes of congenital hyperinsulinism represents a significant new discovery. The development of non-invasive techniques (such as the ^{18}F-fluoro-L-DOPA PET scan) that can accurately identify patients with focal KATPHI and the potential for cure with surgical removal of the lesion are promising advances in the treatment of these children. These and future discoveries should result in continued improvement in outcome in hypoglycemic patients.

REFERENCES

1. Cryer PE (2003). Glucose homeostasis and hypoglycemia. Philadelphia: WB Saunders.
2. Nehlig A (1997). Cerebral energy metabolism, glucose transport and blood flow: changes with maturation and adaptation to hypoglycaemia. Diabetes Metab 23:18.
3. Devaskar SU, Mueckler MM (1992). The mammalian glucose transporters. Pediatr Res 31:1.
4. Scheepers A, Joost HG, Schurmann A (2004). The glucose transporter families SGLT and GLUT: molecular basis of normal and aberrant function. JPEN J Parenter Enteral Nutr 28:364.
5. Kahn BB (1992). Facilitative glucose transporters: regulatory mechanisms and dysregulation in diabetes. J Clin Invest 89:1367.
6. Pardridge WM, Boado RJ, Farrell CR (1990). Brain-type glucose transporter (GLUT-1) is selectively localized to the blood-brain barrier. Studies with quantitative western blotting and in situ hybridization. J Biol Chem 265:18035.
7. Kang L, Routh VH, Kuzhikandathil EV, et al. (2004). Physiological and molecular characteristics of rat hypothalamic ventromedial nucleus glucosensing neurons. Diabetes 53:549.
8. Settergren G, Lindblad BS, Persson B (1980). Cerebral blood flow and exchange of oxygen, glucose ketone bodies, lactate, pyruvate and amino acids in anesthetized children. Acta Paediatr Scand 69:457.
9. De Vivo DC, Trifiletti RR, Jacobson RI, et al. (1991). Defective glucose transport across the blood-brain barrier as a cause of persistent hypoglycorrhachia, seizures, and developmental delay. N Engl J Med 325:703.
10. Fishman RA (1991). The glucose-transporter protein and glucopenic brain injury. N Engl J Med 325:731.
11. Gerich JE (1988). Lilly lecture 1988. Glucose counterregulation and its impact on diabetes mellitus. Diabetes 37:1608.
12. Cryer PE, Gerich JE (1985). Glucose counterregulation, hypoglycemia, and intensive insulin therapy in diabetes mellitus. N Engl J Med 313:232.
13. Menon RK, Sperling MA (1988). Carbohydrate metabolism. Semin Perinatol 12:157.
14. Bloch CA, Ozbun MA, Khan SA (1993). Glycogen phosphorylase: developmental expression in rat liver. Biol Neonate 63:113.
15. (1989). Brain damage by neonatal hypoglycaemia. Lancet 1:882.
16. Lucas A, Morley R, Cole TJ (1988). Adverse neurodevelopmental outcome of moderate neonatal hypoglycaemia. Bmj 297:1304.
17. Haymond MW (1989). Hypoglycemia in infants and children. Endocrinol Metab Clin North Am 18:211.
18. Cornblath M, Schwartz R (1991). Disorders of Carbohydrate Metabolism in Infancy. Boston: Blackwell Scientific.
19. Sperling MA, DeLamater PV, Phelps D, et al. (1974). Spontaneous and amino acid-stimulated glucagon secretion in the immediate postnatal period. Relation to glucose and insulin. J Clin Invest 53:1159.
20. Bloch CA, Sperling MA (1988). Sources and disposition of fetal glucose: studies in the fetal lamb. Am J Perinatol 5:344.
21. Townsend SF, Rudolph CD, Rudolph AM (1991). Cortisol induces perinatal hepatic gluconeogenesis in the lamb. J Dev Physiol 16:71.
22. Kalhan SC, Savin SM, Adam PA (1976). Measurement of glucose turnover in the human newborn with glucose-1-13C. J Clin Endocrinol Metab 43:704.
23. Fukumoto H, Seino S, Imura H, et al. (1988). Characterization and expression of human HepG2/erythrocyte glucose-transporter gene. Diabetes 37:657.
24. Bier DM, Leake RD, Haymond MW, et al. (1977). Measurement of "true" glucose production rates in infancy and childhood with 6,6-dideuteroglucose. Diabetes 26:1016.
25. Sperling MA, Devaskar SU (1989). Insulin action in the fetal-placental unit. New York: Allan R Liss.
26. Hay WW, Jr. (2006). Recent observations on the regulation of fetal metabolism by glucose. J Physiol 572:17.
27. Sperling MA (1982). Integration of fuel homeostasis by insulin and glucagon in the newborn. Monogr Paediatr 16:39.
28. Sperling MA (1994). Carbohydrate metabolism: Insulin and glucagon. Philadelphia: WB Saunders.
29. Hay WW, Jr., Meznarich HK (1986). The effect of hyperinsulinaemia on glucose utilization and oxidation and on oxygen consumption in the fetal lamb. Q J Exp Physiol 71:689.

30. Bloch CA, Menon RK, Sperling MA (1988). Effects of somatostatin and glucose infusion on glucose kinetics in fetal sheep. Am J Physiol 255:E87.

31. Devaskar SU, Ganguli S, Styer D, et al. (1984). Glucagon and glucose dynamics in sheep: evidence for glucagon resistance in the fetus. Am J Physiol 246:E256.

32. Sperling MA, Ganguli S (1983). Pre- and postnatal development of insulin and glucagon receptors: potential role in energy storage and utilization. J Pediatr Gastroenterol Nutr 2 Suppl 1:S46.

33. Menon RK, Bloch CA, Sperling MA (1990). Estimation of glucose kinetics in fetal-maternal studies: potential errors, solutions, and limitations. Am J Physiol 258:E1006.

34. Pagliara AS, Kari IE, De Vivo DC, et al. (1972). Hypoalaninemia: a concomitant of ketotic hypoglycemia. J Clin Invest 51:1440.

35. Sperling MA, Ganguli S, Leslie N, Landt K (1984). Fetal-perinatal catecholamine secretion: role in perinatal glucose homeostasis. Am J Physiol 247:E69.

36. Heck LJ, Erenberg A (1987). Serum glucose levels in term neonates during the first 48 hours of life. J Pediatr 110:119.

37. Frazer TE, Karl IE, Hillman LS, Bier DM (1981). Direct measurement of gluconeogenesis from [2,3]13C2]alanine in the human neonate. Am J Physiol 240:E615.

38. Girard J (1986). Gluconeogenesis in late fetal and early neonatal life. Biol Neonate 50:237.

39. Greengard O (1977). Enzymic differentiation of human liver: comparison with the rat model. Pediatr Res 11:669.

40. Bashan N, Gross Y, Moses S, Gutman A (1979). Rat liver glycogen metabolism in the perinatal period. Biochim Biophys Acta 587:145.

41. Marsac C, Saudubray JM, Moncion A, Leroux JP (1976). Development of gluconeogenic enzymes in the liver of human newborns. Biol Neonate 28:317.

42. Granner D, Andreone T, Sasaki K, Beale E (1983). Inhibition of transcription of the phosphoenolpyruvate carboxykinase gene by insulin. Nature 305:549.

43. Cahill GF, Jr. (1970). Starvation in man. N Engl J Med 282:668.

44. Chaussain JL, Georges P, Olive G, Job JC (1974). Glycemic response to 24-hour fast in normal children and children with ketotic hypoglycemia: II. Hormonal and metabolic changes. J Pediatr 85:776.

45. McGarry JD (1979). Lilly Lecture 1978. New perspectives in the regulation of ketogenesis. Diabetes 28:517.

46. Hirsch HJ, Loo SW, Gabbay KH (1977). The development and regulation of the endocrine pancreas. J Pediatr 91:518.

47. Stanley CA, Baker L (1976). Hyperinsulinism in infants and children: diagnosis and therapy. Adv Pediatr 23:315.

48. Stanley CA, Baker L (1999). The causes of neonatal hypoglycemia. N Engl J Med 340:1200.

49. Cornblath M, Hawdon JM, Williams AF, (2000). Controversies regarding definition of neonatal hypoglycemia: suggested operational thresholds. Pediatrics 105:1141.

50. Lubchenco LO, Bard H (1971). Incidence of hypoglycemia in newborn infants classified by birth weight and gestational age. Pediatrics 47:831.

51. Stanley CA, Anday EK, Baker L, Delivoria-Papadopolous M (1979). Metabolic fuel and hormone responses to fasting in newborn infants. Pediatrics 64:613.

52. Hegardt FG (1999). Mitochondrial 3-hydroxy-3-methylglutaryl-CoA synthase: a control enzyme in ketogenesis. Biochem J 338 (Pt 3):569.

53. Pegorier JP, Chatelain F, Thumelin S, Girard J (1998). Role of long-chain fatty acids in the postnatal induction of genes coding for liver mitochondrial beta-oxidative enzymes. Biochem Soc Trans 26:113.

54. Stanley CA, Gonzales E, Baker L (1983). Development of hepatic fatty acid oxidation and ketogenesis in the newborn guinea pig. Pediatr Res 17:224.

55. Lucas A, Bloom SR, Aynsley-Green A (1978). Metabolic and endocrine events at the time of the first feed of human milk in preterm and term infants. Arch Dis Child 53:731.

56. Farquhar JW (1959). The child of the diabetic woman. Arch Dis Child 34:76.

57. Collins JE, Leonard JV (1984). Hyperinsulinism in asphyxiated and small-for-dates infants with hypoglycaemia. Lancet 2:311.

58. Collins JE, Leonard JV, Teale D, et al. (1990). Hyperinsulinaemic hypoglycaemia in small for dates babies. Arch Dis Child 65:1118.

59. Hoe FM, Thornton PS, Wanner LA, et al. (2006). Clinical features and insulin regulation in infants with a syndrome of prolonged neonatal hyperinsulinism. J Pediatr 148:207.

60. Stanley CA (1997). Hyperinsulinism in infants and children. Pediatr Clin North Am 44:363.

61. Glaser B, Thornton P, Otonkoski T, Junien C (2000). Genetics of neonatal hyperinsulinism. Arch Dis Child Fetal Neonatal Ed 82:F79.

62. Huopio H, Reimann F, Ashfield R, et al. (2000). Dominantly inherited hyperinsulinism caused by a mutation in the sulfonylurea receptor type 1. J Clin Invest 106:897.

63. Thornton PS, MacMullen C, Ganguly A, et al. (2003). Clinical and molecular characterization of a dominant form of congenital hyperinsulinism caused by a mutation in the high-affinity sulfonylurea receptor. Diabetes 52:2403.

64. Magge SN, Shyng SL, MacMullen C, et al. (2004). Steinkrauss L, Ganguly A, Katz LE, Stanley CA: Familial leucine-sensitive hypoglycemia of infancy due to a dominant mutation of the beta-cell sulfonylurea receptor. J Clin Endocrinol Metab 89:4450.

65. Stanley CA, Lieu YK, Hsu BY, et al. (1998). Hyperinsulinism and hyperammonemia in infants with regulatory mutations of the glutamate dehydrogenase gene. N Engl J Med 338:1352.

66. de Lonlay P, Fournet JC, Rahier J, et al. (1997). Somatic deletion of the imprinted 11p15 region in sporadic persistent hyperinsulinemic hypoglycemia of infancy is specific of focal adenomatous hyperplasia and endorses partial pancreatectomy. J Clin Invest 100:802.

67. Clayton PT, Eaton S, Aynsley-Green A, et al. (2001). Hyperinsulinism in short-chain L-3-hydroxyacyl-CoA dehydrogenase deficiency reveals the importance of beta-oxidation in insulin secretion. J Clin Invest 108:457.

68. Molven A, Matre GE, Duran M, et al. (2004). Familial hyperinsulinemic hypoglycemia caused by a defect in the SCHAD enzyme of mitochondrial fatty acid oxidation. Diabetes 53:221.

69. Hussain K, Clayton PT, Krywawych S, et al. (2005). Hyperinsulinism of infancy associated with a novel splice site mutation in the SCHAD gene. J Pediatr 146:706.

70. Finegold DN, Stanley CA, Baker L (1980). Glycemic response to glucagon during fasting hypoglycemia: an aid in the diagnosis of hyperinsulinism. J Pediatr 96:257.

71. Stanley CA, Baker L (1976). Hyperinsulinism in infancy: diagnosis by demonstration of abnormal response to fasting hypoglycemia. Pediatrics 57:702.

72. Levitt Katz LE, Satin-Smith MS, Collett-Solberg P, et al. (1997). Insulin-like growth factor binding protein-1 levels in the diagnosis of hypoglycemia caused by hyperinsulinism. J Pediatr 131:193.

73. Grimberg A, Ferry RJ, Jr., Kelly A, et al. (2001). Dysregulation of insulin secretion in children with congenital hyperinsulinism due to sulfonylurea receptor mutations. Diabetes 50:322.

74. Ferry RJ, Jr., Kelly A, Grimberg A, et al. (2000). Calcium-stimulated insulin secretion in diffuse and focal forms of congenital hyperinsulinism. J Pediatr 137:239.

75. Kelly A, Ng D, Ferry RJ, Jr., et al. (2001). Acute insulin responses to leucine in children with the hyperinsulinism/hyperammonemia syndrome. J Clin Endocrinol Metab 86:3724.

76. Thornton PS, Alter CA, Katz LE, et al. (1993). Short- and long-term use of octreotide in the treatment of congenital hyperinsulinism. J Pediatr 123:637.

77. Muller D, Zimmering M, Roehr CC (2004). Should nifedipine be used to counter low blood sugar levels in children with persistent hyperinsulinaemic hypoglycaemia? Arch Dis Child 89:83.

78. Shilyansky J, Fisher S, Cutz E, et al. (1997). Is 95% pancreatectomy the procedure of choice for treatment of persistent hyperinsulinemic hypoglycemia of the neonate? J Pediatr Surg 32:342.

79. Suchi M, MacMullen C, Thornton PS, et al. (2003). Histopathology of congenital hyperinsulinism: retrospective study with genotype correlations. Pediatr Dev Pathol 6:322.

80. Rahier J, Guiot Y, Sempoux C (2000). Persistent hyperinsulinaemic hypoglycaemia of infancy: a heterogeneous syndrome unrelated to nesidioblastosis. Arch Dis Child Fetal Neonatal Ed 82:F108.

81. de Lonlay-Debeney P, Poggi-Travert F, Fournet JC, et al. (1999). Clinical features of 52 neonates with hyperinsulinism. N Engl J Med 340:1169.

82. Sempoux C, Guiot Y, Dahan K, et al. (2003). The focal form of persistent hyperinsulinemic hypoglycemia of infancy: morphological and molecular studies show structural and functional differences with insulinoma. Diabetes 52:784.

83. Dubois J, Brunelle F, Touati G, et al. (1995). Hyperinsulinism in children: diagnostic value of pancreatic venous sampling correlated with clinical, pathological and surgical outcome in 25 cases. Pediatr Radiol 25:512.

84. Stanley CA, Thornton PS, Ganguly A, et al. (2004). Preoperative evaluation of infants with focal or diffuse congenital hyperinsulinism by intravenous acute insulin response tests and selective pancreatic arterial calcium stimulation. J Clin Endocrinol Metab 89:288.

85. Ribeiro MJ, De Lonlay P, Delzescaux T, et al. (2005). Characterization of hyperinsulinism in infancy assessed with PET and 18F-fluoro-L-DOPA. J Nucl Med 46:560.

86. Otonkoski T, Nanto-Salonen K, Seppanen M, et al. (2006). Noninvasive diagnosis of focal hyperinsulinism of infancy with [18F]-DOPA positron emission tomography. Diabetes 55:13.

87. Hardy O, Hernandez-Pampaloni M, Saffer JR, et al. (2007). Diagnosis and localization of focal congenital hyperinsulinism by 18F-fluorodopa PET scan. J Pediatr 150:140.

88. Ericson LE, Hakanson R, Lundquist I (1997). Accumulation of dopamine in mouse pancreatic B-cells following injection of L-DOPA. Localization to secretory granules and inhibition of insulin secretion. Diabetologia 13:117.

89. Borelli MI, Villar MJ, Orezzoli A, Gagliardino JJ (1997). Presence of DOPA decarboxylase and its localization in adult rat pancreatic islet cells. Diabetes Metab 23:161.

90. Lin YW, MacMullen C, Ganguly A, et al. (2006). A novel KCNJ11 mutation associated with congenital hyperinsulinism reduces the intrinsic open probability of beta-cell ATP-sensitive potassium channels. J Biol Chem 281:3006.

91. Miki Y, Taki T, Ohura T, et al. (2000). Novel missense mutations in the glutamate dehydrogenase gene in the congenital hyperinsulinism-hyperammonemia syndrome. J Pediatr 136:69.

92. MacMullen C, Fang J, Hsu BY, et al. (2001). Hyperinsulinism/hyperammonemia syndrome in children with regulatory mutations in the inhibitory guanosine triphosphate-binding domain of glutamate dehydrogenase. J Clin Endocrinol Metab 86:1782.

93. Huijmans JG, Duran M, de Klerk JB, et al. (2000). Functional hyperactivity of hepatic glutamate dehydrogenase as a cause of the hyperinsulinism/hyperammonemia syndrome: effect of treatment. Pediatrics 106:596.

94. Yorifuji T, Muroi J, Uematsu A, et al. (1999). Hyperinsulinism-hyperammonemia syndrome caused by mutant glutamate dehydrogenase accompanied by novel enzyme kinetics. Hum Genet 104:476.

95. Li C, Matter A, Kelly A, et al. (2006). Effects of a GTP-insensitive mutation of glutamate dehydrogenase on insulin secretion in transgenic mice. J Biol Chem 281:15064.

96. Hsu BY, Kelly A, Thornton PS, et al. (2001). Protein-sensitive and fasting hypoglycemia in children with the hyperinsulinism/hyperammonemia syndrome. J Pediatr 138:383.

97. Raizen DM, Brooks-Kayal A, Steinkrauss L, et al. (2005). Central nervous system hyperexcitability associated with glutamate dehydrogenase gain of function mutations. J Pediatr 146:388.

98. Zammarchi E, Filippi L, Novembre E, Donati MA (1996). Biochemical evaluation of a patient with a familial form of leucine-sensitive hypoglycemia and concomitant hyperammonemia. Metabolism 45:957.

99. Matschinsky FM (2002). Regulation of pancreatic beta-cell glucokinase: from basics to therapeutics. Diabetes 51 Suppl 3:S394.

100. de Lonlay P, Giurgea I, Sempoux C, et al. (2005). Dominantly inherited hyperinsulinaemic hypoglycaemia. J Inherit Metab Dis 28:267.

101. Glaser B, Kesavan P, Heyman M, et al. (1998). Familial hyperinsulinism caused by an activating glucokinase mutation. N Engl J Med 338:226.

102. Christesen HB, Jacobsen BB, Odili S, et al. (2002). The second activating glucokinase mutation (A456V): implications for glucose homeostasis and diabetes therapy. Diabetes 51:1240.

103. Gloyn AL, Noordam K, Willemsen MA, et al. (2003). Insights into the biochemical and genetic basis of glucokinase activation from naturally occurring hypoglycemia mutations. Diabetes 52:2433.

104. Cuesta-Munoz AL, Huopio H, Otonkoski T, et al. (2004). Severe persistent hyperinsulinemic hypoglycemia due to a de novo glucokinase mutation. Diabetes 53:2164.

105. DeBaun MR, King AA, White N (2000). Hypoglycemia in Beckwith-Wiedemann syndrome. Semin Perinatol 24:164.

106. Hussain K, Cosgrove KE, Shepherd RM, et al. (2005). Hyperinsulinemic hypoglycemia in Beckwith-Wiedemann syndrome due to defects in the function of pancreatic beta-cell adenosine triphosphate-sensitive potassium channels. J Clin Endocrinol Metab 90:4376.

107. Bohles H, Sewell AA, Gebhardt B, et al. (2001). Hyperinsulinaemic hypoglycaemia—leading symptom in a patient with congenital disorder of glycosylation Ia (phosphomannomutase deficiency). J Inherit Metab Dis 24:858.

108. de Lonlay P, Cuer M, Vuillaumier-Barrot S, et al. (1999). Hyperinsulinemic hypoglycemia as a presenting sign in phosphomannose isomerase deficiency: A new manifestation of carbohydrate-deficient glycoprotein syndrome treatable with mannose. J Pediatr 135:379.

109. Babovic-Vuksanovic D, Patterson MC, et al. (1999). Severe hypoglycemia as a presenting symptom of carbohydrate-deficient glycoprotein syndrome. J Pediatr 135:775.

110. Marquardt T, Denecke J (2003). Congenital disorders of glycosylation: review of their molecular bases, clinical presentations and specific therapies. Eur J Pediatr 162:359.

111. Salisbury DM, Leonard JV, Dezateux CA, Savage MO (1984). Micropenis: an important early sign of congenital hypopituitarism. Br Med J (Clin Res Ed) 288:621.

112. Lovinger RD, Kaplan SL, Grumbach MM (1975). Congenital hypopituitarism associated with neonatal hypoglycemia and microphallus: four cases secondary to hypothalamic hormone deficiencies. J Pediatr 87:1171.

113. Kaufman FR, Costin G, Thomas DW, et al. (1984). Neonatal cholestasis and hypopituitarism. Arch Dis Child 59:787.

114. Renier WO, Nabben FA, Hustinx TW, et al. (1983). Congenital adrenal hypoplasia, progressive muscular dystrophy, and severe mental retardation, in association with glycerol kinase deficiency, in male sibs. Clin Genet 24:243.

115. Toyofuku T, Takashima S, Takeshita K, Nagafuji H (1986). Progressive muscular dystrophy with congenital adrenal hypoplasia: an unusual autopsy case. Brain Dev 8:285.

116. Clark AJ, Weber A (1994). Molecular insights into inherited ACTH resistance syndromes. Trends Endocr Metab 5:209.

117. Vidnes J, Oyasaeter S (1977). Glucagon deficiency causing severe neonatal hypoglycemia in a patient with normal insulin secretion. Pediatr Res 11:943.

118. Kollee LA, Monnens LA, Cecjka V, Wilms RM, et al. (1978). Persistent neonatal hypoglycaemia due to glucagon deficiency. Arch Dis Child 53:422.

119. Chen YT, Burchell A (1995). Glycogen storage diseases. New York: McGraw-Hill.

120. Greenberg CC, Jurczak MJ, Danos AM, Brady MJ (2006). Glycogen branches out: new perspectives on the role of glycogen metabolism in the integration of metabolic pathways. Am J Physiol Endocrinol Metab 291:E1.

121. Lei KJ, Pan CJ, Shelly LL, et al. (1994). Identification of mutations in the gene for glucose-6-phosphatase, the enzyme deficient in glycogen storage disease type 1a. J Clin Invest 93:1994.

122. Foster JD, Nordlie RC (2002). The biochemistry and molecular biology of the glucose-6-phosphatase system. Exp Biol Med (Maywood) 227:601.

123. Gerin I, Veiga-da-Cunha M, Achouri Y, et al. (1997). Sequence of a putative glucose 6-phosphate translocase, mutated in glycogen storage disease type Ib. FEBS Lett 419:235.

124. Lei KJ, Shelly LL, Pan CJ, et al. (1993). Mutations in the glucose-6-phosphatase gene that cause glycogen storage disease type 1a. Science 262:580.

125. Roe TF, Coates TD, Thomas DW, et al. (1992). Brief report: treatment of chronic inflammatory bowel disease in glycogen storage disease type Ib with colony-stimulating factors. N Engl J Med 326:1666.

126. Nordlie RC, Sukalski KA, Munoz JM, Baldwin JJ (1983). Type Ic, a novel glycogenosis. Underlying mechanism. J Biol Chem 258:9739.

127. Melis D, Parenti G, Gatti R, et al. (2005). Efficacy of ACE-inhibitor therapy on renal disease in glycogen storage disease type 1: a multicentre retrospective study. Clin Endocrinol (Oxf) 63:19.

128. Chen YT, Coleman RA, Scheinman JI, et al. (1988). Renal disease in type I glycogen storage disease. N Engl J Med 318:7.

129. Chen YT, Scheinman JI, Park HK, et al. (1990). Amelioration of proximal renal tubular dysfunction in type I glycogen storage disease with dietary therapy. N Engl J Med 323:590.

130. Rake JP, Visser G, Labrune P, et al. (2002). Glycogen storage disease type I: diagnosis, management, clinical course and outcome. Results of the European Study on Glycogen Storage Disease Type I (ESGSD I). Eur J Pediatr 161 Suppl 1:S20.

131. Moses SW (2002). Historical highlights and unsolved problems in glycogen storage disease type 1. Eur J Pediatr 161 Suppl 1:S2.

132. Bianchi L (1996). Glycogen storage disease I and hepatocellular tumours. Eur J Pediatr 152 Suppl 1:S63.

133. Howell RR, Stevenson RE, Ben-Menachem Y, et al. (1976). Hepatic adenomata with type 1 glycogen storage disease. Jama 236:1481.

134. Limmer J, Fleig WE, Leupold D, et al. (1988). Hepatocellular carcinoma in type I glycogen storage disease. Hepatology 8:531.

135. Greene HL, Slonim AE, O'Neill JA, Jr., Burr IM (1976). Continuous nocturnal intragastric feeding for management of type 1 glycogen-storage disease. N Engl J Med 294:423.

136. Chen YT, Cornblath M, Sidbury JB (1984). Cornstarch therapy in type I glycogen-storage disease. N Engl J Med 310:171.

137. Wolfsdorf JI, Keller RJ, Landy H, Crigler JF, Jr. (1990). Glucose therapy for glycogenosis type 1 in infants: comparison of intermittent uncooked cornstarch and continuous overnight glucose feedings. J Pediatr 117:384.

138. Stanley CA, Mills JL, Baker L (1981). Intragastric feeding in type I glycogen storage disease: factors affecting the control of lactic acidemia. Pediatr Res 15:1504.

139. Yang-Feng TL, Zheng K, Yu J, et al. (1992). Assignment of the human glycogen debrancher gene to chromosome 1p21. Genomics 13:931.

140. Van Hoof F (1967). Amylo-1,6-glucosidase activity and glycogen content of the erythrocytes of normal subjects, patients with glycogen storage disease and heterozygotes. Eur J Biochem 2:271.

141. Fernandes J, Leonard JV, Moses SW, et al. (1988). Glycogen storage disease: recommendations for treatment. Eur J Pediatr 147:226.

142. Goldberg T, Slonim AE (1993). Nutrition therapy for hepatic glycogen storage diseases. J Am Diet Assoc 93:1423.

143. Orho M, Bosshard NU, Buist NR, Gitzelmann R, et al. (1998). Mutations in the liver glycogen synthase gene in children with hypoglycemia due to glycogen storage disease type 0. J Clin Invest 102:507.

144. Weinstein DA, Correia CE, Saunders AC, Wolfsdorf JI (2006). Hepatic glycogen synthase deficiency: an infrequently recognized cause of ketotic hypoglycemia. Mol Genet Metab 87:284.

145. Pithukpakorn M (2005). Disorders of pyruvate metabolism and the tricarboxylic acid cycle. Mol Genet Metab 85:243.

146. Garcia-Cazorla A, Rabier D, Touati G, et al. (2006). Pyruvate carboxylase deficiency: metabolic characteristics and new neurological aspects. Ann Neurol 59:121.

147. Maesaka H, Komiya K, Misugi K, Tada K (1976). Hyperalaninemia hyperpyruvicemia and lactic acidosis due to pyruvate carboxylase deficiency of the liver; treatment with thiamine and lipoic acid. Eur J Pediatr 122:159.

148. Ahmad A, Kahler SG, Kishnani PS, et al. (1999). Artigas-Lopez M, Pappu AS, Steiner R, Millington DS, Van Hove JL: Treatment of pyruvate carboxylase deficiency with high doses of citrate and aspartate. Am J Med Genet 87:331.

149. Holton JB, Gillett MG, MacFaul R, Young R (1981). Galactosaemia: a new severe variant due to uridine diphosphate galactose-4-epimerase deficiency. Arch Dis Child 56:885.

150. Leslie ND (2003). Insights into the pathogenesis of galactosemia. Annu Rev Nutr 23:59.

151. Holton JB, Leonard JV (1994). Clouds still gathering over galactosaemia. Lancet 344:1242.

152. Wong D (2005). Hereditary fructose intolerance. Mol Genet Metab 85:165.

153. Gitzelmann G, Steinmann B, Van den Berghe G (1995). Disorders of fructose metabolism. New York: McGraw-Hill.

154. Steinmann B, Gitzelmann R (1981). The diagnosis of hereditary fructose intolerance. Helv Paediatr Acta 36:297.

155. Vockley J, Singh RH, Whiteman DA (2002). Diagnosis and management of defects of mitochondrial beta-oxidation. Curr Opin Clin Nutr Metab Care 5:601.

156. Hale DE, Bennett MJ (1992). Fatty acid oxidation disorders: a new class of metabolic diseases. J Pediatr 121:1.

157. Stanley CA (1998). Dissecting the spectrum of fatty acid oxidation disorders. J Pediatr 132:384.

158. Andresen BS, Bross P, Vianey-Saban C, et al. (1996). Cloning and characterization of human very-long-chain acyl-CoA dehydrogenase cDNA, chromosomal assignment of the gene and identification in four patients of nine different mutations within the VLCAD gene. Hum Mol Genet 5:461.

159. Stanley CA, DeLeeuw S, Coates PM, et al. (1991). Chronic cardiomyopathy and weakness or acute coma in children with a defect in carnitine uptake. Ann Neurol 30:709.

160. DiMauro S, DiMauro PM (1973). Muscle carnitine palmityltransferase deficiency and myoglobinuria. Science 182:929.

161. Frerman FE, Goodman SI (1995). Nuclear-encoded defects of the mitochondrial respiratory chain, including glutaric acidemia type II. New York: McGraw-Hill.

162. Treem WR, Rinaldo P, Hale DE, Stanley CA, Millington DS, Hyams JS, Jackson S, Turnbull DM: Acute fatty liver of pregnancy and long-chain 3-hydroxyacyl-coenzyme A dehydrogenase deficiency. Hepatology 19:339-345, 1994.

163. Roe CR, Ding JH (2001). Mitochondrial fatty acid oxidation disorders. New York, McGraw-Hill, 200.

164. Ziadeh R, Hoffman EP, Finegold DN, et al. (1995). Medium chain acyl-CoA dehydrogenase deficiency in Pennsylvania: neonatal screening shows high incidence and unexpected mutation frequencies. Pediatr Res 37:675.

165. (1986). Sudden infant death and inherited disorders of fat oxidation. Lancet 2:1073.

166. Ding JH, Roe CR, Iafolla AK, Chen YT (1991). Medium-chain acyl-coenzyme A dehydrogenase deficiency and sudden infant death. N Engl J Med 325:61.

167. Aoyama T, Souri M, Ushikubo S, et al. (1995). Purification of human very-long-chain acyl-coenzyme A dehydrogenase and characterization of its deficiency in seven patients. J Clin Invest 95:2465.

168. Yamaguchi S, Indo Y, Coates PM, et al. (1993). Identification of very-long-chain acyl-CoA dehydrogenase deficiency in three patients previously diagnosed with long-chain acyl-CoA dehydrogenase deficiency. Pediatr Res 34:111.

169. Longo N, Amat di San Filippo C, Pasquali M: Disorders of carnitine transport and the carnitine cycle. Am J Med Genet C Semin Med Genet 142:77.

170. Hsu BY, Iacobazzi V, Wang Z, et al. (2001). Aberrant mRNA splicing associated with coding region mutations in children with carnitine-acylcarnitine translocase deficiency. Mol Genet Metab 74:248-255, 2001.

171. Hug G, Bove KE, Soukup S (1991). Lethal neonatal multiorgan deficiency of carnitine palmitoyltransferase II. N Engl J Med 325:1862.

172. Treem WR, Stanley CA, Finegold DN, et al. (1988). Primary carnitine deficiency due to a failure of carnitine transport in kidney, muscle, and fibroblasts. N Engl J Med 319:1331.

173. Tein I, De Vivo DC, Bierman F, et al. (1990). Impaired skin fibroblast carnitine uptake in primary systemic carnitine deficiency manifested by childhood carnitine-responsive cardiomyopathy. Pediatr Res 28:247.

174. Rinaldo P, Matern D, Bennett MJ (2002). Fatty acid oxidation disorders. Annu Rev Physiol 64:477.

175. Gregersen N (1985). Riboflavin-responsive defects of beta-oxidation. J Inherit Metab Dis 8 Suppl 1:65.

176. Iafolla AK, Thompson RJ, Jr., Roe CR (1994). Medium-chain acyl-coenzyme A dehydrogenase deficiency: clinical course in 120 affected children. J Pediatr 124:409.

177. Stanley CA, Hale DE (1994). Genetic disorders of mitochondrial fatty acid oxidation. Curr Opin Pediatr 6:476.

178. Kelley RI (1994). The role of carnitine supplementation in valproic acid therapy. Pediatrics 93:891.

179. Bressler R (1976). Editorial: The unripe akee—forbidden fruit. N Engl J Med 295:500.

180. Georgiou M, Sianidou L, Hatzis T, et al. (1988). Papadatos J, Koutselinis A: Hepatotoxicity due to Atractylis gummifera-L. J Toxicol Clin Toxicol 26:487.

181. Chappell JB, Crofts AR (1965). The effect of atractylate and oligomycin on the behaviour of mitochondria towards adenine nucleotides. biochem J 95:707.

182. Gordon N, Newton RW (2003). Glucose transporter type1 (GLUT-1) deficiency. Brain Dev 25:477.

183. Wang D, Pascual JM, Yang H, et al. (2005). Glut-1 deficiency syndrome: clinical, genetic, and therapeutic aspects. Ann Neurol 57:111.

184. Klepper J, Voit T (2002). Facilitated glucose transporter protein type 1 (GLUT1) deficiency syndrome: impaired glucose transport into brain—a review. Eur J Pediatr 161:295.

185. Santer R, Schneppenheim R, Dombrowski A, et al. (1997). Mutations in GLUT2, the gene for the liver-type glucose transporter, in patients with Fanconi-Bickel syndrome. Nat Genet 17:324.

186. Santer R, Steinmann B, Schaub J (2002). Fanconi-Bickel syndrome—a congenital defect of facilitative glucose transport. Curr Mol Med 2:213.

187. Yeung CY (1970). Hypoglycemia in neonatal sepsis. J Pediatr 77:812.

188. Wharton B (1970). Hypoglycaemia in children with kwashiorkor. Lancet 1:171.

189. Black VD, Lubchenco LO, Koops BL, et al. (1985). Neonatal hyperviscosity: randomized study of effect of partial plasma exchange transfusion on long-term outcome. Pediatrics 75:1048.

190. McQuarrie I (1954). Idiopathic spontaneously occurring hypoglycemia in infants; clinical significance of problem and treatment. Am J Dis Child 87:399.

191. Cornblath M, Odell GB, Levin EY (1959) Symptomatic neonatal hypoglycemia associated with toxemia of pregnancy. J Pediatr 55:545.

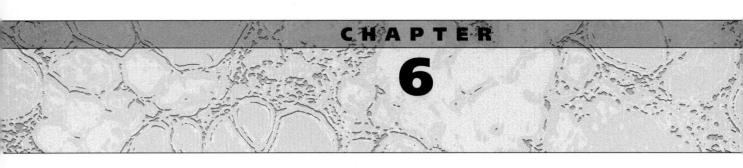

Disorders of the Thyroid in the Newborn and Infant

DELBERT A. FISHER, MD • ANNETTE GRUETERS, MD

Introduction

During the past four decades, understanding of thyroid system ontogenesis and thyroid function and dysfunction in the fetus and newborn have advanced dramatically. Newborn screening for congenital hypothyroidism is now routine throughout most of the industrialized world. Insights regarding fetal and perinatal thyroid function have improved management of complicated pregnancies and thyroid dysfunction in the premature and term infant.

Molecular genetics and technologies now provide di[f]ferential diagnostic approaches to the inborn defects i[n] thyroid hormone metabolism. This chapter reviews ou[r] current understanding of thyroid system ontogenesis an[d] the classification and management of the disorders of thy[]roid function in the fetus and newborn infant. Gene name[s] are abbreviated throughout the text. Complete names ar[e] available according to the Human Gene Nomenclatur[e] Committee at *www.gene.ucl.ac.uk/nomenclature/*.

Thyroid System Embryogenesis

Anatomic development of the hypothalamic-pituitary-thyroid system occurs during the first trimester of gestation.[1-4] The human fetal forebrain and hypothalamus begin to differentiate by 3 weeks of gestation. The hypothalamic cell condensations (destined to become the hypothalamic nuclei) and the interconnecting fiber traits are visible histologically by 15 to 18 weeks gestation, and significant concentrations of thyrotropin releasing hormone (TRH) and dopamine are detectable by 10 to 14 weeks.[5] Forebrain and hypothalamic development are dependent on a series of homeodomain proteins or transcription factors.

Mutations of three homeobox genes [sonic hedgehog (SHH), SIX3, and ZIC1] have been identified in infants with holoprosencephaly.[6-8] HESX1 homeobox gene mutations have been described in siblings with septo-optic dysplasia involving midline brain defects and pituitary hypoplasia.[9] Other homeodomain genes involved in hypothalamic development in the rodent include SF-1, SIM1, SIM2, SIX3, SIX6, PAX6, and BRN2.[4,10]

Anatomically, the pituitary gland develops from two anlagen: a neural component from the floor of the primitive forebrain, and Rathke's pouch (an ectodermal component from the primitive oral cavity). The latter is visible by 5 weeks, evolving to a morphologically mature pituitary gland by 14 to 15 weeks.[1,5] The pituitary-portal blood vessels are present by this time, and further mature through 30 to 35 weeks. In rodent models, the Rathke's pouch gene and pituitary homeobox (PTX1) gene are early factors in a cascade of determinants programming pituitary embryogenesis.[11] Later factors in the cascade include TTF1, LHX3, LHX4, Prop1, and Pit1.[4] TTF1 knockout leads to pituitary gland as well as thyroid aplasia. LHX3 and LHX4 are also essential to normal pituitary embryogenesis. Prop-1 and Pit-1 are terminal factors in the cascade, programming development and function of pituitary cells producing growth hormone, prolactin, TSHβ, and the GHRH receptors.[4] Mutations of Prop-1 or Pit-1 have been described in patients with familial hypopituitarism.[12]

The human thyroid gland develops from a median anlage derived from the primitive pharyngeal floor and paired lateral anlagen from the fourth pharyngobronchial pouch. These structures are visible by day 16 to 17 of gestation.[1,2] By 50 days, the median and lateral anlagen have fused, the buccal stalk has ruptured, and the thyroid gland has migrated to its definitive location in the anterior neck. By 70 days gestation, iodide concentration, TSH receptors, thyroglobulin and thyroid peroxidase mRNA, and protein can be demonstrated within the thyroid gland.

Thyroid embryogenesis is dependent on production of a programmed sequence of homeobox and transcription factors, including thyroid transcription factors NKX2.1 (TTF-1), FOXE-1 (TTF2), and PAX8.[13] NKX2.5 appears to play a role in regulation of NKX2.1, and HOX-A3 and HOX-B3 are important in expression of NKX2.1 and PAX8.[2,14] Targeted disruption of NKX2.1 in mice leads to thyroid gland aplasia. PAX8 gene disruption results in a small thyroid gland composed almost exclusively of C cells.

FOXE-1 null mice manifest thyroid aplasia or an ectopic sublingual thyroid gland.[13] Mutations in these genes, however, account for only approximately 2% of human thyroid dysgenesis.[13]

Placental Iodine and Thyroid Metabolism

Adequate quantities of iodide are essential to fetal thyroid hormone synthesis, and during pregnancy the fetal thyroid competes with the maternal gland for the available iodine supply. In geographic areas of iodine deficiency, this competition is increased by the increased size and iodine-concentrating activity of the maternal thyroid gland. In lower species, the placenta compensates this maternal advantage to some degree by actively transporting iodide in the maternal-to-fetal direction. Studies in the rabbit have shown that the placental iodide transport is capable of generating a fetal serum/maternal serum iodide concentration ratio of 5–9:1.[15] This is not the case in human pregnancy, and cretinism is likely in the neonates of women with large iodine deficiency goiters.[15,16] The human placenta appears freely permeable to iodide, but whether this transfer is carrier mediated (as is chloride or sulfate transfer) is not clear[17] (Figure 6-1).

The placenta imposes a relative barrier to the thyroid hormones and is impermeable to TSH so that the fetal hypothalamic-pituitary-thyroid system develops largely autonomously of the maternal system.[18,19] There are large maternal-to-fetal gradients of total and free thyroxine (T4) and triiodothyronine (T3) across the placenta during most of gestation.[18,20] Near term, the free T4 gradient

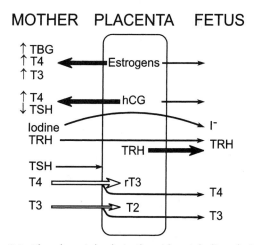

Figure 6-1. The placental role in thyroid metabolism during human pregnancy. The placenta produces estrogens and a human chorionic gonadotropin (hCG), which increase maternal TBG levels and stimulate maternal thyroid hormone production, respectively. Both activities tend to increase maternal T4 and T3 concentrations and inhibit maternal TSH secretion. Iodide and TRH readily cross the placenta. In addition, the placenta synthesizes TRH. The placenta is impermeable to TSH and only partially permeable to T4 and T3. Placental type III iodothyronine monodeiodinase enzymes degrade T4 to reverse T3 and T3 to 3,3′ T2. The placenta is also permeable to the thiourea drugs used to treat maternal Graves' disease.

gradually diminishes as fetal thyroid function matures. However, the marked maternal-to-fetal free T3 gradient persists. The placental barrier is due in part to the presence in placental tissue of an inner ring iodothyronine monodeiodinase (MDI), which converts T4 to inactive reverse T3 and T3 to diiodothyronine (T2).[19] Placental tissue also contains a type II outer ring MDI capable of catalyzing conversion of T4 to active T3.[19]

The net result of the placental metabolism of T4 is that significant maternal T4 does reach the fetus early as well as late in gestation. Significant fetal tissue T4 levels have been documented prior to the advent of fetal thyroid hormone production, and low levels of fetal T4 have been demonstrated in the athyroid human fetus at term.[21,22] Moreover, maternal hypothyroxinemia during the first half of gestation (prior to the activation of fetal thyroid hormone production) is associated with a decreased IQ in the offspring.

The placenta is permeable to the thioureylene antithyroid drugs, and TRH crosses the placenta readily (Figure 6-1). However, little endogenous TRH is normally detected in adult peripheral blood due to the presence of TRH-degrading enzyme systems in the blood.[18,24] Although the sera of pregnant women contain somewhat lower levels of these enzymes than do nonpregnant sera, the nearly immeasurable levels of TRH in the maternal circulation have little effect on fetal thyroid function. The placenta synthesizes a pro-TRH molecule, and fetal gut tissues (particularly pancreas) produce TRH.[18,24] The placental and pancreatic TRH have been isolated and characterized and found to be identical to hypothalamic TRH.

In addition to TRH, the placenta produces thyrotropin-like activity.[15,25] The α-subunit of TSH is identical to that of human chorionic gonadotropin (hCG), and the β-subunit of hCG has structural homology with the β-subunit of TSH. Thus, hCG has some TSH-like bioactivity. However, the biologic potency of hCG is only about 0.01% that of TSH, and hCG normally has little influence on fetal thyroid system development or function. However, the large increase in maternal serum hCG activity that occurs early in pregnancy leads to a transient stimulation of thyroid function with suppression of maternal TSH.

Thyroid System Maturation

Maturation of thyroid function in the fetus can be considered to occur in three phases: hypothalamic, pituitary, and thyroidal. Changes in these systems are complex and superimposed on the increasing production and increasing serum concentration of serum thyroid hormone-binding globulin (TBG), as well as the changing pattern of fetal tissue iodothyronine deiodination. As previously mentioned, the fetal thyroid gland is capable of iodide concentration and iodothyronine synthesis as early as 70 days gestation. However, thyroid hormone production is limited until 18 to 20 weeks. At this time, thyroid follicular cell iodine uptake increases and serum T4 levels begin to increase (Figure 6-2).[26-28] Thereafter, TBG and total T4 concentrations increase steadily until the final weeks of pregnancy.

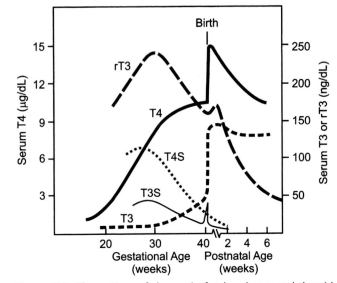

Figure 6-2. The pattern of change in fetal and neonatal thyroid function parameters during pregnancy and extrauterine adaptation. Fetal serum thyroxine (T4) concentrations begin to increase at mid-gestation and increase progressively thereafter to term. This increase is due largely to the increase in thyroxine-binding globulin concentration, but free T4 concentrations (not shown) also increase progressively between 20 and 40 weeks. T4 in the fetus is metabolized predominantly to inactive reverse triiodothyronine (rT3) and sulfated analogues (T4S, T3S). Monodeiodination of T4 to active triiodothyronine (T3) increases at about 30 weeks to levels approximating 50 ng/dL at term. The TSH surge (not shown), which peaks at 25 to 30 minutes after extrauterine exposure, stimulates thyroidal T4 and T3 secretion. Neonatal T4 and T3 peak at 2 to 3 days. Serum T3 concentrations remain at higher postnatal levels due to increased T4-to-T3 conversion mediated by increased type I iodothyronine deiodinase activity in newborn tissues.

The trend of free T4 concentrations has been variable in several studies, increasing progressively to term in the intrauterine studies of Thorpe-Beeston et al. and seeming to plateau in cord blood studies between 24 weeks and term.[27,28] This variation is due at least in part to underestimation of free T4 concentrations in fetal/neonatal premature blood samples in many commercial free T4 immunoassay systems because of the low TBG concentrations in these samples. The fetal serum T3 concentration remains low (<15 ng/dL) until 30 weeks, and then increases in two distinct phases (a prenatal and a postnatal phase). Prenatally, serum T3 increases slowly after 30 weeks gestation—to reach a level of approximately 50 ng/dL (or 0.77 nmol/L) in term cord serum.

The low fetal T3 concentrations are due to low levels of type I iodothyronine monodeiodinase and relatively low rates of T4 to T3 conversion in fetal tissues and to active type III monodeiodinase in placenta and selected fetal tissues degrading T3 to T2.[18,29] Postnatally, T3 and T4 serum concentrations increase two- to sixfold within the first few hours of life—peaking at 24 to 36 hours after birth. These levels then gradually decline to levels characteristic of infancy over the first 4 to 5 weeks of life. The prenatal increase in serum T3 is due to progressive maturation of hepatic type I (phenolic) outer ring iodothyronine deiodinase activity increasing hepatic conversion of T4 to T3, and to decreased placental T3 degradation.[18,29]

Fetal serum TSH increases from a low level at 18 to 20 weeks to a peak value of approximately 7 to 10 mU/L at term. At the time of parturition, in response to neonatal (cold) extrauterine exposure there is an acute release of TSH (the TSH surge)—with blood levels peaking at a mean concentration approximating 70 mU/L at 30 minutes. Circulating TSH remains elevated for 3 to 5 days after birth. TSH secretion in the neonatal period increases to a rate approximating 3 mU/L/min, and the increase in serum T4 levels immediately after birth is TSH dependent.[8,30]

Fetal thyroid gland function develops under the influence of an increasing serum TSH level during the last half of gestation. Serum free T4 levels tend to plateau after 24 weeks, and thus the TSH to free T4 ratio tends to increase—suggesting increasing TRH secretion and changes in pituitary thyrotroph sensitivity to the negative feedback effect of thyroid hormones on TSH secretion and changes in thyroid follicular cell sensitivity to TSH[31] (Figure 6-3). A progressive maturation of the thyroidal response to TSH has been shown in the fetal sheep, and seems likely in the human fetus.[32] The events involved in maturation of the negative feedback control system are complex, probably involving changes in pituitary thyrotroph T3 and TRH receptors, in thyrotroph outer ring iodothyronine deiodinase activity, and nuclear-T3-receptor-mediated action on TSH biosynthesis.[31]

The ontogeny of TRH secretion and function in the human fetus remain somewhat obscure. TRH production from the placenta and gut tissues and relatively high serum TRH levels have been demonstrated in fetal sheep.[24] TRH immunoactivity is detectable in the human fetal pancreas early in gestation and in the hypothalamus by midgestation, increasing markedly in the third trimester after the peak in serum TSH activity is noted (Figure 6-3). Serum TRH levels in the human fetus are relatively high at term due to extrahypothalamic production and to low or absent levels of TRH-degrading activity in fetal blood.[24]

Thyroid function in the premature infant (before 30 to 32 weeks) is characterized by low circulating levels of T4 and free T4, a normal or low level of TSH, and a normal or prolonged TSH response to TRH—indicating a state of physiologic TRH deficiency.[33] The full-term human fetus responds to pharmacologic maternal doses of TRH with a somewhat prolonged increase in TSH, suggesting a degree of relative hypothalamic (tertiary) hypothyroidism. Peripheral sources of TRH (placenta and pancreas) contribute to the elevated circulating levels of fetal and cord blood TRH and may be responsible in part for stimulating TSH release in the fetus prior to the increase in hypothalamic TRH concentration.

In summary, the control of fetal thyroid hormone secretion can be characterized as a balance among increasing hypothalamic TRH secretion, increasing thyroid follicular cell sensitivity to TSH, and increasing pituitary sensitivity to thyroid hormone inhibition of TSH release.[24,33] The fetus progresses from a state of primary (thyroidal) and tertiary (hypothalamic) hypothyroidism in mid-gestation through a state of mild tertiary hypothyroidism during the final weeks of pregnancy. There is a progressive decrease in the TSH to free T4 ratio, suggesting a progressive maturation of the negative feedback hypothalamic-pituitary TSH control axis.[31] The marked cold-stimulated TRH-TSH surge at birth is associated with a marked increase in T4 secretion and free T4 concentration with reequilibration by 1 to 2 months. During infancy and childhood, there is a progressive decrease in T4 secretion rate (on a μg/kg/day basis) correlating with a decreasing metabolic rate—probably reflecting decreasing TRH secretion.[31]

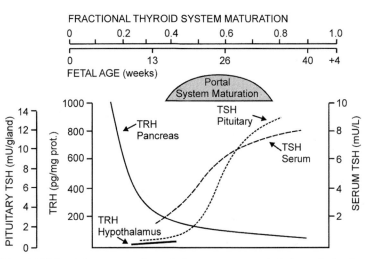

Figure 6-3. Changes in fetal TRH and TSH levels in pancreas, hypothalamus, serum, and pituitary during human gestation. Hypothalamic TRH concentrations increase progressively after mid-gestation, but the pattern of change has not been documented in the human fetus. [Reproduced with permission from Fisher DA, Polk DH (1994). Development of the fetal thyroid system. In Thorburn GD, Harding R (eds.), *Textbook of fetal physiology.* Oxford, UK: Oxford University Press 359–368.]

Maturation of Thyroid Hormone Metabolism and Transport

The thyroid gland is the sole source of T4. Most of the circulating T3 after birth is derived from conversion of T4 to T3 via monodeiodination in peripheral tissues. Deiodination of the iodothyronines is the major route of metabolism, and monodeiodination may occur either at the outer (phenolic) ring or the inner (tyrosyl) ring of the iodothyronine molecule (Figure 6-4).[18,34] Outer ring monodeiodination of T4 produces T3, the active form of thyroid hormone with greatest affinity for the thyroid nuclear receptor.

Inner ring monodeiodination of T4 produces rT3, an inactive metabolite. In adults, between 70 and 90% of circulating T3 is derived from peripheral conversion of T4—and 10 to 30% is derived from direct glandular secretion. Nearly all circulating rT3 derives from peripheral conversion, with only 2 to 3% coming directly from the thyroid gland. T3 and rT3 are progressively metabolized to diiodo, monoiodo, and noniodinated forms of thyroxine—none of which possesses biologic activity.

Two types of outer ring iodothyronine monodeiodinase have been described.[18,34] Type I MDI (predominantly expressed in liver, kidney, and thyroid) is a high-Km enzyme inhibited by propylthiouracil and stimulated by thyroid hormone. Type I MDI is capable of inner ring monodeiodination, particularly of T4 sulfate (to rT3 sulfate) and T3 sulfate (to T2 sulfate).[34-36] Type II MDI [predominantly located in brain, pituitary, placenta, skeletal muscle, heart, thyroid, and brown adipose tissues (BATs)] is a low-Km enzyme insensitive to propylthiouracil and inhibited by thyroid hormone. Types I and II MDI contribute to circulating T3 production, whereas type II acts as well to increase local tissue levels of T3.[34-36] An inner (tyrosyl) ring iodothyronine monodeiodinase (type III

MDI) has been characterized in most fetal tissues, including brain and placenta (and more recently in uterus and fetal skin).[19] This enzyme system catalyzes the conversion of T4 to rT3 and T3 to diiodothyronine.

Types I and II MDI are developmentally and thyroid-state regulated.[34-38] In sheep, a species in which thyroid hormone system maturation closely resembles that in the human, hepatic type I MDI activity increases about 100%—and brain type II MDI activity increases about 50% over the last third of gestation.[39] In the human fetal brain, type II MDI activity in the cortex increases between 13 and 20 weeks gestation and cerebellar activity after mid-gestation.[40] There is a general inverse correlation of type II and type III activities.[38] Both deiodinase species are thyroid hormone responsive.

Hepatic type I MDI activity in the fetal sheep becomes thyroid hormone responsive (i.e., activity decreases with hypothyroidism) only during the final weeks of gestation. Brain type II MDI is responsive (increases with hypothyroidism) throughout the final third of gestation.[39] Thus, in the hypothyroid fetus T4 appears to be shunted from the liver to the brain—where it is preferentially deiodinated to T3 to provide a source of intracellular T3 to those tissues (such as brain and pituitary) dependent on T3 during fetal life. Hepatic type I enzyme activity (to provide increased serum T3 levels) normally increases only during the final weeks of gestation and during postnatal life.

Fetal thyroid hormone metabolism is characterized by a predominance of type III enzyme activity (particularly in liver, kidney, and placenta), accounting for the increased circulating levels of rT3 observed in the fetus.[18,41] However, the persistence of high circulating rT3 levels for several weeks in the newborn indicate that type III MDI activities expressed in nonplacental tissues are important to the maintenance of high circulating rT3 levels. The mixture of type II and type III MDI activities in the

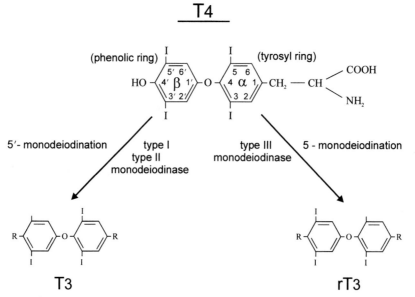

Figure 6-4. The deiodination of thyroxine by types I, II, and III iodothyronine monodeiodinase enzymes. The type I enzyme is also capable of inner ring monodeiodination, particularly of the sulfated conjugates (not shown).

Postnatal thermogenesis is mediated via the BAT prominent in subscapular and perirenal areas in the mammalian fetus and neonate.[66] Heat production in BAT is stimulated by catecholamines via β-adrenergic receptors and is thyroid hormone dependent. The uncoupling protein thermogenin (or UCP-1) unique to BAT is located on the inner mitochondrial membrane and uncouples phosphorylation by dissipating the proton gradient created by the mitochondrial respiratory chain. The type II MDI in BAT mediates local T4 to T3 conversion. Full thermogenin expression in BAT requires both catecholamine and T3 stimulation.[66] BAT matures progressively in the fetus but remains thermoneutral until stimulated by catecholamines in the perinatal period.[39,67]

BAT thermogenesis is immature in small premature infants, and BAT tissue mass decreases in the neonatal period in full-term infants as the capacity for nonshivering thermogenesis develops in other tissues. UCP-2 is found in many tissues, but does not appear to be regulated by β-adrenergic agonists or thyroid hormone.[68] UCP-3 has been cloned and is expressed in muscle and white adipose tissue as well as BAT. Muscle UCP-3 is regulated by β3-adrenergic stimulation and thyroid hormone and probably contributes importantly to nonshivering thermogenesis in adult rats and presumably in humans. UCP-3 mRNA levels are also regulated by dexamethasone, leptin, and starvation, but the regulation differs in BAT and muscle.[68] Starvation increases muscle and decreases BAT UCP-3, suggesting that muscle serves a larger role in thermoregulation during starvation.[68]

The critical role of thyroid hormones is CNS maturation has long been recognized. Nervous system development involves neurogenesis, gliogenesis, neural cell migration, neuronal differentiation, dendritic and axonal growth, synaptogenesis, myelination, and neurotransmitter synthesis.[69] Thyroid hormones have been shown to stimulate a number of developmentally regulated nervous tissue genes, but the role of these factors in the CNS developmental program remains undefined.[69] Available evidence suggests that deficiency or excess of thyroid hormones alters the timing or synchronization of the CNS developmental program, presumably by initiating critical gene actions or other genetic CNS maturation events.

There is increasing evidence for a critical period for thyroid-dependent brain maturation in utero. Early maternal hypothyroxinemia in the rat alters histogenesis and cerebral cortical architecture of the progeny, and maternal hypothyroxinemia in humans is associated with IQ reduction in offspring.[23,70,71] Studies of the timing of iodine supplementation in pregnant women in geographic areas of severe iodine deficiency have suggested a critical period of hormone action on CNS maturation during a narrow interval of time at the beginning of the third trimester of gestation.[72] This period has been likened to the irreversible thyroid-dependent action of thyroid hormone initiating tadpole metamorphosis.[73] Recent studies of the dose and timing of thyroid hormone therapy in infants with congenital hypothyroidism suggest a second critical period of thyroid hormone action during the very early neonatal period, but the period of CNS thyroid hormone dependency extends further (to 3 to 4 years of age).[74]

Thyroid Dysfunction Syndromes in the Premature Infant

Premature infants are defined by gestational age (GA) and weight. By weight, premature infants are classified as low birth weight (LBW, 2,500-1,500 g), very low birth weight (VLBW, 1,500-1,000 g), and extremely low birth weight (ELBW, <1,000 g). They range from 34 to 35 weeks to 23 to 24 weeks GA (the current threshold of viability). Thyroid system control progresses from mid-gestation through early infancy and involves hypothalamic-pituitary-thyroid maturation and tissue responsiveness to thyroid hormones.

VLBW infants (<30 weeks gestation) have relatively immature hypothalamic-pituitary-thyroid systems (Table 6-1) and a high prevalence of neonatal morbidities, including respiratory distress, hypoxia, undernutrition, gastrointestinal and cardiac dysfunction, sepsis, and cerebral pathology.[75-78] As a result, they are predisposed to development of transient primary hypothyroidism and the syndrome of transient hypothyroxinemia of prematurity (THOP)—which probably represents transient hypothalamic-pituitary hypothyroidism and/or nonthyroidal illness (NTI, the low T3 syndrome).[75-78]

TRANSIENT PRIMARY HYPOTHYROIDISM

Transient hypothyroidism in the neonate, characterized by low serum T4 and high TSH concentrations, is more common in Europe than in America—and the prevalence varies geographically relative to iodine intake.[79-81] Transient

TABLE 6-1

Thyroid Disorders and Approximate Prevalences in the Neonatal Period

Disorder	Prevalence
Thyroid Dysgenesis Agenesis Hypogenesis Ectopia	1:4000
Thyroid Dyshormonogenesis Resistance to TSH Sodium/Iodide Symporter Defects Organification Defects in Thyroglobulin Synthesis Iodotyrosine Deiodinase Defect	1:40,000
Hypothalamic-Pituitary Hypothyroidism Hypothalamic-Pituitary Anomaly Panhypopituitarism Isolated TSH Deficiency	1:20,000
Thyroid Hormone Resistance	Rare*
Iodothyronine Monodeiodinase Deficiency	Rare**
Transient Hypothyroidism/ Hyperthyrotropinemia Drug Induced Maternal Antibody Induced Idiopathic TSH Receptor Defect	1:10,000
Congenital Hyperthyroidism	1:50,000
Hormone Transport Defects	1:2000+

*1000 cases reports.
**4 cases reported.
+variable by geography and abnormality (see text).

hypothyroidism in Belgium, an area of moderate iodine deficiency, occurs in 15 to 20% of premature infants (and prevalence is higher with decreasing gestational age).[79] Cord-blood T4 and TSH values in these infants are usually in the normal range for premature infants. Premature infants require higher iodine intake levels than term infants to maintain a positive iodine balance and adequate T4 production in the extrauterine environment, and in iodine-deficient geographic areas they may develop transient iodine deficiency.[79,81]

The primary hypothyroid state develops during the first 1 to 2 weeks of extrauterine life and is often superimposed on the transient hypothyroxinemia characteristic of prematurity. Urinary iodine and thyroid iodine contents are reduced. The hypothyroidism may persist for several weeks, in which case treatment is recommended. T4 or T3 can be prescribed. The average time to recovery of function and discontinuation of treatment in Belgium was 2 months. Iodine treatment also corrects the primary hypothyroid state in such infants.[79]

Premature infants are also susceptible to iodine overload due to the inhibitory effects of iodide excess on thyroidal iodide organification, referred to as the Wolff-Chaikoff effect.[82,83] The fetal thyroid is inordinately sensitive to the inhibitory effect of iodide on hormone synthesis.[81] Excess iodide exposure has occurred via maternal ingestion of iodide- or iodine-containing drugs or via neonatal exposure from iodide-containing disinfectants used for skin cleansing or iodinated contrast dyes used for radiographic studies.[83]

TRANSIENT HYPOTHYROXINEMIA OF PREMATURITY

Relative to term infants at birth, serum TBG and total T4 concentrations in premature infants are lower, the neonatal TSH surge is obtunded, tissue type I monodeiodinase activity and serum T3 levels are lower, postnatal TSH and free T4 concentrations are lower, bioinactive thyroid hormone analogue levels are higher, BAT thermogenic mechanisms are immature, and tissue thyroid hormone response systems are variably immature[75-78] (Table 6-1). The extent of these immaturities is related inversely to GA. In ELBW and VLBW infants less than 30 weeks GA, the TSH surge and the early thyroidal response are limited and are followed by a progressive decrease in serum total T4—with nadir values at 7 to 10 days of postnatal life.[75-77]

The decrease in serum total T4 concentrations is in part due to a decrease in TBG, which reflects neonatal morbidity.[76,84] Free T4 levels are variable, relative to cord blood concentrations, due to variable suppression of TBG-binding capacity and variable sensitivities of the free T4 immunoassay methods employed.[76,77,85] Serum TSH levels do not usually increase in response to the transient hypothyroxinemia, and serum free T4 levels reequilibrate to cord-blood values by 3 to 4 weeks. These very premature infants manifest a negative iodine balance during the early postnatal weeks, suggesting that they are unable to adapt to the extrauterine environment with augmentation of thyroidal iodine uptake and increased T4 secretion as do the larger infants.[81]

The high prevalence of neonatal morbidities in these infants is associated with characteristics of NTI, including a low serum T3 concentration (secondary to a decreased rate of conversion of T4 to T3) and decreased T4 concentrations. Free T4 levels are variable, but are usually in the range of values for healthy premature infants of matched gestational age and weight. TBG levels tend to be low, and there may be an inhibitor of T4 binding to TBG (as described in adults with the low T3 syndrome).[33,76,84] Serum TSH concentrations are normal or low. It is difficult to differentiate the contribution of NTI versus hypothalamic-pituitary immaturity in the pathogenesis of THOP. van Wassenaer and co-workers have shown that a serum free T4 level, measured by immunoassay, below 10 pmol/L (0.78 ng/dL) will trigger an increase in serum TSH concentration in most VLBW infants—suggesting a major contribution of NTI.[84]

The impact of THOP on brain maturation is not clear. In a placebo-controlled treatment study of VLBW infants, van Wassenaer et al. showed that a subgroup of 13 thyroxine-treated ELBW infants 25 to 26 weeks GA manifested a higher DQ at 24 months than 18 placebo control infants.[86] In a later analysis of IQ and neurologic function data at 5.7 years of age, mean IQ in the treated and control children were statistically similar—although some neurologic dysfunction persisted, especially in infants with free T4 levels in the 10.1- to 12.5-pmol/L range.[87] The infant cohorts were small, however, and the results must be considered preliminary. van Wassenaer administered a thyroxine dose of 8 micrograms/kg/day given parenterally over a 6-week period. Earlier dosage studies suggest that a 4- to 5-microgram/kg parenteral dose or a 5- to 6-microgram/kg oral dose of Na-l-thyroxine provides adequate replacement.[33]

Congenital Hypothyroidism

NEWBORN SCREENING

Newborn screening for congenital hypothyroidism (CH) is now routine in most industrialized societies.[60,64,88,89] CH screening tests are usually carried out in dried blood spot samples collected via skin puncture. Although screening program protocols vary, in effect all are screening for elevated serum TSH concentrations as the most reliable indicator of primary hypothyroidism. The threshold value for a significant TSH elevation in most screening programs is 20 to 25 mU/L (20-25 μU/mL). The preferred time for screening sampling is 3 to 5 days after birth. However, many mother-newborn diads are now discharged from the hospital within 3 days of delivery (and some are discharged within 1 day).

Early measurement increases the prevalence of infants demonstrating elevation of blood spot TSH concentrations due to the physiological neonatal TSH surge. Thus, early screening for CH increases false positive results. In most programs, the false positive to confirmed CH case ratio is 2–3:1. The effect of early hospital discharge of mother and infant in one study increased this ratio from 2.5 to 1 to about 5 to 1. The ratio will vary, however, depending on the threshold value established for a significant TSH elevation by the individual program. Some programs have a higher threshold value for infants discharged on day 1.

It has been shown that as many as 5% of CH infants are missed in newborn screening programs.[88] Most of these relate to errors in specimen handling, testing and data analysis, or results reporting. In rare instances the increase in serum TSH concentrations in the affected infant is delayed for several days or weeks after delivery, presumably due to immaturity of the hypothalamic-pituitary axis.[60,88] The prevalence of CH approximates 1 in 4,000 births.[64,89] The etiologies include thyroid dysgenesis (aplasia, hypoplasia, ectopy), thyroid dyshormonogenesis, hypothalamic-pituitary (TSH) deficiency, and transient hypothyroidism (usually iodine, drug, or maternal antibody induced). The proportions approximate 75%, 10%, 5% and 10%, respectively, of the total CH cases (Table 6-1). Modifications of CH screening programs have been introduced to improve detection of infants with delayed increase in serum TSH and those with central hypothyroidism.[60,88-91] Repeat testing at 2 to 6 weeks of age has detected an additional 10% of infants with CH, and addition of a T4 has been shown to detect the 12% to 15% of infants with central hypothyroidism. Some 80% of these manifested multiple pituitary hormone deficiency.[90,91]

THYROID DYSGENESIS

The term *thyroid dysgenesis* describes infants with ectopic or hypoplastic thyroid glands (or both), as well as those with total thyroid agenesis. Thyroid dysgenesis is the etiologic factor in most infants with permanent congenital hypothyroidism detected in newborn screening programs.[60,64,89] Some thyroid tissue is probably present in two-thirds of these infants, and thus they represent a spectrum of severity of thyroid deficiency. A normal or near-normal circulating level of T3 in the face of a low T4 value suggests the presence of residual thyroid tissue, and this can be confirmed by a thyroid scan. A measurable level of serum thyroglobulin (TG) indicates the presence of some thyroid tissue. Athyroid infants have no circulating TG.[89]

Thyroid dysgenesis is usually sporadic, and the mechanism(s) for the defective embryogenesis remains obscure. Dysgenesis is more prevalent in female than in male infants. The female-to-male ratio approximates 2:1. The disorder has been reported to be less prevalent in black (1:32,000) than in white infants, and is more frequent (1:2,000) in Hispanic infants.[64,89] Approximately 2% to 3% of thyroid dysgenesis cases are familial and associated with mutations in the homeobox genes TTF1 (NKF2.1), TTF2 (FOXE1), or PAX8.[13,14,92] More recently, mutations of another transcription factor (GL153) have been described as the cause of a rare syndrome of neonatal diabetes: congenital hypothyroidism and congenital glaucoma.[93] The prevalence of thyroid dysgenesis is increased in infants with Down syndrome.[64,89]

An increased prevalence (8%-10%) of nonthyroid anomalies has been reported in infants with congenital hypothyroidism.[64,89,94] The most prevalent are cardiac, but include anomalies of the nervous, musculoskeletal, digestive and urological systems, cleft palate, and eye anomalies.[94] First-degree relatives of children with thyroid dysgenesis have an increased prevalence of thyroglossal duct cysts, a pyramidal thyroid lobe, thyroid hemiagenesis, and ectopic thyroid.[95] These abnormalities are compatible with an autosomal-dominant mode of inheritance with a low penetrance estimated at 21%, supporting the hypothesis of a genetic predisposition for a larger proportion of congenital hypothyroidism than is accounted for by the homeobox gene syndromes.[95] In rare instances, thyroid dysgenesis has occurred in association with maternal autoimmune thyroiditis. However, this appears to be coincidence. There is no correlation between thyroid dysgenesis and the presence of maternal autoimmune thyroiditis or circulating thyroid antimicrosomal or antithyroglobulin autoantibodies.[89]

THYROID DYSHORMONOGENESIS

General Features

The function of the thyroid gland is to concentrate iodide from the blood and return it to peripheral tissues in a hormonally active form.[96-98] The major substrates for thyroid hormone synthesis are iodide and tyrosine. Tyrosine is not rate limiting even in individuals with phenylketonuria, in whom tyrosine becomes an essential amino acid. Iodine, by contrast, is a trace element that can be rate limiting in thyroid hormone synthesis. The process of thyroid hormone biosynthesis is stimulated by TSH binding to the follicular cell TSH receptor and cAMP activation.

Processes stimulated by cAMP include cell membrane iodide transport, thyroglobulin synthesis, oxidation and organification of trapped iodide, activation of colloid endocytosis and intracellular phagolysosome formation, hydrolysis of thyroglobulin to release the iodotyrosines [monoiodotyrosine (MIT) and diiodotyrosine (DIT)] and iodothyronine (T4 and T3) residues, deiodination of MIT and DIT by an iodotyrosine deiodinase, and release of the T4 and T3 into the circulation. Significant amounts of thyroglobulin also escape from the gland, predominantly via the thyroid lymphatic system. These events are summarized in Figure 6-6. Infants with defects in thyroid hormone metabolism comprise some 10% to 15% of newborns with CH. A defect in TSH binding/action and several functional abnormalities have been described.[96-98]

These involve decreased iodide trapping, defective organification of trapped iodide, abnormalities of thyroglobulin structure, or deficiency of iodotyrosine deiodination and recycling. These disorders are usually transmitted as autosomal-recessive traits. Except for the familial incidence and tendency for affected individuals to develop goiter, the clinical manifestations of congenital hypothyroidism due to a biochemical defect are similar to those in infants with thyroid dysgenesis. Thyroid enlargement may be manifest at birth, but in many patients development of the goiter is delayed. Features of these disorders are summarized in Table 6-2.

Resistance to TSH

The thyroid follicular cell response to TSH involves a series of coordinated steps, including TSH binding to a receptor in the plasma membrane, activation of adenyl

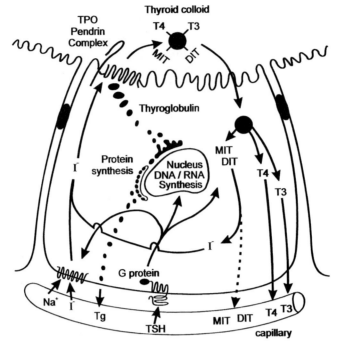

Figure 6-6. The biosynthesis and secretion of thyroid hormones by the thyroid follicular cell. The events of cellular synthesis are shown on the left, and those of secretion on the right. The Pendrin protein is localized with the thyroid peroxidase (TPO) and THOX (not shown) genes at or near the apical cell membrane, facilitating the organification process. With TSH stimulation, thyroid colloid droplets reenter the cell via micropinocytosis. The thyroglobulin-containing vesicles fuse with lysosomes in phagolysosomes, resulting in proteolytic degradation of thyroglobulin and release of T4 and T3, and the iodotyrosines monoiodotyrosine (MIT) and diiodotyrosine (DIT). MIT and DIT are deiodinated via the dehalogenase enzymes (DEHALI) to release and recycle the iodide. Small amounts of MIT and DIT are released into the circulation.

TABLE 6-2

Inborn Abnormalities of Thyroid Hormone Metabolism

Abnormality	Prevalence	Inheritance	Clinical CH	Goiter	T4
Familial TSH Deficiency	Rare	AR	Yes	No	↓
Pit-1 Deficiency Hypopituitarism	Not yet clear	AR	Yes	No	↓
TSH Unresponsiveness	Rare	AR	Yes	No	↓
Iodide Transport Defect	Rare	AR	Yes	Yes	↓
Organification Defects	1:40,000 newborns	AR	Yes	Yes	↓
Pendred Syndrome	1:50,000 children	AR	V	Yes	N,↑
Thyroglobulin Defects	1:40,000 newborns	AR	Yes	Yes	↓
Iodotyrosine Deiodinase Defect	Rare	AR	Yes	Yes	↓
Thyroid Hormone Resistance	1:100,000 newborns?	Autosomal/ dominant or sporadic	V	Yes	↑
Thyroid Hormone Transporter Defect	Rare	X-linked	CNS damage	No	↓
Iodothyronine Deiodinase Deficiency	Rare	Autosomal recessive	No	No	↑
Autosomal Dominant Hyperthyroidism	Rare	Autosomal dominant	No Hyper	Yes	↑

AR = autosomal recessive; CH = congenital hypothyroidism; Tg = serum thyroglobulin; RAIU = thyroid radioactive iodine uptake; T4 and TSH refer to serum concentrations, V = variable.

cyclase, synthesis of cyclic AMP, activation of protein kinase(s), phosphorylation of receptor protein(s), and stimulation of the several intracellular events of thyroid hormone synthesis and release. A defect at one of several sites could lead to an abnormality in thyroid responsiveness to TSH. Only a few patients with TSH nonresponsiveness have been reported. Characteristically, they present with neonatal CH—including low serum T4 and increased TSH concentrations.[97-99] Thyroid radioiodine uptake is low or low normal and unresponsive to TSH.

The TSH receptor is one of the family of G-protein–coupled receptors. It belongs to the superfamily of seven-transmembrane domain receptors coupled to G proteins. The TSH receptor gene is localized to chromosome 14. A long extracellular hormone-binding domain is encoded by 9 exons. A tenth exon codes the seven-transmembrane and intracellular domains of the receptor.[100] Germ-line mutations of the thyrotropin receptor gene have been described recently in association with congenital or acquired thyroid disease. Both loss-of-function and gain-of-function phenotypes have been described.[97,99,101,102] Sixty to 70% of these map to the aminoterminal hormone-binding domain. Others involve the transmembrane and intracellular domains.[102] Most of these defects lead to asymptomatic hyperthyrotropinemia, and most were compound heterozygotes with normal heterozygote parents. A few cases of severe congenital hypothyroidism with absent iodine uptake and thyroid hypoplasia have been reported. These cases tend to have mutations in exon 10 involving the transmembrane domain.[103,104]

Defects in the Gs subunits have been reported in families with dominantly inherited pseudohypoparathyroidism and in patients with Albright hereditary osteodystrophy, and affected subjects may have reduced TSH responsiveness and compensated or decompensated hypothyroidism.[105] It is difficult to assess the severity of hypothyroidism due to TSH resistance in these cases, because the pituitary TRH receptor also is a G-protein–coupled receptor and therefore circulating TSH levels are low rather than high.

Sodium/Iodide Symporter Defects

The transport of iodide across the thyroid follicular cell membrane from plasma to cytosol is the first step in thyroid hormone biosynthesis. Under normal circumstances, the thyroid cell membrane iodide pump generates a thyroid/serum (T/S ratio) concentration gradient in excess of 20 to 30. This gradient can reach several hundredfold when the thyroid gland is stimulated by a low-iodine diet, by TSH, by a variety of thyroid-stimulating immunoglobulins in Graves' disease, or by drugs that impair the efficiency of hormone synthesis. Other tissues (such as the salivary glands, gastric mucosa, mammary glands, ciliary body, choroid plexus, and placenta) are also capable of concentrating iodide against a gradient. However, these tissues are not capable of organifying inorganic iodide.

Fewer than 50 cases have been reported with defective iodide transport.[106,107] The patients present with congenital hypothyroidism. The diagnosis is based on the presence of goiter, limited or absent radioiodine uptake, and

Features				
TSH	Tg	RAIU	Other	Molecular Abnormality
↓	↓	↓	Absent TSH response to TRH	TSHβ gene mutations
N or ↓	↓	↓	GH and PRL deficiencies	Pit-1 gene mutations
↑	↓	N	No RAIU, T4, or Tg response to TSH	TSH receptor gene mutations
↑	↑	↓	Salivary and gastric tissues also fail to concentrate iodide. Hypothyroid state responds to iodide Rx	Defect not characterized
↑	↑	↑	Positive perchlorate discharge test	TPO or THOX mutations
↑	↑	↑	Deaf mutism; positive perchlorate discharge	Pendrin mutations
↑	↓↑	↑	Usually low Tg with no Tg response to TSH	Tg gene mutations (Abent or defective Tg); hyposialylated Tg due do sialyltransferase defect
↑	↑	↑	High RAIU with early discharge: high serum MIT, DIT; failure to deiodinate IV dose of labeled DIT (excretion intact)	DEHAL1 mutations
N,↑	↑	↑	Generalized resistance, TSH N or ↑; Peripheral resistance. TSH ↑; Pituitary resistance TSH ↑ (patient hyperthyroid)	Thyroid nuclear receptor gene mutations (TR beta; TR alpha?)
N,↑	N	N	Increased T3; psychomotor; retardation	Monocarboxylate Transporter MCT8 Gene mutations
↑	N-↑	N-↑	Decrease T3 and increased rT3	SECISBP2 gene mutation
↓	↑	↑	Absence of thyroid autoimmunity	Activating TSH receptor gene mutations

elevated serum TSH. Other iodine-concentrating tissues (salivary glands, gastric mucosa) also fail to concentrate iodide from the circulation. Lugol's solution ameliorates the hypothyroidism by increasing serum iodide to high levels and increasing intrathyroidal inorganic iodide concentration by diffusion. Partial defects have also been described. Thyroid radioiodine uptake was decreased but not absent in these patients and did not respond to TSH. The salivary-to-plasma ratio of radioiodine also was reduced but not entirely absent. Nonetheless, the patients were hypothyroid with mental retardation.[97,98]

Cloning of the gene for the thyroid hormone sodium/iodide symporter (NIS) was reported in 1996.[108,109] Secondary structure prediction suggests a membrane protein with 12 transmembrane helices. The transporter gene is expressed in thyroid and salivary tissues and in gastric mucosa, where functional protein has been demonstrated. Transporter RNA is present in a variety of other tissues that do not show iodide uptake. The functional significance of the symporter mRNA in these tissues is not clear.[110] Several reports have documented mutations in the NIS gene in patients with congenital hypothyroidism.[106,107] Ten mutations were described through 2003, with affected individuals demonstrating homozygous or compound heterozygous mutation patterns.[107] Heterozygous family members were not clinically affected. The timing of onset of hypothyroidism tends to correlate with the genotype-specific residual NID activity.[107] Neonatal onset is likely with mutations associated with lower radioactive iodine uptake.

Peroxidase System Defects (Organification Defects)

Normally, iodide concentrated by the thyroid follicular cell is rapidly oxidized and bound in organic form. Organification of iodide involves two processes: oxidation of iodide and iodination of thyroglobulin-bound tyrosine.[97-99] Trapped iodide is oxidized to an active intermediate, followed by iodination of thyroglobulin-bound tyrosyl residues to form the iodotyrosines MIT and DIT. Two DIT residues are "coupled" to form T4. MIT and DIT couple to form T3. Tyrosyl iodination and coupling are catalyzed by a thyroid peroxidase enzyme system located at the apical membrane of the thyroid follicular cell in association with thyroid (NADPH) oxidases. Thyroid peroxidase is a membrane-bound heme protein that requires peroxide and an acceptor, which in the normal thyroid gland is thyroglobulin but can be albumin or other proteins or peptides. The hydrogen peroxide may be provided by one or more NADPH oxidases.

Some 200 patients with defective organification of iodide have been reported.[97-99] The defects included a quantitative deficiency of thyroid peroxidase (TPO), an abnormal and functionally defective TPO, or a deficiency of hydrogen peroxide generation. The complete defect can be detected by a perchlorate discharge test. Perchlorate is administered 1 to 2 hours after a dose of radioiodine. If organification is impaired, there is a rapid and profound discharge of the thyroidal radioiodine trapped during the following 1- to 2-hour period. Patients with partial TPO deficiency have a lesser discharge. The test is not specific, however, and more definitive testing is necessary for a precise diagnosis.

Thyroid peroxidase is a glycoprotein located at the apical membrane of the thyroid follicular cell. The gene is located on chromosome 2 and contains 3 kilobases of coding sequence over 17 exons coding for a protein of 933 amino acids. Some 20 different mutations have been described, including homozygous and compound heterozygous missence mutations, frame-shift mutations, base pair duplications, and single-nucleotide substitutions.[111,112] The variable molecular defects account for the clinical and biochemical heterogeneity in patients with defective iodine organification. Premature termination codons prevent translation of the protein. Other mutations affect the structure of the protein and perhaps its cellular location. Mutations in exons 8 through 10, which contain the putative hormone-binding histidine residues, produce a dysfunctional protein. Milder or transient organification defects have been associated with compound heterozygosity.[97,98]

Several patients have been described who were euthyroid or mildly hypothyroid but manifested goiter and partial discharge of radioiodine following perchlorate administration.[97,98,112] In these patients, the thyroid gland was found to contain no peroxidase activity—but such activity could be restored by adding hematin, the noncovalently bound prosthetic group of the peroxidase. This suggested an abnormal peroxidase apoenzyme deficient in binding to its heme moiety. In other patients, the organification defect was found to be associated with defective H_2O_2 generation. Iodination capacity in vitro was restored by the addition of riboflavin, FMN, oxidized cytochrome b2, cytochrome C, NADH, or NADPH. A defect in thyroid H_2O_2 generation was postulated to be due to a defect in biosynthesis of FAD from riboflavin.[98]

The H_2O_2 generation defect is rare. Recently, two genes encoding NADPH oxidases have been cloned and referred to as THOX1 and THOX2.[113] They are closely linked on chromosome 15 and predict proteins of 1,551 and 1,558 amino acids, respectively. The proteins colocalize with TPO at the apical membrane of thyroid follicular cells. Activating mutations in THOX2 associated with transient or severe congenital hypothyroidism have been described in four patients, and inactivating mutations in four other patients.[114]

The Pendred Syndrome

The Pendred syndrome, which includes familial goiter and congenital eighth-nerve deafness, is transmitted as an autosomal-recessive trait.[115,116] Approximately 750 cases were reported in some 400 families by 1992. About 6% of deaf mute children in a survey in England were found to be affected.[97,98] The prevalence is estimated to be 1.5 to 3 cases per 100,000 school children. One in 60 persons has one abnormal Pendred gene and is a carrier. The syndrome includes high tone or complete congenital deafness, goiter of variable degree appearing in middle or late childhood, and euthyroidism or mild hypothyroidism. One-third of patients have the complete syndrome. The remainder present with hearing loss or mild goiter.[97,98] The degree of impaired iodide organification is mild to moderate.

Infants with the syndrome are usually not detected unless in an iodine-deficient environment. Goitrous children manifest a positive perchlorate discharge with normal TPO activity. Atypical patients without an abnormal perchlorate discharge have been described.[115] The disorder was recently mapped to chromosome 7, and the gene defect localized to a chloride-iodide transport protein referred to as Pendrin.[116,117] The Pendrin gene contains 21 exons and a predicted open reading frame of 2,343 base pairs. The predicted protein consists of 780 amino acids (86 kilodaltons), including 11 putative transmembrane segments. Molecular studies have been conducted in more than 20 affected families from different geographic areas. In most of these there were independent point mutations and no large deletions. The etiology of the deafness remains controversial. The available information suggests that Pendrin gene mutations can give rise to syndromic or nonsyndromic deafness.[97,117,118]

Defects in Thyroglobulin Synthesis

Thyroglobulin is an essential substrate for organification and is the major protein component of thyroid colloid. It is an iodinated glycoprotein with a molecular weight approximating 650,000 daltons and a sedimentation coefficient of 19.7 (19S). It consists of two monomeric chains, 2,767 amino acids in length, each with 67 tyrosine residues and 20 potential glycosylation sites.[97-99] About one-third of the tyrosine residues are spatially oriented such that they are susceptible to iodination. The thyroglobulin gene is located on chromosome 8. It codes for a 300-kilodalton monomer molecule via an 8- to 9-kilodalton mRNA.

Genetic defects can lead to thyroglobulin deficiency or structural/functional abnormalities of the protein. Thyroglobulin synthesis defects occur in about 1 in 80,000 to 1 in 100,000 newborns.[97,98] Goiter and hypothyroidism are usually manifest at birth, but mild defects are likely to be described in association with later onset. To date, the functional defects have included defective thyroglobulin transport with carbohydrate-deficient thyroglobulin sequestered in golgi or cytoplasmic membranes, thyroglobulin with deficient tyrosine residues or tyrosine residues buried within the molecule and not available for iodination, and sialic-acid-deficient thyroglobulin (due to a sialyltransferase deficiency) containing MIT and DIT but manifesting defective coupling.[97,98,119-121]

Iodotyrosine Deiodinase Defect

Deficiency of the iodotyrosine deiodinase can cause congenital hypothyroidism or a less severe form of familial goiter. Failure to deiodinate thyroid MIT and DIT as they are released from thyroglobulin leads to severe iodine wastage because the non-deiodinated MIT and DIT leak out of the thyroid and are excreted in urine. Iodotyrosine deiodinases are present in both thyroid cells and peripheral tissues, and abnormalities involving both systems have been described.

The patients originally described were cretinous and hypothyroid, with goiters presenting at birth or shortly thereafter. They manifested early rapid thyroid radioiodine uptake and rapid spontaneous discharge. By 48 hours, most of the thyroidal radioiodine was discharged.[97,98] The serum in such patients contains high concentrations of iodotyrosines. They excrete essentially all of an intravenous dose of labeled iodotyrosine directly into urine, whereas normal subjects excrete the label almost entirely as free iodide. Partial defects have been described in thyroid and peripheral tissues, in peripheral tissues only, and in thyroid tissue only. In patients with a mild defect, compensation may be possible in a high-iodine environment. A goiter may appear only if iodine intake is limited.

Recently, the gene encoding the iodothyronine dehalogenase (DEHAL1) was cloned.[122] The cDNA encodes a 289-amino-acid protein member of the nitroreductase family. It contains a putative transmembrane segment and a large extracellular N-terminal region. The gene is also expressed in the kidney. DEHAL1 is localized to the apical thyroid membrane close to the thyroglobulin iodination site, closely linking tyrosine deiodination with the organification process. Mutations of the DEHAL1 gene have been identified in patients with congenital hypothyroidism from three different families. The phenotype is variable, including goiter, mental retardation, or normal mental development despite delayed thyroid hormone substitution.[123]

Iodothyronine Monodeiodinase Deficiency

As discussed previously, iodothyronines are metabolized via three iodothyronine monodeiodinases: MDI type I, MDI type II, and MDI type III[18,34] (Figure 6-5). To date, no defects have been identified in the genes encoding the MDI enzymes. All are selenoproteins requiring the incorporation of selenocysteine (sec) during biosynthesis. Incorporation of selenocysteine into the iodothyronine monodeiodinase enzymes requires several components: a selenocysteine insertion sequence (SECIS) element, a SECIS-binding protein (SECISBP2), and a selenoprotein-specific elongation factor (EFSec) and its transfer RNA tRNA^sec.[124]

Dumitrescu et al. have identified a Bedouin Saudi family with 3 of 7 siblings ages 4, 7, and 14 years with a phenotype of hyperthyroxinemia, decreased T3, increased reverse T3, and mildly increased TSH concentrations. The children were otherwise euthyroid.[124] The parents and four other siblings had normal thyroid function parameters. Patient fibroblasts showed reduced MDI II activity not linked to the MDI II locus, and linkage analysis of the genes involved in MDI synthesis revealed a homozygous missense mutation in SECISBP2. An unrelated Irish child age 6 with a similar phenotype carried compound heterozygous mutations in SECISBP2.[124] The family mutations were in exon 12 (R540Q) of the 17 SECISBP2 exons. The Irish mutations were a paternal K438X and maternal alternative donor splice site in exon 8. In both families, serum selenoprotein levels were low in affected individuals and normal in unaffected individuals.

THYROID HORMONE RESISTANCE

Thyroid Hormone Receptor Defects

Patients with thyroid hormone resistance classically present with increased circulating levels of T4 and T3 with a normal or increased serum TSH concentration.[125,126] Such infants may be detected in newborn screening programs in which TSH in measured directly. TSH levels are mildly to moderately increased, but the increased T4 level would preclude detection in a primary T4, secondary TSH screening program. The prevalence is not yet clear. More than 1,000 cases have been reported.[125] Preliminary data from regional populations suggests a prevalence approximating 1 in 40,000 newborns. They have been classified into three phenotypes: generalized resistance to thyroid hormones (GRTH), pituitary resistance to thyroid hormone (Pit RTH), and peripheral resistance to thyroid hormone (PRTH).

Inheritance has been autosomal dominant in all familial cases except one. Fifteen to 20% of cases appear sporadically. Many patients are asymptomatic or demonstrate nonspecific symptoms. Deafness is observed in 20%, and a syndrome of attention deficit hyperactivity has been documented in half of affected patients.[125-128] Hypothyroid features include growth retardation, delayed bone maturation, and intellectual impairment. Some children exhibit features of thyrotoxicosis, including failure to thrive, accelerated growth, and hyperkinetic behavior.[125,126]

Thyroid hormone action is mediated via nuclear thyroid hormone receptor proteins with zinc-finger DNA-binding regions and thyroid hormone-binding domains. The latter have a 10:1 relative binding affinity for T3/T4. The receptors act as DNA-transactivating factors to stimulate or suppress responsive genes. Two genes coding for the TR proteins have been described: an alpha gene on chromosome 17 and a beta gene on chromosome 3. Each codes for two major transcripts via alternative splicing: TRα1, TRα2, TRβ1, TRβ1. The TRα2 receptors do not bind T3, but have functional DNA-binding domains. The TRβ1 mRNA is distributed in highest concentrations in brain, liver, kidney, and heart.

TRβ2 mRNA is restricted to pituitary, retina, and cochlea. TRα1 and TRα2 mRNA are widely distributed among tissues.[53,54] The molecular defect in all cases studied to date has involved the TRβ1 gene on chromosome 3.[125,126] In most affected subjects, specific TRβ gene mutations have been demonstrated. More than 120 different defects have been described. More than 90% have been single-amino-acid deletions or substitutions involving the hormone-binding domain at the carboxy terminal end of the receptor molecule.[128] A few in-frame deletions and frame-shift insertions have been described.

There has been considerable variation of thyroid effects among tissues within family members with identical TRβ mutations.[125-129] TRs (like other steroid hormone superfamily receptors) bind to DNA response elements as monomers, homodimers, or heterodimers—and heterodimerization can involve another TR, including the TRα2 receptors, or other transactivation factors. The ability of the defective receptor to bind T3, to bind to other TR, or other factors appear to determine the effect of the defective receptor in a given tissue. Affected members of most families studied have one normal and one abnormal TRβ allele. The abnormal TRβ with minimal or reduced T3 binding fails to mediate T3-regulated transcription and may block the action of the normal allele. This has been referred to as a dominant negative effect, presumably mediated by binding of the defective allele with normal TRβ and producing an inactive homodimer.

Recent studies of patients with the PitRTH phenotype have revealed point mutations and decreased T3 binding of TRβ1 receptors similar to defects described in GRTH patients. These observations suggest that the apparent selective pituitary resistance and generalized resistance phenotypes are not qualitatively different syndromes but rather reflect a continuous spectrum of a similar molecular defect with variable tissue resistance.

Thyroid Hormone Membrane Transporter Defects

Carrier-mediated energy-dependent transport of thyroid hormones has recently been demonstrated in many in vitro cell lines involving the Na+/taurochlate co-transporting polypeptide (NTCP), the Na+-independent organic anion transporter (OATP) family, the L-type amino acid transporters, and more recently the monocarboxylate transporter MCT-8.[48] The significance of these several transporter systems in different cell types remains to be clarified. However, mutations in the MCT-8 gene (SLC16A2)—located on the X chromosome and associated with combined thyroid and neurological dysfunction—have been characterized.[48,130-132] The gene encodes a 613-amino-acid protein with 12 predicted transmembrane domains. The N-terminal and 6-terminal domains are located intracellularly.[131]

Nine patients with the MCT-8 thyroid hormone transporter defect have been reported presenting during infancy or childhood with hypotonia, poor head control, involuntary athetoid and dystonic movements, hyperreflexia, nystagmus, and severe mental retardation.[130-132] There were no other signs of hypothyroidism. Serum T3 concentrations were elevated, serum T4 and free T4 were low, and TSH concentrations were normal or slightly elevated. The gene defects have included deletions and missense mutations. Subsequent to these reports, it was recognized that this phenotype resembles that previously characterized as the Allan-Herndon-Dudley syndrome (AHDS)—an X-linked mental retardation syndrome. Recent studies have shown that AHDS is also associated with mutations in the SLC16A2 (MCT-8) gene. By mid 2006, 22 patients from 11 families with AHDS and SLC16A2 mutations had been characterized.[132]

The MCT-8 gene in mice is expressed in brain (choroid plexus, cerebrum, hippocampus, amygdala, striatum, and hypothalamus), liver, kidney, and pituitary and thyroid tissues. In brain tissues, MCT-8 transporters seem localized to neuronal rather than to glial cells.[132] MCT knockout mice have no apparent neurologic phenotype, but hemizygous males have elevated serum T3 and low T4 concentrations with a sevenfold increase in the serum T3/T4 ratio.[132]

Iodothyronine monodeiodinase 2 (MDI-2) activities in the brain and pituitary gland are markedly increased, and brain MDI-3 activity is decreased—supporting the hypothesis that the brain MDI changes in these animals is compensatory to reduced brain T3 levels. MDI-1 activities are increased in liver and kidney, reflecting increased tissue T3 content—suggesting an adequate T3 transport despite the MCT-8 gene inactivation.[132] The thyroid phenotype in human patients is similar to that in the MCT knockout mice and reflects altered T4 monodeiodination patterns due to altered T4 content in various tissues. Much of the brain damage due to decreased neuronal T4 content occurs in utero, and the phenotype resembles that in severe endemic cretinism. There is currently little information regarding effective treatment.

HYPOTHALAMIC-PITUITARY HYPOTHYROIDISM

Infants with central hypothyroidism are relatively uncommon, with a prevalence in the range of 1:20,000 to 1:30,000 newborns.[91,133] These infants are not usually detected in newborn thyroid screening programs because all programs are designed to screen for increased TSH levels. However, some programs also employ initial T4 and/or T4/TBG ratio measurements to detect infants with central hypothyroidism.[91] Hypothalamic-pituitary or central hypothyroidism can result from hypothalamic and/or pituitary dysgenesis or isolated TSH deficiency.

A variety of homeobox (expressed in embryonic stem cells) or transcription factor gene defects have been described in association with hypothalamic-pituitary dysgenesis. SHH, ZIC2, and SIX3 defects have been identified in patients with holoprosencephaly; HESX1 defects in association with septo-optic dysplasia; GL13 mutation in the pallister-hall syndrome; and LHX3, PROP1, PIT1, and POUIFI defects in hypopituitarism.[4-10,97]

Trh Deficiency

The human TRH gene has been mapped to chromosome 3q13.3.-q21, but no human mutations have been described to date. Targeted disruption of the TRH receptor gene in mice led to an unexpected mild phenotype of central hypothyroidism and hyperglycemia.[134,135] To date, only one family with compound heterozygosity for loss-of-function mutations of the TRH receptor gene with central hypothyroidism has been described. The affected patient presented with severe congenital hypothyroidism, short stature, and mental retardation.[136]

Tsh Deficiency

Familial isolated TSH deficiency is a rare disorder best characterized in Japanese patients. Several families have been reported with an autosomal-recessive pattern of inheritance of nongoitrous CH.[137-139] Serum T4 and TSH concentrations are low, whereas other pituitary functions are intact. The thyroid gland responds to TSH. There is no TSH response to TRH. A number of homozygous mutations in the TSHβ subunit gene on chromosome 1 have

been described, including single base substitutions in the CAGYC region of the gene.[137,140] The CAGYC-mutated mRNA codes for an altered beta polypeptide that does not associate with TSH alpha subunits to form active TSH. The most prevalent mutation identified in different populations is derived from a common ancestor and results in severe congenital hypothyroidism.[141] It involves a 1-bp deletion from codon 105 of the βTSH gene (C105V).

Recent studies have characterized at least four different Pit-1 gene mutations associated with a subtype of panhypopituitarism manifesting GH, prolactin, and TSH deficiency.[142] All were single base substitutions blocking Pit-1 synthesis or function. Prop-1 gene mutations also lead to multiple pituitary hormone deficiencies. The clinical spectrum resembles that of Pit-1 deficiency but includes gonadotropin deficiency.[143]

All of these disorders are characterized by a low serum free T4 concentration with a low or normal-range TSH level. If TSH deficiency is suspected, measurements of serum cortisol and GH concentrations may indicate panhypopituitarism. Hypoglycemia is a term neonate suggests ACTH and/or GH deficiency. A CAT scan or NMR scan is useful in characterizing hypothalamic-pituitary anomalies. A subnormal serum TSH response (measured at 30 minutes) to 7-μg/kg TRH infusion confirms a diagnosis of pituitary TSH deficiency. Selective studies measuring the TSH and TSH subunits can help characterize a thyrotropin gene defect. Therapy of the hypothyroidism in these infants is similar to therapy of other CH states. In addition, replacement of other pituitary or end-organ hormone deficiencies is necessary.

TRANSIENT CONGENITAL HYPOTHYROIDISM

Transient CH occurs in 5% to 10% of infants detected in newborn thyroid screening programs. These infants manifest low or normal T4 levels with variably elevated serum TSH concentrations. The most common causes in North America are goitrogenic agents and transplacentally derived TSH receptor-blocking maternal autoantibodies. Autoantibody-mediated CH accounts for 1% to 2% of the total.[144] In areas of endemic iodine deficiency, transient CH is more frequent and is due to a relative iodine deficiency associated with the increased thyroid hormone requirements in the neonatal period.[145] Maternal iodine or potentially antithyroid drug ingestion should be considered in all cases of CH. The presence of a goiter in the infant is supportive evidence of a drug- or goitrogen-induced transient hypothyroidism, but transient hypothyroidism is not usually associated with goiter.

The thyroid scan result varies, depending on the cause. Iodine usually inhibits technetium or radioiodine uptake, whereas drug or dietary goitrogens typically increase uptake and produce a positive scan. Maternal TSH receptor-blocking antibody-induced hypothyroidism should be suspected in any case where the mother has a history of autoimmune thyroid disease.[144,146,147] The presence in maternal or neonatal blood of a high level of TSH receptor-blocking antibody (TBA) is strong supportive evidence. The transient CH in these infants is usually of short duration (1-2 weeks) in the case of drugs, and longer (1-4 months) if related to maternal blocking antibody—the half-life of which approximates 2 weeks. If the CH state persists beyond 1 to 2 weeks, treatment is in order. Feedback control of TSH is normal in these infants, and the serum TSH level is easily suppressed. Measurements of TSH receptor antibody levels can be conducted to determine when to discontinue therapy in TBA-mediated CH.

EUTHYROID HYPERTHYROTROPINEMIA

Asymptomatic hyperthyrotropinemia is a relatively common disorder and may be transient or permanent. The prevalence of transient hyperthyrotropinemia in Europe approximates 1 in 8,000 births, with 50% due to perinatal iodine exposure.[148] Other causes could include defects in TSH or the TSH receptor, a mild intrathyroidal synthetic defect, a hemithyroid, or a resetting of the TSH feedback control system. Germ-line mutations of the thyrotropin receptor gene have been associated with a phenotype of asymptomatic hyperthyrotropinemia. Most were compound heterozygotes with normal heterozygote parents.[101,102]

Transient neonatal hyperthyrotropinemia is a relatively frequent phenomenon in Japan, where it is detected in about 1 in 18,000 newborns.[149] In a recent report of 16 cases followed for 2 to 7 years in Europe, the elevated serum TSH levels at 2 to 7 weeks of age ranged from 17 to 77 mU/L (17-77 μU/mL).[150] Serum T4, T3, and free T4 levels were normal, as were basal metabolic rates and thyroid radioiodine uptake values. All infants had increased TSH responses to exogenous TRH, whereas none had detectable levels of TBA. The elevated TSH values spontaneously normalized in 11 of the 16 infants within 6 months, excluding an abnormal TSH molecule or a TSH receptor defect in these subjects. However, the augmented TSH response to TRH persisted for 3 to 7 years in children.

All infants also had a normal T3 response to TSH, which tends to exclude a hormone synthetic defect. However, small diffuse goiters developed in 3 of 16 cases by 5 to 7 years.[150] The mechanism in these cases remains obscure, but partially inactivating mutations in the TSH receptor gene account for some of the familial cases.[146,147] In Italy, TSH receptor mutations were found in 5 of 42 patients with euthyroid hyperthyrotropinemia.[151] These five were from two families. There were no TSH mutations in the remaining 34 cases. The mutations were in the extracellular portion of the receptor in both families, and TSH levels ranged from 5.2 to 13 mU/L.

Eight families have been studied in Japan.[152] All have the R450H mutation in at least one allele. In four families, the mutation was homozygous—and in four there were compound heterozygotes. With normal serum T4 and free T4 levels, normal thyroid scan results, and absent thyroid antibodies, many such infants are followed expectantly. It is always necessary to rule out primary thyroid disease in such patients. Hyperthyrotropinemia in the newborn is usually treated, but in the presence of free T4 levels in the upper half of the normal range could be managed expectantly. Infants exposed to excess iodine usually recover spontaneously in 3 to 4 weeks.

EVALUATION OF INFANTS WITH PRESUMPTIVE POSITIVE SCREENING RESULTS

A positive screening report for CH in a newborn demands prompt evaluation of the infant, including a history, physical examination, and laboratory testing.[61,64,133] A history of autoimmune thyroid disease in the family suggests the possibility of transient CH, either drug or maternal TSH receptor autoantibody induced. Recurrent CH in the same sibship also suggests maternal autoantibody-mediated disease.[144] A history of familial congenital thyroid disease suggests thyroid dyshormonogenesis, which is usually transmitted as an autosomal-recessive trait.

Physical examination may reveal one of several early and subtle manifestations of hypothyroidism, including a large posterior fontanelle (>1 cm in diameter), prolonged jaundice (hyperbilirubinemia >7 days), macroglossia, hoarse cry, distended abdomen, umbilical hernia, hypotonia, or goiter.[61,133] Less than 5% of infants are diagnosed on clinical grounds before the screening report, but 15% to 20% of CH infants have suggestive signs when carefully examined.

The diagnosis of CH is confirmed by serum measurements of T4 and/or free T4 (FT4) and TSH concentrations. Serum total T4 assays are now quite well standardized but will vary directly with thyroxine-binding globulin concentrations. Automated FT4 immunoassay results vary by method and may underestimate FT4 concentrations in infants with low TBG levels.[153] This is particularly true in premature infants. The gold standard FT4 method is equilibrium dialysis, available in most reference laboratories. Like total T4, FT4 in hypothyroid infants should be maintained in the upper half of the normal range for the assay method employed. In the neonatal period (2-6 weeks), serum T4, FT4, and TSH levels below 84 nmol/L (6.5 μg/dL), 10 pmol/L (0.8 ng/dL), and above 10 mU/L (10 μU/mL), respectively, suggest CH.

In infants with proven CH, 90% have TSH levels above 50 mU/L and 75% have T4 and FT4 concentrations below 84 nmol/L (6.5 μg/dL) and 10 pmol/L (0.8 ng/dL), respectively. Perhaps 20% of CH infants have T4 and FT4 levels in the 84- to 165-nmol/L (6.5-13 μg/dL) and 10- to 25-pmol/L (0.8-1.9 ng/dL) range (respectively)—usually with clearly elevated TSH concentrations (>30 mU/L). A few infants will manifest only modest TSH elevations (7-30 mU/L). Such infants may require repeat examinations in order to establish a diagnosis of CH. Serum T3 or rT3 concentrations have limited practical value in the diagnosis of CH.

Hypothalamic-pituitary hypothyroidism is more difficult to diagnose. Most such infants are missed in screening programs unless a T4/TBG ratio measurement is included as a free T4 surrogate in the testing.[91] The disorder is characterized by a low serum T4 concentration and low T4/TBG ratio, with a normal or low-normal range TSH value. Measurements of serum free T4 concentrations will distinguish these possibilities. An infant or child with a low free T4 concentration and low TSH level should be carefully examined for evidence of hypothyroidism, and other tests of pituitary function should be conducted.[91] A subnormal TSH response to TRH confirms a diagnosis of pituitary TSH deficiency. If the peak level of TSH is normal and/or prolonged, and there is a good 4-hour T4 (thyroid) response to TSH, hypothalamic TRH deficiency is more likely. The TSH deficiency may be isolated or associated with other pituitary hormone deficiencies. In these infants, treatment with T4 raises the serum T4 and free T4 to normal levels.

All infants with proven CH should undergo radionuclide or ultrasound thyroid scanning if possible, using either technetium or I.[123,133] Radioiodine 123 is preferred, if available. Technetium is trapped by thyroid follicular cells but is not organified. Use of radioiodine provides greater isotope concentration, and allows later scanning (2-24 hours) with lower background radioactivity and improved discrimination. The confirmation of an ectopic thyroid gland provides a definitive diagnosis of thyroid dysgenesis. The absence of uptake of radioisotope suggests thyroid gland agenesis, but some infants may have low radioisotope uptake and a nondetectable gland by scan due to a TSH receptor defect, iodide trapping defect, or TSH receptor blockade by maternal TBA. These infants or the mother should have blood drawn for measurement of TBA if there is a history of maternal autoimmune thyroid disease. Thyroid ultrasound will usually confirm thyroid gland dysgenesis.

A normal radioisotope scan and/or a palpable or ultrasound-positive thyroid gland in the presence of hypothyroidism indicates impaired thyroid hormone synthesis. Infants with mild to moderate TBA-mediated transient CH may have normal thyroid scan results. The maternal and family histories should be carefully reviewed in such cases. A serum thyroglobulin measurement may be helpful in infants with absent uptake or normal scans. A very low or absent serum thyroglobulin level indicates thyroid agenesis in an infant with absent radioisotope uptake,

and suggests a defect in thyroglobulin synthesis in infants with a normal imaging study.[154]

Infants with thyroid dysgenesis have elevated serum thyroglobulin levels that relate to the mass of residual thyroid tissue and degree of stimulation. However, levels usually do not exceed 1,000 pmol/L (660 ng/mL). Very high thyroglobulin levels (>1,000 pmol/L) may be observed in infants with CH due to defective thyroxine synthesis not involving the capacity for thyroglobulin production. Serum calcitonin levels are also low in CH infants with thyroid agenesis but offer no advantage over the thyroglobulin measurement in diagnosis. These approaches are summarized in Figure 6-7. Normal thyroid function test results in infants 2 to 6 weeks of age are summarized in Table 6-3. A bone age measurement (x-ray examination of the knee and foot) is also useful as a test for possible intrauterine hypothyroidism.

TREATMENT OF AFFECTED INFANTS

Initial evaluation should be accomplished promptly and should require no more than 2 to 5 days.[64,74,133] In the absence of facilities or funds to conduct scanning, ultrasound, TBA bioassay, or thyroglobulin measurements, treatment should be instituted as soon as the diagnosis is confirmed. The goal of newborn CH screening is the institution of early adequate thyroid hormone replacement therapy. Most of the brain cell thyroid hormone is derived from local T4-to-T3 conversion. Approximately 70% of the T3 in the cerebral cortex is derived via local T4 monodeiodination.[65] Thus, the preferred thyroid hormone preparation for treatment of infants with CH is thyroxine.

Because the focus of screening is early and adequate treatment, the dosage of T4 should normalize the serum T4 level as quickly as possible.[74,133,155,156] To guarantee

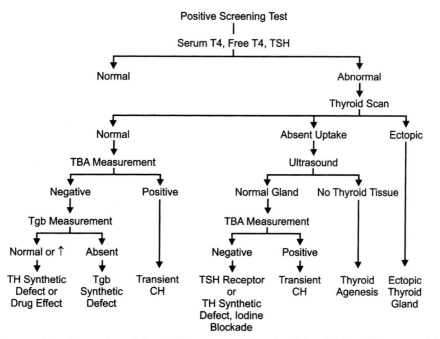

Figure 6-7. Suggested approach to the newborn infant with congenital hypothyroidism. TBA = TSH receptor blocking antibody, Tgb = thyroglobulin, TH = thyroid hormone.

TABLE 6-3

Normal Thyroid Function Parameters

Thyroid Parameter	2-6 Weeks of Age Normal Range
T4	84-210 nmol/L (6.5-16.3 ug/dL)
T3	1.5-4.6 nmol/L (100-300 ng/dL)
Free T4	10-30 pmol/L (0.8-2.2 ng/dL)
TSH	1.7-9.1 mU/L (1.9-9.1 mU/ml)
TBG	160-750 nmol/L (1.0-4.5 mg/dL)
Thyroglobulin	15-375 pmol/L (10-250 ng/mL)

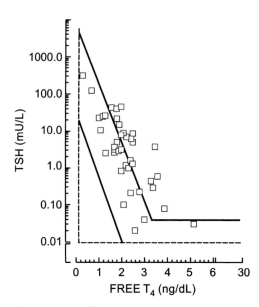

Figure 6-8. Serum third-generation TSH and direct dialysis free T4 measurements in 42 infants 2 to 9 months of age with congenital hypothyroidism on thyroxine replacement therapy. Normal infants plot within the parallel lines demarcating the 99-percentile range characterizing the TSH-free T4 relationship in individuals with a normal hypothalamic-pituitary-thyroid axis. Patients with pituitary resistance to T4 plot to the right of the normal range. Eighteen of the 42 infant values (43%) plot to the right of the 99-percentile range. In treated congenitally hypothyroid children and adolescents 1 year to 20 years of age (data not shown), only 6 of 63 (10%) plot to the right of the normal range. [From Fisher DA, Schoen EJ, LaFranchi S, et al. (2000). The hypothalamic-pituitary-thyroid negative feedback control axis in children with treated congenital hypothyroidism. J Clin Endocrinol Metab 85:2722.]

adequate hormone to all infants, it is desirable to maintain the serum T4 and/or FT4 in the upper half of the normal range during therapy. The 97% upper limit of serum T4 levels in hypothyroid infants may range to 130 nmol/L (10 μg/dL). For these reasons, the initial target range for the total T4 concentration is 130 to 210 nmol/L (10-16.3 μg/dL). This assumes a normal serum TBG concentration. This can be confirmed by measuring a normal-range T3 resin uptake, free thyroxine, or TBG level at the time of the first post-treatment T4 measurement. The initial direct free T4 target concentration should also be in the upper half of the normal infant range and with adequate treatment should transiently range to 40 to 45 pmol/L.[156,157]

To rapidly normalize the serum T4 concentration in the CH infant, an initial dose of Na-L-T4 of 10 to 15 μg/kg/day is recommended.[64,74,133] For the average term infant of 3 to 4.5 kg, an initial dose of 50 μg (0.050 mg) daily is appropriate. Serum TSH concentrations in some treated infants with CH may remain relatively elevated despite normalized levels of T4 or free T4[157] (Figure 6-8). The relative elevation of serum TSH is more marked during the early months of therapy but can persist to some degree in about 10% of patients through the second decade of life.[157] The elevated serum TSH concentration relative to T4 concentration in CH infants is presumably due to a resetting of the feedback threshold for T4 suppression of TSH release in infants with CH.[157] This resetting occurs in utero, but the mechanism remains obscure. Nonetheless, after the first few weeks of treatment serum TSH is the most important marker for therapy management.[74]

Physical growth and development of infants with CH are usually normalized by early adequate therapy, and infants with a delay in bone maturation at the time of diagnosis will normalize their bone by 1 to 2 years of age.[63] IQ values and mental and motor development are also normalized in most infants with CH.[64,158-160] However, low normal or occasionally low IQ values and motor impairments have been reported in treated children with severe CH (very low serum T4 and delayed bone maturation at birth).[161-164] This outcome has been more prevalent in programs employing a relatively low replacement dose of T4 or in infants in whom treatment is delayed.[64,165,166]

This deficit, although variable, amounts to several IQ points for every week of delayed early treatment. Early therapy with 10 to 15 μg/kg/day of levothyroxine reduces the serum TSH level more rapidly and minimizes

the early IQ loss.[74,155,156,161,166] Overtreatment resulting in tachycardia, excessive nervousness, or disturbed sleep patterns may occur but can be eliminated by frequent dosage adjustment and carries little or no risk if transient. Excessive dosage over a prolonged period (3-6 months) may produce osteoporosis, premature synostosis of cranial sutures, and undue advancement of bone age.

Infants with presumed transient hypothyroidism caused by maternal goitrogenic drugs need not be treated unless the low serum T4 and elevated TSH levels persist beyond the second week. Therapy can usually be discontinued after 8 to 12 weeks. Hyperthyroid mothers on antithyroid drugs may breast-feed their infants because the concentrations of drug in breast milk are very low. Infants with transient hypothyroidism secondary to maternal (transplacental) TSH receptor-blocking antibody also require treatment if they are hypothyroxinemic. The half-life of the maternal autoantibody approximates 2 weeks, and depending on the initial level may require several months for degradation. Treatment is usually required for 2 to 5 months.

Infants with thyroid resistance are very difficult to manage, and treatment must be individualized. It is important to detect infants with GRTH as early as possible to manage early relative hypothyroidism and to minimize brain dysfunction, including attention deficit hyperactivity disorder. Some patients will be adequately compensated by the TSH-mediated thyroid hyperplasia and hyperthyroxinemia. Other patients will be poorly compensated, and compensation will vary among tissues.[125,126] The serum TSH level in GRTH patients may be elevated or within the normal range (albeit high in the face of the hyperthyroxinemia).

An elevated TSH level in the absence of clinical evidence for thyrotoxicosis is an indication for treatment. Failure to thrive, delayed developmental milestones, and delayed bone maturation are other indications for treatment. The levothyroxine treatment dose may be three to six times the usual replacement dose. Data from other involved family members may be helpful when available. Patients with predominant PitRTH (and elevated TSH levels) will have variable peripheral tissue responsiveness. TSH-dependent thyrotoxicosis of variable degree usually presents during childhood or adolescence in such patients.

Some infants with GRTH have significant TSH elevation at birth in association with increased serum total and free T4 and T3 concentrations. Figure 6-9 shows pre- and

post-treatment serum TSH, thyroglobulin and total T4 and T3, and free T4 index and reverse T3 in a newborn infant with GRTH treated by Weiss et al.[167] Initial TSH approximated 50 mU/L, and total T4 approximated 650 nmol/L (50 μg/dL). The infant manifested an enlarged thyroid gland, and serum thyroglobulin concentrations measured at 1 month approximated 0.5 nmol/L (330 ng/mL). TSH and T4 levels fell during the first month, but TSH remained elevated and treatment was begun at 34 days. On a levothyroxine dosage of 150 to 250 μg daily, serum TSH plateaued in the 5- to 10-mU/L range—with total T4 approximating 500 nmol/L.

Congenital Hyperthyroidism

FETAL-NEONATAL GRAVES' DISEASE

Neonatal Graves' disease is uncommon because of the low incidence of thyrotoxicosis in pregnancy (1 to 2 cases per 1,000 pregnancies) and because the neonatal disease occurs only in about 1 in 70 cases of thyrotoxic pregnancy.[168-170] The disease is usually due to transplacental passage of TSH receptor-stimulating antibody (TSA) from a mother with active or inactive Graves' disease. It is possible to predict neonatal disease in offspring of women with high TSA titers. In general, TSA titers (measured as cAMP response to TSH as a percentage of control in a thyroid cell bioassay) of 300% to 500% are associated with a high prevalence of neonatal Graves' disease.[168] Rarely, an infant may acquire both TSH receptor-stimulating and TSH receptor-blocking antibodies from the mother. The blocking antibodies may block the effect of the stimulating antibodies for several weeks, and the infant develops late-onset neonatal Graves' disease.[168]

In pregnancies associated with autoimmune thyroid disease and high titers of TSH receptor-stimulating and/or TSH receptor-blocking autoantibodies, fetal-neonatal thyroid dysfunction may develop. In a recent study of 230 Graves' disease pregnancies, Mitsuda and colleagues reported a prevalence of neonatal thyroid dysfunction of 16.3%.[171] Overt or chemical hyperthyroidism accounted for 5.6%, and transient hypothyroidism for 10.7% (Table 6-4). These disorders reflect the effects of TSAs, TSH-receptor blocking antibodies, and the effects of fetal hyperthyroxinemia—which can produce fetal growth retardation, tachycardia, and feedback suppression of the fetal hypothalamic-pituitary-thyroid axis, resulting in long-standing hypothalamic-pituitary hypothyroidism.[172]

Antithyroid drugs used to treat maternal disease readily cross the placenta and can compromise fetal-neonatal thyroid hormone production.[168,169] Fetal hyperthyroidism is a significant risk in a pregnancy complicated by Graves'

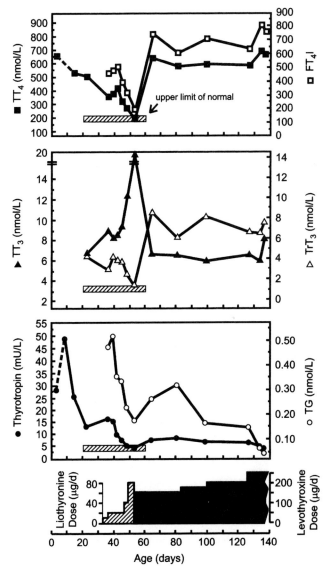

Figure 6-9. Thyroid function parameters in an infant with generalized resistance to thyroid hormone (GRTH). Total T4 (TT4), free T4 index (FT4I), total T3(TT3), total reverse T3(TrT3), thyrotropin (TSH), and thyroglobulin (Tg) levels before and during levothyroxine therapy are shown. [Reproduced with permission from Weiss RE, et al. (1990). Neonatal detection of generalized resistance to thyroid hormone. JAMA 264:2245.]

TABLE 6-4

Thyroid Dysfunction in Neonates of 230 Women with Graves' Disease

Thyroid Disorder	Number of Infants	% Infants
Thyrotoxicosis, neonatal		
Severe	6	2.6
Mild	7	3.0
Hypothyroidism, transient		
Overt	5	2.1
Hyperthyrotropinemia	18	7.8
Central	2	0.8
Total	38	16.3

Data from Mitsuda et al, Obstet Gynecol 80:359, 1992.

disease, and surveillance of the fetus with ultrasound allows detection of fetal goiter. Measurement of maternal serum levels of TSA as TSH binding-inhibiting immunoglobulin (TBII, which measures stimulating and blocking antibodies) or TSH receptor stimulating antibody (TSA) provide useful prognostic information. Levels of TBII in excess of 30% or TSA in excess of 300% of control values are predictive of fetal hyperthyroidism.[168,169]

Cordocentesis remains the method of choice for confirmation of fetal thyroid status. Standards for fetal serum thyroid hormone and TSH concentrations versus GA have been developed[28] (Figure 6-10). Fetal Graves' disease is also suspect if the fetus develops tachycardia. Baseline fetal heart rate averages about 140 beats/min between 21 and 30 weeks gestation, and 135 beats/min between 31 and 40 weeks.[169,173] The currently acceptable normal range during the last 15 weeks of gestation is 120 to 160 beats/min. The baseline rate is defined as the average baseline fetal heart rate in a 10-minute period rounded off to the nearest 5 beats/min. In the reported instances of fetal thyrotoxicosis responding to maternal antithyroid drug treatment, fetal tachycardia exceeding 160 beats/min occurred between 25 and 30 weeks gestation.

Maternal antithyroid drug treatment normalized the fetal heart rate within 2 weeks. Treatment of fetal thyrotoxicosis is accomplished by administration of an antithyroid drug to the mother in a dose of 150 to 300 mg daily. The dose is adjusted at 1- to 2-week internals to maintain the fetal heart rate at 140 beats/min. The antithyroid drug dose can usually be decreased progressively, aiming for

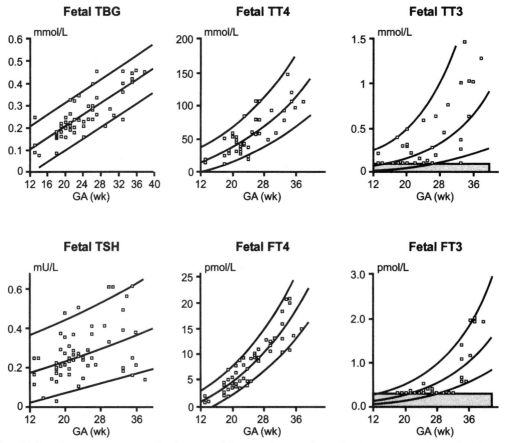

Figure 6-10. Thyroid function test parameters in the normal in utero human fetus. Serum concentrations of TBG, total T4(TT4), total T3(TT3), TSH, free T4(FT4) and free T3(FT3) were measured in blood obtained by cordocentesis or cardiocentesis conducted for prenatal diagnosis of blood disorders, fetal karyotyping, investigation of maternal toxoplasmosis, or fetal blood grouping in red cell isoimmunized pregnancies. These values were derived from fetuses found not to have the disorder or infection in question. The progressive increase in free T4 concentration with increasing gestation age is not in agreement with recent umbilical cord-blood concentrations. [Reproduced with permission from Thorpe-Beeston JG, et al. (1992). Fetal thyroid function. Thyroid 2:207.]

a 75- to 100-mg daily dose near term. In rare circumstances, maternal autoantibodies against thyroxine can produce hyperthyroxinemia in the fetus and neonate and can complicate interpretation of in vitro thyroid function tests.[174] This possibility can be tested if the clinical and laboratory data are incongruent.

Graves' disease in the newborn is manifested by irritability, flushing, tachycardia, hypertension, poor weight gain, thyroid enlargement, and exophthalmos.[169,170] Thrombocytopenia, hepatosplenomegaly, jaundice, and hypoprothrombinemia may occur. Cardiac failure and death may occur if the thyrotoxicity is severe and the treatment inadequate. The suppression of cord-blood TSH to values less than 0.1 mU/L in the presence of normal or elevated levels of T4 and T3 suggests a TSA effect. The diagnosis is confirmed by measuring high levels of T4, free T4, and T3 in postnatal blood.

Cord-blood values may be normal or near normal, but levels at 2 to 5 days may be markedly increased. The serum TSH is low. In some neonates, the onset of symptoms and signs may be delayed as long as 8 to 9 days. This is due both to the postnatal depletion of transplacentally acquired blocking doses of antithyroid drugs, and to the fact that there is an abrupt increase in conversion of T4 to active T3 by liver and other tissues shortly after birth. Neonatal Graves' disease resolves spontaneously as maternal TSA in the newborn is degraded. The half-life approximates 12 days. The usual clinical course of neonatal Graves' disease extends from 3 to 12 weeks.

The treatment of Graves' hyperthyroidism in the newborn includes sedatives and digitalization as necessary.[170] Iodide or antithyroid drugs are administered to decrease thyroid hormone secretion. These drugs have additive effects with regard to inhibition of hormone synthesis. In addition, iodide rapidly inhibits hormone release. Lugol's solution (5% iodine and 10% potassium iodide; 126 mg of iodine per milliliter) is begun in a dose of one drop (about 8 mg) three times daily. Methimazole or propylthiouracil are administered in a dose of 0.5 to 1 mg or 5 to 10 mg, respectively, per kilogram daily in divided doses at 8-hour intervals. A therapeutic response should be observed within 24 to 36 hours. If a satisfactory response is not observed, the dose of antithyroid drug and iodide can be increased by 50%. Adrenal corticosteroids in anti-inflammatory dosage and propranolol (1 to 2 mg per kilogram per day) may also be helpful. Radiographic contrast agents, too, may be useful in treatment (sodium ipodate, 100 mg a day or 0.3 to 0.5 g every 2 to 3 days) either alone or in conjunction with antithyroid drug treatment.[175,176]

AUTOSOMAL-DOMINANT HYPERTHYROIDISM

Several families have been reported with hyperthyroidism segregating as an autosomal-dominant trait in the absence of thyroid autoimmune disease.[101,102,177-181] Some 12 families and 11 children with sporadic occurrence of activating TSH receptor mutations have been reported.[181] The affected individuals present with goiter, increased total and free T4 levels, and suppressed TSH concentrations. In patients treated surgically, the thyroid glands manifest diffuse hyperplasia without lymphocytic infiltration. In two large French cohorts, TSH receptor gene mutations have been characterized involving the third and seventh transmembrane segments of the TSH receptor.[177] Functionally, the transfected mutated receptors demonstrated abnormally increased constitutive cAMP-stimulating activity. Only one constitutively activating mutation (located in the large extracellular domain at position 281) has been identified.[103]

Most of the affected individuals have been detected during childhood or adolescence, but a few infants have been diagnosed before 2 years of age and occasionally at birth.[178,180] Clearly, the abnormality is congenital—and it is possible that some of the earlier reported cases of familial persistent neonatal Graves' disease have been due to unrecognized activating TSH receptor mutations. Treatment of such infants is difficult because the disorder is not transient.[180] Antithyroid drugs and partial or near-total thyroidectomy are the available treatment options.

Disorders of Thyroid Hormone Transport

Several genetic abnormalities of the iodothyronine-binding serum proteins have been described and all are manifest at birth. These include complete TBG deficiency, partial TBG deficiency, TBG excess, transthyretin (TTR) (prealbumin) variants, and familial dysalbuminemic hyperthyroxinemia (FDH).[182-192] Features of these disorders are summarized in Table 6-5. All are associated with a euthyroid state, but the abnormal total thyroxine concentrations can be misleading during neonatal screening and in the assessment of thyroid function.

COMPLETE TBG DEFICIENCY

In 1959, Tanaka and Starr first reported TBG deficiency in a euthyroid male. Since that time, some 14 T4-binding globulin variants have been identified that produce complete deficiency of TBG.[182,183] These include TBG-CD, TBG-CD5, TBG-CD6, TBG-CDJ (Japan), TBG-CDY (Yonago), TBG-CDB (Buffalo), TBG-CDBe (Bedouin), and TBG-CDK (Kankakee). The prevalence of TBG deficiency varies from 1 in 5,000 to 1 in 12,000 newborn infants. This prevalence estimate includes infants with partial TBG deficiency (low TBG). The disorder seems to be transmitted as an X-linked trait. Serum TBG levels measured by immunoassay or T4-binding capacity are very low in affected males and are approximately half-normal in carrier females. Serum T4 levels vary similarly, but affected subjects are euthyroid—with normal serum free T4 concentrations, normal serum TSH levels, and normal serum TSH responses to exogenous TRH.

Male-to-male transmission has not been observed, and there is usually transmission of the trait from affected males to female offspring. Variable phenotypes have been observed in association with selective inactivation of the X chromosome carrying one of the two alleles.[184] The defects have included a single-amino-acid substitution producing abnormal post-translational processing

TABLE 6-5

Thyroid Hormone Binding Protein Abnormalities

					Clinical	
Abnormality	Prevalence	Inheritance	T4	T3	T3RU
Complete TBG Deficiency	1:15,000 Newborns	X-linked	low	↓	↑
Partial TBG Deficiency	1:4,000 to 1:12,000 Newborns	X-linked	↓	↓	↑
TBG Excess	1:25,000 Newborns	X-linked	↑	↑	↓
Transthyretin (TTR) Variants	Rare	Autosomal Dominant	↑ ↓	N N	N N
Familial Dysalbuminemic Hyperthyroxinemia (FDH)	1:100 Newborns?	Autosomal Dominant	↑	N	N

*Manifest in heterozygotes.
**Manifest in heterozygotes or homozygotes depending on mutation.

(TBG-CD5). The other five single-nucleotide substitutions or nucleotide deletions produce truncated molecules caused by early termination of translation.[183] The most recently described defect, TBG-CDK (Kankakee), involved an A-to-G transition in the acceptor splice function of intron II—causing a frame-shift and premature stop codon, predicting a truncated TBG protein lacking 201 amino acids.[183]

PARTIAL TBG DEFICIENCY

A partial TBG deficiency has been described, characterized by diminished but not absent TBG. A number of families have been reported.[182,185] Careful studies indicate that in these families, as in those with very low serum TBG levels, serum free T4 and TSH levels are normal. TBG levels are diminished in affected males, and there is a tendency to decreased concentrations in carrier females. However, the carrier state in females is sometimes difficult to identify because of overlap with affected males or normals.

This abnormality also seems to be transmitted as an X-linked trait. Six variant partial TBG defects have been described associated with altered TBG binding of T4. These defects (including TBG-SD, TBG-G, TBG-M, TBG-A, TBG-Q and TBG-PDJ) are characterized by decreased serum TBG concentrations by immunoassay and increased concentrations of denatured TBG identified on the basis of decreased heat stability.[182]

TBG EXCESS

Congenital TBG excess occurs in from 1 in 6,000 newborns in England to 1 in 40,000 in New York.[182] Subjects with increased levels of TBG have increased total serum T4 concentrations with normal free T4 and TSH levels and are hence euthyroid. Studies in these subjects, as in those with low TBG concentrations, have shown correlation between TBG production rates and serum levels—suggesting that the mechanism for the high TBG concentrations is increased production, presumably by the liver.

TBG levels are increased up to 4.5 times normal in affected individuals, and carrier females have serum concentrations intermediate between normal values and the high levels in affected males. Early reports suggested a dominant mode of inheritance, but subsequent studies and review of the earlier data are compatible with an X-linked mode of inheritance.[182] Mori et al., using gene dosage and in situ hybridization studies, showed that the defect in two Japanese families appears to be due to gene amplification secondary to three copies of the TBG gene on the affected X chromosome.[186]

TRANSTHYRETIN VARIANTS

Moses et al. first reported a 52-year-old euthyroid man with an elevated serum T4 (not corrected by the use of a free T4 index) but with normal free T4, normal total serum T3 and TSH concentrations, and normal TSH and T3 responses to TRH.[187] Serum TBG and albumin levels were normal, but the serum TBPA concentration measured by radioimmunoelectrophoresis was 2.5 to 3.0 times greater than the level in a normal human serum pool. Moreover, 70% of the serum T4 was selectively removed by an anti-TBPA immunoglobulin affinity column. One of the subject's three children had a similar abnormality, but the mode of inheritance was not clearly defined. Several similar patients have been reported.[187-189]

The family recently reported by Refetoff et al. demonstrated dominant inheritance, with serum T4 levels in affected family members 50% above the mean of unaffected relatives.[189] Reverse T3 concentrations were increased, but serum T3 and TSH levels were normal. Four transthyretin variants have been reported (Ser6, Thr109, Met119 and Val109). Only two of these, Thr109 and Val109, demonstrated high enough affinity for T4 to produce consistent hyperthyroxinemia in heterozygous individuals.[189]

FAMILIAL DYSALBUMINEMIC HYPERTHYROXINEMIA AND HYPERTRIIODOTHYRONINEMIA

FDH is the most common cause of inherited euthyroid hyperthyroxinemia in Caucasians. The binding protein abnormality was described by several investigators who

Features			
FT4	Protein Level	Other	Molecular Abnormality
N	TBG<0.5 μg/dl	TBG absent or decreased immunoreactivity; decreased binding affinity	TBG gene mutations
N	↓	TBG decreased immunoreactivity or decreased stability; decreased binding affinity	TBG gene mutations
N	TBG ↑ 3.0-4.5 X		Defect not yet clear
N	N	Increased T4-binding affinity*	TTR gene mutations
N	N	Decreased T4-binding affinity**	TTR gene mutations
N	N	Increased T4-binding affinity	Genetic polymorphism?

studied euthyroid subjects with increased serum T4 concentrations not corrected by the use of the free T4 index correction and with normal free T4, total serum T3, and TSH levels.[190] Wada and co-workers described the defect in Japanese subjects. The thyroid function parameters in these subjects resemble those in the patients with high TBPA reported by Moses et al.[187,191]

Serum thyroxine in affected subjects migrates with albumin by conventional polyacrylamide electrophoresis, and TBPA levels are normal on the basis of saturation-binding studies in vitro. The disorder seems to be transmitted as an autosomal-dominant trait. There is male-to-male transmission and an affected-to-unaffected ratio of 1 or greater in first-degree relatives. A missense mutation in codon 218 of the albumin gene has been described in 11 unrelated families (G to A in Caucasians and G to C in the Japanese family), resulting in arginine-to-histidine and arginine-to-proline amino acid substitutions (respectively) in the albumin molecule.[192]

Familial dysalbuminemic hypertriiodothyroninemia has been reported in a Thai family presenting with high serum total T3 and normal T4 concentrations.[192] The affected patients were euthyroid, with normal free T4, free T3, and TSH concentrations. T3-binding studies showed a 40-fold increased association constant (Ka) of serum albumin in affected subjects, whereas the Ka for T4 was increased only 1.5-fold. The molecular defect was a nucleotide substitution at normal codon 66, resulting in substitution of a cytosine for thymine and replacement of the normal leucine by proline.[192]

The Fetus as Patient

Advances in medical science and technology have paved the way for an increasingly direct approach to the fetus as patient.[169,193,194] Improvements in fetal ultrasound imaging, Doppler ultrasound, and the availability and relative safety of intrauterine cordocentesis now provide new windows on fetal development and metabolism. Fetal therapy via maternal transplacental drug therapy or amniotic fluid instillation are now commonplace. Fetal surgery and fetal gene therapy are being pioneered. One of the first fetal disease states directly addressed in the fetus was thyroid dysfunction.

This effort was frustrated by the failure of measurements of amniotic fluid TSH and iodothyronine concentrations to reliably reflect fetal thyroid function. Currently, fetal thyroid size can be reliably assessed by ultrasound—and normative data for thyroid function tests has been provided for cordocentesis samples during the latter half of gestation. Thus, it is now possible to accurately assess and monitor fetal thyroid function and thyroid-directed therapeutic interventions in the in utero fetus during the latter half of human pregnancy (Figure 6-10).

Possible indications for fetal thyroid assessment include a family history of inborn defects in hypothalamic-pituitary function or thyroid hormone metabolism, maternal drug therapy that might affect fetal thyroid function, or maternal autoimmune thyroid disease. It is clear that maternal or fetal hypothyroidism can be associated with reduction in IQ or with psychomotor dysfunction syndromes, and fetal hyperthyroidism is associated with brain damage, reduced fetal growth, and occasional fetal demise.[23,40,69,170,195] Diagnosis and treatment of fetal hypothyroidism using amniotic injection of levothyroxine and the management of fetal hyperthyroidism via maternal antithyroid drug therapy are now accepted procedures.[170,196-198] Refinements will occur with increasing experience.

REFERENCES

1. Santisteban P (2005). Development and anatomy of the hypothalamic-pituitary-thyroid axis. In Braverman LE, Utiger RD (eds.), The thyroid: Ninth edition. Philadelphia: Lippincott Williams & Wilkins 8–25.
2. Brown RS, Huang SA, Fisher DA (2005). The maturation of thyroid function in the perinatal period and during childhood. In Braverman LE, Utiger RD (eds.), The thyroid: A fundamental and clinical text, Ninth edition. Philadelphia: Lippincott Williams & Wilkins 1013–1033.
3. Polk DH, Fisher DA (2004). Fetal and neonatal thyroid physiology. In Polin RA, Fox WW, Abman SH (eds.), Fetal and neonatal physiology, Third edition. Saunders, Philadelphia: WB Saunders 1926–1933.
4. Fisher DA (2006). Fetal and neonatal endocrinology. In DeGroot LJ, Jameson JL (eds.), Endocrinology, Fifth edition. Philadelphia: Elsevier-Saunders 3369–3386.

5. Grumbach MM, Gluckman PD (1994). The human fetal hypothalamus and pituitary gland: The maturation of neuroendocrine mechanisms controlling secretion of pituitary growth hormone, prolacton, gonadotropins, adrenocorticotropin-related peptides and thyrotropin. In Tulchinsky D, Little AB (eds.), *Maternal Fetal Endocrinology, Second edition.* Philadelphia: WB Saunders 193–261.

6. Roessler E, Belloni E, Gaudenz K, Jay P, et al. (1996). Mutations in the human sonic hedgehog gene cause holoprosencephaly. Nature Genetics 14:356.

7. Wallis DE, Roessler E, Hehr U, Nanni L, et al. (1999). Mutations in the homeodomain of the human SIX-3 gene cause holoprosencephaly. Nature Genetics 22:196.

8. Brown SA, Warburton D, Brown LY, et al. (1998). Holoprosencephaly due to mutation in ZIC2, a homologue of drosphila odd paired. Nature Genetics 20:180.

9. Dattani MT, Martinez-Barbera JP, Thomas PQ, et al. (1998). HESX1: A novel homeobox gene implicated in septo-optic dysplasia. Horm Res 50(3):6.

10. Tran PV, Savage JJ, Ingraham HA, Rhodes SJ (2004). Molecular genetics of hypothalamic-pituitary development. In Pescovitz OH, Eugster EA (eds.), *Pediatric endocrinology.* Philadelphia: Lippincott Williams & Wilkins 63–79.

11. Lanctôt C, Gauthier Y, Drouin J (1999). Pituitary homeobox (Ptx-1) is differentially expressed during pituitary development. Endocrinology 140:1416.

12. Machinis K, Pantel J, Netchine I, et al. (2001). Syndromic short stature in patients with a germline mutation in the LIM homeobox LHX4. Am J Hum Genet 69:961.

13. DeFelice M, DiLauro R (2004). Thyroid development and its disorders: Genetics and molecular mechanisms. Endocrine Rev 25:722.

14. Manley NR, Capecchi MR (1998). HOX group 3 paralogs regulate the development and migration of the thymus, thyroid and parathyroid glands. Dev Biol 195:1.

15. Roti E, Gnudi A, Braverman LE (1983). The placental transport, synthesis and metabolism of hormones and drugs which affect thyroid function. Endocrine Rev 4:131.

16. Buttfield JH, Hetzel BA (1969). Endemic cretinism in Eastern New Guinea. Aust Ann Med 18:217.

17. Sibley CP, Boyd RDH (2004). Mechanisms of transfer across the human placenta. In Polin RA, Fox WW, Abman SH (eds.), *Fetal and neonatal physiology, Third edition.* Philadelphia: WB Saunders 111–122.

18. Burrow GN, Fisher DA, Larsen PR (1994). Maternal and fetal thyroid function. N Engl J Med 331:1072.

19. Huang SA. Physiology and pathophysiology of type 3 monodeiodinase in humans. Thyroid 15:875.

20. Fisher DA, Dussault JH, Sack J, Chopra IJ (1977). Ontogenesis of hypothalamic-pituitary-thyroid function and metabolism in man, sheep and rat. Rec Prog Horm Res 33:59.

21. Contempre B, Jauniaux E, Calvo R, et al. (1993). Detection of thyroid hormones in human embryonic cavities during the first trimester of pregnancy. J Clin Endocrinol Metab 77:1719.

22. Vulsma T, Gons MH, DeVijlder JJM (1989). Maternal fetal transfer of thyroxine in congenital hypothyroidism due to a total organification defect or thyroid agenesis. N Engl J Med 321:13.

23. Haddow JE, Palomaki GE, Allan WC, et al. (1999). Maternal thyroid hormone deficiency during pregnancy and subsequent neuropsychological development of the child. N Engl J Med 341:549.

24. Polk DA, Reviczky A, Lam RW, Fisher DA (1991). Thyrotropin releasing hormone in the ovine fetus; ontogeny and effect of thyroid hormone. Am J Physiol: Endocrinol Metab 23:E53.

25. Parry S, Strauss JF III (2004). Placental hormones. In Polin RA, Fox WW, Abman SH (eds.), *Fetal and neonatal physiology, Third edition.* Philadelphia: WB Saunders 3353–3367.

26. Fisher DA (1989). Development of fetal thyroid system control. In Delong GR, Robbins J, Condliffe PG (eds.), *Iodine and the brain.* New York: Plenum Press 167–176.

27. Hume R, Simpson J, Delahunty C, et al. (2004). Human and cord serum thyroid hormones: developmental trends and interrelationships. J Clin Endocrinol Metab 89:4097.

28. Thorpe-Beeston JG, Nicolaides KH, McGregor AM (1992). Fetal thyroid function. Thyroid 2:207.

29. Santini F, Chiovata L, Ghirri P, et al. (1999). Serum iodothyronines in the human fetus and the newborn: Evidence for an important role of placenta in fetal thyroid hormone homeostasis. J Clin Endocrinol Metab 84:493.

30. de Zegher F, Van hole C, Van den Berghe G, et al. (1994). Properties of thyroid stimulating hormone and cortisol secretion by the human newborn on the day of birth. J Clin Endocrinol Metab 79:576.

31. Fisher DA, Nelson JC, Carlton EI, Wilcox RB (2000). Maturation of human hypothalamic-pituitary-thyroid function and control. Thyroid 10:229.

32. Klein AH, Fisher DA (1980). Thyrotropin releasing hormone stimulated pituitary and thyroid gland responsiveness and 3,5,3' triiodothyronine suppression in fetal and neonatal lambs. Endocrinology 106:697.

33. Fisher DA (1998). Thyroid function in premature infants: The hypothyroxinemia of prematurity. Clin Perinatol 25:999.

34. Kuiper GJM, Kester MHA, Peeters RP, Visser TJ (2005). Biochemical mechanisms of thyroid hormone deiodination. Thyroid 15:787.

35. Maia A, Kim BW, Huang SA, et al. (2005). Type 2 iodothyronine deiodinase is the major source of plasma T3 in euthyroid humans. J Clin Invest 115:2524.

36. Wu SY, Green WL, Huang WS, Hays MT, et al. (2005). Alternate pathways of thyroid hormone metabolism. Thyroid 15:943.

37. Wassen WJS, Klootwijk W, Kaptein E, et al. (2004). Characteristics and thyroid state-dependent regulation of iodothyronine deiodinases in pigs. Endocrinology 145:4251.

38. Richard K, Hume R, Kaptein E, et al. (1998). Ontogeny of iodothyronine deiodinases in human liver. J Clin Endocrinol Metab 83:2868.

39. Fisher DA, Polk DH, Wu SY (1994). Fetal thyroid metabolism: A pluralistic system. Thyroid 4:367.

40. Kester MHA, DeMena RM, Obregon J, et al. (2004). Iodothyronine levels in the human developing brain: Major regulatory roles of iodothyronine deiodinases in different areas. J Clin Endocrinol Metab 89:3117.

41. Koopdonk-Kool JM, DeVijlder JJM, Veenboer GJM, et al. (1996). Type II and type III deiodinase in human placenta as a function of gestational age. J Clin Endocrinol Metab 81:2154.

42. Polk DH, Reviczky A, Wu SY, et al. (1994). Metabolism of sulfoconjugated thyroid hormone derivatives in developing sheep. Am J Physiol 266:E892.

43. Richard K, Hume R, Kaptein E, et al. (2001). Sulfation of thyroid hormone and dopamine during human development: ontogeny of phenol sulfotransferases and arylsulfatase in liver, lung and brain. J Clin Endocrinol Metab 86:2734.

44. Stanley EM, Hume R, Visser TJ, Coughtrie WH (2001). Differential expression of sulfotransferase enzymes involved in thyroid hormone metabolism during human placental development. J Clin Endocrinol Metab 86:5944.

45. Morreale de Escobar G, Obregon MJ, Calvo R, Escobar del Rey F (1993). Effects of iodine deficiency on thyroid hormone metabolism and the brain in iodine deficient rats: The role of the maternal transfer of thyroxine. Am J Clin Nutr Suppl 57:280S.

46. Fowden AL, Silver M (1995). The effects of thyroid hormones on oxygen and glucose metabolism in the sheep fetus during late gestation. J Physiology 482:203.

47. Polk DH (1988). Thyroid hormone effects on neonatal thermogenesis sermin. Perinatal 12:151.

48. Jansen J, Friesema ECH, Milici C, Visser TJ (2005). Thyroid hormone transporters in health and disease. Thyroid 15:757.

49. Incerpi S (2006). Thyroid hormones: Rapid reply by surface delivery only. Endocrinology 146:2861.

50. Bergh JJ, Lin HY, Lansing L, et al. (2006). Integrin $\alpha V\beta 3$ contains a cell surface receptor site for thyroid hormone that is linked to activation of mitogen-activated protein kinase and induction of angiogenesis. Endocrinology 146:2864.

51. Farwell AP, Dubord-Tomaselti SA, Pietrzykowski AZ, Leonard JL (2006). Dynamic nongenomic actions of thyroid hormone in the developing rat brain. Endocrinology 147:2567.

52. Lanni A, Moreno M, Lombardi A, et al. (2005). 3,5-diiodothyronine powerfully reduces adiposity in rats by increasing the burning of fats. FASEBJ online [July, doi:10.1096/fj.05-3977fje] 1–22.

53. Yen P (2005). Genomic and nongenomic actions of thyroid hormones. In Braverman LE, Utiger RD (eds.), *The thyroid, Ninth edition.* Philadelphia: Lippincott Williams & Wilkins 135–150.

54. Flament F, Samarut J (2005). Thyroid hormone receptors: Lessons from knockout and knockin mutant mice. Trends Endocrinol Metab 14:85.

55. Polk DH, Cheromcha D, Reviczky AL, Fisher DA (1989). Nuclear thyroid hormone receptors: Ontogeny and thyroid hormone effects in sheep. Am J Physiol 256:E543.

56. Forhead AJ, Li J, Saunders JC, et al. (2000). Control of ovine hepatic growth hormone and insulin-like growth factor I by thyroid hormones in utero. Am J Physiol Endocrinol Metab 278:E1166.

57. Bernal J, Pekonen F (1984). Ontogenesis of nuclear 3,5,3' triiodothyronine receptors in human fetal brain. Endocrinology 114:677.

58. Gonzales LA, Ballard PL (1981). Identification and characterization of nuclear 3,5,3' triiodothyronine binding sites in fetal human lung. J Clin Endocrinol Metab 53:21.

59. Kilby MD, Gittoes N, McCabe C, et al. (2000). Expression of thyroid receptor isoforms in the human fetal central nervous system and the effects of intrauterine growth restriction. Clin Endocrinol 53:469.

60. LaFranchi SH, Hanna CE, Krainz PL, et al. (1985). Screening for congenital hypothyroidism with specimen collection at two time periods: Results of the Northwest Regional screening program. Pediatrics 76:734.

61. Grant DB, Smith I, Fuggle PW, et al. (1992). Congenital hypothyroidism detected by neonatal screening: Relationship between biochemical severity and early clinical features. Arch Dis Child 67:87.

62. Leger J, Czernichow P (1989). Congenital hypothyroidism, decreased growth velocity in the first weeks of life. Biol Neonate 55:218.

63. Grant DB (1994). Growth in early treated congenital hypothyroidism. Arch Dis Childh 70:464.

64. Delange F (1997). Neonatal screening for congenital hypothyroidism: Results and perspectives. Horm Res 48:51.

65. Calvo R, Obregon MJ, Ruiz de Ona C, et al. (1990). Congenital hypothyroidism as studied in rats: crucial role of maternal thyroxine but not of 3,5,31-triiodothyronine in the protection of the fetal brain. J Clin Invest 86:889.

66. Silva JE, Rabelo R (1997). Regulation of the uncoupling protein gene expression. Eur J Endocrinol 136:251.

67. Klein AH, Reviczky A, Chou P, et al. (1983). Development of brown adipose tissue thermogenesis in the ovine fetus and newborn. Endocrinology 112:1662.

68. Gong DW, He Y, Karas M, Reitman M (1997). Uncoupling protein-3 is a mediator of thermogenesis regulated by thyroid hormone, β3 adrenergic agonists, and leptin. J Biol Chem 272:24129.

69. Morreale de Escobar G, Obregon MJ, Escobar del Ray F (2004). Role of thyroid hormone during early brain development. Eur J Endocrinol 151:U25–U37.

70. Lavado-Autric R, Auso E, Garcia-Velasco JV, et al. (2003). Early maternal hypothyroxinemia alters histogenesis and cerebral cortex cytoarchitecture of progeny. J Clin Invest 111:1073.

71. Kasaltkina EP, Samsonova LN, Ivakhnenko VN, et al. (2006). Gestational hypothyroxinemia and cognitive function in offspring. Neurosci Behavioral Physiol 36:619.

72. Cao XY, Jiang XM, Dou ZH, et al. (1994). Timing of vulnerability of the brain to iodine deficiency in endemic cretinism. N Engl J Med 331:1739.

73. DeLong GR, Xue-Yi C, Xin Min J, et al. (1998). Iodine supplementation of a cross-section of iodine deficient pregnant women: does the human fetal brain undergo metamorphosis? In Stanbury JB, Delange F, Dunn JT, Pandav CS (eds.), Iodine in pregnancy. Calcutta: Oxford University Press 55–78.

74. Bongers Schokking JJ, de Muinck Keizer-Schrama SMPF (2005). Influence of timing and dose of thyroid hormone replacement on mental, psychomotor and behavioral development in children with congenital hypothyroidism. J Pediatr 147:768.

75. Williams FLR, Simpson J, Delahunty C, et al. (2004). Developmental trends in cord and postpartum serum thyroid hormones in preterm infants. J Clin Endocrinol Metab 89:5314.

76. Williams FLR, Ogsten SA, van Toor H, et al. (2005). Serum thyroid hormones in preterm infants: Associations with postnatal illnesses and drug usage. J Clin Endocrinol Metab 90:5954.

77. Biswas S, Buffery J, Enoch H, et al. (2002). A longitudinal assessment of thyroid hormone concentrations in preterm infants younger than 30 weeks gestation during the first 2 weeks of life and their relationship to outcome. Pediatrics 109:222.

78. La Gamma EF, van Wassenaer AG, Golombek SG, et al. (2006). Neonatal thyroxine supplementation for transient hypothyroxinemia of prematurity (THOP): Beneficial or detrimental? Treat Endocrinol 5:335.

79. Delange F, Dahlem A, Bourdoux P et al. (1984). Increased risk of primary hypothyroidism in preterm infants. J Pediatr 105:462.

80. Delange FM, Dunn JT (2005). Iodine insufficiency. In Braverman LE, Utiger RD (eds.), The thyroid, Ninth edition. Philadelphia: Lippincott Williams & Wilkins 264–288.

81. Ares S, Escobar Morreale H, Quero J, et al. (1997). Neonatal hypothyroxinemia: Effects of iodine intake and of premature birth. J Clin Endocrinol Metab 82:1704.

82. Roti E, Vaginakis AG (2005). Effect of excess iodide: Clinical aspects. In Braverman LE, Utiger RD (eds.), The thyroid, Ninth edition. Philadelphia: Lippincott Williams & Wilkins 288–305.

83. Theodoropoulos T, Braverman LE, Vagenakis AG (1979). Iodide induced hypothyroidism: A potential hazard during perinatal life. Science 205:502.

84. van Wassenaer AG, Kok JH, Dekker FW, De Vijlder JJM (1997). Thyroid function in very preterm infants: Influences of gestational age and disease. Pediatr Res 42:604.

85. Rabin CW, Hopper AO, Job L, et al. (2004). Incidence of low free T4 values in premature infants as determined by direct equilibrium dialysis. J Perinatol 24:640.

86. van Wassenaer A, Kok JH, De Vijlder JJM, et al. (1997). Effects of thyroxine supplementation on neurologic development in infants born at less than 30 weeks gestation. N Engl J Med 336:21.

87. van Wassenaer AG, Briet JM, van Baar A, et al. (2002). Free thyroxine levels during the first weeks of life and neurodevelopmental outcome until the age of 5 years in very preterm infants. Pediatrics 109:534.

88. Fisher DA (1987). Effectiveness of newborn screening programs for congenital hypothyroidism: Prevalence of missed cases. Pediatr Clin N Amer 34:881.

89. Fisher DA (1991). Screening for congenital hypothyroidism: Status report. Trends in Endocrinol 2:129.

90. Tylek-Lemanska D, Kumorowicz-Kopiec M, Starzyk J (2005). Screening for congenital hypothyroidism: The value of retesting after four months in neonates with low or very low birth weight. J Med Screening 12:166.

91. van Tijn DA, de Vijlder JJM, Verbeeten B Jr., et al. (2005). Neonatal detection of congenital hypothyroidism of central origin. J Clin Endocrinol Metab 90:3350.

92. Dentice M, Cordeddu V, Rosica A, et al. (2006). Missense mutation in the transcription factor NKX2-5: A novel molecular event in the pathogenesis of thyroid dysgenesis. J Clin Endocrinol Metab 91:1428.

93. Senee V, Chelala C, Duchatelet S, et al. (2006). Mutations in GL153 are responsible for a rare syndrome of neonatal diabetes mellitus and congenital hypothyroidism. Nat Genet 38:682.

94. Olivieri A, Stazi MA, Mastroiacovo P, et al. (2002). A population based study on the frequency of additional congenital malformations in infants with congenital hypothyroidism: Data from the Italian Registry for Congenital Hypothyroidism (1991–1998). J Clin Endocrinol Metab 87:557.

95. Leger J, Marinovic D, Garel C, et al. (2002). Thyroid developmental anomalies in first degree relatives of children with congenital hypothyroidism. J Clin Endocrinol Metab 87:575.

96. Grueters A, Krude H, Biebermann H (2004). Molecular genetic defects in congenital hypothyroidism. Eur J Endocrinol 151:U39.

97. Fisher DA, Grueters A (2007). Thyroid disorders. In Rimoin DL, Korf BR, Pyeritz RE, Connor JA (eds.), Principles and practice of medical genetics, Fifth edition. New York: Churchill Livingstone 1932–1950.

98. Knobel M, Medeiros-Neto G. An outline of inherited disorders of the thyroid hormone generating system. Thyroid 13:771, 2003.

99. Vulsma T, De Vijlder JJM (2005). Genetic defects causing hypothyroidism. In Braverman LE, Utiger RD (eds.), The thyroid, Ninth edition. Philadelphia: Lippincott Williams & Wilkins 714–730.

100. Gross B, Misrahi M, Sar S, Milgrom E (1991). Composite structure of the thyrotropin receptor gene. Biochem Biophys Res Commun 177:679.

101. Duprez L, Parma J, Van Sande J, et al. (1998). TSH receptor mutations and thyroid disease. Trends in Endocrinol 9:133.

102. Corvillain B, Van Sande J, Dumont JE, Vassart G (2001). Somatic and germline mutations of the TSH receptor and thyroid diseases. Clin Endocrinol 55:143.

103. Gruters A, Schonberg T, Bieberman H, et al. (1998). Severe congenital hyperthyroidism caused by a germline neomutation in the extracellular portion of the thyrotropin receptor. J Clin Endocrinol Metab 83:1431.

104. Abramowicz MJ, Duprez L, Parma J, et al. (1997). Familial congenital hypothyroidism due to inactivating mutation of the thyrotropin receptor causing profound hypoplasia of the thyroid gland. J Clin Invest 99:3018.

105. Spiegel AM (1997). The molecular basis of disorders caused by defects in G proteins. Horm Res 47:89.

106. Pohlenz J, Refetoff S (1999). Mutations in the sodium/iodide symporter gene as a cause for iodide transport defects and congenital hypothyroidism. Biochemie 81:469.

107. Szinnai G, Kusugi S, Derriene, et al. (2006). Extending the clinical heterogeneity of iodide transport defect (ITD): A novel mutation R124H of the sodium/iodide symporter gene and review of genotype-phenotype correlations in ITD. J Clin Endocrinol Metab 91:1199.

108. Dai G, Levy O, Carrasco N (1996). Cloning and characterization of the thyroid iodide transporter. Nature 379:458.

109. Smanik PA, Liu Q, Furminger TL, et al. (1996). Cloning of the human sodium iodide symporter. Biochem Biophys Res Commun 226:339.

110. Dohan D, De La Vieja A, Paroder V, Riedel C, Artani M, Reed M, et al. (2003). The sodium/iodide symporter (NID): Characterization, regulation and medical significance. Endocr Rev 24:48.

111. Pannain S, Weiss RE, Jackson CE, et al. (1999). Two different mutations in the thyroid peroxidase gene of a large inbred Amish kindred: Power and limits of homozygosity mapping. J Clin Endocrinol Metab 84:1061.

112. Vassart G, Dumont JE, Refetoff S (1995). Thyroid disorders. In Beudet AL, Sly WS, Valle D (eds.), *The metabolic and molecular bases of inherited disease, Seventh edition.* New York: McGraw Hill 2883.

113. DeDeken X, Wang D, Many MC, et al. (2000). Cloning of two human thyroid cDNAs encoding new members of the NADPH oxidase family. J Biol Chem 275:23227.

114. Moreno JC, Bikker H, Kempers MJE, et al. (2002). Inactivating mutations in the gene for thyroid oxidase 2 (THOX2) and congenital hypothyroidism. N Engl J Med 347:95.

115. Billerbeck AEC, Cavaliere H, Goldberg AC, et al. (1994). Clinical and molecular genetics studies in Pendred's syndrome. Thyroid 4:279.

116. Sheffield VC, Kraiem Z, Beck JC, et al. (1996). Pendred syndrome maps to chromosome 7q 21-34 and is caused by an intrinsic defect in thyroid iodine organification. Nature Genetics 12:424.

117. Scott DA, Wang R, Kremer TM, et al. (1999). The Pendred syndrome gene encodes a chloride-iodide transport protein. Nature Genetics 21:440.

118. Nakiontek V, Borck G, Muller-Forell W, et al. (2004). Intrafamilial variability of the deafness and goiter phenotype in Pendred syndrome caused by a T416P mutation in the SLC26A4 gene. J Clin Endocrinol Metab 89:5347.

119. Targovnik HM, Medeiros-Neto G, Varela V, et al. (1993). A nonsense mutation causes human hereditary congenital goiter with preferential production of a 171-nucleotide-deleted thyroglobulin ribonucleic acid messenger. J Clin Endocr Metab 77:210.

120. Grollman EF, Doi SQ, Weiss P, et al. (1992). Hyposialylated thyroglobulin in a patient with congenital goiter and hypothyroidism. J Clin Endocrinol Metab 74:43.

121. Van de Graaf SAR, Cammenga M, Ponne NJ, et al. (1999). The screening for mutations in the thyroglobulin cDNA from six patients with congenital hypothyroidism. Biochimie 81:425.

122. Gnidehou S, Caillou B, Talbot M, et al. (2004). Iodothyronine dehalogenase (DEHAL1) is a transmembrane protein involved in recycling of iodide close to the thyroglobulin iodination site. FASEBJ 18:1574.

123. Moreno JC, van der Hout C, Klootwijk W, Visser TJ (2006). Functional analysis of DEHAL1 gene mutations in patients with hypothyroidism. Horm Res 65(4):31.

124. Dumitrescu AM, Liao XH, Abdullah MSY, et al. (2005). Mutations in SECISBP2 result in abnormal thyroid hormone metabolism. Nature Genetics 37:1247.

125. Refetoff S (2005). Resistance to thyroid hormone. In Braverman LE, Utiger RD (eds.), *The thyroid: A fundamental and clinical text, Ninth edition.* Philadelphia: Lippincott Williams & Wilkins 1109–1129.

126. Gurnel M, Beck Peccoz P, Chaterjee VK (2006). Resistance to thyroid hormone. In DeGroot LJ, Jameson JL (eds.), *Endocrinology, Fifth edition.* Philadelphia: Elsevier-Saunders 2227–2238.

127. Hauser P, Zametkin AJ, Martinez P et al. (1993). Attention deficit: Hyperactivity disorders in people with generalized resistance to thyroid hormone. N Engl J Med 328:997.

128. Brucker-Davis F, Skarulis MC, Pikus A, et al. (1996). Prevalence and mechanisms of hearing loss in patients with resistance to thyroid hormone. J Clin Endocrinol Metab 81:2768.

129. Adams M, Matthews C, Collingwood TN, et al. (1994). Genetics analysis of 29 kindreds with generalized and pituitary resistance to thyroid hormone. J Clin Invest 94:506.

130. Dumitrescu M, Liao XH, Best TB, et al. (2004). A novel syndrome combining thyroid and neurological abnormalities is associated with mutations in a monocarboxylate transporter gene. Am J Hum Genet 74:168.

131. Friesema ECH, Grueters A, Biebermann H, et al. (2004). Association between mutations in a thyroid hormone transporter and severe x-linked psychomotor retardation. Lancet 364:1435.

132. Friesema ECH, Jansen J, Heuer J, et al. (2006). Mechanisms of disease: Psychomotor retardation and high T3 levels caused by mutations in monocarboxylate transporter 8. Nature Clin Pract 2:512.

133. La Franchi S (1999). Congenital hypothyroidism, etiologies, diagnosis and management. Thyroid 9:735.

134. Yamada M, Saga Y, Shubusawa N, et al. (1997). Tertiary hypothyroidism and hyperglycemia in mice with targeted disruption of the thyrotropin releasing hormone gene. Proc Natl Acad Sci USA 94:10862.

135. Rabelen R, Miltag J, Geffers L, et al. (2004). Generation of thyrotropin releasing hormone receptor 1-deficient mice as an animal model of central hypothyroidism. Mol Endocrinol 18:1450.

136. Collu R, Tang J, Castagne J, et al. (1997). A novel mechanism for isolated central hypothyroidism: Inactivating mutations in the thyrotropin releasing hormone receptor gene. J Clin Endocrinol Metab 82:1562.

137. Hayashizaki Y, Hiraoka Y, Endo Y, Matsubara K (1989). Thyroid stimulating hormone (TSH) deficiency caused by a single base substitution in the CAGYC region of the β subunit. EMBO Journal 8:2291.

138. Hayashizaki Y, Hiraoka Y, Tatsumi K et al. (1990). Deoxyribonucleic acid analysis of five families with familial inherited thyroid-stimulating hormone deficiency. J Clin Endocr Metab 71:792.

139. Docker BM, Pfaffle RW, Pohlenz J, Andler W (1998). Congenital central hypothyroidism due to a homozygous mutation in the thyrotropin β subunit gene follows an autosomal recessive inheritance. J Clin Endocrinol Metab 83:1762.

140. Medeiros-Neto GA, de Laserda L, Wondisford FE (1997). Familial congenital hypothyroidism caused by abnormal and bioinactive TSH due to mutations in the β subunit gene. Trends in Endocrinol 8:15.

141. Brumm J, Pfeufer A, Biebermann H, et al. (2002). Congenital central hypothyroidism due to a homozygous thyrotropin beta 313 delta T mutation is caused by a founder effect. J Clin Endocrinol Metab 87:4811.

142. Parks JS, Kinoshita E, Pfafle RW (1993). Pit-1 and hypopituitarism. Trends Endocrinol Metab 4:81.

143. Rosenbloom AL, Almonte AS, Brown MR, et al. (1999). Clinical and biochemical phenotype of familial anterior hypopituitarism from mutation of the PROP-1 gene. J Clin Endocrinol Metab 84:50.

144. Brown R, Bellisario R, Botero D, et al. (1996). Incidence of transient congenital hypothyroidism due to maternal thyrotropin receptor blocking antibodies in over one million babies. J Clin Endocrinol Metab 81:1147.

145. Glinoer D, Delange F, Laboureur I, et al. (1992). Maternal and neonatal thyroid function at birth in an area of marginally low iodine intake. J Clin Endocrinol Metab 75:800.

146. Matsura N, Yamada Y, Nohara Y et al. (1980). Familial, neonatal transient hypothyroidism due to maternal TSH-binding inhibitor immunoglobulins. N Engl J Med 303:738.

147. Iseki M, Shimizu M, Oikawa T, et al. (1983). Sequential serum measurements of thyrotropin binding inhibiting immunoglobulin G in transient neonatal hypothyroidism. J Clin Endocrinol Metab 57:384.

148. Kohler B, Schnabel D, Biebermann H, Grueters A (1996). Transient congenital hypothyroidism and hyperthyrotropinemia: Normal thyroid function and physical development at the ages of 6-14 years. J Clin Endocrinol Metab 81:1563.

149. Miki J, Nose O, Miyai K, et al. (1989). Transient infantile hyperthyrotropinemia. Arch Dis Childh 64:1177.

150. Tyfield LA, Abusrewil SSA, Jones SR, Savage DCL (1991). Persistent hyperthyrotropinemia since the neonatal period in clinical euthyroid children. Eur J Pediatr 150:308.

151. Tonacchera M, Perri A, DeMarco G, et al. (2004). Low prevalence of thyrotropin receptor mutations in a large series of subjects with sporadic and familial nonautoimmune subclinical hypothyroidism. J Clin Endocrinol Metab 89:5787.

152. Tsunekawa K, Onigata K, Morimura T, et al. (2006). Identification and functional analysis of novel inactivating thyrotropin receptor mutations in patients with thyrotropin resistance. Thyroid 16:471.

153. Sapin R, d'Herbomez M (2003). Free thyroxine measured by equilibrium dialysis and nine immunoassays. Clin Chem 49:1531.

154. Ilicki A, Ericsson UB, Larsson A, et al. (1990). The value of neonatal serum thyroglobulin determination in the follow-up of patients with congenital hypothyroidism. Acta Paediatr Scand 79:769.

155. Selva K, Harper A, Downs A, et al. (2005). Neurodevelopmental outcomes in congenital hypothyroidism: Comparison of initial T4 dose and time to reach target T4 and TSH. J Pediatr 147:775.

156. Bakker B, Kempers MJE, DeVijlder JJM, et al. (2002). Dynamics of the plasma concentrations of TSH, FT4 and T3 following thyroxine supplementation in congenital hypothyroidism. Clin Endocrinol 57:529.

157. Fisher DA, Schoen EJ, LaFranchi S, et al. (2000). The hypothalamic-pituitary-thyroid negative feedback control axis in children with treated congenital hypothyroidism. J Clin Endocrinol Metab 85:2722.

158. Derksen-Lubsen G, Verkerk PH (1996). Neuropsychologic development in early treated congenital hypothyroidism: analysis of literature data. Pediatr Res 39:561.

159. New England Congenital Hypothyroidism Collaborative (1989). Neonatal thyroid screening: Now we are nine. In Delange F, Fisher DA, Glinoer D (eds.), *Research in congenital hypothyroidism.* New York: Plenum Press 291–299.

160. Heyerdahl S, Kase BF, Lie SO (1991). Intellectual development of children with congenital hypothyroidism in relation to recommended thyroxine treatment. J Pediatrics 118:850.

161. Boileau P, Bain P, Rivas S, Toublanc JE (2004). Earlier onset of treatment or increment in LT4 dose in screened congenital hypothyroidism: Which was the more important factor for IQ at 7 years? Horm Res 61:228.

162. Simoneau-Roy J, Marti S, Deal C, et al. (2004). Cognition and behavior at school entry in children with congenital hypothyroidism treated early with high dose levothyroxine. J Pediatr 144:747.

163. Rovet JF (1999). Congenital hypothyroidism: Long term outcome. Thyroid 9:741.

164. Kempers MJE, van der Sluijs L, Nijhuis-van der Sanden MWG, et al. (2006). Intellectual and motor development of young adults with congenital hypothyroidism diagnosed by neonatal screening. J Clin Endocrinol Metab 91:418.

165. Dubuis JM, Glorieux J, Richer F, et al. (1996). Outcome of severe congenital hypothyroidism: Closing the developmental gap with early high dose levothyroxine treatment. J Clin Endocrinol Metab 81:222.

166. Fisher DA (2000). The importance of early management in optimizing IQ in infants with congenital hypothyroidism. J Pediatrics 136:273.

167. Weiss RE, Balzano S, Scherberg NH, et al. (1990). Neonatal detection of generalized resistance to thyroid hormone. JAMA 264:2245.

168. McKenzie JM, Zakarija M (1992). Fetal and neonatal hyperthyroidism and hypothyroidism due to maternal TSH receptor antibodies. Thyroid 2:155.

169. Fisher DA (1997). Fetal thyroid function: Diagnosis and management of fetal thyroid disorders. Clin Obstet Gynecol 40:16.

170. La Franchi S, Hanna CE (2005). Graves' disease in the neonatal period and childhood. In Braverman, Utiger RD (eds.), *The thyroid: A fundamental and clinical text, Ninth edition.* Philadelphia: Lippincott Williams & Wilkins 1049–1057.

171. Mitsuda N, Tamaki H, Amino N, et al. (1992). Risk factors for developmental disorders in infants born to women with Graves' disease. Obstet Gynecol 80:359.

172. Kempers M, van der Sluijs-Veer L, Nijhuis-van der Sanden M, et al. (2003). Central congenital hypothyroidism due to gestational hyperthyroidism: Detection where prevention failed. J Clin Endocrinol Metab 88:5851.

173. Druzin ML, Hutson JM, Edersheim TG (1986). Relationship of baseline fetal heart rate to gestational age and fetal sex. Am J Obstet Gynecol 154:1102.

174. Momotani N, Ito K, Ohnishi H, et al. (1992). Deceptively high thyroid hormone levels in a neonate due to autoantibodies against thyroid hormones transferred from a mother with Graves' disease. J Endocrinol Invest 15:201.

175. Karpman BA, Rappoport B, Filetti S, Fisher DA (1987). Treatment of neonatal hyperthyroidism due to Graves' disease with sodium ipodate. J Clin Endocrinol Metab 64:119.

176. Earles SM, Gerrits PM, Transue DJ (2004). Experience with iopanoic acid in the management of neonatal Graves' disease. J Perinatology 24:105.

177. Vassart G, Van Sande J, Parma J, et al. (1996). Activating mutations of the TSH receptor gene cause thyroid diseases. Annal Endocrinol (Paris) 57:50.

178. Kopp P, Van Sande J, Parma J, et al. (1995). Brief report: Congenital hyperthyroidism caused by a mutation in the thyrotropin receptor gene. N Engl J Med 332:150.

179. Schwab KO, Gerlich M, Brocker M, et al. (1997). Constitutively active germline mutation of the thyrotropin receptor gene as a cause of congenital hyperthyroidism. J Pediatr 131:899.

180. Borgel K, Pohlenz J, Koch HG, Braunswig JH (2005). Long term carbimazole treatment of neonatal nonautoimmune hyperthyroidism due to a new activating TSH receptor gene mutation (Als-428Val). Horm Res 64:203.

181. Claus M, Maier J, Paschke R, et al. (2005). Novel thyrotropin receptor germline mutation (ile568Val) in a Saxonian family with hereditary nonautoimmune hyperthyroidism. Thyroid 15:1089.

182. Refetoff S (1989). Inherited thyroxine binding globulin abnormalities in man. Endocrine Rev 10:275.

183. Carvalho GA, Weiss RE, Refetoff S (1998). Complete thyroxine binding globulin (TBG) deficiency produced by a mutation in acceptor splice site causing frameshift and early termination of translation (TBG Kankakee). J Clin Endocrinol Metab 83:3604.

184. Okamoto H, Mori Y, Tani Y, et al. (1996). Molecular analysis of females manifesting thyroxine binding globulin (TBG) deficiency: Selective x chromosome inactivation responsible for the difference between phenotype and genotype in TBG deficient females. J Clin Endocrinol Metab 81:2204.

185. Janssen OE, Astner ST, Grasberger H, et al. (2000). Identification of thyroxine binding globulin - San Diego in a family from Houston and its characterization by in-vitro expression using xenopus oocytes. J Clin Endocrinol Metab 85:368.

186. Mori Y, Miura Y, Takeuchi H, et al. (1995). Gene amplification as a cause of inherited thyroxine binding excess in two Japanese families. J Clin Endocrinol Metab 80:3758.

187. Moses AAC, Lawlor JF, Haddow JE, Jackson IMD (1982). Familial euthyroid hyperthyroxinemia resulting from increased immunoreactive thyroxine-binding prealbumin (TBPA). N Engl J Med 306:366.

188. Moses AC, Rosen HN, Moller DE, et al. (1990). A point mutation in transthyretin increases affinity for thyroxine and produces euthyroid hyperthyroxinemia. J Clin Invest 86:2025.

189. Refetoff S, Marinov VSZ, Tunca H, et al. (1996). A new family with hyperthyroxinemia caused by transthyretin VAL109 misdiagnosed as thyrotoxicosis and resistance to thyroid hormone: A clinical research study. J Clin Endocrinol Metab 81:3355.

190. Lee WNP, Golden MP, Van Herle AJ, et al. (1979). Inherited abnormal thyroid hormone binding protein causing selective increase in total serum thyroxine. J Clin Endocrinol Metab 49:292.

191. Wada N, Chiba H, Shimizu C, et al. (1997). A novel missense mutation in codon 218 of the albumin gene in a distinct phenotype of familial dysalbuminemic hyperthyroxinemia in a Japanese kindred. J Clin Endocrinol Metab 82:3246.

192. Sunthornthepvarakul T, Likitmaskul S, Ngowngarmratana, et al. (1998). Familial dysalbuminemic hypertriiodothyroninemia: A new, dominantly inherited albumin defect. J Clin Endocrinol Metab 83:1448.

193. Fisher DA (1993). The fetal frontier. Pediatric Res 34:393.

194. Jenkins TM, Wapner RJ (2004). Prenatal diagnosis of congenital disorders. In Creasy RK, Resnik R (eds.), *Maternal fetal medicine, Fifth edition.* Philadelphia: WB Saunders 235–280.

195. Chopra IJ (1992). Fetal and neonatal hyperthyroidism. Thyroid 2:161.

196. Abuhamad A, Fisher DA, Warsof SL, et al. (1995). Antenatal diagnosis and treatment of fetal goitrous hypothyroidism: Case report and review of the literature. Ultrasound Obstet Gynecol 6:368.

197. Ghazi AM, Ordookhani A, Pourafkari M, et al. (2005). Intrauterine diagnosis and management of fetal goitrous hypothyroidism: A report of an Iranian family with three consecutive pregnancies complicated by fetal goiter. Thyroid 15:1341.

198. Polak M, Legac I, Vuillard E, et al. (2006). Congenital hypothyroidism: The fetus as patient. Horm Res 65:235.

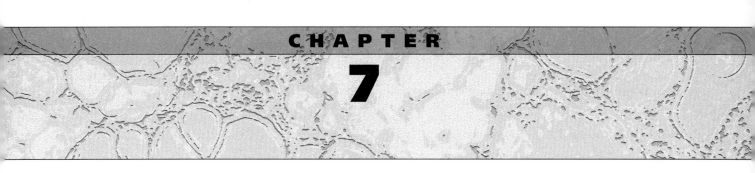

CHAPTER 7

Thyroid Disorders in Childhood and Adolescence

DELBERT A. FISHER, MD • ANNETTE GRUETERS, MD

Introduction

During the last three decades there have been major advances in our understanding of developmental thyroid physiology and important insights and progress in pediatric thyroid disease nosology, diagnosis, and management. Specific etiologic gene mutations have been characterized for pituitary thyroid stimulating hormone (TSH) deficiency,

TSH receptor dysfunction, thyroid dysgenesis, the thyroid dyshormonogenesis syndromes, thyroid hormone resistance, and thyroid neoplasia.[1] Our understanding of the pathophysiology and spectrum of thyroid autoimmune disease has expanded significantly.

Ultrasound and fine-needle aspiration (FNA) cytology have become standard approaches to the assessment of thyroid nodules. Major advances in the menu

227

and efficacy of thyroid function tests have accompanied these advances. Table 7-1 provides a classification of thyroid disorders in children. Thyroid system development, fetal thyroid physiology, thyroid dysfunction in premature infants, and congenital thyroid disorders (including inborn defects in thyroid hormone synthesis, metabolism, and action and thyroid binding protein abnormalities) are discussed in chapter 6.

Metabolism of Iodine

The major thyroid hormone [tetraiodothyronine, or thyroxine (T4)] is approximately 60% iodine by weight, and iodine is the rate-limiting substrate for synthesis of thyroid hormones[2] (Figure 7-1). Iodine is a trace element present in the human body in small amounts (15–20 mg; i.e., 0.02×10^{-3} % of body weight). The recommended dietary allowance of iodine is 100 μg/day for adolescents and adults (150 μg/day in pregnant and lactating women). It is 60 to 100 μg/day for children aged 1 to 10 years, 40 μg/day for infants aged 6 to 12 months, and 30 μg/day for infants 6 months of age or younger. A reevaluation of the iodine requirements in young infants based on iodine balance studies showed that at least in conditions of marginally low iodine intake (as still observed in some parts of Europe) the recommended dietary allowance should be increased to 90 μg for infants aged less than 1 year.[2]

Dietary iodine (I_2) or iodide (I^-) in its ionized form is rapidly absorbed. Iodide is distributed within the extrathyroidal iodide pool, which represents 30% to 40% of body weight. The concentration of iodide in the serum is dependent on iodine intake, and the extrathyroidal pool of iodide is constantly cleared of iodide by two competing mechanisms: active transport into the thyroid cells and excretion by the kidney. The plasma membrane sodium iodide symporter (NIS) confers on the thyroid the ability to concentrate iodide to 20 to 40 times its levels in plasma.[3,4]

TABLE 7-1

Thyroid Disorders in Childhood and Adolescence

Congenital Hypothyroidism
Thyroid Dysgenesis
- Idiopathic (97%-98%)
  - Athyreosis
  - Hypoplasia
  - Ectopia
  - Cryptothyroidism
- Genetic (5%)
  - Athyreosis
    - TTF-1 mutations
    - TTF-2 mutations
  - Hypoplasia
    - PAX-8 mutations
    - TSH receptor mutations

Thyroid Dyshormonogenesis
- Sodium-iodide symporter defect
- Organification defects
- Abnormal thyroglobulin
- Pendrin defect (Pendred syndrome)
- Iodotyrosine deiodinase defect

Hypothalamic-Pituitary Hypothyroidism
- Anencephaly
- Holoprosencephaly
- Septo-optic dysplasia
- Median facial syndromes
- TSHβ mutations
- Pit-1 mutations
- Prop-1 mutations
- LHX3/LHX4 mutations
- Idiopathic

Transient Hypothyroidism
- Maternal TSH receptor-blocking antibody
- Goitrogenic drugs
- Iodine excess or deficiency

Iodine Deficiency Syndromes
- Goiter
- Mental impairment
- Cretinism

Thyroid Hormone Resistance Syndromes
- Thyroid hormone beta receptor (TRβ) mutations
  - Peripheral tissue resistance syndrome
  - Pituitary resistance syndrome
  - Thyroid hormone membrane transport defects

TSH Receptor Mutations
- Loss-of-function hypothyroidism
- Gain-of-function hyperthyroidism

Autoimmune Thyroid Disease
- Hashimoto thyroiditis
- TSH receptor autoantibody disease
  - Stimulating antibody, Graves' disease
  - Blocking antibody, hypothyroidism

Infectious Thyroiditis
- Suppurative thyroiditis
- Subacute thyroiditis

Diffuse Nontoxic Goiter
Non-thyroidal Illness
Thyroid Neoplasia
- Adenoma
  - Nonfunctional
  - Functional
  - Cystic
- Papillary-follicular carcinoma
- Medullary carcinoma
  - MEN 2A, 2B, Ret mutations
  - Sporadic
- Undifferentiated
- Metastatic

Binding Protein Abnormalities
- Complete TBG deficiency
- Partial TBG deficiency
- TBG excess
- Transthyretin variants

Miscellaneous
- G protein mutations (non-autoimmune hyperthyroidism)
- Cystinosis
- Chromosomal disorders

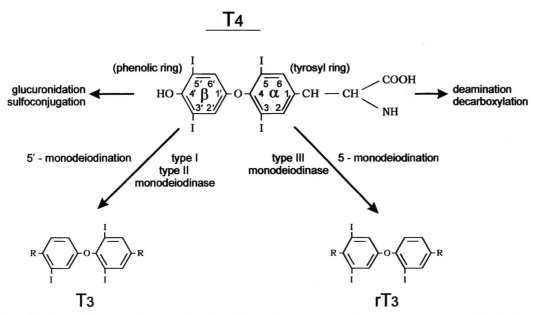

Figure 7-1. The metabolism of thyroxine (tetraiodothyronine). The major metabolic pathway is progressive monodeiodination mediated by the three iodothyronine monodeiodinase enzymes type I, type II, and type III. Outer (phenolic) ring 5'monodeiodination produces active 3,5,3' triiodothyronine. Inner (tyrosyl) ring 5'monodeiodination produces inactive reverse 3,3',5' triiodothyronine. Type I deiodinase is also capable of inner-ring monodeiodination. The alanine side chain of the tyrosyl ring is also subject to degradative reactions, including deamination and decarboxylation. Sulfoconjugation and glucuronide conjugation reactions at the 4' phenolic ring site occur largely in liver tissue.

Under usual conditions, the thyroid clearance of iodide is 10 to 35 mL/min. However, this varies markedly with the dietary intake—increasing in response to low iodine intake and decreasing with high iodine intake. The renal clearance of iodide is about 35 mL/min in normal adults and is not influenced by the dietary intake of iodine. Fecal excretion of iodine under normal conditions is minimal. A small fraction of iodide (1%-2%) is excreted in sweat under basal conditions, which can increase to 5% to 10% with heavy sweating. In conditions of dietary equilibrium, the excretion of iodide in the urine is equal to iodine intake. Thus, intake can be evaluated by the measurement of the daily urinary excretion of iodine.

Biosynthesis of Thyroid Hormones

Thyroid hormones and analogues are tyrosine derivatives. The steps in the synthesis and release of thyroid hormones are as follows.
1. Iodide trapping by the thyroid gland
2. Synthesis of thyroglobulin
3. Organification of trapped iodide as mono and diiodotyrosines (MIT and DIT)
4. Coupling of the iodotyrosines within thyroglobulin to form the iodothyronines [T4 and triiodothyronine (T3)] and storage in follicular colloid
5. Pinocytosis of colloid droplets and hydrolysis of thyroglobulin within the cytoplasmic phagolysosomes to release MIT, DIT, T4, and T3
6. Deiodination of MIT and DIT with intrathyroidal recycling of the iodine

These steps are shown in Figure 7-2, and are reviewed in Chapter 6.

Metabolism of Thyroglobulin

Until recently, thyroglobulin (Tg) was believed to be present only in thyroid tissue. It is now clear that some Tg escapes during golgi processing and appears in serum in association with secreted iodothyronines. It may be incorporated into classic secretory granules or apical vesicles facilitating secretion.[5] The serum concentration of Tg in adults varies from 1 to 30 ng/mL, with a mean of approximately 5 ng/mL. In normal children, serum Tg varies from undetectable values to 80 ng/mL.

Levels in premature infants are high during the first weeks of life, and decrease with age throughout infancy and childhood.[5-8] The control of thyroglobulin synthesis is complex, involving thyroid-specific transcription factors (TTF-1, TTF-2, and PAX-8), TGF-β1, and TSH. However, the secretion of Tg by the thyroid is at least partly under TSH control.[4,5] Circulating Tg levels may be elevated in patients with a variety of thyroid disorders reflecting thyroidal hyperactivity, including endemic goiter, subacute thyroiditis, Graves' disease, and toxic multinodular goiter.[5] In Hashimoto thyroiditis, serum antithyroglobulin antibody precludes reliable measurement of Tg.

Serum Tg concentrations are also increased, often markedly, in patients with thyroid adenoma and papillary follicular carcinoma—although not in those with anaplastic or medullary carcinoma. In iodine deficiency, elevated serum Tg levels in adults and newborns are not entirely due to increased serum TSH but correlate with the serum T3/T4 ratio—suggesting that iodine availability (which affects the degree of thyroglobulin iodination) also influences Tg secretion.[6-8] The average half-life of circulating 19S Tg varies from 4.3 days to 13.8 days. Clearance presumably occurs

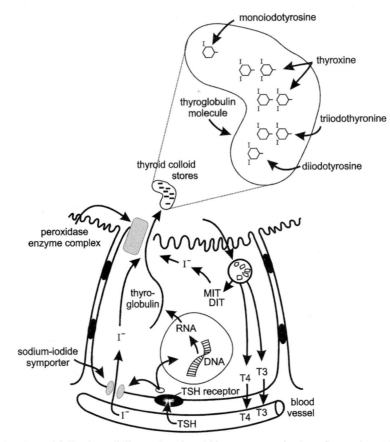

Figure 7-2. Cartoon of the thyroid follicular cell illustrating thyroid hormone synthesis and secretion. TSH regulates the process via the G-protein-linked plasma membrane TSH receptor. TSH binding stimulates thyroglobulin synthesis and sodium-iodide symporter (iodide transporter) uptake of circulating iodide. The iodide diffuses in the cytosol to the apical membrane and is transported to the apical lumen by Pendrin, an anion-bicarconate family exchanger making iodide available to the enzyme organification complex (Pendrin, TPO, THOX). The tyrosine residues of thyroglobulin are iodinated at the apical cell membrane catalyzed by thyroid peroxidase, the organification enzyme. The resulting monoiodotyrosine (MIT) and diiodotyrosine (DIT) residues couple to form the iodothyronines thyroxine (T4) and triiodothyronine (T3) within the stored thyroglobulin molecule. TSH also stimulates micropinocytosis of colloid droplets and progressive thyroglobulin proteolysis within the resulting phagolysosomes. The released T4 and T3 are secreted into the circulation. The uncoupled MIT and DIT are deiodinated by iodotyrosine deiodinase (DEHAL) to release iodide, which is largely recycled within the follicular cell.

within the liver. There is good evidence that Tg reaches the general circulation via thyroidal lymphatics. However, the mechanism of Tg secretion or release remains obscure—and its role in serum or plasma is not known.

Regulation of Thyroid Function

Circulating TSH and iodide levels largely regulate thyroid function. TSH interacts with the thyroid follicular cell at the level of the plasma membrane by binding to TSH receptors, which are coupled to intracellular G proteins.[4,9] TSH activates adenylate cyclase and stimulates the production and accumulation of cyclic adenosine monophosphate (cAMP), which in turn appears to mediate most of the effects of TSH on thyroid metabolism (iodide trapping, iodotyrosine synthesis, Tg synthesis, glucose oxidation, colloid pinocytosis, hormone release, and thyroid growth).

The TSH receptor-stimulating antibodies (TSA) found in the serum of patients with Graves' disease produce the effects of TSH by binding to the TSH receptors. TSH receptor-blocking antibodies (TBA), on the other hand, cause hypothyroidism. A variety of extracellular stimulatory signals have also been implicated in thyroid regulation, including serotonin, epinephrine, histamine, and the prostaglandins.[4,9] However, these agents are much less effective than TSH—and their significance in the control of thyroid function and growth in humans is questionable.

Variations in iodine intake in the physiologic range modulate thyroid membrane iodide trapping, and in pharmacologic doses iodide has been shown to block organification [probably by inhibition of H_2O_2 generation and adenylyl cyclase (the Wolff-Chaikoff effect) followed by decreased Tg synthesis and decreased hormone release].[3] Escape from the Wolff-Chaikoff blockade occurs within days or weeks, mediated by iodide inhibition of NIS mRNA expression and down-regulation of thyroid iodide trapping.[3] Iodide also has an inhibitory effect on the stimulation of cAMP by TSH. TSH functions as a trophic hormone, and removal of the pituitary reduces thyroid cell function to a basal level.

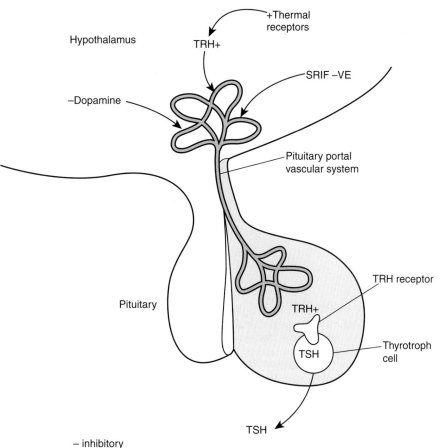

Figure 7-3 Cartoon illustrating the hypothalamic-pituitary TSH axis. Thyrotropin-releasing hormone (TRH) secreted into the pituitary portal vascular system stimulates TSH synthesis and secretion from the pituitary thyrotroph cell. TRH secretion is modulated by central and peripheral thermal sensors. Dopamine or somatostatin (SRIF) can inhibit TSH release.

TSH secretion is modulated by thyrotropin-releasing hormone (TRH), a peptide synthesized in the hypothalamus and secreted into the pituitary portal vascular system for transport to the anterior pituitary thyrotroph cell (Figure 7-3). TRH production is modulated by environmental temperature via peripheral and central (hypothalamic) thermal sensors.[10,11] These sensors modulate neuronal output to the hypothalamic centers regulating TRH secretion. Decreasing environmental and body temperatures increase TRH and increase the tonic level of TSH release. Somatostatin and dopamine can inhibit TSH release, and these transmitters probably contribute to central nervous system modulation of TSH release. Norepinephrine and serotonin may inhibit TSH release, but their significance is not clear. Glucocorticoids inhibit TSH release at the hypothalamic level.

Thyroid Hormone Transport

Thyroid hormones are present in the blood in noncovalent linkage with the carrier proteins: thyroxine-binding globulin (TBG), prealbumin or transthyretin, and albumin. The bound form is in equilibrium with free hormones[12] (Figure 7-4). The major binding protein is TBG, a globulin with an electrophoretic mobility between the α_1- and α_2-globulins. TBG is the most important carrier protein for T4. TBG and albumin seem equally important for T3.

The binding reactions are nearly complete, and thus the euthyroid steady-state concentration of free T4 and T3 approximate 0.03% and 0.30% (respectively) of total hormone concentrations. Absolute mean free T4 and T3 concentrations approximate 10 and 4 pg/mL, respectively. In adolescents and adults, the plasma concentrations of the several binding proteins are 1.0 to 3.0 mg/dL for TBG, 20 to 30 mg/dL for TBPA, and 2 to 5 g/dL for albumin. TBG levels are higher in children than in adults, and decrease progressively to adult levels during adolescence.

Metabolism of Thyroid Hormones

Deiodination is the major pathway of thyroid hormone metabolism.[13] The first step in T4 metabolism is deiodination to T3 or to reverse T3 (rT3) (Figure 7-1). Progressive deiodination of the iodothyronines is mediated via three monodeiodinase enzymes: MDI type I, MDI type II, and MDI type III (Table 7-2). Monodeiodination of the beta or outer ring

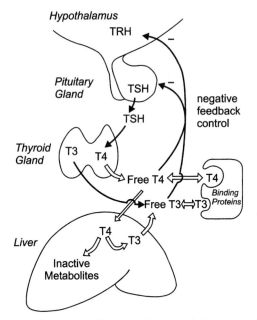

Figure 7-4. Cartoon of the hypothalamic-pituitary-thyroid axis indicating hypothalamic TRH stimulation of pituitary TSH secretion via the pituitary portal vascular system and modulation of hypothalamic-pituitary axis TSH secretion by thyroxine (T4) and triiodothyronine (T3) negative feedback inhibition. The major thyroid gland secretory product is T4, which functions as a prohormone bound to several circulating binding proteins. Only 0.03% of circulating T4 and 0.30% of T3 are free or unbound. Ten to 20% of T3 is secreted by the thyroid gland. The predominant 80% to 90% is derived from monodeiodination of T4 to active T3 in peripheral tissues, here represented by liver. Most of the circulating T3 is produced by liver tissue.

TABLE 7-2

The Iodothyronine Deiodinase Enzymes

Iodothyronine Monodeiodinase Enzymes

Enzyme	Major Tissue	Preferred Substrates	Products
Type I	Liver, kidney, thyroid	rT3, T4, T2S, rT3S	T2, T3, T1S, T2S
Type II	Brain, pituitary, brown adipose tissue Keratinocytes, placenta	T4S, T3S, T4, rT3	rT3S, T2S, T3, T2
Type III	Placenta, brain, epidermis, hemangiomas	T4, T3	rT3, T2

(relative to the alanine side chain) produces T3, which has three to four times the metabolic potency of T4. Monodeiodination of the alpha or inner-ring produces rT3, which is largely inactive metabolically. Under normal circumstances, T3 and rT3 are produced at approximately similar rates.

In most tissues (particularly liver, and excluding brain and brown adipose tissue), T3 and rT3 (generated via T4 monodeiodination) diffuse rapidly from tissue to interstitial fluid to plasma. Significant amounts of T3 and small amounts of rT3 are synthesized and released by the thyroid gland. Thus, the circulating levels of T3 and rT3 reflect both secretion and peripheral production. From 70% to 90% of circulating T3 is derived from peripheral conversion, and 10% to 25% from the thyroid gland. Respective values for rT3 are 96% to 98% and 2% to 4%. Progressive tissue monodeiodination reactions degrade T3 and rT3 to diiodo, monoiodo, and noniodinated thyronine.

The alanine side chain of the inner-ring of the iodothyronines is also subject to degradative reactions, including transmination, deamination, and decarboxylation.[14] Pyruvic acid analogues and small amounts of lactic acid analogues have been observed in urine and bile. These have minimal biologic activity. The acetic acid analogues found in tissue, bile, and urine possess some activity but are rapidly degraded. Thyroid hormones are excreted in urine and stool in both free and conjugated forms. The reactions involve glucuronide conjugation and sulfoconjugation. Glucuronide conjugation occurs mainly in liver via microsomal glycuronyl transferase. Sulfoconjugation is also prominent in liver, and may be an obligatory step for hepatic monodeiodination reactions.[14] Iodothyronine sulfation markedly augments outer-ring deiodination in liver. In the fetus, where outer-ring deiodinase activity is developmentally low, the major thyroid hormone metabolites are sulfate conjugates—which are biologically inactive. (See Chapter 6.)

Actions of Thyroid Hormones

Thyroid hormones influence growth and development, oxygen consumption and heat production, nerve function, and metabolism of lipids, carbohydrates, proteins, nucleic acids, vitamins, and inorganic ions. They also have important effects on other hormone actions.[15-18] The free hormones appear to be transported via plasma membrane iodothyronine transporters belonging to several families of integrin, organic anion, amino acid, and monocarboxylate solute carriers.[19]

T3 is the active hormone, which binds to the nuclear receptors with some 10 times the affinity of T4 (Figure 7-5). T3 also binds to mitochondrial inner-membrane receptors.[20] The major effects of thyroid hormones are mediated via thyroid hormone nuclear receptors (TRs), which are members of the steroid hormone-retinoic acid receptor superfamily and function as DNA transcription factors.[15,16] In humans, there are two genes coding for thyroid hormone nuclear receptors: one on chromosome 17 [designated alpha (TRα)], and one on chromosome 3 [designated beta (TRβ)]. Alternative splicing of expressed mRNA species leads to production of the major thyroid hormone binding transcripts TRα1, TRα2, TRβ1, and TRβ2.[15,16]

The TRs exist as monomers, homodimers, and heterodimers with other nuclear receptor family members (such as the retinoid X receptors). Other receptor transcripts, including TRΔα1 and TRΔα2, have been characterized. These do not bind T3 or DNA but can inhibit TR and retinoid receptor activities. The TRα receptors are expressed in most tissues. TRβ1 is expressed in liver, kidney, heart, lung, brain, cochlea, and pituitary. TRβ2 is

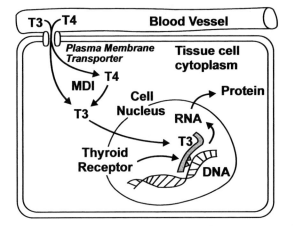

Figure 7-5. Thyroid hormone binding to nuclear receptors. The circulating thyroid hormones appear to be transported into peripheral tissues via iodothyronine plasma membrane transporters. Intracellular T4 is monodeiodinated to triiodothyronine (T3). The cellular cytoplasmic T3 diffuses into the nucleus, where it binds to the thyroid hormone receptors—which in turn bind to DNA and regulate thyroid-hormone-responsive gene transcription.

expressed in pituitary gland, retina, and cochlea. The receptors function redundantly, as indicated by knockout studies in mice. However, predominant effects of one or another TR have been described.[17,18] T3 binding by the TR leads to responsive gene transcription, modulating synthesis of mRNA and proteins—which mediate thyroid hormone effects in various tissues. The effects of thyroid hormones as related to known thyroid actions at the molecular level are summarized in Table 7-3.

Thyroid Function During Infancy and Childhood

IODINE METABOLISM

During the prepubertal and pubertal periods of growth and development, there is a progressive growth of the thyroid gland, a progressive increase in thyroid thyroglobulin and iodothyronine stores, and a progressive increase in thyroxine production rate measured as μg/day.[2,21,22] The iodide space (on a body weight basis) in infants is relatively larger than in older children, adolescents, or adults—and the thyroid iodide clearance rate is nearly three times that of adults (Figure 7-6). Renal iodide clearance is also high in infants and decreases progressively with age. The progressive decrease in thyroid iodide clearance may be at least in part secondary to the change in renal iodide clearance.

During childhood, the growth of the thyroid gland in residents of iodine-sufficient areas roughly parallels body growth. The gland volume, measured by ultrasound, increases in size from about 1.0 g at birth to a mean of about 5 g at 10 years of age (Table 7-4). Average thyroid iodine content increases from 0.3 mg at birth to 16 mg in adolescents and adults.[21] In areas of severe iodine deficiency, the thyroid weight in newborn infants may be 2 to 3 g (and iodine content may be as low as 40 μg).[21]

TABLE 7-3
Effects of Thyroid Hormones

Central Nervous System Development

General
- Stimulation of cell migration and neuronal cell maturation
- Stimulation of dendritic arborization and synaptic density
- Increases myelinogenesis

Gene Products Regulated by T3
- Myelin basic protein
- Nerve growth factor and its receptors
- Neurotropin 3
- Neural cell adhesion molecules
- Cerebellar PCP-2
- Prostaglandin D2 synthase

Effects on Growth and Development
- Stimulation of pituitary growth hormone (GH) synthesis and secretion
- Potentiation of GH stimulation of insulin-like growth factor (IGF) synthesis and action
- Stimulation of growth factor production
  - Epidermal growth factor
  - Nerve growth factor
  - Erythropoietin
- Stimulation of bone metabolism/growth
  - Cartilage response to IGF-I
  - Osteoblastic/osteoclastic bone remodeling

Thermogenic Effects
- Stimulation of mitochondrial enzyme synthesis
- Stimulation of UCP-1 and UCP-3 in brown adipose tissue and muscle
- Stimulation of membrane Na/K ATPase

Metabolic Effects
- Hepatic protein
  - Induction of hepatic lipogenic enzymes
  - Stimulation of hepatic glutamine synthatase and α amino levulinic acid synthetase
  - Potentiation of prolactin stimulation of lactalbumin synthesis
  - Potentiation of GH stimulation of B2 euglobulin synthesis
- Plasma membrane effects
  - Stimulation of glucose transport
  - Stimulation of adrenergic receptor binding

The iodide space also increases progressively in volume with age. However, the relative size (liters per kilogram, expressed as a percentage of body weight) decreases from about 50% of body weight at birth to 40% in 30-kg children (about age 10 years). These values can be compared with the 33% body weight values in 65-kg adults.

Radioiodine uptake and clearance during childhood and adolescence vary with diet and iodine intake. Values during the first two decades have been reported to decrease progressively or remain relatively stable.[22,23] This discrepancy is presumably due to variations in iodine intake. The data showing a decrease with age were from areas of low iodine intake in Europe and Australia. A relatively high iodine intake could tend to mask differences in uptake with age. Thyroid iodine clearance (per gram of thyroid tissue) decreases progressively with age and is associated with a progressive decrease in thyroxine production rate (or turnover) on a μg/kg/day basis (Figure 7-6). Changes in thyroxine kinetics and production

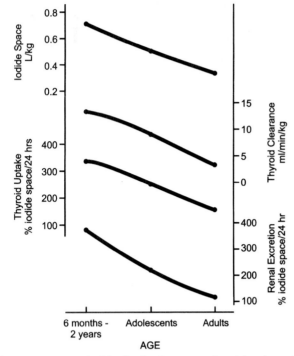

Figure 7-6. Mean iodide distribution space, thyroid and renal iodide clearance rates, and thyroid iodine uptake in infants 6 months to 2 years of age, in adolescents, and in adults. These data were derived from an area of relatively low iodine intake in Belgium. Lower values would be expected in geographic areas with higher mean iodine intake. [From Oliner L, Kohlenbrener RM, Fields T, Kunstadter RH (1957). Thyroid function studies in children: Normal values for thyroidal I131 uptake and PBI131 levels up to the age of 18. J Clin Endocrinol Metab 17:67; and from Beckers C, Malvaux C, De Visscher M (1966). Quantitative aspects of the secretion and degradation of thyroid hormones during adolescence. J Clin Endocrinol Metab 26:202.]

TABLE 7-5

Variation in Peripheral Thyroxine Metabolism with Age*

Thyroxine Kinetic Parameter	Children (3-9 yr)	Adolescents (10-16 yr)	Adults (23-26 yr)
Half-life (d)	5.0 (0.13)	6.0 (0.35)	6.7 (0.30)
Fractional clearance†	0.14 (0.005)	0.12 (0.008)	0.11 (0.004)
Distribution volume (L/kg)	0.16 (0.008)	0.16 (0.014)	0.12 (0.005)
Thyroxine turnover (μg/kg/d)	1.9 (0.09)	1.5 (0.07)	1.1 (0.06)

* Data are means and SE.
† Fraction of extrathyroid pool per day.
[Data from Beckers C, Malvaux C, De Visscher M (1966). Quantitative aspects of the secretion and degradation of thyroid hormones during adolescence. J Clin Endocrinol Metab 1966:26; and from Sterling K, Chodos R (1956). Radiothyroxine turnover studies in myxedema, thyroxicosis and hypermetabolism without endocrine disease. J Clin Invest 1956;35.]

rate (turnover) during childhood and adolescence are summarized in Table 7-5. A high iodine intake can mask certain defects of thyroid hormone biosynthesis [e.g., partial defects of iodotyrosine deiodinase (dehalogenase) activity, which would result in excessive wastage of iodide]. (See Chapter 6.)

SERUM THYROID HORMONE CONCENTRATIONS AND T4 PRODUCTION

Serum total free T4 and T3 concentrations decrease gradually with age[24-27] (Tables 7-6 and 7-7). The decreases in serum total T4 and T3 result largely from a decrease in serum TBG concentrations that is progressive from early childhood through 15 to 16 years of age, when the mean serum TBG concentration is about the same as in adults. Reciprocal changes occur in serum transthyretin concentrations. These changes presumably reflect the effects of gonadal steroids, but other factors may be involved.

Serum free T4 concentrations decrease slightly during childhood and adolescence[25] (Table 7-7). The percentage of iodine-131 labeled protein-bound iodine appearing in blood (percentage of dose per liter per kilogram of body weight) after labeling of the thyroid gland also decreases with age during the first two decades, as does T4 turnover and production rate on a body weight basis (μg/kg/d)[22] (Table 7-4). Estimated T4 turnover or production rate values are 5 to 6 μg/kg/d in infants, 4 μg/kg/d at 1 to 3 years, 2 to 3 μg/kg/d at 3 to 9 years, and 1 μg/kg/d in adults.

The serum concentration of rT3 remains unchanged or increases slightly during childhood and adolescence (Table 7-7). The serum free rT3 index (total rT3 × fractional T3 resin uptake) remains stable or increases slightly. Because circulating rT3 is derived predominantly from peripheral deiodination of T4, these observations and the fact that the mean calculated ratios of serum rT3/serum T4 and free rT3 index/free T4 index increase progressively with age suggest that the relative rate of T4

TABLE 7-4

Variation of Thyroid Gland Volume with Age During Childhood and Adolescence

Average Thyroid Gland Volume (mL)

Age	Male	M and F	Female	Male	Female
1-3 years*		1.00			
5 years*		1.7			
6 years+	3.0		3.0	5.4	5.0
8 years+	4.0		4.0	6.1	6.9
10 years+	4.4		5.0	7.8	9.2
12 years+	5.7		6.3	10.4	11.7
14 years+	7.2		7.6	13.0	14.6

* Chanoine JP, Toppet V, Lagasse R, et al (1991). Determination of thyroid volume by ultrasound from the neonatal period to late adolescence. Eur J Pediatr 150:395.
+ Delange F, Becker G, Caron P, et al (1997). Thyroid volume and urinary iodine in European school children: standardization of values for assessment of iodine deficiency. Eur J Endocrinol 136:180.

TABLE 7-6

Changes with Age in Serum Concentrations of T4, TSH, TBG and Thyroglobulin (Tg)

Age	TSH§ (µU/mL)	T4† (µg/dL)	TBG† (mg/dL)	TG† (ng/mL)
Cord blood	1-20	6.6-15.0	0.8-5.2	15-101
1-7 days	1-39	11-22	0.8-5.2	1-110
1-4 weeks	0.5-6.5	8.2-17	0.6-5.0	11-92
1-12 months	0.5-6.5	5.9-16	1.6-3.6	12-113
1-5 years	0.6-6.3	7.3-15	1.4-2.8	5-72
6-10 years	0.6-6.3	6.4-13	1.4-2.8	3-40
11-15 years	0.6-6.3	5.5-12	1.4-2.8	3-40
16-20 years	0.5-6.0	4.2-12	1.4-2.8	2-36
21-50 years	0.5-6.0	4.3-12	1.2-2.6	2-35

† Mean and 2 SD range; § mean and 95% range. ¶ in Brussels, in moderately iodine deficiency infants.

Compiled from Fisher DA, Vanderschueren-Lodeweycky M (1985). Laboratory tests for thyroid diagnosis in infants and children. In Delange F, Fisher DA (eds). *Pediatric Thyroidology*. Karger Basel 127-142; Walfish PG, Tseng KH (1989). Thyroid physiology and pathology. In Collu R, Ducharme JR, Guyda H (eds). *Pediatric Endocrinology*. New York, Raven 367-448.; Delange, F, Dahlem A, Bourdoux P, et al (1984). Increased risk of primary hypothyroidism in preterm infants. Pediatrics 105:462; Pazzino V, Filetti S, Belfiore A, et al (1981). Serum thyroglobulin levels in the newborn. J Clin Endocrinol Metab 52:3634; and Delange F (1993). Thyroid hormones: Biochemistry and physiology. In Bertrang J, Rappaport, R, Sizonenko PC (eds). *Pediatric Endocrinology*. Baltimore, Williams and Wilkins 242-251.

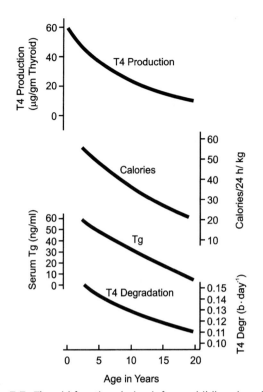

Figure 7-7. Thyroid function during infancy, childhood, and adolescence. There is a progressive decrease in metabolic rate with age (shown as calories/24 h/kg). This is associated with a progressive decrease in T4 production per gram of thyroid, a decreasing T4 degradation rate [as a fraction of the extrathyroidal pool cleared per day (b day-1)], and a progressive fall in serum thyroglobulin (Tg) concentration. [Modified from Fisher DA (1989). Thyroid disease in the neonate and childhood. In DeGroot LJ (ed.), *Endocrinology, Second edition*. Philadelphia: WB Saunders 735.]

TABLE 7-7

Changes with Age in Serum Concentrations of T3, rT3, Free T4, and Free T3

	T3* (ng/dL)	rT3* (ng/dL)	Free T4** (ng/dL)	Free T3** (pg/mL)
Cord blood	14-86	100-501	1.2-2.2	—
4-7 days	36-316	34-258	2.2-5.3	1.3-6.1
1-4 weeks	105-345	26-290	0.9-2.3	2.2-8.0
1-12 months	105-245	11-129	0.8-2.1	2.5-7.0
1-5 years	105-269	15-71	0.8-2.0	2.8-5.2
6-10 years	94-241	17-79	0.8-2.0	2.8-5.2
11-15 years	83-213	19-88	0.8-2.0	2.9-5.6
16-20 years	80-210	25-80	0.8-2.0	2.4-5.0
21-50 years	70-204	30-80	0.9-2.5	2.1-4.4

* Geometric mean and range.
** 2SD range, by tracer dialysis.

Compiled from Delange F (1993). Thyroid hormones Biochemistry and Physiology. In Bertrand J, Rapaport R, Sizonenko PC (eds). *Pediatric Endocrinology*. Baltimore, Williams and Wilkins 242-251; Lucas C, Carayon P, Bellhilehi J, Giraud F (1980). Changes in levels of free thyroid hormones in children from 1 to 16 years. Comparison with other thyroid indices. Pedatric 35:197; and Nelson JC, Clark SJ, Borut DL, Tomei RT, Carlton EI. Age related changes in serum free thyroxine during childhood adolescence. J Pediatr 123:899.

conversion to rT3 increases with age during childhood and adolescence.[24] Direct measurements have not been made. The decreases with age in the ratios of serum T3/serum rT3 and free T3 index/free rT3 index suggests a progressive decrease in the relative conversion of T4 to T3 with age during the first two decades.

The progressive decrease in thyroid T4 production (µg/gm), T4 turnover, serum thyroglobulin, and thyroidal radioiodine uptake indicate a progressive relative decrease in thyroid function with age (Figure 7-7). The decreasing serum TSH concentration with age suggests that these decreases are mediated primarily by reduced TSH secretion. Whether this reflects decreased TRH secretion or non-TRH mechanisms is not clear. A progressive reduction in thyroid gland TSH responsiveness might also be involved.

Acquired Juvenile Hypothyroidism

EXPOSURE TO GOITROGENIC AGENTS

Any food or drug that interferes with thyroid hormone synthesis is a potential cause of goiter and hypothyroidism.[28,29] A partial list of such agents is given in Table 7-8. Dietary goitrogens may be difficult to identify because they

TABLE 7-8

Goitrogenic Agents

Anions
- Iodine (in large amounts)*
- Perchlorate
- Thiocyanate

Cations
- Cobalt (in certain hematinic preparations)
- Arsenic salts
- Lithium salts

Drugs
- Propylthiouracil
- Methimazole
- Carbimazole
- Aminosalicyclic acid
- Aminoglutethimide
- Phenylbutazone
- Amiodarone

Chemicals
- Resorcinol
- 2,4 dinitrophenol
- Polychlorinated biphenyls (PCBs)
- Polybrominated biphenyls (PBBs)

Naturally Occurring Substances
- Cytokines
- Goitrin (1,5-vinyl-2-thiooxazolidone) (present in cabbage and other members of the genus *Brassica*)
- Soybeans (not soybean milk as presently prepared)
- Linamarin (a glycoside in cassava)

* Includes iodinated radiographic contrast agents such as iopanoic acid and ipodate.

may be acquired through devious routes. Epidemiologic evidence suggests that environmental pollutants may be responsible for many goiters. As part of the clinical history, in difficult cases the physician should inquire about intake of known and potential goitrogens and possible environmental or familial occupational contact with PCBs, PBBs, or dinitrophenols. Bacterial contamination of groundwater has been demonstrated, and unidentified goitrogens in groundwater have been postulated. There is also evidence that environmental (region-specific) and immunologic (genetic) factors may be synergistic in goitrogenesis.[29]

THYROID DYSGENESIS

Ectopic thyroid glands in children may first come to attention during childhood because of an enlarging mass at the base of the tongue or along the course of the thyroglossal duct. Generally, thyroid dysgenesis is sporadic and is detected by newborn screening. However, rare familial instances have been reported. An occasional case may be missed by neonatal screening and present during childhood with enlargement of the remnant thyroid and/or hypothyroidism. Remnant enlargement may occur at any age. Commonly, it is accelerated shortly before adolescence. Degrees of hypothyroidism range from barely detectable to severe.

The term *cryptothyroidism,* by analogy with *cryptorchidism,* has been applied for such ectopically located thyroid tissue (Table 7-1). The prevalence of thyroid hemiagenesis approximates 1:2,000 children.[30,31] Such patients are not usually hypothyroid and may be misdiagnosed as having a functioning thyroid nodule as the thyroid lobe enlarges. Complete substitution treatment usually reduces the thyroid tissue enlargement so that surgery can be avoided. Full substitution must be continued for life.

Severe hypothyroidism occasionally follows surgical removal of what has been presumed to be a thyroglossal duct cyst. As with lingual thyroid gland remnants, masses high in the neck may prove to be the only functional thyroid tissue present. In some patients, enlargement of the mass is correlated with failing thyroid function prior to surgery. Some cases of thyroid dysgenesis caused by PAX8 mutations may not have been detected by newborn screening and were diagnosed during childhood as acquired autoimmune hypothyroidism without measurable autoantibodies. (See Chapter 6.)

THYROID DYSHORMONOGENESIS

Most patients whose hypothyroidism is due to defective hormone synthesis are congenitally hypothyroid.[1] (See Chapter 6.) Infants with a compensated defect and normal T4 values may escape detection, however, in a neonatal screening program. Moreover, the appearance of goiter in some of these patients is usually delayed. Hypothyroidism due to the milder Pendred syndrome or other molecular defects producing compensated hypothyroidism may not be detected until later childhood or adolescence.

An increased iodine supply (e.g., by perinatal use of disinfectants or contrast media) can mask milder defects of thyroid hormone biosynthesis, and thus these cases escape diagnosis by newborn screening. In addition, thyroid hormone resistance is usually diagnosed during childhood or adolescence. (See Table 7-1 and Chapter 6.) The goiter in patients with dyshormonogenesis and in those with peripheral resistance to T3 is diffuse, soft, and variable in size. In contrast, Hashimoto glands tend to be firm and bosselated (and only moderately increased in size).

HASHIMOTO (AUTOIMMUNE) THYROIDITIS

Hashimoto thyroiditis (chronic thyroiditis, lymphadenoid goiter, autoimmune thyroiditis) was defined in 1912 when Hashimoto reported four patients with goiter characterized by diffuse infiltration of plasma cells and lymphocytes, fibrosis, parenchymal atrophy, and eosinophilic degeneration in some of the acini. The disease occurs in a genetically predisposed population.[32-34] A family history of thyroid disease is seen in 30% to 40% of patients. The disease also has marked predilection for females. Autoimmune thyroiditis is now the most common cause of nonendemic goiter and of hypothyroidism in children over 6 years of age.[35-40]

The onset of the disorder is usually insidious. Some 5% to 10% of patients (particularly adolescents) may have tachycardia, nervousness, and other signs suggestive of thyrotoxicosis. However, most will have a euthyroid goiter or a goiter with mild hypothyroidism. Only rarely is marked clinically symptomatic hypothyroidism present at diagnosis. The thyroid gland is usually enlarged and firm, with accentuation of the normal lobular architecture (bosselated). Occasionally, the goiter gives rise to the sensation of local pressure and difficulty in swallowing. If left untreated, the course of Hashimoto thyroiditis is variable. Usually, the gland undergoes progressive atrophy—and the patient has acquired hypothyroidism without any recognized period of compensatory hypertrophy. The yearly incidence of hypothyroidism in adult patients with Hashimoto thyroiditis is 5% to 7%. Spontaneous remission may occur in some 30% of adolescent patients.[36,38-40]

The spectrum of autoimmune thyroid disease in childhood and adolescence includes euthyroid goiter, hypothyroid goiter, Graves' disease, Hashitoxicosis, painless postpartum thyroiditis, painless sporadic thyroiditis, and autoimmune polyglandular syndromes (APS2a, 2b).[32-34,41-44] APS2b is the most common polyglandular syndrome and most commonly involves Hashimoto thyroiditis and type 1 diabetes mellitus. Pernicious anemia and vitiligo are associated in 30% to 40% of cases, with other autoimmune manifestations in 10%.[43] APS2a includes adrenocortical insufficiency with thyroiditis and type 1 diabetes. Again, 10% of patients manifest other autoimmune syndromes. APS1, due to mutation of the AIRE (autoimmune regulator) gene, is more rarely associated with thyroid disease. Hypoparathyroidism, mucocutaneous candidasis, diarrhea, and type 1 diabetes are more common.[43] Other autoimmune disorders accompanying autoimmune thyroid disease include antigen-antibody complex nephritis, thrombocytopenia, and celiac disease.[45-47] Approximately 30% of children with diabetes mellitus have thyroid autoantibodies, and approximately 10% have elevated serum TSH levels.[41-44]

Most patients with Hashimoto thyroiditis have detectable circulating antithyroid autoantibodies.[35-41] Several types of thyroid antibodies have been described: antibodies directed against thyroglobulin, against a colloid component other than thyroglobulin, against the thyroid peroxidase enzyme, against the sodium/iodide symporter protein, against thyroid nuclei, and against the thyroid TSH receptor. Antiperoxidase and antithyroglobulin antibodies are most prevalent, and these are the antibodies that to date are the most useful for diagnosis. The thyroid peroxidase is a microsomal enzyme, and there is a high correlation between antimicrosomal and antiperoxidase antibody levels in affected patients. These antithyroid antibodies are not pathognomonic of Hashimoto thyroiditis because in 15% to 20% of cases without evident thyroiditis significant antibody titers are detected. Most of these individuals are genetically predisposed and may not yet have developed thyroiditis. Moreover, thyroid peroxidase and thyroglobulin antibodies are also present in patients with Graves' disease.

Blood from virtually all patients with Hashimoto thyroiditis and Graves' disease can be shown to contain a population of thymus-dependent (T) autoreactive lymphocytes sensitized against the particulate portion of thyroid cells (microsomes and cell membranes).[42,43] T lymphocytes sensitized against thyroidal components and humoral antibodies directed at various thyroidal components produce the thyroid gland pathology

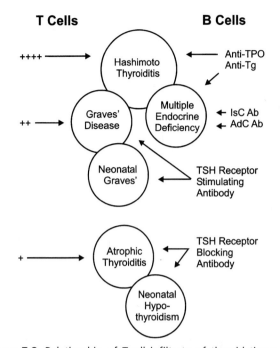

Figure 7-8. Relationship of T-cell infiltrate of thyroid tissue and B-cell antibody production to clinical autoimmune thyroid disease phenotypes. The extent of lymphoid infiltration is shown as + + + + to +. Antibody types are anti-TPO = antiperoxidase antibody and anti-Tg = antithyroglobulin antibody. IsC Ab and AdC Ab are islet cell and adrenal antibodies. The correlations are only approximate.

(Figure 7-8). The latter antibodies are produced by B rather than T lymphocytes, and it is known that the interaction of T and B lymphocytes plays a crucial role in the elaboration of immunoglobulins by B lymphocytes.

Age-specific incidence rates for Graves' disease and Hashimoto thyroiditis show an increasing rate of onset through the fifth decade and a decline thereafter. This has been interpreted as suggesting the existence of a subpopulation of subjects with genetic predisposition who develop thyroid autoimmune disease with increasing exposure to potentiating environmental factors. A genetic predisposition to thyroid autoimmunity is also suggested by observations in twins. There is an approximately 50% concordance for Graves' disease in monozygotic twins, as contrasted with a 5% concordance rate in fraternal twins.[32,48]

There are several reports of monozygotic twins pairs in which one twin manifested Graves' disease and the other Hashimoto thyroiditis. Moreover, thyroid autoantibodies have been reported in some 50% of siblings of patients with Graves' disease. Graves' disease or thyroiditis may occur in the newborn as a result of transplacental passage of maternal thyroid-stimulating immunoglobulins. (See Chapter 6.) In this instance, neonatal Graves' disease is transient—abating as the maternal thyroid stimulator degrades in the newborn.

An increased prevalence of HLA-B8, HLA-DR3, and DQA1-0501 transplantation antigens has been reported in Caucasian patients with Graves' disease. The association has been HLA-DR5 antigen in Japanese patients and HLA-DR9 in Chinese patients with the disorder, but these associations carry a risk ratio of only 3:5.[32,48] Associations have been observed between HLA DR3, DR4, or DR5 and Hashimoto thyroiditis. Linkage to the HLA genes is weak, however, and linkage with other loci on the X chromosome and on chromosomes 14 and 20 have been reported. Responsible genes have not been identified, and multiple genetic factors may be involved. More recently an association with CTLA-4 has been described.[49]

HYPOTHALAMIC-PITUITARY HYPOTHYROIDISM

Hypothalamic or pituitary disorders (including craniopharyngiomas, granulomatous disease, and and meningitis) may be acquired secondary to head-trauma tumors. However, the most frequent causes are irradiation of the neurocranium and chemotherapy in the treatment of malignant disorders (especially brain tumors). Growth failure due to growth hormone (GH) or TSH deficiency is usually the earliest manifestation of pituitary hypofunction, but other features related to the primary disease, neurologic disorder, or hypothalamic dysfunction may be prominent.

Isolated central hypothyroidism is an uncommon disorder associated with subclinical hypothyroidism and short stature in children.[50,51] In children presenting with these clinical symptoms and low free T4 and normal or low serum TSH concentrations without other evidence of pituitary disease, the diagnosis of central hypothyroidism can be considered straightforward. In those with a serum free T4 level in the lower half of the normal range and a normal TSH concentration, however, the diagnosis is difficult to confirm (even if suspected).[50]

These children manifest an abnormal circadian pattern of serum TSH concentration with absence or blunting of their nocturnal TSH surge.[50,51] Testing is accomplished by measuring serum TSH hourly between 2:00 and 4:00 P.M and between 10:00 P.M and 2:00 A.M. Normally, the serum TSH level increases 50% to 300% during sleep. Blunting of the nocturnal surge should lead to a trial of thyroxine treatment in such children. A prevalence of isolated central hypothyroidism of 16% has been reported in a group of 181 children with idiopathic short stature.[50] Autosomal-recessive inheritance of partial loss-of-function mutations of the β-TSH gene also cause central hypothyroidism of childhood onset, but may already be manifest in the newborn period if no residual TSH activity is present. (See Chapter 6.) The prevalence of central hypothyroidism approximates 1 in 20,000 births.[52]

MISCELLANEOUS CAUSES

Hypothyroidism appears to occur with increased frequency in association with several chromosomal disorders, including Turner syndrome, Down syndrome, and Klinefelter syndrome—with autoimmune thyroiditis being the most prevalent cause.[53-56] In Down syndrome, there also is an increased prevalence of thyroid dysgenesis and what has been called euthyroid hyperthyrotropinemia or subclinical hypothyroidism. Recent studies have suggested that newborns and infants with Trisomy 21 benefit from thyroid hormone administration with regard to their psychomotor development.[57] Compensated hypothyroid-

ism occurs frequently and early in children with nephropathic cystinosis, and some children with the disorder manifest overt hypothyroidism.[58] The thyroid glands show extensive destruction and infiltration of the epithelium with cystine crystals.

MANAGEMENT OF ACQUIRED HYPOTHYROIDISM

The possibility of thyroid deficiency should be considered in any child who is not growing normally. A useful aid in recognizing acquired hypothyroidism in childhood is a serial record of growth.[59] Usually, considerable time elapses between the onset of hypothyroidism and the emergence of classic signs of myxedema. If growth records are available, however, the onset of hypothyroidism can readily be documented by a progressive downward deviation from previously normal growth isobar. Weight tends to increase, and in most patients weight for age is proportionately greater than height for age (Figure 7-9).

The retardation of bone age in hypothyroidism almost always equals or exceeds the retardation in linear growth, but delayed bone age is also present in other forms of dwarfism and is not pathognomonic of hypothyroidism. Tooth eruption may be delayed, and in rare cases stippled epiphyses are evident radiographically. The thyroid hormone-deficient patient usually exhibits slowing of the deep tendon reflexes, with a delayed relaxation phase. Varying clinical manifestations of myxedema related to organ hypofunction (e.g., cardiac, hepatic, gut, skin, renal) occur with prolonged or severe hypothyroidism. Rarely, encephalopathy can manifest with signs of intracranial pressure, agitation, reduced vigilance, or seizures (Hashimoto encephalopathy).[60]

Sexual development of most hypothyroid children is delayed in approximate proportion to the retardation of skeletal maturation. However, rare children with severe hypothyroidism present with signs of precocious puberty

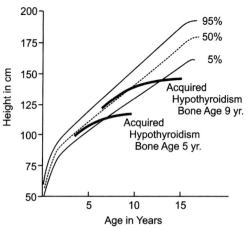

Figure 7-9. Growth failure in acquired hypothyroidism. The evolution of clinical hypothyroidism in childhood and adolescence is usually slow, and the early manifestations are subtle. The earliest sign is a slowing of linear growth, as indicated for two children with thyroid failure at 5 and 9 years, respectively. The rate of bone age maturation also slows markedly, and bone age can be used to estimate the time of onset of the thyroid failure.

(the Van Wyk-Grumbach syndrome).[61-63] Girls manifest precocious menstruation, breast development, and galactorrhea. In boys, this syndrome is associated with excessive enlargement of the penis and testes. Most of these patients lack pubic hair, and bone age is retarded in keeping with the duration of the hypothyroid state. The sella turcica may be enlarged. Serum prolactin and TSH levels are elevated in some children, but the molecular mechanism of precocious puberty is not clear.

The increased serum prolactin levels are probably explained by the fact that TRH stimulates TSH and prolactin release from the pituitary. A paracrine action of the hyperstimulated thyrotropic cells on gonadotrope cells may explain the increased gonadotropin secretion. Because precocious puberty is observed only rarely, it is also possible that these patients have genetic variants of the gonadotropin receptors that can be stimulated by the increased TSH levels.[64] Similar findings have been reported for TSH and FSH receptor variants stimulated by βHCG.[65,66] When the hypothyroid state is alleviated, the manifestations of sexual precocity regress—and normal puberty ensues when the general level of maturity has progressed appropriately.

The diagnosis of Hashimoto thyroiditis is based on a series of characteristic findings. The thyroid gland is moderately enlarged, firm, and bosselated in 80% to 90% of patients. Increased titers of thyroid peroxidase (TPO) or antithyroglobulin antibody occur in 90% to 95% of patients. Serum TSH concentration is elevated in 30% to 40% of patients, who may have an associated low serum T4 concentration, a normal or near normal serum T3 concentration, and an elevated T3/T4 concentration ratio. Minimal documentation should include plasma free T4 and TSH levels. If a goiter exists, antithyroid antibodies should be measured. If antibodies are negative, thyroid ultrasound study or a thyroid scan are useful to exclude thyroid dysgenesis. An elevated TSH level establishes that the disease originates in the thyroid rather than the pituitary gland.

A low T4 (and free T4) with a low serum TSH level indicates hypothalamic or pituitary hypothyroidism. Whenever the latter is suspected, it is mandatory that other pituitary deficiencies be sought by a complete set of pituitary function studies—including provocative tests of ACTH and growth hormone secretion, and the response of TSH to administration of TRH. A CT or MRI scan of the brain and visual field examination should be performed to exclude a pituitary or hypothalamic tumor. Isolated central hypothyroidism should be considered in children with idiopathic short stature if the serum free T4 concentration is low normal.[50,51]

Substitution therapy in older children with hypothyroidism should follow the same guidelines outlined for the treatment of congenital hypothyroidism. Most children respond well to an initial dose of L-thyroxine equivalent to about 100 μg/m² body surface.[59,67-69] If hypothyroidism is longstanding, the dose of Na-L-thyroxine should be increased gradually to prevent cardiac failure. It is also important to exclude Addison disease, and if present to treat it with appropriate glucocorticoid replacement before providing thyroid replacement so as to avoid an Addisonian crisis.

After treatment begins, the hypothyroid child resumes growth at a rate greater than normal (the period of so-called catch-up growth). Indeed, accurate serial height measurements provide assurance that the dosage provided is adequate. If the hypothyroid state is prolonged prior to treatment (>2 years), catch-up growth may be incomplete. Excessive dosage is marked by a disproportionate advancement in skeletal age. This should be avoided because it will hasten the closure of epiphyses and may shorten adult stature. In patients with pituitary TSH deficiency and deficiency of other anterior pituitary hormones, treatment with adrenal glucocorticoids or growth hormone should be provided as necessary.

Non-Thyroidal Illness

Sullivan et al. first described (1973) a selective deficiency of serum and tissue T3 in patients dying with severe prolonged illness. They referred to these patients as the "euthyroid sick." More recently, other terms—including *low T3 syndrome* and *non-thyroidal illness* (NTI)—have been applied. This syndrome of low total and free serum T3; normal, low, or high total serum T4; increased T4 sulfate; normal to high free T4; and normal serum TSH concentrations has now been reported in a variety of situations.[70-72]

These include the premature neonate, patients with protein-calorie malnutrition or anorexia nervosa, fasting subjects, postoperative patients, and patients with a variety of severe acute and chronic illnesses. The latter have included patients with diabetic ketoacidosis, severe trauma, burns, febrile states, cirrhosis, and renal failure. In addition, a number of drugs have been observed to produce a similar syndrome. These drugs include dexamethasone, selected radiographic contrast agents, propylthiouracil, propranolol, and amiodarone.

Three patterns of change in thyroid hormone levels have been described (Table 7-9): low T4, normal T4, and high T4 NTI syndromes. The low serum and tissue T3 levels in this syndrome occur as a result of inhibition of iodothyronine β-ring monodeiodinase-1 activity (MDI-1) and a decreased rate of T3 production from T4 in non-thyroidal tissues.[73,74] In mice, interleukin-1 (IL-1) cytokine inhibition of transcription of iodothyronine monodeiodinase type 1 (MDI-1) results in decreased hepatic T4 to T3 conversion—and this reduction can be reversed by SRC-1 induction of MDI-I.[73] rT3 degradation is decreased because the degradation of rT3 is mediated by the same type I deiodinase enzyme that mediates T4 to T3 conversion. Thus, serum T3 levels fall and rT3 levels tend to remain normal or increase.

TABLE 7-9

Thyroid Function Abnormalities on Non-Thyroidal Illness

Non-Thyroidal Illness Pattern	TSH	T3	rT3	T4
Low T3 syndrome	N	D	N or I	N
Low T4 syndrome				D
High T4 syndrome	N	D	N or I	I

N = normal, D = decreased, I = increased.

In some patients, serum T4 levels also fall (the low T4 syndrome)—and low T4 levels in patients with severe NTI have been associated with increased mortality. TBG levels may be reduced in such patients, and an inhibitor of T4 binding to TBG has been described in the serum and derived from the tissues of such patients. The high T4 NTI syndrome probably involves one or more induced abnormalities in the disposal pathways of T4.

There is no convincing evidence that treatment with thyroid hormones, either T4 or T3, is effective in most patients with NTI. Treatment should be directed to the primary systemic illness. There is also no clear evidence that treatment is disadvantageous, and there is some evidence to suggest that treatment may be beneficial in selected clinical conditions such as postoperative cardiac surgery.[71,75]

Iodine Deficiency Disorders

Iodine deficiency remains the leading cause of hypothyroidism worldwide.[76] During the past 40 years, major efforts to supplement iodine intake in endemic deficiency areas have been highly successful—and the geographic distribution of severe endemic iodine deficiency has been markedly reduced. Residual areas of deficiency include Africa, Southeast Asia, the Western Pacific, and some areas of Europe, the Eastern Mediterranean, and the Americas. It is estimated that some 2 billion individuals remain at risk, with 740 million affected by iodine-deficient goiter and 43 million believed to be mentally handicapped as the result of iodine deficiency.[76] Fifty percent of the world's population are thought to live in countries with iodine deficiency.

Cretinism and severe iodine deficiency are now largely restricted to remote areas of developing countries, but some 40 million individuals in the Americas and 130 million in Europe are exposed to mild to moderate iodine deficiency (largely in more isolated mountainous areas). In Europe in 1989 to 1995, clinically euthyroid school children in iodine-deficient areas were reported to have subtle or overt neuropsychointellectual deficits compared to iodine-sufficient children in the same areas.[76] This is thought to result from transient thyroid failure occurring during fetal or postnatal life during the critical period of brain development.[76] Similar studies have not been conducted in the Americas.

Environmental iodine deficiency leads to a series of thyroid system abnormalities, including increased TSH secretion, increased iodide uptake, reduced thyroglobulin iodination, increased thyroglobulin production and turnover, thyroid colloid depletion, and thyroid gland hypertrophy and hyperplasia.[76] There is an increase in poorly iodinated tyrosine and iodothyronine residues within stored thyroglobulin, resulting in increased MIT/DIT and T3/T4 ratios. As a result, the thyroid T3/T4 secretion ratio is increased and serum T3 levels are increased—whereas serum T4 concentrations fall. T4-to-T3 conversion within the thyroid gland and in peripheral tissues also increases. The result of these changes is a circumstance of compensated euthyroidism manifest by a modest increase in serum TSH, a high normal or increased serum T3 level, a low normal or decreased serum T4 concentration, and thyroidal hyperplasia and hyperactivity.

The increased T3/T4 secretion ratio allows a degree of adaptation to iodine deficiency because T3 possesses four times the metabolic potency of T4 while requiring only 75% as much iodine for synthesis.[76] With severe iodine deficiency, however, such compensation may be inadequate—leading to hypothyroidism of varying degree. In severe endemic goiter areas, goiter and cretinism, decreased fertility, increased perinatal death, increased infant mortality, and varying degrees of mental retardation are observed. In areas of moderate iodine deficiency (<100 μg iodine intake daily) in the absence of overt endemic goiter, thyroid function in adults is normal. However, the prevalence of transient neonatal hypothyroidism is increased, and mental development in euthyroid school children has been shown to be impaired.[77,78]

Consumptive Hypothyroidism

This rare syndrome, first described in 2000, is characterized by excessive ectopic inactivation of thyroid hormone by type III iodothyronine monodeiodinase (MDI III). The syndrome has been associated with massive hemangiomas and hepatic hemangioendotheliomas in children, and by hemangioendothelioma and malignant fibrous tumors in adults.[79-81] The hemangiomata and tumor tissues express high levels of MDI III message and functional activity, which inactivates thyroid hormones at a rate exceeding the production capacity of the thyroid gland. TSH levels are increased, free T4 is decreased, and reverse T3 (rT3) concentrations are increased. The dosage of thyroxine to increase circulating free T4 levels to the normal range is increased severalfold. Treatment includes T4 therapy and management of the causative vascular malformation or tumor.

Diffuse Nontoxic Goiter

A syndrome of euthyroid diffuse goiter has been described during adolescence in nonendemic goiter areas. The prevalence approximates 5% of the population.[82] Many patients with euthyroid goiter have autoimmune thyroiditis, but some have no evidence of thyroid lymphocytic infiltration. A common finding in such patients is a family history of goiter, but detailed tests of thyroid function fail to reveal identifiable defects.[83,84] Recent susceptibility loci have been identified with logarithm of odds (LOD) scores of 1.94 to 2.71.[82] Thyroid volume in affected individuals is positively correlated with age, and older patients are more likely to manifest multinodular goiter.

The genetic pattern in families is suggestive of an autosomal-dominant mode of transmission, with greater expression in the female. Thyroid function tests are normal, and thyroid biopsy in adolescents reveals only "colloid goiter." The thyroid enlargement may regress spontaneously without therapy, but many patients who develop nodular goiters in the third, fourth, and fifth decades of life have a history of mild diffuse thyroid enlargement during childhood or adolescence. There is some evidence for the presence of modest levels of thyroid autoantibodies in the serum of such patients, and thus simple goiter of adolescence may represent a mild form of autoimmune thyroid disease.[83-87]

Subacute Thyroiditis (de Quervain's Syndrome)

In children, subacute thyroiditis is a relatively rare and self-limited inflammation of the thyroid that usually follows or is associated with an upper respiratory illness.[88,89] Patients have been identified with evidence of associated mumps virus infection or with cat-scratch fever. It is likely that a variety of viral agents may be responsible for this condition. The incidence is similar in males and females. The onset is accompanied by fever and pain that may be local or referred to the angles of the jaws.

The thyroid gland may be exquisitely sensitive to palpation or only mildly tender. Characteristically, there is an increase in serum T4 and T3 levels due to release of stored hormone—and signs and symptoms of hyperthyroidism develop. Thyroidal radioiodine uptake at this time is low or absent, indicating thyroid cell damage. Signs and symptoms of hyperthyroidism usually persist for 1 to 4 weeks. After his time, there is a period of transient hypothyroidism as the thyroid gland recovers. The total course runs 2 to 9 months. A syndrome of painless (subacute) thyroiditis has also been described, with a similar pattern of transient hyperthyroidism associated with a low thyroid radioiodine uptake. The "painless thyroiditis" syndrome, however, resembles Hashimoto thyroiditis histologically—and often occurs in the postpartum period in women with a history of autoimmune thyroid disease.

Treatment of subacute painful (viral) thyroiditis includes large doses of acetylsalicylic acid or other anti-inflammatory drugs. In severe cases, corticosteroid medication may be helpful. Most patients do not develop antithyroid antibodies and recover without a residual defect in thyroid function. Subacute thyroiditis may be difficult to distinguish from acute suppurative thyroiditis, but the latter condition is now rare.

Suppurative Thyroiditis

Bacterial infections of the thyroid gland are rare in children and are usually associated with an embryologic remnant and/or a left pyriform sinus tract.[90-92] The left lobe is most often involved. Suppurative thyroiditis may be associated with other head and neck infection. In older children or adolescents, bacterial thyroiditis may be associated with bacteremic spread from distant infection. Children usually present with acute onset of pain (often with dysphagia), and with unilateral or bilateral thyroid enlargement, fever, and local tenderness.

The gland is initially firm and may progress to abscess formation. Leukocytosis is common, and thyroid function tests are usually normal. Early differentiation from subacute thyroiditis may be difficult, but signs and symptoms of hyperthyroidism are uncommon and the course is usually limited to 2 to 4 weeks. The common organisms are *staph-ylococcus aureus, streptococcus pyogenes*, and *streptococcus pneumoniae*. Rarely, *pastuerella, echinococcus,* or *crytococcal* organisms may be causative.[93-95] Thin-needle aspiration and culture are helpful in antimicrobial selection.

Juvenile Hyperthyroidism

GRAVES' DISEASE

Thyrotoxicosis in childhood and adolescence most commonly occurs as a consequence of diffuse thyroid hyperplasia (Graves' disease). Graves' disease is a multisystem autoimmune disease involving hyperthyroidism, eye manifestations, and dermopathy.[96] In children, in contrast to adults the latter manifestations are absent or mild. The disease occurs in preschool children. Rarely, it may begin in infancy. However, the incidence increases sharply as children approach adolescence. Girls are affected six to eight times more often than boys.

Graves' disease, like Hashimoto thyroiditis, has a genetic basis. A high proportion of patients have a family history positive for goiter, hyperthyroidism, or hypothyroidism. It is believed that Graves' disease and Hashimoto thyroiditis arise randomly in a genetically predisposed population. The concordance rate for Graves' disease in monozygotic twins has been reported as 30% to 60%. In dizygotic twins, it is only 3% to 9%. Family studies have disclosed a high percentage of circulating antithyroid antibodies in near relatives. Furthermore, certain HLA haplotypes (such as HLA B8 and Dr3 in Caucasians) and linkage to genetic determinants on the X chromosome and chromosomes 14 and 20 have been reported in affected families.[48,96]

The three principal autoantigens of Graves' disease (the TSH receptor, thyroid peroxidase, and thyroglobulin) have been cloned. The TSH receptor autoantibodies have a major pathogenetic role in Graves' disease. The TSH receptor-stimulating antibodies (TSA) can be identified by bioassay and receptor assay techniques. TSA displaces TSH from membrane TSH receptors and stimulates adenylate cyclase and cAMP production in thyroid follicular cell lines in culture. Current bioassays are available that use TSH receptor-transfected CHO cell lines. These measure cAMP production in response to partially purified serum immunoglobulin moieties. Autoantibodies measured only by displacement of radiolabeled TSH from thyroid cell membrane TSH receptor are referred to as TSH binding-inhibiting immunoglobulin (TBII), or TBIA. The TBII assay measures stimulating and blocking antibodies without differentiation.

The production of TSA by B lymphocytes is probably a secondary response to a cell-mediated immune reaction requiring involvement of T lymphocytes in a manner similar to that postulated for Hashimoto thyroiditis. Cell cultures of lymphocytes from patients with Graves' disease produce immunoglobulins only after stimulation with phytohemagglutinin. Because the latter substance stimulates only T cells (which are incapable of secreting immunoglobulins), it may be inferred that cell-mediated and humoral immune mechanisms are involved in the genesis of the thyrotoxic state. This is supported by recent studies indicating that thyrocytes can be activated by TSA + IGF-I to express powerful T-cell chemoattractants that stimulate T-cell infiltration independently of the TSH receptor.[97]

Clinical Features

The onset of thyrotoxicosis is usually insidious, with a period of increasing nervousness, palpitation, increased appetite, and muscle weakness.[98-101] Marked weight loss occurs in some patients, usually in association with a voracious appetite. Occasionally, children (and especially adolescents) show a weight increase with the onset of the disease. There is a tendency for thyrotoxic children to be in the upper percentile channels for height. Except for exophthalmos and other eye signs, the symptoms of thyrotoxicosis are nonspecific—and for prolonged periods may be mistaken for some other condition.

Behavioral abnormalities, declining school performance, and emotional instability frequently dominate the clinical picture. In other patients, cardiovascular signs are more prominent—and attention is focused on a cardiac murmur or decreased exercise tolerance. Nocturia is due to the increased glomerular filtration rate. Fatigability and objective muscle weakness are observed in 60% to 70% of patients with juvenile thyrotoxicosis. Myopathy varies in severity from fatigability to periodic paralysis, and as in adults may be the most prominent manifestation of the disease. Rarely, juvenile Graves' disease may occur in association with myastenia gravis or another autoimmune disorder such as lupus erythematosis.

Most of the signs and symptoms of Graves' disease are similar to those produced by a hyperactive sympathetic nervous system and can be simulated by anxiety, fright, or acute illness. Even in patients in whom tachycardia is not impressive, the pulse pressure is widened and the precordium overactive. Underlying heart disease is difficult to exclude in the presence of cardiomegaly, ejection murmurs, precordial thrill, and gallop rhythms. Other signs of sympathetic overactivity are tremor, excessive perspiration, rapid tendon reflex relaxation times, and emotional lability. The size of the thyroid gland is highly variable, and the goiter may escape notice in a patient whose gland is only slightly enlarged. The characteristics of the thyroid to be noted on physical examination are size, uniformity, and consistency. A bruit or thrill provides some indication of the degree of hyperplasia but has no specific diagnostic value. During phases of active hyperplasia, the thyroid typically has a resilient bulging characteristic that is lost as recovery takes place.

Severe Graves' ophthalmyopathy is much less common in children than in adults, and malignant exophthalmos is virtually unknown.[101] The eye findings in this disease may be grouped as those due to sympathetic hyperactivity and those due to specific pathologic changes in the orbit. The latter are rarely seen in childhood and adolescence. Those due to sympathetic hyperactivity give the appearance of stare, owing to retraction of the upper eyelid and a wide palpebral aperture. There is also a lag in the descent of the upper eyelid upon looking downward (lid lag), as well as infrequent blinking and absence of forehead wrinkling upon upward gaze. The eyes frequently present a glazed appearance. To a large extent, these findings parallel the severity of the disease and disappear as the patient is rendered euthyroid.

Rarely, there are changes in the orbit due to infiltration of mucopolysaccharides, lymphocytes, and edema fluid within the ocular muscles, lacrimal glands, and retro-orbital fat. These changes can lead to exophthalmos, ophthalmoplegia, chemosis of the conjunctiva, pain, swelling, and irritation. Although the inflammatory changes usually improve with treatment of the hyperthyroid state, the course of the thyroid and eye manifestations may differ. Some degree of exophthalmos tends to remain after recovery from the thyrotoxicosis.

The accumulation of mucopolysaccharides in skin and subcutaneous tissues, referred to as Graves' dermopathy or pretibial myxedema, is also rare in children. Graves' disease and Hashimoto thyroiditis are occasionally encountered in the same patient. These children have clinical and laboratory features of Hashimoto thyroiditis and exhibit thyrotoxicosis and resistance to thyroidal suppression by T3. The somewhat whimsical term *Hashitoxicosis* has been applied to these patients.

Laboratory Diagnosis

The initial laboratory tests should include serum TSH, free T4, and T3 determinations. The serum TSH level is suppressed below the limit of detection of second-generation TSH assays, and is usually below 0.04 mU/L in third-generation ultrasensitive assays. A serum TSH level above 1.0 μU/mL suggests TSH-dependent hyperthyroidism. A measurement of serum levels of TSH receptor autoantibody (TSA and TBII) are confirmatory for the diagnosis.

Treatment

Treatment of thyrotoxicosis must be directed toward reducing the secretory rate of thyroid hormones, and if possible toward blunting the toxic effects produced by high circulating levels. Three principal methods are available for reducing thyroid hormone secretion: subtotal or total ablation of the thyroid gland with radioactive iodine, subtotal surgical thyroidectomy, and blocking thyroid hormone biosynthesis by means of drugs.[102-110]

Treatment with Radioactive Iodine

In terms of ease, cost, efficacy, and short-term safety, treatment with iodine-131 is superior.[102-105] This approach, however, has been used relatively infrequently to date in childhood and adolescence because of the high prevalence of post-treatment hypothyroidism and the potential risks of leukemia, thyroid cancer, and genetic damage. The thyroid glands of young animals are much more susceptible to induction of thyroid carcinoma by ionizing radiation than are those of older animals. Radiation to the neck in infancy has been incriminated as an important cause of thyroid cancer in children, whereas this is infrequent in adults.

Several children treated with radioiodine have been reported to develop thyroid adenomas. This has been attributed to relatively low radioiodine treatment doses in the past. Such low treatment doses (<50 microcuries ^{131}I/gm thyroid tissue) are also associated with the need for additional treatment to achieve euthyroidism and with delayed but eventual hypothyroidism.[103-105] When treating children and adolescents with radioiodine, a dose that will achieve thyroid tissue destruction is recommended. The dosage should be calculated to optimize the thyroid radiation dose while minimizing total body radiation exposure, particularly in young children.[105]

Radioiodine has now been used to treat more than 1,000 reported children and adolescents since 1950, and there have been no recent reports of thyroid neoplasia or other untoward effects.[104,105] Hypothyroidism is expected and requires lifelong management. Most physicians still reserve the use of radioiodine for treatment of thyrotoxicosis in older adolescents who fail to follow a medical regimen and who cannot be adequately prepared for surgical thyroidectomy. However, current evidence suggests that this approach may be safe enough to consider as initial treatment in selected patients—particularly those 10 years of age or older.

Surgical Treatment

With proper preparation of the patient for surgical thyroidectomy, the immediate operative mortality approximates that for other major surgical procedures.[102] With proper surgical management, most patients achieve a rapid and satisfactory remission—and requirements for intensive medical follow-up are less rigorous than in those patients treated exclusively with drugs.

The availability of an experienced thyroid surgeon is an important criterion for successful surgical treatment. The incidences of permanent hypoparathyroidism and recurrent laryngeal nerve damage following subtotal thyroidectomy are still appreciable, and these serious complications will persist and may require lifelong treatment. The surgeon attempts to leave enough thyroid tissue that the patient is euthyroid postoperatively. The patient may, however, have recurrence of the thyrotoxicosis (or, conversely, may develop later hypothyroidism).

Medical Management

Management of Graves' disease patients with antithyroid drugs requires a prolonged period of drug therapy (usually 2 to 5 years), and close supervision by the physician is necessary for years.[98,100,101,110] Even in patients treated successfully, not more than 60% to 70% have permanent remission with drug therapy alone. Combined therapy with an antithyroid drug plus Na-L-thyroxine in replacement dosage has been used to suppress increased serum TSH levels and to minimize the need for frequent adjustment of antithyroid drug dosage. A small percentage of patients are hypersensitive to propylthiouracil (PTU) or methimazole. These reactions are usually mild, and disappear when the drug is withdrawn, but severe drug reactions (including liver failure and agranulocytosis) may occur.[98,103,106]

Approach to Therapy

The choice of therapy in thyrotoxicosis must be individualized, taking into consideration any illnesses, the quality of thyroid surgery available, and the socioeconomic factors that play such a large role in determining the success of a prolonged medical regimen. Patients with weight loss and decreased body mass index (BMI), a large goiter, or a high iodine intake are more resistant to drug therapy.[110] However, in most instances treatment is begun with antithyroid drugs and a decision regarding surgery or radioiodine is made when the patient becomes euthyroid. In severely toxic patients, the β-adrenergic blocking agent propranolol is of value in controlling many of the manifestations of Graves' disease.

The drug is useful in the initial treatment of severely thyrotoxic patients in the interval before specific antithyroid drugs become effective and has proved effective in the preoperative preparation for subtotal thyroidectomy. The antithyroid drugs inhibit oxidation of iodide and thereby block synthesis of thyroid hormone.[106] Neither the release of thyroid hormone nor the effect of TSH on the iodide pump is affected. Of the commonly used drugs, carbimazole and methimazole have a longer half-life of degradation than propylthiouracil—and maintenance therapy with these drugs can sometimes be accomplished with a single daily dose (Table 7-10).

There is always a time lag between institution of drug treatment and achievement of a euthyroid state because the biosynthetic block is not complete and the stores of preformed hormone must first be discharged. The rapidity of response to therapy correlates best with the initial size of the thyroid gland. Those patients with a small gland usually exhibit improvement in a few weeks, whereas those with very large glands may not respond for 2 to 3 months. TSH levels can be suppressed for more than 6 months despite clinical euthyroidism and normal or even low peripheral thyroid hormone levels and are therefore not appropriate in monitoring the success of antithyroid drug treatment.

The initial dose of propylthiouracil varies from 300 to 600 mg daily (175 mg/m^2 or 2-6 mg/kg) in dosages spaced at 6- or 8-hour intervals (Table 7-10). Skin rashes occur in about 2% of patients treated with propylthiouracil or carbimazole, and in 5% of patients treated with methimazole early in the course of therapy. They disappear when the drug is withheld. Often these rashes are

TABLE 7-10

Characteristics of Common Antithyroid Drugs

Drug	Initial Dose (mg/kg /day)	Maintenance Dose (mg/kg /day)	Incidence of Toxic Reactions (%)
Methimazole	0.4-0.6	0.1-0.3	1.4
Carbimazole	0.4-0.6	0.1-0.3	0.5
Propylthiouracil	4-6	1-3	0.9

From Marchant B, Lees JFH, Alexander WD (1979). Antithyroid drugs. In Hershman JM, Bray GA (eds.), *The thyroid: Physiology and treatment of disease*. Oxford: Pergamon Press 209-252.

mild and can be controlled with antihistamines. Severe reactions are rare (0.5%-1.4%). Granulocytopenia, when it occurs, is usually delayed (4-8 weeks of therapy). Protective isolation and antibiotic treatment usually allow recovery. Fatal liver failure has been described in adult patients treated with PTU. Usually, it is necessary to continue drug therapy for 1 to 2 years—and in many instances treatment must be continued for 3 to 6 years before the gland has lost its hyperplastic character.

The best clinical prognostic guide is the size of the thyroid gland. Most patients with continued thyroid enlargement will relapse if antithyroid drugs are discontinued. It is also possible to monitor the levels of circulating TSA. When circulating TSA disappear in a patient in clinical remission on drug treatment, a permanent remission off treatment is more likely. Antithyroid drugs probably have no influence on the fundamental disease process. However, drug treatment does permit the patient to remain euthyroid and in good health until the disease has spontaneously run its course.

Iodide in large doses will block thyroid hormone synthesis, inhibit the release of preformed hormone, and render the gland less vascular. Iodine blockade can be maintained for only a limited period (4-16 weeks) before escape occurs, and a fully euthyroid state may not be achieved. The use of inorganic iodine is reserved for severely toxic patients and for the immediate preoperative preparation of patients who are about to undergo subtotal thyroidectomy. Iodinated radiographic contrast agents (ipodate or iopanoic acid) have been employed successfully in drug treatment of Graves' hyperthyroidism.[107-109] Doses of 0.01 µg/mg/day or 0.04 to 0.05 µg/kg every 3 days have been employed and have maintained remission for 6 to 8 months. There is only limited experience with their use in children. (Neonatal Graves' disease is discussed in Chapter 6.)

TSH-DEPENDENT HYPERTHYROIDISM

Pituitary Tumors

TSH-secreting pituitary tumors associated with clinical hyperthyroidism have been reported in adults and in children.[111,112] In children, the local manifestations of the tumor are prominent. These include visual changes, optic atrophy, hydrocephalus, and amaurosis. Children with hyperthyroidism and measurable serum TSH concentrations (>1 µU/mL or 1 mU/L) should be examined for neurologic dysfunction and visual abnormalities. Skull roentgenograms for careful evaluation of the sella turcica are indicated if this evaluation arouses suspicion or if the serum TSH concentration is normal or elevated.

Selective Pituitary T3 Resistance

Hyperthyroidism with diffuse goiter and elevated serum TSH levels has been reported in several patients without pituitary enlargement.[113-116] These patients manifest resistance to the feedback effect on T3 on TSH release. The TSH response to TRH has been variable. These patients represent selective pituitary resistance to thyroid hormones. Features of thyroid autoimmune disease are absent, and the serum TSH level is inappropriately elevated in relation to the serum T4 and T3 concentrations.

In contrast to patients with pituitary TSH-secreting tumors, the TSH α-subunit level is not elevated and the TSH response to TRH is increased. Treatment of the disorder is difficult. Thyroid ablation controls the hyperthyroidism but aggravates the TSH hypersecretion and increases the risk of development of a pituitary adenoma. Suppression of TSH by exogenous thyroid hormone may aggravate the hyperthyroidism. However, this approach has been successful, and treatment with 3,5,3'-triiodothyroacetic acid (TRIAC) has been proposed.[114,115]

AUTONOMOUS NODULAR HYPERTHYROIDISM

Autonomously functioning thyroid nodules are uncommon in childhood and adolescence. Thyroid function in patients with thyroid nodules is variable. Most patients are euthyroid. Rarely, single or multiple autonomously functioning nodules may be associated with clinical hyperthyroidism.[117-119] Such nodules are true follicular adenomata and nearly always benign. The incidence of thyroid carcinoma in functioning nodules is less than 1%. It is generally felt that function in a thyroid nodule essentially excludes a diagnosis of thyroid carcinoma, but the possibility must be considered.

Small functional nodules usually do not produce clinical thyrotoxicosis. Large nodules (in excess of 3 cm in diameter) are more likely to do so. Somatic gain-of-function mutations of the TSH receptor and gain-of-function mutations of the Gsα-subunit have been found to be a major cause of benign toxic thyroid adenomas.[120] Activating germ-line TSH receptor mutations, by contrast, produce congenital or childhood-onset diffuse thyroid hyperplasia and hyperthyroidism.

Nodular autonomy is usually discerned by thyroid radioiodine scan. A nodule is autonomous if it is the only thyroid tissue showing uptake. If the nodule shows increased radioiodine uptake but the remaining thyroid tissue is still visible on scan, autonomy is likely. Autonomy is confirmed if the serum TSH concentration measured by a highly sensitive method is suppressed. Patients may present euthyroid with normal-range serum T4 and T3 concentrations and suppressed serum TSH. T3-suppression testing has been used to confirm autonomy. Radioiodine uptake in autonomous nodules is not suppressible by exogenous T3. The natural history of functioning thyroid nodules in individual patients is variable.

Most likely, if euthyroid such patients will remain euthyroid. However, there may be a gradual increase in autonomous thyroid hormone production with development of clinical evidence of hyperthyroidism. Nodule enlargement or thyrotoxic symptoms may create the need for ablative therapy. Functioning nodules producing clinical and chemical thyrotoxicosis require surgical removal. Radioiodine treatment now tends to be reserved for older adult patients. Antithyroid drug therapy is considered only for short-term management. Complete lobectomy with preservation of the recurrent laryngeal nerve is the most desirable surgical procedure.

ACTIVATING TSH RECEPTOR MUTATIONS

Several families have been reported with hyperthyroidism segregating as an autosomal-dominant trait in the absence of thyroid autoimmune disease. The affected individuals present with goiter, increased total and free T4 levels, and suppressed TSH concentrations. In patients treated surgically, the thyroid glands manifest diffuse hyperplasia without lymphocytic infiltration. Gain-of-function germline mutations of the TSH receptor have been demonstrated in these patients.[120-123] In vitro studies of cells with transfected mutated receptors demonstrate abnormally increased constitutive cAMP-stimulating activity.

Most of the affected individuals have been detected during childhood or adolescence, but a few infants have been diagnosed before 2 years of age and occasionally in the neonatal period.[122] Clearly, the abnormality is congenital—and it is possible that some of the earlier reported cases of familial persistent neonatal Graves' disease have instead manifested unrecognized activating TSH-receptor mutations. Treatment of such infants is difficult because the disorder is not transient.[122] Antithyroid drugs for short-term management and total or near-total thyroidectomy would seem the therapies of choice at present.

ACTIVATING G-PROTEIN MUTATIONS

The guanine nucleotides (G proteins) are a family of signal-transducing molecules coupling the seven-transmembrane-helix family of cell membrane receptors (including the TSH receptor) to activating cellular effector systems such as adenyl cyclase. Activating mutations of the alpha subunit of the stimulatory G protein, Gs, lead to increased cyclic AMP formation and the associated endocrinopathies of the McCune Albright syndrome.[124] It is postulated that the mutation occurs during embryonic development with a mosaic tissue distribution.

The clinical manifestations relate to the tissues involved and include polyostotic fibrosis, dysplasia of bone, and hyperfunction of one of more endocrine glands. The latter have included ovarian cysts, gonadal hyperfunction and precocious puberty, pituitary adenomas causing adrenal hyperplasia or growth hormone hypersecretion, and hyperthyroidism. The thyroid hyperplasia and hyperthyroidism resemble Graves' disease, but without ophthalmologic features and without autoantibodies. Treatment options for the thyroid disease include antithyroid drugs, surgery, and radioiodine.

Thyroid Neoplasia

CLASSIFICATION

A thyroid neoplasm should be suspected whenever a child is found to have a solitary thyroid mass with a consistency differing from that of the rest of the thyroid gland. A solitary nodule during the first two decades of life has a much greater chance of being malignant than those in older age groups.[125-130] The prevalence of cancer in children with thyroid nodules has been decreasing in North America, presumably due to reduced radiation exposure. Cancer prevalence now approximates 20% of thyroid nodules in children.[127,128] The ratio of girls to boys among children with thyroid cancer varies from 1:6 (F/M) for ages 5 through 9 to 5:2 at ages 15 through 19.[128] Nodular enlargement in boys is somewhat more likely to be cancerous than in girls.

Thyroid cancer accounts for 0.5% of all cancer for all ages and 1% to 1.5% of all childhood cancer. A classification of thyroid neoplasia is shown in Table 7-11. Seventy to 80% of solitary thyroid nodules during childhood prove to be cystic lesions or benign adenomas.[127-130] Hyperfunctioning adenomas are exceedingly uncommon during the first two decades of life. Well-differentiated papillary thyroid carcinoma (PTC) account for more than 60% to 90% of the malignant lesions in this age group. Characterization of the histopathologic type as follicular, papillary, or papillary-follicular carcinoma does not alter therapy.

Other malignant tumors of the thyroid gland during childhood include medullary carcinoma arising in the parafollicular C cells, poorly differentiated thyroid carcinoma, teratomas, lymphoma, and tumors such as metastatic carcinomas arising in other tissues.[125,131,132] The prognosis in these tumors may be worse than in well-differentiated adenocarcinoma of the thyroid. Hence, it is important to establish a tissue diagnosis as early as possible and to design the treatment accordingly. Well-differentiated carcinomas have little tendency to become undifferentiated neoplasms.

RADIATION EXPOSURE

A frequent predisposing cause of the development of differentiated thyroid gland carcinoma during infancy and childhood is radiation exposure involving the neck. In a series of children reported in the 1950s with thyroid cancer, 80% had a history of prior radiotherapy.[133,134] Usually, radiotherapy had been administered during early infancy to the upper mediastinum and neck for control of an "enlarged" thymus gland. Cancer also occurred following irradiation of hypertrophied tonsils and adenoids or acne in older children and adolescents. In those earlier studies, the average time between the irradiation and cancer detection approximated 10 years—and the estimated absolute risk of excess cancers was estimated to be 4.4 per million children per rad of radiation dose (1 rad = 0,01 Gray).

TABLE 7-11
Thyroid Neoplasia in Childhood

Tumors of the Follicular Epithelium
- Follicular adenoma
- Papillary carcinoma
- Follicular carcinoma
- Anaplastic carcinoma

Tumors of Nonfollicular Origin
- Medullary carcinoma
- Metastatic tumors
- Teratoma
- Lymphoma
- Other

The most recent epidemic of radiation-induced thyroid cancer in children followed the Chernobyl nuclear accident in Russia in 1986.[135,136] The radiation dose ranged from 0.5 to 600 rads (0.006–6 Gray) in a group of 107 exposed Russian children detected by 1992, with a mean of 20 rads (0.2 Gray). The age at exposure ranged from 0 to 11 years, and the age at diagnosis 4 to 16 years. The cancers, predominantly papillary adenocarcinoma, developed in most cases within 3 to 5 years. However, the number of cases has continued to increase.

PAPILLARY-FOLLICULAR CARCINOMA

Most children with papillary follicular thyroid carcinoma present with a midneck or lateral neck mass, and most (60%-80%) have one or more palpable neck lymph nodes containing metastatic thyroid cells by histologic examination. One-third to one-half of patients have extracapsular extension, and 10% distant metastases (usually to the lungs). FNA is a helpful diagnostic approach with analysis by an experienced cytopathologist.[130,137] FNA is omitted if malignancy criteria are present. These include a history or radiation to the head or neck, a rapidly growing nodule that is very firm or hard, satellite lymph nodes, hoarseness or dysphagia, and evidence of distant metastases.

Approximately 80% of differentiated thyroid carcinoma is classified as papillary, and 20% as papillary-follicular.[137] Ras mutations are early events in a complex cascade of somatic mutations contributing to many cases of papillary-follicular thyroid carcinoma, and activation of the tyrosine kinase receptors RET (as RET/PTC) and NTRK (as TRK) may be involved.[138] Cytogenetic abnormalities are associated with the RET/PTC and TRK rearrangements or translocations. RET/PTC gene rearrangements are characteristic of papillary carcinoma in adults and are associated with an aggressive clinical course.

RET/PTC mutations and rearrangements are also common in pediatric papillary thyroid carcinoma, varying from 23% to 67% in reported series and averaging about 50%.[139] RET/PTC-3 rearrangements are more prevalent in radiation-induced thyroid papillary carcinoma, whereas RET/PTC-1 and RET/PTC-2 rearrangements are more common in spontaneous papillary carcinoma.[139-142] The radiation-induced thyroid carcinoma in children after the Chernobyl reactor accident was associated with a high prevalence of RET/PTC in the absence of RAS and p53 mutations.[142,143] Raf kinase is a component of the Ras/Raf-MAPK kinase-ERK/MAPK signaling pathway involved in regulation of cell growth and proliferation. The B-type (BRAF) isoform, when constitutively activated, causes tumorigenesis.[144]

BRAF mutations are found in a variety of human cancers, including 29% to 83% of papillary thyroid cancer in adults, and are associated with poorer clinicopathologic outcomes and independently predict recurrence.[144] BRAF mutations are much less common in childhood papillary cancer.[143] Three gene profiles of thyroid nodules (assessing cyclin D, protein convertase 2, and prostate differentiation factor) have been shown to differentiate follicular thyroid carcinoma and adenoma in 114 adult samples, with 97% accuracy. Gene expression profiling methods for differential diagnosis and prognosis are in development.[146,147]

The prognosis in children with papillary-follicular carcinoma is far better than in most other types of childhood cancer.[131] The course is usually indolent, with long periods without progression. However, local or distant recurrence is observed in as many as 35% of patients and constant surveillance is required. Because spread to the lymph nodes has occurred prior to surgery in some patients, the excellent prognosis may be related more to the biologic nature of this form of cancer than to total removal of all cancerous cells at the initial operation.

Thyroid hormone suppression cannot be overemphasized and should be prescribed in doses adequate to suppress serum TSH (as assessed by a high-sensitivity TSH assay) but avoid evidence of toxicity. Mortality in thyroid carcinoma during childhood and adolescence is primarily accounted for by the relatively uncommon instances of medullary carcinoma and undifferentiated carcinoma. In these lesions, more radical surgery combined with radiation or cancer chemotherapy is fully justified.

MEDULLARY CARCINOMA

Medullary thyroid carcinoma (MTC) arises from the parafollicular or C cells of the thyroid gland and accounts for 3% to 9% of thyroid carcinomas.[148-152] There is a distinctive histologic picture, with large deposits of amyloid situated among sheets of pleomorphic epithelial cells. Most patients with MTC have sporadic disease. Hereditary MTC accounts for 25% to 35% of cases and includes multiple endocrine neoplasia type 2A (MEN2A), MEN2B, and familial MTC (FMTC): 80% to 90%, 5%, and 5% to 15% of cases, respectively.[151]

FMTC is a consistent feature of all clinical subtypes (Table 7-12). MEN prevalence approximates 1:30,000 individuals.[151] MEN syndromes (including pheochromocytoma and parathyroid adenoma or hyperplasia) can be distinguished from MEN I (with parathyroid, pituitary, and pancreatic tumors). MEN 2A (Sipple's syndrome) includes MTC, pheochromocytomas, and hyperparathyroidism. MEN 2B (sometimes termed *MEN 3*) includes MTC, pheochromocytomas, and multiple mucosal neuromata. The common feature of all of these tumors is a neuroectodermal origin. Patients with mucosal neuromas usually have a distinctive appearance, with protruding, thick, often bumpy lips; occasionally prognathism; and a marfanoid habitus[148,149,151,152] (Table 7-12).

TABLE 7-12

Classification of Hereditary Medullary Thyroid Cancer

Phenotype	MTC	MN	PCT	HPT
MEN2A	100%	100%	50%	20%
MEN2B	100%	N	50%	N
FMTC	100%	N	N	N

Modified from Kouvaraki MA, Shapiro SE, Perrier NO, et al. (2005). RET proto-oncogene: A review and update of genotype-phenotype correlations in hereditary medullary thyroid cancer and associated endocrine tumors. Thyroid 15:531.
MTC, medullary thyroid carcinoma; MN, mucosal neuromata; PCT, pheochromocytoma; HPT, hyperparathyroidism; N = not present.

The distinctive feature of MTC is excessive secretion of calcitonin. Other substances (including ACTH, chromogranin A, histaminase, serotonin, prostaglandins, somatostatin, and beta endorphin) may be produced. Serum calcitonin is the most reliable biochemical marker for the presence of MTC. Normal levels usually do not exceed 30 pg/mL. C-cell hyperplasia is associated with increased calcitonin secretion, and baseline and pentagastrin- and/or calcium-stimulated serum calcitonin concentrations have been utilized to distinguish C-cell hyperplasia and MTC. Stimulated calcitonin values in the 30- to 100-pg/mL range are generally associated with C-cell hyperplasia, and levels in the 100- to 1,000-pg/mL range with microscopic MTC confined to the thyroid gland. Stimulated calcitonin levels in excess of 10,000 pg/mL are associated with macroscopic MTC, and 20% of these patients manifest distant metastases.[148-150]

MTC is caused by autosomal-dominant gain-of-function mutations in the RET (rearranged during transfection) proto-oncogene on chromosome 10. RET includes 21 exons and encodes a plasma-membrane-bound tyrosine kinase enzyme. The RET receptor is expressed in neuroendocrine and neural cells, including thyroid C cells, adrenal medullary cells, parathyroid cells, and colonic ganglion cells. Extracellular cadherin-like domains are involved in cell-cell signaling. Cysteine-rich extracellular domains are important to receptor dimerization. There are three isoforms with 9,43 or 51 distinct amino acids in the intracellular C-terminal tail. These have different roles in kidney differentiation, in sympathetic neuronal growth and function, and in neuronal signaling.[151] There are four RET ligands mediating receptor dimerization and tyrosine autophosphorylation, activating various signaling pathways.[151] Inactivating RET mutations are associated with congenital megacolon. Activating gain-of-function germ-line mutations are responsible for FMTC and its variants (Figure 7-10, Table 7-13).

A single point mutation at codon 918 of the intracellular tyrosine kinase domain (exon 16) of the RET oncogene has been described in 95% of patients with MEN2B. A codon 634 mutation has been found in 85% of MEN2A patients, and mutations in codons 609, 611, 618, and 620 in 10% to 15%. In the rare cases of sporadic MEN2A, MEN2B and FMTC RET mutations occur de novo on the paternal allele (or rarely on the maternal allele). Somatic RET mutations are found in sporadic MTC.[153] These most frequently occur in codon 918, but a variety of mutations (including multiple mutations) have been characterized.[151,152] Identical germ-line mutations have been observed in association with MEN2A and FMTC[150,151] (Table 7-12).

Prior to 1987, the only available test for detecting MTC in at-risk patients was measurement of serum calcitonin with or without stimulation. Since then, DNA diagnosis has become the procedure of choice. The identification of a mutation of the RET protooncogene indicates that the affected individual has a greater than 90% probability of development of MTC. The optimal treatment strategy is to prevent MTC in children with RET gene mutations by performing early thyroidectomy before malignant transformation occurs.[151]

There is now a large experience correlating RET mutations with MTC aggressiveness, and high-risk mutations have been identified (Table 7-14). These are ranked as

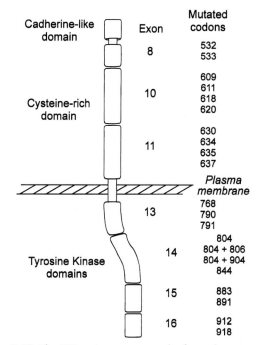

Figure 7-10. The RET proto-oncogene codes for a plasma membrane protein receptor consisting of 21 exons with extracellular, transmembrane, and intracellular tyrosine kinase domains. Activating missense mutations of the indicated codons of exons 8, 10, 11, 13, 14, 15, and 16 predispose to medullary thyroid carcinoma presenting as multiple endocrine neoplasia (MEN) syndromes 2A and 2B or as familial medullary thyroid carcinoma (FMTC). [From Kouvaraki MA, Shapiro SE, Perrier NO, et al. (2005). RET proto-oncogene: A review and update of genotype-phenotype correlations in hereditary medullary thyroid cancer and associated endocrine tumors. Thyroid 15:531.]

TABLE 7-13		
RET Gene Mutations and Associated Syndromes*		
Clinical Syndrome	**Exon**	**Mutated Codons**
MEN2A/ FMTC	10	609, 611, 618, 620
	11	634, 635, 637
	13	790, 791
	14	804
	15	891
FMTC	8	532, 533
	11	630
	13	768
	14	804, 844
	16	912
MEN2B	14	804 + 806
		804 + 904
	15	883
	16	918, 922

From Kouvaraki MA, Shapiro SE, Perrier NO, et al. (2005). RET proto-oncogene: A review and update of genotype-phenotype correlations in hereditary medullary thyroid cancer and associated endocrine tumors. Thyroid 15:531; and from Iler MA, King DR, Ginn-Pease ME, et al. (1999). Multiple endocrine neoplasia, type 2A: A 25 year review. J Pediatr Surg 34:92.

TABLE 7-14

Patient MTC Risk Groups and Recommended Management

	Level 1: High Risk	Level 2: High Risk	Level 3: Highest Risk
Mutated codons	609, 768, 790 791, 804, 891	611, 618, 620 634	883, 918
Phenotype	MEN2A	MEN2A	MEN2B
Recommended management	Thyroidectomy 5-10 yr of age	Thyroidectomy <5 yr of age	Thyroidectomy 1-6 mo of age

From Kouvaraki MA, Shapiro SE, Perrier NO, et al. (2005). RET proto-oncogene: A review and update of genotype-phenotype correlations in hereditary medullary thyroid cancer and associated endocrine tumors. Thyroid 15:531.

levels 1 through 3, with 3 being highest risk. For the highest-risk group (mutated exons 883 or 918 in MEN2B patients), thyroidectomy is recommended before age 6 months (or preferably within the first month of life).[151] For level 2 patients, thyroidectomy before age 5 is indicated, and for level 1 mutations thyroidectomy at 5 to 10 years of age is recommended (Table 7-15). An alternative approach in lower-risk patients is to initiate calcium-pentagastrin testing of gene mutation carriers at age 4 or 5 years, with removal of the thyroid gland at the time of a positive test.

Pheochromocytomas in MEN2 patients, in contrast to sporadic forms, are rarely extra-adrenal or malignant and are diagnosed at a younger age. This has led to the practice of cortex-sparing adrenalectomy to avoid the risk of adrenal insufficiency.[151] The tumors are bilateral in 50% of patients. The risk of recurrent pheochromocytoma in the contralateral gland in patients with unilateral disease is 20% to 30%. Patients with unilateral disease can now be managed via laparoscopic unilateral complete adrenalectomy. For bilateral disease, a unilateral cortical-sparing procedure with removal of the entire centralateral gland is recommended.[151]

Long-term follow-up of hereditary MTC patients is essential to detect recurrence of disease in treated patients or the later appearance of pheochromocytoma or hyperparathyroidism. Pheochromocytoma in MEN patients is diagnosed after MTC in 90% of patients. Parathyroid hyperplasia is associated most commonly with codon 634 mutations and less frequently with codon 609, 611, 618, 620, 790, and 791 mutations.[154] Parathyroid hyperplasia or adenoma in MEN2A patients may be associated with symptoms of hypercalcemia or may be subclinical with only mild increase in serum calcium levels.

FMTC is defined as the presence of MTC in kindreds with four or more affected family members, and the onset of MTC is commonly delayed until 20 to 40 years of age. Thus, in many cases it is difficult to distinguish between MEN2A and FMTC because the FMTC kindreds may have few individuals, incomplete histories, or a predominance of young individuals who have not reached an age for full penetrance of pheochromocytoma or hyperparathyroidism.[151,152] Table 7-15 summarizes available laboratory tests. Details may vary among laboratories.

TABLE 7-15

Laboratory Tests for the Management of MEN2 and FMTC

Test Name	Patient Preparation	Specimen Requirements
Calcitonin (ICMA), post calcium-pentagastrin stimulation	NPO after midnight. With the patient supine, give 20 mg/kg calcium gluconate (2 mg elemental calcium) intravenously over 1 minute, followed by pentagastrin 0.5 μg/kg as a bolus over 5 seconds. Draw blood at 0, 1, 2, 5, and 10 minutes.	3 mL frozen serum (red top tube).
Catecholamines	Avoid alcohol, coffee, tea, tobacco and strenuous exercise prior to specimen collection.	—
Plasma		• 4 mL frozen plasma (green top tube).
Random urine		• 10 mL refrigerated aliquot of 24-hour urine preserved in 25 mL of 6N HCl. Record 24-hour urine volume.
Random urine		• 10-mL refrigerated aliquot of random urine specimen.
Calcium, total, serum	Overnight fasting preferred.	1 mL refrigerated serum (red top tube).
PTH, intact (ICMA)	None.	• 2 mL refrigerated serum (red top tube). • Centrifuge and separate immediately.

MISCELLANEOUS NEOPLASIA

Papillary-follicular carcinoma and medullary carcinoma account for 99% of thyroid cancer during childhood and adolescence. Teratomas rarely present as thyroid tumors in children. Anaplastic carcinoma is an adult disease and is extremely rare in children. Primary thyroid lymphoma or neoplasia metastatic to the thyroid gland is uncommon in adults and is extremely rare in childhood.

MANAGEMENT OF THE SOLITARY NODULE

Thyroid nodules in children are uncommon, with a prevalence of 0.2% to 1.8%. Most are asymptomatic and benign, representing follicular adenomas, colloid cysts, thyroglossal duct cysts, or chronic thyroiditis. The prevalence of malignant disease approximates 20% to 25%.[127,130] Features of the history and physical examination suggesting malignancy are summarized in Table 7-16. Thyroid function tests are usually normal. However, a suppressed serum TSH level and/or an increased serum T3 concentration suggests an autonomous functioning nodule. An elevated serum calcitonin concentration and/or clinical features of MENIIb suggests medullary carcinoma. A bosselated gland in a patient with positive antithyroid peroxidase autoantibodies favors benign pseudonodularity in Hashimoto thyroiditis. Pain or local tenderness suggests suppurative thyroiditis with abscess.

Diagnostic modalities available include ultrasound, thyroid isotopic scan, FNA, and excisional biopsy. Ultrasonography is useful to rule out thyroid developmental abnormalities. FNA is recommended in the absence of malignancy features, only if an experienced aspirationist and cytopathologist are available. In experienced hands, false negative results of FNA are infrequent (2%–5%), and clinical follow-up of patients with a negative FNA result is a reasonable management alternative that is now well accepted in adult patients.[130,137] A positive or suspicious FNA result is followed by surgical excision and histopathologic examination. Radioisotope scanning in useful to confirm an autonomous nodule, and to confirm a cold (nonfunctioning) nodule in questionable cases. Surgical biopsy/excision is recommended if there are features suggesting malignancy (Table 7-16), an autonomous nodule, a positive or suspicious FNA, or a cystic lesion.

The initial approach to therapy of a thyroid nodule is surgical, with simple removal of the affected lobe. No further surgery is necessary if the mass proves to be a cystic lesion or benign adenoma. If a frozen section reveals papillary-follicular or medullary carcinoma, total thyroidectomy should be done because well-differentiated papillary-follicular carcinomas are likely to involve multifocal sites in the thyroid gland. Although accessible regional nodes should be removed, a mutilating neck dissection is not warranted.

Routine use of therapeutic dosages of radioiodine following surgery should be discussed in patients with well-differentiated thyroid carcinoma and no evidence of metastases.[128,129] However, in patients with lymph node involvement or other evidence of metastases postoperative radioiodine is mandatory to ablate any residual func-

TABLE 7-16
Clinical Features Suggesting Malignancy in Children Presenting with a Thyroid Nodule

- History of neck radiation
- Family history of medullary carcinoma
- Rapid growth of nodule
- Firm nodule
- Fixation to adjacent structures
- Vocal cord paralysis
- Enlarged regional lymph nodes
- Evidence of distant metastases

tioning thyroid tissue. Patients are then followed after surgery and radioiodine treatment by measurement of serum thyroglobulin (Tg) concentrations as a reliable tumor marker. Recombinant TSH-stimulated Tg levels greater than 2 ng/mL have been shown in adults to predict metastases 5 years later.[155]

Serum Tg levels of less than 1 ng/mL (1 μg/L) in the absence of Tg antibody in thyroid-ablated patients on thyroxine suppression therapy indicate remission. Higher values suggest metastases.[155] Supplemental whole-body ^{131}I scanning is also utilized to detect metastases. Metastatic disease is usually treated with high-dose radioiodine. Following surgery or surgery and radioiodine, the patient should be maintained on full substitution dosages of exogenous thyroid hormone to protect from any further stimulation by TSH.[128,129]

The management of medullary carcinoma includes total thyroidectomy and aggressive search for involved lymph nodes. Postoperative management includes serum calcitonin monitoring, imaging or scanning procedures [CT, MR or isotope scanning using thallium, metaiodobenzylguanidine (MIBG), and ^{99}Tc-sesta MIBI], postoperative radiation therapy, and surgery for accessible tumor recurrences. In patients without initial distant metastases and with complete tumor resection, the 20-year survival rate free of metastases approximates 80%. Overall, 10- and 20-year survival rates approximate (respectively) 60% and 40%.[156]

Future Directions

Before World War II, the focus of endocrine research was the isoloation, purification, and characterization of the major hormones; the study of their effects; and the description of the clinical syndromes resulting from hormone excess or deficiency.[157] Clinical replacement therapy using thyroid extract and synthetic cortisol were introduced. During the past 50 years, the evolution of radioisotope, immunoassay, imaging, molecular genetic, and pharmaceutic science and technologies transformed basic and clinical endocrinology and metabolism and endocrine oncology—allowing endocrinology as a clinical discipline to move progressively from the academic to the physician office environment.

The impact on pediatric endocrinology is evident comparing Williams and Wilkins' 1952 textbook *The*

Diagnosis and Treatment of Endocrine Disorders in Childhood and Adolescence (Charles C. Thomas, Springfield) with this text. The same technologies facilitating our past progress will fuel future advances: molecular genetics, molecular onology, sophisticated imaging modalities, and evolving molecular- and immunologic-based pharmaceuticals.

Likely advances for thyroid and other endocrine disease management include an expanding spectrum of molecular diagnostic testing for heritable endocrine diseases, further advances in endocrine laboratory diagnostics, improved diagnostic and prognostic genetic and proteomic markers for endocrine cancer, advances in efficacy and availability of diagnostic and management imaging for endocrine diseases, and advances in basic insights and diagnostic testing and therapies for autoimmune endocrine diseases.[157,158] Basic endocrine science is increasingly focused on the cascade of endocrine, paracrine, and autocrine pathways of hormones, growth factors, and second-messenger systems involving receptor system cascades amenable to pharmacologic perturbation.[159-162]

The ability to identify and characterize these receptor systems and to design targeted agonist or antagonist small-molecule drugs have already provided effective endocrine therapies. New molecular and proteomic advances will accelerate the progress and availability of more effective agents. Cellular, organ transplant, stem cell, and gene therapies also offer promise for major therapeutic advances.

REFERENCES

1. Fisher DA, Grueters A (2007). Thyroid disorders. In Rimoin DL, Korf BR, Pyeritz RE, Connor JM (eds.), *Principles and practice of medical genetics, Fifth edition.* New York: Churchill Livingstone 1932–1950.
2. Fisher DA, DeLange FM (1998). Thyroid hormone and iodine requirements in man during brain development. In Stanbury JB, Delange F, Dunn JT, Pandav CS (eds.), *Iodine in pregnancy.* New Delhi: Oxford University Press 1–33.
3. Carrasco N (2005). Thyroid iodine transport. In Braverman LE, Utiger RD (eds.), *The thyroid: A fundamental and clinical text, Ninth edition.* Philadelphia: Lippincott Williams & Wilkins 37–52.
4. Kim P (2006). Thyroid hormone formation. In DeGroot LJ, Jameson JL (eds.), *Endocrinology, Fifth edition.* Philadelphia: Elsevier-Saunders 1823–1836.
5. Arvin P, DiJeso B (2005). Thyroglobulin structure, function and biosynthesis. In Braverman LE, Utiger RD (eds.), *The thyroid: A fundamental and clinical text, Ninth edition.* Philadelphia: Lippincott Williams & Wilkins 77–95.
6. De Nayer P, Cornette C, Vanderschueren M, et al. (1984). Serum thyroglobulin levels in preterm neonates. Clin Endocrinol 21:149.
7. Pezzino V, Vigneri R, Squattito S, Filetti S, Camus M, Palosa P (1978). Increased serum thyroglobulin levels in patients with nontoxic goiter. J Clin Endocrinol Metab 46:653.
8. Sava L, Tomaselli L, Runello F, Belfiore A, Vigneri R (1986). Serum thyroglobulin levels are elevated in newborns from iodine deficient areas. J Clin Endocrinol Metab 62:429.
9. Kopp P (2005). Thyroid hormone synthesis. In Braverman LE, Utiger RD (eds.), *The thyroid: A fundamental and clinical text, Ninth edition.* Philadelphia: Lippincott Williams & Wilkins 52–76.
10. Hollenberg AN (2005). Regulation of thyrotropin secretion. In Braverman LE, Utiger RD (eds.), *The thyroid: A fundamental and clinical text, Ninth edition.* Philadelphia: Lippincott Williams & Wilkins 197–213.
11. Szkudlinski MW, Kazlaukaite R, Weintraub BD (2005). Thyroid stimulating hormone and regulation of the thyroid axis. In DeGroot LJ,

Jameson JL (eds.), *The thyroid: A fundamental and clinical text, Ninth edition.* Philadelphia: Lippincott Williams & Wilkins 1803–1822.
12. Benvenga S (2005). Thyroid hormone transport proteins and the physiology of hormone binding. In Braverman LE, Utiger RD (eds.), *The thyroid: A fundamental and clinical text, Ninth edition.* Philadelphia: Lippincott Williams & Wilkins 97–108.
13. Bianco AC, Larsen PR (2005). Intracellular pathway of iodothyronine metabolism. In Braverman LE, Utiger RD (eds.), *The thyroid: A fundamental and clinical text, Ninth edition.* Philadelphia: Lippincott Williams & Wilkins 109–133.
14. Wu SY, Green WL, Huang WS, et al. (2005). Alternate pathways of thyroid hormone metabolism. Thyroid 15:943.
15. Hollenberg AN, Jameson JL (2006). Mechanisms of thyroid hormone action. In DeGroot LJ, Jameson JL (eds.), *Endocrinology, Fifth edition.* Philadelphia: Elsevier-Saunders 1873–1897.
16. Yen PM (2005). Genomic and nongenomic actions of thyroid hormones. In Braverman LE, Utiger RD (eds.), *The thyroid: A fundamental and clinical text, Ninth edition.* Philadelphia: Lippincott Williams & Wilkins 135–150.
17. Weiss RE, Murata Y, Cua K, et al. (1998). Thyroid hormone action on liver, heart, and energy expenditure in thyroid hormone receptor β-deficient mice. Endocrinology 139:4945.
18. Göthe S, Wang Z, Ng L, et al. (1999). Mice devoid of all known thyroid hormone receptors are viable but exhibit disorders of the pituitary-thyroid axis, growth, and bone maturation. Genes & Devel 13:1329.
19. Jansen J, Friesema ECH, Milici C, Visser J (2005). Thyroid hormone transporters in health and disease. Thyroid 1:757.
20. Goglia F, Moreno M, Lanni A (1999). Action of thyroid hormones at the cellular level: The mitochondrial target. FEBS Letters 452:115.
21. Ponchon G, Beckers C, De Visscher M (1966). Iodine kinetic studies in newborns and infants. J Clin Endocrinol Metab 21:1392.
22. Oliner L, Kohlenbrener RM, Fields T, Kunstadter RH (1957). Thyroid function studies in children: Normal values for thyroidal I131 uptake and PBI131 levels up to the age of 18. J Clin Endocrinol Metab 17:67.
23. Beckers C, Malvaux C, De Visscher M (1966). Quantitative aspects of the secretion and degradation of thyroid hormones during adolescence. J Clin Endocrinol Metab 26:202.
24. Fisher DA, Sack J, Oddie TH, et al. (1977). Serum T4, TBG, T3 uptake, T3, reverse T3 and TSH concentrations in children 1 to 15 years of age. J Clin Endocrinol Metab 45:191.
25. Nelson JC, Clark SJ, Borut DL, et al. (1993). Age related changes in serum free thyroxine during childhood and adolescence. J Pediatr 123:899.
26. Zurakowski D, DiCanzio J, Majzoub JA (1999). Pediatric reference intervals for serum thyroxine, triiodothyronine thyrotropin, and free thyroxine. Clin Chem 45:1087.
27. Sapin R, Schlienger JL, Goichot B, et al. (1998). Evaluation of elecsys free triiodothyronine assay: Relevance of age related reference ranges. Clin Biochem 31:399.
28. Meier CA, Burger AG (2005). Effects of drugs and other substances on thyroid hormone synthesis and metabolism. In Braverman LE, Utiger RD (eds.), *The thyroid: A fundamental and clinical text, Ninth edition.* Philadelphia: Lippincott Williams & Wilkins 229–246.
29. Gaitan E (1986). Environmental goitrogens. In Van Middlesworth L, Givens JR (eds.), *The thyroid gland: A practical clinical treatise.* Chicago: Yearbook 263–280.
30. Shabana W, Delange F, Freson M, et al. (2000). Prevalence of thyroid hemiagensis: Ultrasound screening in normal children. Eur J Pediatr 159:456.
31. Maiorana R, Carta A, Floriddia G, et al. (2003). Thyroid hemiagenesis: Prevalence in normal children and effect on thyroid function. J Clin Endocrinol Metab 88:1535.
32. Weetman A (2005). Chronic autoimmune thyroiditis. In Braverman LE, Utiger RD (eds.), *The thyroid: A fundamental and clinical text, Ninth edition.* Philadelphia: Lippincott Williams & Wilkins 701–713.
33. Amino N, Hidaka Y (2006). Chronic (Hashimoto's) thyroiditis. In DeGroot LJ, Jameson JL (eds.), *Endocrinology, Fifth edition.* Philadelphia: Elsevier-Saunders 2055–2067.
34. Pearce EN, Farwell AP, Braverman LE (2003). Thyroiditis. New Engl J Med 348:2646.

35. Inoue M, Taketani N, Sato T, Nakajima H (1975). High incidence of chronic lymphocytic thyroiditis in apparently healthy school children: Epidemiological and clinical study. Endocrinol Jpn 22:483.

36. Rallison M, Dobyns BM, Keating FR, et al. (1975). Chronic lymphyocytic thyroiditis in children. J Pediatr 86:675.

37. Zois C, Stavrou I, Kalogera C, et al. (2003). The high prevalence of autoimmune thyroiditis in schoolchildren after elimination of iodine deficiency in Northeastern Greece. Thyroid 13:485.

38. Gordin A, Lamberg BA (1981). Spontaneous hypothyroidism in symptomless autoimmune thyroiditis: A long term follow-up study. Clin Endocrinol 15:537.

39. Hayashi Y, Tamai H, Fukata S, et al. (1985). A long term clinical, immunological and histological follow-up of patients with goitrous chronic lymphocytic thyroiditis. J Clin Endocrinol Metab 62:1172.

40. Roth C, Scortea M, Stubbe P, et al. (1997). Autoimmune thyroiditis in childhood: Epidemiology, clinical and laboratory findings in 61 patients. Exp Clin Endocrinol Diabetes 105(4):66–69.

41. Bright GM, Blizzard RM, Kaiser DL, Clarke WL (1982). Organ specific autoantibodies in children with common endocrine diseases. J Pediatr 100:8.

42. Girotra M, Bluestone JA, Herold JC (2006). Immunologic mechanisms causing autoimmune endocrine disease. In DeGroot LJ, Jameson JL (eds.), Endocrinology, Fifth edition. Philadelphia: Elsevier-Saunders 769–797.

43. Maclaren NK (2006). Autoimmune polyglandular syndromes. In DeGroot LJ, Jameson JL (eds.), Endocrinology, Fifth edition. Philadelphia: Elsevier-Saunders 819–835.

44. Holl RW, Böhm B, Loos U, et al. (1999). Thyroid autoimmunity in children and adolescents with type 1 diabetes mellitus. Horm Res 52:113.

45. Jordan SG, Buckingham B, Sakai R, Olson D (1981). Studies of immune complex glomerulonephritis mediated by human thyroglobulin. N Engl J Med 304:1212.

46. Hymes K, Blum M, Lackner H, Karpatkin S (1981). Easy bruising thrombocytopenia, and elevated platelet immunoglobulin G in Graves' disease and Hashimoto's thyroiditis. Ann Intern Med 94:27.

47. Valentino R, Savastano S, Tommaselli AP, et al. (1999). Prevalence of coeliac disease in patients with thyroid autoimmunity. Horm Res 51:124.

48. Pearce SHS, Kendall-Taylor P (2005). Genetic factors in thyroid disease. In Braverman LE, Utiger RD (eds.), The thyroid: A fundamental and clinical text, Ninth edition. Philadelphia: Lippincott Williams & Wilkins 407–421.

49. Christiakov DA, Turakulov RI (2003). CTLA-4 and its role in autoimmune thyroid disease. J Mol Endocrinol 31:21.

50. Rose SR (1995). Isolated central hypothyroidism in short stature. Pediatr Res 38:967.

51. Gruneiro-Papendieck L, Chiesa A, Martinez A, et al. (1998). Nocturnal TSH surge and TRH test response in the evaluation of thyroid axis in hypothalamic pituitary disorders in childhood. Horm Res 50:252.

52. van Tijn DA, de Vijlder JJM, Verbeeten B Jr., et al. (2005). Neonatal detection of congenital hypothyroidism of central origin. J Clin Endocrinol Metab 90:3350.

53. Cutler AT, Benezra-Obeiter R, Brink SJ (1986). Thyroid function in young children with Down Syndrome. Am J Dis Child 140:479.

54. Sharav T, Landau H, Zadik Z, Cinarson TR (1991). Age related patterns of thyroid stimulating hormone response to thyrotropin-releasing hormone stimulation in Down Syndrome. Am J Dis Child 145:172.

55. Ivarsson SA, Ericsson VB, Gustafsson J, et al. (1997). The impact of thyroid autoimmunity in children and adolescents with Down syndrome. Acta Paediatr 86:105.

56. Pai GS, Leach DC, Weiss L, et al. (1977). Thyroid anormalities in 20 children with Turner syndrome. J Pediatr 91:267.

57. van Trotsenburg P, Vulsma T, Rutgers van Rozenburg-Marres S, et al. (2005). The effect of thyroxine treatment started in the neonatal period on development and growth of two-year old Down Syndrome children: A randomized clinical trial. J Clin Endocrinol Metab 90:3304.

58. Lucky AW, Howley PM, Megylesi J, et al. (1977). Endocrine studies in cystinosis: Compensated primary hypothyroidism. J Pediatr 91:204.

59. Van Vliet G (2005). Hypothyroidism in infants, children and adolescents: Acquired hypothyroidism. In Braverman LE, Utiger RD (eds.), The thyroid: A fundamental and clinical text, Ninth edition. Philadelphia: Lippincott Williams and Wilkins 1041–1047.

60. Watenburg N, Greenstein D, Levine A (2006). Encephalopathy associated with Hashimoto thyroiditis: Pediatric perspective. Child Neurol 21:01.

61. Van Wyk JJ, Grumbach MM (1960). Syndrome of precocious menstruation and galacorrhea in juvenile hypothyroidism: An example of hormonal overlap in pituitary feedback. J Pediatr 57:416.

62. Hemady ZS, Siler-Khodr TM, Najjar S (1978). Precocious puberty in juvenile hypothyrodism. Pediatrics 92:55.

63. Chattopadhyay A, Kumar V, Marulaiah M (2003). Polycystic ovaries, precocious puberty and acquired hypothyroidism: The Van Wyk and Grumbach syndrome. J Ped Surg 38:1390.

64. Anasti JN, Flack MR, Frochlich J, et al. (1995). A potential novel mechanism for precocious puberty in juvenile hypothyroidism. J Clin Endocrinol Metab 80:276.

65. Rodien P, Breson C, Sanson L, et al. (1998). Familial gestational hyperthyroidism caused by a mutant thyrotropin receptor hypersensitive to human chorionic gonadotropin. N Engl J Med 17:339.

66. Montanelli M, Delbaere A, Di Carlo C, et al. (2004). A mutation in the follicle-stimulating hormone receptor as a cause of familial spontaneous ovarian hyperstimulation syndrome. J Clin Endocrinol Metab 89:1255.

67. Abbassi V, Aldige C (1977). Evaluation of sodium L-thyroxine (T4) requirement in replacement therapy of hypothyroidism. J Pediatr 90:298.

68. Rezvani IR, DiGeorge AM (1977). Reassessment of the daily dose of oral thyroxine for replacement therapy in hypothyroid children. J Pediatr 90:291.

69. Niimi H, Sasaki N, Inomota H, Nakajima H (1980). Evaluation of L-thyroxine requirement in treatment of congenital hypothyroidism. Endocrinol Jpn 27:733.

70. DeGroot LJ (2006). Nonthyroidal illness syndrome. In DeGroot LJ, Jameson JL (eds.), Endocrinology, Fifth edition. Philadelphia: Elsevier-Saunders 2101–2112.

71. Wiersinga WM (2005). Nonthyroidal illness. In Braverman LE, Utiger RD (eds.), The thyroid: A fundamental and clinical text, Ninth edition. Philadelphia: Lippincott Williams & Wilkins 247–263.

72. Peeters RP, Kester MHA, Wouters PJ, et al. (2005). Increased thyroxine sulfate levels in critically ill patients as a result of adecreased hepatic type 1 deiodinase level. J Clin Endocrinol Metab 90:6460.

73. Yu J, Koenig RJ (2006). Induction of type 1 iodothyronine deiodinase to prevent the nonthyroidal illness syndrome in mice. Endocrinology 147:3580.

74. Peeters RP, van der Geyten S, Wouters PJ, et al. (2005). Tissue thyroid hormone levels in critical illness. J Clin Endocrinol Metab 90:6498.

75. DeGroot LJ (1999). Dangerous dogmas in medicine: The nonthyroidal illness syndrome. J Clin Endocrinol Metab 84:151.

76. Delange FM, Dunn JT (2005). Iodine deficiency. In Braverman LE, Utiger RD (eds.), The thyroid: A fundamental and clinical text, Ninth edition. Philadelphia: Lippincott Williams & Wilkins 264–288.

77. Fenzi GF, Giusti LF, Aghini-Lombardi F, et al. (1990). Neuropsychological assessment in schoolchildren from an area of moderate iodine deficiency. J Endocrinol Invest 13:427.

78. Vermiglio F, Sidoti M, Finocchiaro MD, et al. (1990). Defective neuromotor and cognitive ability in iodine-deficient schoolchildren of an endemic goiter region in Sicily. J Clin Endocrinol Metab 70:379.

79. Huang SA, Tu HM, Harney JW, et al. (2000). Severe hypothyroidism caused by a type 3 iodothyronine deiodinase in infantile hemangiomas. N Engl J Med 343:185.

80. Gaven A, Aygun C, Ince H, et al. (2005). Severe hypothyroidism caused by hepatic hemangioendothelioma in an infant of a diabetic mother. Horm Res 63:86.

81. Ruppe MD, Huang SA, Jan de Beur SM (2005). Consumptive hypothyroidism caused by paraneoplastic production of type 3 iodothyronine deiodinase. Thyroid 15:1369.

82. Bayer Y, Neumann S, Meyer B, et al. (2004). Genome-wide linkage analysis reveals evidence for four new susceptibility loci for familial euthyroid goiter. J Clin Endocrinol Metab 89:4044.

83. Hermus Ad R, Huysmans DA (2005). Pathogenesis of nontoxic diffuse and nodular goiter and clinical manifestations and treatment of nontoxic diffuse and nodular goiter. Braverman LE, Utiger RD (eds.), The thyroid: A fundamental and clinical text,

Ninth edition. Philadelphia: Lippincott Williams & Wilkins 873–885.

84. Drexhage HA, Botazzo GF, Doniach D, et al. (1980). Evidence for thyroid growth stimulating immunoglobulins in some goitrous thyroid diseases. Lancet 2:287.

85. Fisher DA, Pandian PR, Carlton E (1987). Autoimmune thyroid disease: An expanding spectrum. Pediatr Clin N Am 34:907.

86. Smyth PPA, McMullan NM, Grubek-Loebenstein B, O'Donovan DK (1986). Thyroid growth stimulating immunoglobulins in goitrous disease: Relationship to thyroid stimulating immunoglobulins. Acta Endocrinol 111:321.

87. Wadeleux PA, Winand RJ (1986). Thyroid growth modulating factors in the sera of patients with simple non-toxic goiter. Acta Endocrinol 112:502.

88. Guimaraes VC (2006). Subacute and Reidel's thyroiditis. In DeGroot LJ, Jameson JL (eds.), *Endocrinology, Fifth edition.* Philadelphia: Lippincott Williams & Wilkins 2069–2080.

89. Volpé R (1985). Subacute thyroiditis. In Delange F, Fisher DA, Malvaux P (eds.), *Pediatric thyroidology.* Basel: Karger 252–264.

90. Farwell AP (2005). Infectious thyroiditis. In Braverman LE, Utiger RD (eds.), *The thyroid: A fundamental and clinical text, Ninth edition.* Philadelphia: Lippincott Williams & Williams 536–547.

91. Miyauchi A, Matsuzuka F, Kuma K, Takai S (1990). Pyriform sinus fistula: an underlying abnormality common in patients with acute suppurative thyroiditis. World J Surg 14:400.

92. Musharrafieh UM, Nassar NT, Azar ST (2002). Acute suppurative thyroiditis: A forgotten entity, Case report and literature review. The Endocrinologist 12:173.

93. Rauhofer U, Prager G, Hosmann M, et al. (2003). Cystic echinococcosis of the thyroid gland in children and adults. Thyroid 13:497.

94. Auram AM, Sturm CA, Michael CW, et al. (2004). Cryptococcal thyroiditis and hyperthyroidism. Thyroid 14:471.

95. McLanghlin SA, Smith SL, Meek SE (2006). Acute suppurative thyroiditis caused by pasteurella multocida and associated with thyrotoxicosis. Thyroid 16:307.

96. Davies TS (2005). Pathogenesis of Graves' disease. In Braverman LE, Utiger RD (eds.), *The thyroid: A fundamental and clinical text, Ninth edition.* Philadelphia: Lippincott William & Wilkins 457–473.

97. Gianoukakis AG, Douglas RS, King CS, et al. (2006). Immunoglobulin G from patients with Graves' disease induces interleukin-16 and RANTES expression in cultured human thyrocytes: A putative mechanism for T-cell infiltration of the thyroid in autoimmune disease. Endocrinology 147:1941.

98. Zimmerman D, Hayles AB (1985). Hyperthyroidism in children. In Delange F, Fisher DA, Malvaux P (eds.), *Pediatric thyroidology.* Basel: Karger 223.

99. Segni M, Leonardi E, Mazzaoncini B, et al. (1999). Special features of Graves' disease in early childhood. Thyroid 9:881.

100. Perrild H, Grüters-Kieslich A, Feldt-Rasmussen U, et al. (1994). Diagnosis and treatment of thyrotoxicosis in childhood: A European quentionnaire study. Eur J Endocrinol 131:467.

101. Shulman DI, Muhar I, Jorgensen EV, et al. (1997). Autoimmune hyperthyroidism in prepubertal children and adolescents: Comparison of clinical and biochemical features at diagnosis and response to medical therapy. Thyroid 7:755.

102. Hamburger JL (1985). Management of hyperthyroidism in children and adolescents. J Clin Endocrinol Metab 60:1019.

103. Rivkees SA, Sklar C, Freemark M (1998). The management of Graves' disease in children with special emphasis on radioiodine treatment. J Clin Endocrinol Metab 83:3767.

104. Read CH Jr., Tansey MJ, Menda Y (2004). A 36 year retrospective analysis of the efficacy and safety of radioactive iodine in treating young Graves' patients. J Clin Endocrinol Metab 89:4229.

105. Rivkees S (2004). Radioactive iodine use in childhood Graves' disease: Time to wake up and smell the I-131. J Clin Endocrinol Metab 89:4227.

106. Marchant B, Lees JFH, Alexander WD (1979). Antithyroid drugs. In Hershman JM, Bray GA (eds.), *The thyroid: Physiology and treatment of disease.* Oxford: Pergamon Press 209–252.

107. Shen DC, Wu SY, Chopra IJ, et al. (1985). Long term treatment of Graves' hyperthyroidism with sodium ipodate. J Clin Endocrinol Metab 61:723.

108. Wu SY, Shyh TP, Chopra IJ, et al. (1982). Comparison of sodium ipodate (Oragrafin) and propylthiouracil in early treatment of hyperthyroidism. J Clin Endocrinol Metab 54:630.

109. Bal CS, Kumar A, Chandra P (2005). Effect of Iopanoic acid on radioiodine therapy of hyperthyroidism: Long term outcome of a randomized control study. J Clin Endocrinol Metab 90:6536.

110. Glaser NS, Styne DM (1997). Predictors of early remission of hyperthyroidism in children. J Clin Endocrinol Metab 82:1719.

111. Tolis G, Bird C, Bertrand G, et al. (1978). Pituitary hyperthyroidism: Case report and review of the literature. Am J Med 64:177.

112. Beck Peccoz P, Persani L (2005). Thyrotropin-induced thyrotoxicosis. In Braverman LE, Utiger RD (eds.), *The thyroid: A fundamental and clinical text, Ninth edition.* Philadelphia: Lippincott Williams & Wilkins 500–507.

113. Shigakazu S, Nakamura H, Tagami T, et al. (1993). Pituitary resistance to thyroid hormone associated with a base mutation in the hormone binding domain of the human 3,5,3' triiodothyronine receptor β. J Clin Endocrinol Metab 76:1254.

114. Mixson AJ, Renault JC, Ransom S, et al. (1993). Identification of a novel mutation in the gene encoding the β-triiodothyronine receptor in a patient with apparent selective pituitary resistance to thyroid hormone. Clin Endocrinol 38:227.

115. Rosler A, Litvin Y, Hoge C, et al. (1982). Familial hyperthyroidism due to inappropriate thyrotropin secretion successfully treated with triiodothyronine. J Clin Endocrinol Metab 54:76.

116. Beck Peccoz P, Piscitelli G, Cattaneo MG, et al. (1983). Successful treatment of hyperthyroidism due to non-neoplastic pituitary TSH secretion with 2,5,3'-triiodothyroacetic acid (TRIAC). J Endocrinol Invest 6:217.

117. Abe K, Konno M, Sato T, Matsuura N (1980). Hyperfunctioning thyroid nodules in children. Am J Dis Child 134:961.

118. Osburne RC, Goren EN, Bybee DE, Johnsonbaugh RE (1982). Autonomous thyroid nodules in adolescents: Clinical characteristics and results of TRH testing. J Pediatr 100:383.

119. Kaplan MM (2005). Clinical evaluation and management of solitary thyroid nodules. In Braverman LE, Utiger RD (eds.), *The thyroid: A fundamental and clinical text, Ninth edition.* Philadelphia: Lippincott Williams & Wilkins 996–1010.

120. Kopp P, Muirhead S, Jourdain N, et al. (1997). Congenital hyperthyroidism caused by a solitary toxic adenoma harboring a novel somatic mutation (serene 281-isoleucine) in the extracellular domain of the thyrotropin receptor. J Clin Invest 100:1634.

121. Duprez L, Parma J, Van Sande J, et al. (1998). TSH receptor mutations and thyroid disease. Trends in Endocrinol 9:133.

122. Grueters A, Schonberg T, Bieberman H, et al. (1998). Severe congenital hyperthyroidism caused by a germline neomutation in the extracellular portion of the thyrotropin receptor. J Clin Endocrinol Metab 83:1431.

123. Vassart G (2006). Thyroid stimulating hormone receptor mutations. In DeGroot LJ, Jameson JL (eds.), *Endocrinology, Fifth edition.* Philadelphia: Elsevier-Saunders 2191–2200.

124. Weinstein LS, Shenker A, Gejman PV, et al. (1991). Activating mutations of the stimulating G protein in the McCune Albright syndrome. N Engl J Med 325;1688.

125. Pacini F, DeGroot LJ (2006). Thyroid neoplasia. In DeGroot LJ, Jameson JL (eds.), *Endocrinology, Fifth edition.* Philadelphia: Elsevier-Saunders 2147–2180.

126. Schlumberger MJ (1998). Papillary and follicular thyroid carcinoma. N Engl J Med 338:297.

127. Hung W (1999). Solitary thyroid nodules in 93 children and adolescents. Horm Res 52:15.

128. Hung W, Sarlis N (2002). Current controversies in the management of pediatric patients with well differentiated, nonmedullary cancer: A review. Thyroid 8:683.

129. Bauer AJ, Tuttle RM, Francis GL (2002). Differentiated thyroid carcinoma of children and adolescents. The Endocrinologist 12:135.

130. Raab SS, Silverman JF, Elsheikh TM, et al. (1995). Pediatric thyroid nodules: Disease demographics and clinical management as determined by fine needle aspiration biopsy. Pediatrics 95:46.

131. Mechanick JI (1992). Thyroid cancer in the pediatric patient. In Cobin RH, Sirota DK (eds.), *Malignant tumors of the thyroid.* New York: Springer Verlag 45–64.

132. Lam KY, Lo CY, Kwong DLW, et al. (1999). Malignant lymphoma of the thyroid. Am J Clin Pathol 112:263.

133. Shore RE, Hildreth N, Dvoretsky P, et al. (1993). Thyroid cancer among persons given x-ray treatment in infancy for an enlarged thymus gland. Am J Epidemiol 137:1068.

134. Winship T, Rosvoll RV (1970). Thyroid carcinoma in children: Final report and 20 year study. Clin Proc Child Hosp (Washington, DC) 26:327.

135. Robbins J, Schneider AB (1998). Radioiodine induced thyroid cancer: Studies in the aftermath of the accident at chernobyl. Trends in Metabolism 3:87.

136. Astakhova LN, Asnpaugh LR, Beebe GW, et al. (1998). Chernobyl-related thyroid cancer in children of Belarus: A case-control study. Radiation Res 150:349.

137. Khurana KK, Labrador E, Izquierdo R, et al. (1999). The role of fine needle aspiration biopsy in the management of thyroid nodules in children adolescents and young adults: A multi-institutional study. Thyroid 9:383.

138. Learoyd DL, Twigg SM, Zedenius JV, Robinson BG (1998). The molecular genetics of endocrine tumors. J Ped Endocrinol Metab 11:195.

139. Fenton CL, Lukes Y, Nicholson D, et al. (2000). The RET/PTC mutations are common in sporadic papillary thyroid carcinoma of children and young adults. J Clin Endocrinol Metab 85:1170.

140. Motomura T, Nikiforov YE, Namka H, et al. (1998). RET proto-oncogene in Japanese pediatric and adult papillary thyroid cancers. Thyroid 8:485.

141. Klugbauer S, Rabes HM (1999). The transcription coactivator HTIF-1 and a related protein are fused to the RET receptor tyrosine kinase in childhood papillary thyroid carcinomas. Oncogene 18:4388.

142. Pisarchik AV, Ermak G, Fornicheva V, et al. (1998). The RET/PTCI rearrangement is a common feature of chernobyl-associated papillary thyroid carcinomas from Belarus. Thyroid 1998,8:133.

143. Suchy B, Waldmann V, Klughauer S, Rabes HM (1998). Absence of RAS and p53 mutations in thyroid carcinomas of children after chernobyl in contrast to adult thyroid tumors. Brit J Cancer 11:195.

144. Xing M, Westra WH, Tufano RP, et al. (2005). BRAF mutation predicts a poorer clinical prognosis for papillary thyroid cancer. J Clin Endocrinol Metab 90:6373.

145. Penko K, Livezey J, Fenton C, et al. (2005). BRAF mutations are uncommon in papillary thyroid cancer of young patients. Thyroid 4:320.

146. Weber F, Shen L, Aldred MA, et al. (2005). Genetic classification of benign and malignant thyroid follicular neoplasia based on a three gene combination. J Clin Endocrinol Metab 90:2512.

147. Eszlinger M, Wiench M, Jarzab B, et al. (2006). Meta and reanalysis of gene expression profiles of hot and cold thyroid nodules and papillary thyroid carcinoma for gene chips. J Clin Endocrinol Metab 91:1934.

148. Chi DD, Moley JE (1998). Medullary thyroid carcinoma. Surg Oncol Clin N Amer 7:681.

149. Learoyd DL, Lim LC, Robinson BG (2006). Medullary thyroid carcinoma. In DeGroot LJ, Jameson JL (eds.), Endocrinology, Fifth edition. Philadelphia: Elsevier-Saunders 2181–2190.

150. Marsh DJ, Mulligan LM, Eng C (1997). RET proto-oncogene mutations in multiple endocrine neoplasia type 2 and medullary thyroid carcinoma. Horm Res 47:168.

151. Kouvaraki MA, Shapiro SE, Perrier NO, et al. (2005). RET proto-oncogene: A review and update of genotype-phenotype correlations in hereditary medullary thyroid cancer and associated endocrine tumors. Thyroid 15:531.

152. Iler MA, King DR, Ginn-Pease ME, et al. (1999). Multiple endocrine neoplasia, type 2A: A 25 year review. J Pediatr Surg 34:92.

153. Dvorakova S, Vaclavikova E, Sykorova V, et al. (2006). New multiple somatic mutations in the RET proto-oncogene associated with a sporadic medullary thyroid carcinoma. Thyroid 16:311.

154. Rave F, Kraimps JL, Dralle H, et al. (1995). Primary hyperparathyroidism in multiple endocrine neoplasia type 2A. J Intern Med 238:369.

155. Kloos RT, Mazzaferri EL (2005). A single recombinant human thyrotropin-stimulated serum thyroglobulin measurement predicts differentiated thyroid carcinoma metastases three to five years later. J Clin Endocrinol Metab 90:5047.

156. Kaplan EL (2005). Surgery of the thyroid. In DeGroot LJ, Jameson JL (eds.), Endocrinology, Fifth edition. Philadelphia: WB Saunders 2239–2260.

157. Fisher DA (2004). A short history of pediatric endocrinology in North America. Pediatr Res 55:716.

158. Wilson JD (2004). Prospects for research for disorders of the endocrine system. JAMA 285:624.

159. Smith CL, Nawaz Z, O'Malley BW (1997). Coactivator and corepressor regulation of the agonist/antagonist activity of the mixed antiestrogen, 4-hydroxytamoxifen. Mol Endocrinol 11:657.

160. McKenna NJ, Xu J, Nawaz Z, et al. (1999). Nuclear receptor coactivators: Multiple enzymes, multiple complexes, multiple functions. J Steroid Biochem Mol Biol 69:3.

161. Baxter JD, Dillmann WH, Wes BL, et al. (2001). Selective modulation of thyroid hormone receptor action. J Steroid Biochem Mol Biol 76:31.

162. Miner JN, Chang W, Chapman MS, et al. (2007). An orally active selective androgen receptor modulator is efficacious on bone, muscle, and sex function with reduced impact on prostate. Endocrinology 148:363.

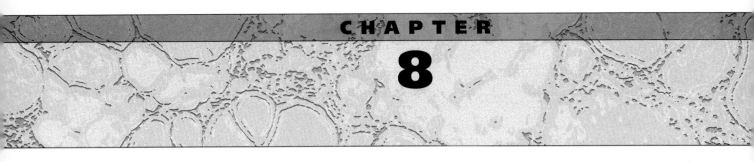

CHAPTER 8

Disorders of Growth Hormone/ Insulin-like Growth Factor Secretion and Action

RON G. ROSENFELD, MD • PINCHAS COHEN, MD

Normal Growth

The most fundamental characteristic of childhood is that it is a time of growth. As multifactorial and complex as the process of growth is, children normally grow in a remarkably predictable manner. Deviation from a normal pattern of growth can be the first manifestation of a wide variety of disease processes, including endocrine and nonendocrine disorders and involving virtually any organ system of the body. Frequent and accurate assessment of growth is, therefore, of primary importance to physicians and nurses caring for children.

MEASUREMENT

Assessment of statural growth necessitates optimizing accuracy in height determinations.[1-3] When feasible, measurement of supine length is employed in children younger than 2 years of age—and that of erect height is done in older children. The inherent inaccuracies involved in measuring length in infants are often obscured by the rapid skeletal growth normally characteristic of this age. For measurement of supine length, it is best to employ a firm box with an inflexible board (against which the head lies) and a movable footboard on which the feet are placed perpendicular to the plane of the supine infant. Optimally, the child needs to be relaxed—with the legs fully extended and the head positioned in the "Frankfurt plane" (with the line connecting the outer canthus of the eyes and the external auditory meatus perpendicular to the long axis of the trunk).

When children are old enough to stand erect (and physically capable of doing so), it is best to employ a wall-mounted "Harpenden" stadiometer similar to that designed by Tanner and Whitehouse for the British Harpenden Growth Study. Freestanding stadiometers are also available but require frequent recalibration. The traditional measuring device of a flexible arm mounted to a weight balance is notoriously unreliable and cannot be counted on to provide accurate serial measurements.

As with length measurements in infants, positioning of the child is critical. The patient should be fully erect, with the head in the Frankfurt plane. The back of the head, thoracic spine, buttocks, and heels should be touching the vertical axis of the stadiometer and one another. Every effort should be made to correct discrepancies related to lordosis or scoliosis. Ideally, serial measurements should be made at the same time of day because diurnal variation in standing height has been observed.[4]

It is critical that height determinations be performed by an individual with proper training, rather than (as is often the case) by an inexperienced member of the staff. We recommend that lengths and heights be measured in triplicate, that variation be no more than 0.3 cm, and that the mean height be recorded. For determination of height velocity, it is obviously best to have the same individual performing the determinations. Even when every effort is made to maximize the precision of height determinations, a minimum interval of 3 months is necessary for accurate height velocity computation. Six months' data are preferable, although it is of note that seasonal variation in height velocity has been reported.[5]

GROWTH CHARTS

Evaluation of a child's height must be done in the context of normal standards. Such standards can be either cross-sectional or longitudinal. Most American pediatric endocrine clinics continue to use the cross-sectional data provided by the National Center for Health Statistics (NCHS), which were originally introduced in 1977 and recently updated.[6-8] Epidemiologic limitations in these growth charts have been noted, however. The data included in the original infant charts, for example, were derived from a private study of a group of subjects who were primarily white, formula-fed, middle-class infants from southwestern Ohio. Data employed for older children came from national health examination surveys conducted from 1963 to 1974.

The NCHS (now a part of the Centers for Disease Control and Prevention) has provided a set of new growth charts, representing revisions of the previous charts, and has introduced new charts for body mass index[9] (Figures 8-1 through 8-8). Interestingly, the new charts show little change in average height over the past 25 years despite the common perception that today's children are taller than peers from 10 to 25 years ago. This is in contrast to other countries (in particular, Holland), where mean height continues to rise in spite of being the tallest in the world—and many current and formerly developing countries in which the population (which was typically shorter than in the Western world) is becoming taller.

Classic percentile-based growth charts are invaluable for plotting growth of children relative to the 3rd or 5th, 10th, 25th, 50th, 75th, 90th, and 95th or 97th percentiles of normal American children. There are, however, two major limitations of these charts. First, they do not satisfactorily define the growth rates of children below the 3rd or above the 97th percentile—the very children for whom it is most critical to accurately describe the degree to which their growth deviates from the normal growth centiles.

The NCHS data can be used to compute standard deviation (SD) scores (or Z scores), which are more helpful because a short child can be described as having a

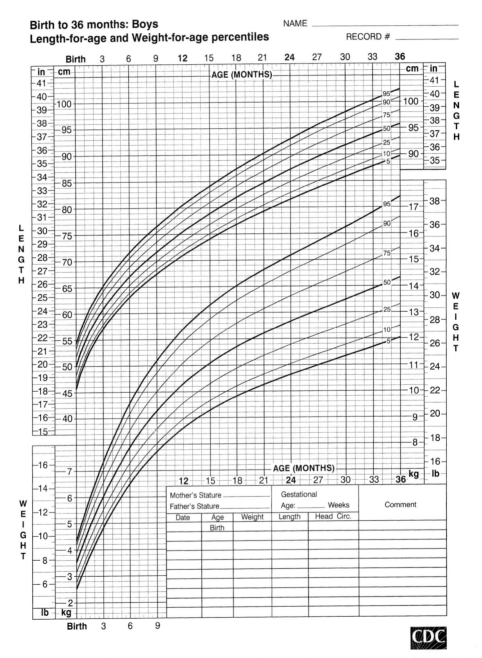

FIGURE 8-1. Length-for-age and weight-for-age percentiles for boys (birth to 36 months). (Developed by the National Center for Health Statistics in collaboration with the National Center for Chronic Disease Prevention and Health Promotion [2000]. http:www.cdc.gov/growthcharts.)

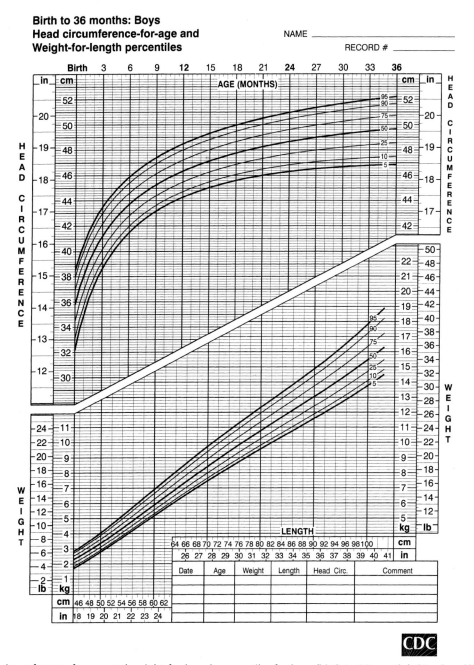

FIGURE 8-2. Head circumference-for-age and weight-for-length percentiles for boys (birth to 36 months). (Developed by the National Center for Health Statistics in collaboration with the National Center for Chronic Disease Prevention and Health Promotion [2000]. http:www.cdc.gov/growthcharts.)

growth rate of (for example) 2 or 2.5 SD from normal. Because these SDs are defined by cross-sectional data, however, SD scores during childhood are not directly comparable with SD scores during adolescence—when great variation in growth rates can be normally observed. Second, cross-sectional data are of greater value during infancy and childhood than in adolescence—when differences in the timing of puberty can introduce considerable variability into normal growth rates. To address this issue, Tanner and colleagues[10] have developed longitudinal growth charts that accommodate the timing of puberty. These charts are of greatest value in assessing

growth during adolescence and puberty, and are probably superior for plotting sequential growth data on any given child.

The data from cross-sectional and longitudinal growth studies have been employed to develop height velocity standards[10] (Figures 8-9 and 8-10). It is important to emphasize that carefully documented height velocity data are invaluable in assessing the child with abnormalities of growth. Although considerable variability exists in the normal height velocity observed in children of different ages, between the age of 2 years and the onset of puberty children normally grow with remarkable fidelity

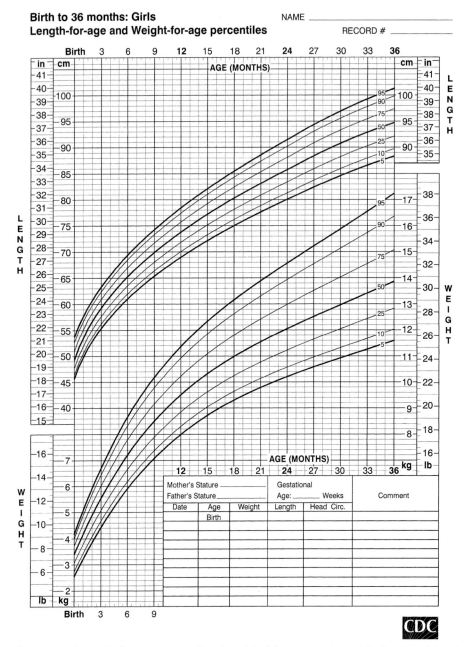

FIGURE 8-3. Length-for-age and weight-for-age percentiles for girls (birth to 36 months). (Developed by the National Center for Health Statistics in collaboration with the National Center for Chronic Disease Prevention and Health Promotion [2000]. http:www.cdc.gov/growthcharts.)

relative to the normal growth curves. Any "crossing" of height percentiles during this age period should be noted by the physician, and abnormal height velocities always warrant further evaluation.

Disease-related growth curves have been developed for a number of clinical conditions associated with growth failure, such as Turner syndrome,[11] achondroplasia,[12] and Down syndrome. Such growth profiles are invaluable for tracking the growth of children with these clinical conditions. Deviation of growth from the appropriate disease-related growth curve suggests the possibility of a second underlying condition.

BODY PROPORTIONS

Many abnormal growth states, including short stature and excessive stature, are characterized by disproportionate growth. The following determinations should be made as part of the evaluation of short stature.
- Occipitofrontal head circumference
- Lower body segment: distance from top of pubic symphysis to the floor
- Upper body segment: sitting height (height of stool should be subtracted from standing height)
- Arm span

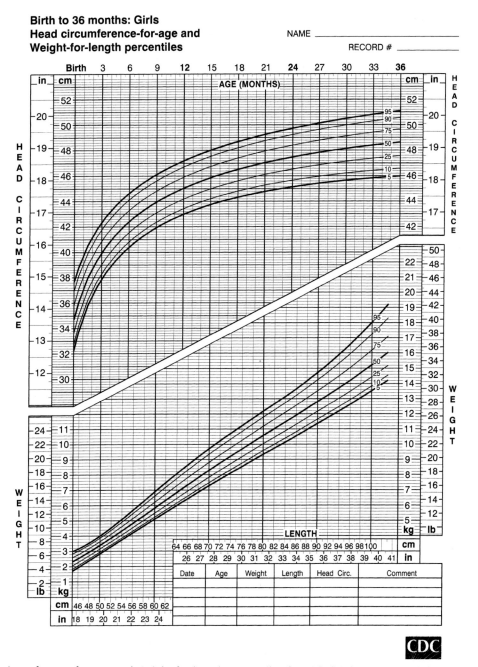

Birth to 36 months: Girls
Head circumference-for-age and
Weight-for-length percentiles

FIGURE 8-4. Head circumference-for-age and weight-for-length percentiles for girls (birth to 36 months). (Developed by the National Center for Health Statistics in collaboration with the National Center for Chronic Disease Prevention and Health Promotion [2000]. http:www.cdc.gov/growthcharts.)

Published standards exist for these body proportion measurements, which must be evaluated relative to the patient's age.[13] The upper segment to lower segment ratio, for example, ranges from 1.7 in the neonate to slightly below 1.0 in the adult.

SKELETAL MATURATION

The growth potential inherent in the tubular bones of the body can be assessed by evaluation of the progression of ossification within the epiphyses. The ossification centers of the skeleton appear and progress in a predictable se-

quence in normal children, and skeletal maturation can therefore be compared with normal age-related standards. This forms the basis of "bone age" or "skeletal age." It is not clear what factors determine this normal maturational pattern, but it is certain that genetic factors and multiple hormones [including thyroxine (T4), growth hormone (GH), and sex steroids] are involved in this process.

Studies in patients with mutations of the gene for the estrogen receptor[14] or for aromatase enzyme[15] have demonstrated that it is estrogen that is primarily responsible for ultimate epiphyseal fusion, although it seems unlikely that estrogen is alone responsible for all skeletal maturation.

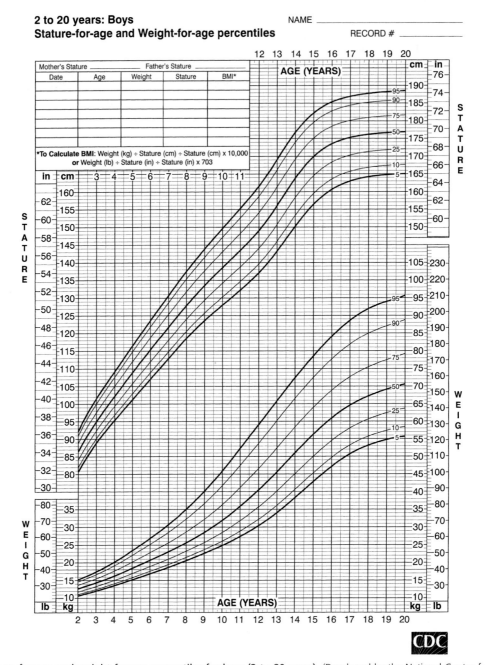

2 to 20 years: Boys
Stature-for-age and Weight-for-age percentiles

FIGURE 8-5. Stature-for-age and weight-for-age percentiles for boys (2 to 20 years). (Developed by the National Center for Health Statistics in collaboration with the National Center for Chronic Disease Prevention and Health Promotion [2000]. http:www.cdc.gov/growthcharts.)

Beyond the neonatal period, a radiograph of the left hand and wrist is commonly used for determination of bone age—which can be related to the published standards of Greulich and Pyle.[16] An alternative method for assessment of bone age from radiographs of the left hand, involving a scoring system for each individual bone, has been developed by Tanner and Whitehouse and their colleagues.[17] The left hand obviously represents a compromise, because radiographs of the entire skeleton would be tedious and expensive and necessitate excessive radiation exposure. It is important to note, however, that the hand obviously does not contribute to the height of an individual and that accurate evaluation of growth potential might necessitate radiographs of the legs and spine.

A number of important caveats concerning bone age must be considered. Experience in determination of bone age is essential, and clinical studies involving bone age generally benefit from having a single reader who does all interpretations. Second, the normal rate of skeletal maturation differs between males and females (and ethnic variability exists). The standards of Greulich and Pyle are divided by sex but were developed in American white children. Finally, the Greulich-Pyle and the Tanner-Whitehouse standards were developed using normal children.[18] They are not necessarily applicable to children with skeletal dysplasias, endocrine abnormalities, or a variety of other causes of growth retardation.

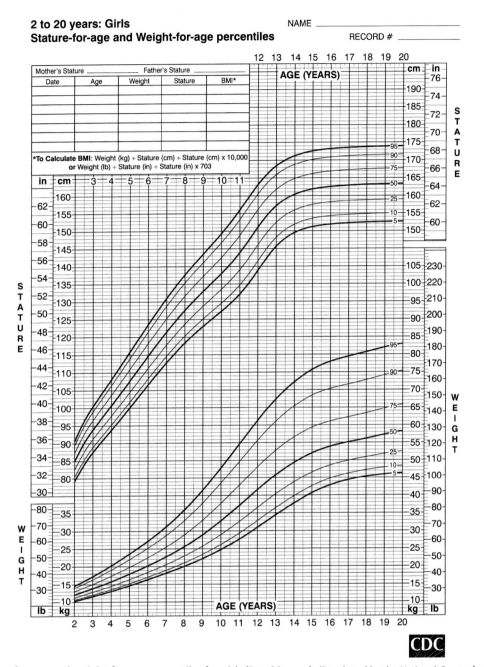

FIGURE 8-6. Stature-for-age and weight-for-age percentiles for girls (2 to 20 years). (Developed by the National Center for Health Statistics in collaboration with the National Center for Chronic Disease Prevention and Health Promotion [2000]. http:www.cdc.gov/growthcharts.)

PREDICTION OF ADULT HEIGHT

The extent of skeletal maturation observed in a patient can be employed to predict the patient's ultimate height potential. Such predictions are based on the observation that the more delayed the bone age (relative to the chronologic age) the greater the length of time before epiphyseal fusion prevents further growth. The classic method for height prediction, based on Greulich and Pyle's *Radiographic Atlas of Skeletal Development*,[16] was developed by Bayley and Pinneau[19] and relies on the patient's bone age and height (Table 8-1).

Additional refinements were introduced by Tanner and colleagues[17,20] (whose system employs height, bone age, and chronologic age) and by Roche and associates,[21] who employ the combination of height, bone age, chronologic age, mid-parental height, and weight. All of these systems are by nature empirical and should never be used as absolute predictors. The more advanced the bone age the greater the accuracy of the adult height prediction, but this is natural because a more advanced bone age places a patient closer to final height.

All of these methods of predicting adult height are based on data from normal children. None of these systems has

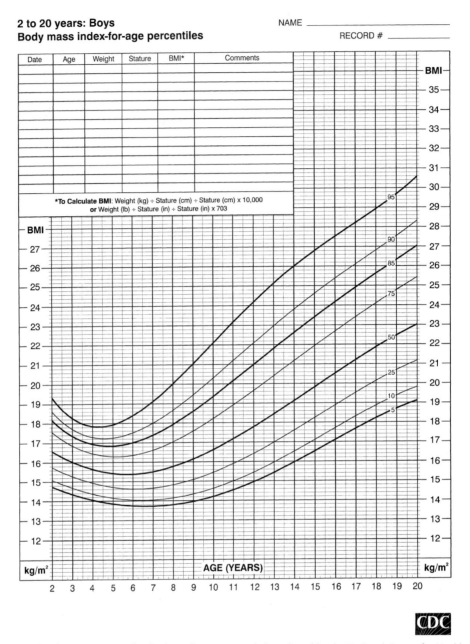

2 to 20 years: Boys
Body mass index-for-age percentiles

NAME _____

RECORD # _____

*To Calculate BMI: Weight (kg) ÷ Stature (cm) ÷ Stature (cm) x 10,000
or Weight (lb) ÷ Stature (in) ÷ Stature (in) x 703

FIGURE 8-7. Body mass index-for-age percentiles for boys (2 to 20 years). (Developed by the National Center for Health Statistics in collaboration with the National Center for Chronic Disease Prevention and Health Promotion [2000]. http:www.cdc.gov/growthcharts.)

been demonstrated to be accurate in children with growth abnormalities. For this type of precision, it would be necessary to develop disease-specific (e.g., achondroplasia, Turner syndrome) atlases of skeletal maturation. Recent retrospective analyses indicate that bone-age-based adult height prediction slightly under-predict female but often over-predict male children's eventual height. Predictions are also notoriously inaccurate in children born small for gestational age.

PARENTAL TARGET HEIGHT

Because genetic factors are of great importance as determinants of growth and height potential, it is always worthwhile to assess a patient's stature relative to that of siblings

and parents. The parental target height can be readily ascertained by calculating the mean parental height and adding or subtracting 6.5 cm for male or female children, respectively. The standard deviation for this calculated parental target height is about 2.5 cm, and the range within which it is likely to occur 95% of the time is approximately 6 to 10 cm. As with predicted adult heights, calculated target heights should be taken as approximations.

Nevertheless, when a child's growth pattern clearly deviates from that of parents or siblings one must seriously consider the possibility of an underlying pathologic process. It is important, when possible, to measure the heights of parents and siblings rather than accepting their own statural claims. In addition, one should recall that it is not always possible to know the heights of the true

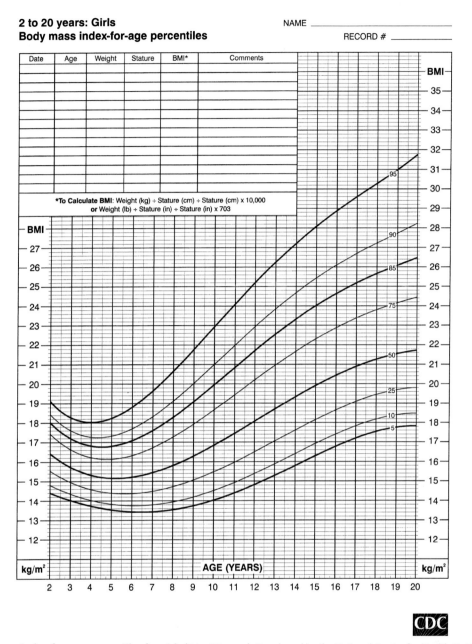

2 to 20 years: Girls
Body mass index-for-age percentiles

NAME _____

RECORD # _____

*To Calculate **BMI**: Weight (kg) ÷ Stature (cm) ÷ Stature (cm) x 10,000
or Weight (lb) ÷ Stature (in) ÷ Stature (in) x 703

FIGURE 8-8. Body mass index-for-age percentiles for girls (2 to 20 years). Developed by the National Center for Health Statistics in collaboration with the National Center for Chronic Disease Prevention and Health Promotion [2000]. http:www.cdc.gov/growthcharts.)

biologic parents (or, sometimes, who the real biologic parents actually are). Finally, short parents are not an excuse to avoid working up a child who is clearly short because this may represent a treatable genetic disorder within the growth hormone signaling cascade.

Endocrine Regulation of Growth

THE PITUITARY

The concept of the pituitary as a "master gland" controlling the endocrine activities of the body has become outdated and has been replaced by an appreciation of the importance of the brain, particularly of the hypothalamus in regulating hormonal production and secretion. Nevertheless, the pituitary gland remains central to our understanding of the regulation of growth.

Embryologically, the pituitary gland is formed from two distinct sources.[22,23] Rathke's pouch, a diverticulum of the primitive oral cavity (stomodeal ectoderm), gives rise to the adenohypophysis. The neurohypophysis originates in the neural ectoderm of the floor of the forebrain, which also develops into the third ventricle. The adenohypophysis normally constitutes 80% of the weight of the pituitary and consists of the pars distalis (also known as the pars anterior or anterior lobe), the pars intermedia (also known as the intermediate lobe), and

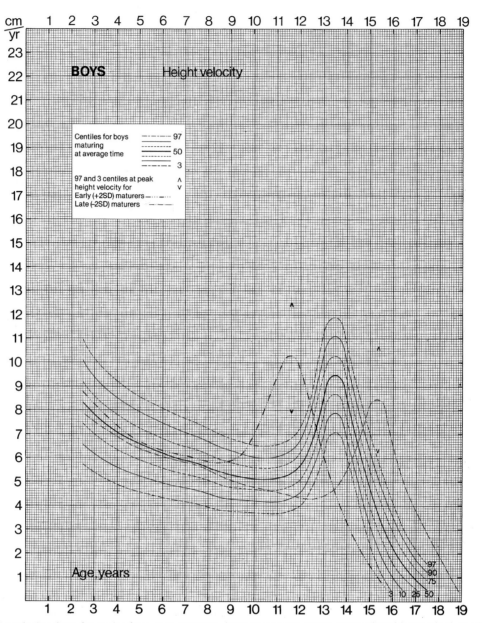

FIGURE 8-9. Height velocity chart for males from 0 to 19 years. (From Tanner JM, Davies SWD: Clinical longitudinal standards for height and height velocity for North American children. J Pediatr 107:312, 1985.)

the pars tuberalis (also known as the pars infundibularis or pars proximalis).

In humans, the pars distalis is the largest portion of the adenohypophysis and houses the great majority of hormone-producing cells. The pars intermedia is, typically, poorly developed and consists of several cystic cavities lined by a single layer of cuboidal epithelium. The pars tuberalis represents an upward extension of the pars distalis onto the pituitary stalk and may contain a limited number of gonadotropin-producing cells. The posterior pituitary (neurohypophysis) consists of the infundibular stem or hypophyseal stalk, the median eminence of the tuber cinereum, and the infundibular process (posterior lobe, neural lobe). It has no known function in the regulation of growth and will not be discussed further in this chapter.

Rathke's pouch, the origin of the adenohypophysis, can be identified in the 3-mm embryo during the third week of pregnancy. GH-producing cells can be identified by 9 weeks of gestation.[24] It is at about this time that the vascular connections between the anterior lobe of the pituitary and the hypothalamus develop,[25,26] although it has been demonstrated that hormonal production by the pituitary can occur in the absence of connections with the hypothalamus. Somatotropic cells in the pituitary are thus frequently demonstrable in the anencephalic newborn. Nevertheless, it appears likely that the initiation of development of the anterior pituitary is dependent on responsiveness of the oral ectoderm to inducing factors from the ventral diencephalon[27-31] (Figure 8-11).

The developing pituitary and hypothalamus are in close anatomic juxtaposition, and their embryonic development

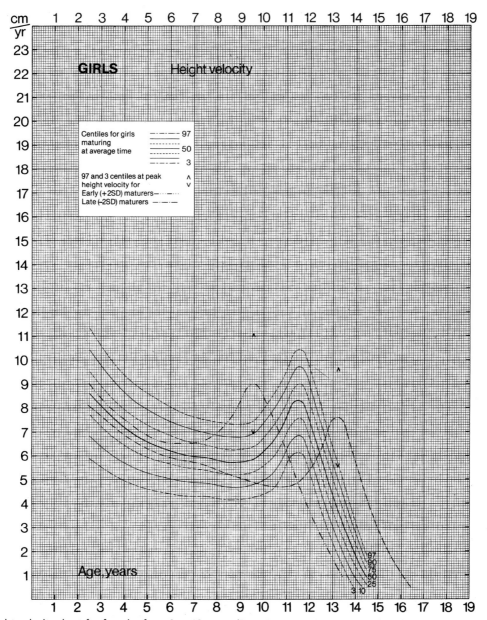

FIGURE 8-10. Height velocity chart for females from 0 to 19 years. (From Tanner JM, Davies SWD: Clinical longitudinal standards for height and height velocity for North American children. J Pediatr 107:312, 1985.)

is likely to be co-dependent.[32] Some of the diencephalic factors identified to be critical in formation and patterning of Rathke's pouch (which in the mouse is initiated on embryonic day 8) are bone morphogenic protein 4 (BMP4), Wnt5a, and fibroblast growth factor 8 (FGF8). Explant studies in the mouse have demonstrated that if Rathke's pouch is removed from the oral ectoderm on embryonic days 12 to 13 and incubated in appropriate culture medium differentiation of each of the pituitary cell types continues, indicating that by that point organogenesis of the anterior pituitary is no longer dependent on hypothalamic signals—although such signals may remain critically involved in pituitary hormone production.

Multiple pituitary-specific transcription factors are involved in the determination of pituitary cell lineages and cell-specific expression of anterior pituitary hormones.[27-31]

To date, several homeodomain transcription factors have been shown to be involved in human anterior pituitary development and differentiation. Defects in each have now been associated with various combinations of pituitary hormone deficiencies (Figure 8-11 and Table 8-2). Because additional gene defects have been implicated in abnormal murine pituitary development, it seems likely that the number of human genetic defects will expand.

In the human adult, the mean pituitary size is 13 by 9 by 6 mm.[33] Mean weight is 600 mg, with a range of 400 to 900 mg. Pituitary weight is slightly greater in women than in men, and typically increases during pregnancy.[34] In the newborn, pituitary weight averages about 100 mg. Infrequently, the craniopharyngeal canal (marking the embryonic migration of Rathke's pouch) remains patent and may contain small nests of adenohypophyseal

TABLE 8-1

Fraction of Adult Height Attained at Each Bone Age

Bone age (yr-mo)	Girls			Boys		
	Retarded	Average*	Advanced	Retarded	Average*	Advanced
6-0	0.733	0.720		0.680		
6-3	0.742	0.729		0.690		
6-6	0.751	0.738		0.700		
6-9	0.763	0.751		0.709		
7-0	0.770	0.757	0.712	0.718	0.695	0.670
7-3	0.779	0.765	0.722	0.728	0.702	0.676
7-6	0.788	0.772	0.732	0.738	0.709	0.683
7-9	0.797	0.782	0.742	0.747	0.716	0.689
8-0	0.804	0.790	0.750	0.756	0.723	0.696
8-3	0.813	0.801	0.760	0.765	0.731	0.703
8-6	0.823	0.810	0.771	0.773	0.739	0.709
8-9	0.836	0.821	0.784	0.779	0.746	0.715
9-0	0.841	0.827	0.790	0.786	0.752	0.720
9-3	0.851	0.836	0.800	0.794	0.761	0.728
9-6	0.858	0.844	0.809	0.800	0.769	0.734
9-9	0.866	0.853	0.819	0.807	0.777	0.741
10-0	0.874	0.862	0.828	0.812	0.784	0.747
10-3	0.884	0.874	0.841	0.816	0.791	0.753
10-6	0.896	0.884	0.856	0.819	0.795	0.758
10-9	0.907	0.896	0.870	0.821	0.800	0.763
11-0	0.918	0.906	0.883	0.823	0.804	0.767
11-3	0.922	0.910	0.887	0.827	0.812	0.776
11-6	0.926	0.914	0.891	0.832	0.818	0.786
11-9	0.929	0.918	0.897	0.839	0.827	0.800
12-0	0.932	0.922	0.901	0.845	0.834	0.809
12-3	0.942	0.932	0.913	0.852	0.843	0.818
12-6	0.949	0.941	0.924	0.860	0.853	0.828
12-9	0.957	0.950	0.935	0.869	0.863	0.839
13-0	0.964	0.958	0.945	0.880	0.876	0.850
13-3	0.971	0.967	0.955		0.890	0.863
13-6	0.977	0.974	0.963		0.902	0.875
13-9	0.981	0.978	0.968		0.914	0.890
14-0	0.983	0.980	0.972		0.927	0.905
14-3	0.986	0.983	0.977		0.938	0.918
14-6	0.989	0.986	0.980		0.948	0.930
14-9	0.992	0.988	0.983		0.958	0.943
15-0	0.994	0.990	0.986		0.968	0.958
15-3	0.995	0.991	0.988		0.973	0.967
15-6	0.996	0.993	0.990		0.976	0.971
15-9	0.997	0.994	0.992		0.980	0.976
16-0	0.998	0.996	0.993		0.982	0.980
16-3	0.999	0.996	0.994		0.985	0.983
16-6	0.999	0.997	0.995		0.987	0.985
16-9	0.9995	0.998	0.997		0.989	0.988
17-0	1.00	0.999	0.998		0.991	0.990
17-3					0.993	
17-6		0.9995	0.9995		0.994	
17-9					0.995	
18-0		1.00			0.996	
18-3					0.998	
18-6					1.00	

* Average: Bone age within 1 year of chronologic age.
Data from Post EM, Richman RA: A condensed table for predicting adult stature. J Pediatr 98:440, 1981, based on the data of Bayley and Pinneau.[19] These tables have been organized in an easy-to-use slide-rule format ("Adult Height Predictor," copyright 1987, Ron G. Rosenfeld).

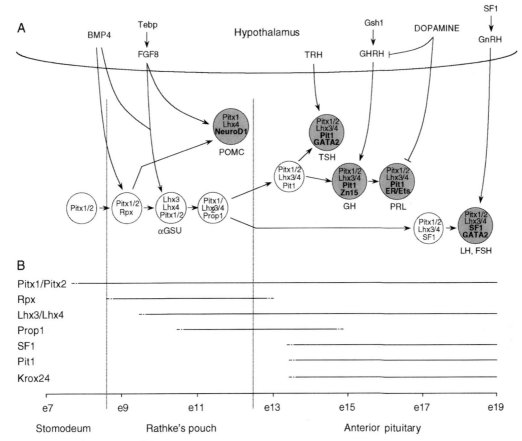

FIGURE 8-11. Development of pituitary cell lineages. A, Schematic representation of pituitary cell precursors showing the expression of prevalent transcription factors at each stage of development. Terminaly differentiated cells are shown as larger and shaded circles together with the hormones produced (lineage-specific transcription factors are highlighted in bold in these cells). The interaction with transcription factors and signaling molecules in the hypothalamus is also noted. Transcription factors are represented in lower case (except for SFI and GATA2), whereas signaling molecules appear in upper case. B, Schema showing the timing of appearance and disappearance of pituitary transcription factors during mouse embryogenesis. BMP4, bone morphogenic protein 4; e, embryonic day; ER, estrogen receptor; FGF8, fibroblast growth factor 8; FSH, follicle-stimulating hormone; GH, growth hormone; GHRH, growth hormone-releasing hormone; GnRH, gonadotropin–releasing hormone; αGSU, α-glycoprotein subunit; LH, luteinizing hormone; POMC, pro-opiomelanocortin; PRL, prolactin; SFI, steroidogenic factor I; TRH, thyrotropin-releasing hormone; TSH, thyroid-stimulating hormone. (From Lopz-Bermejo A, Buckway CK, Rosenfeld RG: Genetic defects of the growth hormone–insulin-like growth factor axis. Trends Endocrinol 11:43, 2000, with permission from Elsevier Science.)

TABLE 8-2

Homeodomain Transcription Factors Involved in Human Pituitary Development and Differentiation

Transcription Factor	Murine Homologue
HESX1 (homeobox gene expression in embryonic stem cells)	Hesx1/Rpx (Rathke's pouch, Homeobox)
PROP1 (prophet of Pit1)	Prop1 (Ames mouse)
POU1F1 (POU domain/Pit 1)	Pit1/Ghf1 (Snell mouse, Jackson mouse)
RIEG (Rieger syndrome)	Rieg/Pitx2
LHX3 (LIM homeodomain protein)	Lhx3

cells—giving rise to a pharyngeal hypophysis that may be capable of hormone synthesis.[35]

Normally, however, the pituitary resides in the sella turcica immediately above and partially surrounded by the sphenoid bone. The volume of the sella turcica provides a good measure of pituitary size, which may be reduced in the child with pituitary hypoplasia.[36] It is important, however, to recognize that considerable variation in pituitary size occurs normally. The pituitary is covered superiorly by the diaphragma sellae, and the optic chiasm is directly above the diaphragma. The anatomic proximity between the optic chiasm and the pituitary is important because hypoplasia of the optic chiasm may occur together with hypothalamic/pituitary dysfunction, as in the condition of septo-optic dysplasia.[37] The patient with congenital blindness or nystagmus should be monitored carefully for hypopituitarism. In addition, suprasellar growth of a pituitary tumor may initially manifest with visual complaints or evidence of decreases in peripheral vision.

The existence of a portal circulatory system within the pituitary is critical to normal pituitary function[25,26] (Figure 8-12). The blood supply of the pituitary derives from the superior and inferior hypophyseal arteries, branches of the internal carotid. The anterior and posterior branches of the superior hypophyseal artery may terminate within the infundibulum and the proximal portion of the pituitary stalk. Hypothalamic peptides, produced in neurons that terminate in the infundibulum, enter the primary plexus of the hypophyseal portal circulation and are transported by means of the hypophyseal portal veins to the capillaries of the anterior pituitary. This portal system thus provides a means of communication between the neurons of the hypothalamus and the hormone-producing cells of the anterior pituitary. The blood supply of the neurohypophysis is separate, deriving from the inferior hypophyseal artery. Regulation of the posterior lobe of the pituitary does not involve the hypophyseal portal circulation but, rather, is mediated through direct neural connections.

GROWTH HORMONE

Chemistry

Human GH is produced as a single-chain 191-amino-acid 22-kd protein (Figure 8-13).[38,39] It is nonglycosylated, but in its mature form contains two intramolecular disulfide bonds. GH is homologous with several other proteins produced by the pituitary or placenta, including prolactin, chorionic somatomammotropin (CS, placental lactogen), and a 22-kd GH variant (hGH-V) secreted only by the placenta.[40] The latter differs from pituitary GH by 13 amino acids. The genes for these proteins have probably descended from a common ancestral gene, even though the genes are now located on different chromosomes (chromosome 6 for prolactin and chromosome 17 for GH).[41]

The genes for GH, prolactin, and placental lactogen share a common structural organization—with four introns separating five exons. The HGH subfamily contains five members, whose genes are all located on a 78-kb

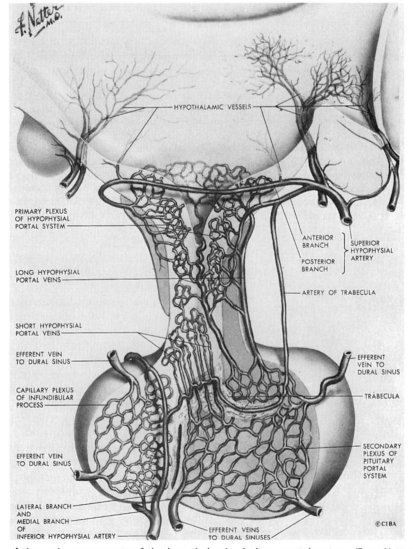

FIGURE 8-12. Illustration of the main components of the hypothalamic-pituitary portal system. (From Netter FH: The Ciba Collection of Medical Illustrations, Vol 4, Endocrine System and Selected Metabolic Diseases. Summit, NJ, CIBA Pharmaceutical, 1965.)

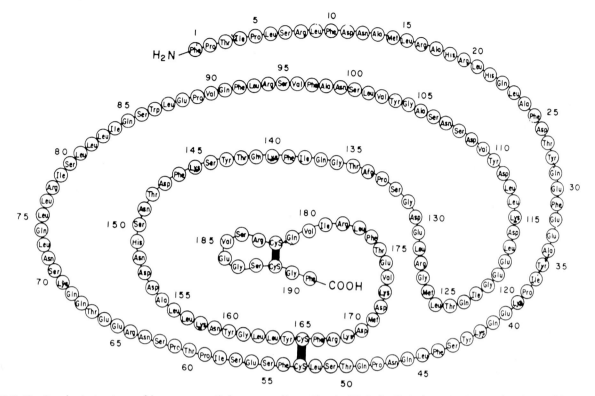

FIGURE 8-13. Covalent structure of human growth hormone. (From Chawla RK, Parks JS, Rudman D: Structural variants of human growth hormone: Biochemical, genetic and clinical aspects. Annu Rev Med 34:519, 1983.)

section of chromosome 17. The 5-prime to 3-prime order of the genes is GH, a CS pseudogene, CS-A, GH-V, and CS-B.[42] Normally, the vast majority of GH produced by the pituitary is of the mature 22-kd form. Alternative splicing of the second codon results in deletion of amino acids 32 through 46, yielding a 20-kd form that normally accounts for less than 10% of pituitary GH.[41-43] The remainder of pituitary GH includes desamidated and N-acetylated forms, as well as various GH oligomers.

Secretion

The pulsatile pattern characteristic of GH secretion largely reflects the interplay of multiple regulators, including two hypothalamic regulatory peptides: GH-releasing hormone (GHRH)[44,45] and somatostatin [somatotropin release–inhibiting factor (SRIF)].[46] The amino terminus of GHRH is required for stimulation of GH secretion. GHRH activity is species specific, presumably reflecting the specificity of binding to a G-protein–related receptor on the pituitary somatotropes.

Regulation of GH production by GHRH is largely transcriptionally mediated and is dependent on stimulation of adenylate cyclase and increases in intracellular cyclic adenosine monophosphate (AMP) concentrations. The GHRH receptor is a member of the G-protein–coupled receptor family B (also called the secretin family) and has partial sequence identity with receptors for vasoactive intestinal polypeptide, secretin, calcitonin, and parathyroid hormone.[47] Solid tumors secreting GHRH are a rare cause of GH excess. GHRH has previously been approved in the United States for treatment of growth hormone deficiency but has been withdrawn from the market for therapeutic purposes. It is still used as a diagnostic, especially for the identification of adult growth hormone deficiency.

Somatostatin actions appear to be related to the timing and amplitude of pulsatile GH secretion, rather than to GH synthesis. The binding of somatostatin to its specific receptor results in an inhibition of adenylate cyclase activity and a reduction in intracellular calcium concentrations.[46] Treatment of cultured somatotropic cells with GHRH and somatostatin has indicated a dominant effect of somatostatin, with reduction of intracellular calcium concentrations and inhibition of GH secretion. The pulsatile secretion of GH observed in vivo is believed to result from a simultaneous reduction in hypothalamic somatostatin release and increase in GHRH activity.[48] Conversely, a trough of GH secretion occurs when somatostatin release is increased in the presence of diminished GHRH activity. Somatostatin analogues are used therapeutically for the treatment of acromegaly, underscoring its role as a GH secretion inhibitor.

The regulation, on a neuronal basis, of this reciprocal secretion of GHRH and somatostatin is imperfectly understood. Multiple neurotransmitters and neuropeptides are involved in regulation of release of these hypothalamic factors, including serotonin, histamine, norepinephrine, dopamine, acetylcholine, g-aminobutyric acid (GABA), thyroid-releasing hormone, vasoactive intestinal peptide, gastrin, neurotensin, substance P, calcitonin, neuropeptide Y, vasopressin, corticotrophin releasing hormone,[49] and galanin.[50] These factors are clearly implicated in the alterations of GH secretion observed in a wide variety of physiologic states (such as stress, sleep, hemorrhage, fasting, hypoglycemia, and exercise) and form the basis for a number of GH-stimulatory tests employed in the evaluation of GH secretory capacity/ reserve.

GH secretion is also impacted by a variety of nonpeptide hormones, including androgens,[51,52] estrogens,[53] thyroxine,[54] and glucocorticoids.[55,56] The precise mechanisms by which these hormones regulate GH secretion are complex, potentially involving actions at the hypothalamic and pituitary levels. Practically speaking, hypothyroidism and glucocorticoid excess may each blunt spontaneous and provocative GH secretion (and therefore should be corrected prior to GH testing). Sex steroids, at the onset of puberty or administered pharmacologically, appear to be responsible for the rise in GH secretion characteristic of puberty.[57]

Synthetic hexapeptides capable of stimulating GH secretion have been developed[58] and termed *GH-releasing peptides* (GHRPs). These peptides, later recognized as analogues of the gastric hormone ghrelin, are capable of directly stimulating GH release and enhancing the GH response to GHRH.[59] These agents have the potential advantage of oral administration, and in the patient with an intact pituitary may be capable of greatly enhancing GH secretion. When these agents were administered chronically to elderly patients and to some GH-deficient children, the amplitudes of GH pulses were significantly increased. Ghrelin-mimetic ligands were used to characterize a common receptor termed the *GH secretagogue receptor* (GHS-R) for the GH-releasing substances. The GHS-R is distinct from the GHRH receptor.[60]

Subsequently, the GHS-R gene was cloned and shown to encode a unique G-protein–coupled receptor with a deduced protein sequence that was 96% identical in human and rat. Three receptor isotypes were isolated from human genomic libraries. Mutations in this receptor could cause variable degrees of GH insufficiency and short stature. Ghrelin is a 28-amino-acid peptide found in hypothalamus and stomach, and has been identified as the endogenous ligand for the growth hormone secretagogue receptor (GHS-R).[61] Ghrelin is a unique gene product that requires acetylation for normal function. Intravenous, intracerebroventricular, and intraperitoneal administration of ghrelin in animal models stimulates food intake and obesity[62] and raises plasma GH concentrations[63]—and to a lesser extent adrenocorticotropic hormone (ACTH) levels. Mutations in the ghrelin receptor have been identified as a possible cause of idiopathic short stature (ISS).[64]

This suggests that ghrelin is an important stimulus for nutrient allocation for growth and metabolism and that it represents a key component of the GH regulatory system. A second peptide encoded by the same gene as ghrelin has been identified and termed *obestatin*. This gene appears to regulate weight but not GH secretion.[65,66] Abnormalities of pituitary-specific transcription factors have been implicated in genetic forms of short stature. POU1F1 (Pit-1) is involved in the developmental regulation not only of somatotropes but of lactotropes and thyrotropes.[67] Abnormalities of POU1F1 expression are therefore associated with multiple pituitary deficiencies, including GH, thyroid-stimulating hormone (TSH), and prolactin.[68,69] Mutations of the POU1F1 gene have

been described in patients with hereditary forms of multiple pituitary hormone deficiencies.

In addition to the complex regulatory processes described previously, the synthesis and secretion of GH are also regulated by feedback by the insulin-like growth factor (IGF) peptides.[70-72] IGF receptors have been identified in the pituitary.[73-75] Inhibition by IGF-1 of GH secretion has been demonstrated in multiple systems.[76] In addition, inhibition of spontaneous GH secretion has been demonstrated in humans treated with subcutaneous injections of recombinant IGF-1.[77,78] GH can be identified in fetal serum by the end of the first trimester. Serum concentrations are lower in term infants than in premature infants, perhaps reflecting feedback by the higher serum levels of IGF peptides characteristic of the later stages of gestation.[79]

Twenty-four hour GH secretion peaks during adolescence,[57] undoubtedly contributing to the very high serum concentrations of IGF-1 characteristic of puberty. GH secretion begins to decline by late adolescence, and continues to fall throughout adult life. Indeed, puberty may be considered with some justification a period of "acromegaly," whereas aging (with its characteristic decrease of GH secretion) has been termed the *somatopause*.[53,80,81]

Twenty-four hour GH production rates for normal men range from 0.25 to 0.52 mg/m^2.[82,83] A wide variety of physiologic conditions, however (in addition to aging) affect GH secretion. These include stage of sleep,[84,85] nutritional status,[86] acute fasting, exercise,[87] stress,[87] and sex steroids.[51,52] Ho and associates[53] have reported that serum estradiol concentrations are the dominant factor affecting GH secretion. Neither age nor sex influenced the integrated serum concentrations of GH when the effects of estradiol were removed from analysis. The effects of testosterone on serum IGF-1 concentrations may be at least in part independent of GH because individuals with mutations of the GH receptor (GHR) still experience a rise in serum IGF-1 during puberty.[88]

The pulsatile nature of GH secretion is readily demonstrable by frequent serum sampling, especially when coupled with sensitive assays for GH.[86] Such assays demonstrate that under normal conditions serum GH concentrations are less than 0.2 ng/mL between bursts of GH secretion. It is consequently impractical to assess GH secretion by random serum sampling. Maximal GH secretion occurs during the night, especially at the onset of the first slow-wave sleep (stages III and IV). Rapid-eye-movement (REM) sleep is, on the other hand, associated with low GH secretion.

Normal young men generally experience 12 GH secretory bursts per 24 hours. Obesity is characterized by decreased GH secretion, reflected by a decreased number of GH secretory bursts.[89] Fasting increases the number and amplitude of GH secretory bursts, presumably reflecting decreased somatostatin secretion. The impact of the pulsatile secretory nature of GH secretion on its biologic actions remains uncertain.

GH Receptor/GH-Binding Protein

The GH receptor is synthesized as a 638-amino-acid peptide, which is later processed into a mature receptor of 620 amino acids and a predicted molecular weight of 70 kDa before glycosylation. The extracellular hormone-binding domain contains 246 amino acids, followed by a single membrane-spanning domain and a cytoplasmic domain of 350 amino acids. In humans, the circulating GH-binding protein (GHBP) appears to derive from proteolytic cleavage of the extracellular domain of the receptor.

The gene for the human GHR has been localized to chromosome 5p13.1-p12, where it spans more than 87 kb.[90,91] In the mouse[92,93] and rat,[94] on the other hand, multiple transcripts for the GHR have been identified. The larger (3.4 to 4.8 kb) transcript codes for the intact receptor, whereas the 1.2- to 1.9-kb transcript codes for the soluble GHBP. The coding and 3-prime untranslated regions of the human GHR are encoded by the nine exons, numbered 2 through 10.[95] Exon 2 corresponds to the secretion signal peptide, whereas exons 3 through 7 encode the extracellular domain. Exon 8 encodes the transmembrane domain. Exons 9 and 10 encode, respectively, the intracellular domain and the 3-prime untranslated region. Exon 3 of the GHR has been shown to be deleted in a substantial number of normal individuals. This delta-3 GHR polymorphism has been shown by some but not all investigators to determine responsiveness to GH and to be associated with birth size and postnatal growth.[96,97]

The GHR has been found to be highly homologous with the prolactin receptor and to share sequence homology with many of the receptors for interleukins, as well as receptors for erythropoietin, granulocyte-macrophage colony-stimulating factor, and interferon.[95] The GHR is a member of the class 1 hematopoietic cytokine family. Recently, a complex of the GH and the GHBP molecule has been shown to be more effective than GH alone—indicating a physiologic and possible therapeutic role for the GHBP.[98] Examination of the crystal structure of the GH-GHR complex revealed that the complex consisted of one molecule of GH bound to two GHR molecules, indicating a GH-induced receptor dimerization—which is necessary in GH action.[99] Interestingly, a genetically engineered fusion complex of GH and the GHR has been recently shown to have a significantly improved efficacy and a dramatically longer half-life compared to growth hormone alone when tested in rodent models.[100]

After binding to its receptor, and inducing receptor dimerization, GH has been demonstrated to stimulate phosphorylation of a protein with an apparent molecular weight of 120 kd. Janus Kinase 2(JAK2) has been identified as a major GHR-associated tyrosine kinase.[101] The presumed sequence of steps in GH action are binding of GH to the membrane-associated GHR, dimerization of the GHR, interaction of the GHR with JAK2, tyrosine phosphorylation of JAK2 and the GHR, changes in cytoplasmic and nuclear protein phosphorylation and dephosphorylation, and stimulation of target gene transcription. The GHR itself appears to have no intrinsic kinase activity. It is likely that colocalization of two JAK2 molecules by the dimerized GHR results in transphosphorylation of one JAK2 by the other, leading to JAK2 activation.[102]

Activated JAK2 then appears to phosphorylate the GHR on multiple tyrosine sites. GH- and JAK2-dependent phosphorylation and activation have been demonstrated for several signal transducers and activators of transcription (STAT); namely, STAT1, STAT3, and STAT5. These cytoplasmic proteins (after forming homodimers or het-erodimers) translocate into the nucleus, bind DNA, and activate transcription.[103] Other GH-activated pathways include mitogen-activated protein kinases (MAPKs), extracellular signal-regulated kinase (ERK)-1 and ERK2, the insulin-signaling pathway [by means of insulin receptor substrate (IRS)-1 and IRS-2], and protein kinase C (PKC). How all of these pathways interact to mediate the various anabolic and metabolic actions of GH remains to be elucidated (Figure 8-14).

The GHBP in human plasma binds GH with high specificity and affinity, but with relatively low capacity.[104-106] The GHBP is in essence the extracellular domain of the GHR and has an apparent molecular weight of approximately 55 kDa. Initial assays for GHBP involved incubation of serum with 125-I-GH and separation of bound from free radioligand by gel filtration, high-pressure liquid chromatography, or dextran-coated charcoal. Carlsson and colleagues[107] developed a ligand-mediated immunofunctional assay (LIFA) that measures GHBP capable of binding GH. Assays of serum concentrations of GHBP have been instrumental in identifying patients with GH insensitivity (GHI) caused by genetic abnormalities of the GHR.[108,109] Patients with GHI from nonreceptor abnormalities, abnormalities of the intracellular portion of the GHR, or inability of the receptor to dimerize may, however, have normal serum concentrations of GHBP.[110]

The inhibition of GH signaling by several members of the GH-inducible suppressors of the cytokine signaling (SOCS) family has been demonstrated.[111] Evidence for the importance of SOCS proteins in controlling growth is derived from SOCS-2 knockout mice, which display gigantism.[112] By contrast, complete inhibition of GH activation of the signal transducer STAT5 and STAT5-dependent transcriptional activity is seen when cellular overexpression of SOCS family members is induced. SOCS also inhibit the GHR-dependent tyrosine phosphorylation of JAK2.[113] Endotoxin and proinflammatory cytokines such as interleukin-1b (IL-1b) and tumor necrosis factor-a (TNFa) induce a state of GH resistance.

All of these agents can also induce SOCS proteins.[114] SOCS-3 induced by IL-1b and TNFa or by endotoxin in vivo may play a role in the GH resistance induced by sepsis.[115] Critically ill patients with septic shock who had been treated with GH were shown to have increased mortality,[116] possibly related to the induction of GH resistance in specific tissues as a consequence of sepsis. Thus, the role of SOCS proteins as intracellular GH signaling antagonists appears to be important in a variety of pathophysiologic states.

GH Actions

According to the somatomedin hypothesis, the anabolic actions of GH are mediated through the IGF peptides.[117,118] Although this hypothesis is at least in part true, it appears that GH is capable of stimulating a variety of effects that are independent of IGF activity. Indeed, the effects of GH and IGF are on occasion contradictory—as evident in the "diabetogenic" actions of GH[119,120] and the glucose-lowering activity of IGFs. Green and colleagues[121] attempted to resolve some of these differences in a "dual-effector" model in which GH stimulates precursor cells, such as prechondrocytes, to differentiate.

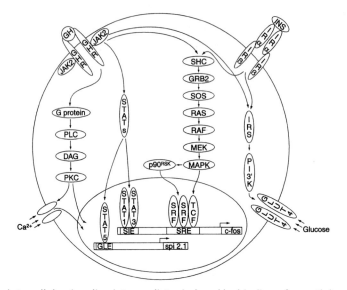

FIGURE 8-14. A model depicting intracellular signaling intermediates induced by binding of growth hormone (GH) with the GH receptor (GHR). DAG, diacylglycerol; ERK, extracellular signal-regulated kinase; GLE, interferon-γ–activated sequence (GAS)–like response element; GLUT, glucose transporter; GRB, growth factor receptor–binding protein; JAK, janus kinase; INS, insulin; Irα, insulin receptor α subunit; MAPK, mitogen-activated protein kinase; MEK, MAPK-ERK kinase; PKC, protein kinase C; PLC, phospholipase C; SHC, SrC homology complex; SIE, sis-inducible element; SOS, son of sevenless; SRE, serum response element; SRF, serum response factor; STAT, signal transducer and activator of transcription; TCF, ternary complex factor. (From Kopchick JJ, Bellush LL, Coschigano KT: Transgenic models of growth hormone action. Annu Rev Nutr 19:437, 1999. With permission, from the Annual Review of Nutrition, Volume 19 © 1999 by Annual Reviews. www.Annual-Reviews.org.)

When differentiated cells or neighboring cells then secrete IGFs, these peptides act as mitogens and stimulate clonal expansion. This hypothesis is based on the ability of IGF peptides to work not only as classic endocrine factors that are transported through the blood but as paracrine or autocrine growth factors. GH also stimulates a variety of metabolic effects, some of which appear to occur independently of IGF production—such as lipolysis,[122] amino acid transport in diaphragm[123] and heart,[124] and production of specific hepatic proteins. Thus, there are multiple sites of GH action—and frequently it is not entirely clear which of these actions are mediated through the IGF system and which might represent IGF-independent effects of GH.[125] These sites of action include the following.

- *Epiphysis:* Stimulation of epiphyseal growth.
- *Bone:* Stimulation of osteoclast differentiation and activity, stimulation of osteoblast activity, and increase of bone mass by endochondral bone formation. Lupu et al.[126] have shown that mice with a complete knockout of IGF-I (making them substantially smaller than wild-type mice) become even smaller when mated into a GH receptor knockout strain, indicating a direct IGF-independent effect of GH on growth.
- *Adipose tissue:* Acute insulin-like effects, followed by increased lipolysis, inhibition of lipoprotein lipase, stimulation of hormone sensitive lipase, decreased glucose transport, and decreased lipogenesis.[127]
- *Muscle:* Increased amino acid transport, increased nitrogen retention, increased lean tissue, and increased energy expenditure.[127]

The concept of IGF-independent actions of GH is supported by in vivo studies, in which IGF-1 cannot duplicate all of the effects of GH (such as nitrogen retention and insulin resistance). The effects of GH in normal human

aging[128] and in catabolic conditions[129] are subjects of active investigation.

INSULIN-LIKE GROWTH FACTORS

Historical Background

The insulin-like growth factors (or somatomedins) constitute a family of peptides that are at least in part GH dependent and that are believed to mediate many of the anabolic and mitogenic actions of GH. Although they were originally identified in 1957 by their ability to stimulate [35S]sulfate incorporation into rat cartilage,[117] it has been established over the ensuing 45 years that they are involved in diverse metabolic activities (Figure 8-15).

In 1957, Salmon and Daughaday[117] first demonstrated that the ability of serum from hypophysectomized rats to stimulate [35S]sulfate incorporation into rat chondrocyte proteoglycans could not be restored by in vitro addition of GH. [35S]sulfate incorporation could be restored by the addition of serum from hypophysectomized rats that had been treated with GH, however, thereby demonstrating the existence of a GH-dependent "sulfation factor."

Concurrent investigations on insulin activity in rat muscle and adipose tissue indicated that only a small component of the insulin-like activity of normal serum could be blocked by the addition of anti-insulin antibodies. The remaining activity was termed *nonsuppressible insulin-like activity* (NSILA) and was subsequently demonstrated to contain two soluble 7-kd forms named *NSILA-I* and *NSILA-II*.[130,131]

A third converging line of investigation arose from studies by Dulak and Temin[132] of the mitogenic nature of bovine serum. Serum-free conditioned media from fetal

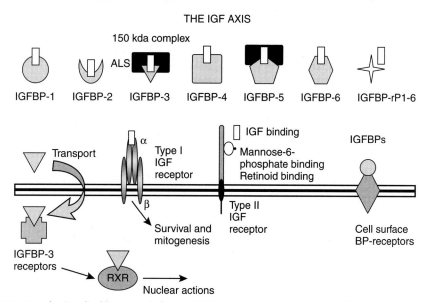

FIGURE 8-15. The insulin-like growth factor (IGF) axis. BP, binding protein; RXR, retinoid X receptor.

Buffalo rat liver cells (BRL-3A) were found to support the growth of cultured cells. The mitogenic factor in the medium was termed *multiplication-stimulating activity* (MSA) and was found to share metabolic and mitogenic activities with sulfation factor and NSILA.

In 1972, the restrictive labels of sulfation factor and NSILA were replaced by the term *somatomedin* (SM).[133] In recognition of the broad metabolic and mitogenic actions of these factors, the following criteria were established: concentration in serum must be GH dependent, must possess insulin-like activity in extraskeletal tissues, must promote the incorporation of sulfate into cartilage, and must stimulate DNA synthesis and cell multiplication.

Purification efforts yielded two legitimate somatomedin peptides: a basic peptide (SM-C) and a neutral peptide (SM-A).[134,135] In 1978, Rinderknecht and Humbel[136,137] isolated two active somatomedins from human plasma that demonstrated a striking structural resemblance to proinsulin. Accordingly, these two peptides were renamed *insulin-like growth factors* (IGFs).

IGF Structure and Molecular Biology

IGF-1, a basic peptide of 70 amino acids, correlates with SM-C—whereas IGF-2 is a slightly acidic peptide of 67 amino acids (Figure 8-16). The two peptides are structurally related, sharing 45 of 73 possible amino acid positions. They have approximately 50% amino acid homology to insulin.[118,136,137] Like insulin, both IGFs have A and B chains connected by disulfide bonds. The connecting

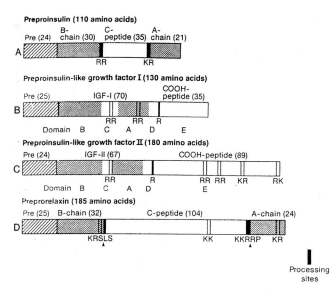

FIGURE 8-16. Schematic representations of the structures of precursors to human insulin, insulin-like growth factor I (IGF-I), IGF-2, and relaxin. *Stippled segments* indicate the homologous B- and A-chain regions. Proteolytic processing sites are indicated by the following amino acid code: K, lysine; L, leucine; P, proline; R, arginines; S, serine. (From Bell GI, Merryweather JP, Sanchez-Pescado R, et al: Sequence of cDNA clone encoding human preproinsulin-like growth factor II. Nature 310:775, 1984, MacMillan Magazines Limited.)

(C-peptide) region is 12 amino acids long for IGF-1 and 8 amino acids long for IGF-2 and bears no homology with the C-peptide region of proinsulin. IGF-1 and IGF-2 also differ from proinsulin in possessing carboxyl-terminal extensions (D-peptides) of 8 and 6 amino acids, respectively. It is clear that this structural homology explains the ability of both IGFs to bind to the insulin receptor and for insulin to bind to the type 1 IGF receptor. On the other hand, structural differences explain the failure of insulin to bind to the IGF-binding proteins.

Two different forms of IGF-1 precursor molecules have been identified.[118] The first 134 amino acids of each are identical, comprising the signal peptide (48 amino acids), the mature IGF-1 molecule (70 amino acids), and the first 16 amino acids of the E domain of the precursor. IGF-1A has an additional 19 amino acids (total 153 residues), whereas IGF-1B has an additional 61 amino acids (total 195 residues).

Alternative splicing of the IGF-1 gene presumably generates the two alternative messenger RNAs (mRNAs). The primary IGF-2 translation product in human, rat, and mouse contains 180 amino acids—including a 24-residue signal peptide, the 67-amino-acid mature IGF-2 sequence, and a carboxyl-terminal E-peptide of 89 amino acids.

Control of IGF gene expression appears to be complex, perhaps explaining variability in tissue expression as well as differential expression in the embryo, fetus, child, and adult.[118,138-140] IGF-1 and IGF-2 are encoded by single large genes, spanning approximately 95 and 35 kb of genomic DNA, respectively. The human IGF-1 gene contains at least six exons. Exons 1 and 2 encode alternative signal peptides, probably each containing several transcription start sites. Exons 3 and 4 encode the remaining signal peptide, the remainder of the mature IGF-1 molecule, and part of the trailer peptide. Exons 5 and 6 encode alternatively used segments of the trailer peptide (resulting in the IGF-1A and IGF-1B forms), as well as 39 untranslated sequences, with multiple different polyadenylation sites. The human IGF-1 gene is located on the long arm of chromosome 12.[141,142]

The human IGF-2 gene is located on the short arm of chromosome 11,[141-143] adjacent to the insulin gene, and spans 35 kb of genomic DNA—containing nine exons. Exons 1 through 6 encode 59 untranslated RNA, including multiple promoter sites. Exon 7 encodes the signal peptide and most of the mature protein, whereas exon 8 encodes the carboxyl-terminal portion of the protein plus the trailer peptide (whose coding is completed in exon 9). The result is that multiple mRNA species exist for both IGF-1 and IGF-2. This permits remarkable complexity in the regulation of gene expression, allowing for tissue-specific expression of specific transcripts as well as ontogenic and hormonal regulation.

Assay Methodologies for the IGF Peptides

Since their first identification in 1957, the IGF peptides have proven to be remarkably difficult to permit accurate measurement. Bioassay methods were often influenced by a variety of other serum factors capable of mimicking or inhibiting IGF action. More importantly, virtually all assays were influenced by the presence of IGF-binding proteins (IGFBPs)—which have been found in all biologic fluids tested to date.

Bioassay methods included stimulation of [35S]sulfate incorporation, using various modifications of the original method described by Salmon and Daughaday.[117,144,145] A wide variety of several bioassays included stimulation of DNA synthesis,[146] RNA synthesis, protein synthesis,[147] glucose uptake,[148] and others. In general, however, such assays were cumbersome, subject to interference by IGFBPs, and unable to distinguish between IGF-1 and IGF-2. When SM-C (and later, IGF-1 and IGF-2) were purified, it became possible to radiolabel the pure proteins and employ them in a variety of radioreceptor assays[149,150] and competitive protein-binding assays.[151,152] It was not until the development of specific antibodies that it became possible to accurately distinguish between IGF-1 and IGF-2 and measure each peptide accurately.[153-156] Current frequently used assays for IGF-I are primarily "double antibody sandwich assays" such as ELISA and have a reasonable accuracy and reproducibility.[157]

Nevertheless, the issue of IGFBPs must be dealt with in any IGF assay.[158] Powell and co-workers,[159] for example, have demonstrated that the discrepant results found in uremic sera assayed for IGF by bioassay, radioreceptor assay, and radioimmunoassay can be entirely attributed to the interference of IGFBPs. Even antibodies with high affinity and specificity will still exhibit interference by IGFBPs. This is particularly true in conditions in which there is a relatively high IGFBP/IGF peptide ratio, or at the clinical extremes of the assay [i.e., GH deficiency (GHD) or acromegaly].

In general, the most effective and reliable way to deal with IGFBPs is their separation from IGF peptides by sizing chromatography under acidic conditions.[160] IGF-1 and IGF-2, each with a molecular weight of approximately 7 kd, can be readily separated from the IGFBPs—whose molecular weights range from 25 to 45 kd (glycosylated form of IGFBP-3). This is, however, a labor-intensive procedure and has been occasionally replaced by the more rapid acid ethanol extraction.[161] Although this method may be reasonably effective for most serum samples, it is problematic in conditions of high IGFBP/IGF peptide ratios—such as conditioned media from cell lines and sera from newborns, GHD, uremia, and so on.

Alternative methodologies include the use of antibodies generated against synthetic peptides, such as the C-peptide region of IGF-1 or IGF-2. In general, such antibodies have high specificity but relatively low affinity. Nevertheless, the radiolabeled peptide does not bind to endogenous IGFBPs—offering an important advantage. An alternative approach, developed by Blum and colleagues,[162] has been the use of an antibody with high specificity for IGF-2—which permits the addition of excess unlabeled IGF-1 to saturate endogenous IGFBPs. Bang and co-workers[163] have bypassed the interference of IGFBPs by employing truncated IGF-1, which has decreased affinity for IGFBPs, as a radioligand.

At present, the most practical and effective way to perform accurate IGF assays that have minimal interference by IGFBPs is to use methodologies similar to the so-called sandwich assay.[164] These assays, which can be performed in enzyme-linked immunosorbent assay or immunoradiometric assay, do not employ a radiolabeled IGF molecule—which can bind to IGFBPs (as in the case of conventional radioimmunoassays) and thereby lead to erroneous readings when IGFBPs are elevated.[165]

Serum Levels of IGF Peptides

In human fetal serum, IGF-1 levels are relatively low and are positively correlated with gestational age (Figure 8-17).[166,167] A correlation between fetal cord serum IGF-1 levels with birth weight has been reported by some groups,[166-168] although others have reported no correlation.[169] IGF-1 levels in human newborn serum are generally 30% to 50% of adult levels. There is a slow, gradual rise in serum concentrations during childhood, with attainment of adult levels at the onset of sexual maturation.[170]

During the process of puberty, IGF-1 concentrations rise to be two to three times the concentrations seen in adults.[171] Thus, concentrations during adolescence correlate better with Tanner stage (bone age) than with chronologic age. Girls with gonadal dysgenesis show no adolescent increase in serum IGF-1, clearly establishing the association of the pubertal rise in IGF-1 with the production of sex steroids.[172-174] It has been suggested that the pubertal rise in sex steroids stimulates IGF-1 production indirectly by first leading to a rise in GH secretion. It is of note, however, that patients with GHI from GHR mutations show a pubertal rise in serum IGF-1 despite a decline in GH levels—thereby implicating a direct effect of sex steroids on IGF-1.[178]

After adolescence, or at least after 20 to 30 years of age, serum IGF-1 concentrations demonstrate a gradual and progressive age-associated decline.[128,175] It has been suggested that this decline may be responsible for the negative nitrogen balance, decrease in body musculature, and osteoporosis characteristic of aging.[128] Although this provocative hypothesis remains unproven at this time, it has generated considerable interest in the potential use of GH and/or IGF-1 therapy in normal aging.

Human newborn levels of IGF-2 are generally 50% of adult levels. By 1 year of age, however, adult concentrations are attained with little if any subsequent decline—even out to the seventh or eighth decade of life. It is of interest that this pattern of IGF-2 concentrations is distinctly different from that in the rat or mouse (in which serum IGF-2 levels are highest in the fetus and rapidly decline postnatally to essentially undetectable levels in the adult).[176,177]

Measurement of IGF Levels in Growth Disorders

The GH dependency of the IGFs was established by the initial report from Salmon and Daughaday.[117] Following the development of sensitive and specific radioimmunoassays that could distinguish between IGF-1 and IGF-2, the relationship of serum IGF levels to GH status has been established.[157] Measurement of each IGF peptide offers its own particular advantages. IGF-1 concentrations are far more GH dependent than are IGF-2 concentrations and are useful in identifying changes in GH secretory patterns. Serum IGF-1 concentrations, however, are greatly influenced by chronologic age, degree of sexual maturation, and nutritional status. As a result, construction of age-defined normative values is critical. IGF-1 levels in normal children younger than 5 years of age may be so low that extensive overlap exists between the normal range and values in GH-deficient children.

Ranke and co-workers[178] performed GH stimulation tests in 400 children with heights below the 5th percentile and assessed the value of IGF-I as a surrogate of the diagnosis of GHD. The children subsequently diagnosed as GH deficient on the basis of standard provocative tests had very low levels of IGF-I. However, significant overlap of serum IGF-1 levels existed between GH-deficient patients and children with other forms of short stature and normal provocative GH levels. It was only in children with bone ages greater than 12 years that serum IGF-1 levels permitted complete discrimination between GHD and normal short children.

Similarly, Rose and colleagues[179] found that in children with low provocative GH or overnight GH concentrations serum IGF-1 concentrations were lower but not dramatically lower compared to children with normal GH

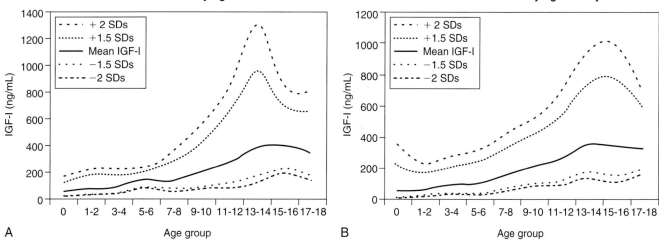

FIGURE 8-17. Serum insulin-like growth factor I (IGF-I) values by age for males *(A)* and females *(B)*. SD, standard deviation.

levels. Rosenfeld and associates[157] evaluated the efficacy of IGF-1 and IGF-2 radioimmunoassays in 68 children with GHD, 197 children of normal stature, and 44 normal short children. Eighteen percent of the GH-deficient children had serum IGF-1 levels within the normal range for age, whereas 32% of normal short children had low IGF-1 concentrations. Low IGF-2 levels were found in 52% of GH-deficient children but also in 35% of normal short children. The use of combined IGF-1/IGF-2 assays provided better discrimination, however, but this is not commonly practiced by pediatric endocrinologists.

The observation that many "normal but short" children have low serum concentrations of IGF-1 or IGF-2 (or both) calls into question the criteria by which the diagnosis of GHD is currently made. Given that provocative GH testing is both arbitrary and nonphysiologic and that inherent variability in GH radioimmunoassays exists, it is not surprising that the correlation between IGF-1 levels and provocative GH levels is imperfect. These points are further supported by observations with radioimmunoassays for IGFBP-3.

IGF Receptors

In the early 1970s, it became apparent that the IGFs could bind (although generally with low affinity) to insulin receptors, thus providing an explanation for their insulin-like activity.[180] Shortly thereafter, Megyesi and associates[181] identified distinct receptors for insulin and IGF in rat hepatic membranes. Specificity studies, employing radiolabeled IGF preparations, demonstrated that at least two classes of IGF receptors existed. Insulin, at high concentrations, could compete for occupancy of one form of IGF receptor but had essentially no affinity for the second form of receptor.

The development of methodologies for structural characterization of these receptors enabled the clear discrimination of two receptor forms[182-185] (Figure 8-15). The type 1 IGF receptor is closely related to the insulin receptor. Both are heterotetramers composed of two membrane-spanning alpha subunits of apparent molecular weight of 130 kd and two intracellular beta subunits of apparent molecular weight of 90 kd. The alpha subunits contain the binding sites for IGF-1 and are linked by disulfide bonds. The beta subunits contain a transmembrane domain, an adenosine triphosphate (ATP)-binding site, and a tyrosine kinase domain, which constitutes the presumed signal transduction mechanism for the receptor. Whereas each alpha-beta heterodimer appears capable of binding one molecule of ligand, it appears that 1 mole of the full heterotetrameric receptor binds only 1 mole of ligand.

Although the type 1 IGF receptor has been commonly referred to as the "IGF-1 receptor," studies indicate that the receptor is capable of binding IGF-1 and IGF-2 with high affinity—and both IGF peptides appear capable of activating tyrosine kinase by binding to this receptor. Affinity of the type 1 receptor for insulin is generally 100-fold less, thereby providing a mechanism for the relatively weak mitogenic effect commonly observed with insulin. Ullrich and co-workers[186] deduced the complete primary structure of the human type 1 IGF receptor

from cDNA cloned from a human placental library. The mature peptide constitutes 1,337 amino acids, with a predicted molecular mass of 152 kd.

The translated alpha-beta heterodimer is subsequently cleaved at an Arg-Lys-Arg-Arg sequence at positions 707 to 710. As is the case with the insulin receptor, the beta subunit has the expected hydrophobic transmembrane domain and the intracellular tyrosine kinase domain and ATP binding site. Although it appears reasonable to presume that insulin and IGF-1 receptors have both evolved from a common ancestor protein, they are encoded by genes on separate chromosomes (chromosome 15 for the type 1 IGF receptor and chromosome 19 for the insulin receptor).

The type 1 IGF receptor mediates IGF actions on all cell types, and these actions are diverse and tissue specific. In general, it is believed that all of the effects of IGF receptor activation are mediated by tyrosine kinase activation and phosphorylation of substrates—which activate specific cellular pathways, leading to various biologic actions. Among these effects is induction of cell growth through activation of the cell cycle machinery, maintenance of cell survival (prevention of apoptosis) mediated by effects on the bcl family members, and induction of cellular differentiation, which occurs by as yet incompletely characterized mechanisms.

The substrates, which are phosphorylated by the IGF receptor, include the members of the insulin receptor substrate family (particularly IRS-1 and IRS-2) because both of the knockout mice models for these genes result in poor growth (as well as insulin resistance).[187] Other IRS molecules may have a negative feedback role in regulating IGF action.[188] In addition, several other signaling molecules respond to IGF receptor activation. Blockade of the IGF-I receptor has been proposed as a cancer therapy, and clinical studies are showing promise in early trials.[189]

It is of particular note that a prototypic molecule for the IGF-1/insulin receptor in nematodes (termed Daf2) is related to longevity, such that mutations of this gene extend the life expectancy of these organisms. This extension of life expectancy in nematodes has also been shown for other components of the GH-IGF system, as well as being demonstrated in several other species including flies and mice.[190] It is unclear, however, what relevance the IGF-1/insulin receptor has for human longevity (though this question is under investigation). The type 2 IGF receptor, however, bears no structural homology with either the insulin or the type 1 IGF receptors. On sodium dodecyl sulfate–polyacrylamide gel electrophoresis, the type 2 IGF-R has been demonstrated to migrate at an apparent molecular weight of 220 kd under nonreducing conditions and 250 kd after reduction—indicating that it is a monomeric protein.

The cloned human type 2 receptor has a predicted molecular mass of 271 kd and is characterized by a lengthy extracellular domain containing 15 repeat sequences of 147 residues each,[191] followed by a 23-residue transmembrane domain and a small cytoplasmic domain consisting of only 164 residues. The receptor does not contain an intrinsic tyrosine kinase domain or any other recognizable signal transduction mechanism. Surprisingly, the type 2 IGF receptor has been found to be identical to the cation-independent mannose-6-phosphate (CIM6P) receptor—a protein involved in the intracellular lysosomal targeting of a variety of acid hydrolases and other mannosylated proteins.[192,193] The majority of these receptors are located on intracellular membranes, where they are in equilibrium with receptors on the plasma membrane.[194]

Why this receptor binds IGF-2 and mannose-6-phosphate–containing lysosomal enzymes remains unresolved. Unlike the type 1 IGF receptor, which binds both IGF peptides with high affinity and insulin with 100-fold lower affinity, the type 2 receptor only binds IGF-2 with high affinity. IGF-1 binds with substantially lower affinity, and insulin not at all.[194] One mole of IGF-2 binds per mole of receptor. The binding sites for IGF-2 and mannose-6-phosphate appear to reside in different portions of the receptor. Nevertheless, the two classes of ligand do show some reciprocal inhibitory effects on receptor binding—suggesting a potential effect of IGF-2 on the sorting of lysosomal enzymes.

Most studies have indicated that the classic mitogenic and metabolic actions of IGF-1 and IGF-2 are mediated through the type 1 IGF receptor, with its tyrosine kinase signal transduction mechanism. Conover and co-workers[195] and Furlanetto and associates[196] have demonstrated that monoclonal antibodies directed against the IGF-1 binding site on the type 1 IGF receptor inhibit the ability of IGF-1 and IGF-2 to stimulate thymidine incorporation and cell replication. Similarly, several groups have shown that polyclonal antibodies capable of blocking IGF-2 binding to the type 2 IGF/mannose-6-phosphate receptor do not block IGF-2 actions.[197-199]

More direct evidence for the role of the type 1 IGF receptor in mediating classic IGF actions of IGF-2 comes from the use of IGF-2 analogues as probes of receptor function. IGF-2 analogues with decreased affinity for the type 1 receptor but preserved affinity for the type 2 receptor were markedly less potent than IGF-2 in stimulating DNA synthesis.[200] In further support of the concept that the type 2 IGF receptor does not mediate the mitogenic actions of IGF-2 it has been shown that the mannose-6-phosphate receptor in hepatic tissues from chicken[201] or frogs[202] does not bind IGF-2. Presumably, IGF-2 mitogenic actions in these species are mediated solely through the type 1 IGF receptor.

Nevertheless, a number of observations are consistent with the possibility of an IGF-2 action mediated via the type 2 IGF receptor. Rogers and Hammerman[203] have suggested that the type 2 receptor is involved in production of inositol triphosphate and diacylglycerol in proximal tubule preparations and canine kidney membranes. Tally and co-workers[204] have reported that IGF-2 stimulates the growth of a subclone of the K562 human erythroleukemia cell line, an action not duplicated by either IGF-2 or insulin. Minniti and co-workers[205] reported that IGF-2 appears capable of acting as an autocrine growth factor and cell motility factor for human rhabdomyosarcoma cells, actions apparently mediated through the type 2 receptor. It has been suggested that IGF-2 can activate a calcium-permeable cation channel by means of the type 2 IGF receptor, perhaps through coupling to a pertussis toxin–sensitive guanine nucleotide–binding protein (Gi protein).[206]

It now appears that the type 2 IGF receptor binds several other molecules in addition to IGF-2. The ability of this receptor to bind mannose-6-phosphate–containing enzymes (such as cathepsin and urokinase) is well recognized and may be important in its ability to remove these enzymes from the cellular environment, thus modulating tissue remodeling.[207] In addition, reports indicate that the type 2 IGF receptor binds retinoic acid and may mediate some of the growth inhibitory effects of retinoids.[208] As discussed later in the chapter, knockout of the type 2 IGF receptor results in excessive growth. It appears that this receptor acts as a growth inhibitory component of the IGF system responding to and mediating multiple antimitogenic systems.[209]

The occasional observation of seemingly anomalous competitive binding results[210] has led to the suggestion that variant or atypical insulin and IGF receptors might exist.[211] One possible explanation for such findings is the existence of hybrid receptors composed of 1 alpha-beta dimer of the insulin receptor and 1 alpha-beta dimer of the type 1 IGF receptor.[212] Ligand-dependent formation of hybrid IGF/insulin receptors has been reported by Treadway and associates,[213] and studies with monoclonal antibodies specific for the insulin or type 1 IGF receptor have suggested that such receptors may develop spontaneously in cells with abundant native receptors.[214] The physiologic significance of such hybrid receptors, however, is entirely speculative.

IGF-Binding Protein Superfamily

Although insulin and the IGFs share significant structural homology, and despite the structural-functional similarity of the insulin and type 1 IGF receptors, the IGFs differ from insulin in one important respect. In contrast to insulin, the IGFs circulate in plasma complexed to a family of binding proteins.[215-217] These carrier proteins extend the serum half-life of the IGF peptides, transport the IGFs to target cells, and modulate the interaction of the IGFs with their surface membrane receptors.

The existence of IGFBPs was initially inferred from chromatographic studies of size distribution of IGF peptides in serum,[218] but it has only been in the decade that the complexity of the interactions among the IGFs, IGFBPs, and IGF receptors has been fully appreciated. The identification and characterization of IGFBPs in body fluids and in conditioned media from cultured cells have been facilitated by the development of a number of biochemical and assay techniques, including gel chromatography, radioreceptor assays, affinity cross-linking, Western ligand blotting,[219] immunoblotting, and recently specific radioimmunoassay and ELISA assays. It has been the study of the molecular biology of the IGFBPs that has provided the most information concerning their structural interrelationship, however.

Six distinct human and rodent IGFBPs have been cloned and sequenced.[216,217,220] Their structural characteristics are summarized in Figure 8-18. The determination of the primary amino acid sequences from the cloned cDNAs of the IGFBPs has revealed important structural relationships among the IGFBPs. Probably the most impressive similarity in structure is the conservation of the

Human Insulin-like Growth Factor Binding Proteins

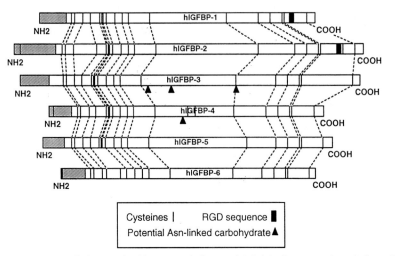

FIGURE 8-18. Schematic representation of the insulin-like growth factor (IGF)–binding proteins. (Adapted from Lamson G, Giudice L, Rosenfeld RG: Insulin-like growth factor binding protein and molecular relationship. Growth Factors 5:19, 1991.)

number and placement of the cysteine residues. The total number of cysteines varies from 16 to 20, and each of the IGFBPs has cysteine-rich regions at the amino and carboxyl termini of the protein. Conservation of the spatial order of the cysteines presumably indicates that the secondary structure of the IGFBPs, which is dependent on disulfide bonding, must also be well maintained. Disulfide bonding establishes the IGF-binding site of each IGFBP. Reduction of the binding proteins results in loss of IGF binding.

Analysis of the amino acid sequences of the IGFBPs also reveals the presence of an arginine-glycine-aspartic acid (RGD) positioned near the carboxyl terminus of IGFBP-1 and IGFBP-2.[221] This sequence has been demonstrated to be the minimum required sequence in many extracellular matrix proteins for their binding by membrane receptors of the integrin protein family. It has been suggested that IGFBPs may associate with the cell surface through such amino acid sequences. On the other hand, IGFBP-3 (which lacks an RGD sequence) also appears capable of specific binding to cell membrane receptors.[222,223] Membrane proteins capable of specifically binding IGFBP-3 have been proposed.[224]

Under most conditions, the IGFBPs appear to inhibit IGF action—presumably by competing with IGF receptors for IGF peptides.[225] This is supported by the observation that IGF analogues with decreased affinity for IGFBPs generally appear to have increased biologic potency.[226-228] In many studies involving transfection of the hIGFBP-3 gene cells, expression of IGFBP-3 resulted in an inhibition of cell growth even in the absence of added IGF—suggesting a direct inhibitory role of the binding protein.[229] Under specific conditions, however, several of the IGFBPs apparently are capable of enhancing IGF action—perhaps by facilitating IGF delivery to target receptors.[230]

Of interest is the recent discovery of several groups of cysteine-rich proteins that contain domains strikingly similar to the amino-terminal domain of the IGFBPs. This has led to the proposal of an IGFBP superfamily,[231] which includes the family of six high-affinity IGFBPs—as well as a number of families of IGFBP-related proteins (IGFBP-rPs). Three of the IGFBP-rPs (Mac25/IGFBP-rP1; connective tissue growth factor, CTGF/IGFBP-rP2; NovH/IGFBP-rP3) have been shown to bind IGFs, although with considerably lower affinity than in the case of IGFBPs. Like the IGFBPs, the IGFBP-rPs are modular proteins—and the highly preserved amino-terminal domain appears to represent the consequence of exon shuffling of an ancestral gene. It is not clear what role, if any, the IGFBP-rPs play in normal IGF physiology. However, it is likely that they can influence cell growth by IGF-independent (and perhaps IGF-dependent) mechanisms.

Evidence indicates that IGFBPs are essentially bioactive molecules that in addition to binding IGF have a variety of IGF-independent functions. These clearly include growth inhibition in some cell types,[232] growth stimulation in other tissues,[233] direct induction of apoptosis,[234] and modulation of the effects of other non-IGF growth factors. These effects of IGFBPs are mediated, undoubtedly, by binding to their own receptors. These IGFBP-signaling pathways are currently being unraveled and involve the interaction of IGFBPs with nuclear retinoid receptors as well as with other molecules on the cell surface and in the cytoplasm.[235] Because IGFBP-3 is regulated by GH, it is intriguing that in vivo IGFBP-3 enhances IGF-I action when given to hypophysectomized rats (rather than inhibiting it).[236] The mechanisms involved in this effect have not been elucidated but may explain the limited effects of IGF-1 therapy on the growth of Laron patients (discussed later in the chapter).

Analysis of IGFBPs is further complicated by the presence of IGFBP proteases, capable of various levels of IGFBP degradation.[237,238] Initially reported in the serum of pregnant women,[237,238] proteases for IGFBP-3, -4, and -5 have already been demonstrated in a variety of biologic fluids—including serum, seminal plasma,[45] cerebrospinal fluid,[239] and urine.[240] Proteolysis of IGFBPs complicates their assay by both Western ligand blotting and radioimmunoassay methodologies and must be taken into consideration when concentrations of the various IGFBPs in biologic fluids are reported.[241] The physiologic significance of limited proteolysis of IGFBPs remains to be determined, although evidence suggests that protease activity results in decreased affinity of the IGFBP for IGF peptides.

The relative amounts of each of the IGFBPs vary among biologic fluids. IGFBP-1 is the major IGFBP in human amniotic fluid.[242] IGFBP-2 is prominent in cerebrospinal fluid[243] and seminal plasma.[244] IGFBP-3 is the major IGFBP in normal human serum and demonstrates clear GH dependence.[245] Among the IGFBPs, IGFBP-3 and IGFBP-5 are unique in that they normally circulates in adult serum as part of a ternary complex consisting of IGFBP-3 or IGFBP-5, an IGF peptide, and an acid-labile subunit.[246]

Specific immunoassays have been developed for the IGFBPs, including IGFBP-1,[242,247,248] IGFBP-2,[249] and IGFBP-3.[241,250,251] Currently, measurement of IGFBP-3 appears to have the greatest potential clinical value because this IGFBP appears to be directly GH dependent (Figure 8-19). Blum and associates[34] have suggested that radioimmunoassay determination of serum concentrations of IGFBP-3 might be more specific (but less sensitive) than IGF-1 assays in the diagnosis of GHD because normal levels of IGF-1 are so low in young children and many "normal" short children have low levels of IGF-1. Because IGFBP-3 determinations reflect not only IGF-1 levels but IGF-2 concentrations, their age dependency is not nearly as striking as that of IGF-1. Even in young children, normal levels are above 500 ng/mL. The use of IGFBP assays in the evaluation of IGF deficiency and GHD is discussed later in this chapter.

Targeted Disruption of Components of the IGF System

The critical role of the IGF system in fetal and postnatal growth was demonstrated in a series of elegant gene knockout studies in mice.[252] Unlike GH and GHR knockouts,[157] which are near normal size at birth, Igf1 null mice have a birth weight 60% of normal.[88] Postnatal growth is

abnormal, and the surviving mice are only 30% of normal size by 2 months of age. A similar prenatal and postnatal growth phenotype has been observed in a reported human case of an IGF-1 gene deletion.[253]

Igf2 null mice (or heterozygous mice carrying a paternally derived mutated Igf2 gene) also have birth weights 60% of normal and remain about 60% of normal size throughout life.[254] When the gene for the IGF-1 receptor is knocked out (Igf1r null mice), the mice are severely growth retarded with a birth weight only 45% of normal and die soon after birth—apparently of respiratory failure.[255] The addition of an Igf1 knockout to the Igf1r knockout does not change the growth characteristics significantly, consistent with the hypothesis that IGF-1 is signaling exclusively (at least from the perspective of growth) through the IGF-1 receptor. On the other hand, the combination of Igf2 and Igf1r knockouts results in further growth retardation (birth weight 30% of normal)—indicating that IGF-2 is signaling through the IGF-1 receptor and a second receptor (probably the insulin receptor).

The relationship between GH and IGF-1 in controlling postnatal growth was analyzed in mouse mutants lacking GHR, IGF-1, or both.[126] This demonstrated that GH and IGF-1 promote postnatal growth by independent and common functions because the growth retardation of double GHR/IGF-1 null mice is more severe than that observed with either class of single mutant. In fact, the body weight of these double-mutant mice is only approximately 17% of normal—indicating IGF-independent GH actions. Thus, the growth control pathway in which the components of the GH/IGF-1 signaling systems participate constitutes the major determinant of body size.

The Igf2 gene has been shown to be maternally imprinted in mice and humans (only the paternal gene is expressed). On the other hand, the gene for the IGF-2 receptor (Igf2r) is paternally imprinted (although only in mice).[256] The phenotypes of Igf2r null mice or of heterozygous mice inheriting a mutated maternal gene are indistinguishable and demonstrate overgrowth, with birth weights 140% of normal. Because this receptor normally degrades IGF-2, increased growth reflects excess IGF-2

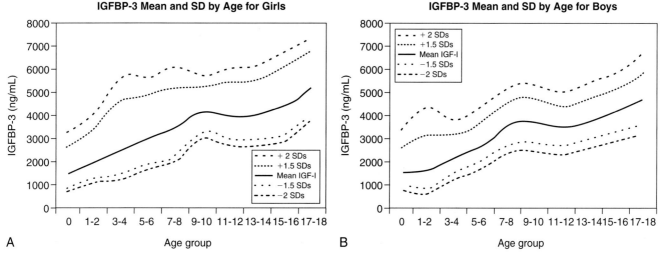

FIGURE 8–19. Insulin-like growth factor–binding protein 3 (IGFBP-3) values by age for males (A) and females (B). SD, standard deviation.

acting through the IGF-1 receptor. As mentioned previously, mice with deletions in GH and GH-receptor-related genes (as well as IGF-1R and downstream signaling genes) display increased life span and reduced oxidative stress.

OTHER GROWTH FACTORS

The FGF Family of Peptides and Receptors

Fibroblast growth factors (FGFs) constitute an important and rapidly expanding family of peptide cytokines, which are important in the regulation of many tissues. Initially, it was suggested that these factors may be specific for cells of stromal lineage. However, it appears that many other cells respond to FGFs as well. There are at least seven different FGFs (FGF-1 through FGF-7) that have been identified, including the best characterized acidic FGF (aFGF or FGF-1), basic FGF (bFGF or FGF-2), and keratinocyte growth factor (KGF or FGF-7).

The FGFs mediate their actions by binding to at least three receptors[257] (FGFR1, FGFR2, and FGFR3), which have distinct tissue distributions.[258] For the most part, FGFs appear to be autocrine-paracrine growth factors that participate in organ growth and differentiation (as well as in carcinogenesis) but not in somatic growth. An exception to this rule is the observation that the genetic form of dwarfism known as achondroplasia is caused by a mutation in the FGFR3 gene, suggesting that normal FGFR3 signaling is essential to the normal growth of long bones.[259] A human mutation in the FGFR2 gene causes craniosynostosis, a condition characterized by abnormal closure of the bones in the skull but normal long bone growth.[260] So far, targeted disruptions of several murine FGF and FGFR genes have been reported—and the phenotypes associated with them include various developmental abnormalities.

The EGF System

Epidermal growth factors (EGFs) and their receptors are ubiquitous in many tissues and participate in developmental processes in mice, such as precocious eyelid opening and tooth eruption. The mitogenic actions of EGF have been extensively explored in cell culture systems, and the receptor for EGF was characterized as a prototype model for signal transduction involving tyrosine kinases. The extensive in vitro data indicate multiple cellular functions of EGF. EGF has been identified in most body fluids of several mammalian species. However, neither EGF antibody administration to newborn animals nor gene targeting of EGF has caused major deleterious effects—as might have been expected from the in vitro studies.[261]

The EGF family of growth factors appears to be important in mammalian development and function, although the precise roles and significance are not yet clear. Members of the EGF family may have a role in embryogenesis and fetal growth because receptors have been identified in fetal tissues. It has been proposed that abnormal EGF-EGF receptor interactions may be instrumental in the development of cancer, but it appears that they are not involved in somatic growth.

Other Growth-Promoting Peptides

An ever-growing number of growth factors are being recognized, and multiple hormones and peptides are being characterized as having growth-promoting activities in certain cell types. In general, these molecules appear to lack somatic growth-promoting effects but play important autocrine-paracrine and endocrine roles. Notable among these molecules are groups of growth factors that have tissue-specific effects. Endothelin, platelet-derived growth factor (PDGF), and vascular-epithelial growth factor (VEGF) regulate angiogenesis and other vascular processes in addition to modulating the function of numerous cultured cells. A variety of hematopoietic growth factors [such as the granulocyte and macrophage colony-stimulating factors (GCSF, MCSF), erythropoietin, and thrombopoietin] promote the growth of the different lineages of the hematopoietic cells.

The growth of various cells of the immune system is stimulated by an array of cytokines, including interleukins and interferons. The complex array of cells that comprise the nervous system is under the regulatory influence of specific growth factors, such as nerve growth factor (NGF), the neurotrophins, and brain- and glial-derived neurotrophic factors (BDNF, GDNF). Other growth factors that have been attributed to specific tissues [e.g., hepatocyte growth factor (HGF)] are being recognized as having a general growth-promoting effect in numerous tissues, and additional organ-specific growth regulatory processes have been described in the gastrointestinal tract and kidneys.

Growth Inhibitory Peptides

Of particular interest is a class of cytokines that can negatively modulate cellular growth. Transforming growth factor-beta (TGFb) can act as an agent that mediates cellular growth and malignant transformation and as a growth inhibitory substance that has the potential of arresting the growth of normal and neoplastic cells. Tumor necrosis factors (TNFs) and other compounds have been reported to have similar effects.

These molecules may regulate the entry of cells into programmed cell death (apoptosis). The growth inhibitory processes of TGFb and other cytokines may prove to be of great importance in the development of cancer treatments. A family of genes/proteins, of which the most important is p53, is also critical to growth and tumor suppression.[262] These tumor suppressors may be involved in fetal growth.

SEX STEROIDS

Whereas androgens and estrogens do not contribute substantially to normal growth before the onset of puberty, the adolescent rise in serum sex steroid concentrations is an important part of the pubertal growth spurt. States of androgen or estrogen excess before epiphyseal fusion are invariably characterized by rapid linear growth and skeletal maturation. Thus, just as growth deceleration requires further evaluation growth acceleration can be just as abnormal and may be a sign of increased sex steroids—as observed in precocious puberty and virilizing congenital adrenal hyperplasia.

A GH-replete state is obligatory for a normal growth response to sex steroids. Children with GHD do not have a normal growth response to either endogenous or exogenous androgens. Although androgens work at least in part by enhancing GH secretion, they must also have a direct effect on IGF-1 production—as observed with the rise in serum IGF-1 concentrations and pubertal growth spurt characteristic of children with mutations of the GHR.[88]

Androgens and estrogens have been shown to increase skeletal maturation. Advancement of skeletal age and epiphyseal fusion appear to be estrogen mediated, as indicated by the report of tall stature with open epiphyses in a patient with a mutation of the estrogen receptor[14] and by similar findings in those with inactivating mutations of the gene regulating aromatase that converts androgens to estrogens.[263] Whatever the mechanism, however, clinical states of androgen or estrogen excess are characterized by disproportionate skeletal maturation and premature epiphyseal fusion. Interestingly, a condition of aromatase excess has been described, resulting from mutations in the propoter region of the gene and leading to early epiphysial closure and gynecomastia.[264]

THYROID HORMONE

Thyroid hormone is a major contributor to postnatal growth, although like GH it is of relatively little importance to growth of the fetus. Hypothyroidism occurring postnatally can, however, result in profound growth failure and virtual arrest of skeletal maturation. In addition to a direct effect on epiphyseal cartilage, thyroid hormone appears to have a permissive effect on GH secretion. Patients with hypothyroidism have decreased spontaneous GH secretion and have a blunted response to GH provocative tests. Treatment with thyroid hormone results in rapid "catch-up" growth, which is typically accompanied by marked skeletal maturation—potentially resulting in overly rapid epiphyseal fusion and compromise of adult height.

Growth Retardation

Systems for classification of growth disorders are problematic because diagnostic categories have not always been sharply defined and frequently overlap. Genetic short stature, for example, may often be associated with constitutional delay of growth and maturation—and both disorders fall under the umbrella of ISS. Because diagnostic criteria for GHD have been problematic, overlap has frequently existed among genetic short stature, constitutional delay, and the vague category of "partial" GHD. In addition, the cause of growth failure in intrauterine growth retardation (IUGR) and various syndromes associated with poor growth has generally remained obscure.

Table 8-3 represents an effort at classification of growth retardation. Growth disorders have been subdivided into primary growth abnormalities, in which the defect(s) appears to be intrinsic to the growth plate; genetic short stature; and secondary growth disorders (i.e., growth

TABLE 8-3
Classification of Growth Retardation

I. Primary Growth Abnormalities
A. Osteochondrodysplasias
B. Chromosomal abnormalities

II. Secondary Growth Disorders
A. Malnutrition
B. Chronic disease
C. Intrauterine growth retardation
D. Endocrine disorders
  1. Hypothyroidism
  2. Cushing syndrome
  3. Pseudohypoparathyroidism
  4. Vitamin D deficient or resistant rickets

III. IGF Deficiency
A. Secondary IGFD
• GH deficiency due to hypothalamic dysfunction
• GH deficiency due to pituitary GH deficiency
B. Primary IGFD (GH insensitivity)
• Primary GH insensitivity
• Secondary GH insensitivity (Stat-5b)
• Primary defects of IGF synthesis
• Primary defects of IGF transport/clearance (ALS)
C. IGF resistance
• Defects of the IGF-1 receptor
• Post-receptor defects

IV. Idiopathic Short Stature
1. Constitutional delay of growth and puberty with normal height prediction
2. ISS with delayed bone age and tempo of puberty
3. ISS with normal bone age and tempo of puberty
4. ISS with a familial component
5. ISS without a familial component

GH, growth hormone; IGF, insulin-like growth factor.

failure resulting from chronic disease or endocrine disorders). In recent years, the category of "IGF deficiency (IGFD)" has become accepted as an overall category encompassing disorders that can result from various causes of GH deficiency (sometimes called secondary IGFD) or GH-insensitivity (sometimes referred to as primary IGFD). The category of "IGF deficiency" takes on special meaning in light of recent recommendations for reevaluation of the diagnosis of GHD and primary IGFD.

PRIMARY GROWTH ABNORMALITIES
Osteochondrodysplasias

The osteochondrodysplasias represent a heterogeneous group of disorders characterized by intrinsic abnormalities of cartilage and/or bone.[265] These conditions share the following features: genetic transmission; abnormalities in the size and/or shape of bones of the limbs, spine, and/or skull; and radiologic abnormalities of the bones (generally). More than 100 osteochondrodysplastic conditions have been identified, based on physical features and radiologic characteristics. The ongoing characterization of biochemical and molecular abnormalities in these conditions will undoubtedly lead to an increase in the number of these disorders.

An international classification for the osteochondrodysplasias was developed.[266] Table 8-4 provides a brief summary of this classification. Of note, the category of dysostoses has been dropped from the classification—which now focuses on developmental disorders of chondro-osseous tissues. Diagnosis of osteochondrodysplasias can be problematic and often relies on careful radiologic evaluation. Although progress has been made in identifying the underlying molecular and biochemical defects in many of these conditions, clinical and radiologic evaluation remains central to the diagnosis at this time. Frequently, the clinical features are obvious—and the diagnosis can then be made at birth (or even prenatally) by ultrasound.

The family history is obviously critical. However, many cases represent fresh mutations—as is generally the case in the classic autosomal-dominant achondroplasia and hypochondroplasia. Careful measurement of body proportions is necessary, including arm span, sitting height, upper/lower body segments, and head circumference. Clinical and radiologic evaluation should be used to determine whether involvement is of the long bones, skull, and/or vertebrae—and whether abnormalities are primarily at the epiphyses, metaphyses, or diaphyses. Two of the more common forms (achondroplasia and hypochondroplasia)

of the more than 100 defined osteochondrodysplasias are discussed in the following sections.

Achondroplasia. This is the most common of the osteochondrodysplasias, with a frequency of approximately 1:26,000 births. Although transmitted as an autosomal-dominant disorder, 90% of cases apparently represent new mutations. Studies have indicated that achondroplasia is caused by a mutation of the gene for fibroblast growth factor receptor 3 (FGFR3), located on the short arm of chromosome 4.[267] Because the overwhelming majority of cases identified represent mutations at a "hot spot" at nucleotide 1138 of FGFR3, and because these mutations create new recognition sites for restriction enzymes, it is easy to test for the mutation.

Infants homozygous for this condition have severe disease, typically dying in infancy of respiratory insufficiency resulting from the small thorax. Short stature may not be evident until after 2 years of age, although the deviation from the normal growth curve is progressive. Mean adult height in males and females is 131 and 124 cm, respectively. Growth curves for achondroplasia have been developed and are of great value in following patients.[12]

With increasing age, the diagnosis of achondroplasia becomes easier because in addition to short stature these patients have other abnormalities of the skeleton—including megalocephaly, low nasal bridge, lumbar lordosis, short trident hand, and rhizomelia (shortness of the proximal legs and arms). Radiologic abnormalities include small cuboid-shaped vertebral bodies with short pedicles and progressive narrowing of the lumbar interpedicular distance. The iliac wings are small, with narrow sciatic notches. The small foramen magnum may lead to hydrocephalus, and spinal cord and/or root compression may result from kyphosis, stenosis of the spinal canal, or disc lesions.

Hypochondroplasia. Hypochondroplasia has been described as a "milder form" of achondroplasia. However, although the two disorders are both transmitted as autosomal-dominant traits they have not been reported to occur in the same family. Hypochondroplasia, however, has been shown to result from a mutation (Asn540Lys) of the FGFR3 gene—the same gene involved in achondroplasia. The facial features characteristic of achondroplasia are absent, and the short stature and rhizomelia are less pronounced.

Adult heights are typically in the 120- to 150-cm range. As in the case of achondroplasia, short stature may not be evident until after 2 years of age—but stature then deviates progressively from normal. Outward bowing of the legs accompanied by genu varum is frequently observed. Lumbar interpedicular distances diminish between L1 and L5, and as with achondroplasia there may be flaring of the pelvis and narrow sciatic notches.

Chromosomal Abnormalities

Abnormalities of the autosomes and sex chromosomes may be characterized by growth retardation. In general, these disorders are also associated with somatic abnormalities and mental retardation—as in deletion of chromosome 5 or trisomy 18 or 13. Such abnormalities, however, may be subtle—and, for example, the diagnosis of

---

TABLE 8-4

Classification of Osteochondrodysplasias

Defects of Tubular (and Flat) Bones and/or Axial Skeleton
Achondroplasia group
   Achondrogenesis
   Spondylodysplastic group (perinatally lethal)
   Metatropic dysplasia group
   Short rib dysplasia group (with/without polydactyly)
   Atelosteogenesis/diastrophic dysplasia group
   Kniest-Stickler dysplasia group
   Spondyloepiphyseal dysplasia group
   Other spondyloepi(meta)physeal dysplasias
   Dysostosis multiplex group
   Spondylometaphyseal dysplasias
   Epiphyseal dysplasias
   Chondrodysplasia punctata (stippled epiphyses) group
   Metaphyseal dysplasias
   Brachrachia (short spine dysplasia)
   Mesomelic dysplasias
   Acromelic/acromesomelic dysplasias
   Dysplasias with significant (but not exclusive) membranous bone involvement
   Bent bone dysplasia group
   Multiple dislocations with dysplasias
   Osteodysplastic primordial dwarfism group
   Dysplasias with increased bone density
   Dysplasias with defective mineralization
   Dysplasias with increased bone density
Disorganized Development of Cartilaginous and Fibrous
   Components of the Skeleton
Idiopathic Osteolyses

Turner syndrome must be considered in any girl with unexplained short stature. In many cases, the precise cause of growth failure in these chromosomal abnormalities is unclear because the genetic defects do not appear to affect known components of the GH-IGF system. It is presumed, then, that the chromosomal defect influences normal tissue growth and/or development or indirectly affects the responsiveness to IGF or to other growth factors yet to be identified.

Down Syndrome. Trisomy 21, or Down syndrome, is probably the most common chromosomal disorder associated with growth retardation—affecting approximately 1 in 600 live births. On average, newborns with Down syndrome have birth weights 500 g below normal and are 2 to 3 cm shorter. Growth failure continues postnatally, and is typically associated with delayed skeletal maturation and a poor delayed pubertal growth spurt. Adult heights range from 135 to 170 cm in males and 127 to 158 cm in women.[268] The cause of growth failure in Down syndrome and in other autosomal defects is unknown. Attempts to find underlying hormonal explanations for growth retardation have been unsuccessful, even though hypothyroidism is more common than normal in Down syndrome and should be excluded. It is likely that growth failure in such conditions reflects a generalized biochemical abnormality of the epiphyseal growth plate.

Turner Syndrome. Short stature is the single most common feature of Turner syndrome, occurring more frequently than delayed puberty, cubitus valgus, and webbing of the neck.[269-271] Reviews of large series of Turner syndrome individuals have indicated that short stature occurs in 95% to 100% of girls with a 45,X karyotype. Several distinct phases of growth have been identified in girls with Turner syndrome by Ranke and colleagues:[272] mild IUGR, with mean birth weights and heights of 2,800 g and 48.3 cm, respectively; normal height gain from birth until 3 years of age; progressive decline in height velocity from 3 years of age until approximately 14 years of age, resulting in a gradual and progressive deviation from normal height percentiles; and a prolonged adolescent growth phase characterized by a partial return toward normal height, followed by delayed epiphyseal fusion.

More recent detailed analyses of longitudinal and cross-sectional growth data from several centers have indicated that growth in girls with Turner syndrome is frequently abnormal in infancy and early childhood and that the majority of cases of Turner syndrome diagnosed before adult life have fallen off the normal growth curve by 2 to 3 years of age.[273,274] Investigations of Turner syndrome from the United States and Europe have indicated mean adult heights ranging from 142.0 to 146.8 cm (lower in Asia).

The cause of growth failure in Turner syndrome is multifactorial, although the loss of one copy of the homeobox gene—SHOX (short stature homeobox-containing gene)—is the major contributor.[275] The SHOX gene covers a 40-kb region of the pseudoautosomal region of the X chromosome, escapes X inactivation, and is highly expressed in osteogenic tissue. Haploinsufficiency for SHOX has been implicated in the short stature of Turner syndrome, as well as several other somatic features. In addition, SHOX mutations appear responsible for the mesomelic growth retardation and Madelung deformity characteristic of Leri-Weil dyschondrosteosis—and complete absence of SHOX is associated with Langer mesomelic dysplasia.

The majority of patients have normal GH levels during childhood. Reports of low GH levels in adolescents with Turner syndrome are likely ascribable to low serum levels of sex steroids.[276] Nevertheless, GH therapy is capable of accelerating short-term growth and increasing adult height in both Turner syndrome and SHOX haploinsufficiency.[173,277-279] Indeed, early initiation of GH therapy at appropriate dosages appears to enable most girls with Turner syndrome to attain heights within the normal adult range.[278,279] Turner syndrome is described in greater detail in Chapter 15. The point is worth repeating, however, that the diagnosis of Turner syndrome should be considered in any phenotypic female with unexplained growth failure.

18q Deletions. Deletion of the long arm of chromosome 18 has an estimated prevalence of 1 in 40,000 live births. In one review of 50 cases, 64% of children (mean age 5.8 years) had heights greater than 2 SD below the mean.[280] Fifteen percent had serum IGF-1 concentrations below 2 SD, and 9% had IGFBP-3 concentrations below 2 SD. Seventy-two percent of children had reduced GH responses to provocative testing, although such testing was not always rigorous.

Intrauterine Growth Retardation

Despite the critical importance of the endocrine system in postnatal growth, normal intrauterine growth is largely independent of fetal pituitary hormones.[281,282] Athyreotic and agonadal infants are of normal length and weight at birth. Based on the normal size of anencephalic fetuses, it has been proposed that even the pituitary is unnecessary for fetal growth.[283,284] Careful documentation of birth size of rats with congenital GHD[285] and of human newborns with mutations of the GH or GHR gene[88] has indicated, however, that fetal pituitary-derived GH makes a small but statistically significant contribution to birth size.

These observations should not be interpreted to mean that the IGF axis is irrelevant in fetal growth. Gene knockout studies have shown that elimination of paracrine/autocrine production of IGF-1 has a major impact on fetal and postnatal growth.[286] A human with an IGF-1 gene deletion had the same growth characteristics as observed in the murine IGF-1 knockout. That is, IUGR and postnatal growth failure that was unresponsive to GH administration.[287] Similarly, several reports of IGF-1 receptor defects associated with IUGR and postnatal growth retardation have appeared, and a family with bioinactive IGF-1 has also been reported.[281-282]

Thus, although the fetus may be largely GH independent the production and activity of IGF-1 is clearly critical for normal intrauterine (as well as postnatal) growth. Human cord lymphocytes have been demonstrated to have increased numbers of IGF receptors[288] and mRNAs because IGF-1 and IGF-2 are abundant in fetal tissues.[289,290] Similarly, the IGFBPs are identifiable in serum and other biologic fluids, although it is of note that the relative serum concentrations of various IGFBPs are different in the fetus and newborn than in the older child or adult.[291] In particular, serum concentrations of IGFBP-3 and acid-labile subunit (ALS)—which together comprise the major serum carriers of IGF peptides in the adult—are much lower in the fetus and newborn.

IUGR is defined on the basis of a birth weight and/or birth length more than 2 SD below the mean for gestational age. Although the majority of such infants show good catch-up growth during the first few years of life, approximately 15% of such children fail to have sufficient catch-up growth to bring them into the normal height range by 4 years of age.[281,282,292] Whereas several studies have demonstrated that infants with IUGR tend to have low serum levels of IGF-1 and IGFBP-3 at birth,[293] it is not entirely clear whether failure of catch-up growth represents the effects of subtle persistent abnormalities of the GH-IGF axis. Barker and colleagues have proposed that in the process of adapting to a limited supply of nutrients in utero IUGR fetuses permanently alter their physiology and metabolism, a reprogramming process that results in physiologic consequences in later life—such as increased risk of coronary artery disease, stroke, hypertension, and diabetes.[294,295]

IUGR can arise from intrinsic abnormalities in the fetus, placental insufficiency, or maternal disorders (Table 8-5). Although it is understandable why uterine constraint or twin pregnancies might result in limited fetal growth, the biochemical and cellular basis for abnormal fetal growth in most cases of IUGR is unclear. It has been proposed that such cases result from reduced cell number or cell size, but the mechanisms for such abnormalities remain to be elucidated. Intrinsic fetal endocrine abnormalities are unlikely explanations for IUGR in most cases.

Congenital thyroid and/or GH deficiencies are typically characterized by near-normal birth size. Recently recognized human mutations in IGF-1 and IGF-1 receptors are associated with IUGR, but circulating IGF-1 levels in IUGR children are highly variable—indicating that there is a large clinical diversity in this condition. Infants with IUGR frequently exhibit poor postnatal growth, particularly when the abnormalities are intrinsic to the fetus. Such conditions have frequently been categorized as "primordial growth failure."

Russell-Silver Syndrome. This condition was independently described by Russell,[296] and later by Silver and associates, in the early 1950s. Although this syndrome probably represents a heterogeneous group of patients, the "common" findings include IUGR, postnatal growth failure, congenital hemihypertrophy, and small triangular facies. Because no genetic or biochemical basis for this disorder has been identified, Russell-Silver syndrome is often used improperly as a designation for IUGR of unknown cause. Other common nonspecific findings include clinodactyly, precocious puberty, delayed closure of the fontanelles, and delayed bone age. Recently, it has been demonstrated that hypermethylation (termed *epimutation*) of the IGF2 gene leading to its decreased expression is associated with the majority of cases of this condition.[297]

Seckel Syndrome. Although originally described by Mann and Russell in 1959,[298] this condition is most commonly termed *Seckel syndrome* or *Seckel birdheaded dwarfism.*[299] An autosomal-recessive condition, Seckel syndrome is characterized by IUGR and severe postnatal growth failure combined with microcephaly, prominent nose, and micrognathia. Final height is typically 91.4 to 106.7 cm, with moderate to severe mental retardation.

Noonan Syndrome. Although this condition shares certain phenotypic features with Turner syndrome, the two disorders are clearly distinct.[300] In Noonan syndrome, several genes have been implicated—including KRAS (Kirsten rat sarcoma 2 viral oncogene homolog)—but the majority of cases are caused by PTP11 (protein tyrosine phosphatase nonreceptor type 11) mutations. Both males and females may be affected, explaining the misleading names "Turner-like syndrome" and "male Turner syndrome." As in Turner syndrome, patients typically have webbing of the neck, a low posterior hairline, ptosis, cubitus valgus, and malformed ears.

Cardiac abnormalities are, however, primarily right-sided (pulmonary valve)—rather than the left-sided lesions (aorta, aortic valve) characteristic of Turner syndrome. Microphallus and cryptorchidism are common, and puberty is frequently delayed or incomplete. Mental retardation is observed in approximately 25% to 50% of patients. In a manner similar to Turner syndrome, Noonan syndrome responds to GH therapy—and this

TABLE 8-5
Etiology of Intrauterine Growth Retardation

Intrinsic fetal abnormalities
  Chromosomal disorders
  Syndromes associated with primary growth failure
    Russell-Silver syndrome
    Seckel syndrome
    Noonan syndrome
    Progeria
    Cockayne syndrome
    Bloom syndrome
    Prader-Willi syndrome
    Rubinstein-Taybi syndrome
  Congenital infections
  Congenital anomalies
  Primary abnormalities of insulin-like growth factor axis
Placental anomalities
  Abnormal implantation of the placenta
  Placental vascular insufficiency; infarction
  Vascular malformations
Maternal disorders
  Malnutrition
  Constraints on uterine growth
  Vascular disorders
    Hypertension
    Toxemia
    Severe diabetes mellitus
  Uterine malformations
  Drug ingestion
    Tobacco
    Alcohol
    Narcotics

From Underwood LE, Van Wyk JJ: Normal and aberrant growth. In Wilson JD, Foster DW (eds): Williams Textbook of Endocrinology, 8th ed. Philadelphia, WB Saunders, 1992; p 1110.

treatment recently resulted in FDA approval in the United States.

Progeria. The senile appearance characteristic of progeria (Hutchinson-Gilford syndrome) typically appears by 2 years of age.[301] There is a progressive loss of subcutaneous fat, accompanied by alopecia, hypoplasia of the nails, joint limitation, and early onset of atherosclerosis—typically followed by angina, myocardial infarction, hypertension, and congestive heart failure. Skeletal hypoplasia results in severe growth retardation, which typically becomes evident by 6 to 18 months of age. The molecular basis of this syndrome, as well as that of the Cockayne syndrome, are described at *http//:www.ncbi.nlm.nih.gov/omim/*.

Cockayne Syndrome. Cockayne syndrome, like progeria, is characterized by a premature senile appearance.[302] Patients also have retinal degeneration, photosensitivity of the skin, and impaired hearing. Growth failure typically appears at 2 to 4 years of age. Transmission is as an autosomal-recessive disorder.

Prader-Willi Syndrome. Growth failure may be evident at birth but is generally more impressive postnatally. The neonatal period is characterized by hypotonia, and in the male by cryptorchidism and microphallus. With advancing age, hyperphagia and obesity become prominent. Hypogonadism may persist into adult life. The cause of growth failure is unclear. Low serum GH concentrations may reflect the impact of obesity and are not necessarily etiologic. On the other hand, low GH secretion and hypogonadism may reflect subtle defects of hypothalamic-pituitary function—and these patients respond well to GH therapy.[303-305] Patients with Prader-Willi syndrome have been found to have deletions of the paternal short arm of chromosome 15, or uniparental disomy of the maternal imprinted region of chromosome 15—a situation equivalent to paternal deletion of that region.

A variety of other syndromes may be associated with moderate-profound growth failure. These include Bloom syndrome, de Lange syndrome, leprechaunism (mutations of the insulin receptor gene), Ellis-van Creveld syndrome, Aarskog syndrome, Rubinstein-Taybi syndrome, mulibrey nanism (Perheentupa syndrome), Dubowitz syndrome, and Johanson-Blizzard syndrome. The syndromes discussed in this section are described in greater detail in Online Mendelian Inheritance in Man (OMIM), a National Institutes of Health–supported regularly updated web site that publishes information on genetic conditions *(http://www.ncbi.nim.nih.gov/omim/)*.

Placental insufficiency and maternal factors may also contribute to poor fetal growth. Whereas such infants have a better growth potential than do cases of "primordial growth failure," postnatal growth is not always normal. Maternal nutrition is an important contributor to fetal growth, impacting not only the size of the fetus but growth during the first year of life.[306] Fetal growth retardation may also result from alcohol consumption during pregnancy,[307-309] as well as from use of cocaine,[310,311] marijuana,[311] and tobacco.[312] The mechanisms for such drug-induced fetal growth retardation are unclear but probably include uterine vasoconstriction and vascular insufficiency, as well as placental abruption and premature rupture of membranes. Although maternal tobacco

use is statistically a major contributor to reduced fetal size, it is unlikely by itself to result in severe IUGR.

The implications of IUGR may extend beyond decreased fetal size. In a retrospective study of 47 children evaluated before puberty for growth failure secondary to IUGR, 23 boys had an adult height of 162 cm and 24 girls an adult height of only 148 cm[313] in the U.S. and Europe. Being SGA and failing to catch up is in an indication of GH therapy. More recent studies have indicated that small-for-gestational-age infants have an increased risk of hypertension, maturity-onset diabetes, and cardiovascular disease.[314] It remains unclear, however, whether IUGR is causally related to these disorders or is a symptom of an underlying inborn metabolic disorder.

Other Genetic Causes of Short Stature

Regulation of skeletal growth involves multiple factors, including hormones and growth factors, nutrition, general health, and a wide variety of other environmental factors. Even when evaluating hereditary aspects of skeletal growth, it is clear that control of growth in childhood (as well as final height) is polygenic by nature. Nevertheless, a direct impact of familial height on an individual subject's growth is normally evident, and evaluation of a child's growth pattern must be placed in the context of familial growth and stature. As described previously, formulas have been developed for determination of a person's target height based on parental heights—and growth curves that relate a child's height to parental height are available.[315] As a general rule, a child who is growing at a rate that is clearly inconsistent with that of siblings or parents warrants further evaluation.

Many organic diseases characterized by growth retardation are genetically transmitted. This list includes many endocrine causes, such as GHI resulting from mutations of the GHR gene, GH gene deletions, mutations of the POU1F1 gene, pseudohypoparathyroidism, and familial thyroid deficiency. Many other nonendocrine diseases characterized by short stature may be genetically transmitted, such as osteochondrodysplasias, dysmorphic syndromes associated with IUGR, diabetes, metabolic disorders, renal disease, thalassemia, and others. Identifying short stature as genetically transmitted thus does not by itself relieve the physician of responsibility for determining the underlying cause of growth failure.

SECONDARY GROWTH DISORDERS

Malnutrition

Given the worldwide presence of undernutrition, it is not surprising that inadequate caloric and/or protein intake represents by far the most common cause of growth failure.[316] Marasmus refers to cases with a global deficiency of calories, although often accompanied by protein insufficiency. Kwashiorkor, on the other hand, refers to inadequate protein intake—although it may also be characterized by caloric undernutrition. Frequently, the two conditions overlap.

The impaired growth characteristic of protein-energy malnutrition is frequently characterized by elevated basal and/or stimulated serum GH concentrations.[317] In generalized malnutrition (marasmus), however, GH concentrations may be normal or even low.[318] In both conditions, nevertheless, serum IGF-1 concentrations are typically reduced.[319,320] Malnutrition may, consequently, be considered a form of GHI in cases in which serum IGF-1 concentrations are reduced in the presence of normal or elevated GH levels. It has been suggested that elevated serum GH concentrations represent an adaptive response whereby protein is spared by the lipolytic and anti-insulin actions of GH. Reduced serum IGF-1 concentrations may represent a mechanism by which precious calories are shifted from use in growth to survival requirements of the organism. These adaptive mechanisms may be further enacted by changes in serum IGFBPs during periods of malnutrition.[321]

Inadequate caloric or protein intake may also complicate many chronic diseases characterized by growth failure. Anorexia is a common feature of renal failure and inflammatory bowel disease but may also be associated with cyanotic heart disease, congestive heart failure, central nervous system (CNS) disease, and other illnesses. Some of these conditions may, furthermore, be characterized by deficiencies of specific dietary components—such as zinc, iron, and various vitamins necessary for normal growth and development.

Undernutrition may also be voluntary, as is the case with dieting and food fads.[322] Caloric restriction is especially common in girls (such as among gymnasts and ballet dancers) during adolescence, when it may be associated with anxiety concerning obesity. Anorexia nervosa and bulimia represent extremes of "voluntary" caloric deprivation and are commonly associated with impaired growth if undernutrition occurs before epiphyseal fusion. Even later in adolescence, these conditions may be characterized by delayed puberty and/or menarche and a variety of metabolic alterations.

Chronic Diseases

Malabsorption. Intestinal disorders associated with inadequate absorption of calories or protein are typically associated with growth failure for many of the reasons cited previously.[323-326] It is not uncommon for growth retardation to predate many of the other manifestations of malabsorption and/or chronic inflammatory bowel disease. Accordingly, such conditions [especially gluten-induced enteropathy (celiac disease) and regional enteritis (Crohn disease)] must be in the differential diagnosis of unexplained growth failure. Serum concentrations of IGF-1 may be reduced,[327] reflecting the malnutrition. It is therefore all the more critical to discriminate these conditions from GHD or related disorders.

Documentation of malabsorption requires demonstration of fecal wasting of calories, especially fecal fat. The diagnosis of celiac disease ultimately requires a biopsy of the small intestine and demonstration of the characteristic flattening of the mucosa. Normalization of jejunal mucosa after gluten withdrawal and reappearance of abnormalities on gluten challenge are necessary to confirm the diagnosis. The use of antigliadin autoantibodies has been disappointing in the diagnosis of celiac disease because of its low specificity, but transglutaminase antibodies are useful.

On the other hand, whereas some have recommended jejunal biopsy to rule out celiac disease in all cases of unexplained growth failure during the first 5 years of life this aggressive an approach is not usually necessary.[328] Generally, an alternative would be to reserve biopsies for children with a history of diarrhea and/or steatorrhea in the first 2 years of life, abnormal D-xylose absorption tests, and positive transglutaminase antibodies.[329] The growth failure characteristic of Crohn disease probably represents a combination of malabsorption, anorexia, chronic inflammation, inadequacy of trace minerals, and use of glucocorticoids.[330] As stated previously, growth retardation may precede other clinical manifestations—such as fever, abdominal pain, and diarrhea. An elevated erythrocyte sedimentation rate is a useful clue, although diagnosis ultimately requires endoscopy and biopsy.

Cardiovascular Disease. Cyanotic heart disease and congestive heart failure may be associated with growth failure.[331,332] Because cardiac defects are usually congenital, many infants have syndromes associated with dysmorphic features and IUGR. Postnatal growth failure is usually attributable to hypoxia and the increased energy demands of a failing heart. These conditions are often accompanied by feeding difficulties that exacerbate the poor growth.

Corrective surgery often results in restoration of normal growth, frequently with a phase of "catch-up" growth. Unfortunately, surgery must on occasion be delayed until the infant has reached an appropriate size—resulting in the conundrum that surgery corrects growth failure but cannot be performed because the infant is too small. In these situations, meticulous attention to caloric support and alleviation of hypoxia and heart failure is necessary to maximize growth before surgery.

Renal Disease. A wide variety of clinical conditions that affect renal function can result in significant growth retardation.[333,334] Uremia, Fanconi syndrome, and renal tubular acidosis can all lead to growth failure before other clinical manifestations become evident. It is probable that renal disease leads to growth retardation through multiple mechanisms, including decreased caloric intake, loss of electrolytes necessary for normal growth, metabolic acidosis, protein wasting, inadequate formation of 1,25-dihydroxycholecalciferol, insulin resistance, chronic anemia, and compromised cardiac function.

Although earlier studies suggested a decrease in serum IGF concentrations in uremia, it is now evident that these erroneous determinations reflected inadequate separation of IGF peptides from IGFBPs before assay.[159] Serum IGF-1 and IGF-2 concentrations are in general within normal limits, but increases in serum IGFBPs (especially IGFBP-1) may lead to inhibition of IGF action. The use of chronic glucocorticoid therapy in the treatment of a variety of nephritic and nephrotic conditions can exacerbate the growth retardation characteristic of renal disease.

The age at onset of renal dysfunction is a factor in the resultant growth failure. Impairment of renal function at an early age typically results in a greater degree of growth failure, probably owing at least in part to the cumulative effects of growth retardation over many years. Subsequent correction of renal failure does not always allow for full catch-up growth. In a study in which renal transplantation was performed before 15 years of age (with a mean age at onset of hemodialysis of 10.6 years and at initial transplantation of 11.8 years), height SD scores did not significantly improve.[335] Approximately 75% of subjects had adult heights below the third percentile.

Although the growth failure of renal disease is not caused by GH or IGF deficiency, GH therapy has proven useful in accelerating skeletal growth. It is likely that such treatment increases the molar ratio of IGF peptides to IGFBPs, potentially overriding the inhibitory actions of IGFBPs.

Hematologic Disorders. Chronic anemias, such as sickle cell disease, are characterized by growth failure.[336-338] The causes of growth retardation probably include impaired oxygen delivery to tissues, increased work of the cardiovascular system, energy demands of increased hematopoiesis, and impaired nutrition. Thalassemia, in addition to the consequences of chronic anemia, can also be characterized by endocrine deficiencies resulting from chronic transfusions and accompanying hemosiderosis.[339,340] Despite vigorous efforts to maintain hemoglobins near normal and to employ chelation therapy, growth failure has remained a common feature of thalassemia—especially in adolescents. It is likely that impaired IGF-1 synthesis,[341,342] hypothyroidism, gonadal failure, and hypogonadotropic hypogonadism—combined with chronic anemia—all contribute to growth failure.

Diabetes Mellitus. Growth failure can be observed in children whose diabetes is under chronically poor control.[71] The so-called Mauriac syndrome[343] describes children with diabetes mellitus, severe growth failure, and hepatomegaly resulting from excess hepatic glycogen deposition. This type of striking growth retardation is unusual in diabetes, and in general growth failure is modest. As with other chronic diseases, growth retardation probably represents a combination of pathophysiologic processes—such as calorie wasting from hyperglycemia or malabsorption secondary to celiac sprue, chronic acidosis, increased glucocorticoid production, and hypothyroidism.

Because IGFBP-1 is normally suppressed by insulin, chronic hypoinsulinemia results in elevated serum IGFBP-1 concentrations—which may inhibit IGF action. In addition, insulin regulates the expression of the GHR—and hypoinsulinemia commonly leads to low IGF-1 levels through this mechanism.[344] Nevertheless, the correlation between glycemic control and skeletal growth is surprisingly unreliable—and many children with apparently marginal control appear to grow well.[345] One can only surmise that such patients are able to attain normal intracellular nutrition despite seeming hypoinsulinemia. It is likely, however, that continued progress in improving glycemic control in diabetes will improve growth in these children.

Inborn Errors of Metabolism. Inborn errors of protein, carbohydrate, and lipid metabolism are often accompanied by growth failure—which can be pronounced. Glycogen storage disease, the mucopolysaccharidoses, glycoproteinoses, and mucolipidoses may all be characterized

by poor growth. Many inborn metabolic disorders are also associated with significant skeletal dysplasia.

Pulmonary Disease. Cystic fibrosis is the classic example of growth failure associated with pulmonary disease, although poor growth undoubtedly represents the combined effects of pulmonary and pancreatic dysfunction.[181] The Cystic Fibrosis Foundation reports that 18% of patients with cystic fibrosis fall below the 5th percentile in height, and 23% fall below the 5th percentile in weight. In addition, the appearance of diabetes, the use of steroids, and the presence of frequent infections all contribute to the poor growth cystic fibrosis. Any condition associated with chronic hypoxemia may result in growth retardation. In children with chronic asthma, the long-term use of glucocorticoids undoubtedly contributes significantly to growth failure.

Chronic Infection. In many developing countries, chronic infestation with intestinal and systemic parasites (such as schistosomiasis, hookworm, and roundworm) contributes to nutritional debilitation and growth failure.[346]

Endocrine Disorders

Hypothyroidism. Many of the clinical features characteristic of adult myxedema are lacking in pediatric patients with acquired hypothyroidism. The most common and prominent manifestation of chronic acquired hypothyroidism is growth failure, which may be profound.[347] Postnatal growth retardation may also be observed in the infant with congenital hypothyroidism, but the development of newborn screening programs for hypothyroidism have generally resulted in prompt diagnosis and treatment of such patients. In acquired hypothyroidism, growth retardation may take several years to become clinically evident. However, once present growth failure is typically severe and progressive.

Rivkees and associates[347] have reported a mean 4.2-year delay between documentation of growth deceleration and the diagnosis of hypothyroidism. At diagnosis, girls were 24.04 SD and boys 23.15 SD below heights for age. (This is one of several situations in which the diagnosis of short stature is more delayed in girls than in boys.) Although chronic hypothyroidism is generally characterized by delayed puberty, precocious puberty and even premature menarche can occur in hypothyroid children—an entity called VanWyk-Grumbach syndrome. In some females with severe primary hypothyroidism, large recurrent ovarian cysts may manifest.[348] Skeletal age is usually markedly delayed.

Confirmation of the diagnosis of primary hypothyroidism is usually straightforward. Serum concentrations of T4 are reduced, and TSH concentrations are elevated. The presence of antithyroid antibodies is consistent with a diagnosis of Hashimoto thyroiditis, the most common cause of acquired hypothyroidism in the United States. Isolated secondary and tertiary hypothyroidism, caused by TSH and TRH deficiency (respectively), are very rare causes of acquired hypothyroidism.

Replacement therapy with levothyroxine is associated with a period of rapid catch-up growth. Despite this gratifying response, however, accelerated growth often does not result in restoration of full growth potential—

largely because of the rapid increase in skeletal age during the first 18 months of treatment. In the study of Rivkees and associates,[347] children treated at an initial mean chronologic age of 11 years had adult heights approximately 2 SD below the means for sex. These final heights were significantly lower than mid-parental heights or initial predicted adult heights based on data of Bayley and Pinneau. The deficit in adult stature correlated significantly with the duration of hypothyroidism before initiation of treatment. Accordingly, it may be appropriate to use lower than usual replacement dosages of levothyroxine and/or to consider delaying puberty and epiphyseal fusion pharmacologically.

Cushing Syndrome. Glucocorticoid excess has a profound effect on skeletal growth[348,349] whether the cause of Cushing syndrome is hypersecretion of ACTH, a primary adrenal tumor, or glucocorticoid therapy. It is assumed that the effects of glucocorticoids are directly at the epiphysis because GH secretion is typically normal and serum concentrations of IGF peptides and IGFBPs are not generally affected. This is supported by the observation that treatment with GH cannot completely overcome the growth inhibiting effects of excess glucocorticoids. The "toxic" actions of glucocorticoids on the epiphysis often persist at least in part after termination of chronic glucocorticoid excess, and patients frequently do not attain their target heights.[350]

The longer the duration and the greater the intensity of glucocorticoid excess the less likely the patient will experience complete catch-up growth. It is therefore important to limit exposure to excess glucocorticoids as much as the underlying condition being treated will allow. This may in part be accomplished by the use of alternate-day steroid therapy. The characteristic signs of Cushing syndrome (such as truncal obesity, decreased muscle mass, striae, easy bruising, thin skin, and osteoporosis) are well known. Adrenal tumors secreting large amounts of glucocorticoids frequently also produce excess androgens, which may mask the growth inhibitory effects of glucocorticoids.

It is also important to note that Cushing syndrome in children may be lacking many of the clinical signs and symptoms associated with the disorder in adults and may present exclusively with growth arrest. On the other hand, Cushing syndrome is an unlikely diagnosis in children presenting with obesity because exogenous obesity is associated with normal or even accelerated skeletal growth—whereas in Cushing syndrome growth deceleration is generally evident by the time other signs appear.

Pseudohypoparathyroidism. This condition is discussed in more detail elsewhere, but it is included here because at time of presentation growth failure is a frequent feature.[351] In its classic form, this condition combines growth failure and characteristic dysmorphic features with hypocalcemia and hyperphosphatemia secondary to end-organ resistance to parathyroid hormone (PTH). Children with pseudohypoparathyroidism are short and truncally obese, with short metacarpals, subcutaneous calcifications, round facies, and mental retardation.

Rickets. Hypovitaminosis D is historically a major cause of abnormal skeletal growth and short stature. Often it is associated with other causes of growth failure, such as malnutrition, prematurity, malabsorption, hepatic disease, and chronic renal failure. When vitamin D deficiency occurs by itself, typically when infants have poor exposure to sunlight and are not being nutritionally supplemented with vitamin D, the characteristic skeletal manifestations of rickets are evident: frontal bossing, craniotabes, rachitic rosary, and bowing of the legs.

Vitamin D–Resistant (Hypophosphatemic) Rickets. This X-linked condition results from decreased renal tubular reabsorption of phosphate. Clinical features are generally more severe in males and include short stature and prominent bowing of the legs, but other rachitic signs may be present.[352] The metabolic and skeletal abnormalities cannot be overcome by vitamin D therapy alone, and thus the name "vitamin D–resistant rickets." Treatment requires oral phosphate replacement, but such therapy often results in poor calcium absorption from the intestine. The addition of vitamin D to oral phosphate increases intestinal phosphate absorption and prevents hypocalcemia. Preliminary studies with GH therapy have indicated (at least in the short term) an enhancement of skeletal growth.

IGF Deficiency. Thyroid hormone and IGF-1 appear to be the major mediators of skeletal growth. Studies involving targeted disruption of genes for various components of the IGF system have established the critical role of the IGF axis in prenatal and postnatal growth.[353] Deficiency of IGF-1 can result in severe growth failure and may result from hypothalamic dysfunction, pituitary GHD, or primary or secondary GHI. It is not always possible to completely discriminate between hypothalamic and pituitary dysfunction because both organs may be involved in the same pathologic process. In addition, embryonic development of the hypothalamus and pituitary appears to be co-dependent.[27-31]

A number of factors produced in the developing ventral diencephalon function as molecular signals for initial formation and development of Rathke's pouch. Subsequent differentiation of each of the various anterior pituitary cell types appears to be primarily regulated by a strict temporal and spatial pattern of pituitary transcription factors.

It thus becomes somewhat of a semantic issue as to whether to label some of the molecular defects "hypothalamic" or "pituitary." Nevertheless, some arbitrary classification decisions have been made. Table 8-6 presents our current classification of molecular defects of the GH-IGF axis, and sites of established and hypothetical defects are shown in Figure 8-20. Figure 8-21 provides a "decision tree" for investigation of genetic defects in patients with IGF deficiency. It is to be anticipated that significant developments will be made in our understanding of these defects over the next few years and that this classification will require frequent updating and modification.

Hypothalamic Dysfunction. Hypothalamic dysfunction can arise from congenital malformations of the brain or hypothalamus, trauma, infections, sarcoid, tumors, or cranial irradiation. Anencephaly results in a pituitary gland that is small or abnormally formed and frequently ectopic. Holoprosencephaly, resulting from abnormal midline development of the embryonic brain, is also typically associated with hypothalamic insufficiency.[354,355]

TABLE 8-6

Established Genetic Defects of the GH-IGF Axis Resulting in IGF Deficiency

Mutant Gene	Inheritance	Phenotype
HPA		Developmental abnormalities
HESX1	AR	Septo-optic dysplasia; variable involvement of pituitary hormones
PROP1	AR	GH, PRL, TSH, LH, FSH deficiencies; variable ACTH deficiency
POU1F1 (Pit1)	AR, AD	GH, PRL deficiency; variable degree of TSH deficiency
RIEG	AD	Rieger syndrome
LHX3	AR	GH, TSH, LH, FSH, prolactin deficiencies
LHX4	AD	GH, TSH, ACTH deficiencies
SOX3	XL	GH deficiency, mental retardation
GLI2	AD	Holoprosencephaly, hypopituitarism
GLI3	AD	Pallister-Hall syndrome, hypopituitarism
Isolated GHD		
GHRHR	AR	IGHD, Type IB form of IGHD
GHS-R	AD	GHD and ISS
GH1	AR	Type IA form of IGHD
	AR	Type IB form IGHD
	AD	Type II form of IGHD
	X-linked	Type III form of IGHD; hypogamma-globulinemia
	AD	Bioinactive GH molecule
GHI		
GHR		
Extracellular domain	AR, AD	IGF-I deficiency; decreased or normal GHBP
Transmembrane	AR	IGF-I deficiency; normal or increased GHBP
Intracellular domain	AD	IGF-I deficiency; normal or increased GHBP
IGF		
IGF1	AR	IGF-I deficiency; IUGR and postnatal growth failure
ALS	AR	IGF-I deficiency; variable postnatal growth failure, delayed puberty

HPA, hypothalamic pituitary; ACTH, adrenocorticotropic hormone (corticotropin); AD, autosomal dominant; AR, autosomal recessive; FSH, follicle-stimulating hormone; GH, growth hormone; GHBP, GH-binding protein; GHRHR, GH-releasing hormone receptor; IGF, insulin-like growth factor; IGHD, isolated GHD; IUGR, intrauterine growth retardation; LH, luteinizing hormone; PRL, prolactin; TSH, thyroid-stimulating hormone; and ALS, acid labile subunit.

GH and IGF signaling

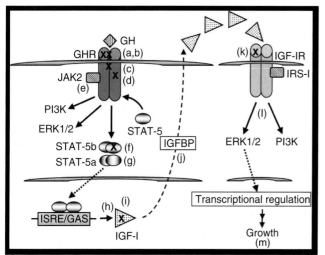

Figure 8-20 Schematic diagram of the GH–IGF axis, showing identified and theoretical defects: (*a*) defects of the extracellular domain of the GHR, affecting binding of GH; (*b*) defects in GHR dimerization; (*c*) defects of the transmembrane domain of the GHR; (*d*) defects of the intracellular domain of the GHR; (*e*) defects of JAK2 (theoretical at this time); (*f*) defects of STAT5b; (*g*) defects of STAT5a (theoretical at this time); (*h*) defects of transcriptional regulation of IGF-I (theoretical at this time); (*i*) defects of the IGF-I gene; (*j*) defects of IGFBPs, affecting IGF availability (theoretical at this time); (*k*) defects of the IGF receptor; (*l*) defects of IGF receptor signal transduction (theoretical at this time); and (*m*) defects at the epiphyseal growth plate, potentially affecting IGF action. GH, growth hormone; GHR, growth hormone receptor; JAK2, janus-family tyrosine kinase 2; PI3K, phosphatidylinositol-3 kinase; ERK, extracellular signal-regulated kinase; STAT, signal transducer and activator of transcription; ISRE, interferon-stimulated response element; GAS, interferon-gamma-activated sequences; IGF, insulin-like growth factor; IGFBP, IGF binding proteins; IGF-IR, IGF-I receptor; and IRS, insulin receptor substrate. [Used with permission from Rosenfeld RG, Hwa V (2004). New molecular mechanisms of GH resistance. Eur J Endocrinol 151(1):S11–S15.]

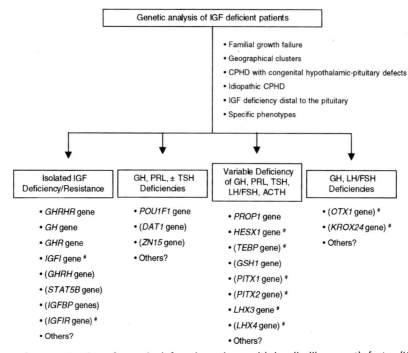

FIGURE 8-21. Decision tree for investigation of genetic defects in patients with insulin-like growth factor (IGF) deficiency. Hypothetical genetic defects are presented in parentheses. Abnormalities in other organs and structures besides the hypothalamus-pituitary-IGF axis are expected to occur as a result of these genetic defects. ACTH, adrenocorticotropic hormone; CPHD, combined pituitary hormone deficiencies; FSH, follicle-stimulating hormone; GH, growth hormone; GHR, growth hormone receptor; GHRHR, GH-releasing hormone receptor; IGFIR,IGF-1 receptor; LH, luteinizing hormone; PRL, prolactin; STAT5, signal transducer and activator of transcription 5; TSH, thyroid-stimulating hormone. (From Lopez-Bermejo A, Buckway CK, Rosenfeld RG: Genetic defects of the growth hormone–insulin-like growth factor axis. Trends Endocrinol 11:43, 2000, with permission from Elsevier Science.)

The clinical spectrum of holoprosencephaly can range from cyclopia to hypertelorism, accompanied by absence of the philtrum or nasal septum and midline clefts of the palate or lip. In these situations, GHD is often accompanied by other pituitary insufficiencies.

Debate continues as to whether the incidence of GHD is increased in cases of simple clefts of the lip and/or palate alone.[356,357] Clearly, children with clefts who are growing abnormally certainly require further evaluation. The syndrome of septo-optic dysplasia in its complete form combines hypoplasia or absence of the optic chiasm and/or optic nerves, agenesis or hypoplasia of the septum pellucidum and/or corpus callosum, and hypothalamic insufficiency.[37,358] The extent of the anatomic abnormalities and hypothalamic/pituitary insufficiency can vary considerably.[359] GHD can occur by itself, or in combination with TSH, ACTH, and/or gonadotropin deficiencies. Accordingly, this diagnosis should be considered in any child with growth failure associated with nystagmus or impaired vision.

Two siblings with septo-optic dysplasia have been reported to have homozygous missense mutations of HESX1, a paired-like homeodomain gene.[360,361] The mutation, which results in an Arg53Cys substitution, appears to totally abrogate DNA binding. Rathke's pouch homeobox (Rpx), the murine homologue, is expressed in the prospective cephalic region earlier during gastrulation. Later, it can be found throughout the prosencephalon—but it is restricted ultimately to Rathke's pouch. Knockout of the Hesx1 gene in the mouse results in phenotypes varying from an embryonic lethal form (with complete absence of Rathke's pouch) to a milder phenotype, with hypoplasia of the anterior lobe of the pituitary.

Molecular Defects of GHRH or the GHRH Receptor. No convincing cases of mutations of the GHRH gene in humans have been identified. This is a somewhat surprising observation, and the GHRH gene must still be considered a candidate gene for familial forms of isolated GHD. Abnormalities of the gene for the GHRH receptor (GHRHR), on the other hand, have been found in at least four kindreds.[362-365] A family from India was found to harbor a nonsense mutation of the GHRHR, resulting from a Glu72 stop mutation in exon 3.[362]

The resulting truncated molecule lacks the transmembrane region and the G-protein–binding sites. An apparently identical mutation has been identified in a family from Sri Lanka,[364] and in 17 members of an inbred kindred in Sindh (Pakistan).[363] The largest kindred with a mutation of GHRHR has been identified in Brazil.[365] A donor splice mutation in position 1 of exon 1 results in a severely truncated GHRHR protein.

Trauma of the Brain and/or Hypothalamus. Trauma to the brain, hypothalamus, pituitary stalk, or anterior pituitary may result in isolated GHD or in multiple deficiencies of the anterior pituitary.[366,367] Many published series of patients with GHD indicate an increased incidence of birth trauma, such as breech deliveries, extensive use of forceps, prolonged labor, or abrupt delivery.[367]

Debate continues as to whether GHD is the consequence of difficult delivery or merely reflects the perinatal consequences of fetal pituitary insufficiency.

Inflammation of the Brain and/or Hypothalamus. Inflammation of the brain (resulting from bacterial, viral, or fungal infections) may result in hypothalamic/pituitary insufficiency.[368,369] The hypothalamus and/or pituitary may also be involved in sarcoidosis.[370]

Tumors of the Brain and/or Hypothalamus. Tumors of the CNS are a major cause of hypothalamic insufficiency.[371] This is especially true for midline brain tumors, such as germinomas, meningiomas, gliomas, colloid cysts of the third ventricle, ependymomas, and gliomas of the optic nerve. Although metastasis from extracranial carcinomas is rarely found in children, hypothalamic insufficiency may result from local extension of craniopharyngeal carcinoma or Hodgkin disease of the nasopharynx. Craniopharyngiomas and histiocytosis may result in hypothalamic dysfunction (discussed under "Pituitary GH Deficiency").

Irradiation of the Brain and/or Hypothalamus. Cranial irradiation continues to emerge as an increasing cause of hypothalamic/pituitary dysfunction.[372-375] Irradiation may directly impair hypothalamic and pituitary function, and it is not always easy to discriminate between damage at each of these levels. In addition, thyroidal and gonadal function may also be directly affected. The degree of pituitary impairment is related to the dose of radiation received. Low doses typically result in isolated GHD. With higher doses, multiple pituitary hormone deficiencies are observed. Two to 5 years after irradiation, 100% of children receiving more than 3000 cGy over 3 weeks to the hypothalamic-pituitary axis showed subnormal GH responses to insulin-provocative tests.[376]

The degree of pituitary deficiency observed is also directly correlated to the length of time since irradiation. Children who test normally at 1 year post-irradiation may still develop pituitary deficiencies at later times. Even when serum GH concentrations after provocative testing are normal, measures of spontaneous GH secretion may indicate an impairment. As little as 1,800 cGy has been shown to affect spontaneous GH secretion in pubertal children.

Decreased GH secretion may be further complicated by the impact of irradiation on spinal growth, which can result in short stature and skeletal disproportion. Surprisingly, cranial irradiation can also result in precocious puberty—with the consequence that epiphyseal fusion occurs at an earlier age than is ideal from the perspective of maximizing growth. Gonadotropin-releasing hormone (GnRH) analogues may be necessary to delay pubertal progression. The endocrinologist observing the child who has received craniospinal irradiation must weigh these three factors: evolving hypopituitarism, decreased spinal growth potential, and early puberty and premature epiphyseal fusion. Care must be taken to maximize the growth potential of the patient without causing skeletal disproportion and without delaying puberty excessively or allowing growth to terminate too early.

Pituitary GH Deficiency. As discussed previously, many of the disease processes that affect hypothalamic regulation of GH secretion also impact pituitary function. Given current diagnostic limitations, it is not in fact always possible to completely discriminate between hypothalamic and pituitary dysfunction. Furthermore, it is likely that many cases of so-called idiopathic GHD will be found to have a molecular basis for the disorder. Indeed, in the past 5 years we have seen an explosion of information concerning genes critically involved in pituitary somatotrope differentiation and function (Tables 8-2 and 8-6).

At this time, however, a clear cause for pituitary GHD is often not identified—hence the term *idiopathic*. An incidence of pituitary GHD in 1:60,000 live births was reported from the United Kingdom.[377] A more recent survey of 48,000 Scottish schoolchildren has indicated an incidence as high as 1:4,000,[378] whereas the best estimate available in the United States population is at least 1:3,480.[379]

It is likely, however, that childhood GHD is an overdiagnosed condition. In particular, the diagnosis of acquired idiopathic isolated GHD should always be suspect. Although one may argue that destructive or inflammatory lesions of the hypothalamus or pituitary may only affect GH secretion, that isolated GHD caused by a mild mutation/deletion of the GHRH receptor gene or GH gene may appear late, or that combined pituitary hormone deficiency (CPHD) may first present with what appears to be isolated GHD, such circumstances appear to be rare. In the absence of anatomic abnormalities evident on imaging studies and/or biochemical evidence of CPHD, the diagnosis of acquired isolated idiopathic GHD demands careful and thorough documentation.

Genetic Abnormalities Resulting in Combined Pituitary Hormone Deficiency. Septo-optic dysplasia and its relationship to HESX1 was discussed previously. The gene PROP1 (standing for prophet of Pit1) is involved in the early determination and differentiation of multiple anterior pituitary cell forms.[380,381] Abnormalities of PROP1 result in CPHD, characterized by variable degrees of deficiency of GH, prolactin, TSH, follicle-stimulating hormone (FSH), luteinizing hormone, and occasionally ACTH.[381-385] In humans, PROP1 abnormalities identified to date include at least three missense and one splicing mutation.

A GA repeat in exon 2 (295-CGA-GAG-AGT-303) has been reported to be a hot spot in PROP1. Any combination of a GA or AG deletion in this repeat region results in a frame-shift in the coding sequence and premature termination at codon 109.[381] Similar abnormalities result from GA or AG deletions at codon 149.[382] Large-scale screening of families with multiple cases of CPHD has suggested that PROP1 mutations may be frequent causes of CPHD (32% of unrelated CPHD-affected patients and 50% of unrelated CPHD-affected families, according to one study).[381]

POU1F1 is the human homologue of the mouse gene pit1 and encodes a transcription factor involved in activation of GH and prolactin genes, regulation of the TSH-b promoter, and specification, proliferation, and survival of the corresponding cell lineages.[69,386] Abnormalities of the POUF1 gene result in deficiency of GH and prolactin and in variable TSH deficiency. CPHD resulting from abnormalities of POU1F1 can be transmitted as an autosomal-recessive or autosomal-dominant trait.[387-389] At least 12 different mutations and a deletion of POU1F1 have been reported in cases of CPHD. The most common mutation is an R271W substitution, which results in production of a protein that remains capable of binding to DNA but acts as a dominant negative inhibitor of transcription.[388] Screening studies suggest that abnormalities of POU1F1 are less common causes of CPHD than are abnormalities of the PROP1 gene.[381,386]

Haploinsufficiency of the homeobox gene RIEG results in Rieger syndrome, an autosomal-dominant disorder that involves abnormal development of the anterior chamber of the eye, teeth, and umbilicus—with an occasional association with GHD.[390,391] The rieg/pitx2 null mouse has been shown to be characterized by multiple pituitary hormone deficiency (MPHD).

Genetic Abnormalities of GH Production and/or Secretion Resulting in Isolated GHD. It has been reported that up to 30% of patients with isolated GHD have an affected parent or sibling. In addition to the abnormalities of the PROP1 and POU1F1 genes described previously, in which abnormalities of GH secretion are associated with decreased secretion of other anterior pituitary hormones, four mendelian forms of isolated GHD have been reported[392,393] (Table 8-6). GH1 is one member of a cluster of five contiguous structurally related genes located on chromosome 17: GH1, CSHP1 (chorionic somatomammotropin pseudogene), CSH1 (chorionic somatomammotropin gene), GH2, and CSH2.

Isolated GHDIA results from deletions (6.7, 7.0, 7.6, and 45 kb deletions have been reported) or mutations of the GH1 gene that totally block GH synthesis or secretion.[394-396] Transmission of isolated GHDIA is autosomal recessive, and patients have profound congenital GHD. Because GH has never been produced by the patient, even in fetal life, patients are immunologically intolerant of GH and typically develop anti-GH antibodies when treated with pituitary-derived or recombinant DNA–derived GH—although development of growth-attenuating antibodies appears to be less frequent with the newer synthetic GH preparations.

When antibodies prevent a patient from responding to GH, GHDIA can be viewed as a form of GHI and the patient is a candidate for IGF-1 therapy. The less severe form of autosomal-recessive GHD (isolated GHDIB) is likely to also be the result of mutations or rearrangements of the GH1 gene, presumably resulting in a GH molecule that retains some function but is perhaps unstable.[397] To date, however, most patients with presumed isolated GHDIB have not demonstrated an alteration of the GH1 gene and the cause of their GHD remains unclear. These patients generally respond to GH therapy, and development of clinically significant anti-GH antibodies is unusual.

Isolated GHDII is transmitted as an autosomal dominant. If such patients also prove to have abnormalities of the GH1 gene, it is likely they function in a dominant negative manner. Isolated GHDIII is transmitted in an X-linked manner. The most common causes of this disorder appear to be splice site and intronic mutations that inactivate the 59-splice donor site of intron 3, resulting in skipping of exon 3. In addition, a missense mutation (Arg183His) has been identified in this phenotype[80]—presumably causing production of an abnormal GH molecule that acts in a

dominant negative manner. Finally, the X-linked hypogammaglobinemia and GHD syndrome (an additional X-linked form of GHD associated with hypogammaglobinemia) has not been found to be associated with mutations of the GH gene.[45]

Congenital Absence or Hypoplasia of the Pituitary. A number of reports have described the association of "idiopathic" GHD with an ectopic neurohypophysis.[398-400] Magnetic resonance imaging (MRI) findings have been described in several series of patients with idiopathic dwarfism. Abrahams and associates[399] studied 35 patients with idiopathic GHD and found that those with MRI findings could be divided into two groups: 43% had an ectopic neurohypophysis (neurohypophysis located near the median eminence), absent infundibulum, and an absence of the normal posterior pituitary bright spot, and 43% had a small anterior pituitary as an isolated finding or combined with an ectopic neurohypophysis.

All in all, an ectopic neurohypophysis was found in 87% of cases with multiple pituitary hormone deficiencies but in only 10% of cases with isolated GHD. Kuroiwa and co-workers[400] suggested that the ectopic neurohypophysis, typically visualized as a bright spot at the median eminence, might be the consequence of perinatal asphyxia.

In other studies, however, high-resolution MRI findings of one or more of the following have been suggested to be sensitive and/or specific indicators of hypopituitarism: a small anterior pituitary, attenuated pituitary stalk, and ectopic posterior pituitary. In one study,[401] pituitary abnormalities were found in 80% with isolated GHD and 93% with MPHD. In patients whose peak growth hormone level was less than 3 ng/mL, 90% had MRI findings—compared with 39% of those with growth hormone levels 3 ng/mL or greater. In another study,[402] the stalk was abnormal in 90% of patients with IGHD and was absent in 96% of patients with MPHD. Thus, MRI abnormalities are common in children with isolated GHD and MPHD and are closely associated with the severity of GHD.

Tumors Involving the Pituitary. Many of the tumors that affect hypothalamic function also directly impact pituitary secretion of GH.[371] In addition, craniopharyngiomas comprise a major cause of pituitary insufficiency.[403,404] These tumors arise from remnants of Rathke's pouch, the diverticulum of the roof of the embryonic oral cavity that normally gives rise to the anterior pituitary. Some consider this tumor a congenital malformation because it is believed to be present at birth, gradually growing over the ensuing years and decades.

The tumor arises from rests of squamous cells at the junction of the adenohypophysis and neurohypophysis. As it enlarges, it forms a cyst that contains degenerated cells and that may calcify but does not undergo malignant degeneration. Clinical signs and symptoms of craniopharyngiomas can arise at any age, from infancy to adulthood, but most typically in mid childhood. The most common presentation is with symptoms of increased intracranial pressure, such as headaches, vomiting, or oculomotor abnormalities. Impaired vision is common. Visual field defects may result from compression of the optic chiasm, and papilledema or optic atrophy may be observed.

Visual and olfactory hallucinations have been reported, as have seizures and dementia. Although short stature is not as common a presenting complaint as are symptoms of increased intracranial pressure, most children with craniopharyngiomas have evidence of growth failure at the time of presentation. GH is the most commonly affected pituitary hormone, but TSH, ACTH, and/or gonadotropin deficiency may also occur—and diabetes insipidus is observed in 25% to 50% of patients.

Lateral skull films often demonstrate enlargement or distortion of the sella turcica, frequently accompanied by suprasellar calcification(s). Nevertheless, some children with craniopharyngiomas will have normal plain films (and alternative radiologic techniques are recommended). Computed tomography is a sensitive technique for identification of small amounts of calcification or cystic abnormalities. MRI is probably the most sensitive technique.

Histiocytosis X consists of three related forms: disseminated (Letterer-Siwe), Hand-Schüller-Christian disease, and the solitary form (eosinophilic granuloma). Although these disorders, (especially Hand-Schüller-Christian disease) are classically associated with diabetes insipidus, approximately 50% of patients have growth failure at the time of presentation.[405] GHD may be isolated, or it may be associated with deficiencies of other pituitary hormones.

Psychosocial Dwarfism. An extreme form of "failure to thrive" is observed in a condition labeled "psychosocial dwarfism" or "emotional deprivation dwarfism."[406,407] Most cases of failure to thrive can be traced back to a poor home environment and inadequate parenting, with improved weight gain and growth observed on removal of the infant from the dysfunctional home. In 1967, Powell and co-workers[406] described a group of children with dramatic behavioral manifestations beyond those observed in the typical infant with failure to thrive. Behavior was characterized by bizarre eating and drinking habits, such as drinking from toilets, social withdrawal, and primitive speech. GH secretion was abnormally low after provocative testing but returned to normal on removal from the home. Concomitantly, when eating and behavioral habits normalized children experienced a period of catch-up growth.

The neuroendocrinologic mechanisms involved in psychosocial dwarfism remain to be elucidated, GH secretion is abnormal, and ACTH and TSH activity may also be reduced—although some patients have been reported to be hypercortisolemic. Even though GH secretion is reduced, treatment with GH is not usually of benefit until the psychosocial situation is improved. It is our experience that whereas failure to thrive is a common cause of poor growth in infancy the constellation of findings described in psychosocial dwarfism is, fortunately, rare.

GH Neurosecretory Dysfunction. Because of concerns that tests of GH secretion after pharmacologic provocation do not accurately reflect normal GH secretion, it has been argued that there exists a group of children with "GH neurosecretory dysfunction"—identified by frequent serum sampling over a 12- to 24-hour period or by continuous serum withdrawal over a similar period of time.[408,409] GH neurosecretory dysfunction is characterized by short stature

and poor growth, normal provocative serum GH concentrations, reduced 24-hour serum GH concentrations, and low serum IGF-1 concentrations. There appears to be little doubt that some children should be considered GH deficient, even if they pass provocative GH testing, although whether such patients should be identified by 24-hour GH sampling or by measures of the IGF axis remains controversial. This subject is discussed later in the chapter.

Acquired Idiopathic Isolated GHD. In most pediatric endocrine centers, many children receiving GH carry a diagnosis of acquired idiopathic isolated GHD. As stated previously, this diagnosis should always be considered somewhat suspect—although it is clear that some of these patients may actually have undiagnosed gene defects in GH production/secretion or have first manifestations of combined pituitary hormone deficiencies. Tauber and colleagues[410] performed GH stimulation tests on 131 young adults who carried the diagnosis of childhood-onset GHD. Of 10 subjects with organic GHD, 90% had peak GH levels less than 5 ng/mL. On the other hand, 67% of 121 subjects carrying a diagnosis of idiopathic GHD had peak GH levels greater than 10 ng/mL and only 17% had peak levels less than 5 ng/mL.

This study also compared retesting results when subjects were divided into complete GHD (defined by an initial peak), stimulated GH level less than 5 ng/mL, and partial GHD (defined by a peak GH level after two stimulation tests of between 5 and 10 ng/mL or one test below 10 ng/mL and a 24-hour GH level below 2.5 ng/mL). Subjects with partial GHD were twice as likely to have normal GH responses on retesting than were those with complete GHD (71% versus 36%, respectively).

In a similar study, Maghnie and co-workers[411] reinvestigated 35 young adults with childhood-onset GHD divided into four groups according to their first pituitary MRI: isolated GHD and normal pituitary volume; isolated GHD and small pituitary volume; isolated GHD or MPHD, together with hypothalamic-pituitary abnormalities on MRI such as pituitary hypoplasia, pituitary stalk agenesis, and posterior pituitary ectopia; and MPHDs secondary to craniopharyngioma. On retesting, all subjects in the first and second groups had normal GH responses to provocative testing, regardless of pituitary size. On the other hand, all subjects in the third and fourth groups had peak GH responses less than 3 ng/mL. These findings and those of a number of similar studies[412] have indicated that the likelihood of sustained GHD is much greater in cases of MPHDs and/or structural abnormalities of the hypothalamus/pituitary.

Bio-inactive GH. Serum GH exists in multiple molecular forms, representing alternative post-transcriptional or post-translational processing of the mRNA or protein, respectively. It is conceivable that different molecular forms of GH may have varying potency in stimulating skeletal growth, although this remains to be rigorously demonstrated. It has been suggested that some cases of short stature may be characterized by serum GH forms that have normal immunopotency but reduced biopotency.[413] Until recently, no completely convincing cases of "bio-inactive GH" had been demonstrated. In 1996, Takahashi and colleagues[414,415] reported two cases that were heterozygous for point mutations in GH1. One patient was characterized by a R77C mutant GH molecule that bound with high affinity to the GHBP but abnormally to the GHR.

The mutant molecule appeared to behave in a dominant negative fashion and could inhibit tyrosine phosphorylation through the GHR. This patient had a partial clinical response to GH, and the father (who was heterozygous for the same mutation) was phenotypically normal—thereby raising some questions about the physiologic significance of this mutation. A second patient, with a D112G mutation, produced a GH molecule that apparently inhibits GHR dimerization. This patient, however, was able to respond to exogenous GH by increasing serum IGF-1 and accelerating growth. Although searches will continue for other examples of GH variants with decreased activity, it seems likely that true "bio-inactive GH" is a rare cause of growth failure.

GH Insensitivity. It is important to consider growth in the context of GH secretion and GH sensitivity, which can operate alone or in combination in a variety of patients—including those with ISS (Figure 8-22). GHI describes patients with the phenotype of GHD but with normal or elevated serum GH concentrations[88,416] (Table 8-7). Primary GHI implies abnormalities of the GHR, including the extracellular GH binding site, the extracellular GHR dimerization site, or the intracellular site; post-receptor abnormalities of GH signal transduction; and primary defects of IGF-1 biosynthesis. Secondary GHI is an acquired condition and includes circulating antibodies to GH, antibodies to the GHR, malnutrition, and hepatic disease.

The initial report, by Laron and colleagues, described ". . . three siblings with hypoglycemia and other clinical and laboratory signs of growth hormone deficiency, but

TABLE 8-7
Proposed Classification of Growth Hormone (GH) Insensitivity

A. Primary GH Insensitivity (Hereditary Defects)
1. GH receptor defect (may be positive or negative for GH-binding protein)
- Extracellular mutation
- Cytoplasmic mutation
- Intracellular mutation
2. GH signal transduction defects (distal to cytoplasmic domain of GH receptor)
Stat-5b mutations
3. Insulin-like growth factor-1 defects
- IGF-1 gene deletion
- IGF-1 transport defect (ALS mutation)
- IGF-1 receptor defect
4. Bioinactive GH molecule (responds to exogenous GH)

B. Secondary GH Insensitivity (Acquired Defects)
- Circulating antibodies to GH that inhibit GH action
- Antibodies to the GH receptor
- GH insensitivity caused by malnutrition, liver disease, catabolic states, diabetes mellitus
- Other conditions that cause GH insensitivity

Definitions:
- *GH insensitivity:* Clinical and biochemical features of IGF-1 deficiency and insensitivity to exogenous GH, associated with GH secretion that would not be considered abnormally low.
- *GH insensitivity syndrome:* GH insensitivity associated with the recognizable dysmorphic features described by Laron.
- *Partial GH insensitivity:* GH insensitivity in the absence of dysmorphic features described by Laron.

with abnormally high concentrations of immunoreactive serum growth hormone."[416] To date, approximately several hundred cases have been identified worldwide.[88] The majority of reported cases come from the Mediterranean region or from Ecuador (in presumed descendants of Spanish "conversos": that is, Jews who converted to Christianity during the Inquisition).[416] These patients have been demonstrated to be unresponsive to exogenous GH in terms of growth, metabolic changes, and alterations in serum concentrations of IGF-1 and IGFBP-3.[417]

Cellular unresponsiveness to GH was demonstrated in vitro by the failure of GH to stimulate erythroid progenitor cells from the peripheral blood of patients.[418] Direct evidence of receptor failure was provided by the demonstration that hepatic microsomes obtained by liver biopsy failed to bind radiolabeled GH.[419] An absence of detectable GHBP activity in the sera of patients with this familial form of GHI was subsequently demonstrated by the reduced ability of serum to bind radiolabeled GH.[108,109]

This observation was rapidly followed by the purification, cloning, and sequencing of the serum GHBP and the demonstration that it was in essence identical to the extracellular domain of the GHR.[90] Initial studies of the GHR gene in Israeli patients indicated that some contained gene deletions.[420] Subsequently, a wide variety of point mutations (missense, nonsense, and abnormal splicing) were identified.[88,421,422] The majority of reported point mutations are in the extracellular domain of the GHR, although there are some at the extracellular domain that

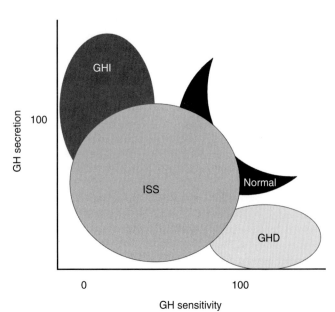

Two-dimensional diagnostic paradigm

Figure 8-22 Dual contributions of GH secretion and action to growth. [From Cohen P (2006). Controversy in clinical endocrinology: Problems with reclassification of IGF-1 production and action disorders. J Clin Endocrinol Metab 91:4235–4236.]

did not affect GH binding but prevented dimerization of the receptor.[423] Such cases may be characterized by normal or even increased serum concentrations of GHBP because the GHBP binding site is intact. There are reports of patients with two separate amino acid substitutions in the intracellular domain.[424]

Woods and associates[425] reported two cousins with severe GHI resulting from a mutation in the 59-splice donor site of intron 8, resulting in a truncated GHR lacking the transmembrane and intracellular domains and leading to increased concentrations of serum GHBP—presumably owing to accelerated release from the cell membrane. A similar defect has been described in a Druse girl with a mutation of the 39-acceptor site of intron 7.[426] Two defects directly affecting the intracellular domain have been reported to result in dominantly inherited GHI. In one, a white girl and her mother (both with short stature and biochemical evidence of GHI) were found to be heterozygous for a single G-to-C transversion in the 39-splice acceptor site of intron 8—resulting in a truncated GHR 1–277 lacking most of the intracellular domain.[427]

A second report described high serum GHBP concentrations in two Japanese siblings and their mother, who were characterized by partial GHI. The patients and their mother had a point mutation that disrupted the 59-splice donor site of intron 9, causing skipping of exon 9 and the appearance of a premature stop codon in exon 10—resulting in the same GHR 1–277 molecule described by Ayling and associates.[427] Under in vitro conditions, the Japanese mutation has been shown to result in a GHR molecule that behaves

in a dominant negative manner—inhibiting GH-induced tyrosine phosphorylation of STAT5.

The clinical features of GHI due to GHR deficiency (GHRD) are identical to those of other forms of severe IGF deficiency, such as congenital GHD.[88] Basal serum GH concentrations are typically elevated in children but may be normal in adults (Figure 8-23). Most patients have decreased serum GHBP concentrations, at least as measured by functional assays. A normal (or even elevated) serum GHBP concentration does not, however, exclude the diagnosis of GHRD because mutations at the GHR dimerization site have been already described, as well as mutations of the intracellular domain of the receptor. Serum IGF-1, IGF-2, and IGFBP-3 concentrations are profoundly reduced in classic GHI (Figure 8-24)—but partial clinical and biochemical phenotypes have been described, typically related to milder mutations of the GHR gene and resulting in only a modest reduction in binding activity and/or receptor action.

GHR Signaling Defects. Although some cases of primary IGFD with normal serum GHBP have proven to have defects of the transmembrane or intracellular domain of the GH receptor, patients have been reported with similar clinical and biochemical phenotypes but with normal sequencing of the GH receptor gene. Until recently, such cases (even when characterized by apparently abnormal activation of the STAT or MAPK pathways) have had no demonstrable molecular basis. Koefed et al.,[428] however, reported a 16-year-old girl with a height of −7.5 SD and markedly low serum concentrations of IGF-I, IGFBP-3 and ALS despite normal serum

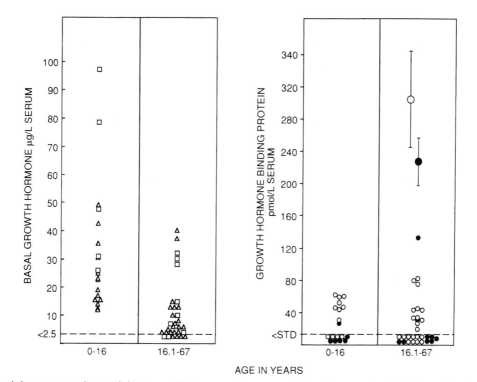

FIGURE 8-23. Growth hormone and growth hormone-binding protein concentrations in sera of patients from Ecuador with GH receptor deficiency. (From Rosenfeld RG, Rosenbloom AL, Guevara-Aguirre J: Growth hormone [GH] insensitivity due to primary GH receptor deficiency. Endocr Rev 15:369, 1994.)

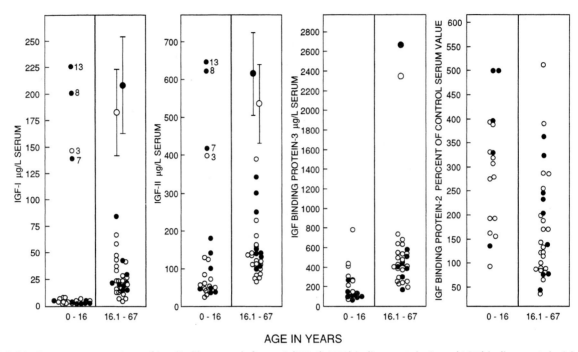

FIGURE 8-24. Serum concentrations of insulin-like growth factor-1 (IGF-1), IGF-binding protein-3, and IGF-binding protein-2 in patients from Ecuador with growth hormone receptor deficiency. (From Rosenfeld RG, Rosenbloom AL, Guevara-Aguirre J: Growth hormone [GH] insensitivity due to primary GH receptor deficiency. Endocr Rev 15:369, 1994.)

concentrations of GHBP and a normal GHR gene sequence.

The patient, born to consanguineous parents, proved to be homozygous for a point mutation resulting in a substitution of proline for alanine at position 630 of the STAT5b gene—with resulting marked decrease in phosphorylation of tyrosine, a critical step in the pathway to STAT activation of IGF-I gene transcription. Subsequent investigations indicated that the mutant STAT5b could not function as a signal transducer or transcription factor, presumably because of an inability to dock with phosophotyrosines on GH-activated receptors as well as an inability to form a stable interaction with DNA. The A630P STAT5b was shown to be characterized by aberrant folding and diminished solubility, resulting in aggregation and formation of cytoplasmic inclusion bodies.

A second case of severe primary IGFD and GH insensitivity resulting from a novel mutation of STAT5b has been reported recently. The patient was shown to be homozygous for a single nucleotide insertion in exon 10 of the STAT5b gene, leading to early protein termination. Because STAT5b is involved in the signaling pathway for multiple cytokines, it is of note that both patients had evidence of immune dysfunction and recurrent pulmonary infections. The growth and clinical characteristics of these two patients strongly support the hypothesis that STAT5b mediates the overwhelming majority, if not all, of GH's effects on IGF-I gene transcription. To date, no convincing mutations of the genes for JAK2 or MAPK have been implicated in primary IGFD and GH insensitivity. It is quite possible that severe mutations of JAK2 (involved in signaling for multiple growth factors and cytokines) are incompatible with life.

ALS Mutations. Markedly reduced serum concentrations of IGF-I and IGFBP-3 have also been observed in two cases involving mutations of the ALS gene.[429] Of note is that in both cases even though serum concentrations of IGF-I and IGFBP-3 were as low as in patients with mutations of the GHR or STAT5b genes growth was only modestly affected. Indeed, the index case actually attained an adult height within the normal range. Whether the relatively normal growth reflects the greater importance of locally produced IGF-I or reflects altered kinetics of serum IGF-I in the face of reduced concentrations of binding proteins remains uncertain.

Growth failure associated with a primary defect of IGF-1 synthesis has also been reported.[287] The first case was a 15-year-old boy who had many of the growth characteristics predicted from mouse knockout models,[286,353,430] including intrauterine and postnatal growth failure. Additional features were mental retardation and sensorineural deafness. The patient was shown to be homozygous for deletions of exons 4 and 5 of the human IGF-1 gene, with both parents being heterozygous carriers and perhaps mildly affected themselves. Although unresponsive to GH therapy, the patient was able to accelerate growth velocity on treatment with IGF-1. Of note is that the patient with IGF-1 gene deletion had in addition to severe growth failure and mental retardation substantial insulin resistance, and that IGF-1 therapy resulted in a marked improvement of insulin sensitivity, reduction of serum insulin, and overall improvement in various aspects of carbohydrate metabolism.[432]

Cases of IGF-1 receptor mutations have also been described.[431] In mouse knockout models, homozygous mutations of the IGF-I receptor result in profound growth failure and neonatal mortality. Heterozygous mutations are phenotypically similar to wild-type mice. In the African Efe pygmies, a series of studies demonstrated extreme insensitivity to the in vitro growth-enhancing effects of IGF-I. Reduced IGF-I receptor transcripts and sites with resultant diminished tyrosine phosphorylation and post-receptor signaling, though no definable receptor mutation, are suggested explanations.

Patients with IUGR and postnatal growth failure associated with defects of the IGF1R have been reported. Clinical findings have included microcephaly and mild mental retardation. Serum IGF-I concentrations were normal to elevated, but binding of IGF-I was shown to be reduced. Whether such mutations will prove to be a common cause of combined IUGR and postnatal growth failure remains to be determined.

In leprechaunism, a syndrome of growth failure and insulin receptor dysfunction, there is variable IGF-I insensitivity. The profound abnormality of the insulin receptor suggests that heterodimeric insulin- and IGF-I receptor combinations could possible lead to failed activation of the IGF-I signaling cascade. As the IGF-I receptor gene resides at 15q26.3, deletions of the distal long arm of chromosome 15 or ring chromosome 15 may lead to hemizygosity for the IGF-I receptor. Although such patients may have intrauterine growth retardation and striking postnatal growth failure, lack of a biologic response to IGF-I has not been conclusively demonstrated. Whether growth failure in such patients is due to altered levels of IGF-I receptor or represents the net effect of the loss of other genes located on 15q remains to be determined.[431]

Clinical Features. Cases of IGF-1 deficiency resulting from hypothalamic dysfunction, decreased pituitary GH secretion, or GHI share a common phenotype. The striking clinical similarity among patients with GHD caused by a GH gene deletion and patients with GHI secondary to mutations of the GHR gene emphasizes the role of IGF-1 in mediating most, if not all, of the anabolic and growth-promoting actions of GH. This point is further supported by the ability of IGF-1 therapy to partially normalize growth in children with mutations of the GHR gene. Accordingly, the clinical features of severe IGF deficiency are shared by all of these conditions. Children with less severe IGF deficiency will generally have milder clinical characteristics. If GH or IGF deficiency is acquired, clinical signs and symptoms will obviously appear at a later age. (See Table 8-8.)

As stated previously, birth size is remarkably normal even in severe forms of congenital GHD or GHI. Birth length and weight are typically within 10% of normal, and severe IUGR is not part of the classic phenotype. Neonatal signs can exist, however, including hypoglycemia and prolonged jaundice.[433] When GHD is combined with ACTH and TSH deficiency, hypoglycemia may be severe. On the other hand, when GHD is combined with gonadotropin deficiency microphallus, cryptorchidism, and hypoplasia of the scrotum may be observed.[434] GHD (or GHI) should therefore be considered in the differential diagnosis of neonatal hypoglycemia or microphallus/cryptorchidism.

Postnatal growth is strikingly abnormal in severe congenital IGF deficiency (Figure 8-25). Although earlier reports suggested that growth in such cases was rela-

---

TABLE 8-8
Clinical Features of Growth Hormone Insensitivity

Growth and Development
Birth weight: near-normal
Birth length: may be slightly decreased
Postnatal growth: severe growth failure
Bone age: delayed, but may be advanced relative to height age
Genitalia: micropenis in childhood; normal for body size in adults
Puberty: delayed 3 to 7 years
Sexual function and fertility: normal

Craniofacies
Hair: sparse before the age of 7 years
Forehead: prominent; frontal bossing
Skull: normal head circumference; craniofacial disproportion due to small facies
Facies: small
Nasal bridge: hypoplastic
Orbits: shallow
Dentition: delayed eruption
Sclerae: blue
Voice: high-pitched

Musculoskeletal/Metabolic/Miscellaneous
Hypoglycemia: in infants and children; fasting symptoms in some adults
Walking and motor milestones: delayed
Hips: dysplasia; avascular necrosis of femoral head
Elbow: limited extensibility
Skin: thin, prematurely aged
Osteopenia

---

tively normal during the first 6 months of life, more recent surveys of GHD and GHI have indicated that growth failure may be observed during the first months of life. By 6 to 12 months of age, the child is clearly growing at an abnormally slow rate and has usually deviated away from the normal growth curve. It is important to emphasize that the single most important clinical manifestation of IGF deficiency is growth failure, and careful documentation of growth rates is critical to making the correct diagnosis. Deviation away from the normal growth curve should always be a cause of concern, and between the ages of 2 years and the onset of puberty growth deceleration (or acceleration) is always pathologic.

Skeletal proportions tend to be relatively normal, although they often correlate better with bone age than with chronologic age. Skeletal age is delayed, often to less than 60% of the chronologic age. In acquired GHD, as from a tumor of the CNS that presents as symptoms resulting from increased intracranial pressure, the skeletal age may approximate the chronologic age and should therefore not be considered a requirement for the diagnosis of GHD. Weight/height ratios tend to be increased, and fat distribution is often "infantile" in pattern.

Musculature is poor, especially in infancy, which may result in significant delays in gross motor development—leading to the erroneous impression of mental retardation. Facial bone growth is particularly retarded, and the nasal bridge may appear underdeveloped (Figure 8-26). Fontanelle closure is often delayed, but the overall

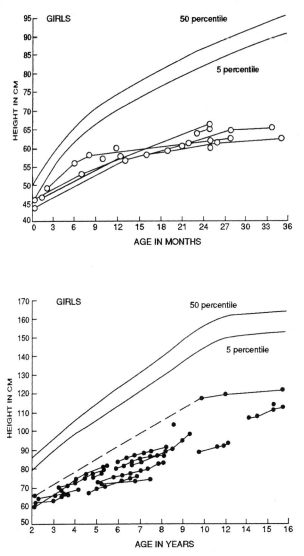

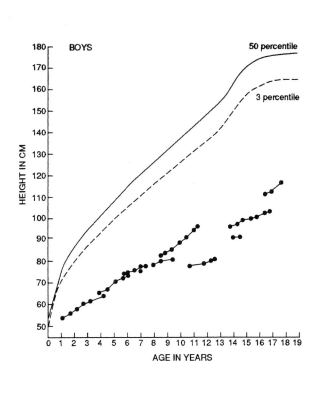

FIGURE 8-25. Height measurements for children from Ecuador with growth hormone receptor deficiency. (From Rosenfeld RG, Rosenbloom AL, Guevara-Aguirre J: Growth hormone [GH] insensitivity due to primary GH receptor deficiency. Endocr Rev 15:369, 1994.)

growth of the skull is normal—leading to cephalofacial disproportion and the appearance of hydrocephalus. The voice remains infantile, owing to hypoplasia of the larynx. Hair growth is sparse and the hair itself is thin, especially during the early years of life. Nail growth is also frequently slow. Even with normal gonadotropin production, the penis is small and puberty is generally delayed.

Diagnosis of IGF Deficiency. The proper means of establishing a diagnosis of GHD continues to be highly controversial.[254] With the availability of highly specific assays for the IGF peptides and binding proteins, and with increasing understanding of the GH-IGF axis, we believe that evaluation of patients with growth failure should rest on a combination of careful auxologic assessment and appropriate measures of the GH-IGF system. Establishment of deficiency of IGF peptides and concomitant alterations in serum concentrations of IGFBPs then necessitates a thorough evaluation of hypothalamic-pituitary-IGF function.

The foundation for the diagnosis of IGF deficiency must be auxology, with careful documentation of serial heights and determination of height velocity. In the absence of other evidence of pituitary dysfunction, it is generally unnecessary to perform tests of GH secretion. Thus, even in children below the 5th percentile in height (which obviously applies to 5% of the population) documentation of a normal height velocity makes the diagnosis of IGF deficiency and GHD highly unlikely.

Assessment of pituitary GH production is problematic because GH secretion is pulsatile throughout the day and night, with the most consistent surges occurring at times of slow-wave electroencephalographic rhythms during phases 3 and 4 of sleep. Regulation of GH secretion is complex, involving two hypothalamic proteins (GHRH and somatostatin) as well as multiple other peptides and neurotransmitters. Spontaneous GH secretion varies significantly with gender, age, and pubertal status—all of which must be factored into any evaluation of GH production.

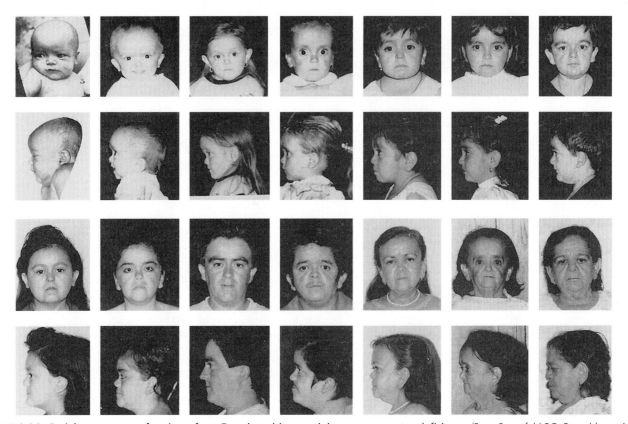

FIGURE 8-26. Facial appearance of patients from Ecuador with growth hormone receptor deficiency. (From Rosenfeld RG, Rosenbloom AL, Guevara-Aguirre J: Growth hormone [GH] insensitivity due to primary GH receptor deficiency. Endocr Rev 15:369, 1994. Photography by Arlan L. Rosenbloom, MD.)

Between normally occurring pulses of GH secretion, serum GH concentrations are normally low—below the limits of sensitivity of most conventional assays. Accordingly, measurement of random serum GH concentrations is virtually useless in establishing a diagnosis of GHD. Measurement of GH "reserve" has therefore relied on the use of physiologic or pharmacologic stimuli, and these "provocative tests" have been the basis for diagnosing GHD for more than 30 years.[254,435]

"Physiologic" stimuli have included fasting, sleep,[436] and exercise[437,438]—whereas pharmacologic stimuli have included levodopa,[439] clonidine,[440] glucagon,[441] propranolol, arginine,[442] and insulin[443,444] (Table 8-9). Stimulation tests have often been divided into "screening tests" (exercise, fasting, levodopa, clonidine)—characterized by ease of administration, low toxicity, low risk, and low specificity—and "definitive tests" (arginine, insulin, glucagon). To improve specificity, provocative tests are customarily combined or given sequentially.[445-447] It has been generally accepted that a child must "fail" provocative tests with at least two separate stimuli to be considered as having GHD. Standard provocative GH tests are summarized in Table 8-9.

Although provocative GH testing has been the foundation for the diagnosis of GHD since GH radioimmunoassays first became available, its use as a determiner of GH status has come under criticism for a number of reasons.[254,448] These issues, as follows, have been summarized in a consensus report on the diagnosis of childhood GHD.[434]

• Provocative GH testing is nonphysiologic.

None of the standard pharmacologic provocative tests satisfactorily mimics the normal secretory pattern of pituitary GH. Even when naturally occurring regulatory peptides are used for stimulation, their dosage, route of administration, and interactions with other regulatory factors are artificial. In addition, because most endocrine centers use several different stimulation tests there is no validated means of resolving conflicting data from two or more provocative tests.[449] In a report of 6,373 GH stimulation tests performed on 3,233 short French children, 11 different pharmacologic tests were employed, 62 of the possible 66 pairs were employed at least once, and the most frequent combination of tests was used in only 12.7% of the patients.[450]

• Arbitrary definitions of "subnormal" response to provocative tests.

Endocrine centers vary in their definition of a "normal" response to stimulation tests. Whereas early reports generally employed a cutoff level of 5 ng/mL, this was gradually increased to 7 ng/mL. With the availability of recombinant DNA–derived hGH, this level was increased to 10 ng/mL—although no data exist for validating any of these arbitrary cutoff levels. The lack of objective confirmation of any defined normal response can be seen in the use of language such as "lack of adequate endogenous growth hormone secretion"[451] and "inadequate secretion of normal endogenous growth hormone."[452] As indicated by Guyda, many of the newer GH assays measure GH concentrations twofold to threefold lower than older assays and yet there

TABLE 8-9

Growth Hormone Stimulation Tests*

Stimulus	Dosage	Samples (Min)	Comments/side Effects
Levodopa (PO)	< 15 kg: 125mg 15-30 kg: 250 mg >30 kg: 500 mg	0, 60, 90	Nausea
Clonidine (PO)	0.15 mg/m²	0, 30, 60, 90	Tiredness, postural hypotension
Arginine HCl (IV)	0.5 g/kg (max 30 g) 10% arginine HCl in 0.9% NaCl over 30 min	0, 15, 30, 45, 60	
Insulin (IV)	0.05-0.1 IU/kg	0, 15, 30, 45, 60, 75, 90, 120	Hypoglycemia; requires supervision†
Glucagon (IM)	0.03 mg/kg (max 1 mg)	0, 30, 60, 90, 120, 150, 180	Nausea

* Tests should be performed after an overnight fast. It is generally recommended by some authorities that prepubertal children be "primed" with sex steroids (e.g., premarin, 5 mg PO the night before and the morning of the test, or ethinyl estradiol, 50 to 100 μg/d for 3 consecutive days before testing; or depot testosterone, 100 mg 3 days before testing). Patients should be euthyroid at time of testing.

† Insulin-induced hypoglycemia is a potential risk of this procedure, which is designed to lower the blood glucose by at least 50%. Documentation of appropriate lowering of blood glucose is recommended. If growth hormone deficiency, the lower dosage of insulin may be advisable, especially in infants. $D_{50}W$ solutions and glucagon should be available.

has been no systematic reevaluation of the "normal" GH cutoff level.

• Age dependency and use of sex steroids.

Serum GH concentrations typically rise during puberty, manifested as an increase in pulse-amplitude but not pulse frequency.[57,453] Immediately before puberty and during the earliest phases of puberty, GH secretion may normally be so low as to blur the distinction between GHD and constitutional delay of growth and maturation.[57,453] There are multiple reports of children who "failed" provocative testing before the onset of puberty but proved to have "normal" GH secretion after puberty or after administration of exogenous sex steroids.[454-457] One study of provocative GH testing in children of normal stature has clearly demonstrated the inherent problems with provocative GH testing and the need for standardization of sex steroid administration during stimulation tests.[458]

When exercise and arginine/insulin stimulation tests were administered to these normal children, the lower limit of normal (2 SD) for peak serum GH concentration in prepubertal children was only 1.9 ng/mL—whereas in children of Tanner stage 5 puberty this level was 9.3 ng/mL. When estrogen was administered before provocative testing, the lower 95% confidence limit for the normal serum GH range rose to 7.2 ng/mL. All in all, when estrogen was not administered 61% of the normal prepubertal children failed to raise their serum GH concentration above 7 ng/mL after three provocative tests. These children could have been erroneously labeled as having GHD.

• GH assays of limited accuracy.

Several studies have demonstrated as much as threefold variability in the measurement of serum GH concentrations by established laboratories.[460,461] This is explained at least in part by the existence of several molecular forms of GH in serum and by the use of monoclonal versus polyclonal antibodies. The inevitable result has been that children labeled as having GHD by one assay would be considered normal by another.

A highly sensitive immunofunctional GH assay has been developed that measures concentrations of GH capable of binding to GHBP. It is not clear, however, that such assays necessarily have any advantages over standard radioimmunoassays for routine GH measurements.[462] When arginine/levodopa or arginine/insulin stimulation tests were used, approximately 50% of normal children had peak GH concentrations less than 7 ng/mL and 30% were less than 5 ng/mL whether GH was measured by immunofunctional assay or enzyme-linked immunosorbent assay.

• Expense, discomfort, and risks of provocative GH testing.

Provocative testing typically requires multiple timed blood samples, and frequently necessitates parenteral administration of drugs. The resulting discomfort to the patient and expense are self-evident. In addition, insulin administration carries the risk of hypoglycemia and seizures and should be performed by experienced medical personnel under appropriate supervision. Death has been reported from insulin-induced hypoglycemia and from its overly vigorous correction with parenteral glucose.[463]

• Poor reproducibility of provocative tests.

The reproducibility of provocative GH tests has never been adequately demonstrated, even when GH concentrations are determined with the same assay.[463] An alternative approach is the measurement of spontaneous GH secretion. This can be done either by multiple sampling (every 5 to 30 minutes) over a 12- to 24-hour period or by continuous blood withdrawal over 12 to 24 hours.[82,408,464,465] The former method allows one to evaluate and characterize GH pulsatility, whereas the latter only permits determination of mean GH concentration. Either approach, however, is subject to many of the same criticisms as provocative GH testing. The potential expense and discomfort of such testing are obvious.

Furthermore, although it has been claimed that this technique is more reproducible than are provocative GH tests variability remains problematic.[343,345,466,467] The ability of such tests to discriminate between GHD and normal short children is also an issue. Rose and colleagues[468] reported that spontaneous GH determinations identified only 57% of children with GHD, defined by provocative testing. In this report, no case of "neurosecretory dysfunction" could be identified in the group of normal short children. Similarly, Lanes and co-workers[469] reported that one-fourth of normally growing children had decreased overnight GH concentrations.

Given the problems with GH testing in general, it is not surprising that provocative tests and 24-hour GH profiles do not correlate perfectly. It is in fact likely that 12- to 24-hour GH profiles can correctly identify the majority of children with GHD and may be superior in sensitivity and specificity to provocative GH testing. With the advent of more routine treatment of ISS with GH, GH testing is no longer the controversial topic it once was— and many experts recognize that a large overlap exists between GHD and ISS as they are commonly defined.

"Neurosecretory dysfunction" probably does exist in children who have had cranial irradiation and likely does describe a subgroup of children with GHD and IGF deficiency. However, the expense and discomfort of frequent overnight or 24-hour sampling combined with many of the problems intrinsic to GH determinations preclude this form of testing for GH deficiency from being the test of choice in establishing the diagnosis of GHD.

The measurement of GH concentrations in urine has provided an alternative means of assessing "integrated" GH secretion (or at least excretion).[470-472] This technique requires anti-GH antibodies of high affinity because urinary GH concentrations are normally low. It also requires timed urine collections. Adequate age- and sex-related standards have not yet been fully developed, and the diagnostic use of urinary GH determinations remains to be adequately evaluated.

Whereas some have interpreted these difficulties in measuring GH as a reason to stop performing GH testing altogether, we strongly recommend continuing use of this testing modality that is nevertheless critical to differentiating GHD from ISS, and secondary from primary IGFD. These conditions are vastly different in a variety of ways. Rather, we believe that the results of the GH testing should not serve as an absolute determinant of the decision to treat with GH (or other drugs, including IGF-I). A complementary approach to the diagnosis of GHD is the use of IGF-related assays.[153,154,157,179] GHD then becomes part of the differential diagnosis of IGF deficiency, which

includes hypothalamic dysfunction, pituitary insufficiency, and GHI.

With the development of sensitive and specific assays for IGFs, as well as for the IGFBPs, it has become apparent that these peptides can reflect the GH status of the patient. Furthermore, they have the advantage that they normally circulate in serum at high concentrations—and thus assay sensitivity is less of an issue. Serum levels of these peptides remain relatively constant during the day, and provocative testing or multiple sampling is not necessary. It is important, however, to recognize the following potential limitations of assays for IGF-1.

- The IGFBPs potentially interfere with radioimmunoassays, radioreceptor assays, and bioassays.[159-161] These binding proteins must be completely removed, as with acid gel chromatography (which is labor intensive),[159-161] or blocked by the addition of excess IGF-2 (which requires a high-affinity antibody with a high degree of specificity for IGF-1).[162] An alternative approach is to employ a radiolabeled IGF-1 analogue with reduced affinity for IGFBPs.[163]

- Serum IGF-1 concentrations are highly age dependent.[155,170,171] They are lowest in young children (<5 years of age), the age at which one most wishes to have a simple diagnostic test.

- Serum IGF-1 concentrations may be reduced in a variety of conditions other than GHD. These include primary and secondary forms of GHI. Malnutrition or any cause of diminished insulin concentration (such as poor food intake; dieting; and malabsorption, such as celiac sprue) will result in low circulating IGF-1 levels. Patients whose weights are less than the 25th percentile for age are likely to have low IGF-1 levels in the range of classic GH deficiency, but their primary problem is malnutrition and not GH deficiency.

- Serum concentrations of IGF-1 (and IGFBP-3) are frequently normal in adult-onset GHD and in children with GHD resulting from brain tumors and/or cranial irradiation.

Even when these caveats are considered, the correlation between serum IGF-1 concentrations and provocative or spontaneous GH measurements is imperfect. Juul and co-workers[473] have reported that in children younger than 10 years of age IGF-1 levels were below 2 SD in only 8 of 15 children with a diagnosis of GHD based on provocative testing (53.3% sensitivity) and were normal in 47 of 48 children with a normal GH response (97.9% specificity).

In one study, 18% of patients with abnormally low provocative GH concentrations had IGF-1 concentrations in the normal range but only 4% of "GHD" patients had normal serum concentrations of IGF-1 and IGF-2. Serum levels of IGF-1 and IGF-2 were reduced in only 0.5% of normal children and in 11% of normal short children.[157] The development of specific immunoassays for IGFBP-3, normally the major serum carrier of IGF peptides, has provided a supplementary means of establishing a diagnosis of IGF deficiency and GHD (Figures 8-19 and 8-27).[241,250,251] Because molar concentrations of IGFBP-3 correlate with the sum of the molar concentrations of IGF-1 and IGF-2, IGFBP-3 determinations offer the following advantages over assays of IGF peptides and other IGFBPs.

Step I—Defining the Risk of GH/IGF Deficiency

Auxologic Abnormalities
• Severe short stature (height SDS <-3 SD)
• Severe growth deceleration (height velocity SDS <-2 SD over 12 months)
• Ht <-2 SD and HV<-1 SD over 12 months
• Ht <-1.5 SD and HV<-1.5 SD over 2 years
• Features of GHD or GHI

Risk Factors

• History of a brain tumor, cranial irradiation, or other documented organic pituitary abnormality
• Incidental finding of pituitary abnormality on MRI

If any of the above exists, proceed to step 2; if not, follow clinically and return to step 1 in 6 months

Step 2—Screening for GH/IGF Deficiency and Other Diseases

A. Order a laboratory panel including assessment of bone age, thyroid function, chromosomes (in females), and nonendocrine tests, and, if indicated, treat diagnosed conditions as appropriate.
And
B. Order an IGF-1 and an IGFBP-3 level.
• If IGF-1/IGFBP-3 are above the mean, follow clinically and return to step 1 in 6 months.
• If IGF-1/IGFBP-3 are low, proceed to step 3; but if the MRI is abnormal, GH stimulation is optional.
• If height <-2,25 SDS proceed to step 3 regardless of the screening tests.

Step 3—Testing GH Secretion

This step can be bypassed if a clear GHD risk factor AND a severe IGF deficiency are identified.
Perform two of the following GH stimulation tests (if appropriate, estrogen prime):

• Clonidine
• Arginine
• Insulin
• Glucagon
• Levodopa
• Propranolol

If both are below 10, go to step 4.
If GH>15, obtain GHBP; if GHBP <-2 SD, consider an IGF-generation test, and, if abnormal, IGF treatment.
If GH>10 and height is <-2.25 SDS consider GH treatment for ISS (Step 5)

Step 4—Evaluating the Pituitary

Perform MRI.
Test HPA, if not already done (CRH stimulation or ITT), and teach cortisol supplementation as needed.

Step 5—Treating for Growth Promotion

Initiate GH therapy (or if GHIS is suspected, consider IGF-1).
Regularly evaluate growth parameters, IGF-1, and IGFBP-3, as well as compliance and safety.
GH secretion should be retested at the end of GH treatment if the diagnosis was GHD.

Figure 8-27 Algorithm of biochemical evaluation of growth failure. CRH, corticotropin-releasing hormone; GH, growth hormone; GHBP, GH-binding protein; HPA, hypothalamic-pituitary axis; HV, height velocity; IGF, insulin-like growth factor; IGFBP-3, IGF-binding protein-3; ITT, insulin tolerance test; MRI, magnetic resonance imaging; SD, standard deviation; and SDS, standard deviation score.

• IGFBP-3 immunoassays are technically simple and do not require any separation of the binding protein from IGF peptides.
• Normal serum concentrations of IGFBP-3 are quite high, typically in the 1- to 5-mg/mL range, and thus assay sensitivity is not an issue.
• Although age dependency exists, serum IGFBP-3 concentrations vary with age to a lesser degree than is the case for IGF-1. Even in infants, serum IGFBP-3 concentrations are normally sufficiently high to allow discrimination of pathologically low values from the normal range.
• Serum IGFBP-3 concentrations are less nutritionally dependent than concentrations of IGF-1, reflecting the "stabilizing" effect of IGF-2 concentrations.
• IGFBP-3 concentrations are clearly GH dependent.

The utility of IGFBP-3 assays in the diagnosis of GHD was evaluated by Blum and colleagues,[251] who found that serum IGFBP-3 concentrations were below the 5th percentile for age in 128 of 132 (97%) of children diagnosed as having GHD by conventional criteria (height <3rd percentile, height velocity <10th percentile, and peak serum GH <10 ng/mL). At the same time, 124 of 130 (95%) of non-GHD short children had normal IGFBP-3 concentrations.

It is likely that Blum's patients largely consisted of children with severe GHD because this degree of correlation between provocative GH testing and serum IGFBP-3 concentrations has not been consistently identified. For example, Hasegawa and associates[474] reported that the sensitivity of the IGFBP-3 radioimmunoassay in complete GHD (peak GH <5 ng/mL) was 93% but was only 43% in cases of partial GHD (peak GH 5 to 10 ng/mL). Smith and co-workers[475] found that 100% of children with severe GHD (peak GH <1 ng/mL) and low serum IGF-1 also had decreased serum IGFBP-3. Four of 8 children with GHD and normal serum IGF-1 levels had reduced IGFBP-3 concentrations, and 10 of 23 (43%) of normal short children had decreased serum IGFBP-3. The addition of a radioimmunoassay for IGFBP-2 further enhanced the ability of IGF axis measures to identify children who had GHD by conventional criteria.

The correlation between IGF-axis determinations and measures of spontaneous GH secretion nevertheless remains imperfect. Even in healthy normal children the correlation between 24-hour GH secretion and serum IGF-1 and IGFBP-3 concentrations is modest (r = 0.78 and r = 0.62, respectively).[475] In the Smith study,[476] 18% of patients were found to have discordant measures of IGFBP-3 and provocative GH response. It is impossible at this time to resolve conflicts between assays of the IGF axis and measurements of GH secretion because there is no way to definitively diagnose GHD. Recent experience in patients with GHRD, however, has provided further evidence in support of the utility of IGF-related determinations.[88,477,478]

Although such patients may have normal or elevated serum GH concentrations, mutations or deletions of the GHR gene render them unresponsive to GH—and such patients may be considered "functionally GH deficient." In the experience in Ecuador, of approximately 70 documented cases of GHR gene mutations all patients were found to have markedly reduced serum concentrations of both IGF-I and IGFBP-3. Even so, IGF-1 and IGFBP-3 correlated significantly with height. Measures of serum concentrations of IGF-1 and IGFBP-3 have been used in other studies of GHI to establish diagnostic criteria.

Ultimately, the diagnosis of GHD (or IGF deficiency) should be made on the basis of combined clinical and laboratory criteria. Short children who have well-documented normal height velocities do not generally require evaluation of GH secretion, and normal (>25%) serum IGF-1 and IGFBP-3 concentrations can be reassuring. Children with Turner syndrome and short stature that is consistent with the expected growth pattern for this syndrome should not be required to undergo GH testing to qualify for GH therapy because such treatment is not predicated on abnormal GH secretion.

On the other hand, the child with documented growth deceleration requires further evaluation—even if tests of GH secretion appear normal. Documentation of decreased serum IGF-1 or IGFBP-3 concentrations would then constitute a diagnosis of IGF deficiency, and the diagnoses of GHD and GHI would need to be considered. The child with a history of cranial irradiation, decreased height velocity, and reduced serum concentrations of IGF-1 and IGFBP-3 should be considered to have GHD (or GHI)—even in the presence of normal provocative tests.

This approach still requires measurements of GH secretion. Such determinations are critical to distinguishing between GHD and GHI as causes of IGF deficiency. Documentation of abnormal pituitary GH secretion alerts the physician to the possibility of intracranial tumors and to the potential for other pituitary hormone deficiencies. Evaluation for GHD allows for concomitant assessment of ACTH secretion, and TSH and gonadotropin determinations can be added where appropriate. Ultimately, however, one must conclude that the single most important parameter in assessment of children with growth failure is careful clinical evaluation—including accurate serial measurements of height and determinations of height velocity.

The possibility of hypothalamic-pituitary dysfunction should always be considered in children with documented growth deceleration, particularly in the presence of a known intracranial pathologic process (e.g., tumors, irradiation, malformations, infection, trauma, blindness, nystagmus). Similarly, the neonate with hypoglycemia and/or microphallus warrants evaluation of pituitary function—and patients with documented TSH, ACTH, ADH, or gonadotropin deficiency are candidates for GHD. For children with proportional short stature and documented growth deceleration, assessment of serum concentrations of IGF-1 and IGFBP-3 is clearly warranted—and based on those results the possibilities of hypothalamic dysfunction, pituitary insufficiency, and GHI can be investigated.

Recommendations by the Growth Hormone Research Society (GRS)[280] for the diagnosis of GHD recognize that there is no "gold standard" for the diagnosis of GHD and suggest that in a child with slow growth whose history and auxology suggest GHD testing for GH/IGF-1 deficiency requires the measurement of IGF-1 and IGFBP-3 levels as well as GH provocation tests (after hypothyroidism has been excluded). In suspected isolated GHD, two GH provocation tests (sequential or on separate days) are required. In those with a defined CNS pathologic process, history of irradiation, MPHD, or genetic defect, one GH test will suffice. In addition, an evaluation of other pituitary function is required. In patients who have had cranial irradiation or malformations of the hypothalamic-pituitary unit, GHD may evolve over years and its diagnosis may require repeat testing of the GH-IGF axis.

It is recognized, however, that some patients with auxology suggestive of GHD may have IGF-1 and/or IGFBP-3 levels below the normal range on repeated tests but GH responses in provocation tests above the cutoff level. These children are not classically GH deficient but may have an abnormality of the GH/IGF axis, and after the exclusion of systemic disorders affecting the synthesis or action of IGF-I could be considered for GH treatment. An MRI (or computed tomographic scan) of the brain with particular attention to the hypothalamic-pituitary region should be carried out in any child diagnosed as having GHD. These GRS recommendations underscore the importance of good clinical judgment rather than specific tests as the key to the diagnosis of GHD.

Testing in the Neonate. The diagnosis of GHD in a newborn is particularly challenging and important. The presence of a micropenis in a male newborn should always be addressed by an evaluation of the GH axis. A GH level should always be measured in the presence of neonatal hypoglycemia in the absence of a metabolic disorder. A GH level in a polyclonal radioimmunoassay of less than 20 mg/L would suggest GHD in the newborn. The use of standard GH stimulation tests is not recommended in newborns, with the exception of the glucagon test (which is safe). In the newborn, although normative data are not available for stimulated serum GH a cutoff of 25 ng/mL is probably appropriate and certainly stimulated values under 20 ng/mL should raise suspicion.

An MRI is essential when the diagnosis is suspected, and results may be available sooner than with serum assays. An IGFBP-3 level is of great value to the diagnosis of GHD in infancy, but IGF-1 levels are rarely helpful.[479] In fact, serum IGFBP-3 should be performed as the test of choice in suspected neonatal GHD. Figure 8-27 provides an algorithm for the biochemical evaluation of growth failure. The diagnosis of IGF and/or GHD should be considered in any child who meets one or more of the criteria listed in Table 8-10.

A child should be considered a candidate for GH therapy if he or she meets one of these criteria, supported by biochemical evidence of GHD based on sex-steroid–primed provocative tests and/or evidence of IGF deficiency based on measurement of IGF-1 and IGFBP-3 concentrations. Such cases need to also have MRI of the hypothalamus-pituitary and assessment of other pituitary hormone deficiencies. It is understood that this approach will result in GH treatment of some children with "idiopathic isolated" GHD or IGF deficiency and that such cases require careful monitoring of both pituitary status and responsiveness to GH treatment. The latter can be assessed relative to recently developed predictive models,[480] and the diagnosis of GHD should be reconsidered in the child with idiopathic isolated GHD, a normal MRI, and a subnormal clinical response to GH.

Diagnosis of GHI. The combination of decreased serum concentrations of IGF-1, IGF-2, and IGFBP-3 plus increased serum concentrations of GH is highly suggestive of a diagnosis of GHI.[88] The possibility of GHRD is supported by a family history consistent with autosomal-recessive transmission. Savage and Rosenfeld[481] devised a scoring system for evaluating short children for the diagnosis of GHRD based on five parameters: basal serum GH greater than 5 ng/mL, serum IGF-1 less than or equal to 50 ng/mL, height SD scores less than –3, serum GHBP less than 10%, and a rise in serum IGF-1 concentrations after a week of GH stimulation of less than twofold the intra-assay variation (approximately 10%).

Blum and colleagues[482] proposed that these criteria could be strengthened by evaluating GH secretory profiles, rather than isolated basal levels; employing an age-dependent range for evaluation of serum IGF-1 concentrations and using the 0.1 centile as the cutoff level; employing highly sensitive IGF-1 radioimmunoassays and defining a failed GH response as the inability to increase serum IGF-1 concentrations by at least 15 ng/mL; and employing basal and GH-stimulated IGFBP-3 concentrations. These criteria fit well with the population of GHRD patients studied in Ecuador, but that is a remarkably homogeneous population of patients who have severe GHI.[88,478] The universal applicability of these criteria remains to be evaluated. An important biochemical marker will be the IGF-1 (and possibly IGFBP-3) response to GH stimulation. Although such tests were first employed in the early 1980s, normal ranges and age-defined responses of serum IGF-1 concentrations have not yet been determined.[483]

Decreased serum concentrations of GHBP are obviously highly suggestive of a diagnosis of GHRD, but it is important to point out that cases of GHRD with normal serum concentrations of GHBP have already been identified.[425,484] Such cases may represent mutations in the site responsible for dimerization of the GHR, or potentially for abnormalities of the intracellular portion of the receptor or of the postreceptor signal transduction mechanism. On the other hand, polymorphisms of the GHR gene without resulting reductions in IGF-1 and IGFBP-3 concentrations should not be considered GHRD. At this point, definitive diagnosis requires the classic phenotype, decreased serum concentrations of IGF-1 and IGFBP-3, and identification of an abnormality of the GHR gene.

Constitutional Delay of Growth and Maturation. The diagnosis of constitutional delay has had different meanings to different clinicians.[485,486] To some, it has consisted of delayed adolescent growth and maturation in the presence of decreased (even if only transiently) GH secretion.[486,487] More commonly, it has been considered a normal variant (characterized by short stature) but with relatively normal growth rates during childhood, delayed puberty, a delayed pubertal growth spurt, and attainment of normal adult height.

TABLE 8-10

Key History and Physical Examination Findings That May Indicate Growth Hormone Deficiency (The GRS 2000 Criteria)*

- In the neonate; hypoglycemia, prolonged jaundice, microphallus, or traumatic delivery
- Cranial irradiation
- Head trauma or central nervous system infection
- Consanguinity and/or an affected family member
- Craniofacial midline abnormalities
- Severe short stature (< – 3 SD)
- Height (< – 2 SD) and a height velocity below over 1 year (< – 1 SD)
- A decrease in height SD of more than 0.5 over in children older than 2 years of age
- A height velocity Below – 2 SD) over 1 year
- A height velocity more than 1.5 SD below the mean sustained over 2 years
- Signs indicative of an intracranial lesion
- Signs of multiple pituitary hormone deficiency
- Neonatal symptoms and signs of growth hormone deficiency

SD, standard deviation; GRS, Growth Hormone Research Society.
* Frasier SD (2000). Editorial. J clin Endocrinol

Most patients with constitutional delay begin to deviate from the normal growth curve during the early years of life and are typically by age 2 years at or slightly below the 5th percentile for height. Such children would be expected to have normal serum IGF-1 and IGFBP-3 concentrations, a normal result of a GH provocative test (if pretreated with sex steroids), and skeletal ages that were delayed (Table 8-11). By definition, children with pure constitutional delay should have bone ages sufficiently delayed to result in normal predicted adult heights (Table 8-11). When constitutional delay is found in the context of familial short stature, however, children may experience a delayed adolescent growth spurt and a short final height. Such children should be considered to have elements of constitutional delay and familial short stature and should be classified as ISS and considered for GH therapy.

As stated previously, some have attributed constitutional delay to a transient GHD or to a "lazy" pituitary. It is likely that much of this experience can be attributed to the inadequacies of GH testing, especially to the failure to pretreat patients with a brief course of sex steroids.[458] Low serum concentrations of IGF-1 and IGFBP-3 and/or a poor GH response to provocative testing (after priming with sex steroids) should mandate an investigation for an underlying pathologic process, such as intracranial tumors.

Idiopathic Short Stature. ISS can be defined as a condition in which the height of an individual is more than 2 SD below the corresponding mean height for a given age, sex, and population group without evidence of systemic, endocrine, nutritional, or chromosomal abnormalities. Specifically, children with ISS have normal birth weight and are growth hormone sufficient. ISS describes a heterogeneous group of children consisting of many presently unidentified causes of short stature. It is estimated that approximately 60% to 80% of all short children at or below −2 SD fit the definition of ISS.

This definition of ISS includes short children labeled with "constitutional delay of growth and puberty" and "familial short stature." The frequency of referral of these children is dependent on the socioeconomic environment. Furthermore, there is a greater perceived disability of short stature in boys compared to girls irrespective of social class. ISS should be subcategorized, principally based on auxological criteria. The main distinction is between children with a familial history of short stature whose heights are within the expected range for parental target height and those children who are short for their parents. The corrected target height standard deviation score (SDS) is calculated as 0.72 multiplied by the average of the father's and mother's height SD scores and the lower limit of the target height range as corrected target height −1.6 SD.

It is generally accepted that on average adult height achieved in children with ISS is below the parental target height. ISS should also be classified by the presence or absence of bone age delay, indicating the probability of delayed growth and puberty. Subcategorization may help to predict adult height, which would be expected to be greater in a child with delayed maturation. Individuals with no family history of short stature generally have a lower adult height in comparison to target height. In situations in which a specific genetic diagnosis associated with short stature is expected (such as Noonan's syndrome or GH insensitivity), the gene(s) of interest should be examined. On-line resources exist, such as Genetest (www.genetests.org), which identify laboratories capable of performing these tests.

Although routine analysis of SHOX should not be undertaken in all patients with ISS, SHOX gene analysis should be considered for any patient with clinical findings compatible with SHOX haploinsufficiency. With currently available data it is difficult to generalize the impact of short stature on psychosocial adaptation. Short stature may be a risk factor for psychosocial problems, such as social immaturity, infantilization, low self-esteem, and being bullied—especially for those referred for evaluation. The large interindividual differences in adaptation to short stature and in the impact of being short may be a function of several risk and protective factors, including parental attitudes and prevailing cultural opinions. Stress experiences may be frequent, but true psychopathology is rare.[459]

Treatment of Growth Disorders

When growth failure is the result of a chronic underlying disease (such as renal failure, cystic fibrosis, or malabsorption), therapy must be directed at treatment of the underlying condition. Although growth acceleration may be observed with GH or IGF-1 therapy, complete catch-up requires correction of the primary medical problem. If treatment of the underlying condition involves glucocorticoids, growth failure may be profound and is unlikely to be correctable until the patient is weaned from steroids.

Correction of growth failure associated with chronic hypothyroidism requires appropriate thyroid replacement. As discussed previously, thyroid therapy results in dramatic catch-up growth but also markedly accelerates skeletal maturation—potentially limiting adult height. More gradual thyroid replacement and/or the use of gonadotropin

---

TABLE 8-11

Criteria for Presumptive Diagnosis of Constitutional Delay of Growth and Maturation

- No history of systemic illness
- Normal nutrition
- Normal physical examination, including body proportions
- Normal thyroid function test results
- Normal renal function test results
- Normal complete blood cell count, erythrocyte sedimentation rate, electrolytes
- Normal stimulated GH
- Height between −2.5 and −1.5 SDS
- Height velocity >−1 SDS
- Delayed puberty:
  - Males: failure to achieve Tanner G2 stage by age 13.8 years or P2 by 15.6 years
  - Females: failure to achieve Tanner B2 stage by age 13.3 years
- Delayed bone age (more than 1 year delayed)
- Normal predicted adult height:
  - Males: >165 cm (65 inches)
  - Females: >153 cm (60 inches)

inhibitors to delay puberty may be necessary to maximize final height.

TREATMENT OF CONSTITUTIONAL DELAY

Constitutional delay is a normal variant, with (by definition) potential for a normal (although delayed) pubertal maturation and a normal adult height. Most cases can be successfully managed by careful examination and evaluation to rule out other causes of delayed puberty and/or abnormal growth, combined with appropriate explanation and psychological counseling. The skeletal age and Bayley-Pinneau table are often helpful in explaining the potential for normal growth. A family history of constitutional delay is also frequently a source of reassurance. On occasion, however, the stigmas of delayed maturation and short stature may be psychologically disabling for the adolescent.

Studies have demonstrated that some adolescents with constitutional delay have poor self-images and limited social involvement.[488] In such patients, there is a role for the judicious use of short-term sex steroids. In males, therapy should generally be limited to adolescents who meet the following criteria: a minimal age of 14 years; height below the 3rd centile; prepubertal or early Tanner G2 stage, with a serum testosterone level less than 100 ng/dL; evidence of poor self-image that does not respond to reassurance alone; and predicted adult height well within the normal range. Therapy in males consists of depot testosterone enanthate, 50 to 200 mg every 3 weeks for a total of four injections.[488,489]

Patients will typically show early secondary sex characteristics by the fourth injection and grow an average of 10 cm in the ensuing year. This brief course of therapy has been shown to not cause overly rapid skeletal maturation, compromise adult height, or suppress pubertal maturation.[490] It is important to emphasize to the patient that he is normal, that therapy is short term and designed to provide him with some pubertal development earlier than he would experience on his own, and that treatment will not increase adult height. In such situations, the combination of short-term androgen therapy plus reassurance and counseling has been helpful in assisting the patient with constitutional delay cope with a difficult adolescence.

Patients must be reevaluated to ensure that they spontaneously enter "true" puberty. One year after testosterone treatment, patients should demonstrate testicular enlargement and a serum testosterone level in the pubertal or adult range. If this is not the case, the diagnosis of pituitary insufficiency should be considered. Although a second course of testosterone may be warranted at this time, it is our experience that most such patients eventually prove to be gonadotropin deficient.

The recent availability of several new forms of testosterone supplementation, which are approved for adults with hypogonadism, provided pediatricians with an opportunity to offer patients a choice among different androgen replacement therapies. Although these new therapies have not been published as efficacious in children with constitutional delay, we have personal experience with their successful use—with an equivalent response to

that obtained with testosterone injections. Testosterone gel is painless and easy to apply, and has proven popular since its release.[491] Testosterone patches also avoid the need for injections but work best when applied to the scrotum and are often accompanied by complaints of itching.[492] The dosing of these alternative forms of therapy in children is not clearly established, and further experience will undoubtedly accumulate on their use in pediatrics in the coming years.

Referrals for constitutional delay are much more common in males than in females, undoubtedly reflecting our cultural values. When constitutional delay is a problem in girls, short-term estrogen therapy can be employed. The use of GH in patients with constitutional delay is discussed later in this chapter.

TREATMENT OF GROWTH HORMONE DEFICIENCY

Patients with proven GHD should be treated with recombinant human GH (rhGH) as soon as possible after the diagnosis is made. The primary objectives of the therapy for GHD are normalization of height during childhood and attainment of normal adult height. Normally growing patients with craniopharyngioma and GHD should be considered for therapy with GH for metabolic and body composition benefits and for enhancement of pubertal growth.

GH exhibits a high degree of species specificity in its actions. Unlike most other hormones, the only GH biologically active in humans is primate GH. For many years, the only practical source of primate GH for treatment of GHD was human cadaver pituitary glands—first employed in the late 1950s. Over the next 25 years, more than 27,000 children with GHD worldwide were treated. In 1985, distribution of pituitary-derived human growth hormone (hGH) in the United States and most of Europe was halted because of concern about a causal relationship with Creutzfeldt-Jakob disease—a rare and fatal spongiform encephalopathy that had been previously reported to be capable of iatrogenic transmission through human tissue.[493,494]

In North America and Europe, this disorder has an incidence of approximately 1 case per million. Noniatrogenic cases are exceedingly rare before the age of 50 years. To date, more than 20 young adults of about 8,000 patients in the United States who had received human cadaver pituitary products have died of Creutzfeldt-Jakob disease. In France, there have been more than 60 cases of Creutzfeldt-Jakob disease among 1,700 human cadaver GH recipients—and in England 32 cases among 1,900 human cadaver GH recipients have been reported.

Fortunately, by the time the risks of pituitary-derived hGH were discovered recombinant DNA–derived hGH had already begun extensive testing for safety and efficacy.[252,495,496] The original form of rhGH included an N-terminal methionine, added for use as a start signal for transcription (met-hGH). This preparation was found to mimic pituitary-derived hGH in its anabolic and metabolic actions. Subsequent rhGH preparations were produced without the additional methionine. Over the next decade, rhGH universally replaced pituitary-derived hGH as the treatment of choice for children with GHD.

Dosing of GH

Despite continued variability and lack of consensus, considerable progress and improvement have been made in the standardization of GH dosage and administration. It is well established that GH administration should be initiated as early as possible in the GH-deficient child to optimize final height outcome.[497] Daily administration of GH is clearly more effective than giving the same total dose three times weekly.[498] GH injections are best administered in the evening, better mimicking natural physiology and achieving higher GH peaks.[499] The hGH should be administered subcutaneously.

The dosage of GH should be expressed in milligrams (or micrograms) per kilogram per day, although consideration should be given to dosing in micrograms per square meter of body surface per day in patients with obesity. GH is routinely used in the range of 25 to 50 mcg/kg/day. A dose-response relationship in terms of height velocity in the first 2 years has been clearly demonstrated within this range (Figure 8-28).[500-502] On this regimen, the typical GH-deficient child accelerates growth from a pretreatment rate of 3 to 4 cm/year to 10 to 12 cm/year in year 1 of therapy and 7 to 9 cm/year in years 2 and 3. This progressive waning of GH efficacy has been observed universally and is still not fully understood. It can, however, be overcome at least in part by increasing the dosage of hGH. In the United States, at a dosage of 50 mcg/kg/day the approximate current cost of hGH therapy for a 20-kg child is $15,000/year. The practice of individualizing treatment according to the specific needs of each GH-deficient child is gaining popularity.

Consensus does not exist as to how to formulate individualized treatment plans. Emerging evidence suggests that mathematical prediction models of growth response may be useful for determination of the optimal individual dose.[480,503,504] Although these models will need further improvement in their predictive power (as well as further validation), their potential utility is considerable. GH dose can be calculated to achieve specific therapeutic aims

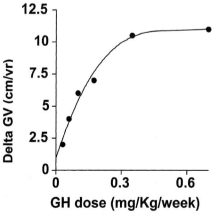

FIGURE 8-28. Meta-analysis of the dose-response relationship between growth hormone (GH) and delta growth velocity (GV) in the first year of treatment of naive GH-deficient children. The lower three doses are from Frasier and colleagues,[501] and the higher three doses are from Cohen and coworkers.[502]

(i.e., catch-up to target height within 2, 3, or 4 years). They can also enable a comparison between observed and predicted growth, hastening identification of causes of suboptimal growth. Further application of these models to specific diseases and conditions in which GH responsiveness varies will allow disease-specific optimization.

Despite the availability of GH therapy, long-term studies have indicated that many patients fail to achieve normal adult heights—and only a few attain their genetic target heights. Although the development of rhGH has solved the problem of supply experienced in the pituitary GH era, delays in diagnosis and initiation of therapy have still compromised adult height. Data from the National Cooperative Growth Study evaluation of adult heights in 121 patients with childhood GHD indicate a mean adult height in male and female patients of <0.7 SD.[505] By multiple-regression analysis, factors found to correlate with enhanced adult height were baseline height, younger age at onset of treatment, longer treatment duration, and a greater growth velocity during the first year of treatment.

In an effort to increase final height of GHD patients, Mauras and associates[506] have evaluated the use of high-dose GH during puberty—with the rationale that GH secretion normally doubles during the pubertal growth spurt (as indicated by the dramatic rise in serum IGF-1 concentrations during puberty) and that the pubertal growth spurt normally accounts for approximately 17% of adult male height and 12% of adult female height. Earlier studies by Stanhope and associates[507] indicated that little difference in height gain could be observed when adolescent patients were treated with 30 versus 15 IU/m²/wk of GH (approximately 0.04 versus 0.02 mg/kg/day).

Mauras and associates[506] evaluated higher doses of GH during puberty (100 versus 50 mcg/kg/day) and found that the higher dosage resulted in a 4.6-cm increase in near-final height (defined as height at a bone age of more than 16 years in males and more than 14 years in females). The mean height SD score at near-final height was higher for the 100-mcg/kg/day group. The higher GH dosage did not result in more rapid acceleration of skeletal maturation.

An alternative approach to maximizing height gain during adolescence is to combine GH treatment with suppression of the hypothalamic-pituitary-gonadal axis by GnRH analogues (or recently, but only in boys, the use of aromatase inhibitors). This combined therapy may lead to significant improvement of final height or predicted adult height of patients, as shown in some studies (but long-term results are still lacking). In addition, the effect of suppression of puberty on bone accretion during the critical pubertal phase (as well as on psychosocial function) has not yet been evaluated adequately. Similar concerns may exist for the combination of GH therapy with aromatase inhibitors, which are designed to prevent the effects of estrogen on epiphyseal fusion.

Novel Modalities for Treatment of GHD

Several novel treatment modalities have emerged (Table 8-12). These include oral secretagogues, GHRH, extended-action depot rhGH preparations, and liquid rhGH formulations. A number of GH-releasing peptides and

---

TABLE 8-12

New and Emerging Modalities for Treatment of Growth Hormone (GH) Deficiency

- Liquid formulations
- Pen-type delivery devices
- Long-acting GH formulations
  - Sustained-release GH formulations
  - Dermal patch delivery of GH
- Oral ghrelin-mimetics

---

nonpeptidyl GH secretagogues have been formulated since their discovery in the 1980s.[508] Although these oral agents would be an attractive potential treatment option for GHD secondary to hypothalamic GRF deficiency, their evaluation remains incomplete at this time.[509,510] GHRH has been demonstrated to be safe and more effective than placebo at increasing height velocity in some GHD children. However, further long-term studies are needed.[511,512]

The development of sustained-release long-acting depot GH formulations may eventually provide a desirable alternative to daily subcutaneous rhGH injections for some patients. Currently, such formulations remain under study in ongoing clinical trials—and although efficacious they appear less effective than daily rhGH therapy. Further studies will be necessary, however, to ascertain whether such preparations can provide the same level of growth acceleration as is seen with daily GH—and whether side effects will not be increased. Liquid rhGH formulations, which eliminate the need for reconstitution, and new delivery devices such as pen systems have been introduced that appear to improve patient compliance.

Additional novel delivery GH strategies remain under active development, including orally inhaled and intranasally administered rhGH formulations. In time and with further experience, novel treatment approaches may emerge as useful alternatives to conventional rhGH therapy. The combination of GH along with IGF-I therapies may also prove to be a useful treatment of growth disorders.

Management of Multiple Pituitary Hormone Deficiency

In the patient with an initial diagnosis of isolated GHD, particularly those with an ectopic posterior pituitary or other developmental abnormalities, the clinician should be alert to the risk of the development of MPHD. This involves regular repeat biochemical testing and consideration of repeat pituitary imaging. If GHD is part of a multiple pituitary insufficiency, it is necessary to address each endocrine deficiency. TSH deficiency is often "unmasked" during the initial phase of hGH therapy, and thyroid tests should be performed both before the onset of therapy and during the first 3 months of hGH treatment.[513] Even if normal initially, thyroid function should be tested subsequently on at least an annual basis.

The pituitary-adrenal axis is customarily evaluated during the insulin stimulation test for GHD. If ACTH secretion

is impaired, patients should be placed on the lowest safe maintenance dose of glucocorticoids—certainly no more than 10 mg/m²/day of hydrocortisone. Higher doses may impair the growth response to hGH therapy but may be necessary during times of stress. An alternative approach is to avoid maintenance glucocorticoids and treat with steroids only during periods of physiologic stress.

Gonadotropin deficiency may be evident in infancy in the child with microphallus. This can usually be treated with three to four monthly injections of 25 to 50 mg of testosterone enanthate.[514] Management of puberty can be more complicated because the physical and psychological benefits of normalizing sexual maturation must be balanced against the risk of epiphyseal fusion. When hGH therapy is initiated in childhood and the child's growth is normalized before adolescence, it is appropriate to begin sex steroid replacement at a normal age (e.g., 11 to 12 in females and 12 to 13 in males).

In males, this can be done by beginning with monthly injections of 100 mg of testosterone enanthate—gradually increasing to 200 mg/month, and eventually moving to the appropriate adult replacement regimen. In girls, therapy involves use of conjugated estrogens or ethinyl estradiol, and eventual cycling with estrogen and progesterone (as described elsewhere in this book). On the other hand, in patients in whom normal or precocious puberty may limit the statural response to hGH it may be appropriate to delay puberty by the use of the GnRH analogue.

Monitoring GH Therapy

Careful monitoring of pediatric patients with GHD is critical. Important aspects of this process are outlined in Table 8-13. The routine follow-up of GHD children should be performed by a pediatric endocrinologist on a 3- to 6-month basis in partnership with the patient's primary care physician. Assessment of the growth response is perhaps the single most important parameter of monitoring. This consists of accurate determination of height velocity and interval height increase (best expressed in terms of the change in height Z score). Establishment of a target height (typically the mid-parental target height) against which the child's progress can be assessed is important. Careful attention must also be directed toward screening for possible adverse effects and toward assessing compliance.

TABLE 8-13

Elements of Monitoring Growth Hormone Therapy

Close follow-up with a pediatric endocrinologist every 3 to 6 months
Determination of growth response (change in height Z-score)
Monitoring serum IGF-1 and IGFBP-3 levels
Screening for potential adverse effects
Evaluation of compliance
Consideration of dose adjustment based on IGF values, growth response, and comparison to growth prediction models

IGF, insulin-like growth factor; IGFBP-3, insulin-like growth factor-binding protein-3.

Monitoring Serum IGF-1 Levels

The emerging consensus is that annual monitoring of serum IGF-1 and IGFBP-3 levels should be an aspect of routine care of the GHD child receiving rhGH therapy.[515] Titration of rhGH dose to maintain these growth factors within age-dependent normal limits is physiologically sound and is standard practice in the treatment of adults with GHD. It is well recognized that IGF-1 and IGFBP-3 levels are low in children with GHD and increase with rhGH injections.[516]

The relationship between the rise in IGF-1 levels and the growth response during therapy has recently been demonstrated in a study that used a GH-dose titration to achieve target IGF-I levels.[517] In that paper, it was demonstrated that at least over the first two years of treatment there is a substantial correlation between the level of the IGF-I achieved and the height gain—and that this correlation was valid for both GHD and ISS patients. Growth factor monitoring certainly has important utility in assessment of compliance issues as well as in the assurance of safety. Several epidemiologic studies have linked serum IGF-1 levels and lower IGFBP-3 levels to increased risk of prostate, breast, and colorectal cancer in otherwise healthy subjects.[515,518,519] Although a causal relationship between serum IGF-1 levels and cancer is not proven, monitoring lifetime exposure to IGF-1 and ensuring that IGF-1 and IGFBP-3 levels in the GH-deficient patient are within age-defined normal limits certainly seem prudent at this time.

Role of Serial Bone Age Assessment

Although a well-established diagnostic tool in the initial evaluation of a GH-deficient patient, bone age assessment no longer has a role in the ongoing management of childhood GHD. Previously, many clinicians have included serial bone age assessment as part of their monitoring of a GH-deficient child's progress on rhGH therapy by comparing the observed to predicted heights and by following the Bailey-Pinneau predicted height calculations.[520,521]

When the wide SDs applied to such measures and the lack of clinical evidence that management is enhanced by their use are considered, they have no sound role in the monitoring of GH therapy.[522] It also appears that whereas GH therapy accelerates bone maturation there may be an initial delay before this is apparent radiographically and height predictions may be skewed as a result.[522] At this time, the role of bone age assessment during GH therapy lies only in determining remaining growth potential in the patient with GHD approaching final height and in assessing children with concerns about rapid progression of puberty.

Assessment of Treatment Efficacy and Optimizing Growth Response

Clearly defined individual treatment goals need to be established for each patient with GHD. During the initial 2 years of therapy, catch-up growth at a rate twofold to fourfold above pretreatment growth velocity and a gain of 1 to 2 SDs in height should be expected in the majority of patients.[523] This will be influenced by age at diagnosis and severity of GHD. The dose may need to be increased if catch-up growth is inadequate. After the initial catch-up phase, growth velocity should be maintained at a rate at or above the 50th percentile for age.

Mathematical prediction models may be used to not only predict growth response to a specific dose but to guide the pediatric endocrinologist in modifying therapy when the observed growth falls short of predicted growth.[504] Prediction models have considerable promise but need to be improved and studied further in a prospective manner before any recommendations regarding their use can be formulated. In instances in which an inadequate response is encountered, it is also important to consider all possible causes—including poor compliance, technical difficulties, underlying hypothyroidism, incorrect diagnosis, poor nutrition, neutralizing antibodies, and intercurrent illness.

It is critically important to maximize height with GH therapy before the onset of puberty. If this is not achieved, modulation of the GH dose during puberty may be considered. As stated previously, the growth response to hGH typically attenuates after the first year—but it should continue to be equal to or greater than the normal height velocity for age throughout treatment. In situations in which the clinical response to hGH is suboptimal, the following possibilities must be considered: poor compliance; improper preparation of hGH for administration or incorrect injection techniques, subclinical hypothyroidism, chronic disease, glucocorticoid therapy, history of irradiation of the spine, epiphyseal fusion, anti-GH antibodies,[524] and incorrect diagnosis of GHD as explanation for growth retardation. Some recipients of rhGH have developed detectable anti-GH antibodies, but growth failure resulting from such antibodies has been exceedingly rare.

Maximal growth response to hGH can be obtained by early diagnosis and initiation of therapy and by careful attention to compliance and psychological support. Thus, although some studies have indicated that as many as 50% of males and 85% of females with idiopathic GHD do not achieve adult heights above the third centile[505,525] it is our belief that normalization of height (i.e., achieving target height) should be achievable in most cases. Despite the efficacy of hGH in accelerating growth in children with GHD, and the ability of such therapy to normalize adult height if treatment is begun sufficiently early, several studies have indicated that the long-term prognosis for such patients is guarded.[526] The educational, vocational, and social outlook for adults with GHD dating from childhood is frequently suboptimal. Whether this reflects subtle intellectual deficits or the consequences of lower expectations of patients, families, or teachers remains to be determined. In any case, patients with GHD clearly require careful and thorough follow-up throughout childhood and adolescence—and possibly adulthood.

Studies have focused on the clinical consequences of GHD in adults and on the potential benefits of hGH therapy in such patients.[527,528] Signs and symptoms of adult GHD have included reduced lean body mass and musculature, increased body fat, reduced bone mineral density, reduced exercise performance, and increased plasma cholesterol. Adults with GHD have been found to have a significantly increased risk of death from cardio-vascular causes, a finding potentially linked to the increase in adiposity and in serum cholesterol.[529]

Adults with GHD have been found to have "impaired psychological well-being and quality of life" characterized by depression, anxiety, reduced energy and vitality, and social isolation. Several placebo-controlled studies have demonstrated that hGH therapy for adults with GHD results in marked alterations in body composition, fat distribution, bone density, and sense of well-being.[530,531] Whether these effects of hGH therapy will be sustained (and if so, what the optimal hGH regimen will be) remains to be determined.

Because of the potential metabolic benefits of treatment of adult GHD, it is necessary to discuss the need for lifelong GH therapy with patients and families at the time of diagnosis. Given the studies that have demonstrated that many (perhaps the majority) of the children diagnosed with childhood GHD demonstrate normal GH levels on repeat provocative testing, it is recommended that on completion of skeletal growth GH therapy be halted for a period of 1 to 3 months and the patient then retested. Toogood and colleagues[532] have reported that the likelihood of GHD persisting in adult life increases with the number of pituitary hormone deficiencies. Approximately 90% of patients with two or three additional pituitary hormone deficiencies had provocative GH levels less than 5 ng/mL. Similarly, patients with documented structural abnormalities of the hypothalamus-pituitary (such as pituitary hypoplasia, pituitary stalk agenesis, posterior pituitary ectopia, or septo-optic dysplasia) have a very high likelihood of retesting as GHD.

A conservative approach would suggest that all children diagnosed as having GHD should be retested by insulin-provocative tests on completion of skeletal growth, and before a commitment is made for long-term adult treatment. An argument can be made, however, that patients with multiple pituitary hormone deficiencies, documented structural abnormalities, or documented hypothalamic-pituitary molecular defects do not necessarily require retesting—or at most should have IGF-1 and IGFBP-3 concentrations determined. On the other hand, the child who has carried a diagnosis of idiopathic isolated GHD should always be retested.

Transition to Adult Management

A suggested algorithm to guide the transition to adult management is displayed in Figure 8-29. After attainment of final height, retesting of the GH-IGF axis using the adult GHD diagnostic criteria as defined by the Growth Hormone Research Society (GRS) Consensus Workshop on Adult GHD should be undertaken by the pediatric endocrinologist.

Standard GH stimulation tests can be performed after an interval of 1 to 3 months off GH therapy.[533] In places where an insulin tolerance test is mandatory for the patient to qualify for further GH therapy, this test should be performed. At the time of retesting, other pituitary hormones and serum IGF-1 and IGFBP-3 levels should be measured.[473] As recommended by the GRS, the opportunity should be taken to assess body composition,

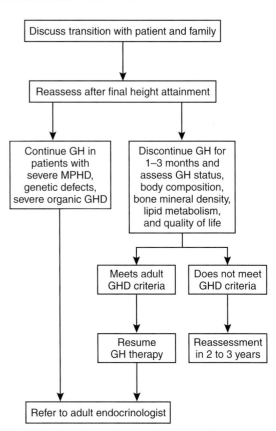

FIGURE 8-29. Algorithm for transition to adult treatment of growth hormone (GH) deficiency. MPHD, multiple pituitary hormone deficiency.

bone mineral density, fasting lipids, insulin, and quality of life before and after discontinuation of GH therapy. Patients with severe long-standing MPHD, those with genetic defects, and those with severe organic GHD can probably be excluded from GH retesting.[411]

When the diagnosis of adult GHD is established, continuation of GH therapy is strongly recommended. Caution should be exercised when considering the decision of continuing GH therapy in conditions where there is a known risk of diabetes or malignancy. Although large patient registries have not seen an increase in the incidence of malignancy in pediatric GH recipients, patients with certain high-risk states (such as Bloom syndrome) may be at an increased risk as a result of long-term GH therapy and such patients should be monitored carefully. The transition to adult GH replacement should be arranged as a close collaboration between the pediatric and adult endocrinologists, who should discuss the re-initiation of treatment with the patient.

GROWTH HORMONE TREATMENT OF OTHER FORMS OF SHORT STATURE

The development of rhGH has provided the capability for a theoretically unlimited supply of hGH. Although treatment of GHD is the one unequivocal indication for "replacement" therapy, the potential use of hGH for treatment of other forms of short stature has been actively explored. Theoretically, any child with open epiphyses should be capable of accelerating growth and achieving heights greater than indicated by genetic potential—as indicated by experience with cases of pituitary gigantism. Whether such therapy can be done safely and whether it justifies the cost and potential risks of hGH are more complicated issues. In addition, questions have been raised about the appropriateness of "cosmetic" hormonal therapy.

Chronic Renal Failure

Several studies have now convincingly demonstrated the ability of hGH to accelerate growth over at least several years of therapy.[534,535] These findings have now been confirmed by several double-blind placebo-controlled investigations. Using an hGH dosage of 0.05 mg/kg/day, Fine and co-workers[536] showed a mean first-year growth rate of 10.7 cm in GH recipients and 6.5 cm in the placebo group. In the second year, GH-treated patients had a mean growth rate of 7.8 cm/year versus 5.5 cm/year in placebo recipients. No deleterious effects on renal function were observed. Longer-term studies will be necessary to determine whether these effects on growth will be sustained and whether they will translate into an improved adult height.

Turner Syndrome

Before the availability of rhGH, a number of uncontrolled studies had produced conflicting data concerning the efficacy of GH therapy in Turner syndrome.[537,538] In 1983, a randomized controlled study of rhGH was initiated.[173,277] First-year results indicated a growth rate of 3.8 cm/year in the control group, 6.6 cm/year in hGH recipients, 7.9 cm/year in oxandrolone recipients, and 9.8 cm/year in subjects receiving hGH plus oxandrolone. At the end of 6 years, heights for 30 subjects who had completed therapy were compared with their projected adult heights[539] based on the growth curves of Lyon and colleagues.[11]

Mean height achieved after 2 to 6 years of treatment was 151.9 cm, compared to a mean projected adult height of only 143.8 cm. Near-adult heights in these subjects showed that girls receiving GH alone had a final height 8.4 cm greater than their projected adult heights. Girls receiving GH plus oxandrolone had a 10.3-cm increase.[278] Sixteen of 17 girls receiving GH alone achieved adult heights above the 50th percentile for Turner syndrome, and 10 of 17 attained heights above the 90th percentile. All 45 girls receiving combination treatment attained heights above the 50th percentile for Turner syndrome, and 23 of 45 had heights above the 90th percentile.

In a subsequent study, GH was employed in combination with estrogen replacement at either 12 or 15 years of age.[540] Earlier initiation of estrogen therapy resulted in accelerated epiphyseal fusion and a compromise in final height attained, a not surprising observation given the critical role of estrogen in skeletal maturation. Girls who began GH therapy before 11 years of age and estrogen at age 15 had the greatest increase in adult height.

Even more dramatic results have been observed in Dutch studies, in which the GH dosage was progressively increased to 0.09 mg/kg/day.[279] At the highest GH dosage, increases in adult height over projected heights averaged

16 cm. Estrogen therapy was withheld until subjects had received at least 4 years of GH treatment and reached a minimum age of 12 years. With this regimen, the majority of girls with Turner syndrome attained adult heights within the normal range.

In light of the detailed historical data that exist on natural growth in Turner syndrome, the results to date provide convincing data that hGH can accelerate growth and increase adult height. Furthermore, early initiation of GH treatment should allow for normalization of growth in childhood—as well as the potential to begin estrogen replacement at a physiologically appropriate age. This subject is discussed in detail in Chapter 15.

Down Syndrome

The encouraging results of hGH trials in Turner syndrome have led to studies of hGH in other chromosomal disorders, such as Down syndrome. Several preliminary studies have confirmed the ability of hGH to accelerate growth in such patients, although ethical issues have been raised concerning the appropriateness of such therapy.[541,542] No convincing data exist that hGH improves neurologic or intellectual function in such patients.

Intrauterine Growth Retardation or Small for Gestational Age

A number of studies, employing pituitary-derived or recombinant DNA–derived hGH, have been performed in children with short stature resulting from IUGR/SGA.[543,544] Such studies are hampered by the inherent heterogeneity of this group of patients, whose poor growth may reflect maternal factors, chromosomal disorders, dysmorphic syndromes, toxins, and so on. Interpretation of the results from such studies are frequently complicated by an accompanying diagnosis of GHD, often lacking stringency in diagnostic criteria.

Coutant and colleagues,[545] for example, compared children treated with GH for a diagnosis of IUGR associated with "idiopathic" GHD and children with IUGR not treated with GH and found no significant differences in adult height. Furthermore, almost 80% of the alleged GH-deficient IUGR children proved to have normal GH levels when reevaluated after cessation of growth. Two studies have examined the effects of two doses of continuous GH treatment administered over a 6-year period.[292,546,547] GH at doses of 0.033 and 0.067 mg/kg/day resulted in 2.0- and 2.7-SD increments in height, respectively. Together, most studies have demonstrated taller final height—leading to approval of the therapy in most countries. The doses commonly used in SGA children are between 50 and 70 mcg/kg/day, and treatment is typically started at age 3 years.[546]

Prader-Willi Syndrome

One form of IUGR/short stature in which GH therapy has been studied fairly extensively is Prader-Willi syndrome. Early studies in a limited number of subjects demonstrated promising short-term results.[304] Lindgren and colleagues[548] demonstrated that patients with Prader-Willi syndrome had lower serum IGF-1 concentrations than did normal obese controls. Prader-Willi subjects treated with GH at a dosage of 0.033 mg/kg/day showed a 1-year increase in height velocity, whereas untreated Prader-Willi subjects experienced a decrease in height velocity.

GH treatment also resulted in a reduction of relative fat mass and an increase in fat-free mass. Carrel and co-workers[125] employed a similar dosage of GH in Prader-Willi patients with reduced clonidine-stimulated GH levels and low serum IGF-1 concentrations and demonstrated an increase in height velocity—whereas untreated controls showed no significant change in height velocity.

Dual-energy x-ray absorptiometry (DEXA) demonstrated a GH-induced reduction in total body fat and increased strength and agility. The Food and Drug Administration has recognized Prader-Willi syndrome to be an accepted diagnosis for GH therapy, even in the absence of demonstrable GHD. This treatment is effective in improving growth and body composition. However, several reports have indicated a possible GH-associated mortality in Prader-Willi patients with massive obesity—perhaps related to tonsillar hypertrophy as a contributory factor.[549]

Osteochondrodysplasias

Therapy with hGH has been studied in several studies of skeletal dysplasias. The largest published study to date in achondroplasia is by Seino and co-workers,[550] who reported on hGH administration to 40 children. During the first year of treatment, the height velocity increased from 3.8 to 6.6 cm/year. In year 2, the height velocity decreased to approximately 5 cm/year. A modest improvement was seen in the ratio of lower limb length to height. Although hGH was well tolerated, it is of note that one patient with atlantoaxial dislocation during hGH therapy has been reported. There has also been limited experience with hGH treatment of other skeletal disorders, such as dyschondrosteosis, hereditary multiple exostoses, osteogenesis imperfecta, and Ellis-van Creveld syndrome.

Idiopathic Short Stature

Several countries, including the United States, have recently approved GH therapy of ISS. It is important to recognize that this is a heterogeneous group of patients, as emphasized by Kelnar and co-workers.[551] Even though they are grouped under the title "normal short children" or as having "idiopathic short stature," this group will include children who have passed provocative GH testing but are nevertheless IGF deficient—reflecting the inadequacies of GH testing.

There is abundant evidence that determination of provocative GH levels does not adequately discriminate between true GHD (IGF deficiency) and ISS. In addition, the group labeled "normal short children" will inevitably contain children with unidentified syndromes and possibly with unidentified chronic illnesses or endocrine disorders. These issues have made it difficult to properly evaluate existing clinical trials. Furthermore, published clinical trials have not contained long-term control groups and have indicated considerable variability in growth response.[552-554]

The majority of normal short children treated with hGH have shown growth acceleration that is generally sustained over the first several years of therapy (although attenuation of the response is seen, just as in all other instances of hGH treatment). Longer-term data are inadequate, however, to address the question of impact of therapy on adult height. Hintz and co-workers[555] treated 80 children with ISS (0.3 mg/kg/wk) for 2 to 10 years and compared results with those in untreated short retrospective control subjects. In children with ISS, GH therapy increased the mean height scores from 2.7 at the start of treatment to 1.4 at final height. The mean increase in final height over the pretreatment predicted adult height was 5.0 cm for boys and 5.9 cm for girls. Concern has been raised that hGH therapy in normal short children may result in an earlier onset of puberty—and as a result, earlier fusion of the epiphyses—and thereby may offset the positive response observed during the early years of hGH treatment.[556]

Other important questions have been raised about the financial, ethical, and psychosocial impact of hGH therapy on normal short children.[557] Given the current cost of hGH, the financial implications of treating normal short children (whether it is the bottom 5, 3, 1, or 0.1%) is considerable and potentially diverts a limited pool of health care dollars away from other needs. The point is well taken that 5% of the population will always be below the 5th percentile whether we treat them with hGH or not. Concern has been raised that focusing on a short child's stature potentially disables an otherwise normal child, handicapping that child psychologically or socially. No convincing data have been presented that hGH treatment of normal short children improves psychological, social, or educational function. Finally, the known and unknown treatment risks of hGH therapy must be considered when treatment of otherwise normal children is an issue.

On the other hand, given the current limitations in our ability to clinically or biochemically discriminate definitively between GHD and normal short stature, our inadequate understanding of neurosecretory defects of GH secretion, our inadequate definition of "partial" GHD, and the need to move to a more global concept of "IGF deficiency" it seems unfair to prevent hGH therapy of short children who do not meet a definition of GHD (i.e., provocative testing) we recognize as inadequate. Many of these children behave clinically and biochemically in a manner identical to those with classic GHD.

The mean improvement in adult height in children with ISS attributable to GH therapy (average duration of 4-7 years) is 3.5 to 7.5 cm compared to initial predicted adult height. Responses are highly variable and are dose dependent. Concern has been raised that in ISS higher GH doses (>50 ug/kg/day) may advance bone age (BA) and the onset of puberty, but this has not been seen in other studies.

Multiple factors affect the growth response to GH in ISS, most of which are unknown. The first-year response is influenced negatively by age at start (and positively by GH dose), weight at start, and difference from target height—and these factors account for approximately 40% of the variance. Adult height outcome is influenced negatively by age at start and positively by mid-parental height, height at start, bone age delay, and the first-year response to growth hormone.[556] The utility of baseline and treatment-related biochemical data including IGF-I has not been validated in long-term studies, but 2-year studies suggest that the rise in IGF-I correlates with short-term height gain.

Children treated with GH should be monitored for height, weight, pubertal development, and adverse effects at 3- to 6-month intervals. Periodic monitoring for scoliosis, tonsillar hypertrophy, papilledema, and slipped femoral capital epiphyses (SCFE) should be performed as part of the regular physical exam during follow-up visits. We recommend that after 1 year the response to therapy be assessed by calculating height velocity SDS as well as the change in height SDS. Bone age may be obtained periodically to reassess height prediction and for consideration of manipulation of the tempo of puberty. IGF-1 levels may be helpful in guiding GH dose adjustment, but the significance of abnormally elevated IGF-1 levels remains unknown. Thus far, no cases of elevated blood glucose in GH treated patients with ISS have been reported—but there is controversy regarding the need for routine monitoring of glucose metabolism.

Dosage is usually selected and adjusted by weight. If the growth response is considered inadequate, the dose may be increased. There are no definitive data concerning the long-term safety of doses higher than 50 ug/kg/day in ISS. The upper limit of GH dosage used in ISS and other indications is approximately 70 ug/kg/day,[546,555] but the possibility of using such doses varies in terms of national health economics. In the future, growth prediction models may improve GH dosing strategies. IGF-1 levels may be helpful in assessing compliance and GH sensitivity. Levels that are consistently elevated (>2.5 SDS) should prompt consideration of GH dose reduction. Recent studies on IGF-based dose adjustments in ISS demonstrated increased short-term growth when higher IGF targets were selected, but this strategy has not been validated in long-term studies in terms of safety or final height effects.

If height prediction is below −2 SDS at the time of pubertal onset in either sex, the addition of GnRH analogues may be considered. Alternatively, in males aromatase inhibitors may also be an option. However, long-term efficacy and safety data are not available for either of these interventions. In addition, the impact of delayed puberty on somatic and psychological development is not known. We do not recommend aromatase inhibitors in girls.

There are two schools of thought about the duration of treatment. One is that treatment should stop when near-adult height is achieved [Ht velocity <2 cm/year and/or bone age >16 years (in boys) and >14 years (in girls)]. Alternatively, therapy can be discontinued when height is in the "normal" adult range (above −2 SD) or has reached another cutoff for the reference adult population (for example, in Australia the 10th percentile; elsewhere, the 50th percentile). Stopping therapy is influenced by patient/family satisfaction with the result of therapy, on-going cost-benefit analysis, and when the child wants to stop for other reasons.

Miscellaneous Causes of Growth Failure

In addition to the clinical conditions described previously, hGH has been employed in treatment of short stature associated with Noonan syndrome, neurofibromatosis, and a variety of other conditions associated with postnatal growth failure. In general, such trials have been uncontrolled and have not included sufficient numbers of subjects for adequate evaluation of efficacy. A review of a large database, however, indicates that many of these conditions might in fact be responsive to GH therapy.[558]

Although this database is uncontrolled, 4-year results of GH treatment of Prader-Willi syndrome, IUGR, Russell-Silver dwarfism, neural tube defects, neurofibromatosis, and familial hypophosphatemic rickets were indistinguishable from those observed with GH treatment of "idiopathic GHD" using comparable dosages of GH. Furthermore, a variety of other conditions (such as Down syndrome, cystic fibrosis, fetal alcohol syndrome, Crohn disease, sickle cell anemia, hypochondroplasia, and thalassemia) responded in a manner comparable to that observed with Turner syndrome.

Although management of such patients is often complex and the use of GH may be characterized by important ethical issues, one must conclude that at least on auxologic grounds it becomes difficult to discriminate among GHD (as currently diagnosed), Turner syndrome, and many other medical conditions characterized by growth failure. If as proposed by Allen and Fost[559] responsiveness to GH rather than GHD should be the most important criterion for GH treatment, these findings indicate that GH therapy for many of these "other" conditions warrants an open-minded appropriately controlled evaluation.

Normal Aging and Other Catabolic States

A lengthy discussion of the potential use of hGH in normal aging is beyond the scope of this chapter.[128] The rationale for therapy is based on the concept of the "somatopause," referring to the fact that GH secretion normally declines progressively after 30 years of age—reflected in decreasing serum concentrations of IGF-1. Aging can be viewed as a catabolic state, with the potential that hGH therapy will reverse or retard the loss of muscle mass and strength and the decrease in bone density characteristic of the older population.

It is also conceivable, however, that aging individuals may be more sensitive to the metabolic changes produced by hGH—resulting in fluid accumulation, carpal tunnel syndrome, and glucose intolerance. Clinical studies are currently in progress. hGH therapy is also being investigated in a variety of catabolic states,[129] such as burns, tumor cachexia, major abdominal surgery, AIDS, sepsis, and hyperalimentation. Although the frontiers of new indications of GH therapy are being explored in well-controlled trials, we believe that aging, catabolic states, and other unapproved indications for GH therapy should not be routinely treated by clinicians outside appropriate clinical studies.

SIDE EFFECTS OF GROWTH HORMONE

Pituitary-derived hGH, which for a quarter of a century had an enviable safety record, proved to be the agent for transmission of the fatal spongiform encephalopathy Creutzfeldt-Jakob disease.[493,554] Although this risk does not exist with recombinant DNA-derived hGH, the experience with pituitary hGH serves as a grim reminder of the potential toxicity that can reside in "normal" products and "physiologic replacement." Nevertheless, 15 years of extensive experience with rhGH has been encouraging. Concerns have been raised, however, about a number of potential complications that clearly required continued follow-up and assessment. This evaluation has been greatly facilitated by the extensive databases established by hGH manufacturers.

Development of Leukemia

In 1988, the development of leukemia as a complication of hGH therapy was reported in 5 cases from Japan.[317] Since then, more than 30 cases of leukemia in hGH-treated patients have been reported—a disproportionate number coming from Japan,[318] but with cases also reported in the United States.[319] One of the difficulties in assessing the role of hGH treatment in these cases was that many children with GHD have clinical conditions that may predispose them to the development of leukemia, such as histories of previous malignancies, histories of irradiation, and underlying syndromes known to predispose to the development of leukemia (Bloom syndrome, Down syndrome, Fanconi anemia).

Patients have included recipients of pituitary-derived and recombinant DNA–derived hGH, and leukemia has occurred both during treatment and after termination of therapy. Cases of leukemia have been also reported in GH-deficient individuals without any history of hGH therapy, suggesting that the GHD state by itself might be a predisposing factor. In a comprehensive set of large cohorts of patients from the United States, Europe, and (most recently) Japan, the concern of increased leukemia risk in patients with GHD without predisposing factors has been dispelled.

In a large series describing the entire Japanese experience, the same authors who first reported the increased incidence of leukemia in GHD reanalyzed their data—together with a much larger number of patients treated since the original report—and showed that the risk for leukemia is the same for GH recipients and controls.[560] At this time, most authorities agree that hGH treatment is not a causative agent in the development of leukemia in individuals without a predisposing condition. The authors recommend that this issue be discussed with all potential recipients of hGH.

Recurrence of CNS Tumors and Occurence of Second Malignancies

Because many recipients of hGH have acquired GHD from CNS tumors or their treatment, the possibility of tumor recurrence is of obvious importance. Extensive analysis of the data on 1,300 American children treated for a CNS malignancy before receiving hGH has not indicated any increased risk. A similar conclusion has emerged from analysis of a European database. However, one study suggests that GH recipients who had a brain tumor have a slightly higher risk of a second malignancy.[561]

Pseudotumor Cerebri

Pseudotumor cerebri (idiopathic intracranial hypertension) has been reported in at least 26 hGH-treated patients, approximately half of whom had classic GHD.[562] The mechanism of hGH action is unclear, but it may reflect changes in fluid dynamics within the CNS. Pseudotumor has also been described after thyroid hormone replacement and may represent restoration of a normal physiologic state. In any case, physicians need to be alert to complaints of headache, nausea, dizziness, ataxia, and visual changes.

Slipped Capital Femoral Epiphysis

The potential association of slipped capital femoral epiphysis (SCFE) and GHD was first suggested by studies in rats.[563] It is clear that SCFE can be associated with hypothyroidism and GHD.[564,565] The potential role of hGH therapy has been more difficult to determine. This is in part because the incidence of SCFE in the normal population varies by age, sex, race, and geographic locale—being variously reported as between 2 and 142 cases per 100,000. Accordingly, although SCFE cannot at this time be definitively attributed to hGH therapy per se complaints of hip and knee pain and/or displaying a limp should receive appropriate evaluation.

Miscellaneous Side Effects

A number of other physical concerns have been raised as possible consequences of hGH treatment. Current data are inadequate to ascribe a causal role to hGH treatment. The potential side effects include prepubertal gynecomastia, increased growth of nevi, behavior changes, scoliosis and kyphosis, worsening of neurofibromatosis, hypertrophy of tonsils and adenoids, and sleep apnea. This list is obviously only partial. It is best for the clinician to remember that GH and the peptide growth factors it stimulates are potent mitogens with diverse metabolic and anabolic actions. All patients receiving hGH treatment, even as replacement therapy, must be carefully monitored for side effects.

For the most part, the side effects of GH are minimal and rare. When they occur, careful history and physical examination are adequate to identify their presence. Management of these side effects may include transient reduction of dosage or temporary discontinuation of GH.[566] The association of GH treatment with insulin resistance is well documented,[567] and one report suggested that there is an increased incidence of development of diabetes in pediatric recipients of GH.[568] Most authorities agree, however, that rather than a side effect of GH this relationship probably represents a common susceptibility of patients to develop growth disorders and diabetes owing to a common genetic trait.[569]

In the absence of other risk factors, there is no evidence that the risk of leukemia, brain tumor recurrence, SCFE, and diabetes is increased in recipients of long-term GH treatment. In any case, any patient receiving GH who has a second major medical condition (such as a tumor survivor receiving GH) should be followed in conjunction with a specialist such as an oncologist or a neurosurgeon when appropriate. Although GH has been shown to increase the mortality of critically ill patients in the intensive care unit,[116] there is no evidence that GH replacement needs to be discontinued during intercurrent illness in children with GHD.

THE QUESTION OF LONG-TERM CANCER RISK

Several epidemiologic studies have been published suggesting an association between high serum IGF-1 levels and the incidence of malignancies.[570,571] In addition, the risk of cancer calculated in those studies was increased for patients with low IGFBP-3 levels. Although additional studies are being conducted to verify or disprove the association between serum IGF-1 and cancer risk, the role of GH in this potential phenomenon should be carefully examined.

In a paper analyzing the risk of colon cancer, it was shown that IGF-1 was not statistically associated with cancer risk. However, the combination of high IGF-1 and low IGFBP-3 was shown to be related to an increased risk (Table 8-14).[572] Notably, GH positively influences both parameters in parallel. This casts doubt on its role as a driving force in the IGF-cancer equation.

Additional epidemiologic data of note involve the risk of malignancy associated with acromegaly. A number of studies have been published that claimed to identify an association between acromegaly and colon cancer risk,[573-575] whereas others did not find significant associations.[576,577] The interpretation of these studies is hampered by their small size, uncontrolled retrospective nature, and multiple possible sources of bias. The largest study to date, reviewing more than a thousand patients, indicated that overall cancer incidence is not increased in acromegaly.[578] The overall incidence of colon cancer was also not shown to be increased in Orme and associates' study, although mortality from colon cancer was higher in this population—suggesting perhaps an effect of GH or IGF-1 on established tumors.[579]

One prospective analysis of colon cancer and colonic polyps in acromegalics using controlled colonoscopies did not observe an association between these two diseases when using autopsy series or prospective colonoscopy screening series for the control population.[580] It is notable that acromegaly is associated with a dramatic increase in the incidence of benign hyperplasia of several organs, including colonic polyps.[581] These findings raise the possibility that the GH-IGF axis may lead to symptomatic benign proliferative disease, which could be associated with symptoms (such as rectal bleeding) that would then lead to a potential detection (or ascertainment) bias.

Children receiving GH have not been shown to have an increased risk of de novo tumors. An earlier concern that leukemia risk was increased has been dispelled by the same authors who first published on this topic, showing in a large cohort that the risk for leukemia is the same for GH recipients and controls.[582] Several studies indicate absolutely no increase in the risk of tumor recurrence in pediatric GH recipients.[583]

In a number of studies, no increased incidence of cancer was found in GH recipients among adults treated for GHD.[584,585] Clearly, these reports represent imperfect uncontrolled studies. However, the experience gained through them demonstrates that even though the IGF-1 levels are normalized GH therapy is not associated with tumor recurrence or with de novo tumors in the absence of other risk factors. The use of IGF-1 and IGFBP-3 in the monitoring of GH recipients, adult and pediatric, has been recommended and endorsed by international bodies such as the GH Research Society.[533]

Until the issue of cancer risk in GH therapy is fully resolved, the most prudent approach appears to be regular monitoring of IGF-1 and IGFBP-3 and modulation of the GH dose to ensure that the theoretical risk profile induced by GH therapy is favorable. This can be done by avoiding the unlikely situation in which a GH-treated patient will have an IGF-1 level at the upper end and IGFBP-3 levels at the lower end. In the twenty-first century, many patients with GHD will receive lifetime GH replacement. In that setting, it is especially important that we monitor serum IGF-1 and IGFBP-3 on a regular basis.

Overall, many controversies still surround the issue of the GH-IGF axis and cancer risk, specifically concerning the safety of GH therapy. In general, the currently approved indications for GH therapy in children and adults do not warrant concern regarding future cancer risk. Although additional research coupled with stringent pharmacovigilance is clearly warranted, the state of the clinical field mandates that patients' physicians be aware of the vast body of evidence regarding the safety of GH in this regard.[586]

TREATMENT OF PRIMARY SEVERE IGFD: USE OF IGF-1

The production of IGF peptides by recombinant DNA technology has permitted clinical trials of IGF therapy. IGF-I administration to normal adult male volunteers as a single intravenous injection of 100 µg/kg caused hypoglycemia within 15 minutes. On a molar basis, IGF-I has approximately 6% of the hypoglycemic potency of insulin. In contrast, intravenous infusions of IGF-I to normal men at a rate of 20 µg/kg/hour resulted in serum IGF-I levels within the normal range and did not produce hypoglycemia—but did

TABLE 8-14

Risk of Future Cancer Relative to Serum IGF-I and IGFBP-3 Tertiles

	IGF-I Lowest Tertile	IGF-I Middle Tertile	IGF-I Upper Tertile
IGFBP-3 upper tertile	—	—	—
IGFBP-3 middle tertile	—	—	—
IGFBP-3 lowest tertile	—	—	Fourfold increased risk

IGF, insulin-like growth factor; IGFBF-3, insulin-like growth factor-binding protein-3.

suppress GH levels, increase creatinine clearance, and decrease plasma urea nitrogen.[77, 587-595]

The most obvious clinical use of IGF-I therapy is in patients with GHI. A number of short-term growth-related studies with IGF-I treatment at varied doses have been reported. Data from 17 patients in a European collaborative trial, treated for at least 4 years, showed an increase in mean height SDS from –6.5 to –4.9—with two adolescents reaching the 3rd percentile. This emphasizes the importance of early diagnosis and initiation of therapy. Side effects included hypoglycemia, headache, convulsions, urolithiasis, and papilledema. The latter, which suggests the possibility of pseudotumor cerebri, resolved spontaneously while receiving IGF-I.

In the longest treatment study, Chernausek and colleagues[589] showed data similar to the European study—with an initial burst of growth followed by slowing to just above baseline by the sixth year of therapy. Height SDS improved from –5.6 to –4.2 by the end of the sixth year (Figure 8-30). A randomized double-blind placebo-controlled trial of IGF-I therapy in GHRD has been performed in Ecuador, probably the only place where the patient population is sufficiently large and homogeneous to permit such investigation.[589] Growth rates in subjects receiving IGF-I increased from 2.9 to 8.6 cm/year over the first year of therapy. The placebo group grew 4.4 cm/year during the same time, and then their growth rate increased to 8.4 cm/year during IGF-I treatment. Incidence of hypoglycemia was equal in the two groups. One recipient of IGF-I developed papilledema, which resolved spontaneously while on treatment.

Although these early studies are promising, little is known about the long-term effects of IGF-I or about the optimal dose or frequency of administration. When all clinical studies are combined, the total number of children treated to date is still only several hundred—and relatively few have been treated for greater than 5 years. Taken together, the IGF-I treatment studies show that although significant the growth response is neither as successful nor as long-lived as that of GHD children treated with exogenous GH. The failure of serum levels of IGFBP-3 to increase with IGF-I administration and the

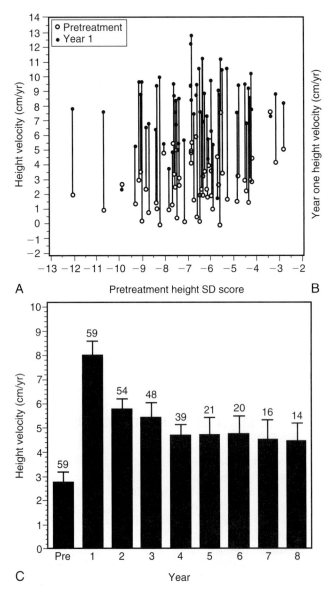

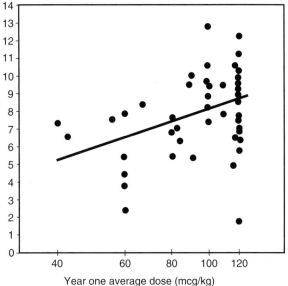

Figure 8-30 Linear growth in response to rhIGF-I treatment. (*A*) Height velocity (centimeters per year) before (open circle) and during first year of therapy (closed circles) for each child is displayed relative to pretreatment height. (*B*) The dose dependency of first-year growth rate is shown. Each point represents a single subject. The equation for the regression line shown is *Height velocity (centimeters per year) = –6.2 + 7.2 log10 rhIGF-I dose (microgram per kilogram, BID)*. (*C*) Average growth rates before and during rhIGF-I for first and subsequent years are shown. Error bar shows upper limit of 95% confidence interval. Number of subjects at each year is indicated. [From Chernausek SD, Backeljauw PF, Frane J, Kuntze J, Underwood LE for the GH Insensitivity Syndrome Collaborative Group (2007). Long-term treatment with recombinant insulin-like growth factor (IGF)-I in children with severe IGF-I deficiency due to growth hormone insensitivity. J Clin Endocrinol Metab 92(3):902–910.]

suppression of endogenous GH secretion underscores the complexity of the treatment. The possibility that local production of IGF-I at the growth plate may be critical to optimal growth also requires consideration. Nevertheless, these data indicate that the IGF peptides (long considered to function as autocrine or paracrine growth factors) can act as classic endocrine hormones.

IGF-I has received FDA approval recently. The drug shows promise in treatment of severe primary IGFD. The use of IGF-I in milder forms of primary IGFD is also the subject of current investigations. Vaccarello and co-workers[78] treated six adults with GHRD for 7 days with subcutaneous IGF-1 at a dosage of 40 mg/kg every 12 hours. Normal serum IGF-1 concentrations were achieved 2 to 6 hours post-injection, followed by a rapid decline—reflecting low serum concentrations of IGFBP-3. No symptomatic hypoglycemia was observed, but mean 24-hour GH levels were significantly suppressed and urinary calcium level was increased. In longer-term studies, Laron and co-workers[590] reported significant growth acceleration—to rates of 8.8 to 13.6 cm/year in five children treated for 3 to 10 months with a single daily injection of 150 mg/kg.

Walker and associates[591] reported an increase in growth rate from 6.5 to 11.4 cm/year in a patient with GHRD treated with twice-daily subcutaneous injections of 120 mg/kg. Wilton and co-workers[592] have reported preliminary data in 30 children, aged 3 to 23 years, with GHI from GHRD or GHD-IA with anti-GH antibodies. The dosage of IGF-1 varied from 40 to 120 mg/kg twice daily. With the exception of the two oldest patients, all subjects increased their growth rates by at least 2 cm/year. These results have been updated and indicate a continued good response by most subjects.[593] Observed side effects included hypoglycemia, headache, convulsions, possible urolithiasis, and papilledema—the last indicating the possibility of pseudotumor cerebri, as has been reported with GH therapy.

A randomized double-blind placebo-controlled trial of IGF-1 therapy in GHRD has been performed in Ecuador, probably the only place where the population is sufficiently large and homogeneous to permit such investigation.[594] Subjects receiving IGF-1 showed a significant increase in growth rate (from 2.9 to 8.6 cm/year), which was sustained over the 1-year course of therapy. The placebo group grew 4.4 cm/year during the placebo phase and increased their height velocity to 8.4 cm/year during the IGF-1 phase. Incidents of hypoglycemia were equal in the two experimental groups. One recipient of IGF-1 developed papilledema, which resolved spontaneously while on treatment.

Longer-term studies of IGF-1 treatment of GHI have indicated a persistent, although progressively waning, effect (Figure 8-30).[595] Data from 17 patients treated for at least 4 years showed a total height gain of 1.7 SD score and emphasize the importance of early initiation of therapy.

As promising as these early studies are, IGF-I therapy is still under active investigation and the exact clinical scenarios in which this therapy is appropriate is still evolving. The failure of serum levels of IGFBP-3 to rise with IGF-1 administration underscores the relevance of the IGFBPs to IGF pharmacokinetics.[78,594] Nevertheless, the early results indicate that the IGF peptides (long considered to function

primarily as autocrine or paracrine growth factors) are capable of acting as classic endocrine hormones.

Excess Growth and Tall Stature

TALL STATURE AND OVERGROWTH SYNDROMES

Although on a statistical basis as many children have heights more than <2 SD as have heights more than 2 SD, referral for evaluation of tall stature is much less common than that for short stature. This referral pattern speaks eloquently to the psychosocial pressure involved in referral patterns of children with "growth disorders." Nevertheless, it is critical to be able to identify situations in which tall stature or an accelerated growth rate provides a clue to an underlying disorder. Table 8-15 provides a listing of causes of statural overgrowth in infancy and during childhood.

OVERGROWTH IN THE FETUS

Maternal diabetes constitutes the most common cause of overgrowth in infants who are large for gestational age. Even in the absence of clinical symptoms or a family

---

TABLE 8-15

Differential Diagnosis of Statural Overgrowth

Fetal Overgrowth
Maternal diabetes mellitus
Cerebral gigantism (Sotos syndrome)
Weaver syndrome
Beckwith-Wiedemann syndrome
Other IGF-2 excess syndromes

Postnatal Overgrowth Leading to Childhood Tall Stature
Familial (constitutional) tall stature
Cerebral gigantism
Beckwith-Wiedemann syndrome
Exogenous obesity
Excess GH secretion (pituitary gigantism)
McCune-Albright syndrome or multiple endocrine neoplasia associated with excess GH secretion
Precocious puberty
Marfan syndrome
Klinefelter syndrome (XXY)
Weaver syndrome
Fragile X syndrome
Homocystinuria
XYY
Hyperthyroidism

Postnatal Overgrowth Leading to Adult Tall Stature
Familia (constitutional) tall stature
Androgen or estrogen deficiency/estrogen resistance (in males)
Testicular feminization
Excess GH secretion
Marfan syndrome
Klinefelter syndrome (XXY)
XYY

GH, growth hormone; IGF, insulin-like growth factor.

history, the birth of an excessively large infant should lead to evaluation for maternal (or gestational) diabetes. A group of disorders associated with excessive somatic growth and growth of specific organs has been described and collectively referred to as overgrowth syndromes.[596] These disorders appear to be caused by excess availability of the IGF-2 encoded by the gene Igf2. The best described of these syndromes is the Beckwith-Wiedemann syndrome, which is an overgrowth malformation syndrome that occurs with an incidence of 1:13,700 births.

It is manifested as a fetal overgrowth syndrome in which hypertrophy dominates the clinical picture. Typically, macroglossia, omphalocele, hepatosplenomegaly, nephromegaly, and hypoglycemia secondary to pancreatic beta cell hyperplasia in an infant who is large for gestational age comprise the clinical picture at birth. An additional complication is that these children are predisposed to a specific subset of childhood neoplasms, among which are Wilms' tumor and adrenocortical carcinoma.

Overexpression of IGF-2 in Beckwith-Wiedemann syndrome may be caused by a number of genetic disruptions, including gene duplication, loss of heterozygosity, and relaxation or loss of imprinting of the Igf2 gene. Various lines of investigation have localized "imprinted" genes involved in Beckwith-Wiedemann syndrome and associated childhood tumors to chromosome 11p. These include (in addition to Igf2) the gene H19, which is involved in Igf2 suppression—as well as the gene WT1 (the Wilms' tumor gene). Mutations in GPC3, a glypican gene that codes for an IGF-2 neutralizing membrane receptor, cause the related Simpson-Golabi-Behmel overgrowth syndrome.[597]

Children with cerebral gigantism (also known as Sotos syndrome) are typically above the 90th percentile for both length and weight at birth, and macrocrania may also be noted at that time.[598] Mutations and deletions of the NSD1 gene (located at chromosome 5q35 and coding for a histone methyltransferase implicated in transcriptional regulation) are responsible for more than 75% of cases. FISH analysis, MLPA, or multiplex quantitative PCR allow the detection of total/partial NSD1 deletions—and direct sequencing allows detection of NSD1 mutations. The large majority of NSD1 abnormalities occur de novo, and there are very few familial cases.

Although most cases are sporadic, several reports of autosomal-dominant inheritance have been described.[598] Growth is rapid, and by 1 year of age affected infants are over the 97th percentile in height. Accelerated growth continues for the first 4 to 5 years and then returns to a normal rate. Puberty usually occurs at the normal time, but may occur slightly early. Adult height is usually in the upper normal range. The hands and feet are large, with thickened subcutaneous tissue. The head is large and dolichocephalic, the jaw is prominent, there is hypertelorism, and the eyes have an antimongoloid slant. Clumsiness and awkward gait are characteristic, and affected children have great difficulty in sports, in learning to ride a bicycle, and in other tasks requiring coordination.

Some degree of mental retardation affects most patients. In some children, perceptual deficiencies may predominate. Osseous maturation is compatible with the patient's height. Results of tests of GH and IGF-1 levels and of other endocrine studies are usually normal. There are no distinctive laboratory or radiologic markers for the syndrome. Abnormal electroencephalograms are common. Imaging studies frequently reveal a dilated ventricular system. Most cases are sporadic. Familial cases are usually consistent with autosomal-dominant inheritance and occasionally with autosomal-recessive inheritance. Affected patients may be at increased risk for neoplasia, particularly hepatic carcinoma—and Wilms', ovarian, and parotid tumors have been reported.

TALL STATURE AND POSTNATAL STATURAL OVERGROWTH

The normal distribution of height predicts that 2.5% of the population will be taller than 2 SD above the mean. The social acceptability and even desirability of tallness ("heightism") makes tall stature an uncommon complaint, however. In North America, it is extremely unusual for males to seek help regarding excessive height—although in Europe it is somewhat more common. Even in females, tall stature has become more socially acceptable—although tall girls may still approach their physician with a desire to curb their growth rate.

DIFFERENTIAL DIAGNOSIS OF TALL STATURE

Table 8-15 lists the causes of tall stature in childhood and adolescence. Of these, the normal variant familial or constitutional tall stature is by far the most common cause. Almost invariably, a family history of tallness can be elicited—and no pathologic process is present. The child is often tall throughout childhood and enjoys excellent health. The parent of the constitutionally tall adolescent may reflect unhappily on his or her own adolescence as a tall teenager. There are typically no abnormalities in the physical examination, and the laboratory studies (if obtained) are always negative.

As was described for the child with growth failure, crossing height percentiles between infancy and the onset of puberty always warrants further evaluation. Although such growth patterns frequently are of no concern to parents, an alert pediatrician will recognize that overly rapid statural growth can indicate a serious underlying problem. Furthermore, as with short stature children with tall stature must be evaluated in the context of their familial growth and pubertal patterns.

Klinefelter syndrome (XXY syndrome) is a relatively common (1:500 to 1:1,000 live male births) abnormality associated with tall stature, mild mental retardation, gynecomastia, and decreased upper to lower body segment ratio. The testes are invariably small, although androgen production by Leydig cells is often at the low normal range. Spermatogenesis and Sertoli cell function are defective, resulting in infertility. XYY syndrome is associated with tall stature and possible behavioral and mental problems.

Marfan syndrome is an autosomal-dominant connective tissue disorder consisting of tall stature, increased arm span, and decreased upper to lower body segment ratio. Additional abnormalities include arachnodactyly, ocular abnormalities, and cardiac anomalies. Homocystinuria is an autosomal-recessive inborn error of amino acid metabolism causing mental retardation when untreated. It has many features resembling Marfan syndrome, particularly ocular manifestations. Hyperthyroidism in adolescence is associated with rapid growth but normal adult height. It is almost always caused by Grave's disease and is much more common in females.

Exogenous obesity is a common condition in childhood and adolescence and may be associated with rapid linear growth and early maturation. This association is so characteristic that the child with obesity and short stature should always be evaluated for an underlying pathologic process such as hypothyroidism, GHD, Cushing syndrome, and various syndromes (such as Prader-Willi). In exogenous obesity, bone age is usually modestly accelerated—and thus puberty and epiphyseal fusion occur early, resulting in normal adult height. As stated, cerebral gigantism and Beckwith-Wiedemann syndrome are associated with rapid perinatal growth but rapid postnatal growth usually ends by early to mid childhood. Nevertheless, these conditions should be considered when tall stature in childhood is accompanied by the characteristic phenotypic features, a history of unexplained fetal overgrowth, or the presence of the childhood tumors mentioned previously.

PRECOCIOUS AND DELAYED PUBERTY

Precocious puberty, whether mediated centrally (increased gonadotropin secretion) or peripherally (increased secretion of androgens, estrogens, or both), results in accelerated linear growth in childhood—mimicking the pubertal growth spurt. Because skeletal maturation is also accelerated, adult height is frequently compromised. The diagnostic evaluation and management of precocious puberty are discussed in Chapters 14 and 16.

Although delayed puberty may be associated with short stature in childhood, as with constitutional delay failure to eventually enter puberty and complete sexual maturation may result in sustained growth during adult life—with ultimate tall stature. The reports of tall stature in men with open epiphyses, resulting from mutations of the estrogen receptor or of the aromatase gene, underscores the fundamental role of estrogen in promoting epiphyseal fusion and termination of normal skeletal growth.[15,263]

DIAGNOSING FAMILIAL TALL STATURE

The purpose of the diagnostic evaluation of tall stature is to distinguish the commonly occurring normal variant constitutional (or familial) variety from the rare pathologic conditions. Often, when the history is suggestive of familial tall stature and the physical examination is entirely normal, no laboratory tests are indicated. It is valuable to obtain a bone age radiograph to be able to predict adult height, which serves as a basis for discussions with the family and for management decisions. If, however, the history is suggestive for any of the previously mentioned disorders or the physical examination reveals

abnormalities additional laboratory tests should be obtained to evaluate for brain disorders, GH excess, chromosomal abnormalities, or other rare causes of tallness.

IGF-1 and IGFBP-3 are excellent screening tests for GH excess and can be verified with a glucose suppression test. Laboratory evidence of GH excess mandates MRI evaluation of the pituitary. Chromosome analysis is useful in males, especially when the upper to lower body segment ratio is decreased or when mental retardation is present. If Marfan syndrome or homocystinuria is suspected from the physical examination, referral to a cardiologist and an ophthalmologist should be made. Thyroid function tests are useful to diagnose or rule out hyperthyroidism when this disorder is suspected.

MANAGEMENT OF CONSTITUTIONAL AND SYNDROMIC TALL STATURE

Reassurance of the family and the patients is the key to the management of normal variant tall stature. The use of the bone age evaluation and a careful assessment of pubertal status to predict adult height may provide some comfort for them, as will general supportive discussions on the social acceptability of this condition. Although treatment is available for girls and boys with excessive growth, its use should be restricted to patients with predicted adult height greater than 3 SD above the mean (198 cm in males or 180 cm in females) and evidence of significant psychosocial impairment.

For the child with extreme familial tall stature (or another condition, such as Marfan syndrome) whose parents feel strongly about treatment, a trial of sex steroids is possible. Such therapy is designed to accelerate puberty and epiphyseal fusion, and is therefore of little benefit when given in late puberty. Therapy is initiated ideally prepubertally or in early puberty. Oral estrogens in various doses have successfully reduced the predicted height of females by 5 to 10 cm on the average.[599]

This is a direct result of the known effects of sex steroids on promoting epiphyseal fusion, and therapy must therefore begin before the bone age has reached 12 years. Oral ethinyl estradiol at a dose of 0.15 to 0.5 mg/day until cessation of growth occurs has been used successfully in girls. If necessary, a progestational agent can be added after 1 year of unopposed estrogen. In boys, treatment should begin before the bone age reaches 14 years. Testosterone enanthate is used at a dose of 500 mg intramuscularly every 2 weeks for 6 months. Whereas no long-term complications of sex steroid therapy have been clearly documented, short-term side effects are common. These include lipid abnormalities, thromboembolism, cholelithiasis, hypertension, nausea, menstrual irregularities, and acne fulminans. The lack of extensive experience with this form of therapy and the risks involved should be carefully weighed and discussed with the family before embarking on therapy.

The mechanism of estrogen action affects both GH and IGF production. Perhaps more important, however, is the action of estrogen on the epiphysis. Studies have demonstrated that it is estrogen that mediates epiphyseal fusion in both females and males. In prepubertal girls, adult height is reportedly decreased by as much as 5 to

6 cm relative to pretreatment predictions. When therapy is initiated after the onset of puberty, the decrement in adult height is not likely to be as large. Therapy in boys with tall stature is even more problematic. For the reasons discussed, estrogen is likely to be most efficacious in accelerating epiphyseal fusion but is obviously undesirable in males. Androgens will also accelerate skeletal maturation, presumably through aromatization to estrogen, but at the price of rapid virilization.

EXCESS GH SECRETION AND PITUITARY GIGANTISM

In young persons with open epiphyses, overproduction of GH results in gigantism. In persons with closed epiphyses, the result is acromegaly. Often, some acromegalic features are seen with gigantism—even in children and adolescents. After closure of the epiphyses, the acromegalic features become more prominent. Famous examples of gigantism include Robert Wadlow (the Alton giant), who stood 271.8 cm at the time of his death in his mid 20s. The well-known Andre Rousimoff (Andre the Giant) was 190.5 cm at age 12 and reached a height of 223.5 cm by adulthood.[600] Pituitary gigantism is rare, and its cause is most often a pituitary adenoma—but gigantism has been observed in a 2.5-year-old boy with a hypothalamic tumor that presumably secreted GHRH. Other tumors, particularly in the pancreas, have produced acromegaly by secretion of large amounts of GHRH with resultant hyperplasia of the somatotrophs.[601]

The cardinal clinical feature of gigantism is longitudinal growth acceleration secondary to the GH excess. The usual manifestations consist of coarse facial features and enlarging hands and feet. In young children, rapid growth of the head may precede linear growth. Some patients have behavioral and visual problems. In most of the recorded cases, the abnormal growth became evident at puberty—but the condition has been established as early as the newborn period in 1 child and at 21 months of age in another. Giants may grow to a height of 243.8 cm or more. Acromegalic features consist chiefly of enlargement of the distal parts of the body, but manifestations of abnormal growth involve all portions.

The circumference of the skull increases, the nose becomes broad, and the tongue is often enlarged—with coarsening of the facial features. The mandible grows excessively, and the teeth become separated. Visual field defects and neurologic abnormalities are common. Signs of increased intracranial pressure appear later. The fingers and toes grow chiefly in thickness. There may be dorsal kyphosis. Fatigue and lassitude are early symptoms. GH levels are elevated and may occasionally exceed 100 ng/mL. There is typically no suppression of GH levels by the hyperglycemia of a glucose tolerance test. IGF-1 and IGFBP-3 levels are consistently elevated in gigantism, whereas other growth factors are not. Gigantism is extremely rare, with only several hundred reported cases. The presentation of gigantism is usually dramatic, unlike the insidious onset of acromegaly in adults.

The tumor mass itself may cause headaches, visual changes from optic nerve compression, and hypopituitarism. About half of the patients also have marked hyperprolactinemia as a result of plurihormonal adenomas that secrete GH and prolactin. This is because mammosomatotrophs are the most common type of GH-secreting cells involved in childhood gigantism. GH-secreting tumors of the pituitary are typically eosinophilic or chromophobe adenomas. Adenomas may compromise other anterior pituitary function through growth or cystic degeneration. Secretion of gonadotropins, thyrotropin, or corticotropin may be impaired. Delayed sexual maturation or hypogonadism may occur. When GH hypersecretion is accompanied by gonadotropin deficiency, accelerated linear growth may persist for decades. In some cases, the tumor spreads outside the sella—invading the sphenoid bone, optic nerves, and brain. GH-secreting tumors in pediatric patients are more likely to be locally invasive or aggressive than are those in adult patients.[602]

The cause of these tumors is uncertain, although recent studies of acromegalics have suggested that many cases result from mutations that generate constitutively activated G proteins with reduced GTPase activity. The resultant rise in intracellular cyclic AMP in the pituitary leads to increased GH secretion. McCune-Albright syndrome, which can also be caused by mutations resulting in constitutively activated G proteins, may also include the presence of somatotrophic tumors and excess GH secretion. In fact, approximately 20% of patients with gigantism are those with McCune-Albright syndrome (commonly consisting of a triad of precocious puberty, café-au-lait spots, and fibrous dysplasia). GH-secreting tumors have also been reported in multiple endocrine adenomatosis and in association with neurofibromatosis, tuberous sclerosis, and Carney complex.[603,604]

Activating mutations of the stimulatory Gsa protein have been found in the pituitary lesions in McCune-Albright syndrome and are believed to be responsible for the other glandular adenomas observed in this condition as well. Somatic point mutations of the Gsa protein have also been identified in somatotrophs of up to 40% of sporadic GH-secreting pituitary adenomas.

DIAGNOSIS OF GH EXCESS

The "gold standard" for making the diagnosis of GH excess is a failure to suppress serum GH levels to less than 5 ng/dL after a 1.75-g/kg oral glucose challenge (maximum, 75 g). This test measures the ability of IGF-1 to suppress GH secretion because the glucose load results in insulin secretion, leading to suppression of IGFBP-1, which results in an acute increase in free IGF-1 levels. The increased free IGF-1 suppresses GH secretion within 30 to 90 minutes.[605] This test can be abnormal in diabetic patients. Note that a single measurement of GH is inadequate because GH is secreted in a pulsatile manner. Therefore, the use of a random GH measurement can lead to both false-positive and false-negative results.

Measurement of serum IGF-1 concentration is a sensitive screening test for GH excess. An excellent linear dose-response correlation between serum IGF-1 levels and 24-hour mean GH secretion has been demonstrated. An elevated IGF-1 level in a patient with appropriate clinical suspicion is almost always indicative of GH excess. Potential confusion may arise when evaluating normal adolescents because significantly higher IGF-1 levels occur during puberty than in adulthood.

For accurate control comparison, the IGF-1 level must be age and gender matched. Serum IGFBP-3 levels may also be useful in the diagnosis of GH excess. In patients with confirmed somatotroph adenomas, increased IGFBP-3 levels have been reported to be a sensitive marker of GH elevations and may be elevated despite normal IGF-1 levels. If laboratory findings suggest GH excess, the presence of a pituitary adenoma should be confirmed using MRI. In rare cases, a pituitary mass may not be identified. This may be an occult pituitary microadenoma or an ectopic tumor. Computed tomography is acceptable when MRI is unavailable.

TREATMENT OF GH OVERSECRETION

The goals of therapy are to remove or shrink the pituitary mass, to restore GH and secretory patterns to normal, to restore IGF-1 and IGFBP-3 levels to normal, to retain the normal pituitary secretion of other hormones, and to prevent recurrence of disease. For well-circumscribed pituitary adenomas, transsphenoidal surgery is the treatment of choice and may be curative.[606] The tumor should be removed completely. The likelihood of surgical cure depends greatly on the surgeon's expertise as well as on the size and extension of the mass. Intraoperative GH measurements can improve the results of tumor resection. Transsphenoidal surgery to resect the tumors has been shown to be as safe in children as in adults. At times, a transcranial approach may be necessary. The primary goal of treatment is to normalize GH levels. GH levels (<1 ng/mL within 2 hours after a glucose load) and serum IGF-1 levels (age-adjusted normal range) are the best tests to define a biochemical cure.

If GH secretion is not normalized by surgery, the options include pituitary radiation and medical therapy. In general, radiation therapy is recommended if GH hypersecretion is not normalized by surgery. Further growth of the tumor is prevented by radiation in more than 99% of the patients. The main disadvantage is the delayed efficacy in decreasing GH levels. GH is reduced approximately 50% from the initial concentration by 2 years and 75% by 5 years, and approaches 90% by 15 years. Hypopituitarism is a predictable outcome, occurring in 40 to 50% of patients 10 years after irradiation.

It is now clear that surgery fails to cure a significant number of patients and therefore medical therapy has taken on a more important role in the management of patients with GH excess. Indeed, the greatest progress in recent years in the treatment of GH excess has been within the realm of medical therapy. Treatment has been improved by the availability of effective and well-tolerated long-acting somatostatin analogues and dopamine agonists, as well as by novel GH antagonists.

The somatostatin analogues have been found to be highly effective in the treatment of patients with GH excess. Octreotide suppresses GH to less than 2.5 ng/mL in 65% of patients with acromegaly, and normalizes IGF-1 levels in 70%. Studies of patients for more than 14 years have shown that the effects of octreotide are well sustained over time. Tumor shrinkage also occurs with octreotide, but it is generally modest. Consistent GH suppression has been obtained with a continuous subcutaneous pump infusion of octreotide in a pubertal boy with pituitary gigantism.[607] New long-acting formulations, including octreotide and lanreotide, have been shown to produce consistent GH and IGF-1 suppression in acromegalics with once-monthly or biweekly intramuscular depot injections. The sustained-release preparations have not been formally tested in children. Octreotide injection in the pediatric population has been used at doses of 1 to 40 mg/kg/day.

Dopamine agonists, such as bromocriptine, bind to pituitary dopamine type 2 (D2) receptors and suppress GH secretion—although the precise mechanism of action remains unclear. Prolactin levels are often adequately suppressed. However, GH levels and IGF-1 levels are rarely normalized with this treatment modality. Less than 20% of patients achieve GH levels less than 5 ng/mL, and less than 10% achieve normalization of IGF-1 levels. Tumor shrinkage occurs in a minority of patients. It is generally used as adjuvant medical treatment for GH excess. Its effectiveness may be additive to that of octreotide.[608]

Long-acting formulations are available. However, data on long-term control of GH and IGF-1 with these agents are not yet available. The dose of bromocriptine needed ranges between 10 and 60 mg orally divided four times a day. Only a minority of patients benefit from doses greater than 20 mg/day. It has been found to be safe when used in children for an extended period of time, but side effects may include nausea, vomiting, abdominal pain, arrhythmias, nasal stuffiness, orthostatic hypotension, sleep disturbances, and fatigue.

A novel GHR antagonist has been approved for use in acromegaly (Pegvisomant). It is an analogue of hGH that functions as a GHR antagonist. It has been shown to effectively suppress GH and IGF-1 levels in patients with acromegaly from pituitary tumors as well as ectopic GHRH hypersecretion.[609] Normalization of IGF-1 levels occurs in up to 90% of patients treated daily with this drug for 3 months or longer.[610] Long-term studies need to be performed. It has not been tested in children. The adult dose is 10 to 30 mg through subcutaneous once-daily injection.

Conclusions

The advancement in our understanding of the molecular mechanisms of growth has resulted in a dramatic enhancement of our ability to diagnose and treat growth disorders. Undoubtedly, in the coming years new and improved methods of identifying specific abnormalities leading to short stature (particularly in the form of genetic tests) will further refine the diagnostic process. In addition, the therapies available to treat growth disorders are also undergoing constant improvements and in the future will surely allow more efficacious, safer, and easier-to-tolerate management of growth abnormalities.

REFERENCES

1. Cameron N (1986). The methods of auxoogical anthropometry. In Falkner F, Tanner JM (eds.), *Human growth: A comprehensive treatise: Volume II, Postnatal growth, neurobiology, Second edition.* , New York: Plenum Press 35–90.

2. Tanner JM (1986). Normal growth and techniques of growth assessment. Clin Endocrinol Metab 15:411.

3. Underwood LE, Tanner JM (1992). Normal and aberrant growth. In Wilson JD, Foster DW (eds.), *Williams textbook of endocrinology, Eighth edition.* Philadelphia: WB Saunders 1079–1138.

4. Whitehouse RH, Tanner JM (1974). Diurnal variation in stature and sitting height in 12–14 year old boys. Ann Hum Biol 1:103.

5. Marshall WA (1971). Evaluation of growth rate in height over periods of less than one year. Arch Dis Child 46:414.

6. Hamill PVV, Drizd TA, Johnson CL, et al. (1979). Physical growth: National Center for Health Statistics percentiles. Am J Clin Nutr 32:607.

7. National Center for Health Statistics (1976). *NCHS Growth Charts, 1976. Monthly Vital Statistics Report.* Rockville, MD, Health Resources Administration, Vol. 25, No 3., Suppl (HRA) 76–1120, June 22.

8. National Center for Health Statistics (1977). *NCHS Growth Curves for Children 0–18 years: United States, Vital and Health Statistics.* Washington, D.C.: Health Resources Administration, U.S. Government Printing Office, Series 11, No. 165.

9. National Center for Health Statistics (2000). CDC Growth Charts. Washington, D.C.: Health Resources Administration, U.S. Government Printing Office.

10. Tanner JM, Davies SWD (1985). Clinical longitudinal standards for height and height velocity for North American children. J Pediatr 107:317.

11. Lyon AL, Preece MA, Grant DB (1985). Growth curve for girls with Turner syndrome. Arch Dis Child 60:932.

12. Horton WA, Rotter JI, Rimoin DL, et al. (1978). Standard growth curves for achondroplasia. J Pediatr 93:435.

13. Bayer LM, Bayley L (1959). *Growth diagnosis.* Chicago: University of Chicago Press 226–231.

14. Smith EP, Boyd J, Frank GR, et al. (1994). Estrogen resistance caused by a mutation in the estrogen-receptor gene in a man. N Engl J Med 331:1056.

15. Morishima A, Grumbach MM, Simpson ER, et al. (1995). Aromatase deficiency in male and female siblings caused by a novel mutation and the physiological role of estrogens. J Clin Endocrinol Metab 80:3689.

16. Greulich WW, Pyle SI (1959). *Radiographic atlas of skeletal development of the hand and wrist, Second edition.* Stanford, CA: Stanford University Press.

17. Tanner JM, Whitehouse RH, Marshall WA, et al. (1975). *Assessment of skeletal maturity and prediction of adult height: TW2 method.* New York: Academic Press.

18. Roche AF, Davila GH, Eyman SL (1971). A comparison between Greulich-Pyle and Tanner-Whitehouse assessments of skeletal maturity. Radiology 98:273.

19. Bayley N, Pinneau SR (1952). Tables for predicting adult height from skeletal age: Revised for use with the Greulich-Pyle hand standards. J Pediatr 40:423.

20. Tanner JM, Whitehouse RH, Marshall WA, et al. (1975). Prediction of adult height from height, bone age, and occurrence of menarche at ages 4–16 with allowance for midparent height. Arch Dis Child 50:14.

21. Roche AF, Wainer H, Thissen D (1975). The RWT method for the prediction of adult stature. Pediatrics 56:1026.

22. Asa SL, Kovacs K (2000). Functional morphology of the human fetal pituitary. Pathol Annu 19(I):275.

23. Ikeda H, Suzuki J, Sasano N, et al. (1988). The development and morphogenesis of the human pituitary gland. Anat Embryol (Berl) 178:327.

24. Goodyear CG (1989). Ontogeny of pituitary hormone secretion. In Collu R, Ducharme JR, Guyda HJ (eds.), *Pediatric endocrinology.* New York: Raven Press 125–169.

25. Stanfield JP (1960). The blood supply of the human pituitary gland. J Anat 94:257.

26. Gorcyzca W, Hardy J (1987). Arterial supply of the human anterior pituitary gland. Neurosurgery 20:369.

27. Treier M, Rosenfeld MG (1996). The hypothalamic-pituitary axis: Co-development of the two organs. Curr Opin Cell Biol 8:833.

28. Parks JS, Adess ME, Brown MR (1997). Genes regulating hypothalamic and pituitary development. Acta Paediatr Suppl 423:28.

29. Burrows HL, Douglas KR, Seasholtz AF, Camper SA (1999). Genealogy of the anterior pituitary gland: Tracing a family tree. Trends Endocrinol Metab 10:343.

30. Cohen LE (2000). Genetic regulation of the embryology of the pituitary gland and somatotrophs. Endocrine 12:99.

31. Lopez-Bermejo A, Buckway CK, Rosenfeld RG (2000). Genetic defects of the growth hormone-insulin-like growth factor axis. Trends Endocrinol Metab 11:39.

32. Ericson J, Norlin S, Jessell TM, Edlund T (1998). Integrated FGF and BMP signaling controls the progression of progenitor cell differentiation and the emergence of pattern in the embryonic anterior pituitary. Development 125:1005.

33. Thorner MO, Vance ML, Horvath E, et al. (1992). The anterior pituitary. In Wilson JD, Foster DW (eds.), *Williams textbook of endocrinology, Eighth edition.* Philadelphia: WB Saunders 221.

34. Scheithauer BW, Sano T, Kovacs K, et al. (1990). The pituitary gland in pregnancy: A clinicopathologic and immunohistochemical study of 69 cases. Mayo Clin Proc 65:461.

35. Boyd JD (1956). Observations on human pharyngeal hypophysis. J Endocrinol 14:66.

36. Underwood LE, Radcliffe WB, Guinto FC (1976). New standards for the assessment of sella turcica volume in children. Radiology 119:651.

37. Hoyt WF, Kaplan SL, Grumbach MM, et al. (1970). Septo-optic dysplasia and pituitary dwarfism. Lancet 1:893.

38. Lewis UJ, Singh RNP, Tutwiler GH, et al. (1980). Human growth hormone: A complex of proteins. Recent Prog Horm Res 36:477.

39. Baumann G (1988). Heterogeneity of growth hormone. In Bercu B (ed.), *Basic and clinical aspects of growth hormone.* New York: Plenum Press 13–31.

40. Frankenne F, Closset J, Gomez F, et al. (1988). The physiology of growth hormones (GHs) in pregnant women and partial characterization of the placental GH variant. J Clin Endocrinol Metab 66:1171.

41. Cook NE, Ray J, Watson MA, et al. (1988). Human growth hormone gene and the highly homologous growth hormone variant gene display different splicing patterns. J Clin Invest 82:270.

42. Miller WL, Eberhardt NL (1983). Structure and evaluation of the growth hormone gene family. Endocr Rev 4(2):97.

43. DeNoto FM, Moore DD, Goodman HM (1981). Human growth hormone DNA sequence and mRNA structure: Possible alternative splicing. Nucleic Acids Res 9:3719.

44. Barinaga M, Yamonoto G, Rivier C, et al. (1983). Transcriptional regulation of growth hormone gene expression by growth hormone-releasing factor. Nature 306:84.

45. Esch FS, Bohlen P, Ling NC, et al. (1983). Primary structure of three human pancreas peptides with growth hormone releasing activity. J Biol Chem 258:1806.

46. Holl RW, Thorner MO, Leong DA (1988). Intracellular calcium concentration and growth hormone secretion in individual somatotropes: Effects of growth hormone-releasing factor and somatostatin. Endocrinology 122:2927.

47. Mayo KE (1992). Molecular cloning and expression of a pituitary-specific receptor for growth hormone-releasing hormone. Mol Endocrinol 6:1734.

48. Hartman ML, Faria ACS, Vance ML, et al. (1991). Temporal sequence of in vivo growth hormone secretory events in man. Am J Physiol 260:E101.

49. Frohman LA (1980). Neurotransmitters as regulators of endocrine function. In Krieger DT, Hughes JC (eds.), *Neuroendocrinology.* Sunderland, MA: Sinauer Associates.

50. Melander T, Hokfelt T, Rokaeus A (1986). Distribution of galanin-like immunoreactivity in the rat central nervous system. J Comp Neurol 218:175.

51. Deller JJ, Plunket DC, Forsham PH (1966). Growth hormone studies in growth retardation: Therapeutic response to administration of androgen. Calif Med 104:359.

52. Zeitler P, Argente J, Chowen-Breede JA, et al. (1990). Growth hormone releasing hormone messenger ribonucleic acid in the hypothalamus of the adult male rat is increased by testosterone. Endocrinology 127:362.

53. Ho KY, Evans WS, Blizzard RM, et al. (1987). Effects of sex and age on the 24-hour profile of growth hormone secretion in man: Importance

of endogenous estradiol concentrations. J Clin Endocrinol Metab 64:51.

54. Katz HP, Youlton R, Kaplan SL, Grumbach MM (1969). Growth and growth hormone: III. Growth hormone release in children with primary hypothyroidism and thyrotoxicosis. J Clin Endocrinol Metab 29:346.

55. Fratz AG, Rabkin MT (1964). Human growth hormone: Clinical measurement, response to hypoglycemia and suppression by corticosteriods. N Engl J Med 271:1375.

56. Thompson RG, Rodriguez A, Kowarski A, Blizzard RM (1972). Growth hormone: Metabolic clearance rates, integrated concentrations, and production rates in normal adults and effect of prednisone. J Clin Invest 51:3193.

57. Martha PM Jr., Rogol AD, Veldhuis JD, et al. (1989). Alterations in the pulsatile properties of circulating growth hormone concentrations during puberty in boys. J Clin Endocrinol Metab 69:563.

58. Bowers CY, Momany F, Reynolds GA, et al. (1984). On the in vitro and in vivo activity of a new synthetic hexapeptide that acts on the pituitary to specifically release growth hormone. Endocrinology 114:1537.

59. Malozowski SS, Hao EH, Ren SG, et al. (1991). Growth hormone (GH) responses to hexapeptide GH-releasing peptide and GH-releasing hormone (GHRH) in the cynomolgus macaque: Evidence for non–GHRH-mediated responses. J Clin Endocrinol Metab 73:314.

60. Smith RG, Palyha OC, Feighner SD, et al. (1999). Growth hormone releasing substances: Types and their receptors. Horm Res 51(3):1.

61. Kojima M, Hosoda H, Date Y, et al. (1999). Ghrelin is a growth hormone–releasing acylated peptide from stomach. Nature 402:656.

62. Tschop M, Smiley DL, Heiman ML (2000). Ghrelin induces adiposity in rodents. Nature 407:908.

63. Hosoda H, Kojima M, Matsuo H, Kangawa K (2000). Purification and characterization of rat des-Gln14-ghrelin, a second endogenous ligand for the growth hormone secretagogue receptor. J Biol Chem 275:1995.

64. Pantel J, Legendre M, Cabrol S, Hilal L, Hajaji Y, Morisset S, et al. (2006). Loss of constitutive activity of the growth hormone secretagogue receptor in familial short stature. J Clin Invest 116(3):760–768.

65. Zhang JV, Ren PG, Avsian-Kretchmer O, Luo CW, Rauch R, Klein C, et al. (2005). Obestatin, a peptide encoded by the ghrelin gene, opposes ghrelin's effects on food intake. Science 310:996–999.

66. Yamamoto D, Ikeshita N, Daito R, Herningtyas EH, Toda K, Takahashi K, et al. (2007). Neither intravenous nor intracerebroventricular administration of obestatin affects the secretion of GH, PRL, TSH and ACTH in rats. Regul Pept 138:141–144.

67. Nelson C, Albert VR, Elsholtz HP, et al. (1988). Activation of cell-specific expression of rat growth hormone and prolactin genes by a common transcription factor. Science 239:1400.

68. Quentien MH, Barlier A, Franc JL, Pellegrini I, Brue T, Enjalbert A (2006). Pituitary transcription factors: From congenital deficiencies to gene therapy. J Neuroendocrinol 18(9):633–642.

69. Li S, Crenshaw III EB, Rawson EJ, et al. (1990). Dwarf locus mutants lacking three pituitary cell types result from mutations in the POU-domain gene pit-1. Nature 347:528.

70. Berelowitz M, Szabo M, Frohman LA, et al. (1981). Somatomedin-C mediates growth hormone negative feedback by effects on both the hypothalamus and pituitary. Science 212:1279.

71. Yamashita S, Melmed S (1986). Insulin-like growth factor I action on rat anterior pituitary cells: Suppression of growth hormone secretion and messenger ribonucleic acid levels. Endocrinology 118:176.

72. Abe H, Molitch M, Van Wyk JJ, et al. (1983). Human growth hormone and somatomedin-C suppress the spontaneous release of growth hormone in unanesthetized rats. Endocrinology 113:1319.

73. Rosenfeld RG, Ceda G, Cutler CW, et al. (1985). Insulin and insulin-like growth factor (somatomedin) receptors on cloned rat pituitary tumor cells. Endocrinology 117:2008.

74. Rosenfeld RG, Ceda G, Wilson DM, et al. (1984). Characterization of high-affinity receptors for insulin-like growth factors-I and -II on rat anterior pituitary cells. Endocrinology 114:1571.

75. Ceda GP, Hoffman AR, Silverberg GD, et al. (1985). Regulation of growth hormone release from cultured human pituitary adenomas by somatomedins and insulin. J Clin Endocrinol Metab 60:1204.

76. Ceda GP, Davis WT, Rosenfeld RG, et al. (1987). The growth hormone (GH) releasing hormone (GHRH)-GH-somatomedin axis: Evidence for rapid inhibition of GHRH-elicited GH release by insulin-like growth factors I and II. Endocrinology 120:1658.

77. Guler HP, Zapf J, Froesch ER (1987). Short-term metabolic effects and half-lives of intravenously administered insulin-like growth factor I in healthy adults. N Engl J Med 317:137.

78. Vaccarello MA, Diamond FB Jr., Guevara-Aguirre J, et al. (1993). Hormonal and metabolic effects and pharmacokinetics of recombinant insulin-like growth factor-I in growth hormone receptor deficiency (GHRD)/Laron syndrome. J Clin Endocrinol Metab 77:273.

79. Gluckman PD, Grumbach MM, Kaplan SL (1981). The neuroendocrine regulation and function of growth hormone and prolactin in the mammalian fetus. Endocr Rev 2:363.

80. Dudl RJ, Ensinck JW, Palmer HE, et al. (1973). Effect of age on growth hormone secretion in man. J Clin Endocrinol Metab 37:11.

81. Rudman D, Kutner MH, Rogers CM, et al. (1981). Impaired growth hormone secretion in the adult population: Relation to age and adiposity. J Clin Invest 67:1361.

82. Thompson RG, Rodriguez A, Kowarski A, Blizzard RM (1972). Growth hormone: Metabolic clearance rates, integrated concentrations, and production rates in normal adults and the effects of prednisone. J Clin Invest 51:3193.

83. MacGillivray MH, Frohman LA, Doe J (1970). Metabolic clearance and production rates of human growth hormone in subjects with normal and abnormal growth. J Clin Endocrinol Metab 30:632.

84. Sassin JF, Parker DC, Mace JW, et al. (1969). Human growth hormone release: Relation to slow-wave sleep and sleep-waking cycles. Science 165:513.

85. Van Cauter E, Kerkhofs M, Van Onderbergen A, et al. (1989). Modulation of spontaneous and GHRH-stimulated growth hormone secretion by sleep. Presented before the 71st annual meeting of the Endocrinology Society, Abstract 220.

86. Veldhuis JD, Carlson ML, Johnson ML (1987). The pituitary gland secretes in bursts: Appraising the nature of glandular secretory impulses by simultaneous multiple-parameter deconvolution of plasma hormone concentrations. Proc Natl Acad Sci USA 84:7686.

87. Schalch DS (1967). The influence of physical stress and exercise on growth hormone and insulin secretion in man. J Lab Clin Med 69:256.

88. Rosenfeld RG, Rosenbloom AL, Guevara-Aguirre J (1994). Growth hormone (GH) insensitivity due to primary GH receptor deficiency. Endocr Rev 15:369.

89. Veldhuis JD, Iranmanesh A, Ho KK, et al. (1991). Dual defects in pulsatile growth hormone secretion and clearance subserve the hyposomatotropism of obesity in man. J Clin Endocrinol Metab 72:519.

90. Leung DW, Spencer SA, Cachianes G, et al. (1987). Growth hormone receptor and serum binding protein: Purification, cloning and expression. Nature 330:537.

91. Trivedi B, Daughaday WH (1988). Release of growth hormone binding protein from IM-9 lymphocytes by endopeptidase is dependent on sulfhydryl group inactivation. Endocrinology 123:2201.

92. Smith WC, Linzer DH, Talamantes F (1988). Detection of two growth hormone receptor mRNAs and primary translation products in the mouse. Proc Natl Acad Sci USA 85:9576.

93. Smith WC, Kuniyoshi J, Talamantes F (1989). Mouse serum growth hormone (GH) binding protein has GH receptor extracellular and substituted transmembrane domains. Mol Endocrinol 3:984.

94. Sadeghi H, Wang BS, Lumunglas AL, et al. (1990). Identification of the origin of the growth hormone-binding protein in rat serum. Mol Endocrinol 4:1799.

95. Kelly PA, Djiane J, Postel-Vinay MC, et al. (1991). The prolactin/growth hormone receptor family. Endocr Rev 12:235.

96. Bougneres P, Goffin V (2007). Growth hormone receptor in growth. Endocrinol Metab Clin North Am; 36:1–16.

97. Jensen RB, Vielwerth S, Larsen T, Greisen G, Leffers H, Juul A (2007). The presence of the d3-growth hormone receptor polymorphism is negatively associated with fetal growth but positively associated with postnatal growth in healthy subjects. J Clin Endocrinol Metab 92:2758–2763.

98. Wilkinson IR, Ferrandis E, Artymiuk PJ, Teillot M, Soulard C, Touvay C, et al. (2007). A ligand-receptor fusion of growth hormone forms a dimer and is a potent long-acting agonist. Nat Med 13(9):1108–1113.

99. de Vos AM, Ultsch M, Kossiakoff AA (1992). Human growth hormone and extracellular domain of its receptor: Crystal structure of the complex. Science 255:306.

100. Wilkinson IR, Ferrandis E, Artymiuk PJ, Teillot M, Soulard C, Touvay C, et al. (2007). A ligand-receptor fusion of growth hormone forms a dimer and is a potent long-acting agonist. Nat Med 13(9):1108–1113.

101. Argetsinger LS, Campbell GS, Yang X, et al. (1993). Identification of JAK2 as a growth hormone receptor-associated tyrosine kinase. Cell 74:237.

102. Argetsinger LS, Carter-Su C (1996). Mechanism of signaling by growth hormone receptor. Physiol Rev 76:1089.

103. Schindler C, Darnell JE Jr. (1995). Transcriptional responses to polypeptide ligands: The JAK-STAT pathway. Annu Rev Biochem 64:621.

104. Baumann G, Stolar MW, Amburn K, et al. (1986). A specific growth hormone-binding protein in human plasma: Initial characterization. J Clin Endocrinol Metab 62:134.

105. Herington AC, Ymer S, Stevenson J (1986). Identification and characterization of specific binding proteins for growth hormone in normal human sera. J Clin Invest 77:1817.

106. Herington AC, Ymer S, Stevenson JL (1986). Affinity purification and structural characterization of a specific binding protein for human growth hormone in human serum. Biochem Biophys Res Commun 138:150.

107. Carlsson LMS, Rowland AM, Clark RG, et al. (1991). Ligand-mediated immunofunctional assay for quantitation of growth hormone binding protein in human blood. J Clin Endocrinol Metab 73:1216.

108. Daughaday WH, Trivedi B (1987). Absence of serum growth hormone binding protein in patients with growth hormone receptor (Laron dwarfism). Proc Natl Acad Sci USA 84:4636.

109. Baumann G, Shaw MA, Winter RJ (1987). Absence of plasma growth hormone-binding protein in Laron-type dwarfism. J Clin Endocrinol Metab 65:814.

110. Buchanan CR, Maheshware HG, Normal MR, et al. (1991). Laron-type dwarfism with apparently normal high affinity serum growth hormone-binding protein. Clin Endocrinol (Oxford) 35:179.

111. Hansen JA, Lindberg K, Hilton DJ, et al. (1999). Mechanism of inhibition of growth hormone receptor signaling by suppressor of cytokine signaling proteins. Mol Endocrinol 13:1832.

112. Metcalf D, Greenhalgh CJ, Viney E, et al. (2000). Gigantism in mice lacking suppressor of cytokine signalling-2. Nature 405:1069.

113. Ram PA, Waxman DJ (1999). SOCS/CIS protein inhibition of growth hormone-stimulated STAT5 signaling by multiple mechanisms. J Biol Chem 274:35553.

114. Colson A, Le Cam A, Maiter D, et al. (2000). Potentiation of growth hormone–induced liver suppressors of cytokine signaling messenger ribonucleic acid by cytokines. Endocrinology 141:3687.

115. Mao Y, Ling PR, Fitzgibbons TP, et al. (1999). Endotoxin-induced inhibition of growth hormone receptor signaling in rat liver in vivo. Endocrinology 140:5505.

116. Takala J, Roukonen E, Webster NR, et al. (1999). Increased mortality associated with growth hormone treatment in critically ill adults. N Engl J Med 341:785.

117. Salmon WDJ, Daughaday WH (1957). A hormonally controlled serum factor which stimulates sulfate incorporation by cartilage in vitro. J Lab Clin Med 49:825.

118. Daughaday WH, Rotwein P (1989). Insulin-like growth factors I and II: Peptide, messenger ribonucleic acid and genetic structures, serum tissue concentrations. Endocr Rev 10:68.

119. Sherwin RS, Schulman GA, Hendler R, et al. (1983). Effect of growth hormone on oral glucose tolerance and circulating metabolic fuels in man. Diabetologia 24:155.

120. Rosenfeld RG, Wilson DM, Dollar LA, et al. (1982). Both human pituitary growth hormone and recombinant DNA-derived human growth hormone cause insulin resistance at a postreceptor level. J Clin Endocrinol Metab 54:1033.

121. Green H, Morikawa M, Nixon T (1985). A dual effector theory of growth hormone action. Differentiation 29:195.

122. Gerich JE, Lorenzi M, Bier DM, et al. (1976). Effects of physiologic levels of glucagon and growth hormone on human carbohydrate and lipid metabolism: Studies involving administration of exogenous hormone during suppression of endogenous hormone secretion with somatostatin. J Clin Invest 57:875.

123. Kostyo JL, Hotchkiss J, Knobil E (1959). Stimulation of amino acid transport in isolated diaphragm by growth hormone added in vitro. Science 130:1653.

124. Hjalmarson A, Isaksson O, Ahmen K (1969). Effects of growth hormone and insulin on amino acid transport in perfused rat heart. Am J Physiol 217:1795.

125. Carrel AL, Allen DB (2000). Effects of growth hormone on body composition and bone metabolism. Endocrine 12:163.

126. Lupu F, Terwilliger J, Lee K, et al. (2001). Roles of growth hormone and insulin-like growth factor 1 in mouse postnatal growth. Dev Biol 229:141.

127. Kaplan SA, Cohen P (2007). The somatomedin hypothesis 2007. Fifty years later. J Clin Endocrinol Metab (E-pub ahead of print).

128. Rudman D, Feller AG, Nagraj HS, et al. (1990). Effects of human growth hormone in men over 60 years old. N Engl J Med 323:1.

129. Horber FF, Haymond MV (1990). Human growth hormone prevents the protein catabolic side effects of prednisone in humans. J Clin Invest 86:265.

130. Burgi H, Muller WA, Humbel RE, et al. (1966). Non-suppressible insulin-like activity of human serum: I. Physiochemical properties, extraction and partial purification. Biochem Biophys Acta 121:349.

131. Froesch ER, Zapf J, Meuli C, et al. (1975). Biological properties of NSILAs. Adv Metab Disord 8:211.

132. Dulak NC, Temin HM (1973). A partially purified polypeptide fraction from rat liver cell conditioned medium with multiplication-stimulating activity for embryo fibroblasts. J Cell Physiol 81:153.

133. Daughaday WH, Hall K, Raben MS, et al. (1972). Somatomedin: Proposed designation for sulphation factor. Nature 235:107.

134. Hall K, Takano K, Fryklund L, et al. (1975). Somatomedins. Adv Metab Disord 8:19.

135. VanWyk JJ, Underwood LE, Hintz RL, et al. (1974). The somatomedins: A family of insulin-like hormones under growth hormone control. Recent Prog Horm Res 30:259.

136. Rinderknecht E, Humbel RE (1978). The amino acid sequence of human insulin-like growth factor I and its structural homology with proinsulin. J Biol Chem 253:2769.

137. Rinderknecht E, Humbel RE (1978). Primary structure on human insulin-like growth factor II. FEBS Lett 89:283.

138. Sussenbach JS (1989). The gene structure of the insulin-like growth factor family. Prog Growth Factor Res 1:33.

139. Lund PK, Moats-Staats BM, Hynes MA, et al. (1986). Somatomedin-C/insulin-like growth factor-I and insulin-like growth factor-II mRNAs in rat fetal and adult tissues. J Biol Chem 261:14539.

140. Brown AL, Graham DE, Nissley SP, et al. (1986). Developmental regulation of insulin-like growth factor II mRNA in different rat tissues. J Biol Chem 261:13144.

141. Brissenden JE, Ullrich A, Francke U (1984). Human chromosomal mapping of genes for insulin-like growth factors I and II and epidermal growth factor. Nature 310:781.

142. Tricoli JV, Rall LB, Scott J, et al. (1984). Localization of insulin-like growth factor genes to human chromosomes 11 and 12. Nature 310:784.

143. Bell GI, Gerhard DS, Fong NM, et al. (1985). Isolation of the human insulin-like growth factor genes: Insulin-like growth factor II and insulin genes are contiguous. Proc Natl Acad Sci USA 82:6450.

144. Hall K (1970). Quantitative determination of the sulphation factor activity in human serum. Acta Endocrinol (Copenh) 63:338.

145. Phillips LS, Herington AC, Daughaday WH (1974). Somatomedin stimulation of sulfate incorporation in porcine costal cartilage discs. Endocrinology 94:856.

146. Garland JT, Lottes ME, Kozak S, et al. (1972). Stimulation of DNA synthesis in isolated chondrocytes by sulfation factor. Endocrinology 90:1086.

147. Garland JT, Buchanan CR (1976). Stimulation of RNA and protein synthesis in isolated chondrocytes by human serum. J Clin Endocrinol Metab 48:842.

148. Meuli C, Froesch ER (1975). Effects of insulin and of NSILA-S on the perfused rat heart: Glucose uptake, lactate production and efflux of 3-O-methyl glucose. Eur J Clin Invest 5:93.

149. Hall K, Takano K, Fryklund L (1974). Radioreceptor assay for somatomedin A. J Clin Endocrinol Metab 39:973.

150. VanWyk JJ, Underwood LE, Baseman JB, et al. (1975). Explorations of the insulin-like and growth-promoting properties of somatomedin C by membrane receptor assays. Adv Metab Disord 8:128.

151. Zapf J, Kaufmann U, Eigenmann EJ, et al. (1977). Determination of nonsuppressible insulin-like activity in human serum by a sensitive protein-binding assay. Clin Chem 23:672.

152. Schalch DS, Heinrich UE, Koch JG, et al. (1978). Nonsuppressible insulin-like activity (NSILA): Development of a new sensitive competitive protein-binding assay for determination of serum levels. J Clin Endocrinol Metab 46:664.

153. Furlanetto RW, Underwood LE, VanWyk JJ, et al. (1977). Estimation of somatomedin-C levels in normals and patients with pituitary disease by radioimmunoassay. J Clin Invest 60:646.

154. Zapf J, Walter H, Froesch ER (1981). Radioimmunological determination of insulin like growth factors I and II in normal subjects and in patients with growth disorders and extrapancreatic tumor hypoglycemia. J Clin Invest 68:1321.

155. Bala RM, Bhaumick B (1979). Radioimmunoassay of a basic somatomedin: Comparison of various assay techniques and somatomedin levels in various sera. J Clin Endocrinol Metab 49:770.

156. Rosenfeld RG, Wilson DM, Lee PDK (1986). Insulin-like growth factors I and II in the evaluation of growth retardation. J Pediatr 109:428.

157. Clemmons DR (2007). Value of insulin-like growth factor system markers in the assessment of growth hormone status. Endocrinol Metab Clin North Am 36(1):109–129.

158. Daughaday WH, Kapadia M, Mariz I (1986). Serum somatomedin binding proteins: Physiologic significance and interference in radioligand assay. J Lab Clin Med 109:355.

159. Powell DR, Rosenfeld RG, Baker BK, et al. (1986). Serum somatomedin levels in adults with chronic renal failure: The importance of measuring insulin-like growth factor (IGF)-1 and -2 in acid chromatographed uremic serum. J Clin Endocrinol Metab 63:1186.

160. Horner JM, Liu F, Hintz RL (1978). Comparison of [125I] somatomedin-A and [125I] somatomedin C radioreceptor assays for somatomedin peptide content in whole and acid-chromatographed plasma. J Clin Endocrinol Metab 47:1287.

161. Daughaday WH, Mariz IK, Blethen SL (1980). Inhibition of access of bound somatomedin to membrane receptor and immunobinding sites: A comparison of radioreceptor and radioimmunoassay of somatomedin in native and acid-ethanol-extracted serum. J Clin Endocrinol Metab 51:781.

162. Blum WF, Ranke MB, Bierich JR (1988). A specific radioimmunoassay for IGF-II: The interference of IGF binding proteins can be blocked by excess IGF-I. Acta Endocrinol (Copenh) 118:374.

163. Bang P, Ericksson U, Sara V, et al. (1991). Comparison of acid ethanol extraction and acid gel filtration prior to IGF-I and IGF-II radioimmunoassays: Improvement of determinations in acid ethanol extracts by the use of a truncated IGF-I as radioligand. Acta Endocrinol (Copenh) 124:620.

164. Khosravi MJ, Diamandi A, Mistry J, Lee PD (1996). Noncompetitive ELISA for human serum insulin-like growth factor-I. Clin Chem 42(8/1):1147.

165. Cohen P (1998). Serum insulin-like growth factor-I levels and prostate cancer risk: Interpreting the evidence. J Natl Cancer Inst 12:876.

166. Bennett A, Wilson DM, Liu F, et al. (1983). Levels of insulin-like growth factor-I and -II in human cord blood. J Clin Endocrinol Metab 57:609.

167. Gluckman PD, Barrett-Johnson JJ, Butler JH, et al. (1983). Studies of insulin-like growth factor I and II by specific radioligand assays in umbilical cord blood. Clin Endocrinol 19:405.

168. Lassare C, Hardouin S, Daffos F, et al. (1991). Serum insulin-like growth factors and their binding proteins in the human fetus: Relationships with growth in normal subjects and in subjects with intrauterine growth retardation. Pediatr Res 29:219.

169. Hall K, Hansson U, Lundin G, et al. (1986). Serum levels of somatomedins and somatomedin-binding protein in pregnant women with type I or gestational diabetes and their infants. J Clin Endocrinol Metab 63:1300.

170. Luna AM, Wilson DM, Wibbelsman CJ, et al. (1983). Somatomedins in adolescence: A cross-sectional study of the effect of puberty on plasma insulin-like growth factor I and II levels. J Clin Endocrinol Metab 57:268.

171. Cara JF, Rosenfield RL, Furlanetto RW (1987). A longitudinal study of the relationship of plasma somatomedin-C concentration to the pubertal growth spurt. Am J Dis Child 147:562.

172. Cuttler L, Van Vliet G, Conte FA, et al. (1985). Somatomedin-C levels in children and adolescents with gonadal dysgenesis: Differences from age-matched normal females and effect of chronic estrogen replacement therapy. J Clin Endocrinol Metab 60:1087.

173. Rosenfeld RG, Hintz RL, Johanson AJ, et al. (1986). Methionyl human growth hormone and oxandrolone in Turner syndrome: Preliminary results of a prospective randomized trial. J Pediatr 109:936.

174. Copeland KC (1988). Effects of acute high dose and chronic low dose estrogen on plasma somatomedin-C and growth in patients with Turner's syndrome. J Clin Endocrinol Metab 66:1278.

175. Johanson AL, Blizzard RM (1981). Low somatomedin-C levels in older men rise in response to growth hormone administration. Johns Hopkins Med J 149:115.

176. Donovan SM, Oh Y, Pham H, et al. (1989). Ontogeny of serum insulin-like growth factor binding proteins in the rat. Endocrinology 125:2621.

177. Glasscock GF, Gelber SE, Lamson G, et al. (1990). Pituitary control of growth in the neonatal rat: Effects of neonatal hypophysectomy on somatic and organ growth, serum insulin-like growth factors (IGF)-I and -II levels, and expression of IGF binding proteins. Endocrinology 127:1792.

178. Ranke MB, Schweizer R, Elmlinger MW, Weber K, Binder G, Schwarze CP, et al. (2000). Significance of basal IGF-I, IGFBP-3 and IGFBP-2 measurements in the diagnostics of short stature in children. Horm Res 54(2):60–68.

179. Nunez SB, Municchi G, Barnes KM, Rose SR (1996). Insulin-like growth factor I (IGF-I) and IGF-binding protein-3 concentrations compared to stimulated and night growth hormone in the evaluation of short children: A clinical research center study. J Clin Endocrinol Metab 81(5):1927–1932.

180. Hintz RL, Clemmons DR, Underwood LE, et al. (1972). Competitive binding of somatomedin to the insulin receptors of adipocytes, chondrocytes, and liver membranes. Proc Natl Acad Sci USA 69:2351.

181. Megyesi K, Kahn CR, Roth J, et al. (1974). Insulin and nonsuppressible insulin-like activity (NSILA-s): Evidence for separate plasma membrane receptor sites. Biochem Biophys Res Commun 57:307.

182. Massague J, Czech MP (1982). The subunit structures of two distinct receptors for insulin-like growth factors I and II and their relationship to the insulin receptor. J Biol Chem 257:5038.

183. Kasuga M, Van Obberghen E, Nissley SP, et al. (1981). Demonstration of two subtypes of insulin-like growth factor receptors by affinity crosslinking. J Biol Chem 256:5305.

184. Chernausek SD, Jacobs S, VanWyk JJ (1981). Structural similarities between receptors for somatomedin C and insulin: Analysis by affinity labeling. Biochemistry 20:7345.

185. Oh Y, Muller HL, Neely EK, et al. (1993). New concepts in insulin-like growth factor receptor physiology. Growth Regul 3:113.

186. Werner H, Le Roith D (1997). The insulin-like growth factor-I receptor signaling pathways are important for tumorigenesis and inhibition of apoptosis. Crit Rev Oncog 8:71.

187. Kadowaki T, Tamemoto H, Tobe K, et al. (1996). Insulin resistance and growth retardation in mice lacking insulin receptor substrate-1 and identification of insulin receptor substrate-2. Diabet Med 13(9/6):S103.

188. Tsuruzoe K, Emkey R, Kriauciunas KM, et al. (2001). Insulin receptor substrate 3 (IRS-3) and IRS-4 impair IRS-1- and IRS-2 mediated signaling. Mol Cell Biol 21:26.

189. Wu JD, Haugk K, Coleman I, Woodke L, Vessella R, Nelson P, et al. (2006). Combined in vivo effect of A12, a type 1 insulin-like growth factor receptor antibody, and docetaxel against prostate cancer tumors. Clin Cancer Res 12(20/1):6153–6160.

190. Yang J, Anzo M, Cohen P (2005). Control of aging and longevity by IGF-I signaling. Exp Gerontol 40:867–872.

191. Morgan DO, Edman JC, Standring DN, et al. (1987). Insulin-like growth factor II receptor as a multifunctional binding protein. Nature 329:301.

192. MacDonald RG, Pfeffer SR, Coussens L, et al. (1988). A single receptor binds both insulin-like growth factor II and mannose-6-phosphate. Science 239:1134.

193. Kornfeld S (1987). Trafficking of lysosomal enzymes. FASEB J 1:462.

194. Rosenfeld RG, Conover CA, Hodges D, et al. (1987). Heterogeneity of insulin-like growth factor-I affinity for the insulin-like growth factor-II receptor: Comparison of natural, synthetic and recombinant DNA-derived insulin-like growth factor-I. Biochem Biophys Res Commun 143:195.

195. Conover CA, Misra P, Hintz RL, et al. (1987). Effect of an anti–insulin-like growth factor I receptor antibody on insulin-like growth factor II stimulation of DNA synthesis in human fibroblasts. Biochem Biophys Res Commun 139:501.

196. Furlanetto RW, DiCarlo JN, Wisehart C, et al. (1987). The type II insulin-like growth factor receptor does not mediate deoxyribonucleic acid synthesis in human fibroblasts. J Clin Endocrinol Metab 64:1142.

197. Mottola C, Czech MP (1984). The type II insulin-like growth factor receptor does not mediate DNA synthesis in H-35 hepatoma cells. J Biol Chem 259:12705.

198. Kiess W, Haskell JF, Lee L, et al. (1987). An antibody that blocks insulin-like growth factor (IGF) binding to the type II IGF receptor is neither an agonist nor an inhibitor of IGF-stimulated biologic response in L6 myoblasts. J Biol Chem 162:12756.

199. Adashi EY, Resnick CE, Rosenfeld RG (1989). Insulin-like growth factor-I (IGF-I) hormonal action in cultured rat granulosa cells: Mediation via type I but not type II IGF receptors. Endocrinology 126:216.

200. Beukers M, Oh Y, Zhang H, et al. (1991). [Leu27] insulin-like growth factor II is highly selective for the type II IGF receptor in binding, cross-linking and thymidine incorporation experiments. Endocrinology 128:1201.

201. Canfield WM, Kornfeld S (1989). The chicken liver cation-independent mannose-6-phosphate receptor lacks the high affinity binding site for insulin-like growth factor II. J Biol Chem 264:7100.

202. Clairmont KB, Czech MP (1989). Chicken and Xenopus mannose 6phosphate receptors fail to bind insulin-like growth factor II. J Biol Chem 264:16390.

203. Rogers SA, Hammerman MR (1988). Insulin-like growth factor II stimulates production of inositol triphosphate in proximal tubular basolateral membranes from canine kidney. Proc Natl Acad Sci USA 85:4037.

204. Tally M, Li CH, Hall K (1987). IGF-2 stimulated growth mediated by the somatomedin type 2 receptor. Biochem Biophys Res Commun 148:811.

205. Minniti CP, Kohn EC, Grubb JH, et al. (1992). The insulin-like growth factor II (IGF-II)/mannose 6-phosphate receptor mediates IGF-II-induced motility in human rhabdomyosarcoma cells. J Biol Chem 267:9000.

206. Nishimoto I, Murayama Y, Katada T, et al. (1989). Possible direct linkage of insulin-like growth factor-II receptor with guanine nucleotide-binding proteins. J Biol Chem 264:14029.

207. Braulke T (1999). Type-2 IGF receptor: A multi-ligand binding protein. Horm Metab Res 31:242.

208. Kang JX, Bell J, Beard RL, Chandraratna RA (1999). Mannose 6phosphate/insulin-like growth factor II receptor mediates the growth-inhibitory effects of retinoids. Cell Growth Differ 10:591.

209. Melnick M, Chen H, Buckley S, et al. (1998). Insulin-like growth factor II receptor, transforming growth factor-beta, and Cdk4 expression and the developmental epigenetics of mouse palate morphogenesis and dysmorphogenesis. Dev Dyn 211:11.

210. Misra P, Hintz RL, Rosenfeld RG (1986). Structural and immunological characterization of insulin-like growth factor II binding to IM-9 cells. J Clin Endocrinol Metab 63:1400.

211. Jonas HA, Cox AJ (1990). Insulin-like growth factor binding to the atypical insulin receptors of a human lymphoid-derived cell line (IM-9). Biochem J 266:737.

212. Feltz SM, Swanson SM, Wemmie JA, et al. (1988). Functional properties of an isolated heterodimeric human placenta insulin-like growth factor I complex. Biochemistry 27:3234.

213. Treadway JL, Morrison BD, Goldfine ID, et al. (1989). Assembly of insulin/insulin-like growth factor-1 hybrid receptors in vitro. J Biol Chem 264:21450.

214. Soos MA, Siddle K (1989). Immunological relationships between receptors for insulin and insulin-like growth factor I. Biochem J 263:553.

215. Rosenfeld RG, Lamson G, Pham H, et al. (1990). Insulin-like growth factor binding proteins. Recent Prog Horm Res 46:99.

216. Lamson G, Giudice L, Rosenfeld RG (1991). The insulin-like growth factor binding proteins: Structural and molecular relationships. Growth Factors 5:19.

217. Rechler MM (1977). Insulin-like growth factor binding proteins. Vitam Horm 47:114.

218. Hintz RL, Liu F (1977). Demonstration of specific plasma protein binding sites for somatomedin. J Clin Endocrinol Metab 45:988.

219. Hossenlopp P, Surin D, Segovia-Quinson B, et al. (1986). Analysis of serum insulin-like growth factor binding proteins using Western blotting: Use of the method for titration of the binding proteins and competitive binding studies. Anal Biochem 154:138.

220. Shimasaki S, Shimonaka M, Zhang HP, et al. (1991). Identification of five different insulin-like growth factor binding proteins (IGFBPs) from adult rat serum and molecular cloning of a novel IGRBP-5 in rat and human. J Biol Chem 266:10646.

221. Brewer MT, Stetler GL, Squires CH, et al. (1988). Cloning, characterization, and expression of a human insulin-like growth factor binding protein. Biochem Biophys Res Commun 152:1289.

222. Oh Y, Muller H, Pham H, et al. (1992). Non-receptor mediated, posttranscriptional regulation of insulin-like growth factor binding protein (IGFBP)-3 in Hs578T human breast cancer cells. Endocrinology 131:3123.

223. Oh Y, Muller H, Lamson G, et al. (1993). Insulin-like growth factor (IGF)-independent action of IGF binding protein (BP)-3 in Hs578T human breast cancer cells: Cell surface binding and growth inhibition. J Biol Chem 268:14964.

224. Oh Y, Muller HL, Pham H, et al. (1993). Demonstration of receptors for insulin-like growth factor binding protein-3 (IGFBP-3) on Hs578T human breast cancer cells. J Biol Chem 268:26045.

225. Ritvos O, Ranta T, Julkanen J, et al. (1988). Insulin-like growth factor (IGF) binding protein from human decidua inhibits the binding and biological action of IGF-I in cultured choriocarcinoma cells. Endocrinology 122:2150.

226. Ross MM, Francis GL, Szabo L, et al. (1989). Insulin-like growth factor (IGF)-binding proteins inhibit the biological activities of IGF-I and IGF-II but not des-(1–3)-IGF-I. Biochem J 258:267.

227. Clemmons DR, Cascieri MA, Camacho-Hubner C, et al. (1990). Discrete alterations of the insulin-like growth factor I molecule which alter its affinity for insulin-like growth factor-binding proteins result in changes in bioactivity. J Biol Chem 265:12210.

228. Okajima T, Nakamura K, Zhang H, et al. (1992). Sensitive colorimetric bioassays for insulin-like growth factor (IGF) stimulation of cell proliferation and glucose consumption: Use in studies of IGF analogs. Endocrinology 130:2201.

229. Cohen P, Lamson G, Okajima T, et al. (1993). Transfection of the human insulin-like growth factor binding protein-3 gene into Balb/c fibroblasts inhibits cellular growth. Mol Endocrinol 7:380.

230. Elgin RC, Busby WH Jr., Clemmons DR (1987). An insulin-like growth factor (IGF) binding protein enhances the biologic response to IGF-I. Proc Natl Acad Sci USA 84:3254.

231. Hwa V, Oh Y, Rosenfeld RG (1999). The insulin-like growth factor binding protein (IGFBP) superfamily. Endocr Rev 20:761.

232. Oh Y, Muller HL, Ng L, Rosenfeld RG (1995). Transforming growth factor-beta-induced cell growth inhibition in human breast cancer cells is mediated through insulin-like growth factor-binding protein-3 action. J Biol Chem 270:13589.

233. Conover CA, Bale LK, Durham SK, Powell DR (2000). Insulin-like growth factor (IGF) binding protein-3 potentiation of IGF action is mediated through the phosphatidylinositol-3-kinase pathway and is associated with alteration in protein kinase B/AKT sensitivity. Endocrinology 141:3098.

234. Rajah R, Valentinis B, Cohen P (1997). Insulin-like growth factor (IGF)-binding protein-3 induces apoptosis and mediates the effects of transforming growth factor-beta 1 on programmed cell death through a p53- and IGF-independent mechanism. J Biol Chem 272:12181.

235. Liu B, Lee HY, Weinzimer SA, et al. (2000). Direct functional interactions between insulin-like growth factor-binding protein-3 and retinoid X receptor-alpha regulate transcriptional signaling and apoptosis. J Biol Chem 275:33607.

236. Clark RG, Mortensen D, Reifsynder D, et al. (1993). Recombinant human insulin-like growth factor binding protein-3 (rhIGFBP-3): Effects on the glycemic and growth promoting activities of rhIGF-1 in the rat. Growth Regul 3:50.

237. Giudice LC, Farrell EM, Pham H, et al. (1990). Insulin-like growth factor binding proteins in the maternal serum throughout gestation and in the puerperium: Effects of a pregnancy-associated protease activity. J Clin Endocrinol Metab 71:1330.

238. Hossenlopp P, Segovia B, Lassaree C, et al. (1990). Evidence of enzymatic degradation of insulin-like growth factor binding proteins in the 150K complex during pregnancy. J Clin Endocrinol Metab 71:797.

239. Muller H, Oh Y, Gargosky SE, et al. (1993). Concentrations of insulin-like growth factor binding protein-3, insulin-like growth factors and IGFBP-3 protease activity in cerebrospinal fluid (CSF) of children with leukemia, brain tumors, or meningitis. J Clin Endocrinol Metab 77:1113.

240. Lee D-Y, Park S-K, Yorgin P, et al. (1994). Alteration in insulin-like growth factor binding proteins (IGFBPs) and IGFBP-3 protease activity in serum and urine from acute and chronic renal failure. J Clin Endocrinol Metab 79:1376.

241. Gargosky SE, Pham H, Wilson KF, et al. (1992). Measurement and characterization of insulin-like growth factor binding protein-3 in human biological fluids: Discrepancies between radioimmunoassay and ligand blotting. Endocrinology 131:3051.

242. Drop SLS, Valiquette G, Guyda HJ, et al. (1979). Partial purification and characterization of a binding protein for insulin-like activity (ILAs) in human amniotic fluid: A possible inhibitor of insulin-like activity. Acta Endocrinol 90:505.

243. Rosenfeld RG, Pham H, Conover CA, et al. (1989). Structural and immunological comparison of insulin-like growth factor (IGF) binding proteins of cerebrospinal and amniotic fluids. J Clin Endocrinol Metab 68:636.

244. Rosenfeld RG, Pham H, Oh Y, et al. (1989). Identification of insulin-like growth factor binding protein-2 (IGF-BP-2) and a low molecular weight IGF-BP in human seminal plasma. J Clin Endocrinol Metab 69:963.

245. Martin JL, Baxter RC (1986). Insulin-like growth factor binding protein from human plasma: Purification and characterization. J Biol Chem 261:8754.

246. Baxter RC (1988). Characterization of the acid-labile subunit of the growth hormone-dependent insulin-like growth factor binding protein complex. J Clin Endocrinol Metab 67:265.

247. Povoa G, Roovete A, Hall K (1984). Cross-reaction of a serum somatomedin-binding protein in a radioimmunoassay developed for somatomedin binding protein isolated from human amniotic fluid. Acta Endrocrinol 107:563.

248. Baxter RC, Cowell CT (1987). Diurnal variation of growth hormone independent binding protein for insulin-like growth factors in humans. Clin Endocrinol Metab 65:432.

249. Cohen P, Peehl DM, Stamey TA, et al. (1993). Elevated levels of insulin-like growth factor binding protein-2 in the serum of prostate cancer patients. J Clin Endocrinol Metab 76:1031.

250. Baxter RC, Martin JL (1986). Radioimmunoassay of growth hormone dependent insulin-like growth factor binding protein in human plasma. J Clin Invest 78:1504.

251. Blum WF, Ranke MB, Kietzmann K, et al. (1990). A specific radioimmunoassay for the growth hormone-dependent somatomedin-binding protein: Its use for diagnosis of GH deficiency. J Clin Endocrinol Metab 70:1292.

252. Rosenfeld RG, Aggarwal BB, Hintz RL, Dollar LA (1982). Recombinant DNA-derived methionyl growth hormone is similar in membrane binding properties to human pituitary growth hormone. Biochem Biophys Res Commun 106:202.

253. Rosenfeld RG (1995). Broadening the growth hormone insensitivity syndrome. N Engl J Med 333:1145.

254. Rosenfeld RG, Albertsson-Wikland K, Cassorla F, et al. (1995). Diagnostic controversy: The diagnosis of childhood growth hormone deficiency revisited. J Clin Endocrinol Metab 80:1532.

255. Rosenfeld RG, Gargosky SE (1996). Assays for insulin-like growth factors and their binding proteins: Practicalities and pitfalls. J Pediatr 128(5/2):S52.

256. Vu TH, Jirtle RL, Hoffman AR (2006). Cross-species clues of an epigenetic imprinting regulatory code for the IGF2R gene. Cytogenet Genome Res. 113(1-4):202–208.

257. Plotnikov AN, Schlessinger J, Hubbard SR, Mohammadi M (1999). Structural basis for FGF receptor dimerization and activation. Cell 98:641.

258. Ladher RK, Anakwe KU, Gurney AL, et al. (2000). Identification of synergistic signals initiating inner ear development. Science 290:1965.

259. Rousseau F, Bonaventure J, Legeai-Mallet L, et al. (1996). Mutations of the fibroblast growth factor receptor-3 gene in achondroplasia. Horm Res 45:108.

260. Cohen MM Jr. (1997). Transforming growth factor betas and fibroblast growth factors and their receptors: Role in sutural biology and craniosynostosis. J Bone Miner Res 12:322.

261. Casci T, Freeman M (1999). Control of EGF receptor signalling: Lessons from fruitflies. Cancer Metastasis Rev 18:181.

262. Sherr CJ (2000). The Pezcoller lecture: Cancer cell cycles revisited. Cancer Res 60:3689.

263. Jones ME, Boon WC, McInnes K, Maffei L, Carani C, Simpson ER (2007). Recognizing rare disorders: Aromatase deficiency. Nat Clin Pract Endocrinol Metab [volume]:414–421.

264. Demura M, Martin RM, Shozu M, Sebastian S, Takayama K, Hsu WT, et al. (2007). Regional rearrangements in chromosome 15q21 cause formation of cryptic promoters for the CYP19 (aromatase) gene. Hum Mol Genet 16:2529–2541.

265. Horton WA, Hall JG, Hecht JT (2007). Achondroplasia. Lancet 370:162–172.

266. Spranger J (1992). International classification of osteochondrodysplasias. Eur J Pediatr 151:407.

267. Shiang R, Thompson LM, Zhu Y-Z, et al. (1994). Mutations in the transmembrane domain of FGFR3 cause the most common genetic form of dwarfism, achondroplasia. Cell 78:335.

268. Cronk C, Crocker AC, Pueschel SM, et al. (1988). Growth charts for children with Down's syndrome: 1 month to 18 years of age. Pediatrics 81:102.

269. Rosenfeld RG, Grumbach MM (eds.) (1990). *Turner syndrome*. New York: Marcel Dekker.

270. Ranke MB, Rosenfeld RG (eds.) (1991). *Turner syndrome: Growth promoting therapies*. Amsterdam: Excerpta Medica.

271. Hibi I, Takano K (eds.) (1993). *Basic and clinical approach to Turner syndrome*. Amsterdam: Excerpta Medica.

272. Ranke MB, Pfluger H, Rosendahl W, et al. (1983). Turner syndrome: Spontaneous growth in 150 cases and review of the literature. Eur J Pediatr 141:81.

273. Davenport ML, Punyasavatsut N, Gunther D, et al. (1999). Turner syndrome: A pattern of early growth failure. Acta Paediatr Suppl 433(8):118.

274. Even L, Cohen A, Marbach N, et al. (2000). Longitudinal analysis of growth over the first 3 years of life in Turner's syndrome. J Pediatr 137:460.

275. Blaschke RJ, Rappold GA (2000). SHOX: Growth, Leri-Weill and Turner syndrome. Trends Endocrinol Metab 11:227.

276. Ross JL, Long LM, Loriauz DL, et al. (1985). Growth hormone secretory dynamics in Turner syndrome. J Pediatr 106:202.

277. Rosenfeld RG, Hintz RL, Johanson AJ, et al. (1988). Three-year results of a randomized prospective trial of methionyl human growth hormone and oxandrolone in Turner syndrome. J Pediatr 113:393.

278. Quigley CA (2007). Growth hormone treatment of non-growth hormone-deficient growth disorders. Endocrinol Metab Clin North Am 36(1):131–186.

279. Sas TC, deMuinck Keizer-Schrama SM, Stignen T, et al. (1999). Normalization of height in girls with Turner syndrome after long-term growth hormone treatment: Results of a randomized dose-response trial. J Clin Endocrinol Metab 84:4607.

280. Hale DE, Cody JD, Baillargeon J, et al. (2000). The spectrum of growth abnormalities in children with 18q deletions. J Clin Endocrinol Metab 85:4450.

281. Saenger P, Czernichow P, Hughes I, Reiter EO (2007). Small for gestational age: Short stature and beyond. Endocr Rev 28(2):219–251.

282. Chernausek SD (2006). Mendelian genetic causes of the short child born small for gestational age. J Endocrinol Invest 29(1):16–20.

283. Gluckman PD, Harding J (1992). The regulation of fetal growth. In Hernandez M, Argente J (eds.), *Human growth: Basic and clinical aspects*. New York: Elsevier 253–276.

284. Cooke PS, Nicoll CS (1983). Hormonal control of fetal growth. Physiologist 26:317.

285. Kim JD, Nanto-Salonen K, Szczepankiewicz JR, et al. (1993). Evidence for pituitary regulation of somatic growth, insulin-like growth factors-I and -II, and their binding proteins in the fetal rat. Pediatr Res 33:144.

286. Liu J-P, Baker J, Perkins AS, et al. (1993). Mice carrying null mutations of the genes encoding insulin-like growth factor I (Igf-1) and type 1 IGF receptor (Igf1r). Cell 75:73.

287. Woods KA, Camacho-Hubner C, Savage MO, Clark AJ (1996). Intrauterine growth retardation and postnatal growth failure associated with deletion of the insulin-like growth factor I gene. N Engl J Med 335:1363.

288. Rosenfeld RG, Thorsson AV, Hintz RL (1979). Increased somatomedin receptor sites in newborn circulating mononuclear cells. J Clin Endocrinol Metab 48:456.

289. D'Ercole AJ (1987). Somatomedins/insulin-like growth factors and fetal development. J Dev Physiol 9:481.

290. Han VK, D'Ercole AJ, Lund PK (1987). Cellular localization of somatomedin (insulin-like growth factor) messenger RNA in the human fetus. Science 236:193.

291. Giudice LC, deZegher F, Gargosky SE, et al. (1995). Insulin-like growth factors and their binding proteins in the term and preterm human fetus and neonate with normal and extremes of intrauterine growth. J Clin Endocrinol Metab 80:1548.

292. Sas T, deWaal W, Mulder P, et al. (1999). Growth hormone treatment in children with short stature born small for gestational age: 5-year results of a randomized, double-blind, dose-response trial. J Clin Endocrinol Metab 84:3064.

293. Giudice L, de Zegher F, Gargosky SE (1995). Insulin-like growth factors and their binding proteins in the term and preterm human fetus with normal and extremes of intrauterine growth. J Clin Endocrinol Metab 80:1548.

294. Simmons RA (2007). Developmental origins of diabetes: The role of epigenetic mechanisms. Curr Opin Endocrinol Diabetes Obes 14(1):13–16.

295. Barker DJP (1995). *Fetal origins of coronary heart disease.* London: BMJ Publishing Group.

296. Russell AA (1954). A syndrome of "intrauterine" dwarfism recognizable at birth with craniofacial dysostosis, disproportionately short arms and other anomalies (5 examples). Proc R Soc Med 47:1040.

297. Gicquel C, Rossignol S, Cabrol S, Houang M, Steunou V, Barbu V, et al. (2005). Epimutation of the telomeric imprinting center region on chromosome 11p15 in Silver-Russell syndrome. Nat Genet 37(9):1003–1007.

298. Mann TP, Russell AA (1959). Study of a microcephalic midget of extreme type. Proc R Soc Med 52:1024.

299. Harper RG, Orti E, Baker RK (1967). Bird-headed dwarfs (Seckel's syndrome): A familial pattern of developmental, dental, skeletal, genital, and central nervous system anomalies. J Pediatr 70:799.

300. Allanson JE (2007). Noonan syndrome. Am J Med Genet C Semin Med Genet 145(3):274–279.

301. Rosenbloom AL, DeBusk FL (1971). Progeria of Hutchinson-Gilford: A caricature of aging. Am Heart J 82:287.

302. MacDonald WB, Fitch KD, Lewis IC (1960). Cockayne's syndrome: An heredo-familial disorder of growth and development. Pediatrics 25:997.

303. Bray GA, Dahms WT, Swerdloff RS, et al. (1983). The Prader-Willi syndrome: A study of 40 patients and review of the literature. Medicine 62:59–80.

304. Lee PDK, Wilson DM, Hintz RL, Rosenfeld RG (1987). Growth hormone treatment of short stature in Prader-Willi syndrome. J Pediatr Endocrinol 2:31.

305. Angulo M, Castro-Magana M, Uly J (1991). Pituitary evaluation and growth hormone treatment in Prader-Willi syndrome. J Pediatr Endocrinol 3:167.

306. Edwards LE, Alton IR, Barrada MI, et al. (1979). Pregnancy in the underweight woman: Course, outcome and growth patterns of the infant. Am J Obstet Gynecol 135:297.

307. Ouellette EM, Rosett HL, Rosman NP, et al. (1977). Adverse effects on offspring of maternal alcohol abuse during pregnancy. N Engl J Med 297:528.

308. Jones KL, Smith DW, Streissguth AP (1974). Outcome in offspring of chronic alcoholic women. Lancet 1:1076.

309. Abel EL (1982). Consumption of alcohol during pregnancy: A review of effects on growth and development of offspring. Hum Biol 54:421.

310. Chasnoff IJ, Griffith DR, MacGregor S, et al. (1989). Temporal patterns of cocaine use in pregnancy: Perinatal outcome. JAMA 261:1741.

311. Zuckerman B, Frank DA, Hingson R, et al. (1989). Effects of maternal marijuana and cocaine use on fetal growth. N Engl J Med 320:762.

312. Abel EL (1980). Smoking during pregnancy: A review of effects on growth and development of offspring. Hum Biol 52:593.

313. Chaussain JL, Colle M, Ducret JP (1994). Adult height in children with prepubertal short stature secondary to intrauterine growth retardation. Acta Paediatr Suppl 399:72.

314. Barker DJP, Gluckman PD, Dodrey KM, et al. (1993). Fetal nutrition and cardiovascular disease in adult life. Lancet 341:938.

315. Tanner JM, Goldstein H, Whitehouse RH (1970). Standards for children's height at ages 2–9 years allowing for height of parents. Arch Dis Child 45:755.

316. Graham GC, Adrianzen T, Rabold J, et al. (1982). Later growth of malnourished children. Am J Dis Child 136:348.

317. Pimstone B, Berbezat G, Hansen JD, et al. (1967). Growth hormone and protein-calorie malnutrition: Impaired suppression during induced hyperglycemia. Lancet 2:1333.

318. Beas F, Contreras I, Maccioni A, et al. (1971). Growth hormone in infant malnutrition: The arginine test in marasmus and kwashiorkor. Br J Nutr 26:169.

319. Grant DB, Hambley J, Becker D, et al. (1973). Reduced sulphation factor in undernourished children. Arch Dis Child 48:596.

320. Soliman AT, Hassan AEHI, Aref MK, et al. (1986). Serum insulin-like growth factors I and II concentrations and growth hormone and insulin responses to arginine infusion in children with protein-energy malnutrition before and after nutritional rehabilitation. Pediatr Res 20:1122.

321. Donovan SM, Atilano LC, Hintz RL, et al. (1991). Differential regulation of the insulin-like growth factors (IGF-I and IGF-II) and IGFbinding proteins during malnutrition in the neonatal rat. Endocrinology 129:149.

322. Pugliese MT, Lifschitz F, Grad G, et al. (1982). Fear of obesity: A cause of short stature and delayed puberty. N Engl J Med 309:513.

323. Preece MA, Law CM, Davies PSW (1986). The growth of children with chronic paediatric disease. Clin Endocrinol Metab 15:453.

324. Groll A, Candy D, Preece M, et al. (1980). Short stature as the primary manifestation of celiac disease. Lancet 2:1097.

325. Mock DM (1980). Growth retardation in chronic inflammatory bowel disease. Gastroenterology 91:1019.

326. Rosenthal SR, Snyder JD, Hendricks KM, et al. (1983). Growth failure and inflammatory bowel disease: Approach to treatment of a complicated adolescent problem. Pediatrics 72:481.

327. Lecornu M, David L, François P (1978). Low serum somatomedin activity in celiac disease. Helv Paediatr Acta 33:509.

328. Greco L, Troncone R, DeVizia B, et al. (1987). Discriminant analysis for the diagnosis of childhood celiac disease. Pediatr Gastroenterol Nutr 6:538.

329. Sblattero D, Berti I, Trevisiol C, et al. (2000). Human recombinant tissue transglutaminase ELISA: An innovative diagnostic assay for celiac disease. Am J Gastroenterol 95:1253.

330. Booth IW, Harries JT (19984). Inflammatory bowel disease in childhood. Gut 25:188.

331. Bayer LM, Robinson SJ (1969). Growth history of children with congenital heart defects. Am J Dis Child 117:573.

332. Feldt RH, Strickler GB, Weidman WH (1969). Growth of children with congenital heart disease. Am J Dis Child 117:573.

333. Holliday MA (1978). Symposium on metabolism and growth in children with kidney disease. Kidney Int 14:299.

334. Rizzoni G, Broyer M, Guest G, et al. (1986). Growth retardation in childhood renal disease: Scope of the problem. Am J Kidney Dis 7:256.

335. Hokken-Koelega AC, van Zaal MA, van Bergen W, et al. (1994). Final height and its predictive factors after renal transplantation in childhood. Pediatr Res 36:323.

336. Platt OS, Rosenstock W, Espeland MA (1984). Influence of sickle hemoglobinopathies on growth and development. N Engl J Med 311:7.

337. Stevens MCG, Maude GH, Cupidore L (1986). Prepubertal growth and sexual maturation in children with sickle cell disease. Pediatrics 78:124.

338. Phebus CK, Gloninger MF, Maciak BJ (1984). Growth patterns in children with sickle cell disease. J Pediatr 105:23.

339. Borgna-Pignatti C, DeStefano P, Zonta L, et al. (1985). Growth and sexual maturation in thalassemia major. J Pediatr 106:150.

340. DeLuca F, Simone E, Corona G, et al. (1987). Adult height in thalassemia major without hormonal treatment. Eur J Pediatr 146:494.

341. Saenger P, Schwartz E, Markenson AL, et al. (1980). Depressed serum somatomedin activity in beta-thalassemia. J Pediatr 96:214.

342. Werther GA, Matthews RN, Burger HG, et al. (1981). Lack of response of non-suppressible insulin-like activity to short-term administration of human growth hormone in thalassemia major. J Clin Endocrinol Metab 53:806.

343. Zadik Z, Chalew SA, McCarter RJ Jr., et al. (1985). The influence of age on the 24-hour integrated concentrations of growth hormone in normal individuals. J Clin Endocrinol Metab 60:153.

344. Menon R, Sperling M (1996). Insulin as a growth factor. Endocrinol Metab Clin North Am 25:633.

345. Zadik Z, Chalew SA, Gilula Z, Kowarski AA (1990). Reproducibility of growth hormone testing procedures: A comparison between 24-hour integrated concentration and pharmacological stimulation. J Clin Endocrinol Metab 71:1127.

346. (1981). Infections as deterrants of growth. Nutr Rev 39:328.

347. Rivkees SA, Bode HH, Crawford JD (1988). Long-term growth in juvenile-acquired hypothyroidism. N Engl J Med 318:599.

348. Van Wyk JJ, Grumbach MM (1960). Syndrome of precocious menstruation and galactorrhea. J Pediatr 57:416–435.

349. Magiakou MA, Mastorakos G, Oldfield EH, et al. (1994). Cushing's syndrome in children and adolescents: Presentation, diagnosis, and therapy. N Engl J Med 331:629.

350. Mosier HD, Smith FG, Schultz MA (1972). Failure of catch-up growth after Cushing's syndrome in childhood. Am J Dis Child 124:251.

351. Schwindinger WF, Levine MA (1994). Albright hereditary osteodystrophy. Endocrinologist 4:17.

352. Chan JCM (1982). Renal hypophosphatemic rickets: A review. Int J Pediatr Nephrol 3:305.

353. Efstratiadis A (1998). Genetics of mouse growth. Int J Dev Biol 42:955.

354. Hintz RL, Menking M, Sotos JF (1968). Familial holoprosencephaly with endocrine dysgenesis. J Pediatr 72:81.

355. Lieblich JM, Rosen SW, Guyda H, et al. (1978). The syndrome of basal encephalocele and hypothalamic pituitary dysfunction. Ann Intern Med 89:910.

356. Roiyman A, Laron Z (1978). Hypothalamo-pituitary hormone deficiency associated with cleft lip and palate. Arch Dis Child 53:852.

357. Rudman D, Davis GT, Priest JH, et al. (1978). Prevalence of growth hormone deficiency in children with cleft lip or palate. J Pediatr 93:378.

358. Izenberg N, Rosenblum M, Parks JS (1984). The endocrine spectrum of septo-optic dysplasia. Clin Pediatr 23:632.

359. Wilson DM, Enzmann DR, Hintz RL, et al. (1984). Cranial computed tomography in septo-optic dysplasia: Discordance of clinical and radiological features. Neuroradiology 26:279.

360. Hermesz E, Mackem S, Mahon KA (1996). Rpx: A novel anterior-restricted homeobox gene progressively activated in the prechordal plate, anterior neural plate, and Rathke's pouch of the mouse embryo. Development 122:41.

361. Dattani MT, Martinez-Barbera JP, Thomas PO, et al. (1998). Mutations in the homeobox gene HESX1/Hesx1 associated with septo-optic dysplasia in human and mouse. Nat Genet 19:125.

362. Wajnrajch MP, Gertner JM, Harbison MD, et al. (1996). Nonsense mutation in the human growth hormone–releasing hormone receptor causes growth failure analogous to the little (litt) mouse. Nat Genet 12:88.

363. Baumann G, Maheshwari H (1997). The dwarfs of Sindh: Severe growth hormone (GH) deficiency caused by a mutation in the GH-releasing hormone receptor gene. Acta Paediatr Suppl 423:33.

364. Netchine I, Talon P, Dastot F, et al. (1998). Extensive phenotypic analysis of a family with growth hormone (GH) deficiency caused by a mutation in the GH-releasing hormone receptor gene. J Clin 83:432.

365. Salvatori R, Hayashida CY, Aguilar-Oliveira MH, et al. (1999). Familial dwarfism due to a novel mutation of the growth hormone-releasing hormone receptor gene. J Clin Endocrinol Metab 84:917.

366. Miller WL, Kaplan SL, Grumbach MM (1980). Child abuse as a cause of post-traumatic hypopituitarism. N Engl J Med 302:724.

367. Craft WH, Underwood LE, Van Wyk JJ (1980). High incidence of perinatal insult in children with idiopathic hypopituitarism. J Pediatr 96:397.

368. Mayfield RK, Levine JH, Gordon L, et al. (1980). Lymphadenoid hypophysitis presenting as a pituitary tumor. Am J Med 69:619.

369. Bartsocas CS, Pantelakis SN (1973). Human growth hormone therapy in hypopituitarism due to tuberculous meningitis. Acta Paediatr Scand 62:304.

370. Stuart CA, Neelon FA, Lebovitz HE (1978). Hypothalamic insufficiency: The cause of hypopituitarism in sarcoidosis. Ann Intern Med 88:589.

371. Costin G (1979). Endocrine disorders associated with tumors of the pituitary and hypothalamus. Pediatr Clin North Am 26:15.

372. Brauner R, Rappaport R, Prevot C, et al. (1989). A prospective study of the development of growth hormone deficiency in children given cranial irradiation and its relation to statural growth. J Clin Endocrinol Metab 68:346.

373. Shalet SM (1986). Irradiation-induced growth failure. Pediatr Clin North Am 15:591.

374. Blatt J, Bercu BB, Gillin JC, et al. (1984). Reduced pulsatile growth hormone secretion in children after therapy for acute lymphoblastic leukemia. J Pediatr 104:182.

375. Stubberfield TG, Byrne GC, Jones TW (1995). Growth and growth hormone secretion after treatment for acute lymphoblastic leukemia in childhood. J Pediatr Hematol Oncol 17:167.

376. Albertsson-Wikland K, Lannering B, Marky I, et al. (1987). A longitudinal study on growth and spontaneous growth hormone (GH) secretion in children with irradiated brain tumors. Acta Paediatr Scand 76:966.

377. Pankin JM (1974). Incidence of growth hormone deficiency. Arch Dis Child 49:904.

378. Vimpani GV, Vimpani AF, Lidgard GP, et al. (1977). Prevalence of severe growth hormone deficiency. BMJ 2:427.

379. Lindsay R, Feldkamp M, Harris D, et al. (1994). Utah Growth Study: Growth standards and the prevalence of growth hormone deficiency. J Pediatr 125:29.

380. Sornson MW, Wu W, Dasen JS, et al. (1996). Pituitary lineage determination by the Prophet of Pit-1 homeodomain factor defective in Ames dwarfism. Nature 384:327.

381. Deladoey J, Fluck C, Buyu K, Gebiz A (1999). Hot spot in the PROP1 gene responsible for combined pituitary hormone deficiency. J Clin Endocrinol Metab 84:1645.

382. Fofanova O, Takamura N, Kinoshita E, et al. (1998). Compound heterozygous deletion of the PROP-1 gene in children with combined pituitary hormone deficiency. J Clin Endocrinol Metab 83:2601.

383. Wu W, Cogan JD, Pfaffle RW, et al. (1998). Mutations in PROP1 cause familial combined pituitary hormone deficiency. Nat Genet 18:147.

384. Brown MR, et al. (1998). Prop-1 mutations and hypopituitarism in Poland. In, Proceedings of the 80th Annual Meeting of the Endocrine Society. [city: publisher].

385. Parks JS, et al. (1998). Natural history and molecular mechanisms of hypopituitarism with large sella turcica. In, Proceedings of the 80th Annual Meeting of the Endocrine Society.

386. Camper SA, Sanders TL, Katz RW, et al. (1990). The Pit-1 transcription factor gene is a candidate for the murine Snell dwarf mutation. Genomics 8:586.

387. Pfaffle RW, DiMattia GE, Parks JS (1992). Mutation of the POU-specific domain of Pit-1 and hypopituitarism without pituitary hypoplasia. Science 257:1118.

388. Radovick S, Nations M, Du Y, et al. (1992). A mutation in the POU-homeodomain of Pit-1 responsible for combined pituitary hormone deficiency. Science 257:1115.

389. Fofanova OV, Takamura N, Kinoshita E, et al. (1998). Rarity of PIT1 involvement in children from Russia with combined pituitary hormone deficiency. Am J Med Genet 77:360.

390. Sadeghi-Nejad A, Senior B (1974). Autosomal dominant transmission of isolated growth hormone deficiency in iris-dental dysplasia (Rieger's syndrome). J Pediatr 85:644.

391. Semina EV, Reiter R, Leysens NJ, et al. (1996). Cloning and characterization of a novel bicoid-related homeobox transcription factor gene, RIEG, involved in Rieger syndrome. Nat Genet 14:392.

392. Phillips JA III, Hjell BL, Seeburg PH, et al. (1981). Molecular basis for familial isolated growth hormone deficiency. Proc Natl Acad Sci USA 78:6372.

393. Phillips JA III, Cogan JD (1994). Genetic basis of endocrine disease: VI. Molecular basis of familial human growth hormone deficiency. J Clin Endocrinol Metab 76:11.

394. Illig R, Prader A, Ferrandez A, et al. (1971). Hereditary prenatal growth hormone deficiency with increased tendency to growth hormone antibody formation: "A-type" of isolated growth hormone deficiency. Acta Paediatr Scand 60:607.

395. Cogan JD, Phillips JA III (1998). Growth disorders caused by genetic defects in the growth hormone pathway. Adv Pediatr 45:337.

396. Wagner JK, Eble A, Hindmarsh PC, Mullis PE (1998). Prevalence of human GH-1 alterations in patients with isolated growth hormone deficiency. Pediatr Res 43:105.

397. Cogan JD, Phillips JA III, et al. (1993). Heterogeneous growth hormone (GH) gene mutations in familial GH deficiency. J Clin Endocrinol Metab 76:1224.

398. Fujisawa I, Kikuchi K, Nishimura K, et al. (1987). Transection of the pituitary stalk: Development of an ectopic posterior lobe assessed with MR imaging. Radiology 165:487.

399. Abrahams JJ, Trefelner E, Boulware SD (1991). Idiopathic growth hormone deficiency: MR findings in 35 patients. Am J Neuroradiol 12:155.

400. Kuroiwa T, Okabe Y, Hasuo K, et al. (1991). MR imaging of pituitary dwarfism. Am J Neuroradiol 12:161.

401. Hamilton J, Blaser S, Daneman D (1998). MR imaging in idiopathic growth hormone deficiency. Am J Neuroradiol 19:1609.

402. Kornreich L, Horev G, Lazar L, et al. (1998). MR findings in growth hormone deficiency: Correlation with severity of hypopituitarism. Am J Neuroradiol 19:1495.

403. Jenkins JS, Gilberg CJ, Ang V (1976). Hypothalamic-pituitary function in patients with craniopharyngiomas. J Clin Endocrinol Metab 43:394.

404. Thomsett MJ, Conte FA, Kaplan SL, et al. (1980). Endocrine and neurologic outcome in childhood craniopharyngioma: Review of effect of treatment in 42 patients. J Pediatr 97:728.

405. Braunstein GD, Kohler PO (1972). Pituitary function in Hand-Schüller-Christian disease: Evidence for deficient growth hormone release in patients with short stature. N Engl J Med 286:1225.

406. Powell GF, Brasel JA, Blizzard RM (1967). Emotional deprivation and growth retardation simulating idiopathic hypopituitarism. N Engl J Med 276:1271.

407. Blizzard RM (1985). Psychosocial short stature. In Lifshitz F (ed.), Pediatric endocrinology. New York: Marcel Dekker 87–107.

408. Spiliotis BE, August GP, Hung W, et al. (1984). Growth hormone neurosecretory dysfunction: A treatable cause of short stature. JAMA 252:2223.

409. Bercu BB, Shulman D, Root AW, et al. (1986). Growth hormone (GH) provocative testing frequently does not reflect endogenous GH secretion. J Clin Endocrinol Metab 63:709.

410. Tauber M, Moulin P, Pienkowski C, et al. (1997). Growth hormone (GH) retesting and auxological data in 131 GH-deficient patients after completion of treatment. J Clin Endocrinol Metab 82:352.

411. Maghnie M, Strigazzi C, Tinelli C, et al. (1999). Growth hormone (GH) deficiency (GHD) of childhood onset: Reassessment of GH status and evaluation of the predictive criteria for permanent GHD in young adults. J Clin Endocrinol Metab 84:1324.

412. Toogood AA, Shalet SM (1997). Diagnosis of severe growth hormone (GH) deficiency in young adults who received GH replacement therapy during childhood. Acta Paediatr Suppl 423:117.

413. Valenta LJ, Sigel MB, Lesniak MA, et al. (1985). Pituitary dwarfism in a patient with circulating abnormal growth hormone polymers. N Engl J Med 312:214.

414. Takahashi Y, Kaji H, Okimura Y, et al. (1996). Brief report: Short stature caused by a mutant growth hormone. N Engl J Med 334:432.

415. Takahashi Y, Shirono H, Arisaka O, et al. (1997). Biologically inactive growth hormone caused by an amino acid substitution. J Clin Invest 100:1159.

416. Laron Z, Pertzelan A, Mannheimer S (1966). Genetic pituitary dwarfism with high serum concentration of growth hormone: A new inborn error of metabolism? Isr J Med Sci 2:152.

417. Rosenbloom AL, Guevara-Aguirre J, Rosenfeld RG, et al. (1990). The little women of Loja: Growth hormone receptor deficiency in an inbred population of southern Ecuador. N Engl J Med 323:1367.

418. Golde DW, Bersch N, Kaplan SA, et al. (1980). Peripheral unresponsiveness to human growth hormone in Laron dwarfism. N Engl J Med 303:1156.

419. Eshet R, Laron Z, Pertzelan A, et al. (1984). Defect of human growth hormone receptors in the liver of two patients with Laron-type dwarfism. Isr J Med Sci 20:8.

420. Godowski PJ, Leung DW, Meacham LR, et al. (1989). Characterization of the human growth hormone receptor gene and demonstration of a partial gene deletion in two patients with Laron-type dwarfism. Proc Natl Acad Sci USA 86:8083.

421. Amselem S, Duquesnoy P, Attree O, et al. (1989). Laron dwarfism and mutations of the growth hormone-receptor gene. N Engl J Med 321:989.

422. Berg MA, Guevara-Aguirre J, Rosenbloom AL, et al. (1992). Mutation creating a new splice site in the growth hormone receptor genes of 37 Ecuadorian patients with Laron syndrome. Hum Mutat 1:24.

423. Amselem S, et al. (1993). Molecular analysis of two families with Laron syndrome and positive growth hormone binding protein. Fourth Joint LWPES/ESPE Meeting, San Francisco [details of publication].

424. Kou K, Lajara R, Rotwein P (1993). Amino acid substitutions in the intracellular part of the growth hormone receptor in a patient with Laron syndrome. J Clin Endocrinol Metab 76:54.

425. Woods KA, Fraser NC, Postel-Vinay MC, et al. (1996). A homozygous splice site mutation affecting the intracellular domain of the growth hormone (GH) receptor resulting in Laron syndrome with elevated GH-binding protein. J Clin Endocrinol Metab 81:1686.

426. Silbergeld A, Dastot F, Klinger B, et al. (1997). Intronic mutation in the growth hormone (GH) receptor gene from a girl with Laron syndrome and extremely high serum GH binding protein: Extended phenotypic study in a very large pedigree. J Pediatr Endocrinol Metab 10:265.

427. Ayling RM, Ross R, Towner P, et al. (1997). A dominant-negative mutation of the growth hormone receptor causes familial short stature. Nat Genet 16:13.

428. Rosenfeld RG, Belgorosky A, Camacho-Hubner C, Savage MO, Wit JM, Hwa V (2007). Defects in growth hormone receptor signaling. Trends Endocrinol Metab 18(4):134–141.

429. Hwa V, Haeusler G, Pratt KL, Little BM, Frisch H, Koller D, et al. (2006). Total absence of functional acid labile subunit, resulting in severe insulin-like growth factor deficiency and moderate growth failure. J Clin Endocrinol Metab 91(5):1826–1831

430. Baker J, Liu JP, Robertson EJ, Efstratiadis A (1993). Role of insulin-like growth factors in embryonic and postnatal growth. Cell 75:73.

431. Walenkamp MJ, Wit JM (2006). Genetic disorders in the growth hormone-insulin-like growth factor-I axis. Horm Res 66(5):221–230.

432. Woods KA, Camacho-Hubner C, Bergman RN, et al. (2000). Effects of insulin-like growth factor I (IGF-1) therapy on body composition and insulin resistance in IGF-1 gene deletion. J Clin Endocrinol Metab 85:1407.

433. Copeland KC, Franks RC, Ramamurthy R (1981). Neonatal hyperbilirubinemia and hypoglycemia in congenital hypopituitarism. Clin Pediatr 20:523.

434. Lovinger RD, Kaplan SL, Grumbach MM (1975). Congenital hypopituitarism associated with neonatal hypoglycemia and microphallus: Four cases secondary to hypothalamic hormone deficiencies. J Pediatr 87:1171.

435. Frasier SD (1974). A review of growth hormone stimulation tests in children. Pediatrics 53:929.

436. Underwood LE, Azumi K, Voina SJ, et al. (1971). Growth hormone levels during sleep in normal and growth hormone deficient children. Pediatrics 48:946.

437. Buckler JMH (1973). Plasma growth hormone response to exercise as a diagnostic aid. Arch Dis Child 48:565.

438. Lacey KA, Hewison A, Parkin JM (1973). Exercise as a screening test for growth hormone deficiency in children. Arch Dis Child 48:508.

439. Collu R, Leboeuf G, Letarte J (1975). Stimulation of growth hormone secretion by levodopa-propranolol in children and adolescents. Pediatrics 56:262.

440. Lanes R, Hurtado E (1982). Oral clonidine: An effective growth hormone-releasing agent in prepubertal subjects. J Pediatr 100:710.

441. Mitchell ML, Bryne MJ, Sanchez Y, Sawin CT (1970). Detection of growth hormone deficiency. N Engl J Med 282:539.

442. Merimee TJ, Rabinowitz D, Fineberg SE (1969). Arginine-initiated release of human growth hormone. N Engl J Med 280:1434.

443. Kaplan SL, Abrams CAL, Bell JJ (1968). Growth and growth hormone: I. Changes in serum levels of growth hormone following hypoglycemia in 134 children with growth retardation. Pediatr Res 2:43.

444. Root AW, Rosenfield RL, Bongiovanni AM, et al. (1967). The plasma growth hormone response to insulin-induced hypoglycemia in children with retardation of growth. Pediatrics 39:844.

445. Penny R, Blizzard RM, Davis WT (1969). Sequential arginine and insulin tolerance tests on the same day. J Clin Endocrinol Metab 29:1499.

446. Fass B, Lippe BM, Kaplan SA (1979). Relative usefulness of three growth hormone stimulation screening tests. Am J Dis Child 133:931.

447. Weldon, Gupta SK, Klingensmith G (1975). Evaluation of growth hormone release in children using arginine and l-dopa in combination. J Pediatr 87:540.

448. Reiter EO, Martha PMJ (1990). Pharmacological testing of growth hormone secretion. Horm Res 33:121.

449. Raiti S, Davis WT, Blizzard RM (1967). A comparison of the effects of insulin hypoglycemia and arginine infusion on release of human growth hormone. Lancet 2:1182.

450. Guyda HJ (2000). Growth hormone testing and the short child. Pediatr Res 48:579.

451. [author/editor] (1994). Physicians' desk reference, Forty-eighth edition. Montvale, NJ: Medical Economics Data Production 1004.

452. [author/editor] (1994). Physicians' desk reference, Forty-eighth edition. Montvale, NJ: Medical Economics Data Production 1228.

453. Martha PM Jr., Gorman KM, Blizzard RM, et al. (1992). Endogenous growth hormone secretion and clearance rates in normal boys, as determined by deconvolution analysis: Relationship to age, pubertal status, and body mass. J Clin Endocrinol Metab 74:336.

454. Lippe B, Wong S-LR, Kaplan SA (1971). Simultaneous assessment of growth hormone and ACTH reserve in children pretreated with diethylstilbestrol. J Clin Endocrinol 33:949.

455. Chernausek SD (1987). Laboratory diagnosis of growth disorders. In Hintz RL, Rosenfeld RG (eds.), Growth abnormalities: Contemporary issues in endocrinology and metabolism. New York: Churchill Livingstone 231.

456. Bourmelen M, Pham-Huu-Trung MT, Girard F (1979). Transient partial GH deficiency in prepubertal children with delay of growth. Pediatr Res 13:221.

457. Cacciari E, Tassoni P, Parisi G, et al. (1974). Pitfalls in diagnosing impaired growth hormone (GH) secretion: Retesting after replacement therapy of 63 children defined as GH deficient. J Clin Endocrinol Metab 74:1284.

458. Marin G, Domene HM, Barnes KM, et al. (1994). The effects of estrogen priming and puberty on the growth hormone response to standardized treadmill exercise and arginine-insulin in normal girls and boys. J Clin Endocrinol Metab 79:537.

459. Lee MM (2006). Clinical practice: Idiopathic short stature. N Engl J Med 354(24):2576–2582.

460. Reiter EO, Morris AH, MacGillivray MH, et al. (1988). Variable estimates of serum growth hormone concentrations by difference radioassay systems. J Clin Endocrinol Metab 66:68.

461. Celniker AC, Chem AB, Wert RM Jr, et al. (1989). Variability in the quantitation of circulating growth hormone using commercial immunoassays. J Clin Endocrinol Metab 68:469.

462. Mauras N, Walton P, Nicar M, et al. (2000). Growth hormone stimulating testing in both short and normal statured children: Use of an immunofunctional assay. Pediatr Res 48:614.

463. Shah A, Stanhope R, Matthews D (1992). Hazards of pharmacological tests of growth hormone secretion in childhood. BMJ 304:173.

464. Eddy RL, Gilliland PF, Ibarra JD Jr., et al. (1974). Human growth hormone release: Comparison of provocative test procedures. Am J Med 56:179.

465. Zadik Z, Chalew SA, Raiti S, et al. (1985). Do short children secrete insufficient growth hormone? Pediatrics 76:355.

466. Tassoni P, Cacciari E, Cau M, et al. (1990). Variability of growth hormone response to pharmacological and sleep tests performed twice in short children. J Clin Endocrinol Metab 71:230.

467. Donaldson DL, Hollowell JG, Pan F, et al. (1989). Growth hormone secretory profiles: Variation on consecutive nights. J Pediatr 115:51.

468. Rose SR, Ross JL, Uriarte M, et al. (1988). The advantage of measuring stimulated as compared with spontaneous growth hormone levels in the diagnosis of growth hormone deficiency. N Engl J Med 319:201.

469. Lanes R (1989). Diagnostic limitations of spontaneous growth hormone measurements in normally growing prepubertal children. Am J Dis Child 143:1284.

470. Hourd P, Edwards R (1994). Current methods for the measurement of growth hormone in urine. Clin Endocrinol 40:155.

471. Albini CH, Quattrin T, Vandlen RL, et al. (1988). Quantitation of urinary growth hormone in children with normal and subnormal growth. Pediatr Res 23:89.

472. Granada ML, Sanmarti A, Lucas A, et al. (1992). Clinical usefulness of urinary growth hormone measurements in normal and short children according to different expressions of urinary growth hormone data. Pediatr Res 32:73.

473. Juul A, Katstrup KW, Pedersen SA, Skakkebaek NE (1997). Growth hormone (GH) provocative retesting of 108 young adults with childhood-onset GH deficiency and the diagnostic value of insulin-like growth factor I (IGF-I) and IGF-binding protein-3. J Clin Endocrinol Metab 82:1195.

474. Hasegawa Y, Hasegawa T, Aso T, et al. (1994). Clinical utility of insulin-like growth factor binding protein-3 in the evaluation and treatment of short children with suspected growth hormone deficiency. Eur J Endocrinol 131:27.

475. Hasegawa Y, Hasegawa T, Aso T, et al. (1992). Usefulness and limitation of measurement of insulin-like growth factor binding protein-3 (IGFBP-3) for diagnosis of growth hormone deficiency. Endocrinol Jpn 39:585.

476. Smith WJ, Nam TJ, Underwood LE, et al. (1993). Use of insulin-like growth factor binding protein-2 (IGFBP-2), IGFBP-3, and IGF-I for assessing growth hormone status in short children. J Clin Endocrinol Metab 77:1294.

477. Savage MO, Blum WF, Ranke MB, et al. (1993). Clinical features and endocrine status in patients with growth hormone insensitivity (Laron syndrome). J Clin Endocrinol Metab 77:1465.

478. Guevara-Aguirre J, Rosenbloom AL, Fielder PJ, et al. (1993). Growth hormone receptor deficiency in Ecuador: Clinical and biochemical phenotype in two populations. J Clin Endocrinol Metab 76:417.

479. Bhala A, Harris M, Cohen P (1998). Insulin-like growth factors and their binding proteins in critically ill neonates. J Pediatr Endocrinol 11:451.

480. Ranke MB, Lindberg A, Chatelain P, et al. (1999). Derivation and validation of a mathematical model for predicting the response to exogenous recombinant human growth hormone (GH) in prepubertal children with idiopathic GH deficiency: Kabi Pharmacia International Growth Study. J Clin Endocrinol Metab 84:1174.

481. Savage MO, Rosenfeld RG (1999). Growth hormone insensitivity: A proposed revised classification. Acta Paediatr Suppl 428:147.

482. Blum WF, Ranke MB, Savage MO, et al. (1992). Insulin-like growth factors and their binding proteins in patients with growth hormone receptor deficiency: Suggestions for new diagnostic criteria. Acta Paediatr 383:125.

483. Rosenfeld RG, Kemp SF, Hintz RL (1981). Constancy of somatomedin response to growth hormone treatment of hypopituitary dwarfism and lack of correlation with growth rate. J Clin Endocrinol Metab 53:611.

484. Douquesnoy P, Sobrier ML, Duriez B, et al. (1994). A single amino acid substitution in the exoplasmic domain of the human growth hormone (GH) receptor confers familial GH resistance (Laron syndrome) with positive GH-binding activity by abolishing receptor homodimerization. EMBO J 13:1386.

485. Bierich JR (1982). Constitutional delay of growth and adolescent development. Eur J Pediatr 139:221.

486. Clayton PE, Shalet SM, Price DA (1988). Endocrine manipulation of constitutional delay in growth and puberty. J Endocrinol 116:321.

487. Eastman CJ, Lazarus L, Stuart MC, et al. (1971). The effect of puberty on growth hormone secretion in boys with short stature and delayed adolescence. Aust NZ J Med 1:154.

488. Rosenfeld RG, Northcraft GB, Hintz RL (1982). A prospective, randomized trial of testosterone treatment of constitutional short stature in adolescent males. Pediatrics 69:681.

489. Richman RA, Kirsch LR (1988). Testosterone treatment in adolescent boys with constitutional delay in growth and development. N Engl J Med 319:1563.

490. Wilson DM, Kei J, Hintz RL, et al. (1988). Effects of testosterone enanthate therapy for pubertal delay. Am J Dis Child 142:96.

491. Wang C, Swerdloff RS, Iranmanesh A, et al. (2000). Transdermal testosterone gel improves sexual function, mood, muscle strength and body composition parameters in hypogonadal men: Testosterone Gel Study Group. J Clin Endocrinol Metab 85:2839.

492. Ahmed SR, Boucher AE, Manni A, et al. (1988). Transdermal testosterone therapy in the treatment of male hypogonadism. J Clin Endocrinol Metab 66:546.

493. Fradkin JE (1993). Creutzfeldt-Jakob disease in pituitary growth hormone recipients. Endocrinologist 3:108.

494. Buchanan CR, Preece MA, Milner RDG (1991). Mortality, neoplasia, and Creutzfeldt-Jakob disease in patients treated with human pituitary growth hormone in the United States. BMJ 302:824.

495. Hintz RL, Rosenfeld RG, Wilson DM, et al. (19982). Biosynthetic methionyl-human growth hormone is biologically active in adult humans. Lancet 1:1276.

496. Kaplan SL, Underwood LE, August GP, et al. (1986). Clinical studies with recombinant-DNA-derived methionyl-hGH in GH deficient children. Lancet 1:697.

497. Grimberg A, Cohen P (1997). Optimizing growth hormone therapy in children. Horm Res 48:11.

498. Albertsson-Wikland K, Westphal O, Westgren U (1986). Daily subcutaneous administration of human growth hormone in growth hormone deficient children. Acta Paediatr Scand 75:89.

499. Jorgensen JO, Muller N, Lauitzen T, et al. (1990). Evening versus morning injections of growth hormone (GH) in GH-deficient patients: Effects on 24-hour patterns of circulating hormones and metabolites. J Clin Endocrinol Metab 70:207.

500. Saggese G, Ranke MB, Saenger P, et al. (1998). Diagnosis and treatment of growth hormone deficiency in children and adolescents: Towards a consensus, Ten years after the availability of recombinant human growth hormone. Horm Res 50:320.

501. Frasier SD, Costin G, Lippe BM, et al. (1981). A dose-response curve for human growth hormone. J Clin Endocrinol Metab 53:1213.

502. Cohen P, Rosenfeld RG for the American Norditropin Trial Group (1997). Dose response effects of growth hormone on auxological and biochemical parameters in GH deficient children. Endocrinol Metab 4S:59.

503. Ranke MB, Schweizer R, Wollmann HA, Schwarze P (1999). Dosing of growth hormone in growth hormone deficiency. Horm Res 50:70.

504. Sudfeld H, Kiese K, Heinecke A, Bramswig JH (2000). Prediction of growth response in prepubertal children treated with growth hormone for idiopathic growth hormone deficiency. Acta Paediatr 89:34.

505. Blethen SL, Baptista J, Kuntze J, et al. (1997). Adult height in growth hormone (GH)-deficient children treated with biosynthetic GH: The Genentech Growth Study Group. J Clin Endocrinol Metab 82:418.

506. Mauras N, Attie KM, Reiter EO, et al. (2000). High dose recombinant human growth hormone (GH) treatment of GH-deficient patients in puberty increases near-final height: A randomized, multicenter trial: Genentech, Inc., Cooperative Study Group. J Clin Endocrinol Metab 85:3653.

507. Stanhope R, Uruena M, Hindmarsh P, et al. (1991). Management of growth hormone deficiency through puberty. Acta Paediatr Scand Suppl 372:47.

508. Bercu BB, Walker RF (1996). Xenobiotic growth hormone secretagogues: Growth hormone releasing peptides. In [editor(s)] eds.), *Growth hormone secretagogues.* New York: Springer 9–28.

509. Svensson J, Bengtsson BA (1999). Clinical and experimental effects of growth hormone secretagogues on various organ systems. Horm Res 51:16.

510. Ghigo E, Arvat E, Camanni F (1998). Orally active growth hormone secretagogues: State of the art and clinical perspectives. Ann Med 30:159.

511. Thorner M, Rochiccioli P, Colle M, et al. (1996). Once daily subcutaneous growth hormone–releasing hormone therapy accelerates growth in growth hormone–deficient children during the first year of therapy: Geref International Study Group. J Clin Endocrinol Metab 81:1189.

512. Duck SC, Rapaport R (1999). Long term treatment with GHRH(1–44) amide in prepubertal children with classical growth hormone deficiency. J Pediatr Endocrinol Metab 12:531.

513. Lippe BM, Van Herle AJ, LaFranchi SH, et al. (1975). Reversible hypothyroidism in growth-hormone deficient children treated with human growth hormone. J Clin Endocrinol Metab 40:612.

514. Guthrie RD, Smith SW, Graham CB (1975). Testosterone treatment for micropenis during early childhood. J Pediatr 83:247.

515. Juul A (1999). Determination of insulin-like growth factor-I in the monitoring of growth hormone treatment with respect to efficacy of treatment and side effects: Should potential risks of cardiovascular disease and cancer be considered? Horm Res 51:141.

516. Cowell CT, Loke KY, Baxter RC (1993). The response of the insulin-like growth factor binding protein 3 complex to growth hormone. Clin Pediatr Endocrinol 2:45.

517. Cohen P, Rogol AD, Howard CP, Bright GM, Kappelgaard AM, Rosenfeld RG (2007). Effects of IGF-based dosing on the efficacy of GH therapy in children: Results of a randomized concentration-controlled study. J Clin Endocrinol and Metab 92:2480–2486.

518. Shim M, Cohen P (1999). IGFs and human cancer: Implications regarding the risk of growth hormone therapy. Horm Res 51:42.

519. Cohen P (1998). Serum insulin-like growth factor-I levels and prostate cancer risk: Interpreting the evidence. J Natl Cancer Inst 90:876.

520. Ranke MB (1995). Growth hormone therapy in children: When to stop? Horm Res 104:122.

521. Kaufman FR, Sy JP (1999). Regular monitoring of bone age is useful in children treated with growth hormone. Pediatrics 104:1039.

522. Wilson DM (1999). Regular monitoring of bone age is not useful in children treated with growth hormone. Pediatrics 104:1036.

523. Guidelines for the use of growth hormone in children with short stature: A report by the Drug and Therapeutics Committee of the Lawson Wilkins Pediatric Endocrine Society. J Pediatr 127:857.

524. Retegui LA, Masson PL, Paladini AC (1985). Specificities of antibodies to human growth hormone (hGH) in patients treated with hGH: Longitudinal study and comparison with the specificities of animal antisera. J Clin Endocrinol Metab 60:184.

525. Burns EC, Tanner JM, Preece MA, et al. (1981). Final height and pubertal development in 55 children with idiopathic growth hormone deficiency, treated for between 2 and 15 years with human growth hormone. Eur J Pediatr 137:155.

526. Dean HJ, McTaggart TL, Fish DG, et al. (1985). The educational, vocational, and marital status of growth hormone-deficient adults treated with growth hormone during childhood. Am J Dis Child 139:1105.

527. Salomon F, Cuneo RC, Hesp R, et al. (1989). The effects of treatment with recombinant human growth hormone on body composition and metabolism in adults with growth hormone deficiency. N Engl J Med 321:1797.

528. Bengtsson B-A, Eden S, Lonn L, et al. (1993). Treatment of adults with growth hormone deficiency with recombinant human growth hormone. J Clin Endocrinol Metab 76:309.

529. Rosen T, Bengtsson B-A (1990). Premature mortality due to cardiovascular disease in hypopituitarism. Lancet 336:285.

530. Sonksen PH, Cuneo RC, Salomon F, et al. (1991). Growth hormone therapy in adults with growth hormone deficiency. Acta Paediatr Scand 379:139.

531. Mardh G, Lundin K, Borg B, et al. (1994). Growth hormone replacement therapy in adult hypopituitary patients with growth hormone deficiency: Combined data from 12 European placebo-controlled clinical trials. Endocrinol Metab 1(A):43.

532. Toogood AA, Beardwell CG, Shalet SM (1994). The severity of growth hormone deficiency in adults with pituitary disease is related to the degree of hypopituitarism. Clin Endocrinol (Oxford) 41:511.

533. Growth Hormone Research Society (1998). Consensus guidelines for the diagnosis and treatment of adults with growth hormone deficiency: Summary statement of the Growth Hormone Research Society Workshop on Adult Growth Hormone Deficiency. J Clin Endocrinol Metab 83:379.

534. Tonshoff B, Mehls O, Heinrich U, et al. (1990). Growth-stimulating effects of recombinant human growth hormone in children with end-stage renal disease. J Pediatr 116:561.

535. Hokken-Koelega ACS, Stijnen T, De Muinck Keizer-Schrama SMPF, et al. (1991). Placebo-controlled, double-blind, cross-over trial of growth hormone treatment in prepubertal children with chronic renal failure. Lancet 338:585.

536. Fine RN, Kohaut EC, Brown D, et al. (1994). Growth after recombinant human growth hormone treatment in children with chronic renal failure: Report of a multicenter randomized double-blind placebo-controlled study. J Pediatr 124:374.

537. Rudman D, Goldsmith M, Kutner M, Blackston D (1980). Effect of growth hormone and oxandrolone singly and together on growth rate in girls with X chromosome abnormalities. J Pediatr 96:132.

538. Forbes AP, Jacobsen JG, Carroll EL, et al. (1962). Studies of growth arrest in gonadal dysgenesis: Response to exogenous human growth hormone. Metabolism 11:56.

539. Rosenfeld RG, Frane J, Attie KM, et al. (1992). Six-year results of a randomized, prospective trial of human growth hormone and oxandrolone in Turner syndrome. J Pediatr 121:49.

540. Chernausek SD, Attie KM, Cara JF, et al. (2000). Growth hormone therapy of Turner syndrome: The impact of age of estrogen replacement on final height. J Clin Endocrinol Metab 85:2439.

541. Anneren G, Sara VR, Hall K, et al. (1986). Growth and somatomedin responses to growth hormone in Down's syndrome. Arch Dis Child 61:48.

542. Torrado C, Bastian W, Wisniewski KE, et al. (1991). Treatment of children with Down syndrome and growth retardation with recombinant human growth hormone. J Pediatr 119:478.

543. Chatelain PG (1993). Auxology and response to growth hormone treatment of patients with intrauterine growth retardation or Silver-Russell syndrome: Analysis of data from the Kabi Pharmacia International Growth Study. Acta Paediatr Suppl 391:79.

544. deZegher F, Maes M, Heinrichs C, et al. (1994). High-dose growth hormone therapy for short children born small for gestational age. Acta Paediatr Suppl 399:77.

545. Coutant R, Carel J-C, Letrait M, et al. (1998). Short stature associated with intrauterine growth retardation: Final height of untreated and growth hormone-treated children. J Clin Endocrinol Metab 83:1070.

546. Clayton PE, Cianfarani S, Czernichow P, Johannsson G, Rapaport R, Rogol A (2007). Management of the child born small for gestational age through to adulthood: A consensus statement of the International Societies of Pediatric Endocrinology and the Growth Hormone Research Society. J Clin Endocrinol Metab 92(3):804–810.

547. de Zegher F, Albertsson-Wikland K, Wollmann HA, et al. (2000). Growth hormone treatment of short children born small for gestational age: Growth responses with continuous and discontinuous regimens over 6 years. J Clin Endocrinol Metab 85:2816.

548. Lindgren AC, Hagenas L, Muller J, et al. (1998). Growth hormone treatment of children with Prader-Willi syndrome affects linear growth and body composition favourably. Acta Paediatr 87:28.

549. Hardin DS, Kemp SF, Allen DB (2007). Twenty years of recombinant human growth hormone in children: Relevance to pediatric care providers. Clin Pediatr 46:279–286.

550. Seino Y, Yamate T, Kanzaki S, et al. (1994). Achondroplasia: Effect of growth hormone in 40 patients. Clin Pediatr Endocrinol 3(4):41.

551. Kelnar CJ, Albertsson-Wikland K, Hintz RL, et al. (1999). Should we treat children with idiopathic short stature? Horm Res 52:150.

552. Van Vliet G, Styne DM, Kaplan SL, et al. (1983). Growth hormone treatment for short stature. N Engl J Med 309:1016.

553. Gertner JM, Henel M, Gianfredi SP, et al. (1984). Prospective clinical trial of human growth hormone in short children without growth hormone deficiency. J Pediatr 104:172.

554. Hopwood NJ, Hintz RL, Gertner JM, et al. (1993). Growth response of children with non-growth hormone deficiency and marked short stature during three years of growth hormone therapy. J Pediatr 123:215.

555. Hintz RL, Attie KM, Baptistra J, Roche A (1999). Effect of growth hormone treatment on adult height of children with idiopathic short stature: Genentech Collaborative. N Engl J Med 340:502.

556. Ranke MB, Lindberg A, Price DA, Darendeliler F, Albertsson-Wikland K, Wilton P, et al. for the KIGS International Board (2007). Age at growth hormone therapy start and first-year responsiveness to growth hormone are major determinants of height outcome in idiopathic short stature. Horm Res 68(2):53–62.

557. Allen DB, Brook CGD, Bridges NA, et al. (1994). Therapeutic controversies: Growth hormone (GH) treatment of non-GH deficient subjects. J Clin Endocrinol Metab 79:1239.

558. Rosenfeld RG, Buckway CK (2000). Should we treat genetic syndromes? J Pediatr Endocrinol Metab 13:971.

559. Allen DB, Fost NC (1990). Growth hormone therapy for short stature: Panacea or Pandora's box? J Pediatr 117:16.

560. Herber SM, Dunsmore IR (1988). Does control affect growth in diabetes mellitus? Acta Paediatr Scand 77:303.

561. Ergun-Longmire B, Mertens AC, Mitby P, Qin J, Heller G, Shi W, et al. (2006). Growth hormone treatment and risk of second neoplasms in the childhood cancer survivor. J Clin Endocrinol Metab 91(9):3494–3498.

562. Malozowski S, Tanner LA, Wysoluski D, et al. (1993). Growth hormone, insulin-like growth factor-I, and benign intracranial hypertension. N Engl J Med 329:665.

563. Harris WR (1950). The endocrine basis for slipping of the upper femoral epiphysis: An experimental study. J Bone Joint Surg 32B:5.

564. Kelsey JL (1973). Epidemiology of slipped capital femoral epiphysis: A review of the literature. Pediatrics 51:1042.

565. Rappaport EB, Fife D (1985). Slipped capital femoral epiphysis in growth hormone-deficient patients. Am J Dis Child 139:396.

566. Consensus guidelines for the diagnosis and treatment of growth hormone (GH) deficiency in childhood and adolescence: Summary statement of the GH Research Society. J Clin Endocrinol Metab 85:3990.

567. Alford FP, Hew FL, Christopher MC, Rantzau C (1999). Insulin sensitivity in growth hormone (GH)-deficient adults and effects of GH replacement therapy. J Endocrinol Invest 22:28.

568. Cutfield WS, Wilton P, Bennmarker H, et al. (2000). Incidence of diabetes mellitus and impaired glucose tolerance in children and adolescents receiving growth-hormone treatment. Lancet 355:610.

569. Wetterau L, Cohen P (2000). New paradigms for growth hormone therapy in children. Horm Res 53:31.

570. Chan JM, Stampfer MJ, Giovannucci E, et al. (1998). Plasma insulin-like growth factor-1 and prostate cancer risk: A prospective study. Science 279:563.

571. Hankinson SE, Willett WC, Colditz GA, et al. (1998). Circulating concentrations of insulin-like growth factor-1 and risk of breast cancer. Lancet 351:1393.

572. Ma J, Pollak MN, Giovannucci E, et al. (1999). Prospective study of colorectal cancer risk in men and plasma levels of insulin-like growth factor (IGF)-1 and IGF-binding protein-3. J Natl Cancer Inst 91:620.

573. Ron E, Gridley G, Hrubec Z, et al. (1991). Acromegaly and gastrointestinal cancer. Cancer 68:1673.

574. Popovic V, Damjanovic S, Micic D, et al. (1998). Increased incidence of neoplasia in patients with pituitary adenomas. Clin Endocrinol (Oxford) 49:44.

575. Bengtsson BA, Eden S, Ernest I, et al. (1988). Epidemiology and long-term survival in acromegaly: A study of 166 cases diagnosed between 1955 and 1984. Acta Med Scand 223:327.

576. Delhougne B, Deneux C, Abs R, et al. (1995). The prevalence of colonic polyps in acromegaly: A colonoscopic and pathological study in 103 patients. J Clin Endocrinol Metab 80:3223.

577. Ladas SD, Thalassinos NC, Ioannides G, Raptis SA (1994). Does acromegaly really predispose to an increased prevalence of gastrointestinal tumours? Clin Endocrinol (Oxford) 41:597.

578. Orme SM, McNally RJ, Cartwright RA, Belchetz PE (1998). Mortality and cancer incidence in acromegaly: A retrospective cohort study. J Clin Endocrinol Metab 83:2730.

579. Sonksen PH, Jacobs H, Orme S, Belchetz P (1997). Acromegaly and colonic cancer. Clin Endocrinol (Oxford) 47:647.

580. Renehan AG, O'Dwyer ST, Shalet SM (2000). Colorectal neoplasia in acromegaly: The reported increased prevalence is overestimated. Gut 46:440.

581. Colao A, Balzano A, Ferone D, et al. (1997). Increased prevalence of colonic polyps and altered lymphocyte subset pattern in the colonic lamina propria in acromegaly. Clin Endocrinol (Oxford) 47:23.

582. Nishi Y, Tanaka T, Takano K, et al. (1999). Recent status in the occurrence of leukemia in growth hormone-treated patients in Japan. J Clin Endocrinol Metab 84:1961.

583. Swerdlow AJ, Reddingius RE, Higgins CD, et al. (2000). Growth hormone treatment of children with brain tumors and risk of tumor recurrence. J Clin Endocrinol Metab 85:4444.

584. Abs R, Bengtsson BA, Hernberg-Stahl E, et al. (1999). GH replacement in 1034 growth hormone deficient hypopituitary adults: Demographic and clinical characteristics, dosing and safety. Clin Endocrinol (Oxford) 50:703.

585. Tuffli GA, Johanson A, Rundle AC, Allen DB (1995). Lack of increased risk for extracranial, nonleukemic neoplasms in recipients of recombinant deoxyribonucleic acid growth hormone. J Clin Endocrinol Metab 80:1416.

586. Cohen P, Clemmons DR, Rosenfeld RG (2000). Does the GH-IGF axis play a role in cancer pathogenesis? Growth Horm IGF Res 10:297.

587. Guler HP, Schmid C, Zapf J, et al. (1989). Effects of recombinant insulin-like growth factor-I on insulin secretion and renal function in normal human subjects. Proc Natl Acad Sci USA 86:2868.

588. Laron Z, Erster B, Klinger B, et al. (1988). Effects of acute administration of insulin-like growth factor-I in patients with Laron-type dwarfism. Lancet 2:1170.

589. Chernausek SD, Backeljauw PF, Frane J, Kuntze J, Underwood LE for the GH Insensitivity Syndrome Collaborative Group (2007). Long-term treatment with recombinant insulin-like growth factor (IGF)-I in children with severe IGF-I deficiency due to growth hormone insensitivity. J Clin Endocrinol Metab 92(3):902–910.

590. Laron Z, Anin S, Klipper-Auerbach Y, et al. (1992). Effects of insulin-like growth factor-I on linear growth, head circumference, and body fat in patients with Laron-type dwarfism. Lancet 339:1258.

591. Walker J, Van Wyk JJ, Underwood LE (1992). Stimulation of statural growth by recombinant insulin-like growth factor-I in a child with growth hormone insensitivity syndrome (Laron type). J Pediatr 121:641.

592. Wilton P for the Kabi Pharmacia Study Group (1992). Treatment with recombinant insulin-like growth factor-I of children with growth hormone receptor deficiency (Laron syndrome). Acta Paediatr 282:137.

593. Savage MO, Wilton P, Ranke MB, et al. (1993). Therapeutic response to recombinant IGF-I in thirty-two patients with growth hormone insensitivity. Pediatr Res 33:S5.

594. Guevara-Aguirre J, Vasconez O, Martinez V, et al. (1995). A randomized, double blind, placebo-controlled trial on safety and efficacy of recombinant human insulin-like growth factor-I in children with growth hormone receptor deficiency. J Clin Endocrinol Metab 80:1393.

595. Ranke MB, Savage MO, Chatelain PG, et al. (1999). Long-term treatment of growth hormone insensitivity syndrome with IGF-I: Results of the European multicentre study. Horm Res 51:128.

596. Morison IM, Becroft DM, Taniguchi T, et al. (1996). Somatic overgrowth associated with overexpression of insulin-like growth factor II. Nat Med 2:311.

597. Sakazume S, Okamoto N, Yamamoto T, Kurosawa K, Numabe H, Ohashi Y, et al. (2007). GPC3 mutations in seven patients with Simpson-Golabi-Behmel syndrome. Am J Med Genet A 143:1703–1707.

598. Saugier-Veber P, Bonnet C, Afenjar A, Drouin-Garraud V, Coubes C, Fehrenbach S, et al. (2007). Heterogeneity of NSD1 alterations in 116 patients with Sotos syndrome. Hum Mutat 28:1098–1107.

599. Sorgo W, Scholler K, Heinze F, et al. (1984). Critical analysis of height reduction in oestrogen-treated tall girls. Eur J Pediatr 142:260.

600. Kunwar S, Wilson CB (1999). Pediatric pituitary adenomas. J Clin Endocrinol Metab 84:4385.

601. Thapar K, Kovacs K, Stefanneanu I, et al. (1997). Overexpression of the growth hormone-releasing hormone gene in acromegaly-associated pituitary tumors. Am J Pathol 151:769.

602. Lafferty AR, Chrousos GP (1999). Pituitary tumors in children and adolescents. J Clin Endocrinol Metab 84:4317.

603. Fuqua JS, Berkovitz GD (1998). Growth hormone excess in a child with neurofibromatosis type 1 and optic pathway tumor: A patient report. Clin Pediatr 37:749.

604. Statakis CA, Carney JA, Lin JP, et al. (1996). Carney complex, a familial multiple neoplasia and lentiginosis syndrome: Analysis of 11 kindreds and linkage to the short arm of chromosome 2. J Clin Invest 97:699.

605. Holl RW, Bucher P, Sorgo W, et al. (1999). Suppression of growth hormone by oral glucose in the evaluation of tall stature. Horm Res 51:20.

606. Abe T, Tara LA, Ludecke DK (1999). Growth hormone–secreting pituitary adenoma in childhood and adolescence: Features and results of transnasal surgery. Neurosurgery 45:1.

607. Nanto-Salonen K, Koskinen P, Sonninen P, Toppari J (1999). Suppression of GH secretion in pituitary gigantism by continuous subcutaneous octreotide infusion in pubertal boy. Acta Paediatr 88:29.

608. Moran A, Pescovitz OH (1994). Long-term treatment of gigantism with combination octreotide and bromocriptine in a child with McCune-Albright syndrome. Endocrine J 2:111.

609. Trainer PJ, Drake WM, Katznelson L, et al. (2000). Treatment of acromegaly with the growth hormone receptor antagonist pegvisomant. N Engl J Med 342:1171.

610. Herman-Bonert VS, Zib K, Scarlett JA, Melmed S (2000). Growth hormone receptor antagonist therapy in acromegalic patients resistant to somatostatin analogs. J Clin Endocrinol Metab 85:2958.

Disorders of the Posterior Pituitary

LOUIS J. MUGLIA, MD, PhD • JOSEPH A. MAJZOUB, MD

Introduction

Maintenance of the tonicity of extracellular fluids within a very narrow range is crucial to proper cell function.[1,2] Extracellular osmolality regulates cell shape as well as intracellular concentrations of ions and other osmolytes. Furthermore, proper extracellular ionic concentrations are necessary for the correct function of ion channels, action potentials, and other modes of intercellular communication. Extracellular fluid tonicity is regulated almost exclusively by the amount of water intake and excretion, whereas extracellular volume is regulated by the level of sodium chloride intake and excretion. In children and adults, normal blood tonicity is maintained over a tenfold variation in water intake by a coordinated interaction among thirst, vasopressin, and renal systems. Dysfunction in any of these systems can result in abnormal regulation of blood osmolality, which if not properly recognized and treated may cause life-threatening dysfunction in neuronal and other cellular activities.

The posterior pituitary, or the neurohypophysis, secretes the nonapeptide hormones vasopressin and oxytocin. Vasopressin controls water homeostasis, and oxytocin regulates smooth-muscle contraction during parturition and lactation. Disorders of vasopressin secretion and action lead to clinically important derangements in water metabolism. In this chapter, the physiology of water and volume regulation is summarized, a symptom-based approach to the differential diagnosis of the diseases of water homeostasis is presented, and a review of the pathology and treatment of disorders involving these systems is provided. (See Chapter 12 for a discussion of defects in mineralocorticoid regulation that result in disturbances in volume regulation.)

Physiology of Osmotic and Volume Regulation

The control of plasma tonicity and intravascular volume involves a complex integration of endocrine, neural, and paracrine pathways. Osmotic sensor and effector

pathways control the regulation of vasopressin release and signal transduction, whereas volume homeostasis is determined largely through the action of the renin-angiotensin-aldosterone system—with contributions from vasopressin and the natriuretic peptide family. An improved understanding of the anatomic structures and molecules involved has developed through detailed molecular biologic and physiologic studies.

Osmotic Sensor and Effector Pathways

VASOPRESSIN AND OXYTOCIN BIOCHEMISTRY

Vasopressin and oxytocin are evolutionarily related peptides (paralogs), having arisen from gene duplication of a phylogenetically common molecule approximately 450 million years ago.[3,4] Both peptides consist of a 6-amino-acid disulfide ring plus a 3-amino-acid tail, with amidation of the carboxy terminus.[5,6] As early as 1895, a potent biologic principle (consisting of vascular pressor activity, "birth quickening," and milk secretory effects) was recognized in neurohypophyseal extracts.[7] The sequences of the individual peptides with pressor and antidiuretic capacity (vasopressin) and oxytocic capacity were determined by Du Vigneaud and colleagues during the mid 1950s,[6] culminating in the synthesis of each hormone in its biologically active form.[8,9]

In most mammals, vasopressin and oxytocin differ in only two amino acids: one substitution within the ring and one within the tail structure (Figure 9-1). Exploration of the structure-function relationship of specific amino acids within vasopressin and oxytocin has allowed characterization of molecules with substantial clinical use. Most notably, by replacement of l-arginine with d-arginine at position 8 of the vasopressin molecule and by amino-terminal deamidation an analogue with enhanced prolonged antidiuretic-to-pressor activity was found [desmopressin (desamino-d-arginine vasopressin; dDAVP); see Figure 9-1].[10] Desmopressin, with an antidiuretic potency

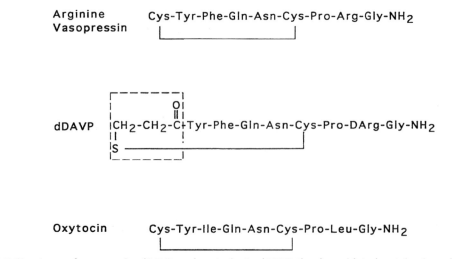

Figure 9-1 Structures of vasopressin, dDAVP, and oxytocin. In dDAVP, the de-amidated cysteine is enclosed in the box.

more than double that of its parent vasopressin, is now routinely used in clinical practice.

The association of vasopressin and oxytocin with specific proteins, the neurophysins, stored in the neurohypophysis was apparent as early as 1900.[11] Subsequent isolation and characterization of the neurophysins revealed two distinct forms: one type exclusively associated with vasopressin and the other exclusively associated with oxytocin.[12,13] Both are single-polypeptide chains of molecular weight 10,000 daltons. Despite extensive biophysical characterization, including crystallography of the oxytocin-neurophysin complex,[14,15] the biologic function of the neurophysins remains unclear. Possible roles for the neurophysins include stabilization against degradation during intracellular storage, more efficient packaging within secretory granules, and enhancement of post-translational processing by the proenzyme convertases.

The common origin of vasopressin and its neurophysin from a single larger precursor was first proposed by Sachs and colleagues,[16,17] who showed increased incorporation of ^{35}S cysteine (infused into canine third ventricle) into vasopressin isolated from the hypothalamus compared with vasopressin isolated from the posterior pituitary. Isolation of the larger precursor from the hypothalamus followed by trypsin-digestion-produced fragments of size similar to those of vasopressin and its neurophysin—with vasopressin immunoreactivity in the 1,000-dalton component.[18,19]

Since 1990, molecular genetic analyses have furthered the understanding of the synthesis, processing, and evolution of the vasopressin and oxytocin preprohormones. Human, mouse, rat, and bovine vasopressin and oxytocin genes consist of three exons (Figure 9-2).[20,21] The first exon encodes the 19-amino-acid signal peptide, followed by vasopressin or oxytocin nonapeptides. This is followed by a 3-amino-acid protease cleavage site leading into the first nine amino acids of neurophysin II (for vasopressin) or neurophysin I (for oxytocin). After interruption of the coding region by an intron, exon 2 continues with neurophysin coding sequences. The third exon completes the sequence of the neurophysin, which for vasopressin only is followed by coding information for an additional 39-amino-acid glycopeptide (copeptin) whose function is unclear. Preprovasopressin contains 16 cysteines, which likely participate in eight disulfide bridges that determine the tertiary structure of the protein (Figure 9-3). One cysteine pair is present in vasopressin peptide, whereas the rest are in neurophysin.

In all mammalian species analyzed thus far, oxytocin and vasopressin genes are adjacent in chromosomal location (chromosome 20 in the human[22]) and linked tail to tail in opposite transcriptional orientation. In the human, they are separated by 12 kb.[22] This likely explains their origin from the ancient duplication of a common ancestral gene.[23] Whether this adjacent linkage is of regulatory significance is under investigation.

Expression of vasopressin and oxytocin genes occurs in the hypothalamic paraventricular and supraoptic nuclei.[18,24] The magnocellular components of each of these nuclei are the primary neuronal populations involved in water balance, with vasopressin synthesized in these areas carried by means of axonal transport to the posterior pituitary, its primary site of storage and release into the systemic circulation (Figure 9-4). The bilaterally paired hypothalamic paraventricular and supraoptic nuclei are separated from one another by relatively large distances

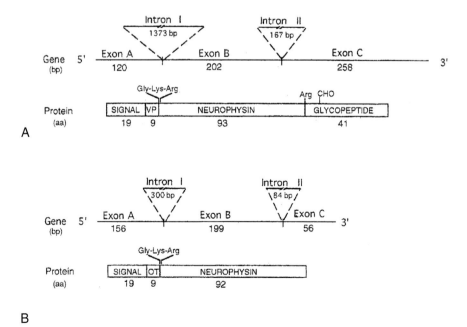

Figure 9-2 Structure of the human genes and peptide products of *(A)* vasopressin (VP) and *(B)* oxytocin (OT). Shown are the sizes of exons and intron in nucleotide base pairs (bp) and peptide products in amino acids (aa). Depicted are the amidation-dibasic cleavage signal (Gly-Lys-Arg) at the carboxy terminus of vasopressin and oxytocin and the monobasic cleavage signal at the end of neurophysin. Signal, signal peptide; VP, vasopressin; OT, oxytocin; and CHO, carbohydrate.

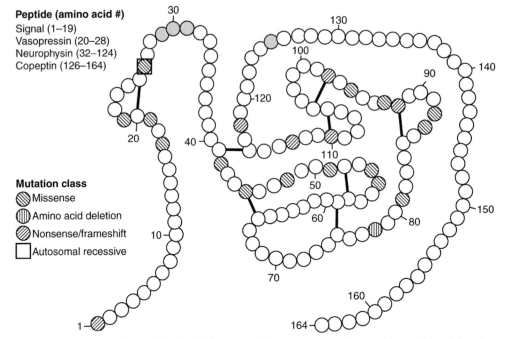

Figure 9-3 Structure of preprovasopressin peptide. The 164-amino-acid preprovasopressin peptide consists of signal peptide, vasopressin, neurophysin, and copeptin. The latter three entities are separated by basic residues (gray), which serve as cleavage sites for proconvertase enzymes. The 16 cysteines are connected by 8 putative disulfide bridges. Amino acid mutations are classified as missense, in-frame deletion, or nonsense/frame-shift mutations. Most mutations are inherited with an autosomal-dominant pattern. The one with an autosomal-recessive pattern is boxed. [Reproduced with permission from Uyeki TM, Barry FL, Rosenthal SM, Mathias RS (1993). Successful treatment with hydrochlorothiazide and amiloride in an infant with congenital nephrogenic diabetes insipidus. Pediatric Nephrology 7:554.

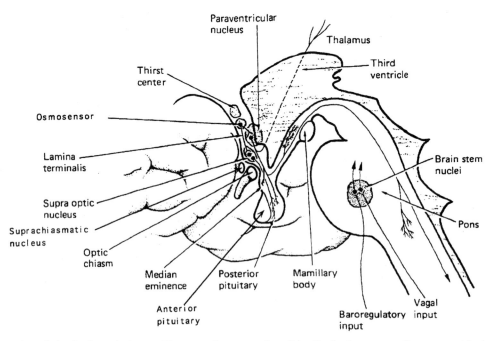

Figure 9-4 Vasopressin cells in the hypothalamus. Diagram of vasopressin cell bodies in the supraoptic, paraventricular, and suprachiasmatic hypothalamic nuclei—and axonal termination in the posterior pituitary and median eminence. Because vasopressin axons terminate at different levels in the pituitary stalk and posterior pituitary, the amount of permanent cell loss following neurosurgical insult is determined by the highest level of damage—which will dictate the degree of vasopressin axon transection and retrograde neuronal degeneration. [Modified with permission from Baylis PH (1989). Vasopressin and its neurophysin. In Degroot LD (ed.), *Endocrinology, Second edition*. Philadelphia: WB Saunders 213.]

(approximately 1 cm). Their axons course caudad, converge at the infundibulum, and terminate at different levels within the pituitary stalk and the posterior pituitary gland (Figure 9-4).

Vasopressin is also synthesized in the parvocellular neurons of the paraventricular nucleus, where it has a role in modulation of hypothalamic-pituitaryadrenal axis activity. In this site, vasopressin is colocalized in cells that synthesize corticotropin-releasing hormone[25,26]—and both are secreted at the median eminence and carried through the portal-hypophyseal capillary system to the anterior pituitary, where together they act as the major regulators of adrenocorticotropic hormone synthesis and release.[27] Vasopressin is also present in the hypothalamic suprachiasmatic nucleus, the circadian pacemaker of the body, where its function is unknown.

REGULATION OF VASOPRESSIN SECRETION AND THIRST

Osmotic Regulation

The rate of secretion of vasopressin from the paraventricular and supraoptic nuclei is influenced by several physiologic variables, including plasma osmolality and intravascular volume—as well as nausea and a number of pharmacologic agents. The major osmotically active constituents of blood are sodium, chloride, and glucose (with insulin deficiency). Normal blood osmolality ranges between 280 and 290 mOsm/kg H_2O.

The work of Verney[28] first demonstrated the relationship of increased vasopressin release in response to increasing plasma osmolality, as altered by infusion of sodium chloride or sucrose. At that time, it was postulated that there existed intracranial sensors sensitive to changes in plasma osmolality. Multiple researchers have subsequently confirmed that plasma vasopressin concentration increases in response to increasing plasma tonicity, although the exact nature of the osmosensor has not been defined.[29,30] Neurons of the supraoptic nucleus can respond directly to hypertonic stimuli with depolarization and vasopressin secretion,[31] but the majority of evidence

indicates that osmosensor- and vasopressin-secreting neurons are anatomically distinct.[32,33]

The osmosensor is likely to reside outside the blood-brain barrier, as implicated by differential vasopressin secretory response to similar changes in plasma osmolality depending on whether the change was induced by salt, sucrose, or urea.[28,34] The organ vasculosum of the lamina terminalis (OVLT) and the subfornical organ (SFO), areas of the preoptic hypothalamus outside the blood-brain barrier, are likely sites of osmosensing because lesions of the OVLT result in impaired vasopressin secretion and hypernatremia.[32,33] In addition, the site of action of angiotensin II infused intracerebrally or peripherally to produce vasopressin secretion and antidiuresis resides within the OVLT.[35-37]

The pattern of secretion of vasopressin into blood has been characterized extensively in normal individuals and in those with abnormalities in water homeostasis. Normally, at a serum osmolality of less than 280 mOsm/kg plasma vasopressin concentration is at or below 1 pg/mL (the lower limit of detection of most radioimmunoassays).[29,30] Above 283 mOsm/kg (the normal threshold for vasopressin release), plasma vasopressin concentration increases in proportion to plasma osmolality—up to a maximum concentration of about 20 pg/mL at a blood osmolality of approximately 320 mOsm/kg (Figure 9-5).

The osmosensor can detect as little as a 1% change in blood osmolality. Plasma concentrations in excess of 5 pg/mL are also found with nausea, hypotension, hypovolemia, and insulin-induced hypoglycemia. However, further increments in urine concentration do not occur because peak antidiuretic effect is achieved at 5 pg/mL. The rate of increase of plasma vasopressin concentration, and thus the sensitivity of the osmosensor, exhibits substantial (as much as tenfold) interindividual variation as plasma osmolality increases.[38] The set-point for vasopressin secretion varies in a single individual in relation to changes in volume status and hormonal environment (e.g., pregnancy[39]) or glucocorticoid status.[40,41]

After the seventh week of gestation, osmotic thresholds for both vasopressin release and thirst are reduced by approximately 10 mOsm/kg (Figure 9-5), such that

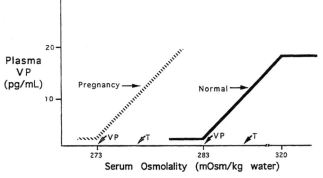

Figure 9-5 Osmotic thresholds for vasopressin and thirst. The threshold for vasopressin release is below that for thirst. In nonpregnant persons, there is linear increase in vasopressin (VP) release up to a serum osmolality of 320 mOsm/kg—after which no further increase occurs. In pregnancy, there is a decreased threshold for vasopressin release and thirst sensation—with no change in the sensitivity (slope) of the vasopressin-osmolality relationship. Vasopressin secretion in pregnancy presumably also plateaus at some level of hyperosmolality, although this has not been studied. Normal nonpregnant persons are indicated with solid line and arrows. Pregnant women are indicated with dashed line and arrows.

normal blood osmolality during pregnancy is approximately 273 mOsm/ kg (serum sodium 135 mEq/L).[39,42] Similarly, thresholds for vasopressin release and thirst during the luteal phase of the menstrual cycle are approximately 5 mOsm/kg lower than those in the follicular phase.[43,44] Human chorionic gonadotropin during pregnancy[45] and luteinizing hormone during the second half of the menstrual cycle may contribute to these changes in osmotic thresholds.

The sensation of thirst, a more integrated cortical activity, is determined by other anatomically distinct hypothalamic neurons—with afferents involving the ventromedial nucleus.[46] The activation of the thirst mechanism is also probably mediated by angiotensin II.[47] Whether the osmosensor for thirst and vasopressin release are the same is not certain, although this is suggested by lesions in the anteroventral region of the third ventricle that abolish thirst sensation and vasopressin release.[48] It makes physiologic sense that the threshold for thirst (293 mOsm/kg) is approximately 10 mOsm/kg higher than that for vasopressin release (Figure 9-5).

Otherwise, during the development of hyperosmolality the initial activation of thirst and water ingestion would result in polyuria without activation of vasopressin release—causing a persistent diuretic state. Immediately after water ingestion, before a change in blood osmolality or volume, vasopressin concentration falls and thirst ceases.[49] The degree of suppression is directly related to the coldness[50] and volume[51] of the ingested fluid. This effect is probably mediated by chemoreceptors present in the oropharynx, which guard against the rapid overdrinking of fluids after intense thirst during the time before the lowering of blood osmolality.

As noted previously, water balance is regulated in two ways: vasopressin secretion stimulates water reabsorption by the kidney (thereby reducing future water loss) and thirst stimulates water ingestion, thereby restoring previous water loss. Ideally, these two systems work in parallel to efficiently regulate extracellular fluid tonicity (Figure 9-6). However, each system by itself can maintain plasma osmolality in the near-normal range. For example, in the absence of vasopressin secretion but with free access to water thirst drives water ingestion up to the 5 to 10 L/m² of urine output seen with vasopressin deficiency. Conversely, an intact vasopressin secretory system can compensate for some degree of disordered thirst regulation. When both vasopressin secretion and thirst are compromised, however, by either disease or iatrogenic means there is great risk of the occurrence of life-threatening abnormalities in plasma osmolality.

Nonosmotic Regulation

Separate from osmotic regulation, vasopressin has been shown to be secreted in response to alterations in intravascular volume. Afferent baroreceptor pathways arising from the right and left atria and the aortic arch (carotid sinus) are stimulated by increasing intravascular volume and stretching of vessel walls, and they send signals through the vagus and glossopharyngeal nerves (respectively) to the brain stem nucleus tractus solitarius.[52,53] Upon stimulation, noradrenergic fibers from the nucleus

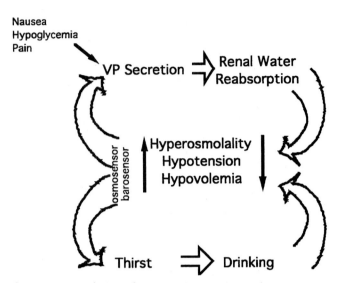

Figure 9-6 Regulation of vasopressin secretion and serum osmolality. Hyperosmolality, hypovolemia, and hypotension are sensed respectively by osmosensors, volume sensors, and barosensors. These stimulate vasopressin (VP) secretion and thirst. Vasopressin, acting on the kidney, causes increased reabsorption of water (antidiuresis). Thirst causes increased water ingestion. The results of these dual negative feedback loops cause a reduction in hyperosmolality or hypotension/hypovolemia. Additional stimuli for vasopressin secretion include nausea, hypoglycemia, and pain.

tractus solitarius synapse on the hypothalamic paraventricular nucleus and the supraoptic nucleus inhibit vasopressin secretion.[54,55] Experimental verification of this pathway has included demonstration of increased vasopressin concentration after interruption of baroreceptor output to the brain stem and decreased plasma vasopressin concentration after mechanical stimulation of baroreceptors, an effect diminished by vagotomy.[56,57]

The pattern of vasopressin secretion in response to volume as opposed to osmotic stimuli is markedly different (Figure 9-7). Although minor changes in plasma osmolality above 280 mOsm/kg evoke linear increases in plasma vasopressin, substantial alteration in intravascular volume is required for alteration in vasopressin output.[58-60] No change in vasopressin secretion is seen until blood volume decreases by approximately 8%. With intravascular volume deficits exceeding 8%, vasopressin concentration increases exponentially. Furthermore, osmotic and hemodynamic stimuli can interact in a mutually synergistic fashion such that the response to either stimulus may be enhanced by the concomitant presence of the other (Figure 9-7). When blood volume (or blood pressure[61-63]) decreases by approximately 25%, vasopressin concentrations are evident of 20- to 30-fold above normal and vastly exceeding those required for maximal antidiuresis. Surprisingly, the use of vasopressin antagonists has suggested that the high concentration of vasopressin observed with hypotension does not contribute to the maintenance of blood pressure in humans.[64]

Nausea (as evoked by apomorphine,[65] motion sickness,[66] and vasovagal reactions) is a very potent stimulus for vasopressin secretion. This effect is likely mediated by afferents from the area postrema of the brain stem and

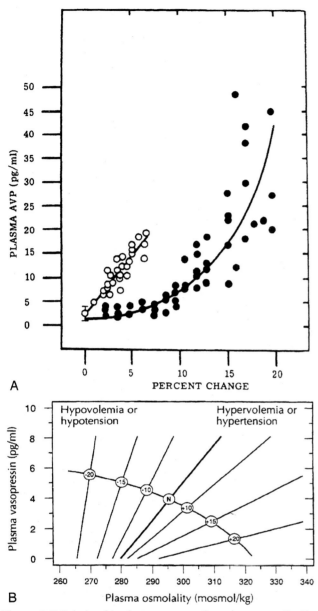

Figure 9-7 Relationships between osmotic and nonosmotic stimuli for vasopressin release. *(A)* Relationship of plasma vasopressin (AVP) concentration to the percent increase in blood osmolality (open circles) or decrease in blood volume (closed circles). *(B)* Alteration of sensitivity of osmotic stimulation of vasopressin secretion by volume or pressure stimuli. [Reproduced with permission from Dunn FL, et al. (1973). The role of blood osmolality and volume regulating vasopressin secretion in the rat. J Clin Invest 52:3212; and from Robertson GL (1985). Regulation of vasopressin secretion. In Seldin DW, Giebisch G (eds.), *The kidney: Physiology and pathophysiology.* New York: Raven Press 869.]

may result in vasopressin concentrations two to three orders of magnitude above basal levels. Nicotine is also a strong stimulus for vasopressin release.[67] These pathways probably do not involve osmotic or hemodynamic sensor systems because blockade of the emetic stimulus with dopamine or opioid antagonists does not alter the vasopressin response to hypernatremia or hypovolemia.

Vasopressin secretion is inhibited by glucocorticoids. Because of this, loss of negative regulation of vasopressin

secretion occurs in the setting of primary or secondary glucocorticoid insufficiency.[68,69] The effects of cortisol loss of both enhancing hypothalamic vasopressin production and directly impairing free water excretion[70] are important considerations in the evaluation of the patient with hyponatremia, as is subsequently discussed.

VASOPRESSIN METABOLISM

Once in the circulation, vasopressin has a half-life of only 5 to 10 minutes owing to its rapid degradation by a cysteine amino-terminal peptidase called vasopressinase. A synthetic analogue of vasopressin, desmopressin, is insensitive to amino-terminal degradation and thus has a much longer half-life of 8 to 24 hours. During pregnancy, the placenta secretes increased amounts of this vasopressinase,[71] resulting in a fourfold increase in the metabolic clearance rate of vasopressin.[72]

Normal women compensate with an increase in vasopressin secretion, but women with preexisting deficits in vasopressin secretion or action[73] or those with increased concentrations of placental vasopressinase associated with liver dysfunction[74] or multiple gestations[75] may develop diabetes insipidus in the last trimester—which resolves in the immediate postpartum period.[76] As expected, this form of diabetes insipidus responds to treatment with desmopressin but not with vasopressin.[77,78]

SITES OF VASOPRESSIN ACTION

Vasopressin Receptors

Vasopressin released from the posterior pituitary and the median eminence affects the function of several tissue types by binding to members of a family of G-protein–coupled cell surface receptors, which subsequently transduce ligand binding into alterations of intracellular second messenger pathways.[79] Biochemical and cell biologic studies have defined at least three receptor types, designated V1, V2, and V3 (or V1b). The major sites of V1 receptor expression are on vascular smooth muscle[80] and hepatocytes,[81-84] where receptor activation results in vasoconstriction[85,86] and glycogenolysis,[87] respectively.

The latter activity may be augmented by stimulation of glucagon secretion from the pancreas.[87] The V1 receptor on platelets also stimulates platelet aggregation.[88] V1 receptor activation mobilizes intracellular calcium stores through phosphatidylinositol hydrolysis.[86,89] Despite its initial characterization as a powerful pressor agent, the concentration of vasopressin needed to significantly increase blood pressure is severalfold higher than that required for maximal antidiuresis,[90] although substantial vasoconstriction in renal and splanchnic vasculature can occur at physiologic concentrations.[91]

The cloning of the V1 receptor[80,81,83] has greatly elucidated the relationship of the vasopressin (and oxytocin[92,93]) receptors, and through sensitive in situ hybridization analysis has further localized V1 expression to the liver and the vasculature of the renal medulla—as well as to many sites within the brain, including the hippocampus, the amygdala, the hypothalamus, and the brain stem.[82,84] The V3 (or V1b) receptor is present on corticotrophs in the anterior pituitary[94] and acts through the phosphatidylinositol pathway[95] to increase adrenocorticotropic hormone secretion. Its binding profile for vasopressin analogues resembles more closely that of the V1 receptor than of the V2 receptor. The structure of this receptor has been determined in humans by cloning of its complementary DNA.[95,96] Its structure is similar to that of the V1 and oxytocin receptors, and it is expressed in the kidney as well as in the pituitary. Recently, mice with deletion of the V1b receptor gene have been created.[97,98] As expected, they have defective activation of the pituitary-adrenal axis following some acute and chronic stressors.

Modulation of water balance occurs through the action of vasopressin on V2 receptors located primarily in the renal collecting tubule, along with other sites in the kidney—including the thick ascending limb of the loop of Henle and periglomerular tubules.[82,84,99] It is also present on vascular endothelial cells in some systemic vascular beds, where vasopressin stimulates vasodilation[100]—possibly through activation of nitric oxide synthase.[101] Vasopressin also stimulates von Willebrand factor, factor VIIIa, and tissue plasminogen activator through V2-mediated actions.

Because of this, desmopressin is used to improve the prolonged bleeding times characteristic of uremia, type I von Willebrand disease, and hemophilia.[102] The V2 receptor consists of 370 amino acids encoding seven transmembrane domains characteristic of the G-protein–coupled receptors.[99,103] These transmembrane domains share approximately 60% sequence identity with the V1 receptor

but substantially less with other members of this family (Figure 9-8). Unlike the V1 and V3 receptors, the V2 receptor acts through adenylate cyclase to increase intracellular cyclic adenosine monophosphate (AMP) concentration. The human V2 receptor gene is located on the long arm of the X chromosome (Xq28),[104,105] at the locus associated with congenital X-linked vasopressin-resistant diabetes insipidus. Mice in which V2R has been deleted have a similar phenotype.[106]

Renal Cascade of Vasopressin Function

Vasopressin-induced increases in intracellular cyclic AMP as mediated by the V2 receptor triggers a complex pathway of events, resulting in increased permeability of the collecting duct to water and efficient water transit across an otherwise minimally permeable epithelium (Figure 9-9).[107] Activation of a cyclic AMP-dependent protein kinase imparts remodeling of cytoskeletal microtubules and microfilaments that culminate in the insertion of aggregates of water channels into the apical membrane.[108] These mechanisms may involve a vesicle-associated membrane protein-2-like protein (VAMP-2; which also regulates synaptic vesicle activity in neuronal terminals[109]) and its associated receptor syntaxin-4.[110]

Insertion of the water channels causes an up to 100-fold increase in water permeability of the apical membrane, allowing water movement along its osmotic gradient into the hypertonic inner medullary interstitium from the tubule

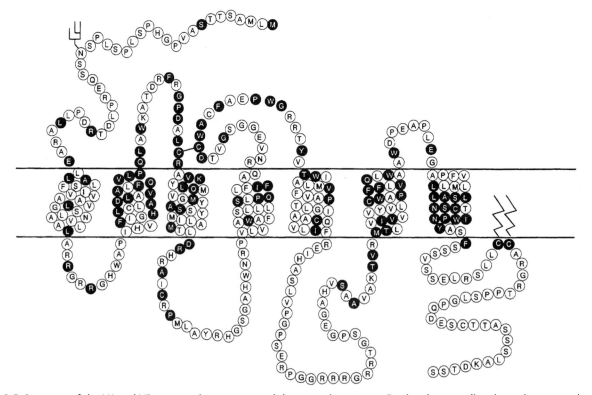

Figure 9-8 Structure of the V1 and V2 vasopressin receptors and the oxytocin receptor. Depicted are predicted membrane topology, with the extracellular domain at the top of the figure and amino acids in the one-letter code. Amino acids in open circles encode the V1 receptor, whereas those in black circles are common to all three receptors. [Reproduced with permission from Bichet DG (1995). The posterior pituitary. In Melmed S (ed.), *The pituitary*. Cambridge: Blackwell Science 277.]

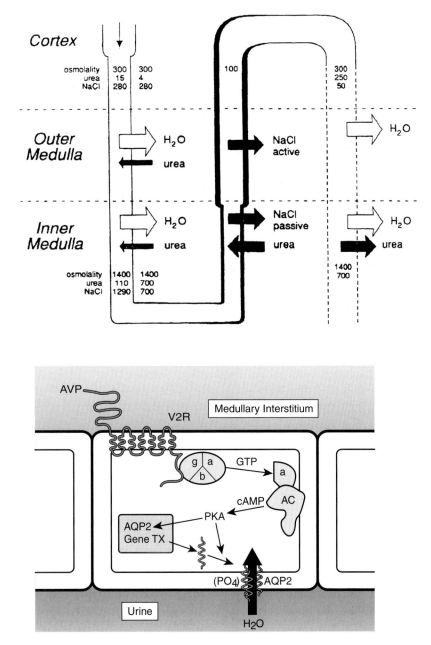

Figure 9-9 Vasopressin action in the kidney. *(A)* Solute and water handling in the kidney. *(B)* Action of vasopressin in the collecting duct cell. Vasopressin (AVP) binds to the V2 receptor (V2R), causing the binding of GTP to the stimulatory alpha G-protein subunit *(α)*. This activates adenylate cyclase (AC), resulting in an increase in cAMP and activation of protein kinase A (PKA). The catalytic subunit of PKA, via phosphorylation of serine 256 of the water channel [aquaporin-2 (AQP2)], causes aggregation of AQP2 homotetramers in membrane vesicles and their fusion with the collecting duct luminal membrane—resulting in an increase in water flow from the urine into the renal medullary interstitium. Demeclocycline, lithium, high calcium, and low potassium interfere with these processes—possibly at the level of cAMP generation and AQP2 synthesis or action. [From Reeves WB, Andreoli TE (1989). Nephrogenic diabetes insipidus. In Scriver CR, Beaudet AL, Sly WS (eds.), *The metabolic basis of inherited disease, Sixth edition.* New York: McGraw-Hill 1985.]

lumen and excretion of a concentrated urine (Figure 9-9). The molecular analysis of the water channels has revealed a family of related proteins (designated aquaporins) that differ in their sites of expression and pattern of regulation.[111] Each protein consists of a single polypeptide chain with six membrane-spanning domains (Figure 9-10). Although functional as monomers, they are believed to form homotetramers in the plasma membrane.[107]

Aquaporin-2 is expressed mostly within the kidney,[112] primarily within the collecting duct.[113] It is also expressed in the vas deferens, at least in the rat, although it is not regulated by vasopressin in this location.[114] Studies with immunoelectron microscopy have demonstrated large amounts of aquaporin-2 in the apical plasma membrane and subapical vesicles of the collecting duct, consistent with the "membrane-shuttling" model of water

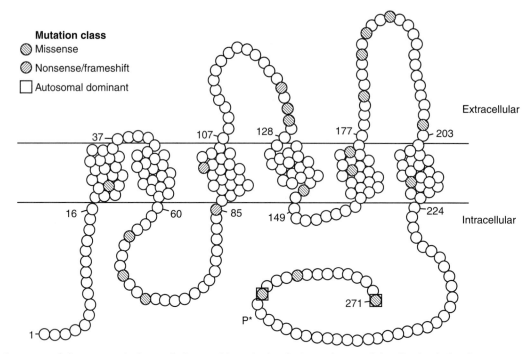

Figure 9-10 Structure of the aquaporin-2 protein inserted into the luminal membrane of the distal tubule. The 271-amino-acid protein consists of five transmembrane domains, four intracellular domains, and three extracellular domains. Amino acid mutations are denoted by filled circles. Most mutations are transmitted with an autosomal-recessive pattern. The two dominant mutations are bounded by squares. Vasopressin-dependent protein-kinase-A-mediated phosphorylation of serine at amino acid 256 (P*) is noted. [Reproduced with permission from Uyeki TM, Barry FL, Rosenthal SM, Mathias RS (1993). Successful treatment with hydrochlorothiazide and amiloride in an infant with congenital nephrogenic diabetes insipidus. Pediatric Nephrology 7:554.]

channel aggregate insertion into the apical membrane after vasopressin stimulation.[114]

Studies analyzing the mechanism by which aquaporin-2 traffics to the apical plasma membrane have demonstrated that vasopressin-induced protein-kinase-A-mediated serine phosphorylation at amino acid 256 is required for its exocytosis,[115] a process also requiring a heterotrimeric G protein of the G_i family.[116] In response to water restriction or desmopressin infusion in humans, the content of urinary aquaporin-2 in both soluble and membrane-bound forms has been found to increase.[117] Mice with targeted deletion of the aquaporin-2 gene have been made.[118] As expected, they have nephrogenic diabetes insipidus that is unresponsive to treatment with vasopressin.

In addition to aquaporin-2, different aquaporins appear to be involved in other aspects of renal water handling. In contrast to the apical localization of aquaporin-2, aquaporin-3 and aquaporin-4 are expressed on the basolateral membrane of the collecting duct epithelium. They appear to be involved in the flow of water and urea from the inside of the collecting duct cell into the extracellular renal medullary space. Mice made genetically deficient in aquaporin-4 demonstrate a mild urinary concentrating defect,[119] whereas those with deficiency of aquaporin-3 alone or together with aquaporin-4 demonstrate more severely impaired urinary concentrating ability.[120] Mice made genetically deficient in aquaporin-1 demonstrate a urinary concentrating defect caused by decreased water permeability in the proximal tubule.[121]

Volume Sensor and Effector Pathways

RENIN-ANGIOTENSIN-ALDOSTERONE SYSTEM

In contrast to the vasopressin system, the classic (peripheral) renin-angiotensin system primarily affects maintenance of intravascular volume as opposed to plasma tonicity. In addition to the well-established endocrine regulatory system, several local renin-angiotensin systems have emerged—with both autocrine and paracrine effects in their tissue of synthesis, whose regulation is independent of the classic system. Finally, brain and pituitary angiotensin systems involved in blood pressure, autonomic function, and fluid balance have been characterized with extensive interaction with the vasopressin system.

ENDOCRINE RENIN-ANGIOTENSIN-ALDOSTERONE SYSTEM

Anatomy and Biochemistry

Renin (which is synthesized by the renal juxtaglomerular apparatus) is a proteolytic enzyme that catalyzes the cleavage of angiotensinogen, synthesized by hepatocytes, into the decapeptide angiotensin I.[122,123] Angiotensin I possesses no intrinsic vasoreactive or mineralocorticoid secretagogue activity but is efficiently cleaved by angiotensin-converting enzyme in the lungs, as well as other peripheral sites, to generate the octapeptide angiotensin II. Angiotensin II is further metabolized to the heptapeptide angiotensin III by removal of one amino-terminal amino acid. Angiotensin II possesses greater vasopressor activity and is present in approximately a fourfold greater amount than angiotensin III. Angiotensins II and III possess equivalent mineralocorticoid secretory activity on the adrenal glomerulosa cells.

Angiotensin II and III act through cell surface receptors (AT_1) on the adrenal glomerulosa cells to activate the phospholipase C/protein kinase C pathway.[124-128] This activation results in increased production of pregnenolone from cholesterol by side-chain cleavage enzyme (20, 22-desmolase) and of aldosterone from corticosterone by the glomerulosa-specific corticosterone methyloxidase I and II activities (18-hydroxylation and dehydrogenation, respectively).[129-132] A distinct receptor subtype for angiotensin II, the AT_2 receptor, is not G protein coupled and is of unclear physiologic significance in the periphery.[133-135]

Aldosterone, the primary and most potent endogenous mineralocorticoid released by the zona glomerulosa, acts on target tissues expressing the nuclear mineralocorticoid (or type I glucocorticoid) receptor to promote sodium absorption and potassium excretion. For control of intravascular volume, the primary target of action of aldosterone is the distal nephron. Here, aldosterone increases synthesis of apical membrane sodium channels, mitochondrial enzymes involved in adenosine triphosphate production, and components of Na^+,K^+ adenosine triphosphatase to cause increased sodium reabsorption and potassium excretion.[136]

Regulation of Secretion

Decreased intravascular volume as sensed by the renal juxtaglomerular apparatus results in release of renin.[122,137] Increased plasma renin activity then allows increased conversion of angiotensinogen to angiotensin I, which in turn is converted peripherally to angiotensins II and III. Increased angiotensin II activity causes vasoconstriction and blood pressure elevation, whereas both angiotensins II and III stimulate aldosterone release from the zona glomerulosa and subsequent salt and water retention and potassium excretion by the distal tubule of the kidney. Conversely, expanded intravascular volume causes decreased renin output and less sodium and water resorption in the kidney—serving to decrease intravascular volume and restore homeostasis.

Changes in vascular volume are not the only regulators of the renin-angiotensin-aldosterone system. Serum potassium concentration directly modulates aldosterone release by the adrenal glomerulosa by its effects on plasma membrane potential and activation of voltage-gated calcium channels.[123,138] Membrane depolarization, the result of increased serum potassium, leads to increased aldosterone synthesis—which promotes renal potassium excretion. Low serum potassium reduces aldosterone synthesis and decreases urinary potassium losses. Pituitary adrenocorticotropin hormone and vasopressin act through their respective receptors on the glomerulosa cells to increase acute aldosterone secretion. These effects are of short duration because long-term chronic infusions do not

chronically elevate aldosterone concentrations. Direct inhibitors of aldosterone secretion (and thus promoters of natriuresis) include atrial natriuretic peptide (ANP),[139,140] somatostatin,[141-143] and dopamine.[144,145]

LOCAL RENIN-ANGIOTENSIN SYSTEMS

Anatomy and Biochemistry

In addition to the well-defined endocrine circuit, the components of the renin-angiotensin system have been found in a wide variety of tissues—including brain, pituitary, arterial wall, heart, ovary, kidney, and adrenal—where paracrine and autocrine regulatory functions[146-150] have been postulated, undergoing regulation independent of the systemic counterpart. From the standpoint of regulation of water and volume homeostasis, the brain renin-angiotensin system merits further description.[151] It has long been known that peripherally synthesized angiotensin II could increase blood pressure by effects on the brain outside the blood-brain barrier at sites such as the OVLT, SFO, area postrema, and median eminence as revealed by ligand-binding studies.[35,151-153] Over the past decade, it has become clear that the complete system for generation of angiotensin II is present within the brain.

Angiotensinogen has been localized to astrocytes by both immunohistochemical peptide localization and in situ hybridization analysis of messenger RNA.[154] In contrast, renin has been found in high concentration in nerve terminals—with enhanced release on nerve depolarization.[155] Angiotensin-converting enzyme has been found within vascular, choroid plexus, and neuronal components of the central nervous system[156-158]—most notably the SFO and many hypothalamic nuclei, sites of endogenous angiotensin II receptor expression (primarily of the AT_1 subtype), and sites not expressing the angiotensin II receptor such as the basal ganglia. The primary effector molecule, angiotensin II, has been localized specifically to neurons and subcellularly to synaptic vesicles.[159] Two of the most significant sites include the circumventricular organs and the paraventricular nucleus of the hypothalamus. Within the paraventricular nucleus, angiotensin II immunoreactivity colocalizes with magnocellular vasopressin—whereas its receptors are within the parvocellular region of the paraventricular nucleus.[160]

Regulation of Secretion

The forebrain angiotensin II pathway, of which the paraventricular nucleus is one component, and circumventricular organ angiotensin II pathway are important control centers for maintenance of osmotic and volume homeostasis.[161] Increased concentration of peripheral angiotensin II, as would be expected in intravascular volume depletion, stimulates drinking behavior.[35] This action of peripheral angiotensin II can be abolished by destruction of the OVLT or SFO, regions whose destruction has long been recognized as causing adipsia.[36]

Further effects of central angiotensin II action include augmentation of sodium appetite and stimulation of vasopressin release, all serving (as with peripheral angiotensin

II) to restore intravascular volume and maintain blood pressure.[35] The signal of hypovolemia is transduced through the vagal nerve from volume sensors to the brain stem and the region of the nucleus tractus solitarius. Efferents from these brain-stem centers project to the median preoptic nucleus and paraventricular nucleus—as does the forebrain angiotensin II pathway, where drinking and pressor effects as well as vasopressin release are elicited.[162-167]

Separate pathways for vasopressin release mediate the response to peripheral angiotensin II or to purely osmotic stimulation of the osmosensors.[168] The release of vasopressin in response to osmotic stimulation is not increased by peripheral angiotensin II, and pure osmotic stimulation does not increase salt appetite. Central angiotensin II, in contrast, may function as a transmitter in the osmosensing circuit—leading to vasopressin release.[169]

THE NATRIURETIC PEPTIDE SYSTEM

In addition to the classic vasopressin and renin-angiotensin-aldosterone systems, the natriuretic peptide families of ligands and their receptors add further potential for modulation of salt and water balance. The interaction of the natriuretic peptide system occurs in the central nervous system through effects on vasopressin secretion and peripherally through its ability to both directly promote natriuresis in the kidney and indirectly inhibit adrenal aldosterone production.

Anatomy and Biochemistry

Atrial natriuretic peptide was initially discovered as a component of cardiac atrial muscle that was able to induce natriuresis, a decrease in blood pressure, and an increase in hematocrit when injected into rats.[170,171] The biologically active form of ANP consists of a 28-amino-acid peptide that includes a 17-amino-acid ring structure[172] (Figure 9-11). The primary sequence of the peptide has been conserved among mammalian species, and in addition to synthesis in cardiac atrial tissue[173] has been detected in brain, spinal cord, pituitary, and adrenal gland.[174-177]

Within the brain, ANP synthesis occurs at several critical neuroendocrine regulatory sites—including the periventricular, arcuate, anteroventral preoptic, and lateral hypothalamic nuclei.[178,179] ANP is synthesized as a 151-amino-acid preprohormone and is stored as a 126-amino-acid prohormone after removal of the signal peptide sequence.[172,180] Coupled with secretion of pro-ANP is its cleavage between amino acids 98 and 99 to yield the mature 28-amino-acid 99-126 fragment.

Subsequent investigation defined a second peptide from porcine brain with structural homology to ANP.[181] This peptide, designated brain natriuretic peptide (BNP), was later found to be secreted by the heart as well—in this case from ventricular and atrial tissue.[182-184] Human BNP consists of a 32-amino-acid processed from a larger preprohormone[185] sharing a central ring structure with ANP (Figure 9-11), although it is less conserved between species than ANP.

A third member of this family, C-type natriuretic peptide (CNP), was also isolated from porcine brain.[186] In brain, CNP is the most abundant member of the natriuretic peptide family. Within the hypothalamus, specific sites of synthesis largely overlap sites of ANP expression.[179] Little CNP can be detected in plasma, and in marked contrast to ANP and BNP CNP does not increase in plasma in the setting of cardiac failure.[187,188] Outside the brain, CNP is synthesized in endothelial and vascular smooth muscle. In tissues capable of CNP gene expression, two forms of the

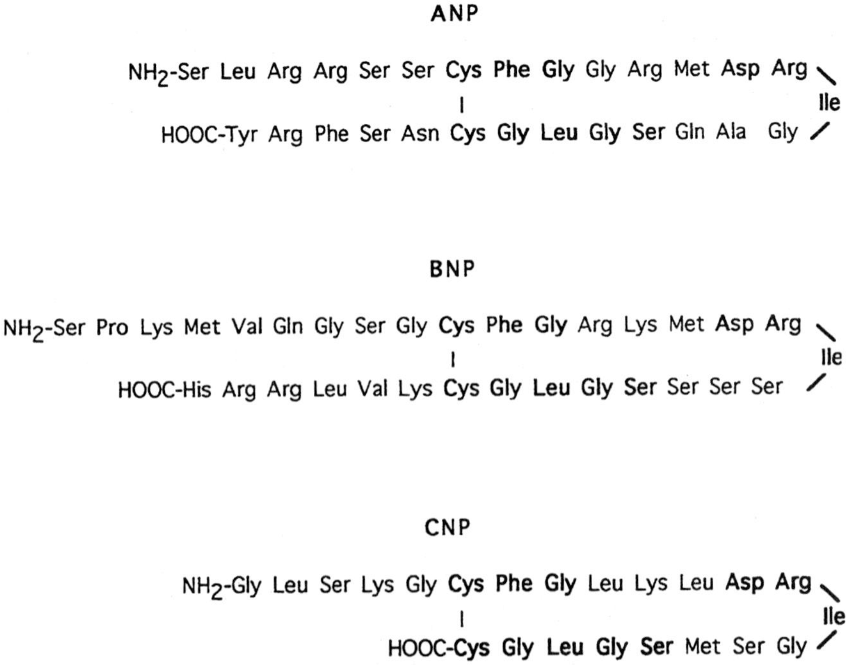

ANP

NH₂-Ser Leu Arg Arg Ser Ser **Cys Phe Gly** Gly Arg Met **Asp Arg**
                                                    | **Ile**
HOOC-Tyr Arg Phe Ser Asn **Cys Gly Leu Gly Ser** Gln Ala Gly

BNP

NH₂-Ser Pro Lys Met Val Gln Gly Ser Gly **Cys Phe Gly** Arg Lys Met **Asp Arg**
                                                            | **Ile**
HOOC-His Arg Arg Leu Val Lys **Cys Gly Leu Gly Ser** Ser Ser Ser

CNP

NH₂-Gly Leu Ser Lys Gly **Cys Phe Gly** Leu Lys Leu **Asp Arg**
                                            | **Ile**
HOOC-**Cys Gly Leu Gly Ser** Met Ser Gly

Figure 9-11 Amino acid composition of the human natriuretic peptides. Amino acids identical among the three peptides are indicated by bold letters, and the disulfide bond between Cys residues is shown.

peptide are produced: a 53-amino-acid peptide and a less abundant 22-amino-acid molecule[189] (Figure 9-11).

Three distinct endogenous receptors exist for the natriuretic peptides. The first of these receptors isolated (NPR-A or GC-A) was cloned by virtue of its homology to sea urchin sperm guanylyl cyclase and was later found to have ANP and BNP as its normal ligands.[190-192] A second guanylyl-cyclase-type receptor (NPR-B) has substantial homology to NPR-A. However, it binds CNP with substantially greater affinity than ANP or BNP.[193] A third receptor (NPR-C[194]) does not possess guanylyl cyclase activity and probably functions to clear all three natriuretic peptides from the circulation.[195] In situ hybridization studies using probes capable of distinguishing the different receptor types have revealed some interspecies discrepancy in distribution. The NPR-A receptor has been localized to kidney, adrenal, pituitary, brain, and heart in monkey—with NPR-B limited to adrenal, pituitary, and brain.[196] In rat, broad tissue distribution of both NPR-A and NPR-B has been described.[197] The NPR-C receptor has similarly been found in adrenal, heart, brain, and pituitary.[196]

Regulation of Secretion and Action

Secretion of ANP by cardiac tissue occurs in response to increasing atrial transmural pressure, from both left and right atria.[188,198] Studies employing intravascular volume expansion, exercise, and hypoxia demonstrate increased plasma concentration of ANP after these stimuli in animal and human paradigms.[187,198-200] In addition, increased heart rate (especially increased atrial contractile frequency) results in increased ANP secretion. In the setting of supraventricular tachycardia, high plasma concentration of ANP and suppressed concentration of vasopressin (both probably caused by an increase in atrial volume and pressure) contribute to the polyuria associated with this syndrome.[201-203] Ventricular production of ANP has also been demonstrated. It is increased in states of left-sided overload associated with ventricular hypertrophy.[183] ANP synthesized within the central nervous system varies in a volume-dependent fashion in a manner similar to peripheral ANP, suggesting similar function.[174]

The physiologic ramifications of increased ANP production are several. Infusion of ANP in the setting of normovolemia causes natriuresis, diuresis, and a small increase in divalent cation excretion.[187,188,204] ANP, through the NPR-A receptor, primarily inhibits sodium reabsorption within the renal inner medullary collecting duct but also opposes the salt-retaining effects of angiotensin II at the level of the proximal tubule.[204] ANP similarly inhibits the actions of vasopressin and aldosterone in the renal tubules.[205-207] Direct cardiovascular effects of ANP include arterial smooth-muscle relaxation, both acutely and with chronic administration. In part, this effect may be mediated through opposition of angiotensin II action.[208]

ANP modulates mineralocorticoid production in a manner that results in the reduction of intravascular volume or pressure. Although direct reduction in plasma renin activity has been described with ANP infusion,[209,210] the most dramatic response to ANP occurs at the level of the adrenal glomerulosa cell. ANP inhibits aldosterone production by inhibiting action of most aldosterone secretagogues, with the most pronounced reduction being angiotensin II activity.[98,187,204] The serum concentration of ANP at which the effects on PRA and aldosterone production occur is within the physiologic range, although the importance of this pathway in normal human physiology remains incompletely defined.

Direct injection of ANP into the central nervous system of animals has suggested an important role for ANP (or CNP) in cardiovascular and salt homeostasis. Vasodepression and bradycardia have both been observed,[211] as has inhibition of vasopressin, adrenocorticotropic hormone, and gonadotropin-releasing hormone secretion.[174,212] Thus, antagonistic action of ANP and angiotensin II on intravascular volume and blood pressure remain congruent between central and peripheral systems.

BNP synthesis and secretion from cardiac ventricular tissue are augmented in congestive heart failure, and as for ANP with hypertension, chronic renal, and chronic liver failure.[184,188] BNP binds the NPR-A receptor, where it is capable of stimulating cyclic guanosine monophosphate production.[190] Infusion of BNP inhibits aldosterone production and results in natriuresis similar to that reported for ANP. With infusion rates generating BNP concentrations tenfold greater than baseline, reduction in blood pressure has also been found.

In contrast to ANP and BNP, CNP expression primarily causes activation of the NPR-B receptor.[193] Plasma concentration of CNP does not change significantly with volume overload, and it is believed that the majority of CNP action occurs in a paracrine fashion within the brain and vasculature.[188] CNP synthesized within vascular endothelium acts on receptors in vascular smooth muscle to cause relaxation.[213] CNP infusions in dogs acutely reduce blood pressure and right atrial pressure but do not result in natriuresis, whereas in humans moderately supraphysiologic doses cause neither hypotension nor natriuresis.[214] In contrast to ANP, intracerebroventricular infusion of CNP leads to a reduction in blood pressure—suggesting a role for CNP in central control of arterial pressure.[215] CNP inhibits angiotensin-II-stimulated vasopressin secretion but stimulates thirst.[216] The overall importance of the CNP central pathways in modulation of water balance in humans remains to be defined.

Approach to the Patient: Differential Diagnosis of Disorders of Water Metabolism

HYPONATREMIA

Hyponatremia (serum sodium of 130 mEq/L or less) in children is usually associated with severe systemic disorders. It is most often caused by intravascular volume depletion or excessive salt loss, and is encountered with hypotonic fluid overload (especially in infants). Inappropriate vasopressin excess is one of the least common causes of hyponatremia in children, except for vasopressin administration for treatment of diabetes insipidus.

In evaluating the cause of hyponatremia, one should first determine whether the patient is dehydrated and hypovolemic. This is usually evident from the physical examination (decreased weight, skin turgor, central venous pressure) and laboratory data (high blood urea nitrogen, renin, aldosterone, uric acid). With a decrease in the glomerular filtration rate, proximal tubular reabsorption of sodium and water will be high—leading to a urinary sodium value less than 10 mEq/L.

Patients with decreased "effective" intravascular volume from congestive heart failure, cirrhosis, nephrotic syndrome, or lung disease will present with similar laboratory data but will also have obvious signs of their underlying disease—which often includes peripheral edema. Patients with primary salt loss will also appear volume depleted. If the salt loss is from the kidney (e.g., diuretic therapy or polycystic kidney disease), the urine sodium level will be elevated—as may urine volume. Salt loss from other regions (e.g., the gut in gastroenteritis or the skin in cystic fibrosis) will cause urine sodium to be low, as in other forms of systemic dehydration. Cerebral salt wasting is encountered with central nervous system insults and results in high serum ANP concentrations, leading to high urine sodium and urine excretion.

The syndrome of inappropriate antidiuresis (SIAD) exists when a primary elevation in vasopressin secretion or inappropriate activation of the vasopressin V2 receptor is the cause of hyponatremia. It is characterized by hyponatremia, an inappropriately concentrated urine (>100 mOsm/kg), normal or slightly elevated plasma volume, and a normal-to-high urine sodium (because of volume-induced suppression of aldosterone and elevation of ANP). Serum uric acid is low in patients with SIAD, whereas it is high in those with hyponatremia caused by systemic dehydration or other causes of decreased intravascular volume.[217]

Measurement of plasma vasopressin is often not very useful because it is elevated in nearly all causes of hyponatremia except for primary hypersecretion of ANP[218] or mutations in the vasopressin receptor that lead to inappropriate regulation of its activity. Because cortisol and thyroid deficiency cause hyponatremia by several mechanisms, discussed subsequently, they should be considered in all hyponatremic patients. Drug-induced hyponatremia should be considered in patients on potentially offending medications, as discussed later. In children with SIAD who do not have an obvious cause, a careful search for a tumor (thymoma, glioma, bronchial carcinoid) should be considered.

POLYURIA, POLYDYPSIA, AND HYPERNATREMIA

In children, it must first be determined whether pathologic polyuria or polydipsia (exceeding 2 L/m²/day) is present. The following questions are asked. Is there a psychosocial reason for either polyuria or polydipsia? Can either be quantitated? Has either polyuria or polydipsia interfered with normal activities? Is nocturia or enuresis present? If so, does the patient also drink after nocturnal awakening? Does the history (including longitudinal growth data) or physical examination suggest other deficient or excessive endocrine secretion or an intracranial neoplasm?

If pathologic polyuria or polydipsia is present, the following should be obtained in the outpatient setting: serum osmolality; serum concentrations of sodium, potassium, glucose, calcium, and blood urea nitrogen; and urinalysis, including measurement of urine osmolality, specific gravity, and glucose concentration. A serum osmolality greater than 300 mOsm/kg, with urine osmolality less than 300 mOsm/kg, establishes the diagnosis of diabetes insipidus. If serum osmolality is less than 270 mOsm/kg, or urine osmolality is greater than 600 mOsm/kg, the diagnosis of diabetes insipidus is unlikely. If upon initial screening the patient has a serum osmolality less than 300 mOsm/kg but the intake/output record at home suggests significant polyuria and polydipsia that cannot be attributed to primary polydipsia (i.e., the serum osmolality is greater than 270 mOsm/kg), the patient should undergo a water deprivation test to establish a diagnosis of diabetes insipidus and to differentiate central from nephrogenic causes.

After a maximally tolerated overnight fast (based on the outpatient history), the child is admitted to the outpatient testing center in the early morning of a day when an 8- to 10-hour test can be carried out with the child deprived of water.[219,220] The physical signs and biochemical parameters shown in the accompanying protocol are measured (Figure 9-12). If at any time during the test the urine osmolality exceeds 1,000 mOsm/kg, or 600 mOsm/kg and is stable over 1 hour, the patient does not have diabetes insipidus. If at any time the serum osmolality exceeds 300 mOsm/kg and the urine osmolality is less than 600 mOsm/kg, the patient has diabetes insipidus. If the serum osmolality is less than 300 mOsm/kg and the urine osmolality is less than 600 mOsm/kg, the test should be continued unless vital signs disclose hypovolemia.

A common error is to stop a test too soon, based on the amount of body weight lost, before either urine osmolality has plateaued above 600 mOsm/kg or a serum osmolality above 300 mOsm/kg has been achieved. Unless the serum osmolality increases above the threshold for vasopressin release, a lack of vasopressin action (as inferred by a nonconcentrated urine) cannot be deemed pathologic. If the diagnosis of diabetes insipidus is made, aqueous vasopressin (Pitressin, 1 U/m²) should be given subcutaneously. If the patient has central diabetes insipidus, urine volume should fall and osmolality should at least double during the next hour compared with the value before vasopressin therapy. If there is less than a twofold increase in urine osmolality after vasopressin administration, the patient probably has nephrogenic diabetes insipidus.

Desmopressin should not be used for this test because it has been associated with water intoxication in small children in this setting.[221] Patients with long-standing primary polydipsia may have mild nephrogenic diabetes insipidus because of dilution of their renal medullary interstitium. This should not be confused with primary nephrogenic diabetes insipidus because patients with primary polydipsia should have a tendency toward hyponatremia, rather than hypernatremia, in the basal state. Patients with a family history of X-linked nephrogenic diabetes insipidus can be evaluated for the disorder in the prenatal or perinatal period by DNA sequence analysis, thus allowing therapy to be initiated without delay.[222]

Water Deprivation Test

ENDOCRINE FUNCTION TEST	Patient Name
DIAGNOSIS: Suspected Diabetes Insipidus	
TEST: Water Deprivation	

Present Health _____ Good _____ Fair _____ Poor

Diet for previous two days (attach diet history), to avoid tobacco, ethanol: _____

_____

Initial period of fast_____hr

Initial body weight_____ kg   Recent Medications: _____

Thirst sensation normal?_____

No	Hour	Interval Minutes	Body weight	Vital signs	Serum			Plasma	Urine			
					Na	OSM	BUN	VP	Na	OSM	S.G.	vol/hr
		-30	Place IV hep lock									
		0	X	X	X	X	X	X	X	X	X	X
		60	X	X	X	X				X	X	X
		120	X	X	X	X			X	X	X	X
		180	X	X	X	X				X	X	X
		240	X	X	X	X		X	X	X	X	X
		300	X	X	X	X				X	X	X
		360	X	X	X	X			X	X	X	X
		420	X	X	X	X				X	X	X
		480	X	X	X	X	X	X*	X	X	X	X

*If patient has DI, last VP sample at last time point before VP admininstration (see below)

AT ANY TIME DURING TEST:

If serum osm <300 (Na<145), urine osm <600, continue test unless vital signs disclose hypovolemia

If urine osm >1000, or >600 and stable (<30 mosm change for 2 time points), stop test = NORMAL

If serum osm >300 and urine osm<600=DIABETES INSIPIDUS.   Give Pitressin, 1U/m2 SQ and measure:

TIME AFTER PITRESSIN ADMINISTRATION:

		0		X						X	X	X
		30		X						X	X	X
		60		X					X	X	X	X

COMMENTS:

_____

_____

_____

Figure 9-12 Protocol for evaluation of diabetes insipidus using water deprivation. IV, intravenous; OSM, osmolality; S.G., urinary specific gravity; and SQ, subcutaneous.

The water deprivation test should be sufficient in most patients to establish the diagnosis of diabetes insipidus and to differentiate central from nephrogenic causes. Plasma vasopressin concentrations may be obtained during the procedure (Figure 9-12), although they are rarely needed for diagnostic purposes in children.[223] They are particularly helpful in differentiating between partial central diabetes insipidus and nephrogenic diabetes insipidus in that they are low in the former and high in the latter situation.[224] If urine osmolality concentrates normally but only after serum osmolality is well above 300 mOsm/kg, the patient may have an altered threshold for vasopressin release (also termed a *reset osmostat*). This may occur after head trauma, neurosurgery, or brain tumors.[225]

Magnetic resonance imaging (MRI) is not very helpful in distinguishing central diabetes insipidus from nephrogenic diabetes insipidus.[226] Normally, the posterior pituitary is seen as an area of enhanced brightness in T1-weighted images after administration of gadolinium.[227] The posterior pituitary "bright spot" is diminished or absent in both forms of diabetes insipidus, presumably because of decreased vasopressin synthesis in central (and increased vasopressin release in nephrogenic) disease.[227-229] In primary polydipsia, the bright spot is normal—probably because vasopressin accumulates in the posterior pituitary during chronic water ingestion,[227] whereas it is decreased in SIADH (presumably because of increased vasopressin secretion).[226] Dynamic fast-frame MRI analysis has allowed estimation of blood flow to the posterior pituitary.[230] With this technique, both central and nephrogenic diabetes insipidus are associated with delayed enhancement in the area of the neurohypophysis.[231]

In the inpatient post-neurosurgical setting, central diabetes insipidus is likely if hyperosmolality (serum osmolality >300 mOsm/kg) is associated with urine osmolality less than serum osmolality. One must beware of intraoperative fluid expansion with subsequent hypo-osmolar polyuria masquerading as diabetes insipidus.

Specific Disorders of Water Metabolism

HYPONATREMIA WITH NORMAL REGULATION OF VASOPRESSIN

Hyponatremia with Appropriate Decreased Secretion of Vasopressin

Increased Water Ingestion (Primary Polydipsia). In a hypo-osmolar state with vasopressin secretion normally suppressed, the kidney can excrete urine with an osmolality as low as 50 mOsm/kg. Under these conditions, a daily solute load of 500 mOsm/m² could be excreted in 10 L/m² of urine per day. Neonates cannot dilute their urine to this degree and are prone to develop water intoxication at levels of water ingestion above 4 L/m²/day (approximately 60 mL/hr in a newborn). This may happen when concentrated infant formula is diluted with excess water, either by accident or in a misguided attempt to make it last longer.[232]

A primary increase in thirst, without apparent cause, leading to hyponatremia has been reported in infants as young 5 weeks of age.[233] In older children, with a normal kidney and the ability to suppress vasopressin secretion, hyponatremia does not occur unless water intake exceeds 10 L/m²/day—a feat almost impossible to accomplish. Long-standing ingestion of large volumes of water will decrease the hypertonicity within the renal medullary interstitium, which will impair water reabsorption and guard against water intoxication.[234] Hyponatremia will occur at lower rates of water ingestion when renal water clearance is impaired, because of inappropriately elevated vasopressin secretion or for other reasons.

The rare patient in whom the osmotic thresholds for thirst and vasopressin release are reversed illustrates the importance of the normal relationship between these two responses to osmotic stimulation.[235] If thirst is activated below the threshold for vasopressin release, water intake and hypo-osmolality will occur and suppress vasopressin secretion—leading to persistent polydipsia and polyuria. As long as daily fluid intake is less than 10 L/m², hyponatremia will not occur. Despite the presence of polyuria and polydipsia, this entity should not be confused with diabetes insipidus because of the absence of hypernatremia. Desmopressin treatment of such a patient may lower serum osmolality below the threshold for thirst, suppressing water ingestion and the consequent polyuria.

Decreased Renal Free Water Clearance. Adrenal insufficiency, primary or secondary, has long been known to result in compromised free water excretion.[40,70] The mechanisms by which glucocorticoids and mineralocorticoids modulate water diuresis have been the subject of substantial investigation. Some studies have demonstrated increased plasma vasopressin activity in the context of glucocorticoid insufficiency,[236,237] consistent with more recent molecular biologic evidence that glucocorticoids inhibit transcription of the vasopressin gene.[238]

Other investigators, however, have failed to detect vasopressin in plasma of patients with adrenal insufficiency and abnormal water clearance.[239] Consistent with vasopressin-independent actions of adrenal steroids on water metabolism, Brattleboro rats with hypothalamic diabetes insipidus manifest impaired excretion of a water load after adrenalectomy.[70] In adrenalectomized Brattleboro rats, glucocorticoid administration restored urine flow rate but did not restore maximal urinary diluting capacity. Conversely, mineralocorticoid administration restored maximal urinary diluting capacity but not flow rate. Thus, both mineralocorticoids and glucocorticoids are required for normal free water clearance. In part, these vasopressin-independent actions of mineralocorticoids and glucocorticoids have been attributed to the increased glomerular filtration rate arising from reexpansion of extracellular fluid volume (reduced owing to salt wasting) and improved cardiovascular tone, respectively.[41,240,241]

By restoring the glomerular filtration rate, more free water is delivered to the distal tubule for excretion. In addition, volume repletion reduces the nonosmotic stimuli for vasopressin release of volume depletion and hypotension. Recently, nitric oxide has been found to stimulate cyclic-guanosine-monophosphate-dependent membrane insertion of aquaporin-2 into renal epithelial cells.[242] Because glucocorticoid has been shown to inhibit endothelial nitric oxide synthase,[243] it is possible that under conditions of glucocorticoid deficiency high levels of nitric oxide synthase result in elevated levels of endothelial nitric oxide in the renal vasculature—which in the distal renal tubule stimulate increased vasopressin-independent aquaporin-2 activity and decreased free water clearance.

Direct effects of glucocorticoid or mineralocorticoid insufficiency on aquaporin expression and function have not been reported. In addition to impairing maximal renal diluting capacity, adrenal insufficiency compromises maximal urine-concentrating capacity.[244] This effect has been shown to result from reduced tubular response to vasopressin.

Thyroid hormone is also required for normal free water clearance, and its deficiency likewise results in decreased renal water clearance and hyponatremia. Although some studies suggest that vasopressin mediates the hyponatremia of hypothyroidism because ethanol increases free water excretion in hypothyroid patients, this effect has not been found in other reports.[245] In severe hypothyroidism, hypovolemia is not present and hyponatremia is accompanied by appropriate suppression of vasopressin.[246] Similar to the consequences of isolated glucocorticoid deficiency described previously, hypothyroidism impairs free water clearance more than maximal urine diluting capacity.[247] This decrease in free water clearance may result from diminished glomerular filtration rate and delivery of free water to the diluting segment of distal nephron, as suggested by animal[248] and human studies.[249]

Given the often subtle clinical findings associated with adrenal and thyroid deficiency, all patients with hyponatremia should be suspected of having these disease states and have appropriate diagnostic tests performed if indicated. Moreover, patients with coexisting adrenal failure and diabetes insipidus may have no symptoms of the latter until glucocorticoid therapy unmasks the need for vasopressin replacement.[250,251] Similarly, resolution of diabetes insipidus in chronically polyuric and polydipsic patients may suggest inadequate glucocorticoid supplementation or noncompliance with glucocorticoid replacement.

Some drugs may cause hyponatremia by inhibiting renal water excretion without stimulating secretion of vasopressin (Table 9-1), an action that could be called nephrogenic SIAD. In addition to augmenting vasopressin release, carbamazepine[252,253] and chlorpropamide[254,255] increase the cellular response to vasopressin. Acetaminophen also increases the response of the kidney to vasopressin.[254] However, this has not been found to cause hyponatremia. High-dose cyclophosphamide treatment (15 to 20 mg/kg intravenous bolus) is often associated with hyponatremia, particularly when it is followed by a forced water diuresis to prevent hemorrhagic cystitis.[256-258] Plasma vasopressin concentrations are normal, suggesting a direct effect of the drug to increase water resorption.[259] Similarly, vinblastine (independent of augmentation of plasma vasopressin concentration or vasopressin action[260]) and cisplatin[261,262] cause hyponatremia. These drugs may damage the collecting duct tubular cells, which are normally highly impermeable to water, or may enhance aquaporin-2 water channel activity and thereby increase water reabsorption down its osmotic gradient into the hypertonic renal interstitium.

Treatment

Hyponatremia due to cortisol or thyroid hormone deficiency reverses promptly after institution of hormone replacement. Because the hyponatremia is often chronic, too rapid an increase in the serum sodium concentration should be avoided if possible (as will be discussed). When drugs that impair free water excretion must be used, water intake should be limited (as if the patient has SIAD) to 1 L/m²/24 hr using the regimen recommended later in the chapter.

HYPONATREMIA WITH APPROPRIATE INCREASED SECRETION OF VASOPRESSIN

Increased vasopressin secretion causing hyponatremia may be an appropriate response or an inappropriate response to a pathologic state. Inappropriate secretion of vasopressin or V2 receptor activity (SIAD) is the much less common of the two entities.[263,264] Whatever the cause, hyponatremia is a worrisome sign often associated with increased morbidity and mortality.[265]

Causes

Systemic Dehydration. Systemic dehydration (water in excess of salt depletion) initially results in hypernatremia, hyperosmolality, and activation of vasopressin secretion (as previously discussed). In addition, the associated fall in the renal glomerular filtration rate results in an increase in proximal tubular sodium and water reabsorption—with a concomitant decrease in distal tubular water excretion. This limits the ability to form a dilute urine, and along with the associated stimulation of the renin-angiotensin-aldosterone system and suppression of ANP secretion results in the excretion of urine very low in sodium.

As dehydration progresses, hypovolemia and/or hypotension become major stimuli for vasopressin release—much more potent than hyperosmolality. This effect, by attempting to preserve volume, decreases free water clearance further and may lead to water retention and hyponatremia—especially if water replacement in excess of salt is given. In many cases, hyponatremia caused by intravascular volume depletion is evident from physical and laboratory signs such as decreased skin turgor, low central venous pressure, hemoconcentration, and elevated blood urea nitrogen levels. The diagnosis may be subtle, however. For example, patients with meningitis may present with hyponatremia for which water restriction has been advocated in the belief that it is due to central SIAD.

Several studies have found that volume depletion, rather than SIAD, is often the cause of the hyponatremia[266,267] and that it resolves more readily when supplemental (rather than restricted) fluid and solute are administered.[268] In patients with hyponatremia after head trauma, volume depletion rather than central SIAD is the cause in approximately one half of cases.[269] Similarly, many patients with gastroenteritis who present with mild hyponatremia and elevated plasma vasopressin levels[270] have these on the basis of systemic dehydration rather than SIAD and benefit from volume expansion rather than fluid restriction.[271] More generally, most hospitalized pediatric patients with hyponatremia benefit from isotonic rather than hypotonic fluid replacement, suggesting that the underlying cause of the electrolyte disturbance is dehydration.[272]

Primary Loss of Sodium Chloride. Salt can be lost from the kidney, such as in patients with congenital polycystic kidney disease, acute interstitial nephritis, and chronic renal failure. Mineralocorticoid deficiency, pseudohypoaldosteronism (sometimes seen in children with

TABLE 9-1

Drugs Impairing Free Water Clearance

Class	Drug	Increases AVP Secretion	Increases AVP Effect	AVP-Independent Renal Effects	Hyponatremia
Angiotensin-converting enzyme inhibitors	Lisinopril	—	—	—	Yes
Anticonvulsants	Carbamazepine/ oxacarbazepine	Yes	Yes	Possibly	Yes
	Valproic acid	—	—	—	Yes
Antineoplastics	Cis-platinum	—	—	Yes	Yes
	Cyclophosphamide	No	—	Yes	Yes
	Vinblastine	Yes	—	Yes	Yes
	Vincristine	Yes	—	—	Yes
Antiparkinsonian	Amantadine, trihexyphenidyl	Yes	—	—	Yes
Antipsychotics	haloperidol, thioridazine	—	—	—	Yes
Antipyretics	Acetaminophen	—	Yes	—	—
Hypolipidemics	Clofibrate	Yes	No	—	—
Oral hypoglycemics	Chlorpropamide, tolbutamide	Yes	Yes	No	Yes
Selective serotonin uptake inhibitors	Fluoxetine, sertraline, others	Likely	—	—	Yes
Tricyclic antidepressants	Imipramine, amitriptyline	Yes	—	—	Yes

Proven actions of the drugs, if known, and whether the drugs have resulted in hyponatremia in humans are indicated.
Adapted from:
Van Amelsvoort T, Bakshi R, Devaux CB, Schwabe S (1994). Hyponatremia associated with carbamazepine and oxcarbazepine therapy: a review. Epilepsia 35:181;
Lozada ES, Gouaux J, Franki N, et al. (1972). Studies of the mode of action of the sulfonylureas and phenylacetamides in enhancing the effect of vasopressin. J Clin Endocrinol Metab 34:704;
Moses AM, Numann P, Miller M (1973). Mechanism of chlorpropamide-induced antidiuresis in man: Evidence for release of ADH and enhancement of peripheral action. Metabolism 22:59;
Zavagli G, Ricci G, Tataranni G, et al. (1988). Life-threatening hyponatremia caused by vinblastine. Med Oncol Tumor Pharmacother 5:67;
Liu BA, Mittman N, Knowles SR, Shear NH (1996). Hyponatremia and the syndrome of inappropriate secretion of antidiuretic hormone associated with the use of selective serotonin reuptake inhibitors: A review of spontaneous reports. Can Med Assoc J 155:519;
Branten AJ, Wetzels JF, Weber AM, Koene RA (1998). Hyponatremia due to sodium valproate. Ann Neurol 43:265;
Jojart I, Laczi F, Laszlo FA, et al. (1987). Hyponatremia and increased secretion of vasopressin induced by vincristine administration in rat. Exp Clin Endocrinol 90:213;
Rider JM, Mauger TF, Jameson JP, Notman DD (1995). Water handling in patients receiving haloperidol decanoate. Ann Pharmacother 29:663;
Settle ECJ (1998). Antidepressant drugs: Disturbing and potentially dangerous adverse effects. J Clin Psychiatry 59:25;
Shaikh ZHA, Taylor HC, Maroo PV, Llerena LA (2000). Syndrome of inappropriate antidiuretic hormone secretion associated with lisinopril. Ann Pharmacother 34:176;
van Laar T, Lammers G-J, Roos RAC, et al. (1998). Antiparkinsonian drugs causing inappropriate antidiuretic hormone secretion. Movement Disorders 13:176.

urinary tract obstruction or infection), diuretic use, and gastrointestinal disease (usually gastroenteritis with diarrhea and/or vomiting) can also result in excess loss of sodium chloride. Hyponatremia can also result from salt loss in sweat in cystic fibrosis, although obstructive lung disease with elevation of plasma vasopressin probably plays a more prominent role (as has been discussed). With the onset of salt loss, any tendency toward hyponatremia will initially be countered by suppression of vasopressin and increased water excretion.

With continuing salt loss, hypovolemia and/or hypotension ensues—causing nonosmotic stimulation of vasopressin. This plus increased thirst, which leads to ingestion of hypotonic fluids with low solute content, results in hyponatremia. Weight loss is usually evident, as is the source of sodium wasting. If it is the kidney, it is accompanied by a rate of urine output and a urine sodium content greater than those associated with most other causes of hyponatremia except a primary increase in ANP secretion.

Decreased Effective Plasma Volume. Congestive heart failure, cirrhosis, nephrotic syndrome, positive pressure mechanical ventilation,[273] severe burns,[274] lung disease (bronchopulmonary dysplasia[275-277] in neonates), cystic fibrosis with obstruction,[278,279] and severe asthma[280,281] are all characterized by a decrease in effective intravascular volume.[245,282] This occurs because of impaired cardiac output, an inability to keep fluid within the vascular space, or impaired blood flow into the heart, respectively.

As with systemic dehydration, in an attempt to preserve intravascular volume water and salt excretion by the kidney are reduced—and decreased barosensor stimulation results in an appropriate compensatory increase in vasopressin secretion, leading to an antidiuretic state and hyponatremia.[283] Because of the associated stimulation of the renin-angiotensin-aldosterone system, these patients also have an increase in total body content of sodium chloride and may have peripheral edema—which distinguishes them from those with systemic dehydration. In patients with impaired cardiac output and elevated atrial volume (e.g., congestive heart failure or lung disease), ANP concentrations are elevated—which contributes to hyponatremia by promoting natriuresis.

Treatment

Patients with systemic dehydration and hypovolemia should be rehydrated with salt-containing fluids such as normal saline or lactated Ringer's solution. Because of activation of the renin-angiotensin-aldosterone system, the administered sodium will be avidly conserved and a water diuresis will quickly ensue as volume is restored and vasopressin concentrations fall.[284] Under these conditions, caution must be taken to prevent too rapid a correction of hyponatremia—which may itself result in brain damage.

Hyponatremia caused by a decrease in effective plasma volume from cardiac, hepatic, renal, or pulmonary dysfunction is more difficult to reverse. The most effective therapy is the least easily achieved: treatment of the underlying systemic disorder. Patients weaned from positive-pressure ventilation undergo a prompt water diuresis and resolution of hyponatremia as cardiac output is restored and vasopressin concentrations fall. The only other effective route is to limit water intake to that required for the renal excretion of the obligate daily solute load of approximately 500 $mOsm/m^2$ and to replenish insensible losses. In a partial antidiuretic state with a urine osmolality of 750 mOsm/kg and insensible losses of 500 mL/m^2, oral intake would have to be limited to approximately 1,200 $mL/m^2/day$.

Because of concomitant hyperaldosteronism, the dietary restriction of sodium chloride needed to control peripheral edema in patients with heart failure may reduce the daily solute load and further limit the amount of water that can be ingested without exacerbating hyponatremia. Hyponatremia in these settings is often slow to develop, rarely causes symptoms, and usually does not need treatment. If the serum sodium falls below 125 mEq/L, water restriction to 1 $L/m^2/day$ is usually effective in preventing a further decline. Because water retention in these disorders is a compensatory response to decreased intravascular volume, an attempt to reverse it with drugs such as demeclocycline or specific V2 receptor antagonists (which induce nephrogenic diabetes insipidus, as discussed earlier) could result in worsening hypovolemia—with potentially dire consequences.[285]

In general, patients with hyponatremia caused by salt loss require ongoing supplementation with sodium chloride and fluids. Initially, intravenous replacement of urine volume with fluid containing sodium chloride (150 to 450 mEq/L, depending on the degree of salt loss) may be necessary. Oral salt supplementation may be required subsequently.[218] This treatment contrasts with that of SIAD, in which water restriction without sodium supplementation is the mainstay.

Precautions in the Emergency Treatment of Hyponatremia

Most children with hyponatremia develop the disorder gradually and are asymptomatic, and thus should be treated with water restriction alone. The development of acute hyponatremia or a serum sodium concentration below 120 mEq/L may be associated with lethargy, psychosis, coma, or generalized seizures—especially in younger children. Acute hyponatremia causes cell swelling owing to the entry of water into cells (Figure 9-13), which can lead to neuronal dysfunction from alterations in the ionic environment or to cerebral herniation because of the encasement of the brain in the cranium. If present for more than 24 hours, cell swelling triggers a compensatory decrease in intracellular organic osmolytes—resulting in the partial restoration of normal cell volume in chronic hyponatremia.[286]

The proper emergency treatment of cerebral dysfunction depends on whether the hyponatremia is acute or chronic.[1,287] In all cases, water restriction should be instituted. If hyponatremia is acute, and therefore probably not associated with a decrease in intracellular organic osmolyte concentration, rapid correction with hypertonic 3% sodium chloride administered intravenously may be indicated. As a general guide, this solution (given in the amount of 12 mL/kg) will result in an increase in serum sodium concentration of approximately 10 mEq/L. If hyponatremia is chronic, hypertonic saline treatment must be undertaken with caution because it may result in cell shrinkage (Figure 9-13) and the associated syndrome of central pontine myelinolysis.[288]

This syndrome, affecting the central portion of the basal pons as well as other brain regions, is characterized by axonal demyelination—with sparing of neurons. It becomes evident within 24 to 48 hours after too rapid correction of hyponatremia, has a characteristic appearance by computed tomography and MRI, and often causes irreversible brain damage.[288-290] If hypertonic saline treatment is undertaken, the serum sodium concentration should be raised only high enough to cause an improvement in mental status—and in no case faster than 0.5 mEq/L/hr or 12 mEq/L/day.[287-290] In the case of systemic dehydration, the increase in serum sodium level may occur very rapidly using this regimen. The associated hyperaldosteronism will cause avid retention of the administered sodium, leading to rapid restoration of volume and suppression of vasopressin secretion and resulting in a brisk water diuresis and an increase in the serum sodium concentration.[284]

Acute treatment of hyponatremia is more difficult in patients with decreased effective plasma volume. This is because the underlying disorder makes it difficult to maintain the administered fluid within the intravascular space and because an associated increase in ANP promotes natriuresis and loss of the administered salt. Furthermore, patients with cardiac disease who are administered hypertonic saline may require concomitant treatment with a diuretic such as furosemide to prevent worsening of heart failure—which will also increase natriuresis.

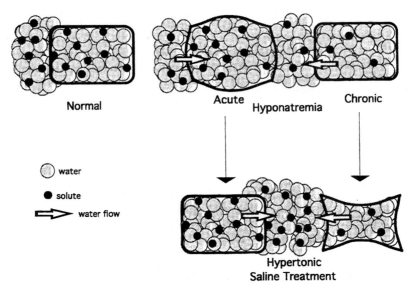

Figure 9-13 Changes in organic osmolytes with hyponatremia and after its correction. Under normal conditions, osmotic balance exists between extracellular and intracellular compartments. With acute hyponatremia, water enters cells—causing cell swelling. After approximately 24 hours of continued hyponatremia, intracellular organic osmolytes decrease—restoring cell volume toward normal. Hypertonic saline treatment of acute hyponatremia results in restoration of normal cell volume, whereas the same treatment of chronic hyponatremia results in cell shrinkage. Large circle, water; closed smaller circle, solute; and arrow, direction of water flow.

Hyponatremia with Abnormal Regulation of Vasopressin

HYPONATREMIA WITH INAPPROPRIATE INCREASED SECRETION OF VASOPRESSIN OR INCREASED VASOPRESSIN V2 RECEPTOR ACTIVITY (SYNDROME OF INAPPROPRIATE ANTIDIURESIS)

Causes of SIAD

SIAD is uncommon in children.[263,264,291] It can occur with encephalitis, brain tumor,[292] head trauma,[269,293] or psychiatric disease[294]; in the postictal period after generalized seizures[295]; and after prolonged nausea,[296,297] pneumonia,[298,299] or AIDS.[300] Many drugs have been associated with impaired free water clearance, as indicated in Table 9-1. Impaired free water clearance can result from alteration in vasopressin release, increased vasopressin effect at the same plasma vasopressin concentration, or vasopressin-independent changes in distal collecting tubule water permeability. Common drugs that have been shown to increase vasopressin secretion and result in hyponatremia include carbamazepine,[253] chlorpropamide,[301] vinblastine,[260] vincristine,[302] and tricyclic antidepressants.[303,304]

Newer sulfonylurea agents, including glyburide, are not associated with SIAD.[305] Other rarer causes of SIAD in children are listed in Table 9-2. Although SIAD has been believed to be the cause of hyponatremia associated with viral meningitis, volume depletion is more commonly the etiology.[266,268] In contrast, the majority of children with tuberculous meningitis have hyponatremia and SIAD—which predict more severe disease and poor outcome.[306-308] SIAD is the cause of the hyponatremic second phase of triple-phase response seen after hypothalamic-pituitary surgery.

Hyponatremia with elevated vasopressin secretion is found in up to 35% of patients 1 week after transsphenoidal pituitary surgery.[309,310] The mechanism is most likely retrograde neuronal degeneration with cell death and vasopressin release. Secondary adrenal insufficiency causing stimulation of vasopressin release[69] may also play a role because hyponatremia most commonly follows the removal of adrenocorticotropin hormone-secreting corticotroph adenomas.[310] In the vast majority of children with SIAD, the cause is the excessive administration of vasopressin—whether to treat central diabetes insipidus,[221,311] or less commonly bleeding disorders[312] (as has been discussed previously), or most uncommonly following dDAVP therapy for enuresis.

Recently, two unrelated infants (with mutations in the vasopressin V2 receptor) who presented with severe hyponatremia in the first months of life have been described.[313] These two infants had missense mutations at codon 137 that converted arginine to cysteine or leucine and led to constitutive activation of the V2 receptor with appropriately suppressed arginine vasopressin plasma concentration. This genetic disorder has been termed *nephrogenic syndrome of antidiuresis*. It remains unclear what portion of isolated early-onset chronic SIAD results from activating mutations of the V2 receptor, although the incidence is likely to be very low. Interestingly, this same codon is also the site of a loss-of-function mutation (R137H) that leads to X-linked nephrogenic diabetes insipidus.[314]

Treatment of SIAD

Chronic SIAD is best treated by chronic oral fluid restriction. Under full vasopressin antidiuretic effect (urine osmolality of 1,000 mOsm/L), a normal daily obligate renal solute load of 500 mOsm/m² would be excreted in 500 mL/m² of water. This plus a daily nonrenal water

TABLE 9-2

Causes of Syndrome of Inappropriate Secretion of Antidiuretic Hormone (Vasopressin)

Central Nervous System	Cancer	Infections	Pulmonary
Head trauma	Small cell of lung	Herpes zoster	Viral pneumonia
Subarachnoid hemorrhage	Duodenum	Respiratory syncytial virus	Bacterial pneumonia
Brain abscess	Pancreas	Tuberculosis	Abscess
Guillain-Barré syndrome	Thymoma	Aspergillosis	
Hydrocephalus	Bladder	Botulism	
Meningitis	Ureter		
	Lymphoma		
	Ewing's sarcoma		

loss of 500 mL/m² would require that oral fluid intake be limited to 1,000 mL/m²/day to avoid hyponatremia, as has been discussed more fully. In young children, this degree of fluid restriction may not provide adequate calories for growth. In this situation, the creation of nephrogenic diabetes insipidus using demeclocycline therapy may be indicated to allow sufficient fluid intake for normal growth.[315]

Demeclocycline is superior to lithium for this purpose.[316] Lithium and demeclocycline, however, are associated with significant toxicities—which may limit their use in pediatric patients. Oral urea has been effectively used to treat adult patients with chronic SIAD by virtue of its ability to induce an effective osmotic diuresis. This therapy was also demonstrated to be safe and effective in four children with chronic SIAD, including two with mutations in the vasopressin V2 receptor.[317] Specific V2 receptor antagonists are also being developed for use in chronic SIAD.[318-320] In a large series of adult patients with euvolemic or hypervolemic hyponatremia, the vasopressin receptor antagonists were effective in sustained elevation of serum sodium concentration.[320] These agents would not be expected to be effective in activating mutations of the V2 receptor unless they interfered with the normal trafficking of the receptor to the cell surface. On that note, some of these V2 receptor antagonists facilitate the proper transport of loss-of-function V2 receptor mutants to the cell surface.[321]

Acute treatment of hyponatremia due to SIAD is only indicated if cerebral dysfunction is present. In that case, treatment is dictated by the duration of hyponatremia and the extent of cerebral dysfunction. Because patients with SIAD have volume expansion, salt administration is not very effective in raising the serum sodium because it is rapidly excreted in the urine due to suppressed aldosterone and elevated atrial natriuretic peptide concentrations.

HYPONATREMIA WITH INAPPROPRIATE DECREASED SECRETION OF VASOPRESSIN DUE TO INCREASED SECRETION OF ATRIAL NATRIURETIC PEPTIDE

Although atrial natriuretic peptide does not usually play a primary role in the pathogenesis of disorders of water metabolism, it may have an important secondary role.[275,322-324]

Patients with SIAD have elevated atrial natriuretic peptide concentrations, probably due to hypervolemia, which may contribute to the elevated natriuresis of SIAD and which decrease as water intake is restricted.[322] Likewise, the suppressed atrial natriuretic peptide concentrations found in central diabetes insipidus, probably due to the associated hypovolemia, rise after dDAVP therapy.[322] However, hyponatremia in some patients (primarily those with central nervous system disorders, including brain tumor, head trauma, hydrocephalus, neurosurgery, cerebral vascular accidents, and brain death) may be due to the primary hypersecretion of atrial natriuretic peptide.[218,325-327]

This syndrome, called cerebral salt wasting, is defined by hyponatremia accompanied by elevated urinary sodium excretion (often more than 150 mEq/L), excessive urine output, hypovolemia, suppressed vasopressin, and elevated atrial natriuretic peptide concentrations (>20 pmol/L). Thus, it is distinguished from SIAD—in which normal or decreased urine output, euvolemia, only modestly elevated urine sodium concentration, and elevated vasopressin concentration occur. Direct measurement of intravascular volume status with a central venous line is often helpful. The distinction is important because the therapies of the two disorders are markedly different.

Treatment of Cerebral Salt Wasting

Treatment of patients with cerebral salt wasting consists of restoring intravascular volume with sodium chloride and water, as with the treatment of other causes of systemic dehydration. The underlying cause of the disorder, which is usually due to acute brain injury, should also be treated if possible.

OTHER CAUSES OF TRUE AND FACTITIOUS HYPONATREMIA

True hyponatremia is associated with hyperglycemia, which causes the influx of water into the intravascular space. Serum sodium will decrease by 1.6 mEq/L for every 100 mg/dL increment in blood glucose above 100 mg/dL. Glucose is not ordinarily an osmotically active agent, and does not stimulate vasopressin release—probably because it is able to equilibrate freely across plasma membranes. However, in the presence of insulin deficiency and hyperglycemia glucose acts as an osmotic agent—presumably because its normal intracellular access to osmosensor sites is prevented.[328]

Under these circumstances, an osmotic gradient exists—and this stimulates vasopressin release. In diabetic ketoacidosis, this (together with the hypovolemia caused by the osmotic diuresis secondary to glycosuria) results in marked stimulation of vasopressin secretion.[329-332] Rapid correction of hyponatremia may follow soon after the institution of fluid and insulin therapy. Whether this contributes to the pathogenesis of cerebral edema occasionally seen following treatment of diabetic ketoacidosis is not known. Elevated concentrations of triglycerides may cause factitious hyponatremia, as can obtaining a blood sample downstream from an intravenous infusion of hypotonic fluid.

Hypernatremia with Inappropriate Decreased Vasopressin Secretion or Action

CENTRAL DIABETES INSIPIDUS

Causes of Central Diabetes Insipidus

Central (hypothalamic, neurogenic, or vasopressin-sensitive) diabetes insipidus can be caused by disorders of vasopressin gene structure; accidental or surgical trauma to vasopressin neurons; congenital anatomical hypothalamic or pituitary defects; neoplasms; infiltrative, autoimmune, and infectious diseases affecting vasopressin neurons or fiber tracts; and increased metabolism of vasopressin. In approximately 10% of children with central diabetes insipidus, the etiology is not apparent.[333,334]

Genetic Causes. Familial autosomal-dominant central diabetes insipidus is manifest within the first half of the first decade of life.[335] Vasopressin secretion, initially normal, gradually declines until diabetes insipidus of variable severity ensues. Patients respond well to vasopressin replacement therapy. The disease has a high degree of penetrance, but may be of variable severity within a family[336] and may spontaneously improve in middle age.[336,337] Vasopressin-containing neurons are absent from the magnocellular paraventricular neurons[338] but present in parvocellular regions.[339] Several different oligonucleotide mutations in the vasopressin structural gene have been found to cause the disease (*www.medcon.mcgill.ca/nephros/avp_npii.html*).

To date, there have been more than 25 mutations detected in the coding region of the vasopressin gene (Figure 9-3). Most mutations are in the neurophysin portion of the vasopressin precursor, except for five in either the signal peptide or vasopressin peptide regions of the gene. This suggests that neurophysin has a valuable function, possibly in the proper intracellular sorting or packaging of vasopressin into secretory granules. There are no disease-causing mutations in the copeptin region of the vasopressin precursor. This suggests either that this region has a low mutation rate or more likely that it does not serve a critical function in vasopressin biology.

A family with a missense mutation within the vasopressin peptide region (Proline→Leucine at amino acid 7)

of the gene, causing markedly reduced biological activity, was reported.[340] The disease in this family is transmitted with an autosomal-recessive pattern. This indicates that haplo-insufficiency is not the basis for the autosomal-dominant nature of the disease in families with the more common mutations in the neurophysin region of the gene. Rather, the abnormal gene product may interfere with the processing and secretion of the product of the normal allele[341] or may cause neuronal degeneration and cell death.[342] In support of this, mutant vasopressin precursors impair the secretion of the normal protein in cell models.[341] In a transgenic mouse model of the disease, a progressive loss of hypothalamic vasopressin-containing neurons occurs as the mice develop diabetes insipidus.[343]

Vasopressin deficiency is also found in the DIDMOAD syndrome, consisting of diabetes insipidus, diabetes mellitus, optic atrophy, and deafness.[344,345] One[346] (but not another[347]) study has suggested that a mitochondrial defect is responsible for the disease. The gene for this syndrome complex, also known as Wolfram syndrome, was localized to human chromosome 4p16 by polymorphic linkage analysis[348] and has recently been isolated.[349] The Wolfram syndrome gene, WFS1, encodes an 890-amino-acid putative transmembrane protein of unknown function.[349] More recent analysis of multiple kindreds with Wolfram syndrome has disclosed a variety of different single-nucleotide mutations in the WFS1 gene, and no mutations in mitochondrial DNA.[350]

Trauma. The axons of vasopressin-containing magnocellular neurons extend uninterrupted to the posterior pituitary over a distance of approximately 10 mm. Trauma to the base of the brain can cause swelling around or severance of these axons, resulting in transient or permanent diabetes insipidus.[351] Permanent diabetes insipidus can occur after seemingly minor trauma. Approximately half of patients with fractures of the sella turcica will develop permanent diabetes insipidus,[352] which may be delayed as long as 1 month following the trauma—during which neurons of severed axons may undergo retrograde degeneration.[353]

Septic shock[354] and postpartum hemorrhage associated with pituitary infarction (Sheehan syndrome)[355,356] may involve the posterior pituitary with varying degrees of diabetes insipidus. Diabetes insipidus is never associated with cranial irradiation of the hypothalamic-pituitary region, although this treatment can cause deficits in all of the hypothalamic-releasing hormones carried by the portal-hypophyseal system to the anterior pituitary (see Chapter 8). Because vasopressin is carried directly to the posterior pituitary via magnocellular axonal transport, radiation may affect hypothalamic-releasing hormone function by interruption of the portal-hypophyseal circulation.

Neurosurgical Intervention. One of the most common causes of central diabetes insipidus is the neurosurgical destruction of vasopressin neurons following pituitary-hypothalamic surgery. It is important to distinguish polyuria associated with the onset of acute postsurgical central diabetes insipidus from polyuria due to the normal diuresis of fluids given during surgery. In both cases, the urine may be very dilute and of high volume, exceeding 200 mL/m²/h. However, in the former case serum osmolality will be high—whereas in the latter case it will be normal. A careful examination of the intraoperative record should also help distinguish between these two possibilities.

Vasopressin axons traveling from the hypothalamus to the posterior pituitary terminate at various levels within the stalk and gland (Figure 9-4). Because surgical interruption of these axons can result in retrograde degeneration of hypothalamic neurons, lesions closer to the hypothalamus will affect more neurons and cause greater permanent loss of hormone secretion. Not infrequently, a "triple-phase" response is seen.[357]

Following surgery, an initial phase of transient diabetes insipidus is observed—lasting 0.5 to 2 days and possibly due to edema in the area interfering with normal vasopressin secretion. If significant vasopressin cell destruction has occurred, this is often followed by a second phase of SIAD—which may last up to 10 days and is due to the unregulated release of vasopressin by dying neurons. A third phase of permanent diabetes insipidus may follow if more than 90% of vasopressin cells are destroyed. Usually, a marked degree of SIAD in the second phase portends significant permanent diabetes insipidus in the final phase of this response.

In patients with coexisting vasopressin and cortisol deficits (e.g., in combined anterior and posterior hypopituitarism following neurosurgical treatment of craniopharyngioma), symptoms of diabetes insipidus may be masked because cortisol deficiency impairs renal free water clearance. In such cases, institution of glucocorticoid therapy alone may precipitate polyuria, leading to the diagnosis of diabetes insipidus.

Congenital Anatomic Defects. Midline brain anatomic abnormalities such as septo-optic dysplasia with agenesis of the corpus callosum,[358] the Kabuki syndrome,[359] holoprosencephaly,[360] and familial pituitary hypoplasia with absent stalk[361] may be associated with central diabetes insipidus. These patients need not have external evidence of craniofacial abnormalities.[360] Central diabetes insipidus due to midline brain abnormalities is often accompanied by defects in thirst perception,[358] suggesting that a common osmosensor may control vasopressin release and thirst perception. Some patients with suspected defects in osmosensor function but with intact vasopressin neurons may have recumbent diabetes insipidus, with baroreceptor-mediated release of vasopressin while upright and vasopressin-deficient polyuria while supine.[362]

Neoplasms. Several important clinical implications follow from knowledge of the anatomy of the vasopressin system. Because hypothalamic vasopressin neurons are distributed over a large area within the hypothalamus, tumors that cause diabetes insipidus must either be very large or infiltrative or be strategically located at the point of convergence of the hypothalamo-neurohypophyseal axonal tract in the infundibulum. Germinomas and pinealomas typically arise near the base of the hypothalamus, where vasopressin axons converge before their entry into the posterior pituitary. For this reason, they are among the most common primary brain tumors associated with diabetes insipidus.

Germinomas causing the disease can be very small,[363,364] and can be undetectable by MRI for several years following the onset of polyuria.[365] For this reason, quantitative measurement of the β subunit of human chorionic gonadotropin (often secreted by germinomas and pinealomas) and regularly repeated MRI scans should be performed in children with idiopathic or unexplained diabetes insipidus. Empty sella syndrome, possibly due to unrecognized pituitary infarction, can be associated with diabetes insipidus in children.[366]

Craniopharyngiomas and optic gliomas can also cause central diabetes insipidus when very large, although this is more often a postoperative complication of the treatment for these tumors. Hematologic malignancies can cause diabetes insipidus. In some cases, such as with acute myelocytic leukemia, the cause is infiltration of the pituitary stalk and sella.[367-369] However, more than 30 patients with monosomy or deletion of chromosome 7 associated with acute blast transformation of myelodysplastic syndrome presented with central diabetes insipidus[370-373] without evidence of infiltration of the posterior pituitary by neoplastic cells—leaving the cause of the diabetes insipidus unresolved.

Infiltrative, Autoimmune, and Infectious Diseases. Langerhans cell histiocytosis and lymphocytic hypophysitis are the most common types of infiltrative disorders causing central diabetes insipidus. Approximately 10% of patients with histiocytosis will have diabetes insipidus. These patients tend to have more serious multisystem disease for longer periods of time than those without diabetes insipidus,[374,375] and anterior pituitary deficits often accompany posterior pituitary deficiency.[376] MRI characteristically shows thickening of the pituitary stalk.[377] One report suggests that in patients with Langerhans cell histiocytosis radiation treatment to the pituitary region within 14 days of onset of symptoms of diabetes insipidus may result in return of vasopressin function in more than a third of affected patients.[378]

Lymphocytic infundibuloneurohypophysitis may account for more than half of patients with "idiopathic" central diabetes insipidus.[379] This entity may be associated with other autoimmune diseases.[380] Image analysis discloses an enlarged pituitary and thickened stalk,[379,381] and biopsy of the posterior pituitary reveals lymphocytic infiltration of the gland, stalk, and magnocellular hypothalamic nuclei.[382] A necrotizing form of this entity has been described that also causes anterior pituitary failure and responds to steroid treatment.[383] Diabetes insipidus can also be associated with pulmonary granulomatous diseases,[384] including sarcoidosis.[385]

Whether antibody-mediated destruction of vasopressin cells occurs is controversial. More than half of patients with central diabetes insipidus of a nontraumatic cause have antibodies directed against vasopressin-containing cells,[386] and patients with other autoimmune diseases have such antibodies without evidence of diabetes insipidus.[387] Many patients with central diabetes insipidus also have anti-vasopressin peptide antibodies, although their appearance usually follows institution of vasopressin treatment.[388] It is very possible that antibodies directed against vasopressin-containing cells or vasopressin are not pathogenetic, but are instead markers of prior neuronal cell destruction.

Infections involving the base of the brain (such as meningococcal,[389] cryptococcal, listeria,[390] and toxoplasmosis[391] meningitis; congenital cytomegalovirus infection[392];

and nonspecific inflammatory disease of the brain[393]) can cause central diabetes insipidus. The disease is often transient, suggesting that it is due to inflammation rather than destruction of vasopressin-containing neurons.

Brain Death. Central diabetes insipidus can appear in the setting of hypoxic brain death.[394] Although its presence has been suggested as a marker for brain death in children,[395] in some studies only a minority of patients with brain death manifest the disorder[396] and up to 15% of patients with cerebral insults and diabetes insipidus ultimately recover brain function.[397] Polyuria in the setting of brain death can be accompanied by high concentrations of plasma vasopressin,[398] suggesting that some cases mistaken for diabetes insipidus are actually due to other causes—such as cerebral salt wasting with polyuria.

Increased Metabolism of Vasopressin. The metabolic clearance rate of vasopressin increases fourfold during pregnancy due to the elaboration of a vasopressinase by the placenta.[72] If the mother cannot respond with a concomitant increase in vasopressin action because of preexisting subclinical central or nephrogenic diabetes insipidus,[73] overt transient disease will appear—usually early in the third trimester. This will resolve within 1 week of delivery.[76,399] Even without prior defects in vasopressin function, an extreme elevation in vasopressinase concentrations in primigravidas (with preeclampsia, liver dysfunction, or multiple gestation[74,75,78,400-402]) may result in development of the syndrome.

Drugs. The most common agent associated with inhibition of vasopressin release and impaired urine concentrating ability is ethanol.[403] Because inhibition of vasopressin release by ethanol can be overcome in the setting of concurrent hypovolemia, clinically important diabetes insipidus due to ethanol ingestion is uncommon.[404] Phenytoin, opiate antagonists, halothane, and α-adrenergic agents have also been associated with impaired vasopressin release.[405,406]

Children with Primary Enuresis. Although normal children have a nocturnal rise in plasma vasopressin associated with an increase in urine osmolality and a decrease in urine volume, those with primary enuresis have a blunted or absent rise in vasopressin and excrete a higher urine volume of lower tonicity.[407,408] This has suggested that enuretic children have a primary deficiency in vasopressin secretion, although the same outcome could be caused solely by excessive water intake in these children. The use of the V2 agonist dDAVP is highly effective in abolishing bed wetting episodes, although relapse is high once therapy is stopped.[409-411] Fluid intake must be limited while a child is exposed to the antidiuretic action of dDAVP to guard against water intoxication. Recently, the FDA has issued an alert stating that intranasal forms of dDAVP are no longer indicated for treatment of primary enuresis and all forms should be used with caution.

Treatment of Central Diabetes Insipidus

Fluid Therapy. Patients with otherwise untreated diabetes insipidus crave cold fluids, especially water. With complete central diabetes insipidus, maximum urine-concentrating ability is approximately 100 mOsm/kg. Because 5 L of urine would be required to excrete an average daily solute load of 500 mOsm/m², fluid intake

must match this to maintain normal plasma tonicity. With an intact thirst mechanism and free access to oral fluids, a person with complete diabetes insipidus can maintain plasma osmolality and sodium in the high normal range—although at great inconvenience. Furthermore, long-standing intake of these volumes of fluid in children can lead to hydroureter[412]—and even in hyperfluorosis in communities that provide fluoridated water.[413]

There are two situations in which central diabetes insipidus may be treated solely with high levels of fluid intake (i.e., without vasopressin). Vasopressin therapy coupled with excessive fluid intake (usually greater than 1 L/m²/day, as discussed subsequently) can result in unwanted hyponatremia. Because neonates and young infants receive all of their nutrition in liquid form, the obligatory high oral fluid requirements for this age (3 L/m²/day) combined with vasopressin treatment are likely to lead to this dangerous complication.[311] Oral tablet or intranasal liquid desmopressin is difficult to accurately administer to infants.

Such neonates may be better managed with fluid therapy alone. A reduced solute load diet will aid in this regard. Human milk is best for this purpose (75 mOsm/kg H_2O), whereas cow's milk is worst (230 mOsm/kg H_2O). For example, in an infant with diabetes insipidus with a fixed urine osmolality of 100 mOsm/kg H_2O 300 mL of urine per day is required to excrete the amount of solute consumed in human milk—whereas 900 mL of urine per day is required to excrete the higher amount of solute consumed in cow's milk. Although children managed with such a regimen may be chronically thirsty, parents may have difficulty keeping up with the voluminous fluid intake and urine output, and poor growth may occur if adequate calories are not provided along with water,[233] these problems are more easily addressed than is life-threatening hyponatremia.

Alternatively, thiazide (chlorthiazide, 5-10 mg/kg/dose) twice daily[414] and/or amiloride diuretics may be added to facilitate renal proximal tubular sodium and water reabsorption[415]—and thereby decrease oral fluid requirements. This therapy may be accompanied by a mild degree of dehydration. More recently, parenteral desmopressin (0.02-0.08 μg/dose given once or twice daily) has been administered subcutaneously in infants with good results—although this has not been approved by the FDA.[416]

Parenteral desmopressin was originally formulated at a concentration of 4 μg/mL, to be used at a dose of 0.3 μg/kg/dose to treat bleeding diatheses such as hemophilia A and von Willebrand's disease type 1. Thus, care must be taken if it is used at 1/40 to 1/4 of this dose to treat infants with diabetes insipidus. In older children on more calorie-dense solid diets, the use of short-acting agents such as arginine vasopressin (Pitressin) or lysine vasopressin (Diapid, lypressin) or longer-acting desmopressin will decrease fluid needs while minimizing the possible occurrence of hyponatremia (see "Vasopressin and Vasopressin Analogues").

In the acute postoperative management of central diabetes insipidus occurring after neurosurgery in children, vasopressin therapy may be successfully employed.[417-419] However, extreme caution must be exerted with its use. While under the full antidiuretic effect of vasopressin, a patient will have a urine osmolality of approximately 1,000 mOsm/kg and become hyponatremic if he or she receives an excessive amount of fluids—depending on the solute load and nonrenal water losses. With a solute excretion of 500 mOsm/m²/day, normal renal function, and nonrenal fluid losses of 500 ml/m²/day, fluid intake of greater than 1 L/m²/day (2/3 of the normal maintenance fluid requirement) will result in hyponatremia. In addition, vasopressin therapy will mask the emergence of the SIAD phase of the triple-phase neurohypophyseal response to neurosurgical injury.

Because of the concerns associated with perioperative vasopressin administration, two different approaches to managing central diabetes insipidus in the surgical patient have been employed. The first approach may be particularly useful in managing acute postoperative diabetes insipidus in young children. It employs fluids alone and avoids the use of vasopressin.[420] This method consists of matching input and output hourly using between 1 and 3 L/m²/day (40 to 120 mL/m²/hr). If intravenous therapy is used, a basal 40 mL/m²/hr should be given as 5% dextrose (D5) in one-fourth normal saline (normal saline = 0.9% sodium chloride)—and the remainder, depending on the urine output, as 5% dextrose in water.

Potassium chloride (40 mEq/L) may be added if oral intake is to be delayed for several days. No additional fluid should be administered for hourly urine volumes under 40 mL/m²/hr. For hourly urine volumes above 40 mL/m²/hr, the additional volume should be replaced with 5% dextrose up to a total maximum of 120 mL/m²/hr. For example, in a child with a surface area of 1 m² (approximately 30 kg), the basal infusion rate would be 40 mL/hr of 5% dextrose in one-fourth normal saline. For an hourly urine output of 60 mL, an additional 20 mL/hr 5% dextrose would be given for a total infusion rate of 60 mL/hr.

For urine outputs above 120 mL/hr, the total infusion rate would be 120 mL/hr. In the presence of diabetes insipidus, this will result in a serum sodium in the 150-mEq/L range and a mildly volume contracted state—which will allow one to assess thirst sensation and the return of normal vasopressin function or the emergence of SIAD. Patients may become mildly hyperglycemic with this regimen, particularly if they are also receiving postoperative glucocorticoids. However, because it does not use vasopressin this fluid management protocol prevents any chance of hyponatremia.

Vasopressin and Vasopressin Analogues. Recent evidence suggests that perioperative use of intravenous vasopressin in children with central diabetes insipidus may be the treatment modality of choice in most situations, resulting in excursions of serum sodium of smaller magnitude and few adverse sequelae.[419] Although intravenous therapy with synthetic aqueous vasopressin (Pitressin) had been shown to be useful in the management central diabetes insipidus of acute onset,[417,418] concern existed as to the safety of its administration in the complex and rapidly changing course of the child recovering from hypothalamic/pituitary surgery. If continuous vasopressin is administered, fluid intake must be limited to 1 L/m²/day or two-thirds maintenance fluid administration (assuming normal solute intake and nonrenal water losses, as described).

The potency of synthetic vasopressin is still measured using a bioassay and is expressed in bioactive units, with one milliunit (mU) equivalent to approximately 2.5 ng of vasopressin. For intravenous vasopressin therapy, 1.5 mU/kg/hr results in a blood vasopressin concentration of approximately 10 pg/mL[421]—twice that needed for full antidiuretic activity.[422] Vasopressin's effect is maximal within 2 hours of the start of infusion,[422] and one must beware of it sticking to intravenous bottles and tubing. Occasionally following hypothalamic (but not trans-sphenoidal) surgery, higher initial concentrations of vasopressin are required to treat acute diabetes insipidus—which may be attributable to the release of a substance related to vasopressin from the damaged hypothalamo-neurohypophyseal system, which acts as an antagonist to normal vasopressin activity.[423] Much higher rates of vasopressin infusion resulting in plasma concentrations above 1,000 pg/mL should be avoided because they may cause cutaneous necrosis,[424] rhabdomyolysis,[424,425] and cardiac rhythm disturbances.[426]

In light of the considerations described in the previous paragraph, an effective and safe algorithm for management of perioperative central diabetes insipidus with central diabetes insipidus has been utilized with encouraging results.[419] This algorithm starts with the child receiving an intravenous infusion of normal saline at two-thirds maintenance or 1 L/m²/day. A tentative diagnosis of intraoperative or postoperative central diabetes insipidus is made by documenting a serum sodium of greater than 145 mEq/L along with urine output of greater than 4 mL/kg/hr. Additional confirmatory evidence includes plasma osmolarity above 300 mOsm/kg H₂O and a relatively hypotonic urine.

When documentation of parameters consistent with central diabetes insipidus is obtained, an intravenous infusion of aqueous vasopressin begins at 0.5 mU/kg/hr—with no change in intravenous fluid administration. The dose of vasopressin is titrated upward in 0.5-mU/kg/hr increments to establish a urine output rate of less than 2 mL/kg/hr at approximately 10-minute intervals. The vasopressin and intravenous fluid administration then remain stable at these rates, with additional normal saline or equivalent volume expanding solutions given only to replace ongoing blood loss or to maintain hemodynamic stability. Postoperatively, this management paradigm requires intensive care unit monitoring—with frequent assessment of electrolytes (hourly initially), urine output and osmolarity/specific gravity, and vital signs.

This management scheme can also be followed for patients with established central diabetes insipidus requiring general surgery and prolonged restriction of oral intake. In this situation, the usual dose of chronic long-acting vasopressin is withheld or reduced immediately prior to surgery—depending on the timing of surgery in relation to the usual administration times. In preparation for surgery, normal saline is infused at two-thirds maintenance (1 L/m²/day). When measures consistent with emergence of central diabetes insipidus due to termination of efficacy of the presurgical dose are obtained, the intravenous vasopressin is initiated and titrated as described previously.

Patients treated with vasopressin for post-neurosurgical diabetes insipidus should be switched from intravenous to oral fluid intake at the earliest opportunity because thirst sensation, if intact, will help regulate blood osmolality. Intravenous dDAVP (Desmopressin) should not be used in the acute management of postoperative central diabetes insipidus because it offers no advantage over vasopressin and because its long half-life (8-12 hr) compared with that of vasopressin (5-10 min) is a distinct disadvantage—as it may increase the chance of causing water intoxication.[221] In fact, the use of intravenous dDAVP (0.3 μg/kg) to shorten the bleeding time in a variety of bleeding disorders has been associated with water intoxication[312]—particularly in young children, who have high obligate oral fluid needs.

A special problem arises when a patient with established central diabetes insipidus must receive a high volume of fluid for therapeutic reasons (e.g., accompanying cancer chemotherapy). Such patients can be managed by discontinuing antidiuretic therapy and increasing fluid intake to 3 to 5 L/m²/day (rendering the patient moderately hypernatremic). Although 5 L/m²/day is typically adequate to maintain serum sodium concentration in the range of 150 mEq/L in children with central diabetes insipidus, this rate may not be adequate in the setting of chemotherapy administration when solute excretion increases due to cell death and release of cellular content.

By using a low dose of intravenous vasopressin (0.08-0.1 mU/kg/hr, approximately one-eighth the full antidiuretic dose, titrated upward as needed), a partial antidiuretic effect allows the administration of higher amounts of fluid without causing hyponatremia.[427] Recent data suggests that excretion of a hypotonic urine, as would occur in patients with diabetes insipidus management with fluids alone, increases the risk of developing nephrotoxicity during therapy with platinum-based antineoplastic agents.[428] By allowing administration of 0.45 normal saline at rates of approximately 3 L/m²/day, the low-dose vasopressin infusion yields a urine osmolarity higher than that achievable with fluids alone[427] and may have the additional benefit of conferring renal protection.

In the outpatient setting, treatment of central diabetes insipidus in older children should begin with oral (see material following) or intranasal dDAVP (10 μg/0.1 mL)—0.025 mL (2.5 μg) given by rhinal tube at bedtime and the dose increased to the lowest amount that gives an antidiuretic effect. If the dose is effective but has too short a duration, it should be increased further—or a second (morning) dose should be added. Patients should escape from the antidiuretic effect for at least 1 hour before the next dose, to ensure that any excessive water will be excreted. Otherwise, water intoxication may occur. dDAVP is also available as a nasal spray in the same concentration, with each spray delivering 10 μg (0.1 mL). This is the standard preparation used for treatment of primary enuresis. Oral dDAVP tablets have recently come into widespread use and have largely replaced intranasal therapy. Although when given orally dDAVP is at least twentyfold less potent than when given via the intranasal route, oral dDAVP in doses of 25 to 300 micrograms every 8 to 12 hours is reported to be highly effective and safe in children.[429-431] Lysine vasopressin (Diapid) nasal spray (50 U/mL) may be used if a duration less than that

of dDAVP is desired. One spray delivers 2 U (0.04 mL), with a duration of action between 2 and 8 hours.

As noted previously, cortisol deficiency may cause decreased free water clearance by stimulating a nitric-oxide-mediated pathway that results in the insertion of aquaporin-2 channels into the apical membranes of collecting duct cells in a vasopressin-independent fashion.[242,243] Conversely, it is possible that excessive amounts of cortisol (due to endogenous release during stress, or to treatment with exogenous drug) may inhibit the insertion of water channels. This may explain why patients with central diabetes insipidus treated with desmopressin become "resistant" and require an increased dosage during times of stress or treatment with glucocorticoids.

In addition to polyuria and polydipsia, decreased bone mineral density has been reported in patients with central diabetes insipidus.[432] The decreased bone density was not corrected by vasopressin analog treatment alone, suggesting that institution of bisphosphonate or other therapies designed to prevent bone loss may be of long-term benefit in the treatment of diabetes insipidus.

NEPHROGENIC DIABETES INSIPIDUS

Causes of Nephrogenic Diabetes Insipidus

Nephrogenic (vasopressin-resistant) diabetes insipidus can be due to genetic or acquired causes. Genetic causes are less common but more severe than acquired forms of the disease, although genetic etiologies are more common in children than in adults.

Genetic Causes

Congenital X-linked Diabetes Insipidus: V2 Receptor Mutations. Congenital X-linked nephrogenic diabetes insipidus is caused by inactivating mutations of the vasopressin V2 receptor. Due to its mode of transmission, it is a disease of males—although rarely females may be affected, presumably due to extreme Lyonization during X chromosome inactivation.[433] In keeping with a germ-line (as opposed to somatic) mutation in the V2 receptor, these patients are deficient in all systemic V2-receptor-mediated actions[434,435] and have intact V1-receptor-mediated responses.[436,437] As expected, the V2 receptor defect is proximal to the activation of renal adenylate cyclase.[438,439] Unlike the function of other G-protein–coupled seven-transmembrane receptors such as the PTH and TSH receptors, that of the V2 receptor is unaffected in patients with pseudohypoparathyroidism (who have inactivating mutations in the alpha subunit of G_s[440]).

Because of vasopressin resistance in congenital nephrogenic diabetes insipidus, the kidney elaborates large volumes of hypotonic urine—with osmolality ranging between 50 and 100 mOsm/kg. Manifestations of the disease are usually present within the first several weeks of life,[441] but may only become apparent after weaning from the breast. The predominant symptoms are polyuria and polydypsia. Thirst may be more difficult to satisfy than in central diabetes insipidus. Many infants initially present with fever, vomiting, and dehydration—often leading to an evaluation for infection. Growth failure in the untreated child may be secondary to the ingestion of large amounts of water, which the child may prefer over milk and other higher-caloric substances.[442]

Mental retardation of variable severity may result from repeated episodes of dehydration.[443] Intracerebral calcification of the frontal lobes and basal ganglia is not uncommon in children with X-linked nephrogenic diabetes insipidus.[444-447] Because this appears early and is not seen in children with central diabetes insipidus of equivalent severity, cerebral calcification is probably unrelated to the level of dehydration or therapeutic intervention. It is possible that elevated vasopressin concentrations, acting via intact V1 or V3 receptors, contribute to some of the unique manifestations of X-linked nephrogenic diabetes insipidus—such as cerebral calcification, intense thirst, vomiting, and growth failure. Older children may present with enuresis or nocturia. They may learn to reduce food intake (and therefore solute load) to decrease polyuria, which may contribute to growth failure. After long-standing ingestion and excretion of large volumes of water, patients may develop nonobstructive hydronephrosis, hydroureter, and megabladder.[412]

Although one founder (arriving in North America from Scotland in 1761 on the ship *Hopewell*) was initially postulated to be the ancestor of most North American subjects with congenital X-linked nephrogenic diabetes insipidus,[448] more than 180 mutations in the V2 receptor have been found—with some appearing to have arisen independently more than once[449-462] (Figure 9-14). These are mostly single base mutations that either result in

amino acid substitutions, translational frame shifts, or termination of peptide synthesis and are distributed fairly evenly throughout the receptor protein (*www.medcon. mcgill.ca/nephros/avpr2.html*). Mutations may affect vasopressin binding, cyclic AMP generation, or possibly transcriptional regulation.[463-467] Patients with different mutations will likely be found to exhibit phenotypic heterogeneity, including in severity of disease and response to treatment. Genetic heterogeneity may underlie the variable response of patients with X-linked diabetes insipidus to dDAVP treatment. In a family with a known mutation, prenatal or early postnatal DNA screening can unambiguously identify affected males—allowing the institution of appropriate therapy.[222]

Congenital Autosomal Nephrogenic Diabetes Insipidus: Aquaporin-2 Mutations. After the initial description of X-linked nephrogenic diabetes insipidus,[468] several patients were reported with similar clinical findings except for autosomal-recessive transmission of the disease[469] or normal V2 receptor function outside the kidney.[470] With the cloning of the complementary DNA for the renal water channel, aquaporin-2, many patients with autosomal-recessive nephrogenic diabetes insipidus have been reported who have a total of 21 mutations different in this gene[464] (*www.medcon.mcgill.ca/nephros/aqp2.html*). Most are missense mutations, although four are nonsense or frame-shift mutations. They are scattered throughout the molecule, including within four of the five transmembrane domains, two of three extracellular domains, and two of four intracellular domains (Figure 9-10).

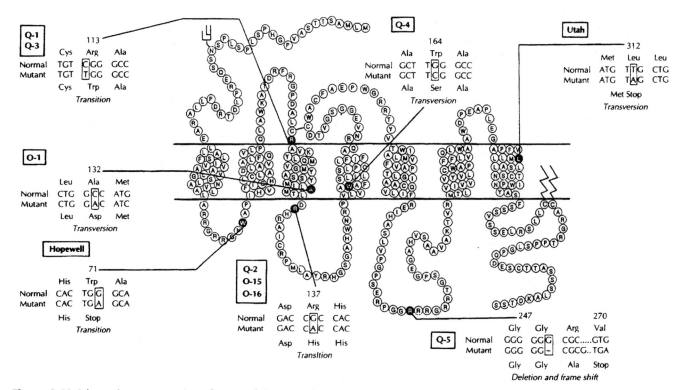

Figure 9-14 Schematic representation of seven of the more than 180 V2 receptor mutations in families with X-linked nephrogenic diabetes insipidus. Q, families from Quebec; F, families from France; and O, other families. [Reproduced with permission from Bichet DG (1995). The posterior pituitary. In Melmed S (ed.), *The pituitary*. Cambridge: Blackwell Science 277.]

Recently, an autosomal-dominant mode of inheritance for nephrogenic diabetes insipidus has been described, associated with mutations in aquaporin-2. One of these dominant mutations results in mixed tetramers of the wild type and mutant alleles being retained in the golgi apparatus.[471] Aquaporin-2 mutations impair the ability of the luminal membrane to undergo an increase in water permeability following signaling through the V2 receptor. They could include patients previously described who had a normal rise in urinary cyclic AMP in response to vasopressin, without a concomitant increase in urine osmolality.[438] Aquaporin-2 protein has recently been shown to be excreted in the urine in both soluble and membrane-bound forms. Aquaporin-2 excretion is low in untreated central and nephrogenic diabetes insipidus, but following dDAVP administration increases markedly in the former (but not the latter) disease.[117] For this reason, its measurement in urine has been suggested as an aid in the differential diagnosis of diabetes insipidus.[117]

Acquired Causes. Acquired causes of nephrogenic diabetes insipidus are more common and less severe than genetic causes. Nephrogenic diabetes insipidus may be caused by drugs such as lithium and demeclocycline, both of which are thought to interfere with vasopressin-stimulated cyclic AMP generation or action. Approximately 50% of patients receiving lithium have impaired urinary concentrating ability, although only 10% to 20% of them develop symptomatic nephrogenic diabetes insipidus—which is almost always accompanied by a reduction in the glomerular filtration rate.[472,473] The risk increases with duration of therapy. Lithium impairs the ability of vasopressin to stimulate adenylate cyclase,[474] resulting in a 90% fall in aquaporin-2 messenger RNA expression in renal collecting duct[475] (which may be the basis for its causing nephrogenic diabetes insipidus).

Demeclocycline treatment causes nephrogenic diabetes insipidus by inhibiting transepithelial water transport.[476] For this reason, it is useful in the treatment of dilutional hyponatremia associated with inappropriate secretion of vasopressin. Other agents that cause nephrogenic diabetes insipidus include hypercalcemia, hyperkalemia, and therapy with foscarnet (used in the treatment of cytomegalovirus infection in immunosuppressed patients),[477,478] clozapine,[478] amphotericin,[479] methicillin,[480] and rifampin.[481] Whether any of these agents causes nephrogenic diabetes insipidus by interfering with the expression or insertion into apical collecting duct membranes of aquaporin-2 water channels is not yet known.

Ureteral obstruction,[482] chronic renal failure, polycystic kidney disease, medullary cystic disease, Sjögren's syndrome,[483] and sickle cell disease can also impair renal concentrating ability. Osmotic diuresis due to glycosuria in diabetes mellitus, or to sodium excretion with diuretic therapy, will interfere with renal water conservation. Primary polydipsia can result in secondary nephrogenic diabetes insipidus because the chronic excretion of a dilute urine lowers the osmolality of the hypertonic renal interstitium, thus decreasing renal concentrating ability. Finally, decreased protein or sodium intake can also lead to diminished tonicity of the renal medullary interstitium and to nephrogenic diabetes insipidus.

Treatment of Nephrogenic Diabetes Insipidus

The treatment of acquired nephrogenic diabetes insipidus focuses on elimination, if possible, of the underlying disorder—such as offending drugs, hypercalcemia, hypokalemia, and ureteral obstruction. Congenital nephrogenic diabetes insipidus is often difficult to treat. The main goals should be to ensure the intake of adequate calories for growth and to avoid severe dehydration. Foods with the highest ratio of caloric content to osmotic load should be ingested, to maximize growth and minimize the urine volume required to excrete urine solute. However, even with the early institution of therapy growth and mental retardation are not uncommon.[484]

Thiazide diuretics in combination with amiloride or indomethacin are the most useful pharmacologic agents in the treatment of nephrogenic diabetes insipidus. Thiazides work by enhancing sodium excretion at the expense of water and by causing a fall in glomerular filtration rate, which results in proximal tubular sodium and water reabsorption.[415,485] Indomethacin (2 mg/kg/day) further enhances proximal tubular sodium and water reabsorption,[415,486,487] although this effect is not mediated by inhibition of cyclo-oxygenase.[488]

The combination of thiazide and amiloride diuretics is the most commonly used regimen for the treatment of congenital X-linked nephrogenic diabetes insipidus because amiloride counteracts thiazide-induced hypokalemia,[441] avoids the nephrotoxicity associated with indomethacin therapy, and is well tolerated (even in infants).[489] In addition, amiloride decreases the uptake of lithium by renal epithelial cells—and for this additional reason has been proposed in combination with thiazide as treatment for lithium-induced nephrogenic diabetes insipidus.[490]

High-dose dDAVP therapy, in combination with indomethacin, has been reported to be helpful in treating some subjects with nephrogenic diabetes insipidus.[491] This treatment may prove to be useful in patients with genetic defects in the V2 receptor that reduce the binding affinity for vasopressin. A therapy that has thus far only been employed in mice and not yet available for humans, in which abnormal stop codons are bypassed,[492] may prove useful in treating patients with nonsense mutations in AVPR2 and AQP2.

Concluding Remarks

Precise regulation of water balance is necessary to the proper function of multiple cellular pathways. Vasopressin released from the posterior pituitary, stimulated by hyperosmolar and nonosmotic factors, acts via the kidney V2 vasopressin receptor to stimulate an increase in aquaporin-2 expression and its insertion into collecting duct luminal membrane—thereby enhancing renal water reabsorption to minimize subsequent water loss. Thirst controls the second major physiologic response to hyperosmolality and results in increased water intake to make up for past water loss. The renin-angiotensin-aldosterone and atrial natriuretic peptide systems also make important contributions to water and volume regulation by modulation of sodium intake and output.

The proper diagnosis of disorders caused by deficient and excessive action of vasopressin requires a thorough understanding of the physiologic regulation of this hormone. Recent advances in molecular medicine have revealed mutations in the vasopressin gene, and in the V2 receptor or aquaporin-2 genes (responsible for familial central and nephrogenic diabetes insipidus, respectively). Molecular methods allow the diagnosis of these disorders in the prenatal or early postnatal periods. Nevertheless, the most frequent cause of central diabetes insipidus remains a destructive lesion of the central nervous system caused by tumor or neurosurgical insult—and pharmacologic toxicity remains the most common cause of nephrogenic diabetes insipidus.

Hyponatremia is a common occurence in childhood, but is rarely due to a primary increase in vasopressin secretion or increase in intrinsic activity of the V2 receptor (SIAD). It is more commonly caused by hypovolemia (primary or secondary to decreased effective vascular volume), salt loss, excessive ingestion of hypotonic fluids, or cortisol deficiency. Hyponatremia due to increased vasopressin action is most commonly caused by excessive vasopressin administration during the treatment of central diabetes insipidus or coagulopathies.

Central diabetes insipidus is best treated in infants with fluid therapy that avoids the administration of vasopressin or its V2 receptor analog, dDAVP—whereas in older children dDAVP is the drug of choice. Nephrogenic diabetes insipidus remains a theraputic challenge. Hyponatremia due to SIAD is best managed by restricting water intake, whereas salt and water replacement are indicated when hyponatremia is due to hypovolemia or excessive secretion of atrial natriuretic peptide (as occurs in cerebral salt wasting). Hyponatremia causing central nervous system dysfunction is a medical emergency. Blood sodium must be raised promptly, but at a rate not greater than 0.5 mEq/L/hr to avoid the occurrence of central pontine myelinolysis.

REFERENCES

1. Strange K (1992). Regulation of solute and water balance and cell volume in the central nervous system. Journal of the American Society of Nephrology 3:12.
2. Vokes TJ, Robertson GL (1988). Disorders of antidiuretic hormone. Endocrinology & Metabolism Clinics of North America 17:281.
3. Acher R (1980). Molecular evolution of biologically active peptides. Proceedings of the Royal Society (London) 210:21.
4. Gorbman A, Dickhoff WW, Vigna SR, et al. (1983). *Comparative endocrinology.* New York: John Wiley & Sons.
5. Turner RA, Pierce JG, Du Vigneaud V (1951). The purification and amino acid content of vasopressin preparation. Journal of Biological Chemistry 191:21.
6. Du Vigneaud V (1954). Hormones of the posterior pituitary gland: Oxytocin and vasopressin. Harvey Lectures 50:1.
7. Oliver G, Schafer EA (1895). On the action of extracts of pituitary body and certain other glandular organs. Journal of Physiology (London) 18:277.
8. Du Vigneaud V, Gish DT, Katsoyannis PG (1954). A synthetic preparation possessing biological properties associated with arginine-vasopressin. Journal of the American Chemical Society 76:4751.
9. Du Vigneaud V, Ressler C, Swan JM, et al. (1953). The synthesis of an octapeptide amide with the hormonal activity of oxytocin. Journal of the American Chemical Society 75:4879.
10. Vavra I, Machova A, Holecek V, et al. (1968). Effect of a synthetic analogue of vasopressin in animals and in patients with diabetes insipidus. Lancet 1:948.
11. Osborne WA, Vincent S (1900). A contribution to the study of the pituitary body. British Journal of Medicine I:502.
12. Acher R, Fromagest C (1957). The relationship of oxytocin and vasopressin to active proteins of posterior pituitary origin. In Heller H (ed.), *The neurohypophysis.* London: Butterworths 39.
13. Pickering BT, Jones CW (1978). The neurophysins. Horm Proteins Peptides 5:103.
14. Chen L, Rose JP, Breslow E, et al. (1991). Crystal structure of a bovine neurophysin II dipeptide complex at 2.8A determined from the single-wave length anomalous scattering signal of an incorporated iodine atom. Proceedings of the National Academy of Sciences of the United States of America 88:4240.
15. Rose JP, Breslow E, Huang HB, Wang BC (1991). Crystallographic analysis of the neurophysin-oxytocin complex: A preliminary report. Journal of Molecular Biology 221:43.
16. Sachs H, Fawcett P, Takabatake Y, et al. (1969). Biosynthesis and release of vasopressin and neurophysin. Recent Progress in Hormone Research 25:447.
17. Sachs H, Takabatake Y (1964). Evidence for a precurosr in vasopresin biosynthesis. Endocrinology 75:943.
18. Brownstein MJ, Russell JT, Gainer H (19980). Synthesis, transport, and release of posterior pituitary hormones. Science 207:373.
19. Takabatake Y, Sachs S (1964). Vasopressin biosynthesis: III. In vitro studies. Endocrinology 75:934.
20. Hara Y, Battey J, Gainer H (1990). Structure of the mouse vasopressin and oxytocin genes. Molecular Brain Research 8:319.
21. Ivell R, Richter D (1984). Structure and comparison of the oxytocin and vasopressin genes from rat. Proceedings of the National Academy of Sciences of the United States of America 81:2006.
22. Summar ML, Phillips JA, Battey J, et al. (1990). Linkage relationships of human arginine vasopressin-neurophysin-II and oxytocin-neurophysin-I to prodynorphin and other loci on chromosome 20. Molecular Endocrinology 4:947.
23. Ruppert SD, Schere G, Schutz G (1984). Recent gene conversion involving bovine vasopressin and oxytocin precursor genes suggested by nucleotide sequence. Nature 308:554.
24. Vandesande F, Dierickx K (1975). Identification of the vasopressin producing and of the oxytocin producing neurons in the hypothalamic magnocellular neurosecretory system of the rat. Cell Tissue Research 164:153.
25. Sawchenko PE, Swanson LW, Vale WW (1984). Co-expression of corticotropin-releasing factor and vasopressin immunoreactivity in parvocellular neurosecretory neurons of the adrenalectomized rat. Proceedings of the National Academy of Sciences of the United States of America 81:1883.
26. Whitnall MH, Mezey E, Gainer H (1985). Co-localization of corticotropin-releasing factor and vasopressin in median eminence neurosecretory vesicles. Nature 317:248.
27. Majzoub JA, Herman M (2002). Adrenocorticotropin. In Melmed S (ed.), *The pituitary, Second edition.* Cambridge (UK): Blackwell Scientific.
28. Verney EB (1947). The antidiuretic hormome and the factors which determine its release. Proceedings of the Royal Society 135:25.
29. Hammer M, Ladefoged J, Olgaard K (1980). Relationship between plasma osmolality and plasma vasopressin in human subjects. American Journal of Physiology 238:E313.
30. Robertson GL, Shelton RL, Athar S (1976). The osmoregulation of vasopressin. Kidney International 10:25.
31. Leng G (1980). Rat supraoptic neurones: The effects of locally applied hypertonic saline. Journal of Physiology (London) 304:405.
32. Bealer SL, Crofton JT, Share L (1983). Hypothalamic knife cuts alter fluid regulation, vasopressin secretion and natriuresis during water deprivation. Neuroendocrinology 36:364.
33. Thrasher TN, Keil LC, Ramsay DJ (1982). Lesions of the organum vasculosum of the lamin terminalis (OVLT) attenuate osmotically-induced drinking and vasopressin secretion in the dog. Endocrinology 110:1837.
34. McKinley MJ, Denton DA, Weisinger RS (1978). Sensors for antidiuresis and thirst-osmoreceptors or CSF sodium detectors? Brain Research 141:89.
35. Phillips MI (1987). Functions of angiotensin in the central nervous system. Annual Review of Physiology 49:413.
36. Simpson JB (1981). The circumventricular organs and the central action of angiotensin. Neuroendocrinology 32:248.

37. Yamaguchi K, Koike M, Hama H (1985). Plasma vasopressin response to peripheral administration of angiotensin in conscious rats. American Journal of Physiology 248:R249.

38. Robertson GL (1977). The regulation of vasopressin function in health and disease. Recent Progress in Hormone Research 33:333.

39. Davison JM, Gilmore EA, Durr J, et al. (1984). Altered osmotic thresholds for vasopressin secretion and thirst in human pregnancy. American Journal of Physiology 246:F105.

40. Boykin J, DeTorrente A, Erickson A, et al. (1978). Role of plasma vasopressin in impaired water excretion of glucocorticoid deficiency. Journal of Clinical Investigation 62:738.

41. Linas SL, Berl T, Robertson GL, et al. (1980). Role of vasopressin in the impaired water excretion of glucocorticoid deficiency. Kidney Int 18:58.

42. Lindheimer MD, Barron WM, Davison JM (1989). Osmoregulation of thirst and vasopressin release in pregnancy. American Journal of Physiology 257:F159.

43. Spruce BA, Baylis PH, Burd J, Watson MJ (1985). Variation in osmoregulation of arginine vasopressin during the human menstrual cycle. Clinical Endocrinology 22:37.

44. Vokes TJ, Weiss NM, Schreiber J, et al. (1988). Osmoregulation of thirst and vasopressin during normal menstrual cycle. American Journal of Physiology 254:R641.

45. Davison JM, Shiells EA, Philips PR, Lindheimer MD (1988). Serial evaluation of vasopressin release and thirst in human pregnancy: Role of human chorionic gonadotrophin in the osmoregulatory changes of gestation. Journal of Clinical Investigation 81:798.

46. Kucharczyk J, Morgenson GJ (1975). Separate lateral hypothalamic pathways for extracellular and intracellular thirst. American Journal of Physiology 228:295.

47. Phillips PA, Rolls BJ, Ledingham JG, et al. (1985). Angiotensin II-induced thirst and vasopressin release in man. Clinical Science 68:669.

48. Gruber KA, Wilkin LD, Johnson AK (1986). Neurohypophyseal hormone release and biosynthesis in rats with lesions of the anteroventral third ventricle (AV3V) region. Brain Research 378:115.

49. Thompson CJ, Burd JM, Baylis PH (1987). Acute suppression of plasma vasopressin and thirst after drinking in hypernatremic humans. American Journal of Physiology 252:R1138.

50. Salata RA, Verbalis JG, Robinson AG (1987). Cold water stimulation of oropharyngeal receptors in man inhibits release of vasopressin. Journal of Clinical Endocrinology & Metabolism 65:561.

51. Williams TD, Seckl JR, Lightman SL (1989). Dependent effect of drinking volume on vasopressin but not atrial peptide in humans. American Journal of Physiology 257:R762.

52. Gauer OH, Henry JP (1963). Circulatory basis of fluid volume control. Physiology Review 43:423.

53. Thrasher TN (1994). Baroreceptor regulation of vasopressin and renin secretion: Low-pressure versus high-pressure receptors. Frontiers in Neuroendocrinology 15:157.

54. Cunningham ET Jr., Sawchenko PE (1991). Reflex control of magnocellular vasopressin and oxytocin secretion. Trends in Neurosciences 14:406.

55. Sawchenko PE, Swanson LW (1981). Central noradrenergic pathways for the integration of hypothalamic neuroendocrine and autonomic responses. Science 214:685.

56. Blessing WW, Sved AF, Reis DJ (1983). Destruction of noradrenergic neurons in rabbit brainstem. Science 217:661.

57. Schrier RW, Berl T, Harbottle JA (1972). Mechanism of the antidiuretic effect associated with interruption of parasympathetic pathways. J Clin Invest 51:2613.

58. Goetz KL, Bond GC, Smith WE (1974). Effect of moderate hemorrhage in humans on plasma ADH and renin. Proceedings of the Society for Experimental Biology & Medicine 145:277.

59. Robertson GL (1976). The regulation of vasopressin function in health and disease. Recent Progress in Hormone Research 33:333.

60. Robertson GL, Athar S (1976). The interaction of blood osmolality and blood volume in regulating plasma vasopressin in man. Journal of Clinical Endocrinology & Metabolism 42:613.

61. Arnauld E, Czernichow P, Fumoux F, Vincent JD (1977). The effects of hypotension and hypovolaemia on the liberation of vasopressin during haemorrhage in the unanaesthetized monkey (Macaca mulatta). Pflugers Archiv/European Journal of Physiology 371:193.

62. Murase T, Yoshida S (1971). Effect of hypotension on levels of antidiuretic hormone in plasma in dogs. Endocrinologia Japonica 18:215.

63. Wiggins RC, Basar I, Slater JD, et al. (1977). Vasovagal hypotension and vasopressin release. Clinical Endocrinology 6:387.

64. Hirsch AT, Majzoub JA, Ren CJ, et al. (1993). Contribution of vasopressin to blood pressure regulation during hypovolemic hypotension in humans. Journal of Applied Physiology 75:1984.

65. Feldman M, Samson WK, O'Dorisio TM (1988). Apomorphine-induced nausea in humans: release of vasopressin and pancreatic polypeptide. Gastroenterology 95:721.

66. Koch KL, Summy-Long J, Bingaman S, et al. (1990). Vasopressin and oxytocin responses to illusory self-motion and nausea in man. Journal of Clinical Endocrinology & Metabolism 71:1269.

67. Seckl JR, Johnson M, Shakespear C, Lightman SL (1988). Endogenous opioids inhibit oxytocin release during nicotine-stimulated secretion of vasopressin in man. Clinical Endocrinology 28:509.

68. Ishikawa S, Fujisawa G, Tsuboi Y, et al. (1991). Role of antidiuretic hormone in hyponatremia in patients with isolated adrenocorticotropic hormone deficiency. Endocrinologia Japonica 38:325.

69. Oelkers W (1989). Hyponatremia and inappropriate secretion of vasopressin (antidiuretic hormone) in patients with hypopituitarism. New England Journal of Medicine 321:492.

70. Green HH, Harrington AR, Valtin H (1970). On the role of antidiuretic hormone in the inhibition of acute water diuresis in adrenal insufficiency and the effects of gluco- and mineralocorticoids in reversing the inhibition. J Clin Invest 49:1724.

71. Viinamaki O, Erkkola R, Kanto J (1986). Plasma vasopressin concentrations and serum vasopressinase activity in pregnant and nonpregnant women. Biological Research in Pregnancy & Perinatology 7:17.

72. Davison JM, Sheills EA, Barron WM, et al. (1989). Changes in the metabolic clearance of vasopressin and in plasma vasopressinase throughout human pregnancy. Journal of Clinical Investigation 83:1313.

73. Iwasaki Y, Oiso Y, Kondo K, et al. (1991). Aggravation of subclinical diabetes insipidus during pregnancy. New England Journal of Medicine 324:522.

74. Kennedy S, Hall PM, Seymour AE, Hague WM (1994). Transient diabetes insipidus and acute fatty liver of pregnancy. British Journal of Obstetrics & Gynaecology 101:387.

75. Katz VL, Bowes WA Jr. (1987). Transient diabetes insipidus and preeclampsia. Southern Medical Journal 80:524.

76. Durr JA, Hoggard JG, Hunt JM, Schrier RW (1987). Diabetes insipidus in pregnancy associated with abnormally high circulating vasopressinase activity. New England Journal of Medicine 316:1070.

77. Davison JM, Sheills EA, Philips PR, et al. (1993). Metabolic clearance of vasopressin and an analogue resistant to vasopressinase in human pregnancy. American Journal of Physiology 264:F348.

78. Krege J, Katz VL, Bowes WA Jr. (1989). Transient diabetes insipidus of pregnancy. Obstetrical & Gynecological Survey 44:789.

79. Jard S (1983). Vasopressin isoreceptors in mammals: Relation to cyclic-AMP dependent and cyclic-AMP-independent transducer mechanisms. Current Topics in Membr Transp 18:225.

80. Hirasawa A, Shibata K, Kotosai K, Tsujimoto G (1994). Cloning, functional expression and tissue distribution of human cDNA for the vascular-type vasopressin receptor. Biochemical & Biophysical Research Communications 203:72.

81. Morel A, O'Carroll AM, Brownstein MJ, Lolait SJ (1992). Molecular cloning and expression of a rat V1a arginine vasopressin receptor. Nature 356:523.

82. Ostrowski NL, Young WS, Knepper MA, Lolait SJ (1993). Expression of vasopressin V1a and V2 receptor messenger ribonucleic acid in the liver and kidney of embryonic, developing, and adult rats. Endocrinology 133:1849.

83. Thibonnier M, Auzan C, Madhun Z, et al. (1994). Molecular cloning, sequencing, and functional expression of a cDNA encoding the human V1a vasopressin receptor. Journal of Biological Chemistry 269:3304.

84. Ostrowski NL, Lolait SJ, Bradley DJ, et al. (1992). Distribution of V1a and V2 vasopressin receptor messenger ribonucleic acids in rat liver, kidney, pituitary and brain. Endocrinology 131:533.

85. Johnson EM, Theler JM, Capponi AM, Vallotton MB (1991). Characterization of oscillations in cytosolic free Ca2+ concentration and measurement of cytosolic Na+ concentration changes evoked

by angiotensin II and vasopressin in individual rat aortic smooth muscle cells: Use of microfluorometry and digital imaging. Journal of Biological Chemistry 266:12618.

86. Takeuchi K, Abe K, Yasujima M, et al. (1992). Phosphoinositide hydrolysis and calcium mobilization induced by vasopressin and angiotensin II in cultured vascular smooth muscle cells. Tohoku Journal of Experimental Medicine 166:107.

87. Spruce BA, McCulloch AJ, Burd J, et al. (1985). The effect of vasopressin infusion on glucose metabolism in man. Clinical Endocrinology 22:463.

88. Inaba K, Umeda Y, Yamane Y, et al. (1988). Characterization of human platelet vasopressin receptor and the relation between vasopressin-induced platelet aggregation and vasopressin binding to platelets. Clinical Endocrinology 29:377.

89. Briley EM, Lolait SJ, Axelrod J, Felder CC (1994). The cloned vasopressin V1a receptor stimulates phospholipase A2, phospholipase C, and phospholipase D through activation of receptor-operated calcium channels. Neuropeptides 27:63.

90. Montani JP, Liard JF, Schoun J, Mohring J (1980). Hemodynamic effects of exogenous and endogenous vasopressin at low plasma concentrations in conscious dogs. Circulation Research 47:346.

91. Altura BM, Altura BT (1984). Actions of vasopressin, oxytocin, and synthetic analogs on vascular smooth muscle. Federation Proceedings 43:80.

92. Kimura T, Tanizawa O, Mori K, et al. (1992). Structure and expression of a human oxytocin receptor. Nature 356:526.

93. Rozen F, Russo C, Banville D, Zingg HH (1995). Structure, characterization, and expression of the rat oxytocin receptor gene. Proceedings of the National Academy of Sciences of the United States of America 92:200.

94. Baertschi AJ, Friedli M (1985). A novel type of vasopressin receptor on anterior pituitary corticotrophs. Endocrinology 116:499.

95. de Keyzer Y, Auzan C, Lenne F, et al. (1994). Cloning and characterization of the human V3 pituitary vasopressin receptor. FEBS Letters 356:215.

96. Sugimoto T, Saito M, Mochizuki S, et al. (1994). Molecular cloning and functional expression of a cDNA encoding the human V1b vasopressin receptor. J Biol Chem 269:27088.

97. Tanoue A, Ito S, Honda K, et al. (2004). The vasopressin V1b receptor critically regulates hypothalamic-pituitary-adrenal axis activity under both stress and resting conditions. J Clin Invest 113:302.

98. Lolait SJ, Stewart LQ, Jessop DS, et al. (2007). The hypothalamic-pituitary-adrenal axis response to stress in mice lacking functional vasopressin V1b receptors. Endocrinology 148:849.

99. Lolait SJ, O'Carroll AM, McBride OW, et al. (1992). Cloning and characterization of a vasopressin V2 receptor and possible link to nephrogenic diabetes insipidus. Nature 357:336.

100. Hirsch AT, Dzau VJ, Majzoub JA, Creager MA (1989). Vasopressin-mediated forearm vasodilation in normal humans: Evidence for a vascular vasopressin V2 receptor. Journal of Clinical Investigation 84:418.

101. Tagawa T, Imaizumi T, Endo T, et al. (1993). Vasodilatory effect of arginine vasopressin is mediated by nitric oxide in human forearm vessels. Journal of Clinical Investigation 92:1483.

102. Kobrinsky NL, Israels ED, Gerrard JM, et al. (1984). Shortening of bleeding time by 1-deamino-8-D-arginine vasopressin in various bleeding disorders. Lancet 1:1145.

103. Birnbaumer M, Seibold A, Gilbert S, et al. (1992). Molecular cloning of the receptor for human antidiuretic hormone. Nature 357:333.

104. Frattini A, Zucchi I, Villa A, et al. (1993). Type 2 vasopressin receptor gene, the gene responsible nephrogenic diabetes insipidus, maps to Xq28 close to the LICAM gene. Biochemical & Biophysical Research Communications 193:864.

105. Seibold A, Brabet P, Rosenthal W, Birnbaumer M (1992). Structure and chromosomal localization of the human antidiuretic hormone receptor gene. American Journal of Human Genetics 51:1078.

106. Yun J, Schoneberg T, Liu J, et al. (2000). Generation and phenotype of mice harboring a nonsense mutation in the V2 vasopressin receptor gene. J Clin Invest 106:1361.

107. Harris HW, Paredes A, Zeidel ML (1993). The molecular structure of the antidiuretic hormone elicited water channel. Pediatric Nephrology 7:680.

108. Harris HW, Strange K, Zeidel ML (1991). Current understanding of the cellular biology and molecular structure of the antidiuretic

hormone-stimulated water transport pathway. Journal of Clinical Investigation 88:1.

109. Nielsen S, Marples D, Birn H, et al. (1995). Expression of VAMP2-like protein in kidney collecting duct intracellular vesicles. J Clin Invest 96:1834.

110. Mandon B, Chou CL, Nielsen S, Knepper MA (1996). Syntaxin-4 is localized to the apical plasma membrane of rat renal collecting duct cells: Possible role in aquaporin-2 trafficking. J Clin Invest 98:906.

111. Knepper MA (1994). The aquaporin family of molecular water channels. Proceedings of the National Academy of Sciences of the United States of America 91:6255.

112. Sasaki S, Fushimi K, Saito H, et al. (1994). Cloning, characterization, and chromosomal mapping of human aquaporin of collecting duct. Journal of Clinical Investigation 93:1250.

113. Deen PM, Verdijk MA, Knoers NV, et al. (1994). Requirement of human renal water channel aquaporin-2 for vasopressin-dependent concentration of urine. Science 264:92.

114. Stevens AL, Breton S, Gustafson CE, et al. (2000). Aquaporin 2 is a vasopressin-independent, constitutive apical membrane protein in rat vas deferens. Am J Physiol 278:C791.

115. Fushimi K, Sasaki S, Marumo F (1997). Phosphorylation of serine 256 is required for cAMP-dependent regulatory exocytosis of the aquaporin-2 water channel. J Biol Chem 272:14800.

116. Valenti G, Procino G, Liebenhoff U, et al. (1998). A heterotrimeric G protein of the Gi family is required for cAMP-triggered trafficking of aquaporin 2 in kidney epithelial cells. J Biol Chem 273:22627.

117. Kanno K, Sasaki S, Hirata Y, et al. (1995). Urinary excretion of aquaporin-2 in patients with diabetes insipidus. New England Journal of Medicine 332:1540.

118. Yang B, Gillespie A, Carlson EJ, et al. (2001). Neonatal mortality in an aquaporin-2 knock-in mouse model of recessive nephrogenic diabetes insipidus. J Biol Chem 276:2775.

119. Ma T, Yang B, Gillespie A, et al. (1997). Generation and phenotype of a transgenic knockout mouse lacking the mercurial-insensitive water channel aquaporin-4. J Clin Invest 100:957.

120. Ma T, Song Y, Yang B, et al. (2000). Nephrogenic diabetes insipidus in mice lacking aquaporin-3 water channels. Proc Natl Acad Sci USA 97:4386.

121. Schnermann J, Chou CL, Ma T, et al. (1998). Defective proximal tubular fluid reabsorption in transgenic aquaporin-1 null mice. Proc Natl Acad Sci USA 95:9660.

122. Gibbons GH, Dzau VJ, Farhi ER, Barger AC (1984). Interaction of signals influencing renin release. Annual Review of Physiology 46:291.

123. Quinn SJ, Williams GH (1988). Regulation of aldosterone secretion. Annual Review of Physiology 50:409.

124. Balla T, Baukal AJ, Eng S, Catt KJ (1991). Angiotensin II receptor subtypes and biological responses in the adrenal cortex and medulla. Molecular Pharmacology 40:401.

125. Murphy TJ, Alexander RW, Griendling KK, et al. (1991). Isolation of a cDNA encoding the vascular type-1 angiotensin II receptor. Nature 351:233.

126. Murphy TJ, Takeuchi K, Alexander RW (1992). Molecular cloning of AT1 angiotensin receptors. American Journal of Hypertension 5:236S.

127. Stromberg C, Tsutsumi K, Viswanathan M, Saavedra JM (1991). Angiotensin II AT1 receptors in rat superior cervical ganglia: Characterization and stimulation of phosphoinositide hydrolysis. European Journal of Pharmacology 208:331.

128. Tsutsumi K, Stromberg C, Viswanathan M, Saavedra JM (1991). Angiotensin-II receptor subtypes in fetal tissue of the rat: autoradiography, guanine nucleotide sensitivity, and association with phosphoinositide hydrolysis. Endocrinology 129:1075.

129. Aguilera G, Catt KJ (1979). Loci of action of regulators of aldosterone biosynthesis in isolated glomerulosa cells. Endocrinology 104:1046.

130. Aguilera G, Menard RH, Catt KJ (1980). Regulatory actions of angiotensin II on receptors and steroidogenic enzymes in adrenal glomerulosa cells. Endocrinology 107:55.

131. Catt KJ, Aguilera G, Capponi A, et al. (1979). Angiotensin II receptors and aldosterone secretion. Journal of Endocrinology 81:37P.

132. Kramer RE, Gallant S, Brownie AC, et al. (1990). Actions of angiotensin II on aldosterone biosynthesis in the rat adrenal cortex: Effects on cytochrome P-450 enzymes of the early and late pathway

discrimination of two angiotensin II receptor subtypes with a selective agonist analogue of angiotensin II, p-aminophenylalanine6 angiotensin II. Journal of Biological Chemistry Biochemical & Biophysical Research Communications 169:997.

133. Bottari SP, de Gasparo M, Steckelings UM, Levens NR (1993). Angiotensin II receptor subtypes: characterization, signalling mechanisms, and possible physiological implications. Frontiers in Neuroendocrinology 14:123.

134. Bottari SP, Taylor V, King IN, et al. (1991). Angiotensin II AT2 receptors do not interact with guanine nucleotide binding proteins. European Journal of Pharmacology 207:157.

135. Speth RC, Kim KH (1990). Discrimination of two angiotensin II receptor subtypes with a selective agonist analogue of angiotensin II, p-aminophenylalanine6 angiotensin II. Biochemical & Biophysical Research Communications 169:997.

136. Morris DJ (1981). The metabolism and mechanism of action of aldosterone. Endocrine Reviews 2:234.

137. Dzau VJ (1988). Molecular and physiological aspects of tissue renin-angiotensin system: Emphasis on cardiovascular control. Journal of Hypertension 6:S7.

138. Chartier L, Schiffrin EL (1987). Role of calcium in effects of atrial natriuretic peptide on aldosterone production in adrenal glomerulosa cells. American Journal of Physiology 252:E485.

139. Chartier L, Schiffrin E, Thibault G, Garcia R (1984). Atrial natriuretic factor inhibits the stimulation of aldosterone secretion by angiotensin II, ACTH and potassium in vitro and angiotensin II-induced steroidogenesis in vivo. Endocrinology 115:2026.

140. Chartier L, Schiffrin EL (1987). Atrial natriuretic peptide inhibits the effect of endogenous angiotensin II on plasma aldosterone in conscious sodium-depleted rats. Clinical Science 72:31.

141. Hausdorff WP, Aguilera G, Catt KJ (1989). Inhibitory actions of somatostatin on cyclic AMP and aldosterone production in agonist-stimulated adrenal glomerulosa cells. Cellular Signalling 1:377.

142. Rebuffat P, Mazzocchi G, Gottardo G, Nussdorfer GG (1989). Further studies on the involvement of dopamine and somatostatin in the inhibitory control of the growth and steroidogenic capacity of rat adrenal zona glomerulosa. Experimental & Clinical Endocrinology 93:73.

143. Robba C, Mazzocchi G, Nussdorfer GG (1986). Further studies on the inhibitory effects of somatostatin on the growth and steroidogenic capacity of rat adrenal zona glomerulosa. Experimental Pathology 29:77.

144. Gallo-Payet N, Chouinard L, Balestre MN, Guillon G (1990). Dual effects of dopamine in rat adrenal glomerulosa cells. Biochemical & Biophysical Research Communications 172:1100.

145. Missale C, Lombardi C, Sigala S, Spano PF (1990). Dopaminergic regulation of aldosterone secretion. Biochemical mechanisms and pharmacology. American Journal of Hypertension 3:93S.

146. Dzau VJ, Hirsch AT (1990). Emerging role of the tissue renin-angiotensin systems in congestive heart failure. European Heart Journal 11(B):65.

147. Ganten D, Paul M, Deboben A, et al. (1984). The brain renin angiotensin system in central cardiovascular control. Contributions to Nephrology 43:114.

148. Hirsch AT, Dzau VJ, Creager MA (1987). Baroreceptor function in congestive heart failure: Effect on neurohumoral activation and regional vascular resistance. Circulation 75:IV36.

149. Tang SS, Stevenson L, Dzau VJ (1990). Endothelial renin-angiotensin pathway: Adrenergic regulation of angiotensin secretion. Circulation Research 66:103.

150. Unger T, Badoer E, Ganten D, et al. (1988). Brain angiotensin: pathways and pharmacology. Circulation 77:I40.

151. Saavedra JM (1992). Brain and pituitary angiotensin. Endocrine Reviews 13:329.

152. Van Houten M, Posner BI (1983). Circumventricular organs: Receptors and mediators of direct peptide hormone action on brain. Advances in Metabolic Disorders 10:269.

153. Van Houten M, Schiffrin EL, Mann JF, et al. (1980). Radioautographic localization of specific binding sites for blood-borne angiotensin II in the rat brain. Brain Research 186:480.

154. Stornetta RL, Hawelu-Johnson CL, Guyenet PG, Lynch KR (1988). Astrocytes synthesize angiotensinogen in brain. Science 242:1444.

155. Paul M, Printz MP, Harms E, et al. (1985). Localization of renin (EC 3.4.23) and converting enzyme (EC 3.4.15.1) in nerve endings of rat brain. Brain Research 334:315.

156. Correa FM, Guilhaume SS, Saavedra JM (1990). Autoradiography of angiotensin-converting enzyme in fixed and unfixed rat brain using the specific enzyme inhibitor [125I]351A or a polyclonal antibody and [125I]staphylococcal protein A. Neuroscience Letters 110:244.

157. Correa FM, Plunkett LM, Saavedra JM (1986). Quantitative distribution of angiotensin-converting enzyme (kininase II) in discrete areas of the rat brain by autoradiography with computerized microdensitometry. Brain Research 375:259.

158. Plunkett LM, Correa FM, Saavedra JM (1985). Quantitative autoradiographic determination of angiotensin-converting enzyme binding in rat pituitary and adrenal glands with 125I-351A, a specific inhibitor. Regulatory Peptides 12:263.

159. Pickel VM, Chan J, Ganten D (1986). Dual peroxidase and colloidal gold-labeling study of angiotensin converting enzyme and angiotensin-like immunoreactivity in the rat subfornical organ. Journal of Neuroscience 6:2457.

160. Castren E, Saavedra JM (1989). Angiotensin II receptors in paraventricular nucleus, subfornical organ, and pituitary gland of hypophysectomized, adrenalectomized, and vasopressin-deficient rats. Proceedings of the National Academy of Sciences of the United States of America 86:725.

161. Andersson B, Leksell LG, Lishajko F (1975). Perturbations in fluid balance induced by medially placed forebrain lesions. Brain Research 99:261.

162. Saavedra JM, Castren E, Gutkind JS, Nazarali AJ (1989). Regulation of brain atrial natriuretic peptide and angiotensin receptors: Quantitative autoradiographic studies. International Review of Neurobiology 31:257.

163. Saper CB, Levisohn D (1983). Afferent connections of the median preoptic nucleus in the rat: anatomical evidence for a cardiovascular integrative mechanism in the anteroventral third ventricular (AV3V) region. Brain Research 288:21.

164. Saper CB, Loewy AD, Swanson LW, Cowan WM (1976). Direct hypothalamo-autonomic connections. Brain Research 117:305.

165. Sawchenko PE (1983). Central connections of the sensory and motor nuclei of the vagus nerve. Journal of the Autonomic Nervous System 9:13.

166. Sawchenko PE, Swanson LW (1983). The organization of forebrain afferents to the paraventricular and supraoptic nuclei of the rat. Journal of Comparative Neurology 218:121.

167. Swanson LW, Sawchenko PE (1983). Hypothalamic integration: organization of the paraventricular and supraoptic nuclei. Annual Review of Neuroscience 6:269.

168. Ishikawa S, Saito T, Yoshida S (1980). Effects of glucose and sodium chloride on the release of vasopressin in response to angiotensin II from the guinea pig. Neuroendocrinology 31:365.

169. Simon-Oppermann C, Gray DA, Simon E (1986). Independent osmoregulatory control of central and systemic angiotensin II concentrations in dogs. American Journal of Physiology 250:R918.

170. de Bold AJ (1982). Tissue fractionation studies on the relationship between an atrial natriuretic factor and specific atrial granules. Canadian Journal of Physiology & Pharmacology 60:324.

171. de Bold AJ, Borenstein HB, Veress AT, Sonnenberg H (1981). A rapid and potent natriuretic response to intravenous injection of atrial myocardial extract in rats. Life Sciences 28:89.

172. Yandle TG (1994). Biochemistry of natriuretic peptides. Journal of Internal Medicine 235:561.

173. Hamid Q, Wharton J, Terenghi G, et al. (1987). Localization of atrial natriuretic peptide mRNA and immunoreactivity in the rat heart and human atrial appendage. Proceedings of the National Academy of Sciences of the United States of America 84:6760.

174. Imura H, Nakao K, Itoh H (1992). The natriuretic peptide system in the brain: Implications in the central control of cardiovascular and neuroendocrine functions. Frontiers in Neuroendocrinology 13:217.

175. Inagaki S, Kubota Y, Kito S, et al. (1986). Atrial natriuretic peptide-like immunoreactivity in the rat pituitary: Light and electron microscopic studies. Regulatory Peptides 14:101.

176. Inagaki S, Kubota Y, Kito S, et al. (1986). Immunoreactive atrial natriuretic polypeptide in the adrenal medulla and sympathetic ganglia. Regulatory Peptides 15:249.

177. Ritter D, Chao J, Needeleman P, et al. (1992). Localization, synthetic regulation, and biology of renal atriopeptin-like prohormone. American Journal of Physiology 263:F503.

178. Grundlach AL, Knobe KE (1992). Distribution of preproatrial natriuretic peptide mRNA in rat brain detected by in situ hybridization of DNA oligonucleotides: Enrichment in hypothalamic and limbic regions. Journal of Neurochemistry 59:758.

179. Herman JP, Langub MC Jr, Watson RE Jr. (1993). Localization of C-type natriuretic peptide mRNA in rat hypothalamus. Endocrinology 133:1903.

180. Lewicki JA, Greenberg B, Yamanaka M, et al. (1986). Cloning, sequence analysis, and processing of the rat and human atrial natriuretic peptide precursors. Federation Proceedings 45:2086.

181. Sudoh T, Kanagawa K, Minamino N, Matsuo H (1988). A new natriuretic peptide in porcine brain. Nature 332:78.

182. Hasegawa K, Fujiwara H, Doyama K, et al. (1993). Ventricular expression of brain natriuretic peptide in hypertrophic cardiomyopathy. Circulation 88:372.

183. Hasegawa K, Fujiwara H, Doyama K, et al. (1993). Ventricular expression of atrial and brain natriuretic peptides in dilated cardiomyopathy: An immunohistocytochemical study of the endomyocardial biopsy specimens using specific monoclonal antibodies. American Journal of Pathology 142:107.

184. Yoshimura M, Yasue H, Okumura K, et al. (1993). Different secretion patterns of atrial natriuretic peptide and brain natriuretic peptide in patients with congestive heart failure. Circulation 87:464.

185. Sudoh T, Maekawa K, Kojima M, et al. (1989). Cloning and sequence analysis of cDNA encoding a precursor for human brain natriuretic peptide. Biochemical & Biophysical Research Communications 159:1427.

186. Sudoh T, Minamino N, Kanagawa K, Matsuo H (1990). C-type natriuretic peptide (CNP): a new member of natriuretic peptide family identified in porcine brain. Biochemical & Biophysical Research Communications 168:863.

187. Cuneo RC, Espiner EA, Nicholls MG, et al. (1986). Renal, hemodynamic, and hormonal responses to atrial natriuretic peptide infusions in normal man, and effect of sodium intake. Journal of Clinical Endocrinology & Metabolism 63:946.

188. Espiner EA (1994). Physiology of natriuretic peptides. Journal of Internal Medicine 235:527.

189. Nakao K, Ogawa Y, Suga S, Imura H (1992). Molecular biology and biochemistry of the natriuretic peptide system. I: Natriuretic peptides. Journal of Hypertension 10:907.

190. Garbers DL, Koesling D, Schultz G (1994). Guanylyl cyclase receptors. Molecular Biology of the Cell 5:1.

191. Schulz S, Singh S, Bellet RA, et al. (1989). The primary structure of a plasma membrane guanylate cyclase demonstrates diversity within this new receptor family. Cell 58:1155.

192. Yamaguchi M, Rutledge LJ, Garbers DL (1990). The primary structure of the rat guanylyl cyclase A/atrial natriuretic peptide receptor gene. Journal of Biological Chemistry 265:20414.

193. Koller KJ, Lowe DG, Bennett GL, et al. (1991). Selective activation of the B natriuretic peptide receptor by C-type natriuretic peptide (CNP). Science 252:120.

194. Fuller F, Porter JG, Arfsten AE, et al. (1988). Atrial natriuretic peptide clearance receptor. Complete sequence and functional expression of cDNA clones. Journal of Biological Chemistry 263:9395.

195. Maack T (1992). Receptors of atrial natriuretic factor. Annual Review of Physiology 54:11.

196. Wilcox JN, Augustine A, Goeddel DV, Lowe DG (1991). Differential regional expression of three natriuretic peptide genes within primate tissues. Molecular and Cellular Biology 11:3454.

197. Tallerico-Melnyk T, Yip CC, Watt VM (1992). Widespread colocalization of messenger RNAs encoding the guanylate cyclase-coupled natriuretic peptide receptors in rat tissues. Biochemical & Biophysical Research Communications 189:610.

198. Espiner EA, Nicholls MG, Yandle TG, et al. (1986). Studies on the secretion, metabolism and action of atrial natriuretic peptide in man. Journal of Hypertension 4:S85.

199. Crozier IG, Nicholls MG, Ikram H, et al. (1986). Atrial natriuretic peptide in humans. Production and clearance by various tissues. Hypertension 8:II11.

200. Yandle TG, Espiner EA, Nicholls MG, Duff H (1986). Radioimmunoassay and characterization of atrial natriuretic peptide in human plasma. Journal of Clinical Endocrinology & Metabolism 63:72.

201. Fujii T, Kojima S, Imanishi M, et al. (1991). Different mechanisms of polyuria and natriuresis associated with paroxysmal supraventricular tachycardia. Am J Cardiol 68:343.

202. Fujii T, Kojima S, Ohe T, et al. (1991). Dominance of blood pressure in natriuresis associated with supraventricular tachycardia. Nephron 57:262.

203. Kaye GC, Bayliss P, Lowry PJ, et al. (1992). Effect of induced supraventricular tachycardias on changes in urine and plasma hormone levels in man. Clin Sci 82:33.

204. Cuneo RC, Espiner EA, Nicholls MG, et al. (1987). Effect of physiological levels of atrial natriuretic peptide on hormone secretion: inhibition of angiotensin-induced aldosterone secretion and renin release in normal man. Journal of Clinical Endocrinology & Metabolism 65:765.

205. Kimura T, Abe K, Shoji M, et al. (1986). Effects of human atrial natriuretic peptide on renal function and vasopressin release. American Journal of Physiology 250:R789.

206. Thrasher TN, Ramsay DJ (1993). Interactions between vasopressin and atrial natriuretic peptides. Annals of the New York Academy of Sciences 689:426.

207. Williams TD, Walsh KP, Lightman SL, Sutton R (1988). Atrial natriuretic peptide inhibits postural release of renin and vasopressin in humans. American Journal of Physiology 255:R368.

208. Bahr V, Sander-Bahr C, Ardevol R, et al. (1993). Effects of atrial natriuretic factor on the renin-aldosterone system: in vivo and in vitro studies. Journal of Steroid Biochemistry & Molecular Biology 45:173.

209. Florkowski CM, Richards AM, Espiner EA, et al. (1994). Renal, endocrine, and hemodynamic interactions of atrial and brain natriuretic peptides in normal men. American Journal of Physiology 266:R1244.

210. Wittert GA, Espiner EA, Richards AM, et al. (1993). Atrial natriuretic factor reduces vasopressin and angiotensin II but not the ACTH response to acute hypoglycaemic stress in normal men. Clinical Endocrinology 38:183.

211. Levin ER, Mills S, Weber MA (1989). Central nervous system mediated vasodepressor acton of atrial natriuretic factor. Life Sciences 44:1617.

212. Yeung VT, Lai CK, Cockram CS, et al. (1991). Atrial natriuretic peptide in the central nervous system. Neuroendocrinology 53(1):18.

213. Wei C, Aarhus LL, Miller VM, Burnett JC (1993). Action of C-type natriuretic peptide in isolated canine arteries and veins. American Journal of Physiology 264:H71.

214. Clavell A, Stingo A, Wei C, et al. (1993). C-type natriuretic peptide: a selective cardiovascular peptide. American Journal of Physiology 264:R290.

215. Charles CJ, Richards AM, Espiner EA (1992). Central C-type natriuretic peptide but not atrial natriuretic factor lowers blood pressure and adrenocortical secretion in normal conscious sheep. Endocrinology 131:1721.

216. Samson WK, Skala KD, Huang FLS (1991). CNP-22 stimulates, rather than inhibits, water drinking in the rat: evidence for a unique biological action of the C-type natriuretic peptides. Brain Research 568:285.

217. Assadi FK, John EG (1985). Hypouricemia in neonates with syndrome of inappropriate secretion of antidiuretic hormone. Pediatric Research 19:424.

218. Ganong CA, Kappy MS (1993). Cerebral salt wasting in children: The need for recognition and treatment. American Journal of Diseases of Children 147:167.

219. Frasier SD, Kutnik LA, Schmidt RT, Smith FG Jr. (1967). A water deprivation test for the diagnosis of diabetes insipidus in children. American Journal of Diseases of Children 114:157.

220. Richman RA, Post EM, Notman DD, et al. (1981). Simplifying the diagnosis of diabetes insipidus in children. American Journal of Diseases of Children 135:839.

221. Koskimies O, Pylkkanen J (1984). Water intoxication in infants caused by the urine concentration test with the vasopressin analogue (DDAVP). Acta Paediatrica Scandinavica 73:131.

222. Bichet DG (1994). Molecular and cellular biology of vasopressin and oxytocin receptors and action in the kidney. Current Opinion in Nephrology & Hypertension 3:46.

223. Milles JJ, Spruce B, Baylis PH (1983). A comparison of diagnostic methods to differentiate diabetes insipidus from primary polyuria: a review of 21 patients. Acta Endocrinologica 104:410.

224. Zerbe RL, Robertson GL (1981). A comparison of plasma vasopressin measurements with a standard indirect test in the differential diagnosis of polyuria. New England Journal of Medicine 305:1539.

225. Andersson B, Leksell LG, Rundgren M (1982). Regulation of water intake. Annual Review of Nutrition 2:73.

226. Papapostolou C, Mantzoros CS, Evagelopoulou C, et al. (1995). Imaging of the sella in the syndrome of inappropriate secretion of antidiuretic hormone. Journal of Internal Medicine 237:181.

227. Moses AM, Clayton B, Hochhauser L (1992). Use of T1-weighted MR imaging to differentiate between primary polydipsia and central diabetes insipidus. American Journal of Neuroradiology 13:[pages].

228. Halimi P, Sigal R, Doyon D, et al. (1988). Post-traumatic diabetes insipidus: MR demonstration of pituitary stalk rupture. Journal of Computer Assisted Tomography 12:135.

229. Maghnie M, Villa A, Arico M, et al. (1992). Correlation between magnetic resonance imaging of posterior pituitary and neurohypophyseal function in children with diabetes insipidus. Journal of Clinical Endocrinology & Metabolism 74:795.

230. Maghnie M, Genovese E, Arico M, et al. (1994). Evolving pituitary hormone deficiency is associated with pituitary vasculopathy: Dynamic MR study in children with hypopituitarism, diabetes insipidus, and Langerhans cell histiocytosis. Radiology 193:493.

231. Sato N, Ishizaka H, Yagi H, et al. (1993). Posterior lobe of the pituitary in diabetes insipidus: Dynamic MR imaging. Radiology 186:357.

232. Medani CR (1987). Seizures and hypothermia due to dietary water intoxication in infants. Southern Medical Journal 80:421.

233. Davidson S, Frand M, Rotem Y (1978). Primary polydipsia in infancy: A benign disorder simulating diabetes insipidus. Clinical Pediatrics 17:419.

234. Kovacs L, Sulyok E, Lichardus B, et al. (1986). Renal response to arginine vasopressin in premature infants with late hyponatraemia. Archives of Disease in Childhood 61:1030.

235. Robertson GL (1987). Dipsogenic diabetes insipidus: a newly recognized syndrome caused by a selective defect in the osmoregulation of thirst. Transactions of the Association of American Physicians 100:241.

236. Ahmed AB, George BC, Gonzalez-Auvert C, Dingman JF (1967). Increased plasma arginine vasopressin in clinical adrenocortical insufficiency and its inhibition by glucosteroids. J Clin Invest 46:111.

237. Dingman JF, Despointes RH (1960). Adrenal steroid inhibition of vasopressin release from the neurohypophysis of normal subjects and patients with Addison's disease. J Clin Invest 39:1851.

238. Iwasaki Y, Oiso Y, Saito H, Majzoub JA (1997). Positive and negative regulation of the rat vasopressin gene promoter. Endocrinology 138:5266.

239. Kleeman CR, Czaczkes JW, Cutler R (1964). Mechanisms of impaired water excretion in adrenal and pituitary insufficiency: IV. Antidiuretic hormone in primary and secondary adrenal insufficiency. J Clin Invest 43:1641.

240. Kamoi K, Tamura T, Tanaka K, et al. (1993). Hyponatremia and osmoregulation of thirst and vasopressin secretion in patients with adrenal insufficiency. Journal of Clinical Endocrinology & Metabolism 77:1584.

241. Laczi F, Janaky T, Ivanyi T, et al. (1987). Osmoregulation of arginine-8-vasopressin secretion in primary hypothyroidism and in Addison's disease. Acta Endocrinologica 114:389.

242. Bouley R, Breton S, Sun T, et al. (2000). Nitric oxide and atrial natriuretic factor stimulate cGMP-dependent membrane insertion of aquaporin 2 in renal epithelial cells. J Clin Invest 106:1115.

243. Wallerath T, Witte K, Schafer SC, et al. (1999). Down-regulation of the expression of endothelial NO synthase is likely to contribute to glucocorticoid-mediated hypertension. Proc Natl Acad Sci USA 96:13357.

244. Schwartz MJ, Kokko JP (1980). Urinary concentrating defect of adrenal insufficiency: Permissive role of adrenal steroids on the hydroosmotic response across the rabbit cortical collecting tubule. Journal of Clinical Investigation 66:234.

245. Schrier RW, Berl T (1975). Nonosmolar factors affecting renal water excretion (first of two parts). New England Journal of Medicine 292:81.

246. Iwasaki Y, Oiso Y, Yamauchi K, et al. (1990). Osmoregulation of plasma vasopressin in myxedema. Journal of Clinical Endocrinology & Metabolism 70:534.

247. Discala VA, Kinney MJ (1971). Effects of myxedema in the renal diluting and concentrating mechanism. Am J Med 50:325.

248. Michael UF, Barenberg RL, Chavez R, et al. (1972). Renal handling of sodium and water in the hypothyroid rat: Clearance and micropuncture studies. J Clin Invest 51:1405.

249. Yount E, Little JM (1955). Renal clearance in patients with myxedema. J Clin Endocrinol Metab 15:343.

250. Iwasaki Y, Kondo K, Hasegawa H, Oiso Y (1997). Osmoregulation of plasma vasopressin in three cases with adrenal insufficiency of diverse etiologies. Horm Res 47:38.

251. Yamada K, Tamura Y, Yoshida S (1989). Effect of administration of corticotropin-releasing hormone and glucocorticoid on arginine vasopressin response to osmotic stimulus in normal subjects and patients with hypocorticotropinism without overt diabetes insipidus. Journal of Clinical Endocrinology & Metabolism 69:396.

252. Kamiyama T, Iseki K, Kawazoe N, et al. (1993). Carbamazepine-induced hyponatremia in a patient with partial central diabetes insipidus. Nephron 64:142.

253. Van Amelsvoort T, Bakshi R, Devaux CB, Schwabe S (1994). Hyponatremia associated with carbamazepine and oxcarbazepine therapy: a review. Epilepsia 35:181.

254. Lozada ES, Gouaux J, Franki N, et al. (1972). Studies of the mode of action of the sulfonylureas and phenylacetamides in enhancing the effect of vasopressin. J Clin Endocrinol Metab 34:704.

255. Moses AM, Numann P, Miller M (1973). Mechanism of chlorpropamide-induced antidiuresis in man: Evidence for release of ADH and enhancement of peripheral action. Metabolism 22:59.

256. Bressler RB, Huston DP (1985). Water intoxication following moderate-dose intravenous cyclophosphamide. Archives of Internal Medicine 145:548.

257. Harlow PJ, DeClerck YA, Shore NA, et al. (1979). A fatal case of inappropriate ADH secretion induced by cyclophosphamide therapy. Cancer 44:896.

258. Larose P, Ong H, du Souich P (1987). The effect of cyclophosphamide on arginine vasopressin and the atrial natriuretic factor. Biochemical & Biophysical Research Communications 143:140.

259. Bode U, Seif SM, Levine AS (1980). Studies on the antidiuretic effect of cyclophosphamide: Vasopressin release and sodium excretion. Medical & Pediatric Oncology 8:295.

260. Zavagli G, Ricci G, Tataranni G, et al. (1988). Life-threatening hyponatremia caused by vinblastine. Med Oncol Tumor Pharmacother 5:67.

261. Hutchison FN, Perez EA, Gandara DR, et al. (1988). Renal salt wasting in patients treated with cisplatin. Annals of Internal Medicine 108:21.

262. Ritch PS (1988). Cis-dichlorodiammineplatinum II-induced syndrome of inappropriate secretion of antidiuretic hormone. Cancer 61:448.

263. Gerigk M, Bald M, Feth F, Rascher W (1993). Clinical settings and vasopressin function in hyponatraemic children. European Journal of Pediatrics 152:301.

264. Judd BA, Haycock GB, Dalton N, Chantler C (1987). Hyponatraemia in premature babies and following surgery in older children. Acta Paediatrica Scandinavica 76:385.

265. Anderson RJ, Chung HM, Kluge R, Schrier RW (1985). Hyponatremia: A prospective analysis of its epidemiology and the pathogenetic role of vasopressin. Annals of Internal Medicine 102:164.

266. Kanakriyeh M, Carvajal HF, Vallone AM (1987). Initial fluid therapy for children with meningitis with consideration of the syndrome of inappropriate anti-diuretic hormone. Clinical Pediatrics 26:126.

267. Padilla G, Ervin MG, Ross MG, Leake RD (1991). Vasopressin levels in infants during the course of aseptic and bacterial meningitis. American Journal of Diseases of Children 145:991.

268. Powell KR, Sugarman LI, Eskenazi AE, et al. (1990). Normalization of plasma arginine vasopressin concentrations when children with meningitis are given maintenance plus replacement fluid therapy. Journal of Pediatrics 117:515.

269. Vingerhoets F, de Tribolet N (1988). Hyponatremia hypo-osmolarity in neurosurgical patients: "Appropriate secretion of ADH" and "cerebral salt wasting syndrome." Acta Neurochirurgica 91:50.

270. Neville KA, Verge CF, O'Meara MW, Walker JL (2005). High antidiuretic hormone levels and hyponatremia in children with gastroenteritis. Pediatrics 116:1401.

271. Neville KA, Verge CF, Rosenberg AR, et al. (2006). Isotonic is better than hypotonic saline for intravenous rehydration of children with gastroenteritis: A prospective randomized study. Arch Dis Child 91:226.

272. Choong K, Kho ME, Menon K, Bohn D (2006). Hypotonic versus isotonic saline in hospitalized children: A systematic review. Arch Dis Child 91:828.

273. Zanardo V, Ronconi M, Ferri N, Zacchello G (1989). Plasma arginine vasopressin, diuresis, and neonatal respiratory distress syndrome. Padiatrie und Padologie 24:297.

274. Potts FL, May RB (1986). Early syndrome of inappropriate secretion of antidiuretic hormone in a child with burn injury. Annals of Emergency Medicine 15:834.

275. Kojima T, Fukuda Y, Hirata Y, et al. (1990). Changes in vasopressin, atrial natriuretic factor, and water homeostasis in the early stage of bronchopulmonary dysplasia. Pediatric Research 27:260.

276. Rao M, Eid N, Herrod L, et al. (1986). Antidiuretic hormone response in children with bronchopulmonary dysplasia during episodes of acute respiratory distress. American Journal of Diseases of Children 140:825.

277. Sulyok E, Kovacs L, Lichardus B, et al. (1985). Late hyponatremia in premature infants: role of aldosterone and arginine vasopressin. Journal of Pediatrics 106:990.

278. Cohen LF, di Sant'Agnese PA, Taylor A, Gill JR Jr. (1977). The syndrome of inappropriate antidiuretic hormone secretion as a cause of hyponatremia in cystic fibrosis. Journal of Pediatrics 90:574.

279. Stegner H, Caspers S, Niggemann B, Commentz J (1986). Urinary arginine-vasopressin (AVP) excretion in cystic fibrosis (CF). Acta Endocrinologica Supplementum. 279:448.

280. Arisaka O, Shimura N, Hosaka A, et al. (1988). Water intoxication in asthma assessed by urinary arginine vasopressin. European Journal of Pediatrics 148:167.

281. Iikura Y, Odajima Y, Akazawa A, et al. (1989). Antidiuretic hormone in acute asthma in children: effects of medication on serum levels and clinical course. Allergy Proceedings 10:197.

282. Schrier RW, Berl T (1975). Nonosmolar factors affecting renal water excretion. New England Journal of Medicine 292:141.

283. O'Rahilly S (1985). Secretion of antidiuretic hormone in hyponatraemia: Not always "inappropriate." British Medical Journal Clinical Research Ed. 290:1803.

284. Kamel KS, Bear RA (1993). Treatment of hyponatremia: a quantitative analysis. American Journal of Kidney Diseases 21:439.

285. Schrier RW (1985). Treatment of hyponatremia. New England Journal of Medicine 312:1121.

286. Videen JS, Michaelis T, Pinto P, Ross BD (1995). Human cerebral osmolytes during chronic hyponatremia: A proton magnetic resonance spectroscopy study. Journal of Clinical Investigation 95:788.

287. Ayus JC, Arieff AI (1993). Pathogenesis and prevention of hyponatremic encephalopathy. Endocrinology & Metabolism Clinics of North America 22:425.

288. Sterns RH, Riggs JE, Schochet SS Jr. (1986). Osmotic demyelination syndrome following correction of hyponatremia. New England Journal of Medicine 314:1535.

289. Ayus JC, Krothapalli RK, Arieff AI (1985). Changing concepts in treatment of severe symptomatic hyponatremia: Rapid correction and possible relation to central pontine myelinolysis. American Journal of Medicine 78:897.

290. Ayus JC, Krothapalli RK, Arieff AI (1987). Treatment of symptomatic hyponatremia and its relation to brain damage: A prospective study. New England Journal of Medicine 317:1190.

291. Sklar C, Fertig A, David R (1985). Chronic syndrome of inappropriate secretion of antidiuretic hormone in childhood. American Journal of Diseases of Children 139:733.

292. Tang TT, Whelan HT, Meyer GA, et al. (1991). Optic chiasm glioma associated with inappropriate secretion of antidiuretic hormone, cerebral ischemia, nonobstructive hydrocephalus and chronic ascites following ventriculoperitoneal shunting. Childs Nervous System 7:458.

293. Padilla G, Leake JA, Castro R, et al. (1989). Vasopressin levels and pediatric head trauma. Pediatrics 83:700.

294. Goldman MB, Luchins DJ, Robertson GL (1988). Mechanisms of altered water metabolism in psychotic patients with polydipsia and hyponatremia. New England Journal of Medicine 318:397.

295. Meierkord H, Shorvon S, Lightman SL (1994). Plasma concentrations of prolactin, noradrenaline, vasopressin and oxytocin during and after a prolonged epileptic seizure. Acta Neurologica Scandinavica 90:73.

296. Edwards CM, Carmichael J, Baylis PH, Harris AL (1989). Arginine vasopressin: A mediator of chemotherapy induced emesis? British Journal of Cancer 59:467.

297. Coslovsky R, Bruck R, Estrov Z (1984). Hypo-osmolal syndrome due to prolonged nausea. Archives of Internal Medicine 144:191.

298. Dhawan A, Narang A, Singhi S (1992). Hyponatraemia and the inappropriate ADH syndrome in pneumonia. Annals of Tropical Paediatrics 12:455.

299. van Steensel-Moll HA, Hazelzet JA, van der Voort E, Neijens HJ (1990). Excessive secretion of antidiuretic hormone in infections with respiratory syncytial virus. Archives of Disease in Childhood 65:1237.

300. Tang WW, Kaptein EM, Feinstein EI, Massry SG (1993). Hyponatremia in hospitalized patients with the acquired immunodeficiency syndrome (AIDS) and the AIDS-related complex. American Journal of Medicine 94:169.

301. Weissman PN, Shenkman L, Gregerman RI (1971). Chlorpropamide hyponatremia: Drug-induced inappropriate antidiuretic-hormone activity. New England Journal of Medicine 284:65.

302. Escuro RS, Adelstein DJ, Carter SG (1992). Syndrome of inappropriate secretion of antidiuretic hormone after infusional vincristine. Cleveland Clinic Journal of Medicine 59:643.

303. Liskin B, Walsh BT, Roose SP, Jackson W (1984). Imipramine-induced inappropriate ADH secretion. Journal of Clinical Psychopharmacology 4:146.

304. Parker WA (1984). Imipramine-induced syndrome of inappropriate antidiuretic hormone secretion. Drug Intelligence & Clinical Pharmacy 18:890.

305. Moses AM, Howanitz J, Miller M (1973). Diuretic action of three sulfonylurea drugs. Annals of Internal Medicine 78:541.

306. Cotton MF, Donald PR, Schoeman JF, et al. (1991). Plasma arginine vasopressin and the syndrome of inappropriate antidiuretic hormone secretion in tuberculous meningitis. Pediatric Infectious Disease Journal 10:837.

307. Cotton MF, Donald PR, Schoeman JF, et al. (1993). Raised intracranial pressure, the syndrome of inappropriate antidiuretic hormone secretion, and arginine vasopressin in tuberculous meningitis. Childs Nervous System 9:10.

308. Hill AR, Uribarri J, Mann J, Berl T (1990). Altered water metabolism in tuberculosis: Role of vasopressin. American Journal of Medicine 88:357.

309. Olson BR, Rubino D, Gumowski J, Oldfield EH (1995). Isolated hyponatremia after transsphenoidal pituitary surgery. Journal of Clinical Endocrinology & Metabolism 80:85.

310. Sane T, Rantakari K, Poranen A, et al. (1994). Hyponatremia after transsphenoidal surgery for pituitary tumors. Journal of Clinical Endocrinology & Metabolism 79:1395.

311. Crigler JF Jr. (1976). Commentary: On the use of pitressin in infants with neurogenic diabetes insipidue. Journal of Pediatrics 88:295.

312. Smith TJ, Gill JC, Ambruso DR, Hathaway WE (1989). Hyponatremia and seizures in young children given DDAVP. American Journal of Hematology 31:199.

313. Feldman BJ, Rosenthal SM, Vargas GA, et al. (2005). Nephrogenic syndrome of inappropriate antidiuresis. N Engl J Med 352:1884.

314. Morello JP, Bichet DG (2001). Nephrogenic diabetes insipidus. Annu Rev Physiol 63:607.

315. Anmuth CJ, Ross BW, Alexander MA, Reeves GD (1993). Chronic syndrome of inappropriate secretion of antidiuretic hormone in a pediatric patient after traumatic brain injury. Archives of Physical Medicine & Rehabilitation 74:1219.

316. Forrest JN Jr., Cox M, Hong C, et al. (1978). Superiority of demeclocycline over lithium in the treatment of chronic syndrome of inappropriate secretion of antidiuretic hormone. New England Journal of Medicine 298:173.

317. Huang EA, Feldman BJ, Schwartz ID, et al. (2006). Oral urea for the treatment of chronic syndrome of inappropriate antidiuresis in children. J Pediatr 148:128.

318. Ohnishi A, Orita Y, Okahara R, et al. (1993). Potent aquaretic agent: A novel nonpeptide selective vasopressin 2 antagonist (OPC-31260) in men. Journal of Clinical Investigation 92:2653.

319. Decaux G (2001). Long-term treatment of patients with inappropriate secretion of antidiuretic hormone by the vasopressin receptor antagonist conivaptan, urea, or furosemide. Am J Med 110:582.

320. Schrier RW, Gross P, Gheorghiade M, et al. (2006). Tolvaptan, a selective oral vasopressin V2-receptor antagonist, for hyponatremia. N Engl J Med 355:2099.

321. Bernier V, Morello JP, Zarruk A, et al. (2006). Pharmacologic chaperones as a potential treatment for X-linked nephrogenic diabetes insipidus. J Am Soc Nephrol 17:232.

322. Kamoi K, Ebe T, Kobayashi O, et al. (1990). Atrial natriuretic peptide in patients with the syndrome of inappropriate antidiuretic hormone secretion and with diabetes insipidus. Journal of Clinical Endocrinology & Metabolism 70:1385.

323. Manoogian C, Pandian M, Ehrlich L, et al. (1988). Plasma atrial natriuretic hormone levels in patients with the syndrome of inappropriate antidiuretic hormone secretion. Journal of Clinical Endocrinology & Metabolism 67:571.

324. Kojima T, Hirata Y, Umeda Y, et al. (1989). Role of atrial natriuretic peptide in the diuresis of a newborn infant with the syndrome of inappropriate antidiuretic hormone secretion. Acta Paediatrica Scandinavica 78:793.

325. Wijdicks EF, Ropper AH, Hunnicutt EJ, et al. (1991). Atrial natriuretic factor and salt wasting after aneurysmal subarachnoid hemorrhage. Stroke 22:1519.

326. Isotani E, Suzuki R, Tomita K, et al. (1994). Alterations in plasma concentrations of natriuretic peptides and antidiuretic hormone after subarachnoid hemorrhage. Stroke 25:2198.

327. Diringer M, Ladenson PW, Borel C, et al. (1989). Sodium and water regulation in a patient with cerebral salt wasting. Archives of Neurology 46:928.

328. Vokes TP, Aycinena PR, Robertson GL (1987). Effect of insulin on osmoregulation of vasopressin. American Journal of Physiology 252:E538.

329. Zerbe RL, Vinicor F, Robertson GL (1979). Plasma vasopressin in uncontrolled diabetes mellitus. Diabetes 28:503.

330. Ishikawa S, Saito T, Okada K, et al. (1990). Prompt recovery of plasma arginine vasopressin in diabetic coma after intravenous infusion of a small dose of insulin and a large amount of fluid. Acta Endocrinologica 122:455.

331. Tulassay T, Rascher W, Korner A, Miltenyi M (1987). Atrial natriuretic peptide and other vasoactive hormones during treatment of severe diabetic ketoacidosis in children. Journal of Pediatrics 111:329.

332. Zerbe RL, Vinicor F, Robertson GL (1985). Regulation of plasma vasopressin in insulin-dependent diabetes mellitus. American Journal of Physiology 249:E317.

333. Greger NG, Kirkland RT, Clayton GW, Kirkland JL (1986). Central diabetes insipidus. 22 years' experience. American Journal of Diseases of Children 140:551.

334. Wang LC, Cohen ME, Duffner PK (1994). Etiologies of central diabetes insipidus in children. Pediatric Neurology 11:273.

335. Pedersen EB, Lamm LU, Albertsen K, et al. (1985). Familial cranial diabetes insipidus. A report of five families: Genetic, diagnostic and therapeutic aspects. Quarterly Journal of Medicine 57:883.

336. Os I, Aakesson I, Enger E (1985). Plasma vasopressin in hereditary cranial diabetes insipidus. Acta Medica Scandinavica 217:429.

337. Toth EL, Bowen PA, Crockford PM (1984). Hereditary central diabetes insipidus: Plasma levels of antidiuretic hormone in a family with a possible osmoreceptor defect. Canadian Medical Association Journal 131:1237.

338. Nagai I, Li CH, Hsieh SM, et al. (1984). Two cases of hereditary diabetes insipidus, with an autopsy finding in one. Acta Endocrinologica 105:318.

339. Bergeron C, Kovacs K, Ezrin C, Mizzen C (1991). Hereditary diabetes insipidus: An immunohistochemical study of the hypothalamus and pituitary gland. Acta Neuropathologica 81:345.

340. Willcutts MD, Felner E, White PC (1999). Autosomal recessive familial neurohypophyseal diabetes insipidus with continued secretion of mutant weakly active vasopressin. Hum Mol Genet 8:1303.

341. Ito M, Yu RN, Jameson JL (1999). Mutant vasopressin precursors that cause autosomal dominant neurohypophyseal diabetes insipidus retain dimerization and impair the secretion of wild-type proteins. J Biol Chem 274:9029.

342. Ito M, Jameson JL (1997). Molecular basis of autosomal dominant neurohypophyseal diabetes insipidus: Cellular toxicity caused by the accumulation of mutant vasopressin precursors within the endoplasmic reticulum. J Clin Invest 99:1897.

343. Russell TA, Ito M, Ito M, et al. (2003). A murine model of autosomal dominant neurohypophyseal diabetes insipidus reveals progressive loss of vasopressin-producing neurons. J Clin Invest 112:1697.

344. Thompson CJ, Charlton J, Walford S, et al. (1989). Vasopressin secretion in the DIDMOAD (Wolfram) syndrome. Quarterly Journal of Medicine 71:333.

345. Grosse Aldenhovel HB, Gallenkamp U, Sulemana CA (1991). Juvenile onset diabetes mellitus, central diabetes insipidus and optic atrophy (Wolfram syndrome)-neurological findings and prognostic implications. Neuropediatrics 22:103.

346. Rotig A, Cormier V, Chatelain P, et al. (1993). Deletion of mitochondrial DNA in a case of early-onset diabetes mellitus, optic atrophy, and deafness (Wolfram syndrome, MIM 222300). Journal of Clinical Investigation 91:1095.

347. Jackson MJ, Bindoff LA, Weber K, et al. (1994). Biochemical and molecular studies of mitochondrial function in diabetes insipidus, diabetes mellitus, optic atrophy, and deafness. Diabetes Care 17:728.

348. Polymeropoulos MH, Swift RG, Swift M (1994). Linkage of the gene for Wolfram syndrome to markers on the short arm of chromosome 4. Nature Genetics 8:95.

349. Inoue H, Tanizawa Y, Wasson J, et al. (1998). A gene encoding a transmembrane protein is mutated in patients with diabetes mellitus and optic atrophy (Wolfram syndrome). Nature Genetics 20:143.

350. Hardy C, Khanim F, Torres R, et al. (1999). Clinical and molecular genetic analysis of 19 Wolfram syndrome kindreds demonstrating a wide spectrum of mutations in WFS1. Am J Hum Genet 65:1279.

351. Labib M, McPhate G, Marks V (1987). Post-traumatic diabetes insipidus combined with primary polydipsia. Postgraduate Medical Journal 63:33.

352. Defoer F, Mahler C, Dua G, Appel B (1987). Posttraumatic diabetes insipidus. Acta Anaesthesiologica Belgica 38:397.

353. Hadani M, Findler G, Shaked I, Sahar A (1985). Unusual delayed onset of diabetes insipidus following closed head trauma. Case report. Journal of Neurosurgery 63:456.

354. Jenkins HR, Hughes IA, Gray OP (1988). Cranial diabetes insipidus in early infancy. Archives of Disease in Childhood 63:434.

355. Piech JJ, Thieblot P, Haberer JP, et al. (1985). [Twin pregnancy with acute hepatic steatosis followed by antehypophyseal insufficiency and diabetes insipidus]. [French]. Presse Medicale 14:1421.

356. Iwasaki Y, Oiso Y, Yamauchi K, et al. (1989). Neurohypophyseal function in postpartum hypopituitarism: Impaired plasma vasopressin response to osmotic stimuli. Journal of Clinical Endocrinology & Metabolism 68:560.

357. Seckl JR, Dunger DB, Lightman SL (1987). Neurohypophyseal peptide function during early postoperative diabetes insipidus. Brain 110:737.

358. Masera N, Grant DB, Stanhope R, Preece MA (1994). Diabetes insipidus with impaired osmotic regulation in septo-optic dysplasia and agenesis of the corpus callosum. Archives of Disease in Childhood 70:51.

359. Tawa R, Kaino Y, Ito T, et al. (1994). A case of Kabuki make-up syndrome with central diabetes insipidus and growth hormone neurosecretory dysfunction. Acta Paediatrica Japonica 36:412.

360. Van Gool S, de Zegher F, de Vries LS, et al. (1990). Alobar holoprosencephaly, diabetes insipidus and coloboma without craniofacial abnormalities: A case report. European Journal of Pediatrics 149:621.

361. Yagi H, Nagashima K, Miyake H, et al. (1994). Familial congenital hypopituitarism with central diabetes insipidus. Journal of Clinical Endocrinology & Metabolism 78:884.

362. Villadsen AB, Pedersen EB (1987). Recumbent cranial diabetes insipidus: Studies in a patient with adipsia, hypernatremia, poikilothermia and polyphagia. Acta Paediatrica Scandinavica 76:179.

363. Ono N, Kakegawa T, Zama A, et al. (1992). Suprasellar germinomas; relationship between tumour size and diabetes insipidus. Acta Neurochirurgica 114:26.

364. Tarng DC, Huang TP (1995). Diabetes insipidus as an early sign of pineal tumor. American Journal of Nephrology 15:161.

365. Appignani B, Landy H, Barnes P (1993). MR in idiopathic central diabetes insipidus of childhood. American Journal of Neuroradiology 14:[pages].

366. Hung W, Fitz CR (1992). The primary empty-sella syndrome and diabetes insipidus in a child. Acta Paediatrica 81:459.

367. Eichhorn P, Rhyner K, Haller D, et al. (1988). [Diabetes insipidus in chronic myeloid leukemia. Remission of hypophyseal infiltration during busulfan treatment]. [German]. Schweizerische Medizinische Wochenschrift Journal Suisse de Me:275.

368. Puolakka K, Korhonen T, Lahtinen R (1984). Diabetes insipidus in preleukaemic phase of acute myeloid leukaemia in 2 patients with empty sella turcica: A report of 2 cases. Scandinavian Journal of Haematology 32:364.

369. Foresti V, Casati O, Villa A, et al. (1992). Central diabetes insipidus due to acute monocytic leukemia: Case report and review of the literature. Journal of Endocrinological Investigation 15:127.

370. de la Chapelle A, Lahtinen R (1987). Monosomy 7 predisposes to diabetes insipidus in leukaemia and myelodysplastic syndrome. European Journal of Haematology 39:404.

371. Kanabar DJ, Betts DR, Gibbons B, et al. (1994). Monosomy 7, diabetes insipidus and acute myeloid leukemia in childhood. Pediatric Hematology & Oncology 11:111.

372. La Starza R, Falzetti D, Fania C, et al. (1994). 3q aberration and monosomy 7 in ANLL presenting with high platelet count and diabetes insipidus. Haematologica 79:356.

373. Ra'anani P, Shpilberg O, Berezin M, Ben-Bassat I (1994). Acute leukemia relapse presenting as central diabetes insipidus. Cancer 73:2312.

374. Dunger DB, Broadbent V, Yeoman E, et al. (1989). The frequency and natural history of diabetes insipidus in children with Langerhans-cell histiocytosis. New England Journal of Medicine 321:1157.

375. Grois N, Flucher-Wolfram B, Heitger A, et al. (1995). Diabetes insipidus in Langerhans cell histiocytosis: Results from the DAL-HX 83 study. Medical & Pediatric Oncology 24:248.

376. Broadbent V, Dunger DB, Yeomans E, Kendall B (1993). Anterior pituitary function and computed tomography/magnetic resonance imaging in patients with Langerhans cell histiocytosis and diabetes insipidus. Medical & Pediatric Oncology 21:649.

377. Tien RD, Newton TH, McDermott MW, et al. (1990). Thickened pituitary stalk on MR images in patients with diabetes insipidus and Langerhans cell histiocytosis. AJNR: American Journal of Neuroradiology 11:703.

378. Minehan KJ, Chen MG, Zimmerman D, et al. (1992). Radiation therapy for diabetes insipidus caused by Langerhans cell histiocytosis. International Journal of Radiation Oncology, Biology, Physics 23:519.

379. Imura H, Nakao K, Shimatsu A, et al. (1993). Lymphocytic infundibuloneurohypophysitis as a cause of central diabetes insipidus. New England Journal of Medicine 329:683.

380. Paja M, Estrada J, Ojeda A, et al. (1994). Lymphocytic hypophysitis causing hypopituitarism and diabetes insipidus, and associated with autoimmune thyroiditis, in a non-pregnant woman. Postgraduate Medical Journal 70:220.

381. Koshiyama H, Sato H, Yorita S, et al. (1994). Lymphocytic hypophysitis presenting with diabetes insipidus: Case report and literature review. Endocrine Journal 41:93.

382. Kojima H, Nojima T, Nagashima K, et al. (1989). Diabetes insipidus caused by lymphocytic infundibuloneurohypophysitis. Archives of Pathology & Laboratory Medicine 113:1399.

383. Ahmed SR, Aiello DP, Page R, et al. (1993). Necrotizing infundibulohypophysitis: A unique syndrome of diabetes insipidus and hypopituitarism. Journal of Clinical Endocrinology & Metabolism 76:1499.

384. Rossi GP, Pavan E, Chiesura-Corona M, et al. (1994). Bronchocentric granulomatosis and central diabetes insipidus successfully treated with corticosteroids. European Respiratory Journal 7:1893.

385. Lewis R, Wilson J, Smith FW (1987). Diabetes insipidus secondary to intracranial sarcoidosis confirmed by low-field magnetic resonance imaging. Magnetic Resonance in Medicine 5:466.

386. Scherbaum WA, Wass JA, Besser GM, et al. (1986). Autoimmune cranial diabetes insipidus: Its association with other endocrine diseases and with histiocytosis X. Clinical Endocrinology 25:411.

387. De Bellis A, Bizzarro A, Amoresano Paglionico V, et al. (1994). Detection of vasopressin cell antibodies in some patients with autoimmune endocrine diseases without overt diabetes insipidus. Clinical Endocrinology 40:173.

388. Vokes TJ, Gaskill MB, Robertson GL (1988). Antibodies to vasopressin in patients with diabetes insipidus. Implications for diagnosis and therapy. Annals of Internal Medicine 108:190.

389. Christensen C, Bank A (1988). Meningococcal meningitis and diabetes insipidus. Scandinavian Journal of Infectious Diseases 20:341.

390. Sloane AE (1989). Transient diabetes insipidus following listeria meningitis. Irish Medical Journal 82:132.

391. Brandle M, Vernazza PL, Oesterle M, Galeazzi RL (1995). [Cerebral toxoplasmosis with central diabetes insipidus and panhypopituitarism in a patient with AIDS]. [German]. Schweizerische Medizinische Wochenschrift Journal Suisse de Me:684.

392. Mena W, Royal S, Pass RF, et al. (1993). Diabetes insipidus associated with symptomatic congenital cytomegalovirus infection. Journal of Pediatrics 122:911.

393. Watanabe A, Ishii R, Hirano K, et al. (1994). Central diabetes insipidus caused by nonspecific chronic inflammation of the hypothalamus: case report. Surgical Neurology 42:70.

394. Arisaka O, Arisaka M, Ikebe A, et al. (1992). Central diabetes insipidus in hypoxic brain damage. Childs Nervous System 8:81.

395. Outwater KM, Rockoff MA (1984). Diabetes insipidus accompanying brain death in children. Neurology 34:1243.

396. Fiser DH, Jimenez JF, Wrape V, Woody R (1987). Diabetes insipidus in children with brain death. Critical Care Medicine 15:551.

397. Barzilay Z, Somekh E (1988). Diabetes insipidus in severely brain damaged children. Journal of Medicine 19:47.

398. Hohenegger M, Vermes M, Mauritz W, et al. (1990). Serum vasopressin (AVP) levels in polyuric brain-dead organ donors. European Archives of Psychiatry & Neurological Sciences 239:267.

399. Durr JA (1987). Diabetes insipidus in pregnancy. American Journal of Kidney Diseases 9:276.

400. Hadi HA, Mashini IS, Devoe LD (1985). Diabetes insipidus during pregnancy complicated by preeclampsia: A case report. Journal of Reproductive Medicine 30:206.

401. Harper M, Hatjis CG, Appel RG, Austin WE (1987). Vasopressin-resistant diabetes insipidus, liver dysfunction, hyperuricemia and decreased renal function: A case report. Journal of Reproductive Medicine 32:862.

402. Frenzer A, Gyr T, Schaer HM, et al. (1994). [Triplet pregnancy with HELLP syndrome and transient diabetes insipidus]. [German]. Schweizerische Medizinische Wochenschrift Journal Suisse de Me:687.

403. Kleeman CR, Rubini ME, Lamdin E, et al. (1955). Studies on alcohol diuresis: II. The evaluation of ethyl alcohol as an inhibitor of the neurohypophysis. J Clin Invest 34:448.

404. Tata PS, Buzalkov R (1966). Vasopressin studies in the rat: III. Inability of ethanol anesthesia to prevent ADH secretion due to pain and hemorrhage. Pfluegers Arch 290:294.

405. Miller M, Moses AM (1977). Clincial states due to alteration of ADH release and action. In Moses AM, Share L (eds.), Neurohypophysis. Basel: Karger 153.

406. Sklar AH, Schrier RW (1983). Central nervous system mediators of vasopressin release. Physiol Rev 63:1243.

407. Rittig S, Knudsen UB, Norgaard JP, et al. (1989). Abnormal diurnal rhythm of plasma vasopressin and urinary output in patients with enuresis. American Journal of Physiology 256:F664.

408. Wille S, Aili M, Harris A, Aronson S (1984). Plasma and urinary levels of vasopressin in enuretic and non-enuretic children. Scandinavian Journal of Urology & Nephrology 28:119.

409. Terho P, Kekomaki M (1984). Management of nocturnal enuresis with a vasopressin analogue. Journal of Urology 131:925.

410. Evans JH, Meadow SR (1992). Desmopressin for bed wetting: length of treatment, vasopressin secretion, and response. Archives of Disease in Childhood 67:184.

411. Steffens J, Netzer M, Isenberg E, et al. (1993). Vasopressin deficiency in primary nocturnal enuresis: Results of a controlled prospective study. European Urology 24:366.

412. Uribarri J, Kaskas M (1993). Hereditary nephrogenic diabetes insipidus and bilateral nonobstructive hydronephrosis. Nephron 65:346.

413. Seow WK, Thomsett MJ (1994). Dental fluorosis as a complication of hereditary diabetes insipidus: studies of six affected patients. Pediatric Dentistry 16:128.

414. Rivkees SA, Dunbar N, Wilson T (2007). The management of central diabetes insipidus in infancy: Desmopressin, low renal solute load formula, thiazide diuretics. Journal of Pediatric Endocrinology and Metabolism [in press].

415. Jakobsson B, Berg U (1994). Effect of hydrochlorothiazide and indomethacin treatment on renal function in nephrogenic diabetes insipidus. Acta Paediatrica 83:522.

416. Blanco EJ, Lane AH, Aijaz N, et al. (2006). Use of subcutaneous DDAVP in infants with central diabetes insipidus. J Pediatr Endocrinol Metab 19:919.

417. McDonald JA, Martha PM, Jr., Kerrigan J, et al. (1989). Treatment of the young child with postoperative central diabetes insipidus. American Journal of Diseases of Children 143:201.

418. Ralston C, Butt W (1990). Continuous vasopressin replacement in diabetes insipidus. Archives of Disease in Childhood 65:896.

419. Wise-Faberowski L, Soriano SG, Ferrari L, et al. (2004). Perioperative management of diabetes insipidus in children. J Neurosurg Anesthesiol 16:14.

420. Muglia LJ, Majzoub JA (1993). In Burg F, Inglefinger J, Wald E (eds.), *Gellis and Kagan's current pediatric therapy, Fourteenth edition.* Philadelphia: WB Saunders 318.

421. Aylward PE, Floras JS, Leimbach WN Jr. (1986). Abboud FM: Effects of vasopressin on the circulation and its baroreflex control in healthy men. Circulation 73:1145.

422. Andersen LJ, Andersen JL, Schutten HJ, et al. (1990). Antidiuretic effect of subnormal levels of arginine vasopressin in normal humans. American Journal of Physiology 259:R53.

423. Seckl JR, Dunger DB, Bevan JS, et al. (1990). Vasopressin antagonist in early postoperative diabetes insipidus. Lancet 335:1353.

424. Moreno-Sanchez D, Casis B, Martin A, et al. (1991). Rhabdomyolysis and cutaneous necrosis following intravenous vasopressin infusion. Gastroenterology 101:529.

425. Pierce ST, Nickl N (1993). Rhabdomyolysis associated with the use of intravenous vasopressin. American Journal of Gastroenterology 88:424.

426. Mauro VF, Bingle JF, Ginn SM, Jafri FM (1988). Torsade de pointes in a patient receiving intravenous vasopressin. Critical Care Medicine 16:200.

427. Bryant WP, O'Marcaigh AS, Ledger GA, Zimmerman D (1994). Aqueous vasopressin infusion during chemotherapy in patients with diabetes insipidus. Cancer 74:2589.

428. Polycarpe E, Arnould L, Schmitt E, et al. (2004). Low urine osmolarity as a determinant of cisplatin-induced nephrotoxicity. Int J Cancer 111:131.

429. Williams TD, Dunger DB, Lyon CC, et al. (1986). Antidiuretic effect and pharmacokinetics of oral 1-desamino-8-D-arginine vasopressin: 1. Studies in adults and children. Journal of Clinical Endocrinology & Metabolism 63:129.

430. Cunnah D, Ross G, Besser GM (1986). Management of cranial diabetes insipidus with oral desmopressin (DDAVP). Clinical Endocrinology 24:253.

431. Stick SM, Betts PR (1987). Oral desmopressin in neonatal diabetes insipidus. Archives of Disease in Childhood 62:1177.

432. Pivonello R, Colao A, Di Somma C, et al. (1998). Impairment of bone status in patients with central diabetes insipidus. J Clin Endocrinol Metab 83:2275.

433. Moses AM, Sangani G, Miller JL (1995). Proposed cause of marked vasopressin resistance in a female with an X-linked recessive V2 receptor abnormality. Journal of Clinical Endocrinology & Metabolism 80:1184.

434. Kobrinsky NL, Doyle JJ, Israels ED, et al. (1985). Absent factor VIII response to synthetic vasopressin analogue (DDAVP) in nephrogenic diabetes insipidus. Lancet 1:1293.

435. Bichet DG, Razi M, Lonergan M, et al. (1988). Hemodynamic and coagulation responses to 1-desamino[8-D-arginine] vasopressin in patients with congenital nephrogenic diabetes insipidus. New England Journal of Medicine 318:881.

436. Knoers VV, Janssens PM, Goertz J, Monnens LA (1992). Evidence for intact V1-vasopressin receptors in congenital nephrogenic diabetes insipidus. European Journal of Pediatrics 151:381.

437. Brink HS, Derkx FH, Boomsma F, et al. (1993). 1-Desamino-8-D-arginine vasopressin (DDAVP) in patients with congenital nephrogenic diabetes insipidus. Netherlands Journal of Medicine 43:5.

438. Ohzeki T (1985). Urinary adenosine 3',5'-monophosphate (cAMP) response to antidiuretic hormone in diabetes insipidus (DI): Comparison between congenital nephrogenic DI type 1 and 2, and vasopressin sensitive DI. Acta Endocrinologica 108:485.

439. Bichet DG, Razi M, Arthus MF, et al. (1989). Epinephrine and dDAVP administration in patients with congenital nephrogenic diabetes insipidus: Evidence for a pre-cyclic AMP V2 receptor defective mechanism. Kidney International 36:859.

440. Moses AM, Weinstock RS, Levine MA, Breslau NA (1986). Evidence for normal antidiuretic responses to endogenous and exogenous arginine vasopressin in patients with guanine nucleotide-binding stimulatory protein-deficient pseudohypoparathyroidism. Journal of Clinical Endocrinology & Metabolism 62:221.

441. Knoers N, Monnens LA (1992). Nephrogenic diabetes insipidus: Clinical symptoms, pathogenesis, genetics and treatment. Pediatric Nephrology 6:476.

442. Vest M, Talbot NB, Crawford JD (1963). Hypocaloric dwarfism and hydronephrosis in diabetes insipidus. American Journal of Diseases of Children 105:175.

443. Macaulay D, Watson M (1967). Hypernatremia in infants as a cause of brain damage. Archives of Disease in Childhood 42:485.

444. Freycon MT, Lavocat MP, Freycon F (1988). [Familial nephrogenic diabetes insipidus with chronic hypernatremia and cerebral calcifications]. [French]. Pediatrie 43:409.

445. Nozue T, Uemasu F, Endoh H, et al. (1993). Intracranial calcifications associated with nephrogenic diabetes insipidus. Pediatric Nephrology 7:74.

446. Schofer O, Beetz R, Kruse K, et al. (1990). Nephrogenic diabetes insipidus and intracerebral calcification. Archives of Disease in Childhood 65:885.

447. Tohyama J, Inagaki M, Koeda T, et al. (1993). Intracranial calcification in siblings with nephrogenic diabetes insipidus: CT and MRI. Neuroradiology 35:553.

448. Bode HH, Crawford JD (1969). Nephrogenic diabetes insipidus in North America: The Hopewell hypothesis. New England Journal of Medicine 280:750.

449. Rosenthal W, Seibold A, Antaramian A, et al. (1992). Molecular identification of the gene responsible for congenital nephrogenic diabetes insipidus. Nature 359:233.

450. Bichet DG, Birnbaumer M, Lonergan M, et al. (1994). Nature and recurrence of AVPR2 mutations in X-linked nephrogenic diabetes insipidus. American Journal of Human Genetics 55:278.

451. Bichet DG, Hendy GN, Lonergan M, et al. (1992). X-linked nephrogenic diabetes insipidus: From the ship Hopewell to RFLP studies. American Journal of Human Genetics 51:1089.

452. Birnbaumer M, Gilbert S, Rosenthal W (1994). An extracellular congenital nephrogenic diabetes insipidus mutation of the vasopressin receptor reduces cell surface expression, affinity for ligand, and coupling to the Gs/adenylyl cyclase system. Molecular Endocrinology 8:886.

453. Holtzman EJ, Kolakowski LF Jr., Geifman-Holtzman O, et al. (1994). Mutations in the vasopressin V2 receptor gene in two families with nephrogenic diabetes insipidus. Journal of the American Society of Nephrology 5:169.

454. Holtzman EJ, Kolakowski LF Jr., O'Brien D, et al. (1993). A null mutation in the vasopressin V2 receptor gene (AVPR2) associated with nephrogenic diabetes insipidus in the Hopewell kindred. Human Molecular Genetics 2:1201.

455. Knoers NV, van den Ouweland AM, Verdijk M, et al. (1994). Inheritance of mutations in the V2 receptor gene in thirteen families with nephrogenic diabetes insipidus. Kidney International 46:170.

456. Yuasa H, Ito M, Oiso Y, et al. (1994). Novel mutations in the V2 vasopressin receptor gene in two pedigrees with congenital nephrogenic diabetes insipidus. Journal of Clinical Endocrinology & Metabolism 79:361.

457. Oksche A, Dickson J, Schulein R, et al. (1994). Two novel mutations in the vasopressin V2 receptor gene in patients with congenital nephrogenic diabetes insipidus. Biochemical & Biophysical Research Communications 205:552.

458. Pan Y, Metzenberg A, Das S, et al. (1992). Mutations in the V2 vasopressin receptor gene are associated with X-linked nephrogenic diabetes insipidus. Nature Genetics 2:103.

459. Tsukaguchi H, Matsubara H, Aritaki S, et al. (1993). Two novel mutations in the vasopressin V2 receptor gene in unrelated Japanese kindreds with nephrogenic diabetes insipidus. Biochemical & Biophysical Research Communications 197:1000.

460. van den Ouweland AM, Dreesen JC, Verdijk M, et al. (1992). Mutations in the vasopressin type 2 receptor gene (AVPR2) associated with nephrogenic diabetes insipidus. Nature Genetics 2:99.

461. Wenkert D, Merendino JJ Jr., Shenker A, et al. (1994). Novel mutations in the V2 vasopressin receptor gene of patients with X-linked nephrogenic diabetes insipidus. Human Molecular Genetics 3:1429.

462. Wildin RS, Antush MJ, Bennett RL, et al. (1994). Heterogeneous AVPR2 gene mutations in congenital nephrogenic diabetes insipidus. American Journal of Human Genetics 55:266.

463. Friedman E, Bale AE, Carson E, et al. (1994). Nephrogenic diabetes insipidus: An X chromosome-linked dominant inheritance pattern with a vasopressin type 2 receptor gene that is structurally normal. Proceedings of the National Academy of Sciences of the United States of America 91:8457.

464. Oksche A, Rosenthal W (1998). The molecular basis of nephrogenic diabetes insipidus. J Mol Med 76:326.

465. Pan Y, Wilson P, Gitschier J (1994). The effect of eight V2 vasopressin receptor mutations on stimulation of adenylyl cyclase and binding to vasopressin. Journal of Biological Chemistry 269:31933.

466. Rosenthal W, Antaramian A, Gilbert S, Birnbaumer M (1993). Nephrogenic diabetes insipidus: A V2 vasopressin receptor unable to stimulate adenylyl cyclase. Journal of Biological Chemistry 268:13030.

467. Rosenthal W, Seibold A, Antaramian A, et al. (1994). Mutations in the vasopressin V2 receptor gene in families with nephrogenic diabetes insipidus and functional expression of the Q-2 mutant. Cellular & Molecular Biology 40:429.

468. Waring AJ, Kajdi L, Tappan V (1945). A congenital defect of water metabolism. Am J Dis Child 69:323.

469. Langley JM, Balfe JW, Selander T, et al. (1991). Autosomal recessive inheritance of vasopressin-resistant diabetes insipidus. American Journal of Medical Genetics 38:90.

470. Knoers N, Monnens LA (1991). A variant of nephrogenic diabetes insipidus: V2 receptor abnormality restricted to the kidney. European Journal of Pediatrics 150:370.

471. Mulders SM, Bichet DG, Rijss JP, et al. (1998). An aquaporin-2 water channel mutant which causes autosomal dominant nephrogenic diabetes insipidus is retained in the Golgi complex. J Clin Invest 102:57.

472. Boton R, Gaviria M, Batlle DC (1987). Prevalence, pathogenesis, and treatment of renal dysfunction associated with chronic lithium therapy. American Journal of Kidney Diseases 10:329.

473. Bendz H, Aurell M, Balldin J, et al. (1994). Kidney damage in long-term lithium patients: A cross-sectional study of patients with 15 years or more on lithium. Nephrology, Dialysis, Transplantation 9:1250.

474. Yamaki M, Kusano E, Tetsuka T, et al. (1991). Cellular mechanism of lithium-induced nephrogenic diabetes insipidus in rats. American Journal of Physiology 261:F505.

475. Marples D, Christensen S, Christensen EI, et al. (1995). Lithium-induced downregulation of aquaporin-2 water channel expression in rat kidney medulla. Journal of Clinical Investigation 95:1838.

476. Hirji MR, Mucklow JC (1991). Transepithelial water movement in response to carbamazepine, chlorpropamide and demeclocycline in toad urinary bladder. British Journal of Pharmacology 104:550.

477. Navarro JF, Quereda C, Quereda C, et al. (1996). Nephrogenic diabetes insipidus and renal tubular acidosis secondary to foscarnet therapy. Am J Kidney Dis 27:431.

478. Bendz H, Aurell M (1999). Drug-induced diabetes insipidus: incidence, prevention and management. Drug Saf 21:449.

479. Hohler T, Teuber G, Wanitschke R, Meyer zum Buschenfeld KH (1994). Indomethacin treatment in amphotericin B induced nephrogenic diabetes insipidus. Clinical Investigator 72:769.

480. Vigeral P, Kanfer A, Kenouch S, et al. (1987). Nephrogenic diabetes insipidus and distal tubular acidosis in methicillin-induced interstitial nephritis. Adv Exp Med Biol 212:129.

481. Quinn BP, Wall BM (1989). Nephrogenic diabetes insipidus and tubulointerstitial nephritis during continuous therapy with rifampin. American Journal of Kidney Diseases 14:217.

482. Kato A, Hishida A, Ishibashi R, et al. (1994). Nephrogenic diabetes insipidus associated with bilateral ureteral obstruction. Internal Medicine 33:231.

483. Nagayama Y, Shigeno M, Nakagawa Y, et al. (1994). Acquired nephrogenic diabetes insipidus secondary to distal renal tubular acidosis and nephrocalcinosis associated with Sjögren's syndrome. Journal of Endocrinological Investigation 17:659.

484. Hartenberg MA, Cory M, Chan JC (1985). Nephrogenic diabetes insipidus: Radiological and clinical features. International Journal of Pediatric Nephrology 6:281.

485. Alon U, Chan JC (1985). Hydrochlorothiazide-amiloride in the treatment of congenital nephrogenic diabetes insipidus. American Journal of Nephrology 5:9.

486. Libber S, Harrison H, Spector D (1986). Treatment of nephrogenic diabetes insipidus with prostaglandin synthesis inhibitors. Journal of Pediatrics 108:305.

487. Rascher W, Rosendahl W, Henrichs IA, et al. (1987). Congenital nephrogenic diabetes insipidus-vasopressin and prostaglandins in response to treatment with hydrochlorothiazide and indomethacin. Pediatric Nephrology 1:485.

488. Vierhapper H, Jorg J, Favre L, et al. (1984). Comparative therapeutic benefit of indomethacin, hydrochlorothiazide, and acetylsalicylic acid in a patient with nephrogenic diabetes insipidus. Acta Endocrinologica 106:311.

489. Uyeki TM, Barry FL, Rosenthal SM, Mathias RS (1993). Successful treatment with hydrochlorothiazide and amiloride in an infant with congenital nephrogenic diabetes insipidus. Pediatric Nephrology 7:554.

490. Batlle DC, von Riotte AB, Gaviria M, Grupp M (1985). Amelioration of polyuria by amiloride in patients receiving long-term lithium therapy. New England Journal of Medicine 312:408.

491. Weinstock RS, Moses AM (1990). Desmopressin and indomethacin therapy for nephrogenic diabetes insipidus in patients receiving lithium carbonate. Southern Medical Journal 83:1475.

492. Welch EM, Barton ER, Zhuo J, et al. (2007). PTC124 targets genetic disorders caused by nonsense mutations. Nature [volume/pages].

493. Liu BA, Mittman N, Knowles SR, Shear NH (1996). Hyponatremia and the syndrome of inappropriate secretion of antidiuretic hormone associated with the use of selective serotonin reuptake inhibitors: A review of spontaneous reports. Can Med Assoc J 155:519.

494. Branten AJ, Wetzels JF, Weber AM, Koene RA (1998). Hyponatremia due to sodium valproate. Ann Neurol 43:265.

495. Jojart I, Laczi F, Laszlo FA, et al. (1987). Hyponatremia and increased secretion of vasopressin induced by vincristine administration in rat. Exp Clin Endocrinol 90:213.

496. Rider JM, Mauger TF, Jameson JP, Notman DD (1995). Water handling in patients receiving haloperidol decanoate. Ann Pharmacother 29:663.

497. Settle ECJ (1998). Antidepressant drugs: Disturbing and potentially dangerous adverse effects. J Clin Psychiatry 59:25.

498. Shaikh ZHA, Taylor HC, Maroo PV, Llerena LA (2000). Syndrome of inappropriate antidiuretic hormone secretion associated with lisinopril. Ann Pharmacother 34:176.

499. van Laar T, Lammers G-J, Roos RAC, et al. (1998). Antiparkinsonian drugs causing inappropriate antidiuretic hormone secretion. Movement Disorders 13:176.

500. Baylis PH (1989). In DeGroot LJ (ed.), Endocrinology. Philadelphia: WB Saunders 213.

501. Dunn FL, Brennan TJ, Nelson AE, et al. (1973). The role of blood osmolality and volume regulating vasopressin secretion in the rat. J Clin Invest 52:3212.

502. Robertson GL (1985). Regulation of vasopressin secretion. In Seldin DW, Giebisch G (eds.), The kidney: Physiology and pathophysiology. New York: Raven Press 869.

503. Bichet DG (1995). The posterior pituitary. In Melmed S (ed.), The pituitary. Cambridge (London): Blackwell Science 277.

504. Reeves WB, Andreoli TE (1989). Nephrogenic diabetes insipidus. In Scriver CR, Beaudet AL, Sly WS (eds.), The metabolic basis of inherited disease. New York: McGraw-Hill.

CHAPTER 10

Diabetes Mellitus

MARK A. SPERLING, MD • STUART A. WEINZIMER, MD
• WILLIAM V. TAMBORLANE, MD

Introduction

Diabetes mellitus is best defined as a syndrome characterized by inappropriate fasting or postprandial hyperglycemia, and its metabolic consequences which include disturbed metabolism of protein and fat. This syndrome results from a deficiency of insulin secretion or its action. Diabetes mellitus occurs when the normal constant of the product of insulin secretion times insulin sensitivity, a parabolic function (Figure 10-1), is inadequate to prevent hyperglycemia and its clinical consequences of polyuria, polydipsia, and weight loss.

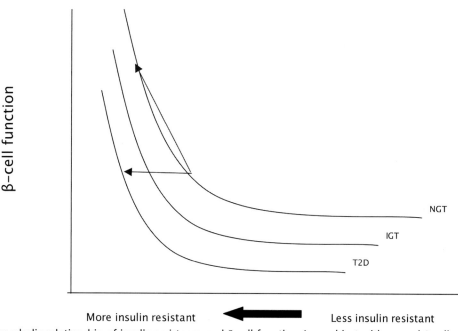

Figure 10-1. The hyperbolic relationship of insulin resistance and β-cell function. In a subject with normal β-cell reserve, an increase in insulin results in increased insulin release and normal glucose tolerance (top arrow). In an individual for whom the capacity to increase insulin release is compromised, increased insulin resistance with no β-cell compensation results in progression from normal glucose tolerance to impaired glucose tolerance to diabetes (bottom arrow). The product of insulin sensitivity (the reciprocal of insulin resistance) and acute insulin response (a measurement β-cell function) has been called "disposition index." This index remains constant in an individual with normal β-cell compensation in response to changes in insulin resistance. IGT, impaired glucose tolerance; NGT, normal glucose tolerance; and T2D, type 2 diabetes. [From Ize-Ludlow D, Sperling MA (2005). The classification of diabetes mellitus: A conceptual framework. Pediatric Clinics of North America 52:1533-1552.]

By simultaneously considering insulin secretion and insulin action in any given individual, it becomes possible to account for the natural history of diabetes in that person (e.g., remission in a patient with T1 diabetes or ketoacidosis in a person with T2DM). Thus, diabetes mellitus may be the result of absolute insulin deficiency, or of absolute insulin resistance, or a combination of milder defects in both insulin secretion and insulin action.[1] Collectively, the syndromes of diabetes mellitus are the most common endocrine/metabolic disorders of childhood and adolescence. The application of molecular biologic tools continues to provide remarkable insights into the etiology, pathophysiology, and genetics of the various forms of diabetes mellitus that result from deficient secretion of insulin or its action at the cellular level.

Morbidity and mortality stem from metabolic derangements and from the long-term complications that affect small and large vessels, resulting in retinopathy, nephropathy, neuropathy, ischemic heart disease, and arterial obstruction with gangrene of extremities.[2] The acute clinical manifestations can be fully understood in the context of current knowledge of the secretion and action of insulin.[3] Genetic and other etiologic considerations implicate autoimmune mechanisms in the evolution of the most common form of childhood diabetes, known as type 1 diabetes.[4,5] Genetic defects in insulin secretion are increasingly recognized and understood as defining the causes of monogenic forms of diabetes such as maturity-onset diabetes of youth (MODY) and neonatal DM and contributing to the spectrum of T2DM.[6]

There is evidence that the long-term complications are related to the degree and duration of metabolic disturbances.[2] These considerations form the basis of standard and innovative therapeutic approaches to this disease that include newer pharmacologic formulations of insulin, delivery by traditional and more physiologic means, and evolving methods to monitor blood glucose to maintain it within desired limits.

Classification

Diabetes mellitus is not a single entity but a heterogeneous group of disorders in which there are distinct genetic patterns as well as other etiologic and pathophysiologic mechanisms that lead to impairment of glucose tolerance.[1,7] Table 10-1 outlines an etiologic classification of diabetes mellitus in children, modified from "Report of the Expert Committee on the Classification and Diagnosis of Diabetes Mellitus," published by the American Diabetes Association in January of 2007.[7]

Our classification is modified to reflect more accurately the major categories in childhood, including the emergence of type 2 diabetes mellitus, cystic fibrosis–related diabetes, and drug-induced diabetes [largely from the antirejection agents cyclosporine and tacrolimus (formerly FK-506)]. Table 10-2 presents a summary of the classification originally proposed in 1979 but incorporates the newer criteria for blood glucose values used to diagnose diabetes, impaired glucose tolerance, and gestational diabetes.

TABLE 10-1

Etiologic Classification of Diabetes Mellitus

I. Type 1 Diabetes (Beta Cell Destruction Ultimately Leading to Complete Insulin Deficiency)
A. Immune mediated
B. Idiopathic

II. Type 2 Diabetes (Variable Combinations of Insulin Resistance and Insulin Deficiency)
A. Typical
B. Atypical

III. Genetic Defects of β-Cell Function
A. MODY syndromes
1. MODY 1 chromosome 20, HNF-4α
2. MODY 2 chromosome 7, glucokinase
3. MODY 3 chromosome 12, HNF-1α, TCF-1
4. MODY 4 chromosome 13, IPF-1
5. MODY 5 chromosome 17, HNF-1β, TCF-2
6. MODY 6 chromosome 2q32, neuro-D1/beta-2
B. Mitochondrial DNA mutations (includes one form of Wolfram syndrome; Pearson syndrome; Kearns-Sayre, diabetes mellitus, deafness)
C. Wolfram syndrome—DIDMOAD (diabetes insipidus, diabetes mellitus, optic atrophy, deafness): WFS1-Wolframin—chromosome 4p
1. Wolfram locus 2—chromosome 4q22-24
2. Wolfram mitochondrial
D. Thiamine responsive

IV. Drug or Chemical Induced
A. Antirejection—cyclosporine
B. Glucocorticoids (with impaired insulin secretion; e.g., cystic fibrosis)
C. L-Asparaginase
D. β-Adrenergic blockers
E. Vacor (rodenticide)
F. Phenytoin (Dilantin)
G. Alfa-Interferon
H. Diazoxide
I. Nicotinic acid
J. Others

V. Diseases of Exocrine Pancreas
A. Cystic fibrosis–related diabetes
B. Trauma—pancreatectomy
C. Pancreatitis—ionizing radiation
D. Others

VI. Infections
A. Congenital rubella
B. Cytomegalovirus
C. Hemolytic-uremic syndrome

VII. Variants of Type 2 Diabetes
A. Genetic defects of insulin action
1. Rabson-Mendenhall syndrome
2. Leprechaunism
3. Lipoatrophic diabetes syndromes
4. Type A insulin resistance—acanthosis
B. Acquired defects of insulin action
1. Endocrine tumors—rare in childhood
A. Pheochromocytoma
B. Cushing
C. Others
2. Anti-insulin receptor antibodies

VIII. Genetic Syndromes with Diabetes and Insulin Resistance/ Insulin Deficiency
A. Prader-Willi syndrome, chromosome 15
B. Down syndrome, chromosome 21
C. Turner syndrome
D. Klinefelter syndrome
E. Others
1. Bardet-Biedel
2. Alstrom
3. Werner

IX. Gestational Diabetes
X. Neonatal Diabetes
A. Transient—chromosome 6q24, KCNJ11, ABCC8
B. Permanent—agenesis of pancreas—glucokinase deficiency, homozygous and KCNJ11, ABCC8

Among the insulin-dependent forms, severe lack of insulin secretion results from presumed autoimmune destruction of islets in genetically predisposed hosts. This form is synonymous with type 1a diabetes, formerly called juvenile-onset diabetes.[5,8,9] Severe insulin-dependent diabetes mellitus, however (clinically indistinguishable from the autoimmune form), may not have any evidence of autoimmunity and can result from mitochondrial or other gene defects that interfere with the generation of intraislet energy required for insulin secretion[10-12] or rarely from pancreatic agenesis.[13]

The more severe forms of the MODY syndromes, subsequently detailed, also may require insulin.[14] Clinically similar forms of diabetes may occur secondary to cystic fibrosis[15] from toxic drugs such as the immunosuppressive agents cyclosporine and tacrolimus,[16,17] the rodenticide Vacor,[18] or streptozotocin as used for certain

pancreatic islet cell tumors;[19] with the hemolytic uremic syndrome;[20] or after pancreatectomy, such as for persistent hyperinsulinemic hypoglycemia in infancy.[21] Childhood insulin-dependent diabetes is generally type 1 diabetes mellitus.

TYPE 1 DIABETES MELLITUS

This condition is characterized by severe insulinopenia and dependence on exogenous insulin to prevent ketosis and to preserve life. Thus, it was called insulin-dependent diabetes mellitus (IDDM). The natural history of this disease indicates that there are preketotic non–insulin-dependent phases before and after the initial diagnosis. Although the onset is predominantly in childhood, the disease may occur at any age.[1] Therefore, such names as "juvenile diabetes," "ketosis-prone diabetes," and "brittle

TABLE 10-2

Summary of Classification of Diabetes Mellitus in Children and Adolescents

Category	Criteria
Diabetes Mellitus	
Type 1	Typical symptoms: glucosuria, ketonuria; random plasma glucose >200 mg/dL
Type 2	Fasting plasma glucose >126 mg/dL with 2-hour intervening value >200 mg/dL on OGTT more than once and in the absence of precipitating factors
Other types	Type 1 or 2 criteria with genetic syndrome, drug therapy; pancreatic disease or other known causes or associations
Impaired fasting glucose	Glucose >110 mg/dL but <126 mg/dL
Impaired glucose tolerance	Fasting plasma glucose <126 mg/dL with 2-hour >140 mg/dL but <200 mg/dL on OGTT
Gestational diabetes	Two or more abnormal fasting plasma glucose levels >105 mg/dL, 1-hour >180 mg/dL, 2-hour >155 mg/dL, 3-hour >140 mg/dL on OGTT
Statistical Risk Classes	
Previous abnormality of glucose tolerance	Normal OGTT with previously abnormal OGTT, spontaneous hyperglycemia, or gestational diabetes
Potential abnormality of glucose tolerance	Genetic propensity (e.g., identical twin with diabetes mellitus); islet cell antibodies

diabetes" have been abandoned in favor of the term *type 1 diabetes.*

Type 1 diabetes is generally distinct by virtue of its association with certain histocompatibility locus antigens (HLAs) and other genetic markers; by the presence of circulating antibodies to cytoplasmic and cell-surface components of islet cells; of antibodies to insulin in the absence of previous exposure to exogenous injection of insulin, of antibodies to glutamic acid decarboxylase (GAD, the enzyme that converts glutamic acid to γ-aminobutyric acid found abundantly in the innervation of pancreatic islets), and of antibodies to IA-2 (an islet cell–associated phosphatase); by lymphocytic infiltration of islets early in the disease; and by coexistence with other autoimmune diseases. Occasionally, markers of autoimmunity are not found and yet there is profound insulinopenia and dependence on insulin without evidence of a mitochondrial or other genetic defect. In these cases, type 1 diabetes is considered idiopathic (type 1b). With the exceptions noted, diabetes in children is usually insulin dependent and fits the type 1 category.[1]

TYPE 2 DIABETES

Persons with this subclass of diabetes [formerly known as "adult-onset diabetes," "maturity-onset diabetes" (MOD), or "stable diabetes"] may not be permanently insulin dependent and only occasionally develop ketosis. Some may, however, need insulin to correct symptomatic hyperglycemia—and ketosis may develop in some during severe infections or other stress. Therefore, this was previously called non–insulin-dependent diabetes mellitus (NIDDM).[1] It is becoming an increasing problem in overweight adolescents, especially those from vulnerable groups such as Africans, Mexicans, Native Indians, and other susceptible ethnic groups.[22,23]

Type 2 diabetes is not a single entity.[1] It may be a primary disorder, with inadequate insulin secretion caused by mutations in one of several genes encoding enzymes or transcription factors important to islet cell development and insulin secretion. These defects are now part of the spectrum of the syndromes commonly associated with MODY, which has a dominant mode of inheritance.[13,24] However, some patients with MODY defects, which some term *monogenic diabetes of youth,* may require insulin from the outset or as they grow older. A defect in the gene regulating glucose transport into the pancreatic beta cell, the GLUT2 transporter, may be responsible for another form of type 2 diabetes.[25]

Defects in glycogen synthase have also been implicated.[26,27] A primary defect in insulin receptors—often associated with acanthosis nigricans,[28] postreceptor defects [including Rad (Ras associated with diabetes)[29]], and milder mitochondrial gene defects[10]—also may result in type 2 diabetes. Secondary causes of type 2 diabetes mellitus include excessive counterregulatory hormones, especially pharmacologic doses of glucocorticoids, antibodies to the insulin receptor, and obesity with impaired insulin secretion.[30-41]

In type 2 diabetes mellitus, the serum concentration of insulin may be increased, normal, or moderately depressed depending on whether the defect is one of insulin action or secretion.[27-41] The onset of type 2 diabetes mellitus occurs in children generally around the time of puberty or shortly thereafter, but we increasingly recognize that it may occur at any age. It is becoming increasingly frequent in childhood and adolescence.[22,23] In some instances, there appears to be adequate secretion of insulin but with resistance to it—and in some individuals it may represent slowly evolving type 1 diabetes mellitus.[6,42,43] As an initial approach, weight reduction is indicated in children who are obese. In type 2 diabetes, there is no association with specific HLA antigens, autoimmunity, or various islet cell antibodies (ICAs).[42] However, several genetic abnormalities regulating insulin secretion are increasingly implicated in T2DM

Type 1 Diabetes Mellitus

EPIDEMIOLOGY

The prevalence of diabetes mellitus is highly correlated with increasing age. Available data indicate a range of 1 case per 1,430 children at 5 years of age to 1 case in

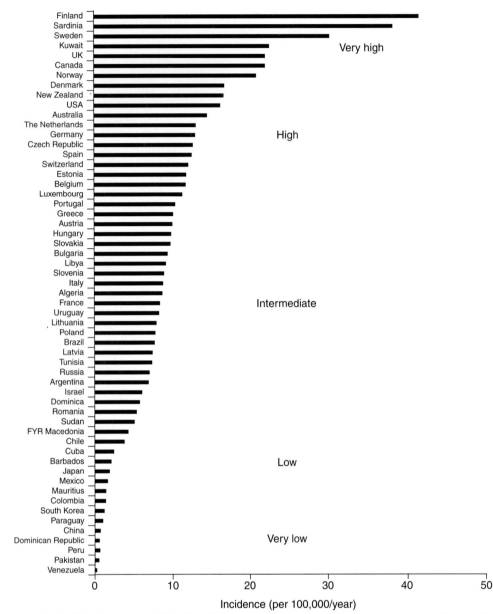

Figure 10-2. Age-standardized incidence (per 100,000/year) of type 1 diabetes in children younger than 14 years of age in 100 populations. Data for boys and girls have been pooled. Countries are arranged in descending order according to the incidence. (Puerto Rico and the Virgin Islands are presented separately from other populations in the United States.) [From Diamond Project Group (2006). Incidence of trends of childhood type 1 diabetes worldwide 1990-1999. Diabetic Medicine 23:857-866.]

360 children at 16 years.[44] Data on incidence in relation to racial or ethnic backgrounds indicate a range of more than 35 new cases annually per 100,000 population in Finland and Sardinia to about 1 per 100,000 in China and parts of South America[45-47] (Figure 10-2). In all examined areas there appears to be an increasing incidence of T1DM of about 2% to 3% per year.

In the United States, the occurrence of type 1 in blacks had previously been reported to be only between one-third and two-thirds of that in whites.[44,47] More recent data suggest that the incidence of diabetes mellitus in African Americans may be as high as in white Americans.[48,49] It is not clear, however, whether this new increase in incidence among African Americans is exclusively type 1 or

includes cases of type 2 presenting in ketoacidosis and thus misclassified.[50] The annual incidence in the United States is 15 to 18 cases per 100,000 of the childhood population[45] (Figure 10-2).

Males and females appear to be almost equally affected. There is no apparent correlation with socioeconomic status. Peaks of presentation occur in two age groups: at 5 to 7 years of age and at the time of puberty. The first peak corresponds to the time of increased exposure to infectious agents coincident with the beginning of school. The latter corresponds to the pubertal growth spurt induced by increased pubertal growth hormone secretion and gonadal steroids that antagonize insulin action. Emotional stresses accompanying puberty have also been implicated.

These possible cause-and-effect relationships remain to be proved but are strongly supported for the role of increased growth hormone secretion at the time of puberty. The incidence of type 1 diabetes is increasing worldwide, most prominently in certain populations (e.g., Finland) and in certain age groups (especially those younger than age 5 years).[45,46] In these younger patients, onset appears to be more abrupt and the extent of immune markers is less apparent than in older children.[51] Type 1 diabetes with abrupt onset, less evidence of autoimmunity, and indicators of viral infection (including evidence of pancreatitis) has been described in Japan.[52,53]

Seasonal and long-term cyclical variations have been noted in the incidence of type 1 diabetes. Newly recognized cases appear to occur with greater frequency in the autumn and winter in the northern and southern hemispheres.[54] Seasonal variations are most apparent in the adolescent years.[54] There is no consistent pattern linking long-term cyclicity with the incidence of viral infections. There is a definite increased incidence of diabetes in children with congenital rubella.[55,56] These changing patterns in incidence and associations with viral infections suggest a potential role for viruses or other microbial agents or their products as direct or indirect triggering mechanisms for inducing T1DM in a susceptible host.[57-60]

ETIOLOGY, PATHOGENESIS, AND GENETICS

The cause of the initial clinical findings in this predominant form of diabetes in childhood is the sharply diminished secretion of insulin. Although basal insulin concentrations in plasma may be normal in newly diagnosed patients, insulin production in response to a variety of potent secretagogues is blunted and usually disappears over a period of months to years (rarely exceeding 5 years). In certain individuals considered at high risk for

the development of type 1 diabetes, such as the nonaffected identical twin of a diabetic, a progressive decline in insulin-secreting capacity has been noted for months to years before the clinical appearance of symptomatic diabetes that usually manifests when insulin-secreting reserve is 20% or less of normal for that individual (Figure 10-3).[7]

The mechanisms that lead to failure of pancreatic beta-cell function point to autoimmune destruction of pancreatic islets in predisposed individuals. Type 1 diabetes has long been known to have an increased prevalence among persons with such disorders as Addison disease and Hashimoto thyroiditis, in whom autoimmune mechanisms are known to be pathogenic.[6] These conditions, as well as type 1 diabetes mellitus, are known to be associated with an increased frequency of certain histocompatibility loci antigens (HLAs)—in particular, DR3 and DR4. Located on chromosome 6, the HLA system is the major histocompatibility complex—consisting of a cluster of genes that code transplantation antigens and play a central role in immune responses.[61-74]

Increased susceptibility to a number of diseases has been related to one or more of the identified HLA antigens. The inheritance of HLA DR3 or DR4 confers a twofold to threefold increased risk for developing type 1 diabetes. When both DR3 and DR4 are inherited, the relative risk for developing diabetes is increased sevenfold to tenfold. Application of newer molecular genetic techniques has revealed further heterogeneity in the HLA D region among individuals with and without diabetes despite possessing the DR3 or DR4 markers, suggesting the participation of other susceptibility loci within these markers.

Among these loci may be the LMP2 and LMP7 genes that occur within the major histocompatibility complex.[61-72] Extensive genome-wide scans of markers associated with type 1 diabetes mellitus have uncovered more than a

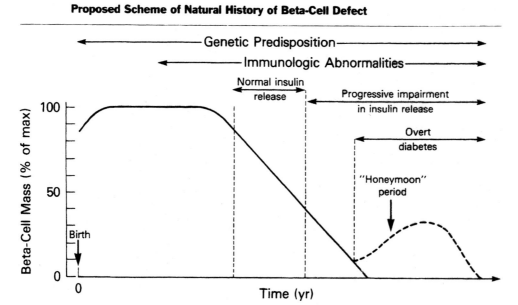

Figure 10-3. Proposed scheme of natural history of the evolution of insulin-dependent diabetes mellitus with progressive beta cell failure. [From Sperling MA (ed.) (1988). *Physician's guide to insulin-dependent (type 1) diabetes mellitus: Diagnosis and treatment.* Alexandria, VA: American Diabetes Association.]

dozen loci considered to confer susceptibility (Table 10-3). Some of these loci are confirmed and replicated by at least three different data sets. Others are suggestive but as yet not definitively linked. The strongest markers are those on chromosomes 6 and 11 (IDDM1 and IDDM2), respectively linked to the HLA DQ β chain and the insulin gene itself.

TABLE 10-3

Summary of Human Susceptibility Loci for Type 1 Diabetes Mellitus

Chromosome	Locus	Linkage Status
6p21	IDDM1; HLA-DQB	Confirmed
11p15.5	IDDM2; INS 59 VNTR	Confirmed
15q26	IDDM3; IGF1R	Suggestive (P,.001, MLS.2.2)
11q13	IDDM4; FGF3	Confirmed (P,2.2310^{25}, MLS.3.6)
6q25	IDDM5; ESR1	Confirmed (P,2.2310^{25}, MLS.3.6)
18q21	IDDM6	
2q31	IDDM7; IL1, HOXD8	Suggestive (P,.001, MLS.2.2)
6q27	IDDM8; IGF2R	Confirmed (P,2.2310^{25}, MLS.3.6)
3q21-q25	IDDM9	
10p11.2-q11.2	IDDM10	
14q24.3	IDDM11	Significant (P,2.2310^{25}, MLS.3.6)
2q33	IDDM12; CTLA-4	
2q34	IDDM13; IGFBP2, IGFBP5	
6p21	IDDM15 (distinct from HLA)	
10q25†	IDDM17	Significant (NPL: P,.002)
7p	Not assigned: GCK, IGFBP1, IGFBP3	
Xq	Not assigned	
Xp‡	Not assigned	Significant (P52.7310^{24}; MLS.3.6)
1q§	Not assigned	Suggestive (MLS53.31)

The IDDM nomenclature is assigned to a locus after linkage has been formally demonstrated, replicated, and confirmed in at least three different data sets. Where functional candidate genes are flanked by or very close to susceptibility markers, they are indicated.
P According to Lander and Kruglyak.
† The evidence for linkage increased substantially (P5.00004) with the higher density of markers and the inclusion of data for additional affected relatives and all unaffected siblings; NPL, nonparametric linkage.
‡ In HLA-DR3–positive patients.
§ This locus colocalizes with loci for systemic lupus enythematosus and ankylosing spondylitis.
MLS, maximum LOD score.
Adapted from Friday RP, Trucco M, Pietropaolo M (1999). Genetics of type 1 diabetes mellitus. Diabetes Nutr Metab 12:3.

TABLE 10-4

HLA DR and DQ Phenotype Frequencies in Patients with Type 1 Diabetes Mellitus and Healthy Control Subjects

Phenotype	Diabetic (%)	Nondiabetic	Odds Ratio (%)
DR (Serology)			
DR3/DR4	33	6	8.3
DR3/DR3	7	1	9.8
DR3/DRX	7	14	0.05
DR4/DR4	26	0	—
DR4/DRX	22	16	1.5
DRX/DRX	4	63	0.02
DQ (Molecular Probes)			
Non-Asp/ non-Asp	96	19	107.2
Non-Asp/Asp	4	46	0.04
Asp/Asp	0	34	0

Based on Morel PA, Dorman JS, Todd JA, et al. (1988). Aspartic acid at position 57 of the HLA-DQ beta chain protects against type 1 diabetes: A family study. Proc Natl Acad Sci USA 85:8111.

In IDDM1, the homozygous absence of aspartic acid at position 57 of the HLA DQ *b* chain (non-Asp/non-Asp) confers an approximately 100-fold relative risk for developing type 1 diabetes. Those who are heterozygous with a single aspartic acid at position 57 (non-Asp/Asp) are less likely to develop diabetes and are no more susceptible than individuals who contain aspartic acid on both DQ *b* chains [i.e., homozygous Asp/Asp (Table 10-4)]. Some studies suggest that type 1 diabetes mellitus is proportional to the gene frequency of non-Asp alleles in that population.[65,74] In addition, arginine at position 52 of the DQ *a* chain confers marked susceptibility to type 1.[61] Position 57 of the DQ *b* and position 52 of the DQ *a* chains are at critical locations of the HLA molecule that permit or prevent antigen presentation to T-cell receptors and activate the autoimmune cascade (Figure 10-4).[65]

IDDM2 is a polymorphic marker near the transcription start site of the insulin gene, giving rise to variable numbers of tandem repeats (VNTR) at the promoter end of the insulin gene on chromosome 11. Each tandem repeat element consists of an approximately 14-bp DNA segment with a consensus nucleotide sequence. The number of repeats ranges from about 25 to about 200, and the three classes of alleles are based on overall size. Class I insulin VNTR consists of 26 to 63 repeats and confers susceptibility, whereas class III consists of 140 to 200 or more repeats and is protective of diabetes. Together, the gene markers on chromosomes 6 and 11 (i.e., IDDM1 and IDDM2) account for 50% to 60% of the heritability of type 1 diabetes. However, combinations of certain DQ alleles in association with certain DR alleles may confer susceptibility or protection to the development of type 1 diabetes (Table 10-5).

In addition, other as yet undefined genetic factors play a role because the same high-risk genotypes are about sixfold more likely to develop diabetes in an individual with a

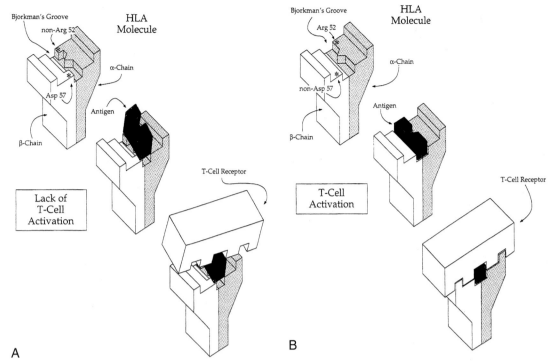

Figure 10-4. Representation of the interaction between antigen presentation in the context of specific HLA-DQ subtypes and the T-cell receptor. *(A)* Presence of aspartic acid at position 57 of the DQ *b* chain and an amino acid other than arginine at position 52 of the *a* chain prevents antigen lodging in the Bjorkman groove. Therefore, antigen presentation to the T-cell receptor is impaired—and in the absence of this "fit" T-cell activation is prevented. *(B)* Lack of aspartic acid at position 57 of the DQ *b* chain and arginine at position 52 of the DQ *a* chain permits antigen to fit and be recognized by the T-cell receptor that is now activated. [From Trucco M (1995). To be or not to be Asp 57, that is the question. Diabetes Care 15:705; and from Faas S, Trucco M (1995). The genes influencing the susceptibility to IDDM in humans. J Endocrinol Invest 17:477.]

TABLE 10-5
Effect of HLA Alleles on Susceptibility of Type 1 Diabetes Mellitus

DQ Alleles	Effect	Associated DR
B1p0302, A1p0301	Susceptible	DR4
B1p0201, A1p0501	Susceptible	DR3
B1p0501, A1p0101	Susceptible	DR1
B1p0201, A1p0301	Susceptible (African Americans)	DR7
B1p0502, A1p0102	Susceptible (Sardinia)	DR2 (DR16)
B1p0303, A1p0301	Susceptible (Japanese)	DR4
B1p0303, A1p0301	Susceptible (Japanese)	DR9
B1p0602, A1p0102	Protective	DR2 (DR15)
B1p0301, A1p0501	Protective	DR5
B1p0600, ?	Neutral	DR6
B1p0201, A1p0201	Neutral	DR7
B1p0303, A1p0301	Neutral	DR4
B1p0301, A1p0301	Neutral	DR4

Adapted from Friday RP, Trucco M, Pietropaolo M (1999). Genetics of type 1 diabetes mellitus. Diabetes Nutr Metab 12:3.

TABLE 10-6
Genetic Risk Estimates for HLA Class II in Type 1 Diabetes Mellitus

High-Risk Genotypes	Risk in an Individual with This Genotype
DQB1p0302 (DQ3.2)	1 in 60
DQ3.2/DQ2 (DR3)	1 in 25
DQB1p03021 family history of IDDM	1 in 10
DQ3.2/DQ2 (DR3)1 family history of IDDM	1 in 4
Complete sharing of both HLA haplotypes	1 in 2*

*Individual is a sibling of patient with T1DM.
Adapted from Nepom GT (1995). Class II antigens and disease susceptibility. Ann Rev Med 46:17; and from Aly TA, et al. Extreme genetic risk for type 1A diabetes. PNAS 103:14, 74-79.

positive family history than in one without a family history without type 1 diabetes (Table 10-6). It was anticipated that as the human genome map and its proteins are increasingly defined more precise knowledge of genetics of type 1 diabetes would become available. Investigation of four genome-wide linkage scans in close to 1,500 families with more than one affected member having T1DM identified several susceptibility loci. Of these, about 40% can still be attributed to allelic variation of HLA loci, and the influence of the VNTR in the insulin gene was confirmed.

In addition, the cytotoxic T-lymphocyte antigen 4 (CTLA4) gene on chromosome 2 and the protein tyrosine phosphatase nonreceptor 22 (PTPN22) gene on chromosome 1p13 were found to contribute significantly to predisposition to T1DM. However, the genome scan identified other potential loci conferring susceptibility on chromosomes 2q31-q33, 10p14-q11, and 16q220q24 and a locus on the long arm of chromosome 6 (6q21) distinct from the HLA region on 6p21. The precise genes in these regions that may predispose to T1DM have not been identified as yet, although some have been excluded[69] and newer candidate genes [such as CBLB interacting with CTLA4,[70] the decay-accelerating factor gene (DAF, a complement inhibitor),[71] and the interleukin 2A receptor IL2RA] are under scrutiny.[63]

These considerations provide a rational framework for the long-recognized association of type 1 diabetes with genetic factors on the bases of the increased incidence in some families, of the concordance rates in monozygotic twins, and of ethnic and racial differences in prevalence.[64-67] From multiple family pedigrees and HLA typing data, it has been estimated that if a sibling shares both HLA D haplotypes with an index case the risk for that individual is 12% to 20%; for a sibling sharing only one haplotype, the risk for IDDM is 5% to 7%; and with no haplotypes in common, the risk is only 1% to 2%.[75] HLA typing is not recommended for routine practice, but for purposes of genetic counseling it can be safely assumed that in whites the overall recurrence risks to siblings is approximately 6% if the proband is younger than 10 years of age and 3% if older at the time of diagnosis. The risk to offspring is 2% to 5%, with the higher risk in the offspring of a diabetic father.[65,74]

Factors other than pure inheritance must also be involved in evoking clinical diabetes. For example, DR3 or DR4 is found in approximately 50% of the general population and (non-Asp/non-Asp) is found in approximately 20% of white nondiabetics in the United States. However, the risk for type 1 diabetes in these subjects is only one-tenth that in an HLA-identical sibling of an index case with type 1 diabetes possessing these markers.[76] Even siblings sharing only one haplotype have a sixfold to tenfold greater risk of developing type 1 compared with the normal population (Table 10-6).

Importantly, approximately 10% of patients with type 1 do not have HLA DR3 or DR4, although almost all white diabetics lack at least one aspartic acid at position 57 of the DQ β chain (Table 10-4).[73] Most compelling is the fact that the concordance rate among identical twins of whom one has insulin-dependent diabetes is only 30% to 50%, suggesting the participation of environmental triggering factors or other genetic factor such as the postnatal selection of certain autoreactive T-cell clones that bear receptors recognizing "self." This postnatal process occurs within the thymus and implies that identical twins are not identical with respect to the T-cell receptor repertoire they possess.

Triggering factors might include viral infections.[48,58,76] In animals, a number of viruses can cause a diabetic syndrome—the appearance and severity of which depend on the genetic strain and immune competence of the species of animal tested. In humans, epidemics of mumps, rubella, and coxsackievirus infections have been associated with subsequent increases in the incidence of type 1 diabetes. The acute onset of diabetes mellitus, presumably induced by coxsackievirus B4, has been described.[57,76] The viruses may act by directly destroying beta cells, by persisting in pancreatic beta cells as slow viral infections, or by triggering a widespread immune response to several endocrine tissues.

A superantigen response may be involved in triggering T cells, bypassing the classic presentation by antigen-presenting cells (APCs) of the processed antigen in the context of restricted HLA molecules to T-cell receptors.[72,77,78] Viruses and certain endotoxins or exotoxins are capable of inducing a superantigen response. In addition, the virus may induce initial beta cell damage—which results in the presentation of previously masked or altered antigenic determinants. It is also possible that the virus shares some antigenic determinants with those present on or in beta cells, including GAD, such that antibodies formed in response to the virus may interact with these shared determinants of beta cells—resulting in their destruction, an example of molecular mimicry.[78]

Early exposure to cow's milk may be a factor in triggering diabetes, thus explaining the reported lower incidence of diabetes among exclusively breast-fed infants. This is the basis for one ongoing primary prevention study: TRIGR (the Trial to Reduce Insulin-dependent Diabetes in Those Genetically at Risk).[79-84] Antecedent stress and exposure to certain chemical toxins have been implicated in the development of type 1 diabetes. Although the rodenticide Vacor has been a cause of diabetes in individuals deliberately or inadvertently poisoned by this agent, some of these patients had islet cell antibodies (ICAs), suggesting that such antibodies are secondary to islet damage or that evolving type 1 disease preceded the drug ingestion. Nitrosamines in cured meat have also been implicated in type 1 diabetes, as have other environmental toxins.[85,86]

Evidence supports an autoimmune basis for the development of type 1 diabetes.[5-8,78] Histologic examination of pancreas from patients with type 1 who die of incidental causes has revealed lymphocytic infiltration around the islets of Langerhans. Later the islets become progressively hyalinized and scarred, a process suggesting an ongoing inflammatory response that is possibly autoimmune. Eighty to 90% of newly diagnosed patients with type 1 diabetes have ICA directed at cell surface or cytoplasmic determinants in their islet cells. The prevalence of these antibodies decreases with the duration of established disease.[87-89] In contrast, after pancreatic transplantation ICA may reappear in patients whose sera had become negative for ICA before transplantation. Taken together, these findings suggest that ICA disappears as the antigens intrinsic to pancreatic islets are destroyed and reappear when fresh antigen (transplanted islets) is presented.[90]

Studies in identical twins and in family pedigrees demonstrate that the existence of ICA may precede by months to years the appearance of symptomatic type 1 diabetes.[6] In vitro, ICA may impair insulin secretion in response to secretagogues and can be shown to be cytotoxic to islet cells—especially in the presence of complement or T cells from patients with type 1 diabetes. As many as 80% of patients may have antibodies to GAD, and 30% to 40% of newly diagnosed patients have spontaneous anti-insulin antibodies at initial diagnosis. These antibodies may be detected months to years before clinical diabetes becomes apparent.[91-94] There is also some evidence of abnormal T-cell function with an alteration in the ratio of suppressor to killer T cells at the onset of the disease.[5-8]

These findings suggest that type 1 diabetes (akin to other autoimmune diseases such as Hashimoto thyroiditis) is a disease of "autoaggression" in which autoantibodies in cooperation with complement, T cells, cytokines, FAS, and FAS's ligand (or other factors) induce apoptosis or destruction of the insulin-producing islet cells.[5-8] Thus, the inheritance of certain genes (such as those associated with the HLA system on chromosome 6 or other immunoregulatory or immunomodulatory genes) appears to confer a predisposition for autoimmune disease—including diabetes—when triggered by an appropriate stimulus such as a virus.[5-8] Evidence of superantigen-triggered T-cell receptor activation was discussed previously.[72,77,95]

Although it is understood that some insulin-dependent diabetic patients have none of the frequently associated HLA antigens, the evidence for an immune basis of islet cell destruction is sufficiently compelling to have fostered several studies of different immunosuppressive agents in the treatment of newly diagnosed diabetics (Table 10-7). None of these immunosuppressive agents has had long-term positive outcome, and some (e.g., cyclosporine) have proven toxic to beta cells. Although newer approaches are being attempted, all must be considered as experimental and not be viewed as established or recommended therapy.[91-94] The Diabetes Prevention Trial for T1DM (DPT1) was a multicenter randomized but non-blinded study using daily subcutaneous insulin and an annual admission for intravenous insulin infusion in first-degree relatives with proven risk factors for developing

---

TABLE 10-7

Immune Intervention Trials in Human Type 1 Diabetes Mellitus

Mycophenolate Mofetil/Daclizumab
This RDBPCCT clinical trial aims at assessing preservation of beta cell function in newly diagnosed patients.

Effect of Rituximab (Anti CD-20)
Aim: Preservation of beta cell function in newly diagnosed patients. Anti CD3 monoclonal antibody

ENDIT
See *http://www.diabetestrialnet.org* for details.

Nutritional Intervention to Prevent (NIP) Type 1 Diabetes Pilot Trial (RDBPCCL)
Test if dietary supplementation with docosahexaenoic acid (DHA) immediately after birth will prevent development of ICA in those genetically at risk for T1DM.

Oral Insulin for the Prevention of Diabetes in Relatives at Risk for Type 1 Diabetes

TRIGR - Trial to Prevent T1DM in Those Genetically at Risk via Cow's Milk Avoidance
Vitamin D supplementation

T1DM. Whereas prediction was highly accurate in identifying those most likely to develop T1DM within 5 years of entering the study, insulin injections had no protective effect to prevent the appearance of T1DM.[95,97,98]

Figure 10-3 is a summary of current concepts of the cause of type 1 diabetes as an autoimmune disease, the tendency for which is inherited and in which autoimmune destruction of beta cells is triggered by an as yet unidentified agent (possibly a virus). The slope of decline in insulin varies, and there may be periods of partial recovery such that the course of decline in insulin secretion is bumpy rather than smooth. The point at which clinical features appear corresponds to approximately 80% destruction of insulin secretory reserve. This process may take months to years in adolescent and older patients, and weeks in the very young patient in whom acute destruction by nonautoimmune mechanisms may play a significant role. Higher titers of spontaneous anti-insulin antibodies and ICA are characteristic of more active islet cell destruction, typically in the younger patient, and may prove useful in predicting evolving diabetes.[88,93]

PREDICTION AND PREVENTION

Although no presently available single marker or test can accurately predict type 1 diabetes mellitus, evidence suggests that a combination of immune and genetic markers for type 1 diabetes may provide predictability.[89-94] Whereas some authorities suggest that type 1 diabetes is a predictable disease, other authorities have raised objections because predictability is not as robust in their studies. Definitive preventive therapy is not available, thereby raising ethical dilemmas, and the majority of new cases occur sporadically in the absence of a positive family history in a first-degree relative.[92]

Most predictive studies have been performed in first-degree relatives of patients with new-onset type 1 diabetes.[89-94] Nevertheless, there is increasing evidence that the presence of high titers of islet cell, GAD, IA2, and insulin autoantibodies combined with a consistently diminished first-phase response of insulin to a pulse of intravenous glucose (corresponding to the fifth percentile or less for age in insulin response) can be used to reliably predict the onset of type 1 disease.[89-94]

Figure 10-5 demonstrates that in a set of first-degree relatives conversion to type 1 diabetes was highly dependent on the number of antibodies detected in their sera. Of those with three antibodies, about half developed clinical diabetes within 5 years of follow-up. First-phase insulin response and genetic (HLA) markers may be used to augment the predictability. For example, Table 10-8 demonstrates that the relative risk of developing clinical diabetes within 4 years of detecting ICA is almost 230 among those who possess all four heterodimers in HLA DQ β that predispose to diabetes (i.e., Asp572/2 and Arg521/1).

As technologic improvements continue, it is likely that population-wide screening for antibody markers (alone or combined with specific genetic markers) will be available to identify those at risk for developing type 1 diabetes. Such population-wide screening would be ethically justified if prevention could be proven effective. Presently, the

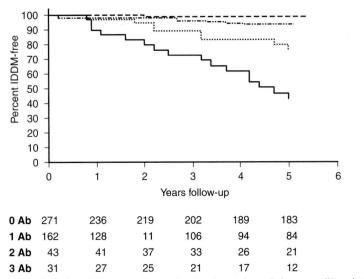

0 Ab	271	236	219	202	189	183
1 Ab	162	128	11	106	94	84
2 Ab	43	41	37	33	26	21
3 Ab	31	27	25	21	17	12

Figure 10-5. Survival analysis showing conversion to insulin-dependent diabetes mellitus (IDDM) in a subset of first-degree relatives according to the presence of 0, 1, 2, or 3 autoantibodies to islet antigens (ICA, GAD65, and IA-2 autoantibodies). [From Rosenbloom AL, Schatz DA, Krischer JP, et al. (2000). Therapeutic controversy: Prevention and treatment of diabetes in children. J Clin Endocrinol Metab 85:494. Copyright © The Endocrine Society.]

data are sufficiently persuasive to have fostered national trials in Europe and the United States to predict and possibly prevent the clinical onset of type 1 diabetes through immune intervention strategies.[91-94,96-102]

The European Nicotinamide Diabetes Intervention Trial (ENDIT) was a multicenter trial that screened approximately 22,000 first-degree relatives of patients with type 1 diabetes to identify 500 considered to be at high risk for developing this disease.[99,100] These at-risk individuals were treated with nicotinamide or a placebo in a double-blind fashion. The purported advantage of nicotinamide is that it is not known to be toxic or harmful in humans at the recommended doses. Its major disadvantage is that its proposed protective effects in delaying diabetes were based on a small sample cohort. A smaller trial in Germany was abandoned as ineffective, and the results of ENDIT were equally disappointing.

The U.S. Diabetes Prevention Trial for T1DM (DPT-I) was based on promising pilot data that suggested preservation of insulin secretion and prevention of progression to diabetes mellitus in at-risk individuals treated with insulin.[97] Daily subcutaneous insulin, coupled with intensive intravenous insulin every 9 months, prevented diabetes for at least 3 years in five subjects considered to be at risk because of genetic markers, islet cell and insulin autoantibodies, and diminished first-phase insulin response.

Among seven similar at-risk subjects who chose not to be treated, six developed insulin-dependent diabetes within 3 years.[97] DPT-1 was concluded in 2001, and there was no difference in the rates of developing diabetes among the placebo and insulin-treated groups. However, the ENDIT and DPT1 studies proved that large-scale multicenter studies could be successfully undertaken and that the prediction of progression to clinical diabetes was remarkably accurate. Thus, in those at highest risk (such as first-degree relatives of patients with T1DM) prediction is feasible and the discovery of a successful means of arresting or reversing progression to clinical diabetes is the subject of intense research.

Another study (TRIGR) involves 3,000 families in whom half will avoid cow's milk for the first 9 months of life to test the hypothesis that the ingestion of breast milk and avoidance of cow's milk formula (with its bovine syrum albumin [BSA]) may protect participants from the appearance of diabetes.[88,102] Several other studies are examining the utility of antibodies to the IL2 receptor, CD3 antibodies, immune suppressors such as mycophenolate mofetil, and immune modulators in preventing diabetes, including oral insulin. These studies are conducted by worldwide consortia of participating institutions (see *http://www2.diabetestrialnet.org*).

In animal models, oral insulin or oral GAD has been successfully used to prevent diabetes.[101] It is postulated

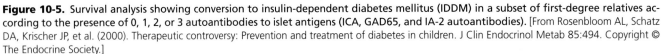

TABLE 10-8

Influence of Diabetic Heterodimers (ASP57neg Arg52pos) and Islet Cell Antibody (ICA) Status on Relative Risk for Developing Diabetes after 4 Years

	ICA Negative				ICA Positive			
Diabetic heterodimers (dH)	0	1	2	4	0	1	2	4
Developed IDDM after 4 years	12	16	37	12	12	18	29	15
Relative risk	1.0	2.9	8.6	25.4	9.0	26.5	78.0	229.3

Adapted from Friday RP, Trucco M, Pietropaolo M (1999). Genetics of type 1 diabetes mellitus. Diabetes Nutr Metab 12:3.

that ingestion of T-lymphocyte–dependent antigens can establish immunologic tolerance. Such oral strategies have been proposed and oral insulin is being tested in humans.[94] The subjects of primary prevention trials and secondary intervention trials to preserve residual insulin secretion at initial diagnosis are of major interest to investigators and clinicians alike. Progress is likely, but at present all of these strategies must be viewed as experimental and not currently in the domain of daily clinical practice.

INSULIN BIOSYNTHESIS

Insulin is synthesized on the ribosomes of pancreatic islet beta cells and released into the circulation as a molecule composed of two separate straight polypeptide chains linked by disulfide bridges between and within these chains.[103-114] The two chains are not synthesized separately but are derived from a larger precursor, proinsulin, a single coiled chain in which the NH_2 terminus of the A chain is linked to the COOH terminus of the B chain by a connecting peptide [C-peptide (Figure 10-6)]. An even larger precursor (preproinsulin, containing an additional peptide chain on the NH_2 terminus of the A chain) is first synthesized, but this additional piece (important to the initiation of synthesis) is rapidly excised. Further processing of proinsulin within the beta cell cleaves the C-peptide, consisting of 31 amino acids, from the insulin molecule at the sites indicated in the figure.

Defects in these cleavage sites are inherited in an autosomal-dominant manner and result in insulin molecules with less-than-normal biologic activity that can give rise to two types of familial hyperproinsulinemia. One defect yields B-C proinsulin, cleaved at site 1 but not at site 2 (Figure 10-6). This intermediate has 50% of the biologic

activity of insulin, which is sufficient to prevent any abnormality in carbohydrate metabolism. The defect at site 1 yields A-C proinsulin, cleaved at site 2 but not at site 1, which has inadequate biologic activity to prevent carbohydrate intolerance. A structural mutation in the proinsulin molecule, between the C-peptide and insulin, has been confirmed.[107,110] In addition, a defect also occurs in the enzymatic conversion of a normal proinsulin molecule to insulin—yielding hyperproinsulinemia and mild carbohydrate intolerance.[103]

The proconvertases responsible for correct conversion of proinsulin to insulin are also involved in the processing of other hormones. Thus, impaired prohormone processing may lead to obesity and secondary hypocortisolism owing to defective processing of pro-opiomelanocortin (POMC) and to hypogonadotropic hypogonadism.[106,111-113] Native proinsulin has less than 5%, whereas C-peptide has none, of the biologic activity of insulin. During synthesis, the role of C-peptide appears to be the provision of the spatial arrangement necessary in the formation of the disulfide bonds. Other defects have been described in insulin biosynthesis involving substitution of amino acids in the B chain that lead to impaired glucose tolerance in the presence of hyperinsulinemia.[106,108]

The insulin gene has been cloned and localized to chromosome 11, and genetic defects in insulin synthesis may be associated with diabetes—especially the syndromes MODY1, -3, -5, and -6 with candidate genes for MODY7.[104,105,114] By some estimates, MODY syndromes may constitute 2% to 5% of all lean persons developing clinical diabetes between the ages of 10 and 30 years. The association of VNTRs in the insulin gene and genetic predisposition for diabetes have been described previously.

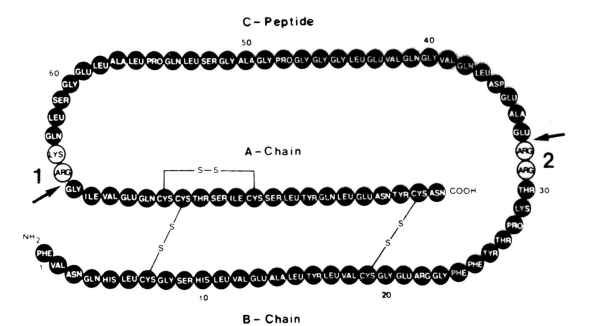

Figure 10-6. Structure of proinsulin. Arrows 1 and 2 indicate the two sites of normal cleavage that yield insulin and C-peptide when the amino acid residues indicated in the open circles are removed. These cleavage points are known mutation sites, are inherited in an autosomal-dominant manner, and can yield two types of familial hyperproinsulinemia. During insulin secretion, equimolar amounts of insulin and C-peptide are released.

Under normal circumstances, only small quantities of proinsulin are released into the circulation—amounting to less than 15% of total insulin as measured by radioimmunoassay (RIA). Even smaller quantities of proinsulin intermediates are also released. However, during insulin secretion induced by all stimuli one molecule of C-peptide is released with each molecule of insulin. Thus, the plasma of normal individuals contains small amounts of proinsulin, proinsulin intermediates, and almost equimolar amounts of insulin and C-peptide. The plasma metabolic half-life of C-peptide is, however, longer than that of insulin. Therefore, the molar ratio of C-peptide to insulin in peripheral plasma is always greater than 1 and the peak of C-peptide secretion or the nadir after suppression of release appears to occur later than that of insulin. Although standard RIA of insulin will also measure proinsulin, C-peptide will not be measured because it is immunologically distinct.

Separation of proinsulin from insulin can be achieved by chromatography to separate the larger proinsulin before assay. This is done with the use of an enzyme that degrades insulin but not proinsulin, or with the use of a C-peptide assay that will also measure proinsulin but not insulin. Because C-peptide is immunologically distinct, RIAs for this substance can be used to assess beta cell secretory reserve even in the presence of insulin antibodies formed in response to injections of bovine-porcine or human insulin.

Endogenous insulin secretion is accompanied by C-peptide release, whereas exogenous insulin administration suppresses endogenous insulin (and therefore C-peptide) secretion in all circumstances except insulinoma. Results of standard RIA with double-antibody precipitation are high in both circumstances. These attributes are important in distinguishing abuse of individuals by injection of exogenous insulin (high insulin, low C-peptide) from insulinomas or dysregulated insulin secretion (high insulin, high C-peptide) in casess of hypoglycemia. Measurements of C-peptide kinetics or of urinary excretion of C-peptide can be used as an index of endogenous insulin secretion.[115]

INSULIN SECRETION

Insulin secretion is governed by the interaction of nutrients, hormones, and the autonomic nervous system. Glucose, as well as certain other sugars metabolized by islets, stimulates insulin release. Basal and peak insulin levels are closely related to the glucose concentration, and prolonged fasting will further reduce glucose and insulin levels—which, however, remain in the measurable range at 2 to 5 mU/mL. There is evidence that a product or products of glucose metabolism may be involved in maintaining insulin secretion and that sugars not metabolized by islet cells do not promote insulin release.

The initial steps of glucose-stimulated insulin release are depicted in Chapter 5 in connection with mutations in the SUR(sulfonylurea receptor)-Kir6 (inward-rectifying potassium channel) complex of the adenosine triphosphate–regulated potassium channel K_{ATP} with the subsequent steps that may cause activation of glucose or amino acid–stimulated insulin secretion. This schema involves glucose transport into the beta cell through the GLUT2 glucose transporter and phosphorylation of glucose by means of glucokinase. Defects in the former are associated with type 2 diabetes, whereas heterozygous mutations in the latter are associated with MODY. Homozygous mutations in glucokinase result in permanent neonatal diabetes mellitus (as described in detail later in the chapter). Glucokinase defects are generally associated with normal insulin release at higher glucose concentrations, and therefore with a milder type of diabetes.[29] During glucose infusion in normal persons, insulin secretion is biphasic—with an initial spike followed by a sustained plateau. It is proposed that the initial spike represents preformed insulin, whereas the sustained plateau represents newly synthesized insulin.

Cyclic adenosine monophosphate (AMP) is involved in stimulating insulin release. Therefore, agents that inhibit phosphodiesterase and reduce cyclic AMP destruction (such as theophylline) augment insulin release. Translocation of calcium ions into the cytoplasm from the exterior as well as from the intracellular organelles plays a key role in the contractile forces that propel insulin to the cell surface.[116] There, the membrane of the insulin vesicle fuses with the cell membrane—allowing extrusion of insulin granules into the surrounding vascular space, a process known as emiocytosis. Other ions, including potassium and magnesium, are involved in the insulin secretion.[117-123] The sulfonylurea receptor is closely linked to potassium channels in the beta cell.[124-128] Amino acids also stimulate insulin release, although the potency of individual amino acids varies. A group of amino acids is more potent than any single one, and the insulin-secretory response is potentiated in the presence of glucose.[129] Free fatty acids and ketone bodies may also stimulate insulin release.[117-121,127]

Insulin responses to oral glucose administration are always greater than responses to intravenous administration of glucose that result in the same blood glucose profile.[128] This has led to the concept that gut factors modulate and increment insulin secretion. Although a variety of gut hormones participate in promoting insulin release,[128] gastrointestinal polypeptide (GIP) pancreatic glucagon and the glucagon-like peptides play a major role in stimulating insulin release. These properties have found application as agents, collectively named incretins, in augmenting insulin secretion in persons with T2DM and in some persons with T1DM. Somatotropin release-inhibiting factor (somatostatin), produced in the delta cells of islets, inhibits insulin and glucagon release and reduces splanchnic blood flow. These properties have found application to reduce insulin secretion in neonates with hyperinsulinemic hypoglycemia of infancy. Together, these factors may finely regulate nutrient intake and its disposition and form an enteroinsular axis for metabolic homeostasis.[117,118]

In addition to these gut hormones, several other hormones modulate insulin secretion. Growth hormone is involved in insulin synthesis and storage. Persons with congenital growth hormone deficiency have subnormal basal and stimulated insulin responses, whereas in acromegaly basal and stimulated insulin levels are increased.[129,130] Human chorionic somatomammotropin (also known as human placental lactogen), structurally related to growth hormone, likewise affects insulin release. The stimulatory effect of each hormone on insulin secretion is antagonized by the anti-insulin effect at the peripheral level, however. Similarly, glucocorticoids and estrogens evoke greater insulin secretion while inducing peripheral insulin resistance—in part by decreasing insulin receptors on target cells.[129]

Insulin secretion is constantly modulated by the autonomic nervous system.[119] The parasympathetic arm, through the vagus, directly stimulates insulin release. Modulation of insulin secretion by the sympathetic arm depends on whether α- or β-adrenergic receptors are activated. Activation of β_2 receptors by agents such as isoproterenol stimulates insulin secretion by a process that involves cyclic AMP generation. Blockade of β-adrenergic receptors by propranolol blunts basal and stimulated insulin release. Conversely, activation of α-adrenergic receptors blunts insulin secretion, and blockade of these receptors by agents such as phentolamine augments basal and glucose-stimulated insulin release. Epinephrine and norepinephrine stimulate predominantly α-adrenergic receptors in islets, resulting in impaired insulin secretion—as observed during stress or in patients with pheochromocytoma.[119]

In summary, in normal humans insulin secretion is constantly modulated by the quantity, quality, and frequency of nutrient intake; by the hormonal milieu; and by autonomic impulses. The ingestion of nutrients, principally carbohydrate and protein, produces intestinal hormonal signals that prime and initiate insulin release. The entry of glucose into the beta cell, the phosphorylation of glucose, and the generation of adenosine triphosphate (ATP) by this or other nutrients result in insulin release. This sequence involves cyclic AMP, β-adrenergic receptors, and ions—principally calcium and potassium. Glucose metabolism within the beta cell provides energy for further synthesis and release of insulin.

INSULIN ACTION

Insulin action on target cells in tissues such as liver, adipocytes, and muscle begins by binding to specific insulin receptors located on the cell membrane. Binding to these receptors is saturable, occurs with a high energy of association (affinity), and is pH and temperature dependent.[27,131-136] The insulin receptor is a heterodimeric glycoprotein consisting of two α and two β subunits linked by disulfide bonds (Figure 10-7). The α subunit, with a molecular mass of approximately 125,000 kd, acts as the binding site—whereas the β subunit, with a molecular mass of approximately 90,000 kd, possesses tyrosine kinase activity for endogenous and exogenous substrates (Figures 10-7 and 10-8).

This ability to phosphorylate proteins may underlie some of the manifold actions of insulin. Among the classes of proteins phosphorylated are insulin receptor substrates 1 through 3 (considered an important insulin-signaling effector molecule) and pp 185, another substrate of the insulin receptor (Figure 10-8).[27,131-136] Other insulin mediators may be involved in insulin action. This action may also be mediated in part by hydrolysis of

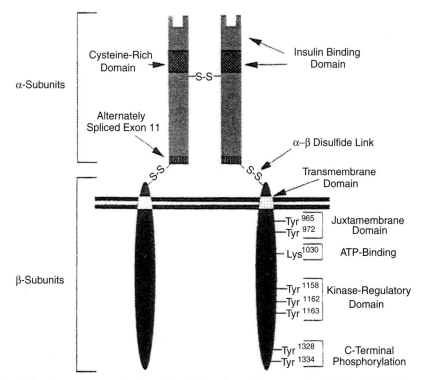

Figure 10-7. Structure of the insulin receptor. ATP, adenosine triphosphate. [From Cheatham B, Kahn CR (1995). Insulin action and the insulin signaling network. Endocr Rev 16:117.]

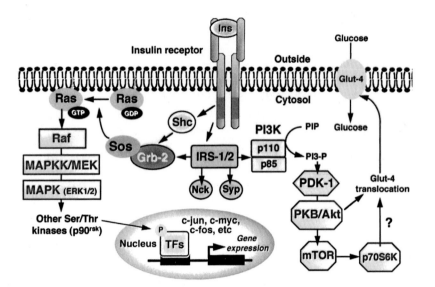

Figure 10-8. Schema of insulin receptor signal transduction pathways. ERK, extracellular regulated kinase; Glut-4, glucose transporter 4; Grb-2, growth factor receptor binding protein 2; Ins, insulin; IRS, insulin receptor substrate; MAPK, mitogen-activated protein kinase; MAPKK, mitogen-activated protein kinase kinase; MEK, map/Erk kinase; mTOR, target of rapamycin; P13K, phosphoinositol-3-kinase; p70S6K, p70S6 kinase (small ribosomal subunit of protein-6-kinase); PDK-1, phospholipid-dependent kinase 1; PKB, protein kinase B; Ras, rat sarcoma; Shc, Sh2 cytosolic adaptor; SOs, son of sevenless; Syp, now called SHP-2 (for SH-2-containing phosphatase). [Courtesy of L. Mandarino, PhD, University of Texas Health Science Center, San Antonio.]

glycan phosphoinositides in the cell plasma membrane.[137,138] The insulin receptor gene has been cloned and localized to chromosome 19, whereas the structurally related insulin-like growth factor-1 (IGF-1) receptor has been localized to chromosome 15.[131]

Under normal conditions, only a small proportion of the total available cell receptors need be occupied to achieve maximal biologic response. Thus, ordinarily there are spare receptors. Insulin receptors display two phenomena: down-regulation (in which high ambient insulin concentrations reduce the number of available receptors) and negative cooperativity, in which the occupancy of a receptor reduces the affinity of adjoining receptor sites. Scatchard analysis of insulin-binding data in in vitro systems reveals curvilinear plots compatible with negative cooperativity or with two classes of receptors: high-affinity/low-capacity and low-affinity/high-capacity. Total receptor number and the affinities of both classes of receptor sites can be calculated with use of these Scatchard plots.

After binding to the cell surface, the receptor-insulin complex is internalized within the cell and processed by lysosomal enzymes, with release of free insulin and potential recycling of the receptor back to the cell membrane. Binding of insulin to the cell surface receptor, perhaps with the participation of internalization that permits insulin action at the level of the nucleus, leads to the complex biochemical processes characteristic of insulin action in a given tissue. The ultimate mechanism or mechanisms by which insulin exerts its effects beyond receptor binding and phosphorylation remain unknown.

With postreceptor events assumed to be normal, however, the biologic response to insulin in a tissue is a function of the number of receptor/insulin complexes formed—which in turn is directly related to the circulat-

ing insulin concentration and to the receptor concentration. Thus, a reduction in receptor number could be compensated for by an increase in insulin concentration as long as the critical number of receptors necessary to produce maximal biologic response remains. Conversely, reduced insulin concentration could be compensated for by an increase in receptor number, provided the minimum amount of insulin necessary to produce a maximal biologic response is present.

Insulin receptors and their signaling proteins (Figures 10-7 and 10-8) are widely distributed in various tissues. Using targeted deletions of individual components or various combinations of components of the insulin receptor pathway has provided remarkable insight into the contribution of liver, muscle, fat, the beta cell, and brain to overall glucose homeostasis.[133-136] Key concepts that have emerged are that the insulin receptor signal cascade on beta cells is critically important in maintaining normal insulin secretion. Thus, mutations causing insulin resistance at the beta cell eventually lead to relative hypoinsulinemia that can interact with the insulin resistance in peripheral tissues to produce the hallmark of type 2 diabetes (i.e., peripheral insulin resistance plus relative insulinopenia).

In addition, studies with targeted deletion of the insulin receptor in the brain—the so-called NIRKO mouse (neuron-specific insulin receptor knockout)—demonstrate that these animals developed obesity, increased body fat, insulin resistance with modest hyperinsulinemia, and elevated levels of triglycerides. Reproductive function in both males and females is impaired as a result of abnormal regulation of luteinizing hormone secretion, and serum leptin levels are elevated.[136] Thus, insulin signaling in the brain joins the emerging list of factors important in regulating energy homeostasis and reproduction.

Clearly, primary defects in insulin receptor number or affinity may produce the same profound derangements

TABLE 10-9

Influence of Feeding (High Insulin) or Fasting (Low Insulin) on Some Metabolic Processes in Liver, Muscle, and Adipose Tissue*

	High Plasma Insulin (Postprandial State)	Low Plasma Insulin (Fasted State)
Liver	Glucose uptake	Glucose production
	Glycogen synthesis	Glycogenolysis
	Absence of gluconeogenesis	Gluconeogenesis
	Lipogenesis	Absence of lipogenesis
	Absence of ketogenesis	Ketogenesis
Muscle	Glucose uptake	Absence of glucose uptake
	Glucose oxidation	Fatty acid and ketone oxidation
	Glycogen synthesis	Glycogenolysis
	Protein synthesis	Proteolysis and amino acid release
Adipose tissue	Glucose uptake	Absence of glucose uptake
	Lipid synthesis	Lipolysis and fatty acid release
	Triglyceride uptake	Absence of triglyceride uptake

*Insulin is considered the major factor governing these metabolic processes. Diabetes mellitus may be viewed as a permanent low-insulin state that if untreated results in exaggerated fasting.

in intermediary metabolism as deficient insulin secretion, and similar disturbances may result despite normal insulin concentration and normal receptor characteristics if postreceptor steps are defective.[29,133-138] Insulin signaling for the regulation of metabolism has been the subject of considerable research and is extensively reviewed.[136,138] Examples of each type of defect in the individual components of this integrated system that comprises insulin biosynthesis, secretion, and action exist and can account for the metabolic abnormalities that characterize diabetes mellitus. An approach based on the principles of insulin biosynthesis secretion and action also permits a rational classification of diabetes mellitus.

PATHOPHYSIOLOGY

Normal insulin secretion in response to feeding is exquisitely modulated by the interplay of neural, hormonal, and substrate-related mechanisms to permit controlled disposition of ingested foodstuff as energy for immediate or future use. Mobilization of energy during the fasted state depends on low plasma levels of insulin. Thus, in normal metabolism there are regular swings between the postprandial high-insulin anabolic state and the fasted low-insulin catabolic state that affect three major tissues: liver, muscle, and adipose tissue (Table 10-9).

Insulin is the key anabolic hormone that promotes the synthesis and storage of carbohydrates, lipids, and proteins while simulataneously restraining their degradation. The uptake of glucose, fatty acids, and amino acids is stimulated—as is the activity or expression of enzymes that promote glycogen, fat, and protein synthesis. Conversely, the activity or expression of enzymes that break down these metabolites is restrained. All of these anabolic actions of insulin are reversed during the low-insulin state of starvation. Type 1 diabetes mellitus, as it evolves, becomes a permanent low-insulin catabolic (starvation) state in which feeding cannot reverse but rather exaggerates these catabolic processes.

It is important to emphasize that liver is more sensitive than muscle or fat to a given concentration of insulin. That is, endogenous glucose production from the liver by means of glycogenolysis and gluconeogenesis can be restrained at insulin concentrations that do not fully augment glucose utilization by peripheral tissues. Consequently, with progressive failure of insulin secretion the initial manifestation is postprandial hyperglycemia. Fasting hyperglycemia is a late manifestation that reflects severe insulin deficiency and indicates excessive endogenous glucose production.[139] Although insulin deficiency is the primary defect, several secondary changes that involve the stress hormones (i.e., epinephrine, cortisol, growth hormone, and glucagon) accelerate and exaggerate the rate and magnitude of metabolic decompensation.

Increased plasma concentrations of these counterregulatory hormones magnify metabolic derangements by further impairing insulin secretion (e.g., epinephrine), by antagonizing its action (e.g., epinephrine, cortisol, and growth hormone), and by promoting glycogenolysis, gluconeogenesis, lipolysis, and ketogenesis (e.g., glucagon, epinephrine, growth hormone, and cortisol) while decreasing glucose utilization and glucose clearance (e.g., epinephrine, growth hormone, and cortisol).[140] With progressive insulin deficiency, especially with concurrently elevated stress hormones, excessive glucose production and impairment of its utilization result in hyperglycemia with glucosuria when the renal threshold of approximately 180 mg/dL is exceeded.

The resultant osmotic diuresis produces polyuria, urinary losses of electrolytes, dehydration, and compensatory polydipsia. These evolving manifestations, especially dehydration, represent physiologic stress—resulting in hypersecretion of epinephrine, glucagon, cortisol, and growth hormone that amplifies and perpetuates metabolic derangements and accelerates metabolic decompensation. The acute stress of trauma or infection may likewise accelerate metabolic decompensation to ketoacidosis in evolving or established diabetes.[140-142] Hyperosmolality, commonly encountered as a result of progressive hyperglycemia, contributes to the symptomatology—especially to cerebral obtundation in diabetic ketoacidosis. Serum osmolality can be estimated with the following formula.

$$\text{Serum osmolality (mOsm/kg)} = (\text{serum Na [mEq/L]} + \text{K [mEq/L]}) \times 2$$
$$+ \text{Glucose mmol/L} = \left(\frac{\text{mg/dl}}{18}\right)$$

Consideration of serum osmolality has important implications in the treatment of diabetic ketoacidosis. The combination of insulin deficiency and elevated plasma values of the counterregulatory hormones is also responsible for accelerated lipolysis and impaired lipid synthesis, with resulting increased plasma concentrations of total lipids, cholesterol, triglycerides, and free fatty acids. The hormonal interplay of insulin deficiency and glucagon excess shunts the free fatty acids into ketone body formation. The rate of formation of these ketone bodies, principally β-hydroxybutyrate and acetoacetate, exceeds the capacity for peripheral utilization and for their renal excretion. Accumulation of these ketoacids results in metabolic acidosis and in compensatory rapid deep breathing in an attempt to excrete excess carbon dioxide (Kussmaul respiration).

Acetone, formed by nonenzymatic conversion of acetoacetate, is responsible for the characteristic fruity odor of the breath. Ketones are excreted in the urine in association with cations and thus further increase losses of water and electrolytes (Figure 10-9, Tables 10-10 and 11-11). With progressive dehydration, acidosis, and hyperosmolality and diminished cerebral oxygen utilization, consciousness becomes impaired—with the patient ultimately becoming comatose. Thus, insulin deficiency produces a profound catabolic state—an exaggerated starvation in which all of the initial clinical features can be explained on the basis of known alterations in intermediary metabolism mediated by insulin deficiency in combination with counterregulatory hormone excess. Because the counterregulatory hormonal

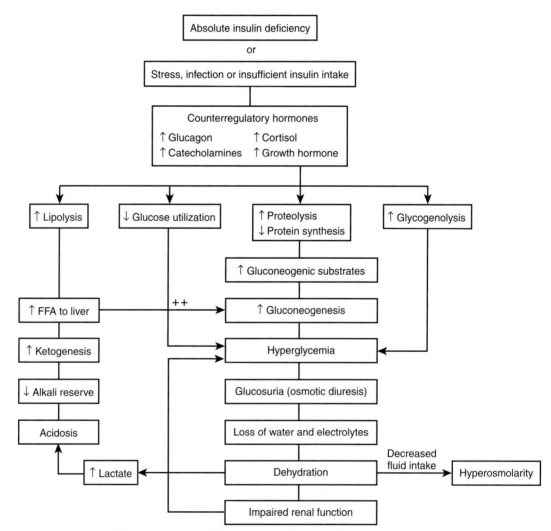

Pathophysiology of Diabetic Ketoacidosis

Figure 10-9. The pathophysiology of diabetic ketoacidosis is illustrated as a function of absolute insulin deficiency or insufficient insulin in the presence of major stress such as an infection, which leads to increases in the four major counter-regulatory hormones. Together, these changes increase glucose production via glycogenolysis and gluconeogenesis which together result in hyperglycemia, osmotic diuresis and dehydration. Simultaneously increase lipolysis leads to ketone body production and acidosis in combination with increased lactic acid from dehydration. See text for greater detail.

TABLE 10-10

Fluid and Electrolyte Maintenance Requirements and Estimated Losses in Diabetic Ketoacidosis

Approximate Daily Maintenance Requirements*		Approximate Accumulated Losses†
Water	1,500 mL/m²	100 mL/kg (range, 60–100 mL/kg)
Sodium	45 mEq/m²	6 mEq/kg (range, 5–13 mEq/kg)
Potassium	35 mEq/m²	5 mEq/kg (range, 4–6 mEq/kg)
Chloride	30 mEq/m²	4 mEq/kg (range, 3–9 mEq/kg)
Phosphate	10 mEq/m²	3 mEq/kg (range, 2–5 mEq/kg)

* Maintenance is expressed in surface area to permit uniformity because fluid requirements change as weight increases.

† Losses are expressed per unit of body weight because the losses remain relatively constant in relation to total body weight.

changes are usually secondary, the severity and duration of the symptoms are a reflection of the extent of primary insulinopenia.[139-143]

CLINICAL MANIFESTATIONS OF DIABETES MELLITUS

The classic presentation of diabetes in children is a history of polyuria, polydipsia, polyphagia, and weight loss. Polyuria may be heralded by the recurrence of bedwetting in a previously toilet trained child and polydipsia by a child constantly requesting fluids to drink. Unexplained weight loss should raise suspicion of the existence of diabetes that should be confirmed or excluded by measurement of blood glucose concentration first in the postprandial and later in the fasting state. The urine should also be checked for the presence of glucosuria. The duration of these symptoms varies but is often less than 1 month.

An insidious onset with lethargy, weakness, and weight loss is also quite common. The loss of weight despite increased dietary intake is readily explicable by the following example. The average healthy 10-year-old child has a daily caloric intake of 2,000 or more calories, of which approximately 50% are derived from carbohydrates. With the development of diabetes, daily losses of water and glucose may be as much as 5 L and 250 g, respectively. This represents 1,000 calories lost in the urine, or 50% of average daily caloric intake. Therefore, despite the child's compensatory increased intake of food and water the calories cannot be utilized, excessive caloric losses continue, and increasing catabolism and weight loss ensue.

Pyogenic skin infections and candidal vaginitis in girls or candidal balanitis in uncircumsized boys are occasionally present at the time of diagnosis of diabetes. They are rarely the sole clinical manifestations of diabetes in children, and a careful history will invariably reveal the coexistence of polyuria, polydipsia, and perhaps weight loss.

Ketoacidosis is responsible for the initial presentation of many (about 25 to 40%) diabetic children. Ketoacidosis is likely to be present more often in children younger than 5 years of age because the diagnosis may not be suspected and a history of polyuria and polydipsia may be difficult to elicit.[144,145] The early manifestations may be relatively mild and consist of vomiting, polyuria, and dehydration.

In more prolonged and severe cases, Kussmaul respiration is present—and there is an odor of acetone on the breath. Kussmaul respiration may be confused with bronchiolitis or asthma and be treated with steroids or adrenergic agents that worsen diabetes. Abdominal pain and/or rigidity may be present and may mimic appendicitis or pancreatitis. Cerebral obtundation and (ultimately) coma ensue and are related to the degree of hyperosmolarity. Laboratory findings include glucosuria, ketonuria, hyperglycemia, ketonemia, and metabolic acidosis. Leukocytosis is common, and nonspecific serum amylase levels may be elevated. The serum lipase level is usually not elevated. In those with abdominal pain, it should not be assumed that these findings are evidence of a surgical emergency before a period of appropriate fluid, electrolyte, and insulin therapy to correct dehydration and acidosis. The abdominal manifestations frequently disappear after several hours of such treatment.

DIAGNOSIS

Children in whom the diagnosis of diabetes mellitus must be considered may, for practical purposes, be divided into three general categories: those who have a history suggestive of diabetes, especially polyuria with polydipsia and failure to gain weight or a weight loss despite a voracious appetite; those who have a transient or persistent glucosuria; and those who have clinical manifestations of metabolic acidosis with or without stupor or coma. In all instances, the diagnosis of diabetes mellitus is dependent on the demonstration of hyperglycemia in association with glucosuria with or without ketonuria. When classic symptoms of polyuria and polydipsia are associated with hyperglycemia and glucosuria, the glucose tolerance test is contraindicated.

Renal glucosuria may be an isolated congenital disorder or a manifestation of the Fanconi syndrome and other renal tubular disorders owing to severe heavy metal intoxication, ingestion of certain drugs (e.g., outdated tetracycline), or inborn errors of metabolism (e.g., cystinosis). When vomiting, diarrhea, and/or inadequate intake of food are complicating factors in any of these conditions, starvation ketosis may ensue and simulate diabetic ketoacidosis. The absence of hyperglycemia eliminates the possibility of diabetes. It is also important to recognize that not all urinary sugar is glucose, and infrequently galactosemia, pentosuria, and the fructosurias will require consideration as diagnostic possibilities.

The discovery of glucosuria, with or without a mild degree of hyperglycemia, during a hospital admission for trauma or infection (or even during the associated emotional upheaval) may herald the existence of diabetes. In most of these instances, the glucosuria remits during recovery.[134] Because this circumstance may indicate a limited capacity for insulin secretion, which is unmasked by elevated plasma concentrations of stress hormones, these patients should be rechecked at a later date for the possibility of hyperglycemia, clinical features of diabetes mellitus, and family history of diabetes.

A strong family history of diabetes mellitus in two preceding generations suggests the possibility of a MODY syndrome. Under these circumstances, a glucose tolerance test may be useful to establish a diagnosis. Glucose tolerance testing should be performed several weeks after recovery from the acute illness, with a glucose loading dose adjusted for weight. Evidence indicates that the test is most likely to be abnormal in those with HLA DR3 and DR4, in whom ICA or insulin autoantibodies are detected, or who have MODY.[147]

Transient hyperglycemia is common in patients with asthma treated with epinephrine and steroids. Further testing in such patients is not indicated. Screening procedures, such as postprandial determinations of blood glucose or oral glucose tolerance tests, have yielded low detection rates in children—even among those considered at risk, such as siblings of diabetic children. Accordingly, such screening procedures are not recommended in children.

DIABETIC KETOACIDOSIS

Diabetic ketoacidosis is a medical emergency and represents a life-threatening decompensation of metabolism that requires prompt recognition and appropriate treatment, with careful monitoring of clinical and biochemical indices. DKA must be differentiated from acidosis and coma from other causes. These include hypoglycemia, uremia, gastroenteritis with metabolic acidosis, lactic acidosis, salicylate intoxication, encephalitis, and other intracranial lesions. Diabetic ketoacidosis exists when there is hyperglycemia (glucose 300 mg/dL), ketonemia (ketones strongly positive at greater than 1:2 dilution of serum), acidosis (pH 7.30 or less and bicarbonate 15 mEq/L or less), glucosuria, and ketonuria in addition to the clinical features of tachypnea (Kussmaul respiration) and cerebral obtundation.

Precipitating factors, even for the initial presentation, include stress (e.g., trauma), infections, vomiting, and major psychological disturbances. Recurrent episodes of ketoacidosis in established diabetics often represent deliberate errors in recommended insulin dosage, unusual stress responses that indicate psychological disturbances, and at times pleas to be removed from a home environment perceived to be stressful or intolerable.[141] Diabetic ketoacidosis should also be distinguished from nonketotic hyperosmolar coma.[142,148,149]

Nonketotic hyperosmolar coma is a syndrome characterized by severe hyperglycemia (blood glucose concentration of more than 600 mg/dL), absence of or only very slight ketosis, nonketotic acidosis, severe dehydration, depressed sensorium or frank coma, and various neurologic signs that may include grand mal seizures, hyperthermia, hemiparesis, and positive Babinski signs. Respiration is usually shallow, but coexistent metabolic (lactic) acidosis may be manifested by Kussmaul breathing. Serum osmolarity is commonly 350 mOsm/kg or higher. This condition usually occurs in middle-aged or elderly individuals who have "mild" diabetes. Among them, mortality rates have been as high as 40% to 70%, possibly in part owing to delays in recognition and institution of appropriate therapy.

In children, this condition is infrequent. Among reported cases, there has been a high incidence of preexisting neurologic damage. The profound hyperglycemia may develop over a period of days, and initially the obligatory osmotic polyuria and dehydration may be partially compensated for by increased fluid intake. With progression, thirst becomes impaired—possibly because of alteration of the hypothalamic thirst center by hyperosmolarity and possibly in some instances because of a preexisting defect in the hypothalamic osmo-regulating mechanism.[142,148-150] More recently, nonketotic hyperglycemia with coma has been a feature of presentation in youth with T2DM and often associated with morbid obesity. Some of these obese patients may present with ketoacidosis as the initial clinical presentation.

The low production of ketones is attributed mainly to the hyperosmolarity, which in vitro blunts the lipolytic effect of epinephrine, and to the concomitant antilipolytic effect of residual insulin. Blunting of lipolysis by the therapeutic use of β-adrenergic blockers may also contribute to the syndrome. The key difference between diabetic ketoacidosis and hyperglycemic hyperosmolar nonketotic coma appears to be the degree of insulinopenia, which is nearly absolute in ketoacidosis but with sufficient residual activity in hyperglycemic hyperosmolar nonketotic coma to limit lipolysis in adipose tissue but inadequate to permit normal peripheral glucose utilization at a time of increased glucose production induced by the stress hormones. As indicated, prerenal azotemia and decreased thirst contribute to this syndrome in adults and in children. Depression of consciousness is closely correlated with the degree of hyperosmolarity in this condition, as well as in diabetic ketoacidosis. Hemoconcentration may also predispose to cerebral arterial and venous thromboses.[142,148-150]

Treatment of nonketotic hyperosmolar coma is directed at repletion of the vascular volume deficit and correction of the hyperosmolar state (see "Diabetic Ketoacidosis" for management). Patients who are hypotensive should be started on isotonic saline (0.9% NaCl) until the condition is stable. Then, treatment should proceed as for DKA—extending the period of repair to 36 to 48 hours. Insulin may be infused as for DKA or at half the amount used in DKA (i.e., 0.05 U/kg/hour. When the blood glucose concentration approaches 300 mg/dL, the hydrating fluid should be changed to 5% dextrose in 0.2N saline. Approximately 20 mEq/L of potassium chloride, or more if indicated, should be added to each of these fluids to prevent hypokalemia. Serum potassium and plasma glucose concentrations should be monitored at 2-hour intervals for the first 12 hours and at 4-hour intervals for the next 24 hours to permit appropriate adjustments of administered potassium and insulin.[142,148-150]

Insulin can be given by continuous intravenous infusion, beginning with the second hour of fluid therapy. Because blood glucose may decrease dramatically with fluid therapy alone, the intravenous loading dose should be 0.05 U/kg of fast-acting insulin followed

TABLE 10-11

Fluid Electrolyte Therapy for Diabetic Ketoacidosis: Recommendations for Replacement of Fluid

Replacement Fluids	Approximate Accumulated Losses with 10% Dehydration	Approximate Requirements for Maintenance (36 Hr)	Approximate Totals for Replacement and Maintenance (36 Hr)
Water (mL)	3,000	2,250	5,500
Sodium (mEq)	180	65	250
Potassium (mEq)	150	50	200
Chloride (mEq)	120	45	165
Phosphate (mEq)	90	15	100

Replacement Schedule (Continuous Intravenous Infusion)

Approximate Duration	Fluid (Composition)	Sodium (mEq)	Potassium (mEq)	Chloride (mEq)	Phosophate (mEq)
Hour 1	500 mL of 0.9% NaCl (isotonic saline)	75	—	75	—
Hour 2p	500 mL of 0.45% NaCl (0.5 isotonic saline) plus 20 mEq of KCl	35	20	55	—
Hour 3–12 (200 mL/hr for 10 hr)	2,000 mL of 0.45% NaCl with 30 mEq/L of potassium phosphate	150	60	150	40
Subtotal initial 12 hr	3,000 mL	260	80	280	40
Next 24 hr 100 mL/hr	2,400 mL of 5% glucose in 0.2% NaCl with 40 mEq/L of potassium phosphate	75	100	75	60
Total over 36 hours	5,400 mL	335	180	355	100

Note: Maintenance requirements remain the same. Losses and for maintenance of a 30-kg (surface area, 1.0 m²) child with assumed 10% dehydration (duration of treatment, 36 hours). All replacement values should be halved if dehydration is estimated to be 5%.
Additional guidelines:
• A diabetic flowsheet with laboratory data appropriately recorded must be maintained in the patient's chart.
• Insulin therapy by continuous low-dose intravenous method: priming dose—bolus injection of 0.1 U/kg of regular insulin IV followed immediately by continuous IV infusion of 0.1 U/kg/hr of regular insulin beginning with second hour.
• Directions for making insulin infusion: Add 50 units of regular insulin to 500 mL of isotonic saline. Flush 50 mL through the tubing to saturate insulin-binding sites. For 30-kg patient, infuse at rate of 30 mL/hr. When the blood glucose concentration approaches 300 mg/dL, continue the insulin infusion at a reduced rate or add glucose to the infusate until acidosis is resolved and then start insulin therapy by subcutaneous injections of 0.2 to 0.4 U/kg of insulin at intervals of 6 hours.
• Bicarbonate therapy: For pH ≥ 7.10, no therapy is necessary. For pH 7.00 to 7.10, 40 mEq/m² of bicarbonate over 2 hours; then reevaluate. For pH ≤ 7.00, 80 mEq/m² of bicarbonate over 2 hours; then reevaluate. For new diabetics younger than 2 years of age with diabetic ketoacidosis and 10% dehydration or any diabetic with pH ≤7.00, coma or blood glucose ≥ 1,000 mg/dL should be managed in an intensive care unit or equivalent setting.

by 0.05 U/kg/hour of the same insulin—rather than 0.1 U/kg/hour as advocated for diabetic ketoacidosis. Some advocate that the initial insulin loading dose be omitted. During the recovery period, therapy with insulin and diet and monitoring of the patient are as described for patients recovering from diabetic ketoacidosis (Table 10-11).

TREATMENT OF DIABETES MELLITUS

The management of type 1 diabetes may be divided into three phases, depending on the initial presentation: ketoacidosis, the postacidotic transition period for establishment of metabolic control, and the continuing phase of guidance of the diabetic child and his or her family for daily living with diabetes integrating insulin regimens, nutritional intake, exercise, and glucose monitoring to achieve as near normal glucose control as is feasible. Each of these phases has separate goals, although in practice they merge into a continuum. For purposes of management, the transition period corresponds to presentations with polyuria, polydipsia, and weight loss but without biochemical decompensation to ketoacidosis.

Treatment of Diabetic Ketoacidosis

The pathophysiology and treatment of diabetic ketoacidosis was extensively reviewed and published as a consensus conference. The views and recommendations are endorsed by the Lawson Wilkins Pediatric Endocrine Society, the European Society for Pediatric Endocrinology, the International Society of Pediatric and Adolescent Diabetes, and others. Similar guidelines for management have now also been recommended by the American Diabetes Association.

The immediate aims of therapy are expansion of intravascular volume; correction of deficits in fluid, electrolyte, and acid-base status; initiation of insulin therapy to correct intermediary metabolism; and the exclusion of a treatable precipitating event such as infection or trauma. Treatment should be instituted as soon as the clinical diagnosis is confirmed by the presence of hyperglycemia and ketonemia. Determinations of blood pH and electrolytes should also be obtained. An electrocardiogram is useful to provide a rapid reference for the existence of hyperkalemia.

If sepsis is suspected as a possible precipitating factor, a blood culture should be obtained and the urine should be examined for the presence of bacteria and leukocytes. A flow sheet is essential to record chronologically the rate and composition of fluid input and urine output, the amount of insulin administered, and the acid-base and electrolyte values of the blood. Catheterization of the bladder is not routinely recommended in children. Bag collection or condom drainage permits an assessment of urinary output, but catheterization may be indicated in comatose patients.[141-154]

Fluid and Electrolyte Therapy. The expansion of reduced intravascular volume and correction of depleted fluid and electrolyte stores are important in the treatment of diabetic ketoacidosis (Tables 10-10 and 10-11). It must be stressed, however, that exogenous insulin is essential to arrest further metabolic decompensation and restore intermediary metabolism.[141-145,154] Dehydration is commonly approximately 10%. Initial fluid therapy can be based on this estimate, with subsequent adjustments to be related to clinical and laboratory data. The initial hydrating fluid should be isotonic saline (0.9%). Because of the hyperglycemia, hyperosmolarity is universal in diabetic ketoacidosis. Thus, even 0.9% saline is hypotonic relative to the patient's serum osmolality.

A gradual decline in osmolality is desirable because too rapid a decline has been implicated in the development of cerebral edema, one of the major complications of therapy in children. For the same reason, the rate of fluid replacement is adjusted to provide the total calculated deficit plus maintenance requirement over 48 hours after the initial rehydration with normal isotonic salinel. In addition, administration of glucose (5% solution in 0.2-0.5 N saline) is initiated when blood glucose concentration approaches 300 mg/dL to limit the decline of serum osmolality in an attempt to reduce the risk of developing cerebral edema (Table 10-11). Insulin should be continued until ketoacidosis is resolved and the pH is equal to or greater than 7.3 or the bicarbonate concentration in plasma equal to or greater than 18 mEq/L because blood glucose corrects more rapidly than ketoacidosis. As long as acidosis persists, insulin infusion should be maintained at the same rate (and, if necessary, with 5% to 10% glucose added to the infusate) to maintain blood glucose at approximately 300 mg/dL.

Cerebral Edema. Cerebral edema is an unusual but potentially devastating complication of diabetic ketoacidosis and its management in childhood. There is considerable debate and several hypotheses have been proposed, but there is presently no consensus as to the precise cause of this syndrome. It remains unproved whether cerebral edema during treatment of diabetic ketoacidosis can be predicted on the basis of clinical and biochemical indices and whether physicians contribute to it by their mode of management through the choice and composition of the hydrating fluid, its rate of administration, and the controlled rate of decline of blood glucose.[144,145,155-160]

The incidence of cerebral edema is reported to occur in 0.5% to 1.5% of all episodes of diabetic ketoacidosis. It is more common in younger children, especially at initial presentation.[144] Duration and severity of symptoms and signs before initiating treatment are the major identifiable factors.[144] If cerebral edema develops during treatment for diabetic ketoacidosis, mortality and morbidity are high. Although mortality has declined from previously reported rates of 40% to 90% to a more recently reported rate of 20%, cerebral edema remains the cause of about one-half of all deaths in children with diabetes mellitus. Morbidity from cerebral edema also remains high. About one-fourth of the survivors may have permanent neurologic sequelae.[144,145,160] Prompt recognition and intervention with mannitol or other hyperosmolar agents, respiratory support by means of endotracheal intubation, and hyperventilation may be lifesaving. Awareness, early recognition, and treatment are responsible for the reported decline in mortality cited previously.[141] Subclinical cerebral edema may be more common than hitherto appreciated.[146]

Randomized prospective trials of management of diabetic ketoacidosis are not ethically feasible, but in the most rigorous and extensive retrospective analysis involving some 6,000 episodes of diabetic ketoacidosis the following risk factors were identified: young age, duration and severity of symptoms before starting treatment, low PCO_2, high serum urea nitrogen, lack of an increase in serum sodium during therapy, and treatment with bicarbonate.[144,145] All of the biochemical risk factors in this study may reflect the initial severity of biochemical derangement. Thus, avoidance of diabetic ketoacidosis (especially in young children) by early recognition of the signs and symptoms of diabetes mellitus is the best way to prevent cerebral edema.

The duration and severity of symptoms before therapy may predispose to cerebral ischemia, to which younger children would be more prone because of the higher metabolic rate and hence higher oxygen requirement of a child's brain relative to an adult's. In addition, there may be a longer time to accumulate so-called idiogenic osmoles in the brain. Many children may have evidence of raised intracranial pressure on imaging studies (e.g., computed tomography), but only a minority develop clinical cerebral edema.[161]

Moreover, early studies in dogs and in adult men demonstrated that intracranial pressure rose in all during fluid replacement therapy for diabetic ketoacidosis.[162,163] Thus, given the hyperbolic pressure/volume relationship of the intracranial space and the likely shift of water into the intracellular compartment during therapy it is considered prudent to advocate the use of normal saline (or equivalent volume expanders) during initial therapy to limit the rate of infusion to no more than twice-daily maintenance requirement and not to exceed 4.0 L/m²/day, to carefully monitor the decline in blood glucose not to exceed about

Ketonemia and ketonuria may persist despite clinical improvement. The nitroprusside reaction routinely used to measure ketones reacts with acetoacetate and weakly with acetone but not with β-hydroxybutyrate. The usual ratio of β-hydroxybutyrate to acetoacetate is approximately 3:1, but is commonly 8:1 or more in diabetic ketoacidosis. With correction of acidosis, β-hydroxybutyrate dissociates to acetoacetate—which is identified by the nitroprusside reaction. Therefore, persistence of ketonuria for 1 or more days may not reliably reflect the clinical improvement and should not be interpreted as an index of poor therapeutic response.

Living with Diabetes

GENERAL PRINCIPLES

Optimal management of the child with diabetes requires an integrated approach, taking into account the overall level of functioning of the child and family, the nutritional and lifestyle patterns specific to that child, and attention to the overall developmental stages of childhood and adolescence. There is no one appropriate insulin regimen or meal plan. The overriding principle should be that the diabetes care plan should fit wherever possible into the surrounding home and school environments, and that the primary childhood tasks of education, socialization, growth, and maturity continue unhindered by the extra responsibilities diabetes care entails.

This potentially daunting task requires a multidisciplinary team, consisting of physicians, nurses, dietitians, and mental health professionals all trained and experienced in the nuances of diabetes care. Children with diabetes should be seen by the team at frequent intervals for assessment of glycemic control, growth and development; evaluation for related disorders and complications, education, troubleshooting, problem solving, and screening for adjustment problems that may affect diabetes and/or the overall health of the child.

GOALS OF THERAPY

As a result of the Diabetes Control and Complications Trial (DCCT) and its follow-up Epidemiology of Diabetes Interventions and Complications (EDIC) study,[168-170] current recommendations mandate that youth with T1DM should aim to achieve plasma glucose and HbA1c levels as close to normal as possible—as early in the course of the disease as possible and with as few severe hypoglycemic events as possible. A particular challenge in the care of children with T1DM is to make the treatment regimens that are employed to achieve these goals of treatment consistent with the general principles of care summarized previously.

Remarkably, a much greater proportion of young patients are able to meet these strict standards of care than imagined possible only a few years ago.[171] Moreover, recent data suggest that an intensive approach to diabetes education and aggressive self-management by patients and families may reduce rather than increase the adverse psychosocial effects of this chronic illness.[172]

TYPES OF INSULIN

Currently available insulins and their duration of action are listed in Table 10-13. They are classified as rapid-, short-, intermediate-, and long-acting and each is available in a concentration of 100 U/mL (U-100). Higher concentrations are available for the unusual patient who has high resistance to insulin. Appropriate dilutions can be prepared for younger patients requiring low doses. The development of recombinant DNA technology to synthesize human insulin and human insulin analogs has changed the face of insulin treatment over the past several years.

The traditional "short-acting" regular insulin has now been supplanted by new insulin analogs with more rapid time-action profiles.[173-176] Lispro (Eli Lilly), aspart (Novo Nordisk) and glulisine (Sanofi Aventis) insulins are produced by amino acid substitutions in the C-terminal region of the B-chain that reduce the affinity for insulin molecules to self-aggregate into hexamers. Consequently, these modifications allow more rapid absorption of the analog into the bloodstream after subcutaneous injection. The advantages of rapid-acting analogs in comparison to regular insulin include more rapid onset, sharper and higher peak concentrations, and shorter duration of action.[177] Thus, insulin is available immediately to cover meal-related glucose excursions and does not persistent as long after the complete absorption of the carbohydrates in the meal. Clinical trials of these analogs have demonstrated improvements in postprandial hyperglycemia and lower rates of hypoglycemia compared to regular insulin.[178] Regular human insulin has been relegated to use in the hospital for intravenous administration.

The pharmaceutical industry has terminated the manufacture of lente insulins, leaving NPH as the only remaining intermediate-acting insulin suspension. Although still employed in some "split-mix" regimens to avoid the need for insulin injections at lunch time or mid-afternoon, the dose-to-dose variability and peaking action of NPH make it less than satisfactory for basal insulin replacement—especially during the overnight period.[179]

TABLE 10-13

Pharmacodynamic Properties of Common Insulin Formulations

Category	Onset (Hr)	Peak (Hr)	Duration (Hr)
Rapid acting insulin lispro, aspart, and glulisine	0.25-0.5	0.5-1	3-5
Short-acting regular	0.5-1	2-4	4-8
Intermediate-acting NPH	2-4	4-10	12-18
Long-acting insulin glargine and detemir	2-4	n/a	18>24
Premixed			
Mix 25 (75% NPH/25% lispro)	0.25-0.5	1-2	12-18
Novolog mix (70% NPH/30% aspart) from living with diabetes	0.25-0.5	1-2	12-18

Glargine (Sanofi Aventis) insulin is a new analog of human insulin with C-terminal elongation of the β-chain by two arginine residues and replacement of asparagine in position A21 by glycine. This molecule is soluble in the acidic solution in which it is packaged but relatively insoluble in the physiologic pH of the extracellular fluid. Consequently, microprecipitates of glargine insulin are formed following subcutaneous injection, which markedly delays its absorption into the systemic circulation.

Pharmacokinetic and pharmacodynamic studies have demonstrated that the insulin analog has a very flat and prolonged time-action profile.[180] Results of preliminary studies of the efficacy and safety of glargine in children and adolescents with diabetes showed modestly lower fasting blood glucose levels and reduced risk of nocturnal hypoglycemia with glargine compared to human NPH insulin, although no differences in HbA1c were noted.[181,182] Because glargine cannot be mixed with other insulins, it has to be given by separate injection—which might affect its acceptability by some youngsters. Detemir (Novo Nordisk) insulin is the second soluble long-acting insulin approved by the FDA.

A prolonged and flat time-action profile was produced with this insulin analog by an amino acid deletion and fatty acid addition that result in extensive binding to albumin in the interstitium and circulation. Compared to glargine, detemir insulin appears to have less day-to-day variability in its pharmacodynamics effects[179] but may have a shorter duration of action.[183] Current experience with this insulin in pediatrics is limited. Because glargine and detemir are not approved for mixing with other insulins, they should be given by separate injection—which might affect their acceptability by some youngsters.

INSULIN REGIMENS

Plasma insulin levels in nondiabetic individuals are characterized by basal levels on which are superimposed meal-related spikes in insulin concentrations (Figure 10-10A). Current intensive treatment regimens attempt to simulate this diurnal pattern of plasma insulin by employing a basal-bolus approach to insulin replacement. Because exogenous insulins are injected or infused subcutaneously rather than directly into the portal vein, their rates of absorption may be variable—and because the dose injected is determined empirically it lacks the precision of endogenously secreted insulin. Therefore, it should be apparent that no insulin replacement regimen will precisely duplicate the pattern of normal insulin secretion—and there will be periods of excessive plasma insulin that may produce hypoglycemia and periods of inadequate insulin that permit hyperglycemia (Figure 10-10B).

Analog-Based Basal-Bolus Regimens

Perhaps the most physiologic approach to insulin replace involves the continuous infusion of rapid-acting insulin via an insulin pump. Originally introduced in the late 1970s,[184,185] this approach to basal bolus therapy only began to be used extensively in pediatrics over the past 7 to 8 years. The pumps are battery powered and about the size of a beeper. Most pumps employ a reservoir

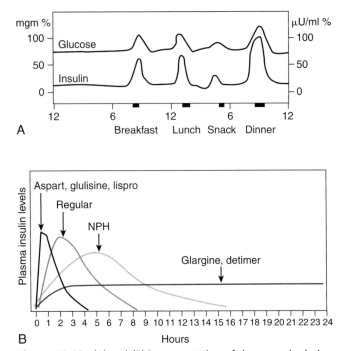

Figure 10-10. *(A)* and *(B)* Representation of the normal relationship between food intake, blood glucose, and serum insulin concentration. Note that glucose concentration is maintained between 80 and 140 mg/dl. Note also the precise release of insulin that has passed through the portal circulation synchronous with and proportional to the food-induced glycemic excursions. Compare and contrast these patterns with the time pattern of insulin action after subcutaneous injection of Aspart/glulisine/lispro, Regular, NPH and glargine/detimer insulins.

(modified syringe) to hold the insulin and the infusion set, which consists of tubing with a small plastic catheter at the end.

The insertion site can be the abdomen or hip area, except in the young child in whom there may not be sufficient subcutaneous tissue in the abdomen. Infusion site catheters should be changed every 2 to 3 days. Initially used with regular insulin, insulin pumps are most often used with the rapid-acting insulin analogs—which are associated with improved meal coverage and less hypoglycemia.[175] The newest "smart pumps" have advanced functions that include bolus dose calculators, record and summarize bolus and blood glucose history, and receive sensor inputs from continuous glucose monitoring systems.[186]

With insulin pump treatment, small amounts of rapid-acting insulin (down to 0.05-0.025 U increments) are infused as a basal rate—and bolus doses are given at each meal or snack.[187] The basal rate can be programmed to change every half hour. Varying the basal rate can be particularly helpful in regulating overnight blood glucose levels because it can be lowered for the early part of the night to prevent hypoglycemia and increased in the hours before dawn to keep glucose from rising. However, younger children may need a higher basal rate during the earlier part of the night—perhaps due to earlier nocturnal peaks of growth hormone in this age group.

Bolus doses are given before meals based on glucose level, carbohydrate content of the meal, and anticipated exercise after the meal. Pump therapy also enhances flexibility in children with variable exercise and meal routines, and temporary basal rates for the evening following vigorous physical activity is a simple means of preventing exercise-related nocturnal hypoglycemia. Most children and parents are encouraged to use carbohydrate counting as a means of adjusting pre-meal bolus doses.

When used correctly, insulin pump therapy has been shown to improve glycemic control in children, reduce severe hypoglycemia, and improve quality of life.[188,189] This is especially true for infants and toddlers, in whom we recently demonstrated durable improvements in HbA1c and risk of hypoglycemia for more than 2 years of treatment.[190] In this group, in whom unpredictable eating and activity patterns make multiple daily injection regimens problematic, part of the usual pre-meal bolus can be given prior to the meal and the rest given at the end of the meal—depending on the actual amount of carbohydrate intake. However, children using insulin pumps and their families must be reminded that because only rapid acting insulin is used in the pump discontinuation of the insulin infusion for more than 4 hours at a time may lead to significant ketoacidosis and preventable hospitalization.[191]

Basal bolus therapy can also be accomplished with multiple daily insulin injections. In this method, once- or twice-daily injections of glargine or detemir provide basal insulin coverage—and meal-related insulin requirements are covered with rapid-acting insulin bolus doses, which may easily be administered with an insulin pen. Multiple daily injection regimens with glargine in children have been associated with lower rates of nocturnal hypoglycemia compared to regimens with NPH.[181,182] Such regimens have become increasingly popular, but the inability to "fine-tune" basal insulin over the course of the day may be a problem.

In addition, the flat time-action profiles of glargine and detemir put a premium on compliance with pre-meal bolus dosing. Indeed, the difficulty of administering 4 to 5 insulin injections daily accounted for the recent finding that adolescents randomized to glargine-based basal-bolus therapy had higher HbA1c levels than those randomized to insulin pumps.[192] Even the added convenience of insulin pumps fails to prevent some adolescents from omitting many of their prescribed pre-meal bolus doses. However, the bolus history function allows clinicians and parents to easily identify such problems with compliance.[187]

NPH-Based Conventional Treatment Regimens

The "split-mixed" regimen consisting of two daily doses of NPH and regular insulin that were mixed together in the same syringe was a standard approach to insulin replacement in pediatrics for many years (Figure 10-11). More recently, the regular insulin component was replaced by rapid-acting insulin analogs. Patients started on this approach generally receive two-thirds of the total daily dose before breakfast and one-third before dinner.[193] Each injection starts with approximately two-thirds NPH and one-third rapid-acting analog. Individual components of the regimen are subsequently adjusted based on blood glucose testing results.

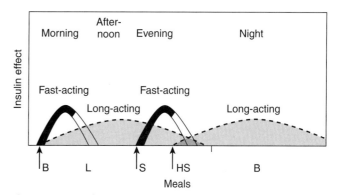

Figure 10-11. Three-dose insulin regimen. The morning dose is composed of a combination short- and intermediate-acting insulin of one-half to two-thirds of the total daily dose. The short-acting dose before supper covers the anticipated glycemic elevation with dinner. The long-acting insulin is not given until bedtime so that the peak effect is delayed. [Redrawn from Schade DS, et al. (1983). *Intensive insulin therapy.* Belle Mead, NJ: Excerptal Medica.]

Although this conventional treatment regimen is almost always inadequate for the patient with T1DM who has no residual endogenous insulin secretion, it may still play a role in the newly diagnosed patient—who frequently goes through a "honeymoon" or partial remission period of diabetes. During the "honeymoon" insulin requirements rapidly decrease and the doses of rapid-acting insulin may even be discontinued due to low pre-lunch and bedtime glucose levels. A major reason the two daily injections regimen is effective during the honeymoon period is that endogenous insulin secretion provides much of the overnight basal insulin requirements, leading to normal fasting blood glucose values. Conversely, increased and more labile pre-breakfast glucose levels often herald the loss of the relatively small amount of residual endogenous insulin secretion required for overnight glucose control.

When residual β-cell function wanes, problems with the two-injection regimen become apparent. One problem is that the peak of the pre-dinner intermediate-acting insulin may coincide with the time of minimal insulin requirements (i.e., midnight to 4:00 a.m.). Subsequently, insulin levels fall off when basal requirements may be increasing (i.e., 4:00 to 8:00 a.m.)—also known as the "dawn phenomenon."[194] Increasing the pre-dinner dose of intermediate-acting insulin to lower fasting glucose values often leads to hypoglycemia in the middle of the night without correcting hyperglycemia before breakfast. Another problem with the conventional two-injection regimen is high pre-dinner glucose levels despite normal or low pre-lunch and mid-afternoon values. This is due in part to eating an afternoon snack when the effects of the pre-breakfast dose of intermediate-acting insulin are waning.

One of the first true multiple daily injection regimens attempted to solve the problem of the dawn phenomenon by moving the pre-dinner NPH to bedtime. A current alternative to this method shown to be effective in children is to retain the pre-breakfast mixture of NPH and rapid-acting insulin, cover dinner with rapid-acting analog, and use glargine or detemir (given before supper or bedtime) for overnight basal replacement.[195] Indeed, some pediatric diabetologists have come full circle back to two shots a day by mixing the rapid and long-acting insulins together in the same syringe at dinner[196]—even though such mixing is not approved by the FDA.

Self-Monitoring of Blood Glucose

The safety and success of any insulin regimen is dependent on frequent monitoring of blood glucose. Intensive diabetes control would have been impossible without the development of inexpensive, accurate, easy-to-use home glucose meters. There are many brands of glucose meters commercially available, most of which are accurate to within about 5% to 10% of laboratory measurements.[197] Current models utilize glucose-oxidase-based electrochemical methods. The meters are fast (results in 5 seconds) and require very small volumes of blood (0.1 mL). The smaller blood volume requirement has allowed alternate site testing (forearm, thigh, calf), which may minimize discomfort and improve adherence to self-monitoring regimens. Alternate site testing has been associated with a time lag under conditions of rapidly changing blood glucose, and thus it should be used for routine testing before instead of after meals or exercise.[198]

Children with diabetes should routinely test the blood glucose four times daily (pre-meal and pre-bedtime) and record the results in a log (written or electronic) for later review by the family and diabetes care team. A target range is established, typically of 80 to 120 mg/dL before meals and <180 mg/dL 2 hours after meals. However, this may be altered based on the age of the child and the ability of the family. Ideally, 80% of the blood glucose values should fall within the target range—but this is rarely the case in current clinical practice. Information gained from frequent testing is used to titrate insulin dosages according to need. Because daily insulin requirements continually increase in growing children over time and may acutely change with the start of a new sports season, it is important that the families be taught to look for trends that indicate a need to alter insulin doses.

Due to the physiologic insulin resistance normally observed during puberty,[199] the adolescent growth spurt is regularly associated with a sharp increase in insulin requirements—which is usually lower when puberty is completed. Virtually all of the meters are equipped with memory functions that record and store the date and time and results of blood glucose test. Although these data are extremely useful with respect to checking the compliance with and accurate reporting of glucose testing, all too often the patient and parents fail to retrieve and review these data for trend analysis.

Dose-to-dose adjustments should also be made based on blood glucose measurements that are outside the target range. In particular, supplemental correction doses of rapid-acting insulin should be given when blood glucose values above the target range are discovered according to a predetermined formula. For example, a younger child with pre-meal blood glucose values outside the goal range may be given an extra 0.5 unit of rapid-acting insulin analog to reduce the blood glucose by 100 mg/dL (in addition to the usual insulin dose at that mealtime)—whereas an adolescent may use 2 to 3 units to "correct"

the glucose by 100 mg/dL.[200] Supplemental blood glucose testing should be performed after correction doses are given, before exercise, or during intercurrent illness.

Even when performed correctly, four (or even six) blood tests daily gives only a limited glimpse into the wide fluctuations in blood glucose that occur during a 24-hour period in children with diabetes. Consequently, the recent introduction of continuous glucose monitoring systems has the potential to be the most important advance in assessing diabetes control in the past 20 years. Nevertheless, the original devices were used for short-term retrospective analysis (the Medtronic MiniMed CGMS) or were too difficult and uncomfortable to use (the GlucoWatch Biographer).[201]

More recently, several new real-time continuous glucose monitoring (RT-CGM) systems have been introduced that have improved accuracy, functionality, and tolerability. Each of these devices employs a glucose-oxidase-based electrochemical probe inserted into the subcutaneous space. Glucose in the interstitial fluid is oxidized by the electrode, and the resultant electric signal is relayed to a monitor (which displays the glucose level). Current sensors require calibration against meter glucose values.[202]

In intensively treated children and adolescents with type 1 diabetes, preliminary results in a relatively small number of children suggest that continuous glucose monitoring will provide a wealth of data regarding postprandial glycemic excursions and asymptomatic nocturnal hypoglycemia that were unavailable from capillary blood glucose measurements.[203] A recent small outcome study in insulin pump-treated children demonstrated improvements in glycemic control and a high level of patient and parent satisfaction with the use of such a device.[204]

Because the error of current devices is considerably higher than conventional glucose meters,[197,205] frequent SMBG is still required for making treatment decisions. Nevertheless, it is likely that these technologic breakthroughs will have a great impact on diabetes management over the next few years as accuracy and performance of these systems improve. Continuous monitoring may be particularly useful in reducing postprandial hyperglycemia, reducing hypoglycemia (particularly at night), and programming overnight basal rates in pump-treated patients.[206]

Ultimately, continuous glucose sensors may be employed as part of a closed-loop system, in which sensor data drives an insulin pump—thus creating an artificial β cell. Urine tests still have a role in management of diabetes. However, these are now restricted to measurements of urine ketone levels when the child is ill, nauseous, or vomiting. Home meters for blood β-hydroxybutyrate levels are also available.[207]

Medical Nutrition Therapy

Proper nutritional management is critical to the short- and long-term health of children with diabetes. Generally, terms such as *diet* should be avoided in favor of *meal plan*—both for the negative connotation associated with the former and for the simple fact that nutritional requirements for normal growth and development are the same in diabetic and nondiabetic children. However, reasonably accurate estimations of the carbohydrate content of meals are important to optimal glycemic control. The increasing popularity of basal-bolus therapies and the use of carbohydrate counting to adjust the dose of rapid-acting insulin taken with each meal have fundamentally changed the treatment paradigm.

The traditional approach of adjusting the patient's lifestyle around fixed insulin doses and fixed amounts of carbohydrate intake with each meal has been replaced by a much more flexible approach that attempts to adjust the insulin regimen to the patient's lifestyle. The day-to-day variations in appetite in children and adolescents make the latter approach much more likely to be successful. It is important to note that in some patients and some families the traditional approach maybe more successful because it fits their personalities and lifestyle better.

The currently favored model of nutritional therapy is carbohydrate counting, based on the conceptual model of matching carbohydrate "doses" to insulin doses.[208,209] As the total carbohydrate content of foods (rather than the type of carbohydrate) has the greatest impact on blood glucose, the amount of carbohydrates ingested per meal or snack needs to be estimated as accurately as possible. Protein and fat intake, although important in the larger context of a healthy meal plan, are not counted (to simplify the procedure). Food labeling requirements have simplified the process, as most foods are clearly labeled with the amount of carbohydrate grams per serving and the serving size. Foods less easily quantified may be weighed or estimated, and eating out may be a particular problem. Although the prohibition of "sweets" has been done away with, we still recommend that patients drink diet rather than regular sodas.

In the flexible approach to nutrition counseling, there is no set intake. Rather, the child and parents decide the meal content. The carbohydrates are counted and an insulin dose is calculated based on a ratio of the number of insulin units per grams of carbohydrate determined by the empirical trial-and-error method. In younger children, a typical insulin-to-carbohydrate ratio is 1 unit to 20 to 30 g—whereas an older child may require 1:15 g, and an insulin-resistant adolescent 1:5-10g. Actual insulin-carbohydrate ratios vary from child to child and even in the same child from meal to meal. Breakfast often requires relatively more insulin than lunch or dinner. Carbohydrate counting can also be used in the traditional approach to dietary treatment to provide consistent carbohydrate servings per meal/snack. Indeed, a very simple approach that stresses consistency in the timing and size of meals may be very effective at the time of diagnosis of diabetes—when parents and patients are too overwhelmed to be able to learn more advanced nutritional concepts.

The American Diabetes Association's recommendations regarding general nutritional principles in diabetes also take into consideration the long-term goal of prevention of macrovascular and microvascular complications of diabetes.[210] Consequently, heart-healthy diets low in cholesterol and saturated fats are encouraged. Long-term goals of nutritional management of diabetes include maintenance of nutrient intake balance of about 50% carbohydrate, 20% protein, and 30% fat (of which no more than 10% should be saturated). Most importantly, growth and weight gain should be monitored—and regular follow-up with a dietitian trained in diabetes management should be encouraged to individualize a meal plan for each child based on his/her needs and food preferences. We face an epidemic of childhood obesity in developed countries, and one of the adverse consequences of intensive insulin treatment in the DCCT was a twofold increase in the risk of becoming overweight. Thus, any tendency for BMI Z scores to increase excessively needs to be dealt with promptly.

Exercise

Establishment and maintenance of an active lifestyle should be a goal for all children, but are especially important for children with diabetes. Exercise and increased physical fitness are associated with improved insulin sensitivity and glucose utilization, the clinical correlates of which are lower insulin requirements in general and frequently less pronounced blood glucose excursions after meals. Improvements in physical fitness are also frequently associated with greater self-esteem and motivation to participate in diabetes care.

Despite its benefits, acute bouts of exercise in children with T1DM actually make regulation of blood glucose levels more difficult. Hypoglycemia is a common complication during exercise, and excessive snacking to prevent hypoglycemia can result in hyperglycemia and negate some of the metabolic and cardiovascular benefits of exercise. These difficulties are compounded by the irregular pattern of physical activity that characterizes most youth (who are not participating in organized sports or regimented training programs) and by conventional methods of diabetes management that feature fixed basal insulin replacement doses. Moreover, antecedent exercise may reduce the counterregulatory hormone responses to subsequent hypoglycemia.[211]

The effects of exercise must be carefully considered in the context of the entire diabetes care plan. Children participating in school sports or other programs should be counseled to monitor blood glucose before, during, and after exercise because the hypoglycemic effects of exercise may be delayed for 7 to 11 hours—markedly increasing the risk of nocturnal hypoglycemia.[212] The delayed fall in glucose levels on nights following exercise appears to be due to an increase in nonoxidative glucose disposal during sleep, which may serve to support repletion of muscle glycogen stores.[213]

In pump patients, simply suspending the basal infusion rate can markedly reduce the risk of hypoglycemia during exercise—and similar benefits may accrue from reducing the overnight basal rates after very active days. Recent studies that have examined methods of managing glycemia during exercise illustrate that there is an almost infinite number of combinations of conditions that need to be considered.[214] Because of this complexity, trial and error remains the principal method of managing glucose levels during and after exercise in children and adolescents with T1DM.

TABLE 10-14

Levels of Treatment: Biochemical and Clinical Characteristics

Minimal
- HbA1c 11.0%-13.0%, GHb 13.0%-15.0%
- Many SMBG values of 300 mg/dL
- Almost constantly positive urine glucose tests
- Intermittent spontaneous ketonuria

Average
- HbA1c 8.0%-9.0%, GHb 10.0%-11.0%
- Premeal SMBG 160-200 mg/dL
- Intermittent positive urine glucose
- Rare ketonuria

Intensive
- HbA1c 6.0%-7.0%, GHb 7.0%-9.0%
- Premeal SMBG 70-120 mg/dL; post-meal SMBG,180 mg/dL
- Essentially no positive urine glucose or ketones

GHb, glycosylated hemoglobin; HbA1c, glycohemoglobin; and SMBG, self-monitored blood glucose.

Residual β-Cell Function (The Honeymoon Period)

After the initiation of insulin treatment in newly diagnosed patients, secretory function of residual β-cells improves and the insulin resistance and glucotoxicity of decompensated diabetes are reversed in most newly diagnosed diabetic children—heralding the onset of the partial remission (honeymoon period) of T1DM. Patients require a progressive reduction in their daily dose of insulin from >1.0 to <0.5 U/kg. Recurrent hypoglycemia is the manifestation that prompts a reduction in the insulin dose. A minority of children (fewer than 5% of patients) can even maintain normoglycemia for a time without any administered insulin. Although opinion varies, we do not discontinue insulin treatment unless a daily dose of 0.1 U/kg still causes hypoglycemia.

The duration of this honeymoon phase is variable. It commonly lasts several months, but may last as long as 1 to 2 years. Residual insulin secretion, measured as C-peptide, is present during this remission period and to some extent in virtually all diabetic children in the initial year of their disease. In less than 20% there will be some measurable C-peptide even up to 3 years.[215] In comparison to patients who are C-peptide negative, patients with residual b-cell function have lower HbA1c levels and total daily insulin doses—as well as a reduced risk of hypoglycemia.[216] These clinical and metabolic benefits serve as a strong rationale for current research involving immune interventions directed at preserving b-cell function in newly diagnosed patients.[217] The levels of treatment intensity with anticipated glucose and HbA1c values are shown in Table 10-14.

HYPOGLYCEMIA

The dark side of intensive treatment regimens effective in lowering HbA1c levels is that they also increase the risk of hypoglycemia. In the DCCT, intensive therapy was associated with an approximate threefold increased risk for severe hypoglycemia versus conventional treatment—and irrespective of treatment group the rate of severe hypoglycemia was >50% higher for adolescents than for adults.[168,169] Hypoglycemia has become the most significant barrier to the pursuit and maintenance of tight glycemic control among people with DM, and effectively managing the risk for hypoglycemia is especially important in the treatment of children and adolescents with this disease.

Biochemical hypoglycemia (with or without symptoms) is defined by the American Diabetes Association as any plasma glucose level ≤70 mg/dL.[218] In nondiabetic adults, this is the plasma glucose level at which counterregulatory hormone responses engage and at which awareness of symptoms normally occurs. It should be noted, however, that such responses may be triggered at higher glucose levels in healthy 8- to 16-year-olds and in children and adolescents with T1DM who have poor glycemic control.[219] Differentiation of hypoglycemic events, based on symptoms and treatment characteristics, is important clinically.

The two main mechanisms that cause symptoms and signs are an outpouring of catecholamines (which results in pallor, sweating, apprehension, trembling, and tachycardia) and the effects of cerebral glucopenia, which include hunger, drowsiness, mental confusion, seizures, and coma. Mood and personality changes plus some abnormal physical patterns may be other more subtle cerebral glucopenic effects that provide an early clue that plasma glucose has fallen to a dangerous level. Symptomatic episodes in which patients are able to treat themselves without the assistance of others are considered minor or mild hypoglycaemia, whereas episodes in which there is sufficient cognitive impairment that treatment requires the assistance of another person are considered major or severe hypoglycemic events. In severe hypoglycemia, ingestion of carbohydrates may be precluded due to loss of consciousness, seizures, or coma—and treatment may require administration of glucagon injection or IV glucose infusion.

In nondiabetic children, the initial response to falling plasma glucose levels is a prompt suppression of insulin secretion. If plasma glucose continues to fall and threshold values for release of anti-insulin counterregulatory hormones are reached, there are abrupt increases in circulating concentrations of glucagon and epinephrine. Plasma growth hormone and cortisol levels also increase, but these hormones are less important in acutely counteracting the effects of insulin. Defective counterregulation occurs in patients with T1DM because exogenously supplied insulin levels do not decrease in response to low blood glucose levels and the ability to secrete glucagon in response to hypoglycemia is lost early in the course of the disease.[220,221] Consequently, patients with T1DM depend on sympathetic nervous system responses—especially increases in plasma epinephrine levels—to prevent hypoglycemia.

Nevertheless, it has been demonstrated that the repeated episodes of mild hypoglycemia that frequently accompany intensive treatment blunt catecholamine responses and symptom awareness to subsequent hypoglycemic challenges. This phenomenon has been called hypoglycemia-associated autonomic failure (HAAF)[221,222]—a major contributing factor to the risk of hypoglycemia in patients whose DM is well controlled. Catecholamine responses to hypoglycemia are also impaired during sleep, which is an important reason most of the severe hypoglycemia events occur during the night.[223] Children and adolescents are also prone to erratic eating behaviors and patterns of bolus dosing. Bouts of exercise in the afternoon sharply increase the risk of hypoglycemia on the following night.[212]

The use of basal-bolus therapy with insulin analogs has reduced frequency of severe hypoglycemia somewhat but has by no means eliminated this problem. It is important that the patient and family recognize early symptoms and signs of hypoglycemia and known precipitating factors. Mild episodes should be immediately treated with 10 to 15 g of carbohydrate (e.g., glucose tablets, juice, or glucose gel). Parents and school nurses also need to be instructed on how to perform injections of glucagon (0.5 to 1.0 mg) when the patient is losing consciousness and unable to swallow exogenous carbohydrate. If exercise has been the precipitating factor, the patient should be instructed about preventive measures.

To avoid more severe events, insulin doses need to be adjusted if there are repetitive patterns of mild hypoglycemia. Physicians caring for patients with type 1 diabetes should be aware of a syndrome of cerebral glucopenia with hypoglycemic encephalopathy. In these patients, prolonged severe hypoglycemia that is not recognized or treated may result in seizures and a coma that lasts for hours despite correction of blood glucose concentration. Such patients are often combative and use profane language. Several hours of glucose therapy may be necessary for recovery in such patients.

SICK DAY MANAGEMENT

Children with intercurrent illnesses, such as infections or vomiting, should be closely monitored for elevations in blood glucose levels and ketonuria. On sick days, blood glucose levels should be checked every 2 hours—and the urine should be checked for ketones with every void. Supplemental doses of rapid-acting insulin (0.1 to 0.3 U per kilogram) should be given every 2 to 4 hours for elevations in glucose and/or ketones. Even in the absence of marked hyperglycemia, the presence of ketones indicates insulin deficiency and therefore the need for supplemental insulin.

Adequate fluid intake is essential to prevent dehydration and hasten the excretion of ketones. Fluids such as flat soda, clear soups, popsicles, and gelatin water are recommended to provide some electrolyte and carbohydrate replacement. In the child tolerating oral rehydration, a fluid "dose" of 1 ounce per year of age per hour serves as a rough guideline—the sugar content of which depends on the serum glucose. For blood glucose values >200 mg/dL, sugar-free fluids should be given. For those levels between 140 and 200 mg/dL, a mixture of sugar-free and sugar-containing fluids should be given. For blood sugar <140 mg/dL, only sugar-containing fluids should be given.

If emesis precludes normal oral intake, the intermediate or long-acting insulin should be discontinued and small frequent doses of short- or rapid-acting insulin should be given. Once the ketones have cleared and the child is tolerating an oral diet, the family may resume the normal routine. If vomiting is persistent and ketones remain moderate or large after several supplemental insulin doses, arrangements should be made for potential hydration and evaluation in the emergency department.

ASSOCIATED AUTOIMMUNE DISEASES

Various autoimmune diseases are frequently associated in patients with type 1 diabetes mellitus. These are detailed in Chapter 18 (Heller-Schatz), in the discussion of multiple endocrine deficiency syndromes. Chronic lymphocytic thyroiditis is frequently associated with type 1 diabetes in children, and as many as one in five may have thyroid antibodies in their serum.[224] Only a small proportion of these patients develop clinical hypothyroidism, however. The interval between the diagnosis of diabetes and that of thyroid disease averages about 5 years. Physicians should anticipate the possibility of hypothyroidism in patients with type 1 diabetes mellitus by periodic examination of the thyroid gland and measurement of serum thyroid-stimulating hormone (TSH) concentration.

When diabetes and thyroid disease coexist, the possibility of adrenal insufficiency should be considered. This may be heralded by decreased insulin requirements, increased pigmentation of the skin and buccal mucosa, salt craving, weakness, and postural hypotension. Rarely, frank Addisonian crisis is the first evidence of adrenal failure. This syndrome generally occurs in the second decade of life or later.

Celiac disease affects from 1.5% to 4.5% of children with T1DM and most of them are not aware of any gastrointestinal symptoms.[225] Early diagnosis requires screening of tissue transglutaminase antibodies, which have high degrees of reproducibility, specificity, and sensitivity if total circulating IgA concentrations are not abnormally low. Antibody-positive children should be referred to a pediatric gastroenterologist for confirmation by small bowel biopsy, as well as for counseling and disease management.

When typical signs and symptoms of malabsorption are present or the patient has frequent hypoglycemia or unexplained behavioral mood swings, dietary intervention is indicated. When symptoms are minimal or absent, the decision to introduce gluten-free diets with their additional restrictive and inconvenient burdens on the patient and family are less clear-cut. To guide their decision, the parents and older children need to be made aware of the risk of bowel malignancies in untreated celiac disease in later life and of other long-term complications of this disease.

ASSOCIATED PSYCHOSOCIAL PROBLEMS

Diabetes in a child affects the lifestyle and interpersonal relationships of the entire family. Guidelines for psychosocial management and support of families with childhood diabetes have recently been published.[226] Feelings of anxiety and guilt are common in parents. Similar feelings, coupled with denial and rejection, are equally common in children—particularly during the rebellious teenage years. These issues are not unique to T1DM but are observed in families with children who have other chronic disorders difficult to treat. Such stresses are often exaggerated in single-parent low-income families and impair their ability to effectively carry out needed self-management tasks, resulting in poor metabolic control.[171]

Language and cultural barriers are additional obstacles in immigrant families. Psychosocial difficulties and conflict between patients and parents may result in nonadherence to instructions regarding nutritional and insulin therapy and in noncompliance with self-monitoring.[227] Deliberate over dosage with insulin resulting in hypoglycemia or omission of insulin, often in association with excesses in nutritional intake resulting in ketoacidosis, may be pleas for psychological help or manipulative events to escape an environment perceived as undesirable or intolerable. Occasionally, they may be manifestations of suicidal intent. Frequent admissions to the hospital for ketoacidosis or hypoglycemia should arouse suspicion of underlying emotional conflict. Overprotection on the part of parents is common and is often not in the best interest of the patient. Feelings of being different and/or of being alone are common and may be justified in view of the restrictive schedules imposed by testing of urine and blood, administration of insulin, and nutritional limitations.

The physician managing a child or adolescent with diabetes should be aware of his or her pivotal role as counselor and advisor and should anticipate the common emotional problems of the patient. When emotional problems are clearly responsible for poor compliance with the medical regimen, referral for psychological help is indicated. In pediatric centers, psychologists form part of the management team for children with diabetes.

OUTPATIENT CARE

The importance of frequent follow-up by the diabetes health care team cannot be overemphasized. Children and adolescents with T1DM should be routinely cared for by a diabetes center that uses a multidisciplinary team knowledgeable about and experienced in the management of young patients. This team should ideally consist of pediatric diabetologists, diabetes nurse specialists, nutritionists, and social workers or psychologists.

The American Diabetes Association has recently published guidelines for care of the child and adolescent with diabetes.[228] Regular follow-up visits with the physician or diabetes nurse specialist/practitioner every 2 to 3 months are recommended for most patients. The main purpose of these visits is to ensure that the patient is achieving primary treatment goals. Routine outpatient visits provide an opportunity to review glucose monitoring, to adjust the treatment regimen, and to assess child and family adjustment. At each visit, the blood glucose records should be reviewed and appropriate dosage or schedule changes should be instituted as needed. Follow-up advice and support are given by the nutritionist and psychologist or social worker.

A detailed interim history should include questions relating to general health, energy, fatigue, polyuria or nocturia, intercurrent illnesses, hypoglycemic episodes, and the presence of symptoms such as abdominal pain, bloating, or diarrhea. It is important to remember the

comorbidities of other autoimmune disorders that occur with an increased frequency in children with T1DM: thyroiditis, adrenal insufficiency, and celiac disease. The child should be weighed and measured at each visit, and blood pressure documented. Physical examination of the child should focus not only on the general organ systems but on examination of the skin and insulin injection/pump insertion sites for signs of lipohypertrophy or pigmentary changes, palpation of the thyroid, and determination of the sexual development stage.

Lipoatrophy was commonly observed in the past but is now a rare complication of insulin therapy.[229] A deceleration in growth, delay in sexual development, or finding of goiter may herald hypothyroidism—which occurs in approximately 5% of children with T1DM. The astute clinician should also consider that frequent unexplained hypoglycemia or reduction in insulin requirements in the absence of exercise or activity may be a subtle indicator of hypothyroidism or adrenal insufficiency. Similarly, although the history of frequent foul-smelling greasy stools are more obvious indicators of celiac disease (which occurs in about 2% to 5% of children with T1DM), the presence of abdominal pain, poor weight gain, and unexplained hypoglycemia may be the first and only signs. Indeed, many patients are asymptomatic and are diagnosed by screening for celiac-related autoantibodies.

There are currently no formal recommendations for screening for thyroid/adrenal autoimmunity and celiac disease for pediatric patients with T1DM. However, because the prevalence of thyroid autoantibodies in children with diabetes may be as high as 21% (and of celiac disease in children with T1DM about 4%), we routinely screen with T4, TSH, and tissue tranglutaminase IgA every 1 to 2 years.

Measurement of glycosylated hemoglobin (HbA_{1c}) provides the gold standard by which to judge the adequacy of the insulin regimen. A variety of methods are available for assaying glycosylated hemoglobin. A simple point-of-service method that can be performed in the office in 6 minutes (i.e., DCA 2000 instrument) offers the opportunity to make immediate changes in the insulin regimen while the patient is being seen.[230] Even more important, the results of this test delivered during face-to-face encounters with the clinician serve as the quarterly "report cards" for the child and the parents.

Teenagers may not be able to identify with the concept of working hard on their diabetes to be healthier many years in the future, but most are able to understand good grades. Thus, the HbA1c level provides a tangible outcome with which they can identify. The goal of treatment is to achieve HbA_{1c} levels as close to normal as possible. Based on DCCT results, our general goal of therapy is to try to keep all patients under 7.5%. HbA_{1c} levels are determined at least every 3 months.

Monitoring of the diabetic child for potential complications is an important function of the clinic visit. Urinary albumin excretion may be measured in a spot sample by comparison to urinary creatinine. Urinary albumin/creatinine ratio should be <30 mg albumin to gm creatinine. Elevated spot samples should be confirmed by collections of first morning void or a timed overnight period to eliminate the confounding variable of benign orthostatic proteinuria. If the first morning void or timed overnight collection demonstrates microalbuminuria (>30 mg albumin to gm creatinine or >30 mg albumin excretion per 24 hours), treatment with angiotensin-converting enzyme inhibitor or angiotensin receptor blocker therapy or referral to pediatric nephrologist may be indicated. All diabetic children with hypertension, regardless of albumin excretion status, should be considered candidates for these medications. Although there are no specific guidelines for diabetic children,[231] current recommendations for nondiabetic children are that blood pressures above the 90th percentile for age warrant lifestyle intervention and those about the 95th merit the use of pharmacologic agents.

Other screening studies for complications of diabetes include measurement of serum lipid concentrations. The current standards of care for adults with diabetes indicate that low-density lipoprotein (LDL) concentrations should be maintained below 100 mg/dL, whereas pharmacologic therapy for dyslipidemia in children with diabetes is not recommended unless dietary interventions fail to lower LDL concentrations below 130 mg/dL. The American Diabetes Association recommends that annual dilated retinal examinations be obtained in patients who are over 10 years or age and have had T1DM for 3 or more years. On the other hand, a recent study from our clinic population indicated that the yield from such examinations is very low in children and adolescents who have normal blood pressure and HbA1c levels that meet current targets and who are without microalbuminuria.[232]

MANAGEMENT DURING SURGERY

Management objectives during surgery are the prevention of hypoglycemia, excessive loss of fluids, and ketosis during anesthesia. The regimens described here are generally applicable, but vigilance and individual adjustments for each patient are necessary to achieve these goals. Evidence-based controlled studies of perioperative care have not been carried out in children, but detailed expert reviews of management have recently been published in the anesthesia and pediatric diabetes literature.[233,234]

The most reliable and straightforward approach to achieving management objectives during major elective or emergency surgeries is to use intravenous infusions of glucose and insulin during the perioperative period. For surgical emergencies that can be briefly delayed, such as acute appendicitis, rehydration and metabolic balance should be restored before the operation. Elective major operations should be performed first thing in the morning, and the glucose and insulin infusions should be started ~2 hours prior to proceeding to the operating room. For elective surgeries, an infusion of 5% glucose in 0.45% or 0.9% saline solution is begun on the morning of surgery—and 1 unit of regular insulin is infused intravenously for each 4 to 6 g of administered glucose. One unit of regular insulin for every 2 to 4 g of exogenous glucose may be required in surgical emergencies due to elevated circulating concentrations of stress hormones or in insulin-resistant obese diabetic patients.

The rate of infusion should provide maintenance fluid requirements plus estimated losses during surgery. The blood glucose concentration should be monitored at periodic intervals before, during, and after surgery. Concentrations of 120 to 150 mg/dL should be the goal. This can be achieved by varying the rate of infusion of the glucose and electrolyte mixture or the rate of insulin administration. The intravenous insulin and glucose infusions can be continued until the patient is awake and capable of taking regular meals, at which time their usual injection or insulin pump regimen can be reinstituted. Most centers do not routinely add potassium to the intravenous fluids until after completion of the surgical procedure.

In patients who receive NHP insulin in the morning and are undergoing surgery of short duration, a standard and effective approach is as follows: on the morning of surgery, one-half of the usual morning dose of NPH insulin is administered subcutaneously, the usual dose of rapid-acting insulin is omitted unless needed to correct hyperglycemia, and a maintenance intravenous infusion of the electrolyte and glucose solution is initiated if needed. Similarly, in patients on insulin pump therapy who are undergoing short procedures the continuous subcutaneous infusion of insulin (CSII) can be continued at the usual or slightly reduced overnight basal rate. Insulin pump-treated patients can also be maintained on CSII for major procedures as long as the integrity of the infusion and infusion site is ensured.

The nighttime dose of glargine or detemir insulin may provide sufficient basal insulin coverage for surgery in patients who receive these long-acting insulins before dinner or bedtime. A reduction in the glargine or detemir dose by 20% to 30% on the night prior to surgery should be considered in patients who have had a tendency to low pre-breakfast plasma glucose levels. With all three regimens, a correction dose of rapid-acting insulin can be given subcutaneously immediately after the procedure if needed for hyperglycemia—and repeated as needed to balance initial oral intake (e.g., carbohydrate-containing clear liquids). When the intravenous infusion is discontinued and the patient is ready to resume regular meals, the usual treatment regimen is reinstituted.

Nonautoimmune Type 1 Diabetes

Not all forms of apparently classic type 1 diabetes mellitus have associated markers of autoimmunity.[235] In one report, among children presenting with newly diagnosed diabetes mellitus fewer of those younger than 5 years of age at diagnosis had positive titers of islet cell and GAD antibodies—and fewer had a honeymoon phase within 6 months—compared with a group with onset at a mean age of 10 years.[51] Similarly, Japanese investigators have reported that some patients with idiopathic type 1 diabetes mellitus have a nonautoimmune fulminant disorder with abrupt onset characterized by absence of circulating antibodies, evidence of insulinitis in pancreatic biopsies, and high concentrations of pancreatic enzymes—suggesting an acute inflammatory process in the pancreas.[52]

MODY syndromes, as discussed in material following, may also be initially considered to be T1DM.[236] However, the strong family history of vertically transmitted DM in three generations, the relatively milder degree of hyperglycemia, and the absence of autoimmune markers should alert the physician to the possibility of a monogenic form of DM.

Type 2 Diabetes Mellitus

TYPICAL

Type 2 diabetes mellitus, formerly known as NIDDM, is a heterogeneous disorder characterized by defective insulin secretion that progressively fails to compensate for insulin resistance.[235] The cause of insulin resistance is usually obesity,[237-242] although agents such as growth hormone and cortisol also antagonize insulin action and may unmask inadequately compensated insulin secretion. The high concentrations of placental growth hormones during mid to late gestation likewise may unmask inadequate insulin secretion, resulting in gestational diabetes—a harbinger of permanent diabetes later in life.

The mechanism of insulin resistance caused by obesity may in part relate to changes in fatty acid metabolism that interfere with normal glucose metabolism, and in part to factors synthesized within fat cells that antagonize insulin action.[35,37,242] Most notable are the recently described hormones adiponectin, leptin, and resistin,[243] which are produced by fat cells and are a likely major link between obesity and diabetes. Thus, in addition to the genetic component(s) responsible for impaired insulin secretion (which are being investigated, progressively identified, and presently cannot be changed[244-247]) the key modifiable factor responsible for the epidemic of type 2 diabetes in children is the epidemic of obesity increasingly recognized throughout the world.[237-242]

Type 2 diabetes mellitus is being recognized in children, particularly obese adolescents and especially but not exclusively in certain ethnic groups such as Native American Indians, African Americans, Mexican Americans, and Southeast Asians in the developing world.[237-242] Here, too, an epidemic of obesity is responsible for a rapid increase in the proportion of patients with type 2 diabetes—representing up to one-third of newly presenting cases in one major medical center in the United States.[248] These patients often have a family history of type 2 diabetes, may have acanthosis nigricans, are more commonly girls, and often have poor metabolic control that predisposes them to the earlier appearance of microvascular and macrovascular complications.[248] They may present initially in diabetic ketoacidosis suggesting type 1 diabetes, but after recovery they may manifest a prolonged "honeymoon phase"—the so-called atypical diabetes mellitus (ADM), or type 2 diabetes, as documented by significant insulin or C-peptide levels not consistent with type 1 diabetes. They also lack markers of islet autoimmunity and the classic HLA associations.[238]

In those with a family history of type 2 diabetes mellitus, insulin resistance (as shown by impaired insulin-stimulated glucose disposal and higher insulin values during oral glucose tolerance or so-called hyperglycemic clamps) is demonstrable in the first decade of life before clinically demonstrable changes in glucose tolerance.[237-244] The site(s) of this presumably genetic impairment in insulin sensitivity is not yet identified but clearly precedes clinical diabetes mellitus brought about by obesity-induced insulin resistance.[237-244] There may be other factors that induce insulin resistance.

There also are an emerging number of newly identified genetic factors associated with impaired insulin secretion and action. Genome-wide scans have consistently identified three major genetic linkages: the ATP-regulated potassium channel KATP, especially the Kir 6.2 subunit encoded by the KCNJ11 gene; the peroxisome proliferator activator receptor γ (PPARG); and transcription factor 7 like 2 (TCF7L2). The development of sophisticated arrays that permit genotyping of literally hundreds of thousands of polymorpisms has revealed additional loci of genetic markers in T2DM, including a polymorphism in the zinc transporter SLC30A8 (expressed only on pancreatic β cells) and genes potentially involved in pancreatic development (IDE, KIF11, HHEX) or function (EXT2-ALX4).[244-247,250-252]

These sophisticated genetic screening approaches are likely to identify more of the complex genetic traits that underlie T2DM. From a practical point of view, type 2 diabetes mellitus in children and adolescents should be viewed as a major public health issue—and without effective lifestyle interventions (such as weight reduction combined with regular exercise) treatment options are limited and only modestly successful.[237,238] Exogenous insulin may be necessary to control blood glucose initially, but its appetite-stimulating effects challenge attempts at weight reduction. Sulfonylureas may be temporarily helpful, as may meglitinide—which acutely increase insulin secretion.

Metformin, which sensitizes tissue to insulin action and diminishes hepatic glucose production, is the most frequently used agent for treating type 2 diabetes in children. It has been approved for use by the U.S. Food and Drug Administration for those over 10 years of age. The thiozolidinediones (glitazones) that sensitize tissue to insulin are not approved for use in children by the U.S. Food and Drug Administration but nevertheless have reportedly been used.[237,238] These agents are potentially hepatotoxic, and the original product was withdrawn for this reason. Newer glitazones (such as Rosiglitazone) are under investigation in adolescents with T2DM, although Rosiglitazone itself is under scrutiny for potential harmful effects on cardiac function.[253] Alpha-glucosidase inhibitors that slow carbohydrate absorption and lipase inhibitors to diminish fat absorption are available, but none has undergone clinical trials in children/adolescents for efficacy and compliance. This represents a major deficiency in our ability to treat type 2 diabetes mellitus in children.[237]

GENETIC DEFECTS OF BETA CELL FUNCTION

MODY Syndromes

Although MODY was originally conceptualized as a form of maturity-onset (i.e., type 2) diabetes, the MODY syndromes are best considered a group of disorders of monogenic defect in beta cell function. Affected patients may have modest elevation of glucose, may remain asymptomatic for many years, and may become clinically apparent during intercurrent illness or pregnancy that unmasks the limited insulin secretion.[13] Clinical criteria used to establish the diagnosis include the following.

- Dominant inheritance with at least two (and preferably three) consecutive affected generations
- Onset before age 25 to 30 years
- Evidence of significant but impaired residual insulin secretion reflected in C-peptide levels whether or not the patient is being treated with insulin

As of this time, six specific genetic defects have been identified. (see Table 10-15) Of these genetic defects that together account for no more than 2 to 5% of type 2 diabetes, about two-thirds (65%) are MODY 3 (HNF1α), 10% are MODY 2 (glucokinase defect), and the remainder constitute the other defects. Mild stable hyperglycemia may be present from birth and not require treatment except during stress, such as infections in an infant or child or pregnancy in a young adult.

With glucokinase deficiency, microvascular complications of diabetes are rare. In the other forms of MODY, however, onset is usually in the early teens to 20s, glucose intolerance may become progressively worse and hence require treatment, and microvascular complications may develop. Renal cysts or other reno-pelvic anomalies may occur in MODY 5 (HNF1βb). Notably, if the genetic defect in IPF1 (insulin promoter factor-1, MODY 4) is homozygous pancreatic agenesis results and this is a cause for permanent neonatal diabetes associated with exocrine as well as endocrine insufficiency. Likewise, homozygous mutations in glucokinase have been associated with congenital diabetes. By contrast, gain-of-function mutations in glucokinase cause persistent hyperinsulinemic hypoglycemia of infancy (see Chapter 5). Thus, the MODY syndromes are monogenic defects of islet cell formation (MODY 4) or of transcription factors (MODY 1, 3, 5, and 6)—or a defect in the functional glucose sensor glucokinase (MODY 2).[13,236,254]

Table 10-16 compares and contrasts the four most common types of diabetes found in adolescents: type 1, type 2, atypical diabetes mellitus, and MODY. The monogenic MODY syndromes have been extensively reviewed

in terms of chemical, biochemical, and molecular analyses.[13,254] Other monogenic defects reportedly associated with a type 2 clinical picture include mutation in GLUT2 and the glycogen synthase genes.[255,256]

Other Forms of Monogenic Diabetes

Mitochondrial Diabetes. Mitochondrial genetic defects that cause diabetes are commonly but not invariably associated with neuromuscular disorders, including deafness, migraine, seizures, and mental retardation. For example, the MELAS (mitochondrial encephalopathy, lactic acidosis, and stroke-like episodes) syndrome may initially present in childhood with short stature, go on to deafness in teen years, and develop diabetes and encephalopathy in midlife. Diabetes mellitus maybe the only manifestation of a mitochondrial disorder encoded by a gene defect within the mitochondria (all of which are maternally inherited) or a nuclear DNA-encoded gene necessary to the oxidative phosphorylation sequence within mitochondria.

This defective energy pathway leads to progressive impairment of insulin secretion, and thus an initially mild hyperglycemia may progressively worsen. This is the case with the most common form of diabetes caused by a mitochondrial gene mutation at nucleotide pair 3243 of the mitochondrial genome, often associated with deafness. Remarkably, this same genetic defect may be associated with the MELAS syndrome. Initially, patients with np 3243 mutations can be controlled by diet alone but later may require insulin. Diabetes mellitus presenting in infancy and severe from the outset and requiring insulin may be associated with mitochondrial DNA deletions, as seen in the Kearns-Sayre syndrome and Pearson syndrome.[257] Figure 10-12 identifies the critical role of energy production by the mitochondrial oxidative phosphorylation pathway for normal insulin secretion.

Defects in this pathway may be responsible for transient or permanent neonatal diabetes mellitus, especially those that involve activating mutations in the KATP channel subunits Kir 6.2 and its regulatory subunit sulfonylurea receptor SUR1. Inactivating mutations in the KATP

TABLE 10-15

Protein/Gene Mutations Causing Maturity-Onset Diabetes of the Young

MODY Type	Protein Mutated	Gene/Gene Location	Gene Function with Respect to the Beta Cell
MODY 1	Hepatocyte nuclear factor-4α	HNF4α; 20q12-q13.1	Binds to HNF1α and IPF1 promoter; regulates HNF1α and IPF1 gene transcription
MODY 2	Glucokinase	GCK; 7p15-p13	Catalyzes conversion of glucose to glucose 6-phosphate
MODY 3	Hepatocyte nuclear factor-1α	HNF1α; 12q24.2	Binds to A3/A4 box of insulin gene promoter; regulates insulin gene transcription
MODY 4	Insulin promoter factor-1	IPF1; 13q12.1	Binds to A5, A3/A4, A2, and A1 boxes of insulin gene promoter; regulates insulin gene transcription
MODY 5	Hepatocyte nuclear factor-1β	HNF1β, TCF2; 17cen-q21.3	Regulates HNF4α gene transcription
MODY 6	Neuro-D1/beta-2	Neuro-D1; 2q32; beta-2	Transcription factor for normal insulin secretion and normal development of pancreatic islets

TCF2, Transcription factor-2, hepatic; also known as LF-B3, variant hepatic nuclear factor.
From Winter WE, Nakamura M, Hause D (2001). Monogenic diabetes mellitus in youth. Endocrinol Metab Clin North Am 28:765; and from Fajans SS, Bell GI, Polonsky KS (2001). Molecular mechanisms and clinical pathophysiology of maturity-onset diabetes of the young. N Engl J Med 345:971.

TABLE 10-16

Comparison of the Common Forms of Youth-Onset Diabetes

Characteristic	Type 1 Diabetes	Type 2 Diabetes	Classic MODY	Atypical Diabetes Mellitus
Age at onset	Peaks at 5 and 15 years old	Teenage years, young adults	<25 years old	>40 years old
Predominant ethnic groups affected	White	Hispanic, African American, Native American	White	African American
Male to female ratio	1:1:1	1:1.5	1:1	1:3
Severity at onset	Acute, severe, insulin required	Subtle, insulin not required	Subtle, insulin not required	Acute, severe, insulin required
Islet autoimmunity	Present	Absent	Absent	Absent
HLA-DR3, -DR4	Very common	No increased frequency	No increased frequency	No increased frequency
Ketosis, DKA	Common	Uncommon	Rare	Common at onset
Long-term course	Insulin-dependent	Non insulin-dependent	Non insulin-dependent	Non-insulin-dependent
Prevalence of obesity	Uncommon	≥90%	Uncommon	40%
Proportion of cases of 100% youth-onset diabetes	Most common form of youth-onset diabetes	Rising in frequency; ± as common as type 1 diabetes in specific populations	≤5% of youth-onset diabetes in whites	≤10% of cases of youth-onset diabetes in African-Americans
Percentage of probands with an affected first-degree relative	≤15%	Variable but common	100%	>75%
Mode of inheritance	Nonmendelian, generally sporadic	Nonmendelian but strongly familial	Autosomal dominant	Autosomal dominant
Number of genes controlling inheritance	Polygenic	Polygenic	Monogenic	Monogenic
Pathogenesis	Autoimmune beta cell destruction: insulinopenia	Insulin resistance plus relative insulinopenia	Insulinopenia	Insulinopenia

DKA, diabetic ketoacidosis; and MODY, maturity-onset diabetes of the young.
Adapted from Winter WE, Nakamura M, Hause D (1999). Monogenic diabetes mellitus in youth. Endocrinol Metab Clin North Am 28:765-785.

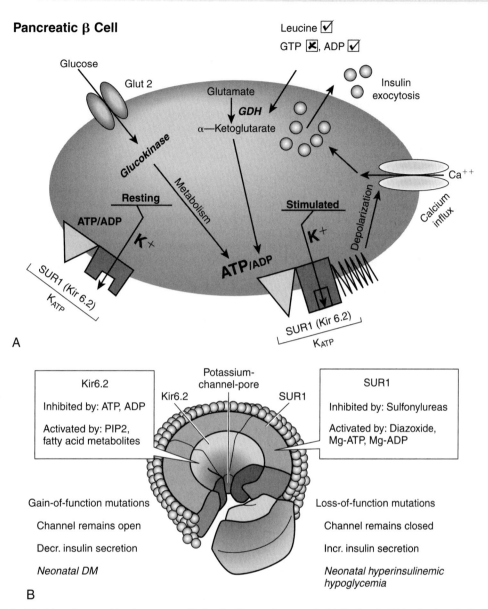

Figure 10-12. *(A)* Model of insulin secretion by pancreatic β cell. Glucose transported into the β cell by the insulin-independent glucose transporter (Glut 2) undergoes phosphorylation by glucokinase and is metabolized. This results in an increase in the ATP/ADP ratio with subsequent closure of the KATP channel and initiation of a cascade of events that is characterized by decreased flux of potassium across the membrane, membrane depolarization, calcium influx, and release of insulin from storage granules. Leucine stimulates insulin secretion by allosterically activating glutamate dehydrogenase (GDH) and by increasing the oxidation of glutamate; this increases the ATP/ADP ratio and closure of the KATP channel. Check mark sign (√) indicates stimulation of insulin secretion; cross sign (x) indicates inhibition of insulin secretion. Diazoxide inhibits insulin secretion by interacting with the sulfonylurea receptor; somatostatin and calcium channel blockers interfere with calcium signaling. *(B)* Regulation of Insulin Secretion. The Kir6.2–SUR1 complex and its regulation and genetic variability. The panel shows the detailed subunit structure of the KATP channel, which is composed of four small subunits, Kir6.2, that surround a central pore and four larger regulatory subunits constituting SUR1. In the normal resting state, the potassium channel is open, modulated by the ratio of ATP to ADP. PIP2 denotes phosphatidylinositol-4,5-bisphosphate. Kir6.2 denotes the inward rectifying potassium channel 6.2; SUR1 denotes the sulfonylurea receptor 1. ADP is adenosine diphosphate; ATP is adenosine triphosphate. As noted, in gain of function mutations, the channel remains open leading to decreased insulin secretion so that neonatal diabetes may result. With loss of function mutations the channel remains closed, leading to persistent insulin secretion and hence is a cause of neonatal hyperinsulinemic hypoglycemia. Redrawn from Sperling MA, New Engl J Med 2006; 355:507-510.

subunits cause neonatal hyperinsulinemic hypoglycemia of variable severity, as described in detail in Chapter 5. Diabetes in the mitochondrial syndromes is generally well controlled by exogenous insulin.[257]

Wolfram Syndrome. Wolfram syndrome is characterized by diabetes insipidus, diabetes mellitus, optic atrophy, and deafness (DIDMOAD).[258] There is a selective loss of beta cells, which is responsible for the diabetes mellitus. Genetic linkage studies in consanguineous families with autosomal-recessive inheritance led to the positional cloning of a gene on the short arm of chromosome 4 (termed *WFS1*, and now identified as Wolframin).

Although the function of this gene is not entirely understood, it is expressed in many tissues (most abundantly in beta cells, compared with the exocrine pancreas). Mutations in Wolframin have been identified in many families with Wolfram syndrome. Affected individuals are usually compound heterozygotes. The Wolframin gene may have a role in beta cell and neural tissue survival, and there does not appear to be a correlation between the observed mutation and severity of disease. Defects in Wolframin have been implicated in the idiopathic common nonimmune form of type 1 diabetes mellitus.[257] A second locus of Wolfram syndrome has been mapped to the long arm of chromosome 4 in several consanguineous Jordanian families.[258] In these patients, diabetes insipidus was not a feature—but upper gastrointestinal bleeding and ulceration were prominent.

Although a mitochondrial form of Wolfram syndrome has been proposed, a defect in mitochondrial DNA could not be confirmed in one large cohort.[260] It has been suggested that diabetes mellitus (before age 15) and progressive optic atrophy are highly predictive of Wolfram syndrome. The sequence of appearance of the stigmata is nonautoimmune type 1 diabetes in the first decade of life, central diabetes insipidus and sensorineural deafness in two-thirds to three-fourths of the patients in the second decade, renal tract anomalies in approximately one-half in the third decade, and neurologic complications such as cerebellar ataxia and myoclonus in one-half to two-thirds in the fourth decade. Other features include primary gonadal atrophy in the majority of males and a progressive neurodegenerative course with neurorespiratory death at a median age of 30 years. Depression has been reported as a frequent feature of relatives of patients with Wolfram syndrome.[236,258-260]

Thiamine-Responsive Diabetes Mellitus (Roger Syndrome). This syndrome is characterized by megaloblastic anemia, diabetes mellitus, and sensorineural deafness—all of which may respond to vitamin B_1 (thiamine). Diabetes mellitus is mild to moderate, insulin secretion may improve with thiamine therapy, and there are no associated autoimmune markers. It may be caused by a defect in the thiamine transporter,[261,262] which has now been identified as being caused by mutations in the SLC19A gene. This gene encodes the membrane-bound thiamine transporter THTR-1.

Uptake of thiamine by the combined pathways of an active high-affinity carrier and a passive low-affinity carrier leads to accumulation of intracellular thiamine, which is then converted to its active form thiamine pyrophosphate. This cofactor enables proper function of transketolase which is important in the pentose phosphate shunt which

is key to ribose synthesis and hence nucleic acid production and of pyruvate dehydrogenase, α ketoglutarate dehydrogenase, and branched chain acid dehydrogenase—all of which are key to oxidative decarboxylation. Mutations in the high-affinity transporter THTR-1 lead to cell death in those cells that have a high rate of nucleic acid turnover (such as bone marrow cells) and activity (such as pancreatic β cells), thereby explaining the association of thiamine-responsive anemia with diabetes in those affected by this mutation.

Drug or Chemical Induced. A number of drugs and chemical agents may be toxic to the beta cell. Best known for the diabetogenic effects are the immunosuppressive agents cyclosporine and tacrolimus, which are toxic to beta cells—causing insulin-dependent diabetes in a significant proportion of patients treated with these agents for organ transplantation. Their toxicity to pancreatic beta cells is compounded by the use of immunosuppressive glucocorticoids, which antagonize insulin action to unmask diabetes.

Streptozotocin and the rodenticide Vacor are also beta cell toxic, causing diabetes. Table 10-1 lists other agents that may induce diabetes. Among these, L-asparaginase (used in chemotherapy for leukemia) and diazoxide (used to treat persistent hyperinsulinemic hypoglycemia in infancy) may cause diabetes. All of these agents, especially glucocorticoids, may combine to unmask clinical diabetes mellitus.[262]

Diseases of the Exocrine Pancreas. Cystic fibrosis (CF) is one of the most common inborn errors of metabolism, involving the chloride channel encoded on chromosome 7 and affecting approximately 1 in 2,500 live-born white infants. The increasing survival of patients with CF and the increased use of glucocorticoids to suppress bronchopulmonary inflammation have brought to the fore an entity termed *cystic fibrosis–related diabetes* (CFRD), characterized by variable impairment of carbohydrate intolerance.

Some have mild diabetes mellitus clinically apparent only while receiving steroids, whereas others require insulin for a nonimmune form of insulinopenic diabetes mellitus. Up to 75% of adults with CF have CFRD. Islet amyloid is prominent, both insulin secretion and insulin sensitivity may be impaired, and diabetic ketoacidosis may occur—as may microvascular complications. When fasting hyperglycemia (7 mM = 126 mg/dL or higher) is documented, therapy with insulin is indicated. Insulin also facilitates optimal nutrition and growth and hence promotes a sense of well-being. The diagnostic and management criteria for CFRD have been extensively reviewed.[15,266]

Ionizing Radiation to the Abdomen. Ionizing radiation to the abdomen in childhood for a condition such as nephroblastoma has been associated with the development of diabetes mellitus some 20 years later in 5% to 10% of children so treated.[264]

Pancreatectomy. Extensive pancreatectomy performed for the management of severe hyperinsulinemic hypoglycemia of infancy is associated with diabetes in approximately 50% or more of long-term survivors.[21]

Virus Infections. Several viruses have been implicated in the cause of type 1 diabetes mellitus in children. Coxsackievirus B_4 has been shown in one case report as likely fulfilling Koch's postulates for a direct beta cell toxic effect in causing acute fulminant diabetes mellitus. In other cases of coxsackievirus infections (as well as with the established association among rubella, cytomegaloviruses, and enteroviruses), molecular mimicry between antigenic determinants in the virus and certain islet cell antigens has been implicated as the mechanism leading to an autoimmune form of type 1 diabetes mellitus. Finally, a superantigen-triggered immune response has been suggested for some viral infections and may be the mechanism related to the acute onset of diabetes mellitus with the hemolytic-uremic syndrome.[20,58,268,269]

Variants of Type 2 Diabetes

GENETIC DEFECTS IN INSULIN ACTION

Type A Insulin Resistance with Acanthosis Nigricans

This syndrome is characterized by severe insulin resistance, acanthosis nigricans in the absence of obesity, or lipoatrophy. Affected females also have hyperandrogenism, possibly as a secondary manifestation of the hyperinsulinemia with stimulation of androgen synthesis by ovarian theca cells. Glucose intolerance is variable and includes symptomatic diabetes. The hyperandrogenism presents as clinical and biochemical findings suggestive of polycystic ovary syndrome.

Some patients (predominantly black females with obesity, acanthosis nigricans, and accelerated growth suggestive of gigantism) may represent insulin resistance owing to obesity, with down-regulation of the insulin receptor. The gigantism may represent a "spillover" effect of insulin acting through the insulin-like growth factor-1 receptor rather than the insulin receptor.[270,271]

Type B Insulin Resistance

Type B insulin resistance is a rare syndrome associated with evidence of immune dysfunction (such as the defined autoimmune disease rheumatoid arthritis) or of nonspecific features of autoimmunity (such as elevated sedimentation rate or high levels of antinuclear antibodies). As with other autoimmune disorders, females are predominantly affected. An insulin-resistant diabetes develops together with acanthosis nigricans and features of PCOS (such as hirsutism).

The syndrome is due to serum autoantibodies against the insulin receptor whose function becomes impaired. However, the receptor may be activated by the presumed conformational changes induced by the antibody and cause severe hypoglycemia rather than diabetes. Treatment may require high doses of insulin to try to control the hyperglycemia, along with immunosuppressive drugs to suppress antibody production.

Leprechaunism (Donohue's Syndrome). Leprechaunism is a syndrome characterized by intrauterine growth retardation, fasting hypoglycemia, and postprandial hyperglycemia in association with profound resistance to insulin in a patient whose serum concentrations of insulin may be 100-fold that of comparable age-matched infants during an oral glucose tolerance test. Various defects of the insulin receptor have been described, thereby attesting to the important role of insulin and its receptor in fetal growth and possibly in morphogenesis. Even a probable complete absence of functional insulin receptors caused by homozygous inheritance of missense mutation in the insulin receptor, however, resulted in normal organogenesis and a liveborn infant who had a severe form of leprechaunism. Most of these patients die during the first year of life.[272]

Rabson-Mendenhall Syndrome. The Rabson-Mendenhall syndrome is defined by clinical features that appear to be intermediate between those of acanthosis nigricans with insulin resistance type A and leprechaunism. Features include extreme insulin resistance, acanthosis nigricans, abnormalities of the teeth and nails, and pineal hyperplasia. It is not clear whether this syndrome is entirely distinct from leprechaunism. However, patients with Rabson-Mendenhall syndrome tend to live beyond the first year of life. Defects in the insulin receptor gene have been described in this syndrome.[273]

Lipoatrophic Diabetes. Lipoatrophic diabetes presents an interesting paradox. Whereas classic type 2 diabetes mellitus is generally associated with an excess of fat and its metabolic consequences (as described previously), a paucity of fat also causes severe insulin resistance and marked metabolic disturbances. Table 10-17 lists the genetic syndromes associated with lipoatrophic diabetes. A primary cause has been identified in the form called familial partial lipoatrophy (also known as Dunnigan syndrome). This is a gene defect localized to chromosome 1q21-22 and its product lamin A/C.

This autosomal disease usually manifests peripubertally as subcutaneous fat in the extremities and trunk but with progressively more fat in the face and neck as puberty progresses. Visceral and interfascicular fat also increases. Females seem to develop diabetes mellitus and dyslipidemia earlier and more severely than males. Why and how the lamin A/C mutations cause this lipoatrophy syndrome is unclear, especially as mutations in this gene also are associated with a progressive form of muscular dystrophy (Emery-Dreifuss syndrome), cardiomyopathy, and cardiac conduction defects.[274,275] Recently, the gene altered in Berardinelli-Seip congenital lipodystrophy has been localized to chromosome 11q13.274.[275] In addition, defects in genes encoding the enzyme AGPAT2, the endoprotease ZMPSTE24, the kinase AKT2, the nuclear receptor PPARγ, and the protein BSCL 2 have been found in patients with lipodystrophies.[274,275]

ACQUIRED DEFECTS IN INSULIN ACTION

These defects range from hormonal disorders such as pheochromocytoma and Cushing syndrome that antagonize insulin action to disease to drug-acquired forms of lipodystrophy. Anti-insulin receptor antibodies may be found in some collagen vascular disorders and can cause a type 2 diabetes mellitus syndrome characterized by acanthosis nigricans and severe insulin resistance. This is generally referred to as acanthosis nigricans with insulin resistance type B. The type A syndrome consists of a variety of insulin receptor mutations, some of which were described above. The type B syndrome is rarely described in childhood.[276]

TABLE 10-17

Genetic Syndromes of Lipoatrophy

Syndrome	Lipoatrophy	Gene/Locus	Inheritance	OMIM
Primary Lipoatrophy Syndromes				
Congenital generalized lipoatrophy (Seip-Berardinelli)	Generalized See text for details.	9q34 Gmg3lg; 11q13p	AR	269700
Dunnigan syndrome	Familial partial See text for details.	1q21-22 Lamin A/C	AD	151660
Others	Numerous distributions	Unknown	AD/AR	N/A
Complex Syndromes Associated with Lipoatrophy				
Mandibuloacral dysplasia	Congenital, partial Involves extremities	Unknown	AR	248370
Werner syndrome	Congenital, partial Involves extremities	8p12 Werner's helicase	AR	277700
Cockayne syndrome	Congenital, partial Involves extremities	5 CSA	AR	216400
Carbohydrate-deficient glycoprotein syndrome	Transient, partial Buttocks	16p13.3 PMM1 and 2	AR	212065
SHORT syndrome†	Generalized, congenital	Unknown	AR	269880
AREDYLD syndrome‡	Generalized, congenital	Unknown	Unknown	207780

Evidence for genetic heterogeneity.
† Short stature, hyperextensibility, hernia, ocular depression, Rieger anomaly, and teething delay.
‡ Acrorenal field defect, ectodermal dysplasia, and lipoatrophic diabetes; not clear if this is a variation of Seip-Berardinelli syndrome.
AD, autosomal dominant; AR, autosomal recessive; OMIM, Online Mendelian Inheritance in Man, database providing information about genetic syndromes; and PMM1, PMM2, phosphomannomutase 1 and 2.
From Ariouglu E, et al. (2000). Lipoatrophy syndromes. Pediatr Diabetes 1:155; and from Magre J, Delepine M, Khallouf E, et al. (2001). Identification of the gene altered in Berardinelli-Seip congenital lipodystrophy on chromosome 11q13. Nat Genet 28:365.

Genetic Syndromes with Diabetes and Insulin Resistance and/or Insulin Deficiency

A number of genetic syndromes are associated with diabetes mellitus. In children, four relatively common genetic syndromes may be associated with diabetes. In trisomy 21 (Down syndrome) and Turner syndrome (a single normal X chromosome) there is an increased incidence of autoimmune disorders, especially of the thyroid. Type 1 diabetes mellitus also has a higher prevalence in patients with Down syndrome than in the general population.

In Turner syndrome, insulin secretory reserve may be limited such that treatment with growth hormone (now common) can result in impaired glucose tolerance or a type 2 diabetes. In Klinefelter syndrome (XXY), insulin resistance is a major feature—but autoimmune associations have been described. In Prader-Willi syndrome, the reported high frequency of diabetes mellitus may not be caused simply by the insulin resistance as part of the obesity of this syndrome but possibly by a primary defect in insulin secretion.[277-280]

Alstrom syndrome consists of retinal dystrophy, sensorineural deafness, obesity and associated diabetes, cardiomyopathy, hypertriglyceridemia, liver disease, and urological abnormalities. Severe insulin resistance may lead to acanthosis and diabetes. Mutations in the gene ALMS1 have been identified in these patients.[281] Bardet-Biedel syndrome also has atypical retinitis pigmentosa as a key feature, along with central obesity, polydactyly, mental retardation, hypogonadism, and renal dysfunction. Eleven loci have been linked to this syndrome, with abnormalities in celia-like structures a central theme.[281,282] The association of these and other syndromes with diabetes (listed in Table 10-1) can be ascertained by searching the Online Mendelian Inheritance in Man database (OMIM, available at *www.ncbi.nlm.nih. gov/omim/*).

Gestational Diabetes

Gestational diabetes is a disease of the second and third trimesters of pregnancy that is due to congenital or acquired defects in insulin secretion that result in the inability to compensate for the increased demands of insulin as a result of the counter-insulin effects of placental growth hormones.[283]

Neonatal Diabetes

Recent discoveries in the molecular basis for pancreas formation and regulation of insulin secretion have propelled the syndromes of neoanatal diabetes from the backwater of rarity to the forefront of research. These syndromes probably occur more frequently than previously

TABLE 10-18

Classification of Neonatal Diabetes Mellitus

Permanent	Transient

• PDX-1/IPF-1 *1
• Glucokinase-GCK *2
• HNF-1β*3
• FOX P3 (IPEX syndrome)
• EIF$_2$AK$_3$ (Wolcott-Rallison syndrome)
• K$_{ATP}$ KIR 6.2 or Sur1
• Others (PTF1)
	• ZAC/PLAGL1-HYMA1 mutations
	  • Human
	  • Transgenic mouse
	• KCNJ11 or ABCC8, mild activating

*Homozygous mutations cause permanent neonatal diabetes heterozygous mutations cause maturity-onset diabetes of youth (MODY). 1 = MODY 2; 3 = MODY 5.

considered, and may have an overall incidence of about 1:100,000 births.[284-291] Moreover, some of those with activating mutations in KATP channel subunits Kir 6.2 or SUR1 lend themselves to treatment with oral sulfonylurea hypoglycemic drugs such as glibenclamide—which results in endogenous insulin secretion with near-normal glycemic control and at least partial reversal of neuromuscular manifestations.[285-288]

Mutations in these genes also may contribute to T2DM in adults by impairing the ability to secrete adequate amounts of insulin to overcome insulin resistance.[289] Table 10-18 outlines the common entities responsible for neonatal diabetes, which clinically present as a transient form in the neonate (followed by remission and then recurrence in the second to fourth decade) or permanent diabetes mellitus from the outset. Both forms share the following clinical features. Most affected infants are intrauterine growth retarded (IUGR), reflecting the critical role of insulin as an in utero growth factor. Clinical features include polyuria with glucosuria, dehydration, failure to thrive, and occasionally diabetic ketoacidsis. When measured, insulin and IGF-1 levels are low.

Dysmorphic features in some include mental retardation, muscle weakness, and epilepsy. These features are found only in the permanent severe forms.[284-289] Treatment with insulin results in dramatic catch-up growth, and after several weeks to months insulin may be withdrawn in about one-half of cases. These constitute cases of transient neonatal diabetes, of whom about one-half or more have recurrence of DM several years later. About 50% of cases of neonatal DM have the permanent form from the outset.[284]

TRANSIENT

Onset of persistent insulin-dependent diabetes before the age of 6 months is very unusual and had previously been estimated to occur in only 1:500,000 births.[292] The syndrome of diabetes mellitus in a newborn has its onset in the first 6 weeks to months of life. The transient form may spontaneously recover within 3 to 6 months, at which time the insulin response to stimuli are brisk.[293] This syndrome should be distinguished from severe hyperglycemia, which sometimes occurs in hypertonic de-

hydration in infants beyond the newborn period. Such infants promptly respond to rehydration, with minimal requirement for insulin.

During the active phase of transient diabetes of the newborn, administration of insulin is mandatory. From 1 to 2 U/kg/24 hours of an intermediate-acting insulin in two divided doses usually results in dramatic improvement, accelerated growth, and weight gain. Pump therapy has also proven to be highly successful in neonatal diabetes and is likely superior in providing flexibility and precision in managing such patients.[292] As the syndrome resolves beyond 2 to 3 months of age, the recurrent hypoglycemia permits a gradual reduction and discontinuation in exogenous insulin.[292]

A gene for transient neonatal diabetes mellitus has been localized to the long arm of chromosome 6 at 6q24.[285,293] Transient neonatal diabetes mellitus is associated with paternal uniparental disomy of chromosome 6 or paternal duplications in this region. Differential methylation of a subportion of this region has been demonstrated in patients with transient neonatal diabetes whether they do or do not have uniparental disomy or paternal duplications of chromosome 6.[294] These findings suggest that transient neonatal diabetes mellitus may be associated with a specific methylation imprint on chromosome 6 that must be paternally expressed. In one extensive investigation of 30 patients with neonatal transient diabetes, only 6 had no methylation rearrangement in chromosome 6. The role of this imprinted region on 6q24 is not fully understood, but it has been suggested that this gene may have an important function in normal pancreatic development.

To date, defects of this gene have not been found in permanent neonatal diabetes. The imprinted gene in this region is most likely ZAC (Zfinger protein regulating Apoptosis and Cell cycle arrest). A transgenic mouse model expressing the human region of 6q24 has been generated.[295] This mouse model recapitulates many of the human findings and has provided insights into the sequence of events that characterize the human condition (i.e., neonatal diabetes, followed by remission and then recurrence in later life).[295] In addition to the locus on 6q24, some activating mutations in KCNJ11 (which codes for the potassium channel pore) and in ABCC8 (which codes for the sulfonylurea receptor regulatory subunit of the K$_{ATP}$ channel on beta cells) (Figure 10-12) can result in a transient neonatal DM followed by remission and recurrence. However, mutations in the K$_{ATP}$ units are the most common cause of permanent neonatal DM.[284-290]

PERMANENT

The permanent forms of neonatal DM are outlined in Table 10-18. Diabetes mellitus in the newborn period will be permanent if associated with the rare syndrome of pancreatic agenesis. In one such case, there was homozygous mutation of the gene for insulin promoter factor-1 (IPF1)[296]—also known as PDX-1 because it is a pancreas duodenum homeobox gene involved in the formation of the exocrine plus endocrine pancreas and the duodenum. Hence, patients with this cause of neonatal DM have exocrine manifestations (such as malabsorption) and the endocrine manifestations of severely diminished insulin secretion.

Heterozygous mutations of PDX-1/IPF1 are the cause of MODY 4 and have been implicated as a cause of some forms of late-onset type 2 diabetes mellitus.[297] Likewise, homozygous mutations in the glucokinase gene are associated with permanent neonatal diabetes—whereas the heterozygous forms are the cause of MODY 2.[285,298] Severe mutation in hepatic nuclear factor 1β (HNF-1β) can cause permanent or transient neoanatal DM and is associated with renal cysts.[285] FoxP3 is a human gene that is the ortholog of the mouse scurfy gene and responsible for the IPEX (immune dysregulation, polyendocrinopathy, enteropathy, X-linked) syndrome. Autoimmunity may not be the sole factor in causing DM.[285,291]

The Wolcott-Rallison syndrome is a disorder characterized by the appearance of permanent insulin-requiring diabetes mellitus within 3 months of life. It is associated with multiple epiphyseal or spondyloepiphyseal dysplasia, renal and hepatic impairment, ectodermal dysplasia, cardiac anomalies, and poor prognosis. Inheritance is consistent with an autosomal-recessive pattern. The eukaryotic translation-initiation factor-2-alpha kinase-3 (E1F2AK3) was mutated in two consanguineous families with this syndrome. This factor, highly expressed in islets, has a role in protein translation that may account for the multiple manifestations of this syndrome.[43,44,300]

The most common forms of permanent neoantal DM are caused by mutations in the Kir6.2 (KCNJ11) and SUR1 (ABCC8) subunits of the KATP channel.[284-291] Severe mutations, especially of KCNJ11, may be associated with the DEND (developmental delay, epilepsy, and neonatal diabetes) syndrome. The pathophysiology of these syndromes has been elucidated, and the relationship of the severity of mutation in terms of channel activity has been correlated with the clinical manifestations. Remarkably, the KCNJ11 and ABCC8 mutations may be responsive to pharmacologic doses of the oral sulfonylurea glibenclamide—with restoration of endogenous insulin secretion, ability to discontinue insulin injections, and marked improvement in overall metabolic control. In addition, some improvement in neuromuscular activity has been reported.[284-289] Some of the mutations in KCNJ11 have been reported to occur in T2DM, and hence these mutations might be selectively targeted for treatment with sulfonylurea drugs.[289]

Impaired Glucose Tolerance

The term *impaired glucose tolerance* is used to characterize individuals who have a plasma glucose concentration in excess of 140 mg/dL at 2 hours after initiation of the standard oral glucose tolerance test but do not have symptoms of diabetes or fasting hyperglycemia. Such a constellation may represent the earliest phase of a gene defect in insulin secretion or action or be a step in evolving diabetes mellitus type 1. The hyperglycemia may be a chance discovery during an intercurrent illness, during therapy with corticosteroids, or as part of

a screening of close relatives of patients with defined genetic syndromes.

In those who have impaired glucose tolerance but do not have fasting hyperglycemia, repeated oral glucose tolerance tests are not recommended. Investigations in such children indicate that the degree of impaired glucose tolerance tends to remain stable except in those who have markedly subnormal insulin response.[3] The arbitrarily designated response that identifies impaired glucose tolerance is defined as a fasting plasma glucose value of less than 110 mg/dL and a value at 2 hours of more than 140 mg/dL. The determination of serum insulin responses during the glucose tolerance test is not a prerequisite for reaching a diagnosis. Because the magnitude of the insulin response may have prognostic value, however, insulin determination is performed by some investigators.[237]

Pancreas and Islet Transplantation

In an attempt to cure insulin-dependent diabetes, transplantation of a segment of the pancreas or of isolated islets has been increasingly performed in humans.[302,303] These procedures are technically demanding and associated with the risks and complications of rejection and its treatment by immunosuppression. Therefore, segmental pancreas transplantation is generally performed in association with transplantation of a kidney for a patient with end-stage renal disease owing to diabetic nephropathy in whom the immunosuppressive regimen is indicated for the renal transplant.

Several thousand such transplants have been performed worldwide during the past 25 years. With experience and newer immunosuppressive agents, functional survival of the pancreatic graft may be achieved for as long as several years—during which patients may be in metabolic control with no or minimal exogenous insulin and reversal of some of the microvascular complications. Because children and adolescents with diabetes mellitus are not likely to have end-stage renal disease as a result of diabetes, however, pancreas transplantation as a primary treatment cannot be recommended (nor its risks justified) in children.

Attempts to transplant isolated islets have been equally challenging because of techniques to harvest sufficient islets and the issue of rejection.[303] Some of the newer antirejection drugs, notably cyclosporine and tacrolimus, are toxic to the islets of Langerhans—impairing insulin secretion and even causing diabetes.[304] The Edmonton protocol for islet transplantation avoids steroid and uses an anti-IL-2 receptor antibody and tacrolimus instead of other immunosuppressants.[303] Initial success had been promising, but long-term survival of the graft beyond 3 to 5 years is most unusual—and there have been serious side effects of the procedure as well as failure to restore hypoglycemia unawareness.[303] Hence, this islet transplantation protocol cannot be recommended in children.

Research continues to improve techniques for the yield, viability, and loss of immunogenicity of islets of Langerhans for transplantation. Transplantation has been investigated of islets coated or microencapsulated with a film of protective chemicals that permit diffusion of insulin and nutrients but prevent T-cell contact and therefore avoid rejection.[305] These novel approaches have been frustrated in the long term by overgrowth of fibroblasts that progressively impair glucose sensing by the islets and insulin diffusion from them. Should these technical problems be overcome, or methods to avoid rejection become established, transplantation of pancreas or islets as primary treatment for diabetes may be entertained after their risks are carefully compared with and weighed against potential benefits—especially in children. Islet regeneration by modulating the immune response is also under scrutiny.[306,307]

Conclusions

Progress continues to be spectacular in understanding and treating diabetes mellitus. We have moved from a glimmer of understanding that diabetes is a syndrome of broad categories (insulin dependent and non–insulin dependent) to an understanding of disease susceptibility and disease causality at a molecular level. Type 1 diabetes is acknowledged to be an autoimmune disease with major susceptibility loci in the HLA complex. Positional cloning techniques have identified other gene markers, and we now recognize the importance of mitochondrial gene defects in some types of insulin-dependent diabetes that may not be autoimmune.

More spectacular has been the unraveling of the molecular basis of neonatal diabetes and its treatment, including the use of sulfonylureas. Not surprisingly, this knowledge is being rapidly applied to predict the likelihood of disease appearance in individuals whose susceptibility can be quantified by the presence of certain antibodies and by limitations in first-phase insulin response. Population surveys in individuals not known to be at risk for diabetes have just begun. We are in the early stages of attempts to prevent the disease, reminiscent of the early trials examining the relationship between control and microvascular complications.

The monumental DCCT and European studies have irrefutably established the link, requiring new standards of care. Progress and understanding of insulin secretion and insulin action have been equally spectacular for the insights provided in defining non–insulin-dependent forms of diabetes at physiologic, biochemical, and molecular levels. Therapy with human insulin is now standard. Trials with improved insulin-delivery systems, including computerized artificial pancreas as well as pancreas and islet transplantation, are in progress. The beneficiaries of these advances are our patients, whose interests will continue to be best served by bidirectional scientific inquiry from bench to bedside.

REFERENCES

1. Ize-Ludow D, Sperling MA (2005). The classification of diabetes Mellitus: A conceptual Framework. Pediatr Clin N Am 52:1533–1552.
2. Pambianco G, Cousacou T, Ellis D, et al. (2006). The 30 year natural history of type 1 diabetes complications: The Pittsburgh Epidemiology of Diabetes Complications Study experience. Diabetes 55:1463–1469.
3. Saltiel AR, Kahn CR (2001). Insulin signaling and the regulation of glucose and lipid metabolism. Nature 414:799–806.
4. Daneman D (2006). Type 1 diabetes. Lancet 367:847–858.
5. Eisenbarth GS (2007). Update in type 1 diabetes. J Clin Endocrinol Metab 92:2403–2407.
6. Hattersley A, Bruining J, Shield J, et al. (2006). ISPAD Clinical Practice Consensus Guidelines 2006-2007: The diagnosis and management of monogenic diabetes in children. Pediatric Diabetes 7:352–360.
7. American Diabetes Association (2007). Diagnosis and classification of diabetes mellitus. Diabetes Care 30:S42–S47.
8. Wang J, Miao D, Babu S, et al. (2007). Prevalence of autoantibody-negative diabetes is not rare at all ages and increases with older age and obesity. J Clin Endocrinol Metab 92:88–92.
9. Trucco M, Giannoukakis N (2007). Immunoregulatory dendritic cells to prevent and reverse new-onset type 1 diabetes mellitus. Expert Opin Biol Ther 7:951–963.
10. Stark R, Roden M (2007). ESCI Award 2006, Mitochondrial function and endocrine disease. Eur J Clin Invest 37:236–248.
11. Chinnery P, Howell N, Andrews R, Turnbull D (1999). Clinical mitochondrial genetics. J Med Genet 36:425–436.
12. Maassen JA, Tafrechi RS J, Raap AK, et al. (2006). New insights in the molecular pathogenesis of the maternally inherited diabetes and deafness syndrome. Endocrinol Metab Clin N Am 35:385–396.
13. Fajans SS, Bell GI, Polonsky JS (2001). Molecular mechanisms and clinical pathophysiology of maturity-onset diabetes of the young. N Engl J Med 345:971–980.
14. Rosenecker J, Eichler I, Kuhn L, et al. (1995). Genetic determination of diabetes mellitus in patients with cystic fibrosis. J Pediatr 127:441–443.
15. Mackle AD, Thornton SJ, Edenborough FP (2003). Cystic fibrosis-related diabetes. Diabet Med 20:425–436.
16. Heit JJ (2007). Calcineurun/NFAT signaling in the beta cell: From diabetes to new therapeutics. Bioessays 29:1011–1021.
17. David-Neto E, Lemos FC, Fadel LM, et al. (2007). The dynamics of glucose metabolism inder calcineurin inhibitors in the first year after renal transplantation in nonobese patients. Transplantation 84:50–55.
18. Esposti MD, Ngo A, Myers MA (1996). Inhibition of mitochondrial complex 1 may account for IDDM induces by intoxication with therodenticide Vacor. Diabetes 45:1531–1534.
19. Strosberg J, Hoffe S. Gardner N, et al. (2007). Effective treatment of locally advanced endocrine tumors of the pancreas with chemoradiotherapy. Neuroendocrinology 85:216–220.
20. Nesmith JD, Ellis E (2007). Childhood hemolyic uremic syndrome is associated with adolescent-onset mellitus. Pediatr Nephrol 22:294–297.
21. de Lonlay–Debeney P, Poggi-Travert F, Fournet JC, et al. (1999). Clinical features of 52 neonates with hyperinsulinism. N Engl J Med 340:1169–1175.
22. Dabelea D, Pettitt DJ, Jones KL, Arslanian SA (1999). Type 2 diabetes in minority children and adolescents. Endocrinol Metab Clin North Am 28:709–729.
23. Writing Group for the SEARCH for Diabetes in Youth Study Group, et al. (2007). Incidence of diabetes in youth in the United States. JAMA 297:2716–2724.
24. Slingerland AS (2006). Monogenic diabetes in children and young adults: Challenges for researcher, clinician and patient. Rev Endocr Metab Disord 7:171–185.
25. Santer R, Schneppenheim R, Dombrowski A, et al. (1997). Mutations in GLUT2, the gene for the liver-type glucose transporter, in patients with Fanconi-Bickel syndrome. Nat Genet 17:324–326.
26. Zouali H, Velho G, Frouguel P (1993). Polymorphism of the glycogen synthase gene and non-insulin dependent diabetes mellitus. N Engl J Med 328:1568.

27. Henriksen EJ, Dokken BB (year). Role of glycogen synthase kinase-3 in insulin resistance and type 2 diabetes. Curr Drug Targets 7:1435–1441.

28. Taylor SI, Cama A, Accili D, et al. (1992). Mutations in the insulin receptor gene. Endocr Rev 13:566–595.

29. Reynet C, Kahn CR (1993). Rad: A member of the Ras family over-expressed in muscle of type 2 diabetic humans. Science 262: 1441–1444.

30. Polonsky KS (1995). The beta-cell in diabetes: From molecular genetics to clinical research. Diabetes 4:705–717.

31. Polonsky KS, Sturis JP, Bell GI (1996). Non–insulin-dependent diabetes mellitus: A genetically programmed failure of the beta cell to compensate for insulin resistance. N Engl J Med 334: 777–783.

32. Permutt MA, Chiu K, Ferrer J, et al. (1998). Genetics of type 2 diabetes. Recent Prog Horm Res 53: 201–216.

33. Kahn BB (1998). Type 2 diabetes: When insulin secretion fails to compensate for insulin resistance. Cell 92: 593–596.

34. Saltiel AR (2001). New perspectives into the molecular pathogenesis and treatment of type 2 diabetes. Cell 104:517–529.

35. Almind K, Doria A, Kahn CR (2001). Putting the genes for type 2 diabetes on the map. Nat Med 7:277–279.

36. Froguel P, Velho G (2001). Genetic determinants of type 2 diabetes. Recent Prog Horm Res 56:91–105.

37. Bergman RN, Ader M (2000). Free fatty acids and pathogenesis of type 2 diabetes mellitus. Trends Endocrinol Metab 11:351–356.

38. Duggirala R, Blangero J, Almasy L, et al. (2001). A major locus for fasting insulin concentrations and insulin resistance on chromosome 6q with strong pleiotropic effects on obesity-related phenotypes in nondiabetic Mexican-Americans. Am J Hum Genet 68:1149–1164.

39. Flier JS (2001). Diabetes: The missing link with obesity? Nature 409:292–293.

40. Unger RH, Zhou YT (2001). Lipotoxicity of beta-cells in obesity and in other causes of fatty acid spillover. Diabetes 50(1):S118–S121.

41. Sladek R, Rocheleau G, Rung J, et al. (2007). A genome-wide association study identifies novel risk loci for type 2 diabetes. Nature 445:881–885.

42. Schranz DB, Bekris L, Landin-Olsson M, et al. (2000). Newly diagnosed latent autoimmune diabetes in adults (LADA) is associated with low level glutamate decarboxylase (GAD65) and IA-2 autoantibodies. Horm Metab Res 32:133–138.

43. Libman IM, Becker DJ (2003). Coexistence of type 1 and type 2 diabetes mellitus: "Double" diabetes? Pediatr Diabetes 4:110–113.

44. Lipman TH, Jawad AF, Murphy KM, et al. (2006). Incidence of type 1 diabetes in Philadelphia is higher in black than white children from 1995 to 1999. Epidemic or misclassification? Diabetes Care 29:2391–2395.

45. The DIAMOND Project Group (2006). Incidence and trends of Childhood type 1 diabetes worldwide 1990–1999. Diabetic Medicine 23:857–866.

46. EURODIAB Study Group (2000). Variation and trends in incidence of childhood diabetes in Europe. Lancet 355:873–876.

47. Libman IM, LaPorte RE (2005). Changing trends in epidemiology of type 1 diabetes mellitus throughout the world: How far have we come and where do we go from here? Pediatric Diabetes 6:119–121.

48. Soltesz G, Patterson CC, Dahlquist G, et al. (2007). Worldwide childhood type 1 diabetes incidence: What can we learn from epidemiology? Pediatric Diabetes 8:6–14.

49. Libman IM, LaPorte RE, Becker DJ, et al. (1998). Was there an epidemic of diabetes in nonwhite adolescents in Allegheny County, Pennsylvania? Diabetes Care 21:1278–1281.

50. Pinhas-Hamiel O, Zeitler P (2007). Acute and chronic complications of type 2 diabetes mellitus in children and adolescents. Lancet 369: 1823–1831.

51. Hathout EH, Sharkey J, Racine M, et al. (2000). Diabetic autoimmunity in infants and pre-schoolers with type 1 diabetes. Pediatr Diabetes 1:131–134.

52. Imagawa A, Hanafusa T, Miyagawa JI, et al. (2000). A novel sub-type of type 1 diabetes mellitus characterized by a rapid onset and an absence of diabetes-related antibodies. N Engl J Med 342: 301–307.

53. Urakami T, Inami I, Morimoto S, et al. (2002). Clinical characteristics of non-immune-mediated, idiopathic type 1 (Type 1B) diabete mellitus in Japanese children and adolescents. J Pediatr Endocrinol Metab 15:283–288.

54. Knip M, Veijola R, Virtanen SM, et al. (2005). Enviromental triggers and determints of type 1 diabetes. Diabetes 54(2):S125–S136.

55. Menser MA, Forrest JM, Bransby RD (1978). Rubella infection and diabetes mellitus. Lancet 1:57–60.

56. Ou D, Mitchell LA, Metzger DL, et al. (2000). Cross-reactive rubella virus and glutamic acid decarboxylase (65 and 67) protein determinants recognized by T cells of patients with type 1 diabetes mellitus. Diabetologia 43:750–762.

57. Yoon JW, Austin M, Onodera T, Notkins AL (1979). Isolation of a virus from the pancreas of a child with diabetic ketoacidosis. N Engl J Med 300:1173–1179.

58. The TEDDY Study Group (2007). The Environmental Determinants of Diabetes in the Young (TEDDY) study: Study design. Pediatr Diabetes 8:286–298.

59. Hiemstra HS, Schloot NC, van Veelen PA, et al. (2001). Cytomegalovirus in autoimmunity: T cell cross reactivity to viral antigen and autoantigen glutamic acid decarboxylase. Proc Natl Acad Sci USA 98:3988–3991.

60. Lammi N, Karvonen M, Tuomilehto J (2005). Do microbes have a casual role in type 1 diabetes? Med Sci Monit 11:RA63–RA69.

61. Khalil I, d'Auriol L, Gobet M, et al. (1990). A combination of HLA-DQ beta Asp57-negative and HLA-DQ alpha ARG52 confers susceptibility to insulin-dependent diabetes mellitus. J Clin Invest 85:1315–1319.

62. Deng GY, Muir A, Maclaren NK, She JX (1995). Association of LMP2 and LMP7 genes within the major histocompatibility complex with insulin-dependent diabetes mellitus. Am J Hum Genet 56:528–534.

63. Loew CE, Cooper JD, Brusko T, et al. (2007). Large-scale genetic fine mapping and genotype-phenotype association implicates polymorphism in the IL2RA region in type 1 diabetes. Nat Genet 39:1074–1082.

64. Friday RP, Trucco M, Pietropaolo M (1999). Genetics of type 1 diabetes mellitus. Diabetes Nutr Metab 12:3–26.

65. Kulmala P, Rahko J, Savola K, et al. (2001). Beta-cell autoimmunity, genetic susceptibility, and progression to type 1 diabetes in unaffected schoolchildren. Diabetes Care 24:171–173.

66. Reed P, Cucca F, Jenkins S, et al. (1997). Evidence for a type 1 diabetes susceptibility locus (IDDM10) on human chromosome 10p11-q11. Hum Mol Genet 6:1011–1016.

67. Ilonen J, Reijonen H, Green A, et al. for the Childhood Diabetes in Finland Study Group. (2000). Geographical differences within Finland in the frequency of HLA-DQ genotypes associated with type 1 diabetes susceptibility. Eur J Immunogenet 27:225–230.

68. Concannon P, Erlich HA, Julier C (2005). Type 1 diabetes: Evidence for susceptibility loci from four genome-wide linkage scans in 1,435 multiplex families. Diabetes 54: 2995–3001.

69. Nejentsev S, Smink LJ, Smyth D, et al. (2007). Sequencing and association analysis of the type 1 diabetes-linked region on chromosome 10p12-q11. BMC Genet 8:24.

70. Payne F, Cooper JD, Walker NM, et al. (2007). Interaction analysis of the CBLB and CTLA4 genes in type 1 diabetes. J Leukoc Biol 81:581–583.

71. Taniguchi H, Lowe CE, Cooper JD, et al. (2006). Discovery, linkage disequilibrium and association analyses of polymorphisms of the immune complement inhibitor, decay-accelerating factor gene (DAF/CD55) in type 1 diabetes. BMC Genet 7:22.

72. Todd JA (2006). Statistical false positive or true disease pathway? Nat Genet 38:731–733.

73. Dorman J, LaPorte R, Stone R, Trucco M (1990). Worldwide differences in the incidence of type 1 diabetes are associated with amino acid variation at position 57 of the HLA-DQ beta chain. Proc Natl Acad Sci USA 87:7370–7374.

74. Allen C, Palta M, D'Alessio DJ (1991). Risk of diabetes in siblings and other relatives of IDDM subjects. Diabetes 40:83–86.

75. Siljander HT, Veijola R, Reunanen A, et al. (2007). Prediction of type 1 diabetes among siblings of affected children and in the general population. Diabetologia (E-pub ahead of print).

76. Skyler JS (2007). Prediction and prevention of type 1 diabetes: Progress, problems and prospects. Clin Pharmacol Ther 81: 768–771.

77. van der Werf N, Kroese FG, Rozing J, Hillebrands JL (2007). Viral infections as potential triggers of type 1 diabetes. Diabetes Metab Res Rev 23:169–183.

78. Sonderstrup G, McDevitt HO (2001). DR, DQ, and you: MHC alleles and autoimmunity. J Clin Invest 107:795–796.

79. Karjalainen J, Martin JM, Knip M, et al. (1992). A bovine albumin peptide as a possible trigger of insulin-dependent diabetes mellitus. N Engl J Med 327:302–307.

80. Atkinson MA, Bowman MA, Kao KJ, et al. (1993). Lack of immune responsiveness to bovine serum albumin in insulin-dependent diabetes. N Engl J Med 329:1853–1858.

81. Norris JM, Beaty B, Klingensmith G, Yu Liping, et al. for the Diabetes Autoimmunity Study in the Young (DAISY) (1996). Lack of association between early exposure to cow's milk protein and beta-cell autoimmunity. JAMA 276:609–614.

82. Vaarala O (2006). Is it dietary insulin? Ann NY Acad Sci 1079: 350–359.

83. Knip M (2003). Cow's milk antibodies in patients with newly diagnosed type 1 diabetes: Primary or secondary? Pediatr Diabetes 4:155–156.

84. Tiittanen M, Paronen J, Savilahti E, Virtanen SM, et al. (2006). Dietary insulin as an immunogen and tolerogen. Pediatr Allergy Immunol 17:538–543.

85. Symon DN, Hennessy ER, Smail PJ (1984). Smoked foods in the diets of mothers of diabetic children. Lancet 2:514.

86. Hathout EH, Beeson WL, Nahab F, Rabadi A, et al. (2002). Role of exposure to air pollutants in the development of type 1 diabetes before and after 5 yr of age. Pediatr Diabetes 3:184–188.

87. Maclaren N, Lan M, Coutant R, et al. (1999). Only multiple autoantibodies to islet cells (ICA), insulin, GAD65, IA-2 and IA-2 beta predict immune-mediated (type 1) diabetes in relatives. J Autoimmun 12:279.

88. Pietropaolo M, Yu S, Libman IM, Pietroapolo SL, et al. (2005). Cytoplasmic islet cell antibodies remain valuable in defining risk of progression to type 1 diabetes in subjects with other islet autoantibodies. Pediatr Diabetes 6:184–192.

89. Knip M (1998). Prediction and prevention of type 1 diabetes. Acta Paediatr Suppl 425:54.

90. Sibley RK, Sutherland DE, Goetz F, Michael AF (1985). Recurrent diabetes mellitus in the pancreas iso- and allograft: A light and electron microscopic and immunohistochemical analysis of four cases. Lab Invest 53:132–144.

91. Pietropaolo M, Becker DJ (2001). Type 1 diabetes intervention trials. Pediatr Diabetes 2:2.

92. Lipton RB (2001). Is now the time for an intervention to prevent autoimmune type 1 diabetes? Pediatr Diabetes 2:12.

93. Verge CF, Gianani R, Kawasaki E, et al. (1996). Prediction of type 1 diabetes in first-degree relatives using a combination of insulin, GAD, and ICA512bdc/IA-s autoantibodies. Diabetes 45:926.

94. Wilson DM, Buckingham B (2001). Prevention of type 1a diabetes mellitus. Pediatr Diabetes 2:17.

95. Conrad B, Trucco M (1994). Superantigens as etiopathogenetic factors in the development of insulin-dependent diabetes mellitus. Diabetes Metab Rev 10:309.

96. Keller RJ, Eisenbarth GS, Jackson RA (1993). Insulin prophylaxis in individuals at high risk of type 1 diabetes. Lancet 341:927.

97. Diabetes Prevention Trial – Type 1 Diabetes Study Group (2002). Effects of insulin in relatives of patients with type 1 diabetes mellitus. N Engl J Med 346:1685–1691.

98. Gale EA (2002). Can we change the course of beta-cell destruction in type 1 diabetes? N Engl J Med 346:1740–1742.

99. Gale EA, Bingley PJ, Emmett CL, Collier T, et al. (2004). European Nicotinamide Diabetes Intervention Trial (ENDIT): A randomized controlled trial of intervention before the onset of type 1 diabetes. The Lancet 363:925–931.

100. Wang PH (2004). Commentary: Growing pains in the pursuit of diabetes prevention. The Lancet 363:901.

101. Barker JM, Eisenbarth GS (2007). Primary prevention of type 1A diabetes: Are we there yet? Pediatr Diabetes 8:115–116.

102. Barker JM, McFann KK, Orban T (2007). Effect of oral insulin on insulin autoantibody levels in the Diabetes Prevention Trial Type 1 oral insulin study. Diabetologia 50:1603–1606.

103. The TRIGR Study Group (2007). Study design of the Trial to reduce IDDM in the Genetically at Risk (TRIGR). Pediatric Diabetes 8:117–137.

104. Gruppuso PA, Gorden P, Kahn CR, et al. (1984). Familial hyperproinsulinemia due to a proposed defect in conversion of proinsulin to insulin. N Engl J Med 311:629–634.

105. Tager HS (1984). Abnormal products of the human insulin gene. Diabetes 33:693–699.

106. O'Rahilly S, Gray H, Humphreys PJ, et al. (1995). Impaired processing of prohormones associated with abnormalities of glucose homeostasis and adrenal function. N Engl J Med 333:1386–1390.

107. Gabbay KH (1980). The insulinopathies. N Eng J Med 302: 165–167.

108. Steiner DF, Tager HS, Chan SJ, et al. (1990). Lessons learned from molecular biology of insulin-gene mutations. Diabetes Care 13:600–609.

109. Steiner DF (2004). The proinsulin C-peptide: A multirole model. Exp Diabesity Res 5:7–14.

110. Steiner DF, James DE (1992). Cellular and molecular biology of the beta cell. Diabetologia 35(2):S41–S48.

111. Jackson RS, Creemers JWM, Ohagi S, et al. (1997). Obesity and impaired prohormone processing associated with mutations in the human prohormone convertase 1 gene. Nat Genet 16:30–63.

112. Boitard C, Efendic S, Ferrannini E, et al. (2005). A tale of two cousins: Type 2 and type 2 diabetes. Diabetes 54(2):S1–S3.

113. Wardlaw SL (2001). Obesity as a neuroendrocrine disease: Lessons to be learned from pro-opiomelanocortin and melanocortin receptor mutations in mice and men. J Clin Endocrinol Metab 86:1442–1446.

114. Nanjo K, Miyano M, Kondo M, et al. (1987). Insulin Wakayama: Familial mutant insulin syndrome in Japan. Diabetologia 30:87–92.

115. Polonsky KS, Licinio-Paixae J, Given BD, et al. (1986). Use of biosynthetic human C-peptide in the measurement of insulin secretion rates in normal volunteers and type 1 diabetic patients. J Clin Invest 77:98–105.

116. Takasawa S, Nata K, Yonekura H, et al. (1993). Cyclic ADP-ribose in insulin secretion from pancreatic beta-cells. Science 259: 370–373.

117. Felig P, Wahren J, Sherwin R, et al. (1976). Insulin, glucagon, and somatostatin in normal physiology and diabetes mellitus. Diabetes 25:1091–1099.

118. Unger RH, Orci L (1981). Glucagon and the A cell: Physiology and pathophysiology. N Engl J Med 304:1575–1580.

119. Woods SC, Porte D Jr. (1974). Neural control of the endocrine pancreas. Physiol Rev 54:596–619.

120. Ashcroft FM (2005). ATP-sensitive potassium channelopathies: Focus on insulin secretion. J Clin Invest 115:2047–2058.

121. Seaquist ER, Walseth TF, Redmon JB (1994). G protein regulation of insulin secretion. J Lab Clin Med 123:338–345.

122. Wallace TM, Matthews DR (2000). Assessment of the effects of insulin secretagogues in humans. Diabetes Obes Metab 2:271–283.

123. McClenaghan NH, Flatt PR (1999). Physiological and pharmacological regulation of insulin release: Insights offered through exploitation of insulin-secreting cell lines. Diabetes Obes Metab 1:137–150.

124. Aguilar-Bryan L, Nichols CB, Wechsler SW (1995). Cloning of the beta cell high-affinity sulfonylurea receptor: A regulator of insulin secretion. Science 268:423–426.

125. Philipson LH, Steiner DF (1995). Pas de deux or more: The sulfonylurea receptor and K^1 channels. Science 268:372–373.

126. Thomas PM, Cote GJ, Wohlik N, et al. (1995). Mutations in the sulfo-nylurea receptor gene in familial persistent hyperinsulinemic hypoglycemia of infancy. Science 268:426–429.

127. Liang Y, Matschinsky FM (1994). Mechanisms of action of nonglucose insulin secretagogues. Annu Rev Nutr 14:59–81.

128. Drucker DJ, Nauck MA (2006). The incretin system: glucagon-like peptide-1 receptor agonists and dipeptidase-4 inhibitors in type 2 diabetes. Lancet 368:1696–1705.

129. Amori RE, Lau J, Pittas AG (2007). Efficacy and safety of incretin therapy in type 2 diabetes: Systematic review and meta-analysis. JAMA 298:194–205.

130. Porte A, Baskin DG, Schwartz MW (2005). Insulin signaling in the central nervous system: A critical role in metabolic homeostasis and disease from C. elegans to humans. Diabetes 54:1264–1276.

131. Cheatham B, Kahn CR (1995). Insulin action and the insulin signaling network. Endocr Rev 16:117–142.

132. Kido Y, Nakae J, Accili D (2001). Clinical review 125: The insulin receptor and its cellular targets. J Clin Endocrinol Metab 86: 972–979.

133. Bevan P (2001). Insulin signaling. J Cell Sci 114:1429–1430.

134. Taniguchi CM, Emanuelli B, Kahn CR (2006). Critical nodes in signalling pathways: insights into insulin action. Nat Rev Mol Cell Bio 7:85–96.

135. Bruning JC, Gautam D, Burks DJ, et al. (2000). Role of brain insulin receptor in control of body weight and reproduction. Science 289:2122–2125.

136. Biddinger SB, Kahn CR (2006). From mice to men: Insights into the insulin resistance syndromes. Annu Rev Physiol 68:123–158.

137. Brady MJ, Saltiel AR (2001). The role of protein phosphatase-1 in insulin action. Recent Prog Horm Res 56:157–173.

138. Chang L, Chiang SH, Saltiel AR (2004). Insulin signaling and the regulation of glucose transport. Mol Med 10:65–71.

139. Rizza RA, Mandarino LJ, Gerich JE (1981). Dose-response characteristics for effects of insulin on production and utilization of glucose in man. Am J Physiol 240:E630–E639.

140. Schade DS, Eaton RP (1980). The temporal relationship between endogenously secreted stress hormones and metabolic decompensation in diabetic man. J Clin Endocrinol Metab 50:131–136.

141. Wolfsdorf J, Glaser N, Sperling M for the American Diabetes Association (2006). Diabetes Ketoacidosis in infants, children and adolescents: A consenus statement from the American Diabetes Association. Diabetes Care 29:1150–1159.

142. Wolfsdorf J, Craig ME, Daneman D, et al. (2007). Diabetes ketoacidosis. Pediatr Diabetes 8:28–43.

143. Foster DW, McGarry JD (1983). The metabolic derangements and treatment of diabetic ketoacidosis. N Engl J Med 309:159–169.

144. Glaser N, Barnett P, McCaslin I, et al. (2001). Risk factors for cerebral edema in children with diabetic ketoacidosis. N Engl J Med 344:264–269.

145. Glaser N (2006). New perspectives on the pathogenesis of cerebral edema complicating diabetic ketoacidosis in children. Pediatr Endocrinol Rev 3:379–386.

146. Sperling MA (2006). Cerebral edema in diabetes ketoacidosis: An underestimated complication? Pediatr Diabetes 7:73–74.

147. Cody D (2007). Infant and toddler diabetes. Arch Dis Child 92:716–719.

148. Rosenbloom AL (2005). Hyperglycemic comas in children: New insights into pathophysiology and management. Rev Endocr Metab Disord 6:297–306.

149. Fourtner SH, Weinzimer SA, Levitt Katz LE (2005). Hyperglycemic hyperosmolar non-ketotic syndrome in children with type 2 diabetes. Pediatr Diabetes 6:129–135.

150. Rosenbloom AL (2007). Hyperglycemia crises and their complications in children. J Pediatr Endocrinol Metab 20:5–18.

151. Adrogue HJ, Wilson H, Boyd AE, et al. (1982). Plasma acid-base patterns in diabetic ketoacidosis. N Engl J Med 307:1603–1610.

152. Arieff AI (1989). Pathogenesis of lactic acidosis. Diabetes Metab Rev 5:637–649.

153. Assadi FK, John EG, Fornell MT, et al. (1982). Falsely elevated serum creatinine concentration in ketoacidosis. J Pediatr 107:562–564.

154. White NH (2000). Diabetic ketoacidosis in children. Endocrinol Metab Clin North Am 29:657–682.

155. Halperin ML, Maccari C, Kamel KS, et al. (2006). Strategies to diminish the danger of cerebral edema in a pediatric patient presenting with diabetes ketoacidosis. Pediatr Diabetes 7:191–195.

156. Hoorn EJ, Carlotti AP, Costa LA, et al. (2007). Preventing a drop in effective plasma osmolality to minmize the likelihood of cerebral edema during treatment of children with diabetes ketoacidosis. J Pediatr 150:467–473.

157. Rosenbloom AL (1990). Intracerebral crisis during treatment of diabetic ketoacidosis. Diabetes Care 13:22–33.

158. Bello FA, Sotos JF (1990). Cerebral edema in diabetic ketoacidosis in children. Lancet 336:64.

159. Carlotti AP, Bohn D, Jankiewicz N, et al. (2007). A hyperglycaemic hyperosmolar state in a young child: Diagnostic insights from a quantitative analysis. QJM 100:125–137.

160. Muir AB, Quisling RG, Yang MC, et al. (2004). Cerebral edema in childhood diabetis ketoacidosis: Natural history, radiographic findings and early identification. Diabetes Care 27:1541–1546.

161. Krane EJ, Rockoff MA, Wallman JK, et al. (1985). Subclinical brain swelling in children during treatment of diabetic ketoacidosis. N Engl J Med 312:1147.

162. Rosenbloom AL, Finberg L, Muir A (2000). Cerebral edema in diabetic ketoacidosis. J Clin Endocrinol Metab 85:507–513.

163. Clements RS Jr., Blumenthal SA, Morrison AD, Winegrad AI (1971). Increased cerebrospinal-fluid pressure during treatment of diabetic ketosis. Lancet 2:671–675.

164. Winter RJ, Harris CJ, Phillips LS, et al. (1979). Diabetic ketoacidosis: Induction of hypocalcemia and hypomagnesemia by phosphate therapy. Am J Med 67:897–900.

165. Dunger DB, Sperling MA, Acerini CL, et al. (2004). ESPE/LWPES consensus statement on diabetic ketoacidosis in children and adolescents. Arch Dis Child 89:188–194.

166. Latif KA, Freire AX, Kitabchi AE, et al. (2002). The use of alkali therapy in severe diabetic ketoacidosis. Diabetes Care 25:2113–2114.

167. Schade DS, Eaton RP (1977). Dose response to insulin in man: Differential effects on glucose and ketone body regulation. J Clin Endocrinol Metab 44:1038–1053.

168. Diabetes Control and Complications Trial Research Group (1993). The effect of intensive treatment of diabetes on the development and progression of long-term complications in insulin-dependent diabetes mellitus. N Engl J Med 329:977–986.

169. Diabetes Control and Complications Trial Research Group (1994). Effect of intensive diabetes treatment on the development and progression of long-term complications in adolescents with insulin-dependent diabetes mellitus: Diabetes Control and Complications Trial. J Pediatr 125:177–188.

170. White NH, Cleary PA, Dahms W, Goldstein D, Malone J, Tamborlane WV (2001). Diabetes Control and Complications Trial (DCCT) / Epidemiology of Diabetes Interventions and Complications (EDIC) Research Group. Beneficial effects of intensive therapy of diabetes during adolescence: Outcomes after the conclusion of the Diabetes Control and Complications Trial (DCCT). J Pediatr 139:804–812.

171. Springer D, Dziura J, Tamborlane WV, Steffen AT, Ahern JH, Vincent M, et al. (2006). Optimal control of type 1 diabetes in youth receiving intensive treatment. J Pediatr 149:227–232.

172. Grey M, Boland EA, Davidson M, Li J, Tamborlane WV (2000). Coping skills training for youth on intensive therapy has long lasting effects on metabolic control and quality of life. J Pediatr 137:107–114.

173. Tamborlane WV, Bonfig W, Boland E (2001). Recent advances in the treatment of youth with type 1 diabetes: Better care through technology. Diabetic Medicine 18:864–870.

174. Andersen JH Jr., Brunelle RL, Koivisto VA, Trautmann ME, Vignati L, DiMarchi R for the Multicenter Insulin Lispro Study Group (1997). Improved mealtime treatment of diabetes mellitus using an insulin analogue. Clin Ther 19:62–71.

175. Zinman B, Tildesley H, Chiasson JL, Tsui E, Strack T (1997). Insulin lispro in CSII, results of a double-blind study. Diabetes 46:440–443.

176. Raskin P, Guthrie RA, Leiter L, Riis A, Jovanovic L (2000). Use of insulin aspart, a fast-acting insulin analog, as the mealtime insulin in the management of patients with type 1 diabetes. Diabetes Care 23:583–588.

177. Howey DC, Bowsher RR, Brunelle RL, Woodworth JR (1994). [Lys(B28),Pro(B29)]-human insulin: A rapidly absorbed analogue of human insulin. Diabetes 43:396–402.

178. Vajo Z, Fawcett J, Duckworth WC (2001). Recombinant DNA technology in the treatment of diabetes: Insulin analogs. Endocr Rev 22: 706–717.

179. Heise T, Nosek L, Ronn BB, Endahl L, Heinemann L, Kapitza C, et al. (2004). Lower within-subject variability of insulin detemir in comparison to NPH insulin and insulin glargine in people with type 1 diabetes. Diabetes 53:1614–1620.

180. Lepore M, Pampanelli S, Fanelli C, Porcellati F, Bartocci L, Di Vincenzo A, et al. (2000). Pharmacokinetics and pharmacodynamics of subcutaneous injection of long-acting human insulin analog glargine, NPH insulin, and ultralente human insulin and continuous subcutaneous infusion of insulin lispro. Diabetes 49:2142–2148.

181. Schober E, Schoenle E, Van Dyk J, Wernicke-Panten K, for the Pediatric Study Group of Insulin Glargine (2002). Comparative trial between insulin glargine and NPH insulin in children and adolescents with type 1 diabetes mellitus. J Pediatr Endocrinol Metab 15:369–376.

182. Murphy NP, Keane SM, Ong KK, Ford-Adams M, Edge JA, Acerini CL, et al. (2003). Randomized cross-over trial of insulin glargine plus lispro or NPH insulin plus regular human insulin in adolescents with type 1 diabetes on intensive insulin regimens. Diabetes Care 26:799–804.

183. Porcellati F, Rossetti P, Busciantella NR, Marzotti S, Lucidi P, Luzio S, et al. (2007). Comparison of pharmacokinetics and dynamics of

the long-acting insulin analogs glargine and detemir at steady state in type 1 diabetes: a double-blind, randomized, crossover study. Diabetes Care 30:2447–2452.

184. Tamborlane WV, Sherwin RS, Genel M, Felig P (1979). Reduction to normal of plasma glucose in juvenile diabetics by subcutaneous administration of insulin with a portable infusion pump. N Engl J Med 300:573–578.

185. Pickup JC, Keen H, Parsons JA, Alberti KG (1978). Continuous subcutaneous insulin infusion: an approach to achieving normoglycemia. Br Med J 1:204–207.

186. Weinzimer S, Doyle EA, Steffen AT, Sikes KA, Tamborlane WV (2004). Rediscovery of insulin pump treatment of childhood type 1 diabetes. Minerva Medica 95:85–92.

187. Sikes KA, Ahern J, Weinzimer SA, Tamborlane WV (2005). Practical aspects of insulin pump therapy in children with diabetes mellitus: The Yale experience. Infusystems USA 4:25–28.

188. Boland EA, Grey M, Fredrickson L, Tamborlane WV (1999). CSII: A "new" way to achieve strict metabolic control, decrease severe hypoglycemia and enhance coping in adolescents with type I diabetes. Diabetes Care 22:1779–1894.

189. Ahern JA, Boland EA, Doane R, Ahern JJ, Rose P, Vincent M, et al. (2002). Insulin pump therapy in pediatrics: A therapeutic alternative to safely lower therapy HbA1c levels across all age groups. Pediatric Diabetes 3:10–15.

190. Weinzimer SA, Ahern JH, Doyle EA, Dzuria J, Steffen AL, Tamborlane WV (2004). Persistence of benefits of continuous subcutaneous insulin infusion (CSII) in very young children with type 1 diabetes mellitus. Pediatrics 114:1601–1605.

191. Attia N, Jones TW, Holcombe J, Tamborlane WV (1998). Comparison of human regular and lispro insulins after interruption of continuous subcutaneous insulin infusion and in the treatment of acutely decompensated IDDM. Diabetes Care 21:817–821.

192. Doyle EA, Weinzimer SA, Steffen AL, Ahern JH, Vincent M, Tamborlane WV (2004). A randomized, prospective trial comparing continuous subcutaneous insulin infusion and with multiple daily injections using insulin glargine in youth with type 1 diabetes mellitus. Diabetes Care 27:1554–1558.

193. Weinzimer SA, Tamborlane WV (2006). Diabetes mellitus in children and adolescents. In Fonseca V (ed.), Clinical diabetes. [city]: Saunders Elsevier 505–521.

194. Edge JA, Matthews DR, Dunger DB (1990). The dawn phenomenon is related to overnight growth hormone release in adolescent diabetics. Clin Endocrinol 33:729–737.

195. Chase HP, Dixon B, Pearson J, Fiallo-Scharer R, Walravens P, Klingensmith G, et al. (2003). Reduced hypoglycemic episodes and improved glycemic control in children with type 1 diabetes using insulin glargine and neutral protamine Hagedorn insulin. J Pediatr 143:737–740.

196. Kaplan W, Rodriguez LM, Smith OE, Haymond MW, Heptulla RA (2004). Effects of mixing glargine and short-acting insulin analogs on glucose control. Diabetes Care 27:2739–2740.

197. The Diabetes Research in Children Network Study Group (2005). Accuracy of newer generation home blood glucose meters in a Diabetes Research in Children Network (DirecNet) inpatient exercise study. Diabetes Technol Ther 7:675–680.

198. Bina DM, Anderson RL, Johnson ML, Bergenstal RM, Kendall DM (2003). Clinical impact of prandial state, exercise, and site preparation on the equivalence of alternative-site blood glucose testing. Diabetes Care 26:981–985.

199. Amiel SA, Sherwin RS, Simonson DC, Lauritano AA, Tamborlane WV (1986). Impaired insulin action in puberty: A contributing factor to poor glycemic control in adolescents with diabetes. N Engl J Med 315:215–219.

200. Weinzimer S, Doyle EA, Steffen AT, Sikes KA, Tamborlane WV (2004). Rediscovery of insulin pump treatment of childhood type 1 diabetes. Minerva Medica 95:85–92.

201. The Diabetes Research in Children Network Study Group (2005). A randomized multicenter trial comparing the GlucoWatch Biographer with standard glucose monitoring in children with type 1 diabetes. Diabetes Care 1101–1106.

202. Weinzimer S, Tamborlane WV, Chase HP, Garg SK (2004). Continuous glucose monitoring and new insulin regimens in type 1 diabetes. Current Diabetes Reports 4:95–100.

203. Boland EA, DeLucia M, Brandt C, Grey MJ, Tamborlane WV (2001). Limitations of conventional methods of self blood glucose monitoring: Lessons learned from three days of continuous glucose monitoring in pediatric patients with type I diabetes. Diabetes Care 24: 1858–1862.

204. The Diabetes Research in Children Network Study Group (2007). Positive impact of FreeStyle Navigator continuous glucose sensor use in children with type 1 DM. J Pediatr 151:388–393.

205. The Diabetes Research in Children Network Study Group (2007). The accuracy of the Freestyle Navigator continuous glucose sensor in the inpatient and outpatient setting in children with type 1 diabetes. Diabetes Care 30:59–64.

206. Tamborlane WV (2006). Fulfilling the promise of insulin pump treatment in childhood diabetes. Pediatric Diabetes 7(4):4–10.

207. Rewers A, McFann K, Chase HP (2006). Bedside monitoring of blood beta-hydroxybutyrate levels in the management of diabetic ketoacidosis in children. Diabetes Technol & Ther 8:671–676.

208. Gregory RP, Davis DL (1994). Use of carbohydrate counting for meal planning in type 1 diabetes. Diabetes Educator 20:406.

209. Aslander-van Vliet, Smart C, Waldron S (2007). Nutrition management of childhood and adolescent diabetes. Pediatric Diabetes 8:323–339.

210. American Diabetes Association Task Force for Writing Nutrition Principles and Recommendations for the Management of Diabetes and Related Complications (2002). American Diabetes Association position statement: Evidence-based nutrition principles and recommendations for the treatment and prevention of diabetes and related complications. J Amer Diet Assoc 102:109.

211. Sandoval DA, Guy DLA, Richardson MA, Ertl AC, Davis SN (2004). Effects of low and moderate exercise on counterregulatory responses to subsequent hypoglycemia in type 1 diabetes. Diabetes 53:1798–1806.

212. The Diabetes Research in Children Network Study Group (2005). Impact of exercise on overnight glycemic control in children with type 1 diabetes. J Pediatr 147:528–534.

213. McMahon SK, Ferreira LD, Davey RJ, Youngs LM, Davis EA, Fournier PA, et al. (2007). Glucose requirements to maintain euglycemia following moderate intensity afternoon exercise in adolescents with type 1 diabetes are increased in a biphasic manner. J Clin Endocrinol Metab 92:963–968.

214. Tamborlane WV (2007). Triple jeopardy for hypoglycemia on nights following exercise in youth with type 1 diabetes. J Clin Endocrinol Metab 92:815–816.

215. The DCCT Research Group (1987). Effects of age, duration and treatment of IDDM on residual ß-cell function: A study of the DCCT population. J Clin Endocrinol Metab 65:30–36.

216. The DCCT Research Group (1998). The effect of intensive diabetes treatment in the DCCT on residual insulin secretion in IDDM. Ann Int Med 28:517–523.

217. Herold KC, Hagopian W, Auger JA, Poumian-Ruiz E, Taylor L, Donaldson D, et al. (2002). Anti-CD3 monoclonal antibody in new-onset type 1 diabetes mellitus. N Engl J Med 346:1692–1698.

218. American Diabetes Association Workgroup on Hypoglycemia (2005). Defining and reporting hypoglycemia in Diabetes. Diabetes Care 28:1245–1249.

219. Jones TW, Boulware SD, Kraemer DT, Caprio S, Sherwin RS, Tamborlane WV (1991). Independent effects of youth and poor diabetes control on responses to hypoglycemia in children. Diabetes 40:358–363.

220. Ryan C, Gurtunca N, Becker D (2005). Hypoglycemia: A complication of diabetes therapy in children. Pediatr Clin N Am 52:1705–1733.

221. Cryer PE (2005). Mechanisms of hypoglycemia-associated autonomic failure and its component syndromes in diabetes. Diabetes 54:3592–3601.

222. Cryer PE (2004). Diverse causes of hypoglycemia-associated autonomic failure in diabetes. N Engl J Med 350:2272–2279.

223. Jones TW, Porter P, Sherwin RS, Davis EA, O'Leary P, Frazer F, et al. (1998). Decreased epinephrine responses to hypoglycemia during sleep. N Engl J Med 338:1657–1662.

224. Kordonouri O, Klinghammer A, Lang EB, et al. (2002). Thyroid autoimmunity in children and adolescents with type 1 diabetes. Diabetes Care 25:1346–1350.

225. Freemark M, Levitsky LL (2003). Screening for celiac disease in children with type 1 diabetes: Two views of the controversy. Diabetes Care 26:1932–1939.

226. Delamater AM (2007). Psychological care of children and adolescents with diabetes: ISPAD Clinical Practice Consensus Guidelines 2006–2007. Pediatric Diabetes 8:340–348.

227. Kovacs M, Kass RE, Schnell TM, et al. (1989). Family functioning and metabolic control of school-aged children with IDDM. Diabetes Care 12:409.

228. Silverstein J, Klingensmith G, Copeland K, Plotnick L, Kaufman F, Deeb L, et al. (2005). Care of children and adolescents with type 1 diabetes: A statement of the American Diabetes Association. Diabetes Care 28:186–212.

229. Griffin ME, Feder A, Tamborlane WV (2001). Lipoatrophy associated with lispro insulin in insulin pump therapy: An old complication, a new cause? Diabetes Care 24:174.

230. The Diabetes Research in Children Network Study Group (2005). Comparison of A1c levels assayed by the DCA 2000 and the DCCT/EDIC Central Laboratory: A Diabetes Research in Children Network study. Pediatric Diabetes 6:13–16.

231. Update on the 1987 task force report on high blood pressure in children and adolescents: A working group report for the national high blood pressure education program. 1996 Pediatrics 98: 649–657.

232. Huo B, Steffen AT, Swan K, Sikes K, Weinzimer SA, Tamborlane WV (2007). Clinical outcomes and cost-effectiveness of retinopathy screening in youth with type 1 diabetes mellitus. Diabetes Care 30:362–363.

233. Rhodes ET, Ferrari LR, Wolsdorf JI (2005). Perioperative management of pediatric surgical patients with diabetes mellitus. Anesth Analg 101:986–999.

234. Betts P, Brink SJ, Swift PGF, Silink M, Wolfsdorf J, Hanas R (2007). Management of children with diabetes requiring surgery. Pediatric Diabetes 8:242–247.

235. Iserman B, Ritzel R, Zorn M, et al. (2007). Autoantibodies in diabetes mellitus: Current utility and perspectives. Exp Clin Endocrinol Diabetes 115:483–490.

236. Barrett TG (2007). Differential diagnosis of type 1 diabetes: Which genetic syndrome need to be considered? Pediatric Diabetes 8:15–23.

237. Libman IM, Arslanian SA (2007). Prevention and treatment of type 2 diabetes in youth. Horm Res 67:22–24.

238. Gungor N, Hannon T, Libman, et al. (2005). Type 2 diabetes mellitus in youth: The complete picture to date. Pediatr Clin A Am 1579–1609.

239. Weiss R, Caprio S (2006). Altered glucose metabolism in obese youth. Pediatric Endocrinol Rev 3:233–238.

240. Savoye M, Shaw M, Dziura J, et al. (2007). Effects of a weight management program on body composition and metabolic parameters in overweight children: A randomized controlled trial. JAMA 297:2697–2704.

241. Weiss R, Dziura J, Burgert TS, et al. (2004). Obesity and the metabolic syndrome in children and adolescents. N Engl J Med 350:2362–2374.

242. Weiss R, Caprio, Trombetta, et al. (2005). Beta-cell function across the spectrum of glucose tolerance in obese youth. Diabetes 54:1735–1743.

243. Kralisch S, Sommer G, Deckert CM, et al. (2007). Adipokines in diabetes and cardiovascular diseases. Minerva Endocrinol 32:161–171.

244. Owen KR, McCarthy MI (2007). Genetics of type 2 diabetes. Curr Opin Genet Dev 17:239–244.

245. Sladek R, Rocheleau G, Rung J, et al. (2007). A genome-wide association study identifies novel risk loci for type 2 diabetes. Nature 445:881–885.

246. Zeggini E, Weedon MN, Lindgren CM, et al. (2007). Replication of genome-wide association signals in UK samples reveals risk loci for type 2 diabetes. Science 316:1336–1341.

247. Scott LJ, Mohlke KL, Bonnycastle LL, et al. (2007). A genome-wide association study of type 2 diabetes in Finns detects multiple susceptibility varients. Science 316:1341–1345.

248. Pinhas-Hamiel O, Standiford D, Hamiel D, et al. (1999). A setting for development and treatment of adolescent type 2 diabetes mellitus. Arch Pediatr Adolesc Med 153: 1063–1067.

249. Rosenbloom AL (2007). Distinguishing type 1 and type 2 diabetes at diagnosis: What is the problem? Pediatr Diabetes 8:51–52.

250. Frayling TM (2007). Genome-wide assoication studies provide new insights into type 2 diabetes aetiology. Nat Rev Genet 8:657–662.

251. Hattersley AT (2007). Prime suspect: The TCF7L2 gene and type 2 diabetes risk. J Clin Invest 117:2077–2079.

252. Salonen JT, Uimari P, Aalto JM, et al. (2007). Type 2 diabetes whole-genome association study in four populations: the DiaGen consortium. Am J Hum Genet 81:338–345.

253. Solomon DH, Winkelmayer WC (2007). Cardiovascular risk and the thiazoiidinediones: Deja vu all over again? JAMA 98:1216–1218.

254. Hattersley AT, Pearson ER (2006). Pharmacogenetics and beyond: The interaction of therapeutic response, beta-cell physiology, and genetics in diabetes. Endocrinology 147:2657–2663.

255. Berry GT, Baynes JW, Wells-Knecht KJ, et al. (2005). Elements of diabetec nephropathy in a patient with GLUT 2 deficiency. Mol Genet Metab 4: 473–477.

256. Macaulay K, Dobie BW, Patel S, et al. (2007). Glycogen synthase kinase 3alpha-specific regulation of murine hepatic glycogen metabolism. Cell Metab 6: 329–337.

257. Whittaker RG, Schaeffer AM, McFarland R, et al. (2007). Diabetes and deafness: Is it sufficient to screen foe the mitochondrial 3243A>G mutation alone? Diabetes Care 30:2238–2239.

258. Mancuso M, Filosto M, Choub A, et al. (2007). Mtochondrial DNA-related disorders. Biosci Rep 27:31–37.

259. Khanim F, Kirk J, Latif F, et al. (2001). WFS1/wolframin mutations, Wolfram syndrome, and associated diseases. Hum Mutat 17:357–367.

260. Barrett TG, Scott-Brown M, Seller A, et al. (2000). The mitochondrial genome in Wolfram syndrome. J Med Genet 37:463–466.

261. Labay V, Raz T, Baron D, et al. (1999). Mutations in SLC19A2 cause thiamine-responsive megaloblastic anaemia associated with diabetes mellitus and deafness. Nat Genet 22:300–304.

262. Olsen BS, Hahnemann JM, Schwartz M, et al. (2007). Thiamine-responsive megalobastic anaemia: A cause of syndromic diabetes in childhood. Pediatr Diabetes 8:239–241.

263. Ferner RE (2006). Drug-induced diabetes. Baillieres Clin Endocrinol Metab 6:849–866.

264. Penfornis A, Kury-Pauliln S (2006). Immonosuppressive drug-induced diabetes. Diabetes Metab 32:539–546.

265. Dufresne RL (2007). Weighing in: Emergent diabetes mellitus and second-generation antipsychotis. Ann Pharmacother 41:1725–1727.

266. Costa M, Potvin S, Bethiaume Y, et al. (2005). Diabetes: A major co-morbidity of cystic fibrosis. Diabetes Metab 31:221–232.

267. Teinturier C, Tournade MF, Caillat-Zucman S, et al. (1995). Diabetes mellitus after abdominal radiation therapy. Lancet 346:633–634.

268. Jun HS, Yoon JW (2003). A new look at viruses in type 1 diabetes. Diabetes Metab Res Rev 19:8-31.

269. Andreoli S, Bergstein J (1987). Exocrine and endocrine pancreatic insufficiency and calcinosis after hemolytic uremic syndrome. J Pediatr 110:816–817.

270. Low L, Chernausek SD, Sperling MA (1989). Acromegaloid patients with type A insulin resistance: Parallel defects in insulin and insulin-like growth factor-1 receptors and biological responses in cultured fibroblasts. J Clin Endocrinol Metab 69:329–337.

271. Flier JS, Moller, Moses AC, et al. (1993). Insulin-mediated pseudo-acromegaly: Clinical and biochemical characterization of a syndrome of selective insulin resistance. J Clin Endocrinal Metab 76:1533–1541.

272. Chernausek SD (2006). Mendelian genetic causes of the short child born small for gestational age. J Endocrinol Invest 29:16–20.

273. Musso C, Cochran E, Moran SA, et al. (2004). Clinical course of genetic diseases of the insulin receptor (type A and Rabson-Mendenhall syndromes): A 30-year prospective. Medicine (Baltimore) 83:209–222.

274. Hegele RA, Joy TR, Al-Attar SA, et al. (2007). Lipodystrophies: Windows on adipose biology and metabolism. J Lipid Res 48:1433–1444.

275. Agrwal AK, Garg A (2006). Genetic basis of lipodystrophies and management of metabolic complications. Annu Rev Med 57:297–311.

276. Flier JS, Kahn CR, Roth J (1979). Receptors, antireceptor antibodies and mechanisms of insulin resistance. N Engl J Med 300:413–419.

277. Crino A, DiGiorgio G, Manco M, et al. (2007). Effects of growth hormone therapy on glucose metabolism and insulin sensitivity indices in prepubertal children with Prader-Willi syndrome. Horm Res 68:83–90.

278. Gillespie KM, Dix RJ, Williams AJ, et al. (2006). Islet autoimmunity in children with Down's syndrome. Diabetes 55:3185–3188.

279. Bakalov VK, Cooley MM, Quon MJ, et al. (2004). Impaired insulin secretion in the Turner metabolic syndrome. J Clin Endocrinol Metab 89:3516–3520.

280. Aoki N (1999). Klinefelter's syndrome, autoimmunity and associated endocrinopathies. Intern Med 38:838–839.

281. Minton JA, Owen KR, Ricketts CJ, et al. (2006). Syndromic obesity and diabetes: Changes in body composition wih age and mutation analysis if ALMS1 in 12 United Kingdom kindreds with Alstrom syndrome. J Clin Endocrinol Metab 91:3110–3116.

282. Benzinou M, Walley A, Lobbens S, et al. (2006). Bardet-Biedl syndrome gene variants are associated with both childhood and adult common obesity in French Caucasians. Diabetes 55:2876–2882.

283. Buchanan TA, Xiang AH (2005). Gestational diabetes mellitus. J Clin Invest 115:485–491.

284. Sperling MA (2006). ATP-sensitive potassium channels-neonatal diabetes mellitus and beyond. N Engl J Med 355:507–510.

285. Sperling MA (2006). The genetic basis of neonatal diabetes mellitus. Pediatr Endocrinol Rev 4:71–75.

286. Gloyn AL, Pearson ER, Antcliff JF, et al. (2004). Activating mutations in the gene encoding the ATP-sensitive potassium-channel subunit Kir6.2 and permanent neonatal diabetes. N Eng J Med 350:1838–1849.

287. Pearson ER, Flechtner I, Njolstad PR, et al. (2006). Switching from insulin to oral sulfonyurease in patients with diabetes due to Kir6.2 mutations. N Engl J Med 355:467–477.

288. Babenko AP, Polak M, Cave H, et al. (2006). Activating mutations in the ABCC8 gene in neonatal diabetes mellitus. N Engl J Med 355:456–466.

289. Hattersley AT, Ashcroft FM (2005). Activating mutations in Kir6.2 and neonatal diabetes: New clinical syndromes, new scientific insights and new therapy. Diabetes 54:2503–2513.

290. Ellard S, Flanagan Se, Girard CA, et al. (2007). Permanent neonatal diabetes caused by dominant, recessive or compound heterozygous SUR1 mutations with opposite functional effects. Am J Hum Genet 81:375–382.

291. Nakhla M, Polychronakos C (2005). Monogenic and other unusual causes of diabetes mellitus. Pediatr Clin North Am 52:1637–1650.

292. Olinder AL, Kernell A, Smide B (2006). Treatment with CSII in two infants with neonatal diabetes mellitus. Pediatr Diabetes 7:284–288.

293. Hermann R, Laine AP, Johansson C, et al. (2000). Transient but not permanent neonatal diabetes mellitus is associated with paternal uniparental isodisomy of chromosome 6. Pediatrics 105:49–52.

294. Varrault A, Bilanges B, Mackay DJ, et al. (2001). Characterization of the methlaton-sensitive promoter of the imprinted zac gene supports its role in transient neonatal diabetes mellitus. J Biol Chem 276:18653–18656.

295. Hattersley AT (2004). Unlocking the secrets of the pancreatic beta cell: Man and mouse provide the key. J Clin Invest 114:314–316.

296. Verwest AM, Poelman M, Dinjens WN, et al. (2000). Absence of a PDX-1 mutation and normal gastroduodenal immunohistology in a child with pancreatic agenesis. Virchows Arch 437:680–684.

297. Hani EH, Stoffers DA, Chevre JC, et al. (1999). Defective mutations in the insulin promoter factor-1 (IPF-1) gene in late-onset type 2 diabetes mellitus. J Clin Invest 104:R41–R48.

298. Njolstad PR, Sovik O, Cuesta-Munoz A, et al. (2001). Neonatal diabetes mellitus due to complete glucokinase deficiency. N Engl J Med 344:1588–1592.

299 Thornton CM, Carson DJ, Stewart FJ (1997). Autopsy findings in the Wolcott-Rallison syndrome. Pediatr Pathol Lab Med 17:487–496.

300. Zhang W, Feng D, Li Y, et al. (2006). PERK EIF2AK3 control of pancreatic beta cell differentiation and proliferation is required for postnatal glucose homeostasis. Cell Metab 4:491–497.

301. Zimmet P, Alberti KG, Kaufman F, et al. (2007). The metabolic syndrome in children and adolescents: An IDF consensus report. Pediatr Diabetes 8:299–306.

302. Robertson RP, Davis C, Larsen J, et al. (2006). Pancreas and islet transplantation in type 1 diabetes. Diabetes Care 29:935.

303. Shapiro AM, Ricordi C, Hering BJ, et al. (2006). International trial of the Edmonton protocol for islet transplantation. N Eng J Med 355:1318–1330.

304. Haddad EM, McAllister VC, Renouf E, et al. (year). Cyclosporin versus tacrolimus for liver transplanted patients. Cochrane Database Syst Rev Oct 18:CD005161.

305. Beck J, Angus R, Madsen B, et al. (2007). Islet encapsulation: strategies to enhance islet cell functions. Tissue Eng 13:589–599.

306. Trucco M (2005). Regeneration of the pancreatic beta cell. J Clin Invest 115:5–12.

307. Voltarelli JC, Couri CE, Stracieri AB, et al. (2007). Autologous non-myeloablative hematopoietic stem cell transplantation in newly diagnosed type 1 diabetes mellitus. JAMA 297:1568–1576.

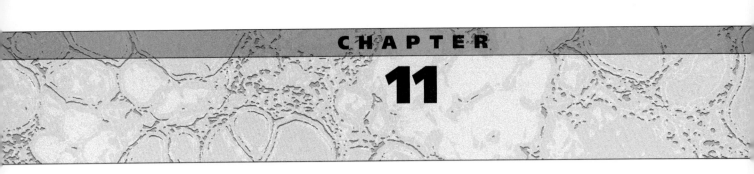

CHAPTER 11

Hypoglycemia in the Infant and Child

DAVID R. LANGDON, MD • CHARLES A. STANLEY, MD
• MARK A. SPERLING, MD

Introduction

Hypoglycemia in later infancy and childhood is less common than hyperglycemia. However, the evaluation is more complex—and the consequences of delayed diagnosis or inadequate management may be more harmful to a developing brain.[1] This chapter describes a diagnostic approach grounded in the physiology of glucose homeostasis, in which the key to diagnosis is identification of which system(s) of metabolism is failing to maintain a normal fuel supply.

The transition from continual intrauterine glucose supply to an extrauterine life of alternating periods of postprandial glucose influx and fasting glucose production requires a series of adaptations (see Chapter 5). Once this transition is complete, the mechanisms of glucose homeostasis remain the same throughout life—although higher rates of glucose utilization in infants and children compared to adults impose a greater dependence on glycogenolysis, gluconeogenesis, and fatty acid oxidation for maintenance of an adequate fuel supply during fasting.[2] As feeding intervals increase in late infancy, disorders of these processes can produce hypoglycemia. The developing brain is susceptible to hypoglycemic damage.[1,3,4]

In infants and children, hypoglycemia is a medical emergency demanding immediate investigation and treatment. When the cause of hypoglycemia is obvious, such as intercurrent illness in a child with known adrenal insufficiency, management may immediately focus on rapid reversal. However, when the cause is not readily apparent discovery of hypoglycemia should prompt immediate taking of "critical samples" of blood and urine to enable diagnosis[3] (Table 11-1).

The principal mechanisms of defense against hypoglycemia are outlined in Chapter 5. The focus of this chapter is on disorders of glucose metabolism in postneonatal infants and older children. Many hypoglycemic disorders may present during or after 1 month of age, and those conditions discussed in Chapter 5 in detail are briefly described.

Definition of Hypoglycemia

There has been controversy over the definition of *hypoglycemia*, especially in infancy, for five decades.[4-7] For the purposes of this chapter, two different definitions of hypoglycemia are used: a diagnostic level and a therapeutic level. For diagnostic purposes, hypoglycemia is a plasma glucose value of less than 50 mg/dL (<2.8 mmol/L). Whole-blood glucose levels tend to be 10% to 15% less than plasma.[8] This level differs from the level of 70 mg/dL, which is the lowest level acceptable during therapy for hypoglycemia. That is, the goal of therapy is to maintain plasma glucose levels in the normal range of 70 to 100 mg/dL most of the time. Failure to do so warrants modification of therapy.

Methods of measuring glucose levels in hospitals include bedside glucose meters originally designed for diabetes management. These monitors are adequate for management of hyperglycemia, but are not accurate for measurement of hypoglycemia. Recent developments in bedside monitoring have improved the technology, but none is sufficiently accurate to establish a diagnosis of hypoglycemia. These meters are most useful as screening tests, and any meter blood glucose level less than 60 mg/dL should be confirmed by a more accurate laboratory determination of blood or plasma glucose concentration.[9,10]

Symptoms and Signs of Hypoglycemia

Most clinical features of hypoglycemia fall into one of two categories (Table 11-2). Adrenergic manifestations (sweating, tachycardia, anxiety) include symptoms

---

TABLE 11-1

The Critical Sample: Acute Blood and Urine Tests at Time of Hypoglycemia

Blood
- Chemistry panel with bicarbonate
- Insulin, C-peptide
- Cortisol, growth hormone
- Free fatty acids, b-hydroxybutyrate, acetoacetate
- Lactate, ammonia
- Total and free carnitine
- Acyl carnitine profile
- Save serum tube

Urine
- Dip for ketones
- Organic acids

TABLE 11-2

Symptoms of Spontaneous Hypoglycemia

Symptoms Caused in Part by Activation of Autonomic Nervous System and Epinephrine Release (Usually Associated with Rapid Decline in Blood Glucose Level)
- Sweating
- Shakiness, trembling
- Tachycardia
- Anxiety, nervousness
- Weakness
- Hunger
- Nausea, vomiting

Symptoms Caused by Decreased Cerebral Glucose Use (Usually Associated with Slow Decline in Blood Glucose Level and/or Severe or Prolonged Hypoglycemia)
- Headache
- Visual disturbances
- Lethargy, lassitude
- Restlessness, irritability
- Difficulty with speech and thinking, inability to concentrate
- Mental confusion
- Somnolence, stupor, prolonged sleep
- Loss of consciousness, coma
- Hypothermia
- Twitching, convulsions, "epilepsy"
- Bizarre neurologic signs
- Motor disturbances
- Sensory disturbances
- Loss of intellectual ability
  - Personality changes
  - Bizarre behavior
  - Outburst of temper
- Psychological disintegration
  - Manic behavior
  - Depression
  - Psychoses
- Permanent mental or neurologic damage

associated with the activation of epinephrine release that occur as the blood glucose concentration declines below 60 to 70 mg/dL.[11] Neuroglycopenic manifestations (lethargy, confusion, seizures) result from decreased cerebral glucose utilization, and are usually associated with glucose levels below the adrenergic activation threshold. Epinephrine release may become blunted or absent in patients with recurrent hypoglycemia, such that neuroglycopenic effects may be the sole clinical presentation. In some children, signs and symptoms are minimal despite prolonged hypoglycemia. However, it cannot be assumed that asymptomatic hypoglycemia carries no risk of harm.

Physiologic Adaptation of Glucose Metabolism During Infancy and Childhood

CHANGES IN GLUCOSE PRODUCTION

Glucose utilization rates per kilogram of body weight are markedly higher in infants than in adults because of their larger brain size relative to body weight. As a result, normal infants and children may develop hypoglycemia after 24 to 36 hours of fasting, whereas normal adults can fast for 48 to 72 hours without hypoglycemia. Stable isotope measurements of glucose turnover rates indicate that the brains of infants and children use glucose at rates of 4 to 6 mg/kg/min, equivalent to almost all of endogenous glucose production during fasting.[2]

The rate of glucose production by the liver is remarkably correlated with estimated brain weight at all ages. Because brain growth is nearly complete as the body weight reaches 40 kg (at 11-12 years of age), little additional glucose production is needed as an adult body mass is achieved (Figure 11-1).[12] Because the greater proportion of brain growth occurs in the first 2 years of life, hypoglycemia occurring during this time may cause significant and permanent neurologic damage. Although hypoglycemia occurring after the first 2 years of life has less likelihood of causing brain damage, its investigation and treatment continue to be crucial.

From the studies of Bier and co-workers it is clear that the glucose requirement per unit of body mass in infants is greater than that of adults, yet the muscle bulk of young children is substantially smaller relative to body mass than that of adults.[2] Because gluconeogenic precursors are derived primarily from muscle, the ability of children to maintain glucose levels through gluconeogenesis while fasting is limited by their smaller muscle mass.

The ability of the infant and child to maintain glucose above 70 mg/dL during a prolonged fast gradually improves with age. Infants from 1 week to 1 year of age should be able to tolerate 15 to 18 hours of fasting. By 1 year of age, a normal child should be able to fast up to 24 hours.[13,14] By 5 years of age, a fast of up to 36 hours may be tolerated. Hypoglycemia induced by fasting of shorter duration should alert the clinician to the possibility of an underlying disorder.

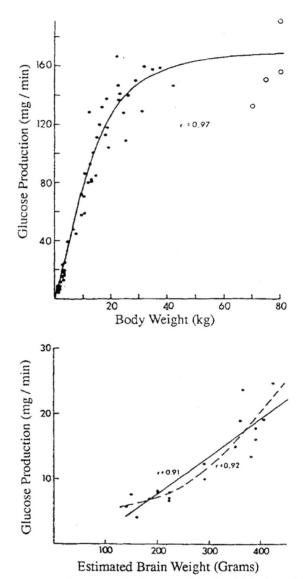

Figure 11-1 Glucose production as a function of body weight (top) and estimated brain weight (bottom). Note the change in slope at approximately 40 kg of body weight when brain growth is complete. [From Bier DM, Leake RD, Haymond MW, et al. (1977). Measurement of "true" glucose production rates in infancy and childhood, with 6,6-dideuteroglucose. Diabetes 20:1016.]

FASTING ADAPTATION

With feeding, serum insulin concentrations rise from fasting values of 3 to 10 µU/mL to peaks of 20 to 50 µU/mL that serve to activate glycogen synthesis, inhibit gluconeogenesis, and enhance peripheral (muscle) glucose uptake. Simultaneously, lipid synthesis is activated and lipolysis and ketogenesis are curtailed. In the postabsorptive state, glucose levels decline and insulin secretion is reduced. Coupled with a rise in counterregulatory hormones during fasting, the fall in insulin levels serves to reverse the anabolic pathways to ensure adequate supplies of glucose, fatty acids, and ketones (Table 11-3). The mobilized fatty acids and the generated ketones serve as alternative fuels for muscle, including cardiac muscle, thereby sparing glucose for brain metabolism.[13]

TABLE 11-3

Hormonal Regulation of Fasting Metabolic Systems

Hormone	Hepatic Glycogenolysis	Hepatic Gluconeogenesis	Adipose Tissue Lipolysis	Hepatic Ketogenesis
Insulin	Inhibits	Inhibits	Inhibits	Inhibits
Glucagon	Stimulates			Stimulates
Cortisol		Stimulates		
Growth hormone		Stimulates	Stimulates	
Epinephrine	Stimulates	Stimulates	Stimulates	Stimulates

The first stage in the defense against hypoglycemia is glycogenolysis. In infants, glycogen stores may provide glucose for up to 4 hours. As the child grows older, glycogen stores are greater and may provide glucose for up to 8 hours of fasting. Glucagon and epinephrine in the presence of lowered insulin levels trigger glycogenolysis. Deficiency of these hormones is very unusual, other than in children on β-blocker drugs. Therefore, hypoglycemia occurring early in fasting suggests either excess insulin secretion or a primary disorder in glycogenolysis.

As glycogen stores become depleted, there is a greater reliance on gluconeogenesis to maintain plasma glucose levels. The main gluconeogenic precursors are amino acids, especially alanine, most of which is generated from skeletal muscle. To prevent excessive breakdown of muscle protein, adipose tissue provides an additional fuel source in the form of triglycerides hydrolyzed to free fatty acids. Mitochondrial fatty acid oxidation (FAO) in the liver produces ketone bodies (β-hydroxybutyrate and acetoacetate) that can be used by the brain and muscle, including cardiac muscle, for energy production. This decreases glucose utilization by these organs and helps ensure an adequate supply of glucose to tissues (e.g., red blood cells) that use only glucose as fuel. Breakdown of adipose tissue triglycerides (lipolysis) is triggered by secretion of the counterregulatory hormones [epinephrine and growth hormone (GH)] and by declining levels of insulin. In infants, ketones appear in the urine 12 to 18 hours into fasting. In older children, ketonuria may not appear until 18 to 24 hours of fasting have been completed. Cortisol, produced during stress, can further accelerate gluconeogenesis.

Defects in gluconeogenesis will usually become manifest only after glycogen stores have been depleted and will thus not occur in the recently fed state. FAO disorders can be triggered by more prolonged fasting. In the first months of life, feeding intervals gradually increase from the typical 2- to 3-hour interval of the on-demand breast-fed infant to 4 hours, and eventually to 8 to 12 hours as nighttime feedings are omitted. For this reason, disorders of gluconeogenesis and FAO rarely present as hypoglycemia in the newborn period when feeding is frequent, but rather later in infancy as fasting is prolonged. Congenital or acquired deficiencies of the counterregulatory hormones that facilitate these processes may also result in hypoglycemia—in the newborn period if congenital and severe or later in infancy as longer fasting occurs. Combined deficiency of cortisol [adrenocorticotropic hormone (ACTH)] and GH in

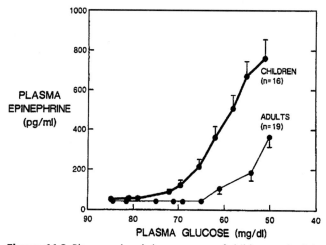

Figure 11-2 Plasma epinephrine response of children and adults to step decreases in blood glucose concentration during a hyperinsulinemic clamp procedure. Note that the increase in epinephrine concentration occurs at a significantly higher glucose concentration in children than in adults. In addition, at comparable glycemia of less than 60 mg/dL epinephrine responses in children are approximately threefold higher than in adults. [From Jones TW, Borg WP, Boulware SD, et al. (1995). Enhanced adrenomedullary response and increased susceptibility to neuroglycopenia: Mechanisms underlying the adverse effects of sugar ingestion in healthy children. J Pediatr 126:171.]

hypopituitarism may produce earlier or more severe hypoglycemia than occurs with isolated hormone deficiencies (Figure 11-2).

Major Causes of Hypoglycemia in the Infant and Child

HYPERINSULINISM

Hyperinsulinism is the most common and the most severe form of hypoglycemia in early infancy.[16] Although less common in later infancy and childhood, it continues to be a significant cause of newly diagnosed hypoglycemia. The hypoglycemia of hyperinsulinism is particularly dangerous because it is associated with inadequate amounts of all brain fuels (low plasma ketones and glucose), thus amplifying the risk of brain damage.[1] As noted in Chapter 5, 60% of patients with hyperinsulinism present in the first week of life. Those infants with the most severe forms tend to present earliest.

Milder forms of hyperinsulinism may become evident beyond the first months of life, when the feeding intervals lengthen and night feedings are omitted. Such infants may present with seizures or early-morning lethargy. Many will have a history of hypoglycemia in the newborn period that was not fully appreciated or will have a history of previous seizures. Some of these children may have unexplained developmental delay. In dominant forms of hyperinsulinism, a parent or other relative may report a more subtle history of hypoglycemia.[14] Defects of the KATP channel are the most common form of congenital hyperinsulinism, but a growing number of other defects in insulin secretion are being identified. As outlined in Chapter 5, all of the genetic causes of hyperinsulinism may initially present in the older infant and child.[15-18]

Hypoglycemia due to hyperinsulinism after the neonatal period is likely to present as recurrent episodes of neuroglycopenic symptoms in an otherwise well child. The hypoglycemia may be mild or severe, occurring after overnight fasting or in a "reactive" pattern 2 to 3 hours after a meal. Obvious adrenergic signs (pallor, perspiration) are common but not invariably present. The diagnosis of hyperinsulinism is suggested when hypoglycemia is accompanied by absence of ketosis. A critical specimen obtained during hypoglycemia that demonstrates measurable amounts of insulin, C-peptide, and/or proinsulin (Table 11-4) can be conclusive. However, it is not always easy to demonstrate elevated insulin levels.

Note also that standard insulin assays may not detect exogenous insulin analogs such as lispro, aspart, glargine, glulisine, and detemir. Plasma free fatty acids and beta-hydroxybutyrate are inappropriately low during hypoglycemia due to hyperinsulinism, as is insulin-like growth-factor-binding protein-1 (IGFBP1).[21] A glycemic response

to glucagon at the time of hypoglycemia is strong evidence of hyperinsulinism as well.[3,21,22] Because of the increased glucose utilization of hyperinsulinism, a glucose infusion rate above 8 mg/kg/min may be needed to maintain glucose above 70 mg/dL in young infants. However, this is usually more difficult to demonstrate or is inconsistently present in older children.

Katp Channel Hyperinsulinism

Two genes, SUR1 and Kir6.2, encode the two proteins of the adenosine triphosphate (ATP)-sensitive potassium channel (KATP channel) in the plasma membrane of the beta cell. Potassium flow through this channel is a key regulator of insulin secretion (Figure 11-3), and defects that impede flow cause excessive insulin secretion. As described in Chapter 5, three distinct defects of these genes are known to cause hyperinsulinism.

- Autosomal-recessive inheritance of two KATP mutations produces a severe neonatal onset of disease that is unresponsive to diazoxide. These mutations are associated with diffuse histologic changes in the pancreatic islets.[19]

TABLE 11-4
Criteria for Diagnosing Hyperinsulinism Based on Critical Samples
Critical sample must be drawn at time fasting hypoglycemia (plasma glucose <50 mg/dL)
• Detectable insulin (>2 mIU/mL)
• Low free fatty facids (<1.5 mmol/L)
• Low ketones (plasma β-hyrdoxybutyrate, (<2.0 mmol/mL)
Inappropriate glycemic response to 1 mg intravenous glucogen at time of fasting hypoglycemia (glucose rise >30 mg/dL in 20 minutes)

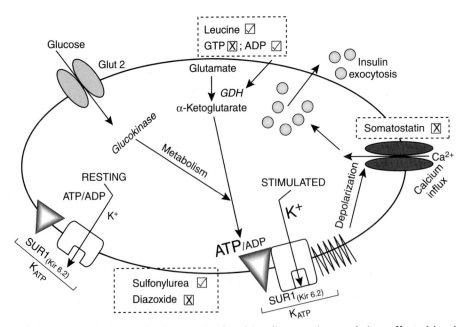

Figure 11-3 Diagram of the pancreatic beta cell, glucose-stimulated insulin secretion, and sites affected by the potassium-channel, SUR1(Kir6.2), glucokinase, and glucose dehydrogenase (GDH) mutations. ADP, adenosine diphosphate; ATP, adenosine triphosphate; and GTP, guanosine triphosphate.

- A clone of beta cells possessing a single recessive mutation on the paternal chromosome may lose the normal maternal allele, resulting in homozygosity for a recessive KATP channel mutation.[17] This "two-hit defect" produces a focal area of adenomatosis in the pancreas.
- A rarer dominantly inherited autosomal mutation causes a milder form of KATP hyperinsulinism, which usually presents after infancy and often responds to diazoxide.[16,24]

The first two forms of KATP hyperinsulinism account for more than 90% of cases of postneonatal endogenous hyperinsulinism in infancy and are clinically similar in their clinical manifestations. Both may require surgery to maintain safe glucose levels. After confirmation of hyperinsulinemic hypoglycemia by the criteria of Table 11-4 and exclusion of the rarer forms described in material following, a KATP channel defect can be presumed the most likely diagnosis. While blood is being tested for specific mutations (e.g., to Athena Diagnostics, *www.athenadiagnostics.com*), management may proceed without molecular confirmation. Treatment measures able to maintain blood glucose levels above 70 mg/dL without surgery are referred to as "medical management" (Table 11-5).

Diazoxide is the first-line drug, but is often ineffective for KATP hyperinsulinism. Octreotide may be given by subcutaneous injection or infusion at up to 20 ug/kg/day.[20] Calcium channel blockers have occasionally been tried.[22] If this approach does not maintain the plasma glucose concentration greater than 60 mg/dL with a normal feeding schedule, surgery may be necessary. Surgical treatment for focal KATP hyperinsulinism is curative, whereas for diffuse disease even a 95% to 99% pancreatectomy may not cure the hypoglycemia (and diabetes is a frequent sequela).[21] PET scanning may distinguish the two types of disease preoperatively, but definitive differentiation of focal and diffuse disease is made intraoperatively by repeated examination of frozen sections.[22] This difficult procedure requires a patient surgeon and a dedicated team of histopathologists.[23-25]

Glutamate Dehydrogenase Hyperinsulinism

Hyperinsulinism can also be caused by activating mutations in the gene (GLUD1 on 10q) for glutamate dehydrogenase (GDH).[18] This disorder, also known as the hyperinsulinism-hyperammonemia syndrome, is a milder form of hyperinsulinism than KATP hyperinsulinism and is more likely to present in late infancy and early childhood than in the newborn period.[26,27] Mutations in GDH cause disease in an autosomal-dominant fashion, but up to 80% cases may be de novo mutations. Severity may vary within a family from seizures in infancy to mild postprandial hypoglycemia in adults. Ingestion of protein without carbohydrate may be especially likely to depress the blood glucose.

Activating mutations of GDH in the beta cell amplify leucine-triggered production of ATP, independent of glucose levels, which then causes closure of KATP channels and insulin release. In the liver, the same mutation increases oxidation of glutamate to a-ketoglutarate with the production of ammonia (Figure 11-4). In addition to increased ammonia production, the low levels of glutamate impair the production of N-acetylglutamate, an important allosteric activator of the urea cycle. Thus, the same mutation causes excessive insulin production in the pancreas and excessive ammonia production (with impaired urea synthesis) in the liver.

The diagnosis of GDH hyperinsulinism is similar to that of KATP hyperinsulinism. In addition to the usual laboratory findings of hyperinsulinism, however, persistently elevated ammonia levels (typically 50 to 200 μmol/L, median 135) are diagnostic of this disorder.[28] Most patients respond to diazoxide, and surgery is unnecessary.[26,29] High ammonia levels do not appear to cause problems in GDH hyperinsulinism because the hyperammonemia is not associated with elevated glutamine, the substance thought to be principally responsible for the central nervous system (CNS) toxicity evident with other forms of hyperammonemia.[30]

TABLE 11-5

Selective Drugs for Hypoglycemic Disorders

Intravenous Glucose Rescue Doses
- Dextrose emergency bolus: IV push 0.2 g/kg bolus (2 mL/kg of dextrose 10%), followed by D10 continuous infusion of 5 mL/kg/hr
- If plasma glucose not corrected after 15 minutes, bolus 2 mL/kg dextrose 10% and increase continuous infusion by 25% to 50%

Glucagon (Emergency Treatment Only in Case of Insulin-Induced Hypoglycemia)
- 1 mg intramuscularly or intravenously
- Side effects: vomiting and rebound hypoglycemia

Diazoxide (Use in Hyperinsulinism or Sulfonylurea Overdose)
- 5-15 mg/kg/day divided into two or three doses (if given by IV route, must be given over 15 minutes to avoid hypotension)
- Start with maximum dose (15 mg/kg to test), then lower as possible (responders usually require 10 mg/kg or less)
- Side effects: fluid and sodium retention, hypertrichosis

Octreotide
- Start at 2 to 5 mg/kg/day and increase to 20 mg/kg/day SC divided q6-8h
- Continuous IV infusion, 510 mg/kg/24 hr
- Side effects: transient diarrhea, abdominal discomfort, gallstones, transient growth impairment

Cornstarch
- 1-2 g/kg/dose (freshly prepare each dose by suspending in cold sugar-containing liquid)
- Effect lasts 4 to 6 hr
- Not well absorbed in infancy
- Side effect: diarrhea

Carnitine (For Plasma Membrane Carnitine Transporter Defect)
- 100 mg/kg/day divided into three or four doses
- Side effects: diarrhea and fishy body odor

IV, intravenous; and SC, subcutaneous.

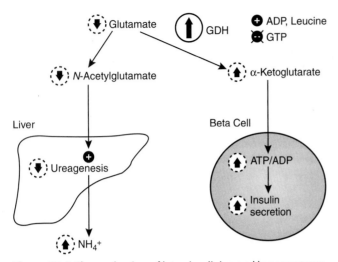

Figure 11-4 The mechanism of hyperinsulinism and hyperammonemia in glucose dehydrogenase (GDH) hyperinsulinism. GDH enzyme activity is increased as a result of mutations that interfere with the inhibitory allosteric effector, guanosine triphosphate (GTP) pancreatic beta cells. This leads to increased oxidation of glutamate to α-ketoglutarate and excessive release of insulin. Simultaneously, in the liver the increase in GDH activity lowers the pool of glutamate—leading to reduced synthesis of N-acetylglutamate. This results in less stimulation of carbamoyl phosphate synthetase (the first step in ureagenesis), and thus in hyperammonemia (NH_4^+). ADP, adenosine diphosphate; and ATP, adenosine triphosphate.

Glucokinase Hyperinsulinism

Glucokinase is the enzyme that serves as the glucose sensor in the beta cells of the pancreas. Gain-of-function mutations can result in a lower glucose threshold for insulin secretion, leading to persistent hypoglycemia. At least six different dominantly expressed mutations have been reported. Enzyme activities, glucose thresholds, and clinical severity of these mutations can vary widely. The most severe mutations have produced neonatal hypoglycemia eventually requiring pancreatic surgery to stabilize glucose levels. Milder mutations have presented as hypoglycemic seizures in childhood, or even reactive hypoglycemia in older relatives.[31] Like the KATP forms of hyperinsulinism, glucokinase mutations can cause apparently transient neonatal hypoglycemia that recurs later in life.

Glucokinase hyperinsulinism resembles KATP hyperinsulinism in the laboratory. In the two GCK-HI patients in whom it was tested, the insulin response to intravenous glucose was greater than is usually seen with KATP hyperinsuinism. Ammonia levels are normal. Mild and moderate mutations have responded to diazoxide treatment, but pancreatectomy was required in two of the more severe cases.[32]

Schad Hyperinsulinism

Short-chain 3-hydroxyacyl-CoA dehydrogenase (SCHAD) is an enzyme of mitochondrial fatty acid oxidation. Recessive loss-of-function SCHAD mutations have been associated with a few cases of familial congenital hyperinsulinism. Some cases have displayed severe hypoglycemia as

newborn infants, but at least one showed no signs of hypoglycemia until several months of age.[33] SCHAD hyperinsulinism resembles other forms of hyperinsulinism more than it resembles other fatty acid oxidation disorders. Elevated levels of 3-hydroxybutyryl-carnitine in blood and 3-hydroxyglutarate in urine led to the diagnosis in the patients described. Treatment with diazoxide was effective.[34,35]

Exercise-associated Hyperinsulinemic Hypoglycemia

A small number of children (infants to adolescents) have been found to suffer hypoglycemic seizures or syncope due to hyperinsulinism occurring with anaerobic exercise.[36] The condition has been inherited in an autosomal-dominant pattern, but the specific molecular defect has not been established. Intravenous pyruvate infusion stimulated excessive insulin release in these cases, suggesting that the defect may involve inappropriate expression of a plasma membrane pyruvate transporter on the beta cells.

Carbohydrate-deficient Glycoprotein Hyperinsulinism

Hypoglycemia due to hyperinsulinism has also been reported in children with the carbohydrate-deficient glycoprotein syndrome (also known as congenital disorders of glycosylation). The hyperinsulinism typically causes hypoglycemia in the newborn period, but in some cases hypoglycemia was not apparent until later infancy. Unlike other forms of hyperinsulinism, CDG usually causes major impairment of other organ systems—especially the brain, liver, gut, and skeleton.[37] The diagnosis is usually confirmed by identification of hyposialylated serum transferrin by isoelectric focusing.[38]

Factitious Hyperinsulinism

Rare instances of factitious hyperinsulinism have been reported in infants or children, typically the result of a caregiver administering the medication to gain attention. This is a form of child abuse often referred to as Munchausen by proxy or Meadow syndrome. In most reported cases, the parent was a nurse or other medical professional—or family members used insulin or sulfonylureas for diabetes.[39-41] This syndrome of child abuse may be lethal. The diagnosis is difficult to make unless suspected.

Insulin administration may be difficult to detect, particularly because the more recent insulin analogs (lispro, aspart, glargine, glulisine, detemir) may not be detected by conventional insulin assay. Typically, classic symptoms of hyperinsulinism are present on an irregular basis. Fasting studies in the absence of the caregivers will be normal. As in other forms of excessive insulin, hypoglycemia will be accompanied by suppression of free fatty acids, ketones, and a positive response to glucagon—indicating that glycogen deposits are abundant and their release inhibited by insulin.

In cases in which regular or NPH insulin have been given, insulin levels may be remarkably high at the times of hypoglycemia. The most conclusive evidence of exogenous insulin is the suppression of C-peptide to undetectable levels at the time other evidence indicates insulin excess, indicating that endogenous insulin production has been suppressed.[42] Insulinomas may secrete high insulin levels, but proinsulin levels will also be persistently elevated.

Oral hypoglycemic agents that induce insulin secretion, especially sulfonylureas, will cause elevation of both insulin and C-peptide.[43] Because they induce endogenous insulin secretion, their use will be difficult to detect unless suspected. Routine toxicology screens on blood and urine may not detect sulfonylureas, but if a sample of the suspected drug can be supplied specific testing can be arranged.

Insulinoma

Insulin-secreting adenomas of the pancreas are rare in young children but become a more common cause of hyperinsulinism by adolescence. They present in a similar manner to the genetic causes of hyperinsulinism but at a later age. One peculiarity of adenomas is that they may cause exercise-induced hypoglycemia. An insulinoma should be suspected when insulin-induced hypoglycemia occurs in older children. Fasting usually produces inappropriate elevation of insulin and proinsulin, but even basal levels of both may be elevated.[44] Routine imaging of the pancreas often fails to reveal the tumor, especially when it is less than 1 to 2 cm in size. Spiral computed tomography, magnetic resonance imaging, and abdominal ultrasound are most often negative. Endoscopic ultrasonography may be most useful before surgery.

Portal venous sampling is invasive and technically challenging in children. In adults, Doppman has demonstrated that pancreatic arterial stimulation with calcium and venous sampling (PASVS) of insulin levels may localize the tumor to a region of the pancreas. This technique has been refined to identify focal KATP hyperinsulinism and equally well to localize insulinomas in infants and children.[45] However, the procedure is invasive and localization is imprecise. Intraoperative ultrasonography is most useful in diagnosing pancreatic insulinomas, with a sensitivity of more than 90%. Islet-cell adenomas are treated by surgical excision. Rarely, isolated insulinomas in childhood may be malignant and metastatic.

Most childhood insulinomas are sporadic, but familial forms should be considered—especially in families with multiple endocrine neoplasia type 1 (MEN 1, Werner syndrome).[46] This disorder is characterized by functioning or nonfunctioning adenomas of the parathyroids, pituitary, and pancreas and is inherited in an autosomal-dominant fashion. MEN 1 is caused by mutation of the gene, localized on chromosome 11, that codes for a protein named menin.

Autoimmune Hypoglycemia

Autoimmune hypoglycemia can result from antibodies directed against insulin or against the insulin receptors. Early cases of hypoglycemia due to anti-insulin antibodies mainly described Japanese women, but cases have been reported in both sexes, all ages, and from all geographic areas.[47,48] The hypoglycemia is most often reactive, but may be fasting. The metabolic features resemble those of hyperinsulinism in most adult cases, with low ketone and fatty acid levels, but intermittent ketosis accompanying severe hypoglycemia was reported in two of the affected children.

Measured levels of insulin can be high, but C-peptide levels are usually low—such that the findings can suggest exogenous hyperinsulinism. Most older patients with this condition have other autoimmune diseases. Among treatments reported to improve the hypoglycemia have been courses of glucocorticoids, plasma exchange, and intravenous immunoglobulin infusions.

Autoimmune hypoglycemia due to antibodies that bind insulin receptors rather than insulin have occurred almost exclusively in adults, usually in association with a malignancy or severe inflammatory disorder, but at least one case in an infant has been described.[49] C-peptide and insulin levels (with some exceptions) are typically undetectable. An even rarer form of autoimmune hypoglycemia has been postulated to involve antibodies directed against surface antigens on beta cells, resulting in stimulation of inappropriate insulin release.[50]

KETOTIC HYPOGLYCEMIA

Ketotic hypoglycemia is a common clinical category of childhood hypoglycemia, with a well-characterized presentation and course but an incompletely understood etiology.[12,51,52] Usually, this condition begins as recurrent episodes of morning hypoglycemia in the second or third year of life—but onset as early as 6 months has been reported. The condition usually remits spontaneously by the age of 8 to 9 years. The classic history is of a child who eats poorly or completely avoids an evening meal, is difficult to rouse from sleep the next morning, and displays neuroglycopenic symptoms that may range from lethargy to seizure or unconsciousness by mid morning. Hypoglycemic episodes are especially likely to occur during periods of intercurrent illness, when food intake is limited.

At the time of documented hypoglycemia, high levels of ketones are found in blood and urine—and plasma insulin concentrations are low (typically under 2 mIU/mL using a high-sensitivity assay). Although ketotic hypoglycemia was described as a clinical entity more than 40 years ago, it remains unsettled whether these children display an accelerated or exaggerated but qualitatively normal metabolic response to fasting (i.e., one tail of the normal distribution) or whether ketotic hypoglycemia is a heterogeneous group of metabolic disorders of substrate availability awaiting further delineation.[53]

Several studies have shown that the hypoglycemia reflects underproduction rather than overutilization of glucose.[54] Children with ketotic hypoglycemia have plasma alanine concentrations that are markedly reduced in the basal state after an overnight fast and that fall still farther with prolonged fasting.[13] Alanine is the only amino acid significantly at lower levels in children with ketotic hypoglycemia. Infusions of alanine produce a rapid rise in plasma glucose concentration without significant changes in blood lactate or pyruvate levels, indicating that the entire gluconeogenic pathway from the level of pyruvate is intact. This suggests that a deficiency of substrate rather than a defect in gluconeogenesis is involved.

The intact nature of the gluconeogenic pathways in affected children is further supported by the normal glycemic response to infusion of fructose and glycerol. Plasma glycerol levels are normal in these children, in both the fed and fasted states. Glycogenolytic pathways are also intact because glucagon induces a normal glycemic response in affected children during the fed state but not at the time of hypoglycemia. The metabolic response to infusion of β-hydroxybutyrate does not differ from that of normal children. Finally, the levels of hormones that counter hypoglycemia are appropriately elevated—whereas insulin levels are appropriately low.[51]

Quantitatively, alanine is the major gluconeogenic amino acid precursor whose formation and release from muscle during periods of caloric restriction are enhanced by the presence of a glucose-alanine cycle, as well as by de novo formation from other substrates within the muscle (principally branched-chain amino acid catabolism). Glutamine may also contribute significantly to these gluconeogenic events. Thus, defects in any of the complex steps involved in protein catabolism, oxidative deamination of amino acids, transamination, alanine synthesis, or alanine or glutamine efflux from muscle could contribute to ketotic hypoglycemia.

Nevertheless, in the majority of children with ketotic hypoglycemia no specific defects can be demonstrated. It was pointed out in the original description of this syndrome that children with ketotic hypoglycemia are frequently smaller than age-matched controls and often have a history of transient neonatal hypoglycemia. Thus, a compromised supply of gluconeogenic substrate may simply reflect the reduced reserve of a small muscle mass at a time when glucose demands per unit of body weight are relatively high.

Ketosis represents the attempt at switching to an alternate fuel supply. Those with ketotic hypoglycemia may represent the low end of the spectrum of capacity to tolerate fasting. Similar relative intolerance to fasting is present in normal children, who cannot maintain blood glucose levels after 30 to 36 hours of fasting (compared with the capacity of adults for prolonged fasting). Spontaneous remission by age 8 to 9 years might be explained by the increase in muscle bulk, with a resultant increase in the supply of endogenous substrate and the relative decrease in glucose requirement per unit of body mass with increasing age.

The diagnosis of ketotic hypoglycemia is one of exclusion, as episodic hypoglycemia with ketosis can occur with deficiencies of several hormones or a variety of defects of gluconeogenesis or glycogen metabolism. The diagnosis of ketotic hypoglycemia is confirmed by a supervised fast. Hypoglycemia with elevated plasma free fatty acids, β-hydroxybutyrate, and acetoacetate associated with ketonuria develops within 14 to 24 hours in most of these children—whereas normal children of similar age can withstand fasting without developing hypoglycemia for at least 24 hours. A ketogenic-provocative diet was formerly recommended but is no longer considered necessary.[55,56]

Treatment of ketotic hypoglycemia consists of frequent feedings of a high-carbohydrate diet. The overnight fast should be shortened, with a carbohydrate bedtime snack and breakfast. During intercurrent illnesses, parents should test the child's urine for the presence of ketones—the appearance of which precedes the hypoglycemia by several hours. In the presence of ketonuria, high-carbohydrate liquids should be offered to the child. If these cannot be tolerated, the child should be admitted to the hospital for intravenous glucose administration. A letter of explanation and treatment recommendation may help ensure an appropriate emergency department response.

HORMONE DEFICIENCY

Although several hormones (including cortisol, GH, glucagon, and epinephrine) are involved in maintaining blood glucose levels or can produce hyperglycemia in excess, deficiencies of only cortisol and GH are common causes of clinically significant hypoglycemia in childhood. Deficiency of both GH and ACTH can occur in congenital hypopituitarism. In the newborn period, hypopituitarism can produce hypoglycemia requiring a glucose infusion rate high enough to resemble congenital hyperinsulinism. In males, a microphallus may provide a clue to coexistent pituitary gonadotropin deficiency. Neonatal jaundice is a common accompaniment of congenital hypopituitarism and may result from either indirect or combined hyperbilirubinemia. Cholestatic jaundice with liver enzyme elevation is especially suggestive of septo-optic dysplasia.

Although fasting hypoglycemia can occur in all forms of glucocorticoid deficiency, ACTH deficiency or unresponsiveness is more likely to produce hypoglycemia than primary adrenal failure—in which the mineralocorticoid deficiency is typically the presenting problem. An increasing number of conditions resulting in ACTH deficiency have been identified in the last decade. Congenital ACTH deficiency presenting with early hypoglycemia has been reported with several rare mutations in genes involved in pituitary development (POU1F1, PROP1, TPIT).[68-70] Some of the patients have had other pituitary deficiencies. In some of them, ACTH insufficiency was not clinically apparent in early infancy. Red hair and early-onset obesity are better known than ACTH deficiency in POMC mutations, but at least one death has been described.[57] Hypoglycemia in an infant due to ACTH deficiency has been attributed to a defect of prohormone cleavage.[58]

Idiopathic ACTH deficiency can be acquired in childhood, adolescence, or later adult life. Circumstantial evidence such as an association with autoimmune thyroiditis suggests autoimmune hypophysitis as a common cause. In some instances, antipituitary antibodies have been demonstrated. ACTH deficiency has been reported in many other conditions of pituitary damage, such as cranial radiation, head trauma, and pituitary infarction.

Iatrogenic suppression of adrenal function is one of the most common causes of glucocorticoid insufficiency, but may be overlooked because the obvious electrolyte abnormalities of mineralocorticoid deficiency are absent. An adrenal crisis with prostration, vomiting, hypotension, and hypoglycemia can be triggered by a stressful event in a child recently weaned from high-dose glucocorticoid therapy. More subtle manifestations may be caused by inhaled and nasal glucocorticoid preparations, which have become the mainstay of allergy treatment for millions of otherwise healthy children. Although most tolerate it well, ongoing combined use of topical and inhaled glucocorticoid preparations can cause enough adrenal suppression to produce episodic hypoglycemia and interference with growth in older children.[59] Absence of the 0800 cortisol peak in a child receiving topical or inhaled glucocorticoids suggests this possibility.

Although hypoglycemia is common in adrenal insufficiency secondary to CRH or ACTH deficiency, it is an infrequent manifestation of primary diseases of the adrenal glands themselves (congenital adrenal hyperplasia or hypoplasia, Addison disease). Nevertheless, a number of clues warrant consideration of primary adrenal insufficiency. Hyperpigmentation may be subtle, but commonly accompanies Addison disease—with increased ACTH and its inherent melanocyte-stimulating hormone activity and adrenal unresponsiveness to ACTH due to a defect in the adrenal receptor for ACTH.[60,61] Childhood Addison disease often occurs in combination with other disorders of immunity or autoimmunity.

In polyglandular autoimmunity type 1 (PGA1), adrenal insufficiency is usually preceded by chronic mucocutaneous candidiasis and/or hypoparathyroidism. PGA1 is now known to be caused by defects in the autoimmune regulator gene (AIRE) and is inherited in an autosomal-recessive fashion. In PGA2 (Schmidt syndrome), Addison disease is associated with diabetes and hypothyroidism: frequent hypoglycemia and an unexplained reduction of insulin requirement is the expected manifestation of adrenal failure in a person with type 1 diabetes. Adrenoleukodystrophy should also be considered in the differential diagnosis of primary Addison disease in children. Neurologic abnormalities may precede or follow the adrenal failure. It is an X-linked disease, and although females may be affected few develop adrenal insufficiency.

Morning hypoglycemia with ketosis is a potential presenting indicator of isolated idiopathic GH deficiency without ACTH deficiency in young children. Low GH levels at the time of hypoglycemia are suggestive, although low levels are occasionally found in normal infants or in children with other causes of hypoglycemia. Insulin levels are quite low, and glycemic response to glucagon during spontaneous hypoglycemia is poor. Poor growth and low IGF-1 levels may be the principal clues after recovery from hypoglycemia. Acquired GH deficiency severe enough to cause hypoglycemia in older children is uncommon. Even though many actions of insulin-like growth factor 1 (IGF-1) on carbohydrate metabolism are opposite those of GH, hypoglycemia is described as common in infants with IGF-1 deficiency (also known as Laron dwarfism).[62]

Hypoglycemia may occur in cortisol and GH deficiency as a result of several factors. Decreased gluconeogenic enzymes are associated with cortisol deficiency. Increased glucose utilization occurs from lack of the antagonistic effects of GH on insulin action and from failure to supply endogenous gluconeogenic substrate in the form of alanine and lactate. Finally, loss of the compensatory breakdown of fat and generation of ketones result in ongoing hypoglycemia during prolonged fasting.

The prominence of epinephrine and glucagon in the counterregulatory responses to hypoglycemia suggests that isolated deficiency of either hormone would be likely to cause hypoglycemia,[63] but few well-demonstrated cases of hypoglycemia caused by isolated chronic deficiency of either hormone have been described in children. Although there have been case reports of reduced epinephrine excretion in patients with hypoglycemia, evidence from patients with diabetes suggests that repeated hypoglycemia is more likely to cause diminished epinephrine excretion than vice versa. A reduction in insulin-induced hypoglycemia restores normal catecholamine responses.

Hypoglycemia is rare in patients after bilateral adrenalectomy, provided they receive adequate glucocorticoid replacement. Consequently, the role of disordered sympathetic activity in childhood ketotic hypoglycemia remains unresolved. Theoretically, epinephrine deficiency may contribute to the hypoglycemia of adrenal insufficiency because cortisol is essential to the stimulation of phenylethanolamine N-methyl transferase (PNMT)—the enzyme that converts norepinephrine to epinephrine in the adrenal medulla. Diminished epinephrine secretion has been documented in patients with congenital adrenal hyperplasia, who have decreased endogenous cortisol secretion.[64]

Perhaps the best candidate for an example of hypoglycemia caused by epinephrine deficiency in childhood is the occasional episode of severe hypoglycemia, usually fasting, occurring in a young child taking propranolol or another beta blocker (either therapeutically or accidentally).[65] Impaired glucagon secretion also increases the vulnerability to hypoglycemia of people with type 1 diabetes, but no well-documented case of childhood hypoglycemia due to isolated glucagon deficiency has been reported. Even the case traditionally cited has since been recognized as having been due to familial SCHAD hyperinsulinism. The major clinical setting in which inadequate glucagon secretion contributes to hypoglycemia remains the combined deficiency of catecholamines and glucagon that occurs in long-standing insulin-dependent diabetes.

GLYCOGEN STORAGE DISEASES

Although glycogen storage diseases (GSDs)—along with hyperinsulinism, hypopituitarism, and fatty acid oxidation defects—are among the main causes of persistent hypoglycemia in the newborn period, most cases of GSD present in later infancy and childhood.[66] Despite the severity of the hypoglycemia in the GSDs, they usually present with failure to thrive and hepatomegaly. There are four main types of GSDs that cause hypoglycemia: GSD 1, GSD 3, GSD 6, and GSD 9. In addition, defects in glycogen synthesis from glycogen synthetase deficiency may be an under-recognized cause of hypoglycemia (GSD 0).

Glucose 6-phosphatase Deficiency (Types 1a And 1b Gsd)

Deficiency of the enzyme that hydrolyzes glucose 6-phosphate to free glucose, the final step in the glycogenolytic and gluconeogenic pathways (Figure 11-5),

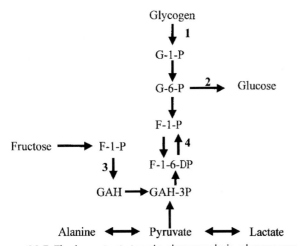

Figure 11-5 The important steps in glycogenolysis, gluconeogenesis, and the metabolism of fructose are shown. (1) Debrancher enzyme (GSD III), (2) glucose 6-phosphatase (GSD I), (3) fructoaldolase (HFI), and (4) FDPase. DP, diphosphate; F, fructose; G, glucose; GAH, glyceraldehyde; and P, phosphate.

results in severe hypoglycemia from early infancy. In its classic form (type 1A, with an estimated incidence of 1:100,000), affected children present with marked hepatomegaly—resulting in a protuberant abdomen that produces an appearance of exaggerated lordosis. Eruptive xanthomas reflect hypertriglyceridemia and hypercholesterolemia in serum, which may be grossly lipemic. Metabolic acidosis is common and is caused by marked lactic acidosis and mild ketosis. Serum triglycerides are markedly elevated and may cause grossly lipemic serum. Hyperuricemia, hypophosphatemia, anomalies in platelet adhesiveness, and severe growth failure are also characteristic features of this form of GSD.

Affected children display a remarkable tolerance to their chronic hypoglycemia. Blood glucose values in the range of 20 to 50 mg/dL are not associated with typical symptoms of hypoglycemia, reflecting the adaptation of the CNS to alternative sources of fuel (lactate). However, the hypoglycemia provokes the appropriate increased secretion of counterregulatory hormones—including GH, glucagon, cortisol, and catecholamines—as well as the suppression of insulin secretion. Thus, glucagon and GH are elevated threefold to fourfold above their normal fasting concentrations—whereas insulin concentrations are suppressed.

These hormonal changes cause increased glycogenolysis and gluconeogenesis to the point of glucose 6-phosphate, with lactic acidosis representing increased formation and decreased utilization of lactate. The hormonal changes also promote exaggerated lipolysis, resulting in fatty liver and hypertriglyceridemia hyperlipidemia and in both the substrate and hormonal settings for accelerated hepatic ketogenesis. Depletion of hepatic ATP and inorganic phosphate as a consequence of glucose phosphorylation ATP consumption during glycogenolysis and resulting excess glycolysis increases the rate of uric acid production by stimulating the degradation of preformed nucleotides.

Endogenous hyperglucagonemia probably contributes substantially to this evolution of hyperuricemia because infusion of exogenous glucagon to patients with type-1 GSD exaggerates the decrease in hepatic ATP and glycogen content while increasing hepatic phosphorylase enzyme activity. Hyperuricemia also reflects decreased renal clearance of urate, which competes with the elevated lactate and ketone concentrations for a common shared renal tubular secretory site. The defect in platelet adhesiveness and resulting clotting abnormalities are consequences of the hypertriglyceridemia and may be the consequence of ATP depletion. Although the liver is laden with glycogen and triglycerides, results of liver function tests remain essentially normal other than mild elevations of serum aspartate aminotransferase levels.

The kidney renal tubules and intestinal mucosa also express the enzyme glucose 6-phosphatase. Renal biopsy reveals excessive glycogen deposition. Long-term renal dysfunction can occur with histologic findings remarkably similar to those found in diabetes (focal glomerular sclerosis). Renal manifestations include kidney enlargement, glomerular hyperfiltration, hypercalciuria, and a mild tubular acidosis.[67] Late renal complications may include Fanconi syndrome, nephrocalcinosis, and progressive proteinuria—leading to end-stage renal failure.[78-80] There are no characteristic gastrointestinal symptoms, but diarrhea has occasionally been reported. Nodular liver enlargement and hepatoma formation have also been reported.

Hepatic glucose 6-phosphatase is now known to be a multicomponent system whose enzyme activity is tightly linked to the inner aspect of the endoplasmic reticular membrane.[68] In addition to glucose-6-phosphatase itself, three translocase systems that allow entry of glucose 6-phosphate (T1), exit of phosphate (T2), and exit of glucose (T3) from the lumen of the endoplasmic reticulum complete the pathway of glycogenolysis. Classic deficiency of enzyme activity is termed *type 1A1a*, whereas deficiency of translocase T1 is termed *type 1B1b*. Both types typically present in infants and children, and have been implicated in sudden infant death syndrome. However, they may present in adults with hepatomegaly and hypoglycemia. Deficiencies of the T2 and T3 transporters as the cause of GSD (types 1c and 1d) have been postulated but not definitively documented.

The genes for human glucose-6-phosphatase and glucose-6-phosphate transporter have been identified on 17q21 and 11q23, respectively. Complementary DNA, its gene, and its expressed protein have been characterized and reported.[69-71] This development has already allowed identification of mutations that inactivate enzyme activity and has demonstrated that the mutations are responsible for type 1A but not types 1B and 1C variants. Mutation analysis for the most common variants is now available commercially.

Type 1b occurs in children with biochemical features that are similar to those of type 1a, but with the addition of neutrophil deficiency, oral lesions, perianal abscesses attributed to the neutropenia, and chronic enteritis indistinguishable from Crohn disease. Treatment with granulocyte-macrophage colony-stimulating factor to increase the neutrophil count ameliorates the enteritis.[72,73]

Diagnosis of GSD 1 is suspected in children with growth failure, protuberant abdomen due to massive hepatomegaly, or hypoglycemia with lactic acidosis. A finding of elevated lactate levels with hypoglycemia combined with an abnormal fed glucagon stimulation test clinches the diagnosis. In the normal child, a 2-hour postprandial (fed) glucagon stimulation test will cause a rise in glucose and no change in lactate. In a patient with GSD 1, lactate rises (but not glucose). Fructose 1,6-diphosphatase deficiency resembles GSD 1, but the fed glucagon stimulation test will be normal.

The previously cited clinical physiologic tests are usually sufficient for a presumptive diagnosis of GSD 1. Liver biopsy with estimation of glucose-6-phosphatase activity has previously been the classic means of definitive diagnosis, but this can often be avoided because of the discovery of the genetic defect—which, as noted, permits genetic testing for the GSD1a and 1b1 genes.

Treatment regimens have transformed the prognostic outlook for duration and quality of life and have resulted in reversal of most of the metabolic disturbances in GSD1. Acceptance of these regimens, including passage of a nasogastric tube for nocturnal provision of glucose, is excellent—and the long-term outcome of this innovative approach is promising. Patients are fed every 2 hours during the day, and have a continuous supply of glucose through a nasogastric tube overnight. The rate of glucose infusion is tailored to the individual but is usually 6 to 8 mg/kg/min (slightly greater than normal hepatic glucose production). Cornstarch therapy has been successfully used in patients older than 1 year of age. Uncooked cornstarch is given in doses of 1 to 2 g/kg every 4 hours, and in some children every 6 hours overnight.

Long-term therapy with uncooked cornstarch and overnight tube feedings has led to improved linear growth and diminution of osteoporosis. Most patients require treatment with allopurinol for hyperuricemia. Although there are no controlled trials of the effect of good metabolic control of GSD on renal disease, some evidence supports the hypothesis that good control lessens the degree of renal impairment. This is assumed from an apparent trend toward later onset of renal disease since the adoption of more effective current treatments.[74] Liver transplantation is not routinely recommended but offers promise of long-term cure for patients who develop liver nodules that become malignant.[66,75,76]

Amylo-1,6-glucosidase Deficiency (Debrancher Deficiency, Gsd Type 3)

Deficiency of this enzyme results in the inability to degrade glycogen beyond the 1:4/1:6 branch point, with the result that only the outer 5% to 10% of glucose residues can be released and the remaining glycogen accumulates as a limit dextrin accumulates. The capacity to generate free glucose from glycogen is therefore markedly impaired, although some free glucose results from the action of liver phosphorylase. However, the gluconeogenic pathways for glucose production from lactate, amino acids, and glycerol are intact. Thus, spontaneous symptomatic hypoglycemia is much less common and less severe than in GSD type 1.[66]

During prolonged fasting, hypoglycemia and a marked compensatory ketonemia and ketonuria appear. Because gluconeogenic pathways are intact, infusions of fructose, galactose, or alanine produce a normal glycemic response. Unlike GSD 1, lactic acidemia at times of hypoglycemia is not a feature of GSD3. Similarly, there is no hyperuricemia in GSD3. Lack of persistent hypoglycemia (and therefore the lack of a rise in counterregulatory hormones) prevents the lipemia, ketonemia, and hyperuricemia. In the fed state, glucagon evokes a normal glycemic response in GSD3 through its activation of phosphorylase enzyme.

When liver glycogen reaches the limit dextrin stage after moderate fasting, glucagon no longer elicits a glycemic response because phosphorylase cannot work on a limit dextrin. Thus, GSD3 (and the related disorders, GSD0, GSD6, and GSD9) can be suspected clinically by features of abbreviated fasting tolerance, hyperketonemia, and absence of fasting lactic acidemia. These defects are also associated with an abnormal rise in blood lactate following oral glucose loading.

Children with this disease usually present with hepatomegaly and growth retardation. Liver function tests (especially transaminases) may be markedly increased, possibly due to cellular responses to accumulated limit dextrin. In addition to the liver, debrancher enzyme is normally present in muscle, kidney, and leukocytes. Consequently, progressive muscle weakness, myotonias, and cardiomyopathy have occasionally been described and may be associated with more severe forms of enzyme deficiency. Cardiomyopathy may be fatal, and severe muscle weakness may appear after the first decade of life.

Creatinine phosphokinase is elevated in these children. Assay of the debrancher enzyme activity in leukocytes has been used to identify affected individuals and presumed heterozygote carriers. Considerable genetic heterogeneity in this enzyme's activity in liver, muscle, or leukocytes among affected individuals and their families precludes the use of leukocytes for the identification of the heterozygous state. The gene locus is on 1p21, and mutation analysis (at least for common mutations) is available from commercial labs. Immunoblot analysis of this enzyme with the use of a monoclonal antibody has been reported.

Two dietary regimens have been advocated for GSD type 3.[77] For those with liver involvement alone, frequent feedings and uncooked cornstarch have been recommended in the expectation that avoidance of prolonged fasting will be sufficient to prevent hypoglycemia and improve growth.[78] However, in patients with liver and muscle involvement the use of a low-carbohydrate high-protein diet has been advocated—with the argument that providing glucose by gluconeogenesis from protein precursors reduces the need to deplete muscle alanine stores. There are no large controlled trials comparing the efficacies of the two approaches. Nasogastric or intravenous glucose infusions may occasionally be indicated if caloric intake cannot be maintained during intercurrent illness.

Liver Phosphorylase Deficiency (Gsd Types 6 And 9)

Normal liver glycogen phosphorylase activity involves a complex cascade of events that activates the enzyme capacity to degrade liver glycogen before and after the debranching step.[66] Consequently, low hepatic phosphorylase activity may result from a defect in any of the steps of activation. Not surprisingly, a variety of defects have been described. In its "classic" form, hepatomegaly, excessive deposition of glycogen in liver, some growth retardation, and occasional symptomatic hypoglycemia occur.

A frequent feeding program with cornstarch overnight is usually adequate therapy, but some authorities also recommend a high-protein diet. Variants of this condition include a presumed defect in the hormonal activating system for phosphorylase, deficiency of the cyclic adenosine monophosphate-dependent protein kinase that activates phosphorylase, and deficiency of the phosphorylase-b kinase that activates phosphorylase-a activity.[79] Patients with GSD 6 and 9 generally do very well, but there has been a report of liver cirrhosis in a patient with GSD type 9.[80]

Glycogen Synthetase Deficiency

An inability to synthesize glycogen appears to be a rare occurrence, but hepatic glycogen synthetase deficiency (GSD 0) has been confirmed through metabolic studies, enzyme assay of liver biopsy material in vivo, and most recently genetic studies identifying mutations in the glycogen synthetase locus (12p12.2.84-86). Infants and children with GSD 0 may have symptoms of fasting-induced hypoglycemia and hyperketonemia from infancy, but may also demonstrate hyperglycemia with glucosuria after meals.[81]

During fasting hypoglycemia, levels of the counterregulatory hormones, including catecholamines, are appropriately elevated or normal—whereas insulin levels are appropriately low. Exogenously administered glucagon produces a glycemic response soon after meals but no response after a 12-hour fast. Gluconeogenic capacity is intact. There is often no hepatomegaly. Glycogen synthetase activity is markedly reduced in liver but normal in muscle. In the index case, protein-rich feedings at frequent intervals resulted in dramatic clinical improvement, including improved growth. Since the initial case reports, more patients have been described. Treatment with uncooked cornstarch has been helpful. Although the majority of cases are recessive mutations, one pedigree has been reported in whom the mother of two affected children had some hypoglycemia. This condition mimics the syndrome of ketotic hypoglycemia and should be considered in the differential diagnosis of that syndrome.[82]

DISORDERS OF GLUCONEOGENESIS

Disorders of gluconeogenesis causing hypoglycemia include a variety of enzyme defects and inborn errors of metabolism, but also some exogenous agents and infections.

Genetic Defects

Hypoglycemia may occur with several inborn errors of organic acid metabolism. In a few of these conditions, the hypoglycemia is a common manifestation (SCHAD deficiency, fatty acid oxidation defects)—whereas in most of the others it is atypical, infrequent, or mild. In the disorders described in the material following, hypoglycemia is attributed mainly to impaired gluconeogenesis—whereas in others the precise mechanism of hypoglycemia is not apparent even though some clinical features are common to most of them.

Hypoglycemia usually occurs during episodes of encephalopathic metabolic decompensation, sometimes spontaneous and sometimes triggered by a stressful illness or starvation. Vomiting and sometimes tachypnea may be prominent symptoms. Many of the conditions result in impairment of physical growth or neuromuscular development even when severe episodes are infrequent. The major clue to diagnosis is usually a pattern of characteristically abnormal organic acids in the urine. In most cases, management (or at least hypoglycemia prevention) consists of providing intravenous glucose at the onset of illness or decompensation.

The major enzymatic defects in gluconeogenesis that are responsible for hypoglycemia include deficiencies in fructose 1-phosphate aldolase (hereditary fructose intolerance), fructose 1,6-diphosphatase, phosphoenol pyruvate carboxykinase (PEPCK), and pyruvate carboxylase. Gluconeogenesis can also be transiently impaired by exogenous agents such as alcohol and salicylates.

In the past, much has been made of the possibility that galactosemia causes significant hypoglycemia. In theory, this is possible because of the role of galactose-1-phosphate and the phosphate pool. Hypoglycemia will occur in galactosemia only when the patient is in extremis with liver failure. Hypoglycemia also occurs in association with advanced liver disease in neonatal hemochromatosis, tyrosinosis type 1, S-adenosylhomocysteine hydrolase deficiency, type 3 glycogenosis, and some of the disorders of mitochondrial function.

Pyruvate carboxylase, despite its pivotal role in gluconeogenesis, will also theoretically cause severe hypoglycemia (but rarely does). Severe lactic acidosis, ketosis, and even hyperammonemia are the primary biochemical disturbances. Hypoglycemia accompanied by ketosis and lactic acidosis has also been reported in late-onset maple syrup urine disease, glycerol kinase deficiency, and phosphenopyruvate carboxykinase (PEPCK) deficiency. In disorders of ketolysis (deficiencies of succinyl CoA transferase and 3-ketothiolase), ketone levels may be quite high but lactic acidosis may not be present.

Fanconi-bickel Syndrome (Glut-2 Deficiency). Mutations of GLUT2 (the gene for the glucose transporter protein 2) can result in hypoglycemia, hepatorenal glycogen accumulation, and a combination of features described as the Fanconi-Bickel syndrome. GLUT2 is a monosaccharide transporter occurring in the plasma membranes of beta cells, renal tubule cells, and hepatocytes, among other tissues. Defective function leads to glycogen accumulation, enlargement of liver and kidneys, and impairment of gluconeogenesis and renal tubular function. Fasting hypoglycemia, hyperuricemia, hypertriglyceridemia, and postprandial hyperglycemia suggest impairment of gluconeogenesis—whereas reduced glucose sensing by beta cells may contribute to postprandial hyperglycemia. Glucosuria, phosphaturia, aminoaciduria, metabolic acidosis, and hypophosphatemic rickets result from the renal tubular effects. Growth failure can be severe.[83,84]

Hereditary Fructose Intolerance. Hereditary fructose intolerance (HFI) was first described as an idiosyncrasy to fructose[85] and later determined to be caused by an inability to split fructose 1-phosphate.[86] It may present in infancy and children with the onset of fructose exposure in the diet, which often occurs from 3 to 4 months onward. After a fructose ingestion (the greater the amount the worse the symptoms) there is an acute onset of vomiting, abdominal pain, and diarrhea that may progress to hypoglycemia, shock, and acute liver failure.

Chronic low-level ingestion causes failure to thrive and liver and kidney failure. Acute treatment of hypoglycemia by intravenous glucose infusions may reverse all symptoms if fructose exposure is discontinued. Aversion to fructose-containing feeds is the hallmark of infants who survive the first episode. Chronic treatment is the avoidance of all fructose-containing food. Classically, older children and adults who survive infancy have no dental caries owing to their avoidance of sweet foods.[87]

Fructose 1,6-diphosphatase Deficiency. Fructose 1, 6-diphosphatase (FDPase) is a rare cause of hypoglycemia first described in 1970 by Baker and Winegrad.[88] The enzyme catalyzes the irreversible splitting of fructose 1,6-diphosphate to fructose-6-phosphate. It is a key enzyme in the process of gluconeogenesis from lactate, alanine, and glycerol and plays an important role in the utilization of ingested fructose by gluconeogenesis.

FDPase presents typically in the first days of life, but up to 50% of cases present later than this. Typical manifestations include hyperventilation from lactic acidosis and ketoacidosis, seizures and coma from hypoglycemia, and hepatomegaly. Attacks are precipitated in infancy and childhood by prolonged fasting and intercurrent illness. Unlike in hereditary fructose intolerance, liver dysfunction and renal tubular dysfunction are rare. Uric acid is elevated. The diagnosis is suspected in children with fasting-induced hypoglycemia and lactic acidosis, and is confirmed by enzyme studies from liver biopsy material. It may be differentiated from GSD type 1 by the fed glucagon stimulation test. Acute treatment is by intravenous glucose and bicarbonate infusion. Chronic treatment is avoidance of prolonged fasting and a reduction but not total elimination of fructose from the diet.

Diarrhea

Hypoglycemia may occur in infants and children with severe diarrhea. It is uncommon in previously healthy children with acute gastroenteritis (e.g., rotavirus) unless there has been a period of starvation (as occurs after prolonged use of water or sugar-free fluids).[89] Hypoglycemia in this setting is usually ketotic and has a good outcome. However, it is important that the history of prolonged starvation be confirmed and disorders of FAO ruled out, as hypoglycemia is uncommon in healthy children. In one survey of sequential emergency department patients, 28% had a significant unsuspected metabolic or hormonal disorder.[90]

In cases of diarrhea in patients with malnutrition, such as occurs during cholera outbreaks in the Third World or in areas of severe poverty, hypoglycemia is a grave and dangerous problem. During severe malnutrition, gluconeogenic substrates such as alanine and lactate are significantly reduced, the capacity to generate glucose by gluconeogenesis is markedly diminished, and alternative fuels such as ketones and lactate are also reduced. In this situation, almost one-half of patients with hypoglycemia plus diarrhea died with an encephalopathic picture—indicating that hypoglycemia in the malnourished child is a poor prognostic sign.[91,92]

Malaria

Hypoglycemia has been described as occurring in approximately one-third of children with severe malaria. As in those with diarrhea and hypoglycemia, there is increased mortality in children with malaria associated with hypoglycemia. Insulin levels in such children were reported to be appropriately low, whereas ketones, lactate, and alanine levels were high—suggesting impaired gluconeogenesis. Provision of glucose is therefore indicated for such patients.[93] In addition, the therapy for malaria (in particular, quinine) may cause hypoglycemia because of its ability to stimulate insulin release.

DEFECTS IN FATTY ACID OXIDATION

The key steps in carnitine uptake, mitochondrial transport, and oxidation of fatty acids are outlined in Figure 11-5. The spectrum of these disorders is remarkably wide, and improved diagnostic methods and population screening are proving them more common than previously suspected. For example, medium-chain acyl CoA dehydrogenase (MCAD) deficiency has been reported to be as common as 1:9,000 births—a frequency comparable to that of phenylketonuria and half as common as that of primary hypothyroidism, justifying the trend toward inclusion in neonatal screening programs.[94] Although the salient features of this group of disorders were discussed in Chapter 5, their importance merits emphasis of key points.

FAO provides a significant proportion of energy required for sustained gluconeogenesis. Therefore, defects in FAO are especially likely to become clinically apparent during prolonged fasting or the accelerated starvation of catabolic illness associated with vomiting. Because FAO and ketone body generation is impaired, hypoglycemia associated with FAO disorders is usually hypoketotic.

Many affected individuals first manifest the illness at age 6 months to 2 years. The hypoglycemia may be accompanied by an encephalopathy that has mimicked

Reye syndrome and does not always immediately respond to glucose.[95,96] Unrecognized, such episodes may be fatal and may resemble sudden infant death syndrome. Diagnosis requires a high index of suspicion and can be established by analysis of plasma acyl carnitine profiles; by urine analysis for pattern of organic acids (especially dicarboxylic aciduria); by complex metabolic studies of liver tissue or cultured fibroblasts; and in certain cases (such as medium-chain acyl CoA dehydrogenase) by molecular analysis or genotyping.[97]

Cardiac and skeletal muscle weakness is a prominent feature with certain defects, principally long-chain acyl CoA dehydrogenase, carnitine transport deficiency, and carnitine transferase deficiency. In patients with carnitine transport deficiency, supplementation with carnitine may improve the clinical features—including improvement in the cardiomyopathy over a period of weeks to months.[98] The biochemical and clinical indicators of disorders of fatty acid metabolism are summarized in Table 11-6.

The primary treatment of these disorders of FAO is avoidance of fasting. In older children, fasting of as long as 10 to 12 hours may be possible without the manifestations. Once an index case has been identified, acute illness with fasting should be treated by rapid institution of intravenous glucose to reverse an evolving episode or to prevent its occurrence.

Several drugs or chemicals that interfere with FAO may mimic the features of inherited defects in FAO, including hypoglycemia. Principal among these is the use of valproic acid, which has been associated with unusual episodes of hypoglycemia with a Reye-like syndrome and hypoketosis. Elevation of ammonia levels and secondary carnitine deficiency may make this side effect appear similar to an FAO defect, leading some to recommend carnitine as a supplement for infants receiving valproic acid.[99] Urine organic acids and acyl carnitine profile will easily distinguish these conditions.

Plant toxins can occasionally produce hypoglycemia by impairing fatty acid oxidation as well. Hypoglycine, a component of unripe ackee fruit found in the Caribbean and Africa, causes hypoglycemia by interfering with FAO.[100] Atractyloside, found in certain Mediterranean plants, uncouples oxidative phosphorylation in the mitochondria.[101]

NONPANCREATIC TUMOR HYPOGLYCEMIA

Certain non insulin-secreting tumors are sometimes associated with hypoglycemia, usually in adults. Initial reports described large retroperitoneal tumors, often of mesodermal origin, in association with hypoglycemia. It has been postulated that extraction of glucose across the tumor vascular bed was responsible for the hypoglycemia. Subsequently, it became apparent that an insulin-like factor was likely involved because the hypoglycemia was associated with fasting, diminished lipolysis and decreased circulating fatty acids, increased glucose utilization, and impaired glucose production. Insulin-like growth factor (IGF)-2 has been demonstrated in the sera of affected patients.

TABLE 11-6

Clinical Manifestations of Inherited Disorders of Fatty Acid Oxidation

Enzyme/Transporter Deficiency	Hepatic	Cardiac	Acute	Chronic
Carnitine Cycle				
• Carnitine transporter (CTD)	+	+		+
• Carnitine palymityl transferase-1 (CPT-1)	+			
• Carnitine/acylcarnitine translocase (TRANS)	+	+		+
• Carnitine palmityl transferase-2 (CPT-2)	+	+	(+)	+
b-Oxidation Cycle				
• Acyl-CoA dehydrogenases				
• Very long-chain (VLCAD)	+	+		+
• Medium-chain (MCAD)	+			
• Short-chain (SCAD)				+
• 3-Hydroxyacyl-CoA dehydrogenases				
• Long-chain (LCHAD)	+	+	+	
• Short-chain (SCHAD)				+
• Medium-chain ketoacyl-CoA thiolase			+	+
• 2,4-Dienoyl-CoA reductase (DER)				+
Electron Transfer				
• Electron transfer flavoprotein (ETF)	+	+	+	+
• ETF dehydrogenase (ETF-DH)	+	+	+	+
Ketone Synthesis				
• HMG-CoA synthase		+		
• HMG-CoA lyase		+		

HMG-CoA, 3-hydroxy-3-methylglutaryl coenzyme A.

Interestingly, one form of IGF-2 is "big"—and serum and tumor contain a large proportion of the "big" form of IGF-2. Big IGF-2 stimulates the IGF-1 receptor and cross activates the insulin receptor, causing hypoglycemia. Stimulation of the IGF-1 receptor causes down-regulation of GH secretion. This reduces IGFBP3 secretion, which in turn lessens the binding capacity of free IGFs and thus increases the potential of the abnormal and dysregulated production of big IGF-2 to cause hypoglycemia. Treatment with GH causes increased IGFBP3, which reduces the free IGF pool and thereby decreases hypoglycemia on a temporary basis until definitive treatment is completed.[102] Removal of the tumor by surgical resection or by chemotherapy/radiotherapy may be required to resolve the hypoglycemia completely. A trial of diazoxide therapy was not successful.

Hypoglycemia caused by hepatoblastoma and Wilms' tumor has been described in children and adolescents. A nonendocrine tumor that causes hypoglycemia is Hodgkin disease, with antibodies to the insulin receptor that bind and stimulate the receptor (mimicking the effects of insulin).[103,104]

LATE DUMPING (ALIMENTARY HYPOGLYCEMIA)

Hypoglycemia occurring in infants and children with a combination of Nissen fundoplication and gastrostomy tube placement is common.[105] Feeding glucose-containing fluid results in a rapid rise of glucose levels, followed by a rapid rise of insulin. The combination of rapid completion of glucose absorption and high insulin levels causes the glucose level to plummet to hypoglycemic levels 1 to 2 hours later. There are usually none of the classic gastrointestinal symptoms of dumping. A critical sample obtained at the time of hypoglycemia may suggest hyperinsulinism, but the tolerance for fasting is usually normal and the patient does not develop hypoglycemia after slow weaning from a continuous infusion.[106]

This condition, known as late dumping or glucose dumping, may occur in up to 33% of patients with fundoplication and gastric tubes. Unfortunately, it is often not recognized and seizures are attributed to the neurologic condition that necessitated the surgery. Treatment is not always completely effective, and various remedies have been suggested—including calcium channel blockers[107] and octreotide. A combination of acarbose in doses of 12 to 75 mg per feeding and a complex carbohydrate formula may be successful.[106,108]

REACTIVE HYPOGLYCEMIA

Reactive hypoglycemia is the term used by endocrinologists for any form of symptomatic hypoglycemia occurring 2 to 4 hours after a meal.[109] Other doctors and many other people use the term to refer to autonomic symptoms of any cause occurring a few hours after a meal, with or without demonstrably low blood glucose. The gap between these usages has turned many an endocrine clinic consultation into an exercise in bilateral frustration.

The latter form of "hypoglycemia" is the most common form of hypoglycemia known to most parents and is covered extravagantly on a myriad of Internet sites. The fundamental concept is simple, but the nature of the condition has been a source of controversy for more than 80 years. Within a decade of the first successful diagnosis and surgical cure of an insulinoma in 1929,[110] it became clear that not all patients with symptoms of hypoglycemia had demonstrable insulinomas curable with surgery.

Seale Harris (who began to compile cases) postulated that in some people an exaggerated insulin response to meals could cause transient hypoglycemia 2 to 4 hours after a meal.[111] In such patients, low glucose levels could be demonstrated several hours after a meal or after a standard oral glucose tolerance test (OGTT), and symptoms could be alleviated by frequent eating. The condition, and the use of the OGTT to diagnose it, became embedded in American culture.[112] A wide array of treatment regimens, ranging from benign (frequent snacks, avoiding sugar) to pernicious (elaborate dietary restrictions, expensive supplements or "adrenal extracts" of uncontrolled composition), have been offered to the public. Self-diagnosed patients describing such symptoms present regularly to pediatric and internist endocrinologists.

Much research has demonstrated that few of the self-diagnosed patients have demonstrable abnormalities of glucose metabolism, either when glucose is measured during symptoms or in response to the most rigorous test of metabolic competency (an extended diagnostic fast).[109,113] The OGTT is of little value in this condition, as many healthy children and adults will have glucose levels below 60 mg/dL several hours after a glucose load (with little or no relation to either symptoms or glucose levels after meals).[114] In fact, the diagnostic test with the strongest demonstrated association with hypoglycemic symptoms has been the Minnesota Multiphasic Personality Test.[115]

These problems have led some endocrinologists to reject the entire concept of reactive or "functional hypoglycemia" as illusory or at least completely unrelated to glucose metabolism, preferring the term *idiopathic postprandial syndrome* as a more accurate descriptor. The American Diabetes Association and the Endocrine Society formulated a position statement in 1973 supporting the need to demonstrate low glucose values at the time of symptoms, as well as improvement after glucose ingestion, in order to validate a diagnosis of hypoglycemia (the Whipple criteria).[116]

Management of children and families arriving at the endocrine clinic with this diagnosis is a challenge in tact and communication. Most of the patients are adolescent or preadolescent girls, and mothers often share the complaint. The oral glucose tolerance test should be avoided as of no value (akin to "using a hammer to slice bread"), and other testing will likely produce normal results. Although the idea of sending the patient home with a glucose meter is intuitively appealing, the physician must be prepared to deal with the inevitable low numbers that will be reported.

The endocrinologist will rarely be able to "take away" a reactive hypoglycemia diagnosis without offering another way to understand and deal with the non-imaginary symptoms. Many parents will accept an explanation that the symptoms may not be due to a measurable low blood sugar (and thus will never be dangerous) but patterns of eating may affect our mood and energy[117] and the best approach may be continued family experimentation with snacks and/or sugar avoidance within healthy boundaries.

Several other conditions are far more common than hypoglycemia as causes of spells in adolescents.[118] Orthostatic hypotension, vasovagal syncope, hyperventilation, and panic attacks all have characteristic histories and features. Management measures are simple, and just identifying the cause of the spells as real but not dangerous often provides considerable relief. Spells occurring with exercise, however, warrant a cardiology evaluation for dangerous arrhythmias.

Reactive hypoglycemia with measurably low glucose levels does occur in several circumstances in both young childen and adolescents. Many forms of hyperinsulinism, from channel defects to insulinomas, may cause hypoglycemia in the postprandial period. When one of these latter types of hypoglycemia is suspected, the correct tool is a fasting study in experienced hands.[119]

HYPOGLYCEMIA IN ORGAN FAILURE AND CRITICAL ILLNESS

Hypoglycemia is common in critically ill patients of all ages,[120] and can occur in failure or severe disease of nearly every major organ system: sepsis,[121] head injury,[122] cyanotic congenital heart disease, congestive heart failure,[123] chronic renal failure,[124,125] acute hepatic necrosis and failure,[126] pancreatitis,[127] severe enteritis, and multiple-organ failure. Hypoglycemia in these patients is often multifactorial, involving substrate depletion, accelerated glucose consumption, undernutrition, impaired gluconeongenesis, cytokine effects, adrenal insufficiency, misplaced infusion lines, and/or drug effects—as well as processes specific to certain diseases. The treating physician should not forget the possibility that an acute illness is unmasking a previously compensated disorder of glucose metabolism, especially in a young child.[90]

HYPOGLYCEMIA INDUCED BY EXOGENOUS AGENTS

In addition to diabetes medications, many less obvious drugs and other exogenous agents have been reported to cause hypoglycemia in individual patients.[53] In children these may represent accidental ingestions or overdoses. Ethanol, salicylates, quinine, and beta-blockers such as propranolol are the most frequent single agents implicated in childhood hypoglycemia. Hypoglycemia has also been reported with sulfonamide and cotrimoxazole use in children, as well as in acetaminophen overdose. Pentamidine is one of the most common nondiabetes medications reported to cause hypoglycemia in adults in therapeutic doses.

Alcohol-induced Hypoglycemia

The liver oxidizes ethanol as a preferred fuel, consuming nicotinamide adenine dinucleotide (NAD$^+$) in the process. Depletion of NAD$^+$ slow oxidation of lactate to pyruvate,

thereby impairing gluconeogenesis. Hypoglycemia may ensue if glycogen stores are depleted by starvation or by preexisting abnormalities in glycogen metabolism. In children who have been fasting for some time, even the consumption of small quantities of alcohol can precipitate these events.

In addition, the use of rubbing alcohol in infants or swallowing mouthwash in children has been associated with hypoglycemia.[128] Three to 5% of children with alcohol intoxication will also have hypoglycemia.[129] The hypoglycemia responds promptly to intravenous glucose, which should always be given to a child at initial presentation of coma or seizure after taking a blood sample for glucose determination. A careful history allows the diagnosis to be made and may avoid needless and expensive hospitalization and investigation.[126]

Salicylate Intoxication

Hyperglycemia and hypoglycemia have been reported to occur in children with salicylate intoxication. Accelerated utilization of glucose due to augmentation of insulin secretion by salicylates and possible interference with gluconeogenesis may contribute to hypoglycemia.[130] Infants appear to be more susceptible than older children. Monitoring of blood glucose levels with appropriate glucose infusion in the event of hypoglycemia should form part of the therapeutic approach to salicylate intoxication in childhood.

Artifactual Hypoglycemia

When a low glucose level is unexpectedly reported in a "well" child who has an outpatient chemistry profile drawn for reasons unrelated to carbohydrate metabolism, it is easy to suspect it is a misleading result. The most common cause of post-phlebotomy artifactual hypoglycemia is glucose consumption during a long delay before measurement.[131] This can be reduced but not eliminated by chilling the specimen, and by newer tubes designed to sequester cells from serum. Fluoride tubes also reduce but do not eliminate glucose consumption. However, they may not be practical for small specimens when other tests are needed.

Even with fluoride, glucose levels may decline by 20% or more when processing is delayed for even a few hours.[132] Unfortunately, post-phlebotomy glycolysis consumes a higher proportion of glucose when the specimen contains a low level when drawn. Blood glucose meters are also prone to higher proportional errors when used to measure blood glucose levels at the low end of normal. The physician must also remember the possibility that a "fluke" lab test has revealed a chronic but asymptomatic hypoglycemic condition such as a glucokinase mutation.

Fasting System Approach to Diagnosis

Understanding the pathophysiology of fasting and the intricate balance of hormonal changes and their effects on intermediary metabolites is the key to discovering the cause of hypoglycemia. From the outline of normal fasting physiology given previously, it is clear that normal infants, children, and adults may develop hypoglycemia if fasted long enough. At the time of hypoglycemia, a blood and urine sample (the critical sample) should demonstrate the normal adaptive changes that occur with time. In an infant or child who presents with unexplained hypoglycemia, the testing of this hypoglycemic sample may be pivotal in making the diagnosis and may avoid prolonged dangerous and expensive testing.

HISTORY

The first element in the diagnostic approach to a patient with hypoglycemia is the history. The timing of hypoglycemia in relation to fasting is an important feature. Hypoglycemia occurring in the immediate postprandial period suggests a defect in glycogenolysis or excess insulin secretion. Hypoglycemia occurring later into fasting suggests disorders of FAO, of gluconeogenesis, or of the hormones that control these processes. The presence of sulfonylureas or alcohol in the household suggests an effect of exogenous substances.

CLINICAL EXAMINATION

The second diagnostic step is physical examination. Hepatomegaly may be suggestive of a GSD or an FAO disorder. Short stature and failure to thrive often occur in a GSD, Fanconi-Bickel syndrome, and hypopituitarism. Neuromuscular signs may occur in association with FAO disorders and adrenoleukodystrophy. Midline defects such as central cleft lip and palate, single central incisor, or optic nerve atrophy are associated with pituitary hormonal deficiencies (as is micropenis).

CRITICAL SAMPLE

Finally, the third stage revolves around the critical sample (Table 1-1). The key feature to assess is the presence or absence of acidosis (Figure 11-6). This can be determined from basic studies before the results of the intermediary metabolites. A chemistry panel with measurement of bicarbonate levels and a urine dip for ketones will be immediately available in most centers. In addition, a lactate level should be easily available.

Acidosis with elevated lactate and absent ketones suggests disorders of glycogenolysis or gluconeogenesis. GSD type 1 and fructose 1,6-diphosphatase (FDPase) deficiency may be difficult to differentiate, and a fed glucagon stimulation test may help. There will be a rise in lactate and no rise in glucose in GSD type 1, with a rise in glucose in FDPase deficiency. An intravenous fructose tolerance test may be required. In the older child, lactic acidosis and hypoglycemia may suggest alcohol ingestion. Normal newborns in the first days of life may present with similar features of lactic acidosis and hypoglycemia.

Acidosis with ketones occurs in normal fasting children, idiopathic ketotic hypoglycemia, and GSD types 3, 6, 9, and glycogen synthetase deficiency. Ketones also may be present in deficiencies of GH and cortisol. Disorders of FAO may sometimes present as small to moderate ketones in the urine, particularly when the patient is dehydrated. Some forms (such as the short-chain length disorders, the disorders of electron transport, and HMG-CoA lyase deficiency) may also have mild ketosis.

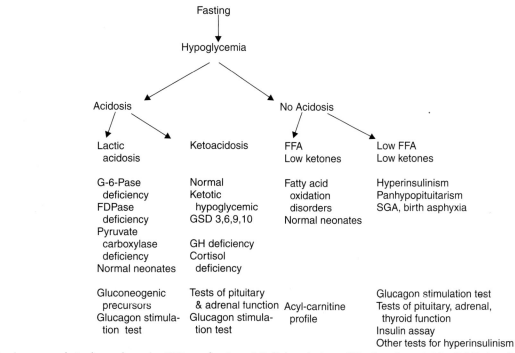

Figure 11-6 An algorithmic approach to hypoglycemia. FDPase, fructose 1,6-diphosphatase; FFA, free fatty acids; G-6-Pase, glucose 6-phosphatase; GH, growth hormone; GSD, glycogen storage disorder; and SGA, small for gestational age.

No acidosis or ketones in the urine is strongly suggestive of hyperinsulinism caused by genetic defects, insulinoma, accidentally administered excess insulin, deliberately administered insulin with intent to harm, or oral hypoglycemic agents. FAO defects will often be hypoketotic, but some forms may have trace or small ketones in the urine. Hyperinsulinism will have neither elevated free fatty acids nor elevated ketones, whereas FAO will have elevated free fatty acids and low ketones. FAO may be diagnosed by acyl-carnitine profile or by urine organic acid measurement. Hyperinsulinism owing to genetic defects and insulinoma can be differentiated from insulin administration by the presence of C-peptide in the plasma at the time of hypoglycemia. Oral hypoglycemic agents will have elevated insulin and C-peptide, and the diagnosis will be missed unless suspected and unless urine toxicology with a request for the specific drug to be sought is performed.

Emergency Treatment of Hypoglycemia

Once the critical sample has been obtained, a mini-bolus of 0.2 g/kg of dextrose should be administered by intravenous infusion over 1 minute (2 mL/kg of 10% dextrose; Table 11-5). This should be followed by a continuous intravenous infusion of 8 mg/kg/min using dextrose 10% solution. This rate of glucose administration may be rapidly and conveniently calculated by using the simple formula that 5 mL/kg/hr of a 10% dextrose solution provides approximately 8 mg/kg/min of glucose. Glucose levels should be determined 15 minutes after the bolus has been given and while the maintenance glucose infusion is running. If hypoglycemia recurs, a bolus of 0.5 g/kg may be given (5 mL/kg of dextrose 10%) and the glucose infusion increased by 25 to 50%. For details of specific treatments of individual disorders, see the sections on each condition.

Conclusions

Since the first edition of this textbook, there have been remarkable changes in one particular area of hypoglycemia-hyperinsulinism. Formerly, it was sufficient to diagnose hyperinsulinism as the cause of hypoglycemia. It is now clear that defects of at least five genes can produce hyperinsulinism. However, it is also known that defects in one of these genes [the sulfonylurea receptor (SUR1)] may be inherited in three different mechanisms (dominant, recessive, and loss of heterozygosity). The association of recessive mutations in SUR1 with diffuse disease and loss of heterozygosity with focal disease is clear. Innovative approaches to identifying focal from diffuse disease have led to the use of partial pancreatectomy with cure in focal disease. New forms of hyperinsulinism continue to be discovered.

Advances in molecular biology allow us to diagnose many conditions without invasive biopsies or prolonged cell cultures. As gene testing expands, even conditions in which there are not common mutations will be easily di-agnosed by a simple blood test. Despite all of these advances, one thing is clear: hypoglycemia is a sign and not a diagnosis. No neonate, infant, or child should ever be labeled as having hypoglycemia as a conclusive diagnosis. Rather, the discovery of hypoglycemia should be the first step in the investigative pathway that ends with a diagnosis and a child no longer at risk of brain damage.

REFERENCES

1. Menni F, de Lonlay P, Sevin C, Touati G, Peigne C, Barbier V, et al. (2001). Neurologic outcomes of 90 neonates and infants with persistent hyperinsulinemic hypoglycemia. Pediatrics 107(3):476–479.
2. Bier DM, Leake RD, Haymond MW, Arnold KJ, Gruenke LD, Sperling MA, et al. (1977). Measurement of "true" glucose production rates in infancy and childhood with 6,6-dideuteroglucose. Diabetes 26(11):1016–1023.
3. Stanley CA, Baker L (1976). Hyperinsulinism in infancy: Diagnosis by demonstration of abnormal response to fasting hypoglycemia. Pediatrics 57(5):702–711.
4. Cornblath M, Schwartz R, Aynsley-Green A, Lloyd JK (1990). Hypoglycemia in infancy: The need for a rational definition. Pediatrics 85(5):834–837.
5. Koh TH, Eyre JA, Aynsley-Green A (1988). Neonatal hypoglycaemia: The controversy regarding definition. Arch Dis Child 63(11):1386–1388.
6. Koh TH, Aynsley-Green A, Tarbit M, Eyre JA (1988). Neural dysfunction during hypoglycaemia. Arch Dis Child 63(11):1353–1358.
7. Cornblath M, Hawdon JM, Williams AF, Aynsley-Green A, Ward-Platt MP, Schwartz R, et al. (2000). Controversies regarding definition of neonatal hypoglycemia: Suggested operational thresholds. Pediatrics 105(5):1141–1145.
8. Tustison WA, Bowen AJ, Crampton JH (1966). Clinical interpretation of plasma glucose values. Diabetes 15(11):775–777.
9. Clarke WL, Cox D, Gonder-Frederick LA, Carter W, Pohl SL (1987). Evaluating clinical accuracy of systems for self-monitoring of blood glucose. Diabetes Care 10(5):622–628.
10. Gama R, Anderson NR, Marks V (2000). "Glucose meter hypoglycaemia": Often a non-disease. Ann Clin Biochem 37(5):731–732.
11. Cryer PE (1997). *Hypoglycemia: Pathophysiology, diagnosis, and treatment.* New York: Oxford University Press.
12. Haymond MW (1989). Hypoglycemia in infants and children. Endocrinol Metab Clin North Am 18(1):211–252.
13. Pagliara AS, Karl IE, De Vivo DC, Feigin RD, Kipnis DM (1972). Hypoalaninemia: A concomitant of ketotic hypoglycemia. J Clin Invest 51(6):1440–1449.
14. Thornton PS, Satin-Smith MS, Herold K, Glaser B, Chiu KC, Nestorowicz A, et al. (1998). Familial hyperinsulinism with apparent autosomal dominant inheritance: Clinical and genetic differences from the autosomal recessive variant. J Pediatr 132(1):9–14.
15. Thomas P, Ye YY, Lightner E (1996). Mutations of the pancreatic islet inward rectifier Kir6.2 also leads to familial persistent hyperinsulinemic hypoglycemia of infancy. Hum Mol Genet 5:1809–1812.
16. Glaser B, Kesavan P, Heyman M, Davis E, Cuesta A, Buchs A, et al. (1998). Familial hyperinsulinism caused by an activating glucokinase mutation. N Engl J Med 338(4):226–230.
17. Ryan F, Devaney D, Joyce C, Nestorowicz A, Permutt MA, Glaser B, et al. (1998). Hyperinsulinism: Molecular aetiology of focal disease. Arch Dis Child 79:445–447.
18. Stanley CA, Lieu YK, Hsu BY, Burlina AB, Greenberg CR, Hopwood NJ, et al. (1998). Hyperinsulinism and hyperammonemia in infants with regulatory mutations of the glutamate dehydrogenase gene. N Engl J Med 338(19):1352–1357.
19. Thomas PM, Cote GJ, Wohllk N, Haddad B, Mathew PM, Rabl W, et al. (1995). Mutations in the sulfonylurea receptor gene in familial persistent hyperinsulinemic hypoglycemia of infancy. Science 268:426–429.
20. Thornton PS, Alter CA, Katz LE, Baker L, Stanley CA (1993). Short- and long-term use of octreotide in the treatment of congenital hyperinsulinism. J Pediatr 123(4):637–643.
21. de Lonlay-Debeney P, Poggi-Travert F, Fournet JC, Sempoux C, Dionisi Vici C, Brunelle F, et al. (1999). Clinical features of 52 neonates with hyperinsulinism. N Engl J Med 340:1169–1175.

22. Hardy OT, Hernandez-Pampaloni M, Saffer JR, Suchi M, Ruchelli E, Zhuang H, et al. (2007). Diagnosis and localization of focal congenital hyperinsulinism by 18F-fluorodopa PET scan. J Pediatr 150(2):140–145.

23. Rahier J, Sempoux C, Fournet JC, Poggi F, Brunelle F, Nihoul-Fekete C, et al. (1998). Partial or near-total pancreatectomy for persistent neonatal hyperinsulinaemic hypoglycaemia: The pathologist's role. Histopathology 32(1):15–19.

24. Smith VV, Malone M, Risdon RA (2001). Focal or diffuse lesions in persistent hyperinsulinemic hypoglycemia of infancy: Concerns about interpretation of intraoperative frozen sections. Pediatr Dev Pathol 4(2):138–143.

25. Suchi MT, Stanley CA, Ruchelli ED (2001). Hyperinsulinism: Are there only two histologic forms? Mod Pathol 14:5P.

26. Weinzimer SA, Stanley CA, Berry GT, Yudkoff M, Tuchman M, Thornton PS (1997). A syndrome of congenital hyperinsulinism and hyperammonemia. J Pediatr 130(4):661–664.

27. Zammarchi E, Filippi L, Novembre E, Donati MA (1996). Biochemical evaluation of a patient with a familial form of leucine-sensitive hypoglycemia and concomitant hyperammonemia. Metabolism 45:957–960.

28. Hsu BY, Kelly A, Thornton PS, Greenberg CR, Dilling LA, Stanley CA (2001). Protein-sensitive and fasting hypoglycemia in children with the hyperinsulinism/hyperammonemia syndrome. J Pediatr 138(3):383–389.

29. Huijmans JGM, Duran M, DeKlerk JBC, Rovers MJ, Scholte HR (2000). Functional hyperactivity of hepatic glutamate dehydrogenase as a cause of the hyperinsulinism/hyperammonemia syndrome: Effect of treatment. Pediatrics 106:596–600.

30. Stanley CA (2004). Hyperinsulinism/hyperammonemia syndrome: Insights into the regulatory role of glutamate dehydrogenase in ammonia metabolism. Mol Genet Metab 81(1):S45–S51.

31. Christesen HB, Gloyn AL (2004). Glucokinase-linked hypoglycemia: Clinical aspects of activating glucokinase mutations. In MA Matschinsky (ed.) *Glucokinase and glycemic disease: From basics to novel therapeutics.* Basel: Karger.

32. Cuesta-Munoz AL, Huopio H, Otonkoski T, Gomez-Zumaquero JM, Nanto-Salonen K, Rahier J, et al. (2004). Severe persistent hyperinsulinemic hypoglycemia due to a de novo glucokinase mutation. Diabetes 53(8):2164–2168.

33. Molven A, Matre GE, Duran M, Wanders RJ, Rishaug U, Njolstad PR, et al. (2004). Familial hyperinsulinemic hypoglycemia caused by a defect in the SCHAD enzyme of mitochondrial fatty acid oxidation. Diabetes 53(1):221–227.

34. Eaton S, Chatziandreou I, Krywawych S, Pen S, Clayton PT, Hussain K (2003). Short-chain 3-hydroxyacyl-CoA dehydrogenase deficiency associated with hyperinsulinism: A novel glucose-fatty acid cycle? Biochem Soc Trans 31(6):1137–1139.

35. Clayton PT, Eaton S, Aynsley-Green A, Edginton M, Hussain K, Krywawych S, et al. (2001). Hyperinsulinism in short-chain L-3-hydroxyacyl-CoA dehydrogenase deficiency reveals the importance of beta-oxidation in insulin secretion. J Clin Invest 108(3):457–465.

36. Meissner T, Otonkoski T, Feneberg R, Beinbrech B, Apostolidou S, Sipila I, et al. (2001). Exercise induced hypoglycaemic hyperinsulinism. Arch Dis Child 84(3):254–257.

37. Bohles H, Sewell AA, Gebhardt B, Reinecke-Luthge A, Kloppel G, Marquardt T (2001). Hyperinsulinaemic hypoglycaemia: Leading symptom in a patient with congenital disorder of glycosylation Ia (phosphomannomutase deficiency). J Inherit Metab Dis 24(8):858–862.

38. Fang J, Peters V, Assmann B, Korner C, Hoffmann GF (2004). Improvement of CDG diagnosis by combined examination of several glycoproteins. J Inherit Metab Dis 27(5):581–590.

39. Editorial (1983). Meadow and Munchausen. Lancet 1(8322):456.

40. Price WA, Zimmer B, Conway R, Szekely B (1986). Insulin-induced factitious hypoglycemic coma. Gen Hosp Psychiatry 8(4):291–293.

41. Marks V, Teale JD (1999). Hypoglycemia: Factitious and felonious. Endocrinol Metab Clin North Am 28(3):579–601.

42. Sperling MA (1980). Insulin biosynthesis and C-peptide: Practical applications from basic research. Am J Dis Child 134(12):1119–1121.

43. Marks V, Teale JD (1999). Drug-induced hypoglycemia. Endocrinol Metab Clin North Am 28(3):555–577.

44. Hirshberg B, Livi A, Bartlett DL, Libutti SK, Alexander HR, Doppman JL, et al. (2000). Forty-eight-hour fast: The diagnostic test for insulinoma. J Clin Endocrinol Metab 85(9):3222–3226.

45. Stanley CA, Thornton PS, Ganguly A, MacMullen C, Underwood P, Bhatia P, et al. (2004). Preoperative evaluation of infants with focal or diffuse congenital hyperinsulinism by intravenous acute insulin response tests and selective pancreatic arterial calcium stimulation. J Clin Endocrinol Metab 89(1):288–296.

46. Greenberg LW, Badosa F, Niakosari A, Schneider A, Zaeri N, Schindler AM (2000). Clinicopathologic exercise: Hypoglycemia in a young woman with amenorrhea. J Pediatr 136(6):818–822.

47. Goldman J, Baldwin D, Rubenstein AH, Klink DD, Blackard WG, Fisher LK, et al. (1979). Characterization of circulating insulin and proinsulin-binding antibodies in autoimmune hypoglycemia. J Clin Invest 63(5):1050–1059.

48. Redmon JB, Nuttall FQ (1999). Autoimmune hypoglycemia. Endocrinol Metab Clin North Am 28(3):603–618.

49. Elias D, Cohen IR, Schechter Y, Spirer Z, Golander A (1987). Antibodies to insulin receptor followed by anti-idiotype: Antibodies to insulin in child with hypoglycemia. Diabetes 36(3):348–354.

50. Wilkin TJ, Hammonds P, Mirza I, Bone AJ, Webster K (1988). Graves' disease of the beta cell: glucose dysregulation due to islet-cell stimulating antibodies. Lancet 2(8621):1155–1158.

51. Pagliara AS, Karl IE, Haymond M, Kipnis DM (1973). Hypoglycemia in infancy and childhood. J Pediatr 82(3):365–379.

52. Pagliara AS, Karl IE, Haymond M, Kipnis DM (1973). Hypoglycemia in infancy and childhood. J Pediatr 82(4):558–577.

53. Stanley CA (2006). Parsing ketotic hypoglycaemia. Arch Dis Child 91(6):460–461.

54. Bodamer OA, Hussein K, Morris AA, Langhans CD, Rating D, Mayatepek E, et al. (2006). Glucose and leucine kinetics in idiopathic ketotic hypoglycaemia. Arch Dis Child 91(6):483–486.

55. Chaussain JL (1973). Glycemic response to 24 hour fast in normal children and children with ketotic hypoglycaemia. J Pediatr 82(3):438–443.

56. Chaussain JL, Georges P, Olive G, Job JC (1974). Glycemic response to 24-hour fast in normal children and children with ketotic hypoglycaemia: Hormonal and metabolic changes. J Pediatr 85(6):776–781.

57. Krude H, Biebermann H, Luck W, Horn R, Brabant G, Gruters A (1998). Severe early-onset obesity, adrenal insufficiency and red hair pigmentation caused by POMC mutations in humans. Nat Genet 19(2):155–157.

58. Nussey SS, Soo SC, Gibson S, Gout I, White A, Bain M, et al. (1993). Isolated congenital ACTH deficiency: A cleavage enzyme defect? Clin Endocrinol (Oxford) 39(3):381–385.

59. Pinney SH, Heltzer M, Brown-Whitehorn T, Langdon DR (2007). Hypoglycemia and growth failure due to inhaled corticosteroids. The Endocrine Society 89th Annual Meeting, Toronto.

60. Clark A (1994). Molecular insights into inherited ACTH resitance syndromes. Trends Endocrinol Metab 5:209.

61. Guo W, Mason JS, Stone CG Jr., Morgan SA, Madu SI, Baldini A, et al. (1995). Diagnosis of X-linked adrenal hypoplasia congenita by mutation analysis of the DAX1 gene. JAMA 274(4):324–330.

62. Laron Z (2004). Laron syndrome (primary growth hormone resistance or insensitivity): The personal experience 1958–2003. J Clin Endocrinol Metab 89(3):1031–1044.

63. Cryer PE, Binder C, Bolli GB, Cherrington AD, Gale EA, Gerich JE, et al. (1989). Hypoglycemia in IDDM. Diabetes 38(9):1193–1199.

64. Merke DP, Chrousos GP, Eisenhofer G, Weise M, Keil MF, Rogol AD, et al. (2000). Adrenomedullary dysplasia and hypofunction in patients with classic 21-hydroxylase deficiency. N Engl J Med 343(19):1362–1368.

65. McBride JT, McBride MC, Viles PH (1973). Hypoglycemia associated with propranolol. Pediatrics 51(6):1085–1087.

66. Chen YT (2001). Glycogen storage diseases. In CRS Scriver (ed.), *The metabolic and molecular bases of inherited disease, Eighth edition.* New York: McGraw-Hill 1521–1553.

67. Chen YT, Coleman RA, Scheinman JI, Kolbeck PC, Sidbury JB (1988). Renal disease in type I glycogen storage disease. N Engl J Med 318(1):7–11.

68. Burchell A, Jung RT, Lang CC, Bennet W, Shepherd AN (1987). Diagnosis of type 1a and type 1c glycogen storage diseases in adults. Lancet 1(8541):1059–1062.

69. Lei KJ, Pan CJ, Shelly LL, Liu JL, Chou JY (1994). Identification of mutations in the gene for glucose-6-phosphatase, the enzyme deficient in glycogen storage disease type 1a. J Clin Invest 93(5):1994–1999.

70. Lei KJ, Shelly LL, Lin B, Sidbury JB, Chen YT, Nordlie RC, et al. (1995). Mutations in the glucose-6-phosphatase gene are associated with glycogen storage disease types 1a and 1aSP but not 1b and 1c. J Clin Invest 95(1):234–240.

71. Lei KJ, Shelly LL, Pan CJ, Sidbury JB, Chou JY (1993). Mutations in the glucose-6-phosphatase gene that cause glycogen storage disease type 1a. Science 262(5133):580–583.

72. Kilpatrick L, Garty BZ, Lundquist KF, Hunter K, Stanley CA, Baker L, et al. (1990). Impaired metabolic function and signaling defects in phagocytic cells in glycogen storage disease type 1b. J Clin Invest 86(1):196–202.

73. McCawley LJ, Korchak HM, Douglas SD, Campbell DE, Thornton PS, Stanley CA, et al. (1994). In vitro and in vivo effects of granulocyte colony-stimulating factor on neutrophils in glycogen storage disease type 1B: Granulocyte colony-stimulating factor therapy corrects the neutropenia and the defects in respiratory burst activity and Ca2+ mobilization. Pediatr Res 35(1):84–90.

74. Wolfsdorf JI, Laffel LM, Crigler JF Jr. (1997). Metabolic control and renal dysfunction in type I glycogen storage disease. J Inherit Metab Dis 20(4):559–568.

75. Bianchi L (1993). Glycogen storage disease I and hepatocellular tumours. Eur J Pediatr 152(1):S63–S70.

76. Limmer J, Fleig WE, Leupold D, Bittner R, Ditschuneit H, Beger HG (1988). Hepatocellular carcinoma in type I glycogen storage disease. Hepatology 8(3):531–537.

77. Goldberg T, Slonim AE (1993). Nutrition therapy for hepatic glycogen storage diseases. J Am Diet Assoc 93(12):1423–1430.

78. McCallion NI, Naughten E, Thornton PS (1998). Uncooked corn flour compared to high protein diet in the treatment of GSD type III. J Inherit Metab Dis 21(2):93.

79. Hendrickx J, Coucke P, Dams E, Lee P, Odievre M, Corbeel L, et al. (1995). Mutations in the phosphorylase kinase gene PHKA2 are responsible for X-linked liver glycogen storage disease. Hum Mol Genet 4(1):77–83.

80. Kagalwalla AF, Kagalwalla YA, al Ajaji S, Gorka W, Ali MA (1995). Phosphorylase b kinase deficiency glycogenosis with cirrhosis of the liver. J Pediatr 127(4):602–605.

81. Aynsley-Green A, Williamson DH, Gitzelmann R (1977). Hepatic glycogen synthetase deficiency: Definition of syndrome from metabolic and enzyme studies on a 9-year-old girl. Arch Dis Child 52(7):573–579.

82. Weinstein DA, Correia CE, Saunders AC, Wolfsdorf JI (2006). Hepatic glycogen synthase deficiency: An infrequently recognized cause of ketotic hypoglycemia. Mol Genet Metab 87(4):284–288.

83. Santer R, Schneppenheim R, Suter D, Schaub J, Steinmann B (1998). Fanconi-Bickel syndrome: The original patient and his natural history, historical steps leading to the primary defect, and a review of the literature. Eur J Pediatr 157(10):783–797.

84. Santer R, Groth S, Kinner M, Dombrowski A, Berry GT, Brodehl J, et al. (2002). The mutation spectrum of the facilitative glucose transporter gene SLC2A2 (GLUT2) in patients with Fanconi-Bickel syndrome. Hum Genet 110(1):21–29.

85. Chambers RA, Pratt RT (1956). Idiosyncrasy to fructose. Lancet 2(6938):340.

86. Hers HG, Joassin G (1961). Anomaly of hepatic aldolase in intolerance to fructose. Enzymol Biol Clin (Basel) 1:4–14.

87. Marthaler TM, Froesch ER (1967). Hereditary fructose intolerance: Dental status of eight patients. Br Dent J 123(12):597–599.

88. Baker L, Winegrad AI (1970). Fasting hypoglycaemia and metabolic acidosis associated with deficiency of hepatic fructose-1,6-diphosphatase activity. Lancet 2(7662):13–16.

89. Reid SR, Losek JD (2005). Hypoglycemia complicating dehydration in children with acute gastroenteritis. J Emerg Med 29(2):141–145.

90. Weinstein DAB, Raymond K, Korson MS, Weiner DL, Wolfsdorf JI (2001). High incidence of unrecognized metabolic and endocrinologic disorders in acutely ill children with previously unrecognized hypoglycemia (abstract P2-525). Pediatr Res 49(suppl2): 88A.

91. Bennish ML, Azad AK, Rahman O, Phillips RE (1990). Hypoglycemia during diarrhea in childhood: Prevalence, pathophysiology, and outcome. N Engl J Med 322(19):1357–1363.

92. Haymond MW (1990). Diarrhea, malnutrition, euglycemia, and fuel for thought. N Engl J Med 322(19):1390–1391.

93. White NJ, Miller KD, Marsh K, Berry CD, Turner RC, Williamson DH, et al. (1987). Hypoglycaemia in African children with severe malaria. Lancet 1(8535):708–711.

94. Ziadeh R, Hoffman EP, Finegold DM, Hoop RC, Brackett JC, Strauss AW, et al. (1995). Medium chain acyl-CoA dehydrogenase deficiency in Pennsylvania: Neonatal screening shows high incidence and unexpected mutation frequencies. Pediatr Res 37:675–678.

95. Roe CRD (2001). Mitochondrial fatty acid oxidation disoders. In CRS Scriver (ed.), *The metabolic and molecular bases of inherited disease, Eighth edition.* New York: McGraw-Hill 2297–2326.

96. Hale DE, Bennett MJ (1992). Fatty acid oxidation disorders: A new class of metabolic diseases. J Pediatr 121(1):1–11.

97. Iafolla AK, Thompson RJ, Roe CR (1994). Medium-chain acyl-coenzyme A dehydrogenase deficiency: Clinical course in 120 affected children. J Pediatr 124:409–415.

98. Treem WR, Stanley CA, Finegold DN, Hale DE, Coates PM (1988). Primary carnitine deficiency due to a failure of carnitine transport in kidney, muscle, and fibroblasts. N Engl J Med 319(20):1331–1336.

99. Kelley RI (1994). The role of carnitine supplementation in valproic acid therapy. Pediatrics 83:891–892.

100. Bressler R (1976). The unripe akee: Forbidden fruit. N Engl J Med 295(9):500–501.

101. Georgiou M, Sianidou L, Hatzis T, Papadatos J, Koutselinis A (1988). Hepatotoxicity due to Atractylis gummifera-L. J Toxicol Clin Toxicol 26(7):487–493.

102. Agus MS, Katz LE, Satin-Smith M, Meadows AT, Hintz RL, Cohen P (1995). Non-islet-cell tumor associated with hypoglycemia in a child: Successful long-term therapy with growth hormone. J Pediatr 127(3):403–407.

103. Walters EG, Tavare JM, Denton RM, Walters G (1987). Hypoglycaemia due to an insulin-receptor antibody in Hodgkin's disease. Lancet 1(8527):241–243.

104. Braund WJ, Naylor BA, Williamson DH, Buley ID, Clark A, Chapel HM, et al. (1987). Autoimmunity to insulin receptor and hypoglycaemia in patient with Hodgkin's disease. Lancet 1(8527):237–240.

105. Samuk I, Afriat R, Horne T, Bistritzer T, Barr J, Vinograd I (1996). Dumping syndrome following Nissen fundoplication, diagnosis, and treatment. J Pediatr Gastroenterol Nutr 23(3):235–240.

106. Thornton PS (2005). Hypoglycemia. In Thomas Moshang J (ed.), *Pediatric endocrinology: The requisites in pediatrics.* St. Louis: Elsevier Mosby.

107. Sanke T, Nanjo K, Kondo M, Nishi M, Moriyama Y, Miyamura K (1986). Effect of calcium antagonists on reactive hypoglycemia associated with hyperinsulinemia. Metabolism 35(10):924–927.

108. Ng D, Ferry RJ, Weinzimer SA, Stanley CA, Levitt Katz LE (2002). Acarbose treatment of postprandial hypoglycemia in children after Nissen fundoplication. J Pediatr 139:877–879.

109. Service FJ (1999). Classification of hypoglycemic disorders. Endocrinol Metab Clin North Am 28(3):501–517.

110. Howland G, Campbev WR, Maltby EJ, Robinson WL (1929). Dysinsulinism: Convulsions, coma due to islet-cell tumor of the pancreas with operation and cure. JAMA 93:674–679.

111. Harris S (1932). Hyperinsulinism and dysinsulinism (insulinogenic hypoglycemia) with a chronologic review of cases reported in the United States and Canada. Internat Clin 1(42):9–29.

112. Yager J, Young RT (1974). Non-hypoglycemia is an epidemic condition. N Engl J Med 291(17):907–908.

113. Hofeldt FD (1989). Reactive hypoglycemia. Endocrinol Metab Clin North Am 18(1):185–201.

114. Lev-Ran A, Anderson RW (1981). The diagnosis of postprandial hypoglycemia. Diabetes 30(12):996–999.

115. Ford CV, Bray GA, Swerdloff RS (1976). A psychiatric study of patients referred with a diagnosis of hypoglycemia. Am J Psychiatry 133(3):290–294.

116. American Diabetes Association, et al. (1973). Special report from the American Diabetes Association, The Endocrine Society, and the American Medical Association: Statement on hypoglycemia. Diabetes 22:137.

117. Jones TW, Borg WP, Boulware SD, McCarthy G, Sherwin RS, Tamborlane WV (1995). Enhanced adrenomedullary response and increased susceptibility to neuroglycopenia: Mechanisms underlying

the adverse effects of sugar ingestion in healthy children. J Pediatr 126(2):171–177.

118. Franklin W (2006). Syncope. Adolesc Health Update 18(3):1–8.

119. Permutt MA, Kelly J, Berstein R, Alpers DH, Siegel BA, Kipnis DM (1973). Alimentary hypoglycemia in the absence of gastrointestinal surgery. N Engl J Med 288(23):1206–1210.

120. Fischer KF, Lees JA, Newman JH (1986). Hypoglycemia in hospitalized patients: Causes and outcomes. N Engl J Med 315(20):1245–1250.

121. Miller SI, Wallace RJ Jr., Musher DM, Septimus EJ, Kohl S, Baughn RE (1980). Hypoglycemia as a manifestation of sepsis. Am J Med 68(5):649–654.

122. Deloof T, Berre J, Genette F, Van de Steene A, Mouawad E (1979). Disturbances of the carbohydrate metabolism in acute head trauma. Acta Neurochirurgica 28(1):113–114.

123. Benzing G III, Schubert W, Sug G, Kaplan S (1969). Simultaneous hypoglycemia and acute congestive heart failure. Circulation 40(2):209–216.

124. Peitzman SJ, Agarwal BN (1977). Spontaneous hypoglycemia in end-stage renal failure. Nephron 19(3):131–139.

125. Arem R (1989). Hypoglycemia associated with renal failure. Endocrinol Metab Clin North Am 18(1):103–121.

126. Arky RA (1989). Hypoglycemia associated with liver disease and ethanol. Endocrinol Metab Clin North Am 18(1):75–90.

127. Nigro G (1991). Pancreatitis with hypoglycemia-associated convulsions following rotavirus gastroenteritis. J Pediatr Gastroenterol Nutr 12(2):280–282.

128. Bradford D (1981). Ethanol poisoning in children. Br J Alcohol Alcoholism 16:27.

129. Ernst AA, Jones K, Nick TG, Sanchez J (1996). Ethanol ingestion and related hypoglycemia in a pediatric and adolescent emergency department population. Acad Emerg Med 3(1):46–49.

130. Fang V, Foye WO, Robinson SM, Jenkins HJ (1968). Hypoglycemic activity and chemical structure of the salicylates. J Pharm Sci 57(12):2111–2116.

131. Horwitz DL (1989). Factitious and artifactual hypoglycemia. Endocrinol Metab Clin North Am 18(1):203–210.

132. de Pasqua A, Mattock MB, Phillips R, Keen H (1984). Errors in blood glucose determination. Lancet 2(8412):1165.

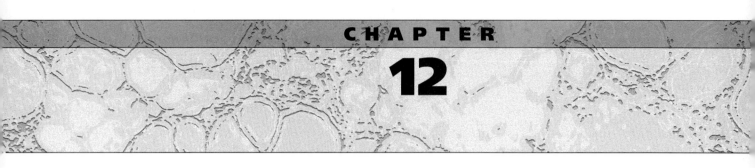

CHAPTER 12

The Adrenal Cortex and Its Disorders

WALTER L. MILLER, MD • JOHN C. ACHERMANN, MD
• CHRISTA E. FLÜCK, MD

History, Embryology, and Anatomy

The adrenal cortex produces three principal categories of steroid hormones that regulate a wide variety of physiologic processes from fetal to adult life. Mineralocorticoids (principally aldosterone) regulate renal retention of sodium and thus profoundly influence electrolyte balance, intravascular volume, and blood pressure. Glucocorticoids (principally cortisol) are named for their carbohydrate-mobilizing activity, but are ubiquitous physiologic regulators influencing a wide variety of bodily functions.

Adrenal androgens serve no known physiologic role but do mediate some secondary sexual characteristics in women (e.g., pubic and axillary hair), and their overproduction may result in virilism. Thus, the adrenal cortex is of considerable interest because of the widespread effects of its secretions and because derivatives of these secreted steroids are widely used as pharmacologic agents.[1] Disorders of the adrenal cortex, once thought to be rare, are being recognized with increasing frequency. The severe congenital adrenal hyperplasias affect nearly 1 in 10,000 persons, and the very mild forms may affect as many as 1 in 100 in some populations. Cushing disease, once regarded as a true rarity in pediatrics, may affect as many children as adults.

HISTORY

The adrenal glands apparently were first described in 1563 by the Italian anatomist Bartolomeo Eustaccio, better known for his description of the eustacian tube of the ear. Medical interest in the adrenals as something other than an anatomic curiosity began in the mid-nineteenth century with Addison's classic description of adrenal insufficiency and Brown-Séquard's experimental creation of similar disorders in animals subjected to adrenalectomy. The signs and symptoms of glucocorticoid excess due to adrenal tumors were well known by 1932, when Cushing described the pituitary tumors that cause what is now known as Cushing disease.[2] Effects of adrenalectomy on salt and water metabolism were reported in 1927, and by the late 1930s Selye had proposed the terms *glucocorticoid* and *mineralocorticoid* to distinguish the two broad categories of actions of adrenal extracts.[3]

Numerous adrenal steroids were painstakingly isolated and their structures determined during the 1930s in the laboratories of Reichstein[4] and Kendall,[5] leading to their sharing the 1950 Nobel Prize in Medicine. Many of these steroids were synthesized chemically, providing pure material for experimental purposes. The observation in 1949 that glucocorticoids ameliorated the symptoms of rheumatoid arthritis[6] greatly stimulated interest in synthesizing new pharmacologically active analogues of naturally occurring steroids. The structures of the various adrenal steroids suggested precursor/product relationships, leading in 1950 to the first treatment of congenital adrenal hyperplasia with cortisone by Wilkins[7] and by Bartter.[8] This opened a vigorous era of clinical investigation of the pathways of steroidogenesis in a variety of inherited adrenal and gonadal disorders.

The association of cytochrome P450 with 21-hydroxylation was made in 1965,[9] and some of the steroidogenic enzymes were then isolated in the 1970s. However, it was not until the genes for most of these enzymes were cloned in the 1980s that it became clear which proteins participated in which steroidal transformations.[10] The identification of these genes (Table 12-1) then led to an

understanding of the genetic lesions causing heritable disorders of steroidogenesis. At the same time, studies of steroid hormone action led to the discovery of steroid hormone receptors in the 1960s. However, it was not until they were cloned in the 1980s that their biology had begun to be understood.[11]

EMBRYOLOGY

The cells of the adrenal cortex are of mesodermal origin, in contrast to cells of the adrenal medulla, which are derived from the neuroectoderm. In human embryos, adreno-gonadal progenitor cells first appear at around the fourth week of gestation as a thickening of the coelomic epithelium, or intermediate mesoderm, between the urogenital ridge and dorsal mesentery (Figure 12-1).

TABLE 12-1

Physical Characteristics of Human Genes Encoding Steroidogenic Enzymes

Enzyme	No. of Genes	Gene Size (kb)	Chromosomal Location	Exons (n)	mRNA Size (kb)
P450scc	1	>20	15q23-q24	9	2.0
P450c11	2	9.5	8q21-22	9	4.2
P450c17	1	6.6	10q24.3	8	1.9
P450c21	2	3.4	6p21.1	10	2.0
P450aro	1	>52	15q21.2	10	3.5, 2.9
3β-HSD-I and -II	2	8	1p13	4	1.7
11β-HSD-I	1	7	1	6	1.6
11β-HSD-II	1	6.2	16p22	5	1.6
17β-HSD-I	2	3.3	17q21	6	1.4, 2.4
17β-HSD-II	1	>40	16q24	5	1.5
17β-HSD-III	1	>60	9q22	11	1.4
Adrenodoxin	1	>30	11q22	5	1.0, 1.4, 1.7
Adrenodoxin Reductase	1	11	17q24-q25	12	2.0
P450 Oxidoreductase	1	69	7q11.2	16	2.5
5α-Reductase - Type 1	1	>35	5p15	5	2.4
5α-Reductase - Type 2	1	>35	2p23	5	2.4

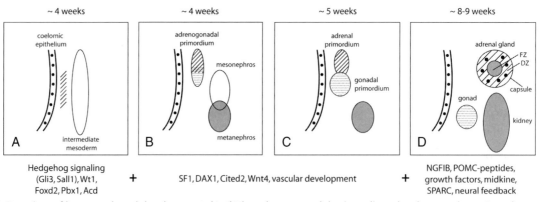

Figure 12-1 Overview of human adrenal development. (A-C) The adrenogonadal primordium develops at about 4 weeks gestation, after which the adrenal primordium becomes a distinct structure that then migrates retroperitoneally to the cranial pole of the mesonephros. (D) By 8 to 9 weeks gestation, the adrenal gland is encapsulated, contains chromaffin cells (black), and has distinct fetal (FZ) and definitive zones (DZ). Some of the signaling molecules, transcription factors, and growth factors implicated in adrenal development are shown below, although the exact timing and interaction of many of these factors remains poorly understood at present. [Adapted with permission from 14. Else T, Hammer GD (2005). Analysis of absence: Adrenal agenesis, aplasia and atrophy. Trends Endocrinol Metab 16:458-468.]

These progenitor cells give rise to the steroidogenic cells of the gonads and to the adrenal cortex.

The adrenal and gonadal cells then separate, with the adrenal cells migrating retroperitoneally to the cranial pole of the mesonephros and the gonadal cells migrating caudally. Between the seventh and eighth week of development, the adrenal primordium is invaded by sympathetic cells derived from the neural crest that give rise to the adrenal medulla. By the end of the eighth week, the rudimentary adrenal has become encapsulated and is clearly associated with the upper pole of the kidney, which at this time is much smaller than the adrenal.[12]

The fetal adrenal cortex consists of an outer "definitive" zone (the principal site of glucocorticoid and mineralocorticoid synthesis) and a much larger "fetal" zone, which makes androgenic precursors (DHEA, DHEAS) for the placental synthesis of estriol throughout pregnancy. A putative "transitional" zone exists between these regions toward the end of fetal development, but its functional role (if any) is unclear. The fetal adrenal glands are huge in proportion to other structures, and continue to grow well into the third trimester (Figure 12-2). At birth, the adrenals weigh 8 to 9 g (about the same size of adult adrenals) and represent approximately 0.4% of total body weight. However, the fetal adrenal zone rapidly involutes following birth and has virtually disappeared by 6 to 12 months of postnatal life. Thereafter, adrenal growth is comparatively slow and thus the adrenal glands represent only 0.01% of body weight in the adult.

The complex mechanisms regulating adrenal development are still relatively poorly understood. However, important insight into key factors has been obtained from studies of transgenic mice and from patients with disorders of adrenal development.[13] For example, the early stages of adrenal differentiation and development involve a number of signaling pathways (hedgehog/GLI3, WNT3/WNT4/WNT11, midkine), transcription factors [SALL1, FOXD2, PBX1, WT1, SF1 (NR5A1), DAX1 (NR0B1)], coregulators (CITED2), matrix proteins (SPARC), and regulators of telomerase activity (ACD).[14] Subsequent fetal adrenal growth is highly dependent on the tropic effects of adrenocorticotropin (ACTH), its receptor (MC2R), and its downstream signaling pathways, as well as on growth-factor-signaling pathways such as insulin-like growth factor II (IGFII), basic fibroblast growth factor (bFGF), and epidermal growth factor (EGF).

ANATOMY

The adrenals, once termed *suprarenal glands,* derive their name from their anatomical location of sitting on top of the upper pole of each kidney. Unlike most other organs, the arteries and veins serving the adrenal do not run in parallel. Arterial blood is provided by several small arteries arising from the renal and phrenic arteries, the aorta, and sometimes the ovarian and left spermatic arteries. The veins are more conventional, with the left adrenal vein draining into the left renal vein and the right adrenal vein draining directly into the vena cava.

Arterial blood enters the sinusoidal circulation of the cortex and drains toward the medulla, so that medullary chromaffin cells are bathed in very high concentrations of steroid hormones. High concentrations of cortisol are required for expression of medullary phenylethanol-amine-N-methyltransferase, which converts norepinephrine to epinephrine, linking the adrenal cortical and medullary responses to stress.[15]

The adrenal cortex consists of three histologically recognizable zones: the glomerulosa is immediately below the capsule, the fasciculata is in the middle, and the reticularis lies next to the medulla. The glomerulosa, fasciculata, and reticularis constitute respectively about 15%, 75%, and 10% of the adrenal cortex of the older child and adult. These zones appear to be distinct functionally as well as histologically, but considerable overlap exists and

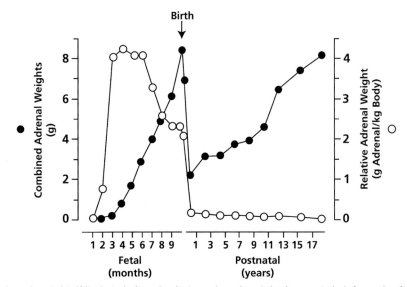

Figure 12-2 Combined adrenal weight (filled circles) and relative adrenal weight (open circles) from the first trimester through early adulthood. [Reprinted with permission from 170. Mesiano S, Jaffe RB (1997). Role of growth factors in the developmental regulation of the human fetal adrenal cortex. Steroids 62:62-72.]

immunocytochemical data show that the zones physically interdigitate. After birth, the large fetal zone begins to involute and disappears by about 6 months of age.

The definitive zone simultaneously enlarges, but two of the adult zones, glomerulosa and fasciculate, are not fully differentiated until about 3 years of age, and the reticularis may not be fully differentiated until about 15 years of age. The origin of the distinct adrenocortical zones and the mechanisms that regulate their proliferation are still poorly understood. One model suggests that a population of undifferentiated stem cells exists between the zona glomerulosa and zona fasciculata, which represents a pool of common precursor cells that can contribute to the inner or outer zones. In contrast, the "cell migration" theory proposes that a subcapsular population of stem cells exists. In this model, precursor cells first differentiate within the zona glomerulosa but change their characteristics as they migrate centripetally into the zona fasciculata then zona reticularis.

Steroid Hormone Synthesis

EARLY STEPS: CHOLESTEROL UPTAKE, STORAGE, AND TRANSPORT

Much is now known about steroid biosynthesis.[16] The human adrenal can synthesize cholesterol de novo from acetate, but most of its supply of cholesterol comes from plasma low-density lipoproteins (LDLs) derived from dietary cholesterol.[17] Rodent adrenals derive most of their cholesterol from high-density lipoproteins via a receptor termed SR-B1, but this pathway appears to play a minor role in human steroidogenesis.[18] Adequate concentrations of LDL will suppress 3-hydroxy-3-methylglutaryl co-enzyme A (HMGCoA) reductase, the rate-limiting enzyme in cholesterol synthesis.

ACTH, which stimulates adrenal steroidogenesis, also stimulates the activity of HMG CoA reductase, LDL receptors, and uptake of LDL cholesterol. LDL cholesterol esters are taken up by receptor-mediated endocytosis and then stored directly or converted to free cholesterol and used for steroid hormone synthesis.[19] Cholesterol can be esterified by acyl-CoA:cholesterol transferase (ACAT), stored in lipid droplets, and accessed by activation of hormone-sensitive lipase (HSL). ACTH stimulates HSL and inhibits ACAT, thus increasing the availability of free cholesterol for steroid hormone synthesis.

STEROIDOGENIC ENZYMES

Cytochrome P450

Most steroidogenic enzymes are members of the cytochrome P450 group of oxidases. *Cytochrome P450* is a generic term for a group of oxidative enzymes, all of which have about 500 amino acids and contain a single heme group.[20] They are termed *P450* (pigment 450) because all absorb light at 450 nm in their reduced states. It is sometimes stated that certain steroidogenic enzymes are "P450-dependent" enzymes. This is a misnomer, as it implies a generic P450 cofactor to a substrate-specific enzyme. However, the P450 binds the steroidal substrate and achieves its catalysis on an active site associated with the heme group.

Human beings have genes for 57 cytochrome P450 enzymes,[21,22] of which 7 are targeted to mitochondria and 50 are targeted to the endoplasmic reticulum—especially in the liver, where they metabolize countless endogenous and exogenous toxins, drugs, xenobiotics, and environmental pollutants. Each P450 enzyme can metabolize multiple substrates, catalyzing a broad array of oxidations. This theme recurs with each adrenal P450 enzyme.

Five distinct P450 enzymes are involved in adrenal steroidogenesis (Figure 12-3). Mitochondrial P450scc is the cholesterol side-chain cleavage enzyme catalyzing the series of reactions formerly termed *20,22 desmolase*. Two distinct isozymes of P450c11, P450c11β and P450c11AS; also found in mitochondria, catalyze 11β-hydroxylase, 18-hydroxylase, and 18-methyl oxidase activities. P450c17, found in the endoplasmic reticulum, catalyzes 17α-hydroxylase and 17,20 lyase activities, and P450c21 catalyzes the 21-hydroxylation of glucocorticoids and mineralocorticoids. In the gonads and elsewhere, P450aro in the endoplasmic reticulum catalyzes aromatization of androgens to estrogens.

Hydroxysteroid Dehydrogenases

The hydroxysteroid dehydrogenases have molecular masses of about 35 to 45 kDa, do not have heme groups, and require NAD^+ or $NADP^+$ as cofactors. Whereas most steroidogenic reactions catalyzed by P450 enzymes are due to the action of a single form of P450, each of the reactions catalyzed by hydroxysteroid dehydrogenases can be catalyzed by at least two, often very different, isozymes. Members of this family include the 3α- and 3β-hydroxysteroid dehydrogenases, the two 11β-hydroxysteroid dehydrogenases, and a series of 17β-hydroxysteroid dehydrogenases. The 5α-reductases are unrelated to this family.

Based on their structures, these enzymes fall into two groups: the short-chain dehydrogenase reductase (SDR) family, characterized by a Rossman fold, and the aldoketo reductase (AKR) family, characterized by a triose-phosphate isomerase (TIM) barrel motif.[23] The SDR enzymes include 11β-HSDs 1 and 2 and 17β-HSDs 1, 2, 3, and 4. The AKR enzymes include 17β-HSD5, which is important in extraglandular activation of androgenic precursors. Based on their activities, it is physiologically more useful to classify them as dehydrogenases or reductases. The dehydrogenases use NAD^+ as their cofactor to oxidize hydroxysteroids to ketosteroids, and the reductases mainly use NADPH to reduce ketosteroids to hydroxysteroids. Although these enzymes are typically bidirectional in vitro, they tend to function in only one direction in intact cells, with the direction determined by the cofactor(s) available.[23]

P450scc

Conversion of cholesterol to pregnenolone in mitochondria is the first rate-limiting and hormonally regulated step in the synthesis of all steroid hormones. This involves three distinct chemical reactions: 20α-hydroxylation,

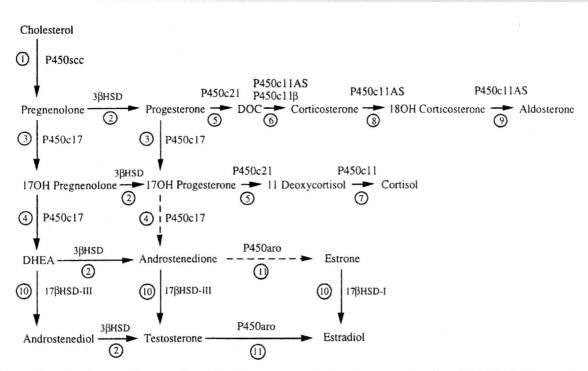

Figure 12-3 Principal pathways of human adrenal steroid hormone synthesis. Other quantitatively and physiologically minor steroids are also produced. The names of the enzymes are shown by each reaction, and the traditional names of the enzymatic activities correspond to the circled numbers. Reaction 1: Mitochondrial cytochrome P450scc mediates 20α-hydroxylation, 22-hydroxylation, and scission of the C20-22 carbon bond. Reaction 2: 3βHSD mediates 3β-hydroxysteroid dehydrogenase and isomerase activities, converting Δ^5 steroids to Δ^4 steroids. Reaction 3: P450c17 catalyzes the 17α-hydroxylation of pregnenolone to 17OH-pregnenolone and of progesterone to 17OH-progesterone. Reaction 4: The 17,20 lyase activity of P450c17 converts 17OH-pregnenolone to DHEA (only insignificant amounts of 17OH-progesterone are converted to Δ^4 androstenedione by human P450c17, although this reaction occurs in other species). Reaction 5: P450c21 catalyzes the 21-hydroxylation of progesterone to DOC and of 17OH-progesterone to 11-deoxycortisol. Reaction 6: DOC is converted to corticosterone by the 11-hydroxylase activity of P450c11AS in the zona glomerulosa and by P450c11β in the zona fasciculata. Reaction 7: 11-deoxycortisol undergoes 11β-hydroxylation by P450c11β to produce cortisol in the zona fasciculata. Reactions 8 and 9: The 18-hydroxylase and 18-methyl oxidase activities of P450c11AS convert corticosterone to 18OH-corticosterone and aldosterone, respectively, in the zona glomerulosa. Reactions 10 and 11 are found principally in the testes and ovaries. Reaction 10: 17βHSD-III converts DHEA to androstenediol and androstenedione to testosterone, whereas 17βHSD-I converts estrone to estradiol. Reaction 11: Testosterone may be converted to estradiol and androstenedione may be converted to estrone by P450aro.

22-hydroxylation, and scission of the cholesterol side chain to yield pregnenolone and isocaproic acid. Because 20-hydroxycholesterol, 22-hydroxycholesterol, and 20, 22-dihydroxycholesterol could all be isolated from bovine adrenals in significant quantities, it was previously thought that three separate enzymes were involved.

However, a single protein, termed *P450scc*, where SCC refers to the side-chain cleavage of cholesterol, encoded by a single gene on chromosome 15[24] catalyzes all steps between cholesterol and pregnenolone.[10,25] These three reactions occur on a single active site that is in contact with the hydrophobic bilayer membrane. Deletion of the gene for P450scc in the rabbit[26] or mouse[27] eliminates all steroidogenesis, indicating that all steroidogenesis is initiated by this one enzyme.

Transport of Electrons to P450scc: Adrenodoxin Reductase and Adrenodoxin

P450scc functions as the terminal oxidase in a mitochondrial electron transport system.[28] Electrons from NADPH are accepted by a flavoprotein, termed *adrenodoxin*

reductase, that is loosely associated with the inner mitochondrial membrane. Adrenodoxin reductase transfers the electrons to an iron/sulfur protein termed *adrenodoxin,* which is found in the mitochondrial matrix or loosely adherent to the inner mitochondrial membrane. Adrenodoxin then transfers the electrons to P450scc (Figure 12-4).

Adrenodoxin reductase and adrenodoxin serve as generic electron transfer proteins for all mitochondrial P450s, and not just for those involved in steroidogenesis. Hence, these proteins are also termed *ferredoxin reductase* and *ferredoxin.* Adrenodoxin forms a 1:1 complex with adrenodoxin reductase and then dissociates, subsequently reforming an analogous 1:1 complex with a mitochondrial P450 such as P450scc or P450c11, thus functioning as an indiscriminate diffusable electron shuttle mechanism. Adrenodoxin reductase is a membrane-bound mitochondrial flavoprotein that receives electrons from NADPH. The human genes for adrenodoxin reductase[29,30] and adrenodoxin[31] are expressed in all tissues,[32,33] indicating they may have other roles. Human mutations in these genes have not been described.

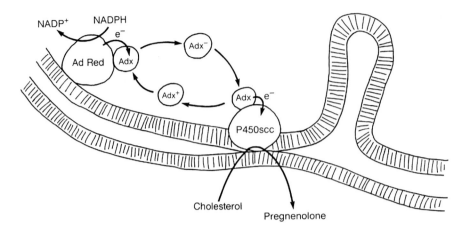

Figure 12-4 Electron transport to mitochondrial forms of cytochrome P450. Adrenodoxin reductase (AdRed), a flavoprotein loosely bound to the inner mitochondrial membrane, accepts electrons (e^-) from NADPH, converting it to $NADP^+$. These electrons are passed to adrenodoxin (Adx), an iron-sulfur protein in solution in the mitochondrial matrix that functions as a freely diffusable electron shuttle mechanism. Electrons from charged adrenodoxin (Adx^-) are accepted by any available cytochrome P450 such as P450c11 (or P450scc, shown here). The uncharged adrenodoxin (Adx^+) may then be again bound to adrenodoxin reductase to receive another pair of electrons. For P450scc, three pairs of electrons must be transported to the P450 to convert cholesterol to pregnenolone. The flow of cholesterol into the mitochondria is facilitated by StAR, which is not shown in this diagram.

Mitochondrial Cholesterol Uptake: The Steroidogenic Acute Regulatory Protein (StAR)

ACTH regulates steroidogenic capacity (chronic regulation) by inducing the transcription of genes for steroidogenic enzymes,[34] but acute regulation (wherein steroids are released within minutes of a stimulus) is at the level of cholesterol access to P450scc.[35,36] When steroidogenic cells or intact rats are treated with inhibitors of protein synthesis such as cycloheximide, the acute steroidogenic response is eliminated, suggesting that a short-lived cycloheximide-sensitive protein acts at the level of the mitochondrion[25] as the specific trigger to the acute steroidogenic response.

This factor was first identified as short-lived 30- and 37-kDa phosphoproteins that were rapidly synthesized when steroidogenic cells were stimulated with tropic hormones[37-39] and then cloned from mouse Leydig MA-10 cells, and named the steroidogenic acute regulatory protein, StAR.[40] The central role of StAR in steroidogenesis was proven by finding that mutations of StAR caused congenital lipoid adrenal hyperplasia.[41,42] Thus, StAR is the acute trigger required for the rapid flux of cholesterol from the outer to the inner mitochondrial membrane that is needed for the acute response of aldosterone to angiotensin II, of cortisol to ACTH, and of sex steroids to an LH pulse.

Some adrenal steroidogenesis is independent of StAR. When nonsteroidogenic cells are transfected with StAR and the P450scc system, they convert cholesterol to pregnenolone at about 14% of the StAR-induced rate.[41,42] Furthermore, the placenta utilizes mitochondrial P450scc to initiate steroidogenesis[43] but does not express StAR.[44] The mechanism of StAR-independent steroidogenesis is unclear. It may occur without a triggering protein, or some other protein may exert StAR-like activity to promote cholesterol flux but without StAR's rapid kinetics.

Substantial data indicate that the action of StAR also requires the peripheral benzodiazepine receptor on the outer mitochondrial membrane.[45-47] The mechanism of StAR's action is unknown, but it is clear that StAR acts on the outer mitochondrial membrane and does not need to enter the mitochondria to be active.[36,48] The interaction with the outer mitochondrial membrane induces structural changes required for StAR's activity, probably permitting it to take up and discharge cholesterol.[36,49,50]

3β-Hydroxysteroid Dehydrogenase/$\Delta^5 \rightarrow \Delta^4$ Isomerase

Once pregnenolone is produced from cholesterol, it may undergo 17α-hydroxylation by P450c17 to yield 17-hydroxypregnenolone, or it may be converted to progesterone—the first biologically important steroid in the pathway. A single 42-kDa microsomal enzyme, 3β-hydroxysteroid dehydrogenase (3βHSD), catalyzes both conversion of the hydroxyl group to a keto group on carbon 3 and the isomerization of the double bond from the B ring (Δ^5 steroids) to the A ring (Δ^4 steroids).[51-53] Thus, a single enzyme (3βHSD) converts pregnenolone to progesterone, 17α-hydroxypregnenolone to 17α-hydroxyprogesterone, dehydroepiandrosterone (DHEA) to androstenedione, and androstenediol to testosterone, all with the same enzymologic efficiency (Km and Vmax).[54]

As is typical of hydroxysteroid dehydrogenases, there are two isozymes of 3βHSD, encoded by separate genes. These isozymes have 93.5% amino acid sequence identity and are enzymatically very similar. The enzyme-catalyzing 3βHSD activity in the adrenals and gonads is the type 2 enzyme,[55,56] whereas the type 1 enzyme, encoded by a closely linked gene with identical intron/exon organization, catalyzes 3βHSD activity in placenta, breast, and "extraglandular" tissues.[55,57] Ultrastructural data surprisingly show that bovine 3βHSD can be found in the endoplasmic reticulum and in mitochondria.[58] It is not clear if this is also true for human 3βHSD, or if this subcellular distribution differs in various types of steroidogenic cells. However, this could be a novel point regulating the direction of steroidogenesis.[59]

P450c17

Pregnenolone and progesterone may undergo 17α-hydroxylation to 17α-hydroxypregnenolone and 17α-hydroxyprogesterone (17OHP), respectively. 17α-hydroxyprogesterone may also undergo scission of the C17,20 carbon bond to yield DHEA. However, very little 17OHP is converted to androstenedione because the human P450c17 enzyme catalyzes this reaction at only 3% of the rate for conversion of 17α-hydroxypregnenolone to DHEA.[60,61] These reactions are all mediated by a single enzyme, P450c17. This P450 is bound to smooth endoplasmic reticulum, where it accepts electrons from P450 oxidoreductase.

As P450c17 has both 17α-hydroxylase activity and 17,20 lyase activity, it is the key branch point in steroid hormone synthesis. Neither activity of P450c17 is present in the adrenal zona glomerulosa, and hence pregnenolone is converted to mineralocorticoids. In the zona fasciculata, the 17α-hydroxylase activity is present but 17,20 lyase activity is not. Hence, pregnenolone is converted to the glucocorticoid cortisol. In the zona reticularis, both activities are present and thus pregnenolone is converted to sex steroids (Figure 12-3).

17α-hydroxylase and 17,20 lyase were once thought to be separate enzymes. The adrenals of prepubertal children synthesize ample cortisol but virtually no sex steroids (i.e., have 17α-hydroxylase activity but not 17,20 lyase activity), until adrenarche initiates production of adrenal androgens (i.e., turns on 17,20 lyase activity).[62] Furthermore, patients had been described lacking 17,20 lyase activity but retaining normal 17α-hydroxylase activity.[63] However, studies of pig P450c17 showed that 17α-hydroxylase and 17,20 lyase activities reside in a single protein[64,65] and that cells transfected with a vector expressing P450c17 cDNA acquire 17α-hydroxylase and

17,20 lyase activities.[66,67] P450c17 is encoded by a single gene on chromosome 10q24.3[68,69] that is structurally related to the genes for P450c21 (21-hydroxylase).[70]

Thus, the distinction between 17α-hydroxylase and 17,20 lyase is functional and not genetic or structural. Human P450c17 catalyzes 17α-hydroxylation of pregnenolone and progesterone equally well, but the 17,20 lyase activity of human P450c17 strongly prefers 17OH pregnenolone and not 17OH progesterone, consistent with the large amounts of DHEA secreted by the fetal and adult adrenal. Furthermore, the 17α-hydroxylase reaction occurs more readily than the 17,20 lyase reaction. The principal factor regulating the 17,20 lyase reaction is electron transport from NADPH.

Electron Transport to P450c17: P450 Oxidoreductase and Cytochrome b₅

P450c17 and P450c21 receive electrons from a membrane-bound flavoprotein, termed *P450 oxidoreductase*, which is a different protein from the mitochondrial flavoprotein adrenodoxin reductase.[28] P450 oxidoreductase receives two electrons from NADPH and transfers them one at a time to the P450.[71,72] Electron transfer for the lyase reaction is promoted by the action of cytochrome b₅ as an allosteric factor rather than as an alternative electron donor.[61] 17,20 lyase activity also requires the phosphorylation of serine residues on P450c17 by a cAMP-dependent protein kinase[73-75] (Figure 12-5).

The availability of electrons determines whether P450c17 performs only 17α-hydroxylation or also performs 17,20 bond scission. Increasing the ratio of P450 oxidoreductase or cytochrome b₅ to P450c17 in vitro or in vivo increases the ratio of 17,20 lyase activity to 17α-hydroxylase activity. Competition between P450c17 and P450c21 for available 17-hydroxyprogesterone (17OHP) does not appear to be important in determining whether 17OHP undergoes 21-hydroxylation or 17,20 bond scission.[76] Thus, the regulation of 17,20 lyase activity, and consequently of DHEA production, depends on factors that facilitate the flow of

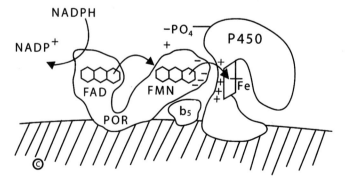

Figure 12-5 Electron transport to microsomal forms of cytochrome P450. NADPH interacts with P450 oxidoreductase (POR), bound to the endoplasmic reticulum, and gives up a pair of electrons (e⁻)—which are received by the FAD moiety. Electron receipt elicits a conformational change, permitting the isoalloxazine rings of the FAD and FMN moieties to come close together so that the electrons pass from the FAD to the FMN. Following another conformational change that returns the protein to its original orientation, the FMN domain of POR interacts with the redox partner binding site of the P450. Electrons from the FMN domain of POR reach the heme group to mediate catalysis. The interaction of POR and the P450 is coordinated by negatively charged acidic residues on the surface of the FMN domain of POR and by positively charged basic residues in the concave redox-partner binding site of the P450. The active site containing the steroid lies on the side of heme ring (Fe) opposite the redox partner binding site. In the case of human P450c17, this interaction is facilitated by the allosteric action of cytochrome b₅ and by the serine phosphorylation of P450c17. [Copyright W L Miller.]

electrons to P450c17: high concentrations of P450 oxido-reductase, the presence of cytochrome b5, and serine phosphorylation of P450c17.[77]

P450c21

After the synthesis of progesterone and 17OHP, these steroids are hydroxylated at the 21 position to yield respectively deoxycorticosterone (DOC) and 11-deoxycortisol (Figure 12-3). The nature of the 21-hydroxylating step has been of great clinical interest because disordered 21-hydroxylation causes more than 90% of all cases of congenital adrenal hyperplasia. The clinical symptoms associated with this common genetic disease are complex and devastating. Decreased cortisol and aldosterone synthesis often lead to sodium loss, potassium retention, and hypotension, which will lead to cardiovascular collapse and death usually within a month after birth if not treated appropriately. Decreased synthesis of cortisol in utero leads to overproduction of ACTH and consequent overstimulation of adrenal steroid synthesis. As the 21-hydroxylase step is impaired, 17OHP accumulates because P450c17 converts only miniscule amounts of 17OHP to androstenedione.

However, 17-hydroxypregnenolone also accumulates and is converted to DHEA, and subsequently to androstenedione and testosterone, resulting in severe prenatal virilization of female fetuses.[78-81] Congenital adrenal hyperplasia (CAH) has been extensively studied clinically. Variations in the manifestations of the disease, and especially the identification of patients without apparent defects in mineralocorticoid activity, suggested that there were two separate 21-hydroxylating enzymes differentially expressed in the zones of the adrenal specifically synthesizing aldosterone or cortisol. However, characterization of the P450c21 protein[82] and gene cloning show that there is only one 21-hydroxylase encoded by a single functional gene on chromosome 6p21.[83-85] As this gene lies in the middle of the major histocompatibility locus, disorders of adrenal 21-hydroxylation are closely linked to specific HLA types.[86]

Adrenal 21-hydroxylation is mediated by P450c21 found in smooth endoplasmic reticulum. P450c21 employs the same P450 oxidoreductase used by P450c17 to transport electrons from NADPH. 21-hydroxylase activity has also been described in a broad range of adult and fetal extra-adrenal tissues.[87] However, extra-adrenal 21-hydroxylation is not mediated by the P450c21 enzyme found in the adrenal.[88] At least three hepatic P450 enzymes can catalyze 21-hydroxylation in vitro,[89] but the significance of this activity in clinical situations is unclear. As a result, patients having absent adrenal 21-hydroxylase activity may still have appreciable concentrations of 21-hydroxylated steroids in their plasma.

P450c11β and P450c11AS

Two closely related enzymes, P450c11β and P450c11AS, catalyze the final steps in the synthesis of glucocorticoids and mineralocorticoids.[90,91] These two isozymes have 93% amino acid sequence identity[92] and are encoded by tandemly duplicated genes on chromosome 8q21-22. Like P450scc, the two forms of P450c11 are found on the inner mitochondrial membrane and use adrenodoxin and adrenodoxin reductase to receive electrons from NADPH.[93] By far the more abundant of the two isozymes is P450c11β, which is the classic 11β-hydroxylase that converts 11-deoxycortisol to cortisol and 11-deoxycorticosterone to corticosterone. The less abundant isozyme, P450c11AS, is found only in the zona glomerulosa, where it has 11β-hydroxylase, 18-hydroxylase, and 18-methyl oxidase aldosterone synthase activities. Thus, P450c11AS is able to catalyze all reactions needed to convert DOC to aldosterone.[94,95]

P450c11β, which is principally involved in synthesis of cortisol, is encoded by a gene (CYP11B1) that is primarily induced by ACTH via cAMP and is suppressed by glucocorticoids. The existence of two distinct functional genes is confirmed by the identification of mutations in each that cause distinct genetic disorders of steroidogenesis. Thus, patients with disorders in P450c11β have classic 11β-hydroxylase deficiency but can still produce aldosterone[96], whereas patients with disorders in P450c11AS have rare forms of aldosterone deficiency, so-called corticosterone methyl oxidase deficiency, while retaining the ability to produce cortisol.[97-99]

17β-Hydroxysteroid Dehydrogenase

Androstenedione is converted to testosterone, DHEA is converted to androstenediol, and estrone is converted to estradiol by the 17β-hydroxysteroid dehydrogenases (17βHSDs), sometimes also termed *17-oxioreductase* or *17-ketosteroid reductase*.[100,101] The terminologies for these enzymes vary, depending on the direction of the reaction being considered. There is confusion in the literature about the 17βHSDs because: (i) there are several different 17βHSDs; (ii) some are preferential oxidases whereas others are preferential reductases; (iii) they differ in their substrate preference and sites of expression; (iv) there is inconsistent nomenclature, especially with the rodent enzymes; / (v) and some proteins termed *17βHSD* actually have very little 17βHSD activity and are principally involved in other reactions.[102]

Type 1 17βHSD (17βHSD1), also known as estrogenic 17βHSD, is a 34-kDa cytosolic reductive SDR enzyme, first isolated and cloned from the placenta, where it produces estriol, and is also expressed in ovarian granulosa cells, where it produces estradiol.[52,103-105] 17βHSD1 uses NADPH as its cofactor to catalyze reductase activity. It acts as a dimer and only accepts steroid substrates with an aromatic A ring, and thus its activity is confined to activating estrogens. The three-dimensional structure of human 17βHSD1 has been determined by x-ray crystallography.[106,107] No genetic deficiency syndrome for 17βHSD1 has been described.

17βHSD2 is a microsomal oxidase that uses NAD+ to inactivate estradiol to estrone and testosterone to Δ4 androstenedione. 17βHSD2 is found in the placenta, liver, small intestine, prostate, secretory endometrium, and ovary. In contrast to 17βHSD1, which is found in placental synctiotrophoblast cells, 17βHSD2 is expressed in endothelial cells of placental intravillous vessels, consistent with its apparent role in defending the fetal circulation from transplacental passage of maternal estradiol or testosterone.[108] No deficiency state for 17βHSD2 has been reported.

17βHSD3, the androgenic form of 17βHSD, is a microsomal enzyme apparently expressed only in the testis.[109] This is the enzyme that is disordered in the classic syndrome of male pseudohermaphroditism that is often termed *17-ketosteroid reductase deficiency*.[109,110]

An enzyme termed *17βHSD4* was initially identified as an NAD⁺-dependent oxidase with activities similar to 17βHSD2,[111] but this peroxisomal protein is primarily an enoyl-CoA hydratase and 3-hydroxyacyl-CoA dehydrogenase.[112,113] Deficiency of 17βHSD4 causes a form of Zellweger syndrome, in which bile acid biosynthesis is disturbed but steroidogenesis is not.[113]

17βHSD5, originally cloned as a 3α-hydroxysteroid dehydrogenase,[114] is an AKR enzyme that catalyzes the reduction of Δ^4 androstenedione to testosterone.[115] The 17βHSD activity of 17βHSD5 is quite labile in vitro,[115] and hence its activity in androgen biosynthesis has been less clear. However, it appears to be responsible for low levels of testosterone synthesis in the adrenal and adipose tissue and may convert androstenedione to testosterone in muscle.

Steroid Sulfotransferase and Sulfatase

Steroid sulfates may be synthesized directly from cholesterol sulfate or may be formed by sulfation of steroids by cytosolic sulfotransferase (SULT) enzymes.[116,117] At least 44 distinct isoforms of these enzymes have been identified belonging to five families of SULT genes. Many of these genes yield alternately spliced products, accounting for the large number of enzymes. The SULT enzymes that sulfonate steroids include SULT1E estrogens, SULT2A1 nonaromatic steroids, and SULT2B1 sterols. SULT2A1 is the principal sulfotransferase expressed in the adrenal, where it sulfates the 3βhydroxyl group of Δ5 steroids, pregnenolone, 17OH-pregnenolone, DHEA, androsterone, but not of cholesterol. SULT2B1a will also sulfonate pregnenolone but not cholesterol, whereas cholesterol is the principal substrate for SULT2B1b in the skin, liver, and elsewhere.

It is not clear whether most steroid sulfates are simply inactivated forms of steroid or if they serve specific hormonal roles. Knockout of the mouse SULT1E1 gene is associated with elevated estrogen levels, increased expression of tissue factor in the placenta, and increased platelet activation, leading to placental thrombi and fetal loss that could be ameliorated by anticoagulant therapy.[118] Mutations ablating the function of human SULT enzymes have not been described, but single-nucleotide polymorphisms that alter the amino acid sequences and catalytic activity affecting drug activity are well described. African Americans have a high rate of polymorphisms in SULT2A1, apparently influencing plasma ratios of DHEA and DHEAS, which may correlate with risk of prostatic and other cancers.[119]

Steroid sulfates may also be hydrolyzed to the native steroid by steroid sulfatase. Deletions in the steroid sulfatase gene on chromosome Xp22.3 cause X-linked ichthyosis.[120,121] In the fetal adrenal and placenta, diminished or absent sulfatase deficiency reduces the pool of free DHEA available for placental conversion to estrogen, resulting in low concentrations of estriol in the maternal blood and urine. The accumulation of steroid sulfates in the stratum corneum of the skin causes the ichthyosis. Steroid sulfatase is also expressed in the fetal rodent brain, possibly converting peripheral DHEAS to active DHEA.[122,123]

Aromatase: P450aro

Estrogens are produced by the aromatization of androgens, including adrenal androgens, by a complex series of reactions catalyzed by a single microsomal aromatase (P450aro).[124,125] This typical cytochrome P450 is encoded by a single gene on chromosome 15q21.1. This gene uses several different promoter sequences, transcriptional start sites, and alternatively chosen first exons to encode aromatase mRNA in different tissues under different hormonal regulation. Aromatase expression in the extraglandular tissues, especially adipose tissue, can convert adrenal androgens to estrogens.

Aromatase in the epiphyses of growing bone converts testosterone to estradiol. The tall stature, delayed epiphyseal maturation, and osteopenia of males with aromatase deficiency and the rapid reversal of these conditions with estrogen replacement indicate that estrogen (not androgen) is responsible for epiphyseal maturation in males.[125] Although it has traditionally been thought that aromatase activity is needed for embryonic and fetal development, infants and adults with genetic disorders in this enzyme have been described recently, demonstrating that feto-placental estrogen is not needed for normal fetal development.[126,127]

5α-Reductase

Testosterone is converted to the more potent androgen dihydrotestosterone by 5α-reductase, an enzyme found in testosterone's target tissues. There are two distinct forms of 5α-reductase. The type 1 enzyme, found in the scalp and other peripheral tissues, is encoded by a gene on chromosome 5. The type 2 enzyme, the predominant form found in male reproductive tissues, is encoded by a structurally related gene on chromosome 2p23.[128] The syndrome of 5α-reductase deficiency, a disorder of male sexual differentiation, is due to a wide variety of mutations in the gene encoding the type 2 enzyme.[129]

The types 1 and 2 genes show an unusual pattern of developmental regulation of expression. The type 1 gene is not expressed in the fetus, is then expressed briefly in the skin of the newborn, and then remains unexpressed until its activity and protein are again found after puberty. The type 2 gene is expressed in fetal genital skin, in the normal prostate, and in prostatic hyperplasia and adenocarcinoma. Thus, the type 1 enzyme may be responsible for the pubertal virilization seen in patients with classic 5α-reductase deficiency, and the type 2 enzyme may be involved in male-pattern baldness.[128]

11β-Hydroxysteroid Dehydrogenase

Although certain steroids are categorized as glucocorticoids or mineralocorticoids, cloning and expression of the "mineralocorticoid" glucocorticoid type 2 receptor shows it has equal affinity for aldosterone and cortisol.[130] However, cortisol does not act as a mineralocorticoid in vivo, even though cortisol concentrations can exceed aldosterone concentrations by 100- to 1,000-fold. In mineralocorticoid-responsive tissues such as the kidney, cortisol is enzymatically converted to cortisone, a metabolically inactive steroid.[131]

The interconversion of cortisol and cortisone is mediated by two isozymes of 11β-hydroxysteroid dehydrogenase 11βHSD, each of which has oxidase and reductase activity, depending on the cofactor available, $NADP^+$ or $NADPH$.[132] The type 1 enzyme 11βHSD1 is expressed mainly in glucocorticoid-responsive tissues such as the liver, testis, lung, and proximal convoluted tubule. 11βHSD1 can catalyze the oxidation of cortisol to cortisone using $NADP^+$ as its cofactor K_m 1.6 μM and can catalyze the reduction of cortisone to cortisol using $NADPH$ as its cofactor K_m 0.14 μM. The reaction catalyzed depends on which cofactor is available, but the enzyme can only function with high micromolar concentrations of steroid.[133,134]

11βHSD2 catalyzes only the oxidation of cortisol to cortisone using $NADH$, and can function with low nanomolar-concentrations of steroid (K_m 10-100 nM).[135,136] 11βHSD2 is expressed in mineralocorticoid-responsive tissues and thus serves to "defend" the mineralocorticoid receptor by inactivating cortisol to cortisone so that only "true" mineralocorticoids, such as aldosterone or deoxycorticosterone, can exert a mineralocorticoid effect. Thus, 11βHSD2 prevents cortisol from overwhelming renal mineralocorticoid receptors.[131] In the placenta and other fetal tissues, 11βHSD2[137,138] also inactivates cortisol.

The placenta also has abundant $NADP^+$ favoring the oxidative action of 11βHSD1, and thus in placenta both enzymes protect the fetus from high maternal concentrations of cortisol.[132] 11βHSD1 is located on the luminal side of the endoplasmic reticulum, and hence is not in contact with the cytoplasm. In this unusual cellular location, 11βHSD1 receives $NADPH$ provided by the action of hexose-6-phosphate dehydrogenase.[139] This links 11βHSD1 to the pentose monophosphate shunt, providing a direct paracrine link between local glucocorticoid production and energy storage as fat.[140]

FETAL ADRENAL STEROIDOGENESIS

Adrenocortical steroidogenesis begins early in embryonic life, about week 7 of gestation. Steroidogenic enzymes are immunocytochemically detected, principally in the fetal zone, at 50 to 52 days postconception; by 8 weeks postconception the adrenal contains cortisol and responds to ACTH in primary culture systems.[141] This cortisol synthesis is under the regulation of pituitary ACTH and involves transient expression of adrenal 3βHSD2. Following the ninth week postconception, expression of 3βHSD2 and synthesis of cortisol wane. 3βHSD2 is

barely detectable at 10 to 11 weeks and is absent at 14 weeks.[141]

At the same time, the fetal adrenal also produces 17βHSD5[141], which can convert androstenedione to testosterone. Thus, the fetal adrenal makes cortisol at the same time during gestation that fetal testicular testosterone is virilizing the genitalia of the normal male fetus. This fetal adrenal cortisol apparently suppresses ACTH, which otherwise would drive adrenal testosterone synthesis via 17βHSD5.

Fetuses affected with genetic lesions in adrenal steroidogenesis can produce sufficient adrenal androgen to virilize a female fetus to a nearly male appearance, and this masculinization of the genitalia is complete by week 12 of gestation.[142] The definitive zone of the fetal adrenal produces steroid hormones according to the pathways shown in Figure 12-3. By contrast, the large fetal zone of the adrenal is relatively deficient in 3βHSD2 activity after 12 weeks.[143] The fetal adrenal has relatively abundant 17,20 lyase activity of P450c17. Low 3βHSD and high 17,20 lyase activity account for the abundant production of DHEA and its sulfate DHEAS by the fetal adrenal, which are converted to estrogens by the placenta.

The fetal adrenal also has considerable sulfotransferase activity but little steroid sulfatase activity, also favoring conversion of DHEA to DHEAS. The resulting DHEAS cannot be a substrate for adrenal 3βHSD2. Instead, it is secreted, 16α-hydroxylated in the fetal liver, and then acted on by placental 3βHSD1, 17βHSD1, and P450aro to produce estriol. Alternatively, the substrates can bypass the liver to yield estrone and estradiol. Placental estrogens inhibit adrenal 3βHSD activity, providing a feedback system to promote production of DHEAS.[144] Fetal adrenal steroids account for 50% of the estrone and estradiol and 90% of the estriol in the maternal circulation.

Although the feto-placental unit produces huge amounts of DHEA, DHEAS, and estriol (as well as other steroids), they do not appear to serve an essential role. Successful pregnancy is wholly dependent on placental synthesis of progesterone, which suppresses uterine contractility and prevents spontaneous abortion. However, fetuses with genetic disorders of adrenal and gonadal steroidogenesis develop normally, reach term gestation, and undergo normal parturition and delivery. Mineralocorticoid production is only required postnatally. Estrogens are not required, and androgens are only needed for male sexual differentiation.[145] It appears that human fetal glucocorticoids are needed at about 8 to 12 weeks,[141] but it is not clear that they are needed thereafter. If they are, the small amount of maternal cortisol that escapes placental inactivation suffices.[145-147]

The regulation of steroidogenesis and growth of the fetal adrenal are not fully understood, but both are related to ACTH. ACTH effectively stimulates steroidogenesis by fetal adrenal cells in vitro,[148,149] and excess ACTH is clearly involved in the adrenal growth and overproduction of androgens in fetuses affected with congenital adrenal hyperplasia. Prenatal treatment of such fetuses by administering pharmacologic doses of dexamethasone to the mother at 6 to 10 weeks gestation can significantly reduce fetal adrenal androgen production and thus reduce the virilization of female fetuses. Thus, the hypothalamic-pituitary-adrenal axis functions very early in fetal life.[150] By contrast, however, anencephalic fetuses lacking pituitary ACTH have adrenals that contain a fairly normal complement of steroidogenic enzymes and retain their capacity for steroidogenesis. Thus, fetal adrenal steroidogenesis may be regulated by ACTH-dependent and ACTH-independent mechanisms.

Regulation of Steroidogenesis

THE HYPOTHALAMIC-PITUITARY-ADRENAL AXIS

Hypothalamus: CRF and AVP

The principal steroidal product of the human adrenal is cortisol, which is mainly secreted in response to adrenocorticotropic hormone (ACTH, corticotropin) produced in the pituitary. Secretion of ACTH is stimulated primarily by corticotropin-releasing factor (CRF) from the hypothalamus. Hypothalamic CRF is a 41-amino-acid peptide synthesized mainly by neurons in the paraventricular nucleus. These same hypothalamic neurons also produce the decapeptide arginine vasopressin AVP, also known as antidiuretic hormone or ADH.[151] CRF and AVP are proteolytically derived from larger precursors, with the AVP precursor containing the sequence for neurophysin, which is the AVP-binding protein.

CRF and AVP travel through axons to the median eminence, which releases them into the pituitary portal circulation, although most AVP axons terminate in the posterior pituitary.[152] AVP is co-secreted with CRF in response to stress, and CRF and AVP stimulate the synthesis and release of ACTH but appear to do so by different mechanisms.[153] CRF binds to a G-protein–coupled receptor on the membranes of pituitary corticotropes and activates adenylyl cyclase, increasing cAMP, which activates the PKA signaling pathway.

PKA triggers ACTH secretion by concerted regulation of cellular potassium and calcium fluxes, and enhances pro-opiomelanocortin (POMC) gene transcription. AVP binds to its G-protein–coupled receptor and activates phospholipase C, which leads to the release of intracellular Ca^{++} and to the activation of protein kinase C (PKC). AVP seems to amplify the effects of CRF on ACTH secretion without affecting synthesis. However, CRF is the more important physiologic stimulator of ACTH release, although maximal doses of AVP can elicit a maximal ACTH response. When given together, CRF and AVP act synergistically, as would be expected from their independent mechanisms of action.

Pituitary: ACTH and POMC

Pituitary ACTH is a 39-amino-acid peptide derived from POMC, a 241-amino-acid protein. POMC undergoes a series of proteolytic cleavages, yielding several biologically active peptides[154,155] (Figure 12-6). The N-terminal glycopeptide (POMC 1-75) can stimulate steroidogenesis and may function as an adrenal mitogen.[156] POMC 112-150 is ACTH 1-39, POMC 112-126 and POMC 191-207 constitute respectively α- and β-MSH melanocyte-stimulating hormone, and POMC 210-241 is β-endorphin. POMC is also produced in small amounts by the brain, testis, liver, kidney, and placenta. However, this extrapituitary POMC does not contribute significantly to circulating ACTH.

Malignant tumors will commonly produce ectopic ACTH in adults and rarely in children. This ACTH derives from ectopic biosynthesis of the same POMC precursor.[154] Only the first 20 to 24 amino acids of ACTH are needed for its full biological activity, and synthetic ACTH 1-24 is widely used in diagnostic tests of adrenal function. However, these shorter forms of ACTH have a shorter half-life than does native ACTH 1-39. POMC gene transcription is stimulated by CRF and inhibited by glucocorticoids.[157]

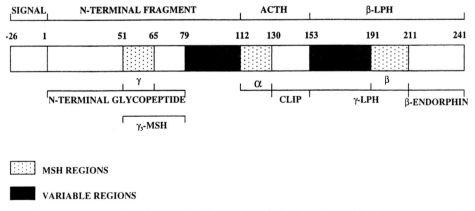

Figure 12-6 Structure of human pre-proopiomelanocortin. The numbers refer to amino acid positions, with no. 1 assigned to the first amino acid of POMC after the 26-amino-acid signal peptide. The α-, β-, and γ- MSH regions (which characterize the three "constant" regions) are indicated by diagonal lines. The "variable" regions are solid. The amino acid numbers shown refer to the N-terminal amino acid of each cleavage site. Because these amino acids are removed, the numbers do not correspond exactly with the amino acid numbers of the peptides as used in the text. ACTH, adrenocorticotropic hormone; CLIP, corticotropin-like intermediate lobe peptide; LPH, lipotropic hormone; and MSH, melanocyte-stimulating hormone.

Actions of ACTH

ACTH stimulates the G-protein–coupled melanocortin 2 receptor (MCR2), which is located almost exclusively in the adrenal cortex. Activation of MCR2 triggers the production of cAMP, activating PKA that catalyzes the phosphorylation of many proteins involved in steroidogenesis, thereby modifying their activity. ACTH elicits acute and long-term effects. ACTH stimulates the biosynthesis of LDL receptors and the uptake of LDL, which provides most of the cholesterol used for steroidogenesis[17], and stimulates transcription of the gene for HMGCoA reductase, the rate-limiting step in cholesterol biosynthesis. However, adrenal biosynthesis of cholesterol is quantitatively much less important than the uptake of LDL cholesterol.[19]

Cholesterol is stored in steroidogenic tissues as cholesterol esters in lipid droplets. ACTH stimulates the activity of cholesterol esterase while inhibiting cholesterol ester synthetase, thus increasing the intracellular pool of free cholesterol, the substrate for P450scc.[158,159] The esterase is similar to gastric and lingual lipases.[160] Finally, ACTH facilitates transport of cholesterol into mitochondria by stimulating the synthesis and phosphorylation of StAR, thus increasing the flow of free cholesterol into the mitochondria. All of these actions are mediated by cAMP and occur within minutes, constituting the "acute" effect of ACTH on steroidogenesis. The adrenal contains relatively modest amounts of steroid hormones. Thus, release of preformed cortisol does not contribute significantly to the acute response to ACTH. Acute responses occur by the rapid provision of large supplies of cholesterol to mitochondrial P450scc.[35,161]

The long-term "chronic" effects of ACTH are mediated directly at the level of the steroidogenic enzymes. ACTH via cAMP stimulates the accumulation of the steroidogenic enzymes and their mRNAs by stimulating the transcription of their genes.[34] ACTH also increases adrenal blood flow, increasing the influx of oxygen and metabolic fuel and the delivery of newly secreted hormones to the circulation.[162] Thus, ACTH increases the uptake of the cholesterol substrate and its conversion to steroidal products. The stimulation of this steroidogenesis occurs at each step in the pathway, not just at the rate-limiting step (P450scc).

The role of ACTH and other peptides derived from POMC in stimulating growth of the adult adrenal remains uncertain.[163,164] However, lack of pituitary POMC causes severe adrenal hypoplasia[165,166] and chronic ACTH excess causes adrenal hyperplasia. In the fetal adrenal, ACTH stimulates the local production of insulin-like growth factor II,[149,167] basic fibroblast growth factor,[168] and epidermal growth factor.[169] These, and possibly other factors, work together to mediate ACTH-induced growth of the fetal adrenal.[170]

Diurnal Rhythms of ACTH and Cortisol

Plasma concentrations of ACTH and cortisol tend to be high in the morning and low in the evening. Peak ACTH levels are usually seen at 4:00 to 6:00 AM, and peak cortisol levels follow at about 8:00 AM ACTH and cortisol are released episodically in pulses every 30 to 120 minutes throughout the day, but the frequency and amplitude of these is much greater in the morning. The basis of this diurnal rhythm is complex and poorly understood. The hypothalamic content of CRF itself shows a diurnal rhythm with peak content at about 4:00 AM.

At least four factors appear to play a role in the rhythm of ACTH and cortisol: intrinsic rhythmicity of synthesis and secretion of CRF by the hypothalamus, light/dark cycles, feeding cycles, and inherent rhythmicity in the adrenal, possibly mediated by adrenal innervation.[171] These factors are clearly interdependent and related. Dietary rhythms may play as large a role as light/dark cycles.[172,173] Animal experiments show that altering the time of feeding can overcome the ACTH/cortisol periodicity established by a light/dark cycle. In normal human subjects, cortisol is released before lunch and supper. However, it is not release at these times in persons eating continuously during the day. Thus, glucocorticoids, which increase blood sugar, appear to be released at times of fasting and are inhibited by feeding.[174,175]

As all parents know, infants do not have a diurnal rhythm of sleep or feeding. Infants acquire such behavioral rhythms in response to their environment long before they acquire a rhythm of ACTH and cortisol. The diurnal rhythms of ACTH and cortisol begin to be established at 6 to 12 months and are often not well established until after 3 years of age.[176] Once the rhythm is well established in the older child or adult, it is changed only with difficulty. When people move to different parts of the world, their ACTH/cortisol rhythms generally take 15 to 20 days to adjust appropriately.

Physical stress (such as major surgery, severe trauma, blood loss, high fever, or serious illness) can increase the secretion of both ACTH and cortisol, but minor surgery and minor illnesses (such as upper respiratory infections) have little effect on ACTH and cortisol secretion.[177,178] Infection, fever, and pyrogens can stimulate the release of cytokines (such as IL-1 and IL-6), which stimulate secretion of CRH and stimulate IL-2 and TNF, which stimulate release of ACTH, providing further stimulus to cortisol secretion during inflammation.[179] Conversely, glucocorticoids inhibit cytokine production in the immune system, providing a negative feedback loop. Most psychoactive drugs, such as anticonvulsants, neurotransmitters, and antidepressants, do not affect the diurnal rhythm of ACTH and cortisol, although cyproheptidine, a serotonin antagonist, effectively suppresses ACTH release.

Adrenal: Glucocorticoid Feedback

The hypothalamic-pituitary-adrenal axis is a classic example of an endocrine feedback system. ACTH increases production of cortisol, and cortisol decreases production of ACTH.[157,180] Cortisol and other glucocorticoids exert feedback inhibition of CRF, ACTH, and AVP principally through the glucocorticoid receptor. Like the acute and chronic phases of the action of ACTH on the adrenal, there are acute and chronic phases of the feedback inhibition of ACTH and presumably CRF.[180]

The acute phase, which occurs within minutes, inhibits release of ACTH and CRF from secretory granules. With prolonged exposure, glucocorticoids inhibit ACTH synthesis by directly inhibiting the transcription of the gene for POMC and AVP. Some evidence also suggests that glucocorticoids can directly inhibit steroidogenesis at the level of the adrenal fasciculata cell itself, but this appears to be a physiologically minor component of the regulation of cortisol secretion.

MINERALOCORTICOID SECRETION: THE RENIN-ANGIOTENSIN SYSTEM

Renin is a serine protease enzyme synthesized primarily by the juxtaglomerular cells of the kidney, but it is also produced in a variety of other tissues, including the glomerulosa cells of the adrenal cortex.[181] The role of adrenally produced renin is not well established. It appears to maintain basal levels of P450c11AS, but it is not known if angiotensin II is involved in this action.[182] Renin is synthesized as a precursor of 406 amino acids that is cleaved to pro-renin, 386 amino acids, and finally to the 340-amino-acid protein found in plasma.[183] Decreased blood pressure, upright posture, sodium depletion, vasodilatory drugs, kallikrein, opiates, and β-adrenergic stimulation all promote release of renin.

Renin enzymatically attacks angiotensinogen, the renin substrate, in the circulation. Angiotensinogen is a highly glycosolated protein and therefore has a highly variable molecular weight, from 50,000 to 100,000 da. Renin proteolytically releases the amino-terminal 10 amino acids of angiotensinogen, referred to as angiotensin I. This decapeptide is biologically inactive until converting enzyme, an enzyme found primarily in the lungs and blood vessels, cleaves off its two carboxy-terminal amino acids to produce an octapeptide termed *angiotensin II*. Angiotensin II binds to specific membrane receptors located in the zona glomerulosa of the adrenal cortex to stimulate aldosterone production. Angiotensin-converting enzyme can be inhibited by captopril and related agents. Alternatively, angiotensin II receptors may be blocked by pharmacologic agents such as irbesartan for the diagnosis and treatment of hyperreninemic hypertension.

Angiotensin II has two principal actions, both of which increase blood pressure. It directly stimulates arteriolar vasoconstriction within a few seconds and it stimulates synthesis and secretion of aldosterone within minutes.[184] Increased plasma potassium is also a powerful and direct stimulator of aldosterone synthesis and release.[185,186] Aldosterone, secreted by the glomerulosa cells of the adrenal cortex, has the greatest mineralocorticoid activity of all naturally occurring steroids. Aldosterone causes renal sodium retention and potassium loss, with a consequent increase in intravascular volume and blood pressure.

Expansion of the blood volume provides the negative feedback signal for regulation of renin and aldosterone secretion. Angiotensin II functions through receptors that stimulate production of phosphatidylinositol, mobilize intracellular and extracellular Ca^{++}, and activate PKC.[187] These intracellular second messengers then stimulate transcription of the P450scc gene by means independent of those employed by ACTH and cAMP.[188] Potassium ion increases uptake of Ca^{++}, with consequent hydrolysis of phosphoinositides to increase phosphotidylinositol. Thus, angiotensin II and potassium work at different levels of the same intracellular second-messenger pathway. However, these differ fundamentally from the action of ACTH.

Although the renin-angiotensin system is clearly the major regulator of mineralocorticoid secretion, ACTH and possibly other POMC-derived peptides such as γ_3-MSH can also promote secretion of aldosterone when used in high concentrations in animal systems.[189,190] Relevance of physiological concentrations in human beings has not been established. Ammonium ion, hyponatremia, dopamine antagonists, and some other agents can also stimulate secretion of aldosterone, and atrial natriuretic factor is a potent physiologic inhibitor of aldosterone secretion.[191]

ADRENAL ANDROGEN SECRETION AND THE REGULATION OF ADRENARCHE

DHEA, DHEAS, and androstenedione which are almost exclusively secreted by the adrenal zona reticularis are generally referred to as adrenal androgens because they can be peripherally converted to testosterone. However, these steroids have little if any capacity to bind to and activate androgen receptors and are hence only androgen precursors and not true androgens. The fetal adrenal secretes large amounts of DHEA and DHEAS, and these steroids are abundant in the newborn. However, their concentrations fall rapidly as the fetal zone of the adrenal involutes following birth. After the first year of life, the adrenals of young children secrete very small amounts of DHEA, DHEAS, and androstenedione until the onset of adrenarche, usually about age 7-8, preceding the onset of puberty by about 2 years.

Adrenarche is independent of puberty, the gonads, or gonadotropins, and the mechanism by which the onset of adrenarche is triggered remains unknown.[62] The secretion of DHEA and DHEAS continue to increase during and after puberty and reach maximal values in young adulthood, following which there is a slow and gradual decrease in the secretion ("adrenopause") of these steroids in the elderly (Figure 12-7).[192]

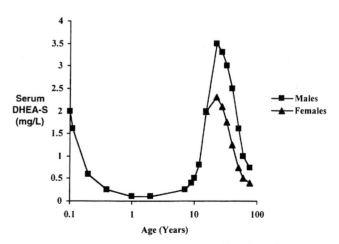

Figure 12-7 Concentrations of DHEAS as a function of age. Note that the X axis is on a log scale.

Throughout much of adult life, adrenal secretion of DHEAS exceeds that of cortisol. In adult women, adrenal secretion of androgen precursors and androgens is equal to their secretion from the ovary. Despite the huge increases in the adrenal secretion of DHEA and DHEAS during adrenarche, circulating concentrations of ACTH and cortisol do not change with age. Thus, ACTH plays a permissive role in adrenarche but does not trigger it. Searches for hypothetical polypeptide hormones that might specifically stimulate the zona reticularis have been unsuccessful.[193,194] Adrenarche is a unique phenomenon confined to a few higher primates such as chimpanzees and orangutans, but the significance of adrenarche remains unknown.[195]

Recent studies of adrenarche have focused on the roles of 3βHSD and P450c17. The abundance of 3βHSD protein in the zona reticularis appears to decrease with the onset of adrenarche,[196-198] and the adrenal expression of cytochrome b_5 (which fosters the 17,20 lyase activity of P450c17) is almost exclusively confined to the zona reticularis.[199,200] Both of these factors would strongly favor the production of DHEA.[201] The phosphorylation of P450c17 also increases 17,20 lyase activity,[73-75] but the kinase has not been identified and hence its role in adrenarche remains uncertain.

Premature and exaggerated adrenarche may be associated with insulin resistance, and girls with premature exaggerated adrenarche appear to be at much higher risk of developing the polycystic ovary syndrome as adults, characterized by hyperandrogenism, fewer ovulatory cycles, insulin resistance, and hypertriglyceridemia.[202-204] Recent evidence suggests that infants born small for gestational age may be at increased risk for this syndrome.[205] Some evidence is accumulating to suggest that replacing the DHEA lost during adrenopause may improve memory and a sense of well-being in the elderly,[206] but this remains controversial.[207] Thus, studies of physiology, biochemistry, and clinical correlates of adrenarche are pointing to premature adrenarche as an early sign of a metabolic disorder.

Plasma Steroids and Their Disposal

STRUCTURE AND NOMENCLATURE

All steroid hormones are derivatives of pregnenolone, whose structure is shown in Figure 12-8. Pregnenolone and its derivatives, which contain 21 carbon atoms, are often termed *C21 steroids*. Each carbon atom is numbered, indicating the location at which the various steroidogenic reactions occur (e.g., 21-hydroxylation, 11-hydroxylation). The 17,20 lyase activity of P450c17 cleaves the bond between carbon atoms 17 and 20, yielding C19 steroids, which include all the androgens. P450aro converts C19 androgens to C18 estrogens. With the exception of estrogens, all steroid hormones have a single unsaturated carbon-carbon double bond. Steroids having this double bond between carbon atoms 4 and 5, including all principal biologically active steroids, are termed *Δ⁴ steroids*. Their precursors (having a double bond between carbon atoms 5 and 6) are

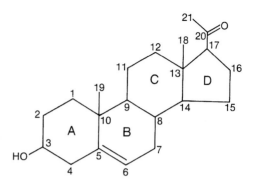

Figure 12-8 Structure of pregnenolone. The carbon atoms are indicated by numbers and the rings are designated by letters according to standard convention. Pregnenolone is derived from cholesterol, which has a 6-carbon side chain attached to carbon 21. Pregnenolone is a "Δ⁵ compound" having a double bond between carbons 5 and 6. The action of 3β-hydroxysteroid dehydrogenase/isomerase moves this double bond from the B ring to carbons 4 and 5 in the A ring, forming Δ⁴ compounds. All of the major biologically active steroid hormones are Δ⁴ compounds.

termed *Δ⁵ steroids*. The two isozymes of 3βHSD convert Δ⁵ to Δ⁴ steroids.

A rigorous logically systematic and unambiguous chemical terminology has been formulated to describe accurately the structure of all steroid hormones and their conceivable derivatives. However, this terminology is unbelievably cumbersome (e.g., cortisol is 11β,17α,21-trihydroxy-pregn-4-ene-3,20-dione, and dexamethasone is 9α-fluoro-11β,17α,21-trihydroxyprena-1,4-diene-3,20-dione). Therefore, we use only the standard "trivial names." Before the structures of the steroid hormones were determined in the 1930s, Reichstein, Kendall, and others identified them as spots on paper chromatograms and designated them A, B, C, and so on. Unfortunately, some persist in using this outmoded terminology more than 60 years later. Thus, corticosterone is sometimes termed *compound B*, cortisol *compound F*, and 11-deoxycortisol *compound S*. This archaic terminology obfuscates the precursor-product relationships of the steroids and confuses students, and should be discarded.

CIRCULATING STEROIDS

Although more than 50 different steroids have been isolated from adrenocortical tissue, the main pathways of adrenal steroidogenesis include only a dozen or so steroids, of which only a few are secreted in sizable quantities. The adult secretion of DHEA and cortisol are each about 20 mg/24 hr, and the secretion of corticosterone, a weak glucocorticoid, is about 2 mg/24 hr.[208] Although glucocorticoids, such as cortisol, and mineralocorticoids, such as aldosterone, are both needed for life and hence are of equivalent physiologic importance, diagrams such as Figure 12-3 fail to indicate that these steroids are not secreted in molar equivalents.

The adult secretion rate of aldosterone is only about 0.1 mg/24 hr. This 100- to 1,000-fold molar difference in the secretory rates of cortisol and aldosterone must be borne in mind when considering the effects of steroid-binding proteins in plasma and when conceptualizing the physiologic manifestations of incomplete defects in steroidogenesis due to single amino acid changes causing the partial loss of activity of a steroidogenic enzyme.

Most circulating steroids are bound to plasma proteins, including corticosteroid-binding globulin (CBG, also termed *transcortin*), albumin, and α_1 acid glycoprotein.[209,210] CBG has a very high affinity for cortisol but a relatively low binding capacity. Albumin has a low affinity and high capacity, and α_1 acid glycoprotein is intermediate for both variables. The result is that about 90% of circulating cortisol is bound to CBG and a little more is bound to other proteins. These steroid-binding proteins are not transport proteins because the biologically important steroids are water soluble in physiologically effective concentrations and because absence of CBG does not cause a detectable physiological disorder. However, these plasma proteins do act as a reservoir for steroids.

This ensures that all peripheral tissues will be bathed in approximately equal concentrations of cortisol, which greatly diminishes the physiologic effect of the great diurnal variation in cortisol secretion. Most synthetic glucocorticoids used in therapy do not bind significantly to CBG and bind poorly to albumin, partially accounting for their increased potencies, which are also associated with increased receptor-binding affinities. Aldosterone is not bound well by any plasma protein. Hence, changes in plasma protein concentration do not affect plasma aldosterone concentrations but greatly influence plasma cortisol concentrations. Estradiol and testosterone bind strongly to a different plasma protein, termed *sex-steroid-binding globulin,* and bind weakly to albumin.

Because steroids are hormones, it is often thought that the concentration of "free" (i.e., unbound) circulating steroids determines biologic activity. However, the target tissues for many steroid hormones contain enzymes that modify those steroids. Thus, many actions of testosterone are actually due to dihydrotestosterone produced by local 5α-reductase. Cortisol will have differential actions on various tissues due to the presence or absence of the two isozymes of 11βHSD, which can inactivate cortisol to cortisone or reactivate cortisone back to cortisol. Similar peripheral metabolism occurs via "extraglandular" 21-hydroxylase, P450aro, 3βHSD, and 17βHSD. Thus, circulating steroids are both classic hormones and precursors of locally acting autocrine or paracrine factors.

STEROID CATABOLISM

Only about 1% of circulating plasma cortisol and aldosterone are excreted unchanged in the urine. The remainder is metabolized by the liver. A large number of hepatic metabolites of each steroid are produced. Most contain additional hydroxyl groups and are linked to a sulfate or glucuronide moiety, rendering them more soluble and readily excretable by the kidney. A great deal is known about the various urinary metabolites of the circulating steroids because their measurement in pooled 24-hour urine samples has been an important means of studying adrenal steroids. Although the measurement of urinary steroid metabolites by modern mass spectrometric techniques remains an important research tool,[211-213] the development of separation techniques and of specific and highly sensitive radioimmunoassays for each of the plasma steroids has greatly reduced the need to measure their excreted metabolites in clinical practice.

Clinical and Laboratory Evaluation of Adrenal Function

CLINICAL EVALUATION

Astute clinical evaluation can generally reveal the presence of primary adrenal deficiency or hypersecretion before performing laboratory tests. Thomas Addison described adrenal insufficiency in 1849, long before immunoassays became available. Virtually all patients with chronic adrenal insufficiency will have weakness, fatigue, anorexia, weight loss, hypotension, and hyperpigmentation. Patients with acute adrenal insufficiency may have hypotension, shock, weakness, apathy, confusion, anorexia, nausea, vomiting, dehydration, abdominal or flank pain, hyperthermia, and/or hypoglycemia.

Deficient adrenal androgen secretion will compromise the acquisition of virilizing secondary sexual characteristics, pubic and axillary hair, acne, axillary odor, in female adolescents. Early signs of glucocorticoid excess include increased appetite, weight gain, and growth arrest without a concomitant delay in bone age. Chronic glucocorticoid excess in children results in typical Cushingoid facies, but the "buffalo hump" and centripetal distribution of body fat characteristic of adult Cushing disease are seen only in long-standing undiagnosed disease. Mineralocorticoid excess is mainly characterized by hypertension, but patients receiving very low sodium diets (e.g., the newborn) will not be hypertensive because mineralocorticoids increase blood pressure primarily by retaining sodium and thus increasing intravascular volume.

Moderate hypersecretion of adrenal androgens is characterized by mild signs of virilization, whereas substantial hypersecretion of adrenal androgens is characterized by accelerated growth with a disproportionate increase in bone age, increased muscle mass, acne, hirsutism, deepening of the voice, and more profound degrees of virilism. A key feature of any physical examination of a virilized male is careful examination and measurement of the testes. Bilaterally enlarged testes suggest true (central) precocious puberty. Unilateral testicular enlargement suggests testicular tumor. Prepubertal testes in a virilized male indicate an extratesticular source of androgen, such as the adrenal.

Imaging studies are of limited utility in adrenal cortical disease. Computed tomography (CT) will only rarely detect pituitary tumors hypersecreting ACTH, and magnetic resonance imaging (MRI) will detect less than half of these, even with gadolinium enhancement. The small size, odd shape, and location near other structures also compromise the use of imaging techniques for the adrenals. Patients with Cushing disease or congenital adrenal hyperplasia will have modestly enlarged adrenals, but such enlargement is not detectable by imaging techniques with any useful degree of certainty. The gross enlargement of the adrenals in congenital lipoid adrenal hyperplasia, their hypoplasia in adrenal hypoplasia congenita or in the hereditary ACTH unresponsiveness syndrome, and many malignant tumors can be usefully diagnosed by imaging studies. However, many adrenal adenomas are too small to be detected. Thus, imaging studies may establish the presence of pituitary or adrenal tumors but they can never establish their absence.

LABORATORY EVALUATION

The diagnostic evaluation of adrenal function is essentially chemical. The nonspecificity of many of the clinical signs described previously and the disappointing results with imaging studies remind us that any proper evaluation of hypothalamic-pituitary-adrenal function must rely on a series of carefully performed physiologic maneuvers associated with hormonal assays. In the past, these tests relied principally on the physiologic effects of adrenal hormones such as the effects of cortisol on glucose metabolism as seen during a glucose tolerance test. However, the development of highly specific and exquisitely sensitive immunoassays that can be done on small volumes of plasma now permits the direct examination of virtually every hormone involved in adrenal metabolism.

Plasma Concentrations of Cortisol and Other Steroids

Plasma cortisol is measured routinely by a variety of techniques, including radioimmunoassay, immunoradiometric assay, and high-pressure liquid chromatography (HPLC). Other procedures, such as fluorimetric assays and competitive protein binding assays, are useful research tools but are not in general clinical use. It is of considerable importance to know what procedure one's laboratory is employing and precisely what it is measuring. All immunoassays have some degree of cross-reactivity with other steroids. Most cortisol immunoassays will detect cortisol and cortisone. By contrast, these are readily distinguished by HPLC.

Because the newborn's plasma contains mainly cortisone rather than cortisol during the first few days of life, comparison of newborn data obtained by HPLC to published standards obtained by immunoassays may incorrectly suggest adrenal insufficiency. Tables 12-1 and 12-3 summarize the normal plasma concentrations for a variety of steroids. With the notable exception of dehydroepiandrosterone sulfate, most adrenal steroids exhibit a diurnal variation based on the diurnal rhythm of ACTH. Because the stress of illness or hospitalization can increase adrenal steroid secretion and because diurnal

TABLE 12-2

Mean Sex Steroid Concentration in Infants and Children

	PROG	17OHP	DHEA	DHEA-S	Δ^4-A	E1	E2	T (M)	T (F)	DHT (M)	DHT (F)
Cord blood	1100	62	21	6,400	3.0	52	30	1.0	0.9	0.2	0.2
Prematures	11	8.1	28	11,000	7.0			4.2	0.4	1.0	0.1
Term newborns		1.1	20	4,400	5.2			6.9	1.4	0.9	0.3
Infants	1.0	1.0	3.8	820	0.7	<0.1	<0.1	6.6	<0.4	1.4	<0.1
Children 1–6 y			1.0	270	0.9	<0.1	<0.1	0.2		0.1	
6–8 y			3.1	540	0.9	<0.1	<0.1	0.2		0.1	
8–10 y			5.6	1,400	0.9	<0.1	<0.1	0.2		0.1	
Males Pubertal stage I	0.6	1.3	5.6	950	0.9	0.0	0.0	0.2		<0.1	
II	0.6	1.6	10	2,600	1.6	0.1	0.0	1.4		0.3	
III	0.8	2.0	14	3,300	2.4	0.1	0.1	6.6		0.7	
IV	1.1	2.6	14	5,400	2.8	0.1	0.1	13		1.2	
V	1.3	3.3	17	6,300	3.5	0.1	0.1	19		1.6	
Adult	1.1	3.3	16	7,300	4.0	0.1	0.1	22		1.7	
Females Pubertal stage I	0.6	1.0	5.6	1,100	0.9	0.1	0.0		0.2		0.1
II	1.0	1.6	11	1,900	2.3	0.1	0.1		0.7		0.3
III	1.3	2.3	14	2,500	4.2	0.1	0.1		0.9		0.3
IV	9.2	2.9	15	3,300	4.5	0.1	0.2		0.9		0.3
V	5.1	3.6	19	4,100	6.0	0.2	0.4		1.0		0.3
Adult Follicular	1.0	1.5	16	4,100	5.8	0.2	0.2		1.0		0.3
Luteal	24	5.4	16	4,100	5.8	0.4	0.5		1.0		0.3

PROG = progesterone; 17OHP = 17-hydroxyprogesterone; DHEA = dehydroepiandrosterone; DHEA-S = DHEA sulfate; Δ^4-A = androstenedione; E$_1$ = estrone; E$_2$ = estradiol; T = testosterone; DHT = dihydrotestosterone; M = male; and F = female.
All values are in nmol/L. To convert these values to ng/dL, multiply nmol/L times the following values: androstenedione, 28.6; DHEA, 28.8; DHT, 29.0; E$_1$, 27.0; E$_2$, 27.2; Prog, 31.5; 17OHP, 33.1. To convert DHEA-S to μg/dL, multiply by .0368.
Data adapted from Endocrine Sciences, Tarzana, California.

TABLE 12-3

Mean Glucocorticoid and Mineralocorticoid Concentrations

	Cortisol	DOC	Corticosterone	18OH Corticosterone	Aldosterone	Plasma Renin Activity
Cord blood	360	5.5	19		2.4	50
Prematures	180			5.5	2.8	222
Newborns	140		6.6	9.7	2.6	58
Infants	250	0.6	16	2.2	0.8	33
Children (8 AM)						
1-2 yr	110-550			1.8	0.8	15
2-10 yr	As adults	0.3		1.2	0.3→0.8[a]	8.3
10-15 yr	As adults			0.7	0.1→0.6[a]	3.3
Adults (8 AM)	280-550	0.2	12	0.6	0.2→0.4[a]	2.8→4.0[a]
(4 PM)	140-280		3.8			

DOC = deoxycorticosterone.

All values in nmol/L except plasma renin activity (μg/L/s). To convert cortisol to μg/dL, multiply by 0.0363. To convert other values to ng/dL, multiply nmol/L times the following values: corticosterone, 34.7; 18OH corticosterone, 36.2; aldosterone, 36.0; DOC, 33.1.

[a] Two values separated by an arrow indicate those in supine and upright posture.

rhythms may not be well established in children under 3 years of age, it is best to obtain two or more samples for the measurement of any steroid.[214,215]

As shown in Tables 12-2 and 12-3, data exist for the concentrations of a large number of steroid hormones throughout normal infancy, childhood, and adolescence. Not all endocrine laboratories perform all of these assays, and depending on the assay procedures employed various laboratories may have different "normal" values. Most central hospital and commercial laboratories are designed primarily to serve adult, rather than pediatric, patients. Thus, it is important to know whether the available assays will be sufficiently sensitive with small volumes of blood to be useful in measuring pediatric values. This is especially true for the measurement of sex steroids (and gonadotropins), which can exhibit pathologic elevations in children and still remain below the limit of detection of most "adult" assays.

Plasma Renin

Renin is not generally measured directly but is assayed by its enzymatic activity. Plasma renin activity (PRA) is simply an immunoassay of the amount of angiotensin I generated per milliliter of serum per hour at 37° C. In normal serum, the concentration of both renin and angiotensinogen (the renin substrate) are limiting. Therefore, another test [plasma renin content (PRC)] measures the amount of angiotensin I generated in 1 hour at 37° C in the presence of excess concentrations of angiotensinogen. Immunoassays for renin itself have been developed but are not yet widely used.

Plasma renin activity is sensitive to dietary sodium intake, posture, diuretic therapy, activity, and sex steroids. Because PRA values can vary widely with these variables, it is best to measure renin twice: once in the morning after overnight supine posture and then again after maintenance of upright posture for 4 hours.[216] A simultaneous 24-hour urine for total sodium excretion is generally needed to interpret PRA results. Decreased

dietary and urinary sodium, decreased intravascular volume, diuretics, and estrogens will increase PRA. Sodium loading, hyperaldosteronemia, and increased intravascular volume decrease PRA.

The greatest use of renin measurements is in the evaluation of hypertension and in the management of CAH. However, several additional situations require assessment of the renin-angiotensin system. Children with simple virilizing adrenal hyperplasia who do not have clinical evidence of urinary salt wasting (hyponatremia, hyperkalemia, acidosis, hypotension, shock) may nevertheless have increased PRA, especially when dietary sodium is restricted. This was an early clinical sign that this form of 21-hydroxylase deficiency was simply a milder form of the more common (severe) salt-wasting form.

Treatment of simple virilizing 21-hydroxylase deficiency with sufficient mineralocorticoid to suppress PRA into the normal range will reduce the child's requirement for glucocorticoids, thus maximizing final adult height. Children with CAH need to have their mineralocorticoid replacement therapy monitored routinely by measuring PRA. Measurement of angiotensin II is also possible in some research laboratories, but most antibodies to angiotensin II strongly cross-react with angiotensin I. Thus, PRA remains the most useful way of evaluating the renin-angiotensin-aldosterone system.

Urinary Steroid Excretion

The measurement of 24-hour urinary excretion of steroid metabolites is one of the oldest procedures for assessing adrenal function and is still useful. Examination of the total 24-hour excretion of steroids eliminates the fluctuations seen in serum samples as a function of time of day, episodic bursts of ACTH and steroid secretion, and transient stress (such as a visit to the clinic or difficult venepuncture). Collection of a complete 24-hour urinary sample can be quite difficult in the infant or small child. Two consecutive 24-hour collections should be obtained, and each should be assayed for creatinine to monitor the completeness of the collection. Because of the diurnal and episodic nature of steroid secretion, one should never obtain 8- or 12-hour collections and attempt to infer the 24-hour excretory rate from such partial collections.

The analytic procedures for urinary steroid analysis typically rely on a chromatographic procedure for separating steroids followed by a colorimetric, immunologic, or other assay. Failure to employ a chromatographic separation step is the most common source of error. Such classic analyses of urinary steroids are now being replaced by gas chromatography followed by mass spectrometry (GC/MS). Recent advances in these techniques permit very sensitive and specific assays of urinary steroids. However, each secreted steroid is metabolized to multiple forms before being excreted in urine, and this metabolism can vary with age and sex in pediatric populations. The analyses are complex and require specialized expertise that is not yet widely available. Thus, analysis of urinary steroids by GC/MS is typically employed only in research settings.

Urinary 17-hydroxycorticosteroids (17OHCS), assayed by the colorimetric Porter-Silber reaction, measure 17, 21-dihydroxy-20-ketosteroids by the generation of a colored compound after treatment with phenylhydrazine.[217] The reaction is highly specific for the major urinary metabolites of cortisol and cortisone. It will also measure metabolites of 11-deoxycortisol, which will be increased in 11-hydroxylase deficiency or after treatment with metyrapone, a commonly used diagnostic agent (see material following).

Urinary 17OHCS secretion is increased in obesity, hyperthyroidism, and anorexia nervosa. It is decreased in starvation, hypothyroidism, renal failure, liver disease, and pregnancy. Drugs that induce hepatic enzymes, such as phenobarbital, can give low urinary 17OHCS values by stimulating hepatic metabolism of circulating steroids to excreted compounds not detected by the Porter-Silber reaction. Other drugs (including phenothiazines, spironolactone, hydroxyzine, and some antibiotics) can interfere with the colorimetric assay directly, giving falsely elevated values.

Measurement of 17OHCS should be replaced by measurement of urinary free cortisol, thus avoiding the nonspecificity and drug interference problems inherent in 17OHCS. In adults, this test is highly reliable in the diagnosis of Cushing syndrome. Free cortisol is extracted from the urine and measured by immunoassay or HPLC, providing the advantage of specificity. Excretion of urinary free cortisol and of total cortisol metabolites (typically 11 ± 5 μg/m^2/day) is closely correlated with age, body surface area, and adiposity.[218,219] Values vary substantially among different reference laboratories, reflecting variations in assay technologies. Thus, it is essential to utilize a laboratory with good data for normal children. It remains important to measure urinary creatinine to monitor the completeness of the collection. Some clinical experience indicates that urinary 17OHCS may be more reliable for the diagnosis of Cushing disease in children, possibly due to greater experience with 17OHCS.[220]

Urinary 17-ketosteroids (17KS), assayed by the Zimmerman reaction, measure 17-ketosteroids by the generation of a colored compound after treatment with meta-dinitrobenzine and acid.[221] The reaction principally measures metabolites of DHEA and DHEA sulfate and thus correlates with adrenal androgen production. Androstenedione will contribute significant 17KS, and if an alkali extraction is not used estrone will also contribute. The principal androgens, testosterone and dihydrotestosterone, have hydroxyl rather than keto groups on carbon 17. Hence, their metabolic products are not measured as 17KS. A wide variety of drugs (including penicillin, nalidixic acid, spironolactone, and phenothiazines, as well as nonspecific urinary chromagens) can spuriously increase values of 17KS. Measurement of urinary 17KS remains a useful inexpensive screening test, and some clinicians prefer to follow 17KS to monitor therapy of CAH. However, measurements of plasma steroids have now replaced the use of urinary 17KS in most centers.

Urinary 17-ketogenic steroids (17KGS) are occasionally confused with urinary 17-ketosteroids because of the similarity of the names. However, 17KGS are used to measure urinary metabolites of glucocorticoids (not sex steroids). Urinary 17KGS are assayed by oxidation of a variety of C-21 steroids to C-19 17-ketosteroids, which are then measured by the Zimmerman reaction as 17KS. All 17OHCS plus a number of other urinary steroids (including the 17KS) are measured, but the basal 17KS values are subtracted. In addition to all of the problems of specificity and drug interference previously described for 17OHCS and 17KS, a major disadvantage of 17KGS is that they will also detect pregnanetriol (the principal urinary metabolite of 17-hydroxyprogesterone). This is the steroid that shows the greatest elevations in congenital adrenal hyperplasia. Although some laboratories continue to perform measurements of 17KGS, this obsolete assay no longer has a place in modern pediatric practice.

Plasma ACTH and Other POMC Peptides

Accurate routine immunoassay of plasma ACTH is now available in most centers, but its measurement remains more difficult and variable than the assays for most other pituitary hormones.[222] Handling of the samples must be done with care. Samples must be drawn into a plastic syringe containing heparin or ethylenediaminetetraacetic acid (EDTA) and quickly transported in plastic tubes on ice because ACTH adheres to glass and is quickly inactivated.

Thus, elevated plasma ACTH concentrations can be highly informative, but most assays cannot detect low or low-normal values and such values can be spurious if the samples are handled badly. In adults and older children who have well-established diurnal rhythms of ACTH, normal 8:00 AM values rarely exceed 50 pg/mL—whereas 8:00 PM values are usually undetectable. Patients with Cushing disease often have normal morning values, but the diagnosis can be suggested by consistently elevated afternoon and evening values. Patients with the ectopic ACTH syndrome can have values anywhere from 100 to 1,000 pg/mL.

The carboxy portion of POMC, termed β-LPH (POMC 153-241), is released from POMC in equimolar amounts with ACTH. β-LPH has a longer circulating plasma half-life than ACTH, is more stable in the laboratory, and is easier to assay than ACTH.[223] Investigational use of such assays indicates that they may be a useful adjunct to ACTH assays, but routine measurement of β-LPH is not available.

Secretory Rates

The secretory rates of cortisol and aldosterone (or other steroids) can be measured by administering a small dose of tritiated cortisol or aldosterone and measuring the specific activity of one or more known metabolites in a 24-hour urine collection. This procedure permitted measurement of certain steroids, such as aldosterone, before specific immunoassays became available. These procedures have also provided much information about the normal rate of production of various steroids. Based on this procedure, most authorities have agreed that children and adults secrete about 12 mg of cortisol per square meter of body surface area per day. However, more recent studies indicate a rate of 6 to 9 mg/m² in children and adults.[224,225] Such differences are of considerable importance in estimating "physiologic replacement" doses of glucocorticoids.

Dexamethasone Suppression Test

Administration of dexamethasone, a potent synthetic glucocorticoid, will suppress secretion of pituitary ACTH and of adrenal cortisol. Originally described by Liddle in 1960,[226] the dexamethasone suppression test remains the most useful procedure for distinguishing whether glucocorticoid excess is due primarily to pituitary disease or adrenal disease. As dexamethasone also suppresses adrenal androgen secretion, this test is useful for distinguishing between adrenal and gonadal sources of sex steroids.

A complete formal dexamethasone suppression test requires the measurement of basal values and those obtained in response to low- and high-dose dexamethasone. This is described in the section on the evaluation of Cushing syndrome. Variations of this test are commonly used, notably the single-dose 1.0-mg in adults[227] or 0.3 mg/m² in children.[228] This is a useful outpatient screening procedure for distinguishing Cushing syndrome from exogenous obesity. It can be useful for the same purpose in adolescents and older children, but is otherwise of limited utility in pediatrics. An overnight high-dose dexamethasone suppression test is probably more reliable than the standard 2-day high-dose test in differentiating adults with Cushing disease from those with the ectopic ACTH syndrome. However, the utility of this test in pediatric patients has not been established.

Stimulation Tests

Direct stimulation of the adrenal with ACTH is a rapid, safe, and easy way to evaluate adrenocortical function. The original ACTH test consisted of a 4- to 6-hour infusion of 0.5 U/kg of ACTH(1-39). This will maximally stimulate adrenal cortisol secretion, and thus effectively distinguish primary adrenal insufficiency Addison disease, in which the adrenal is incapable of responding, from secondary adrenal insufficiency due to hypopituitarism. In secondary adrenal insufficiency, some steroidogenic capacity is present. Therefore, some cortisol is produced in response to the ACTH. Thus, cortisol secretion is less than normal but greater than the negligible values seen in primary adrenal insufficiency.

The 4- to 6-hour intravenous ACTH test has been replaced in clinical practice by the 60-minute test, wherein a single bolus of ACTH(1-24) is administered intravenously and cortisol and possibly other steroids are measured at 0 and 60 minutes.[229] Normal responses to a 60-minute test are shown in Table 12-4.[230] Synthetic ACTH(1-24) (cosyntropin) is preferred, as it has a more rapid action and shorter half-life than ACTH(1-39). The usual dose is 15 μg/kg in children up to 2 years of age and 0.25 mg for adults and for children older than 2 years. All of these doses are pharmacologic. A very-low-dose (1 μg) test may be useful in assessing adrenal recovery from glucocorticoid suppression.[231]

Newer data show that maximal steroidal responses can be achieved after only 30 minutes, but the best available standards are for a 60-minute test. One of the widest uses of intravenous ACTH tests in pediatrics is in diagnosing congenital adrenal hyperplasia (CAH). Stimulating the adrenal with ACTH increases steroidogenesis, resulting in

TABLE 12-4

Responses of Adrenal Steroids to a 60-Minute ACTH Test

	Infants		Prepubertal		Pubertal	
	Basal	Stimulated	Basal	Stimulated	Basal	Stimulated
17OH-pregnenolone	6.8		1.7	9.6	3.6	24
17OHP	0.8	5.8	1.5	5.8	1.8	4.8
DHEA	1.4		2.4	4.3	9.0	19
11-deoxycortisol	2.3		1.8	5.8	1.7	4.9
Cortisol	280	830	360	830	280	690
DOC	0.6	2.4	0.2	1.7	0.2	1.7
Progesterone	1.1	3.2	1.1	4.0	1.9	4.8

All values are mean values in nmol/L. Conversion factors to English units are given in Tables 12-2 and 12-3.
Data adapted from Endocrine Sciences, Tarzana, California.

accumulation of steroids proximal to the disordered enzyme. For example, inspection of Figure 12-3 shows that impaired activity of P450c21 (21-hydroxylase) should lead to the accumulation of progesterone and 17-hydroxyprogesterone (17OHP). However, progesterone does not accumulate in appreciable quantities because it too is converted to 17OHP.

In routine practice, measuring the response of 17OHP to a 60-minute challenge with intravenous ACTH is the single most powerful and reliable means of diagnosing 21-hydroxylase deficiency. Genetic testing can provide a useful confirmation. Comparing the patient's basal to ACTH-stimulated values of 17OHP against those from large numbers of well-studied patients usually permits the discrimination of normal persons, heterozygotes, patients with nonclassic CAH, and patients with classical CAH, although inevitably there is some overlap between groups[232] (Figure 12-9). Measurement of testosterone or Δ^4 androstenedione in response to ACTH can distinguish normal persons from patients with classical CAH, but heterozygotes and patients with cryptic CAH have values overlapping both normals and classic CAH (Figure 12-9).

Longer ACTH tests of up to 3 days have also been employed to evaluate adrenal function. It is important to remember that ACTH has both acute and chronic effects. Thus, short tests measure only the acute effects of ACTH; that is, the maximal stimulation of preexisting steroidogenic machinery. By contrast, a 3-day test will examine the more chronic effects of ACTH to stimulate increased capacity for steroidogenesis by increasing the synthesis of steroidogenic machinery. Few situations exist for which a 3-day intramuscular ACTH test is indicated, although it is useful in diagnosing the rare syndromes of hereditary unresponsiveness to ACTH.[233]

Insulin-induced hypoglycemia is another commonly used test. Insulin (0.1 U/kg/IV) is administered and blood is obtained at 0, 30, 45, and 60 minutes. The insulin-induced hypoglycemia will stimulate the release of counterregulatory hormones that have actions to increase plasma glucose concentrations: ACTH and cortisol, growth hormone (GH), epinephrine, and glucagon. Because of the inherent risk of convulsions as a result of hypoglycemia, an experienced physician must be in attendance, not merely "available", throughout the entire course of the test. Blood glucose must fall to half the initial value or to 45 mg/dL to achieve an adequate test, and it is wise to terminate the test if values of 30 mg/dL are reached. Most patients will experience hunger, irritability, diaphoresis, and tachycardia. When these are followed by drowsiness or sleep, blood sugar levels are likely below acceptable limits. If this occurs, a blood sample should be obtained and 2 mL/kg of 20% to 25% glucose given intravenously (to a maximum of 100 mL).[234]

Metyrapone Test

Metyrapone blocks the action of P450c11β, and to a much lesser extent of P450scc. It is thus a chemical means of inducing a transient deficiency of 11-hydroxylase activity, which results in decreased cortisol secretion and subsequent increase in ACTH secretion. Metyrapone testing is done to assess the capacity of the pituitary to produce ACTH in response to a physiologic stimulus. This test is useful in evaluating the hypothalamic-pituitary axis in the presence of central nervous system lesions after neurosurgery or long-term suppression by glucocorticoid therapy.[235] Patients with a previous history of hypothalamic, pituitary, or adrenal disease or those who have been withdrawn from glucocorticoid therapy should be re-evaluated with a metyrapone test or with an insulin tolerance test. A normal response indicates recovery of the hypothalamic-pituitary-adrenal axis and predicts that the patient will respond normally to the stress of surgery.

Metyrapone is generally given orally as 300 mg/m² every 4 hours for a total of six doses 24 hours. Unlike many other drugs, it is appropriate to continue to increase the dose in older or overweight patients, but the total dose should not exceed 3.0 g.[236] Blood should be obtained for cortisol, 11-deoxycortisol, and ACTH before and after the test, and a 24-hour urine collection should be obtained for 17OHCS before and during the test. In a normal response to metyrapone, cortisol decreases, ACTH increases, and 11-deoxycortisol, the substrate for P450c11β, increases greatly to about 5 μg/dL. Metabolites of 11-deoxycortisol result in a doubling in urinary 17OHCS excretion. Adults and older children can be tested with the administration of a single oral dose of 30 mg/kg at midnight, given with food to reduce gastrointestinal irritation.[236] Blood samples are drawn at 8:00 AM the mornings before and after administering the drug.

CRF Testing

CRF is now generally available as a test of pituitary ACTH reserve.[237] At the present time, CRF testing remains experimental in adults, and little experience has accumulated in children. It is not yet clear what role CRF testing will assume, although early data suggest it may be useful for distinguishing hypothalamic from pituitary causes of ACTH deficiency and may be a useful adjunct in establishing the diagnosis of Cushing disease.[238]

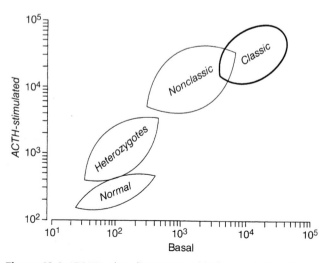

Figure 12-9 17OHP values (in ng/100 mL) before and after stimulation with ACTH in normals, patients with CAH, and heterozygotes.

Genetic Lesions in Steroidogenesis

Autosomal-recessive genetic disorders disrupt each of the steps in the pathway shown in Figure 12-3. Most of these result in diminished synthesis of cortisol. In response to adrenal insufficiency, the pituitary synthesizes increased amounts of POMC and ACTH, which promotes increased steroidogenesis. ACTH and possibly other peptides derived from the amino terminal end of POMC also stimulates adrenal hypertrophy and hyperplasia. Thus, the term *congenital adrenal hyperplasia* refers to a group of diseases traditionally grouped on the basis of the most prominent finding at autopsy.

In theory, the congenital adrenal hyperplasias are easy to understand. A genetic lesion in one of the steroidogenic enzymes interferes with normal steroidogenesis. The signs and symptoms of the disease derive from deficiency of the steroidal end product and the effects of accumulated steroidal precursors proximal to the blocked step. Thus, reference to the pathways in Figure 12-3 and knowledge of the biologic effects of each steroid should permit one to deduce the manifestations of the disease.

In practice, the congenital adrenal hyperplasias can be confusing both clinically and scientifically. The key clinical, laboratory, and therapeutic features of each form of CAH are summarized in Table 12-5. Because each steroidogenic enzyme has multiple activities and many extra-adrenal tissues contain enzymes that have similar activities, the complete elimination of a specific adrenal enzyme may not result in the complete elimination of its steroidal products from the circulation. In the past, disorders of steroidogenic enzymes had to be studied by examining their steroid metabolites in serum and urine, an indirect approach that led to numerous misconceptions about the steroidogenic processes. The cloning of the genes for the steroidogenic enzymes has now permitted the direct study of these diseases, permitting an accurate understanding of their disordered physiology.

CONGENITAL LIPOID ADRENAL HYPERPLASIA

Lipoid CAH is the most severe genetic disorder of steroid hormone synthesis. This disorder is characterized by the absence of significant concentrations of all steroids, high basal ACTH and plasma renin activity, an absent steroidal response to long-term treatment with high doses of ACTH or hCG, and grossly enlarged adrenals laden with cholesterol and cholesterol esters.[239-242] These findings indicate a lesion in the first step in steroidogenesis: the conversion of cholesterol to pregnenolone. It was initially thought that the lesion was in an enzyme involved in this conversion, and before the role of P450scc was understood lipoid CAH was misnamed 20,22-desmolase deficiency.[242-247]

However, the gene for P450scc is normal in these patients[247], as are the mRNAs for adrenodoxin reductase and adrenodoxin.[247] Furthermore, placental steroidogenesis persists in lipoid CAH, permitting normal term gestation, which would not happen if P450scc were involved.[248] The normal P450scc system plus the accumulation of cholesterol esters in the affected adrenal suggested that the lesion lay in an upstream factor involved in cholesterol transport into mitochondria. This factor was identified by cell biologic studies,[37-39] cloned and named StAR,[40] quickly found to be expressed in the adrenal and gonad but not in the placenta, and then identified as the disordered step in lipoid CAH.[41,42,249]

Lipoid CAH is a StAR gene knockout experiment of nature, revealing the complex physiology of the StAR protein.[250] StAR promotes steroidogenesis by increasing the movement of cholesterol into mitochondria, but in the absence of StAR steroidogenic cells make steroids at about 14% of the StAR-induced level.[41,42,161,249] This observation led to the two-hit model of lipoid CAH[42] (Figure 12-10). The first hit is the loss of StAR itself, leading to a loss of most but not all steroidogenesis, leading to a compensatory rise in ACTH and LH. These hormones increase cellular cAMP, which increases biosynthesis of LDL receptors, their consequent uptake of LDL cholesterol, and de novo synthesis of cholesterol. In the absence of StAR, this increased intracellular cholesterol accumulates as in a storage disease, causing the second hit, which is the mitochondrial and cellular damage caused by the accumulated cholesterol, cholesterol esters, and their autooxidation products.[42]

The two-hit model explains the unusual clinical findings in lipoid CAH. In the fetal testis, which normally makes large amounts of testosterone in fetal life,[251] the Leydig cells are destroyed early in gestation, eliminating testosterone biosynthesis. Hence, an affected 46,XY fetus does not undergo normal virilization and is born with female external genitalia and a blind vaginal pouch. However, Wolffian duct derivatives are well developed, indicating the presence of some testosterone synthesis early in fetal life,[252] as predicted by the two-hit model. The undamaged Sertoli cells produce Müllerian inhibitory hormone, and thus the phenotypically female 46,XY fetus has no cervix, uterus, or fallopian tubes.

The steroidogenically active fetal zone of the adrenal is similarly affected, eliminating most DHEA biosynthesis and hence eliminating the feto-placental production of estriol. Thus, mid-gestation maternal and fetal estriol levels are very low.[248] The definitive zone of the fetal adrenal, which differentiates into the zonae glomerulosa and fasciculata, normally produces very little aldosterone, and because fetal salt and water metabolism are maintained by the placenta stimulation of the glomerulosa by angiotensin II generally does not begin until birth. Consistent with this, many newborns with lipoid CAH do not have a salt-wasting crisis until after several weeks of life, when chronic stimulation then leads to cellular damage.[42,253]

The two-hit model also explains the spontaneous feminization of affected 46,XX females who are treated in infancy and reach adolescence.[254,255] The fetal ovary makes little or no steroids and contains no steroidogenic enzymes after the first trimester.[251] Consequently, the ovary remains largely undamaged until it is stimulated by gonadotropins at the time of puberty, when it then produces some estrogen by StAR-independent steroidogenesis. Continued stimulation results in cholesterol accumulation and cellular damage, and thus biosynthesis of progesterone in the latter part of the cycle is impaired.

TABLE 12-5

Clinical and Laboratory Findings in the Congenital Adrenal Hyperplasias

Enzyme Deficiency	Presentation	Laboratory Findings	Therapeutic Measures
Lipoid CAH (StAR or P450scc)	• Salt-wasting crisis • Male pseudohermaphroditism	• Low/absent levels of all steroid hormones • Decreased/absent response to ACTH • Decreased/absent response to hCG in male pseudohermaphroditism • ↑ ACTH and PRA	• Glucocorticoid and mineralocorticoid replacement, salt supplementation • Estrogen replacement at age ≧12 years • Gonadectomy of male pseudohermaphrodite
3β-HSD	• Salt-wasting crisis • Male and female pseudohermaphroditism	• ↑Δ⁵ steroids before and after ACTH • ↑Δ⁵/Δ⁴ serum steroids • Suppression of elevated adrenal steroids after glucocorticoid administration • ↑ ACTH and PRA	• Glucocorticoid and mineralocorticoid replacement • Salt supplementation • Surgical correction of genitalia • Sex hormone replacement as necessary
P450c21	• Classic form: • Salt-wasting crisis • Female pseudohermaphroditism • Pre- and postnatal virilization • Nonclassic form: • Premature adrenarche, menstrual irregularity, hirsutism, acne, infertility	• ↑ 17OHP before and after ACTH • ↑ Serum androgens and urine 17KS • Suppression of elevated adrenal steroids after glucocorticoid Rx • ↑ ACTH and PRA	• Glucocorticoid and mineralocorticoid replacement • Salt supplementation • Surgical repair of female pseudohermaphroditism
P450c11β	• Female pseudohermaphroditism • Postnatal virilization in males and females	• ↑ 11-deoxycortisol and DOC before and after ACTH • ↑ Serum androgens and urine 17KS • Suppression of elevated steroids after glucocorticoid administration • ↑ ACTH and ↓ PRA • Hypokalemia	• Glucocorticoid administration • Surgical repair of female pseudohermaphroditism
P450c11AS	• Failure to thrive • Weakness • Salt loss	• Hyponatremia, hyperkalemia • ↑ Corticosterone • ↓ Aldosterone ↑ PRA	• Mineralocorticoid replacement • Salt supplementation
P450c17	• Male pseudohermaphroditism • Sexual infantilism • Hypertension	• ↑ DOC, 18-OHDOC, corticosterone, 18-hydroxycorticosterone • Low 17α-hydroxylated steroids and poor response to ACTH • Poor response to hCG in male pseudohermaphroditism • Suppression of elevated adrenal steroids after glucocorticoid administration • ↑ ACTH and ↓ PRA • Hypokalemia	• Glucocorticoid administration • Surgical correction of genitalia and sex steroid replacement in male pseudohermaphroditism consonent with sex of rearing • Estrogen replacement in female at ≧12 years • Testosterone replacement if reared as male (rare)
POR	• Male and female pseudohermaphroditism • Antley-Bixler syndrome • Infertility in adults	• ↑ ACTH, prog, 17OHP • ↓ DHEA, andro, T • Normal electrolytes	• Glucocorticoid and sex steroid replacement • Surgical correction of skeletal anomalies

ACTH, adrenocorticotropic hormone (corticotropin); DOC, deoxycorticosterone; hCG, human chorionic gonadotropin; PRA, plasma renin activity; 17OHP, 17-hydroxyprogesterone; 17KS, 7-ketosteroids; and 18-OHDOC, 18-hydroxydeoxycorticosterone.

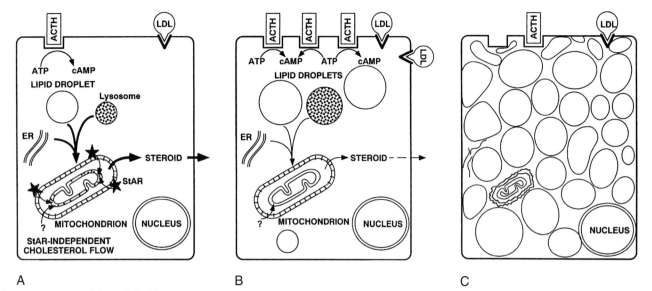

A   B   C

Figure 12-10 Two-hit model of lipoid CAH. (*A*) In a normal adrenal cell, cholesterol is primarily derived from LDL by receptor-mediated endocytosis and is processed in lysosomes before entering the cellular pool. However, cholesterol can also be synthesized de novo from acetyl CoA. Cholesterol from both sources is stored as cholesterol esters in lipid droplets. Cholesterol reaches the mitochondria by poorly defined processes, and then travels from the outer to inner mitochondrial membrane by both StAR-dependent and StAR-independent mechanisms. (*B*) In early lipoid CAH, the absence of StAR reduces cholesterol flow and steroidogenesis. However, some steroidogenesis persists via the StAR-independent pathway. The decreased secretion of cortisol leads to increased ACTH, which stimulates further cholesterol uptake and synthesis. This cholesterol accumulates in lipid droplets. (*C*) Accumulating lipid droplets damage the cell through physical disruption of cytoarchitecture and by the chemical action of auto-oxidation products, eventually destroying all steroidogenic capacity. In the ovary, follicular cells remain unstimulated and undamaged until they are recruited at the beginning of each cycle. They can then produce small amounts of estradiol, as in panel B, leading to feminization and anovulatory cycles in affected females.

Because gonadotropin stimulation only recruits individual follicles and does not promote steroidogenesis in the entire ovary, most follicles remain undamaged and available for future cycles. Cyclicity is determined by the hypothalamic-pituitary axis, and remains normal. With each new cycle, a new follicle is recruited and more estradiol is produced by StAR-independent steroidogenesis. Although net ovarian steroidogenesis is impaired, enough estrogen is produced, especially in the absence of androgens, to induce breast development, general feminization, monthly estrogen withdrawal, and cyclic vaginal bleeding.[42,254]

However, progesterone synthesis in the latter half of the cycle is disturbed by the accumulating cholesterol esters, with the result that the cycles are anovulatory. Measurements of estradiol, progesterone, and gonadotropins throughout the cycle in affected adult females with lipoid CAH confirms this model.[255] Similarly, examination of StAR-knockout mice confirms the two-hit model.[256] Thus, examination of patients with lipoid CAH has elucidated the physiology of the StAR protein in each steroidogenic tissue.

Genetic analysis of patients with lipoid CAH has revealed numerous mutations in the StAR gene.[42,257] Lipoid CAH is common in Japan, and about 65% to 70% of affected Japanese alleles and virtually all affected Korean alleles carry the mutation Q258X.[41,42,242,257-259] The carrier frequency for this mutation appears to be about 1 in 300,[42,258] and 1 in every 250,000 to 300,000 newborns in these countries is affected, for a total of about 500 patients in Japan and Korea. Other genetic clusters are found among Palestinian Arabs, most of whom carry the mutation R182L,[42] in eastern Saudi Arabia carrying R188C[253] and in Switzerland carrying the mutation L260P.[260]

Deletion of only 10 carboxy-terminal residues reduces StAR activity by half,[261] and deletion of 28 carboxy-terminal residues by the common Q258X mutation eliminates all activity. By contrast, deletion of the first 62 amino terminal residues has no effect on StAR activity even though this deletes the entire mitochondrial leader sequence and forces StAR to remain in the cytoplasm.[261] Physical studies and partial proteolysis indicate that residues 63-193 of StAR (i.e., the domain that lacks most of the crucial residues identified by missense mutations) are protease resistant and constitute a "pause-transfer" sequence that permits the bioactive loosely folded carboxy-terminal molten globule domain to have increased interaction with the outer mitochondrial membrane.[49]

The clinical findings in most patients with lipoid CAH are quite similar. An infant with normal-appearing female genitalia experiences failure to thrive and salt loss in the first weeks of life.[42,242,257] However, more recent studies have revealed other clinical presentations, including apparent sudden infant death syndrome (SIDS)[262] and late initial presentation of salt loss at about 1 year of age.[253] An attenuated disease caused by mutations that retain about 20% to 25% of normal StAR activity has been described recently and is called nonclassic lipoid CAH.[263] These children initially experienced symptoms of adrenal insufficiency at 2 to 4 years of age, and two 46,XY patients had normal-appearing male external genitalia.

Thus, the spectrum of clinical presentation of congenital lipoid adrenal hyperplasia is substantially broader than initially appreciated.

Mutations in several other genes can produce a clinical phenotype that is essentially indistinguishable from that caused by StAR mutations, but these disorders should not be called congenital lipoid adrenal hyperplasia. Several patients have now been described with mutations in P450scc.[264-267] It would seem logical that elimination of all P450scc activity would be incompatible with term gestation because the placenta, a fetal tissue, must produce progesterone in the second half of pregnancy to suppress maternal uterine contractions and thus prevent miscarriage.[268]

It is most likely that these few fetuses with P450scc mutations reached term gestation because of unusually protracted maintenance of the maternal corpus luteum of pregnancy, which normally involutes in the second trimester. However, this has not been investigated directly. Three patients have also been described carrying mutations in the gene for steroidogenic factor 1 (SF1), a transcription factor required for adrenal and gonadal but not for placental expression of genes for the steroidogenic enzymes.[269-271] Two of these patients were 46,XY with a female phenotype and had adrenal failure, thus resembling lipoid CAH.

Treatment of lipoid CAH is straightforward if the diagnosis is made. Physiologic replacement with glucocorticoids, mineralocorticoids, and salt will permit survival to adulthood.[241,242] The glucocorticoid requirement is less than in the virilizing adrenal hyperplasias because it is not necessary to oversuppress excess adrenal androgen production. Thus, growth in these patients should be normal.[242] Genetic males have female external genitalia and should undergo orchiectomy and be raised as females.[42,241,242]

3β-HYDROXYSTEROID DEHYDROGENASE DEFICIENCY

3βHSD deficiency is a rare cause of glucocorticoid and mineralocorticoid deficiency that is fatal if not diagnosed early in infancy.[272] In its classic form, genetic females have clitoromegaly and mild virilization because the fetal adrenal overproduces large amounts of DHEA, a small portion of which is converted to testosterone by extra-adrenal 3βHSD1. Genetic males also synthesize some androgens by peripheral conversion of adrenal and testicular DHEA, but the concentrations are insufficient for complete male genital development and thus these males have a small phallus and severe hypospadias.

There are two functional human genes for 3βHSD: the type 1 gene is expressed in the placenta and peripheral tissues[55,57] and the type 2 gene is expressed in the adrenals and gonads.[273,274] Genetic and endocrine studies of 3βHSD deficiency show that the gonads and the adrenals are affected as a result of a single mutated 3βHSD2 gene expressed in both tissues. However, hepatic 3βHSD1 activity persists in the face of complete absence of adrenal and gonadal 3βHSD2 activity, thus complicating the diagnosis. Genetic studies have identified numerous mutations causing 3βHSD deficiency, all found in the type 2 gene.[275-279] Mutations have never been found in 3βHSD1,

presumably because this would prevent placental biosynthesis of progesterone and result in a spontaneous first-trimester abortion.

The presence of peripheral 3βHSD activity complicates the hormonal diagnosis of this disease. One would expect that affected infants should have low concentrations of 17OHP, yet some newborns with 3βHSD deficiency have very high concentrations of serum 17OHP approaching those seen in patients with classical 21-hydroxylase deficiency.[280] The high 17OHP concentrations are due to extra-adrenal 3βHSD1. The adrenal of a patient with 3βHSD2 deficiency will secrete very large amounts of three principal Δ^5 steroids: pregnenolone, 17-hydroxypregnenolone, and DHEA.

Some of the secreted 17-hydroxypregnenolone is then converted to 17OHP by 3βHSD1. This 17OHP is not effectively picked up by the adrenal for subsequent conversion to cortisol because the circulating concentrations are below the K_m of P450c17, which is 1 μM 17OHP, or about 40,000 ng/dL. The ratio of Δ^5 to Δ^4 compounds remains high, consistent with the adrenal and gonadal deficiency of 3βHSD.[280] Thus, the principal diagnostic test in 3β-HSD deficiency is intravenous administration of ACTH with measurement of the three Δ^5 compounds and the corresponding Δ^4 compounds. Unlike the case of 21-hydroxylase deficiency, in which heterozygotes can be diagnosed by the response of 17OHP to ACTH, steroidal responses to ACTH cannot be used to identify carriers of 3βHSD deficiency.[281]

Mild or "partial" defects of adrenal 3βHSD activity have been reported on the basis of ratios of Δ^5 steroids to Δ^4 steroids following an ACTH test that exceed 2 or 3 standard deviations above the mean. These patients are typically young girls with premature adrenarche or young women with a history of premature adrenarche and complaints of hirsutism, virilism, and oligomenorrhea.[282-284] However, the 3βHSD2 genes are normal in these patients, and even patients with mild 3βHSD2 mutations have ratios of Δ^5 to Δ^4 steroids that exceed 8 standard deviations above the mean.[278,285-288] The basis of the mildly elevated ratios of Δ^5 to Δ^4 steroids in these hirsute individuals with normal 3βHSD genes is unknown. In adult women, the hirsutism can be ameliorated and regular menses can be restored by suppressing ACTH with 0.25 mg of dexamethasone given orally each day, but such treatment is contraindicated in girls who have not yet reached their final adult height.

17α-HYDROXYLASE/17,20-LYASE DEFICIENCY

P450c17 is the single enzyme that catalyzes 17α-hydroxylase and 17,20-lyase activities. 17-hydroxylase deficiency has been studied in detail at both clinical and genetic levels[289] and appears to be especially common in Brazil.[290] Deficient 17α-hydroxylase activity and deficient 17,20-lyase activity have been described as separate genetic diseases, but it is now clear that they represent different clinical manifestations of different lesions in the same gene. Deficient 17α-hydroxylase activity results in decreased cortisol synthesis, overproduction of ACTH, and stimulation of the steps proximal to P450c17.

These patients may have mild symptoms of glucocorticoid deficiency, but this is not life-threatening because the lack of P450c17 results in the overproduction of corticosterone which also has glucocorticoid activity. This is similar to the situation in rodents, whose adrenals lack P450c17[291] and consequently produce corticosterone as their glucocorticoid. Affected patients also typically overproduce DOC in the zona fasciculata, which causes sodium retention, hypertension, and hypokalemia and suppresses plasma renin activity and aldosterone secretion from the zona glomerulosa, although the suppression of aldosterone is rather variable. When P450c17 deficiency is treated with glucocorticoids, DOC secretion is suppressed and plasma renin activity and aldosterone concentrations rise to normal.[292]

The absence of 17α-hydroxylase and 17,20-lyase activities in complete P450c17 deficiency prevents the synthesis of adrenal and gonadal sex steroids. As a result, affected females are phenotypically normal but fail to undergo adrenarche and puberty[293] and genetic males have absent or incomplete development of the external genitalia (male pseudohermaphroditism).[294] The classic presentation is that of a teenage female with sexual infantilism and hypertension.[294] The diagnosis is made by finding low or absent 17-hydroxylated C-21 and C-19 plasma steroids, which respond poorly to stimulation with ACTH. Serum levels of DOC, corticosterone, and 18-OH-corticosterone are elevated, hyperresponsive to ACTH, and suppressible with glucocorticoids.

The gene for P450c17[70] is located on chromosome 10q24.3.[68,69] The molecular basis of 17α-hydroxylase deficiency has been determined in numerous patients by the cloning and sequencing of the mutated gene, which have identified more than 50 distinct mutations. Four mutations appear recurrently: a duplication of four nucleotides causing a frame-shift is found among descendents of Dutch Frieslanders,[295] in-frame deletion of residues 487 through 489 is found throughout Southeast Asia,[296] and a deletion of phenylalanine at position 53 or 54[297] and the common W406R and R362C mutations are found respectively among Brazilians of Spanish and Portuguese ancestry.[290] The genetic lesions identified include 12 mutations that cause frame-shifts or premature translational termination. As expected, none of these mutants has any detectable 17α-hydroxylase or 17,20-lyase activity. Eleven missense and in-frame mutations have been found, most of which also eliminate all activity, whereas others, such as P342T, reduce both activities by 80%.

Selective deficiency of the 17,20-lyase activity of P450c17 has been reported in about a dozen cases,[298] which initially led to the incorrect conclusion that 17α-hydroxylase and 17,20-lyase are separate enzymes. One of the original patients was studied at the genetic level, showing two wholly inactivating mutations[299], which led to a corrected diagnosis of the patient as having complete 17α-hydroxylase deficiency.[300] Because the 17α-hydroxylase and 17,20 lyase activities of P450c17 are catalyzed on the same active site, it was not clear that a syndrome of isolated 17,20 lyase deficiency could exist until two patients with genital ambiguity, normal excretion of 17OHCS, and markedly reduced production of C$_{19}$ steroids were studied at the molecular genetic level.[301]

One patient was homozygous for the P450c17 mutation R347H, and the other was homozygous for R358Q. Both mutations changed the distribution of surface charges in the redox partner binding site of P450c17.[301] When assayed in vitro, both mutants retained nearly normal 17α-hydroxylase activity but had no detectable 17,20 lyase activity[301,302], and enzymatic competition experiments showed that the substrate binding site remained normal.[302] When an excess of P450 oxidoreductase and cytochrome b$_5$ was provided, some 17,20 lyase activity was restored, demonstrating that the loss in lyase activity was caused by impaired electron transfer.[302] Several additional patients have been described with similar mutations,[303] and an active site mutation causing isolated 17,20 lyase deficiency has been described.[304]

Computational modeling of P450c17 predicts the effects of all known mutations, including those with partial retention of both activities and those causing selective 17,20 lyase deficiency.[305] The model identifies Arg 347 and Arg 358 and several other arginine and lysine residues in the redox partner binding site. Mutation of these residues causes varying degrees of selective loss of 17,20 lyase activity.[301,302,305,306] Another example of the critical nature of redox partner interactions comes from the sole reported case of cytochrome b$_5$ deficiency. This patient was a male pseudohermaphrodite, but was not evaluated hormonally.[307] Thus, the central role of electron transfer in 17,20 lyase activity is now well established.

21-HYDROXYLASE DEFICIENCY

21-hydroxylase deficiency, which is due to mutations in the gene encoding adrenal P450c21, is one of the most common inborn errors of metabolism and accounts for about 95% of all forms of CAH. Because of success in diagnosis and treatment in infancy, many patients with severe forms of 21-hydroxylase deficiency have now reached adulthood, indicating that management issues in CAH concern all age groups. Detailed reviews of the complex physiology and molecular genetics of this disorder are available.[78-81,150,308]

Pathophysiology

For patients with a complete absence of P450c21, the clinical manifestations can be deduced from Figure 12-3. Inability to convert progesterone to DOC results in aldosterone deficiency, causing severe hyponatremia (Na$^+$ often below 110 mEq/L), hyperkalemia (K$^+$ often above 10 mEq/L), and acidosis (pH often below 7.1), with concomitant hypotension, shock, cardiovascular collapse, and death in an untreated newborn infant. High concentrations of cortisol in the adrenocortical capillary effluent that bathes the medulla are needed for the conversion of norepinephrine to epinephrine. Hence, children with CAH have low epinephrine concentrations, which may exacerbate the hypoglycemia associated with cortisol deficiency.[309] Because the control of fluids and electrolytes in the fetus can be maintained by the placenta and the mother's kidneys, this salt-losing crisis develops only after birth, usually during the second week of life.

The inability to convert 17OHP to 11-deoxycortisol results in cortisol deficiency, which impairs postnatal carbohydrate metabolism and exacerbates cardiovascular collapse because a permissive action of cortisol is required for full pressor action of catecholamines. Although the role of cortisol in fetal physiology is not well established,[141,145] cortisol deficiency is manifested prenatally. Low fetal cortisol stimulates ACTH secretion, which stimulates adrenal hyperplasia and transcription of the genes for all steroidogenic enzymes, especially for P450scc, the rate-limiting enzyme in steroidogenesis. This increased transcription increases enzyme production and activity, with consequent accumulation of non-21-hydroxylated steroids, especially 17OHP. As the pathways in Figure 12-3 indicate, these steroids are converted to testosterone.

In the male fetus, the testes produce large amounts of mRNA for the steroidogenic enzymes, and concentrations of testosterone are high in early to midgestation.[251] This testosterone differentiates external male genitalia from the pluripotential embryonic precursor structures. In the male fetus with 21-hydroxylase deficiency, the additional testosterone produced in the adrenals has little if any demonstrable phenotypic effect. In a female fetus, the ovaries lack steroidogenic enzyme mRNAs and are quiescent.[251] No sex steroids or other factors are needed for differentiation of the female external genitalia.[310]

The testosterone inappropriately produced by the adrenals of the affected female fetus causes varying degrees of virilization of the external genitalia. This can range from mild clitoromegaly with or without posterior fusion of the labioscrotal folds to complete labioscrotal fusion that includes a urethra traversing the enlarged clitoris Figure 12-11. These infants have normal ovaries, fallopian tubes, and a uterus but have ambiguous external genitalia or may be sufficiently virilized so that they appear to be male, resulting in errors of sex assignment at birth.

The diagnosis of 21-hydroxylase deficiency is suggested by genital ambiguity in females, a salt-losing episode in either sex, or rapid growth and virilization in males or females. Plasma 17OHP is markedly elevated at >2,000 ng/dL after 24 hr of age in an otherwise healthy full-term infant and hyperresponsive to stimulation with ACTH (Figure 12-9). Measurement of 11-deoxycortisol, 17OHP, DHEA, and androstenedione is important to distinguish among the forms of CAH and because adrenal or testicular tumors can also produce 17OHP.[311] Similarly, ACTH will induce a substantial rise in serum 21-deoxycortisol in all forms of 21-hydroxylase deficiency but not in normals, providing a useful adjunctive test when this steroid can be measured.[312] High newborn 17OHP values that rise further after ACTH can also be seen in 3βHSD and P450c11 deficiencies.[280]

17OHP is normally high in cord blood but falls to normal newborn levels after 12 to 24 hours (Figure 12-12), and thus assessment of 17OHP levels should not be made in the first 24 hours of life. Premature infants and term infants under severe stress (e.g., with cardiac or pulmonary disease) may have persistently elevated 17OHP concentrations with normal 21-hydroxylase, although longitudinal studies of 17OHP values in the premature have not been reported. Newborn screening programs for CAH are being instituted throughout the world based on 17OHP measurements on the "Guthrie cards" typically used for newborn screening of metabolic disorders. The technologies employed and "cutoff" values used vary substantially in different health care systems. In general, when testing is done on full-term infants more than 24 hours after birth the screening is highly reliable. Each endocrinologist and neonatologist must become familiar with local assays and the values found in the extremely premature, which may be read as false positives for CAH.

Clinical Forms of 21-Hydroxylase Deficiency

There is a broad spectrum of clinical manifestations of 21-hydroxylase deficiency, depending on the particular mutations of the gene for P450c21. These different forms

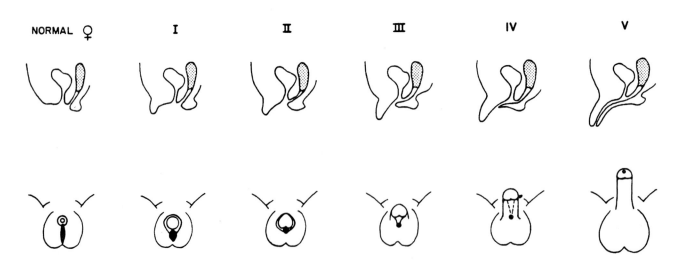

Figure 12-11 Virilization of the external genitalia. A continuous spectrum is shown from normal female to normal male in both saggital section (above) and perineal views (below), using the staging system of Prader. Disorders of external genitalia can occur either by the virilization of a normal female, as in congenital adrenal hyperplasia, or due to an error in testosterone synthesis in the male. In females with congenital adrenal hyperplasia due to 21-hydroxylase deficiency, the degree of virilization correlates poorly with the presence or absence of clinical signs of salt loss.

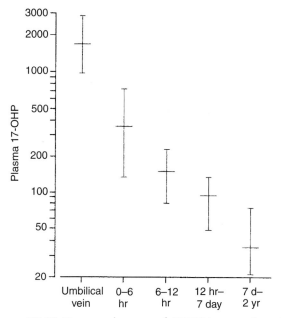

Figure 12-12 Means and ranges of 17OHP in normal newborns (data are in ng/100 mL). Note that values can be very high and quite variable for the first 24 hours of life.

of 21-hydroxylase deficiency are not different diseases because there is a continuous spectrum of manifestations, ranging from the severe salt-wasting form to clinically inapparent forms that may be normal variants. Thus, the typical disease forms discussed in the material following are mainly a clinical convenience.

Salt-Wasting CAH. Salt-wasting CAH is due to a complete deficiency of P450c21 activity, effectively eliminating glucocorticoid and mineralocorticoid synthesis. Females with this disorder are frequently diagnosed at birth because of masculinization of the external genitalia. After appropriate resuscitation of the cardiovascular collapse, acidosis, and electrolyte disorders, the mineralocorticoids and glucocorticoids can be replaced orally and the ambiguous genitalia can be corrected with a series of plastic surgical procedures. The steroidal replacement management is difficult because of the rapidly changing needs of a growing infant or child. Drug doses must be adjusted frequently, and there is considerable individual variability in what constitutes "physiologic" replacement.

As an underdosage of glucocorticoids can be life-threatening, especially during illness, most pediatricians have tended to err on the "safe side" and thus these children usually receive inappropriately large doses of glucocorticoids. It is not possible to compensate for the growth lost during the first 2 years of life, when growth is fastest, and thus these children almost always end up shorter than predicted from their genetic potential. Female survivors may have sexual dysfunction, marry with a low frequency, be more reluctant to form intimate relationships, and have decreased fertility.[313-316] Prenatal androgens appear to affect behavior but not sexual identity.[317] Males with this disorder are generally undiagnosed at birth and either come to medical attention during the

salt-losing crisis that follows 5 to 15 days later or die, invariably with an incorrect diagnosis.

Simple Virilizing CAH. Virilized females who have elevated concentrations of 17OHP but who do not suffer a salt-losing crisis have long been recognized as having the "simple virilizing" form of CAH. Males with this disorder often escape diagnosis until age 3 to 7 years, when they come to medical attention because of early development of pubic, axillary, facial hair, and phallic growth. An astute physician can readily differentiate boys with sexual precocity caused by CAH from boys with true central precocious puberty, as the testes remain of prepubertal size in CAH whereas gonadotropic stimulation in true precocious puberty results in pubertal-size testes.

These children grow rapidly and are tall for their age when diagnosed, but their epiphyseal maturation (bone age) advances at a disproportionately rapid rate so that their ultimate adult height is invariably compromised. Untreated or poorly treated children with CAH may fail to undergo normal puberty, and boys may have small testes and azoospermia because of the feedback effects of the adrenally produced testosterone. When treatment is begun at several years of age, suppression of adrenal testosterone secretion may remove tonic inhibition of the hypothalamus, occasionally resulting in true central precocious puberty requiring treatment with a GnRH agonist.

High concentrations of ACTH in some poorly treated boys may stimulate the enlargement of adrenal rests in the testes. These enlarged testes are usually nodular, unlike the homogeneously enlarged testes in central precocious puberty. Because the adrenal normally produces 100 to 1,000 times as much cortisol as aldosterone, mild defects, or amino acid replacement mutations, in P450c21 are less likely to affect mineralocorticoid secretion than cortisol secretion. Thus, patients with simple virilizing CAH simply have a less severe disorder of P450c21. This is reflected physiologically by the increased plasma renin activity seen in these patients after moderate salt restriction.

Nonclassic CAH. Many people have very mild forms of 21-hydroxylase deficiency. These forms may be evidenced by mild to moderate hirsutism, virilism, menstrual irregularities, and decreased fertility in adult women, so-called late-onset CAH,[318-320] or there may be no phenotypic manifestations at all other than an increased response of plasma 17OHP to an intravenous ACTH test, so-called cryptic CAH.[321] Despite the minimal manifestations of this disorder, these individuals also have hormonal evidence of a mild impairment in mineralocorticoid secretion as predicted from the existence of a single adrenal 21-hydroxylase.[322]

There is some inconsistency in classifying patients into these three categories because each diagnostic category is not a separate disease but represents a typical picture in a continuous spectrum of disease caused by a broad spectrum of genetic lesions in the P450c21 gene. Furthermore, because some mutant P450c21 alleles are common in the general population most patients are compound heterozygotes, carrying a different mutation on the allele inherited from each parent. Finally, factors other than the specific mutations found in P450c21 will influence the clinical phenotype, including the presence of extra-adrenal 21-hydroxylases other than P450c21, undiagnosed

P450c21 promoter mutations, and variations in androgen metabolism and sensitivity. These discordances between genotype and phenotype are to be expected.

Incidence of 21-Hydroxylase Deficiency

Perinatal screening for elevated concentrations of serum 17OHP in several countries has shown that the incidence of classic CAH (i.e., salt-wasting and simple virilizing CAH) is about 1 in 14,000, yielding a heterozygous carrier rate of 1 in 60.[323] The screening of 1.9 million newborns in Texas yielded an overall incidence of 1 in 16,000, including incidences of 1 in 15,600 Caucasians, 1 in 14,500 Hispanics, primarily Mexican Americans of indigenous American ancestry, and 1 in 42,300 African Americans.[324] Because about 20% of the African American gene pool is of European descent, the calculated incidence in individuals of wholly sub-Saharan African ancestry is about 1 in 250,000.

Nonclassical CAH is clearly much more common, but these data are also variable. One group has reported very high incidences: 1 in 27 for Ashkenazi Jews, 1 in 53 for Hispanics, 1 in 63 for Yugoslavs, 1 in 333 for Italians, and 1 in 1,000 for other whites.[325-327] These data would indicate that one-third of Ashkenazi Jews, one-fourth of Hispanics, one-fifth of Yugoslavs, one-ninth of Italians, and one-fourteenth of other Caucasians are heterozygous carriers. However, other studies have shown carrier rates of 1.2%[319] to 6%[328,329] for Caucasian populations that were not subdivided further. The considerable differences in the reported incidences reflect differences in the small populations examined and the errors in distinguishing nonclassic CAH from heterozygous carriers of classic CAH when an ACTH test is not performed.

In homozygotes for classic and nonclassic CAH, serum concentrations of 21-deoxycortisol rise in response to ACTH. However, ACTH-induced 21-deoxycortisol remains normal in heterozygotes for classic and nonclassic CAH.[312] These studies have, however, classified individuals by hormonal phenotype without examining the P450c21 genes directly to establish these incidences. Therefore, the diagnosis of nonclassic CAH requires family studies because the hormonal data, 17OHP responses to ACTH, in these individuals may be indistinguishable from those for unaffected heterozygous carriers of the more severe forms. The high incidence, lack of mortality, and lack of decreased fertility in most individuals with nonclassic CAH indicate that this is probably a variant of normal and is not a disease in the classic sense. Nevertheless, patients with nonclassic CAH may seek help for complaints of virilism and menstrual disorders.

Genetics of the 21-Hydroxylase Locus

21-Hydroxylase Genes. There are two 21-hydroxylase loci: a functional gene (formally termed *CYP21A2*) and a nonfunctional pseudogene (formally termed *CYP21A1P*).[330] These genes, generally termed *P450c21B* (functional gene) and *P450c21A* (pseudogene), are duplicated in tandem, with the C4A and C4B genes encoding the fourth component of serum complement[331,332] (Figure 12-13). Although the P450c21A locus is transcribed, the resultant RNAs do not encode protein,[333] only the P450c21B gene

encodes 21-hydroxylase. The P450c21 genes consist of 10 exons, are about 3.4 kb long, and differ in only 87 or 88 of these bases.[83-85]

This high degree of sequence similarity indicates that these two genes are evolving in tandem through intergenic exchange of DNA. The P450c21 genes of mice[334] and cattle[335,336] are also duplicated and linked to leukocyte antigen loci. However, wheras only the P450c21B gene functions in human beings only the P450c21A gene functions in mice[337,338], and both genes function in cattle.[339] Sequencing of the gene duplication boundaries shows that the human locus was duplicated after mammalian speciation,[340] consistent with data that indicate that other mammals have single P450c21 gene copies.[341]

HLA Linkage. The 21-hydroxylase genes lie within the class III region of the human major histocompatibility complex (MHC) (Figure 12-13). Thus, HLA typing has been widely used for prenatal diagnosis and to identify heterozygous family members. Statistical associations (linkage disequilibrium) are well established between CAH and specific HLA types. Salt-losing CAH is associated with HLA-B60 and HLA-40 in some populations,[342] and the rare HLA type Bw47 is very strongly associated with salt-losing CAH.[343,344]

HLA-Bw51 is often associated with simple virilizing CAH in some populations,[345] and 30% to 50% of haplotypes for nonclassic CAH carry HLA-B14.[346] HLA-B14 is often associated with a duplication of the C4B gene.[347,348] By contrast, all HLA-B alleles can be found linked to CAH. HLA-identical individuals in a single family may have different clinical features of CAH despite HLA identity,[349-352] possibly representing extra-adrenal 21-hydroxylation, de novo mutations, or multiple genetic crossover events.

Other Genes in the 21-Hydroxylase Locus. The tandemly duplicated C4A and C4B loci produce isoforms of complement component C4 that can be distinguished functionally and immunologically. The C4B protein has substantially more hemolytic activity despite greater than 99% sequence identity with C4A.[353] The C4A gene is always 22 kb long, but there are long (22 kb) and short (16 kb) forms of C4B due to a variation in one intron.[354] The 3' ends of the C4 genes are only 2466bp upstream from the transcriptional start sites of the P450c21 genes. Promoter sequences needed for the transcription of the human P450c21B gene lie within intron 35 of the C4B gene.[355,356] In addition to the P450c21 and C4 genes, there are several other genes within 100 kb of the P450c21 gene, including the genes for complement factor C2 and properdin factor Bf (Figure 12-13). Lying just 3' of the Bf gene on the opposite strand of DNA from P450c21 is the STK19 gene, also variously called RD, RP, and G11, which encodes a nuclear serine/threonine kinase.[357]

A pair of genes, termed *XA* and *XB*, is duplicated with the C4 and P450c21 genes. These genes lie on the strand of DNA opposite the C4 and P450c21 genes and overlapping the 3' end of P450c21. The last exon of XA and XB lies within the 3' untranslated region of exon 10 in P450c21A and P450c21B, respectively.[358] The XA gene was truncated during the duplication of the ancestral C4-P450c21-X genetic unit, but is transcribed in the adrenal.[340] The XB gene encodes a large extracellular matrix protein called Tenascin X, which is expressed in most

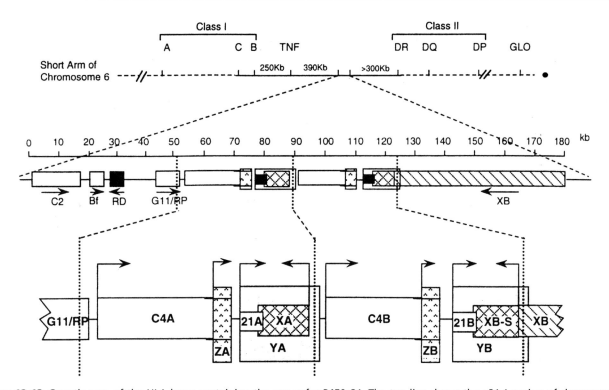

Figure 12-13 Genetic map of the HLA locus containing the genes for P450c21. The top line shows the p21.1 region of chromosome 6, with the telomere to the left and the centromere to the right. Most HLA genes are found in the class I and class II regions. The class III region containing the P450c21 genes lies between these two. The second line shows the scale (in kilobases) for the diagram immediately below, showing (from left to right) the genes for complement factor C2, properedin factor Bf, and the RD and G11/RP genes of unknown function. Arrows indicate transcriptional orientation. The bottom line shows the 21-hydroxylase locus on an expanded scale, including the C4A and C4B genes for the fourth component of complement, the inactive CYP21A gene (21A), and the active CYP21B gene (21B) that encodes P450c21. XA, YA, and YB are adrenal-specific transcripts that lack open reading frames. The XB gene encodes the extracellular matrix protein tenascin-X. XB-S encodes a truncated adrenal-specific form of the tenascin-X protein, whose function is unknown. ZA and ZB are adrenal-specific transcripts that arise within the C4 genes and have open reading frames. However, it is not known if they are translated into protein. Nevertheless, the promoter elements of these transcripts are essential components of the CYP21A and CYP21B promoters. The arrows indicate transcriptional orientation. The vertical dotted lines designate the boundaries of the genetic duplication event that led to the presence of A and B regions.

tissues, especially connective tissue.[359,360] The XB gene spans about 65 kb of DNA and includes 43 exons encoding a 12-kb mRNA.[359,361]

The XB gene also encodes a short truncated form of Tenascin X having unknown function and arising from an intragenic promoter.[362] Identification of a CAH patient with a "contiguous gene syndrome" comprising a deletion of the P450c21B and XB genes demonstrated that Tenascin X deficiency results in Ehlers-Danlos syndrome (EDS).[363] Most forms of EDS are caused by autosomal-dominant mutations in collagen genes. The recessive forms are caused by mutations in genes for collagen-modifying enzymes, including Tenascin-X, which is associated with and stabilizes collagen fibrils.[364,365] Tenascin-X deficiency causes a clinically distinct, somewhat more severe, recessive form of Ehlers-Danlos syndrome, with or without associated 21-hydroxylase deficiency.[366]

P450c21 Gene Lesions Causing 21-Hydroxylase Deficiency

21-hydroxylase deficiency can be caused by P450c21B gene deletions, gene conversions, and apparent point mutations. Most of the point mutations in the P450c21B

gene are actually small gene conversion events,[78,79,367] and thus gene conversions account for about 85% of the lesions in 21-hydroxylase deficiency. The P450c21 genes are autosomal, and hence each person has two alleles, one contributed by each parent.

Most patients with 21-hydroxylase deficiency are compound heterozygotes, having different lesions on their two alleles. Because gene deletions and large conversions eliminate all P450c21B gene transcription, in the homozygous state these lesions will cause salt-losing CAH. Some microconversions, such as those creating premature translational termination, are also associated with salt-losing CAH. Milder forms, such as simple virilizing and nonclassic CAH, are associated with amino acid replacements in the P450c21 protein caused by gene microconversion events. Patients with these forms of CAH are usually compound heterozygotes bearing a severely disordered allele and a mildly disordered allele and thus the clinical manifestations are based on the nature of the mildly disordered allele.

Mapping of P450c21 Genes in Normals and in CAH. Although the P450c21B and P450c21A loci differ by only 87 or 88 nucleotides, they can be distinguished by restriction endonuclease digestion and Southern blotting. Two unusual and related features of the 21-hydroxylase locus complicate its analysis. First, the gene deletions in this locus are most unusual in that they extend 30 kb from one of several points in the middle of P450c21A to the precisely homologous point in P450c21B. Thus, the 15% of alleles that carry deletions do not yield a typical Southern blotting pattern with a band of a size different from that of one of the normal unless one uses very rarely cutting enzymes and analyzes the resulting large DNA fragments by pulsed-field gel electrophoresis. The second unusual feature of this locus is that gene conversions are extremely common.[368,369]

Gene Conversions. If a segment of gene A replaces the corresponding segment of the related gene B, the structure of recipient gene B is said to be "converted" to that of donor gene A. The hallmark of gene conversion is that the number of closely related genes remains constant, whereas their diversity decreases. Two types of gene conversions commonly cause 21-hydroxylase deficiency: large gene conversions that can be mistaken for gene deletions and small microconversions that resemble point mutations. The relative frequency of large gene conversions versus gene deletions was formerly controversial, principally because initial studies used relatively small groups of patients from single locations or ethnic groups.

A compilation of the world literature on the genetics of CAH found that 19% of mutant alleles had gene deletions, 8% had large gene conversions, 67% had microconversions, and 6% had uncharacterized lesions[79] (Figure 12-14). However, such statistics must be viewed with caution because there is considerable ascertainment bias in favor of the more severely affected patients[348] and because some studies excluded mildly affected patients. Thus, the previously cited statistics are weighted in favor of gene deletions and large conversions, which can only yield a phenotype of salt-wasting CAH.

Point Mutations Microconversions Causing CAH. About 75% of mutated P450c21 genes appear to be structurally intact by Southern blotting and thus appear to carry point mutations.[348,368] Many mutant P450c21B genes

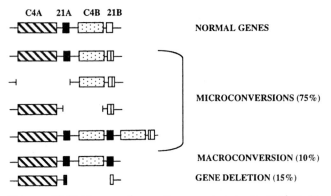

Figure 12-14 Classes of genetic rearrangements causing 21-hydroxylase deficiency. Deletions or duplications of the C4A and C4B genes can occur with or without associated lesions in the P450c21B gene. Note that virtually all "point mutations" in P450c21B are actually microconversion. Many authors combine the gene deletion and macroconversion groups because these are difficult to distinguish by Southern blotting in that both result in a loss of the P450c21B gene. However, the genotypes are clearly distinct (as shown).

TABLE 12-6

Microconversions of the P450c21B Gene That Cause 21-Hydroxylase Deficiency

Mutation	Location	Associated Phenotypes	Activity
Pro 30→Leu	Exon 1	NC/SV	30%-60%
A→G	Intron 2	SV/SW	minimal
8 bp deletion	Exon 3	SW	0
Ile 172→Asn	Exon 4	SV	3%-7%
Ile 236→Asp			
Val 237→Glu	Exon 6	SW	
Met 239→Lys			
Val 281→Leu	Exon 7	NC	18% ± 9%
Gly 292→Ser	Exon 7	SW	
T insertion @ 306	Exon 7	SW	0
Gly 318→Stop	Exon 8	SW	0
Arg 339→His	Exon 8	NC	20%-50%
Arg 356→Trp	Exon 8	SV/SW	2%
Pro 453→Ser	Exon 10	NC	20%-50%
GG→C @ 484	Exon 10	SW	0

causing CAH have been cloned and sequenced (Table 12-6), revealing that a relatively small number of mutations cause CAH, virtually all of which are also found in the P450c21A pseudogene. These observations indicate that most CAH alleles bearing apparent point mutations actually carry microconversions.[78,79,367]

Three changes in the P450c21A pseudogene (8bp deletion, exon 3; T insertion, exon 7; Gly 318 stop, exon 8) render its product nonfunctional. Each change results in an altered reading frame and/or premature stop codon, eliminating all activity. All of these have been found in P450c21B alleles that cause severe salt-losing CAH. Three closely clustered base changes alter the normal amino acid sequence Ile-Val-Glu-Met at codons 236 to 239 in exon 6 to Asn-Glu-Glu-Lys in P450c21A and in a small number of genes causing severe salt-losing CAH.

The most common lesion in classic CAH is an A→G change in the second intron, 13 bases upstream from the normal 3→ splice acceptor site of this intron, a microconversion found in more than 25% of severely affected CAH alleles. This intronic mutation causes abnormal splicing of the mRNA precursor, destroying activity. However, a small portion of this mRNA may be spliced normally in some patients, with the result that the phenotypic presentation is variable. Most such patients are salt losers, but some have non–salt-losing CAH.

This intron 2 microconversion is often associated with the Ser/Thr polymorphism at codon 268. This is a true polymorphism because S268T does not alter enzymatic activity.[370] The microconversion R356W, which is found in about 10% of severely affected alleles,[371] eliminates all detectable activity[372], apparently because it changes a residue in the binding site for P450 oxidoreductase.[305] This mutation may retain slight activity and has been found in simple virilizing CAH. Other extremely rare mutations have been described in single individuals.[373-375]

Missense Mutations Causing Simple Virilizing and Nonclassic CAH. The microconversion I172N is the most common cause of simple virilizing CAH.[372,376,377] Ile 172 is conserved in the other known mammalian proteins and may contribute to the hydrophobic interactions needed to maintain the correct conformation of the enzyme. When Ile 172 was changed to Asn, Leu, Gln, or His and the constructed mutants were expressed in mammalian cells, the mutant constructions yielded only 3% to 7% of the 21-hydroxylase activity of normal P450c21.[372,378] The intron 2 microconversion is occasionally seen in simple virilizing CAH. The microconversion P30L is generally associated with nonclassic CAH but is found in some patients with simple virilizing CAH.

The most common mutation causing nonclassic CAH is V281L. This microconversion is seen in all patients with the form of nonclassic CAH linked to HLA-B14 and HLA-DR1 but is also found in patients with other HLA types. This mutation does not alter the affinity of the enzyme for substrate but drastically reduces its V_{max}.[379] The microconversion P30L is found in about 15% to 20% of nonclassic alleles. In addition, the mutations R339H and P453S have been associated with nonclassic CAH.[380,381] Initial surveys of the mutations in P450c21A failed to reveal these mutations, suggesting that they are bona fide point mutations rather than gene microconversions. However, examination of large numbers of P450c21A pseudogenes shows that at least the P453S mutation is polymorphic in about 20% of P450c21A pseudogenes, and hence also represents a microconversion event.

Structure-Function Inferences from P450c21 Mutations

Each P450c21 missense mutation appears to occur in a functional domain of P450c21. By analogy with the computationally inferred structure of the closely related enzyme P450c17,[305] Arg 356 may be part of the redox partner binding site. Val 281 appears to participate in coordinating the heme moiety, and Cys 428 is the crucial cystine residue in the heme-binding site found in all cytochrome P450 enzymes. The N-terminal region of P450c21, including Pro30, appears to be required for membrane insertion and enzyme stability.[382]

Finding most mutations in the amino terminal portion of P450c21 is consistent with finding most gene conversion and gene deletion events occurring in exons 1 through 8 of the P450c21B gene. Changes in exons 9 and 10 are very rare, possibly as a result of evolutionary pressure to retain the 3′ untranslated and 3′ flanking DNA of the P450c21B gene because this DNA also contains the 3′ end of the XB gene.[358,359]

Prenatal Diagnosis of CAH

The prenatal diagnosis of 21-hydroxylase deficiency has been approached by several tactics. First, the steroids produced by the disordered adrenal of the CAH fetus, 17OHP[383-385] and Δ⁴-androstenedione[386], can be measured in amniotic fluid, but these assays are reliable only for identifying fetuses with severe salt-losing CAH because these steroids may not be elevated above the broad range of normal in non–salt-losing or nonclassic CAH.[387,388] Second, the intimate HLA linkage of the

CYP21 genes means that HLA typing of fetal amniocytes can be informative.

This would require previous linkage analysis of an affected index case and parents. However, only HLA-A and HLA-B can be determined reliably in cultured amniocytes, some HLA-B alleles are expressed weakly in these cells, and there is a relatively high incidence of HLA-B homozygosity among CAH patients. These and other technical considerations have substantially limited the usefulness of HLA typing for prenatal diagnosis. Third, if the genetic lesion in a previously affected sibling is established, DNA-based diagnosis (including DNA sequencing) provides the most reliable tactic. However, the complex genetics of the 21-hydroxylase locus described previously can still render this approach problematic.

Diagnosis

Genital ambiguity or a salt-losing crisis will generally alert pediatricians to most cases of severe 21-hydroxylase deficiency. Salt-losing crises generally occur in the second week of life, and the child presents with vomiting, diarrhea, dehydration, hyperkalemia, and hyponatremia. Occasionally, such infants are thought to have viral syndromes or gastrointestinal obstructions. Such a failure to make the diagnosis can result in the infant's death. Similarly, boys with simple virilizing CAH often escape diagnosis until they are 3 to 7 years old, when they present with isosexual precocity, advanced bone age, and characteristically prepubertal testes. Teenage and adult females with nonclassic CAH may consult an internist, obstetrician, or dermatologist for virilism, hirsutism, menstrual irregularity, infertility, or acne.

The key diagnostic maneuver in all forms of 21-hydroxylase deficiency is the measurement of the 17OHP response to intravenous synthetic ACTH. The usual doses are 15 μg/kg in children up to 2 years of age and 0.25 mg in older children and adults. 17OHP and cortisol should be measured at 0 and 60 minutes. Individual patient responses must be compared to age- and sex-matched data from normal children.[230] Normal responses are outlined in Table 12-4 and shown in Figure 12-9. Both basal and stimulated levels of 17OHP are markedly elevated in patients with salt-losing and simple virilizing forms of 21-hydroxylase deficiency. Basal levels are usually greater than 2,000 ng/dL and increase to more than 5,000 to 10,000 ng/dL after ACTH (Figure 12-9).

Patients with the milder late-onset or cryptic forms typically have normal to mildly elevated basal levels but have supranormal responses to ACTH stimulation (i.e., 1,500 to >10,000 ng/dL).[232,389] The cortisol response to ACTH is absent or subnormal in patients with the classic forms of CAH and is normal in patients with late-onset and cryptic forms. Basal plasma ACTH levels reflect the extent of 21-hydroxylase and cortisol deficiency, i.e., they are markedly elevated in severe forms and may be normal in patients with the milder forms who are not overtly adrenal insufficient.

Other ancillary tests are listed in Table 12-5. Urinary excretion of 17-ketosteroids will generally be elevated, but this test is more useful for monitoring the efficacy of suppressive therapy than for initial diagnosis. When urinary steroids are measured, a complete 24-hour sample must be obtained, and a concomitant measurement of creatinine excretion is required to monitor the completeness of the collection. Less than 24-hour urine collections are not accurate because of diurnal variations in steroid excretion.

Plasma renin activity and its response to salt restriction constitute an especially useful test. Most patients with simple virilizing 21-hydroxylase deficiency have high plasma renin activity, which increases further on sodium restriction, confirming that these patients are partially mineralocorticoid deficient and can maintain normal serum sodium only by hyperstimulation of the zona glomerulosa.

Treatment

Although Wilkins[7] and Bartter[8] first demonstrated effective treatment of 21-hydroxylase deficiency with cortisone in 1950, the management of this disorder remains difficult. Overtreatment with glucocorticoids causes delayed growth even when the degree of overtreatment is insufficient to produce signs and symptoms of Cushing syndrome. Undertreatment results in continued overproduction of adrenal androgens, which hastens epiphyseal maturation and closure, again resulting in compromised growth and other manifestations of androgen excess.

Doses of glucocorticoids should be based on the expected normal cortisol secretory rate. Widely cited classic studies have reported that the secretory rate of cortisol is 12.5 ± 3 mg/m^2 per day[390-392] and have led most authorities to recommend doses of 10 to 20 mg of hydrocortisone (cortisol)/m^2 per day. However, the actual cortisol secretory rate is substantially lower, at 6 to 7 ± 2 mg/m^2/per day.[224,225] Although no single formula can be applied to all patients and extensive experience and judgment are needed, we consider the cortisol secretory rate to be about 6 to 8 mg/m^2 per day. It must be stressed, however, that newly diagnosed patients, especially newborns, will require substantially higher initial dosages to suppress their hyperactive CRH-ACTH-adrenal axis.

The glucocorticoid used is important. Most tables of glucocorticoid dose equivalencies are based on their equivalence in anti-inflammatory assays. However, the growth-suppressant equivalences of various glucocorticoids do not parallel their anti-inflammatory equivalencies.[393] Thus, long-acting synthetic steroids such as dexamethasone have a disproportionately greater growth-suppressant effect and hence must be avoided in treating growing children and adolescents (Table 12-7). Most authorities favor the use of oral hydrocortisone or cortisone acetate in three divided daily doses in growing children. However, adults and older teenagers whose epiphyses are already fused may be managed very effectively with prednisone or dexamethasone.

Mineralocorticoid therapy in these patients returns plasma volume to normal and eliminates the hypovolemic drive to ACTH secretion. Thus, mineralocorticoid therapy often permits the use of lower doses of glucocorticoids in patients with simple virilizing CAH, optimizing growth in children and diminishing unwanted weight gain in adults.

Only one oral mineralocorticoid preparation, fludrocortisone (9α-fluorocortisol), is generally available. When the oral route is not available in severely ill patients, mineralocorticoid replacement is achieved through intravenous hydrocortisone plus sodium chloride. About 20 mg of hydrocortisone has a mineralocorticoid effect of about 0.1 mg of 9α-fluorocortisol (Table 12-7). Mineralocorticoids are unique in pharmacology in that their doses are not based on body mass or surface area. In fact, newborns are quite insensitive to mineralocorticoids, as reflected by their high serum aldosterone concentrations (Figure 12-14), and often require larger doses than do adults (0.15 to 0.30 mg/day, depending on the sodium supplementation).

In older children, the replacement dose of 9α-fluorocortisol is 0.05 to 0.15 mg daily. It must be emphasized that a mineralocorticoid is essentially useless unless adequate sodium is presented to the renal tubules. Thus, additional salt supplementation, usually 1 to 2 g NaCl/day in the newborn, is also needed. Patients with severe salt-losing congenital adrenal

TABLE 12-7

Potency of Various Therapeutic Steroids (Set Relative to the Potency of Cortisol)

Steroid	Anti-inflammatory Glucocorticoid Effect	Growth-retarding Glucocorticoid Effect	Salt-retaining Mineralocorticoid Effect	Plasma Half-life (min)	Biological Half-life (hr)
Cortisol (hydrocortisone)	1.0	1.0	1.0	80-120	8
Cortisone acetate (oral)	0.8	0.8	0.8	80-120	8
Cortisone acetate (IM)	0.8	1.3	0.8		18
Prednisone	4	5	0.25	200	16-36
Prednisolone	4		0.25	120-300	16-36
Methyl prednisolone	5	7.5	0.4		
Betamethasone	25		0	130-330	
Triamcinolone	5		0		
Dexamethasone	30	80	0	150-300	36-54
9α-fluorocortisone	15		200		
DOC acetate	0		20		
Aldosterone	0.3		200-1,000		

hyperplasia can in some cases discontinue mineralocorticoid replacement and salt supplementation as adults. Perhaps adults become more sensitive to the mineralocorticoid action of hydrocortisone via a developmental decrease in renal 11βHSD activity, which normally inactivates cortisol to cortisone.

Long-term management is difficult to monitor and requires careful clinical and laboratory evaluation. Measurements of growth should be made at 3- to 4-month intervals in children, along with an annual assessment of bone age. Each visit should be accompanied by measurement of blood pressure, plasma renin activity, and serum Δ^4-androstenedione, DHEA, DHEA sulfate, and testosterone. Measurement of urinary 17-KS and plasma 3α-androstenediol glucuronide may also be useful. In general, plasma 17OHP is not a useful indicator of therapeutic efficacy because of its great diurnal variation and hyperresponsiveness to stress (e.g., clinic visits).

Experimental Prenatal Treatment of CAH

Because the treatment of CAH involves administering a glucocorticoid to suppress the hypothalamic-pituitary-adrenal axis, this approach has been proposed for treating the affected fetus by administering glucocorticoids to the mother. Female fetuses affected with CAH begin to become virilized at about 6 to 8 weeks gestation, the same time at which the testes of normal male fetuses produce testosterone, causing fusion of the labioscrotal folds, enlargement of the genital tubercle into a phallus, and the formation of the phallic urethra.[310] The adrenals of female fetuses with CAH may produce concentrations of testosterone that approach those of a normal male, resulting in varying degrees of masculinization of the external genitalia. If fetal adrenal steroidogenesis is suppressed in a female fetus with CAH, the virilization can theoretically be reduced or eliminated. Thus, some authorities have advocated administering dexamethasone to the mother as soon as pregnancy is diagnosed.[394-398]

This can be done only when the parents are known to be heterozygotes by having already had an affected child. However, even in such pregnancies, only one in four fetuses will have CAH. Furthermore, as no prenatal treatment is needed for male fetuses affected with CAH only one in eight pregnancies of heterozygous parents would harbor an affected female fetus that might potentially benefit from prenatal treatment. However, treatment must be started at about 6 weeks postconception (8 weeks of amenorrhea), but prenatal diagnosis cannot be done until 12 to 13 weeks and at least a week is required for the assays. Thus, seven of eight pregnancies must be treated needlessly to treat one affected female fetus.

The efficacy, safety, and desirability of such prenatal treatment remain highly controversial.[79,150,385,397-410] The rationale is that dexamethasone, which is not metabolized by placental 11βHSD2, will cross the placenta, suppress fetal ACTH, and consequently suppress adrenal steroidogenesis. However, it is not known precisely when the fetal hypothalamus begins to produce CRH, when the fetal pituitary begins to produce ACTH, whether all fetal ACTH production is regulated by CRH, or whether these hormones are suppressible by dexamethasone in the early fetus.

Although there is considerable evidence that pharmacologic doses of glucocorticoids do not harm pregnant women, few data exist for the fetus. Pregnant women with diseases such as nephrotic syndrome and systemic lupus erythematosus are generally treated with prednisone, which does not reach the fetus because it is inactivated by placental 11βHSD. Treatment of a fetus with CAH requires the use of fluorinated steroids that escape metabolism by these enzymes, and few data are available about the long-term use of such agents throughout gestation. The available preliminary studies also indicate that the response of the fetal genital anatomy to treatment is generally good if the treatment is started very early, before week 6. Thereafter, the virilization is reduced. However, it may not be eliminated, and thus at least one reconstructive surgical procedure may still be needed in the infant.[150,384,397,398,405,411]

Successful treatment requires dexamethasone doses of 20 μg/kg of maternal body weight. For a 70-kg woman, this is 1.4 mg, which is equivalent to that in the low-dose dexamethasone suppression test and is at least three times physiologic replacement. However, the fetus normally develops in the presence of very low cortisol concentrations of only about 20 to 60 nmol/L (0.7 to 2.0 μg/dL)[266,412], which is only about 10% of the corresponding maternal level. Thus, the doses used in prenatal treatment appear to achieve effective concentrations of active glucocorticoid that may be up to 60 times physiologic for the fetus. Treatment of pregnant rats with 20 μg/kg dexamethasone predisposes the fetuses to hypertension in adulthood,[413] and some studies indicate that even moderately elevated concentrations of glucocorticoids can be neurotoxic.[414-417]

The potential benefits of prenatal treatment are reduction or elimination of the genital virilization, reducing the risk of gender confusion and the need for surgery. The advocates of prenatal treatment report modest Cushingoid features in the mother and no untoward effects in the offspring, including the seven of eight fetuses in whom the treatment is stopped once the diagnosis is made.[397,409,418] However, there are concerns based on studies using comparable doses of dexamethasone showing reduced weight and growth and adult hypertension in rats.[419,420] Furthermore, short-term high-dose glucocorticoids cause hippocampal damage in monkeys[421] and in newborn children.[408,422]

However, a recent study of 26 dexamethasone-exposed children aged 8 to 17 years and a matched control group showed that the short-term treated children without CAH had poorer working memory and poorer self-perception of scholastic competence (both at p = 0.003) and increased self-rated social anxiety (p = 0.026).[410] If confirmed, such negative outcomes in unaffected children treated needlessly would indicate that prenatal treatment with dexamethasone should not be pursued and obviate the suggestion that dosing can be reduced in the second half of pregnancy. Alternative approaches, such as preimplantation genetic diagnosis,[423] should be considered, although this also carries some risk.

Experimental Postnatal Treatment of CAH

Children with CAH tend to be short. A meta-analysis of 18 studies of growth in CAH showed final height about 1.4 standard deviations below target height. Most notably, every one of these studies showed a height loss of at least 0.8 standard deviations.[424] Adequacy of salt supplementation appears to have an underappreciated influence on growth.[425] The loss of height in CAH is partially due to the effect of sex steroids on epiphyseal closure and partially due to glucocorticoid-induced resistance to the action of GH. Consequently, multiple studies have addressed optimizing the final height of children with CAH.

Antiandrogens and Aromatase Inhibitors. Antiandrogens and aromatose inhibitors have been tried in the presence of lower doses of glucocorticoids.[426] This approach derives from its successful use in slowing the rapid advancement of bone age found in gonadotropin-independent male sexual precocity (familial testotoxicosis).[427] Estrogen, not androgen, is the key hormone in promoting epiphyseal fusion.[125] Hence, inhibiting the conversion of androgen to estrogen with testolactone promotes growth, whereas antiandrogen treatment ameliorates virilization.

The principal benefit of this approach is that it permits the use of physiologic replacement doses of glucocorticoids (8 mg/m^2/day of hydrocortisone, rather than the traditional supraphysiologic dose of 12 to 15 mg/m^2/day), thus further promoting normal growth. Two-year follow-up data show normal growth and bone maturation,[428] but final heights have not been reported. The drugs are also expensive and not approved for this use, and the child needs to take a very large number of pills, making compliance an issue. Nevertheless, this approach appears to hold great promise, especially if improved aromatase inhibitors and antiandrogens are developed.

Adrenalectomy. Adrenalectomy has been proposed in severe CAH. Because the adrenal carrying severe P450c21 mutations (e.g., gene deletions) cannot produce aldosterone or cortisol, it has been argued that these affected glands do more harm than good and should be removed.[429] The advent of laparoscopic adrenalectomy has made this suggestion feasible without undue trauma to the patient. Among 18 adrenalectomized patients, 5 had adrenal crises when therapy was suboptimal and 2 became hypoglycemic during intercurrent illnesses.[430]

These risks are similar to those faced by children with CAH who do not receive stress-dose steroids. The concern that adrenalectomy will predispose to hypoglycemia because of the removal of adrenal medullary tissue has not been borne out. It should be noted that children with CAH are typically deficient in epinephrine.[309] Thus, although adrenalectomy is an extreme measure it may be appropriate in selected cases.[430]

Growth Hormone and GnRH Agonist Therapy. GH and GnRH agonist therapy have been proposed in children near the age of puberty.[431] Pharmacologic GH therapy may partially overcome the effects of higher doses of glucocorticoids, and GnRH agonist will delay the progression of puberty, permitting more time to grow. Preliminary results with a small group of 14 children experimentally treated with both agents for about 4 years showed an improvement in final height of 0.8 standard deviations compared to historic controls.[432] Both agents are expensive, and further studies are needed to assess the safety and efficacy of this approach.

P450 OXIDOREDUCTASE DEFICIENCY

P450 oxidoreductase (POR) deficiency is a newly recognized form of CAH.[433-438] POR is the protein that transfers electrons from NADPH to all 50 microsomal forms of cytochrome P450, including P450c17, P450c21, and P450aro, and to the drug-metabolizing P450 enzymes of the liver. Because POR participates in so many functions, its mutation might be expected to yield a very severe phenotype. POR-deficient mice die during fetal development.[439,440] However, beginning in 1985 several patients were described with apparent combined deficiencies of P450c17 and P450c21[441-445] and it was suggested that a mutation in POR was responsible,[446] but this was not proven until 2004.[433]

A wide array of POR mutations has now been described, affecting various P450 enzymes to differing degrees, apparently explaining the great variability in the clinical and hormonal findings in POR deficiency.[437] The serum and urinary steroids indicate defects in P450c17 and P450c21, and clinical findings vary from severely affected infants with ambiguous genitalia, cortisol deficiency, and the Antley-Bixler skeletal malformation syndrome (ABS) to mildly affected women who appear to have a form of polycystic ovary syndrome or mildly affected men with gonadal insufficiency. ABS is characterized by craniosynostosis, brachycephaly, radioulnar or radiohumeral synostosis, bowed femora, arachnodactyly, midface hypoplasia, proptosis, and choanal stenosis.

When ABS is seen in association with abnormal steroids and ambiguous genitalia in either sex, the cause is an autosomal-recessive mutation in POR.[433,435-437] By contrast, when ABS is seen without a lesion in steroidogenesis or genital development the cause is an autosomal-dominant gain-of-function mutation in fibroblast growth factor receptor 2.[437,438] Thus, the term *Antley-Bixler syndrome* should be reserved for the phenotypic description of the skeletal malformations and should not be equated with POR deficiency, which may or may not be associated with ABS.[433,434,437,438]

Patients with POR deficiency will typically have normal electrolytes and mineralocorticoid function, nearly-normal levels of cortisol that respond poorly to stimulation with ACTH, high concentrations of 17OHP that respond variably to ACTH, and low levels of C19 precursors to sex steroids. A remarkable feature of POR deficiency is that there is genital ambiguity in both sexes. Females may be virilized, and males may be underdeveloped, although there is considerable variation among individuals. As the 17,20 lyase activity of P450c17 is especially sensitive to perturbations in electron transport,[28,301,302] defects in fetal testicular steroidogenesis leading to incompletely developed external genitalia in 46,XY males is the predicted outcome.

By contrast, the partial virilization seen in 46,XX genetic females appears to be due to two causes. First, placental aromatase (P450aro) requires POR. Some mothers of infants with POR deficiency experience virilization during pregnancy[433,437,438] similar to that experienced by women carrying a fetus with P450aro deficiency.[125,127] The fetus normally disposes of large amounts of adrenal C19 steroids by excreting them through the placenta, which aromatizes them to the maternal estrogens of pregnancy.[145] A defect in this placental aromatase activity, from mutation of POR or P450aro itself, will permit large amounts of fetal C19 steroids to enter and virilize the mother. This is evidenced by the low estriol values seen in women carrying a fetus with POR deficiency.[447,448]

Second, an alternative "backdoor" pathway of androgen biosynthesis has been described in fetal marsupials in which 17OHP is eventually converted to dihydrotestosterone without utilizing androstenedione and testosterone as intermediates.[449,450] Analysis of urinary steroids from patients with POR deficiency suggests that this pathway also applies to the human fetus.[141,435,438,447,448] The relative importance of these two distinct mechanisms for virilizing the fetus with POR deficiency remains unresolved.

The incidence of POR deficiency is unknown. Because the disorder is newly described, it may seem rare. However, the rapid description of large numbers of patients[437,438] and the potentially very subtle clinical manifestations in individuals carrying mutations with partial activity suggest that POR deficiency may be fairly common. Two mutations are especially common: A287P, the predominant mutation in patients of European ancestry, and R457H, the predominant mutation in patients of Japanese ancestry. Because few patients have been studied in the newborn period, it has not been established whether newborn screening of 17OHP designed to detect 21-hydroxylase deficiency will also detect POR deficiency.

The mechanism linking defective POR activity to the ABS skeletal phenotype remains unclear, although this may be related to the POR-associated defect in cholesterol synthesis. Whereas mice harboring POR defects confined to the liver metabolize drugs poorly and accumulate hepatic lipids,[451,452] similar problems have not yet been described in patients with POR deficiency, although it has been suggested that the presence of POR deficiency in a fetus may render maternally ingested fluconazole teratogenic.[438] Thus, much remains to be learned about POR deficiency.

LESIONS IN ISOZYMES OF P450c11

11β-Hydroxylase Deficiency

There are two distinct forms of 11-hydroxylase. P450c11β mediates the 11β-hydroxylation of 11-deoxycortisol to cortisol and that of DOC to corticosterone in the zonae fasciculata and glomerulosa. P450c11AS (aldosterone synthase) is found only in the zona glomerulosa and mediates 11β-hydroxylation, 18-hydroxylation, and 18-oxidation; thus, it is the sole enzyme required to convert DOC to aldosterone. P450c11β is found in the glomerulosa and fasciculata, and mediates 11β-hydroxylation and some 18-hydroxylation but has no 18-methyl oxidase activity.

Deficient P450c11β activity is a rare cause of CAH in persons of European ancestry but accounts for about 15% of cases in Muslim and Jewish Middle Eastern populations.[453]

Severe deficiency of P450c11β decreases the secretion of cortisol, causing CAH and virilization of affected females. The defect in the pathway to cortisol results in accumulation of 11-deoxycortisol, and the defect in the 17-deoxy pathway in the synthesis of corticosterone in the fasciculata may lead to overproduction of DOC. Because DOC is a mineralocorticoid, these patients can retain sodium. Although DOC is less potent than aldosterone, it is secreted at high levels in 11β-hydroxylase deficiency. Thus, salt is retained and serum sodium remains normal.

Overproduction of DOC frequently leads to hypertension. As a result, 11β-hydroxylase deficiency is often termed the *hypertensive form of CAH* when detected in older children. However, newborns often manifest mild transient salt loss,[453,454] presumably as a result of the normal newborn resistance to mineralocorticoids (Figure 12-15). This may lead to incorrect diagnosis and treatment. Thus, there may be a poor correlation among DOC concentrations, serum potassium, and blood pressure or between the degree of virilization in affected females and the electrolyte and cardiovascular manifestations.[455]

Newborns may also have elevated concentrations of 17OHP, presumably as a "backup" phenomenon of high concentrations of 11-deoxycortisol inhibiting P450c21. Thus, P450c11β deficiency may be detected in newborn screening for P450c21 deficiency.[324] The diagnosis is established by demonstrating elevated basal concentrations of DOC and 11-deoxycortisol, which hyperrespond to ACTH. A normal or suppressed plasma renin activity is also a hallmark of this disease.[456]

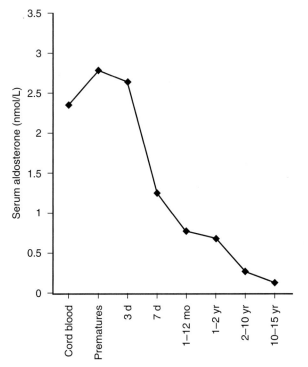

Figure 12-15. Concentrations of aldosterone as a function of age.

The genetic lesions causing 11β-hydroxylase deficiency are in the CYP11B1 gene that encodes P450c11β. In a study of Sephardic Jews of Moroccan ancestry, 11 of 12 affected alleles bore the mutation R448H.[96] However, several other mutations have been described in other populations.[90] A milder nonclassic form of 11β-hydroxylase deficiency analogous to nonclassic 21-hydroxylase deficiency has been reported in otherwise asymptomatic women with hirsutism, virilism, and menstrual irregularities.[453,457]

However, true nonclassic 11β-hydroxylase deficiency is rare. Only two of five hyperandrogenemic women who had 11-deoxycortisol values more than three times higher than the 95th percentile in response to stimulation with ACTH had mutations of P450c11β, all of whom retained 15% to 37% of normal activity.[458] Repeated ACTH testing in two of the three women who lacked mutations showed much lower (but still elevated) 11-deoxycortisol values. Thus, just as in the case of nonclassic 3βHSD deficiency an abnormal steroid response to ACTH is not sufficient to diagnose a genetic lesion.

Corticosterone Methyl Oxidase Deficiencies

P450c11AS, the isozyme of P450c11β that is 93% identical in its amino acid sequence, is expressed exclusively in the zona glomerulosa, where it catalyzes 11β-hydroxylase, 18-hydroxylase, and 18 methyl oxidase activities. P450c11AS and P450c11β are expressed in the human zona glomerulosa, and both can convert DOC to corticosterone. However, the conversion of corticosterone to 18OH-corticosterone and subsequently to aldosterone is exclusively performed by P450c11AS. Disorders of P450c11AS cause the so-called corticosterone methyl oxidase (CMO) deficiencies, wherein aldosterone biosynthesis is impaired but the zona fasciculata and reticularis continue to produce corticosterone and DOC.

The absence of aldosterone biosynthesis will generally result in a salt-wasting crisis in infancy, at which time the normal secretory rate of DOC is insufficient to meet the newborn's mineralocorticoid requirements similarly to the newborn with P450c11β deficiency. Thus, these infants typically present with hyponatremia, hyperkalemia, and metabolic acidosis. However, the salt-wasting syndrome is typically less severe than in patients with 21-hydroxylase deficiency or lipoid CAH because of the persistent secretion of DOC. These patients may recover spontaneously and grow to adulthood without therapy. This probably reflects the increasing sensitivity to mineralocorticoid action with advancing age in childhood, as reflected by the usual age-related decrease in serum aldosterone (Figure 12-15). Consistent with this, plasma renin activity is markedly elevated in affected children but may be normal in affected adults.[459]

CMOI deficiency results from a complete loss of P450c11AS activity, and thus no 18-hydroxylase or 18 methyl oxidase activity persists, eliminating the biosynthesis of 18OH-corticosterone and aldosterone while preserving the biosynthesis of corticosterone by P450c11β. Thus, the diagnosis for CMOI deficiency is usually based on an increased ratio of corticosterone to 18OH corticosterone.[98] Only three cases of CMOI deficiency have been fully characterized genetically, including a frame-

shift mutation,[460] a premature stop codon,[461] and the missense mutation R384P.[462]

CMOII deficiency results from amino acid replacement mutations in P450c11AS that selectively delete the 18 methyl oxidase activity while preserving the 18-hydroxylase activity. The diagnosis of CMOII deficiency requires an increased 18OH corticosterone and very low aldosterone concentration. CMOII deficiency is common in Sephardic Jews of Iranian origin, where all affected individuals appear to be homozygous for two different mutations, R181W and V385A.[97] Family members who were homozygous for only one of these mutations were clinically unaffected; both mutations are required to cause disease.

The distinction between CMOI and CMOII is not always clear. One patient with the clinical history and hormonal phenotype of CMOII had two mutations on each parental allele.[99] The mother's allele carried R181W and a deletion/frame-shift mutation that deleted all activity; the father's allele carried T318M and V386A. Thr318 is predicted to be the universally conserved Thr residue in all P450 enzymes that participates in cleavage of the dioxygen bond of O_2 to create the iron-oxy intermediate required for P450 catalysis. When the T318M/V386A double mutant was recreated in vitro, there was no detectable activity.[99] These data would have predicted the CMOI phenotype instead of the patient's CMOII phenotype. Similarly, another patient was homozygous for the missense mutations E198A and V386A. When recreated in vitro, the double mutant enzyme behaved similarly to the mutant enzyme found in the Iranian Jewish CMOII patients. However, the patient's clinical phenotype was CMOI.[463] This patient also carried R173K, but that is a normally occurring polymorphism that has no effect on the enzyme's K_m or V_{max}.[464] Thus, the distinction between CMOI and CMOII is not precise, and these disorders should be regarded as different degrees of severity on a continuous clinical spectrum, just as the various forms of 21-hydroxylase deficiency are part of a broad clinical spectrum.

Although rats have four CYP11B genes encoding three P450c11 enzymes, it is clear that there are only two CYP11B genes in the human genome, encoding P450c11β and P450c11AS.[465] This genetic anatomy is reminiscent of the P450c21A and P450c21B genes. Although gene conversion can cause CMO II deficiency,[466] gene conversion appears to be much rarer than in the P450c21 locus. This may be due to the higher recombinational frequency in the HLA region carrying the P450c21 genes, or it may be related to the abundant antisense transcripts produced in the P450c21 locus.[333,467]

Glucocorticoid-Suppressible Hyperaldosteronism

Although gene conversions events in the P450c11 locus are rare, an unusual gene duplication causes glucocorticoid-suppressible hyperaldosteronism.[468-470] This homologous recombination event creates a third CYP11B gene that fuses the 5 flanking DNA of the CYP11B1 gene for P450c11β onto the CYP11B2 gene for P450c11AS. In two such patients, the genetic crossover occurred in intron 2, and in two other patients it occurred in intron 3 or exon

4.[469] All of these hybrid genes produce a hybrid P450c11 that retains aldosterone synthase activity. However, as the hybrid gene has P450c11β regulatory regions its transcription is induced by ACTH and cAMP, as is the normal gene for P450c11β. Thus, these patients make P450c11AS in response to physiology that should stimulate P450c11β. The excess P450c11AS causes hyperaldosteronism and hypertension. This is then suppressible by glucocorticoid suppression of ACTH, which normally suppresses P450c11β.

It is conceivable that localized microconversions, similar to those that cause most cases of 21-hydroxylase deficiency, could insert sequences crucial for aldosterone synthase activity into the gene encoding P450c11β. Expression of chimeric proteins produced in vitro identified the residues Ser288 and Val320 as important to this activity.[471] Similarly, activating mutations that increase the aldosterone synthase activity of P450c11AS have been created in vitro.[472] However, examination of large numbers of patients with low-renin hypertension has failed to show mutations in this gene system other than the gene conversions described previously that cause glucocorticoid-suppressible hypertension.[464,473,474]

LESIONS IN ISOZYMES OF 11β-HYDROXYSTEROID DEHYDROGENASE

Cortisone and prednisone are inactive pro-hormones that must be reduced to cortisol or prednisolone in order to bind to and activate the glucocorticoid receptor. The interconversion of these keto- and hydroxysteroids is catalyzed by the two isozymes of 11β-hydroxysteroid dehydrogenase, 11βHSD1 and 11βHSD2. Both enzymes are reversible in vitro, and hence both can act as an oxidase or reductase, depending on the availability of cofactors. However, under physiologic situations 11βHSD1 generally acts to activate cortisone to cortisol and 11βHSD2 reverses this activation.[23,475]

Thus, 11βHSD1 is primarily expressed in liver and fat[476] and 11βHSD2 is expressed in mineralocorticoid-responsive tissues, where it inactivates cortisol, permitting low concentrations of aldosterone to activate mineralocorticoid receptors, which also bind cortisol. 11βHSD2 is inactive against aldosterone, DOC, and fludrocortisol. Interest in these enzymes extends far beyond their deficiency states, as they play central roles in metabolism.[476,477]

Lesions in 11βHSD1—Apparent Cortisone Reductase Deficiency

Defects in 11βHSD1 impair cortisol feedback at the hypothalamic/pituitary axis, increasing the secretion of ACTH and consequently increasing adrenal C19 steroid secretion, resulting in hyperandrogenism, sexual precocity, and polycystic ovaries. Only about 10 such patients have been described.[475] A similar clinical picture is seen in disorders of hexose-6-phosphate dehydrogenase (H6PDH), which generates the NADPH used by 11βHSD1 in the lumen of the endoplasmic reticulum.[139,478] Both disorders are diagnosed from urinary steroids, which show a marked reduction in ratio of metabolites of cortisol to those of cortisone. Variations in 11βHSD1 appear

to make a relatively minor contribution to the common forms of polycystic ovary syndrome.[479-481]

Lesions in 11βHSD2—Apparent Mineralocorticoid Excess

Patients with apparent mineralocorticoid excess (AME) have hypervolemic hypertension, salt retention, and hypokalemic alkalosis—the classic picture of hyperaldosteronism, but with suppressed plasma renin activity and without measurable serum mineralocorticoids due to recessive mutations of 11βHSD2.[132] About 30 different mutations in 11βHSD2 have been described in about 60 patients with AME.[482,483] Preliminary evidence suggests that heterozygous carriers may have an increased risk of hypertension.[484]

Typical features of children with AME include failure to thrive, delayed puberty, polydipsia, polyuria, muscle weakness, and hypertension. The hypertension is severe, often causing end-organ damage at an early age. Diagnosis is made from the high ratio of urinary metabolites of cortisol to cortisone. Treatment includes antagonism of the mineralocorticoid receptor with spironolactone, correction of the hypokalemia, low-salt diets, and diuretics. Treatment is only partially successful, and 10% of patients die from cerebrovascular accidents.[485]

Adrenal Insufficiency

Many conditions will cause adrenal insufficiency, including CAH, hypopituitarism with ACTH deficiency, and primary adrenal disorders. Primary adrenal insufficiency is commonly termed *Addison disease,* but this is a vague term that encompasses many disorders. Up to World War II, most patients with "Addison disease" had tuberculosis of the adrenal, but more than 80% of contemporary adult patients have autoimmune adrenalitis. Therefore, the term *Addison disease* is now widely used to indicate an autoimmune or idiopathic cause.[486]

The spectrum of adrenal disorders presenting in infants, children, and adolescents differs from that presenting in adulthood (Table 12-8). CAH and autoimmune adrenal disease represent the largest proportions of cases, but some of the inherited developmental and metabolic causes of adrenal failure are also fairly common.[486,487] Diagnosing some of these disorders is important to assessing potential associated features, initiating long-term management, and instituting genetic counseling.[488] Adrenal disorders are typically divided into chronic and acute causes, but many acute presentations reflect an undiagnosed underlying chronic or developmental process (Table 12-9). Acute presentations may be triggered by intercurrent illness, trauma, or surgery, with poor fluid and sodium intake.

ACUTE PRIMARY ADRENAL INSUFFICIENCY

Acute adrenal crisis occurs most commonly in the child with undiagnosed chronic adrenal insufficiency who is subjected to an additional severe stress such as major illness, trauma, or surgery. The major presenting symptoms and signs include abdominal pain, fever, hypoglycemia

TABLE 12-8

Causes of Adrenal Insufficiency

Primary Adrenal Insufficiency
- Congenital adrenal hyperplasia
- Autoimmune disorders
  - Autoimmune adrenalitis
  - Autoimmune polyglandular syndromes
- Adrenal hypoplasia congenita
  - X-linked adrenal hypoplasia
  - Other (SF1, IMAGe syndrome)
- ACTH resistance syndromes
  - Familial glucocorticoid deficiencies, types 1 and 2
  - Triple A (Allgrove) syndrome
- Metabolic disorders
  - Adrenoleukodystrophy
  - Peroxisome biogenesis disorders (e.g., Zellweger)
  - Cholesterol metabolism (Smith-Lemli-Opitz, Wolman)
  - Mitochondrial (Kearn-Sayres, mitochondrial deletions)
- Infectious disorders
  - Sepsis
  - Tuberculosis
  - Fungal infections
  - Viral
- Infiltrative/destructive causes
  - Hemorrhage
  - Amyloidosis, sarcoidosis, metastases
- Drugs inhibiting steroid biosynthesis

Secondary Adrenal Insufficiency
- Hypothalamic tumors, radiation or surgery
- Hypopituitarism
- Isolated ACTH insufficiency
- Defects in POMC synthesis and processing
- Withdrawl from glucocorticoid therapy

TABLE 12-9

Signs and Symptoms of Adrenal Insufficiency

Features Shared by Acute and Chronic Insufficiency
- Anorexia
- Apathy and confusion
- Dehydration
- Fatigue
- Hyperkalemia
- Hypoglycemia
- Hyponatremia
- Hypovolemia and tachycardia
- Nausea and vomiting
- Postural hypotension
- Prolonged neonatal jaundice
- Salt craving
- Weakness

Features of Acute Insufficiency (Adrenal Crisis)
- Abdominal pain
- Fever

Features of Chronic Insufficiency (Addison Disease)
- Decreased pubic and axillary hair
- Diarrhea
- Hyperpigmentation
- Low-voltage electrocardiogram
- Small heart on x-ray
- Weight loss

CHRONIC PRIMARY ADRENAL INSUFFICIENCY

Autoimmune Disorders

Autoimmune adrenalitis is most commonly seen in adults 25 to 45 years old, about 60% to 70% of whom are women. The prevalence in adults is about 1 in 25,000.[492] Autoimmune destruction of other endocrine tissues is frequently associated with autoimmune adrenalitis. Chronic adrenal insufficiency is suggested by poor weight gain or weight loss, weakness, fatigue, anorexia, hypotension, hyponatremia, hypochloremia, hyperkalemia, frequent illnesses, nausea, and vague gastrointestinal complaints (Table 12-9), reflecting chronic deficiency of glucocorticoids and mineralocorticoids.

Early in the course of autoimmune adrenalitis, one may see signs of glucocorticoid deficiency (weakness, fatigue, weight loss, hypoglycemia, anorexia) without signs of mineralocorticoid deficiency (hyponatremia, hyperkalemia, acidosis, tachycardia, hypotension, low voltage on EKG, small heart on chest x-ray) or evidence of mineralocorticoid deficiency without glucocorticoid deficiency. Thus, an initial clinical presentation that spares one category of adrenal steroids does not mean it will be spared in the long run. The symptoms listed in Table 12-9 can be seen in primary or secondary chronic adrenal insufficiency. In primary chronic adrenal insufficiency, the low concentrations of plasma cortisol stimulate the hypersecretion of ACTH and other POMC peptides, including the various forms of melanocyte-stimulating hormone (MSH). Consequently, chronic primary adrenal insufficiency is

with seizures, weakness, apathy, nausea, vomiting, anorexia, hyponatremia, hypochloremia, acidemia, hyperkalemia, hypotension, shock, cardiovascular collapse, and death. Treatment consists of fluid and electrolyte resuscitation, ample doses of glucocorticoids, chronic glucocorticoid and mineralocorticoid replacement, and treatment of the precipitating illness.

Massive adrenal hemorrhage with shock due to blood loss can occur in large infants who have had a traumatic delivery.[489] A flank mass is usually palpable and can be distinguished from renal vein thrombosis by microscopic rather than gross hematuria. The diagnosis is then confirmed by CT or ultrasonography.[490] Massive adrenal hemorrhage is more commonly associated with meningococcemia (Waterhouse-Friderichsen syndrome). Meningitis is often present. The characteristic petechial rash of meningococcemia can progress rapidly to large ecchymoses. The blood pressure drops and respirations become labored, frequently leading rapidly to coma and death. Immediate intervention with intravenous fluids, antibiotics, and glucocorticoids is not always successful. A similar adrenal crisis may also occur rarely with septicemia from *Streptococcus, Pneumococcus, Pseudomonas,* diphtheria, and methicillin-sensitive and -resistant isolates of *Staphylococcus aureus.*[491] Adrenal hemorrhage has also been reported with the antiphospholipid syndrome and in patients on anticoagulant therapy.

also characterized by hyperpigmentation of the skin and mucous membranes, whereas secondary adrenal insufficiency is not.

Such hyperpigmentation is most prominent in skin exposed to sun and in flexor surfaces such as knees, elbows, and knuckles. The diagnosis is suggested by the previosly cited signs and symptoms, verified by a low morning cortisol level with a high ACTH and confirmed by a minimal response of cortisol to a 60-minute intravenous ACTH test. Hyponatremia, hyperkalemia, low aldosterone, and elevated PRA suggest a disturbance in mineralocorticoid production. Associated findings may include the appearance of a small heart on chest x-ray, anemia, azotemia, eosinophilia, lymphocytosis, and hypoglycemia. Treatment of chronic primary adrenal insufficiency consists of physiologic glucocorticoid and mineralocorticoid replacement therapy.

Autoimmune adrenalitis is strongly associated with specific HLA haplotypes and with polymorphisms in the gene for cytotoxic T-lymphocyte-associated antigen 4 (CLTA 4), which may be broadly involved in susceptibility to autoimmune disease.[493-495] The diagnosis of autoimmune chronic adrenal insufficiency is based largely on finding circulating antibodies directed against adrenal cells or adrenal cellular content. In many cases, the adrenal antigens are steroidogenic cytochrome P450 enzymes, especially P450scc, P450c17, and P450c21.[492,496,497]

It is not clear how these enzymes reach immune cells to elicit an antibody response, but autopsy studies show infiltration of the adrenal cortex.[486] Thus, it is likely that cell-mediated immunity is responsible for destruction of adrenocortical cells, resulting in a secondary discharge of cellular content including P450 enzymes into the circulation, with subsequent development of secondary "marker" antibodies against these P450s. About half of adult patients with lymphocytic adrenalitis will also have autoimmune disease of another endocrine tissue with high titers of antibodies directed against specific content of the affected tissue. This finding has led to the definition of specific autoimmune polyendocrine syndromes (APS), some of which are more prevalent in childhood.

Type 1 Autoimmune Polyendocrine Syndrome. Type 1 autoimmune polyendocrine syndrome (APS1), also known as autoimmune polyendocrinopathy-candidiasis-ectodermal dysplasia (APECED), is characterized by chronic mucocutaneous candidiasis, autoimmune Addison disease, and hypoparathyroidism.[492,498] At least two of these features must be present to make the diagnosis, and their age of onset can be highly variable. In general, chronic mucocutaneous candidiasis appears in early childhood and affects the mouth and nails. Acquired hypoparathyroidism can present with clinical hypocalcemia during mid or late childhood, although in some cases hypocalcemia may be masked by untreated adrenal insufficiency. The adrenal disorder usually presents in childhood or adolescence. Autoimmune adrenal disease may be a presenting feature in about 5% of cases.[498]

Additional autoimmune features of this condition include alopecia and vitiligo; gastritis, chronic diarrhea, and malabsorption with or without pernicious anemia; hypergonadotropic hypogonadism, especially in women; and less commonly hepatitis, thyroiditis, interstitial nephritis,

myositis, dental enamel hypoplasia, acquired asplenia, and type 1 diabetes mellitus. Keratoconjunctivitis is an important associated feature that requires careful monitoring and treatment to prevent blindness. Oral or esophageal squamous cell carcinoma occurs in 10% of individuals as adults.[498] APS1 is rare in most populations, but is common among people of Finnish (1:15,000), Sardinian, and Iranian Jewish (1:9,000) ancestry.[486]

APS1 is caused by recessively inherited mutations in a 58-kDa transcription factor called AIRE for autoimmune regulator.[499,500] More than 50 different mutations in this gene have been described, although the homozygous or compound heterozygous R257X change is especially common in the Finnish population. The AIRE gene is widely expressed in developing tissues of the immune system. The specific mechanisms by which these mutations result in the pleotropic findings of APS1 are not yet clear, although deletion of AIRE in mice results in ectopic expression of peripheral tissue antigens in thymic medullary epithelial cells, resulting in the development of an autoimmune disorder similar to APS1/APECED.[501,502]

Type 2 Autoimmune Polyendocrine Syndrome. Type 2 autoimmune polyendocrine syndrome (APS2), also known as Schmidt's syndrome, refers to the relatively common association of autoimmune adrenalitis with thyroiditis and/or type 1 diabetes.[492] APS2 is more common in females (3:1 ratio), is HLA linked, and is generally seen in young or middle-aged adults. However, it can present at almost any age. Primary (hypergonadotropic) ovarian failure is seen in up to one-quarter of postpubertal females with APS2, but primary testicular failure is rare.[486] Pernicious anemia, hepatitis, vitiligo, and alopecia may also be seen, but the hypoparathyroidism and mucocutaneous candidiasis typical of APS1 are not seen in APS2. APS2 is associated with the same HLA markers as idiopathic autoimmune adrenalitis, which may simply be a form of APS2.

Adrenal Hypoplasia Congenita

Adrenal hypoplasia congenita, also known as congenital adrenal hypoplasia, is a disorder of adrenal development resulting in primary adrenal insufficiency. This condition can occur with several different inheritance patterns, and with a variety of associated or syndromic features.

X-Linked Adrenal Hypoplasia Congenital. Adrenal hypoplasia congenital (AHC) is caused by mutations of the DAX1 (NR0B1) gene on chromosome Xp21. It is the most prevalent form of primary adrenal hypoplasia, with more than 200 individuals or families identified to date.[503,504] In AHC, the definitive zone of the fetal adrenal does not develop, and the fetal zone is vacuolated and cytomegalic. About half of boys with AHC present with salt loss and glucocorticoid insufficiency in early infancy. The rest present more insidiously with chronic adrenal insufficiency throughout childhood.[487] Hypogonadotropic hypogonadism or arrested puberty is an associated feature, although early puberty with subsequent pubertal arrest has been reported in rare cases. An underlying defect in spermatogenesis may also be present.

DAX1 encodes a nuclear transcription factor involved in adrenal and testicular development, as well as being expressed in the pituitary gonadotropes. About two-thirds of boys with AHC have DAX1 point mutations.[487,504] The other third have DAX1 gene deletions either in isolation or as part of a contiguous gene deletion syndrome involving a telomeric X-linked mental retardation locus (IL1RAPL1) and/or centromeric loci for glycerol kinase deficiency (GKD), and sometimes ornithine transcarbamylase (OTC) and Duchenne muscular dystrophy (DMD). An adult-onset form of AHC due to point mutations in DAX1 has also been described in several patients.[505]

Boys with AHC respond well to glucocorticoid and mineralocorticoid replacement therapy; sexual maturation with testosterone is required in adolescence. Spontaneous fertility is rare, and attempts to induce spermatogenesis with gonadotropins are rarely successful. Alternative forms of fertility treatment such as intracytoplasmic sperm injection have not been reported. Female carriers of DAX1 mutations or deletions are unaffected, but half of their sons will be affected. Close monitoring and genetic counseling can help prevent life-threatening adrenal crises in other family members or future pregnancies.[506] Thus, a family history of adrenal failure, unexplained death, or pubertal abnormalities in the male relatives of a boy with adrenal insufficiency should suggest AHC. Indeed, a substantial proportion of boys with sporadic adrenal hypoplasia have DAX1 mutations.[487]

Autosomal Forms of Adrenal Hypoplasia. Autosomal forms of adrenal hypoplasia exist, but the underlying basis for these conditions is poorly understood. Heterozygous or homozygous mutations in the nuclear receptor steroidogenic factor-1 (SF1, NR5A1) have been reported in 46,XY phenotypic females with spontaneous or recessively inherited primary adrenal failure, and a heterozygous SF1 mutation has been described in a 46,XX girl with adrenal dysfunction.[269-271] However, SF1 mutations have not been found in phenotypic males with adrenal hypoplasia or adrenal steroidogenic defects.[487]

Primary adrenal failure has been associated with Pena-Shoekir syndrome type I, pseudotrisomy 13, Meckel syndrome, Pallister-Hall syndrome (GLI3), and defects in WNT3.[14] Primary adrenal hypoplasia also appears to be part of the IMAGE (intrauterine growth retardation, metaphyseal dysplasia, adrenal hypoplasia, genitourinary anomalies) syndrome.[507] A number of individuals and families with this syndrome have now been reported, but the underlying etiology of this condition remains unknown.[508]

ACTH Resistance Syndromes

Hereditary unresponsiveness to ACTH (familial glucocorticoid deficiency) can present as an acute adrenal crisis precipitated by an intercurrent illness in an infant or with the signs and symptoms of chronic adrenal insufficiency in childhood. A number of distinct recessively inherited causes of FGD have been identified and mutations in these genes have been found in over half the patients with these conditions.[509]

Unlike individuals with autoimmune adrenalitis, adrenal hypoplasia, or other forms of destruction of adrenal tissue patients with hereditary unresponsiveness to ACTH typically continue to produce mineralocorticoids because production of aldosterone by the adrenal zona glomerulosa is regulated principally by the renin-angiotensin system. Thus, the presenting picture consists of failure to thrive, lethargy, pallor, hyperpigmentation, and hypoglycemia, often associated with seizures. Rare cases may also entail electrolyte abnormalities or increased plasma renin activity, leading to misdiagnosis as a different form of adrenal insufficiency.[510]

Familial Glucocorticoid Deficiency Type 1. Familial glucocorticoid deficiency type 1 results from autosomal recessive mutations in the G-protein–coupled ACTH receptor (MC2R).[233,509,511] More than 20 MC2R mutations have been reported in more than 40 individuals or families, accounting for approximately 25% of cases of ACTH resistance. The mutation S74I is especially prevalent. Individuals with FGD1 have the typical presentation of glucocorticoid deficiency; hypoglycemia is common, and ACTH levels can be markedly elevated with consequent hyperpigmentation. Tall stature and increased head circumference have been reported in several cases.[511,512] Treatment with replacement doses of glucocorticoids typically prevents adrenal crises, but may not suppress elevated ACTH levels completely. Nevertheless, the use of supraphysiologic doses of steroids to suppress ACTH should be avoided.[509]

Familial Glucocorticoid Deficiency Type 2. Familial glucocorticoid deficiency type 2 is clinically indistinguishable from FGD1 and is caused by mutations in the melanocortin 2 receptor accessory protein, MRAP,[509,513] accounting for about 20% of cases of ACTH resistance. The MRAP protein (α-isoform) is expressed in a variety of tissues, where it seems to play a role in trafficking the ACTH receptor from the endoplasmic reticulum to the cell membrane. Whether the MRAP protein plays a role in the trafficking of other melancortin receptors, or whether and extended phenotype exists, remains to be seen. Additional genetic loci for other forms of FGD are under investigation (e.g., FGD3, 8q12.1-21.2).[509]

Triple A (Allgrove) Syndrome. Triple A (Allgrove) syndrome consists of ACTH-resistant adrenal (glucocorticoid) deficiency (80% of individuals), achalasia of the cardia (85%), and alacrima (90%).[514] Mineralocorticoid insufficiency is reported in about 15% of cases, and many patients have progressive neurologic symptoms such as intellectual impairment, sensorineural deafness, peripheral and cranial neuropathies, optic atrophy, Parkinsonism, and autonomic dysfunction.[233,515,516] Triple A syndrome is caused by autosomal-recessive mutations in AAAS, which encodes a WD-repeat protein termed *ALADIN*.[517,518] This protein localizes to the cytoplasmic side of the nuclear pore, where it may play a role in nuclear import.[519] Clinical findings can be quite variable even within the same family. Adrenal insufficiency is rarely the presenting feature. Thus, a detailed family history of achalasia, alacrima, or neurologic disorders is important when evaluating a patient with primary adrenal failure.

Metabolic Disorders

Metabolic disorders can also cause chronic primary adrenal insufficiency, including adrenoleukodystrophy (Schilder disease), peroxisome biosynthesis disorders (e.g.,

Zellweger syndrome spectrum), disorders of cholesterol synthesis and metabolism (e.g., Wolman disease, cholesterol ester storage disease, Smith-Lemli-Opitz syndrome), and mitochondrial disorders (e.g., Kearns-Sayre syndrome).

Adrenoleukodystrophy. Adrenoleukodystrophy (ALD) is the most common metabolic disorder causing adrenal failure. Most cases are caused by mutations in the peroxisomal membrane protein ALDP (ABCD1, Xq28),[520,521] which belongs to the superfamily of ATP-binding cassette transporters. The prevalence of this condition is generally reported to be between 1:20,000 and 1:100,000, although the overall frequency may be as high as 1:17,000.[522] A rare autosomal-recessive form of this condition also exists, which usually presents in infancy. ALDP imports activated acyl-CoA derivatives (VLCFA-CoA) into peroxisomes, where they are shortened by β-oxidation.[523,524] Consequently, ALD is characterized by high ratios of C26 to C22 very-long-chain fatty acids in plasma and tissues, permitting the diagnosis of individual patients and affected fetuses.[525] Carriers can usually be detected by very-long-chain fatty acid screening, although genetic analysis may be necessary in some cases. Symptoms of X-linked ALD commonly develop in midchildhood, but a variant of the disorder, termed *adrenomyeloneuropathy*, presents in adulthood.[526] The same ALDP mutation can cause adrenoleukodystrophy and adrenomyeloneuropathy, and hence it is likely that other genetic loci are involved.[527] Earliest findings are associated with the central nervous system leukodystrophy and include behavioral changes, poor school performance, dysarthria, and poor memory progressing to severe dementia.

Symptoms of adrenal insufficiency usually appear after symptoms of white matter disease, but adrenal insufficiency may be the initial finding in up to 20% of children or young adults.[522,528,529] By contrast, adrenomyeloneuropathy typically begins with adrenal insufficiency in childhood and adolescence, and signs of neurologic disease follow 10 to 15 years later. About 1% to 3% of female carriers of X-linked ALD may develop neurologic symptoms or adrenal dysfunction. Because screening is accurate and the diagnosis has long-term implications, very-long-chain fatty acids should be analyzed in all boys presenting with adrenal failure where the diagnosis is not clear. Dietary therapy with so-called Lorenzo's oil, a 4:1 mixture of glyceryl-trioleate and glyceryl-trierucate, improves VLCFA levels, but it has been ineffective for the treatment of established cerebral disease, although a role in preventing the onset of cerebral disease is being evaluated.[522,527] Other therapeutic options include hematopoietic stem cell transplantation for early cerebral disease and lovastatin.[522,524]

Peroxisome Biogenesis Disorders. Peroxisome biogenesis disorders (PBDs) are a group of autosomal-recessive conditions caused by mutations in PEX proteins that include Zellweger syndrome (ZS), neonatal adrenoleukodystrophy (NALD), infantile Refsum's disease (IRD), and rhizomelic chondrodysplasia punctata (RCDP).[530,531] ZS, NALD, and IRD form the "Zellweger spectrum" and are clinically distinct from RCDP. These disorders are characterized by developmental delay, hypotonia, neurosensory deafness, optic atrophy, and dysmorphic facial development. The diagnosis can be confirmed by the presence of C26:1, increased C26:0, and an increased ratio of C26:C22 and C24:C22 very-long-chain fatty acids. Most children with the severe forms of ZS and NALD do not survive past 2 years, although other variants of the Zellweger spectrum are associated with longer survival.[532]

Wolman Disease. Wolman disease or primary xanthomatosis, and cholesterol ester storage disease are disorders in the secreted form of lysosomal acid lipase (cholesterol esterase) that mobilizes cholesterol esters from adrenal lipid droplets.[533] The gene for this enzyme, LIPA, has been cloned and mutations causing Wolman disease have been identified.[534] Because insufficient free cholesterol is available to P450scc, there is adrenal insufficiency.

The disease is less severe than congenital lipoid adrenal hyperplasia with respect to steroidogenesis, and patients may survive for several months after birth. However, the disease affects all cells, not just steroidogenic cells, as all cells must store and utilize cholesterol. Hence, the disorder is relentless and fatal. Vomiting, steatorrhea, failure to thrive, and hepatosplenomegaly are the usual presenting findings. Characteristic bilateral adrenal calcification may be seen on pre- or postnatal ultrasound scan. The diagnosis is established by bone marrow aspiration yielding foam cells containing large lysosomal vaccuoles engorged with cholesterol esters, and is confirmed by finding absent cholesterol esterase activity in fibroblasts, leukocytes, or bone marrow cells. Cholesterol ester storage disease appears to be a milder defect in the same enzyme, generally presenting in childhood or adolescence among the few reported cases.

Smith-Lemli-Opitz Syndrome. Smith-Lemli-Opitz syndrome is a defect in cholesterol biosynthesis, resulting from abnormalities in the sterol Δ-7-reductase gene DHCR7.[535] Associated features of this condition include microcephaly, developmental delay, a typical facial appearance, proximal thumbs and syndactyly of the second and third toes, cardiac abnormalities, and underdeveloped genitalia in males. Adrenal insufficiency is present in a proportion of cases, especially during times of stress or when LDL-derived cholesterol sources are inadequate (e.g., dietary insufficiency/bile salt depletion).[536] Biochemical analysis of sterol Δ-7-reductase activity, coupled with genetic analysis, can confirm the diagnosis.

Mitochondrial Disorders. Mitochondrial disorders can be associated with primary adrenal dysfunction.[537] Typical clinical features include lactic acidosis, cataracts, sensorineuronal deafness, and myopathy/ophthalmoplegia. The Kearns-Sayre syndrome results from large-scale deletions of mitochondrial DNA and can be associated with additional endocrinopathies such as hypothyroidism, hypogonadism, diabetes, growth failure, and hypoparathyroidism.

Other Causes

Chronic adrenal insufficiency may result from other causes. Hemorrhage and infections, discussed previously as causes of acute primary adrenal insufficiency, may spare some adrenal tissue, leaving severely compromised rather than totally absent adrenal function. The result, as with autoimmune adrenalitis, is a chronic disorder with insidious onset of the broad range of nonspecific findings described previously. Tuberculosis, fungal infections (e.g., histoplasmosis, coccidiomycosis), viral infections (e.g., HIV, CMV), metastases, amyloidosis, and sarcoidosis may cause a similar clinical picture. Cortisol biosynthesis can also be inhibited by aminoglutethimide, etomidate, suramin, and ketoconazole.

SECONDARY ADRENAL INSUFFICIENCY

ACTH is required for adrenal cellular growth and for transcription of genes for steroidogenic factors. Hence, any impairment of ACTH synthesis or release can cause secondary adrenal insufficiency. Examples include hypothalamic defects, hypopituitarism, disorders of POMC synthesis and processing, and suppression of the hypothalamic-pituitary axis following exogenous steroid treatment.

Most forms of secondary adrenal insufficiency affect glucocorticoid and androgen synthesis rather than mineralocorticoid release because angiotensin II is the primary drive to the zona glomerulosa. However, the clinical and biochemical assessment may be complicated because glucocorticoids are necessary for renal free water clearance and concomitant vasopression (AVP, ADH) insufficiency may be present. In fact, treatment of secondary adrenal insufficiency can unmask a previously inapparent deficiency of antidiuretic hormone (ADH) and thus precipitate diabetes insipidus. Therefore, close attention must be given to fluid and electrolyte balance when steroid replacement is introduced. Conversely, the hypothyroidism resulting from TSH deficiency will result in slowed metabolism of the small amount of cortisol produced and therefore protect the patient from the symptoms of adrenal insufficiency. Treatment of hypothyroidism with thyroxine will accelerate metabolism of these small amounts of cortisol, thus unmasking adrenal insufficiency due to ACTH deficiency and on occasion precipitating an acute adrenal crisis. Therefore, careful evaluation of the pituitary-adrenal axis is required in hypopituitarism with secondary hypothyroidism.

Many clinicians will choose to "cover" a patient with small doses of glucocorticoids (one-fourth to one-half of physiologic replacement) during initial treatment of such secondary hypothyroidism. Finally, it is important to appreciate that combined deficiency of GH and ACTH will strongly predispose the patient to hypoglycemia because both hormones act to raise plasma glucose. This effect is especially important in infancy and early childhood, when children are vulnerable to hypoglycemia during periods of prolonged fasting.

Hypothalamic Causes

Hypothalamic causes of ACTH insufficiency include tumors and radiotherapy. Tumors, such as craniopharyngioma,[538] are associated with ACTH deficiency in about 25% of patients.[539,540] The frequency may be higher in tumors such as germinoma and astrocytoma.[541] Adrenal

insufficiency is rarely the presenting complaint but may contribute to the clinical picture. After surgery and/or radiation therapy, the great majority of patients with hypothalamic tumors will have ACTH deficiency as part of their surgical or radiation-induced hypothalamic-pituitary damage. Therefore, all such patients should receive glucocorticoid coverage during treatment irrespective of the status of the hypothalamic-pituitary-adrenal axis at the time the tumor is identified.

Because treatment of secondary adrenal insufficiency can precipitate diabetes insipidus, close attention to water balance is essential. ACTH insufficiency can also result following whole-brain irradiation for brain tumors and other central malignancies. This may involve both hypothalamic and pituitary mechanisms. The frequency of ACTH insufficiency in such cases is much lower than following the treatment of hypothalamic tumors, but may manifest some years after treatment.[542]

ACTH Deficiency

ACTH may be deficient as part of a multiple pituitary hormone deficiency (MPHD, panhypopituitarism) or as isolated ACTH insufficiency. MPHD can result from pituitary surgery or radiotherapy, from an infiltrative process (e.g., Langerhans cell histiocytosis), or from a poorly understood form of hypothalamic dysfunction. In most cases, GH secretion is lost first, followed in order by gonadotropins, TSH, and ACTH. Thus, ongoing vigilance and assessment of these patients is required for many years. MPHD can also result from disorders of hypothalamic-pituitary development involving transcription factors such as HESX1, LHX4, and SOX3. Associated features such as optic nerve hypoplasia (HESX1) and cerebellar abnormalities (LHX4) may help to focus the diagnosis. Impaired ACTH secretion has also been described in individuals with PROP1 mutations, one of the most frequent genetic causes of MPHD. This finding can occur many years after presentation with GH, TSH, and gonadotropin deficiency, highlighting the importance of long-term follow-up of patients with pituitary disorders.[543,544]

Patients with MPHD often have a relatively mild form of adrenal insufficiency. Mineralocorticoid secretion is normal, whereas cortisol secretion is reduced but not absent. However, adrenal reserve is severely compromised by the chronic understimulation of steroidogenic enzyme biosynthesis. Because some cortisol synthesis continues, the diagnosis may not be apparent unless a CRF or metyrapone test of pituitary ACTH production capacity and an intravenous ACTH test of adrenal reserve are performed. This can be especially true when TSH deficiency is a component of hypopituitarism, as outlined previously. Treatment of secondary hypothyroidism with thyroxine will accelerate metabolism of these small amounts of cortisol, thus unmasking adrenal insufficiency due to ACTH deficiency and, on occasion, precipitating an acute adrenal crisis.

Isolated ACTH insufficiency is a rare condition that can be caused by recessively inherited mutations in TPIT (TBX19). TPIT encodes a T-box factor that regulates transcription of the POMC promoter in corticotropes.[545] These patients usually present with severe early-onset ACTH insufficiency.[546,547] Hypoglycemia and prolonged jaundice are frequently present, and neonatal death may result.[548] Because this defect is confined to POMC synthesis in the corticotropes, the additional features of generalized POMC deficiency outlined in material following are not present. TPIT mutations are not found in approximately half of patients with isolated ACTH insufficiency, suggesting that other causes are yet to be found. Hypocortisolemia due to isolated ACTH insufficiency has also been described with hippocampal (memory) defects and hair abnormalities (alopecia) as part of the triple H syndrome, a possible autoimmune association.[549]

Disorders of POMC

Defects in POMC synthesis and processing can also cause abnormal ACTH production and action. Recessively inherited mutations or deletion of the POMC gene will affect multiple POMC peptides, including MSH and β-endorphin. Thus, red hair, pale skin, and obesity are associated features of this form of secondary adrenal insufficiency.[165] These clinical signs may be more subtle in individuals with naturally dark hair and pigmented skin, or red hair may darken in adulthood.[550] Mutations in prohormone convertase 1 (PC1, PCSK1), required for the processing of POMC to ACTH, cause abnormal cleavage and processing of several hormone systems, including the generation of bioactive ACTH from POMC.[551] Patients with this rare recessive disorder can have hypocortisolemia together with abnormal glucose metabolism, obesity, hypogonadotropic hypogonadism, and persistent malabsorptive diarrhea.[551,552]

Long-Term Steroid Therapy

Long-term glucocorticoid therapy can suppress POMC gene transcription and the synthesis and storage of ACTH. Furthermore, long-term therapy apparently decreases the synthesis and storage of CRF and diminishes the abundance of receptors for CRF in the pituitary. Therefore, recovery of the hypothalamic-pituitary axis from long-term glucocorticoid therapy entails recovery of multiple components in a sequential cascade and hence often requires considerable time (see section on glucocorticoid therapy and withdrawal). Patients successfully withdrawn from glucocorticoid therapy or successfully treated for Cushing disease may exhibit a fairly rapid normalization of plasma cortisol values while continuing to have diminished adrenal reserve for more than 6 months.

Inhaled steroids, nasal sprays, and even steroid eye drops can cause suppression of the adrenal axis. Thus, vigilance may be needed following their withdrawal or at time of additional stress (e.g., surgery, intercurrent illness).[553-555] Although treatment with cortisone and prednisone during pregnancy will result in minimal suppression of the fetal adrenal, because of the protective effects of placental 11βHSD, dexamethasone treatment in pregnancy can affect fetal adrenal steroidogenesis.

Adrenal Excess

CUSHING SYNDROME

The term *Cushing syndrome* describes any form of glucocorticoid excess. Cushing disease designates hypercortisolism due to pituitary overproduction of ACTH. The related disorder caused by ACTH of nonpituitary origin is termed the *ectopic ACTH syndrome*. The term *Cushing syndrome* is sometimes used to refer specifically to hypersecretion of cortisol from adrenal tumors, but this is ambiguous and should be avoided. Other causes of Cushing syndrome include adrenal adenoma, adrenal carcinoma, and multinodular adrenal hyperplasia. All of the previously cited conditions are distinct from iatrogenic Cushing syndrome, which is the clinical constellation resulting from administration of supraphysiologic quantities of ACTH or glucocorticoids.

Although generally described in great detail and illustrated with striking photographs in endocrine texts, Cushing disease is fairly rare in adults.[556] Furthermore, about 25% of patients referred to large centers for Cushing disease are children. Thus, it is becoming increasingly clear that pediatric Cushing disease is more common than previously recognized. Many patients first seen as adults actually experience the onset of symptoms in childhood or adolescence. Harvey Cushing's original patient was a young woman of only 23 years whose history and clinical features indicated long-standing disease.[2] Hence, many patients with Cushing syndrome can be detected in the pediatric age group.

In adults and children over 7 years of age, the most common cause of Cushing syndrome is true Cushing disease, adrenal hyperplasia due to hypersecretion of pituitary ACTH.[557] Boys are more frequently affected than girls in the prepubertal period, although the sex ratios are equal during adolescence and women have a higher incidence of Cushing disease in adulthood.[558] In infants and children under 7 years, adrenal tumors predominate. Among 60 infants under 1 year of age with Cushing syndrome, 48 had adrenal tumors[559] (Table 12-10).

TABLE 12-10

Etiology of Cushing Syndrome in Infancy

	Males	Females
Adrenal tumors (n = 48)		
Carcinoma	5	20
Adenoma	4	16
Not defined	2	1
Ectopic ACTH syndrome	1	1
Nodular adrenal hyperplasia	1	4
Undefined adrenal hyperplasia	2	2
ACTH-producing tumor	1	0
TOTAL	16	44

Data from Miller WL, Townsend JJ, Grumbach MM, Kaplan SL (1979). An infant with Cushing's disease due to an adrenocorticotropin-producing pituitary adenoma. J Clin Endocrinol Metab 48:1017–1025.

Clinical Findings

The physical features of Cushing syndrome are familiar to virtually all physicians. Central obesity, "moon facies," hirsutism, and facial flushing are seen in more than 80% of adults with Cushing syndrome. Striae, hypertension, muscular weakness, back pain, "buffalo hump" fat distribution, psychological disturbances, acne, and easy bruising are also very commonly described (35% to 80%). However, these are the signs and features of advanced Cushing disease. When annual photographs of such patients are available, it is often apparent that these features can take 5 years or longer to develop. Thus, the classic "Cushingoid appearance" will usually not be the initial picture seen in the child with Cushing syndrome. The earliest and most reliable indicators of hypercortisolism in children are weight gain and growth arrest[560] (Table 12-11).

Cumulative data from three large studies of pediatric Cushing disease identified weight gain at presentation in 91/97 (94%) cases and growth failure in 82/95 (86%) cases.[560-562] Thus, any overweight child who stops growing should be evaluated for Cushing syndrome. Glucocorticoids suppress growth by increasing hypothalamic secretion of somatostatin, by suppressing GH receptor and insulin-like growth factor 1 production, and by acting directly on the epiphyses to inhibit sulfation of cartilage, inhibit mineralization, and inhibit cell proliferation. By contrast, children with simple dietary obesity often grow more rapidly and are tall for their age, presumably due to chronic secondary hyperinsulinism. The obesity of Cushing disease in children is initially generalized rather than centripetal, and a buffalo hump is evidence of long-standing disease.

Psychological disturbances, especially compulsive overachieving behavior, are seen in about 40% of children and adolescents with Cushing disease[560] and are distinctly different from the depression typically seen in adults.[563] Emotional lability has been described in approximately 30% of cases.[562] An underappreciated aspect of pediatric Cushing disease is the substantial degree of bone loss and undermineralization in these patients.[560,564,565] It is likely that Cushing disease is generally regarded as a disease of young adults because the diagnosis was missed, rather than absent, during adolescence. Rarely, Cushing syndrome caused by adrenal carcinoma or the ectopic ACTH syndrome can produce a rapid fulminant course.

Cushing Disease

The recent development of transsphenoidal surgical approaches to the pituitary has led to pituitary exploration in large numbers of patients with Cushing disease. Among adults, more than 90% of such patients have identifiable pituitary microadenomas.[563,566] These tumors are generally 2 to 10 mm in diameter, are not encapsulated, have ill-defined boundaries, and are frequently detectable with a contrast-enhanced pituitary MRI. These tumors are often identifiable only by minor differences in their appearance and texture from surrounding tissue. Thus, the frequency of surgical cure is correlated with the technical skill of the surgeon. Although histologic techniques may not distinguish the tumor from normal tissue, molecular biologic techniques confirm increased synthesis of POMC in these tissues.[567]

Among children and adolescents, about 80% to 85% of those with Cushing disease have surgically identifiable microadenomas.[220,560,568] Although removal of the tumor usually appears curative, 20% of such "cured" patients suffer relapse and again manifest Cushing disease within about 5 years. The net cure rate is thus 65% to 75%.[560-562,569,570] Transsphenoidal surgery offers the best initial approach for rapid and complete cure of most patients, but alternative approaches may be necessary in younger children if sphenoid sinus aeration has not yet occurred.

Control of hypercortisolemia is important in the perioperative period. Careful monitoring for recovery of the hypothalamic-pituitary-adrenal axis is necessary over several months because stress responses may be diminished despite normal basal cortisol secretion. Short-term consequences of transsphenoidal surgery include transient diabetes insipidus and cerebrospinal fluid rhinorrhea.[561,562,571] Persistent panhypopituitarism is rare, but the effects of hypercortisolism on GH secretion may remain for 1 to 2 years after treatment, and GH deficiency can occur even in those children who have not received irradiation.[561,562,571] Final height may be reduced by 1.5 to 2.0 standard deviations by the long-term hypercortisolism.[560,572] Treatment with GH may ameliorate this growth loss in patients with GH insufficiency.[573,574]

The high cure rate of transspenoidal microadenomectomy in Cushing disease indicates that the majority of such patients have primary disease of the pituitary itself, rather than secondary hyperpituitarism resulting from hyperstimulation of the pituitary by CRF or other agents. Careful follow-up studies of these patients confirm this.[560,568,569] In most postoperative patients, the circadian rhythms of ACTH and cortisol return to normal, ACTH and cortisol respond appropriately to hypoglycemia, cortisol is easily

TABLE 12-11

Findings in 39 Children with Cushing Disease

Sign/Symptom	No. of Patients	%
Weight gain	36/39	92
Growth failure	31/37	84
Ostopenia	14/19	74
Fatigue	26/39	67
Hypertension	22/35	63
Delayed or arrested puberty	21/35	60
Plethora	18/39	46
Acne	18/39	46
Hirsutism	18/39	46
Compulsive behavior	17/39	44
Striae	14/39	36
Bruising	11/39	28
Buffalo hump	11/39	28
Headache	10/39	26
Delayed bone age	2/23	13
Nocturia	3/39	8

Data from Devoe DJ, Miller WL, Conte FA, Kaplan SL, Grumbach MM, Rosenthal SM, et al. (1997). Long-term outcome of children and adolescents following transsphenoidal surgery for Cushing disease. J Clin Endocrinol Metab 82:3196–3202.

suppressed by low doses of dexamethasone, and the other hypothalamic-pituitary systems return to normal.

However, some patients with Cushing disease have no identifiable microadenoma, and some "cured" patients relapse. This suggests that this smaller population of patients may have a primary hypothalamic disorder, or that the region of the pituitary responsible for ACTH hypersecretion was not excised. Effective treatment of Cushing disease with cyproheptidine, a serotonin antagonist, has been reported in adults, further suggesting a hypothalamic disturbance. Thus, present clinical investigation suggests that Cushing disease is usually caused by a primary pituitary adenoma but can sometimes be caused by hypothalamic dysfunction. Microsurgery can be curative in the former but not the latter. Unfortunately, no diagnostic maneuver is available to distinguish the two possibilities. Thus, transsphenoidal exploration remains the preferred initial therapeutic approach to the patient with Cushing disease.

The management of nonresponsive or relapsed Cushing disease is challenging. Repeat transsphenoidal surgery is typically the first approach, especially if there is evidence of a distinct lesion or unilateral hypersecretion of ACTH. Second-line approaches include hypophysectomy, gamma-knife irradiation, cyproheptidine, adrenalectomy, and drugs that inhibit adrenal function. All have significant disadvantages, especially in children.

Hypophysectomy will also eliminate pituitary secretion of GH, TSH, and gonadotropins, causing growth failure, hypothyroidism, and failure to progress in puberty respectively. Although hypothyroidism is easily treated with oral thyroxine replacement, GH deficiency requires very expensive replacement therapy. Sex steroid replacement can be used to achieve secondary sexual characteristics at the age of puberty. However, gonadotropin replacement or pulsatile gonadotropin-releasing hormone therapy will be needed to achieve fertility. Pituitary irradiation has been touted to avoid many of these problems and is effective in treating Cushing disease, but GH deficiency occurs in most cases and additional endocrinopathies can occur with time.[575] The interval from radiotherapy to cure can be more than 1 year, during which time therapeutic blockage of hypercortisolemia is necessary to prevent the ongoing effects of Cushing disease on growth, weight, and bone mineralization. Furthermore, large doses of radiation increase the risk of cerebral arteritis, leukoencephalopathy, leukemia, glial neoplasms, and bone tumors involving the skull. Stereotactic radiotherapy may reduce these potential effects, but few data exist yet in children. Cyproheptidine has met with virtually no success in pediatric Cushing disease, in part due to the unacceptable side effects (weight gain, irritability, hallucinations) often seen with the needed doses.

Adrenalectomy is the preferred approach in our centers when two transsphenoidal procedures fail. In addition to the obvious effects of eliminating normal production of glucocorticoids and mineralocorticoids, removal of the adrenal eliminates the physiologic feedback inhibition of the pituitary. In some adults, this results in the development of pituitary macroadenomas, producing very large quantities of ACTH. These can expand and impinge on the optic nerves and can produce sufficient POMC to yield enough MSH to produce profound darkening of the skin (Nelson syndrome). However, this is rarely seen in children.

There is relatively little pediatric experience with ketoconazole and other drugs that inhibit steroidogenesis, but these may provide a useful form of therapy for selected patients or for controlling hypercortisolemia in the short term.[576] Metyrapone is not useful for long-term therapy. Ortho-para DDD (mitotane), an adrenolytic agent, may be used to effect a "chemical adrenalectomy." However, its side effects of nausea, anorexia, and vomiting are severe. Etomidate may be useful in the acute setting for severe or life-threatening Cushing disease prior to surgery.[577,578]

Other Causes of Cushing Syndrome

Ectopic ACTH Syndrome. Ectopic ACTH syndrome is commonly seen in adults with oat cell carcinoma of the lung, carcinoid tumors, pancreatic islet cell carcinoma, and thymoma. Ectopically produced POMC and ACTH are derived from the same gene that produces pituitary POMC,[154] but the ectopic form is not sensitive to glucocorticoid feedback in the malignant cells. This phenomenon permits distinction between pituitary and ectopic ACTH by suppressibility of the former by high doses of dexamethasone. Although the ectopic ACTH syndrome is rare in children, it has been described in infants younger than 1 year of age. Associated tumors have included neuroblastoma, pheochromocytoma, and islet cell carcinoma of the pancreas.[579]

The ectopic ACTH syndrome is typically associated with ACTH concentrations 10 to 100 times higher than those seen in Cushing disease. However, both adults and children with this disorder may show little or no clinical evidence of hypercortisolism, probably due to the typically rapid onset of the disease and to the general catabolism associated with malignancy. Unlike patients with Cushing disease, adults and children with the ectopic ACTH syndrome frequently have hypokalemic alkalosis, presumably because the extremely high levels of ACTH stimulate the production of DOC by the adrenal fasciculata and may also stimulate the adrenal glomerulosa in the absence of hyperreninemia.[579]

Adrenal Tumors. Adrenal tumors, especially adrenal carcinomas, are the more typical cause of Cushing syndrome in infants and small children[580] (Table 12-10). These tend to occur with much greater frequency in girls. The reason for this is unknown.[581] Adrenal adenomas almost always secrete cortisol, with minimal secretion of mineralocorticoids or sex steroids. By contrast, adrenal carcinomas tend to secrete both cortisol and androgens and are often associated with progressive virilization.[582,583] Adrenal adenoma or carcinoma may be associated with congenital bodily asymmetry (hemihypertrophy), sometimes as part of the Beckwith-Wiedemann syndrome, or with germ-line mutations or loss-of-heterozygocity of the tumor suppressor gene p53, sometimes as part of the Li-Fraumeni syndrome.[584]

CT and MRI are useful in the diagnosis of adrenal tumors, and steroid analysis can be informative at the time of presentation and for monitoring for potential relapse. The treatment for both adenoma and carcinoma is surgical, and complete resection is needed for cure. In some cases, the histologic differentiation of adrenal adenomas and carcinomas is difficult. However, a worse prognosis is associated with increased tumor size, capsular and/or vascular invasion, or metastases.[583,585,586] Although a few patients with residual or metastatic disease have done well with adjunctive therapy with ortho-para DDD or other chemotherapeutic strategies, the general prognosis is poor.

ACTH-Independent Multinodular Adrenal Hyperplasia. ACTH-independent multinodular adrenal hyperplasia, also called primary pigmented adrenocorticoid disease (PPNAD), is a rare entity characterized by the secretion of cortisol and adrenal androgens.[587,588] It is seen in infants, children, and young adults, with females affected more frequently. It is usually seen as part of the Carney complex, which is a form of multiple endocrine neoplasia (MEN) consisting of pigmented lentigines and blue nevi on the face, lips, and conjunctiva and a variety of tumors, including schwannomas and atrial myxomas, and occasionally GH-secreting pituitary adenomas, Leydig cell tumors, calcifying Sertoli cell tumors (which may secrete estrogens), and medullary carcinoma of the thyroid.[588,589]

Typical features of Cushing syndrome are often seen in the pediatric population.[590] The adrenals are not truly hyperplastic but consist of discrete pigmented nodules surrounded by atrophic tissue, which permits their identification by MRI or CT. Because the hypercortisolism is resistant to suppression with high doses of dexamethasone and because both glucocorticoids and sex steroids are produced, this entity was difficult to distinguish from the ectopic ACTH syndrome before plasma ACTH assays became routinely available. Complete adrenalectomy is usually indicated, although some successes have been reported with subtotal resections.

Carney complex, like other MEN disorders, is typically autosomal dominant. Loss of heterozygosity and mutations in a regulatory subunit of protein kinase (PRKAR1A) on chromosome 17q22-24 have been found in about 40% of patients with Carney complex,[591-593] or as sporadic germ-line or somatic events in adrenal tumors.[594] Mutations in the gene encoding phosphodiesterase 11A4 (PDE11A) have also been reported in individuals with adrenocortical hyperplasia.[595] Together with reports of multinodular adrenal hyperplasia due to gain-of-function G-protein (GNAS) mutations in the McCune-Albright syndrome, it is becoming clear that abnormalities in signaling pathways play an important role in adrenal hyperplasia and even tumorigenesis.[596]

Differential Diagnosis

The suspicion of Cushing syndrome in children is usually raised by weight gain, growth arrest, mood change, and change in facial appearance (plethora, acne, hirsutism). The diagnosis in children may be subtle and difficult when it is sought at a relatively early point in the natural history of the disease. Absolute elevations above the upper limits of normal for concentrations of plasma ACTH and cortisol are often absent. Rather than finding morning concentrations of cortisol >20 μg/dL or of ACTH >50 pg/mL, it is more typical to find mild and often equivocal elevations in the afternoon and evening values. This loss of the diurnal rhythm, evidenced by continued secretion of ACTH and cortisol throughout the afternoon, evening, and nighttime, is usually the earliest reliable laboratory index of Cushing disease. A single plasma cortisol measurement obtained at midnight from an in-dwelling venous catheter while the patient remains asleep should be less than 2 μg/dL in normal individuals and more than 2 μg/dL in Cushing disease.[597] By contrast, the values for ACTH and cortisol are typically extremely high in the ectopic ACTH syndrome, whereas cortisol is elevated but ACTH suppressed in adrenal tumors and in multinodular adrenal hyperplasia (Table 12-12).

Petrosal sinus sampling is widely used in adults with Cushing disease to distinguish pituitary Cushing disease from the ectopic ACTH syndrome. The smaller vascular bed in children increases the risk of this procedure, but inferior petrosal venous sampling has been used with some success in adolescents in an attempt to localize pituitary adenomas prior to surgery.[598] Such approaches should only be undertaken in specialist centers. Jugular venous sampling may provide an alternative approach, although extensive data in the pediatric population are not available.[599]

In all forms of Cushing syndrome, monitoring of the 24-hour urinary free cortisol assists in deciding whether further investigations are warranted in the obese child. Several repeat collections should be taken, and it is important to use normal ranges adjusted for size as well as age because children with simple obesity have higher cortisol secretion rates.

Low- and high-dose dexamethasone suppression tests can be useful when done with care. To achieve reliable results in pediatric patients, children should be hospitalized, preferably on a "metabolic ward" or pediatric clinical research ward. Two days of baseline (control) data should be obtained. Low-dose dexamethasone (20 μg/kg/day, up to a maximum of 2.0 mg) should be given, divided into equal doses given every 6 hours for 2 days followed by high-dose dexamethasone (80 μg/kg/d) given in the same fashion. Eight AM and 8:00 PM (or midnight) values for ACTH and cortisol and 24-hour urine collections for 17OHS, 17KS, free cortisol, and creatinine (to monitor the completeness of the collection) should be obtained on each of the 6 days of the test.

Measurements of either urinary free cortisol or 17OHCH are probably equally reliable if the laboratory has established good pediatric standards. Because of variations due to episodic secretion of ACTH, the 8:00 AM and 8:00 PM blood values should be drawn in triplicate at 8:00, 8:15, and 8:30. In patients with exogenous obesity or other non-Cushing disorders, cortisol, ACTH, and urinary steroids will be suppressed readily by low-dose dexamethasone. Plasma cortisol should be less than 5 μg/dL, ACTH less than 20 pg/mL, and 24-hour urinary 17OHS less than 1 mg/g of creatinine. Patients with adrenal adenoma, adrenal carcinoma, or the ectopic ACTH syndrome will have values relatively insensitive to both low- and high-dose dexamethasone, although some patients with multinodular adrenal hyperplasia may respond to high-dose suppression, and a

TABLE 12-12

Diagnostic Values in Various Causes of Cushing Syndrome

Test		Normal Values	Adrenal Carcinoma	Adrenal Adenoma	Nodular Adrenal Hyperplasia	Cushing Disease	Ectopic ACTH Syndrome
Plasma cortisol concentration	AM	>14	↑	↑	↑	±	↑↑
	PM	<8	↑	↑	↑	↑	↑↑
Plasma ACTH concentration	AM	<100	↓	↓	↓	↑	↑↑
	PM	<50	↓	↓	↓	↑	↑↑
Low-dose dex suppression	Cortisol	<3	No Δ	No Δ	No Δ	±	No Δ
	ACTH	<30	No Δ	No Δ	No Δ	±	No Δ
	17OHCS	<2	No Δ	No Δ	No Δ	±	No Δ
High-dose dex suppression	Cortisol	↓↓	No Δ	No Δ	Δ	↓	No Δ
	ACTH	↓↓	No Δ	No Δ	Δ	↓	No Δ
	17OHCS	↓↓	No Δ	No Δ	Δ	↓	No Δ
IV ACTH test	Cortisol	>20	No Δ	± ↑	± ↑	↑	No Δ
Metyrapone test	Cortisol	↓	± ↓	No Δ	± ↓	↓	± ↓
11 Deoxycortisol		↑	± ↑	No Δ	± ↑	↑	± ↑
	ACTH	↑	No Δ	No Δ	± ↑	↑	No Δ
	17OHCS	↑	No Δ	No Δ	±	↑	No Δ
24-hour urinary excretion (basal)	17OHCS		↑↑	↑	↑	↑	↑
	17KS		↑↑	± ↑	↑	↑	↑
Plasma concentration DHEA or DHEA-S			↑↑	↓	± ↑	↑	↑

Cortisol concentration in μg/dL.
ACTH concentration in pg/mL.
Dex = dexamethasone.
17OHCS in mg/24 hr.
AM typically refers to 8:00 AM PM refers to 4:00 PM

paradoxical rise in cortisol following dexamethasone has been reported with the Carney complex.[589,600]

Patients with Cushing disease classically respond with a suppression of ACTH, cortisol, and urinary steroids during the high-dose treatment but not during the low-dose treatment. However, some children, especially those early in the course of their illness, may exhibit partial suppression in response to low-dose dexamethasone. Thus, if the low dose that is given exceeds 20 μg/kg/day or if the assays used are insufficiently sensitive to distinguish partial from complete suppression false negative tests may result. In general, the diagnosis of Cushing disease is considerably more difficult to establish in children than in adults.

VIRILIZING AND FEMINIZING ADRENAL TUMORS

Most virilizing adrenal tumors are adrenal carcinomas producing a mixed array of androgens and glucocorticoids. Virilizing and feminizing adrenal adenomas are quite rare. Virilizing tumors in boys will have a presentation similar to that of simple virilizing congenital adrenal hyperplasia. There will be phallic enlargement, erections, pubic and axillary hair, increased muscle mass, deepening of the voice, acne, and scrotal thinning. However, the testicular size will be prepubertal. Elevated concentrations of testosterone in young boys alter behavior, with increased irritability, rambunctiousness, hyperactivity, and rough play, but without evidence of libido. Diagnosis is based on hyperandrogenemia unsuppressable by glucocorticoids. The treatment is surgical. All such tumors should be handled as if they are malignant, with care exerted not to cut the capsule and seed cells onto the peritoneum. The pathologic distinction between adrenal adenoma and carcinoma is difficult.

Feminizing adrenal tumors are extremely rare in either sex. P450aro, the enzyme aromatizing androgenic precursors to estrogens, is not normally found in the adrenals but is found in peripheral tissues such as fat. It is not known whether most feminizing adrenal tumors exhibit ectopic adrenal production of this enzyme, whether some other enzyme mediates aromatization in the tumor, or whether these are truly androgen-producing virilizing tumors occurring in a setting where there is unusually effective peripheral aromatization of adrenal androgens.

Feminizing adrenal or extra-adrenal tumors can be distinguished from true central precocious puberty in girls by the absence of increased circulating concentrations of gonadotropins and by a prepubertal response of luteinizing hormone to an intravenous challenge of gonadotropin-releasing hormone (LRF, GnRH). In boys, such tumors will cause gynecomastia, which will resemble the benign gynecomastia that often accompanies puberty. However, as with virilizing adrenal tumors, testicular size and the gonadotropin response to LRF testing will be prepubertal. The diagnosis of a feminizing tumor in a pubertal boy can be extremely difficult, but it is usually suggested by an arrest in pubertal progression and can be proved by the persistence of circulating plasma estrogens after administration of testosterone.

OTHER DISORDERS

Conn Syndrome

Conn syndrome, characterized by hypertension, polyuria, hypokalemic alkalosis, and low plasma renin activity due to an aldosterone-producing adrenal adenoma, is well described in adults but is exquisitely rare in children. The diagnostic task is to differentiate primary aldosteronism from physiologic secondary hyperaldosteronism occurring in response to another physiologic disturbance. Any loss of sodium, retention of potassium, or decrease in blood volume will result in hyperreninemic secondary hyperaldosteronism. Renal tubular acidosis, treatment with diuretics, salt-wasting nephritis, and hypovolemia due to nephrosis, ascites, or blood loss are typical settings for physiologic secondary hyperaldosteronism. Primary aldosteronism is characterized by hypertension and hypokalemic alkalosis. The cause is a small adrenal adenoma, usually confined to one adrenal. Both adrenals need to be explored surgically because adrenal vein catheterization is not possible in children and is difficult in adults.

Familial Glucocorticoid Resistance

Familial glucocorticoid resistance is a very rare disorder caused by mutations in the α-isoform of the glucocorticoid receptor. Decreased glucocorticoid action results in grossly increased ACTH secretion, which in addition to stimulating the production of cortisol stimulates the production of other adrenal steroids. Thus, these patients may present with fatigue, hypertension, and hypokalemic alkalosis, suggesting a mineralocorticoid excess syndrome but may also have hyperandrogenism.[601] Circadian rhythmicity is maintained and resistance to dexamethasone suppression is observed. Patients have been described who are homozygous for missense mutations[602] or who are heterozygous for a gene deletion.[603] Thus, in each case some receptor activity remains. Heterozygous point mutations with incomplete dominant negative activity or multiple effects on GRα action have also been described.[604] About 10 different GRα mutations have been reported, half of which are familial and half of which appear sporadic. These point mutations may interfere with GRα-dependent transcriptional regulation through altered DNA binding, impaired ligand binding, delayed nuclear localization, abnormal nuclear aggregation, and

disrupted interaction with coactivators, depending on the position of the mutation.[601] No patients have been described with homozygous deletion of this receptor. However, glucocorticoid receptor-knockout mice also have disordered hepatic gluconeogenesis, absent adrenomedullary chromaffin cells, and die from neonatal respiratory distress syndrome.[605] Thus, familial glucocorticoid resistance is a syndrome of only partial resistance to the action of glucocorticoids.

Pseudohypoaldosteronism

Pseudohypoaldosteronism (PHA) is a rare salt-wasting disorder of infancy characterized by hyponatremia, hyperkalemia, and increased plasma renin activity in the face of elevated aldosterone concentrations. The more common autosomal-recessive form of PHA (pseudohypoaldosteronism type II) is caused by inactivating mutations in any of the three subunits (α, β, γ) of the amiloride-sensitive sodium channel ENaC.[606] This condition is often associated with lower respiratory tract disease consisting of chest congestion, cough, and wheezing, but not pulmonary infections, because ENaC mutations increase the volume of pulmonary fluid.[607] This disease persists into adulthood, requiring vigorous salt-replacement therapy throughout life. Gain-of-function mutations due to carboxy-terminal truncation of β-ENaC cause Liddle's syndrome, an autosomal-dominant form of salt-retaining hypertension.[606]

Autosomal-dominant type 1 pseudohypoaldosteronism (PHA type I) is caused by inactivating mutations in the mineralocorticoid receptor.[608] Approximately 20 different mutations have been found in this receptor, which interfere with mineralocorticoid binding and gene transcription.[609] This disease is milder than the recessive forms of PHA caused by ENaC mutations and remits with age, but requires sodium replacement therapy in infancy and childhood. Rarely, point mutations in the mineralocorticoid receptor have been found in association with an autosomal-dominant form of severe hypertension, which begins in adolescence and worsens in pregnancy.[610] In these cases, alterations in the structure of the ligand-binding domain of the mineralocorticoid receptor result in mild constitutive activation as well as permitting binding and activation of the receptor by progesterone.

An acquired transient form of PHA is often seen in infants with obstructive uropathy, especially shortly following surgical relief of the obstruction.[611] The lesion is renal tubular[612] and thus mineralocorticoid treatment is generally ineffective. Salt replacement generally suffices while the renal lesion resolves.

Glucocorticoid Therapy and Withdrawal

Since their introduction into clinical medicine in the early 1950s, glucocorticoids have been used to treat virtually every known disease.[613] At present their rational use falls into two broad categories: replacement in adrenal insufficiency and pharmacotherapeutic use. The latter category is largely related to the anti-inflammatory properties of glucocorticoids but also includes their actions to lyse leukemic leukocytes, lower plasma calcium concentrations, and reduce increased intracranial pressure.

Virtually all of these actions are mediated through glucocorticoid receptors, which are found in most cells. Because there appears to be only one major type of glucocorticoid receptor, clearly all glucocorticoids will affect all tissues containing such receptors. Thus, with the exception of the distinction between glucocorticoids and mineralocorticoids, tissue-specific, disease-specific, or response-specific analogues of naturally occurring glucocorticoids cannot be produced. The only differences among the various glucocorticoid preparations are their ratio of glucocorticoid to mineralocorticoid activity, their capacity to bind to various binding proteins, their molar potency, and their biologic half-life. Dexamethasone is commonly used in reducing increased intracranial pressure and brain edema. Neurosurgical experience indicates that the optimal doses are 10 to 100 times those that would thoroughly saturate all available receptors, suggesting that this action of dexamethasone may not be mediated through the glucocorticoid receptor.

Glucocorticoids are so termed because of their major actions to increase plasma concentrations of glucose. This occurs by their induction of the transcription of the genes encoding the enzymes of the Embden-Meyerhof glycolytic pathway and other hepatic enzymes that divert amino acids, such as alanine, to the production of glucose. Thus, the coordinated action to increase the transcription of these genes can result in increased plasma concentrations of glucose, obesity, and muscle wasting. The other features of Cushing syndrome are similarly attributable to the increased transcriptional activity of specific glucocorticoid-sensitive genes.

REPLACEMENT THERAPY

Glucocorticoid replacement therapy is complicated by undesirable side effects with even minor degrees of overtreatment or undertreatment. Overtreatment can cause the signs and symptoms of Cushing syndrome; and even minimal overtreatment can impair the growth of children. Undertreatment will cause the signs and symptoms of adrenal insufficiency (Table 12-9) only if the extent of undertreatment (dose and duration) are considerable. However, undertreatment may impair the individual's capacity to respond to stress. Glucocorticoid replacement therapy is most commonly employed in congenital adrenal hyperplasia. However, in this setting undertreatment will lead to overproduction of adrenal androgens, which will hasten epiphyseal maturation and closure and thus compromise ultimate adult height. Therefore, when formulating a program of adrenal replacement therapy for the growing child, it is crucial to mimic the normal endogenous production of glucocorticoids.

To optimize pediatric glucocorticoid replacement therapy, astute physicians have gauged their therapy to resemble the endogenous secretory rate of cortisol. Based on studies from the 1960s, most authorities recommend treatment equivalent to a secretory rate of 12.5 mg of cortisol/m² of body surface area per day. It is important to remember that when this value was determined experimentally it was reported as 12.5 ± 3.0 mg/m²/day, and thus the normal

range of requirements was 9.5 to 15.5 mg/m²/day. Thus, the range of normal values varies considerably, indicating that therapy must be tailored and individualized for each patient to achieve optimal results. More recent data suggest that the time-honored value of 12.5 mg/m² may be too high, and that appropriate replacement might be as low as 6 mg/m² in younger children and 9 mg/m² in older children and adolescents.[224,225]

The management of this delicate balance between overtreatment and undertreatment of the child requiring replacement therapy is thus confounded by considerable variation in the "normal" cortisol secretory rate among different children of the same size and the probability that most conventional guidelines err on the side of overtreatment. However, several additional factors must be considered in tailoring a specific child's glucocorticoid replacement regimen.

The specific form of adrenal insufficiency being treated significantly influences therapy. When treating autoimmune adrenalitis or any other form of "Addison disease," it is prudent to err slightly on the side of undertreatment. This will eliminate the possibility of glucocorticoid-induced iatrogenic growth retardation and will permit the pituitary to continue to produce normal to slightly elevated concentrations of ACTH. This ACTH will continue to stimulate the remaining functional adrenal steroidogenic machinery and will provide a fairly convenient means of monitoring the effects of therapy. By contrast, when treating severe virilizing congenital adrenal hyperplasia, the adrenal should be suppressed more completely because essentially all adrenal steroidogenesis will result in the production of unwanted androgens, with their consequent virilization and rate of advancement of bony maturation that is more rapid than the rate of advancement of height. As stated previously, however, overtreatment will also compromise growth.

The presence or absence of associated mineralocorticoid deficiency is an important variable. Children with mild degrees of mineralocorticoid insufficiency, such as those with "simple virilizing" congenital adrenal hyperplasia, may continue to have mildly elevated ACTH values, suggesting insufficient glucocorticoid replacement in association with elevated PRA. In some children, the ACTH is elevated in response to chronic compromised hypovolemia, attempting to stimulate the adrenal to produce more mineralocorticoid. In these children, who do not manifest overt signs and symptoms of mineralocorticoid insufficiency, treatment with mineralocorticoid replacement may permit one to decrease the amount of glucocorticoid replacement needed to suppress plasma ACTH and urinary 17KS. This reduction in glucocorticoid therapy reduces the likelihood that adult height will be compromised.

The specific formulation of glucocorticoid used is also of great importance. Extremely potent long-acting glucocorticoids, such as dexamethasone or prednisone, are preferred in the treatment of adults but are rarely appropriate for replacement therapy in children. Because children are continually growing and changing their weights and body surface areas, it is necessary to adjust their dose frequently. Small incremental changes are more easily done with relatively weaker glucocorticoids. It is easy to change from 25 to 30 mg of hydrocortisone but virtually impossible to change from an equivalent 0.5 to 0.6 mg of dexamethasone. Tablets are not available in 0.1-mg increments.

The efficacy of attempting to mimic the physiologic diurnal variation in steroid hormone secretion remains controversial. Because ACTH and cortisol concentrations are high in the morning and low in the evening, it is intellectually and logically appealing to attempt to duplicate this circadian rhythm in replacement therapy. However, the results do not clearly indicate that better growth is achieved by giving relatively larger doses in the morning and lower doses at night. This probably reflects the fact that ACTH and cortisol secretion are episodic throughout the day and that this well-established circadian variation is not smooth. The pattern of high in the morning and low in the evening is only an averaged result. Furthermore, the adrenal releases cortisol episodically throughout the day in response to various physiologic demands such as hypoglycemia, exercise, stress, etc. Thus, under normal circumstances, the plasma concentrations are high when the clearance and disposal rates are also high. A planned program of replacement therapy cannot possibly anticipate these day-to-day variations.

Finally, dosage equivalents among various glucocorticoids can be misleading. Virtually all handbooks of therapy publish tables of equivalency for the most commonly used pharmaceutical preparations of glucocorticoids. A similar set of equivalencies is outlined in Table 12-7. Because most preparations of glucocorticoids are intended for pharmacotherapeutic use rather than replacement therapy, and because the most common indication for pharmacologic doses of glucocorticoids is for their anti-inflammatory properties, virtually all tables of glucocorticoid equivalencies are based on anti-inflammatory immunosuppressive equivalencies.

However, the differences in the plasma half-life and ability to bind to plasma proteins result in different biologic equivalencies when one assesses, for example, anti-inflammatory versus growth-suppressant equivalencies. For example, dexamethasone is widely reported as being 25 to 30 times more potent than cortisol when its anti-inflammatory capacities are measured. However, the growth-suppressant activity of dexamethasone is about 80 times that of cortisol[393] (Table 12-7). Thus, all of the variables discussed previously explain why there is little unanimity in recommendations for designing a glucocorticoid replacement regimen. However, an understanding of these variables will permit appropriate monitoring of the patient and encourage the physician to vary the treatment according to the responses and needs of the individual child.

COMMONLY USED GLUCOCORTICOID PREPARATIONS

Numerous chemical derivatives and variants of the naturally occurring steroids are commercially available in a huge array of dosage forms, vehicles, and concentrations, all carrying confusing and uninformative brand names. Choosing the appropriate product can be simplified by considering only the most widely used steroids listed in Table 12-7. As indicated in the table, there are four relevant considerations in the choice of which drug to use.

First, the glucocorticoid potency of the various drugs is generally calculated and described according to the anti-inflammatory potency. The pharmaceutical industry has chosen this standard for convenience and because the majority of their sales are to physicians using pharmacologic doses of these steroids to achieve anti-inflammatory effects.

Second, the growth-suppressant effect of a glucocorticoid preparation may be significantly different from its anti-inflammatory effect. This is due to differences in half-life, metabolism and protein binding, and receptor affinity potency but is not due to receptor specificity because all known receptor-mediated effects of glucocorticoids are mediated through a single type of receptor.

Third, the mineralocorticoid activity of various glucocorticoid preparations varies widely. Glucocorticoid and mineralocorticoid hormones can bind to glucocorticoid (type I) and mineralocorticoid (type II) receptors, and most authorities now regard these as two different types of glucocorticoid receptors and find that there is no true specific mineralocorticoid receptor. Mineralocorticoid activity is intimately related to the activity of 11βHSD, which metabolizes glucocorticoids but not mineralocorticoids to a form that cannot bind the receptor. Thus, the relative mineralocorticoid potency of various steroids is determined by their affinity for the type II receptor and their resistance to the activity of 11βHSD. An understanding that some commonly used glucocorticoids, such as cortisol, cortisone, prednisolone, and prednisone, have significant mineralocorticoid activity is especially important when large doses of glucocorticoids are used as "stress doses" in a patient on replacement therapy. Such stress doses of the glucocorticoid preparation may provide sufficient mineralocorticoid activity to meet physiologic needs. Therefore, mineralocorticoid supplementation is not needed.

Fourth, the plasma half-life and biological half-life of the various preparations may be discordant and will vary widely. This is mainly related to binding to plasma proteins, hepatic metabolism, and hepatic activation. For example, cortisone and prednisone are biologically inactive, and even have mild steroid antagonist actions until they are metabolized by hepatic 11βHSD-I to their active forms (cortisol and prednisolone). Thus, the relative glucocorticoid potency of these preparations will also be affected by hepatic function. Cortisone and prednisone are cleared more rapidly in patients receiving drugs such as phenobarbital or phenytoin, which induce hepatic enzymes and are cleared more slowly in patients with liver failure.

In addition to these chemical considerations in the choice of glucocorticoid, the route of administration is a critical variable. Glucocorticoids are available for oral, intramuscular, intravenous, intrathecal, intra-articular, inhalant, and topical use. Topical preparations include those designed for use on skin, mucous membranes, and conjunctiva. Each preparation is designed to deliver the maximal concentration of steroid to the desired tissue while delivering less steroid systemically. However, all such preparations are absorbed to varying extents, and thus the widely used inhalant preparations used to treat asthma can, in sufficient doses, cause growth retardation and other signs of Cushing syndrome.

In general, and in contradistinction to many other drugs, orally administered steroids are absorbed rapidly but incompletely, whereas intramuscularly administered steroids are absorbed slowly but completely. Thus, if the secretory rate of cortisol is 8 mg/m^2 of body surface area, the intramuscular or intravenous replacement dose of cortisol (hydrocortisone) would be 8 mg/m^2. However, because only about one-half of an oral dose is absorbed intact, the oral equivalent would be about 15 to 20 mg of hydrocortisone. The efficiency of absorption of glucocorticoids can vary considerably depending on diet, gastric acidity, bowel transit time and other individual factors. This emphasizes that the dosage equivalents listed in Table 12-7 and similar tables are only general approximations. The equivalencies shown are estimated biologic equivalencies with a broad range of variability and are not physical chemical equivalents.

ACTH can also be used for glucocorticoid therapy by its action to stimulate endogenous adrenal steroidogenesis. Although intravenous and intramuscular ACTH are extremely useful in diagnostic tests of adrenal function, the use of ACTH as a therapeutic agent is no longer favored, principally because it will stimulate synthesis of mineralocorticoids and adrenal androgens as well as glucocorticoids. Furthermore, the need to administer ACTH parenterally further diminishes its usefulness.

Intramuscular ACTH 1-39 in a gel form is the treatment of choice for infantile spasms and possibly for other forms of epilepsy in infants resistant to conventional anticonvulsants. Whether this action is mediated by ACTH itself, by other peptides in the biologic preparation, by ACTH-induced adrenal steroids, or by ACTH-responsive synthesis of novel "neurosteroids"[614] in the brain has not been determined. When pharmacologic doses of ACTH are used therapeutically, as in infantile spasms, the patient should be given a low-sodium diet to ameliorate steroid hypertension. Although greatly elevated concentrations of ACTH as in the ectopic ACTH syndrome will cause pituitary suppression, treatment with daily injections of ACTH results in less hypothalamic-pituitary suppression than does treatment with equivalent doses of oral glucocorticoids, presumably because the effect on the adrenal is transient. In addition, adrenal suppression obviously does not occur in ACTH therapy. Because the effects of ACTH on adrenal steroidogenesis are highly variable it is even more difficult to determine dosage equivalencies for ACTH and oral steroid preparations than it is among the various steroids. A very rough guide from studies in adults is that 40 units of ACTH(1-39) gel are approximately equivalent to 100 mg of cortisol.

PHARMACOLOGIC THERAPY

Pharmacologic doses of glucocorticoids are used in a variety of clinical situations, including immune suppression in organ transplantation, tumor chemotherapy, treatment of "autoimmune" collagen vascular and nephrotic syndromes, regional enteritis, and ulcerative colitis. Asthma,

pseudotumor cerebri, dermatitis, certain infections, neuritis, and certain anemias are also often treated with glucocorticoids. The choice of glucocorticoid preparation to be used is guided by the pharmacologic parameters described previously and listed in Table 12-7, and by custom (e.g., the use of betamethasone rather than dexamethasone to induce fetal lung maturation in impending premature deliveries). There is substantial variation in the relative glucocorticoid and mineralocorticoid activities of each steroid, depending on the assay used.[615] Hence, Table 12-7 is an integration of multiple studies and can only be taken as a rough guide.

Pharmacologic doses of glucocorticoids administered for more than 1 or 2 weeks will cause the signs and symptoms of iatrogenic Cushing syndrome. These are similar to the glucocorticoid-induced findings in Cushing disease but may be more severe because of the high doses involved (Table 12-13). Iatrogenic Cushing syndrome is also not associated with adrenal androgen effects, and mineralocorticoid effects are rare. Alternate-day therapy can decrease the toxicity of pharmacologic glucocorticoid therapy, especially suppression of the hypothalamic-pituitary-adrenal axis and suppression of growth. The basic premise of alternate-day therapy is that the disease state can be suppressed with intermittent therapy, while there is significant recovery of the HPA axis during the "off" day. Thus, alternate-day therapy requires the use of a relatively short-acting glucocorticoid administered only once in the morning of each therapeutic day to ensure that the off day is truly "off." Long-acting glucocorticoids, such as dexamethasone, should not be employed for alternate-day therapy. Results are best with oral prednisone or methyl prednisolone.

WITHDRAWAL OF GLUCOCORTICOID THERAPY

Withdrawal of glucocorticoid therapy can be difficult and can lead to symptoms of glucocorticoid insufficiency. When glucocorticoid therapy has been used for only 1 week or 10 days, therapy can be discontinued abruptly, even if high doses have been used.[616] Although only one

TABLE 12-13

Complications of High-Dose Glucocorticoid Therapy

Short-Term Therapy	Long-Term Therapy
Gastritis	Gastric ulcers
Growth arrest	Short stature
↑ Appetite	Weight gain
Hypercalciuria	Osteoporosis, fractures
Glycosuria	Slipped ephiphises
Immune suppression	Ischemic bone necrosis
Masked symptoms of infection, esp. fever and inflammation	Poor wound healing
Toxic psychosis	Catabolism
	Cataracts
	Bruising (capillary fragility)
	Adrenal/pituitary suppression
	Toxic psychosis

or two doses of glucocorticoid are needed to suppress the hypothalamic-pituitary-adrenal axis, this axis recovers very rapidly from short-term suppression.

When therapy has persisted for 2 weeks or longer, recovery of hypothalamic-pituitary-adrenal function is slower and tapered doses of glucocorticoids are indicated. Acute discontinuation of therapy in such patients will lead to symptoms of glucocorticoid insufficiency, the so-called steroid withdrawal syndrome. This symptom complex does not include salt loss because adrenal glomerulosa function, regulated principally by the renin-angiotensin system, remains normal. However, blood pressure can fall abruptly because glucocorticoids are required for the action of catecholamines in maintaining vascular tone. The most prominent symptoms of the steroid withdrawal syndrome include malaise, anorexia, headache, lethargy, nausea, and fever. In reducing pharmacologic doses of glucocorticoids, it might appear logical to reduce the dosage precipitously to "physiologic" replacement doses. However, this is rarely successful and is occasionally disastrous.

Even when given physiologic replacement, patients who have been receiving pharmacologic doses of glucocorticoids will experience steroid withdrawal. Although the mechanism is not known with certainty, it is most likely that long-term pharmacologic glucocorticoid therapy inhibits transcription of the gene(s) for glucocorticoid receptors, thus reducing the number of receptors per cell. If this is so, physiologic concentrations of glucocorticoids will elicit subphysiologic cellular responses, resulting in the steroid withdrawal syndrome. Thus, it is necessary to taper gradually from the outset. The duration of glucocorticoid therapy is a critical consideration in designing a glucocorticoid withdrawal program. Therapy for a couple of months will completely suppress the hypothalamic-pituitary-adrenal axis but will not cause adrenal atrophy. Therapy of years' duration may result in almost total atrophy of the adrenal fasciculata/reticularis, and hence may require a withdrawal regimen that takes months.

Procedures for tapering steroids are empirical. Their success is determined by the length and mode of therapy and by individual patient responses. Patients who have been on alternate-day therapy can be withdrawn more easily than those receiving daily therapy, especially in cases of daily therapy with a long-acting glucocorticoid such as dexamethasone. In patients on long-standing therapy, a 25% reduction in the previous level of therapy is generally recommended weekly. A patient with a body surface area of 1 m² will have a secretory rate of cortisol of about 9 mg/day, equivalent to 20 mg/day of orally administered cortisone acetate. If the patient has been on daily therapy equivalent to 100 mg of cortisone acetate for many months, a tapering protocol over 8 to 10 weeks may be needed. A protocol of 75% of the previous week's dose would thus be 75 mg/day for the first week, 56 mg/day for the second, and then 42, 31.5, 24, 18, 13.5, 10, 7.5, and 5.5 mg/day and then off treatment. A more practical regimen based on the sizes of tablets available would be 75, 50, 37.5, 25, 17.5, 12.5, 10, 7.5, and 5 mg/day. Most patients can be tapered more rapidly, but all patients need to be followed closely. When withdrawal is done with steroids other than cortisone or cortisol, measurement of morning cortisol values can be a useful adjunct. Morning cortisol values of 10 μg/dL or greater indicate that the dose can be reduced safely.

Even after the successful discontinuation of therapy, the hypothalamic-pituitary-adrenal axis is not wholly normal. Just as in the patient successfully treated for Cushing disease, the hypothalamic-pituitary-adrenal axis may be incapable of responding to severe stress for 6 to 12 months after successful withdrawal from long-term high-dose glucocorticoid therapy. Thus, evaluation of the hypothalamus and pituitary by a CRF or metyrapone test, and evaluation of adrenal responsiveness to pituitary stimulation with an intravenous ACTH test, should be done at the conclusion of a withdrawal program and 6 months thereafter. The results of these tests will indicate if there is a need for "steroid coverage" in acute surgical stress or illness.

STRESS DOSES OF GLUCOCORTICOIDS

The cortisol secretory rate increases significantly during physiologic stress such as trauma, surgery, or severe illness. Patients receiving glucocorticoid replacement therapy or those recently withdrawn from pharmacologic therapy need coverage with "stress doses" of steroids. However, the specific indications for this coverage and the appropriate dosage are controversial and difficult to establish. Most practitioners prefer to err on the "safe" side of steroid overdosage. This is the safest tactic in the short term, but it can have a significant effect on growth over a period of years.

It is generally said that doses 3 to 10 times physiologic replacement are needed for the stress of surgery. The stress accompanying a surgical procedure can vary greatly. Modern techniques of anesthesiology; better anesthetic, analgesic, and muscle-relaxing drugs; and increased awareness of the particular needs of children in managing intraoperative fluids and electrolytes have greatly reduced the stress of surgery. In the past, a significant portion of such stress had to do with pain and hypovolemia, but these are less important in contemporary pediatric services. Similarly, part of the stress of acute illness is fever and fluid loss, factors now familiar to all pediatricians. Although it remains appropriate and necessary to give about three times physiologic requirements during such periods of stress, it is probably not necessary to give much higher doses. Similarly, it is not necessary to triple a child's physiologic replacement regimen during simple colds, upper respiratory infection, and otitis media or after immunizations.

The preparation of the hypoadrenal patient on replacement therapy for surgery is simple if planned in advance. Although stress doses of steroids can be administered intravenously by the anesthesiologist during surgery, this may be suboptimal. Doses administered as an intravenous bolus are short acting and may not provide coverage throughout the procedure. The transition from hospital ward to surgical theater to recovery room usually involves a transition among three or more teams of personnel, increasing the risk for error. Because intramuscularly administered cortisone acetate has a biologic half-life of about 18 hours, we recommend intramuscular administration of twice the day's physiologic requirement at 18 hours before surgery and again at 8 hours before surgery. This provides the patient with a body reservoir of glucocorticoid throughout the surgical and immediate postoperative period. Regular therapy at two to three times physiologic requirements can then be reinstituted on the day after the surgical procedure.

MINERALOCORTICOID REPLACEMENT

Replacement therapy with mineralocorticoids is indicated in salt-losing congenital adrenal hyperplasia and in syndromes of adrenal insufficiency that affect the zona glomerulosa. Only one mineralocorticoid, 9α-fluorocortisol (Fluorinef), is currently available. There is no parenteral mineralocorticoid preparation, hydrocortisone plus salt must be used.

Mineralocorticoid doses used are essentially the same irrespective of the size or age of the patient. In fact, newborns are quite insensitive to mineralocorticoids and may require larger doses than adults. The replacement dose of 9α-fluorocortisol is usually 0.05 to 0.10 mg daily. Sodium must be available to the nephrons for mineralocorticoids to promote reabsorption of sodium. Thus, the newborn with salt-losing congenital adrenal hyperplasia must be treated with mineralocorticoids and sodium chloride. Similarly, mineralocorticoids will cause hypertension only by retaining sodium.

Cortisol has significant mineralocorticoid activity. Approximately 20 mg of cortisol or cortisone intravenously has a mineralocorticoid action equivalent to 0.1 mg of 9α-fluorocortisol. Thus, when cortisol or cortisone is given in stress doses it provides adequate mineralocorticoid activity and mineralocorticoid replacement can be interrupted. This is frequently seen when patients with salt-losing congenital adrenal hyperplasia undergo surgery. The stress doses of intramuscular cortisone acetate and the intravenous saline solutions administered during and after surgery suffice for the patient's mineralocorticoid requirements. Additional 9α-fluorocortisol is not needed until the supraphysiologic stress doses of cortisol are decreased. Because 9α-fluorocortisol can be administered only orally and because this may not be possible in the postoperative period, the appropriate drug for glucocorticoid replacement is cortisol or cortisone, which have mineralocorticoid activity, rather than synthetic steroids such as prednisone or dexamethasone, which have little mineralocorticoid activity.

Concluding Remarks

Because the adrenal cortex is principally concerned with steroid synthesis, most of its disorders reflect genetic lesions in adrenal development and steroidogenesis. Overproduction and underproduction of steroids having varied and complex physiologic actions lead to complex phenotypes and clinical presentations. These primary genetic disorders typically present themselves in infancy and childhood. By contrast, secondary disorders such as Cushing disease (usually a disorder of the pituitary) and Addison disease (usually a disorder of cellular immunity) may be seen at any age.

Thus, the pediatric endocrinologist must have a detailed understanding of the cell biology, genetics, and biochemistry of steroid hormone biosynthesis. Future refinements improving the speed, efficiency, accuracy, and economy of DNA sequencing will eventually permit direct genetic diagnosis of genetic diseases. However, it is unlikely that measurements of steroid hormones will become obsolete in the forseeable future, and an understanding of steroid physiology will always be needed to understand clinical presentations, formulate differential diagnoses, choose genes for study, and monitor therapy. Thus, genetics will continue to enhance clinical physiology but will not replace it.

REFERENCES

1. Miller WL, Chrousos GP (2001). The adrenal cortex. In P. Felig and L. Frohman (eds.), *Endocrinology and metabolism.* New York: McGraw-Hill 386–524.
2. Cushing H (1932). The basophil adenomas of the pituitary body and their clinical manifestations. Bull Johns Hopkins Hosp 50:137–195.
3. Seyle H (1946). The general adaptation syndrome and the diseases of adaptation. J Clin Endocrinol 6:117–230.
4. Steiger M, Reichstein T (1937). Desoxy-cortico-steron (21-oxyprogesterone) aus Δ 5-3 -xoy-atio-cholensaure. Helv Chim Acta 20:1164.
5. Kendall EC, Mason HL, McKenzie BF, Myers CS, Koelsche GA (1934). Isolation in crystalline form of the hormone essential to life from the supranetal cortex: Its chemical nature and physiologic properties. Trans Assoc Am Physicians 49:147.
6. Hench PS, Kendall EC, Slocumb CH, Polley HF (1949). The effect of a hormone of the adrenal cortex (17-hydroxy-11-dehydrocorticosterone compound E) and of pituitary adrenocorticotropic hormone on rheumatoid arthritis. Proc Staff Meet Mayo Clin 24:181–197.
7. Wilkins L, Lewis RA, Klein R, Rosenberg E (1950). The supression of androgen secretion by cortisone in a case of congenital adrenal hyperplasia. Bull Johns Hopkins Hosp 86:249–252.
8. Bartter FC, Forbes AO, Leaf A (1950). Congenital adrenal hyperplasia associated with the adrenogenital syndrome: An attempt to correct its disordered hormonal pattern. J Clin Invest 29:797.
9. Cooper DY, Levin S, Narasimhulu S, Rosenthal O, Estabrook RW (1965). Photochemical action spectrum of the terminal oxidase of mixed function oxidase systems. Science 145:400–402.
10. Miller WL (1988). Molecular biology of steroid hormone synthesis. Endocr Rev 9:295-318.
11. Evans RM (1988). The steroid and thyroid hormone receptor superfamily. Science 240:889–895.
12. Mesiano S, Jaffe RB (1997). Developmental and functional biology of the primate fetal adrenal cortex. Endocr Rev 18:378–403.
13. Hammer GD, Parker KL, Schimmer BP (2005). Transcriptional regulation of adrenocortical development. Endocrinology 146:1018–1024.
14. Else T, Hammer GD (2005). Analysis of absence: Adrenal agenesis, aplasia and atrophy. Trends Endocrinol Metab 16:458–468.
15. Axelrod J, Reisine TD (1984). Stress hormones: Their interaction and regulation. Science 224:452–459.
16. Auchus RJ, Miller WL (2005). The principles, pathways and enzymes of human steroidogenesis. In LJ DeGroot and JL Jameson (eds.), *Endocrinology.* Philadelphia: WB Saunders 2263–2285.
17. Gwynne JT, Strauss JF III (1982). The role of lipoproteins in steroidogenesis and cholesterol metabolism in steroidogenic glands. Endocr Rev 3:299–329.
18. Ikonen E (2006). Mechanisms for cellular cholesterol transport: Defects and human disease. Physiol Rev 86:1237–1261.
19. Brown MS, Kovanen PT, Goldstein JL (1979). Receptor-mediated uptake of lipoprotein-cholesterol and its utilization for steroid synthesis in the adrenal cortex. Rec Prog Horm Res 35:215–257.
20. Gonzalez FJ (1989). The molecular biology of cytochrome P450s. Pharmacol Rev 40:243–288.
21. Ventner JC, et al. (2001). The sequence of the human genome. Science 291:1304–1351.
22. Lander ES, Linton LM, Birren B (2001). Initial sequencing and analysis of the human genome. Nature 409:860.

23. Agarwal AK, Auchus RJ (2005). Cellular redox state regulates hydroxysteroid dehydrogenase activity and intracellular hormone potency. Endocrinology 146:2531–2538.

24. Chung B, Matteson KJ, Voutilainen R, Mohandas TK, Miller WL (1986). Human cholesterol side-chain cleavage enzyme, P450scc: cDNA cloning, assignment of the gene to chromosome 15, and expression in the placenta. Proc Natl Acad Sci USA 83:8962–8966.

25. Simpson ER (1979). Cholesterol side-chain cleavage, cytochrome P450, and the control of steroidogenesis. Mol Cell Endocrinol 13:213–227.

26. Yang X, Iwamoto K, Wang M, Artwohl J, Mason JI, Pang S (1993). Inherited congenital adrenal hyperplasia in the rabbit is caused by a deletion in the gene encoding cytochrome P450 cholesterol side-chain cleavage enzyme. Endocrinology 132:1977–1982.

27. Hu M-C, Hsu N-C, Ben El Hadj B, Pai C-I, Chu H-P, Wang C-KL, et al. (2002). Steroid deficiency syndromes in mice with targeted disruption of Cyp11a1. Mol Endocrinol 16:1943–1950.

28. Miller WL (2005). Regulation of steroidogenesis by electron transfer. Endocrinology 146:2544–2550.

29. Solish SB, Picado-Leonard J, Morel Y, Kuhn RW, Mohandas TK, Hanukoglu I, et al. (1988). Human adrenodoxin reductase: Two mRNAs encoded by a single gene on chromosome 17cen → q25 are expressed in steroidogenic tissues. Proc Natl Acad Sci USA 85:7104–7108.

30. Lin D, Shi Y, Miller WL (1990). Cloning and sequence of the human adrenodoxin reductase gene. Proc Natl Acad Sci USA 87:8516–8520.

31. Chang C -Y, Wu D -A, Lai C -C, Miller W L, Chung B (1988). Cloning and structure of the human adrenodoxin gene. DNA 7:609–615.

32. Picado-Leonard J, Voutilainen R, Kao L, Chung B, Strauss JF III, Miller WL (1988). Human adrenodoxin: Cloning of three cDNAs and cycloheximide enhancement in JEG-3 cells. J Biol Chem 263:3240–3244.

33. Brentano ST, Black SM, Lin D, Miller WL (1992). cAMP posttranscriptionally diminishes the abundance of adrenodoxin reductase mRNA. Proc Natl Acad Sci USA 89:4099–4103.

34. Hum DW, Miller WL (1993). Transcriptional regulation of human genes for steroidogenic enzymes. Clin Chem 39:333–340.

35. Stocco DM, Clark BJ (1996). Regulation of the acute production of steroids in steroidogenic cells. Endocr Rev 17:221–244.

36. Miller WL (2007). StAR search: What we know about how the steroidogenic acute regulatory protein mediates mitochondrial cholesterol import. Mol Endocrinol 21:589–601.

37. Pon LA, Hartigan JA, Orme-Johnson NR (1986). Acute ACTH regulation of adrenal corticosteroid biosynthesis: Rapid accumulation of a phosphoprotein. J Biol Chem 261:13309–13316.

38. Epstein LF, Orme-Johnson NR (1991). Regulation of steroid hormone biosynthesis: identification of precursors of a phosphoprotein targeted to the mitochondrion in stimulated rat adrenal cortex cells. J Biol Chem 266:19739–19745.

39. Stocco DM, Sodeman TC (1991). The 30-kDa mitochondrial proteins induced by hormone stimulation in MA-10 mouse Leydig tumor cells are processed from larger precursors. J Biol Chem 266:19731–19738.

40. Clark BJ, Wells J, King SR, Stocco DM (1994). The purification, cloning and expression of a novel luteinizing hormone-induced mitochondrial protein in MA-10 mouse Leydig tumor cells: Characterization of the steroidogenic acute regulatory protein (StAR). J Biol Chem 269:28314–28322.

41. Lin D, Sugawara T, Strauss JF III, Clark BJ, Stocco DM, Saenger P, et al. (1995). Role of steroidogenic acute regulatory protein in adrenal and gonadal steroidogenesis. Science 267:1828–1831.

42. Bose HS, Sugawara T, Strauss III JF, Miller WL (1996). The pathophysiology and genetics of congenital lipoid adrenal hyperplasia. New England J Med 335:1870–1878.

43. Moore CCD, Hum DW, Miller WL (1992). Identification of positive and negative placental-specific basal elements, a transcriptional repressor, and a cAMP response element in the human gene for P450scc. Mol Endocrinol 6:2045–2058.

44. Sugawara T, Holt JA, Driscoll D, Strauss III JF, Lin D, Miller WL, et al. (1995). Human steroidogenic acute regulatory protein (StAR): Functional activity in COS-1 cells, tissue-specific expression, and mapping of the structural gene to 8p11.2 and an expressed pseudogene to chromosome 13. Proc Natl Acad Sci USA 92:4778–4782.

45. Papadopoulos V (1993). Peripheral-type benzodiazepine/diazepam binding inhibitor receptor: Biological role in steroidogenic cell function. Endocr Rev 14:222–240.

46. Hauet T, Yao ZX, Bose HS, Wall CT, Han Z, Li W, et al. (2005). Peripheral-type benzodiazepine receptor-mediated action of steroidogenic acute regulatory protein on cholesterol entry into Leydig cell mitochondria. Mol Endocrinol 19:540–554.

47. Liu J, Rone MB, Papadopoulos V (2006). Protein-protein interactions mediate mitochondrial cholesterol transport and steroid biosynthesis. J Biol Chem 281:38879–38893.

48. Bose HS, Lingappa VR, Miller WL (2002). Rapid regulation of steroidogenesis by mitochondrial protein import. Nature 417:87–91.

49. Bose HS, Whittal RM, Baldwin MA, Miller WL (1999). The active form of the steroidogenic acute regulatory protein, StAR, appears to be a molten globule. Proc Natl Acad Sci USA 96:7250–7255.

50. Baker BY, Yaworsky DC, Miller WL (2005). A pH-dependent molten globule transition is required for activity of the steroidogenic acute regulatory protein, StAR. J Biol Chem 280:41753–41760.

51. Thomas JL, Myers RP, Strickler RC (1989). Human placental 3β-hydroxy-5-ene-steroid dehydrogenase and steroid 5 → 4-ene-isomerase: Purification from mitochondria and kinetic profiles, biophysical characterization of the purified mitochondrial and microsomal enzymes. J Steroid Biochem 33:209–217.

52. Luu-The V, Lechance Y, Labrie C, Leblanc G, Thomas JL, Strickler RC, et al. (1989). Full length cDNA structure and deduced amino acid sequence of human 3β-hydroxy-5-ene steroid dehydrogenase. Mol Endocrinol 3:1310–1312.

53. Lorence MC, Murry BA, Trant JM, Mason JI (1990). Human 3β-hydroxysteroid dehydrogenase/$\Delta^5 \rightarrow \Delta^4$ isomerase from placenta: Expression in nonsteroidogenic cells of a protein that catalyzes the dehydrogenation/isomerization of C21 and C19 steroids. Endocrinology 126:2493–2498.

54. Lee TC, Miller WL, Auchus RJ (1999). Medroxyprogesterone acetate and dexamethasone are competitive inhibitors of different human steroidogenic enzymes. J Clin Endocrinol Metab 84:2104–2110.

55. Lachance Y, Luu-The V, Labrie C, Simard J, Dumont M, de Launoit Y, et al. (1990). Characterization of human 3β-hydroxysteroid dehydrogenase/Δ^5-Δ^4-isomerase gene and its expression in mammalian cells. J Biol Chem 265:20469–20475.

56. Rhéaume E, Lachance Y, Zhao HL, Breton N, Dumont M, de Launoit Y, et al. (1991). Structure and expression of a new complementary DNA encoding the almost exclusive 3β-hydroxysteroid dehydrogenase/Δ^5-Δ^4-isomerase in human adrenals and gonads. Mol Endocrinol 5:1147–1157.

57. Lorence MC, Corbin CJ, Kamimura N, Mahendroo MS, Mason JI (1990). Structural analysis of the gene encoding human 3β-hydroxysteroid dehydrogenase/$\Delta^5 \rightarrow \Delta^4$ isomerase. Mol Endocrinol 4:1850–1855.

58. Cherradi N, Rossier MF, Vallotton MB, Timberg R, Friedberg I, Orly J, et al. (1997). Submitochondrial distribution of three key steroidogenic proteins (steroidogenic acute regulatory protein and cytochrome P450scc and 3β-hydroxysteroid dehydrogenase isomerase enzymes) upon stimulation by intracellular calcium in adrenal glomerulosa cells. J Biol Chem 272:7899–7907.

59. Chapman JC, Polanco JR, Min S, Michael SD (2005). Mitochondrial 3 beta-hydroxysteroid dehydrogenase (HSD) is essential for the synthesis of progesterone by corpora lutea: An hypothesis. Reprod Biol Endocrinol 3:11.

60. Lin D, Black SM, Nagahama Y, Miller WL (1993). Steroid 17α-hydroxylase and 17,20 lyase activities of P450c17: Contributions of serine[106] and P450 reductase. Endocrinology 132:2498–2506.

61. Auchus RJ, Lee TC, Miller WL (1998). Cytochrome b5 augments the 17,20 lyase activity of human P450c17 without direct electron transfer. J Biol Chem 273:3158–3165.

62. Sklar CA, Kaplan SL, Grumbach MM (1980). Evidence for dissociation between adrenarche and gonadarche: Studies in patients with idiopathic precocious puberty, gonadal dysgenesis, isolated gonadotropin deficiency, and constitutionally delayed growth and adolescence. J Clin Endocrinol Metab 51:548–556.

63. Zachmann M, Vollmin JA, Hamilton W, Prader A (1972). Steroid 17,20 desmolase deficiency: A new cause of male pseudohermaphroditism. Clin Endocrinol 1:369–385.

64. Nakajin S, Hall PF (1981). Microsomal cytochrome P450 from neonatal pig testis: Purification and properties of a C21 steroid side-chain cleavage system (17α-hydroxylase-C17,20 lyase). J Biol Chem 256:3871–3876.

65. Nakajin S, Shinoda M, Haniu M, Shively JE, Hall PF (1984). C21 steroid side-chain cleavage enzyme from porcine adrenal microsomes:

Purification and characterization of the 17α-hydroxylase/C$_{17,20}$ lyase cytochrome P450. J Biol Chem 259:3971–3974.

66. Zuber MX, Simpson ER, Waterman MR (1986). Expression of bovine 17α-hydroxylase cytochrome P450 cDNA in non-steroidogenic (COS-1) cells. Science 234:1258–1261.

67. Lin D, Harikrishna JA, Moore CCD, Jones KL, Miller WL (1991). Missense mutation Ser[106]→Pro causes 17α-hydroxylase deficiency. J Biol Chem 266:15992–15998.

68. Matteson KJ, Picado-Leonard J, Chung B, Mohandas TK, Miller WL (1986). Assignment of the gene for adrenal P450c17 (17α-hydroxylase/17,20 lyase) to human chromosome 10. J Clin Endocrinol Metab 63:789–791.

69. Fan YS, Sasi R, Lee C, Winter JSD, Waterman MR, Lin CC (1992). Localization of the human CYP17 gene (cytochrome P450 17α) to 10q24.3 by fluorescence in situ hybridization and simultaneous chromosome banding. Genomics 14:1110–1111.

70. Picado-Leonard J, Miller WL (1987). Cloning and sequence of the human gene encoding P450c17 (steroid 17α-hydroxylase/17,20 lyase): Similarity to the gene for P450c21. DNA 6:439–448.

71. Yamano S, Aoyama T, McBride OW, Hardwick JP, Gelboin HV, Gonzalez FJ (1989). Human NADPH-P450 oxidoreductase: Complementary DNA cloning, sequence, vaccinia virus-mediated expression, and localization of the CYPOR gene to chromosome 7. Mol Pharmacol 35:83–88.

72. Wang M, Roberts DL, Paschke R, Shea TM, Masters BSS, Kim JJP (1997). Three-dimensional structure of NADPH-cytochrome P450 reductase: Prototype for FMN- and FAD-containing enzymes. Proc Natl Acad Sci USA 94:8411–8416.

73. Zhang L, Rodriguez H, Ohno S, Miller WL (1995). Serine phosphorylation of human P450c17 increases 17,20 lyase activity: Implications for adrenarche and for the polycystic ovary syndrome. Proc Natl Acad Sci USA 92:10619–10623.

74. Pandey AV, Mellon SH, Miller WL (2003). Protein phosphatase 2A and phosphoprotein SET regulate androgen production by P450c17. J Biol Chem 278:2837–2844.

75. Pandey AV, Miller WL (2005). Regulation of 17,20 lyase activity by cytochrome b$_5$ and by serine phosphorylation of P450c17. J Biol Chem 280:13265–13271.

76. Yanagibashi K, Hall PF (1986). Role of electron transport in the regulation of the lyase activity of C-21 side-chain cleavage P450 from porcine adrenal and testicular microsomes. J Biol Chem 261:8429–8433.

77. Miller WL, Auchus RJ, Geller DH (1997). The regulation of 17,20 lyase activity. Steroids 62:133–142.

78. Miller WL, Morel Y (1989). Molecular genetics of 21-hydroxylase deficiency. Ann Rev Genet 23:371–393.

79. Morel Y, Miller WL (1991). Clinical and molecular genetics of congenital adrenal hyperplasia due to 21-hydroxylase deficiency. Adv Hum Genet 20:1–68.

80. Speiser PW, White PC (2003). Congenital adrenal hyperplasia. New England J Med 349:776–788.

81. Forest MG (2004). Recent advances in the diagnosis and management of congenital adrenal hyperplasia due to 21-hydroxylase deficiency. Hum Reprod Update 10:469–485.

82. Kominami S, Ochi H, Kobayashi Y, Takemori S (1980). Studies on the steroid hydroxylation system in adrenal cortex microsomes: Purification and characterization of cytochrome P450 specific for steroid 21 hydroxylation. J Biol Chem 255:3386–3394.

83. Higashi Y, Yoshioka H, Yamane M, Gotoh O, Fujii-Kuriyama Y (1986). Complete nucleotide sequence of two steroid 21-hydroxylase genes tandemly arranged in human chromosome: A pseudogene and genuine gene. Proc Natl Acad Sci USA 83:2841–2845.

84. White PC, New MI, Dupont B (1986). Structure of the human steroid 21-hydroxylase genes. Proc Natl Acad Sci USA 83:5111–5115.

85. Rodrigues NR, Dunham I, Yu CY, Carroll MC, Porter RR, Campbell RD (1987). Molecular characterization of the HLA-linked steroid 21-hydroxylase B gene from an individual with congenital adrenal hyperplasia. EMBO J 6:1653–1661.

86. Dupont B, Oberfield SE, Smithwick ER, Lee TD, Levine LS (1977). Close genetic linkage between HLA and congenital adrenal hyperplasia (21-hydroxylase deficiency). Lancet ii:1309–1312.

87. Casey ML, MacDonald PC (1982). Extra-adrenal formation of a mineralocorticoid: Deoxycorticosterone and deoxycorticosterone sulfate biosynthesis and metabolism. Endocr Rev 3:396–403.

88. Mellon SH, Miller WL (1989). Extra-adrenal steroid 21-hydroxylation is not mediated by P450c21. J Clin Invest 84:1497–1502.

89. Yamazaki H, Shimada T (1997). Progesterone and testosterone hydroxylation by cytochromes P450 2C19, 2C9 and 3A4. Arch Biochem Biophys 346:161–169.

90. White PC, Curnow KM, Pascoe L (1994). Disorders of steroid 11β-hydroxylase isozymes. Endocr Rev 15:421–438.

91. Fardella CE, Miller WL (1996). Molecular biology of mineralocorticoid metabolism. Ann Rev Nutrition 16:443–470.

92. Mornet E, Dupont J, Vitek A, White PC (1989). Characterization of two genes encoding human steroid 11β-hydroxylase (P45011β). J Biol Chem 264:20961–20967.

93. Chua SC, Szabo P, Vitek A, Grzeschik K-H, John M, White PC (1987). Cloning of cDNA encoding steroid 11β-hydroxylase, P450c11. Proc Natl Acad Sci USA 84:7193–7197.

94. Curnow KM, Tusie-Luna M, Pascoe L, Natarajan R, Gu J, Nadler JL, et al. (1991). The product of the CYP11B2 gene is required for aldosterone biosynthesis in the human adrenal cortex. Mol Endocrinol 5:1513–1522.

95. Kawamoto T, Mitsuuchi Y, Toda K, Yokoyama Y, Miyahara K, Miura S, et al. (1992). Role of steroid 11β-hydroxylase and 18-hydroxylase in the biosynthesis of glucocorticoids and mineralocorticoids in humans. Proc Natl Acad Sci USA 89:1458–1462.

96. White PC, Dupont J, New MI, Lieberman E, Hochberg Z, Rösler A (1991). A mutation in CYP11B1 (Arg 448→His) associated with steroid 11β-hydroxylase deficiency in Jews of Moroccan origin. J Clin Invest 87:1664–1667.

97. Pascoe L, Curnow K, Slutsker L, Rösler A, White PC (1992). Mutations in the human CYP11B2 (aldosterone synthase) gene causing corticosterone methyloxidase II deficiency. Proc Natl Acad Sci USA 89:4996–5000.

98. Ulick S, Wang JZ, Morton H (1992). The biochemical phenotypes of two inborn errors in the biosynthesis of aldosterone. J Clin Endocrinol Metab 74:1415–1420.

99. Zhang G, Rodriguez H, Fardella CE, Harris DA, Miller WL (1995). Mutation T318M in P450c11AS causes corticosterone methyl oxidase II deficiency. Am J Hum Genet 57:1037–1043.

100. Labrie F, Luu-The V, Lin SX, Labrie C, Simard J, Breton R, Bélanger A (1997). The key role of 17β-hydroxysteroid dehydrogenases in sex steroid biology. Steroids 62:148–158.

101. Moghrabi N, Andersson S (1998). 17β-hydroxysteroid dehydrogenases: Physiological roles in health and disease. Trends Endocrinol Metab 9:265–270.

102. Penning TM (1997). Molecular endocrinology of hydroxysteroid dehydrogenases. Endocr Rev 18:281–305.

103. Peltoketo H, Isomaa V, Mäenlavsta O, Vihko R (1988). Complete amino acid sequence of human placental 17β-hydroxysteroid dehydrogenase deduced from cDNA. FEBS Lett 239:73–77.

104. Gast MJ, Sims HF, Murdock GL, Gast PM, Strauss AW (1989). Isolation and sequencing of a complementary deoxyribonucleic acid clone encoding human placental 17 β-estradiol dehydrogenase: Identification of the putative cofactor binding site. Am J Obstet Gynecol 161:1726–1731.

105. Tremblay Y, Ringler GE, Morel Y, Mohandas TK, Labrie F, Strauss JF III, et al. (1989). Regulation of the gene for estrogenic 17-ketosteroid reductase lying on chromosome 17cen→q25. J Biol Chem 264:20458–20462.

106. Ghosh D, Pleteu VZ, Zhu DW, Wawarzak Z, Duax WL, Plaugborn W, et al. (1995). Structure of human estrogenic 17β-hydroxysteroid dehydrogenase at 2.2 Å resolution. Structure 3:503–513.

107. Sawicki MW, Erman M, Puranen T, Vihko P, Ghosh D (1999). Structure of the ternary complex of human 17β-hydroxysteroid dehydrogenase type 1 with 3-hydroxyestra-1,3,5,7-tetraen-17-one (equilin) and NADP+. Proc Natl Acad Sci USA 96:840–845.

108. Takeyama J, Sasano H, Suzuki T, Iinuma K, Nagura H, Andersson S (1998). 17β-hydroxysteroid dehydrogenase types 1 and 2 in human placenta: An immunohistochemical study with correlation to placental development. J Clin Endocrinol Metab 83:3710–3715.

109. Geissler WM, Davis DL, Wu L, Bradshaw KD, Patel S, Mendonça BB, et al. (1994). Male pseudohermaphroditism caused by mutations of testicular 17β-hydroxysteroid dehydrogenase 3. Nature Genet 7:34–39.

110. Andersson S, Geissler WM, Wu L, Davis DL, Grumbach MM, New MI, et al. (1996). Molecular genetics and pathophysiology of 17 β-hydroxysteroid dehydrogenase 3 deficiency. J Clin Endocrinol Metab 81:130–136.

111. Adamski J, Normand T, Leenders F, Montae D, Begue A, Staehelin D, et al. (1995). Molecular cloning of a novel widely expressed

human 80 kDa 17 β-hydroxysteroid dehydrogenase IV. Biochem J 311:437–443.

112. Leenders F, Tesdorpf JG, Markus M, Engel T, Seedorf U, Adamski J (1996). Porcine 80-kDa protein reveals intrinsic 17 β-hydroxysteroid dehydrogenase, fatty acyl-CoA-hydratase/dehydrogenase, and sterol transfer activities. J Biol Chem 271:5438–5442.

113. van Grunsven EG, van Berkel E, Ijlst L, Vreken P, De Klerk JBC, Adamski J, et al. (1998). Peroxisomal D-hydroxyacyl-CoA dehydrogenase deficiency: Resolution of the enzyme defect and its molecular basis in bifunctional protein deficiency. Proc Natl Acad Sci USA 95:2128–2133.

114. Lin HK, Jez JM, Schlegel BP, Peehl DM, Pachter JA, Penning TM (1997). Expression and characterization of recombinant type 2 3 α-hydroxysteroid dehydrogenase (HSD) from human prostate: demonstration of bifunctional 3 α/17 β-HSD activity and cellular distribution. Mol Endocrinol 11:1971–1984.

115. Dufort I, Rheault P, Huang XF, Soucy P, Luu-The V (1999). Characteristics of a highly labile human type 5 17β-hydroxysteroid dehydrogenase. Endocrinology 140:568–574.

116. Falany CN (1997). Enzymology of human cystolic sulfotransferases. FASEB J 11:206–216.

117. Stroh CA (2002). Sulfonation and molecular action. Endocr Rev 23:703–732.

118. Tong MH, Jiang H, Liu P, Lawson JA, Brass LF, Song W-C (2005). Spontaneous fetal loss caused by placental thrombosis in estrogen sulfutransferase-deficient mice. Nature Medicine 11:153–159.

119. Nowell S, Falany CN (2006). Pharmacogenetics of human cytosolic sulfotransferases. Oncogene 25:1673–1678.

120. Yen PH, Allen E, Marsh B, Mohandas T, Shapiro LJ (1987). Cloning and expression of steroid sulfatase cDNA and the frequent occurrence of deletions: Implications for X-Y interchange. Cell 49:443–454.

121. Ballabio A, Shapiro LJ (1995). Steroid Sulfatase deficiency and X-linked icthiosis. In JL Goldstein, MS Brown, and CR Scriver (eds.), The metabolic and molecular basis of inherited disease. New York: Mc-Graw-Hill 2999–3022.

122. Compagnone NA, Salido E, Shapiro LJ, Mellon SH (1997). Expression of steroid sulfatase during embryogenesis. Endocrinology 138:4768–4773.

123. Compagnone NA, Mellon SH (1998). Dehydroepiandrosterone: A potential signalling molecule for neocortical organization during development. Proc Natl Acad Sci USA 95:4678–4683.

124. Simpson ER, Mahendroo MS, Means GD, Kilgore MW, Hinshelwood MM, Graham-Lorence S, et al. (1994). Aromatase cytochrome P450, the enzyme responsible for estrogen biosynthesis. Endocr Rev 15:342–355.

125. Grumbach MM, Auchus RJ (1999). Estrogen: Consequences and implications of human mutations in synthesis and action. J Clin Endocrinol Metab 84:4677–4694.

126. Ito Y, Fisher CR, Conte FA, Grumbach MM, Simpson ER (1993). Molecular basis of aromatase deficiency in an adult female with sexual infantilism and polycystic ovaries. Proc Natl Acad Sci USA 90:11673–11677.

127. Conte FA, Grumbach MM, Ito Y, Fisher CR, Simpson ER (1994). A syndrome of female pseudohermaphrodism, hypergonadotropic hypogonadism, and multicystic ovaries associated with missense mutations in the gene encoding aromatase (P450arom). J Clin Endocrinol Metab 78:1287–1292.

128. Thigpen AE, Silver RI, Guileyardo JM, Casey ML, McConnell JD, Russell DW (1993). Tissue distribution and ontogeny of steroid 5α-reductase isozyme expression. J Clin Invest 92:903–910.

129. Wilson JD (1999). The role of androgens in male gender role behavior. Endocr Rev 20:726–737.

130. Arriza JL, Weinberger C, Cerelli G, Glaser TM, Handelin BL, Housman DE, et al. (1987). Cloning of human mineralocorticoid receptor DNA: Structural and functional kinship with the glucocorticoid receptor. Science 237:268–275.

131. Funder JW, Pearce PT, Smith R, Smith I (1988). Mineralocorticoid action: Target tissue specificity is enzyme, not receptor, mediated. Science 242:583–585.

132. White PC, Mune T, Agarwal AK (1997). 11β-hydroxysteroid dehydrogenase and the syndrome of apparent mineralocorticoid excess. Endocr Rev 18:135–156.

133. Agarwal AK, Tusie-Luna M-T, Monder C, White PC (1990). Expression of 11β-hydroxysteroid dehydrogenase using recombinant vaccinia virus. Mol Endocrinol 4:1827–1832.

134. Moore CCD, Mellon SH, Murai J, Siiteri PK, Miller WL (1993). Structure and function of the hepatic form of 11β-hydroxysteroid dehydrogenase in the squirrel monkey, an animal model of glucocorticoid resistance. Endocrinology 133:368–375.

135. Brown RW, Chapman KE, Edwards CRW, Seckl JR (1993). Human placental 11 β-hydroxysteroid dehydrogenase: evidence for and partial purification of a distinct NAD+-dependent isoform. Endocrinology 132:2614–2621.

136. Rusvai E, Náray-Fejes-Tóth A (1993). A new isoform of 11β-hydroxysteroid dehydrogenase in aldosterone target cells. J Biol Chem 268:10717–10720.

137. Krozowski Z, MaGuire JA, Stein-Oakley AN, Dowling J, Smith RE, Andrews RK (1995). Immunohistochemical localization of the 11 β-hydroxysteroid dehydrogenase type II enzyme in human kidney and placenta. J Clin Endocrinol Metab 80:2203–2209.

138. Hirasawa G, Sasono H, Suzuki T, Takeyama J, Muramatu Y, Fukushima K, et al. (1999). 11β-hydroxysteroid dehydrogenase type 2 and mineralocorticoid receptor in human fetal development. J Clin Endocrinol Metab 84:1453–1458.

139. Hewitt KN, Walker EA, Stewart PM (2005). Hexose-6-phosphate dehydrogenase and redox control of 11β-hydroxysteroid dehydrogenase type 1 activity. Endocrinology 146:2539–2543.

140. McCormick KL, Wang X, Mick GJ (2006). Evidence that the 11β-hydroxysteroid dehydrogenase (11βHSD-1) is regulated by pentose pathway flux. J Biol Chem 281:341–347.

141. Goto M, Hanley KP, Marcos J, Wood PJ, Wright S, Postle AD, et al. (2006). In humans, early cortisol biosynthesis provides a mechanism to safeguard female sexual development. J Clin Invest 116:953–960.

142. Miller WL, Levine LS (1987). Molecular and clinical advances in congenital adrenal hyperplasia. J Pediatr 111:1–17.

143. Voutilainen R, Ilvesmaki V, Miettinen PJ (1991). Low expression of 3β-hydroxy-5-ene steroid dehydrogenase gene in human fetal adrenals in vivo; adrenocorticotropin and protein kinase C-dependent regulation in adrenocortical cultures. J Clin Endocrinol Metab 72:761–767.

144. Fujieda K, Faiman C, Feyes FI, Winter JSD (1982). The control of steroidogenesis by human fetal adrenal cells in tissue culture: IV. The effects of exposure to placental steroids. J Clin Endocrinol Metab 54:89–94.

145. Miller WL (1998). Steroid hormone biosynthesis and actions in the materno-feto-placental unit. Clin Perinatol 25:799–817.

146. Pasqualini JR, Nguyen BL, Uhrich F, Wiqvist N, Diczfalvay E (1970). Cortisol and cortisone metabolism in the human fetoplacental unit at midgestation. J Steroid Biochem 1:209–219.

147. Kari MA, Raivio KO, Stenman U-H, Voutilainen R (1996). Serum cortisol, dehydroepiandrosterone sulfate, and sterol-binding globulins in preterm neonates: Effects of gestational age and dexamethasone therapy. Pediatr Res 40:319–324.

148. DiBlasio AM, Voutilainen R, Jaffe RB, Miller WL (1987). Hormonal regulation of mRNAs for P450scc (cholesterol side-chain cleavage enzyme) and P450c17 (17α-hydroxylase/17,20 lyase) in cultured human fetal adrenal cells. J Clin Endocrinol Metab 65:170–175.

149. Voutilainen R, Miller WL (1987). Coordinate tropic hormone regulation of mRNAs for insulin-like growth factor II and the cholesterol side-chain cleavage enzyme, P450scc, in human steroidogenic tissues. Proc Natl Acad Sci USA 84:1590–1594.

150. New MI, Wilson RC (1999). Steroid disorders in children: congenital adrenal hyperplasia and apparent mineralocorticoid excess. Proc Natl Acad Sci USA 96:12790–12797.

151. Sawchenko PE, Swanson LW, Vale WW (1984). Co-expression of corticotropin-releasing factor and vasopressin immunoreactivity in parvocellular neurosecretory neurons of the adrenalectomized rat. Proc Natl Acad Sci USA 81:1883–1887.

152. Whitnall MH, Mezey E, Gainer H (1985). Co-localization of corticotropin-releasing factor and vasopressin in median eminence neurosecretory vesicles. Nature 317:248–250.

153. Aguilera G, Harwood JP, Wilson JX, Morell J, Brown JH, Catt KJ (1983). Mechanisms of action of corticotropin-releasing factor and other regulators of corticotropin release in rat pituitary cells. J Biol Chem 258:8039–8045.

154. Miller WL, Johnson LK, Baxter JD, Robert JL (1980). Processing of the precursor to corticotropin and β-lipotropin in man. Proc Natl Acad Sci USA 77:5211–5215.

155. Whitfeld PL, Seeburg PH, Shine J (1982). The human pro-opiomelanocortin gene: Organization, sequence, and interspersion with repetitive DNA. DNA 1:133–143.

156. Lowry PJ, Silas L, McLean C, Linton EA, Estivariz FE (1983). Pro-gamma-melanocyte-stimulating hormone cleavage in adrenal gland undergoing compensatory growth. Nature 306:70–73.

157. Lundblad JR, Roberts JL (1988). Regulation of proopiomelanocortin gene expression in pituitary. Endocr Rev 9:135–158.

158. Strauss JF, III, Miller WL (1991). Molecular basis of ovarian steroid synthesis. In SG Hillier (eds.), *Ovarian endocrinology.* Oxford (UK): Blackwell Scientific 25–72.

159. Jefcoate CR, McNamara BC, DiBartolomeis MS (1986). Control of steroid synthesis in adrenal fasciculata. Endocr Res 12:315–350.

160. Anderson RA, Sando GN (1991). Cloning and expression of cDNA encoding human lysosomal acid lypase/cholesterol ester hydrolase. J Biol Chem 266:22479–22484.

161. Miller WL, Strauss III JF (1999). Molecular pathology and mechanism of action of the steroidogenic acute regulatory protein, StAR. J Steroid Biochem Mol Biol 69:131–141.

162. Ehrhart-Bornstein M, Hinson JP, Bornstein SR, Scherbaum WA, Vinson GP (1998). Intraadrenal interactions in the regulation of adrenocortical steroidogenesis. Endocr Rev 19:101–143.

163. Dallman MF (1985). Control of adrenocortical growth in vivo. Endocr Rev 10:213–242.

164. Townsend S, Dallman MF, Miller WL (1990). Rat insulin-like growth factors-I and -II mRNAs are unchanged during compensatory adrenal growth but decrease during ACTH-induced adrenal growth. J Biol Chem 265:22117–22122.

165. Krude H, Biebermann H, Luck W, Horn R, Brabant G, Gruters A (1998). Severe early-onset obesity, adrenal insufficiency and red hair pigmentation caused by POMC mutations in humans. Nat Genet 19:155–157.

166. Yaswen L, Diehl N, Brennan MB, Hochgeschwender U (1999). Obesity in the mouse model of pro-opiomelanocortin deficiency responds to peripheral melanocortin. Nature Medicine 5:1066–1070.

167. Voutilainen R, Miller WL (1988). Developmental and hormonal regulation of mRNAs for insulin-like growth factor and steroidogenic enzymes in human fetal adrenals and gonads. DNA 7:9–15.

168. Mesiano S, Mellon SH, Gospodarowicz D, Di Blasio AM, Jaffe RB (1991). Basic fibroblast growth factor expression is regulated by corticotropin in the human fetal adrenal: A model for adrenal growth regulation. Proc Natl Acad Sci USA 88:5428–5432.

169. Mesiano S, Mellon SH, Jaffe RB (1993). Mitogenic action, regulation, and localization of insulin-like growth factors in the human fetal adrenal gland. J Clin Endocrinol Metab 76:968–976.

170. Mesiano S, Jaffe RB (1997). Role of growth factors in the developmental regulation of the human fetal adrenal cortex. Steroids 62:62–72.

171. Moore-Ede MC, Czeisler CA, Richardson GS (1983). Circadian timekeeping in health and disease. Part 1. Basic properties of circadian pacemakers. New England J Med 309:469–476.

172. Follenius M, Brandenberger G, Hietter B (1982). Diurnal cortisol peaks and their relationships to meals. J Clin Endocrinol Metab 55:757–761.

173. Goldman J, Wajchenberg BL, Liberman B, Nery M, Achando S, Germek OA (1985). Contrast analysis for the evaluation of the circadian rhythms of plasma cortisol, androstenedione, and testosterone in normal men and the possible influence of meals. J Clin Endocrinol Metab 60:164–167.

174. Quigley ME, Yen SS (1979). A mid-day surge in cortisol levels. J Clin Endocrinol Metab 49:945–947.

175. Wallace WH, Crowne EC, Shalet SM, Moore C, Gibson S, Littley MD, et al. (1991). Episodic ACTH and cortisol secretion in normal children. Clin Endocrinol (Oxford) 34:215–221.

176. Onishi S, Miyazawa G, Nishimura Y, Sugiyama S, Yamakawa T, Inagaki H, et al. (1983). Postnatal development of circadian rhythm in serum cortisol levels in children. Pediatrics 72:399–404.

177. Dempsher DP, Gann DS (1983). Increased cortisol secretion after small hemorrhage is not attributable to changes in adrenocorticotropin. Endocrinology 113:86–93.

178. Udelsman R, Norton JA, Jelenich SE, Goldstein DS, Linehan WM, Loriaux DL, et al. (1987). Responses of the hypothalamic-pituitary-adrenal and renin-angiotensin axes and the sympathetic system during controlled surgical and anesthetic stress. J Clin Endocrinol Metab 64:986–994.

179. Chrousos GP (1995). The hypothalamic-pituitary-adrenal axis and immune-mediated inflammation. N Engl J Med 332:1351–1362.

180. Keller-Wood ME, Dallman MF (1984). Corticosteroid inhibition of ACTH secretion. Endocr Rev 5:1–24.

181. Deschepper CF, Mellon SH, Cumin F, Baxter JD, Ganong WF (1986). Analysis by immunocytochemistry and in situ hybridization of renin and its mRNA in kidney, testis, adrenal, and pituitary of the rat. Proc Natl Acad Sci USA 83:7552–7556.

182. Sander M, Ganten D, Mellon SH (1994). Role of adrenal renin in the regulation of adrenal steroidogenesis by ACTH. Proc Natl Acad Sci USA 91:148–152.

183. Hardman JA, Hort YJ, Catanzaro DF, Tellam JT, Baxter JD, Morris BJ, et al. (1984). Primary structure of the human renin gene. DNA 3:457–468.

184. Kramer RE, Gallant S, Brownie AC (1980). Actions of angiotensin II on aldosterone biosynthesis in the rat adrenal cortex. J Biol Chem 255:3442–3447.

185. McKenna TJ, Island DP, Nicholson WE, Liddle GW (1978). The effects of potassium on early and late steps in aldosterone biosynthesis in cells of the zona glomerulosa. Endocrinology 105:1411–1416.

186. Farese RV, Larson RE, Sabir MA, Gomez-Sanchez CE (1983). Effects of angiotensin II, K^+, adrenocorticotropin, serotonin, adenosine 3',5'-monophosphate, A23187, and EGTA on aldosterone synthesis and phospholipid metabolism in the rat adrenal zona glomerulosa. Endocrinology 113:1377–1386.

187. Barrett PQ, Bollag WB, Isales CM, McCarthy RT, Rasmussen H (1989). The role of calcium in angiotensin II-mediated aldosterone secretion. Endocrin Rev 10:496–518.

188. Moore CCD, Brentano ST, Miller WL (1990). Human P450scc gene transcription is induced by cyclic AMP and repressed by 12-O-tetradecanolyphorbol-13-acetate and A23187 by independent cis-elements. Mol Cell Biol 10:6013–6023.

189. Gullner HG, Gill JR Jr. (1983). Beta endorphin selectively stimulates aldosterone secretion in hypophysectomized, nephrectomized dogs. J Clin Invest 71:124–128.

190. Yamakado M, Franco-Saenz R, Mulrow PJ (1983). Effect of sodium deficiency on beta-melanocyte-stimulating hormone stimulation of aldosterone in isolated rat adrenal cells. Endocrinology 113:2168–2172.

191. Atarashi K, Mulrow PJ, Franco-Saenz R (1985). Effect of atrial peptides on aldosterone production. J Clin Invest 76:1807–1811.

192. Orentreich N, Brind JL, Rizer RL, Vogelman JH (1984). Age changes and sex differences in serum dehydroepiandrosterone sulfate concentrations throughout adulthood. J Clin Endocrinol Metab 59:551–555.

193. Mellon SH, Shively JE, Miller WL (1991). Human proopiomelanocortin (79-96), a proposed androgen stimulatory hormone, does not affect steroidogenesis in cultured human fetal adrenal cells. J Clin Endocrinol Metab 72:19–22.

194. Penhoat A, Sanchez P, Jaillard C, Langlois D, Begeot M, Saez JM (1991). Human proopiomelanocortin (79-96), a proposed cortical androgen stimulating hormone, does not affect steroidogenesis in cultured human adult adrenal cells. J Clin Endocrinol Metab 72:23–26.

195. Arlt W, Martens JWM, Song M, Wang JT, Auchus RJ, Miller WL (2002). Molecular evolution of adrenarche: Structural and functional analysis of P450c17 from four primate species. Endocrinology 143:4665–4672.

196. Endoh A, Kristiansen SB, Casson PR, Buster JE, Hornsby PJ (1996). The zona reticularis is the site of biosynthesis of dehydroepiandrosterone and dehydroepiandrosterone sulfate in the adult human adrenal cortex resulting from its low expression of 3β-hydroxysteroid dehydrogenase. J Clin Endocrinol Metab 81:3558–3565.

197. Gell JS, Carr BR, Sasano H, Atkins B, Margraf L, Mason JI, et al. (1998). Adrenarche results from development of a 3β-hydroxysteroid dehydrogenase-deficient adrenal reticularis. J Clin Endocrinol Metab 83:3695–3701.

198. Dardis A, Saraco N, Rivarola MA, Belgorosky A (1999). Decrease in the expression of the 3β-hydroxysteroid dehydrogenase gene in human adrenal tissue during prepuberty and early puberty: Implications for the mechanism of adrenarche. Pediatr Res 45:384–388.

199. Yanase T, Sasano H, Yubisui T, Sakai Y, Takayanagi R, Nawata H (1998). Immunohistochemical study of cytochrome b₅ in human adrenal gland and in adrenocortical adenomas from patients with Cushing's syndrome. Endocr J 45:89–95.

200. Mapes S, Corbin CJ, Tarantal A, Conley A (1999). The primate adrenal zona reticularis is defined by expression of cytochrome b$_5$, 17α-hydroxylase/17,20-lyase cytochrome P450 (P450c17) and NADPH-cytochrome P450 reductase (reductase) but not 3β-hydroxysteroid dehydrogenase/Δ5-4 isomerase (3β-HSD). J Clin Endocrinol Metab 84:3382–3385.

201. Miller WL (1999). The molecular basis of premature adrenarche: An hypothesis. Acta Pediatrica Suppl 433:60–66.

202. Ibañez L, Potau N, Virdis R, Zampolli M, Terzi C, Gussinyé M, et al. (1993). Postpubertal outcome in girls diagnosed of premature pubarche during childhood: Increased frequency of functional ovarian hyperandrogenism. J Clin Endocrinol Metab 76:1599–1603.

203. Oppenheimer E, Linder B, DiMartino-Nardi J (1995). Decreased insulin sensitivity in prepubertal girls with premature adrenarche and acanthosis nigricans. J Clin Endocrinol Metab 80:614–618.

204. Ibañez L, Potau N, Zampolli M, Prat N, Virdis R, Vicnes-Calvert E, Carrascosa A (1996). Hyperinsulinemia in postpubertal girls with a history of premature pubarche and functional ovarian hyperandrogenism. J Clin Endocrinol Metab 81:1237–1243.

205. Ibañez L, Potau N, Marcos MV, de Zegher F (1998). Exaggerated adrenarche and hyperinsulinism in adolescent girls born small for gestational age. J Clin Endocrinol Metab 84:4739–4741.

206. Arlt W, Callies F, van Vlijmen JC, Koehler I, Reincke M, Bidlingmaier M, et al. (1999). Dehydroepiandrosterone replacement in women with adrenal insufficiency. New England J Med 341:1013–1020.

207. Nair KS, Rizza RA, O'Brien P, Dhatariya K, Short KR, Nehra A, et al. (2006). DHEA in elderly women and DHEA or testosterone in eldery men. New England J Med 355:1647–1659.

208. Zumoff B, Fukushima DK, Hellman L (1974). Intercomparison of four methods for measuring cortisol production. J Clin Endocrinol Metab 38:169–175.

209. Hammond GL (1990). Molecular properties of corticosteroid binding globulin and the sex-steroid binding proteins. Endocr Rev 11:65–79.

210. Rosner W (1990). The functions of corticosteroid-binding globulin and sex hormone-binding globulin: Recent advances. Endocr Rev 11:80–91.

211. Shackleton CH, Gustafsson JA, Mitchell FL (1973). Steroids in newborns and infants: The changing pattern of urinary steroid excretion during infancy. Acta Endocrinol (Copenh) 74:157–167.

212. Stewart PM, Corrie JET, Shackleton CHL, Edwards CRW (1988). Syndrome of apparent mineralocorticoid excess: A defect in the cortisol-cortisone shuttle. J Clin Invest 82:340–349.

213. Fu GK, Lin D, Zhang MYH, Bikle DD, Shackleton CHL, Miller WL, et al. (1997). Cloning of human 25-hydroxy vitamin D-1α-hydroxylase and mutations causing vitamin D-dependant rickets type I. Mol Endocrinol 11:1961–1970.

214. Weitzman ED, Fukushima D, Nogeire C, Roffwarg H, Gallagher TF, Hellman L (1971). Twenty-four hour pattern of the episodic secretion of cortisol in normal subjects. J Clin Endocrinol Metab 33:14–22.

215. Veldhuis JD, Iranmanesh A, Johnson ML, Lizarralde G (1990). Amplitude, but not frequency, modulation of adrenocorticotropin secretory bursts gives rise to the nyctohemeral rhythm of the corticotropic axis in man. J Clin Endocrinol Metab 71:452–463.

216. Laragh JH, Sealey J, Brunner HR (1972). The control of aldosterone secretion in normal and hypertensives man abnormal renin aldosterone patterns in low renin hypertension. Am J Med 53:649–663.

217. Porter CC, Silber RH (1950). A quantitative color reaction for cortisone and related 17,21-dihydroxy-ketosteroids. J Biol Chem 185:201–207.

218. Dimitriou T, Maser-Gluth C, Remer T (2003). Adrenocortical activity in healthy children is associated with fat mass. Am J Clin Nutr 77:731–736.

219. Remer T, Maser-Gluth C, Boye KR, Hartmann MF, Heinze E, Wudy SA (2006). Exaggerated adrenarche and altered cortisol metabolism in Type 1 diabetic children. Steroids 71:591–598.

220. Styne DM, Grumbach MM, Kaplan SL, Wilson CB, Conte FA (1984). Treatment of Cushing's disease in childhood and adolescence by transcriptional microadenomectomy. New England J Med 310:889–894.

221. Appleby JI, Gibson G, Normyberski JK, Stubbs RD (1955). Indirect analysis of corticosteroids: The determination of 17-hydroxycorticosteroids. Biochem J 60:453–460.

222. Raff H, Findling JW (1989). A new immunoradiometric assay for corticotropin evaluated in normal subjects and patients with Cushing's syndrome. Clin Chem 35:596–600.

223. Gibson S, Crosby SR, White A (1993). Discrimination between beta-endorphin and beta-lipotrophin in human plasma using two-site immunoradiometric assays. Clin Endocrinol (Oxford) 39:445–453.

224. Linder BL, Esteban NV, Yergey AL, Winterer JC, Loriaux DL, Cassorla F (1990). Cortisol production rate in childhood and adolescence. J Pediatr 117:892–896.

225. Kerrigan JR, Veldhuis JD, Leyo SA, Iranmanes HA, Rogol AD (1993). Estimation of daily cortisol production and clearance rates in normal pubertal males by deconvolution analysis. J Clin Endocrinol Metab 76:1505–1510.

226. Liddle GW (1960). Tests of pituitary-adrenal suppressibility in the diagnosis of Cushing's syndrome. J Clin Endocrinol Metab 20:1539–1560.

227. Tyrrell JB, Findling JW, Aron DC, Fitzgerald PA, Forsham PH (1986). An overnight high-dose dexamethasone suppression test for rapid differential diagnosis of Cushing's syndrome. Ann Intern Med 104:180–186.

228. Hindmarsh PC, Brook CG (1985). Single dose dexamethasone suppression test in children: Dose relationship to body size. Clin Endocrinol (Oxford) 23:67–70.

229. Dickstein G, Shechner C, Nicholson WE, Rosner I, Shen-Orr Z, Adawi F, et al. (1991). Adrenocorticotropin stimulation test: effects of basal cortisol level, time of day, and suggested new sensitive low dose test. J Clin Endocrinol Metab 72:773–778.

230. Lashansky G, Saenger P, Fishman K, Gautier T, Mayes D, Berg G, et al. (1991). Normative data for adrenal steroidogenesis in a healthy pediatric population: Age and sex-related changes after ACTH stimulation. J Clin Endocrinol Metab 73:674–686.

231. Crowley S, Hindmarsh PC, Holownia P, Honour JW, Brook CG (1991). The use of low doses of ACTH in the investigation of adrenal function in man. J Endocrinol 130:475–479.

232. New MI, Lorenzen F, Lerner AJ, Kohn B, Oberfield S, Pollack M, et al. (1983). Genotyping steroid 21-hydroxylase deficiency: Hormonal reference data. J Clin Endocrinol Metab 57:320–326.

233. Clark AJ, Weber A (1998). Adrenocorticotropin insensitivity syndromes. Endocr Rev 19:828–843.

234. Shah A, Stanhope R, Matthew D (1992). Hazards of pharmacological tests of growth hormone secretion in childhood. Brit Med J 304:173–174.

235. Avgerinos PC, Yanovski JA, Oldfield EH, Nieman LK, Cutler GB Jr. (1994). The metyrapone and dexamethasone suppression tests for the differential diagnosis of the adrenocorticotropin-dependent Cushing syndrome: A comparison. Ann Intern Med 121:318–327.

236. Spiger M, Jubiz W, Meikle AW, West CD, Tylor FH (1975). Single-dose metyrapone test: Review of a four-year experience. Arch Intern Med 135:698–700.

237. Chrousos GP, Schuermeyer TH, Doppman J, Oldfield EH, Schulte HM, Gold PW, et al. (1985). NIH conference: Clinical applications of corticotropin-releasing factor. Ann Intern Med 102:344–358.

238. Riddick L, Chrousos GP, Jeffries S, Pang S (1994). Comparison of adrenocorticotropin and adrenal steroid responses to corticotropin-releasing hormone versus metyrapone testing in patients with hypopituitarism. Pediatr Res 36:215–220.

239. Sandison AT (1955). A form of lipoidosis of the adrenal cortex in an infant. Arch Dis Childh 30:538–541.

240. Prader A, Siebenmann RE (1957). Nebenniereninsuffizienz bie kongenitaler Lipoidhyperplasie der Nebennieren. Helv Paed Acta 12:569–595.

241. Kirkland RT, Kirkland JL, Johnson CM, Horning MG, Librik L, Clayton GW (1973). Congenital lipoid adrenal hyperplasia in an eight-year-old phenotypic female. J Clin Endocrinol Metab 36:488–496.

242. Hauffa BP, Miller WL, Grumbach MM, Conte FA, Kaplan SL (1985). Congenital adrenal hyperplasia due to deficient cholesterol side-chain cleavage activity (20,22 desmolase) in a patient treated for 18 years. Clin Endocrinol (Oxford) 23:481–493.

243. Camacho AM, Kowarski A, Migeon CJ, Brough A (1968). Congenital adrenal hyperplasia due to a deficiency of one of the enzymes involved in the biosynthesis of pregnenolone. J Clin Endocrinol Metab 28:153–161.

244. Degenhart HJ, Visser KHA, Boon H, O'Doherty NJD (1972). Evidence for deficiency of 20α cholesterol hydroxylase activity in adrenal tissue of a patient with lipoid adrenal hyperplasia. Acta Endocrinologia 71:512–518.

245. Koizumi S, Kyoya S, Miyawaki T, Kidani H, Funabashi T, Nakashima H, et al. (1977). Cholesterol side-chain cleavage enzyme activity and cytochrome P450 content in adrenal mitochondria of a patient with congenital lipoid adrenal hyperplasia (Prader disease). Clin Chim Acta 77:301–306.

246. Matteson KJ, Chung B, Urdea MS, Miller WL (1986). Study of cholesterol side chain cleavage (20,22 desmolase) deficiency causing congenital lipoid adrenal hyperplasia using bovine-sequence P450scc oligodeoxyribonucleotide probes. Endocrinology 118:1296–1305.

247. Lin D, Gitelman SE, Saenger P, Miller WL (1991). Normal genes for the cholesterol side chain cleavage enzyme, P450scc, in congenital lipoid adrenal hyperplasia. J Clin Invest 88:1955–1962.

248. Saenger P, Klonari Z, Black SM, Compagnone N, Mellon SH, Fleischer A, et al. (1995). Prenatal diagnosis of congenital lipoid adrenal hyperplasia. J Clin Endocrinol Metab 80:200–205.

249. Tee MK, Lin D, Sugawara T, Holt JA, Guiguen Y, Buckingham B, et al. (1995). T→A transversion 11 bp from a splice acceptor site in the gene for steroidogenic acute regulatory protein causes congenital lipoid adrenal hyperplasia. Hum Mol Genet 4:2299–2305.

250. Miller WL (1997). Congenital lipoid adrenal hyperplasia: The human gene knockout of the steroidogenic acute regulatory protein. J Mol Endocrinol 19:227–240.

251. Voutilainen R, Miller WL (1986). Developmental expression of genes for the steroidogenic enzymes P450scc (20,22 desmolase), P450c17 (17α-hydroxylase/17,20 lyase) and P450c21 (21-hydroxylase) in the human fetus. J Clin Endocrinol Metab 63:1145–1150.

252. Ogata T, Matsuo N, Saito M, Prader A (1989). The testicular lesion and sexual differentiation in congenital lipoid adrenal hyperplasia. Helv Paediatr Acta 43:531–538.

253. Chen X, Baker BY, Abduljabbar MA, Miller WL (2005). A genetic isolate of congenital lipoid adrenal hyperplasia with atypical clinical findings. J Clin Endocrinol Metab 90:835–840.

254. Bose HS, Pescovitz OH, Miller WL (1997). Spontaneous feminization in a 46,XX female patient with congenital lipoid adrenal hyperplasia caused by a homozygous frame-shift mutation in the steroidogenic acute regulatory protein. J Clin Endocrinol Metab 82:1511–1515.

255. Fujieda K, Tajima T, Nakae J, Sageshima S, Tachibana K, Suwa S, et al. (1997). Spontaneous puberty in 46,XX subjects with congenital lipoid adrenal hypreplasia. J Clin Invest 99:1265–1271.

256. Hasegawa T, Zhao L, Caron KM, Majdic G, Suzuki T, Shizawa S, et al. (2000). Developmental roles of the steroidogenic acute regulatory protein (StAR) as revealed by StAR knockout mice. Mol Endocrinol 14:1462–1471.

257. Nakae J, Tajima T, Sugawara T, Arakane F, Hanaki K, Hotsubo T, et al. (1997). Analysis of the steroidogenic acute regulatory protein (StAR) gene in Japanese patients with congenital lipoid adrenal hyperplasia. Hum Mol Genet 6:571–576.

258. Yoo HW, Kim GH (1998). Molecular and clinical characterization of Korean patients with congenital lipoid adrenal hyperplasia. J Pediatr Endocrinol Metab 11:707–711.

259. Bose HS, Sato S, Aisenberg J, Shalev SA, Matsuo N, Miller WL (2000). Mutations in the steroidogenic acute regulatory protein (StAR) in six patients with congenital lipoid adrenal hyperplasia. J Clin Endocrinol Metab 85:3636–3639.

260. Flück CE, Maret A, Mallet D, Portrat-Doyen S, Achermann JC, Leheup B, et al. (2005). A novel mutation L260P of the steroidogenic acute regulatory protein gene in three unrelated patients of Swiss ancestry with congenital lipoid adrenal hyperplasia. J Clin Endocrinol Metab 90:5304–5308.

261. Arakane F, Sugawara T, Nishino H, Liu Z, Holt JA, Pain D, et al. (1996). Steroidogenic acute regulatory protein (StAR) retains activity in the absence of its mitochondrial targeting sequence: Implications for the mechanism of StAR action. Proc Natl Acad Sci USA 93:13731–13736.

262. Gassner HL, Toppari J, Quinteiro Gonzalez S, Miller WL (2004). Near-miss apparent SIDS from adrenal crisis. J Pediatr 145:178–183.

263. Baker BY, Lin L, Kim CJ, Raza L, Smith CP, Miller WL, et al. (2006). Non-classic congenital lipoid adrenal hyperplasia: A new disorder of the steroidogenic acute regulatory protein with very late presentation and normal male genitalia. J Clin Endocrinol Metab 91:4781–4785.

264. Tajima T, Fujieda K, Kouda N, Nakae J, Miller WL (2001). Heterozygous mutation in the cholesterol side chain cleavage enzyme (P450scc) gene in a patient with 46,XY sex reversal and adrenal insufficiency. J Clin Endocrinol Metab 86:3820–3825.

265. Katsumata N, Ohtake M, Hojo T, Ogawa E, Hara T, Sato N, Tanaka T (2002). Compound heterozygous mutations in the cholesterol side-chain cleavage enzyme gene (CYP11A) cause congenital adrenal insufficiency in humans. J Clin Endocrinol Metab 87:3808–3813.

266. Hiort O, Holterhus P-M, Werner R, Marschke C, Hoppe U, Partsch J, et al. (2005). Homozygous disruption of P450 side-chain cleavage (CYP11A1) is associated with prematurity, complete 46,XY sex reversal, and severe adrenal failure. J Clin Endocrinol Metab 90:538–541.

267. al Kandari H, Katsumata N, Alexander S, Rasoul MA (2006). Homozygous mutation of P450 side-chain cleavage enzyme gene (CYP11A1) in 46,XY patient with adrenal insufficiency, complete sex reversal, and agenesis of corpus callosum. J Clin Endocrinol Metab 91:2821–2826.

268. Miller WL (1998). Why nobody has P450scc (20, 22 desmolase) deficiency (letter). J Clin Endocrinol Metab 83:1399–1400.

269. Achermann JC, Ito M, Ito M, Hindmarsh PC, Jameson JL (1999). A mutation in the gene encoding steroidogenic factor-1 causes XY sex reversal and adrenal failure in humans. Nat Genet 22:125–126.

270. Biason-Lauber A, Schoenle EJ (2000). Apparently normal ovarian differentiation in a prepubertal girl with transcriptionally inactive steroidogenic factor 1 (NR5A1/SF-1) and adrenocortical insufficiency. Am J Hum Genet 67:1563–1568.

271. Achermann JC, Ozisik G, Ito M, Orun UA, Harmanci K, Gurakan B, et al. (2002). Gonadal determination and adrenal development are regulated by the orphan nuclear receptor steroidogenic factor-1, in a dose-dependent manner. J Clin Endocrinol Metab 87:1829–1833.

272. Bongiovanni AM, Kellenbenz G. (1962). The adrenogenital syndrome with deficiency of 3β-hydroxysteroid dehydrogenase. J Clin Invest 41:2086–2092.

273. Lachance Y, Luu-The V, Verreault H, Dumont M, Leblanc G, Labrie F (1991). Characterization and expression of human type II 3β hydroxysteroid dehydrogenase /Δ5-Δ4 isomerase (3β-HSD) gene, the almost exclusive 3β-HSD species expressed in the adrenals and gonads. DNA Cell Biol 10:701–711.

274. Rhéaume E, Lachance Y, Zhao H, Boeton N, Dumont M, DeLaunoit Y, et al. (1991). Structure and expression of a new cDNA encoding the major 3β-hydroxysteroid dehydrogenase/Δ5-Δ4 isomerase. Mol Endocrinol 5:1147–1157.

275. Rhéaume E, Simard J, Morel Y, Mebarki F, Zachmann M, Forest MG, et al. (1992). Congenital adrenal hyperplasia due to point mutations in the type II 3β-hydroxysteroid dehydrogenase gene. Nat Genet 1:239–245.

276. Chang YT, Kappy MS, Iwamoto K, Wang X, Pang S (1993). Mutations in the type II 3β-hydroxysteroid dehydrogenase gene in a patient with classic salt-wasting 3β-HSD deficiency congenital adrenal hyperplasia. Pediatr Res 34:698–700.

277. Simard J, Rhéaume E, Sanchez R, Laflamme N, de Launoit Y, Luu-The V, et al. (1993). Molecular basis of congenital adrenal hyperplasia due to 3β-hydroxysteroid dehydrogenase deficiency. Mol Endocrinol 7:716–728.

278. Morel Y, Mébarke F, Rhéaume E, Sanchez R, Forest MG, Simard J (1997). Structure-function relationships of 3β-hydroxysteroid dehydrogenase: Contribution made by the molecular genetics of 3β-hydroxysteroid dehydrogenase deficiency. Steroids 62:176–184.

279. Moisan AM, Ricketts ML, Tardy V, Desrochers M, Mebarki F, Chaussain JL, et al. (1999). New insight into the molecular basis of 3β-hydroxysteroid dehydrogenase deficiency: identification of eight mutations in the HSD3B2 gene eleven patients from seven new families and comparison of the functional properties of twenty-five mutant enzymes. J Clin Endocrinol Metab 84:4410–4425.

280. Cara JF, Moshang T Jr., Bongiovanni AM, Marx BS (1985). Elevated 17-hydroxy-progesterone and testosterone in a newborn with 3β-hydroxysteroid dehydrogenase deficiency. New Engl J Med 313:618–621.

281. Pang S, Carbunaru G, Haider A, Copeland KC, Chang YT, Lutfallah C, et al. (2003). Carriers for type II 3β-hydroxysteroid dehydrogenase (HSD3B2) deficiency can only be identified by HSD3B2 genotype study and not by hormone test. Clin Endocrinol 58:323–331.

282. Rosenfield RL, Rich BH, Wolfsdorf JI, Cassorla F, Parks JS, Bongiovanni AM, et al. (1980). Pubertal presentation of congenital Δ5-3β hydroxysteroid dehydrogenase deficiency. J Clin Endocrinol Metab 51:345–353.

283. Pang S, Levine LS, Stoner E, Opitz JM, Pollack MS, Dupont B, et al. (1983). Nonsalt-losing congenital adrenal hyperplasia due to

3β-hydroxysteroid dehydrogenase deficiency with normal glomerulosa function. J Clin Endocrinol Metab 56:808–818.

284. Pang SY, Lerner AJ, Stoner E, Levine LS, Oberfield SE, Engel I, et al. (1985). Late-onset adrenal steroid 3β-hydroxysteroid dehydrogenase deficiency. I. A cause of hirsutism in pubertal and postpubertal women. J Clin Endocrinol Metab 60:428–439.

285. Chang YT, Zhang L, Alkaddour HS, Mason JI, Lin K, Yang X, et al. (1995). Absence of molecular defect in the Type II 3β-hydroxysteroid dehydrogenase (3β-HSD) gene in premature pubarche children and hirsute female patients with moderately decreased adrenal 3β-HSD activity. Pediatr Res 37:820–824.

286. Sakkal-Alkaddour H, Zhang L, Yang X, Chang YT, Kappy M, Slover RS, et al. (1996). Studies of 3β-hydroxysteroid dyhydrogenase genes in infants and children manifesting premature pubarche and increased adrenocorticotropin-stimulated Δ⁵-steroid levels. J Clin Endocrinol Metab 81:3961–3965.

287. Pang S (1998). The molecular and clinical spectrum of 3β-hydroxysteroid dehydrogenase deficiency disorder. Trends Endocrinol Metab 9:82–86.

288. Lutfallah C, Wang W, Mason JI, Chang YT, Haider A, Rich B, et al. (2002). Newly proposed hormonal criteria via genotypic proof for type II 3β-hydroxysteroid dehydrogenase deficiency. J Clin Endocrinol Metab 87:2611–2622.

289. Auchus RJ (2001). The genetics, pathophysiology, and management of human deficiencies of P450c17. Endocrinol Metab Clin North America 30:101–119.

290. Costa-Santos M, Kater CE, Auchus RJ (2004). Two prevalent CYP17 mutations and genotype-phenotype correlations in 24 Brazilian patients with 17-hydroxylase deficiency. J Clin Endocrinol Metab 89:49–60.

291. Voutilainen R, Tapanainen J, Chung B, Matteson KJ, Miller WL (1986). Hormonal regulation of P450scc (20,22-desmolase) and P450c17 (17α-hydroxylase/17,20-lyase) in cultured human granulosa cells. J Clin Endocrinol Metab 63:202–207.

292. Scaroni C, Opocher G, Mantero F (1986). Renin-angiotensin-aldosterone system: A long-term follow-up study in 17α-hydroxylase deficiency syndrome. Hypertension (Clin Exp Theory Pract) A8: 773–780.

293. Biglieri EG, Herron MA, Brust N (1966). 17α-hydroxylation deficiency in man. J Clin Invest 15:1945–1954.

294. New MI, Suvannakul L (1970). Male pseudohermaphroditism due to 17α-hydroxylase deficiency. J Clin Invest 49:1930–1941.

295. Imai T, Yanase T, Waterman MR, Simpson ER, Pratt JJ (1992). Canadian Mennonites and individuals residing in the Friesland region of the Netherlands share the same molecular basis of 17α-hydroxylase deficiency. Hum Genet 89:95–96.

296. Lam CW, Arlt W, Chan CK, Honour JW, Lin CJ, Tong SF, et al. (2001). Mutation of proline 409 to arginine in the meander region of cytochrome P450c17 causes severe 17α-hydroxylase deficiency. Mol Genet Metab 72:254–259.

297. Miura K, Yasuda K, Yanase T, Yamakita N, Sasano H, Nawata H, et al. (1996). Mutation of cytochrome P-45017 α gene (CYP17) in a Japanese patient previously reported as having glucocorticoid-responsive hyperaldosteronism: With a review of Japanese patients with mutations of CYP17. J Clin Endocrinol Metab 81:3797–3801.

298. Yanase T, Simpson ER, Waterman MR (1991). 17α-hydroxylase/17,20 lyase deficiency: From clinical investigation to molecular definition. Endocr Rev 12:91–108.

299. Yanase T, Waterman MR, Zachmann M, Winter JSD, Simpson ER, Kagimoto M (1992). Molecular basis of apparent isolated 17,20-lyase deficiency: Compound heterozygous mutations in the C-terminal region (Arg496→Cys, Gln461→Stop) actually cause combined 17α-hydroxylase/17,20-lyase deficiency. Biochim Biophys Acta 1139:275–279.

300. Zachmann M, Kenpken B, Manella B, Navarro E (1992). Conversion from pure 17,20 desmolase to combined 17,20-desmolase/17α-hydroxylase deficiency with age. Acta Endocrinol (Copenh.) 127:97–99.

301. Geller DH, Auchus RJ, Mendonça BB, Miller WL (1997). The genetic and functional basis of isolated 17,20 lyase deficiency. Nat Genet 17:201–205.

302. Geller DH, Auchus RJ, Miller WL (1999). P450c17 mutations R347H and R358Q selectively disrupt 17,20-lyase activity by disrupting interactions with P450 oxidoreductase and cytochrome b₅. Mol Endocrinol 13:167–175.

303. VanDenAkker EL, Koper JW, Boehmer AL, Themmen AP, Verhoef-Post M, Timmerman MA, et al. (2002). Differential inhibition of 17α-hydroxylase and 17,20 lyase activities by three novel missense CYP17 mutations identified in patients with P450c17 deficiency. J Clin Endocrinol Metab 87:5714–5721.

304. Sherbet DP, Tiosano D, Kwist KM, Hochberg Z, Auchus RJ (2003). CYP17 mutation E305G causes isolated 17,20 lyase deficiency by selectively altering substrate binding. J Biol Chem 278:48563–48569.

305. Auchus RJ, Miller WL (1999). Molecular modeling of human P450c17 (17α-hydroxylase/17,20-lyase): Insights into reaction mechanisms and effects of mutations. Mol Endocrinol 13:1169–1182.

306. Lee-Robichaud P, Akhtar ME, Akhtar M (1998). Control of androgen biosynthesis in the human through the interaction of Arg³⁴⁷ and Arg³⁵⁸ of CYP17 with cytochrome b₅. Biochem J 332:293–296.

307. Giordano SJ, Kaftory A, Steggles AW (1994). A splicing mutation in the cytchrome b₅ gene from a patient with congenital methemoglobinemia and pseudohermaphrodism. Hum Genet 93:568–570.

308. Merke DP, Bornstein SR (2005). Congenital adrenal hyperplasia. Lancet 365:2125–2136.

309. Merke DP, Chrousos GP, Eisenhofer G, Weise M, Keil MF, Rogol AD, et al. (2000). Adrenomedullary dysplasia and hypofunction in patients with classic 21-hydroxylase deficiency. New England J Med 343:1362–1368.

310. Grumbach MM, Conte FA (1998). Disorders of sex differentiation. In JD Wilson, DW Foster, HM Kronenberg, and PR Larsen (eds.), *Williams textbook of endocrinology, Ninth edition.* Philadelphia PA: WB Saunders 1303–1425.

311. Solish SB, Goldsmith MA, Voutilainen R, Miller WL (1989). Molecular characterization of a Leydig cell tumor presenting as congenital adrenal hyperplasia. J Clin Endocrinol Metab 69:1148–1152.

312. Gourmelen M, Gueux B, Pham-Huu-Trung MT, Fiet J, Raux-Demany MC, Girard F (1987). Detection of heterozygous carriers for 21-hydroxylase deficiency by plasma 21-deoxycortisol measurement. Acta Endocrinol 116:507–512.

313. Dittmann RW, Kappes ME, Kappes MH (1992). Sexual behavior in adolescent and adult females with congenital adrenal hyperplasia. Psychoneuroendorinology 17:153–170.

314. Mulaikal RM, Migeon CJ, Rock JA (1987). Fertility rates in female patients with congenital adrenal hyperplasia due to 21-hydroxylase deficiency. New England J Med 316:178–182.

315. Zucker KJ, Bradley SJ, Oliver G, Blake J, Fleming S, Hood J (1996). Psychosexual development of women with congenital adrenal hyperplasia. Horm Behavior 30:300–318.

316. Dessens AB, Slijper FM, Drop SL (2005). Gender dysphoria and gender change in chromosomal females with congenital adrenal hyperplasia. Arch Sex Behav 34:389–397.

317. Meyer-Bahlburg HF, Dolezal C, Baker SW, Carlson AD, Obeid JS, New MI (2004). Prenatal androgenization affects gender-related behavior but not gender identity in 5-12-year-old girls with congenital adrenal hyperplasia. Arch Sex Behav 33:97–104.

318. Migeon CJ, Rosenwask Z, Lee PA, Urban MD, Bias WB (1980). The attenuated form of congenital adrenal hyperplasia as an allelic form of 21-hydroxylase deficiency. J Clin Endocrinol Metab 51:647–649.

319. Chrousos GP, Loriaux DL, Mann DL, Cutler GB (1982). Late-onset 21-hydroxylase deficiency mimicking idiopathic hirsutism or polycystic ovarian disease: An allelic variant of congenital virilizing adrenal hyperplasia with a milder enzymatic defect. Ann Intern Med 96:143–148.

320. Kohn B, Levine LS, Pollack MS, Pang S, Lorenzen F, Levy D, et al. (1982). Late-onset steroid 21-hydroxylase deficiency: A variant of classical congenital adrenal hyperplasia. J Clin Endocrinol Metab 51:817–827.

321. Levine LS, Dupont B, Lorenzen F, Pang S, Pollack MS, Oberfield SE, et al. (1981). Genetic and hormonal characterization of the cryptic 21-hydroxylase deficiency. J Clin Endocrinol Metab 53:1193–1198.

322. Fiet J, Gueux B, Gourmelen M, Kuttenn F, Vexiau P, Cuillin P, et al. (1988). Comparison of basal and adrenocorticotropin-stimulated plasma 21-desoxycortisol and 17-hydroprogesterone values as biological markers of late-onset adrenal hyperplasia. J Clin Endocrinol Metab 66:659–667.

323. Pang S, Wallace MA, Hofman L, Thuline HC, Dorche C, Lyon ICT, et al. (1988). Worldwide experience in newborn screening for classical congenital adrenal hyperplasia due to 21-hydroxylase deficiency. Pediatrics 81:866–874.

324. Therrell BL Jr., Berenbaum SA, Manter-Kapanke V, Simmank J, Korman K, Prentice L, et al. (1998). Results of screening 1.9 million Texas newborns for 21-hydroxylase-deficient congenital adrenal hyperplasia. Pediatrics 101:583–590.

325. Speiser PW, Dupont B, Rubinstein P, Piazza A, Kastelan A, New MI (1985). High frequency of nonclassical steroid 21-hydroxylase deficiency. Am J Hum Genet 37:650–667.

326. Sherman SL, Aston CE, Morton NE, Speiser PW, New MI (1988). A segregation and linkage study of classical and nonclassical 21-hydroxylase deficiency. Am J Hum Genet 42:830–838.

327. Dumic M, Brkljacic L, Speiser PW, Wood E, Crawford C, Plavsic V, et al. (1990). An update on the frequency of nonclassic deficiency of adrenal 21-hydroxylase in the Yugoslav population. Acta Endocrinol 122:703–710.

328. Chetkowski RJ, DeFazio J, Shamonki I, Judd HL, Chang RJ (1984). The incidence of the late-onset congenital adrenal hyperplasia due to 21-hydroxylase deficiency among hirsute women. J Clin Endocrinol Metab 58:595–598.

329. Kuttenn F, Couillin P, Girard F, Billaud L, Vincens M, Boucekkine C, et al. (1985). Late-onset adrenal hyperplasia in hirsutism. New England J Med 313:222–231.

330. Nebert DW, Nelson DR, Coon MJ, Estabrook RW, Feyereisen R, Fujii-Kuriyama Y, et al. (1991). The P450 superfamily: Update on new sequences, gene mapping, and recommended nomenclature. DNA Cell Biol 10:1–14.

331. Carroll MC, Campbell RD, Porter RR (1985). Mapping of steroid 21-hydroxylase genes to complement component C4 genes in HLA, the major histocompatibility locus in man. Proc Natl Acad Sci USA 82:521–525.

332. White PC, Grossberger D, Onufer BJ, Chaplin DD, New MI, Dupont B, et al. (1985). Two genes encoding steroid 21-hydroxylase are located near the genes encoding the fourth component of complement in man. Proc Natl Acad Sci USA 82:1089–1093.

333. Bristow J, Gitelman SE, Tee MK, Staels B, Miller WL (1993). Abundant adrenal-specific transcription of the human P450c21A "pseudogene". J Biol Chem 268:12919–12924.

334. Amor M, Tosi M, Duponchel C, Steinmetz M, Meo T (1985). Liver cDNA probes disclose two cytochrome P450 genes duplicated in tandem with the complement C4 loci of the mouse H-2S region. Proc Natl Acad Sci USA 82:4453–4457.

335. Chung B, Matteson KJ, Miller WL (1985). Cloning and characterization of the bovine gene for steroid 21-hydroxylase (P450c21). DNA 4:211–219.

336. Skow LE, Womack JE, Petresh JM, Miller WL (1988). Synteny mapping of the genes for steroid 21-hydroxylase, alpha-A-crystallin, and class I bovine leukocyte antigen (BoLA) in cattle. DNA 7:143–149.

337. Parker KL, Chaplin DD, Wong M, Seidman JG, Smith JA, Schimmer BP (1985). Expression of murine 21-hydroxylase in mouse adrenal glands and in transfected Y1 adrenocortical tumor cells. Proc Natl Acad Sci USA 82:7860–7864.

338. Chaplin DD, Galbraith LJ, Seidman JG, White PC, Parker KL (1986). Nucleotide sequence analysis of murine 21-hydroxylase genes: Mutations affecting gene expression. Proc Natl Acad Sci USA 83:9601–9605.

339. John ME, Okamura T, Dee A, Adler B, John MC, White PC, et al. (1986). Bovine steroid 21-hydroxylase: Regulation of biosynthesis. Biochemistry 25:2846-2853.

340. Gitelman SE, Bristow J, Miller WL (1992). Mechanism and consequences of the duplication of the human C4/P450c21/gene X locus. Mol Cell Biol 12:2124–2134.

341. Geffrotin C, Chardon P, DeAndres-Cara DR, Feil R, Renard C, Vaiman M (1990). The swine steroid 21-hydroxylase gene (CYP21): Cloning and mapping within the swine leukocyte antigen locus. Animal Genet 21:1–13.

342. Partanen J, Koskimies S, Sipila I, Lipsanen V (1989). Major histocompatibility-complex gene markers and restriction fragment analysis of steroid 21-hydroxylase (CYP21) and complement C4 genes in classical adrenal hyperplasia patients in a single population. Am J Hum Genet 44:660–670.

343. Dupont B, Pollack MS, Levine LS, O'Neill GJ, Hawkins BR, New MI (1981). Congenital adrenal hyperplasia: Joint report from the eight international histocompatibility workshop. In PI Terasaki (eds.), Histocompatibility testing 1980. Berlin: Springer Verlag 693–706.

344. Fleischnick E, Awdeh ZL, Raum D, Granados J, Alosco SM, Crigler JR Jr. et al. (1983). Extended MHC haplotypes in 21-hydroxylase

deficiency congenital adrenal hyperplasia: Shared genotypes in unrelated patients. Lancet i:152–156.

345. Holler W, Scholz S, Knorr D, Bidlingmaier F, Keller E, Ekkehard DA (1985). Genetic differences in the salt-wasting, simple virilizing, and nonclassical types of congenital adrenal hyperplasia. J Clin Endocrinol Metab 60:757–763.

346. Pollack MS, Levine LS, O'Neill GL (1981). HLA linkage and B14, DR1, BfS haplotype association with the genes for late onset and cryptic 21-hydroxylase deficiency. Am J Hum Genet 33:540–550.

347. Speiser PW, New MI, White P (1988). Molecular genetic analysis of nonclassical steroid 21-hydroxylase deficiency associated with HLA-B14DR1. New England J Med 319:19–23.

348. Morel Y, Andre J, Uring-Lambert B, Hauptman G, Bétuel H, Tosi M, et al. (1989). Rearrangements and point mutations of P450c21 genes are distinguished by five restriction endonuclease haplotypes identified by a new probing strategy in 57 families with congenital adrenal hyperplasia. J Clin Invest 83:527–536.

349. Rosenbloom NR, Smith DW (1966). Varying expression for salt-losing in related patients with congenital adrenal hyperplasia. Pediatrics 38:215–219.

350. Stoner E, DiMartina J, Kuhnle U, Levine LS, Oberfield SE, New MI (1986). Is salt-wasting in congenital adrenal hyperplasia genetic? Clin Endocrinol 24:9–20.

351. Morel Y, David M, Forest MG, Betuel H, Hauptman G, Andre J, et al. (1989). Gene conversions and rearrangements cause discordance between inheritance of forms of 21-hydroxylase deficiency and HLA types. J Clin Endocrinol Metab 68:592–599.

352. Sinnott PJ, Dyer PA, Price DA, Harris R, Strachan T (1989). 21-hydroxylase deficiency families with HLA identical affected and unaffected sibs. J Med Genet 26:10–17.

353. Law SKA, Dodds AW, Porter RR (1984). A comparison of the properties of two classes, C4A and C4B, of the human complement component C4. EMBO J 3:1819–1823.

354. Yu CY, Belt KT, Giles CM, Campbell RD, Porter RR (1986). Structural basis of the polymorphism of the human complement components C4A and C4B: Gene size, reactivity and antigenicity. EMBO J 5:2873–2881.

355. Tee MK, Babalola GO, Aza-Blanc P, Speek M, Gitelman SE, Miller WL (1995). A promoter within intron 35 of the human C4A gene initiates adrenal-specific transcription of a 1kb RNA: Location of a cryptic CYP21 promoter element? Hum Mol Genet 4:2109–2116.

356. Wijesuriya SD, Zhang G, Dardis A, Miller WL (1999). Transcriptional regulatory elements of the human gene for cytochrome P450c21 (steroid 21-hydroxylase) lie within intron 35 of the linked C4B gene. J Biol Chem 274:38097–38106.

357. Gomez-Escobar N, Chou C-F, Lin W-W, Hsieh S-L, Campbell RD (1998). The G11 gene located in the major histocompatibility complex encodes a novel nuclear serine/threonine protein kinase. J Biol Chem 273:30954–30960.

358. Morel Y, Bristow J, Gitelman SE, Miller WL (1989). Transcript encoded on the opposite strand of the human steroid 21-hydroxylase/complement component/C4 gene locus. Proc Natl Acad Sci USA 86:6582–6586.

359. Bristow J, Tee MK, Gitelman SE, Mellon SH, Miller WL (1993). Tenascin-X: A novel extracellular matrix protein encoded by the human XB gene overlapping P450c21B. J Cell Biol 122:265–278.

360. Burch GH, Bedolli MA, McDonough S, Rosenthal SM, Bristow J (1995). Embryonic expression of tenascin-X suggests a role in limb, muscle, and heart development. Dev Dynamics 203:491–504.

361. Speek M, Barry F, Miller WL (1996). Alternate promoters and alternate splicing of human Tenascin-X, a gene with 5' and 3' ends buried in other genes. Hum Mol Genet 5:1749–1758.

362. Tee MK, Thomson AA, Bristow J, Miller WL (1995). Sequences promoting the transcription of the human XA gene overlapping P450c21A correctly predict the presence of a novel, adrenal-specific, truncated form of Tenascin-X. Genomics 28:171–178.

363. Burch GH, Gong Y, Liu W, Dettman RW, Curry CJ, Smith L, et al. (1997). Tenascin-X deficiency is associated with Ehlers-Danlos syndrome. Nature Genet 17:104–108.

364. Elefteriou F, Exposito JY, Garrone R, Lethias C (1997). Characterization of the bovine Tenascin-X. J Biol Chem 272:22866–22874.

365. Lethias C, Carisey A, Comte J, Cluzel C, Exposito J-Y (2006). A model of tenascin-X integration within the collagenous network. FEBS Lett 580:6281–6285.

366. Schalkwijk J, Zweers MC, Steijlen PM, Dean WB, Taylor G, van Vlijmen IM, et al. (2001). A recessive form of the Ehlers-Danlos syndrome caused by tenascin-X deficiency. New England J Med 345:1167–1175.

367. White PC, Tusie-Luna MT, New MI, Speiser PW (1994). Mutations in steroid 21-hydroxylase (CYP21). Hum Mutat 3:373–378.

368. Matteson KJ, Phillips JA III, Miller WL, Chung B, Orlando PJ, Frisch H, et al. (1987). P450XXI (steroid 21-hydroxylase) gene deletions are not found in family studies of congenital adrenal hyperplasia. Proc Natl Acad Sci USA 84:5858–5862.

369. Miller WL (1988). Gene conversions, deletions, and polymorphisms in congenital adrenal hyperplasia. Am J Hum Genet 42:4–7.

370. Donohoue PA, Neto RS, Collins MM, Migeon CJ (1990). Exon 7 Nco I restriction site within CYP21B (steroid 21-hydroxylase) is a normal polymorphism. Mol Endocrinol 4:1354–1362.

371. Higashi Y, Hiromasa T, Tanae A, Miki T, Nakura J, Kondo T, et al. (1991). Effects of individual mutations in the P-450(C21) pseudogene on P-450(C21) activity and their distribution in patient genomes of congenital steroid 21-hydroxylase deficiency. J Biochem 109:638–644.

372. Chiou SH, Hu MC, Chung B-C (1990). A missense mutation of Ile^{172}→Asn or Arg^{356}→Trp causes steroid 21-hydroxylase deficiency. J Biol Chem 256:3549–3552.

373. Wedell A, Ritzen EM, Haglund-Stengler B, Luthman H (1992). Steroid 21-hydroxylase deficiency: Three additional mutated alleles and establishment of phenotype-genotype relationships of common mutations. Proc Natl Acad Sci USA 89:7232–7236.

374. Wedell A, Luthman H (1993). Steroid 21-hydroxylase (P450c21): A new allele and spread of mutations through the pseudogene. Hum Mol Genet 91:236–240.

375. Wedell A, Luthman H (1993). Steroid 21-hydroxylase deficiency: Two additional mutations in salt-wasting disease and rapid screening of disease-causing mutations. Hum Mol Genet 2:499–504.

376. Amor M, Parker KL, Globerman H, New MI, White PC (1988). Mutation in the CYP21B gene (Ile-172-Asn) causes steroid 21-hydroxylase deficiency. Proc Natl Acad Sci USA 85:1600–1604.

377. Urabe K, Kimura A, Harada F, Iwanage T, Sasazuki T (1990). Gene conversion in steroid 21-hydroxylase genes. Am J Hum Genet 46:1178–1186.

378. Hu MC, Chung B-C (1990). Expression of human 21-hydroxylase (P450c21) in bacterial and mammalian cell: A system to characterize normal and mutant enzymes. Mol Endocrinol 4:893–898.

379. Wu DA, Chung B (1991). Mutations of P450c21 (steroid 21-hydroxylase) at Cys^{428}, Val^{281}, or Ser^{268} result in complete, partial, or no loss of enzymatic activity. J Clin Invest 88:519–523.

380. Helmburg A, Tusie-Luna M, Tabarelli M, Kofler R, White PC (1992). R339H and P453S: CYP21 mutations associated with nonclassic steroid 21-hydroxylase deficiency that are not apparent gene conversion. Mol Endocrinol 6:1318–1322.

381. Owerbach D, Sherman L, Ballard AL, Azziz R (1992). Pro453 to Ser mutation in CYP21 is associated with non-classic steroid 21-hydroxylase deficiency. Mol Endocrinol 6:1211–1215.

382. Hsu LC, Hu MC, Cheng HC, Lu JC, Chung B (1993). The N-terminal hydrophobic domain of P450c21 is required for membrane insertion and enzyme stability. J Biol Chem 268:14682.

383. Forest MG, Bétuel H, Couillin P, Boué A (1981). Prenatal diagnosis of congenital adrenal hyperplasia (CAH) due to 21-hydroxylase deficiency by steroid analysis in the amniotic fluid of mid-pregnancy: Comparison with HLA typing in 17 pregnancies at risk for CAH. Prenatal Diagnosis 1:197–207.

384. Forest MG, Bétuel H, David M (1989). Prenatal treatment in congenital adrenal hyperplasia due to 21-hydroxylase deficiency: Update 88 of the French multicentric study. Endocr Res 15:277–301.

385. Pang SY, Clark A (1990). Newborn screening, prenatal diagnosis, and prenatal treatment of congenital adrenal hyperplasia due to 21-hydroxylase deficiency. Trends Endocrinol Metab 1:300–307.

386. Pang S, Levine LS, Cederqvist LL, Fuentes M, Riccard VM, Holcombe JH, et al. (1980). Amniotic fluid concentrations of Δ^5 and Δ^4 steroids in fetuses with congenital adrenal hyperplasia due to 21-hydroxylase deficiency and in anencephalic fetuses. J Clin Endocrinol Metab 51:223–229.

387. Pang S, Pollack MS, Loo M, Green O, Nussbaum R, Clayton G, et al. (1985). Pitfalls of prenatal diagnosis of 21-hydroxylase

388. Hughes IA, Dyas J, Riad-Fahmy D, Laurence KM (1992). Prenatal diagnosis of congenital adrenal hyperplasia: Reliability of amniotic fluid steroid analysis. J Med Genet 24:344–347.

389. Laue L, Cutler GB Jr. (1992). 21-Hydroxylase deficiency: Overview of treatment. The Endocrinologist 2:291.

390. Kenny FM, Preeyasombat C, Migeon CJ (1966). Cortisol production rate: II. Normal infants, children and adults. Pediatrics 37:34–42.

391. Kenny FM, Taylor FH, Richards C (1970). Reference standards for cortisol production and 17-hydroxy corticosteroid excretion during growth: Variation in the pattern of excretion of radiolabled cortisol metabolites. Metabolism 19:280–290.

392. Peterson KE (1980). The production of cortisol and corticosterone in children. Acta Paediatri Scand Suppl 281:2–38.

393. Styne DM, Richards GE, Bell JJ, Conte FA, Morishima A, Kaplan SL, et al. (1977). Growth patterns in congenital adrenal hyperplasia: Correlation of glucocorticoid therapy with stature. In P Lee, L Plotnick, A Kowarski, and C. Migeon (eds.), Congenital adrenal hyperplasia. Baltimore: University Park Press 247–261.

394. Forest MG, David M, Morel Y (1993). Prenatal diagnosis and treatment of 21-hydroxylase deficiency. J Steroid Biochem Mol Biol 45:75–82.

395. Speiser PW, New MI (1994). Prenatal diagnosis and management of congenital adrenal hyperplasia. Clin Perinatol 21:631–645.

396. Mercado AB, Wilson RC, Cheng KC, Wei JQ, New MI (1995). Prenatal treatment and diagnosis of congenital adrenal hyperplasia owing to 21-hydroxylase deficiency. J Clin Endocrinol Metab 80:2014–2020.

397. Forest MG, Morel Y, David M (1998). Prenatal treatment of congenital adrenal hyperplasia. Trends Endocrinol Metab 9:284–289.

398. Lajic S, Wedell A, Bui T-H, Ritzen EM, Holst M (19998). Long-term somatic follow-up of prenatally treated children with congenital adrenal hyperplasia. J Clin Endocrinol Metab 83:3872–3880.

399. White PC (1994). Genetic diseases of steroid metabolism. Vitam Horm 49:131–195.

400. Seckl JR, Miller WL (1997). How safe is long-term prenatal glucocorticoid treatment? JAMA 277:1077–1079.

401. Miller WL (1998). Prenatal treatment of congenital adrenal hyperplasia: A promising experimental therapy of unproven safety. Trends Endocrinol Metab 9:290-293.

402. Ritzen EM (1998). Prenatal treatment of congenital adrenal hyperplasia: A commentary. Trends Endocrinol Metab 9:293–295.

403. Miller WL (1999). Dexamethasone treatment of congenital adrenal hyperplasia: An experimental therapy of unproven safety. J Urol 162:537–540.

404. Migeon CJ (1990). Comments about the need for prenatal treatment of congenital adrenal hyperplasia due to 21-hydroxylase deficiency. J Clin Endocrinol Metab 70:836.

405. Pang S, Pollack MS, Marshall RN, Immken LD (1990). Prenatal treatment of congenital adrenal hyperplasia due to 21-hydroxylase deficiency. New England J Med 322:111–115.

406. Seckl JR (2004). Prenatal glucocorticoids and long-term programming. Eur J Endocrinol 151:U49–U62.

407. Lajic S, Nordenstrom A, Ritzén EM, Wedell A (2004). Prenatal treatment of congenital adrenal hyperplasia. Eur J Endocrinol 151:U63–U69.

408. Sloboda DM, Challis JRG, Moss TJM, Newnham JP (2005). Synthetic glucocorticoids: Antenatal administration and long-term implications. Curr Pharma Des 11:1459–1472.

409. Nimkarn S, New MI (2007). Prenatal diagnosis and treatment of congenital adrenal hyperplasia. Hormone Res 67:53–60.

410. Hirvikoski T, Nordenstrom A, Lindholm T, Lindblad F, Ritzén EM, Wedell A, et al. (2007). Cognitive functions in children at risk for congenital adrenal hyperplasia treated prenatally with dexamethosone. J Clin Endocrinol Metab 92:542–548.

411. Speiser PW, Laforgia N, Kato K, Pareira J, Khan R, Yang SY, et al. (1990). First trimester prenatal treatment and molecular genetic diagnosis of congenital adrenal hyperplasia (21-hydroxylase deficiency). J Clin Endocrinol Metab 70:838–848.

412. Gitau R, Fisk NM, Teixeira JMA, Cameron A, Glover V (2001). Fetal hypothalamic-pituitary-adrenal stress responses to invasive procedures are independent of maternal responses. J Clin Endocrinol Metab 86:104.

413. Benediktsson R, Lindsay R, Noble J, Seckl JR, Edwards CRW (1993). Glucocorticoid exposure in utero: A new model for adult hypertension. Lancet 341:339–341.

414. Wolkowitz OM (1994). Prospective controlled studies of the behavioral and biological effects of exogenous corticosteroids. Psychoneuroendocrinology 19:233–255.

415. Trautman PD, Meyer-Bahlburg HFL, Postelnek J, New MI (1995). Effects of early prenatal dexamtheasone on the cognitive and behavioral development of young children: Results of a pilot study. Psychoneuroendocrinology 20:439–449.

416. Seeman TE, McEwen BS, Singer BH, Albert MS, Rowe JW (1997). Increase in urinary cortisol excretion and memory declines: MacArthur studies on successful aging. J Clin Endocrinol Metab 82:2458–2465.

417. Kalmijn S, Launer LJ, Stolk RP, de Jong FH, Pols HAP, Hofman A, et al. (1998). A prospective study on cortisol, dehydroepiandrosterone sulfate, and cognitive function in the elderly. J Clin Endocrinol Metab 83:3487–3492.

418. New MI, Carlson A, Obeid J, Marshall I, Cabrera MS, Goseco A, et al. (2001). Extensive personal experience: Prenatal diagnosis for congenital adrenal hyperplasia in 532 pregnancies. J Clin Endocrinol Metab 86:5651–5657.

419. Benediktsson R, Calder AA, Edwards CR, Seckl JR (1997). Placental 11 beta-hydroxysteroid dehydrogenase: A key regulator of fetal glucocorticoid exposure. Clin Endocrinol (Oxford) 46:161–166.

420. Celsi G, Kistner A, Aizman R, Eklöf A-C, Ceccatelli S, de Santiago A, et al. (1998). Prenatal dexamethasone causes oligonephria, sodium retention, and higher blood pressure in the offspring. Pediatr Res 44:317–322, 1998.

421. Uno H, Lohmiller L, Thieme C, Kemnitz JW, Engle MJ, Roeker EB, et al. (1990). Brain damage induced by prenatal exposure to dexamethasone in fetal rhesus macaques. I. Hippocampus. Devel Brain Res 53:157–167.

422. Yeh TF, Lin YJ, Lin HC, Huang CC, Hsieh WS, Lin CH, et al. (2004). Outcomes at school age after postnatal dexamethasone therapy for lung disease of prematurity. New England J Med 350:1304–1313.

423. Verlinsky Y, Cohen J, Munne S, Gianaroli L, Simpson JL, Ferraretti AP, et al. (2004). Over a decade of experience with preimplantation genetic diagnosis: A multicenter report. Ferti Steril 82:292–294.

424. Eugster EA, DiMeglio LA, Wright JC, Freidenberg GR, Seshadri R, Pescovitz OH (2001). Height outcome in congenital adrenal hyperplasia caused by 21-hydroxylase deficiency: A meta-analysis. J Pediatr 138:26–32.

425. Gallagher MP, Levine LS, Oberfield SE (2005). A review of the effects of therapy on growth and bone mineralization in children with congenital adrenal hyperplasia. Growth Horm IGF Res 15:S26–S30.

426. Laue L, Merke DP, Jones JV, Barnes KM, Hill S, Cutler GB (1996). A preliminary study of flutamide, testolactone, and reduced hydrocortisone dose in the treatment of congenital adrenal hyperplasia. J Clin Endocrinol Metab 81:3535–3539.

427. Laue L, Kenigsberg D, Pescovitz OH, Hench KD, Barnes KM, Loriaux DL, et al. (1989). Treatment of familial male precocious puberty with spironolactone and testolactone. New England J Med 320:496–502.

428. Merke DP, Keil MF, Jones JV, Fields J, Hill S, Cutler GB Jr. (2000). Flutamide, testolactone, and reduced hydrocortisone dose maintain normal growth velocity and bone maturation despite elevated androgen levels in children with congenital adrenal hyperplasia. J Clin Endocrinol Metab 85:1114–1120.

429. Van Wyk JJ, Gunther DF, Ritzén EM, Wedell A, Cutler GB Jr., Migeon CJ, et al. (1996). The use of adrenalectomy as a treatment for congenital adrenal hyperplasia. J Clin Endocrinol Metab 81:3180–3189.

430. Van Wyk JJ, Ritzén EM (2003). The role of bilateral adrenalectomy in the treatment of congenital adrenal hyperplasia. J Clin Endocrinol Metab 88:2993–2998.

431. Quintos JBQ, Vogiatzi MG, Harbison MD, New MI (2001). Growth hormone therapy alone or in combination with gonadotropin-releasing hormone analog therapy to improve the height deficit in children with congenital adrenal hyperplasia. J Clin Endocrinol Metab 86:1511–1517.

432. Lin-Su K, Vogiatzi MG, Marshall I, Harbison MD, Macapagal MC, Betensky B, et al. (2005). Treatment with growth hormone and luteinizing hormone releasing hormone analog improves final adult height in children with congenital adrenal hyperplasia. J Clin Endocrinol Metab 90:3318–3325.

433. Flück CE, Tajima T, Pandey AV, Arlt W, Okuhara K, Verge CF, et al. (2004). Mutant P450 oxidoreductase causes disordered steroidogenesis with and without Antley-Bixler syndrome. Nat Genet 36:228–230.

434. Miller WL (2004). P450 oxidoreductase deficiency. A new disorder of steroidogenesis with multiple clinical manifestations. Trends Endocrinol Metab 15:311–315.

435. Arlt W, Walker EA, Draper N, Ivison HE, Ridle JP, Hammer F, et al. (2004). Congenital adrenal hyperplasia caused by mutant P450 oxidoreductase and human androgen synthesis: analytical study. Lancet 363:2128–2135.

436. Fukami M, Horikawa R, Nagai T, Tanaka T, Naiki Y, Sato N, et al. (2005). Cytochrome P450 oxidoreductase gene mutations and Antley-Bixler syndrome with abnormal genitalia and/or impaired steroidogenesis: Molecular and clinical studies in 10 patients. J Clin Endocrinol Metab 90:414–426.

437. Huang N, Pandey AV, Agrawal V, Reardon W, Lapunzina PD, Mowat D, et al. (2005). Diversity and function of mutations in P450 oxidoreductase in patients with Antley-Bixler syndrome and disordered steroidogenesis. Am J Hum Genet 76:729–749.

438. Flück CE, Miller WL (2006). P450 oxidoreductase deficiency: A new form of congenital adrenal hyperplasia. Curr Opin Pediatr 18:435–441.

439. Shen AL, O'Leary KA, Kasper CB (2002). Association of multiple developmental defects and embryonic lethality with loss of microsomal NADPH-cytochrome P450 oxidoreductase. J Biol Chem 277:6536–6541.

440. Otto DM, Henderson CJ, Carrie D, Davey M, Gundersen TE, Blomhoff R, et al. (2003). Identification of novel roles of the P450 system in early embryogenesis: Effects on vasculogenesis and retinoic acid homeostasis. Mol Cell Biol 23:6103–6116.

441. Peterson RE, Imperato-McGinley J, Gautier T, Shackleton CHL (1985). Male pseudohermaphroditism due to multiple defects in steroid-biosynthetic microsomal mixed-function oxidases: A new variant of congenital adrenal hyperplasia. New England J Med 313:1182–1191.

442. Malunowicz E, Romer TE, Szarras-Czapnik M, Mielniczuk Z, Gajewka D (1987). Combined deficiency of 17 α-hydroxylase and 21-hydroxylase in an 8 years-old girl. Endokrynol Pol 38:117–124.

443. Augarten A, Pariente C, Gazit E, Chayen R, Goldfarb H, Sack J (1992). Ambiguous genitalia due to partial activity of cytochromes P450c17 and P450c21. J Steroid Biochem Mol Biol 41:37–41.

444. Lieberman E, Hershkovitz E, Lauber-Biason A, Phillip M, Zachmann M (1997). Subnormal cortisol response to adrenocorticotropin in isolated partial 17,20-lyase activity. J Pediatr Endocrinol Metab 10:387–390.

445. Adachi M, Tachibana K, Asakura Y, Suwa S, Nishimura G (1999). A male patient presenting with major clinical symptoms of glucocorticoid deficiency and skeletal dysplasia, showing a steroid pattern compatible with 17 α-hydroxylase/17/20 lyase deficiency, but without obvious CYP17 gene mutations. Endocr J 46:285–292.

446. Miller WL (1986). Congenital adrenal hyperplasia. New England J Med 314:1321–1322.

447. Shackleton C, Marcos J, Arlt W, Hauffa BP (2004). Prenatal diagnosis of P450 oxidoreductase deficiency (ORD): A disorder causing low pregnancy estriol, maternal and fetal virilization, and the Antley-Bixler syndrome phenotype. Am J Med Genet 129A:105–112.

448. Fukami M, Hasegawa T, Horikawa R, Ohashi T, Nishimura G, Homma K, et al. (2006). Cytochrome P450 oxidoreductase deficiency in three patients initially regarded as having 21-hydroxylase deficiency and/or aromatase deficiency: Diagnostic value of urine steroid hormone analysis. Pediatr Res 59:276–280.

449. Wilson JD, Auchus RJ, Leihy MW, Guryev OL, Estabrook RW, Osborn SM, et al. (2003). 5α-androstane-3α,17β-diol is formed in tammar wallaby pouch young testes by a pathway involving 5α-pregnane-3α,17α-diol-20-one as a key intermediate. Endocrinology 144:575–580.

450. Auchus RJ (2004). The backdoor pathway to dihydrotestosterone. Trends Endocrinol Metab 15:432–438.

451. Gu J, Weng Y, Zhang QY, Cui H, Behr M, Wu L, et al. (2003). Liver-specific deletion of the NADPH-cytochrome P450 reductase gene: Impact on plasma cholesterol homeostasis and the function and regulation of microsomal cytochrome P450 and heme oxygenases. J Biol Chem 278:25895–25901.

452. Henderson CJ, Otto DM, Carrie D, Magnuson MA, McLaren AW, Rosewell I, et al. (2003). Inactivation of the hepatic cytochrome P450 system by conditional deletion of hepatic cytochrome P450 reductase. J Biol Chem 278:13480–13486.

453. Zachmann M, Tassinari D, Prader A (1983). Clinical and biochemical variability in congenital adrenal hyperplasia due to 11β-hydroxylase deficiency. J Clin Endocrinol Metab 56:222–229.

454. Holcombe JH, Keenan BS, Nichols BL, Kirkland RT, Clayton GW (1980). Neonatal salt loss in the hypertensive form of congenital adrenal hyperplasia. Pediatrics 65:777–781.

455. New MI, White P, Pang S, Dupont B, Speiser PW (1989). The adrenal hyperplasias. In CR Scriver, AL Beaudet, WS Sly, and D Valle (eds.), *The metabolic basis of inherited disease*. New York: McGraw-Hill 1881–1917.

456. Sonino N, Levine LS, Vecsci P, New MI (1980). Parallelism of 11- and 18-hydroxylation demonstrated by urinary free hormones in man. J Clin Endocrinol Metab 51:557–560.

457. Azziz R, Boots LR, Parker CR, Jr., Bradley E Jr., Zacur HA (1991). 11 β-hydroxylase deficiency in hyperandrogenism. Fertil Steril 55:733–741.

458. Joehrer K, Geley S, Stasser-Wozak E, Azziz R, Wollmann A, Schmitt K, et al. (1997). CYP11B1 mutations causing non-classic adrenal hyperplasia due to 11β-hydroxylase deficiency. Hum Mol Genet 6:1829–1834.

459. Rösler A (1984). The natural history of salt-wasting disorders of adrenal and renal origin. J Clin Endocrinol Metab 59:689–700.

460. Mitsuuchi Y, Kawamoto T, Miyahara K, Ulick S, Morton DH, Naiki Y, et al. (1993). Congenitally defective aldosterone biosynthesis in the humans: Inactivation of the P-450c18 gene (CYP11B2) due to nucleotide deletion in CMO I deficient patients. Biochem Biophys Res Commun 190:864–869.

461. Peter M, Fawaz L, Drop S, Visser H, Sippell W (1997). Hereditary defect in biosynthesis of aldosterone: Aldosterone synthase deficiency 1964-1997. J Clin Endocrinol Metab 82:3525–3528.

462. Geley S, Jöhrer K, Peter M, Denner K, Bernhardt R, Sippell WG, Kofler R (1995). Amino acid substitution R384P in aldosterone synthase causes corticosterone methyloxidase type I deficiency. J Clin Endocrinol Metab 80:424–429.

463. Portrat-Doyen S, Tourniaire J, Richard O, Mulatero P, Aupetit-Faisant B, Curnow KM, et al. (1998). Isolated aldosterone synthase deficiency caused by simultaneous E198D and V386A mutations in the CYP11B2 gene. J Clin Endocrinol Metab 83:4156–4161.

464. Fardella CE, Rodriguez H, Montero J, Zhang G, Vignolo P, Rojas A, et al. (1996). Genetic variation in P450c11AS in Chilean patients with low renin hypertension. J Clin Endocrinol Metab 81:4347–4351.

465. Zhang G, Miller WL (1996). The human genome contains only two CYP11B (P450c11) genes. J Clin Endocrinol Metab 81:3254–3256.

466. Fardella CE, Hum DW, Rodriguez H, Zhang G, Barry F, Bloch CA, Miller WL (1996). Gene conversion in the CYP11B2 gene encoding aldosterone synthase (P450c11AS) is associated with, but does not cause, the syndrome of corticosterone methyl oxidase II deficiency. J Clin Endocrinol Metab 81:321–326.

467. Speek M, Miller WL (1995). Hybridization of complementary mRNAs for P450c21 (steroid 21-hydroxylase) and Tenascin-X is prevented by sequence-specific binding of nuclear proteins. Mol Endocrinol 9:1655–1665.

468. Lifton R, Dluhy RG, Powers M, Rich GM, Cook S, Ulick S, et al. (1992). A chimaeric 11β-hydroxylase/aldosterone synthase gene causes glucocorticoid-remediable aldosteronism and human hypertension. Nature 335:262–265.

469. Pascoe L, Curnow K, Slutsker L, Connel JMC, Speiser PW, New MI, et al. (1992). Glucocorticoid-suppressible hyperaldosteronism results from hybrid genes created by unequal crossover between CYP11B1 and CYP11B2. Proc Natl Acad Sci USA 89:8327–8331.

470. Dluhy RG, Lifton RP (1999). Glucocorticoid-remediable aldosteronism. J Clin Endocrinol Metab 84:4341–4344.

471. Curnow KM, Mulatero P, Emeric-Blanchouin N, Aupetit-Faisant B, Corvol P, Pascoe L (1997). The amino acid substitutions Ser288Gly and Val320Ala convert the cortisol producing enzyme, CYP11B1, into an aldosterone producing enzyme. Nat Struct Biol 4:32–35.

472. Fardella CE, Rodriguez H, Hum DW, Mellon SH, Miller WL (1995). Artificial mutations in P450c11AS (aldosterone synthase) can increase enzymatic activity: A model for low-renin hypertension? J Clin Endocrinol Metab 80:1040–1043.

473. Mulatero P, Curnow KM, Aupetit-Faisant B, Foekling M, Gomez-Sanchez C, Veglio F, et al. (1998). Recombinant CYP11B genes encode enzymes that can catalyze conversion of 11-deoxycortisol to cortisol, 18-hydroxycortisol, and 18-oxocortisol. J Clin Endocrinol Metab 83:3996–4001.

474. Takeda Y, Furukawa K, Inaba S, Miyamori I, Mabuchi H (1999). Genetic analysis of aldosterone synthase in patients with idiopathic hyperaldosteronism. J Clin Endocrinol Metab 84:1633–1637.

475. Tomlinson JW, Walker EA, Bujalska IJ, et al. (2004). 11 beta-hydroxysteroid dehydrogenase type 1: A tissue specific regulator of glucocorticoid response. Endocr Rev 25:831–866.

476. Seckl JR, Morton NM, Chapman KE, Walker BR (2004). Glucocorticoids and 11β-hydroxysteroid dehydrogenase in adipose tissue. Rec Prog Horm Res 59:359–393.

477. Walker EA, Stewart PM (2003). 11β-hydroxysteroid dehydrogenase: Unexpected connections. Trends Endocrinol Metab 14:334–339.

478. Draper N, Walker EA, Bujalska IJ, et al. (2003). Mutations in the genes encoding 11β-hydroxysteroid dehydrogenase type 1 and hexose-6-phosphate dehydrogenase interact to cause cortisone reductase deficiency. Nat Genet 34:434–439.

479. San Millan JL, Botela-Carretero JI, Alvarez-Blasco F, et al. (2005). A study of the hexose-6-phosphate dehydrogenase gene R453Q and 11beta-hydroxysteroid dehydrogenase type 1 gene 83557insA polymorphisms in the polycystic ovary syndrome. J Clin Endocrinol Metab 90:4157–4162.

480. White PC (2005). Genotypes at 11beta-hydroxysteroid dehydrogenase type IIB1 and hexose-6-phosphate dehydrogenase loci are not risk factors for apparent cortisone reductase deficiency in a large population-based sample. J Clin Endocrinol Metab 90:5880–5883.

481. Gambineri A, Vicennati V, Genghini S, et al. (2006). Genetic variation in 11beta-hydroxysteroid dehydrogenase type 1 predicts adrenal hyperandrogenism among lean women with polycystic ovary syndrome. J Clin Endocrinol Metab 91:2295–2302.

482. Dave-Sharma S, Wilson RC, Harbison MD, Newfield R, Azar MR, Krozowski ZS, et al. (1998). Examination of genotype and phenotype relationships in 14 patients with apparent mineralocorticoid excess. J Clin Endocrinol Metab 83:2244–2254.

483. Wilson RC, Nimkarn S, New MI (2001). Apparent mineralocorticoid excess. Trends Endocrinol Metab 12:104–111.

484. Quinkler M, Stewart PM (2003). Hypertension and the cortisol-cortisone shuttle. J Clin Endocrinol Metab 88:2384–2392.

485. Palermo M, Quinkler M, Stewart PM (2004). Apparent mineralocorticoid excess syndrome: An overview. Arq Bras Endocrinol Metab 48:687–696.

486. Perry R, Kecha O, Paquette J, Huot C, Van Vliet G, Deal C (2005). Primary adrenal insufficiency in children: Twenty years experience at the Sainte-Justine Hospital, Montreal. J Clin Endocrinol Metab 90:3243–3250.

487. Lin L, Gu W-X, Ozisik G, To WS, Owen CJ, Jameson JL, et al. (2006). Analysis of DAX1 (NR0B1) and steroidogenic factor-1 (SF1/Ad4BP, NR5A1) in children and adults with primary adrenal failure: Ten years' experience. J Clin Endocrinol Metab 91:3048–3054.

488. Lin L, Achermann JC (2004). Inherited adrenal hypoplasia: Not just for kids! Clin Endocrinol 60:529–537.

489. Black J, Williams DI (1973). Natural history of adrenal haemorrhage in the newborn. Arch Dis Child 48:183–190.

490. Dahlberg PJ, Goellner MH, Pehling GB (1990). Adrenal insufficiency secondary to adrenal hemorrhage: Two case reports and a review of cases confirmed by computed tomography. Arch Intern Med 150:905–909.

491. Adem PV, Montgomery CP, Husain AN, Koogle TK, Arangelovich V, Humilier M, et al. (2005). Staphylococcus aureus sepsis and the Waterhouse-Friderichsen syndrome in children. New England J Med 353:1245–1251.

492. Betterle C, Dal Pra C, Mantero F, Zanchetta R (2002). Autoimmune adrenal insufficiency and autoimmune polyendocrine syndromes: Autoantibodies, autoantigens, and their applicability in diagnosis and disease prediction. Endocr Rev 23:327–364.

493. Donner H, Braun J, Seidl C, Rau H, Finke R, Ventz M, et al. (1997). Codon 17 polymorphism of the cytotoxic T lymphocyte antigen 4 gene in Hashimoto's thyroiditis and Addison's disease. J Clin Endocrinol Metab 82:4130–4132.

494. Ueda H, Howson JM, Esposito L, et al. (2003). Association of the T-cell regulatory gene CTLA4 with susceptibility to autoimmune disease. Nature 423:506–511.

495. Ghaderi M, Gamelunghe G, Tortoioli C, et al. (2006). MHC2TA single nucleotide polymorphism and genetic risk for autoimmune adrenal insufficiency. J Clin Endocrinol Metab 91:4107–4111.

496. Uibo R, Aavik E, Peterson P, Perheentupa J, Aranko S, Pelkonen R, et al. (1994). Autoantibodies to cytochrome P450 enzymes P450scc, P450c17, and P450c21 in autoimmune polyglandular disease types I and II and in isolated Addison's disease. J Clin Endocrinol Metab 78:323–328.

497. Colls J, Betterle C, Volpato M, Prentice L, Smith BR, Furmaniak J (1995). Immunoprecipitation assay for autoantibodies to steroid 21-hydroxylase in autoimmune adrenal diseases. Clin Chem 41:375–380.

498. Perheentupa J (2006). Autoimmune polyendocrinopathy-candidiasis-ectodermal dysplasia. J Clin Endocrinol Metab 91:2843–2850.

499. Nagamine K, Peterson P, Scott HS, Kudoh J, Minoshima S, Heino M, et al. (1997). Positional cloning of the APECED gene. Nature Genet 17:393–398.

500. Finnish-German APECED Consortium (1997). An autoimmune disease, APECED, caused by mutations in a novel gene featuring two PHD-type zinc finger domains. Nature Genet 17:399–403.

501. Su MA, Anderson MS (2004). AIRE: An update. Curr Opin Immunol 16:746–752.

502. Villasenor J, Benoist C, Mathis D (2005). IARE and APECED: Molecular insights into an autoimmune disease. Immunol Rev 204:156–164.

503. Zanaria E, Muscatelli F, Bardoni B, Strom TM, Guioli S, Guo W, et al. (1994). An unusual member of the nuclear hormone receptor superfamily responsible for X-linked adrenal hypoplasia congenita. Nature 372:635–641.

504. Phelan JK, McCabe ER (2001). Mutations in NR0B1 (DAX1) and NR5A (SF1) responsible for adrenal hypoplasia congenita. Hum Mutation 18:472–487.

505. Tabarin A, Achermann JC, Recan D, Bex V, Bertagna X, Christin-Maitre S, et al. (2001). A novel muation in DAX1 causes delayed-onset adrenal insufficiency and incomplete hypogonadotropic hypogonadism. J Clin Invest 105:321–328.

506. Achermann JC, Silverman BL, Habiby RL, Jameson JL (2000). Presymptomatic diagnosis of X-linked adrenal hypoplasia congenita by analysis of DAX1. J Pediatr 137:878–881.

507. Vilain E, Le Merrier M, Lecointre C, Desangles F, Kay MA, Maroteaux P, et al. (1999). IMAGE, a new clinical association of intrauterine growth retardation, metaphyseal dysplasia, adrenal hypoplasia congenita, and genital anomalies. J Clin Endocrinol Metab 84:4335–4340.

508. Bergada I, Del Ray G, Lapunzina PD, Bergada C, Fellous M, Copelli S (2005). Familial occurrence of the IMAGe association: Additional clinical variants and a proposed mode of inheritance. J Clin Endocrinol Metab 90:3186–3190.

509. Clark AJL, Metherell LA, Cheetham ME, Huebner A (2005). Inherited ACTH insensitivity illuminates the mechanisms of ACTH action. Trends Endocrinol Metab 16:451–457.

510. Lin L, Hindmarsh PC, Metherell LA, Alzyoud M, Al-Ali M, Brain CE, et al. (2007). Severe loss-of-function mutations in the adrenocorticotropin receptor (ACTHR, MC2R) can be found in patients with apparent mineralocorticoid insufficiency. Clin Endocrinol 66:205–210.

511. Flück CE, Martens JWM, Conte FA, Miller WL (2002). Clinical, genetic and functional characterization of ACTH receptor mutations using a novel receptor assay. J Clin Endocrinol Metab 87:4318–4323.

512. Elias LL, Huebner A, Metherell LA, Canas A, Warne GL, Bitti ML, et al. (2000). Tall stature in familial glucocorticoid deficiency. Clin Endocrinol 53:423–430.

513. Metherell LA, Chapple JP, Cooray S, David A, Becker C, Ruschendorf F, et al. (2005). Mutations in MRAP, encoding a new interacting partner of the ACTH receptor, cause familial glucocorticoid deficiency type 2. Nat Genet 37:166–170.

514. Allgrove J, Clayden GS, Grant DB, Macaulay JC (1978). Familial glucocorticoid deficiency with achalasia of the cardia and deficient tear production. Lancet 1:1284–1286.

515. Grant DB, Barnes ND, Dumic M, Ginalska-Malinowska M, Milla PJ, von Petrykowski W, et al. (1993). Neurological and adrenal dysfunction in the adrenal insufficiency/alacrima/achalasia (3A) syndrome. Arch Dis Child 68:779–782.

516. Houlden H, Smith S, de Carvalho M, Blake J, Mathias C, Wood NW, et al. (2002). Clinical and genetic characterization of families with triple A (Allgrove) syndrome. Brain 25:2681–2690.

517. Tullio-Pelet A, Salomon R, Hadj-Rabia S, Mugnier C, de Laet M-H, Chaouachi B, et al. (2000). Mutant WD-repeat protein in triple-A syndrome. Nat Genet 26:332–335.

518. Handschug K, Sperling S, Yoon SJ, Hennig S, Clark AJ, Huebner A (2001). Triple A syndrome is caused by mutations in AAAS, a new WD-repeat protein gene. Hum Mol Genet 10:281–290.

519. Cronshaw JM, Matunis MJ (2003). The nuclear pore complex protein ALADIN is mislocalized in triple A syndrome. Proc Natl Acad Sci USA 100:5823–5827.

520. Ligtenberg MJ, Kemp S, Sarde CO, van Geel BM, Kleijer WJ, Barth PG, et al. (1995). Spectrum of mutations in the gene encoding the adrenoleukodystrophy protein. Am J Hum Genet 56:44–50.

521. Watkins PA, Gould SJ, Smith MA, Braiterman LT, Wei HM, Kok F, et al. (1995). Altered expression of ALDP in X-linked adrenoleukodystrophy. Am J Hum Genet 57:292–301.

522. Moser HW, Raymond GV, Dubey P (2005). Adrenoleukodystrophy: New approaches to a neurodegenerative disease. JAMA 294:3131–3134.

523. McGuinness MC, Lu J-F, Zhang H-P, Dong G-X, Heinzer AK, Watkins PA, et al. (2003). Role of ALDP (ABCD1) and mitochondria in X-linked adrenoleukodystrophy. Mol Cell Biol 23:744–753.

524. Kemp S, Wanders RJA (2007). X-linked adrenoleukodystrophy: Very long-chain fatty acid metabolism, ABC half-transporters and the complicated route to treatment. Mol Genet Metab 90:268-276.

525. Watkins PA, Naidu S, Moser HW (1987). Adrenoleukodystrophy: biochemical procedures in diagnosis, prevention and treatment. J Inherit Metab Dis 10:46–53.

526. Moser HW, Moser AE, Singh I, O'Neill BP (1984). Adrenoleukodystrophy: Survey of 303 cases: biochemistry, diagnosis, and therapy. Ann Neurol 16:628–641.

527. Moser HW (1995). Adrenoleukodystrophy. Curr Opin Neurol 8:221–226.

528. Sadeghi-Nejad A, Senior B (1990). Adrenomyeloneuropathy presenting as Addison's disease in childhood. New England J Med 322:13–16.

529. Laureti S, Casucci G, Santeusanio F, Angeletti G, Aubourg P, Brunetti P (1996). X-linked adrenoleukodystrophy is a frequent cause of idiopathic Addison's disease in young adult male patients. J Clin Endocrinol Metab 81:470–474.

530. Steinberg S, Chen L, Wei L, Moser A, Moser H, Cutting G, et al. (2004). The PEX gene screen: Molecular diagnosis of peroxisome biogenesis disorders in the Zellweger syndrome spectrum. Mol Genet Metab 83:252–263.

531. Wanders RJ, Waterham HR (2005). Peroxisomal disorders I: biochemistry and genetics of peroxisome biogenesis disorders. Clin Genet 67:107–133.

532. Mandel H, Korman SH (2003). Phenotypic variability (heterogeneity) of peroxisomal disorders. Adv Exp Med Biol 544:9–30.

533. Assmann G, Seedorf U (1995). Acid lipase deficiency: Wolman disease and cholesteryl ester storage disease. In JL Goldstein, MS Brown, and CR Scriver (eds.), The metabolic basis of inherited disease. New York: McGraw-Hill 2563–2587.

534. Anderson RA, Byrum RS, Coates PM, Sando GN (1994). Mutations at the lysosomal acid cholesteryl ester hydrolase gene locus in Wolman disease. Proc Natl Acad Sci USA 91:2718–2722.

535. Correa-Cerro LS, Porter FD (2005). 3beta-hydroxysterol delta-7 reductase and the Smith-Lemli-Opitz syndrome. Mol Genet Metab 84:112–126.

536. Andersson HC, Frentz J, Martinez JE, Tuck-Muller CM, Bellizaire J (1999). Adrenal insufficiency in Smith-Lemli-Optiz syndrome. Am J Med Genet 82:382–384.

537. Nicolino M, Ferlin T, Forest M, Godinot C, Carrier H, David M, et al. (1997). Identification of a large-scale mitochondrial deoxyribonucleic acid deletion in endocrinopathies and deafness: Report of two unrelated cases with diabete mellitus and adrenal insufficiency, respectively. J Clin Endocrinol Metab 82:3063–3067.

538. Thomsett MJ, Conte FA, Kaplan SL, Grumbach MM (1980). Endocrine and neurologic outcome in childhood craniopharyngioma: Review of effect of treatment in 42 patients. J Pediatr 97:728–735.

539. De Vile CJ, Grant DB, Hayward RD, Stanhope R (1996). Growth and endocrine sequelae of craniopharyngioma. Arch Dis Child 75:108–114.

540. Karavitaki N, Brufani C, Warner JT, Adams CB, Richards P, Ansorge O, et al. (2005). Craniopharyngiomas in children and adults: Systematic analysis of 121 cases with long-term follow-up. Clin Endocrinol 62:397–409.

541. Sklar CA, Grumbach MM, Kaplan SL, Conte FA (1981). Hormonal and metabolic abnormalities associated with central nervous system germinoma in children and adolescents and the effect of therapy: Report of 10 patients. J Clin Endocrinol Metab 52:9–16.

542. Rose SR, Danish RK, Kearney NS, Schrieber RE, Lustig RH, Burghen GA, et al. (2005). ACTH deficiency in childhood cancer survivors. Pediatr Blood Cancer 45:808–813.

543. Mendonça BB, Osorio MG, Latronico AC, Estefan V, Lo LS, Arnhold IJ (1999). Longitudinal hormonal and pituitary imaging changes in two patients with combined pituitary hormone deficiencies due to deletion of A301, G302 in the PROP1 gene. J Clin Endocrinol Metab 84:942–945.

544. Pernasetti F, Toledo SP, Vasilyev VV, Hayashida CY, Cogan JD, Ferrar C, et al. (2000). Impaired adrenocorticotropin-adrenal axis in combined pituitary hormone deficiency caused by a two-base pair deletion (301-302delAG) in the prophet of Pit-1 gene. J Clin Endocrinol Metab 85:390–397.

545. Lamolet B, Pulichino AM, Lamonerie T, Gauthier Y, Brue T, Enjalbert A, et al. (2001). A pituitary cell-restricted T box factor, Tpit, activates POMC transcription in cooperation with Pitx homeoproteins. Cell 104:849–859.

546. Pulichino AM, Vallette-Kasic S, Couture C, Gauthier Y, Brue T, David M, et al. (2003). Human and mouse TPIT gene mutations cause early onset pituitary ACTH deficiency. Genes Dev 17:711–716.

547. Metherell LA, Savage MO, Dattani M, Walker J, Clayton PE, Farooqi IS, et al. (2004). TPIT mutations are associated with early-onset, but not late-onset isolated ACTH deficiency. Eur J Endocrinol 151:463–465.

548. Vallette-Kasic S, Brue T, Pulichino AM, Gueydan M, Barlier A, David M, et al. (2005). Congenital isolated adrenocorticotropin deficiency: An underestimated cause of neonatal death, explained by TPIT gene mutations. J Clin Endocrinol Metab 90:1323–1331.

549. Farooqi IS, Jones MK, Evans M, O'Rahilly S, Hodges JR (2000). Triple H syndrome: A novel autoimmune endocrinopathy characterized by dysfunction of the hippocampus, hair follicle, and hypothalamic-pituitary-adrenal axis. J Clin Endocrinol Metab 85:2644–2648.

550. Krude H, Biebermann H, Schnabel D, Tansek MZ, Theunissen P, Mullis PE, et al. (2003). Obesity due to proopiomelanocortin deficiency: Three new cases and treatment trials with thyroid hormone and ACTH4-10. J Clin Endocrinol Metab 88:4633–4640.

551. Jackson RS, Creemers JW, Ohagi S, Raffin-Sanson ML, Sanders L, Montague CT, et al. (1997). Obesity and impaired prohormone processing associated with mutations in the human prohormone convertase 1 gene. Nat Genet 16:303–306.

552. Jackson RS, Creemers JW, Farooqi IS, Raffin-Sanson ML, Varro A, Dockiny GJ, et al. (2003). Small intestinal dysfunction accompanies the complex endocrinology of human proprotein convertase 1 deficiency. J Clin Invest 112:1550–1560.

553. Kannisto S, Korppi M, Remes K, Voutilainen R (2000). Adrenal suppression, evaluated by a low dose adrenocorticotropin test, and growth in asthmatic children treated with inhaled steroids. J Clin Endocrinol Metab 85:652–657.

554. Todd GR, Acerini CL, Ross-Russell R, Zahra S, Warner JT, McCance D (2002). Survey of adrenal crisis associated with inhaled corticosteroids in the United Kingdom. Arch Dis Child 87:455–456.

555. Paton J, Jardine E, McNeill E, Beaton S, Galloway P, Young D, et al. (2006). Adrenal responses to low dose synthetic ACTH (Synacthen) in children receiving high dose inhaled fluticasone. Arch Dis Child 91:808–813.

556. Carpenter PC (1988). Diagnostic evaluation of Cushing's syndrome. Endocrinol Metab Clin North Am 17:445–472.

557. McArthur RG, Cloutier MD, Hayles AB, Sprague RG (1972). Cushing's disease in children: Findings in 13 cases. Mayo Clin Proc 47:318–326.

558. Storr HL, Isidori AM, Monson JM, Besser GM, Grossman AB, Savage MO (2004). Prepubertal Cushing's disease is more common in males, but there is no increase in severity at diagnosis. J Clin Endocrinol Metab 89:3818–3820.

559. Miller WL, Townsend JJ, Grumbach MM, Kaplan SL (1979). An infant with Cushing's disease due to an adrenocorticotropin-producing pituitary adenoma. J Clin Endocrinol Metab 48:1017–1025.

560. Devoe DJ, Miller WL, Conte FA, Kaplan SL, Grumbach MM, Rosenthal SM, et al. (1997). Long-term outcome of children and

561. Kanter AS, Diallo AO, Jane JA Jr., Sheehan JP, Asthagiri AR, Oskouian RJ, et al. (2005). Single-center experience with pediatric Cushing's disease. J Neurosurg 103:413–420.

562. Joshi SM, Hewitt RJ, Storr HL, et al. (2005). Cushing's disease in children and adolescents: 20 years of experience in a single neurosurgical center. Neurosurgery 57:281–285.

563. Tyrrell JB, Brooks RM, Fitzgerald PA, Cofoid PB, Forsham PH, Wilson CB (1978). Cushing's disease. Selective trans-sphenoidal resection of pituitary microadenomas. New England J Med 298:753–758.

564. Hermus AR, Smals AG, Swinkels LM, Huysmans DA, Pieters GF, Sweep CF, et al. (1995). Bone mineral density and bone turnover before and after surgical cure of Cushing's syndrome. J Clin Endocrinol Metab 80:2859–2865.

565. Leong GM, Abad V, Charmandari E, Reynolds JC, Hill S, Chrousos GP, et al. (2007). Effects of child- and adolescent-onset endogenous Cushing syndrome on bone mass, body composition, and growth: A 7-year prospective study into young adulthood. J Bone Miner Res 22:110–118.

566. Boggan JE, Tyrrell JB, Wilson CB (1983). Transsphenoidal microsurgical management of Cushing's disease. Report of 100 cases. J Neurosurg 59:195–200.

567. Miller WL, Johnson LK (1982). Synthesis and glycosylation of proopiomelanocortin in a Cushing tumor. J Clin Endocrinol Metab 55:441–446.

568. Magiakou MA, Mastorakos G, Oldfield EH, Gomez MT, Doppman JL, Cutler GB Jr. et al. (1994). Cushing's syndrome in children and adolescents: Presentation, diagnosis, and therapy. New England J Med 331:629–636.

569. Leinung MC, Kane LA, Scheithauer BW, Carpenter PC, Laws ER Jr., Zimmerman D (1995). Long term follow-up of transsphenoidal surgery for the treatment of Cushing's disease in childhood. J Clin Endocrinol Metab 80:2475–2479.

570. Storr HL, Afshar F, Matson M, Sabin I, Davies KM, Evanson J, et al. (2005). Factors influencing cure by transsphenoidal selective adenomectomy in paediatric Cushing's disease. Eur J Endocrinol 152:825–833.

571. Massoud AF, Powell M, Williams RA, Hindmarsh PC, Brook CG (1997). Transsphenoidal surgery for pituitary tumors. Arch Dis Child 76:398–404.

572. Magiakou MA, Mastorakos G, Chrousos GP (1994). Final stature in patients with endogenous Cushing's syndrome. J Clin Endocrinol Metab 79:1082–1085.

573. Lebrethon MC, Grossman AB, Afshar F, Plowman PN, Besser GM, Savage MD (2000). Linear growth and final height after treatment for Cushing's disease in childhood. J Clin Endocrinol Metab 85:3262–3265.

574. Davies JH, Storr HL, Davies K, Monson JP, Besser GM, Afshar F, et al. (2005). Final adult height and body mass index after cure of paediatric Cushing's disease. Clin Endocrinol 92:466–472.

575. Storr HL, Plowman PN, Carroll PV, Francois I, Krassas GE, Afshar F, et al. (2003). Clinical and endocrine responses to pituitary radiotherapy in pediatric Cushing's disease: An effective second-line treatment. J Clin Endocrinol Metab 88:34–37.

576. Nieman LK (2002). Medical therapy of Cushing's disease. Pituitary 5:77–82.

577. Schulte HM, Benker G, Reinwein D, Sippell WG, Allolio B (1990). Infusion of low dose etomidate: Correction of hypercortisolemia in patients with Cushing's syndrome and dose-response relationship in normal subjects. J Clin Endocrinol Metab 70:1426–1430.

578. Greening JE, Brain CE, Perry LA, Mushtaq I, Sales Marques J, Grossman AB, et al. (2005). Efficient short-term control of hypercortisolaemia by low-dose etomidate in severe paediatric Cushing's disease. Hormone Res 64:140–143.

579. Styne DM, Isaac R, Miller WL, Leisti S, Connors M, Conte FA, Grumbach MM (1983). Endocrine, histological, and biochemical studies of adrenocorticotropin-producing islet cell carcinoma of the pancreas in childhood with characterization of proopiomelanocortin. J Clin Endocrinol Metab 57:723–731.

580. Loridan L, Senior B (1969). Cushing's syndrome in infancy. J Pediatr 75:349–359.

581. Gilbert MG, Cleveland WW (1970). Cushing's syndrome in infancy. Pediatrics 46:217–229.

582. Perry RR, Nieman LK, Cutler GB Jr., Chrousos GP, Loriaux DL, Doppman JL, et al. (1989). Primary adrenal causes of Cushing's syndrome: Diagnosis and surgical management. Ann Surg 210:59–68.

583. Michalkiewicz E, Sandrini R, Figueiredo B, Miranda EC, Caran E, Oliveira-Filho AG, et al. (2004). Clinical and outcome characteristics of children with adrenocortical tumors: A report from the International Pediatric Adrenocortical Tumor Registry. J Clin Oncol 22:838–845.

584. Ribeiro RC, Sandrini F, Figueiredo B, Zambetti GP, Michalkiewicz E, Lafferty AR, et al. (2001). An inherited p53 mutation that contributes in a tissue-specific manner to pediatric adrenal cortical carcinoma. Proc Natl Acad Sci USA 98:9330–9335.

585. Wolthers OD, Cameron FJ, Scheimberg I, Honour JW, Hindmarsh PC, Savage MO, et al. (1999). Androgen secreting adrenocortical tumors. Arch Dis Child 80:46–50.

586. Wieneke JA, Thompson LD, Heffess CS (2003). Adrenal cortical neoplasms in the pediatric population: A clinicopathologic and immunophenotypic analysis of 83 patients. Am J Surg Pathol 27:867–881.

587. Young WF Jr., Carney JA, Musa BU, Wulffraat NM, Lens JW, Drexhage HA (1989). Familial Cushing's syndrome due to primary pigmented nodular adrenocortical disease: Reinvestigation 50 years later. New England J Med 321:1659–1664.

588. Stratakis CA (2000). Cushing syndrome and Addison disease. In IA Hughes and AJL Clark (eds.), Adrenal disease in childhood: Clinical and molecular aspects. Basel, Switzerland: Karger 150–173.

589. Stratakis CA, Kirschner LS, Carney JA (2001). Clinical and molecular features of the Carney complex: Diagnostic criteria and recommendations for patient evaluation. J Clin Endocrinol Metab 86:4041–4046.

590. Storr HL, Mitchell H, Swords FM, Main KM, Hindmarsh PC, Betts PR, et al. (2004). Clinical features, diagnosis, treatment and molecular studies in paediatric Cushing's syndrome due to primary nodular adrenocortical hyperplasia. Clin Endocrinol 61:553–559.

591. Kirschner LS, Carney JA, Pack SD, Taymans SE, Giatzakis C, Cho YS, et al. (2000). Mutations of the gene encoding the protein kinase A type 1-alpha regulatory subunit in patients with the Carney complex. Nat Genet 26:89–92.

592. Kirschner LS, Sandrini F, Monbo J, Lin JP, Carney JA, Stratakis CA (2000). Genetic heterogeneity and spectrum of mutations in the PRKARIA gene in patients with Carney complex. Hum Mol Genet 9:3037.

593. Bossis I, Stratakis CA (2004). RPKAR1A: Normal and abnormal functions. Endocrinology 145:5452–5458.

594. Bourdeau I, Matyakhina L, Stergiopoulos SG, Sandrini F, Boikos S, Stratakis CA (2006). 17q22-24 chromosomal losses and alterations of protein kinase a subunit expression and activity in adrenocorticotropin-independent macronodular adrenal hyperplasia. J Clin Endocrinol Metab 91:3626–3632.

595. Horvath A, Boikos S, Giatzakis C, Robinson-White A, Groussin L, Griffin KJ, et al. (2006). A genome-wide scan identifies mutations in the gene encoding phosphodiesterase 11A4 (PDE11A) in individuals with adrenocortical hyperplasia. Nat Genet 38:794–800.

596. Kirk JM, Brain CE, Carlson DJ, Hye JC, Grant DB (1999). Cushing's syndrome caused by nodular adrenal hyperplasia in children with McCune-Albright syndrome. J Pediatr 134:789–792.

597. Newell-Price J, Trainer P, Besser M, Grossman A (1998). The diagnosis and differential diagnosis of Cushing's syndrome and pseudo-Cushing's states. Endocr Rev 19:647.

598. Lienhardt A, Grossman AB, Dacie JE, Evanson J, Huebner A, Afshar F, et al. (2001). Relative contributions of inferior petrosal sinus sampling and pituitary imaging in the investigation of children and adolescents with ACTH-dependent Cushing's syndrome. J Clin Endocrinol Metab 86:5711–5714.

599. Ilias I, Chang R, Pacak K, Oldfield EH, Wesley R, Doppman J, Nieman LK (2004). Jugular venous sampling: An alternative to petrosal sinus sampling for the diagnostic evaluation of adrenocorticotropic hormone-dependent Cushing's syndrome. J Clin Endocrinol Metab 89:3795–3800.

600. Stratakis CA, Sarlis N, Kirschner LS, Carney JA, Doppman JL, Nieman LK, et al. (1999). Paradoxical response to dexamethasone in the diagnosis of primary pigmented nodular adrenocortical disease. Ann Intern Med 131:585–591.

601. Charmandari E, Kino T, Chrousos GP (2004). Familial/sporadic glucocorticoid resistance: Clinical phenotype and molecular mechanisms. Ann NY Acad Sci 1024:168–181.

602. Hurley DM, Accili D, Stratakis CA, Karl M, Vamvakopoulos N, Rorer E, et al. (1991). Point mutation causing a single amino acid substitution in the hormone binding domain of the glucocorticoid receptor in familial glucocorticoid resistance. J Clin Invest 87:680–686.

603. Karl M, Lamberts SW, Detera-Wadleigh SD, Encio IJ, Stratakis CA, Hurley DM, et al. (1993). Familial glucocorticoid resistance caused by a splice-site deletion in the human glucocorticoid receptor gene. J Clin Endocrinol Metab 76:683–689.

604. Kino T, Strauber RH, Resau JH, Pavlakis GN, Chrousos GP (2001). Pathologic human GR mutant has a transdominant negative effect on the wild-type GR by inhibiting its translocation into the nucleus: Importance of the ligand-binding domain for intracellular GR trafficking. J Clin Endocrinol Metab 86:5600–5608.

605. Cole TJ, Blendy JA, Monaghan AP, Krieglstein K, Schmid W, Aguzzi A, et al. (1995). Targeted disruption of the glucocorticoid receptor gene blocks adrenergic chromaffin cell development and severely retards lung maturation. Genes Dev 9:1608–1621.

606. Chang SS, Grunder S, Hanukoglu A, Rosler A, Mathew PM, Hanukoglu I, et al. (1996). Mutations in subunits of the epithelial sodium channel cause salt wasting with hyperkalaemic acidosis, pseudohypoaldosteronism type 1. Nat Genet 12:248–253.

607. Kerem E, Bistritzer T, Hanukoglu A, Hofman T, Zhou ZQ, Bennett W, et al. (1999). Pulmonary epithelial sodium-channel dysfunction and excess airway liquid in pseudohypoaldosteronism. New England J Med 341:156–162.

608. Geller DS, Rodriguez-Soriano J, Boado AV, Schifter S, Bayer M, Chang SS, et al. (1998). Mutations in the mineralocorticoid receptor gene cause autosomal dominant pseudohypoaldosteronism. Nat Genet 19:279–281.

609. Sartorato P, Lapeyraque AL, Armanini D, et al. (2003). Different inactivating mutations of the mineralocorticoid receptor in fourteen families affected by type I pseudohypoaldosteronism. J Clin Endocrinol Metab 88:2508–2517.

610. Geller DS, Farhi A, Pinkerton N, Fradley M, Moritz M, Spitzer A, et al. (2000). Activating mineralocorticoid receptor mutation in hypertension exacerbated by pregnancy. Science 289:119–123.

611. Rodriguez-Soriano J, Vallo A, Oliveros R, Castillo G (1983). Transient pseudohypoaldosteronism secondary to obstructive uropathy in infancy. J Pediatr 103:375–380.

612. Chandar J, Abitbol C, Zilleruelo G, Gosalbez R, Montane B, Strauss J (1996). Renal tubular abnormalities in infants with hydronephrosis. J Urol 155:660–663.

613. Tyrrell JB (1995). Glucocorticoid therapy. In [editor(s)] (eds.), Endocrinology and metabolism. New York: McGraw-Hill 855–882.

614. Mellon SH (1994). Neurosteroids: Biochemistry, modes of action, and clinical relevance. J Clin Endocrinol Metab 78:1003–1008.

615. Grossman C, Scholz T, Rochel M, Bumke-Vogt C, Oelkers W, Pfeiffer AFH, et al. (2004). Transactivation via the human glucocorticoid and mineralocorticoid receptor by therapeutically used steroids in CV-1 cells: A comparison of their glucocorticoid and mineralocorticoid properties. Eur J Endocrinol 151:397–406.

616. Streck WF, Lockwood DH (1979). Pituitary adrenal recovery following short-term suppression with corticosteroids. Am J Med 66:910–914.

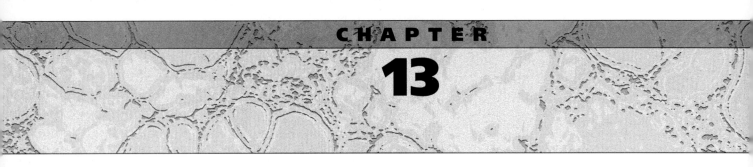

Pheochromocytoma and the Multiple Endocrine Neoplasia Syndromes

STEVEN D. CHERNAUSEK, MD • CHARIS ENG, MD, PhD

Introduction

The multiple endocrine neoplasia (MEN) syndromes and pheochromocytomas are fascinating disorders with an intricate network of genetic etiologies. The field has advanced tremendously over the past decade, including the identification of additional genetic causes of pheochromocytoma, the ability to risk-stratify patients with MEN 2 based on genotype, and the ability to use such information to drive management decisions—all accompanied by a firmer understanding of the underlying pathophysiology. In cases of pheochromocytoma, the type of operation selected may depend on whether there is a germ-line mutation and in what particular gene.

For families with MEN 2, the timing of thyroidectomy is dictated in part by the specific *RET* mutation involved. Therefore, it is now essential that the evaluation and management of these patients involve experts in cancer genetics and include formal genetic counseling. Gene testing should be offered and performed in the setting of a cancer genetic consultation that includes pre-test and post-test genetic counseling. Subsequently, once a family-specific mutation is found the genetics consultant can offer mutation-specific predictive testing to all appropriate relatives of the proband.

Pheochromocytoma

Pheochromocytomas are catecholamine-producing tumors that arise from the chromaffin cells of the adrenal medulla or sympathetic ganglia.* Chromaffin cells, named because of the characteristic staining observed with chromium salt treatment, are neural crest derivatives that

---

* Some use the term paraganglioma for the extra-adrenal forms.

populate the adrenal medulla and sympathetic ganglia. Although most often found in the adrenal, pheochromocytomas can arise anywhere in the sympathetic chain and can produce a wide variety of symptoms.[1] Often, extra-adrenal pheochromocytomas that may not secrete catecholamines are referred to as paragangliomas. The tumors are usually sporadic, but they sometimes appear as a component of a familial syndrome such as multiple endocrine neoplasia type 2, von Hippel-Lindau disease, pheochromocytoma-paraganglioma syndrome, and rarely type 1 neurofibromatosis.

Pheochromocytomas are very rare, with a reported incidence of approximately 1 case per 100,000 patient-years.[2] In a report of 520 cases, only 50 were under age 16 years.[3] Although infrequent, appreciation of the diagnosis and treatment is important because the disease can be deadly if unrecognized. In one autopsy series,[4] the diagnosis was made antemortem only 24% of the time, even though 90% of the patients had symptoms of catecholamine excess.

Pheochromocytoma was traditionally described as a tumor of 90s: 90% are found in the adrenal, 90% are benign, 90% are sporadic, and 90% are unilateral.[5] However, in children the percentages differ—with approximately 70% being unilateral and 70% confined to the adrenal (the majority of the remainder arise in abdominal sympathetic ganglia).[6,7] and a greater likelihood of malignancy.[8,9] In addition, those earlier studies underestimated the frequency of pheochromocytomas occurring in association with specific genetic syndromes.

More recent data indicate that up to 25% of individuals with apparently sporadic pheochromocytomas actually harbor germ-line mutations in one of six genes known to predispose to pheochromocytoma formation.[10] Heritable pheochromocytomas, whether apparently sporadic or familial, frequently occur in the context of multiple endocrine neoplasia type 2 (MEN 2),[11,12] von Hippel-Lindau disease,[13,14] the pheochromocytoma-paraganglioma syndrome,[10,15] and rarely neurofibromatosis type 1.[16,17] It is important to realize that pheochromocytoma, especially in the pediatric setting, may be the initial or sole clinical manifestation of any of four heritable cancer syndromes caused by six distinct susceptibility genes (Table 13-1).

BIOSYNTHESIS AND ACTIONS OF CATECHOLAMINES

The pathophysiology of pheochromocytoma is best appreciated with an understanding of catecholamine biochemistry. The synthesis and metabolism of the catecholamines are illustrated in Figure 13-1. The conversion of tyrosine to dihydroxyphenylalanine (DOPA), catalyzed by the enzyme tyrosine hydroxylase, is the rate-limiting step in catecholamine biosynthesis within chromaffin tissue. Subsequent enzymatic steps yield norepinephrine, the neurotransmitter of the sympathetic nervous system.

The high concentrations of glucocorticoids in the adrenal medulla (reflecting cortical production) induce the enzyme phenylethanolamine-N-methyl transferase—which is responsible for converting norepinephrine to epinephrine in the adrenal medulla (the only location in the sympathetic chain in which this conversion occurs).[18] The catecholamines are stored in granules and released by exocytosis. Norepinephrine released by sympathetic neurons normally undergoes rapid reuptake by the presynaptic neurons. Nonresorbed norepinephrine and secreted epinephrine are enzymatically catabolized, as shown in Figure 13-1. Measurement of epinephrine and norepinephrine and their catabolic products is very useful in defining catecholamine hypersecretion and is the cornerstone of diagnosing pheochromocytoma.

The actions of the catecholamines are mediated by the α- and β-adrenergic receptors (Table 13-2).[19] The initial classification was based on the dissimilar responses of the vasculature to catecholamine exposure. The α-receptors are excitatory for smooth muscle, whereas the β-receptors are inhibitory. Subsequent subtypes (α_1, α_2, β_1, and β_2) were identified by differing responses to catecholamine analogues. The α_1-receptors are postsynaptic excitatory receptors present in the smooth muscle of the vasculature, gut, and genitourinary system as well as cardiac muscle.

TABLE 13-1

Genetic Causes of Pheochromocytoma

Syndrome	Gene	Function	Other Component Features
MEN 2	RET	Growth factor receptor	Medullary thyroid carcinoma; hyperparathyroidism
von Hippel-Lindau	VHL	Tumor suppressor	Cerebellar hemangioblastoma, retinal angioma, renal cell carcinoma
Neurofibromatosis	NF1	Tumor suppressor	Café-au-lait spots, neurofibromas, Optic nerve glioma
Familial paraganglioma	SDHD	Mitochondrial complex II subunit	Parasympathetic paraganglioma, especially in head and neck location
Familial paraganglioma	SDHB	Mitochondrial complex II subunit	Parasympathetic paraganglioma, renal cell carcinoma, papillary thyroid cancer
Familial paraganglioma	SDHC	Mitochondrial complex II subunit	Parasympathetic paraganglioma

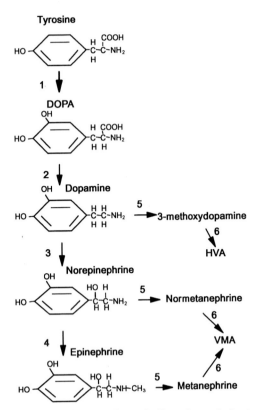

Figure 13-1 Biosynthesis and metabolism of catecholamines. The specific enzymes in the synthetic pathway are (1) tyrosine hydroxylase, (2) aromatic L-amino acid decarboxylase, (3) dopamine ß-hydroxylase, (4) phenylethanolamine N-methyl transferase, (5) catechol-O-methyl transferase, and (6) monoamine oxidase. DOPA, dihydroxyphenylalanine; HVA, homovanillic acid; and VMA, vanillylmandelic acid. [Data from Keiser HR (1995). Pheochromocytoma and related tumors. In DeGroot LJ (ed.), *Endocrinology, Third edition*. Philadelphia: WB Saunders 1853; and from Lefkowitz RJ, et al. (1990). Neurohumoral transmission: The autonomic and somatic motor nervous systems. In Gilman AG, et al. (eds.), *The pharmacologic basis of therapeutics*. New York: Pergamon Press 187.]

The α_1-receptor acts via phospholipase C and produces increases in intracellular calcium. The α_2-receptors are presynaptic and are responsible for feedback inhibition of norepinephrine secretion. Ligand binding by α_2-receptors inhibits adenylyl cyclase by interacting with the inhibitory G protein G_i. The β_1-receptors are found in the myocardium, whereas β_2-receptors are found in most other sites. A β_3-receptor, identified through molecular cloning, is present in adipose tissue. All β-receptor subtypes act by stimulating adenylyl cyclase via the stimulatory G protein G_s. Specific agonists and antagonists characterize the receptor subtype and are useful therapeutic agents.[20]

CLINICAL PRESENTATION

The clinical presentation of pheochromocytoma is highly variable. Symptoms may be absent or unrecognized in the early phase of the disease, as demonstrated by the results of screening families with MEN 2 and by studies that show many pheochromocytomas are first discovered at autopsy.[4] For patients with symptoms, adrenergic paroxysms with headache, palpitations, hypertension, and sweating constitute the classic presentation.

In adults, the hypertension is sustained in approximately 50% and typically responds poorly to standard antihypertensive agents, especially β-blockers.[5] Many patients have orthostatic changes in blood pressure upon physical examination. In children, the most frequent symptom is headache (75%), followed by sweating in two-thirds and nausea and vomiting in one-half of patients.[7,21] Hypertension appears to be uniformly present and is sustained in 80% to 90% of affected children at the time of diagnosis.[7,22,23]

DIAGNOSIS

The diagnosis of pheochromocytoma is typically made by demonstrating increased catecholamine secretion in a patient with suspicious symptoms or known to be at risk

TABLE 13-2			
Adrenergic Receptor Classification, Function, and Pharmacology			
Adrenergic Receptor Type	**Pharmacologic Agonist**	**Pharmacologic Antagonist**	**Major Biologic Effect**
α_1	Phenylephrine	Prazosin, phenoxybenzamine, phentolamine	Arteriolar constriction
α_2	Clonidine, methyldopa	Yohimbine, phenoxybenzamine, phentolamine	Mediates presynaptic feedback inhibition of norepinephrine release; decreases insulin secretion
β_1	Dobutamine	Atenolol, metoprolol, propranolol	Increases cardiac rate and contractility
β_2	Terbutaline, albuterol	Propranolol	Arteriolar and venous dilation; relaxation of tracheobronchial muscles

Data from articles by Lefkowitz and colleagues[19] and Hoffman and Lefkowitz.[20,21]

because of family history or genetic syndrome. Most show increases in a variety of urinary catecholamines and metabolites in a 24-hour specimen.[5,24] Determination of fractionated metanephrines (i.e., separate measures of metanephrine and normetaphrine), in plasma or urine, is the test of choice and is recommended for initial evaluation.[25,26] These o-methylated metabolites are released from chromafin tumors independently of the catecholamines in a more or less continuous manner.

The consistency of production enhances sensitivity, which approaches 100% (97%–99%) for detecting pheochromocytoma while maintaining acceptable specificity (70%–90%).[27,28] It is best if patients receive no medications during the tests, but several antihypertensive agents (e.g., diuretics, calcium channel blockers, angiotensin-converting enzyme inhibitors) do not materially affect results.[5] Special diets are not usually necessary. Recommendations for plasma free metanephrine collections include samplings in the fasting state from a patient who has maintained a supine position for 20 minutes.[25] In a recent study, plasma free metanephrines were elevated in all children diagnosed with pheochromocytoma.[28]

Diagnosis in the few patients with episodic hypertension can be problematic. Normal catecholamine excretion may not exclude a tumor if an episode does not occur during the collection period. Instructing the patient to collect a timed urine specimen after an episode has been proposed as a method of diagnosing such patients.[5] In young children in particular, neuroblastoma enters into the differential diagnosis of increased catecholamine excretion. In such cases, hypertension is usually minimal and homovanillic acid (HVA) is the dominant metabolite in the urine.

GENETIC DIFFERENTIAL DIAGNOSIS

The genetic differential diagnosis of pheochromocytoma comprises von Hippel-Lindau disease (VHL), MEN 2, pheochromocytoma-paraganglioma syndrome, and NF 1. (MEN 2 is discussed in detail in subsequent sections.) An ill-recognized genetic differential diagnosis for paraganglioma is MEN 1, although this is an uncommon neoplasia for this syndrome.

VHL is a heritable disorder predisposing to retinal angiomas, central nervous system hemangiomas and hemangioblastomas, renal cell carcinoma, pheochromocytoma, pancreatic islet cell tumors, and endolymphatic sac tumors.[29] It has an estimated birth incidence of 1 in 36,000 per year and is inherited in an autosomal-dominant manner with a high degree of inter- and intrafamilial variability. The VHL susceptibility gene, VHL, encodes a tumor suppressor. Approximately 28% of mutations in the VHL gene are partial or complete deletions. The remaining 72% are small deletions/insertions or point mutations. Therefore, genetic testing for VHL should use methods that detect both abnormalities (i.e., Southern blot analysis and DNA sequencing). The sensitivity of this combined approach is nearly 100% when performed on patients with a clinical diagnosis of VHL.[30]

Relatively clear genotype-phenotype correlations have been described for VHL. VHL families are categorised into two subtypes based on a low (type 1) or high (type 2) risk of pheochromocytoma. VHL type 2 has been further di-

vided based on a low risk (type 2A) or high risk (type 2B) of renal cell carcinoma. In a third subtype, VHL 2C, pheochromocytoma is the only manifestation. Among those with VHL type 1, 50% will have large deletions or truncating mutations—whereas the majority (~95%) of patients with VHL type 2 (with pheochromocytoma) have missense mutations. Interestingly, when a population-based study of families fitting the VHL type 2C description (isolated pheochromocytoma with no other syndromic features) was conducted 11% had a germ-line VHL mutation.[10] Of the 11% found to have germ-line VHL mutations, ¾ presented with pheochromocytoma under the age of 20 years.

Three new susceptibility genes for pheochromocytoma and paranganglioma have been isolated within the last decade.[31-33] These three genes (SDHB, SDHC, and SDHD) are autosomal genes encoding three of the four subunits of succinate dehydrogenase (SDH) or mitochondrial complex II. SDH is the enzyme that participates in the electron transport chain and the Krebs cycle. Interestingly, whereas homozygous or compound heterozygous mutations in SDHA cause Leigh syndrome heterozygous mutations in SDHB, C, or D cause heritable pheochromocytoma-paraganglioma syndrome.[15] In a population-based registry of apparently sporadic symptomatic pheochromocytoma or paraganglioma presentations, approximately 15% to 20% were found to carry a germ-line mutation in one of the three SDH genes.[10,34] None of those presenting with adrenal pheochromocytoma were found to carry SDHC mutations.[35] Among those found to be SDH mutation positive, approximately 25% to 30% present before the age of 20 years.[10]

Genotype-phenotype relationships are still being refined for these SDH-associated pheochromocytoma-paraganglioma syndromes. SDHC and SDHD mutations tend to be associated with head and neck paragangliomas, whereas SDHB is associated with intra-abdominal disease and malignant pheochromocytomas.[10,34-36] SDHB mutations seem to also predispose to non-paraganglial neoplasias such as very-early-onset (<30 years) renal cell carcinoma and perhaps epithelial thyroid carcinomas.[37] NF 1 is a rare cause of heritable pheochromocytoma. Among 27 population registry-based cases of apparently sporadic pheochromocytomas who were mutation negative at SDHB/C/D, VHL, and RET, only 1 (4%) was found to carry a germ-line mutation in NF1.[17]

TUMOR LOCALIZATION

Imaging studies (Figure 13-2) that localize a suspected pheochromocytoma should take place after excessive catecholamine secretion has been demonstrated. Most silent adrenal masses are not pheochromocytomas. A report of incidentally discovered adrenal masses in 1,000 adults found pheochromocytoma 4% of the time. Only half had hypertension, but the majority had increased catecholamine production.[38]

Computed tomography (CT) and magnetic resonance imaging (MRI) are most helpful in localizing pheochromocytomas. The average diameter of a pheochromocytoma is approximately 5 cm at the time of diagnosis, and the sensitivity of CT or MRI approaches 100%—although the specificity is substantially lower.[39] Scintigraphy with radiolabeled metaiodobenzylguanidine (^{131}I or ^{123}I-MIBG)

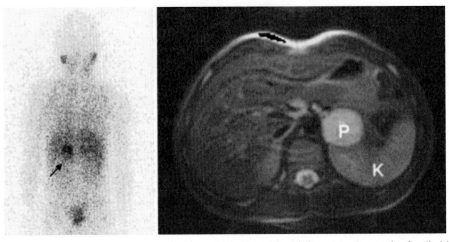

Figure 13-2 Imaging studies in pheochromocytoma. The patient was a 5-year-old with hypertension and a family history of pheochromocytoma. Urinary catecholamines were as follows: norepinephine = 728 μg/24 hr (upper limit 65), epinephrine = 8 μg/24 hr (upper limit 10), and metanephrines = 4.7 mg/24 hr (upper limit 1.3). Left: MIBG imaging, posterior view. Right: MRI, transaxial view. Pheochromocytoma is indicated as P. K denotes kidney.

is very specific for pheochromocytoma, with increased uptake of the compound evident in 90% to 100% of pheochromocytomas.[40,41]

The test is more difficult to perform and slightly less sensitive than CT and MRI.[41] However, a positive MIBG scan provides an independent confirmation of the diagnosis and may reveal disease that is more extensive than that observed by CT or MRI.[42] Therefore, some recommend combining MIBG scanning with CT or MRI to provide additional diagnostic information about adrenal masses found with conventional techniques.[25] Given these available and precise imaging techniques, arteriography and selective venous sampling (which place the patient at greater risk) are almost never indicated.

MANAGEMENT

Surgical removal of a pheochromocytoma was first performed by Charles Mayo in 1926[43] and remains the treatment of choice for this disorder. Nowadays,

endocopic removal of a solitary and bilateral pheochromocytomas is effective and safe in the hands of experienced surgeons and is preferred for most patients.[44] However, there is always the potential for disaster when anesthesia and surgery are applied to patients harboring pheochromocytomas.

Hypertensive crises, myocardial dysfunction, arrhythmias, hypotension, and shock can occur during the perioperative period and result from the acute and chronic effects of the catecholamine excess. In 1963, Stackpole and colleagues[7] reported a 22% intraoperative mortality in a review of 100 children with pheochromocytoma. Careful attention to intravenous fluid management and pharmacotherapy before and during the procedure (Table 13-3) has improved the outcome, and thus intraoperative deaths are now rare.[45] Even so, one study[46] found that 4 of 15 children undergoing pheochromocytoma removal had complications—including myocardial failure in 2 patients.

Preoperative treatment to control blood pressure is recommended, but there is no consensus on which

TABLE 13-3

Useful Agents in the Management of Pheochromocytomᵃ

Drug	Mechanism of Action	Comments
Phenoxybenzamine	α1 and α2 antagonist	Preoperative α-adrenergic blockade
Prazocin	α1 antagonist	Preoperative α-adrenergic blockade
Labetalol	Combined α- and β-adrenergic blockade	Fixed ratio α:β effect disadvantageous
Propranolol	β1 and β2 antagonist	Adjunctive for cardiac effects
Nifedipine	Calcium channel blocker	
Metyrosine	Inhibits catecholamine synthesis	Adjunctive therapy
Phentolamine	α1 and α2 antagonist	Intravenous intraoperative therapy, diagnostic tests, treat hypertensive crisis
Nitroprusside	Nonspecific vasodilation, nitric oxide generation	Intraoperative blood pressure control

Data from Keiser HR (1995). Pheochromocytoma and related tumors. In DeGroot LJ (ed.), *Endocrinology, Third edition*. Philadelphia: WB Saunders 1853-1877.

regimen is best.[26,47] Preoperative α-blockade with phenoxybenzamine remains a widely accepted method of preparing patients for surgery.[24,47] Treatment is begun at least 1 to 2 weeks before planned surgery (dosage, 5 to 10 mg b.i.d.; 0.25 to 1.0 mg/kg/day in divided doses). The dose is increased gradually until the patient's hypertension and symptoms have substantially improved. Because the initial dose may induce or worsen postural hypotension, it is typically given in the evening before bedtime.

Propranolol can be added if tachycardia or arrhythmias occur during phenoxybenzamine therapy, but it must not be used in the absence of α-receptor antagonists. Such preoperative α-blockade appears to work well in children.[22] The α-adrenergic receptor antagonist prazosin, the calcium channel blocker nifedipine, labetalol (a combined α- and β-receptor antagonist), and metyrosine (α-methyl tyrosine, an inhibitor of catecholamine synthesis) have also been used alone or adjunctively to prepare patients for surgery.[5,47]

The reported experience in children treated with these various regimens is necessarily limited. In the study by Deal and colleagues,[22] patients who had no complications during surgery typically had resolution of the signs and symptoms of catecholamine excess with preoperative medical therapy. Although preoperative treatment is commonly used, there are reports of good results in selected patients using principally intraoperative blood pressure control with nitroprusside, nitroglycerin, or both without preoperative α-blockade.[45]

Intraoperative severe hypertension can be managed with phentolamine or nitroprusside. Hypotension that occurs after tumor removal reflects the relaxation of the vascular tone that has maintained a volume-contracted state and should correct with judicious replacement of fluids. Careful and intense monitoring of the patient's status throughout the perioperative period is imperative. Some patients may develop pulmonary edema, possibly as a result of impaired myocardial function and the inability to tolerate the intravenous fluids.

Most patients with solitary adrenal pheochromocytomas are cured by the operation. However, the risk of developing a second primary in the contralateral adrenal is high in those with heritable forms. All pheochromocytoma presentations, especially under the age of 20, have a high likelihood of being heritable irrespective of other features or family history.[10] Therefore, adrenocortical sparing surgery is highly recommended in patients at substantial risk for bilateral disease so that they may avoid the requirement of lifelong glucocorticoid therapy and the risks that accompany adrenal insufficiency.[44,48,49] Finding a gene mutation usually mandates a conservative approach and adrenal-sparing surgery. Depending on the gene involved, different organs are at risk for different neoplasias.[10]

Pheochromocytomas are reported to be malignant in 12% to 47% of pediatric cases.[23,50] The prognosis for malignant pheochromocytoma is variable. Some patients die within months from metastatic disease, whereas others live for decades.[51,52]

SUMMARY OF PHEOCHROMOCYTOMA

Pheochromocytoma is rare but important to diagnose and treat appropriately. In perhaps one in two affected children, the tumor is caused by an underlying diagnosable genetic abnormality with health implications for family members. Indeed, the penetrance of pheochromocytoma/paraganglioma may approach 100% in *RET, VHL,* and *SDH* mutation carriers. All presentations of pheochromocytoma should be offered genetic testing in the setting of a genetics consultation that includes genetic counseling. Measurement of catecholamine metabolites (metanephrines) is the cornerstone of diagnosis, followed by CT imaging or MRI for localization.

Because of its low frequency, the evaluation should generally be limited to children who have hypertension and symptoms suggestive of pheochromocytoma, who have symptoms strongly suggestive of pheochromocytoma in the absence of hypertension, or who are at increased risk for pheochromocytoma because of an inherited condition (Table 13-4). The treatment of choice is surgical removal after successful pharmacotherapy to block the effects of the catecholamines. The procedure should take place in a hospital, with the capability for intense intraoperative and postoperative monitoring and therapy.

MEN Syndromes

The MEN syndromes are genetic disorders in which there is a propensity to develop glandular hyperplasia and malignant neoplasia of endocrine organs (Table 13-5).[53-55] Patients with MEN syndromes suffer from the consequences of glandular hypersecretion and the mass effects of tumors. Untreated, the diseases cause significant morbidity and excess mortality. Because of this, much effort has been directed toward identifying susceptible individuals, screening them for the presence of disease, and preventing and treating their endocrine or

---

TABLE 13-4

Indications for Pheochromocytoma Evaluation

- Triad of episodic headache, diaphoresis, and tachycardia with or without hypertension
- Family history of pheochromocytoma, VHL or MEN 2 syndrome
- Clinical features compatible with MEN 2, VHL, or pheochromocytoma-paraganglioma syndrome
- Known germ-line mutation in a pheochromocytoma-predisposing gene in the patient and/or his family
- An undefined adrenal tumor
- Hypertension unexplained and poorly responsive to standard therapies
- Significant hypertension and tachycardia in response to general anesthesia, surgery, or drugs known to provoke attacks in patients with pheochromocytomas

Data from Bravo EL (1991). Pheochromocytoma: New concepts for future trends. Kidney Int 40:544.

TABLE 13-5

Classification of MEN Syndromes

Syndrome	Principal Endocrine Disorder	Additional Features	Etiology
MEN 1	Parathyroid hyperplasia, pituitary adenomas, islet cell tumors	Carcinoid, adrenocortical hyperplasia, lipoma, cutaneous collagenoma	*MEN1* mutation
MEN 2A	Medullary thyroid carcinoma, parathyroid hyperplasia, pheochromocytoma		*RET* mutation
MEN 2B	Medullary thyroid carcinoma, pheochromocytoma	Marfanoid habitus, mucosal neuromas	*RET* mutation
FMTC	Medullary thyroid carcinoma		*RET* mutation

FMTC, familial medullary thyroid carcinoma; and MEN, multiple endocrine neoplasia.

neoplastic disease very early in order to improve their health and prolong their lives.

In most cases, it is now possible to establish a specific molecular diagnosis in affected individuals and then use the information to identify susceptible relatives. Recommendations as to whom genetic testing should be applied and how such information should be used depend on the specific clinical syndrome in question.

This chapter reviews the pathophysiology, diagnosis, and management of multiple endocrine neoplasia types 1 and 2 and the Carney complex. These specific syndromes were selected because the endocrine manifestations predominate and they are among the most relevant to pediatrics. They share several characteristics. They are inherited as Mendelian autosomal-dominant traits with high penetrance. A specific subset of glands is affected with multicentric and recurrent disease. The diseases become manifest over decades of life. Despite these obvious similarities, there are important differences. For example, MEN 2 is caused by a relatively few specific gain-of-function mutations of a growth factor receptor (RET) and prophylactic surgery is recommended for children with the mutant gene. In contrast, MEN 1 is caused by a variety of inactivating mutations in a tumor suppressor gene. Biochemical monitoring, rather than prophylactic surgery, is the standard approach.

In the text that follows, the clinical features of these syndromes are described—along with their putative pathogenic mechanisms. Newer information from research into the molecular genetic aspects of the conditions has been incorporated as possible. Because this field of medicine is in rapid evolution, the reader should continue to seek the most current information for important clinical decisions.

MULTIPLE ENDOCRINE NEOPLASIA 1 (MEN 1)

MEN 1 is typified by hyperplasia/neoplasia of parathyroid, pituitary, and pancreatic islet cells.[53,56-58] Additional features include carcinoid tumors, adrenal cortical hyperplasia, and lipomas. Extra-adrenal paragangliomas may be

rare components of MEN 1 as well. Cutaneous lesions (collagenomas, facial angiomata) are very common features, being found in nearly 90% of patients in one series.[59] Genetic linkage analysis among families with MEN 1 first localized the inherited abnormality to a small region on the long arm of chromosome 11 (11q13),[60,61] which ultimately led to identification of germ-line mutations in several families with typical MEN 1.[62,63]

The gene, aptly named *MEN1,* encodes MENIN* (a protein unlike any other known biological molecule at that time). Menin was subsequently shown to be expressed by a wide variety of tissues and localized to the nucleus.[64-66] It interacts with specific intracellular proteins involved in growth control pathways [67] and plays a broad role in the transcriptional regulation (including chromatin modification) of many genes.[68,69]

A large body of evidence, experimental and clinical, indicates that menin functions as a "tumor suppressor."[70] Mice lacking one copy of *MEN1* develop tumors in the same organs affected in the MEN1 syndrome.[71] In vitro, reduction of *MEN1* expression results in enhanced cell proliferation—whereas overexpression of menin triggers apoptosis.[70] The proposed mechanism of disease is illustrated in Figure 13-3. Patients with MEN1 carry one normal and one inactive mutant allele of the *MEN1* gene in all cells (a germline mutation).[72] This in itself is insufficient to induce tumor formation. Subsequently, loss of heterozygosity (a "second hit") in a single somatic cell deletes the only normally functioning *MEN1* gene and the ordinary constraints on cell growth from MENIN are attenuated. Tumor growth is thus initiated from a single clone of cells.

The mutations found in MEN 1 families show that they are both various and widely distributed throughout the gene (Figure 13-4), frequently truncating the translation product.[62,73,74] Thus, these are inactivating mutations and are consistent with the tumor suppressor role.

Clinical Presentation

There is significant variation in clinical presentations among and between families affected by MEN 1.[57,58,75-78] The typical patient presents in the third to fifth decades

---

*Menin as all caps refers to human protein, other species are lowercase.

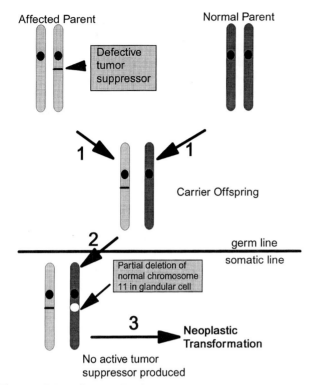

Figure 13-3 Pathogenesis of MEN 1. (1) Affected parent passes mutant MEN1 gene to offspring, who inherits a normal gene from the other parent. (2) Loss of heterozygosity in a somatic cell deletes remaining normal *MEN1* gene. (3) The absence of the tumor suppressor activity in specific cells accompanied by some other cellular event (a "second hit") leads to tumor formation.

of life with single or multiple manifestations of the condition. Hyperparathyroidism is the most common endocrine abnormality and thus hypercalcemia is usually the first sign of disease.[58,75,77,78] It is followed by lesions of the pancreatic islet and pituitary in frequency. Skin lesions are also commonly found in adults with MEN 1. The preva-

lence of cutaneous angiofibromas and collagenomas is reported to be 88% and 72%, respectively, with more lesions tending to occur in older patients.[59] The penetrance of disease in carriers of the *MEN1* genetic abnormality approaches 100% over a lifetime.[77,79]

Patients who undergo routine biochemical screening are diagnosed much earlier than those who present with symptoms (Figure 13-5). It appears that affected patients can be detected by routine biochemical screening approximately 10 years prior to the onset of symptoms. A large study evaluated the age-related penetrance in 63 unrelated kindreds with MEN 1 and found <1% penetrance in gene carriers before age 5 years, 7% penetrance by age 10 years, and 28% and 52% penetrance by ages 15 and 20 years, respectively.[73] Thus, even though MEN 1 is generally considered a disease of adults under careful surveillance nearly half of the gene carriers manifest biochemical signs within the pediatric age range.

The treatment of the various conditions and tumors that arise in MEN 1 syndrome are covered in other parts of this textbook. However, it is appropriate to discuss certain aspects that relate particularly to the MEN 1 syndrome.

Hyperparathyroidism

This is the most common manifestation of MEN 1 and occurs in nearly all affected patients. The disease differs from that of sporadic primary hyperparathyroidism in that there is a slow but inexorable progression of hyperparathyroidism over time, with development of oligoclonal adenomas/hyperplasia in multiple glands.[80,81] These features form the basis of the recommendation that patients at risk be screened with annual serum calcium and intact parathyroid hormone measurements, and receive treatment when there is evidence of clinically significant hyperparathyroidism and/or when there is an increasing trend of ionized calcium levels.

Subtotal parathyroidectomy of three and a half glands or total parathyroidectomy with reimplantation represent

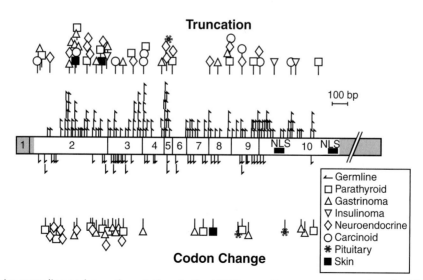

Figure 13-4 Representative germ-line and somatic mutations in the *MEN1* gene. Gene exons are numbered, with the hatched area demarcating untranslated regions. Mutations listed above the gene are those that would result in a truncated mRNA that would either yield a highly abnormal protein or be unstable (e.g., nonsense mutations, frame-shifting deletions/insertions). Those below are missense changes. [Used with permission from Marx, SJ et al. (1999). The gene for multiple endocrine neoplasia type 1: Recent findings. Bone 25:119.]

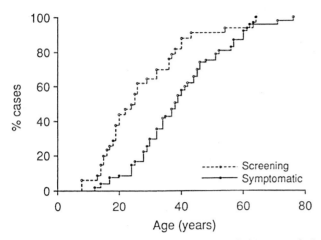

Figure 13-5 Age-related onset of multiple endocrine neoplasia type 1. Patients were divided into those detected by a biochemical screening versus those identified because of symptoms of MEN 1 disease. Data indicate that screening detects individuals with MEN1 before symptoms at almost all ages and decreases the average age at detection by approximately 10 years. The graph was constructed from data for 87 patients. [Graph from Thakker RV (1993). The molecular genetics of multiple endocrine neoplasia syndromes. Clin Endocrinol 38:1.]

the standard treatment, but could be considered palliative because the recurrence rate approximates 20%.[82] Mallette[81] recommended total parathyroidectomy with autologous transplantation of a portion of one of the parathyroid glands in the forearm. This allows a much simpler reoperation if hypercalcemia recurs. Others suggest that subtotal parathyroidectomy is sufficient and perhaps results in a lower rate of postoperative permanent hypoparathyroidism.[83,84] Regardless of the surgical approach selected, it must deal with all parathyroid glands because disease in multiple glands is the rule.

Because the first manifestation of MEN 1 in the large majority of cases is hyperparathyroidism, it would be important to consider the genetic differential diagnosis of parathyroid disease. Although only 2% to 3% of patients presenting with primary HPT have MEN 1,[85] in familial isolated hyperparathyroidism 20% of probands harbor a germ-line *MEN1* mutation.[86] Also important in the differential diagnosis is the hyperparathyroidism-jaw tumor syndrome caused by germ-line mutations in *HRPT2* on 1q25-q31.[87]

Enteropancreatic Islet Cell Tumors

These tumors are the second most common manifestation of MEN 1, being found in up to 60% to 80% of affected patients over their lifetimes.[58,79,88] Approximately half are gastrinomas, and a third are β-cell tumors.[78,89,90] Tumors that secrete pancreatic polypeptide are also found.[88] The elevated circulating concentrations of pancreatic polypeptide do not appear to produce significant symptoms or functional abnormalities, although they may be sign of clinically important pancreatic tumors. Clinically silent lesions can also be detected by endoscopic ultrasonography. In one prospective study, 41% of MEN 1 patients with lesions detected by ultrasound were asymptomatic.[91]

It is important to note the significant morbidity and mortality that results from pancreatic islet cell disease in MEN 1. About half of patients with MEN 1 die from a MEN-1-related condition, most often from peptic ulcers (the Zollinger-Ellison syndrome) or from the mass effects of a malignant islet cell tumor.[76] Multiple insulinomas are frequent, and partial pancreatectomy may be required.[92] Although there are suggestions that earlier detection of the tumors and subsequent removal may improve long-term survival,[93] this is not clearly established at this time.

The major genetic differential diagnosis of islet cell tumors is MEN 1. It is important to recognize that a third of all patients with Zollinger-Ellison syndrome will have MEN 1.[94] Islet cell tumors can also be components of VHL and NF 1. In VHL, pancreatic cysts are common—and approximately 10% to 15% will have islet cell tumors, the latter of which have a high likelihood of malignancy. Surgery is indicated when VHL-related pancreatic islet cell tumors are >3 cm, whereas lesions <1 cm can be safely monitored.

Pituitary Tumors

Approximately 15% to 50% of individuals with MEN 1 develop a pituitary tumor.[95] Two-thirds are microadenomas (<1.0 cm in diameter), and the majority are prolactin secreting.[96] Among patients with pituitary tumors, the prevalence of MEN 1 is 2.5% to 5%[96,97] (but as high as 14% in patients with prolactinoma).[96] These results underscore the importance of carefully taking a thorough medical and family history in patients with a diagnosis of an MEN-1-associated endocrine tumor, even seemingly in isolation. Even so, there are rare cases and families that appear to have MEN 1 or a MEN ½ overlap who do not have *MEN1* or *RET* mutations.[98] For example, probands with only pituitary and parathyroid disease harbor germ-line *MEN1* mutations only 7% of the time.[98]

Screening

At the present time, there is no specific treatment that will prevent the disease manifestations—nor do any prophylactic therapies appear to be warranted. Thus, the goal of screening in MEN 1 is to detect clinical manifestations before there has been spread of tumors or serious ramifications from excess hormone secretion. Prior studies have described results of episodic biochemical screening programs designed to meet this end.[75,77,78,88] However, because of the long latency for disease manifestation many unaffected individuals were required to undergo years of episodic testing.

It is possible to use molecular genetic methods to determine carrier status, although the wide range of genetic mutations (more than 400 germ-line mutations identified) means that it may be necessary to sequence the entire gene to identify the abnormality in the index case. A mutation within the *MEN1* gene can be detected in 70% or more of typical MEN 1 cases with this approach.[99] It is believed that the remainder also bear *MEN1* mutations that affect *MENIN* abundance. They are just not detected by PCR-based sequencing of the coding region.[55]

Genetic testing should be offered to index cases with familial endocrinopathies consistent with MEN 1 or apparently sporadic cases with two or more MEN-1-type tumors.[100] Once a mutation is identified in the index case, the optimal ages for offering genetic testing, beginning screening for disease, and determining the frequency and extent of testing for relatives are not clearly established. Certainly, genetic testing in the young (if clearly negative) would avoid unnecessary biochemical and other monitoring. Consensus guidelines, published in 2001, suggested that screening begin at age 5—with annual biochemical testing for insulinoma and anterior pituitary disease and less frequent imaging studies.[100]

Testing for gastrinoma, other enteropancreatic tumors, and carcinoid could be delayed until age 20. It is important to remember that morbidity from MEN 1 in preadolescence is very rare,[101] even though biochemical abnormalities may be detected. Furthermore, establishing a molecular diagnosis presently offers no therapeutic advantage to the affected. Therefore, some advocate waiting until the patient is old enough to give informed consent before performing genetic testing to determine risk status. Acknowledging the caveats, the authors believe that combining molecular genetic testing with periodic biochemical assessment is the most rational approach.

Useful screening tests are listed in Table 13-6. Probably the minimal requirements in the pediatric population would be history and physical examinations on an annual basis beginning at age 5, and basal ionized calcium, prolactin, and IGF-I measurements every 1 to 2 years thereafter in patients at risk. Whether the patient was at risk would be determined by assessment of *MEN1* gene mutation carrier status, in the setting of genetic counseling, at the age biochemical screening was contemplated. When abnormalities are found on screening tests, further studies (including imaging) are warranted to confirm the diagnosis and to determine the course of therapy.

MULTIPLE ENDOCRINE NEOPLASIA 2

Multiple endocrine neoplasia type 2 (MEN 2) serves as the paradigm for the practice of clinical cancer genetics. Historically, MEN 2 encompasses at least three subtypes: MEN 2A, MEN 2B, and familial medullary thyroid carcinoma (FMTC).[102-104] Each subtype is characterized by C-cell hyperplasia, which progresses to multicentric MTC. Patients with MEN 2A and 2B also develop pheochromocytomas. Parathyroid hyperplasia/adenomata occur in MEN 2A but are rare in MEN 2B.

TABLE 13-6

Major Clinical Features of MEN 1

Organ	Neoplasia	Symptomatic Manifestation	Clinical Detection	Comments
Parathyroid	Hyperparathyroidism	Arthralgia, bone pain, renal stone	Plasma Ca^{2+}, PTH	Present in 95%
Pituitary	Prolactinoma	Galactorrhea, hypogonadism	Plasma prolactin	60% of pituitary tumors in MEN 1
	GH or GH/Prl-secreting tumor	Acromegaly-gigantism	IGF-I, GH	25% of pituitary tumors in MEN 1
Pancreas	Insulinoma	Hypoglycemia	Glucose/insulin	One third of pancreatic tumors in MEN 1
	Gastrinoma	Zollinger-Ellison syndrome	Gastrin	Most common; principal cause of death
	PP producing VIP producing	Usually asymptomatic Diarrhea	Plasma PP, imaging	

GH, growth hormone; IGF-I, insulin-like growth factor-I; PP, pancreatic polypeptide; Prl, prolactin; PTH, parathyroid hormone; and VIP, vasoactive intestinal polypeptide.
Data from Thakker RV (1995). Multiple endocrine neoplasia type 1. In DeGroot LJ (ed.), *Endocrinology, Third edition*. Philadelphia: WB Saunders.

TABLE 13-7

Principal Glandular Diseases in MEN 2

Organ	Neoplasia	Clinical Manifestation	Clinical Detection	Frequency
Thyroid	Medullary carcinoma	Neck mass	Plasma calcitonin	>90%[p]
Parathyroid	Hyperplasia	Arthralgia, bone pain, renal stone	Plasma Ca^{2+}, parathyroid hormone	15% to 20% in MEN 2A
Adrenal	Pheochromocytoma	Hypertension, headache, adrenergic paroxysms	Catecholamine measurement and/or imaging	About 50%

[p] Determined through biochemical screening.
Data from Gagel RF (1995). Multiple endocrine neoplasia type 2. In DeGroot LJ (ed.), *Endocrinology, Third edition*. Philadelphia: WB Saunders.

Germ-line RET Proto-oncogene Mutations Cause MEN 2

All three clinical subtypes of MEN 2 are caused by germ-line mutations of the *RET* proto-oncogene on 10q11.2.[105] Pathogenic gain-of-function germ-line *RET* mutations are found in more than 95% of patients with the MEN 2A or MEN 2B clinical phenotype—and in ~85% of individuals with FMTC.[100,104,106] As might be expected, the *RET* proto-oncogene is expressed by and plays a prominent role during the development of neural crest and its derivatives as well as the parathyroid anlage.[107,108]

The 21-exon *RET* proto-oncogene encodes the RET protein, which is structured like many other cell surface growth factor receptors with an extracellular binding domain and an intracellular tyrosine kinase (Figure 13-6). The RET receptor tyrosine kinase mediates the signals of the glial-derived neurotrophic factor family of peptide growth factors (GDNF), which are involved in the regulation of neural tissue development—including that of the peripheral and enteric nervous systems.[109] Family members include GDNF, neuturin, persephin, and artemin. Rather than binding directly to RET, these ligands need to interact with RET and one of the latter's four membrane-bound coreceptors—known as the GDNF family receptor α family (GFRA1-4 encoding GFRα1-4)—to elicit autophosphorylation of RET and phosphorylation of cytoplasmic signal-transducing molecules.[104] Each member of the GDNF family appears to bind predominantly to a specific GFRα. Thus, the GFRα coreceptor appears to be responsible for the specificity of *RET* signaling.[110]

The specific germ-line mutations found in the *RET* proto-oncogene dictate to a large extent the phenotype of patients and the aggressiveness of the MTC.[100,111] Nearly all *RET* mutations reported in patients with MEN 2A involve missense mutations that replace one of the six extracellular cysteine residues close to the transmembrane domain of the RET protein (Figure 13-6).[105,112,113] Codon 634 mutations (in particular, C634R) are highly associated with the MEN 2A phenotype.[104,106,114] Mutations associated with FMTC are more evenly distributed across the hot-spot cysteine codons, usually favoring the more N-terminal ones. In addition, mutations in some intracellular residues appear to favor FMTC—although rarely MEN 2A phenotype is seen. Although there is a clear genotype-phenotype association in MEN 2, the correlations are imperfect. For example, an identical germ-line RET mutation may produce FMTC in one family and MEN 2A in another. The basis for this remains unclear, but is thought to be due to the influence of additional genetic modifiers within *RET* itself as well as other loci.[104,115]

The great majority (>98%) of MEN 2B appears to be produced by two specific missense mutations in the tyrosine kinase domain of the *RET* proto-oncogene. These are M918T (>95% of MEN 2B) and A883F (2%-3%).[104,116-118] Unlike loss-of-function mutations (e.g., MEN 1), gain-of-function mutations typically occur at select loci. This is precisely the case for the *RET* mutations associated with MEN 2. As noted previously, ligand-induced receptor dimerization followed by autophosphorylation and activation of an intracellular tyrosine kinase domain are mechanisms that operate commonly among growth factor receptors (e.g., receptors for EGF and PDGF).

The mutations that characterize MEN 2A and most FMTC appear to force ligand-independent dimerization because unpaired cysteine residues in the mutant receptor form inter-receptor disulfide bridges that yield stable functional homodimers that maintain an activated state

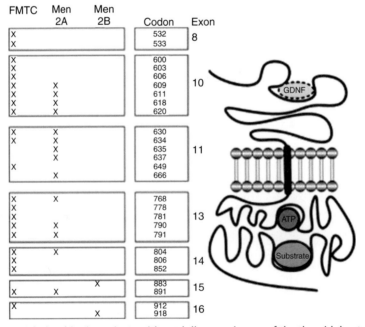

FMTC	Men 2A	Men 2B	Codon	Exon
X			532	8
X			533	
X			600	10
X			603	
X			606	
X	X		609	
X	X		611	
X	X		618	
X	X		620	
X	X		630	11
X	X		634	
	X		635	
	X		637	
X			649	
	X		666	
X	X		768	13
X			778	
X			781	
X	X		790	
X	X		791	
X	X		804	14
X			806	
X			852	
		X	883	15
X	X		891	
X			912	16
		X	918	

Figure 13-6 Genotype-phenotype relationships in patients with medullary carcinoma of the thyroid due to germ-line *RET* mutations. RET protein structure is shown with ligand glial-derived neurotrophic factor (GDNF). Positions (codon numbers) where missense mutations alter amino acid in families with MEN 2A, familial medullary carcinoma of the thyroid (FMTC), and MEN 2B are shown. [Used with permission from You YN, Lakhani V, Wells SA Jr. (2006). Medullary thyroid carcinoma. Surg Oncol Clin North Am 15:644.]

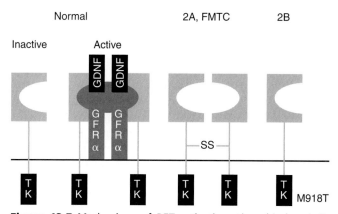

Figure 13-7 Mechanisms of RET activation. Ligand-induced dimerization stabilizes the dimeric form of the receptor in which the tyrosine kinase is active. In the case of MEN2A and familial medullary thyroid carcinoma (FMTC), disulfide bridges form between monomers—yielding a stable (active) homodimer. In MEN 2B, mutation in the intracellular catalytic domain constitutively activates the receptor. TK, tyrosine kinase; and GDNF, glial-derived neurotrophic factor.

(Figure 13-7). C634R (the most common MEN 2A mutation) has been shown to be the most transforming in vitro compared to mutations in the more 5' cysteines.[119] Very rarely, non-cysteine missense mutations have been found in MEN 2A/FMTC, but the mechanism is usually similar (e.g., a small deletion or splice mutation removes one or more of the cysteines, resulting in the same intermolecular disulfide bridging).[120]

The mechanism differs for MEN-2B-related *RET* germline mutations, but the result is similar. The most common MEN 2B mutation, M918T, occurs within the catalytic domain at the heart of the residues dictating substrate specificity. The replacement of methionine by threonine at codon 918 causes RET to favor substrates normally used by cytoplasmic kinases, instead of its native receptor tyrosine kinase substrates, and to lose responsiveness to normal autoinhibitory feedback signals.[121,122]

Constitutive activation or enhanced function of the RET protein (receptor) over time leads to hyperplasia and, in the context of other oncogenic events, subsequent malignant transformation.[119,121,122]

An important clue to RET function in endocrine neoplasia development came from the observation of the coexistence of MEN 2A or FMTC with Hirschsprung disease (HSCR). Germline loss-of-function mutations in *RET* have been found to cause familial and sporadic HSCR in some cases.[123]

Finding MEN 2A/FTMC with HSCR in an individual or segregating in a family appeared paradoxical at the molecular level in that MEN 2 resulted from RET superfunction whereas HSCR was due to attenuated RET signaling.

This conundrum remained until further functional analyses demonstrated that missense mutations that are more 5' in the gene [i.e., mutations in cysteines 611, 618, and 620 (exon 10)[124]] resulted in RET receptors that were trapped in the golgi and never reached the cell surface, resulting in functional haploinsufficiency.[125] Based on these data, the coexistence of MEN 2A/FMTC and HSCR can be explained by the fact that neoplasia results from

constitutive activation of RET whereas normal development of the enteric ganglia is dependent on adequacy of RET dosage. Similarly, the phenotypic variation of MEN 2A and FMTC can be explained by the balance between constitutive RET signaling and the number of RET receptors generating the signals.[104] Thus, C634R is associated with the most fulminant disease—resulting in MTC, pheochromocytoma, and hyperparathyroidism compared to missense mutations in C609 and C611 in FMTC with the lowest penetrance and later onsets.[106]

Calcitonin and C Cells

The parafollicular (C) cells originate from the neural crest and migrate during development into the thyroid gland of humans and higher vertebrates. In lower vertebrates, such as fish, these cells constitute the ultimobranchial body. The C cells secrete calcitonin, a 32-amino-acid single-chain peptide that has calcium-lowering properties in vivo. Calcitonin is synthesized as part of a larger precursor containing katacalcitonin, which is cleaved from calcitonin proper before secretion.

In addition, calcitonin-gene-related peptide is produced by alternate splicing during transcription of the calcitonin gene. Calcitonin is abundant only in the thyroid.[126] Calcitonin-gene-related peptide is most abundant in the nervous system[127] but is also secreted by medullary thyroid carcinomas[128] (a C-cell malignancy). The degree of elevation of the plasma concentration of calcitonin is the traditional marker of medullary carcinoma of the thyroid.[129]

In MEN 2, the C cells are believed to undergo progressive changes—beginning with simple hyperplasia and ending with malignancy. MTC frequently spreads to regional lymph nodes but eventually may metastasize to liver, lung, and bone. Medullary carcinoma of the thyroid is the principal MEN-related cause of death in patients with MEN 2A,[130] which results from the distant metastases or local complications.[102]

Clinical Presentation

MEN 2A/FMTC. The majority of patients present because they were the first to develop MCT in their family or have a relative affected with the disease. The mean age for diagnosis of a C-cell abnormality by biochemical screening is approximately 15 years,[131] whereas palpable tumors are not typically evident until many years later.[130] Increased calcitonin secretion in response to stimulation, reflecting C-cell hyperplasia or carcinoma *in situ,* is evident by the age of 30 years in nearly all individuals bearing the disease gene.[131,132]

Approximately 50% of those with MEN 2A eventually develop pheochromocytomas,[133] usually after detection of a C-cell abnormality. MEN-2A-related hyperparathyroidism is less common, being found in between 15 and 35% of patients—depending on the thoroughness of the investigating physician and the age of the patient because there appears to be a clear age-related penetrance.[114] Studies whose cohorts are very mature have a higher frequency of hyperparathyroidism in MEN 2A cases than in those who have shorter follow-up times. The mean age at diagnosis of symptomatic pheochromocytoma is 36 years, with occasional patients presenting with pheochromocytoma first.[10]

MEN 2B. MEN 2B is much less common, and most patients (60%) with MEN 2B represent de novo mutations rather than being members of large kindreds. In addition, MEN 2B patients have a distinctive appearance with marfanoid body habitus, unusual facies, and multiple mucosal neuromas (Figures 13-8 and 13-9). These neuromas are classically described as occurring on the tongue but in fact occur throughout the oromucocutaneous ragions and gastrointestinal tract—and are frequently associated with gastrointestinal symptoms.

In many patients, the poor intestinal function appears to mimic HSCR—and GI symptoms with failure to thrive may be the presenting symptoms even in the neonatal period.[134] Mucosal neuromas, gastrointestinal symptoms secondary to ganglioneuromatosis of the gut, and other characteristic physical traits are frequently the key features that lead to the diagnosis of MEN 2B.[135] Hypertrophy of the corneal nerves can be observed with slit-lamp examination and can be helpful in establishing the diagnosis.[136,137] Hyperparathyroidism is rare with MEN 2B, and some believe that clinically evident parathyroid disease never occurs in MEN 2B.

Of great importance is the fact that MEN-2B-related MTC occurs on average 10 years earlier than that in MEN 2A and is more aggressive.[130,138] It follows that prophylactic thyroidectomy is recommended at the youngest

age (<1 year) once the molecular or clinical diagnosis of MEN 2B is established.

Indications and Use of Molecular Genetic Testing. Identification of a *RET* gene mutation within a MEN 2 family is of great benefit for those affected because MTC can be prevented or cured when prophylactic thyroidectomy is performed at an early stage[133,139-141] and because biochemical monitoring for pheochromocytoma allows its early detection and therapy. It is obvious that any family with hereditary MTC with or without pheochromocytoma needs testing. Individuals with apparently sporadic MTC should be tested as well because the prevalence of unexpected germ-line *RET* mutations is approximately 5% to 10%.

When the prevalence of germ-line mutations is in this range and/or if testing gives significant information, the American Society of Clinical Oncology Guidelines for Cancer Genetic Testing recommends offering genetic analysis in the setting of genetic counseling.[142] Individuals with pheochromocytoma, especially the familial forms, should also be offered *RET* analysis (see previous section on pheochromocytomas).

RET gene analysis is widely available and generally straightforward because of the limited number of mutations that produce MEN 2/FMTC. Once a germ-line mutation is identified, the approach is partly determined by the particular mutation involved. For those at highest risk for an aggressive form of MTC (MEN 2B; codon 883, 918, and 922 mutations), prophylactic thyroidectomy in infancy is recommended. For those at intermediate risk of aggressive MTC (codon 611, 618, 620, or 634), thyroidectomy by age 5 years is recommended. Children with *RET* mutations with the lowest risk (typically those associated with FMTC) should also have thyroidectomy by age 5 to 10.

Circulating concentrations of calcitonin following stimulation were formerly used as an index of C-cell disease and to identify carriers.[143,144] The superiority of molecular genetic testing became evident shortly after the discovery that MEN 2 was caused by mutations of the *RET* proto-oncogene and molecular biological techniques were used to determine carrier status.[145-147] Lips and colleagues[146] studied 300 subjects in four families segregating MEN 2A. Most of the patients had been previously screened with stimulated calcitonin measurements. Of the patients with abnormal stimulation tests who underwent thyroid surgery, all with histologically diagnosed medullary carcinoma of the thyroid were shown to have the characteristic germ-line mutations of the RET proto-oncogene.

Of special interest were eight children with normal calcitonin stimulation tests who underwent thyroidectomies because they harbored the RET proto-oncogene mutation. Each had microscopic medullary carcinoma of the thyroid. In addition, there were six patients who underwent thyroidectomies because of positive stimulation tests. These were subsequently shown not to be carriers of the mutation. These patients all showed C-cell hyperplasia (known to affect 3% to 5% of the normal population) without medullary carcinoma of the thyroid.

Pheochromocytoma. The pheochromocytomas associated with MEN 2 are usually diagnosed in the third to fifth decades of life and are frequently bilateral.[148,149] Malignant pheochromocytoma is rare. Annual screening through measurement of fractionated metanephrines (urine or plasma) is

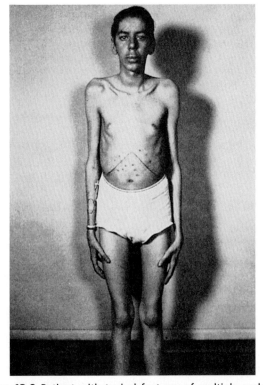

Figure 13-8 Patient with typical features of multiple endocrine neoplasia type 2B. Note the Marfanoid body habitus, thickened lips due to mucosal neuromas, and abdominal scars that reflect surgery for pheochromocytoma. [From Melvin KEW, Tashjian AH Jr., Miller HH (1972). Studies in familial [medullary] thyroid carcinoma. Recent Progr Horm Res 28:399.]

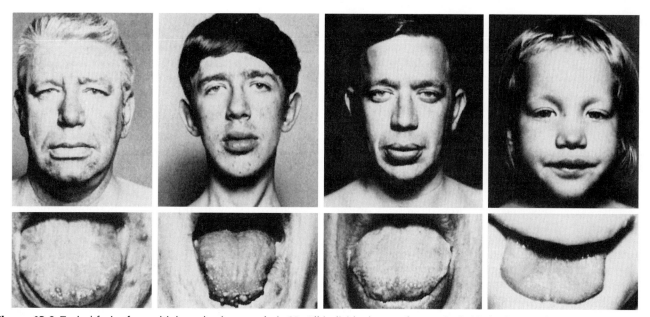

Figure 13-9 Typical facies for multiple endocrine neoplasia 2B. All individuals were from a single kindred. Note the thickened lips, ganglioneuromas of the tongue, and thickened eyelids. [From Sizemore GW, Heath H III, Carney JA (1980). Multiple endocrine neoplasia type-II. Clin Endocrinol Metab 9:299.]

indicated, even though some patients with pheochromocytoma present with radiographic abnormalities before increased excretion of catecholamines.[150] This is probably a reflection of the adrenal medullary hyperplasia (the presumed precursor to the pheochromocytoma) found in many patients with MEN 2.[151] Any child at risk for MEN 2 who develops signs and symptoms of pheochromocytoma (such as headache, irritability, or hypertension) should be completely evaluated (as outlined in the previous section).

The pharmacologic preparation of patients for pheochromocytoma surgery was reviewed earlier in this chapter. If the disease appears to be unilateral at the time of operation, only the affected gland is operated on—even though patients with MEN 2 syndrome have a 40% to 50% chance of developing a second primary in the contralateral adrenal.[133,149,150] A decade may pass before the appearance of a second pheochromocytoma.[133,150] As noted previously, partial adrenalectomy with preservation of adrenal cortical function is recommended in MEN 2.[49,152]

RET Testing and Hirschsprung Disease. HSCR is common in pediatric practice. Because HSCR is a genetically complex trait, performing genetic testing specifically for management of HSCR is currently not recommended. Instead, what is commonly done is to look for RET mutations that also confer risk of MEN 2A—such as germ-line mutations in C620 and C618 and in C609 and C611.[106,153] It is estimated that in MEN 2 cases with C620 or C618 mutations, approximately ⅓ to ½ may actually have HSCR as well.

Carney Complex

Carney complex is a genetic condition that leads to endocrine gland tumors and hyperfunction by mechanisms analogous to those involved in the other conditions reviewed in this chapter.[154] It is characterized by the development of myxomas in multiple tissues (skin, heart, and breast), endocrine tumors/hyperfunction, primary pigmented nodular adrenal hyperplasia (PPNAD)-associated Cushing syndrome, and acromegaly differentiated epithelial thyroid carcinoma and spotty, pigmentation of the skin in select areas.[155]

Molecular Genetics. Two distinct genetic loci are associated with Carney complex. One is found on chromosome 2 (2p16), but that susceptibility gene is yet to be identified.[156] The other is the gene (PRKAR1A) encoding a regulatory subunit of protein kinase A on chromosome 17.[157] The germ-line mutations found in PRKAR1A are characteristically loss-of-function, and it is postulated that PRKAR1A functions as a "tumor suppressor." Most of the germ-line mutations in this gene are truncating, and interestingly lead to nonsense-mediated decay of the mRNA transcript.

Clinical Presentation. No clinical features appear to distinguish the two genetic forms. The diagnosis may be made at any age, usually because of myxoma development. The main sites for these tumors are the skin and heart, with cardiac myxomas being a major cause of morbidity. Thyroid nodules, large-cell calcifying Sertoli cell tumors, and PPNAD (see material following) may also develop during childhood. The lentigenes (spotty skin pigmentation), which may be present at birth, appear primarily around the lips, eyes, and genital mucosa in the postpubertal period. Pigmentation on the ocular canthae is relatively specific for Carney complex. This sign is rarely seen in other pigmentary disorders, such as Peutz-Jeghers syndrome.

Endocrine Manifestations. Acromegaly and Cushing syndrome due to PPNAD are the most common. PPNAD is a form of ACTH-independent hypercortisolism found in approximately one in four patients with Carney complex. Most patients with PPNAD are diagnosed in the second and third decades of life, but some cases appear in early childhood. Many show an unusual response during standard dexamethasone testing, with an increase in cortisol excretion.[158]

Acromegaly is due to GH-producing adenomas and is said to be clinically subtle. Thyroid function is normal, but thyroid neoplasms (follicular adenoma, differentiated nonmedullary thyroid cancer) are common, with up to 75% of patients having nodular disease by ultrasound.

Management. Once the syndrome is identified, the patients must be monitored for the development of the tumors and endocrine disorders characteristic of the syndrome. This should include periodic thyroid and cardiac ultrasonography and measures of adrenocortical function. The pathways for diagnosis of Cushing syndrome and acromegaly and the management of thyroid nodules are described elsewhere in this textbook. As noted previously, a paradoxical response for cortisol excretion during standard suppression testing should be a clue that one may be dealing with PPNAD. The treatment for symptomatic PPNAD at present is bilateral adrenalectomy.

Pediatrics and the MEN Syndromes

The preceding sections describe the clinical manifestations of the MEN syndromes and their therapies. It is relatively uncommon for a child to present with clinical disease. However, when a child does present with an endocrine neoplasia the possibility of a genetic etiology is high. In pediatric practice, the question of MEN more often arises when the relative of an otherwise healthy child is discovered to have a glandular lesion suspicious for an MEN syndrome. For patients with a pedigree clearly demonstrating either the MEN 1 or MEN 2 phenotype, the approach to screening and treatment is as described.

More problematic is the child whose relative, frequently not first degree, has an endocrine neoplasm that may or may not reflect a heritable MEN syndrome. In light of the value of screening and prophylactic therapies, it is imperative that the possibilities be investigated fully. A detailed family history is the first step. It is very important to emphasize that if the presence or absence of disease in the pedigree is based solely on symptomatic clinical manifestations and not on biochemical or genetic screening a MEN syndrome might be present even though only one individual appears to be affected. This is because of the relatively advanced age characteristic of clinical disease in the MEN syndromes. Thus, the best strategy and current standard of care involves molecular examination of the affected relative to determine whether he or she carries a typical germ-line mutation. Although it is possible to analyze the unaffected relatives (e.g., the child in question) without examining the proband, it is generally better when possible to determine whether the affected individual bears a characteristic mutation. Many medical centers have programs for genetic cancer assessment, and a few centers specialize in MEN patients. Consultation with physicians at such centers is indicated for diagnosis and management.

Summary and Future Developments

The advent of new molecular tactics changed the way physicians manage patients with the diseases discussed in this chapter. The utility of using molecular genetic testing to more efficiently and effectively address serious clinical problems can hardly be more evident than in the MEN 2 situation. In the last seven years, the genetic etiologies of pheochromocytoma and paraganglioma have expanded such that this armamentarium is also available for routine clinical management. With these advances in genomic medicine, accurate molecular diagnosis and predictive testing are possible. Furthermore, gene-guided medical management has become possible. Typically, these involve surveillance strategies and prophylactic surgery.

Despite these encouraging developments, problems remain. There are two broad issues. The first is metastatic disease and the second is the effective treatment of the benign neoplasias with the fewest side effects. Metastatic neuroendocrine tumors are not amenable to standard cytotoxic therapies. For example, patients with metastatic MTC are particularly difficult to treat because standard chemotherapy and radiation are ineffective[159] and subsequent surgical cure difficult.[129] Patients with hyperparathyroidism frequently end up with permanent hypoparathyroidism or have recurrent disease.

There are recent therapeutic advances that may prove helpful in these situations. A new class of molecular targeted therapies that inhibit tyrosine kinases have been developed and shown to be efficacious in certain cancers, and show some promise in preclinical models of MTC.[160,161] In addition, calcimimetic agents[162] (calcium-sensing receptor agonists) have the potential to slow the development of parathyroid hyperplasia and theoretically could delay the need for parathyroidectomy in MEN 1. Thus, there are good reasons to expect further improvements in the health and quality of life of probands and their families who are affected by these conditions.

REFERENCES

1. Bravo EL (1994). Evolving concepts in the pathophysiology, diagnosis, and treatment of pheochromocytoma. Endocrine Rev 15:356–368.
2. Beard CM, Sheps SG, Kurland LT, Carney JA, Lie JT (1983). Occurrence of pheochromocytoma in Rochester, Minnesota, 1950 through 1979. Mayo Clin Proc 58:802–804.
3. Beltsevich DG, Kuznetsov NS, Kazaryan AM, Lysenko MA (2004). Pheochromocytoma surgery: Epidemiologic peculiarities in children. World J Surg 28:592–596.
4. Sutton MG, Sheps SG, Lie JT (1981). Prevalence of clinically unsuspected pheochromocytoma. Mayo Clin Proc 56:354–360.
5. Keiser HR (1995). Pheochromocytoma and related tumors. In DeGroot LJ (ed.), *Endocrinology, Third edition.* Philadelphia: WB Saunders 1853–1877.
6. Hume DM (1963). Pheochromocytoma in the adult and in the child. Am J Surg 99:458–496.
7. Stackpole RH, Melicow MM, Uson AC (1963). Pheochromocytoma in children. J Pediatr 63:315–330.
8. Khafagi FA, et al. (1991). Phaeochromocytoma and functioning paraganglioma in childhood and adolescence: Role of iodine 131 metaiodobenzylguanidine. Eur J Nucl Med 18:191–198.
9. Perel Y, et al. (1997). Pheochromocytoma and paraganglioma in children: A report of 24 cases of the French Society of Pediatric Oncology. Pediatr Hematol Oncol 14:413–422.

10. Neumann HP, et al. (2002). Germ-line mutations in nonsyndromic pheochromocytoma. N Engl J Med 346:1459–1466.

11. Casanova S, et al. (1993). Phaeochromocytoma in multiple endocrine neoplasia type 2 A: Survey of 100 cases. Clin Endocrinol (Oxford) 38:531–537.

12. Eng C, et al. (1995). Mutations in the RET proto-oncogene and the von Hippel-Lindau disease tumour suppressor gene in sporadic and syndromic phaeochromocytomas. Journal of Medical Genetics 32:934–937.

13. Latif F, et al. (1993). Identification of the von Hippel-Lindau disease tumor suppressor gene. Science 260:1317–1320.

14. Neumann HP, et al. (1993). Pheochromocytomas, multiple endocrine neoplasia type 2, and von Hippel-Lindau disease. N Engl J Med 329:1531–1538.

15. Eng C, Kiuru M, Fernandez MJ, Aaltonen LA (2003). A role for mitochondrial enzymes in inherited neoplasia and beyond. Nature Reviews 3:193–202.

16. Riccardi VM (1991). Neurofibromatosis: Past, present, and future. N Engl J Med 324:1283–1285.

17. Bausch B, et al. (2006). Comprehensive mutation scanning of NF1 in apparently sporadic cases of pheochromocytoma. J Clin Endocrinol Metab 91:3478–3481.

18. Merke DP, et al. (2000). Adrenomedullary dysplasia and hypofunction in patients with classic 21-hydroxylase deficiency. N Engl J Med 343:1362–1368.

19. Lefkowitz RJ, Hoffman BB, Taylor (1996). Neurotransmission: The autonomic and somatic motor nervous systems. In Hardman JG, Gilman AG, Limbird LE (eds.), Goodman and Gilman's The pharmacologic basis of therapeutics. New York: McGraw-Hill 105–139.

20. Hoffman BB, Lefkowitz RJ (1996). Catecholamines, sympathomimetic drugs, and adrenergic receptor antagonists. In Hardman JG, Gilman AG, Limbird LE (eds.), The Pharmocologic Basis of Therapeutics, Ninth edition. New York: McGraw-Hill 199–248.

21. Hoffman BB, Lefkowitz RJ (1990). Adrenergic receptor antagonists. In Gilman AG, Nies AS, Rall TW, Taylor P (eds.), The pharmocologic basis of therapeutics, Eighth edition. New York: Pergamon Press 221–243.

22. Deal JE, Sever PS, Barratt TM, Dillon MJ (1990). Phaeochromocytoma: Investigation and management of 10 cases. Arch Dis Child 65:269–274.

23. Barontini M, Levin G, Sanso G (2006). Characteristics of pheochromocytoma in a 4- to 20-year-old population. Annals of the New York Academy of Sciences 1073:30–37.

24. Loggie JMH (1992). Catecholamine-producing tumors that cause hypertension: Diagnosis and management. In Loggie LMH (ed.), Pediatric and adolescent hypertension. Cambridge (UK): Blackwell 301–313.

25. Grossman A, et al. (2006). Biochemical diagnosis and localization of pheochromocytoma: Can we reach a consensus? Annals of the New York Academy of Sciences 1073:332–347.

26. Pacak K, et al. (2007). Pheochromocytoma: recommendations for clinical practice from the First International Symposium, October 2005. Nature Clinical Practice 3:92–102.

27. Sawka AM, Jaeschke R, Singh RJ, Young WF Jr. (2003). A comparison of biochemical tests for pheochromocytoma: Measurement of fractionated plasma metanephrines compared with the combination of 24-hour urinary metanephrines and catecholamines. J Clin Endocrinol Metab 88:553–558.

28. Weise M, Merke DP, Pacak K, Walther MM, Eisenhofer G (2002). Utility of plasma free metanephrines for detecting childhood pheochromocytoma. J Clin Endocrinol Metab 87:1955–1960.

29. Maher ER, Eng C (2002). The pressure rises: Update on the genetics of phaeochromocytoma. Hum Mol Genet 11:2347–2354.

30. Stolle C, et al. (1998). Improved detection of germline mutations in the von Hippel-Lindau disease tumor suppressor gene. Human Mutation 12:417–423.

31. Astuti D, et al. (2001). Gene mutations in the succinate dehydrogenase subunit SDHB cause susceptibility to familial pheochromocytoma and to familial paraganglioma. Am J Hum Genet 69:49–54.

32. Baysal BE, et al. (2000). Mutations in SDHD, a mitochondrial complex II gene, in hereditary paraganglioma. Science 287:848–851.

33. Niemann S, Muller U (2000). Mutations in SDHC cause autosomal dominant paraganglioma, type 3. Nat Genet 26:268–270.

34. Neumann HP, et al. (2004). Distinct clinical features of paraganglioma syndromes associated with SDHB and SDHD gene mutations. JAMA 292:943–951.

35. Schiavi F, et al. (2005). Predictors and prevalence of paraganglioma syndrome associated with mutations of the SDHC gene. JAMA 294:2057–2063.

36. Benn DE, et al. (2006). Clinical presentation and penetrance of pheochromocytoma/paraganglioma syndromes. J Clin Endocrinol Metab 91:827–836.

37. Vanharanta S, et al. (2004). Early-onset renal cell carcinoma as a novel extraparaganglial component of SDHB-associated heritable paraganglioma. Am J Hum Genet 74:153–159.

38. Mantero F, et al. for the Study Group on Adrenal Tumors of the Italian Society of Endocrinology. (2000). A survey on adrenal incidentaloma in Italy. J Clin Endocrinol Metab 85:637–644.

39. Glazer GM, Francis IR, Quint LE (1988). Imaging of the adrenal glands. Invest Radiol 23:3–11.

40. Hanson MW, Feldman JM, Beam CA, Leight GS, Coleman RE (1991). Iodine 131-labeled metaiodobenzylguanidine scintigraphy and biochemical analyses in suspected pheochromocytoma. Arch Int Med 151:1397–1402.

41. Maurea S, et al. (1993). Iodine-131-metaiodobenzylguanidine scintigraphy in preoperative and postoperative evaluation of paragangliomas: Comparison with CT and MRI. J Nucl Med 34:173–179.

42. Chatal JF (1993). Can we agree on the best imaging procedures for localization of pheochromocytomas? J Nucl Med 34:180–181.

43. Mayo CH (1927). Paroxysmal hypertension with tumor of retroperitoneal nerve: Report of case. JAMA 89:1047–1050.

44. Walz MK, et al. (2006). Laparoscopic and retroperitoneoscopic treatment of pheochromocytomas and retroperitoneal paragangliomas: Results of 161 tumors in 126 patients. World J Surg 30:899–908.

45. Ulchaker JC, Goldfarb DA, Bravo EL, Novick AC (1999). Successful outcomes in pheochromocytoma surgery in the modern era. J Urol 161:764–767.

46. Turner MC, Lieberman E, DeQuattro V (1992). The perioperative management of pheochromocytoma in children. Clin Ped 31:583–589.

47. Mannelli M (2006). Management and treatment of pheochromocytomas and paragangliomas. Annals of the New York Academy of Sciences 1073:405–416.

48. Diner EK, Franks ME, Behari A, Linehan WM, Walther MM (2005). Partial adrenalectomy: The National Cancer Institute experience. Urology 66:19–23.

49. Neumann HP, Reincke M, Bender BU, Elsner R, Janetschek G (1999). Preserved adrenocortical function after laparoscopic bilateral adrenal sparing surgery for hereditary pheochromocytoma. J Clin Endocrinol Metab 84:2608–2610.

50. Pham TH, et al. (2006). Pheochromocytoma and paraganglioma in children: A review of medical and surgical management at a tertiary care center. Pediatrics 118:1109–1117.

51. Mornex R, Badet C, Peyrin L (1992). Malignant pheochromocytoma: a series of 14 cases observed between 1966 and 1990. J Endocrinol Invest 15:643–649.

52. Schlumberger M, et al. (1992). Malignant pheochromocytoma: Clinical, biological, histologic and therapeutic data in a series of 20 patients with distant metastases. J Endocrinol Invest 15:631–642.

53. Thakker RV (2000). Multiple endocrine neoplasia type 1. Endocrinol Metab Clin North Am 29:541–567.

54. Hoff AO, Cote GJ, Gagel RF (2000). Multiple endocrine neoplasias. Annu Rev Physiol 62:377–411.

55. Marx SJ (2005). Molecular genetics of multiple endocrine neoplasia types 1 and 2. Nature Reviews 5:367–375.

56. Wermer P (1954). Genetic aspects of adenomatosis of endocrine glands. Am J Med 16:363–371.

57. Wermer P (1974). Multiple endocrine adenomatosis: Multiple hormone-producing tumors, a familial syndrome. Clin Gastroenterol 3:671–684.

58. Ballard HS, Frame B, Hartsock RJ (1964). Familial multiple endocrine adenoma-peptic ulcer complex. Medicine 43:481–516.

59. Darling TN, et al. (1997). Multiple facial angiofibromas and collagenomas in patients with multiple endocrine neoplasia type 1. Arch Dermatol 133:853–857.

60. Nakamura Y, et al. (1989). Localization of the genetic defect in multiple endocrine neoplasia type 1 within a small region of chromosome 11. Am J Hum Genet 44:751–755.

61. Thakker RV (1993). Linkage analysis of 7 polymorphic markers at chromosome 11p11.2-11q13 in 27 multiple endocrine neoplasia type 1 families. Ann Hum Genet 57:17–25.

62. Agarwal SK, et al. (1997). Germline mutations of the MEN1 gene in familial multiple endocrine neoplasia type 1 and related states. Hum Mol Genet 6:1169–1175.

63. Chandrasekharappa SC, et al. (1997). Positional cloning of the gene for multiple endocrine neoplasia-type 1. Science 276:404–407.

64. Guru SC, et al. (1998). Identification and characterization of the multiple endocrine neoplasia type 1 (MEN1) gene. J Intern Med 243:433–439.

65. Guru SC, et al. (1998). Menin, the product of the MEN1 gene, is a nuclear protein. Proc Natl Acad Sci USA 95:1630–1634.

66. Guru SC, et al. (1999). Isolation, genomic organization, and expression analysis of Men1, the murine homolog of the MEN1 gene. Mamm Genome 10:592–596.

67. Agarwal SK, et al. (1999). Menin interacts with the AP1 transcription factor JunD and represses JunD-activated transcription. Cell 96:143–152.

68. Agarwal SK, et al. (2007). Distribution of menin-occupied regions in chromatin specifies a broad role of menin in transcriptional regulation. Neoplasia 9:101–107.

69. Hughes CM, et al. (2004). Menin associates with a trithorax family histone methyltransferase complex and with the hoxc8 locus. Molecular Cell 13:587–597.

70. Yang Y, Hua X (2007). In search of tumor suppressing functions of menin. Molecular and Cellular Endocrinology 265–266: 34–41.

71. Bertolino P, Tong WM, Galendo D, Wang ZQ, Zhang CX (2003). Heterozygous Men1 mutant mice develop a range of endocrine tumors mimicking multiple endocrine neoplasia type 1. Molecular Endocrinology 17:1880–1892.

72. Thakker RV (1994). The role of molecular genetics in screening for multiple endocrine neoplasia type 1. Endocrinol Metab Clin North Am 23:117–135.

73. Bassett JH, et al. (1998). Characterization of mutations in patients with multiple endocrine neoplasia type 1. Am J Hum Genet 62:232–244.

74. Marx SJ, et al. (1998). Germline and somatic mutation of the gene for multiple endocrine neoplasia type 1 (MEN1). J Intern Med 243:447–453.

75. Benson L, Sverker L, Akerstrom G, Oberg K (1987). Hyperparathyroidism presenting as the first lesion in multiple endocrine neoplasia type 1. Am J Med 82:731–737.

76. Wilkinson S, et al. (1993). Cause of death in multiple endocrine neoplasia type 1. Arch Surg 128:683–690.

77. Marx SJ, et al. (1986). Multiple endocrine neoplasia type I: assessment of laboratory tests to screen for the gene in a large kindred. Medicine 65:226–241.

78. Vasen HFA, Lamers CBHW, Lips CJM (1989). Screening for the multiple endocrine neoplasia syndrome type I. Arch Int Med 149:2717–2722.

79. Machens A, et al. (2007). Age-related penetrance of endocrine tumours in multiple endocrine neoplasia type 1 (MEN1): A multicentre study of 258 gene carriers. Clin Endocrinol (Oxford) 67(4):613–622.

80. Marx SJ (2001). Multiple endocrine neoplasia type 1. In Scriver CR, Beaudet AL, Sly WS, Valle D (eds.), *The metabolic and molecular basis of inherited disease*. New York: McGraw-Hill 943–966.

81. Mallette LE (1994). Management of hyperparathyroidism in the multiple endocrine neoplasia syndromes and other familial endocrinopathies. Endocrinol Metab Clin North Am 23:19–36.

82. Carling T, Udelsman R (2005). Parathyroid surgery in familial hyperparathyroid disorders. J Intern Med 257:27–37.

83. Hubbard JG, Sebag F, Maweja S, Henry JF (2006). Subtotal parathyroidectomy as an adequate treatment for primary hyperparathyroidism in multiple endocrine neoplasia type 1. Arch Surg 141:235–239.

84. O'Riordan DS, et al. (1993). Surgical management of primary hyperparathyroidism in multiple endocrine neoplasia types 1 and 2. Surgery 114:1031–1037.

85. Uchino S, et al. (2000). Screening of the Men1 gene and discovery of germ-line and somatic mutations in apparently sporadic parathyroid tumors. Cancer Res 60:5553–5557.

86. Pannett AA, et al. (2003). Multiple endocrine neoplasia type 1 (MEN1) germline mutations in familial isolated primary hyperparathyroidism. Clin Endocrinol (Oxford) 58:639–646.

87. Carpten JD, et al. (2002). HRPT2, encoding parafibromin, is mutated in hyperparathyroidism-jaw tumor syndrome. Nat Genet 32:676–680.

88. Skogseid B, et al. (1991). Multiple endocrine neoplasia type 1: A 10-year prospective screening study in four kindreds. J Clin Endocrinol Metab 73:281–287.

89. Marx SJ, et al. (1991). Heterogeneous size of the parathyroid glands in familial multiple endocrine neoplasia type 1. Clinical Endocrinology 35:521–526.

90. Grama D, et al. (1992). Pancreatic tumors in multiple endocrine neoplasia type 1: Clinical presentation and surgical treatment. World J Surg 16:611–618.

91. Thomas-Marques L, et al. (2006). Prospective endoscopic ultrasonographic evaluation of the frequency of nonfunctioning pancreaticoduodenal endocrine tumors in patients with multiple endocrine neoplasia type 1. The American Journal of Gastroenterology 101:266–273.

92. Demeure MJ, Klonoff DC, Karam JH, Duh QY, Clark OH (1991). Insulinomas associated with multiple endocrine neoplasia type I: The need for a different surgical approach. Surgery 110:998–1004.

93. Kouvaraki MA, et al. (2006). Management of pancreatic endocrine tumors in multiple endocrine neoplasia type 1. World J Surg 30:643–653.

94. Roy PK, et al. (2001). Gastric secretion in Zollinger-Ellison syndrome: Correlation with clinical expression, tumor extent and role in diagnosis. A prospective NIH study of 235 patients and a review of 984 cases in the literature. Medicine 80:189–222.

95. Skogseid B, Rastad J, Oberg K (1994). Multiple endocrine neoplasia type 1: Clinical features and screening. Endocrinol Metab Clin North Am 23:1–18.

96. Corbetta S, et al. (1997). Multiple endocrine neoplasia type 1 in patients with recognized pituitary tumours of different types. Clin Endocrinol (Oxford) 47:507–512.

97. Scheithauer BW, et al. (1987). Pituitary adenomas of the multiple endocrine neoplasia type I syndrome. Seminars in Diagnostic Pathology 4:205–211.

98. Ozawa A, et al. (2007). The parathyroid/pituitary variant of multiple endocrine neoplasia type 1 usually has causes other than p27Kip1 mutations. J Clin Endocrinol Metab 92:1948–1951.

99. Klein RD, Salih S, Bessoni J, Bale AE (2005). Clinical testing for multiple endocrine neoplasia type 1 in a DNA diagnostic laboratory. Genet Med 7:131–138.

100. Brandi ML, et al. (2001). Guidelines for diagnosis and therapy of MEN type 1 and type 2. J Clin Endocrinol Metab 86:5658–5671.

101. Stratakis CA, et al. (2000). Pituitary macroadenoma in a 5-year-old: An early expression of multiple endocrine neoplasia type 1. J Clin Endocrinol Metab 85:4776–4780.

102. Gagel RF (1995). Multiple endocrine neoplasia type 2. In DeGroot LJ (ed.), *Endocrinology, Third edition*. Philadelphia: WB Saunders 2832–2845.

103. Eng C (1999). RET proto-oncogene in the development of human cancer. J Clin Oncol 17:380–393.

104. Zbuk KM, Eng C (2007). Cancer phenomics: RET and PTEN as illustrative models. Nature Reviews 7:35–45.

105. Mulligan LM, et al. (1993). Germ-line mutations of the RET proto-oncogene in multiple endocrine neoplasia type 2A. Nature 363:458–460.

106. Eng C, et al. (1996). The relationship between specific RET proto-oncogene mutations and disease phenotype in multiple endocrine neoplasia type 2: International RET mutation consortium analysis. JAMA 276:1575–1579.

107. Avantaggiato V, et al. (1994). Developmental expression of the RET protooncogene. Cell Growth Differ 5:305–311.

108. Pachnis V, Mankoo B, Costantini F (1993). Expression of the c-ret proto-oncogene during mouse embryogenesis. Development 119:1005–1017.

109. Baloh RH, Enomoto H, Johnson EM Jr., Milbrandt J (2000). The GDNF family ligands and receptors: Implications for neural development. Curr Opin Neurobiol 10:103–110.

110. de Groot JW, Links TP, Plukker JT, Lips CJ, Hofstra RM (2006). RET as a diagnostic and therapeutic target in sporadic and hereditary endocrine tumors. Endocrine Rev 27:535–560.

111. Kouvaraki MA, et al. (2005). RET proto-oncogene: A review and update of genotype-phenotype correlations in hereditary medullary thyroid cancer and associated endocrine tumors. Thyroid 15:531–544.

112. Donis-Keller H, et al. (1993). Mutations in the RET proto-oncogene are associated with MEN 2A and FMTC. Hum Mol Genet 2:851–856.

113. Xue F, et al. (1994). Germline RET mutations in MEN 2A and FMTC and their detection by simple DNA diagnostic tests. Hum Mol Genet 3:635–638.

114. Schuffenecker I, et al. (1998). Risk and penetrance of primary hyperparathyroidism in multiple endocrine neoplasia type 2A families with mutations at codon 634 of the RET proto-oncogene: Groupe D'etude des Tumeurs a Calcitonine. J Clin Endocrinol Metab 83:487–491.

115. Vanhorne JB, et al. (2005). A model for GFR alpha 4 function and a potential modifying role in multiple endocrine neoplasia 2. Oncogene 24:1091–1097.

116. Carlson KM, et al. (1994). Single missense mutation in the tyrosine kinase catalytic domain of the RET protooncogene is associated with multiple endocrine neoplasia type 2B. Proc Natl Acad Sci USA 91:1579–1583.

117. Eng C, et al. (1994). Point mutation within the tyrosine kinase domain of the RET proto-oncogene in multiple endocrine neoplasia type 2B and related sporadic tumours. Hum Mol Genet 3:237–241.

118. Hofstra RMW, et al. (1994). A mutation in the RET proto-oncogene associated with multiple endocrine neoplasia type 2B and sporadic medullary thyroid carcinoma. Nature 367:375–376.

119. Santoro M, et al. (1995). Activation of RET as a dominant transforming gene by germline mutations of MEN2A and MEN2B. Science 267:381–383.

120. Beldjord C, et al. (1995). The RET protooncogene in sporadic pheochromocytomas: Frequent MEN 2-like mutations and new molecular defects. J Clin Endocrinol Metab 80:2063–2068.

121. Gujral TS, Singh VK, Jia Z, Mulligan LM (2006). Molecular mechanisms of RET receptor-mediated oncogenesis in multiple endocrine neoplasia 2B. Cancer Res 66:10741–10749.

122. Songyang Z, et al. (1995). Catalytic specificity of protein-tyrosine kinases is critical for selective signalling. Nature 373:536–539.

123. Edery P, et al. (1994). Mutations of the RET proto-oncogene in Hirschsprung's disease. Nature 367:378–380.

124. Mulligan LM, et al. (1994). Diverse phenotypes associated with exon 10 mutations of the RET proto-oncogene. Hum Mol Genet 3:2163–2167.

125. Pelet A, et al. (1998). Various mechanisms cause RET-mediated signaling defects in Hirschsprung's disease. The Journal of Clinical Investigation 101:1415–1423.

126. MacIntyre I (1995). Calcitonin: Physiology, biosynthesis, secretion, metabolism, and mode of action. In DeGroot LJ (ed.), Endocrinology, Third edition. Philadelphia: WB Saunders 978–989.

127. Amara SG, et al. (1985). Expression in brain of a messenger RNA encoding a novel neuropeptide homologous to calcitonin gene-related peptide. Science 229:1094–1097.

128. Steenbergh PH, Hoppener JW, Zandberg J, Lips CJ, Jansz HS (1985). A second human calcitonin/CGRP gene. FEBS Letters 183:403–407.

129. Chi DD, Moley JF (1998). Medullary thyroid carcinoma: Genetic advances, treatment recommendations, and the approach to the patient with persistent hypercalcitoninemia. Surg Oncol Clin N Am 7:681–706.

130. Kakudo K, Carney JA, Sizemore GW (1985). Medullary carcinoma of thyroid. Cancer 55:2821–2828.

131. Easton DF, et al. (1989). The clinical and screening age-at-onset distribution for the MEN-2 syndrome. Am J Hum Genet 44:208–215.

132. Gagel RF, et al. (1982). Age-related probability of development of hereditary medullary thyroid carcinoma. J Pediatr 101:941–946.

133. Gagel RF, et al. (1988). The clinical outcome of prospective screening for multiple endocrine neoplasia 2a. N Eng J Med 318:478–484.

134. Smith VV, Eng C, Milla PJ (1999). Intestinal ganglioneuromatosis and multiple endocrine neoplasia type 2B: Implications for treatment. Gut 45:143–146.

135. Gordon C, et al. (1998). Four cases of mucosal neuroma syndrome: Multiple endocrine neoplasm 2B or not 2B? J Clin Endocrinol Metab 83:17–20.

136. Friedhelm R, Frank-Rau K, Grauer A (1994). Multiple endocrine neoplasia type 2. Endocrinol Metab Clin North Am 23:137–156.

137. Melvin KEW, Tashjian AHJ, Miller HH (1972). Studies in familial (medullary) thyroid carcinoma. Recent Prog Horm Res 28:399–470.

138. Norton JA, Froome LC, Farrell RE, Wells SA (1979). Multiple endocrine neoplasia type IIb: the most aggressive form of medullary thyroid carcinoma. Surg Clin North Am 59:109–118.

139. Decker RA (1992). Long-term follow-up of a large North American kindred with multiple endocrine neoplasia type 2A. Surgery 112:1066–1072.

140. Graze K, et al. (1978). Natural history of familial medullary thyroid carcinoma. N Eng J Med 299:980-985.

141. Vasen HFA, et al. (1987). Multiple endocrine neoplasia syndrome type 2: The value of screening and central registration. 83:847.

142. American Society of Clinical Oncology (2003). Policy statement update: Genetic testing for cancer susceptibility. J Clin Oncol 21:2397–2406.

143. Wells SA Jr., et al. (1978). Provocative agents and the diagnosis of medullary carcinoma of the thyroid gland. Ann Surg 188:139–141.

144. Wells SA Jr., Dilley WG, Farndon JA, Leight GS, Baylin SB (1985). Early diagnosis and treatment of medullary thyroid carcinoma. Arch Int Med 145:1248–1252.

145. Chi DD, Toshima K, Donis-Keller H, Wells SAJ (1994). Predictive testing for multiple endocrine neoplasia type 2A (MEN 2A) based on the detection of mutations in the RET protooncogene. Surgery 116:124–133.

146. Lips CJM, et al. (1994). Clinical screening as compared with DNA analysis in families with multiple endocrine neoplasia type 2A. N Eng J Med 331:828–835.

147. Wells SA Jr., et al. (1994). Predictive DNA testing and prophylactic thyroidectomy in patients at risk for multiple endocrine neoplasia type 2A. Ann Surg 220:237–250.

148. Machens A, Brauckhoff M, Gimm O, Dralle H (2006). Risk-oriented approach to hereditary adrenal pheochromocytoma. Annals of the New York Academy of Sciences 1073:417–428.

149. Evans DB, Lee JE, Merrell RC, Hickey RC (1994). Adrenal medullary disease in multiple endocrine neoplasia type 2. Endocrinol Metab Clin North Am 23:167–176.

150. Jansson S, et al. (1988). Early diagnosis of and surgical strategy for adrenal medullary disease in MEN II gene carriers. Surgery 103:11–18.

151. DeLellis RA, et al. (1994). Adrenal medullary hyperplasia. Am J Pathol 83:177–196.

152. de Graaf JS, Lips CJ, Rutter JE, van Vroonhoven TJ (1999). Subtotal adrenalectomy for phaeochromocytoma in multiple endocrine neoplasia type 2A. Eur J Surg 165:535–538.

153. Butter A, et al (2007). Prophylactic thyroidectomy in pediatric carriers of multiple endocrine neoplasia type 2A or familial medullary thyroid carcinoma: mutation in C620 is associated with Hirschsprung's disease. J Pediatr Surg 42:203–206.

154. Boikos SA, Stratakis CA (2006). Carney complex: Pathology and molecular genetics. Neuroendocrinology 83:189–199.

155. Carney JA, Gordon H, Carpenter PC, Shenoy BV, Go VL (1985). The complex of myxomas, spotty pigmentation, and endocrine overactivity. Medicine 64:270–283.

156. Stratakis CA, et al. (1996). Carney complex, a familial multiple neoplasia and lentiginosis syndrome: Analysis of 11 kindreds and linkage to the short arm of chromosome 2. The Journal of Clinical Investigation 97:699–705.

157. Kirschner LS, et al. (2000). Mutations of the gene encoding the protein kinase A type I-alpha regulatory subunit in patients with the Carney complex. Nat Genet 26:89–92.

158. Stratakis CA, et al. (1999). Paradoxical response to dexamethasone in the diagnosis of primary pigmented nodular adrenocortical disease. Ann Intern Med 131:585–591.

159. Wells SA Jr., Franz C (2000). Medullary carcinoma of the thyroid gland. World J Surg 24:952–956.

160. Ball DW (2007). Medullary thyroid cancer: Therapeutic targets and molecular markers. Current Opinion in Oncology 19:18–23.

161. Strock CJ, et al. (2006). Activity of irinotecan and the tyrosine kinase inhibitor CEP-751 in medullary thyroid cancer. J Clin Endocrinol Metab 91:79–84.

162. Steddon SJ, Cunningham J (2005). Calcimimetics and calcilytics: Fooling the calcium receptor. Lancet 365:2237–2239.

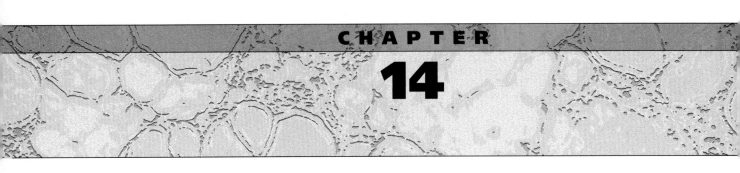

Puberty and Its Disorders in the Female

ROBERT L. ROSENFIELD, MD • DAVID W. COOKE, MD
• SALLY RADOVICK, MD

Introduction

Puberty is the stage of development during which secondary sexual characteristics appear and there is a transition from the sexually immature to the sexually mature stage. Adolescence is widely used as a generally synonymous term for puberty, but it is often used to convey an added cultural connotation as a psychosocial coming of age.

By the mid 1960s, a general concept of the major factors involved in the initiation of puberty was established (Figure 14-1).[1,2] A decrease in sensitivity of the brain "gonadostat" to sex hormone negative feedback was thought to be the primary event. This signaled the hypothalamus to discharge neurohumors (then unidentified), which in turn stimulated the pituitary to release gonadotropins. The resultant rise in secretion of the gonadotropins, luteinizing hormone (LH) and follicle-stimulating hormone (FSH), was thought to account directly for increased estrogen production by the ovary. A mature relationship was thought to develop in which the blood levels of estrogen and gonadotropins were regulated reciprocally via the gonadostat,[3] much as a furnace is regulated by a thermostat. The pineal was identified as having gonadal-

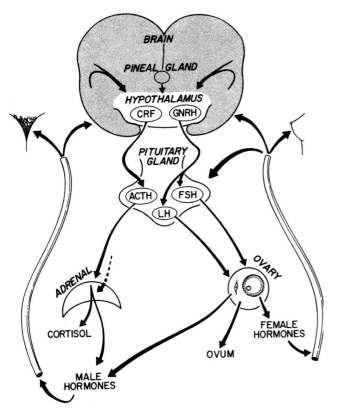

Figure 14-1 Schematic representation of the neuroendocrine-ovarian axis involved in normal pubertal development. ACTH, adrenocorticotropic hormone; CRF, corticotropin-releasing factor; GnRH, gonadotropin-releasing hormone; FSH, follicle-stimulating hormone; and LH, luteinizing hormone.

suppressive properties. The increased adrenocortical secretion of 17-ketosteroids (17-KS), which becomes apparent at about the time of puberty (adrenarche), was thought to be due to a pituitary factor stimulating adrenal androgens in synergism with adrenocorticotropic hormone (ACTH).[4]

The rapid scientific advances since 1965 have permitted this concept to be tested in increasingly sophisticated ways. In the subsequent decade, radioimmunoassay (RIA)—originally developed by Yalow and Berson—was applied to the measurement of gonadotropins and sex steroids. The gonadotropin-releasing hormone (GnRH) for both LH and FSH was isolated, identified, and synthesized by Guillemin's and Schally's groups. Cyclic adenosine-3',5'-monophosphate (cAMP), postulated by Sutherland to mediate the action of peptide hormones, was found to mediate gonadotropin effects on the ovarian follicle. The initial steps in the mechanism of action of steroid hormones were defined by Jensen, Gorski, and their groups. The landmark nature of many of these discoveries has been recognized by the awarding of Nobel Prizes in Medicine to Sutherland in 1971 and to Yalow, Schally, and Guillemin in 1977.

Our present view of the mechanisms controlling puberty is more refined and complex than it once was, although the previously cited schema is correct in a general sense. The gonadostat is a patently oversimplistic concept for but one aspect of a complex system that regulates the hypothalamic GnRH pulse generator, a functionally interconnected and synchronized network of GnRH neurons.[5] The gonadostat setting seems to change throughout childhood in a biphasic manner. This concept is illustrated in Figure 14-2.[6,7] During fetal and perinatal life, the gonadostat is insensitive to negative feedback by sex hormones. At this time, the nascent neuroendocrine-gonadal axis functions at a pubertal level. The gonadostat becomes increasingly sensitive to negative feedback during infancy but does not become highly sensitive until mid-childhood, at which time GnRH pulse generator activity is minimal.

During late prepuberty, the gonadostat begins to relinquish its inhibition. This permits the onset of puberty. The changing set-point initially permits increasing episodic secretion of GnRH. Increasing sensitivity of the pituitary gonadotropic cells to GnRH follows. The change in LH and FSH secretion is first detectable at night. Gradually, the gonads become increasingly sensitized to gonadotropin stimulation, grow at an increased rate, and bring about sustained rises in plasma sex hormone levels. Some of these phenomena synergize with others, and thus autoamplification occurs and the pace of change accelerates. Eventually, the set-point for gonadotropin release comes to vary sufficiently to encompass a positive feedback mechanism.

The data on which this model is based are presented in material following. The most recent data on the hormonal milieu and accompanying physical stages of normal puberty are then presented. Abnormal puberty is subsequently discussed: causes, differential diagnosis, and management.

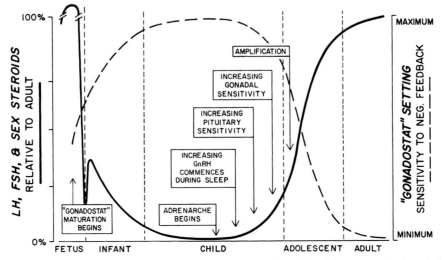

Figure 14-2 The changing pattern of serum gonadotropins and sex hormones from fetal life to maturity in relationship to the apparent sensitivity of the central nervous system "gonadostat" to the negative feedback effect of sex hormones and the underlying hormonal events. FSH, follicle-stimulating hormone; GnRH, gonadotropin-releasing hormone; and LH, luteinizing hormone. [Modified from Grumbach M, Grave C, Mayer F (eds.), *The control of the onset of puberty.* New York: John Wiley & Sons.]

Development of the Female Reproductive System

MATURATION OF THE NEUROENDOCRINE OVARIAN AXIS

Fetus

Neuroendocrine Unit. The anterior lobe of the pituitary gland (of stomal ectodermal origin) and the posterior lobe (of neural origin) differentiate by 11 weeks' gestational age.[8] By this time, GnRH neurons have migrated from the olfactory placode into place in the medial basal hypothalamus.[9] Hypothalamic GnRH rises in parallel with fetal pituitary and serum LH and FSH from this time.[10] All peak at about 20 to 24 weeks, as the connections of the pituitary portal system become complete, to levels not again seen until the mature midcycle surge.[11,12]

Serum LH and FSH levels are higher in female than male fetuses.[11] In rats, GnRH-containing neurons develop earlier in females than in males[13] and there are sexual dimorphisms in the degree of synapsing of specific tracts with dendritic spines in the preoptic nucleus—one of the major GnRH-containing areas of the hypothalamus.[14,15] These differences may be determined by gonadal sex hormone output. In sheep fetuses, secretion of LH (particularly LH pulse frequency) is permanently desensitized to estradiol negative feedback by high fetal testosterone.[16]

In late gestation, fetal hypothalamic GnRH and pituitary gonadotropin secretion fall to low levels. These changes seem explicable by the negative feedback effect of the high sex steroids produced by the fetoplacental unit. In addition, maturation of the central nervous system (CNS) tracts that inhibit hypothalamic GnRH secretion appears to progress throughout gestation.[12]

The production of gonadotropins by the fetal pituitary seems to facilitate normal ovarian development. Hypophysectomy of rhesus fetuses has been reported to reduce the number of germ cells and oocytes as well as the integrity of the rete ovarii.[17] Therefore, it seems that survival of gametes depends on the secretions of the fetal pituitary. The mechanism is unclear. This pituitary effect may be mediated through accelerated atresia, lack of support of the rete system, or lack of stimulation of the follicle.

Ovary. The ovaries differentiate in the urogenital ridge adjacent to the anlage of adrenal cortex and the kidney. The granulosa cells are the homologues of the Sertoli cells of the testes. The theca, interstitial, and hilus cells are the homologues of the Leydig cells. Hilus cells may even contain crystalloids, like Leydig cells. Adrenocortical rests have occasionally been found in the hilus of the ovary.[18] Conversely, ovarian rests have been identified in the adrenal glands.[19]

The primitive germ cells migrate into the ovary from the yolk sac endoderm during the first month of gestation. The WT-1, LIM-1, SF-1, and possibly DAX-1 genes are known to play roles in the formation of the ovaries.[20] The ovaries begin to become distinguishable from testes by 8 weeks of gestation.[21] In the absence of testicular development being switched on by the SRY gene on the Y chromosome,[22] Wnt-4 signaling sustains oocyte and granulosa cell development, and suppresses Sertoli and Leydig cell differentiation,[23] critical steps in ovarion differentiation. Mitotic division of oogonia is maximum before the third month and comes to an end by the seventh month. Oogonia then undergo oogenesis, entering the prophase of meiosis to become primary oocytes during the final 5 to 6 months of gestation.[24] The number of oocytes reaches a peak at the fifth month, when there are 6.8 million germ cells—of which 80% appear to be viable (Figure 14-3).[25]

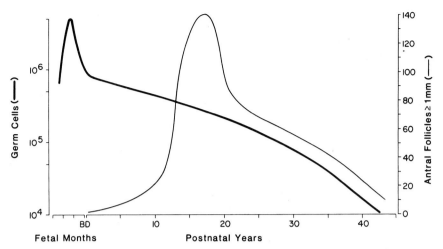

Figure 14-3 The development of ovarian follicles from fetal life to maturity. Curves for total number of viable germ cells (thick line) and large antral follicles (thin line) smoothed from the data of Baker and Block. The number of germ cells is maximal at the fifth month of fetal life. The loss of germ cells is exponential throughout postnatal life. At puberty, a marked shift occurs in the pattern of development of follicles. An increased fraction grows to large antral size.

When oocytes enter the diplotene stage of meiotic prophase they must be furnished with granulosa cells to form a primordial follicle. Otherwise, they undergo atresia.[26]

Primordial follicles appear in the fourth month, when the epithelium of the secondary sex cords provides granulosa cells to the oocytes—and they peak in number between the fifth and ninth months. They become primary follicles when the encircling granulosa cells become cuboidal. Primordial and small primary follicles (Figure 14-4)[27,28] are resting follicles that are the major repository of germ cells.[29] This stock of germ cells is depleted only very slowly during childhood (Figure 14-3).

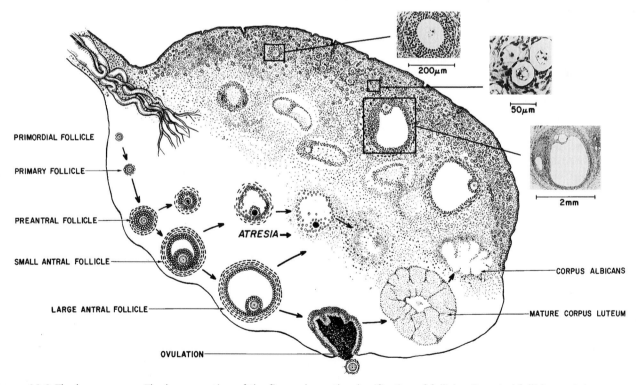

Figure 14-4 The human ovary. The lower portion of the figure shows the classification of follicles. Preantral follicles contain as many as 300 granulosa cells, and their diameter ranges from 50 to 200 m. The oocyte diameter increases from 25 or less to 80 m. Antral (graafian, tertiary, or vesicular) follicles have a fluid-filled antrum and a full-grown oocyte, are lined with more than 300 granulosa cells, and have a well-developed theca. They are greater than 200 m in diameter. The dimensions of the mature ovary are approximately 1.25 x 2.75 4 cm. The upper portion of the figure illustrates the histologic appearance of the perimenarcheal ovary. [Photomicrographs of ovarian details are reproduced from Peters H (1979). The human ovary in childhood and early maturity. Eur J Obstet Gynecol Reprod Biol 9(3):137.]; modified from Ross GT, Schreiber JR (1978). The ovary. In Yen SSC, Jaffe R (eds.), *Reproductive endocrinology*. Philadelphia: WB Saunders 63.]

Secondary follicles and preantral follicles, characterized respectively by a larger granulosa cell population and organization of theca, then appear successively. After the seventh month, antral (Graafian) follicles appear.[28,30,31] Typically, one or two antral follicles of 1 to 2 mm in diameter are present in the ovary by term, at which time the number of small preantral follicles is at its peak. At birth, ovarian follicle development is complete[28,30,31] and the complement of ova is greater than at any other time during postnatal life (Figure 14-3)—totaling 2 million, of which half appear atretic.[25,32]

Both X-chromosomes are active in oocytes,[33] and these are necessary for the full induction of the granulosa cell layer necessary to oocyte survival.[30,34] Oocyte-derived growth differentiation factor-9 is critical to signaling by the specialized granulosa cells of the cumulus to induce the theca cell layer, which in turn through the production of other autosomally determined paracrine factors, including several other members of the TGF-β superfamily, is necessary to the survival of oocytes and the further differentiation and growth of follicles.[35-39] Because ovarian germ cells, unlike male ones, are a nonrenewing population the regulation of atresia is a critical determinant of follicle number.[40] The endowment of follicles may be influenced by environmental factors such as toxins,[41] thymic factors,[42] and placental insufficiency.[43] There has also been considerable interest in the possibility that placental insufficiency, via hypoxemia and resultant overactivation of fetal prostaglandin production and cortisol secretion, is a factor predisposing to postnatal insulin resistance[44] (which has consequences for reproductive function in later life).

The major source of sex hormones in the female fetus is the fetoplacental unit. Theca-interstitial cells of the fetal primordial follicle appear to form androstenedione and dehydroepiandrosterone as early as 3 months in man, but estradiol formation probably does not occur until antral follicular development begins.[21,45] The contribution of the ovaries to fetal sex steroid levels is probably relatively low, however.

Testis. In males, the physiologic consequences of the increase in the levels of gonadotropins and sex steroid hormones include differentiation of male internal and external genitalia and descent of the testes to their scrotal position, as discussed in other chapters.

Infant and Child

Neuroendocrine Unit. The neonate undergoes a transient activation of the hypothalamic-pituitary-gonadal axis. The mechanism of gonadotropin secretion in the neonate, like that governing the onset of central activation during pubertal development, is unknown. There is reason to suspect that some of the regulatory processes may be different.[46-50] Serum FSH and LH are low in cord blood and remain so until estrogen concentrations fall from inhibitory levels upon disruption of the fetoplacental unit at birth. The LH and FSH levels of neonates then promptly begin to rise in pulsatile fashion to early pubertal levels in the first week of life (Figure 14-5).[7,11,51-54]

Serum LH rises less in girls than in boys, possibly because of lesser prenatal androgen accentuation of GnRH pulsatility.[55,56] Responses to GnRH and GnRH agonist are

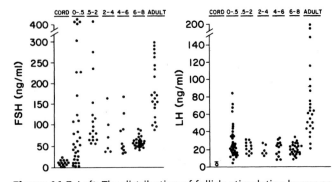

Figure 14-5 Left: The distribution of follicle-stimulating hormone (FSH). Right: Luteinizing hormone (LH) levels from infancy through adulthood (age in years). Umbilical cord level of LH measured by -subunit-specific radioimmunoassay. Pubertal values given in Figures 14-8 and 14-12. Standard LER-907: 100 ng equivalent to 2 mIU FSH and 6 mIU LH of the First International Reference Preparation of human pituitary gonadotropin for bioassay. [Data from Winter J, Faiman C, Hobson W, Prasad A, Reyes F (1975). Pituitary-gonadal relations in infancy: I. Patterns of serum gonadotropin concentrations from birth to four years of age in man and chimpanzee. J Clin Endocrinol Metab 40:545; from Kaplan S, Grumbach M, Aubert M (1976). The ontogenesis of pituitary hormones and hypothalamic factors in the human fetus. Recent Prog Horm Res 32:161; from Nilsson E, Skinner MK (2001). Cellular interactions that control primordial follicle development and folliculogenesis. J Soc Gynecol Investig 8:S17–S20; from Dissen GA, Romero C, Hirshfield AN, Ojeda SR (2001). Nerve growth factor is required for early follicular development in the mammalian ovary. Endocrinology 142:2078–2086 and from Pru JK, Tilly JL (2001). Programmed cell death in the ovary: insights and future prospects using genetic technologies. Mol Endocrinol 15:845–853.]

early pubertal (Figure 14-6).[12,57-60] In congenital agonadism, gonadotropins reach postmenopausal levels.[61] Prematurely born girls develop serum LH and FSH levels that transiently rise into the post-menopausal range, and fall to pubertal levels by about 40 weeks postconceptional age.[12] These gonadotropins appear to be bioactive judging from the reports of ovarian hyperstimulation in preterm infants.[61a] They also have higher prolactin levels than normal adults. These phenomena seem to be related to immaturity of the CNS tracts that will increasingly come to inhibit these pituitary functions in older infants.

Gonadotropin levels then begin to gradually fall after about 4 months of age (Figure 14-5). FSH is higher in girls than in boys, a tendency that tends to persist into early childhood.[51,62] This appears to be related to an intact negative feedback system for the inhibin-B/activin-A system, with higher activin-A and lower inhibin-B levels in girls than in boys.[63] Immunoreactive GnRH excretion also tends to be greater in girls than in boys at this time.[64]

The subsequent decline in gonadotropins may well be related to an increase in hypothalamic estrogen receptors. Hypothalamic estradiol receptors increase in a pattern reciprocal to the fall in serum gonadotropins in the rat (Figure 14-7),[65] as do hypothalamic dihydrotestosterone (DHT) receptors.[66] These changes in the seeming efficiency with which the hypothalamus can recognize sex hormones could account for its increasing sensitivity to the inhibitory effect of small amounts of circulating estradiol and testosterone. However, another mechanism for the fall in gonadotropins seems to be the further

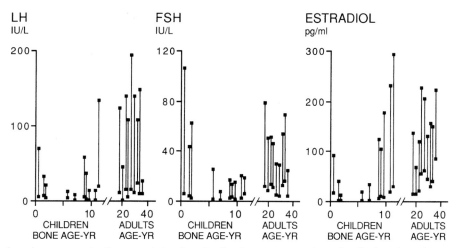

Figure 14-6 Basal and peak responses to the gonadotropin-releasing hormone agonist nafarelin (1µg/kg subcutaneously) during development. Lines connect the basal and peak responses in control children. The responses are related to bone age in children and chronologic age in adults. Note the biphasic pattern of the responses. They are high in infancy, lower in mid-childhood, and rise again during puberty. The peak gonadotropin responses occur at approximately 4 hours, and peak estradiol responses occur at 20 hours. FSH, follicle-stimulating hormone; and LH, luteinizing hormone. [From Rosenfield RL, Burstein S, Cuttler L, et al. (1989). Use of nafarelin for testing pituitary-ovarian function. J Reprod Med 34:1044.]

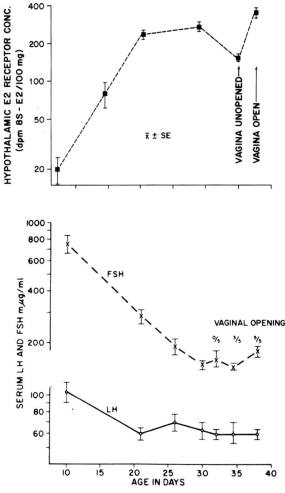

Figure 14-7 Relationship of maturation of hypothalamic estrogen receptors (top) to serum gonadotropin levels (bottom) in the developing female rat. FSH, follicle-stimulating hormone; and LH, luteinizing hormone. [From Rosenfield RL (1977). Hormonal events and disorders of puberty. In Givens JR (ed.), *Gynecologic endocrinology*. Chicago: Year Book Medical. By permission of Mosby-Year Book.]

maturation of neural tracts that conduct inhibitory signals from the CNS to the hypothalamus.

A nadir in both serum gonadotropins occurs by about 6 years of age (Figures 14-2 and 14-5). At this age, the LH and FSH response to GnRH is minimal—apparently because gonadotropes are sluggish from lack of GnRH stimulation. Furthermore, at this stage agonadism is seldom reflected in a rise in serum gonadotropins or gonadotropin reserve.[7,61]

However, gonadotropin production is not completely suppressed in mid-childhood. Gonadotropins have been detected in the urine of young prepubertal children, at the limits of sensitivity of classic bioassays. LH excretion averaged 3% and FSH 15% of the adult amounts.[67] Polyclonal RIA shows that gonadotropins in serial urine specimens rise intermittently.[67,68] The more specific monoclonal antibody-based assays have revealed that the very small amounts of gonadotropins produced at this age are secreted in pulses at intervals of 1 to 2 hours, rise in association with sleep, and fall to less than about 0.15 U/L during the day.[69] The gonadotropins detected by these methods also appear to be bioactive, judging from their sensitivity to estradiol negative feedback in the primate[70] and the active formation of antral follicles during childhood—which indicates gonadotropin stimulation, as discussed in the following section on the adult.

Between 7 and 10 years of age, even girls that remain prepubertal experience a doubling in the output of LH and a lesser increase in that of FSH.[71] This change corresponds with rising excretion of immunoreactive GnRH.[64] These data indicate that the hormonal secretory pattern of the prepubertal 10-year-old child is different from that of the 7-year-old and indicate that the hormonal changes signaling the development of puberty are found late in the first decade of life, antedating by some time the development of secondary sex characteristics.

Ovary. The ovary of the infant and child is not quiescent. Reinitiation of growth and development of resting follicles occurs throughout an individual's life span, although restrained by postnatal expression of anti-Müllerian hormone (AMH).[72] The neonatal ovary typically contain an antral follicle with thecal luteinization.[73,74] Follicles start to grow, and many reach the antral stage at all ages.[26]

By 7 years of age, the number of large antral follicles approximately doubles over that in infancy—and quadruples by 9 years (Figure 14-3). The ovaries of normal girls have up to five antral follicles 4 to 9 mm in diameter in mid-childhood. More begin to appear just before the onset of puberty.[26,75-78] However, all of these large antral follicles normally undergo atresia in childhood—and this augments the amount of stroma.[26] As a result, throughout childhood ovarian volume increases (up to 4 cc by 7 years and 5.5 cc in late prepuberty).

During the first few months of life, early pubertal blood levels of ovarian hormones are found as part of the transient activation of the hypothalamic-pituitary-gonadal axis that occurs in the newborn. Plasma estradiol levels parallel those of FSH. In the neonatal period, they begin rising to early pubertal levels, remain there for the first several months of life, and fall gradually thereafter (Figure 14-8).[57] According to an ultrasensitive recombinant cell bioassay, girls' estrogen levels in late infancy are severalfold greater than those of boys, averaging 1 pg/mL and ranging up to 3 pg/mL.[79]

On occasion, there may be subclinical but detectable estrogen effects on urogenital cytology.[80] Provocation of an acute but transient increase in endogenous gonadotropins by GnRH agonist testing elicits a prompt, though tiny, rise in estradiol secretion in midchildhood.[81,82] As girls begin to experience increasing diurnal production of gonadotropins in late prepuberty, estradiol levels rise in diurnal fashion to peaks of about 6 to 12 pg/mL at mid-morning.[71,83] FSH sometimes reaches the adult range in childhood (Figure 14-5). The reason more ovaries do not secrete pubertal amounts of estrogen is probably because the FSH reaches a pubertal height only episodically and/ or because LH levels are not coincidentally high enough to stimulate sufficient synthesis of estradiol precursors.

Adolescent

The endocrinologic changes of puberty actually begin in late preadolescence, before secondary sex characteristics appear. The underlying basic event is increasing secretion of hypothalamic GnRH. The current concept is that puberty results when the hypothalamus begins to release GnRH with increasing frequency and amplitude, first only at night and then gradually throughout the day.

Increased GnRH secretion in man was initially deduced when Kastin et al. demonstrated that preadolescent children had GnRH-releasable pituitary stores of LH and FSH (Figures 14-6 and 14-9).[84] Subsequently, it was reported that in man the excretion of an immunoreactive fragment of GnRH increases to adult levels during puberty.[64,85] Studies in the rat suggest that hypothalamic GnRH granules increase through puberty.[86]

Knobil subsequently showed that puberty can be induced in the immature female rhesus monkey by administering GnRH in hourly pulses that yield blood levels of about 2,000 pg/mL.[87] Prolonged administration of GnRH according to this regimen first gradually brings about transient increases in LH and FSH. This then induces

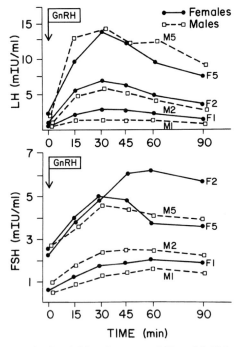

Figure 14-9 The luteinizing hormone (LH) and follicle-stimulating hormone (FSH) responses to gonadotropin-releasing hormone (GnRH) bolus (50 µg/kg/day) in males (M) and females (F) in prepuberty (age 5 to 6 years: F1, M1), early puberty (F2, M2), and later puberty (F5, M5). The responses to GnRH tend to progress with advancing puberty. However, early pubertal girls have a readily releasable FSH pool that is greater than that of more advanced adolescents. The peak responses of girls tend to be somewhat greater than those of boys at comparable stages. [Data from Dickerman Z, Prager-Lewin R, Laron Z (1976). Response of plasma LH and FSH to synthetic LHRH in children at various pubertal stages. Am J Dis Child 130:634.]

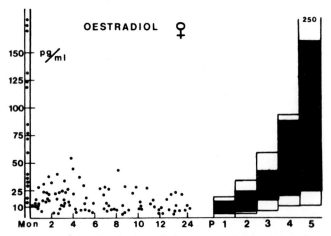

Figure 14-8 The distribution of plasma estradiol levels in infant females compared with pubertal and adult female levels. The columns represent the normal ranges for the various stages of puberty. The area between 10th and 90th percentiles is dark. Stage P1 includes all prepubertal girls older than 2 years. The values between the ordinates were found between 2 and 5 days of age. [From Bidlingmeier F, Knorr D (1978). Oestrogens: Physiological and clinical aspects. Pediatr Adolesc Endocrinol 4:43.]

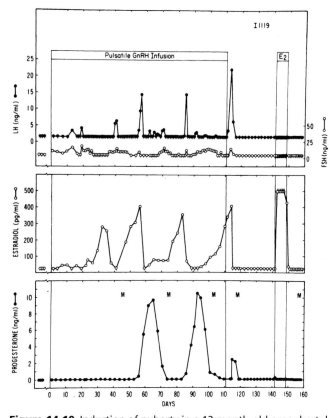

Figure 14-10 Induction of puberty in a 13-month-old prepubertal rhesus monkey by an unvarying pulsatile gonadotropin-releasing hormone (GnRH) regimen (1 μg/min × 6 min hourly). Luteinizing hormone (LH), folliclestimulating hormone (FSH), estradiol (E2), and progesterone were undetectable before the GnRH infusion. On GnRH infusion, a rise in FSH was the first change detectable by mid-morning sampling midway between GnRH pulses. A substantial E2 surge occurred approximately 1 month later. The subsequent LH surge was too modest to elicit ovulation, but menses (M) occurred a few days after subsidence of the week-long E2 surge—menarche resulting from an anovulatory cycle. Continuation of the GnRH led to the sustained occurrence of ovulatory menstrual cycles at 28-day intervals. An identical outcome results if an arcuate-lesioned adult animal undergoes this GnRH regimen. The third of the LH surges occurred 2 days after GnRH was discontinued. Progesterone secretion from the corpus luteum was blunted and transient in the absence of sustained LH secretion. A subsequent increase in plasma E2 produced by E2 implantation subcutaneously failed to elicit a gonadotropin surge, indicating that the animal had reverted to an immature state. Menarche eventually spontaneously recurred in such animals at the usual age (approximately 27 months). Small vertical lines beneath data points indicate values below the sensitivity of the assay. Note that gonadotropins and E2 were often undetectable (prepubertal range) during the induced puberty. [From Knobil E (1980). The neuroendocrine control of the menstrual cycle. Recent Prog Horm Res 36:53.]

cyclic follicular development. The resultant moderate estradiol surge is of such magnitude as to result in menarche due to withdrawal menstrual bleeding in an anovulatory cycle (Figure 14-10). Continuation of the same GnRH regimen leads to development of normal monthly ovulatory menstrual periods. Physiologic pulses of GnRH in man probably attain lower concentrations (200 pg/mL) and occur at slightly wider intervals than in monkeys.[88]

Consequently, LH pulses in mature women occur at intervals of approximately 1 to 1.5 hours during the follicular phases—slowing during the luteal phase.[89]

Puberty begins in girls when serum FSH begins to rise disproportionately to the level of LH.[51,90] In part, FSH predominates because the relatively infrequent GnRH pulses of very early puberty favor the accumulation of FSH because of its slower clearance. FSH also seems to become less regulated by GnRH.[69] The possible explanations for differential regulation of FSH and LH are discussed later in this chapter. This early predominance of FSH has important biologic consequences. It leads to relatively selective growth and development of the follicular compartment of the ovary. Furthermore, the pubertal gonadotropin changes seem to become cyclic well before menarche[7,91] and are capable of inducing cyclic estrogen production.[80,91] Our working model of the nature of pituitary-ovarian dynamics in early puberty is illustrated in Figure 14-11.

Puberty progresses as LH rises. Whereas serum FSH levels rise about 2.5-fold over the course of puberty, LH levels rise 25-fold or more.[69] The initial change in LH secretion at the beginning of puberty is a nightly increase in LH secretion that begins within 20 minutes of the onset of sleep. Subsequently, LH increases more with the onset of sleep, stays up longer, and falls less during waking hours. As the child approaches menarche, the daytime LH levels continue to increase until the diurnal rhythm is typically lost. FSH levels follow a similar pattern, although the FSH changes are less striking. The gonadotropin diurnal rhythm is more resistant to acute sleep reversal than is that of growth hormone (GH).[92] There is a delay of about 12 hours between the peak LH level during sleep and the estradiol zenith, and thus estradiol levels are maximal at mid-morning.[83] The gonadotropin and estradiol rhythms in an early pubertal girl are shown in Figure 14-12.[93]

Augmentation of the bioactivity of plasma LH seems to occur during puberty. Plasma LH bioactivity rises nearly fivefold more during the course of puberty than does LH as measured by polyclonal RIA (Figure 14-13).[94,95] The change in bioactive LH is mirrored well by the third-generation ("pediatric") monoclonal antibody-based immunometric assays, which have very high specificity for bioactive LH epitopes. However, disparities in the ratio of bioactive to immunoreactive LH (B/I) persist with these assays, for reasons related to the molecular microheterogeneity of gonadotropins (discussed later in the chapter). Serum FSH rises during puberty by immunoassay more than by bioassay.[96]

Estradiol output increases rapidly in the year approaching menarche.[97] This seems to be the result of a variety of autoamplification phenomena that facilitate puberty, maturation of the dominant follicle, and ovulation. These are summarized in Table 14-1.[98-111] These phenomena occur at all levels of the axis. The CNS is stimulated by preovulatory levels of estradiol to increase GnRH pulse size. At the pituitary level, there is the self-priming effect of GnRH whereby a pulse of GnRH sensitizes the pituitary to have a greater LH response to a subsequent identical GnRH pulse. Critical patterns of estradiol and progesterone secretion enhance the pituitary LH and FSH responsiveness to GnRH. At the gonadal level, the cascade of events is

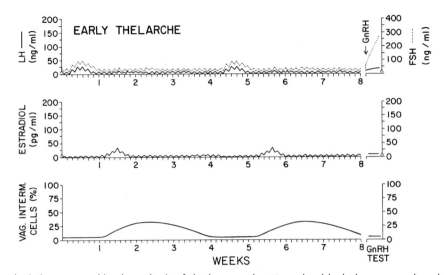

Figure 14-11 Diagram depicting our working hypothesis of the hormonal patterns in girls during very early puberty. We conceptualize this pattern as occurring both cyclically in the earliest stage of normal puberty and occasionally in unsustained sexual precocity (i.e., most U.S. cases of idiopathic premature thelarche). Daytime and nighttime serum concentrations of hormones (gonadotropins relative to the LER-907 standard) and the percentage of intermediate cells on vaginal smear are shown. The typical response to a gonadotropin-releasing hormone (GnRH) test is illustrated. Subclinical hormonal cycles lasting approximately 1 month result from a few days of increased follicle-stimulating hormone (FSH) and luteinizing hormone (LH) secretion. Because the drive to gonadotropin release is relatively weak, FSH and LH production are suppressed promptly and for long periods of time by the resultant modest amounts of estradiol (E2) secretion. Estradiol is detectable in plasma for only a few days a month. Maturation of the vaginal mucosa, however, is detectable for approximately 2 weeks after E2 production has waned.

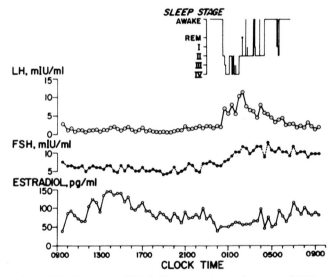

Figure 14-12 The patterns of serum luteinizing hormone (LH), follicle-stimulating hormone (FSH), and estradiol (E2) typical of early female puberty. Note that daytime gonadotropin levels are in the prepubertal range. Note also the episodic nature of LH release at intervals of 1 to 3 hours. Estradiol levels are seen to fluctuate considerably in the course of the daytime, rising to peak levels about 12 hours after the maximum nocturnal gonadotropin surges. [From Boyar RM, Wu RHK, Roffwarg H, et al. (1976). Human puberty: 24-hour estradiol patterns in pubertal girls. J Clin Endocrinol Metab 43:1418.]

augmented by the FSH induction of aromatase activity and progestin production in granulosa cells—phenomena in which androgens play a synergistic role. Furthermore, FSH stimulates granulosa cell mitosis and induces LH receptors—phenomena in which estradiol may play a synergistic role. Subsequently, LH is able to further enhance the aromatase and progesterone effects. Progesterone itself plays a synergistic role in stimulating granulosa cell progesterone and prostaglandin synthesis in concert with FSH and LH. In the rat, ovarian GnRH receptor sites also diminish just before ovulation[112]—and at about this time the ovary changes its pattern of metabolism so that the secretion of androstanediol-3β-monosulfate decreases to levels that are no longer inhibitory to LH secretion.[113]

The preovulatory gonadotropin surge occurs when all of these cascading processes culminate in activation of the positive feedback mechanism, the hallmark of sexual maturity in the female. "Positive feedback" refers to the

TABLE 14-1

Autoamplification Processes Involved in Pubertal Progression, Follicle Maturation, and Ovulation

Central nervous system GnRH secretion increases[98,99] via:
- E2-inducing progesterone receptors[100]
- Progesterone synergization with E2[101]

Pituitary LH and FSH responsiveness to GnRH increases via:
- GnRH self-priming[102]
- Critical patterns of E2 secretion-stimulating LH/FSH responsiveness,[103-105]
- Progesterone synergization with E2[104-106]
- LH bioactivity increases[94]

Gonadal responsiveness to FSH and LH increases via:
- FSH-inducing aromatase and progesterone in granulosa cells: androgens and progesterone synergization with this effect[107-109]
- FSH-stimulated granulosa meiosis[29] and FSH-inducing granulosa LH receptors; IGF-1 synergization[110]

E2, estradiol; FSH, follicle-stimulating hormone; GnRH, gonadotropin-releasing hormone; IGF-1, insulin-like growth factor-1; and LH, luteinizing hormone.

neuroendocrine system acquiring the ability to secrete a midcycle surge of LH when the ovary signals via increasing estrogen secretion that it is prepared for ovulation.

Menarche does not necessarily indicate full maturation of the neuroendocrine-ovarian axis. As the studies of Knobil illustrate (Figure 14-10), the first menstruation can be due to estrogen-withdrawal bleeding (half of the time) but ovulatory cycles may follow in short order. General characteristics of the mature ovary are shown in Figure 14-4.

The morphology of the normal adolescent ovary has long been considered polycystic, and histologic exami-

nation has typically shown thecal luteinization.[73,114] In the perimenarcheal period, the combination of a high number of follicles and mature gonadotropin stimulation leads to a greater number of large antral follicles than at any other stage (Figure 14-3). Ultrasound imaging has shown that about one-quarter of normal adolescents develop "multifollicular" ovaries (containing four to ten follicles of 4-10 mm diameter in the maximum plane without increased ovarian stroma),[115,116] which are considered to be a variation of normal. Polycystic ovaries (over ten follicles and/or increased size) occur in only 10% of regularly menstruating schoolgirls.[116a] Regression of polycystic ovaries probably occurs in fewer than 10% of cases.[76,117] The ovary normally achieves adult size and ultrasound morphology by 14 years of age.[115,117]

Adult

Normal Menstrual Cycle: Hormone Patterns. In many respects, puberty is recapitulated during the follicular phase of each menstrual cycle. The pattern of gonadotropin and steroid hormone levels is shown in Figure 14-14.[118,119] Gonadotropin and sex hormone levels are low during the premenstrual phase of the mature cycle (Figure 14-14A). Gonadotropin concentrations then increase at the time of menstruation, FSH predominating in the early follicular phase while nocturnal LH pulsation is slow[120] (Figure 14-14B). Luteinizing hormone pulsation increases to a circhoral pattern around a stable baseline, and estradiol production slowly begins (Figure 14-14C). Estradiol levels gradually increase, and serum FSH levels fall reciprocally (Figure 14-14D). The subsequent geometric increase in plasma estradiol

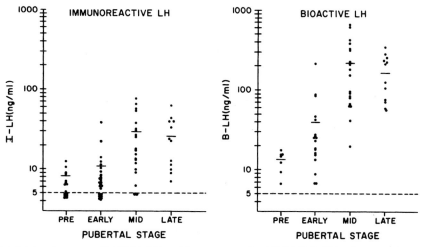

Figure 14-13 Bioactive luteinizing hormone (B-LH) (right) and immunoreactive LH (I-LH) (left) in the same daytime serum samples of girls 10 to 16 years of age at various pubertal stages. The dashed lines indicate the limit of sensitivity of the assays. B-LH rises relatively more than I-LH in the course of puberty. The peak in the apparent biopotency of LH, estimated from the ratio of B-LH to I-LH, occurs at about the time of menarche. "Late" indicates early follicular phase normally menstruating postmenarcheal girls. Standard LER-907: 100 ng equivalent to 6 mIU LH of First International Reference Preparation of human pituitary gonadotropin. The disparity between immunoreactivity and bioactivity is principally due to the presence of different proportions of immunoreactive and bioactive LH moieties in serum and standards. The ratio of bioactivity to immunoreactivity is closer to unity when sera are assayed against highly purified standards (like the first and second IRP of human luteinizing hormone), which have about fivefold higher specific activity and yield dose response relationships with serum LH that are more linear. [Data from Lucky AW, Rich BH, Rosenfield RL, et al. (1980). LH bioactivity increases more than immunoreactivity during puberty. J Pediatr 97:205; and from Rosenfield RL, Helke J (1992). Is an immunoassay available for the measurement of bioactive LH in serum? J Androl 13:1.]

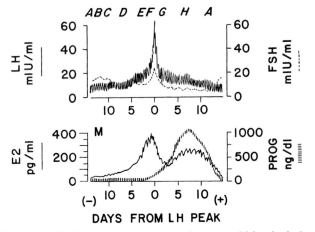

Figure 14-14 Mean gonadotropin and sex steroid levels during the normal menstrual cycle. The data are centered in reference to days before or after the day of the luteinizing hormone (LH) peak (day 0). Letters A through F above the top panel correspond to stages of follicular development in Figure 14-15. G and H are discussed in text. M (bottom panel) shows time of menses. E2, estradiol; FSH, follicle-stimulating hormone; and PROG, progesterone. (Data from Abraham GE (1974). Ovarian and adrenal contributions to peripheral androgens during the menstrual cycle. J Clin Endocrinol Metab 39:340; and from Ross GT, Cargille CM, Lipsett MB, et al. (1970). Pituitary and gonadal hormones in women during spontaneous and induced ovulatory cycles. Recent Prog Horm Res 26:1.]

concentrations then selectively amplifies the pituitary's LH response to GnRH as estradiol reaches about 90 pg/mL for longer than 3 days[103-105] (Figure 14-14E).

When the plasma estradiol rises to greater than 200 to 300 pg/mL for 36 hr, the positive feedback mechanism is activated and the midcycle gonadotropin surge commences (Figure 14-14F). Estradiol then induces progesterone receptor (PR) expression in the hypothalamus and pituitary.[100] Progesterone increasing to 100 ng/dL facilitates the LH surge, shortens the duration of time over which estradiol is required for the surge to 24 hours, and brings about an FSH surge. The mechanism of progesterone action involves inhibition of GnRH cleavage.[106] Androgens may also play a role in facilitating FSH and GnRH release.[121,122] The LH surge is then primarily responsible for luteinizing the preovulatory ovarian follicle (Figure 14-14F). At this time, LH pulses become larger in amplitude but slower in frequency and their apparent bioactivity increases. Ovulation then results.

Estrogen levels fall when the follicle is disrupted (Figure 14-14G). As the corpus luteum begins to form, progesterone increases steadily to be sustained at very high levels for several days—along with lesser but substantial increases in estradiol and 17-hydroxyprogesterone levels (Figure 14-14H). In response to the high progesterone level, gonadotropin pulsation slows.[120] In the absence of increasing human chorionic gonadotropin (hCG) from a conceptus, the corpus luteum's life span is exhausted and its production of progesterone and estradiol wanes. Subsequently, FSH begins to rise out of proportion to LH. Shortly after the sex steroids withdraw from the scene, the endometrium sloughs—giving rise to menstrual flow. Meanwhile, the follicular

growth induced earlier by FSH begins to gain momentum and the next cycle begins.

Follicular (Proliferative) Phase Ovary. The hormonal functions of the follicle have dual purposes that must be closely coordinated: to change the milieu of the ovum to prepare for ovulation and to signal the pituitary to send the signal to ovulate (the LH surge). Thus, the ovary is the zeitgeber for the cycle: the normal cyclic pattern of ovarian hormone secretion induces the midcycle surge of pituitary gonadotropins in the presence of unchanging circhoral pulses of GnRH.[87] The processes triggered also autoamplify the gonadotropin signal (Table 14-1). Ovarian hormones also play a facilitating role in this event by augmenting the amplitude of the GnRH response,[98-101] thereby "guaranteeing" a preovulatory gonadotropin surge.

Ovarian follicular development and steroid secretion in relationship to changing gonadotropin levels are illustrated in Figure 14-15.[29,35,123,124] FSH and LH play major roles in granulosa and thecal cell differentiation, respectively, whereas a host of local factors modulate gonadotropin action. For example, follicular maturation in response to gonadotropins is enhanced by insulin-like growth factors (IGFs), transforming growth factor (TGF)-β, and fibroblast growth factor—whereas it is inhibited by TGF-α, epidermal growth factor, and other factors.

Primordial follicle growth and development is gonadotropin independent. Subsequently, granulosa cells of preantral follicles develop FSH receptors—and theca cells, which encircle granulosa cells, develop LH receptors (Figure 14-15A). Activin can cause FSH-independent upregulation of FSH receptors in preantral follicles,[111] although it opposes FSH stimulation of antral follicle development.[29] The forkhead transcription factor Foxo3a seems to be an important suppressor of early follicle growth, and in its absence follicles initially overgrow and then undergo premature atresia.[125] Fetal undernutrition has been suspected of restricting the follicular endowment.[126]

The initiation of antrum formation is promoted by the presence of FSH, although it is unclear in man whether FSH is absolutely required or is required in only trace amounts (Figure 14-15B).[29,127-129] FSH stimulates androgen receptor expression in primary follicles.[130] Androgen action is necessary to the early stages of follicular growth and development of a full complement of follicles, and androgen excess stimulates excessive follicle number.[131,132] Luteinizing hormone stimulates the appearance in thecal cells of the enzymes necessary to androgen biosynthesis.[133] Androgens in turn stimulate further expression of FSH receptors and the early stages of follicular growth.[130] Some theca cells of small antral follicles are also capable of producing small amounts of estradiol.[134]

As antral follicles reach approximately 1 mm in diameter, their granulosa cells begin to form estradiol from androgen supplied by theca cells (Figure 14-15C).[135-139] Androgen production at low levels may synergize with FSH to stimulate aromatase activity within the granulosa cells.[107,140,141]

For growth beyond 2 mm in diameter, follicles are increasingly FSH dependent and consequently uniformly FSH responsive.[29,127] Antral follicles do not develop without the FSH receptor,[142] and do not grow over 5 mm in diameter without FSH.[129] IGF-I is required for follicular growth

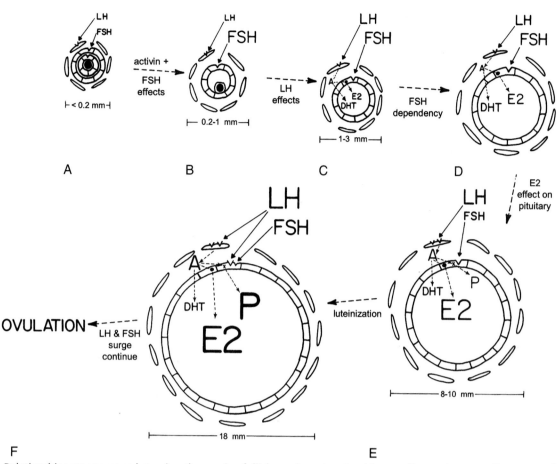

Figure 14-15 Relationships among gonadotropins, the ovarian follicle, and ovarian steroids according to the two-cell two-gonadotropin model of ovarian steroidogenesis. A through F: Stages of ovarian follicular development found during the times of the menstrual cycle designated by the corresponding letters on Figure 14-14. The size of the letters designating hormones relates to the magnitude of their serum and/or follicular concentrations. (A) Preantral follicle with luteinizing hormone (LH) and follicle-stimulating hormone (FSH) receptors in theca and granulosa cells, respectively. There is no antrum surrounding the ovum (stippled in center). (B) Small antral follicle. This appears to develop in response to FSH. The ovum, which becomes eccentric, is not shown in larger antral follicles. (C) Large antral follicle (1 mm or larger). Aromatase activity (.) has been induced in granulosa cells. Interactions between theca and granulosa cells, the former producing androgens (androstenedione: A), result in increasing estradiol (E2) and dihydrotestosterone (DHT) synthesis. A small amount of E2 secretion probably also occurs in theca cells at this stage (not shown). (D) FSH-dependent follicular growth results in more E2 synthesis. (E) Estradiol enhances pituitary LH secretion in response to GnRH, while at the same time inhibiting pituitary FSH secretion. The increased LH induces more theca LH receptors and stimulates androgen production. Androgens serve as substrate for E2 formation and synergize with FSH to stimulate progesterone (P) secretion. (F) In the preovulatory follicle, FSH induces LH receptors on the granulosa cell—which completes luteinization. Steroid secretion is augmented further. Then, increasing progesterone amplifies the positive feedback effect of E2 to initiate the preovulatory gonadotropin surge.

beyond the early antral stage in response to FSH.[143] By the mid-follicular phase, the proliferation of FSH-responsive granulosa cells results in an accelerating rate of estradiol production and preferential conversion of androstenedione to estradiol rather than to DHT by these cells (Figure 14-15D).[135-137,139,144,145] Estradiol itself clearly stimulates proliferation of granulosa cells in rats, and estrogen receptors are necessary to postpubertal maintenance of granulosa cell differentiation and oocyte survival in mice.[146] Recent evidence suggests that estradiol promotes antral growth independently of LH in humans, too.[146a]

A dominant follicle is selected at the beginning of the menstrual cycle from a crop of follicles that were recruited 2.5 months prior.[29] Recruitment of a group of follicles is normally promoted by the midcycle FSH surge and regresses with increasing corpus luteum progester-

one secretion. Another wave of follicle growth in the late luteal phase is promoted by the rise of FSH as luteal progesterone and estradiol secretion wanes. The selected follicle is the one most sensitivite to FSH (lowest "FSH threshold"). FSH is critically important during the follicular phase for optimal development of this dominant follicle. By the mid-follicular phase of the cycle, this follicle becomes virtually the sole source of estradiol (Figure 14-15E). Typically, there is only one such follicle. Only this follicle continues to grow, reaching a diameter of 10 mm or larger. All other gonadotropin-dependent follicles undergo atresia.

At this stage, the rising estradiol level is suppressing FSH secretion and augmenting pituitary LH responsiveness to GnRH. FSH is more bioactive in the dominant follicle because it is more efficiently concentrated[144] and because local factors increase ovarian responsiveness to FSH. The increased LH causes further proliferation of thecal cells and an increase in their LH receptor content.[108] Androgen production is consequently increased. This synergizes with FSH to augment aromatase activity and bring about increasing progesterone secretion by the well-estrogenized granulosa cells of these follicles. Progesterone then enhances the synthesis of itself and of estradiol.[108,109] The increased thecal androstenedione production is diverted much more to estradiol than to dihydrotestosterone biosynthesis. Antral fluid steroid concentrations reflect these changes (Figure 14-16).[135,136,144] Activin acts to prevent premature luteinization of granulosa cells, and activin tone seems to wane as the preovulatory phase approaches.[29,111]

FSH next induces LH receptors in the granulosa cells (Figure 14-15F).[110] These luteinized granulosa cells are capable of augmenting estradiol and progestin production in response to LH as well as FSH. The LH and FSH surge then occurs in response to the positive feedback action of estradiol at both the CNS and pituitary levels, an effect amplified by the rising levels of progesterone. The final steps in follicle maturation ensue rapidly: the LH surge induces granulosa cell PR and prostaglandin synthase while inhibiting cyclin gene transcription. These are all critical steps in preparing for ovulation. In their absence, ovulation and follicular rupture do not occur.[147]

The follicle then promptly becomes desensitized to LH and FSH and ceases to grow.[148] This is followed by an inflammatory-type response. Protease activity, prostaglandin production, plasminogen activitor production, and vascular permeability increase; the intercellular spaces fill with mucopolysaccharides; and cell junctions loosen. Meiosis resumes in response to a specific phosphodiesterase,[149] forming the haploid gamete (secondary oocyte) and the first polar body in response to the LH surge.[150] (A premature LH surge in a subject with an unripe follicle will not result in ovulation.) Ovulation then occurs. Meiosis will go to completion, and the second polar body will be extruded only in response to contact with a sperm.

The processes stimulating dominant follicle emergence are delicately balanced by those preventing it. It seems critical that the intraovarian concentration of androgens not become excessive or no follicles will remain viable beyond about the 8-mm stage.[137] Androgen excess seems to prevent the emergence of dominant follicles by antagonizing granulosa cell proliferation and development.[151] The mechanisms involved include inhibition of aromatase in situations of low FSH activity[107,140] and antagonism of LH receptor formation and action.[109,152] Follicles arrested in their growth become atretic, and atretic follicles contain relatively high concentrations of androgens (Figure 14-16). Progesterone also suppresses further differentiation of nondominant follicles[153] by some of the same mechanisms.[154] High concentrations of estrogen play a critical role in inhibiting selection of the dominant follicles in primates.[155] If there is interference with estrogenization, multiple large cystic follicles develop that are impaired in their abiity to ovulate and undergo androgen-dependent atresia.[156-158]

AMH and inhibins have recently emerged as other important follicular factors important to the direct and indirect regulation of follicular development. Granulosa cells of preantral and small antral follicles produce AMH, which exerts a paracrine negative feedback effect on the differentiation of primordial follicles and inhibits aromatase activity.[72,159-161] They also produce inhibins, which are regulated by FSH in a negative feedback loop and up-regulate thecal steroidogenesis (discussed later in the chapter). Inhibin-B is the predominant form of inhibin. Inhibin-A is a product of the preovulatory follicle (and corpus luteum) that responds to LH and FSH.[162,163]

Atresia is the fate of all except the few hundred follicles chosen for ovulation during an individual's life span. Most follicles beyond the primordial stage become atretic. Atresia occurs by the process of programmed cell death.[29] This apoptotic process has diverse determinants, including cell death inducer and repressor genes.[40,124] FSH support becomes increasingly necessary to survival as the follicle matures, and it is normally only the follicle that has the lowest FSH threshold that escapes atresia.

Luteal (Secretory) Phase Ovary. Following ovulatory rupture of the Graafian follicle, capillaries and fibroblasts from the theca proliferate and break down the separating

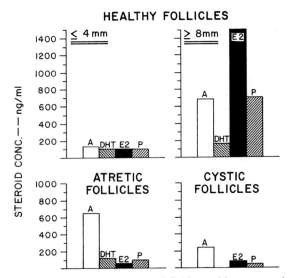

HEALTHY FOLLICLES

Figure 14-16 Normal human antral fluid steroid concentrations. Healthy follicles are well populated by granulosa cells (50% or more of maximal complement). Healthy follicles seem capable of further development because many of them (75%) contain healthy-appearing oocytes (histologically intact germinal vesicles), 96% of which are viable in culture. Moderately large follicles (8 mm or larger in diameter) make their appearance only in the mid-follicular phase of the cycle and contain follicle-stimulating hormone. Data are shown only for those large follicles well populated by granulosa cells, only one of which usually arises in the follicular phase of each menstrual cycle. Atretic follicles are small follicles beginning to show degenerative changes in the number of granulosa cells and appearance of the oocyte. Cystic follicles tend to be larger follicles with only a sparse granulosa cell lining. The testosterone content of antral fluid is about a third that of dihydrotestosterone (DHT) owing to the pattern of granulosa cell metabolism of androstenedione (A). E2, estradiol; and P, progesterone. [Interpolation based on the data of McNatty KP, Makris A, Reinhold VN, et al. (1979). Steroids 34:429. J Clin Endocrinol Metab 49:851, 1979.]

basement membrane. The luteinized granulosa and theca cells then intermingle and complete the luteinization process. These two cell types contribute about equally to corpus luteum steroidogenesis.[164] Histologically, luteinization is a process of lipid accumulation. The biochemical hallmark of luteinization is the capacity for progesterone biosynthesis in response to LH. This is accompanied by increased estrogen secretion in man.[165,166]

During its functional life span the corpus luteum is normally the major source of the sex hormones secreted by the ovary. Corpus luteum function reaches its peak about 4 days after ovulation and begins to wane about 4 days before menstruation (Figure 14-14H). Loss of sensitivity to LH and estradiol heralds luteal senescence. Regression of the corpus luteum-luteolysis occurs if pregnancy does not provide chorionic gonadotropin (hCG). Luteolysis is probably mediated by prostaglandin. Transformation of the corpus luteum into an avascular scar, the corpus albicans, then occurs.

Early luteal-phase increases in secretion of estradiol and progesterone cause secretory transformation and hyperplasia of the endometrium. Later falloff in secretion of female hormones to a level insufficient to maintain the endometrium results in menstruation. Withdrawal of progesterone is specifically responsible for constriction of spiral arteries, local prostaglandin accumulation, and subsequent ischemic necrosis of the endometrium. Normal menstrual flow then results from a complete slough of the secretory endometrium.

A major determinant of normal corpus luteum formation and function is optimal development of the corpus luteum predecessor, the dominant follicle. Experimental lowering of FSH levels in the early follicular phase has been shown to impair subsequent corpus luteum function.[167]

REGULATION OF THE NEUROENDOCRINE-OVARIAN AXIS

Factors Controlling the Onset of Puberty

The mechanisms by which neuroendocrine and genetic factors control pubertal development remain unknown. Epidemiologic studies indicate that nutrition and environmental chemicals, as well as ethnicity and genetic factors, are important in the pubertal process.[168] Evidence that there are genetic factors involved at the time of puberty comes from multiple studies.[169-179] It has been estimated that between 50% and 80% of the variation in the timing of puberty is determined by genes. Hypogonadotropic hypogonadism has been associated with mutations in single genes, including GnRHR, KAL-1, FGFR-1, GPR54, and LHX3.[180-182a]

Although mutations in these genes have been shown to cause physiologic interruptions in development, their role in the initiation of puberty remains unknown. Single nucleotide polymorphisms (SNPs) for GnRH and GnRH receptor genes used to detect associations with late pubertal development have not accounted for variations in the timing of puberty in the general population.[183] The key in the initiation of puberty is the activation of the hypothalamic GnRH pulse generator. The molecular events that control the pulse generator include a complex interplay between inhibitory and stimulatory factors. The

mechanism of central activation of puberty first appears to be a consequence of a removal of a restraint mechanism, with a rise in gonadotropin secretion (initially nocturnally).[46]

This restraint in the GnRH pulse generator is independent of the presence of gonads[61] and is more intense in males.[184] However, the high levels of testosterone to which the male fetus was exposed during the period of sexual differentiation may be responsible for the more prolonged suppression of GnRH release in males than in females. A role for decreased estrogen feedback sensitivity by the hypothalamic pulse generator near the time of puberty has also been shown.[185] Several factors have been shown to have a role in restraining the GnRH pulse generator. They include GnRH itself, NPY, GABA, leptin, and TGF-alpha, and their receptors.

Recent evidence points to an important role for GPR54 (a G-protein–coupled receptor) and its ligand (kisspeptin) as a signal for pubertal GnRH release. Expression of both proteins has been found to increase prior to pubertal resurgence associated with the increase in GnRH pulse generator activity in the hypothalamus.[49] Activation of GPR54 by kisspeptin stimulates LH and FSH release via the activation of GnRH. This activation can be abolished by GnRH antagonists. Mutations in the GPR54 gene result in hypogonadotropic hypogonadism.[181,186,187] However, mutations in GPR54 have not been found in boys with pubertal delay. Nor have polymorphic sequences been associated with delay of pubertal development.[188]

Elegant studies in primates have demonstrated an increase in kisspeptin in pubertal development, with a corresponding increase in GPR54 associated with an increase in LH. However, whether this increase is dependent on activation of the neuronal pulse generator is unclear. The maximum level of expression of kisspeptin and GPR54 in the hypothalamus in both males and females occurs at puberty.[47,189] Chronic administration of kisspeptin to immature female rats induces precocious activation of the central axis.[189] In addition, chronic treatment with kisspeptin restores pubertal development in a rat model of undernutrition.[190] Kisspeptin may thus influence the priming of puberty and the integration of nutritional and energy status. Although it is clear that kisspeptin activation of GnRH neurons occurs at puberty and that GnRH is increasingly sensitive to kisspeptin activation during development,[191] it is unknown whether kisspeptin is the trigger of mammalian puberty or the effector of higher regulatory substances.

Initiation of puberty involves coordinated changes in transsynaptic and glial-neuronal communication.[48] The major inhibitory systems are GABAergic and opioidergic, whereas the major excitatory systems involve glutamate and kisspeptin—with glial cells facilitating GnRH secretion in diverse ways (Figure 14-17). Decreased GABA signaling via GABA$_A$ receptors and increased glutamate signaling via glutamate receptors of several types (ionotropic and metabotropic) are the major proximate changes in neurotransmission involved in the onset of puberty.[46,48,184] Glial cells facilitate the process through elaboration of transforming growth factors (TGFs), other growth factors, prostaglandin E$_2$, and the elaboration of enzymes that control the concentration

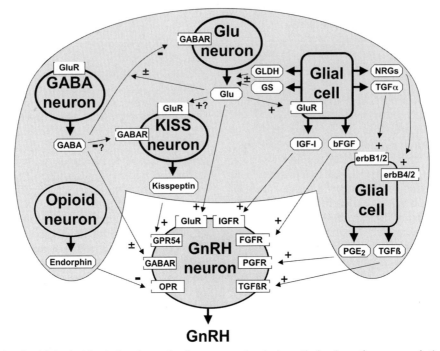

Figure 14-17 The molecular biological basis for the major known proximate hypothalamic pathways regulating GnRH secretion. The left-hand column depicts the major inhibitory pathways, which involve GABA signaling through the GABA receptor and opiodergic signaling through the endorphin receptor (OPR). The central column depicts the major excitatory pathways, which involve glutamate (Glu) signaling through the family of glutamate receptors and kisspeptin (KISS) signaling through GPR54. The right-hand column shows the major glial factors that facilitate GnRH release. These include the elaboration of the enzymes glutamic dehydrogenase (GLDH) and glutamine synthase (GS), which regulate the concentration of glutamate and the elaboration of a variety of growth factors. The KISS neuron has not been isolated at this time, and thus its illustrated signaling pathways are based on indirect evidence. bFGF = basic fibroblast growth factor, erbB 1-4 are subunits for the TGFα and NRG receptors, IGF-I = insulin -like growth factor, NRG = neuroregulins, PGE = prostaglandin E, R = receptor, TGFα = tumor growth factor-α, TGFß = tumor growth factor ß, + = positive stimulation, - = inhibition, ± = either, and ? = unknown. [Modified from Ojeda SR, Lomniczi A, Mastronardi C, Heger S, Roth C, Parent AS, et al. (2006). The neuroendocrine regulation of puberty: Is the time ripe for a systems biology approach? Endocrinology 147:1166–1174.]

of glutamate [glutamic dehydrogenase (which catalyzes the synthesis of glutamate) and glutamine synthase, which converts glutamate to glutamine].

The basis of the change in neurotransmitter balance is becoming clearer. A second tier of control seems to be modulation of these processes by increased hypothalamic expression at puberty of tumor-suppressor genes that act to integrate glial-neuronal interactions. A yet higher echelon of candidate hypothalamic genes has been identified. These are transcriptional regulators of the second-tier genes. These genes include Oct-2 (a regulator of the POU-domain homeobox genes), EAP-1 (enhanced at puberty-1), and thyroid transcription factor-I (TTF-1)—knockout of which delays puberty and decreases fertility in mice.

Genes contiguous with elastin appear to be involved in the pace of puberty. Deletion of chromosome 7q11.23 in Williams syndrome typically leads to an early normal onset but rapid pace of puberty, with an abbreviated pubertal growth spurt.[192] Lesioning studies suggest that two sets of tracts carrying opposing stimuli are involved. Inhibitory tracts mainly seem to be routed through the posterior hypothalamus, and stimulatory tracts through the anterior hypothalamic preoptic area.[1,193]

An overview of the systems involved in regulating the initiation of puberty is shown in Figure 14-18. Pubertal maturation and skeletal maturation seem to have common

determinants. Abundant clinical evidence indicates that sex hormones are one of these.[194,195] Thus, genes involved in sex hormone metabolism and action are candidate regulators of the onset of puberty—and there has been speculation that fetal or early childhood exposure to hormonally active environmental chemicals (environmental disruptors) may influence the onset of puberty.[168]

The GH-IGF system is another determinant. GH facilitates the onset and tempo of puberty.[196] Experimental studies suggest that this occurs through GH or IGF actions at all levels of the neuroendocrine-ovarian axis.[197,198] Girls generally enter puberty when they achieve a pubertal bone age. Pubertal stage normally correlates better with bone age (r = 0.82) than with chronologic age (r = 0.72, unpublished data), particularly as menarche approaches.[199] Skeletal age correlates better with menarche than with chronologic age, height, or weight—and its variance at menarche is half that of chronologic age.[200]

The bone age at the onset of breast development averages about 10.75 years, and that at menarche averages about 13.0 years. Disorders that accelerate bone maturation, such as congenital adrenal hyperplasia or hyperthyroidism, tend to advance the age of onset of true puberty.[201] Disorders that retard skeletal maturation (such as GH deficiency, hypothyroidism, and anemia) tend to delay the onset of puberty.[202] On the other hand, some data suggest that factors linked to intrauterine growth

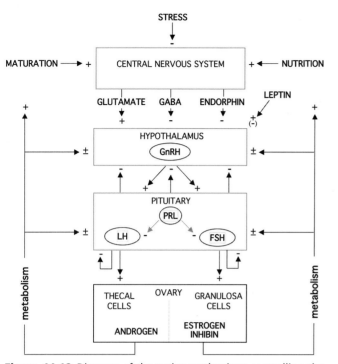

Figure 14-18 Diagram of the major mechanisms controlling the development and function of sex hormone secretion by the unripe antral follicle. Regulation may be either stimulatory (+) or inhibitory (−). The central nervous system (CNS) influences gonadatropin-releasing hormone (GnRH) secretion both negatively and positively. For the CNS to relinquish its inhibitory control over GnRH secretion, it must achieve a high level of maturity. Even after this is achieved, psychological or physical stress may negatively influence the system. Nutrition must be optimal. Its effects are reversible. Leptin is a critical mediator of the nutrition effect. Sex steroids have a maturing effect. Whether efferent tracts from the hypothalamus to the cerebrum play a role in reproductive function is unknown. Pineal secretion of melatonin and other substances are known to exert inhibitory influences on GnRH in lower animals (not shown). GnRH stimulates luteinizing hormone (LH) and follicle-stimulating hormone (FSH). Paracrine and autocrine feedback of the gonadatropins on GnRH release and their own release, respectively, are shown. Prolactin (PRL) has multiple effects on gonadotropin secretion. In unripe antral follicles, LH acts on thecal and interstitial cells and FSH acts on granulosa cells. Androstenedione and testosterone secreted by the theca cells are aromatized by the granulosa cell, under the influence of FSH, to estradiol. The granulosa cell is also the site of production of the FSH inhibitor inhibin B. Estradiol has a diphasic effect on the mature pituitary and on hypothalamic GnRH release as well. Androgens seem normally to be of minor importance in regulating gonadotropin release in females. Intraovarian mechanisms seem to modulate LH action so as to coordinate thecal formation of androgens with granulosa cell formation of estrogens. Paracrine and autocrine factors, including insulin-like growth factors, are involved. GABA, gamma-aminobutyric acid.

retardation (although not necessarily the growth retardation itself) predispose to sexual precocity.[168]

Optimal nutrition is clearly necessary to initiation and maintenance of normal menstrual cycles. The hypothesis that body fat is the weight-related trigger for pubertal development originated with the discovery by Frisch and co-workers that weight correlated with initiation of the pubertal growth spurt, peak growth velocity, and menarche better than with chronologic age or height.[203] Mid-childhood may be a critical period for weight to influence the onset of puberty.[168] Suboptimal nutrition related to socioeconomic factors is more of an important factor in the later onset of puberty in underdeveloped than in developed countries.[168] Conversely, obesity appears to be an important factor in advancing the onset of puberty in the United States.[204,205]

Leptin appears to be an important link between nutrition and the attainment and maintenance of reproductive competence.[184,206,207] Leptin deficiency causes obesity and gonadotropin deficiency. Paradoxically, prolonged leptin excess down-regulates GnRH release.[208] Leptin is secreted by fat cells. It acts on the hypothalamus to reduce appetite and to stimulate gonadotropin secretion. Inhibition of hypothalamic neuropeptide Y formation mediates part of the leptin effect.[209] A critical threshold level appears to signal that nutritional stores are sufficient for mature function of the GnRH pulse generator and are thus permissive of puberty. Blood leptin levels rise throughout childhood and puberty to reach higher levels in girls than in boys.[210] Leptin-binding protein, a truncated form of the leptin receptor, falls as puberty begins—which suggests that circulating leptin becomes more bioavailable at this time. Whether leptin has a direct role in the pubertal activation of the GnH pulse generator is unknown. In models of leptin insufficiency, the administration of kisspeptin-induced LH secretion indicates that the role of leptin in the initiation of puberty is upstream of kisspeptin.[189]

Other factors link nutrition and gonadotropic function. Other cues that provide information on nutritional status to the central reproductive axis may include glucose,[211] ghrelin,[212] and insulin.[213] The effect of these factors on LH pulstility may be mediated directly at the level of the gonadotroph or indirectly by changes in GnRH secretion. There is little evidence for the role of pineal secretions in human reproduction that is found in lower animals.[214, 215]

The essential element for the onset of puberty is an increase in pulsatile hypothalamic GnRH secretion that is regulated by a complex interplay of excitatory and inhibitory signals that have yet to be fully understood or elucidated.[48] During childhood the activity of the GnRH pulse generating system is restrained for reasons that are unclear. An awakening of the pulse generator occurs gradually during late childhood with an increasing tempo during early puberty. The mechanism for the increasing GnRH neuronal activation at the initiation of puberty is also unknown. The pubertal diminution in tone of the CNS centers that inhibit hypothalamic GnRH secretion during childhood has traditionally been considered to result from decreasing sensitivity of a "gonadostat" to negative feedback by sex steroids.[6,216,217] However, this now seems an overly simplistic concept for a mechanism that seems to involve a change in the balance of neural inhibitory and stimulatory signals that impinge upon the GnRH neuron.

Many studies have been performed to help understand the initiating developmental events or the "trigger" for pubertal onset. In fact, it is becoming increasingly clear that there is no single 'trigger' for puberty, but a gradual increase in GnRH pulsatility associated with a complex interplay of factors and hypothalamic developmental programs. The integration of hypothalamic signaling systems along with the developmental changes in the control of GnRH neuronal function converge to trigger the onset of puberty. Thus, the apparent "sensitivity of the gonadostat" seems increasingly likely to reflect the degree of activity of the GnRH neuron. That is, when GnRH secretory activity is attenuated the pulse generator is easily inhibited. When the GnRH neuron is active, the pulse generator is relatively insensitive to negative feedback.

Regulation of Gonadotropin Secretion

An essential feature of the mature hypothalamic-pituitary-gonadal axis is the long-loop negative feedback control of gonadotropin secretion by gonadal secretory products, as depicted in Figure 14-18. The generally tonic nature of gonadotropin secretion is punctuated by two types of periodicity: two- to threefold pulsations of LH above trough levels at 1.5- to 2.0-hour intervals, and in the sexually mature female by a transient midcycle preovulatory gonadotropin surge. The latter is characterized by a greater than tenfold rapid rise of LH and a lesser rise of FSH. This surge is brought about by positive feedback when a critical level of estradiol, facilitated by a modest rise in progesterone, is achieved for a critical period of time (as discussed in relation to Figure 14-14).

Estradiol, in concert with inhibin, reciprocally regulates FSH in a sensitive, log-dose, negative-feedback arrangement.[251] Progesterone in high (luteal phase) concentrations appears to be the major negative regulator of GnRH-LH pulse frequency.[100] Androgens at normal levels do not contribute to long-loop negative feedback regulation of gonadotropins.

Estradiol exerts triphasic, and progesterone biphasic, effects on gonadotropin secretion. As estradiol rises into the late follicular phase range it reduces FSH levels, at preovulatory levels it transiently induces positive feedback, and at sustained high levels it suppresses gonadotropins. As progesterone reaches a preovulatory level, it enhances the estradiol positive feedback effect, but at sustained high levels it suppresses LH pulse frequency while enhancing LH pulse amplitude.[100]

The GnRH neurons primarily responsible for maintenance of the reproductive cycle are those of the arcuate (infundibular) nucleus (Figure 14-19).[87] GnRH neurons are inherently pulsatile.[219] Synchrony is promoted by fluxes of ionic calcium into these cells and autocrine GnRH inhibitory feedback. GnRH secretion is modulated by the variety of neurotransmitters and growth factors involved in initiating puberty.[48] Synchrony of the network of GnRH neurons that comprises the pulse generator is conferred when the hypothalamic concentration of GABA periodically falls from levels inhibitory to GABA$_A$ receptors in the presence of an excitatory neurotransmitter.[220,221]

Sex steroid signals are in part conveyed to GnRH neurons indirectly from higher centers. Regulation of GnRH secretion by estrogen also involves induction of PRs in the hypothalamus.[100,222] GnRH neuronal cell lines have been studied in which estradiol has been shown to directly stimulate and inhibit GnRH gene expression under different experimental conditions.[223,224] Progesterone also exerts its main inhibitory effect on GnRH secretion.[225,226] Prolactin suppresses both hypothalamic and gonadotropin GnRH receptor expression.[227,228]

Other clinically relevant factors affecting GnRH release are endorphins (endogenous opioids) and interleukins. Endorphins are important physiologic regulators of

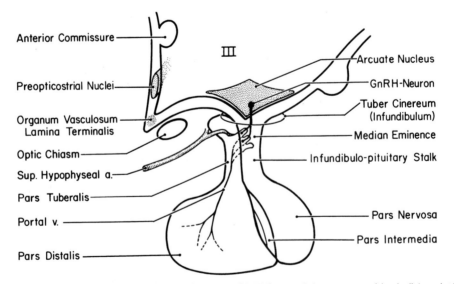

Figure 14-19 The location of major gonadotropin-releasing hormone (GnRH)-containing neurons (shaded) in relation to the hypothalamus and pituitary gland. The neurons are of greatest density in the arcuate nuclei and in the periventricular wall of the medial basal hypothalamus. These neurons project to the adjacent median eminence, the second most dense population of GnRH neurons lies in the preopticostrial area. The development of some is altered by early androgenization. Some are connected by the stria terminalis to the amygdalae. Other projections from this area appear to connect indirectly with the median eminence, perhaps via the organum vasculosum lamina terminalis—a midline structure that resembles the median eminence. The pituitary portal veins transport blood rich in releasing factors to sinusoids engulfing anterior pituitary cells.

GnRH release after puberty has begun. Hypothalamic β-endorphin suppresses oophorectomy-initiated GnRH secretion, and opiate antagonists reverse this effect. The inhibitory effect of stress on gonadotropin release appears to be mediated by β-endorphin released from proopiomelanocortin in response to corticotrophin-releasing hormone.[229] Interleukins inhibit gonadotropin release.[230]

A variety of other neuropeptides influence GnRH release.[5,209,231] Neuropeptide-Y (NPY) is a potent appetite-stimulating member of the pancreatic polypeptide family that stimulates appetite and directly inhibits GnRH release during food deprivation.[209] However, on a background of estrogenization it stimulates GnRH release—an effect mediated by a different neural network acting on a different NPY receptor subtype on the GnRH neuron.[232] Other peptides may also be involved in facilitating the LH surge.[233]

GnRH receptors are maintained in an optimally active state only when GnRH is delivered in pulses approximately 1 to 2 hours apart in man.[87,234,235] Pulses substantially less frequent result in a hypogonadotropic state. Paradoxically, continuous administration of an initially stimulatory dose of GnRH results in down-regulation of gonadotropin production after an initial burst of gonadotropin release. This is the physiologic basis for the success of long-acting gonadotropin agonists in suppressing puberty in children with true central precocious puberty. Pituitary GnRH receptors appear to be directly and indirectly down-regulated by GnRH, inhibins, and sex steroid.[235] LH and FSH themselves inhibit GnRH release (short-loop feedback) and inhibit their own release (ultra-short-loop or autocrine feedback).[236,237]

How is differential regulation of LH and FSH release accomplished in response to a single GnRH pulse? Considerable research has been devoted to potential modulators of the GnRH signal. The frequency of the GnRH pulse is one determinant. Slowing this signal moderately stimulates FSH β-subunits and suppresses follistatin gene expression, raising the FSH/LH ratio.[238] Pituitary-adenylate-cyclase-activating polypeptide amplifies LH responses to GnRH while blocking its effect on FSH.[239]

The sex hormone milieu is also clearly a major differential modulator of LH and FSH release.[87,240-243] FSH is more sensitive than LH to inhibition by estrogen. This effect of modest levels of estradiol is of rapid onset and is sustained. LH is the more sensitive to the stimulatory effects of higher estradiol levels. This effect is of later onset and is short-lived. Similar relationships pertain to aromatase null mice. Estrogen receptor (ER) null mice have identified estrogen receptor alpha as the predominant receptor isoform that conveys negative feedback regulation to the gonadotroph.[244] Progesterone exerts both negative and positive feedback effects at the pituitary level, and these effects are antagonized by androgen. The progesterone metabolite 3β-hydroxyprogesterone suppresses FSH release.[245]

Inhibins of gonadal origin seem to be the major nonsteroidal-specific negative feedback regulator of pituitary FSH synthesis and secretion.[246,247] Inhibins may not only inhibit FSH release at the pituitary level but may act at a higher level.[248] Serum levels of both inhibins rise upon FSH stimulation.[162,163] Inhibin-B, produced by small developing follicles in response to FSH, is virtu-

ally the only inhibin moiety in blood during puberty. Its blood levels rise during the early follicular phase and then fall thereafter except for a small postovulatory peak, generally paralleling the changes in serum FSH. The latter peak may function to attenuate the FSH surge. Serum inhibin-A, a marker of the preovulatory follicle and corpus luteum, begins to rise in the late follicular phase and thereafter parallels those of progesterone. Its fall late in the luteal phase appears to contribute to the early follicular phase rise in the FSH level.

Inhibins also have important local effects, and the structurally related activins seem to be normally important entirely as regulators of both pituitary and ovary function.[249] The primary role of activin in the pituitary is to signal the release of FSH. It is formed by gonadotropes themselves, as is the activin binding protein follistatin.[209,250] It also stimulates the secretion of follistatin within folliculostellate cells of the anterior pituitary. Follistatin, by competitively inhibiting binding of activin to its receptor, specifically inhibits activin stimulation of FSH secretion.[251]

Regulation of Ovarian Secretion

Ovarian secretion results from the combined actions of LH and FSH (Fig. 14-20), as discussed previously in regard to Figures 14-14 and 14-15. Androstenedione is the most abundant steroid formed in the ovary, and it is secreted by the theca-interstitial-stromal (thecal) cell compartment in response to LH. Estrogen is predominantly formed from precursor androgen in response to FSH in granulosa cells. FSH also stimulates granulosa cells to secrete inhibins. Androgen formation by the ovary is primarily regulated by LH. As by-products of the secretion of both ovarian estradiol and adrenal cortisol, androgens do not normally contribute to negative feedback regulation of gonadotropins. However, they have a biphasic effect on gonadotropin secretion: modest elevations increase GnRH pulse frequency by interfering with progesterone negative feedback[252,253] and very high levels directly inhibit gonadotropin secretion.

The regulation of the intraovarian androgen concentration is critical to ovarian function.[254] Androgens are obligate substrates for estradiol biosynthesis and promote the growth of small follicles. However, in excess they appear to interfere with the process of follicular maturation—preventing the emergence of the dominant follicle and committing the follicle to atresia, as well as interfering with LH action on luteinized granulosa cells. Therefore, androgen synthesis must be kept to the minimum necessary to optimize follicular development. This means that the synthesis of ovarian androgens must be coordinated with the needs of the follicle. This is achieved by intraovarian intracrine, autocrine, and paracrine modulation of LH action.

A model of the interaction among some of the major factors regulating steroidogenesis is shown in Figure 14-20.[255] Stimulation of androgen secretion by LH appears to be augmented by specific intraovarian FSH-dependent factors, such as inhibins and IGF's.[129] These processes seem to normally be counterbalanced by other FSH-dependent processes that down-regulate androgen formation as LH stimulation increases. Androgens and

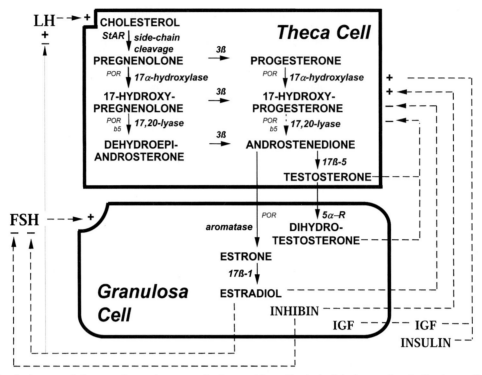

Figure 14-20 Major factors regulating ovarian androgen and estrogen biosynthesis depicted according to the two-cell two-gonadotropin model. Luteinizing hormone (LH) stimulates androgen formation within theca cells by means of the steroidogenic pathway common to the gonads and adrenal glands. Follicle-stimulating hormone (FSH) regulates estradiol biosynthesis from androgen by granulosa cell. Estradiol at early to mid-follicular phase levels does not exert a long-loop negative feeback effect on LH. Androgen formation in response to LH appears to be modulated by intraovarian and endocrine feedback at multiple levels, prominently including 17-hydroxylase and 17,20-lyase—both of which may be activities of cytochrome P-450c17 and side-chain cleavage. Androgen (via dihydrotestosterone) and estradiol inhibit (_), and inhibin, insulin, and insulin-like growth factors (IGFs) stimulate (_) enzyme activities. The sites of aromatase and IGF gene expression appear to vary with the stage of follicular development. Other peptides probably also modulate the steroidogenic response to LH. 3_, _5-Isomerase-3_-hydroxysteroid dehydrogenase (HSD): 17β-HSD5, type 5 17β-HSD; 5α-R, 5α-reductase. [Modified from Ehrmann DA, Barnes RB, Rosenfield RL (1995). Polycystic ovary syndrome as functional ovarian hyperandrogenism due to dysregulation of androgen secretion. Endocr Rev 16:322.]

estrogens themselves seem to mediate at least a portion of this desensitization to LH, with estrogens being critical through an ERα-dependent mechanism.[243]

Insulin and insulin-like growth factors are important co-regulators of ovarian function. The entire IGF system is represented in the ovary. The IGF system is essential to full FSH action. Indeed, IGF-I augments FSH receptor expression.[143, 256] Insulin is a potent augmentor of androgen and estrogen biosynthesis in response to gonadotropins, and insulin receptor mRNA is ubiquitous in all ovarian compartments at all phases of the cycle. In addition, insulin may exert its effects indirectly by its interactions with the IGF system in multiple ways. These include binding to the IGF-I receptor, up-regulating that receptor, and lowering the concentration of IGF binding protein-1 in the blood. GH also promotes granulosa cell steroidogenesis.[257,258]

Many other peptides modulate ovarian cell growth or function in response to gonadotropins.[254,255] Inhibin stimulates ovarian androgen production, whereas androgens reciprocally stimulate ovarian inhibin production. Activin opposes the inhibin effect. A variety of other ovarian peptides are also capable of modulating thecal androgen synthesis.[255] Stimulators include catecholamines (for which an intraovarian system exists[259]), prostaglan-

din, and angiotensin. Inhibitors include leptin, corticotrophin-releasing hormone, epidermal growth factor, tumor necrosis factor, TGF-β, and growth differentiation factor-9.[36] Leptin antagonizes IGF-1 effects.[260]

TGF-β is particularly interesting because it suppresses androgen biosynthesis and stimulates aromatase activity. It also stimulates meiotic maturation of the oocyte.[261] Other peptides acting on granulosa cells include cytokines (which have diverse effects)[256] and AMH, which inhibits aromatase.[159] GnRH is also capable of modulating thecal steroidogenesis. A GnRH-like protein has been described in the ovary that may act through ovarian GnRH receptors to suppress steroidogenesis in the human ovary.[262,263] It inhibits FSH induction of progesterone secretion, aromatase activity, and LH receptors in granulosa cells; down-regulates LH receptors; and inhibits the hCG stimulation of progesterone secretion by luteal cells.[110,123]

Prolactin has complex effects on steroidogenesis. In low concentrations, it enhances ovarian estradiol and progesterone secretion by increasing LH receptors.[264] On the other hand, high levels of prolactin inhibit ovarian estradiol and progesterone biosynthesis.[265] Prolactin also stimulates adrenal androgen production.[266]

ADRENARCHE AND THE REGULATION OF ADRENAL ANDROGEN SECRETION

Adrenarche is the onset of the adrenal androgen production that gradually begins in mid-childhood well before the pubertal maturation of the neuroendocrine-gonadal axis.[267,268] It represents a change in the pattern of adrenal secretory response to ACTH (Figure 14-21). It is characterized by disproportionate rises in the responses to ACTH of the Δ^5-3β-hydroxysteroids 17-hydroxypregnenolone and dehydroepiandrosterone (DHEA), whereas cortisol secretion does not change. Dehydroepiandrosterone sulfate (DHEAS) is the predominant marker for adrenarche. A DHEAS level greater than 40 µg/dL is usually considered adrenarcheal. Other plasma androgens and precursors are ordinarily at the upper end of the prepubertal range at the onset of adrenarche.

Adrenarche reflects the development of the adrenocortical zona reticularis. This zone becomes continuous at about 6 years of age and enlarges steadily over the subsequent decade. Its increasing development correlates with DHEAS levels. This zone's secretion pattern results from a unique enzyme expression profile: it expresses low 3β-hydroxysteroid dehydrogenase type 2 (3βHSD2) but high cytochrome b5 (an enhancer of the 17,20-lyase activity of cytochrome P450c17) and steroid sulfotransferase (SULT2A1) activities.

The zona reticularis may originate from persistent cells of the fetal adrenocortical zone that have failed to undergo involution. A pituitary hormone ("adrenarche factor") may well be required to bring about their adrenarcheal development.[4] It has been postulated to be an ACTH-related hormone distinct from ACTH because adrenal androgen production is more sensitive to glucocorticoid suppression than is cortisol production,[269] falls more slowly than cortisol after dexamethasone administration,[118] and rises more sluggishly after its withdrawal.[270] Candidates for a dexamethasone-suppressible adrenarchal factor include pro-ACTH-related peptides and corticotropin-releasing hormone (CRH). However, the data have not been convincing.[271] Prolactin may be involved.[272]

Currently, the only established adrenal-androgen-stimulating hormone in postnatal life is ACTH. Because the adrenarchal secretion pattern represents a change in the pattern of steroidogenic response to ACTH, an adrenarche factor need only control the growth and differentiation of the zona reticularis or regulate its unique pattern of steroidogenic enzyme expression. A number of factors are known to enhance adrenal androgen output. Insulin and IGF-I particularly stimulate expression of adrenal 3β and P450c17 activities. Leptin has been reported to stimulate P450c17 activity.[273] In addition, interleukin-6 is strongly expressed in the zona reticularis and stimulates DHEA secretion.[274] Whereas gonadal dysgenesis is associated with earlier adrenarche,[275] paradoxically ovariectomy precipitates an early decline in DHEAS levels that is not reversed by estrogen replacement.[276]

Whether adrenarche plays a more fundamental role in puberty than contributing to the growth of sexual hair is unknown. Adrenal androgen formation may serve as a "safety valve" that protects against hypercortisolism by providing an alternate pathway for steroidogenesis. DHEAS and an immediate precursor, pregnenolone sulfate, have been found to be stimulatory neuroactive steroids.[277] Adrenal androgens may contribute to cortical bone accrual,[278] whereas their effect on mid-childhood growth is unclear.[279] DHEA has been suspected of having a number of other functions, but these seem inconsistent. Whether they differ from those of low-dose testosterone remains to be established.[280,281]

HORMONAL SECRETION, TRANSPORT, METABOLISM, AND ACTION

Peptide Hormones

Peptide hormones act after binding to specific receptors located in the plasma membranes of target cells. GnRH receptors and gonadotropin receptors are members of the 7-transmembrane receptor family. These receptors are necessary to the actions of their cognate hormones. However, receptors expressed in nonclassic sites are not necessarily functionally mature.[282] Mature receptors signal after coupling to the guanine nucleotide (G-protein) subunit cluster (Figure 14-22).[5,233,234,283,284] Two modes of signal transduction are then utilized. G proteins activate adenylate cyclase or phospholipase C. The first mode signals via phosphodiesterase-regulated cAMP levels to activate protein kinase A.

The second mode signals via protein kinase C and Ca^{2+}, the latter of which may be mobilized by other factors that influence ion channels. Tyrosine kinase signaling may also be involved in gonadotropin action.[285]

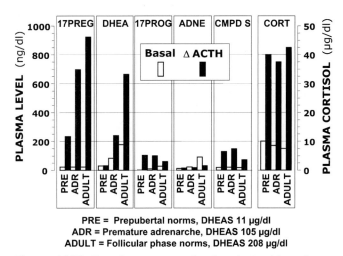

PRE = Prepubertal norms, DHEAS 11 µg/dl
ADR = Premature adrenarche, DHEAS 105 µg/dl
ADULT = Follicular phase norms, DHEAS 208 µg/dl

Figure 14-21 Changing pattern of adrenal steroidogenic response to adrenocorticotropic hormone with maturation. Shown are plasma steroid levels before (basal, 8:00 a.m. after dexamethasone 1 mg/m²) and the rise (Δ) 30 minutes after cosyntropin (ACTH) administration (10 µg/m²) in healthy prepubertal children, children with premature adrenarche as an isolated phenomenon, and follicular phase adult women. Note that 17-hydroxypregnenolone (17PREG) and dehydroepiandrosterone (DHEA) responses of children with premature adrenarche are intermediate between prepubertal and adult responses. 17PROG, 17-hydroxyprogesterone; ADIONE, androstenedione; CMPD S, 11-deoxycortisol; and DHEAS, DHEA sulfate. [Based on data from Rich BH, Rosenfield RL, Lucky AW, Helke JC, Otto P (1981). Adrenarche: Changing adrenal response to adrenocorticotropin. J Clin Endocrinol Metab 52:1129.]

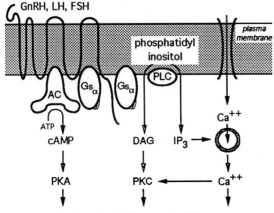

Figure 14-22 Overview of the pathways established to mediate gonadotropin-releasing hormone (GnRH) and gonadotropin action. The receptors for these hormones are members of the seven-transmembrane family of receptors. Hormone-receptor binding alters receptor configuration. One consequence is to couple the receptor to adenylate cyclase (AC) via the stimulatory α-subunit of G protein (GSα). This permits the efficient generation of cyclic adenosine monophosphate (cAMP) from adenosine triphosphate (ATP). Another consequence is to couple phospholipase C (PLC) to the receptor through another subtype of GS_. PLC is a phosphodiesterase that hydrolyzes phosphatidyl inositol to diacylglycerol (DAG) and inositol-1,4,5-triphosphate (IP3). DAG stimulates the calcium-sensitive protein kinase C (PKC). IP3 mobilizes ionic calcium (Ca_2_) from intracellular organelles and stimulates Ca_2_ influx through calcium ion channels. PKA, PKC, and Ca_2_ then bring about cellular responses through protein phosphorylations. FSH, follicle-stimulating hormone; and LH, luteinizing hormone.

Phosphorylation of various cytoplasmic and nuclear proteins is ultimately thought to mediate the action of the peptide hormones. The diversity among target cells in their responses to the action of protein kinases in part relates to diversity and type of kinase, intracellular compartmentalization, substrate availability, and other factors determined by the genome of the target cell.

Gonadotropin-releasing hormone is a decapeptide [pyro]Glu-His-Trp-Ser-Tyr-Gly-Leu-Arg-Pro-Gly-NH$_2$.[233] One gene encodes the single precursor protein for GnRH and prolactin release-inhibiting factor.[286] Gonadotropin-releasing hormone not only effects prompt release of preformed gonadotropins (the readily releasable pool) but stimulates the synthesis of gonadotropins (the reserve pool).[287] Repeated administration of GnRH augments the pituitary responsiveness to subsequent GnRH pulses (self-priming).[102] This has been ascribed partly to up-regulation of GnRH receptors. Gonadotropin-releasing hormone has important paradoxical effects. As discussed previously, it acutely stimulates gonadotropin secretion. However, upon protracted continuous administration it down-regulates pituitary gonadotropin secretion.

An evolutionarily conserved form of GnRH (GnRH-II) was recently discovered that acts primarily through the type 2 GnRH receptor.[288] GnRH-II and the type 2 GnRH receptor are products of unique genes, rather than being modified products of the GnRH or type 1 GnRH receptor genes.[289] The cell bodies of the GnRH-II neurons lie pre-

dominantly in the midbrain and only a minority project to the hypothalamic-pituitary area. Its function in humans is unknown, but it may be more important as a neurotransmitter involved in sexual behavior than in reproduction.

Luteinizing hormone and FSH are synthesized in a single type of cell, and both are sometimes identified within the same cell.[290] A vestigial population of hCG-secreting pituitary cells has been described.[291] Luteinizing hormone, FSH, and hCG are glycoprotein hormones that consist of two chains.[292] After synthesis of these hormones on the ribosomes, the carbohydrate moieties (which constitute about 16% of the weight) are added in the rough endoplasmic reticulum and golgi apparatus. The α chains of LH, FSH, hCG, and thyroid-stimulating hormone (TSH) are identical in amino acid sequence (92 amino acids).

Although the β chain of each hormone is different in both primary amino acid sequence and length, these β chains nevertheless share considerable amino acid homology (ranging from 30% to 80%). The α and β subunits contain a cystine knot structure like other growth factors such as platelet-derived growth factor and nerve growth factor. Biological activity is conferred when an α and β chain are glycosylated and assemble within the cell. The αβ dimer is stabilized by a β−subunit-derived "seatbelt" β-subunit-derived that wraps around the α subunit. Neither the isolated α nor the β glycosylated protein subunit exhibits biologic activity unless noncovalently bound in a heterodimer.

The gonadotropins exhibit considerable molecular heterogeneity. The major basis for this is variation in glycosylation, which confers differing degrees of in vitro and in vivo bioactivity.[95,293-295] Mutations in the LH-β and FSH-β subunits that affect gonadotropin bioactivity have also been described.[296] There are also reports of polymorphisms in amino acid sequence of the LH-β and hCG-β genes, which may affect the expression or bioactivity of LH or hCG.[297-299]

Different LH and FSH standards contain different proportions of immunoreactive material, which is of low bioactivity. The immunoreactive isoforms in the pituitary and serum also contain different proportions of bioactive material, and the isoform distribution differs with reproductive status. Androgens increase and estrogens decrease the apparent LH biopotency by altering LH sialylation.[300,301] The apparent FSH biopotency is reduced after treating women with GnRH antagonist.

One corollary of the molecular heterogeneity is that the antibodies generated from these gonadotropin moieties detect heterogeneous epitopes that are not necessarily bioactive. Indeed, some may even act as gonadotropin antagonists.[302] These factors combine to cause the B/I gonadotropin ratio to vary in a wide variety of circumstances.[95,293] The purest of standards, even recombinant ones, interact very differently in the diverse immunoassay systems. Likewise, the putative level of LH or FSH in a serum sample differs substantially among assays.

This is principally because of lack of specificity of immunoassays for bioactive LH and FSH. However, bioactivity assessments vary with the bioassay model system.[95,303] Monoclonal antibody-based immunometric assays yields results that correlate with but are not necessarily equivalent to those results derived by bioassay.[95,304] The best of these third-generation immunometric assays have the advantage of being more sensitive and specific for low levels of gonadotropins in serum than polyclonal-antiserum-based RIA, but B/I discrepancy remains considerable.

Luteinizing hormone is cleared more rapidly from the blood than FSH or hCG.[305,306] Luteinizing hormone disappears from blood in an exponential pattern. RIA indicates that the half-life of the initial component is about 20 minutes and the half-life of the second component about 4 hours (the bioactive LH half-life is about one-third shorter).[307] These respective components for FSH are 4 and 70 hours. Those for hCG are 11 and 23 hours. Gonadotropins are primarily metabolized by the liver after the removal of the terminal sialic acid residues, which retard clearance. About 10% to 15% of gonadotropins are excreted in urine.[308] Only about a third of this is in a biologically active form.[309] The metabolic clearance rate of LH is 35 L/day, and that of FSH is 20 L/day. Hormone production rates in follicular phase women, which approximate mid-pubertal values, are given in Table 14-2.[310-316] During the luteal phase of the menstrual cycle, estradiol production doubles[315] and progesterone production rises fifteenfold or more.[317]

Prolactin has structural and functional similarities to GH and placental lactogen. Prolactin has a considerable degree of structural heterogeneity. This results from genetic and post-translational events within pituitary cells as well as metabolic processes such as glycosylation in the periphery.[318] Lactotroph growth and prolactin secretion are stimulated by estrogens. Prolactin release from the anterior pituitary is primarily under the control of hypothalamic inhibition, probably mediated by dopamine[319] and prolactin release-inhibiting factor.[286] The latter is contained within the same precursor protein as GnRH, thus providing a potential mechanism for reciprocal control of these two peptides. Prolactin secretion is also inhibited by thyroxine and is directly responsive to thyrotropin-releasing hormone (TRH). Estrogen and suckling are stimulatory. These signals may be positively mediated by α-melanocyte-stimulating hormone.

Inhibins and activins are members of the TGF-β superfamily, and signal accordingly.[249,320] Inhibin was discovered as the result of the search for the nonsteroidal gonadal hormone capable of specifically suppressing FSH. Activin was serendipitously discovered as the FSH-stimulating activity in the side fractions in these studies. These hormones are formed by the differential disulfide-linked dimerization of two of three subunits (α β$_A$, and β$_B$), each encoded by a distinct gene. The combination of an α- and β-subunit yields inhibin-A (αβ$_A$) and inhibin-B (αβ$_B$). Activins are dimers of β-subunits β$_A$β$_A$, β$_B$β$_B$, and β$_A$β$_B$ (activin-A, -B, and -AB). Inhibin antagonizes all known actions of activin. The genes for all three subunits are differentially expressed in a wide variety of tissues. Furthermore, these factors (particularly activin) have proven to exert effects not only on gonadotropes but within other pituitary cells and the gonads and in nonsexual target tissues.

Steroid Hormones

The ovary and adrenal cortex share the core of the steroid biosynthesis pathway (Figure 14-23).[254,321] Low-density and high-density lipoproteins are used as steroidogenic substrates.[322] Most steroidogenic steps are mediated by cytochrome P450 family members, which are the terminal enzymes in electron transfer chains.[323] The initial step in the biosynthesis of all steroid hormones is the conversion of cholesterol to pregnenolone. This is a two-stage process. The rapidity of the process depends on the transport of cholesterol from the outer to the inner mitochondrial membrane by the steroidogenic acute regulatory protein (StAR). The conversion itself is carried out by the cholesterol side chain cleavage activity (scc) of cytochrome P450scc.

The next step is the Δ^5-isomerase-3β-hydroxysteroid dehydrogenase (3β-HSD) step or 17α-hydroxylation. The conversion of Δ^5-3β-hydroxysteroids to steroids with the Δ^4-3-keto configuration (e.g., pregnenolone to progesterone, 17-hydroxypregnenolone to 17-hydroxyprogesterone, or DHEA to androstenedione) is accomplished by 3β-HSD. This step is obligatory in the synthesis of all potent steroid hormones. The type 2 3β-HSD isozyme accounts for the vast majority of the 3β activity in the human ovary and adrenal. The type 1 isozyme accounts for 3β-HSD activity in liver and skin.[324]

Pregnenolone alternatively undergoes a two-step conversion to the 17-ketosteroid DHEA along the Δ^5-steroid pathway. This conversion is accomplished via cytochrome P450c17. P450c17 is a single enzyme with 17α-hydroxylase and 17, 20-lyase activities, the latter being of lesser efficient and critically dependent on electron transfer from P450 oxido-reductase (POR) activity and cytochrome b. Progesterone undergoes a parallel transformation to androstenedione

TABLE 14-2

Average Hormone Blood Production Rates in Mid-follicular Phase Women[a]

Hormone	Production Rate	Pertinent References
Luteinizing hormone	615 IU/day[†]	310
Follicle-stimulating hormone	215 IU/day[†]	311
Androstenedione	3.4 mg/day	312
Dehydroepiandrosterone	7.0 mg/day	312
Dehydroepiandrosterone sulfate	7.0 mg/day[‡]	313, 314
Dihydrotestosterone	0.06 mg/day	312
Estradiol	0.1 mg/day	315
Estrone	0.1 mg/day	315
Progesterone	1.1 mg/day	316
17-OH-progesterone	1.2 mg/day	316
Testosterone	0.2 mg/day	312

[a]These production rates are roughly equivalent to those in mid-puberty. The average daily production of those hormones that fluctuate cyclically is substantially greater. For example, E$_2$ production transiently peaks to about 0.5 mg/day, and thus the average production over the monthly cycle is about 0.2 mg/day or 6 mg/mo.

[†] In terms of second International Reference Preparation, human menopausal gonadotropin.

[‡] Approximate urinary production rate, expressed as unconjugated dehydroepiandrosterone.

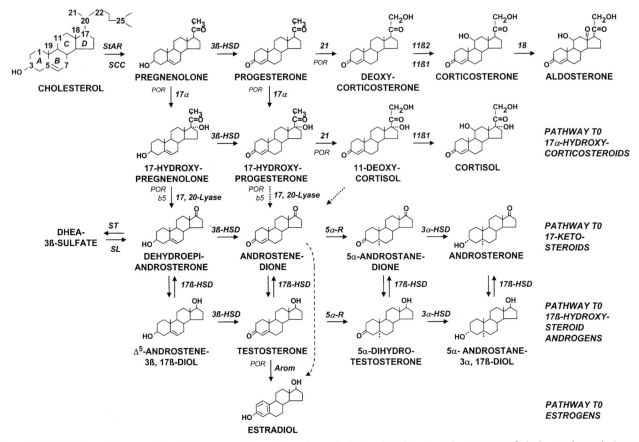

Figure 14-23 Major pathways of steroid hormone biosynthesis from cholesterol. Relevant carbon atoms of cholesterol are designated by conventional numbers. Rings are denoted by letters. The flow of hormonogenesis is generally downward and to the right. The top line shows the pathway to progestins and mineralocorticoids, the second line the pathway to glucocorticoids, the third line the pathway to 17-ketosteroids, and the fourth line to androgens. The bottom and dotted lines indicate the pathways to estrogen [the long dotted line involves the 17-keto-estrogen estrone (not shown) as an intermediate]. The steroidogenic enzymes are italicized. Cytochrome P450 enzyme steps are: side-chain cleavage (scc); 17α-hydroxylase/17,20-lyase; 21 hydroxylase (21); 11β-hydroxylase (11β2); 18-hydroxylase-dehydrogenase (aldosterone synthase, 11β1,18); and aromatase (arom). Non-P450 enzyme steps are steroidogenic acute regulatory protein (StAR); Δ5-isomerase-3β-hydroxysteroid dehydrogenase (3β); 17β-hydroxysteroid dehydrogenase (17β); sulfotransferase (ST), and sulfokinase (SK). Clinically relevant electron transfer enzymes are P450 oxidoreductase (POR) and cytochrome b5 (b5). [Modified from Rosenfield RL, Lucky AW, Allen TD (1980). The diagnosis and management of intersex. Curr Prob in Pediatr 10:1.]

in the Δ4-steroid path. 17α-hydroxylation of progesterone by P450c17 forms 17-hydroxyprogesterone, but in humans P450c17 does not efficiently utilize 17-hydroxyprogesterone as a substrate for 17,20-lyase activity and thus P450c17 seems to form little if any androstenedione.

There is some evidence for the existence of a P450c17-independent Δ4-pathway to androstenedione, but most seems to be formed from DHEA by the action of 3β-HSD.[325] The conversion of 17-ketosteroids to 17β-hydroxysteroids by 17β-HSD is essential to the formation of the potent sex steroids, testosterone, dihydrotestosterone, and estradiol. In the ovary, androstenedione is the major precursor for sex steroids. Testosterone is formed by 17β-HSD type 5[326] and estradiol by aromatase. Cytochrome P450arom carries out aromatase activity.[327] Alternate promoters are utilized by the P450arom gene in the gonads, placenta, and adipose tissue—which yields alternatively spliced forms of aromatase.

The ovary normally accounts for about 25% of testosterone secretion in the mature female (0.06 mg daily), but it secretes about 30 times as much androstenedione

(1.6 mg daily).[312] These amounts are similar to those secreted by the adrenal. However, the ovary secretes less than 10% as much DHEA as the adrenal. The "production rate" of a hormone equals its secretion rate plus (in the case of hormones formed outside of endocrine glands) the rate of formation of the hormone by peripheral conversion of secreted precursors. The "blood production rate" is calculated as metabolic clearance rate (MCR) multiplied by plasma concentration. This is because in the steady state the amount of hormone irreversibly leaving the plasma compartment equals the amount entering it.

Because of extensive steroid interconversions, the quantity of these hormones excreted in urine is not necessarily proportional to the amount reaching target tissues.[312] For example, so large a fraction of urinary testosterone glucuronide is formed directly from androstenedione by compartmentalized metabolism within the liver that the range of urinary excretion of testosterone in women overlaps that in men (Figure 14-24).[328] Estrone sulfate, like DHEAS in the androgen pathway, forms a circulating reservoir of inactive estrogen that can be returned to the active pool by

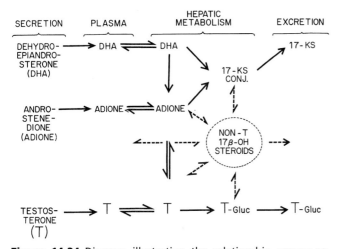

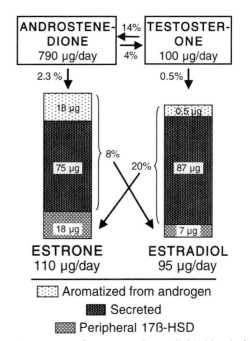

Figure 14-24 Diagram illustrating the relationship among secreted, plasma, and urinary steroids. 17-ketosteroid (17-KS) excretion does not reflect accurately the excretion of the most important plasma androgens. Only 25% or less of testosterone is excreted as 17-KS metabolites. Therefore, important changes in testosterone production may not appreciably affect urinary 7-KS excretion. Futhermore, even the major 17-KS (the sulfate of DHA) is excreted poorly until its production rate becomes quite high. On the other hand, about 50% of the Zimmermann chromogens are not identifiable as 17-KS, and 2 mg daily results from hydrocortisone metabolism. In additon, 17-KS metabolism differs in the child and adult. Testosterone glucuronide excretion does not accurately reflect the plasma testosterone level. Less than 2% of testosterone appears in the urine as such. In addition, plasma 17-KS (such as androstenedione) may be converted to testosterone glucuronide without ever circulating as unconjugated testosterone. [From Rosenfield RL (1973). Relationship of androgens to female hirsutism and infertility. J Reprod Med 11:87.]

Figure 14-25 Sources of estrone and estradiol in blood of follicular phase premenopausal women. Estrogen is derived from direct secretion by the gonad, aromatization of androgen, or conversion of an estrogen precursor by 17ß-HSD activities. The percentage of substrate converted per day and total approximate production in micrograms per day are noted for each source. [Modified from Alonso LC and Rosenfield RL (2002). Oestrogens and puberty. Best Pract Res Clin Endocrinol Metab 16:13.]

desulfation in the liver.[329] The blood production rates of representative steroid hormones are given in Table 14-2 and are shown for estrogens in Figure 14-25.

Sex hormones also have environmental origins. Natural biologic estrogens include equine estrogens and plant-derived phytoestrogens. Synthetic estrogens include pharmacologic compounds such as ethinyl estradiol, diethylstilbestrol, selective estrogen receptor modulators (SERMs), and some industrial chemicals such as organochlorines and plasticizers. Environmental estrogens act as "endocrine disrupters" by activating diverse estrogenic pathways in animal models.[329]

Peripheral conversion of secreted prehormones by non-endocrine organs accounts for a major portion of sex hormone production. The ovary and the adrenal cortex are the sources of prehormones as well as secreted hormones. About 50% of plasma testosterone (0.1 mg daily) is normally formed indirectly by peripheral conversion. Although 85% of normal estrogen production in women arises by secretion in midcycle, 50% of estrogen production can arise from extraglandular sources during the low-estrogen phases of the menstrual cycle.[330] Peripheral formation of active steroids occurs in a wide number of sites, including liver, fat, and target organs.[254,331] For example, the liver has high levels of 3α-, 3β-, and 17β-hydroxysteroid dehydrogenase and 5α-reductase activities (Figure 14-23).

Peripheral steroid metabolism is not tightly regulated. It seems determined to some extent by the perinatal an-

drogenic milieu,[332] the effect of which is possibly mediated by GH.[333] Postnatally it is influenced by the sex hormone binding globulin level (SHBG) and the state of nutrition. Adipose tissue becomes a major site of conversion of androstenedione to estrone and testosterone in the obese.[334] Cytochrome P450 mixed-function oxidases, some of which are inducible by drugs or nutritional status, form hydroxylated steroid metabolites of varying potency.[335] Phytoestrogens increase estradiol bioavailability by inhibiting hepatic sulfotransferase.[336]

Plasma steroids mainly reach their sites of action and metabolism by simple diffusion from the vascular compartment.[337] The bioactive portion of plasma testosterone seems to be the free testosterone and a portion of the albumin-bound testosterone that differs among tissues according to characteristics of the vascular bed.[338,339] About 98% of plasma testosterone and estradiol are bound to albumin and SHBG. The SHBG concentration determines the fraction of plasma testosterone and other ligands that are free or bound to albumin. It is also a major determinant of ligand egress from plasma (Figure 14-26).[340] Recent data indicate that the SHBG may exert independent effects.[341] For example, the SHBG-bound sex steroid complex may stimulate growth after SHBG binding to membrane receptors and activation of adenylate cyclase.[342] A number of physiologic and pathologic states affect the SHBG level. It is increased by estrogen and thyroid hormone excess. It is decreased by androgen, insulin, glucocorticoid, and GH.[339,343]

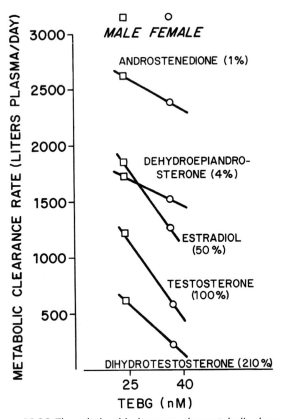

Figure 14-26 The relationship between the metabolic clearance rate (MCR) and binding of sex hormones to sex hormone binding globulin (TEBG). The MCR of each steroid has been related to the mean TEBG levels of men and women. The approximate affinity of each steroid for TEBG relative to testosterone is indicated in parentheses. [From Rosenfield RL (1975). Studies of the relation of plasma androgen levels to androgen action in women. J Steroid Biochem 6:695.]

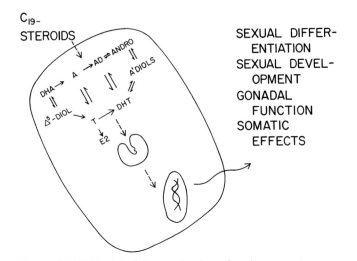

Figure 14-27 Model of the mechanism of androgen action emphasizing the effect of steroid metabolism within a target cell on the mode of action. Solid arrows indicate pathways of steroid metabolism from 17-ketosteroid precursors as laid out in Figure 14-23. Broken arrow indicates transport. The cell-specific intracellular pattern of C19-steroid metabolism determines the relative availability of testosterone or dihydrotestosterone (DHT) to the cytosol receptor for translocation to the nucleus. In cells such as the rat granulosa cell in which $\Delta^5,3\beta$-hydroxysteroid dehydrogenase activity is high, androstenediol (Δ^5-diol) is as potent as testosterone. The human sebaceous gland has a similar pattern of steroid metabolism. A, androstenedione; AD, androstanedione; and DHA, dehydroepiandrosterone. [From Nimrod A, Rosenfield, RL, Otto P (1980). Relationship of androgen action to androgen metabolism in isolated rat granulosa cells. J Steroid Biochem 13:1015, with permission from Elsevier Science.]

Target cell metabolism influences the cell's response to the steroid hormones that reach it (Figure 14-27).[344] Although transformation is not fundamental to the mode of action of estradiol, estradiol effectiveness can be influenced by target cell metabolism. The induction of 17β-hydroxysteroid oxidation in target tissues by progesterone, resulting in conversion of estradiol to the less potent estrogen estrone, counterbalances estrogenization.[345] The intracellular conversion of testosterone to dihydrotestosterone by one of the two isozymes of 5α reductase is important to many but not all effects of testosterone,[346] dependent on the tissue-specific pattern of steroid metabolism. An important mode of testosterone action is via estradiol, notably within the brain. There is also evidence that novel steroid metabolites exert tissue-specific effects.[347,348]

Within target cells, all steroid hormones activate the genome similarly—starting with binding to high-affinity intracellular receptors (Figure 14-28).[349,350] The steroid hormone receptors belong to the superfamily of nuclear hormone receptors. The estrogen, progesterone, and androgen receptors are thus homologous. Classic sex hormone effects are exerted by the interaction of steroid with receptor, not by either alone. Steroid binding triggers the dissociation of inhibitory chaperone heat shock proteins from the receptor.[351] The active receptor-ligand

complex then undergoes noncovalent dimerization and binding to its specific hormone response element on the gene. The DNA-bound steroid-receptor complex acts as a transcriptional regulator of the target gene promoter. Sensitivity to steroids is also modulated by molecular chaperone proteins that influence receptor configuration, intracellular trafficking, and receptor turnover—all of which are determinants of steroid action.[352,353]

The binding properties of steroids to their cognate receptors are the initial determinants of steroid action (Figure 14-28).[349,350] Ligand-based selectivity is one element of this interaction. Estradiol is a more potent estrogen than estrone and estriol partly because it binds best to the steroid-binding domain of the estrogen receptor.[354] Dihydrotestosterone is an inherently more potent androgen than testosterone, mainly because of its higher association rate constant and its lower dissociation rate constant.[355]

The antiestrogens tamoxifen and clomiphene and the antiandrogens cyproterone acetate and spironolactone competitively inhibit the active ligands from binding to their specific receptor sites by weakly and transiently occupying receptor sites. These differences result from potent agonists fitting into the binding pocket more snugly, which induces a receptor conformation different from that of antagonist-bound receptor. One such change is the C-terminal tail of the receptor flipping over to "close the door" when a potent agonist enters. This simultaneously provides a different outer surface for interaction with co-regulator proteins.

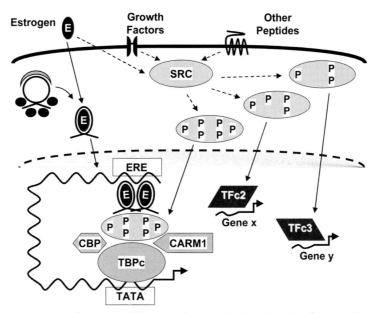

Figure 14-28 A model for the mechanism of estrogen (E) action that emphasizes the role of interaction of the estrogen receptor with co-regulators and other signaling pathways. Estrogen causes the 4S subunit and heat-shock proteins to dissociate from the unliganded estrogen receptor. Then estrogen entry into the binding pocket causes a conformational change in the receptor. Estrogen also stimulates steroid receptor coactivator (SRC) phosphorylation (P) in a specific pattern and recruits it to the nuclear DNA steroid-receptor complex with the estrogen response element (ERE). SRC in turn recruits other coactivators [such as the dual-function cAMP response element binding protein-binding protein (CBP) and coactivator-associated methyltransferase (CARM1)] to the hormone binding complex. This aggregate then interacts with the TATA binding protein initiation complex (TBPc) to initiate estrogen-specific gene transcription. The effect is modified by the effects of environmental signals on other cell-specific transcription factors (TF), some of which involve differentially phosphylated SRC complexes (TFc) in gene activation. Fine dotted lines indicate diverse kinase pathways. ER recycling is not shown. [Modified from Katzenellenbogen BS, Montano MM, Ediger TR, Sun J, Ekena K, Lazennec G, et al. (2000). Estrogen receptors: Selective ligands, partners, and distinctive pharmacology. Recent Prog Horm Res 55:163–193; and from O'Malley BW (2005). A life-long search for the molecular pathways of steroid hormone action. Mol Endocrinol 19:1402–1411.]

Thus, ligand-based selectivity arises not only because of tighter ligand binding but because alternative ligands produce intermediate and unique conformational changes in the receptor—which in turn induce altered receptor interactions with co-regulator proteins that result in a spectrum of activities.[356] Thus, steroids do not simply switch receptors on. They induce selective functions that depend on the nature of the co-regulators that are recruited to the complex.[357-360] In part, this selectivity arises because different domains of these receptors mediate these different functions. For example, the AF-1 domain of the ER mediates interactions with MAP kinase and TGF-β3—whereas the AF-2 domain mediates interactions with co-regulator proteins.[361] Coactivators in turn regulate alternative splicing, gene activation and repression (in some cases via their dual enzymatic functions), and ubiquitin-proteosome-mediated turnover of the receptor-coregulator complex.[362] They also determine cell-specific site-based actions,[350] as discussed in material following.

Receptor-based selectivity is a second element in steroid action. There are now known to be two isoforms of each of the sex steroid receptors. The α and β forms of the estrogen receptor, though homologous, are coded by separate genes.[156] A and B forms of the progesterone and androgen receptors exist.[363,364] These forms of the PR arise by transcription from alternative promoters within the same gene, whereas those of the androgen receptor arise from post-translational modification of a single mRNA. These isoforms have variously been shown to manifest a differential tissue expression pattern and respond differentially to antagonists. Interactions of a steroid with different forms of receptor can regulate some target genes differentially.

One role of ERβ is apparently to modulate ERα activity. ERα and ERβ can have opposite actions at AP-1 and SP-1 sites, and studies of transcriptional activity in bone and breast tissue of mice indicate a restraining effect of ERβ on responses to estradiol.[156,365] Thus, different target tissues exposed to the same hormone may respond selectively because of a distinct repertoire of receptor isoform expression. Some examples are notable. Although both forms of estrogen receptor are expressed in most target tissues, the classic form of the estradiol receptor (ERα) plays the key role in regulation of LH and estrogen actions on the uterus, breasts, sex-specific behavior, and bone.[156,243,366,367]

In the mouse ovary, knockout experiments show that ERα is expressed in thecal cells—where it prevents androgen excess in response to LH. In contrast, ERβ is expressed only in granulosa cells—where its inhibition of androgen receptor expression is critical in preventing premature follicular atresia.[158] Both forms of the receptor are necessary to oocyte survival and the ability of preovulatory follicles to rupture. Furthermore, loss of both causes transdifferentiation of granulosa cells to Sertoli-like cells and massive oocyte death.[146] Liganded progesterone receptor$_A$ is essential to ovulation[368] and is the more effective antagonist of estrogen receptor action.[349] In addition, sequence variation in hormone response elements contributes to differential gene regulation.[369]

Effector-site-based selectivity is a third variable in sex hormone action. In other words, the potency and character of a response to a ligand-receptor complex is not simply an inherent property of the complex. Rather, they depend on the array of effector molecules present in the site of action. Thus, the array of genes expressed locally and the relative expression level of co-regulators (coactivators and co-repressors) are extremely important in the determination of appropriate and graded responses to a ligand by a target cell.[349,370] Heterodimerization of the estrogen receptor with other nuclear receptors can modulate its action.[371] Androgens appear to exert some of their genomic effects by directly complexing with transcription factors other than the androgen receptor.[372] Estrogen and androgen appear to exert antiapoptotic effects in osteoblasts and osteocytes by activating a ligand-dependent but nongenomic kinase-mediated signaling pathway.[373]

Nuclear receptor coactivators are critical in sensing cell-specific environmental signals and to coordinate signals emanating from membrane receptors with nuclear receptor action.[350] Surface receptors send signals through kinase pathways that result in specific serine/threonine phosphorylation patterns of coactivators. These phosphorylation patterns serve as a code for the coactivator to preferentially bind and activate distinct sets of downstream transcription factors (Figure 14-28). Overexpression of steroid receptor coactivator-3 (SRC-3) is as important in the pathogenesis of some breast cancers as is estrogen receptor positivity.

The effects of a given ligand-ER complex often differ from those of the E2-ER complex among cell types. This is the basis for the development of SERMs. These compounds mediate variable effects in a tissue-specific manner, depending on the cell context.[349,356] The chemical structure of a SERM (or any ER ligand, for that matter) determines the configuration of the ER, resulting in a spectrum of activities from agonist to antagonist—depending on which co-regulators are available for recruitment in the target cell. Raloxifene is an estradiol agonist in bone and epiphyseal cartilage but is antiestrogenic in uterus and breast. Tamoxifen is estrogenic in uterus but antiestrogenic in breast and bone. Both appear to retain neural and endothelial estrogenic activity.[374,375]

Sex steroid receptor responsiveness can also be altered by signals emanating from the cell membrane.[376] In some cases, activation occurs independently of ligand binding.[377] For example, epidermal growth factor activates phosphorylation of the estrogen receptor and simulates diverse estrogen effects.[378] In addition, various cell surface signals activate unliganded estrogen receptor and cause it to act as a co-regulator.[379] This may be involved in the mechanism by which ERα represses expression of the androgenic 17β-HSD testicular isoform in the ovary.[243]

Sex steroids also exert rapid (within seconds to minutes) nongenomic effects by membrane signaling in a variety of cells. These can mediate cell proliferation, apoptosis, migration in cell-specific ways. E2 nongenomic actions can be mediated by binding to nuclear ER in plasma membrane domains provided by such scaffolding proteins as caveolin.[373,380,381] On such platforms, the E2-ER complex acts like a membrane receptor—coupling with G proteins and activating cytoplasmic pathways involving SRC and MAP kinase. Androgens appear to act similarly.[373,382,383] Nongenomic actions of nuclear PR have been reported.[384] Signaling also has recently been identified via specific G-protein coupled transmembrane receptors for E2 and progesterone.[385,385a]

Steroids that act by binding to membrane-bound receptors in the brain are termed *neuroactive*.[277] Neuroactive steroids synthesized in the brain are termed *neurosteroids*.[386-388] The best documented of these effects are on neurotransmitters that control ion channels. Allopregnanolone (3α-hydroxy-5α-tetrahydroprogesterone) is an inhibitor of the GABA$_A$ receptor and thus has sedative properties. Pregnenolone sulfate and DHEAS have the opposite effect, being GABA$_A$ receptor agonists. The former is also a positive regulator of the NMDA receptor. Receptors for 5-hydroxytryptamine have been implicated in mediating some of effects of sex steroids and certain of their metabolites.[389,390] Some estrogen effects in brain are membrane mediated.[391]

The tissue-specific post-transcriptional events involved in sex steroid signaling are poorly understood. Estradiol and progesterone modulate the actions of each other through effects on their specific receptors. Increased estrogens in the preovulatory phase of the cycle induce target organ receptors for estradiol and progesterone. Luteal phase levels of progesterone then suppress the production of both receptors.[392,393] However, estrogen prevents bone loss by blocking the production of proinflammatory cytokines.[394] Androgen action seems to involve the arachidonic acid cascade in genitalia[395] and peroxisome proliferator-activated receptors in sebaceous cells,[396] whereas in epiphyseal cartilage testosterone stimulates the IGF-I system.[397]

MATURATION OF SEX HORMONE TARGET ORGANS

Genital Tract

The Müllerian system of the embryo gives rise to the uterus, cervix, upper vagina, and fallopian tubes in the absence of AMH secretion by fetal testes during the first trimester of gestation.[321] Diethylstilbestrol induces dysplasia of the genital tracts.[398] Estrogen receptors are expressed in the labia minora, prepuce, and glans in females, but not in the homologous structures of males.[399] Genital swelling develops to engulf the base of the penis-like clitoris between 11 and 20 weeks gestation in parallel with the development of the ovarian follicular system.[400] In addition, antiestrogen has been reported to cause genital ambiguity.[401] These data suggest that estrogen may play a direct role in female genital tract differentiation. However, knockout of estrogen receptors has no obvious effect on genital tract differentiation.[146]

The infantile uterus and cervix enlarge under the influence of estrogen during puberty. The endometrium and cervical glands then undergo cyclic changes in concert with cyclic ovarian function. In response to estrogen during the follicular phase of the cycle, the endometrial epithelium and stroma proliferate. The uterine glands increase in number and lengthen.

Endometrial hyperplasia is inhibited by hyperandrogenemia.[402] In response to progesterone secretion after ovulation, the endometrium increases in thickness. Stromal edema occurs, and the uterine glands enlarge, become sacculated, and secrete a glycogen-rich mucoid fluid. The coiled arteries lengthen further during this time and become increasingly spiral. These changes are critical to implantation. Antiprogestin therapy is an effective postcoital contraceptive.[403] High-dose progestin is effective in preventing implantation if taken within 3 days of unprotected intercourse.[404]

The major cyclic change in the cervix is in the secretion of the endocervical glands, which lubricate the vaginal vault. The endocervical mucus is scanty and relatively thin during the low-estrogen phase of the cycle. The increase in mucus flow with advancing follicular development seems to require tissue-specific stimulation of the cystic fibrosis transmembrane regulator by estrogen.[405] This mucus becomes more viscous and elastic as estrogens rise in the later follicular phase of the cycle. The extent to which it can be stretched into a long spindle (spinnbarkeit) is a function of the estrogen level.

The mucosa of the vagina and the urogenital tract consists of hormone-responsive stratified squamous epithelium (Figure 14-29).[2] The basal layer is the regenerative area. In the absence of estrogen, there is only a parabasal layer of cells over this—and the vagina is thin, with a tendency to alkalinity [which predisposes it to local infection (nonspecific vaginitis)].[406] In response to estrogen, epithelial proliferation occurs—with formation of successive intermediate and superficial layers. With this maturation, the cytoplasm of each cell first expands—leading to formation of small intermediate cells. With further estrogenization, the nuclei become pyknotic and large intermediate cells form.

Greater estrogenization brings about their transformation to superficial cells. The cytoplasm changes from basophilic to acidophilic with the accumulation of glycogen. Resistance to infection of the fully developed vaginal mucosa results from its thickness and from its acid pH, which occurs from the fermentation of the glycogen of the superficial cells. In response to luteal phase progesterone, degenerative changes appear in vaginal mucosal cells: superficial cells decrease, the cytoplasm assumes a "crinkled" appearance, cells degenerate, and bacterial proliferation increases.

Vaginal smears show the characteristic cyclic changes in the cell types comprising the vaginal epithelium (Figure 14-29).[407] In the prepubertal years, parabasal cells predominate—and characteristically 10% or less are small intermediate cells. A pattern consisting entirely of intermediate cells is typical of early puberty. The early follicular phase of the menstrual cycle is characterized by the predominance of large intermediate cells with few, if any, superficial cells. Peak maturation is reached at midcycle, at which time 35% to 85% of the cells seen on vaginal smear are superficial. The remainder are large intermediate cells. This cornification develops over a 1-week period in response to estradiol levels of about 70 pg/mL and persists 1 to 2 weeks after estrogen withdrawal (Figure 14-11).[408] Many normal variations have been recognized in the appearance of the hymen. The transverse diameter increases with age.[409,410]

Mammary Glands

Multiple rudimentary branching mammary ducts are found beneath the nipple in infancy. They grow and branch very slowly during the prepubertal years.[411] Estrogen stimulates the nipples to grow, mammary terminal duct branching to progress to the stage at which ductules are formed, and fatty stromal growth to increase until it constitutes about 85% of the mass of the breast. GH (via IGF-I) and glucocorticoids play a permissive role.[412, 413]

These hormones interact with breast stroma and local growth factors to stimulate the development of breast epithelium. Lobulation appears around menarche, when multiple blind saccular buds form by branching of the terminal ducts. These effects are presumably due to the presence of progesterone. The breast stroma swells cyclically during each luteal phase. Full alveolar development normally only occurs during pregnancy under the influence of additional progesterone and prolactin. Prolactin does not play a role in breast growth without priming by female hormones.[414]

Estrogen and progesterone also play a role in breast cancer susceptibility. The BRCA1 gene normally restrains mammary growth (at least in part) by inhibiting expression of ERα and PRs, and cancer-related mutations reverse these processes.[415]

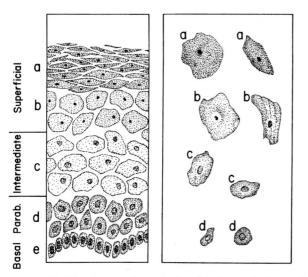

Figure 14-29 The layers of vaginal epithelium of the well-estrogenized adult. The superficial layer contains surface cells that are cornified (squamous) with eosinophilic cytoplasm and pyknotic nuclei (a) as well as large intraepithelial cells that are also karyopyknotic but basophilic (b). The intermediate zone contains basophilic cells that have less cytoplasm and intermediate-size nuclei (c). The basal and parabasal cells have a relatively small amount of basophilic cytoplasm and relatively vesicular nuclei (d, e). [Redrawn from Wilkins L (1968). *The diagnosis and treatment of endocrine disorders in childhood and adolescence.* Springfield, IL: Charles C Thomas.]

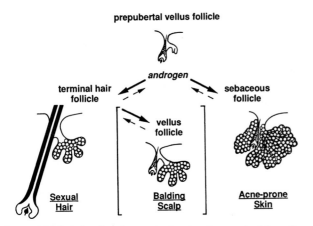

Figure 14-30 Role of androgen in the development of the pilosebaceous unit. Androgens (solid lines) are responsible for the patterned differentiation of the pilosebaceous unit at puberty. Dotted lines indicate effects of antiandrogens. Hairs are depicted only in the anagen (growing) phase of the growth cycle. In balding scalp (bracketed area), terminal hairs not previously dependent on androgen regress to vellus hairs under the influence of androgen. [From Rosenfield RL, Deplewski D (1994). Role of androgens in the developmental biology of the pilosebaceous unit. Am J Med 97(5A):80.]

Pilosebaceous Unit

The pilosebaceous unit (PSU) with but few exceptions consists of a piliary and a sebaceous component.[416] Androgens are a prerequisite for the growth and development of PSUs in their characteristic pattern. Before puberty, the androgen-dependent PSU consists of a prepubertal vellus follicle in which the hair and sebaceous gland components are virtually invisible to the naked eye (Figure 14-30). Under the influence of androgens, in the sexual hair areas the PSU switches to producing a type of terminal hair follicle. This androgen effect seems to be mediated via its action on the dermal papilla.

The difference in the apparent density of sexual hair between men and women is due to differences in the density of fully terminal hairs. In acne-prone areas, androgen causes the prepubertal vellus follicle to develop into a sebaceous follicle. In the balding-prone area of scalp in individuals genetically predisposed to pattern alopecia, PSUs respond to androgen by changing to a mature vellus follicle. Adrenarchal levels of androgens suffice to successively initiate sebaceous gland development and the growth of pubic hair. Progressively greater amounts of androgen are in general required to stimulate terminal hair development along a pubic to cranial gradient. All of these effects of androgen are reversible by antiandrogens.

Estrogens have a modest stimulating effect on hair growth. This may well be due to induction of androgen receptors by estrogen. They are also direct inhibitors of sebum secretion. GH synergizes with androgen action on the PSU, possibly by acting through insulin-like growth factor-I. Retinoic acid receptor agonists antagonize the effects of androgen on the sebaceous gland. To a great extent, this is due to inhibition of sebocyte proliferation and differentiation. Prolactin, glucocorticoids, thyroxine, and catecholamines also play roles in PSU growth, development, and function.

Bone

Increased secretion of sex hormones clearly initiates the pubertal growth spurt. About half of this effect of sex hormones is due to their stimulation of the GH-IGF axis.[417] The remainder of the effects of sex steroids on growth are direct.[418,419] Differences between the actions of sex hormones contribute to women's bones being shorter and narrower than men's.[420,421] The bases for these differences are complex and only beginning to emerge, with studies showing diverse effects on cortical and cancellous bone and periosteal bone formation.

Estrogen and androgen both stimulate epiphyseal growth. However, estradiol is the critical hormone that brings about epiphyseal closure.[419] Estrogen is also particularly effective in reducing bone turnover. To some extent, these effects may be prenatally programmed.[422] Bone accrual during puberty is a major determinant of adult fracture risk. Menarche after 15 years carries a 1.5-fold increase in fracture risk, and the risk rises with age of menarche.[423]

Adipose Tissue

Women have a greater percentage of body fat than men.[210,424] Serum levels of the adipocyte hormone leptin rise throughout puberty to reach higher levels in females than in males. Women have both more and larger fat cells than men in the lower body. Adipose tissue from different body sites has different metabolic activities and responses to sex steroids, with androgens generally promoting lipolysis and upper body (visceral) fat accumulation and estrogen promoting lipogenesis and a lower body (gluteofemoral) fat distribution.[425-427] In addition, androgens lower the antilipolytic adipocytokine adiponectin.[428] The lipolytic effect of androgenic progestins in contraceptives appears to account for their induction of insulin resistance.[429] Paradoxically, estrogen deficiency underlies the increased fat stores of hypogonadism.[156]

Central Nervous System

Considerable evidence supports the possibility that sex hormone exposure prenatally or during the period of transient activation of the hypothalamic-pituitary-gonadal axis of the neonate organizes neural substrates in a sexually dimorphic manner that predisposes to sex-typical behavior or function to become manifest when the child is exposed to the sex-specific pubertal hormonal milieu.[430] However, other factors (biologic, social, and psychological) seem equally important determinants of gender-related aspects of human behavior.[431,432]

Several human brain structures are sexually dimorphic, some becoming so at puberty.[432-434] In lower species, sexually dimorphic nuclei develop only if the brain is exposed to androgen during a critical time in the newborn period—but not if the androgen exposure is too late or too little. For example, in rats the preoptic nucleus of the hypothalamus is larger in males due to prevention of apoptosis in a site-specific fashion—and treatment of newborn females with testosterone or estradiol permanently increases neuronal development and causes subsequent masculinized sexual behavior and anovulation.[14,434]

This and many other such effects appear to be mediated by intraneuronal aromatization of testosterone to estradiol in a manner that is regulated in site-specific fashion by androgen and estrogen.[435, 436] Thus, it has been postulated that low levels of estradiol promote the development of the brain. Greater amounts, as males normally form from secreted testosterone in neurons containing androgen receptors, masculinize it. Estrogen receptor-α knockout in female mice reduces sexual behavior and parental behavior while increasing aggressiveness.[437] On the other hand, some masculinizing effects of testosterone on behavior are androgen specific.[438]

Androgen has been shown to up-regulate brain 5α-reductase and aromatase only in the perinatal period.[439,440] There is also sexual dimorphism in cerebral progestin receptors, and progesterone attenuates the testosterone effect on the brain and reduces the number of estrogen receptors in the cerebral cortex.[441,442]

Sex hormones also have diverse effects on those areas of the adult brain that exhibit apoptosis-mediated morphologic plasticity in synaptic patterns and are involved in reproductive behavior and function and nonreproductive functions such as memory and learning. Estrogen, for example, alters the pattern of synaptic connections in spatially specific and precise patterns, that appear to fine-tune the sensitivity of certain regions of the brain to excitatory and inhibitory aminoacids.[443, 444] Hypothalamic changes in synaptic remodeling have been correlated with the preovulatory surge of GnRH. Androgen stimulation of androgen receptor levels and nuclear size of sexually dimorphic hypothalamic areas of the brain have been shown to occur in adult animals.[445,446]

On average, women tend to perform better than men on tasks that involve verbal skills, processing speed and accuracy, and fine-motor skills—whereas men tend to excel in visual-spatial memory and mathematical ability. The sexes do not differ in vocabulary skills.[430,447,448] These differences are quantitatively modest, of the order of 0.4 to 1.0 standard deviations. The male advantage in visual-spatial skills is established by 4.5 years of age. Because both boys and girls who are congenitally sex hormone deficient are relatively poor in visual-spatial abilities, and sex hormone treatment at puberty does not ameliorate these deficits, this difference seems to be the result of estrogen-mediated patterning in both sexes.

A wide variety of sexual behaviors are found in young children, but normally they have a different character than in adults.[449] Gender identity is established by 3 years of age, and sexual orientation is established by 10 years of age.[432,450] The extent to which this is dependent on subclinical adrenarcheal or pubertal changes is unknown. Early pubertal amounts of androgen or estrogen have little effect on sexual behavior but increase some aspects of aggressive behavior.[451,452] Only later in puberty is there activation of the sex drive, which has been organized in early development.

A male level of androgen acting through the androgen receptor pre- or perinatally seems to be an important determinant of male gender role behavior and mildly disruptive to female gender identity.[431,432] Differences in the size of specific brain structures in men with gender identity disorders has raised the possibility that these disorders similarly have a biologic basis. In homosexuals, the human homologue of the rat preoptic nucleus is smaller (as in females)[453] and the anterior commissure is larger than that of men or women.[454] In male-to-female transsexuals, a nucleus within the stria terminalis is female-sized.[455] Male homosexuals have a pattern of nuclear activation in response to pheromone-like chemosignals (like heterosexual women) rather than like heterosexual men, and homosexual women have an intermediate type of activation.[456]

Androgen and estrogen metabolites in sweat and urine have been found to exert sexually dimorphic activation of the anterior hypothalamus that is independent of their odor.[456] Therefore, they have been postulated to act as pheromone-equivalent chemosignals. It is likely that a dedicated population of olfactory receptors act as pheromone receptors that project to GnRH neurons.[457]

Other Targets of Sex Hormone Action

It is now clear that sex hormones exert effects in a wide variety of tissues. Estrogen down-regulates blood levels of the inflammatory cytokine interleukin-6.[458] Estrogens and progestins also exert hemostatic effects associated with increased resistance to the anticoagulant action of activated protein C.[459]

The cardiovascular effects of estrogen include up-regulation of estrogen and progesterone receptors in vascular tissue and nongenomic effects on endothelial nitric oxide synthase.[460] Although estrogen is generally cardioprotective and the disturbed endothelial dysfunction of young hypogonadal women is improved by estrogen, unexpected risks of conjugated estrogen use with and without medroxyprogesterone have recently emerged in postmenopausal women.[461] Whether or not these risks translate into risks in premenopausal females or to other forms of estrogen and/or progestin replacement is unclear. It has been suggested that estrogen protects against the development of atherosclerosis, having deleterious effects after atherosclerosis has formed.[462] This is an area of controversy and active research.

Normal Sexual Maturation: Hormonal and Physical Stages

THE FETUS AND NEONATE

Hormone levels through puberty are outlined in Table 14-3.[268,463-465] The fetus grows in a richer steroidal milieu than the pubertal female owing to the function of the fetoplacental unit. Concentrations of estrogens in fetal serum are extremely high. The umbilical cord plasma free testosterone level is modestly greater than that in normal adult females.[312] Dehydroepiandrosterone sulfate is at an adrenarchal level. Daily 17-keto steroid (KS) excretion may be as high as 2.5 mg at birth.

The newborn shows some signs of this hormonal stimulation. Hypertrophic labia minora and superficial cell transformation of the urogenital epithelium are

TABLE 14-3

Typical Normal Ranges for Ovarian and Adrenal Function Tests[a]

	E2 (pg/mL)	Estrone (pg/mL)	Testosterone (ng/dL)	Androstenedione (ng/dL)	DHEA (ng/dL)	17PROG (ng/dL)	17PREG (ng/dL)	DHEA-S (µg/dL)
Baseline (8:00 a.m.)								
Umbilical cord	3,000-29,000	3,800-31,000	15-45	30-150		900-5,000		110-410
Children, 1-5 yr old	<10	<20	<20	10-50	20-130	5-115	10-105	5-35
Children, 6-10 yr old	<10	<40	<20	10-75	20-345	5-115	10-200	10-115
Early pubertal	<10-125	10-95	10-35	40-175	40-600	15-220	35-350	35-130
Adult, follicular phase	25-250	15-100	20-60	60-200	100-850	15-150b	55-360	75-255
Peak After ACTH₁₋₂₄ (30-60 minutes after ≥10 µg/m² IV)								
Children, 1-5 yr old	—	—	<20	15-70	25-100	50-270	45-350	5-35
Children, 6-10 yr old	—	—	<20	25-100	70-320	85-300	60-650	10-115
Early pubertal	—	—	10-35	55-230	70-725	90-400	150-750	35-130
Adult, follicular phase	—	—	20-60	60-250	250-1470	35-160b	150-1070	75-255
Peak After GnRH agonist (leuprolide acetate 10 µg/kg SC)							**LH (U/L)**	**FSH (U/L)**
Prepubertal, 6-9 yr old	<10-55	—	—	—	—	20-40	1.0-9.0	8.0-40
Early pubertal, 9-13 yr old	45-350	—	—	—	—	20-155	5-100	15-40
Post-menarcheal, foll. phase	70-300	—	<10-40	45-200	60-450	25-150	30-135	15-50
Conversion multipliers to SI units	3.67 (pmol/L)	3.70 (pmol/L)	0.0347 (pmol/L)	0.0349 (nmol/L)	0.0347 (nmol/L)	0.0303 (nmol/L)	0.0316 (nmol/L)	0.0271 (µmol/L)

[a]. Ranges for radioimmunoassay after preparatory chromatography, except for cortisol and DHEAS. Values differ slightly among laboratories. Data from Rosenfield et al. and co-workers;[268,463,464] Winter and Faiman;[51] Forest;[465] Esoterix, Tarzana, CA and Quest Laboratories, San Juan Capistrano, CA.

[b]. 17-hydroxyprogesterone early and mid-follicular phase baseline levels >140 ng/dL are found in normal women who are heterozygous for 21-hydroxylase deficiency, and they often have responses to ACTH greater than those shown. 17PROG begins rising in the preovulatory phase and peaks as high as 400 ng/dL in the luteal phase of the cycle.

consistently observed estrogen effects, and a palpable breast bud appears at term in one-third of babies.[465] Menstrual bleeding and colostrum production sometimes occur in neonates as the baby is withdrawn from the estrogenic environment. Sebaceous gland hypertrophy results from the androgenic state,[466] and the clitoral shaft is sometimes prominent—particularly in small premature babies.[400]

The transient activation of the hypothalamic-pituitary-gonadal axis of the newborn that occurs before the neuroendocrine-gonadal axis comes under CNS inhibition (Figures 14-5 through 14-8) is maximal at approximately 3 to 4 months of age. This may be sufficient to sustain breast development through early infancy. These phenomena then regress gradually over the first 2 years of life as the inhibitory tone of the neuroendocrlne-gonadal axis undergoes juvenile maturation. Whether this transient activation has an influence on subsequent puberty remains unclear.[50]

CHILDHOOD

As the neuroendocrine-gonadal axis becomes quiescent and the fetal zone of the adrenal cortex regresses, steroid hormone levels fall through infancy to reach a nadir in mid-childhood (Table 14-3). Although their levels fall, there is considerable evidence for the secretion of bioactive gonadotropins at low levels (Figure 14-13). Although there is seldom obvious sexual development as a consequence of these changes, there is evidence of a low level of ovarian activity and occasional evidence of transient estrogen secretion.[467]

ADOLESCENCE

Typical Developmental Pattern

Hormonal. The earliest hormonal changes of puberty occur in late preadolescence. Clinically prepubertal 10-year-olds have greater average gonadotropin and sex hormone levels than do prepubertal 7-year-olds.[71] The earliest change in the late preadolescent years is the adrenarchal rise in DHEAS (Table 14-3).

In the average girl, serum gonadotropins begin to rise gradually after 9 years of age. However, the chronologic age at which this rise occurs varies considerably among children. Therefore, the pubertal rise in gonadotropins is best appreciated by relating gonadotropin levels to pubertal stage. Daytime serum LH rises 25-fold from prepuberty to late puberty according to bioassay, but this rise is underestimated by polyclonal radioimmunoassay (Figure 14-13).[94] Third-generation immunometric assays, using monoclonal antibodies and a more purified standard than earlier radioimmunoassays, shows a rise similar to that found by bioassay.[69,71]

The hallmark of early puberty is a sleep-related increase in LH (Figure 14-12).[71,93.] Daytime sampling underestimates the rise in gonadotropins in early puberty because it does not detect most of this sleep-related increase. In early puberty, third-generation assays show that LH rises during sleep to reach peaks in the lower adult range (generally above 1.0 U/L) and then typically falls during the

day to 0.6 U/L or less.[71,468,468a] A single daytime sample does not necessarily truly represent a child's pubertal status because it does not account for episodic and cyclic changes in gonadotropin secretion (Figure 14-12).[68,91]

The serum LH response to GnRH is more characteristic of the pubertal status than a daytime basal sample (Figure 14-9).[84,468,468a] A peak LH response to GnRH over 4.2 U/L is indicative of the onset of puberty in girls, although some early pubertal girls have lesser responses. The response of LH to GnRH or GnRH agonist administration increases more than that of FSH during puberty, with a resultant increase in the LH:FSH ratio.[69,81] GnRH agonists add a dimension to GnRH testing: they provide a sufficiently potent and prolonged stimulus to LH and FSH release to bring about an increase in ovarian estradiol secretion in pubertal girls.[81] These responses likewise increase characteristically with sexual maturation (Figure 14-6).[59]

Sex hormone levels rise further as the consequence of ovarian and adrenal maturation. Pubertal levels are intermediate between those of prepubertal and sexually mature individuals. Table 14-3 outlines typical normal ranges for serum levels of the major steroid hormones. Once pubertal levels of estrogens and androgens are achieved, their effects ordinarily become obvious within 6 months. Serum prolactin rises moderately in females at about 14 years of age.[469] This may be a response to estrogen secretion because it does not occur in boys.

Clinical. The first physical sign of puberty is usually breast development (breast stage 2, thelarche) but may be pubic hair development (pubic hair stage 3, pubarche). Thelarche represents a response to estrogen, and pubarche a response to androgen. The stages of breast and pubic hair development are shown in Figure 14-31.[470,471] Tanner stage 1 is prepubertal. Breast development stage 2 (B2) is appreciated as a palpable subareolar bud before it can be seen as an elevation. Stage B3 is obvious enlargement and elevation of the entire breast. Stage B4, the phase of areolar mounding, is very transient and may not necessarily appear. Stage B5 is the stage of attainment of mature breast contour.

Presexual pubic hairs (PH2) (i.e., short, light, and straight) are often not obvious except upon close examination and may be related to hypertrichosis rather than puberty. Sexual pubic hair (PH3; long, dark, and curly hairs) subsequently appears, usually commencing

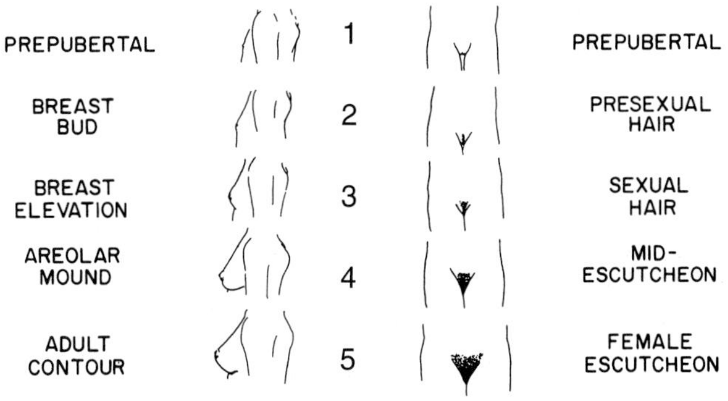

Figure 14-31 The stages of breast and pubic hair development. [Redrawn from Ross GT, Vande Wiele R (1974). The ovary. In Williams RH (ed.), *Textbook of endocrinology, Fifth edition.* Philadelphia, WB Saunders.]

on the labia majora before spreading to the pubis. Pubic hair then gradually progresses to the mature female escutcheon (inverted triangle pattern, stage 5). Axillary hair usually appears about a year later than pubic hair and passes through similar stages.

The age at which pubertal milestones are normally attained is not known with certainty. There has been considerable debate about the normalcy of pubertal changes between 6.0 and 8.0 years of age.[168,178,472] The debate stems from office practice observations that breast and pubic hair development were found more frequently than expected in black girls in this age range, whereas the age of menarche was unremarkable. The increasing prevalence of obesity interacting with ethnic factors now appears to be a major factor in this early onset of puberty.[204,205,464,473]

The prevalence of pubertal milestones has been estimated for the general U.S. population by modeling data collected on children 8.0 years of age and older by the National Health and Nutrition Examination Survey III (NHANES III).[173,174,474] Although NHANES III data has sampling advantages, the quality of the data for early breast and pubic hair development is questionable—and modeling assumptions that permit extrapolation to younger ages may not be valid.[474-476] The ages at which the major pubertal milestones are currently attained in normal-weight U.S. girls according to this database are given in Table 14-4.[474] It appears that puberty begins before 8.0 years in <5% of the normal general female population, while the appearance of breasts is normal in 7 year-old Blacks and Mexican-Americans.

An important normal variable is the span of time between the onset of breast development (B2) and menarche. The concept that this is constant at 2.3 ± 1.0 year regardless of the age at which B2 occurs[470] has recently been challenged. In several normal populations of girls observed longitudinally, the onset of puberty was only weakly correlated with the age at menarche, and the earlier puberty began, the longer its duration and the greater the incremental growth so that height potential was preserved.[477,478,479] These studies suggest that the factors governing the onset of puberty and its tempo differ. However, longitudinal studies reach conflicting conclusions on whether excess adiposity advances the onset or the tempo of puberty.[477-479a] A sub-group of early maturers with a history of intrauterine growth retardation seems to have an unusually rapid tempo of puberty and lose height potential.[479,480]

The onset of puberty is more closely related to an individual's bone age than to chronologic age. This is particularly important in the case of subjects who are later than average in entering puberty, as discussed previously. The great majority of girls can be expected to begin puberty by the time their skeletal age reaches 12.5 years, and to experience menarche by the time skeletal age reaches 14 years.

The pubertal growth spurt occurs during early adolescence. The peak of linear growth velocity corresponds most closely with stage B2,[481] and the increase in serum alkaline phosphatase levels with B3.[482] Fat accumulation increases and fat distribution changes as well.[477] As a consequence of these pubertal changes occurring out of phase with chronologic age, girls begin to differ considerably in size and habitus during the ninth year of life.

Normal Variations in Pubertal Development

Although the onset of breast development (stage B2) characteristically precedes the appearance of sexual pubic hair (PH3) and the onset of menses substantially (Table 14-4), there is normally considerable variation in the sequence of these events. Pubic hair may appear before breasts begin to develop, a situation arising from lack of direct linkage between adrenarche and gonadarche. Menarche may occur within months after the appearance of breasts. However, this is so unusual that its occurrence demands exclusion of an abnormal hyperestrogenic state.

A common normal variant is the unilateral onset of breast development. Unilateral breast development may exist up to 2 years before the other breast becomes palpable. This phenomenon seems related to an asymmetry that normally persists into adulthood. Excisional biopsy of a normal unilateral breast papilla in search of a nonexistent tumor should be avoided because such a procedure

TABLE 14-4			
Pubertal Milestone Attainment in Normal BMI Girls (Estimated Age in Years, 95% CI).*[474]			
Stage	5%	50%	95%
Breast Stage 2	8.25 (7.8, 8.6)	10.2 (9.9, 10.4)	12.1 (11.8, 12.5)
Pubic Hair Stage 3	9.25 (8.9, 9.6)	11.6 (11.3, 11.9)	13.9 (13.3, 14.7)
Menarche	11.0 (10.7, 11.3)	12.6 (12.4, 12.8)	14.1 (13.8, 14.6)

a. Breasts appear before age 8.0 years in 12-19% and sexual pubic hair in ≤3% of normal-BMI non-Hispanic Black and Mexican-American girls. Menarcheal milestones are attained at similar ages in these ethnic groups except for the 5th percentile being significantly earlier in Blacks (10.5 yr, 9.9, 10.9) than non-Hispanic Whites (11.3 yr, 9.9, 10.9).

Adapted from Rosenfeld RL, Lipton RB, Drum ML. Pubertal milestone attainment in normal-weight girls. Pediatric Academic Society Annual Meeting, Toronto, Canada, May 3-8, 2007; E-PAS2007:61:7914.11.

excises the entire breast anlage. Two extreme variations of normal are the most common causes of premature sexual development.[483] These are the isolated appearance of breast development (idiopathic premature thelarche) and the isolated appearance of sexual hair (idiopathic premature pubarche).

Premature Thelarche. Breast development before 8 years usually seems to be due to idiopathic subtle over-function of the pituitary-ovarian axis, occurring in those girls whose FSH levels tend to be sustained about the upper end of the prepubertal normal range.[467] Average serum levels of FSH at baseline and in response to GnRH are significantly increased, whereas those of LH are not. Intermittent low-grade estrogenization of the urogenital mucosa or slight or intermittent elevation of the plasma estradiol is sometimes found (Figure 14-11).[79] Examination via ovarian ultrasound shows an increased prevalence of antral follicles (microcysts). Nevertheless, a growth spurt does not occur, the bone age does not advance abnormally, and menses does not appear until the usual age.

In infants the syndrome seems to be due to a lag in inhibition of the transient activation of the hypothalamic-pituitary-gonadal axis of the newborn and is usually unsustained. In older children, the breast development is more likely to persist. A subgroup with "exaggerated thelarche" has an increased growth rate with relatively proportionate bone age advancement. Their unsustained or intermittent neuroendocrine activation seems to lie on a spectrum between ordinary premature thelarche and true sexual precocity (Figure 14-32).[484] However, the McCune-Albright syndrome mutation is found in the peripheral blood of about 25% of such patients.[485] Premature thelarache may be the first sign of transient autonomously functioning ovarian cysts, complete precocious puberty, or occasionally polycystic ovary syndrome. Therefore, follow-up of these patients is indicated.

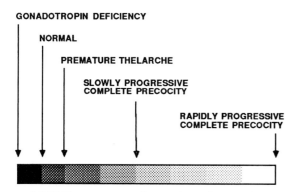

Figure 14-32 The spectrum of gonadotropin secretion in girls. Normal girls are conceptualized as having a small amount of pituitary-ovarian axis activation, which is more than that of congenitally hypogonadotropic girls. Premature thelarche, exaggerated thelarche, slowly progressive precocity, and rapidly progressive precocity fall along a spectrum of increasing activation of the axis—with deterioration of height potential occurring only in those near the most activated end. [From Kreiter ML, Cara JF, Rosenfield RL (1993). Modifying the outcome of complete precocious puberty: To treat or not to treat. In Grave GD, Cutler GB (eds.), *Sexual precocity: Etiology, diagnosis, and management.* New York: Raven Press 109–120.]

Premature Pubarche. Pubarche before 9 years of age usually occurs at adrenarcheal androgen levels (e.g., DHEAS 40-130 µg/dL; Table 14-3), which is termed *premature adrenarche.*[268] However, it may occur at androgen levels that are lower (idiopathic premature pubarche) or higher. The androgen excess is ordinarily so subtle that the only other sign of increased androgen production may be microcomedonal acne and apocrine body odor. There is no obvious growth spurt, the bone age typically does not advance abnormally, and there are no other signs of sexual maturation.

Exaggerated adrenarche is an extreme type of premature adrenarche. These girls have clinical features that suggest subtle androgen excess (e.g., significant bone age advancement but not clitoromegaly) or insulin resistance (e.g., central adiposity or acanthosis nigricans). Such children generally have a slightly advanced onset of true puberty, but height potential is not compromised. Adrenal steroid levels are in the mid- or late pubertal range (e.g., DHEA-S >130–185 µg/dL, androstenedione >75–99 ng/dL, or post-ACTH 17-hydroxypregnenolone >750 ng/dL). Testosterone does not exceed the lower end of the adult female range.

It is unclear whether premature adrenarche is simply a normal variant due to advanced onset of normal zona reticularis development or an early manifestation of the steroidogenic dysregulation of polycystic ovary syndrome (PCOS). Carriers for congenital adrenal hyperplasia may be overrepresented in this group.[486,487] Premature pubarche appears to carry about a 15- to 20% risk of developing PCOS. It seems likely that the risk is relatively high in those with exaggerated adrenarche. Thus, girls with premature adrenarche should be followed through puberty.

Constitutional Delay of Pubertal Development. By statistical definition, puberty can be considered delayed in 3% of girls. Most of these girls are otherwise normal, in which case this is termed *constitutional delay of growth and pubertal development* (which is often familial). Girls do not usually become concerned about this until they enter high school at 14 years of age and realize that not only has pubertal development not begun but most of their friends are menstruating. When puberty does ensue in such subjects, it is perfectly normal in tempo. Endocrinologic status is normal for the stage of puberty. It may be difficult to distinguish constitutional delay of growth and pubertal development from gonadotropin deficiency, as discussed under that heading.

Physiologic Adolescent Anovulation. About half of menstrual cycles are anovulatory during the first two postmenarcheal (gynecologic) years.[488] This causes considerable variation in the length of time it takes for a girl to establish a menstrual pattern that is normal by adult standards. Cycles in the early years tend to be a few days longer than in adults, and long phases of irregularity of menses may occur (Figure 14-33).[489,489a] Nevertheless, even within the first year after menarche it is abnormal to have bleeding that is excessive or lasts over 7 days or occurs more frequently than every 21 days (dysfunctional uterine bleeding) or cycles that occur less frequently than every 90 days, i.e., missing more than 4 cycles per year (oligomenorrhea). By five gynecologic years the menstrual cycle is virtually sexually mature, with approximately 80 per cent

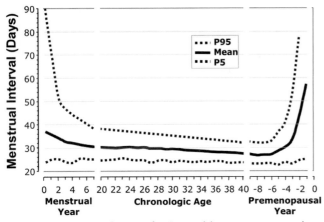

Figure 14-33 Normal range for interval between menstrual cycles. Note that cycle intervals averaging more than 90 days or fewer than 22 days are abnormal at any age. P5 and P95 = 5th and 95th percentiles, respectively. [Modified from Treloar A, Boynton R, Benn B, Brown B (1967). Variation of human menstrual cycle through reproductive life. Int J Fertil 12:77–84.]

menstrual periods for 6 months or more after initially menstruating.

Serum LH, testosterone, and androstenedione levels are significantly higher in adolescents with anovulatory than those with ovulatory cycles.[490,491] It is unclear whether this is the cause or the result of the anovulation. However, if hyperandrogenemia is found it seldom regresses.[117] The distinction between multicystic ovaries, which are usually a variation of normal, and polycytic ovaries (which are not) is often subjective and problematic.[492,493] Failure to establish a normal adult menstrual pattern by 2 postmenarcheal years or to sustain a normal pattern for 2 years after one has been established carries a greater than two-thirds risk of persistent oligoovulation (Figure 14-34).[494] Thus, failure to establish regular cycles by this time is an indication to investigate the cause.

Other. There is considerable variation in the amount of acne, hirsutism, and adiposity among normal adolescent girls—most of which is related to familial factors. Three-quarters of adolescent girls experience some degree of acne, and one-quarter experience inflammatory acne.[495] The initiation of acne is more closely related to blood levels of DHEAS than to blood levels of other androgens.

Profound psychological changes occur during adolescence. Sexually immature girls tend to be socially immature, and the onset of puberty is associated with increased independence and profound changes in outlook

of cycles being ovulatory. At this point, it is abnormal to miss more than 4 periods per year (oligomenorrhea). Primary amenorrhea is defined as failure to begin menses at a normal age (by 15 years of age or within 3 years of thelarche), and *secondary amenorrhea* as cessation of

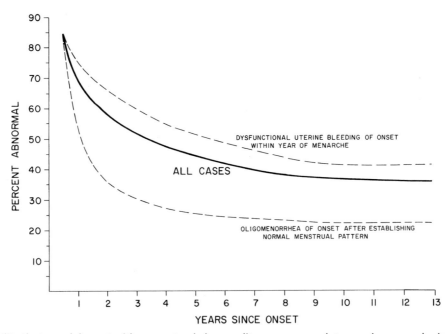

Figure 14-34 Probability that an adolescent with a menstrual abnormality severe enough to require gynecologic consultation will have continued menstrual abnormality. The lines show the cumulative rates at which subjects with menstrual abnormalities converted to normal patterns. The heavy curve shows the overall incidence of continued menstrual abnormality in adolescents when considering both types of anovulatory manifestation (dysfunctional uterine bleeding and oligomenorrhea) regardless of time of onset. The dotted lines show those subgroups that differ most from the overall pattern. Other subgroups fall within approximately 5% of the mean for the entire group. Note that dysfunctional uterine bleeding of onset within 1 year of menarche carries the worst prognosis for continuing menstrual abnormality (upper dotted line). Note also that oligomenorrhea of relatively short duration occurring after a normal menstrual pattern has been established carries the best overall prognosis. Nevertheless, it can be seen that if the menstrual abnormality persists for 2 years there is a 67% probability that the patient will not spontaneously evolve to normal cycles. That is, of the 60% of patients with an abnormal menstrual pattern of 2 years' duration, two-thirds (40% of the total group) will continue to have abnormal periods. Similarly, if the problem persists for 5 years there is an 80% likelihood of persistence of the abnormality. [Redrawn from Southam AL, Richart EM (1966). The prognosis for adolescents with menstrual abnormalities. Am J Obstet Gynecol 94:637.]

on life and in intellectual capacity. The extent to which these developments occur in reaction to the physical changes of puberty and the extent to which they are direct effects of sex hormones are unknown. Masculine tomboyish traits usually have no clear hormonal basis, although there is some evidence that they may have prenatal hormonal determinants. Social interactions have effects on these aspects of development. They affect even the synchrony of the menstrual cycle.[496]

Normal Variations in Mature Menstrual Cycles

The cyclic changes of LH, FSH, estradiol, and progesterone during the menstrual cycle are shown in Figure 14-14.[118,119] Some diurnal and episodic fluctuations are superimposed on these, as noted in the related discussion. Because testosterone and androstenedione have both adrenal and ovarian origins, their levels fluctuate to some extent in cyclic, diurnal, and episodic patterns. For example, testosterone levels tend to be 20% greater in the morning than in the evening—and to rise 50% to 100% in midcycle.[118,497] Normal ranges for most of the important sex hormone levels of women during the early follicular phase of the menstrual cycle are outlined in Table 14-3.

Progesterone levels are below 100 ng/dL until the periovulatory phase of the cycle, and then peak to greater than 500 ng/dL in the mid-luteal phase. Hormonal production rates for the mid-follicular phase in women are given in Table 14-2. Serum prolactin increases transiently in midcycle with maximum ovarian estradiol secretion.[498] Prolactin levels also transiently rise in response to mammary stimulation and psychological factors.[499]

The menstrual cycle of young adults averages 28 days in length (90% confidence limits, 22 to 40 days by the fifth gynecologic year).[489] The variation in cycle length is almost entirely due to differences in the duration of the follicular phase. The luteal phase, the time between ovulation and the onset of menses, invariably lasts 14 ± 1 (standard deviation) days.[119]

Recent evidence indicates that human pheromones modulate the timing of ovulation[500] and mood.[501] Unusual steroids, such as androst-4,16-diene-3-one, have been incriminated in this regard. Uterine cramping is characteristic of ovulatory cycles, presumably as a result of prostaglandins released within the endometrium upon the withdrawal of progesterone.

Abnormal Puberty

ABNORMAL DEVELOPMENT

Disorders of Sex Development

Patients with disorders of sex development (DSD, formerly termed *intersex*)—those whose genitalia are ambiguous or inappropriate for their gonadal sex as a result of endocrinopathy—may come to a physician's attention for the first time at puberty. These syndromes are termed *ovotesticular DSD* (true hermaphroditism), *46, XX DSD* (female pseudohermaphroditism), *46, XY DSD* (male pseudohermaphroditism), *46, XX testic-*ular DSD* (XX male), and *46, XY complete gonadal dysgenesis.*[432]

Patients with any of these disorders may undergo inappropriate puberty. They may present with clitoromegaly and be found upon examination to have a degree of genital ambiguity previously overlooked. Virilization beginning at puberty is sometimes the presenting complaint. Ovotesticular DSD and 46, XX DSD due to congenital adrenal hyperplasia are compatible with fertility.[321] Androgen insensitivity syndrome may present as primary amenorrhea in an otherwise normal adolescent girl. The disorders of sexual differentiation are reviewed in detail in Chapter 4.

Other Dysgenetic Disorders

Failure of the onset of menses can result from structural abnormalities of the genital tract that do not have an endocrinologic basis. The vagina may be aplastic or have an imperforate hymen. If the uterus is intact, hydrometrocolpos will occur. The uterus may be congenitally aplastic. Uterine synechiae develop as the consequence of endometritis, which may result from infection or irradiation (Asherman's syndrome). Congenital absence of the vagina may be associated with varying degrees of uterine aplasia. This is the Rokitansky-Kustner-Hauser syndrome.[502] This syndrome seems to occur as a single gene defect or as an acquired teratogenic event involving mesodermal development and the mesonephric kidney, the latter resulting in abnormalities of the genital tract and sometimes the urinary tract. A subtype due to *Wnt 4* gene defects is associated with hyperandrogenism.[502a]

PRECOCIOUS PUBERTY

Causes

When breast development begins before the age of 8 years, sexual pubic hair before 8 years, or menses before the age of 9.5, puberty is traditionally considered precocious (premature). Puberty can occur prematurely as an extreme variation of normal because of a disturbance in the hormonal axis normally involved in sexual maturation or because of a disturbance outside that axis. Depending on which part of this hormonal axis is involved, different forms of precocious puberty are distinguished. A classification of the causes of premature puberty together with typical findings is given in Table 14-5.

It is important to distinguish between true precocious puberty and pseudoprecocious puberty. In true precocious puberty maturation is "complete." Breasts and pubic hair develop as the result of CNS activating pituitary secretion of the respective gonadotropins FSH and LH (although breast development may be the sole manifestation of early complete precocity for as long as 6 to 12 months). Thus, "central" is another term applied to this type of precocity. Patients with true precocious puberty have *isosexual* precocity because the secondary sexual characteristics are appropriate for the sex of the child.

In pseudoprecocious puberty, maturation is incomplete—with only one type of secondary sexual characteristic developing early. Pseudoprecocious puberty has diverse causes

TABLE 14-5

Typical Findings in Female Sexual Precocity

Locus	Type	HA*	BA*	Estrogens†	Androgens†	LH/FSH†	Pathology	Characteristics
Complete Precocity								
NeuroendoCrine	Isosexual	+	++	+	+	+	Idiopathic Neurogenic Advanced somatic maturation	95% of female cases
Incomplete Precocity								
Normal variant	Isosexual	−	−	±	−	±	None	Thelarche
	Isosexual	−	−	−	±	−	None	Pubarche/adrenarche
Neuroendocrine	Contrasexual	+	++	−	+	+/+++	LH/hCG excess	Familial or tumor
	Isosexual	Low	Low	−	−	+	Hypothyroid	Growth arrest
Ovary	Isosexual/contrasexual	+	++	+/+++	+/+++	−	Tumor	
	Isosexual	+	++	+/+++	−	±	McCune-Albright	Bone lesions ± nevi ± ovarian cysts
Adrenal	Contrasexual	+	++	±	+++	−	Congenital adrenal hyperplasia	Dexamethasone suppressible
	Contrasexual/ isosexual	+	++	+/+++	+/+++	−	Tumor	
Exogenous	Contrasexual/ isosexual	±	±	−	−	−	Steroid ingestion	
End organ	Isosexual/contrasexual	−	−	−	−	−	Vaginal foreign body, abuse, tumor	
Ectopic	Isosexual	+	++	−/+++	−	−	Aromatase excess	

* HA (height for age) and BA (bone age); − normal; + advanced; ++ markedly advanced.
† Hormone levels; − normal prepubertal; + pubertal level; ++ adult level; +++ abnormally high.
FSH, follicle-stimulating hormone; hCG, human chorionic gonadotropin; LH, luteinizing hormone.

and is not mediated by pubertal pituitary gonadotropin secretion. In some patients with pseudoprecocity, pubertal development is isosexual. In others it is "contrasexual," meaning that characteristics of the opposite sex are manifested.

Complete Precocious Puberty. True isosexual precocity results from pubertal function of the hypothalamic-pituitary-gonadal axis. About 95% of true precocity in girls is idiopathic. Idiopathic true sexual precocity seems usually to be due to premature triggering of the normal pubertal mechanism. Pubertal development is usually qualitatively and quantitatively normal except for its early occurrence. Progressive puberty with a growth spurt ensues when activation of the pituitary-ovarian axis is sustained. However, puberty is not necessarily intense enough or sustained enough to cause the inexorable progression of normal puberty or to cause deterioration of height potential.[503]

The predominance of the idiopathic syndrome in females and its benign nature are compatible with the likelihood that this disorder is an extreme exaggeration of the normal tendency of girls to have relatively high gonadotropin levels. Most cases are sporadic, a few familial. The majority of these patients seem to go on to have normal menstrual cycles.[504] Pregnancy has been documented to occur as early as 4 years of age. This is reminiscent of the experimental model in which certain hypothalamic lesions in rats cause premature puberty followed by constant estrus.[1] Rare causes of true sexual precocity include maternal uniparental disomy of chromosome 14, which causes the combination of intrauterine growth retardation and sexual precocity[505]—as well as hyperglycinemia.[506] A genetic variant of a hepatic mixed-function oxidase has been associated with the precocious onset of puberty in girls.[335]

Any type of intracranial disturbance can cause true isosexual precocity. These neurogenic disturbances are presumed to cause true sexual precocity by increasing the prevalence of excitatory inputs or by interfering with neurogenic inhibition of hypothalamic GnRH secretion.[507] These include congenital brain dysfunction (such as cerebral palsy and hydrocephalus) and acquired disorders, such as irradiation, trauma, chronic inflammatory disorders, and masses in the region of the hypothalamus. The activation of GnRH release by hypothalamic injury may be mediated by TGF-α elaborated by reactive astrocytes. An empty sella is occasionally found.[508]

The precocity of neurofibromatosis type I (von Recklinghausen disease) usually results from an optic glioma, which is often a low-grade malignancy, or from a hamartoma[509]—although occasionally from neither.[510] Hamartoma of the hypothalamus may cause sexual precocity by acting as an "accessory hypothalamus" that releases pulses of GnRH into the pituitary portal circulation[511] or by producing TGF-α.[512] Figure 14-35 shows a hypothalamic hamartoma.

A small proportion of pineal tumors cause true sexual precocity.[513, 514] The incidence of sexual precocity is about 3.5 times as great in nonparenchymatous neoplasms (such as gliomas and teratomas) as in parenchymatous pineal tumors. This suggests that these tumors cause sexual precocity via absence of a normal pineal inhibitory factor rather than via destructive effects on inhibitory tracts. Although pineal masses may cause paralysis of upward gaze by pressure on the corpora quadrigemina, this sign is present in only a minority of cases.

Advancement of somatic maturation due to noncentral endocrine disorders that advance the bone age to a pubertal level sometimes causes true sexual precocity. Thus, true puberty may begin after correction of virilizing or feminizing disorders that have advanced the bone age to 10 to 12 years.[194,195] The hypergonadotropinism of premature ovarian failure has been reported to cause sexual precocity or rapid progression of puberty prior to premature menopause.[515,516] The possibility must be considered that true sexual precocity may very occasionally be the first manifestation of polycystic ovary syndrome.[517-519]

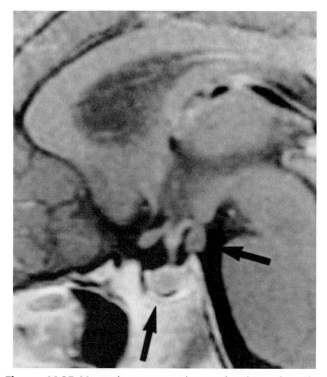

Figure 14-35 Magnetic resonance image showing a hypothalamic hamartoma (right-hand arrow) as the cause of true sexual precocity in a 2.5-year-old girl. The hamartoma is hanging from the floor of the hypothalamus just posterior to the pituitary infundibulum. The sella turcica (bottom arrow) contains a normal pituitary gland with pituitary stalk hanging from the infundibulum.

Incomplete Precocity. The most common causes of incomplete sexual precocity in girls are the extreme variants of normal premature thelarche and premature pubarche. These are incomplete forms of sexual precocity in which either breast development (thelarche) or sexual hair development (pubarche) is of a degree appropriate for an early stage of adolescence and hence isosexual. Isolated prepubertal menses is a rare disorder, which like premature thelarche has been attributed to transient ovarian activity.[520]

Girls with hCG-producing tumors rarely have sexual precocity.[521] Nevertheless, true sexual precocity has been reported in association with pineal or hypothalamic hCG-secreting germ cell tumors.[522,523] Because hCG is a LH receptor agonist, possible explanations for this unusual situation are disinhibition of hypothalamic GnRH release due to a mass effect, the weak FSH effect of massive elevation of hCG, and the capacity of some dysgerminomas to secrete not only hCG but estradiol.[524]

As with hCG-secreting tumors, one would not expect an isolated elevation of LH to cause precocious puberty. However, isolated elevation of LH has been reported as an unusual cause of contrasexual precocious puberty:[525] Mild virilizing signs were reported in siblings with isolated elevation of LH, one of whom was a girl. She developed pubic hair and clitoral hypertrophy at 4 years, with slight to moderate advances in height and bone age in association with an adrenarchal level of DHEAS and a moderately elevated testosterone level (91 ng/dL).

The van Wyk-Grumbach syndrome is one of the most puzzling pediatric complexes.[526] This is an unusual syndrome of sexual precocity associated with juvenile hypothyroidism. A case is illustrated in Figure 14-36. This syndrome is often characterized by galactorrhea, which is often subtle. The breasts must be specifically manipulated in order to express the few drops of milky fluid that may be present. Multicystic ovaries are often demonstrable by ultrasonography.[527] There is little, if any, sexual hair development. There is another clinically unique feature about the sexual precocity of hypothyroidism: it is the only form of sexual precocity in which growth is arrested rather than stimulated.

Van Wyk and Grumbach postulated that this syndrome resulted from hormonal "overlap" in the negative feedback regulation of pituitary hormone secretion, with overproduction of gonadotropins and TSH in response to the thyroid deficiency. The specific nature of hormonal overlap has been considerably clarified in recent years. The increases in plasma TSH and prolactin that characterize the syndrome could well be accounted for by common neurohumoral control systems, TRH stimulating and dopamine inhibiting both hormones.

Although the gonadotropins share a common alpha-subunit with TSH and seem to be elevated according to the early generation of polyclonal radioimmunoassays, they do not appear to be GnRH responsive or bioactive.[528,529] Furthermore, most children with prolonged hypothyroidism have delayed sexual maturation—as would be expected from the maturational retardation characteristic of states with delayed bone ages. Recently, the syndrome has been postulated to arise from the weak intrinsic FSH activity of extreme TSH elevation[530]—which

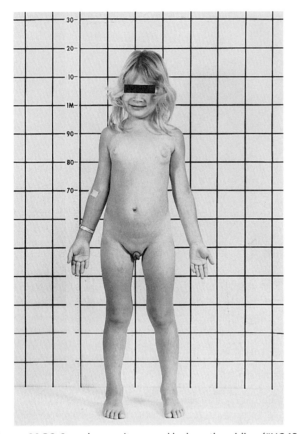

Figure 14-36 Sexual precocity caused by hypothyroidism (#UC 133-33-55-4) in a 9.1-year-old with breast development since 7 years and menarche at 9.0 years. Growth failure had occurred, and her height age was 6 years. In addition to breast enlargement and galactorrhea, the labia minora were noted to be enlarged and pigmented. There was no sexual hair or clitoromegaly. Rectal examination revealed an enlarged and palpable cervix without adnexal masses. There were typical physical findings of hypothyroidism. Bone age was 6.2 years. Thyroxine was less than 1 μg/dL. Thyrotropin-stimulating hormone was 438 μgU/mL. Prolactin was 66 ng/mL. Serum estrogens were 72 to 182 pg/mL. Vaginal smear showed 45% superficial cells and 55% large intermediate cells. Immunoreactive luteinizing hormone (LH) and follicle-stimulating hormone were 300 and 174 ng LER-907/mL, respectively. However, bioactive LH was undetectable. Immunoreactive gonadotropins failed to suppress upon estrogen administration. Their response to a 100-_g gonadtropin-stimulating hormone bolus was minimal, and they seemed responsive to thyrotropin-releasing hormone. All of these hormonal findings were not obviously different from those of hypothyroid girls without sexual precocity except for the higher estrogens. Patient had withdrawal bleeding and evidence of regression of breast development within the first 3 months of thyroid hormone replacement treatment. After 6 months' treatment, normal puberty began. Menarche occurred at 12.5 years of age.

would be analogous to the similarly rare ovarian hyperstimulation syndrome in adults.[531]

The concommittent hyperprolactinemia may play a role in the sexual precocity of hypothyroidism. It seems unlikely to be the primary cause, however, because prolactin levels do not correspond with pubertal development in normal or hypothyroid children. However, induced hyperprolactinemia causes sexual precocity in female rats.[264] Ovarian estrogen and progesterone re-

sponsiveness to hCG is increased by prolactin, possibly by its induction of ovarian LH receptors. Mean LH levels do not change, although an increase in episodic gonadotropin secretion has not been ruled out. Suppression of hyperprolactinemia in experimental hypothyroidism blocks the ovarian cyst formation characteristic of hypothyroidism.[532] These data suggest that hyperprolactinemia sensitizes the ovaries to the trace amounts of gonadotropin present prepubertally.

McCune-Albright syndrome is one of the most intriguing disorders causing incomplete isosexual feminization.[533,534] This is a syndrome of precocious puberty involving cafe-au-lait pigmentation occurring in nevi that have an irregular ("coast of Maine") border and polyostotic fibrous dysplasia. The disorder is caused by a somatic activating mutation in the alpha-subunit of the G protein that couples transmembrane receptors to adenylate cyclase. The syndrome occurs in incomplete and expanded forms. Precocious puberty or monoostotic bone lesions may occur in the absence of cutaneous pigmentation. Not all patients have sexual precocity. The disorder has been recognized predominantly in females. The sexual precocity is of the gonadotropin-independent type. Luteinized follicular cysts within the ovaries function autonomously. Pituitary adenomas capable of secreting excess LH, FSH, GH, and/or prolactin have been reported. Patients may have Cushing syndrome and hyperthyroidism due to autonomous multinodular hyperplasia. These girls may be at increased risk of breast carcinoma.[535] Nonendocrine abnormalities include cardiopulmonary disease, hypertension, and hepatobiliary disease.

Molecular studies have shown an R201H mutation in more than 90% of cases in which an affected tissue could be studied, but in only 50% of blood samples.[536] Because of the variation in the number and degree of tissue involvement in individual patients, due in large part to the extent of mosaicism present, precocious puberty may be the only feature present in an individual who is mosaic for the activating mutation of G_s-alpha. Thus, these mutations have been found in blood samples from 25% to 33% of subjects with isolated gonadotropin-independent precocity or exaggerated thelarche.[485,536]

Congenital adrenal hyperplasia (CAH) is a well-known cause of premature pubarche. Nonclassic CAH, a form of the disorder so mild that there is no genital defect, or poor control of classic CAH may be responsible. Each form has on occasion been reported to mimic true sexual precocity.[537,538]

The most common tumor associated with isosexual feminization is the benign ovarian follicular cyst.[539] The cells lining these cysts are often luteinized. Estrogen production is modest to marked. Testosterone levels tend to be in the adult female range (about 40 ng/dL). Some of these cysts may occur in the course of intermittent or unsustained true sexual precocity. They may be gonadotropin dependent. A case is illustrated in Figure 14-37. The second most common ovarian feminizing neoplasm in girls is the granulosa cell tumor.[540,541] These are on a spectrum that includes variable degrees of sex cord elements and stromal tissue. Granulosa cell tumors are

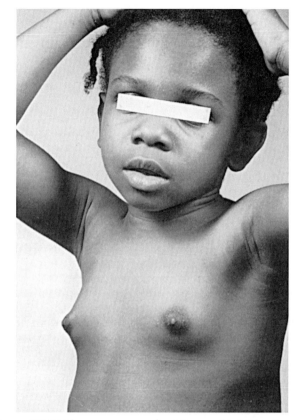

Figure 14-37 The appearance of a 5.2-year-old child with complete isosexual precocity caused by a luteinized follicular cyst. Her breast development is no different from that of girls with idiopathic premature thelarche. She presented at 4.7 years with a 2-week history of breast development. Height and bone ages were 5 years. Over a 5-month follow-up period, breast development progressed, she developed sexual pubic hair and presexual axillary hair, and menstrual flow commenced at 3- to 5-week intervals. Four weekly determinations of plasma unconjugated estrogens (estradiol and estrone) showed them to consistently range between 158 and 215 pg/mL. Luteinizing hormone and follicle-stimulating hormone averaged 50 and 13 ng LER-907/mL, respectively, by radioimmunoassay. Testosterone was 37 ng/dL, and dehydroepiandrosterone sulfate (DHEAS) was 82 μg/dL. Exploratory laparotomy was performed when she was 5.2 years old. Her height age was 5.8 years, and her bone age was 7.5. The laparotomy revealed a right ovarian cyst about 5 cm in diameter, which was removed. Subsequently, there was a rapid fall in plasma estrogens and testosterone to prepubertal levels. However, DHEAS was unchanged. Menses ceased, but intermittent vaginal cornification (maturation index 90/10/0 to 0/90/10) was repeatedly found. Breast enlargement and sexual hair development resumed at 8.5 years, with normal pubertal sex hormone levels. Menarche occurred at 9.5 years.

usually benign. They may produce hCG, AMH, and inhibin;[541,542] a variety of non-specific tumor markers are rarely reported. They are occasionally associated with mesodermal dysplasia syndromes.[543] Granulosa-theca cell tumor has been reported in the adrenal, presumably arising in an ovarian rest.[544] Some ovarian sex cord-stromal tumors may be caused by loss of a tumor-suppressor gene, as in Peutz-Jeghers syndrome,[545] and others by activating mutations of stimulatory G proteins.[546]

Masculinizing tumors of the ovary (characteristically Leydig-Sertoli cell tumors or arrhenoblastomas) are unusual

before the teenage years. The abnormal differentiation that underlies tumor formation typically leads to an abnormal pattern of steroid secretion, with androstenedione predominating over testosterone secretion.[547] Rare causes of masculinization and feminization are respectively granulosa-theca cell and interstitial cell tumors. Thecomas (luteomas) are unusual in children and are generally benign. Dysgerminomas virilize only if they have interstitial cell elements. Gonadoblastomas are virilizing tumors virtually confined to individuals with dysgenetic gonads with Y-chromosomal material in their genome. Adrenal rest and hilus cell tumors of the ovary are extremely rare causes of masculinization in childhood.[18,312]

Lipid cell tumors must be considered in the differential diagnosis of late-onset congenital adrenal hyperplasia because they tend to produce 17-hydroxyprogesterone and respond to ACTH and LH.[548] Some ovarian tumors are of adrenal origin.[549] Adrenal disorders cause pseudoprecocity, as discussed in Chapter 12 Adrenocortical tumors typically cause a rapid virilizing disorder characterized by very high DHEAS production, although androstenedione may instead be the predominant androgen secreted. A case discussion is given with Figure 14-38. On occasion, adrenal tumors cause feminization. When adrenal tumors secrete androgen and estrogen, the clinical picture may resemble complete isosexual precocity.[550] Structural abnormalities of chromosome 11p15 and mutations of the tumor suppressor p53 are fairly common in pediatric adrenocortical tumors.[551]

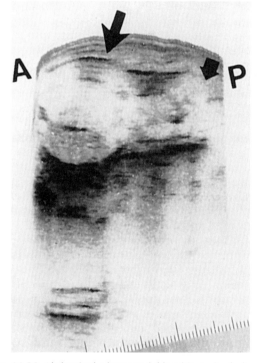

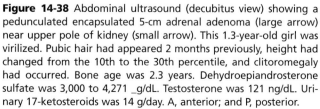

Figure 14-38 Abdominal ultrasound (decubitus view) showing a pedunculated encapsulated 5-cm adrenal adenoma (large arrow) near upper pole of kidney (small arrow). This 1.3-year-old girl was virilized. Pubic hair had appeared 2 months previously, height had changed from the 10th to the 30th percentile, and clitoromegaly had occurred. Bone age was 2.3 years. Dehydroepiandrosterone sulfate was 3,000 to 4,271 _g/dL. Testosterone was 121 ng/dL. Urinary 17-ketosteroids was 14 g/day. A, anterior; and P, posterior.

Exogenous steroids can cause sexual precocity. Estrogen-containing contraceptive pills and creams are widely available. Some cases of precocious thelarche may be caused by ingesting food contaminated with artificial estrogens.[552] Soy formulas are potential sources of phytoestrogens, as are many commonly consumed foods herbs and topicals.[553,554,544a] It has been proposed that childhood exposure to estrogenic chemical contaminants in underdeveloped countries predisposes to sexual precocity when children emigrate to developed countries.[168] Premature pubarche or acne can result from anabolic steroid use. Topical nonprescription androgen use by a parent, such as for sexual dysfunction or anabolic effects, can cause premature pubarche without necessarily being detectable by standard tests.[555]

Vaginal bleeding as an isolated phenomenon suggests a foreign body, sexual abuse, or tumors of the genital tract. Malodorous discharge is highly suggestive of a foreign body. A hymenal opening of greater than 5 mm and posterior notches are compatible with sexual abuse.[409,410] Neurofibromas have been reported to simulate breast development and clitoral hypertrophy. Aromatase excess syndrome has been reported to cause feminization of both sexes.[556] This is an autosomal-dominant disorder that results from aberrant aromatase gene transcription.

Differential Diagnosis

A physician need not be experienced in endocrinology to diagnose and manage most female patients presenting with early breast or pubic hair development. For the most part, the isolated appearance of one of these signs is due to the benign processes of premature thelarche and premature pubarche, respectively. An otherwise normal history and physical examination, together with a normal bone age, constitutes sufficient workup.

In the history, the physician should inquire about the possibility of exposure or access to exogenous steroids in the form of unusual creams, pills, or diet. The possibility of sexual abuse, vaginal infection, or a foreign body must be kept in mind when evaluating the child with isolated vaginal bleeding. In the examination, the physician should search for nevi, acanthosis nigricans, and signs that might suggest intracranial, abdominal, or pelvic disease. The child's height and weight should be carefully recorded and the growth curve examined.

If no other abnormalities are found upon physical examination, only a bone age determination is indicated to check whether the symptom is indeed an isolated phenomenon or whether appreciable hormone excess exists. If the skeletal age is not abnormally advanced relative to height age, it is likely that the presenting symptom is an isolated and benign extreme variant of normal that requires no treatment.[467,557] Support for this impression may be obtained if the serum level of the relevant female or male hormones is low (estradiol less than 10 pg/mL and testosterone less than 25 ng/dL).

To confirm the diagnosis of these benign nonprogressive disorders, the child must be similarly reevaluated after 6 months. The importance of this recheck is illustrated by the patient shown in Figure 14-37. If the results are still negative, the family can be reassured with a high degree of confidence that true puberty (including menses) will not occur until the usual age.

If more than one sign of precocious puberty is present or develops, if the growth is accelerated, or if the bone age is advanced more than 2 standard deviations above the mean for age (particularly if height potential is compromised), a more extensive investigation should be undertaken to rule out a discrete lesion affecting some part of the hormonal axis controlling puberty. For example, if a young girl with early breast development begins to grow pubic hair (or vice versa) something more than premature thelarche or premature adrenarche is involved. The same is true if she develops signs of a growth spurt, her bone age advances inordinately over the 6-month interval of initial observation, or if she begins menstruating. These additional signs indicate the need for more extensive studies. Isolated vaginal bleeding suggests sexual abuse, a foreign body, or tumor. Only rarely does it indicate isolated menarche. Cytology, anaerobic culture, plasma estradiol, and in some cases pelvic ultrasound examinations are indicated.

One must be particularly aware that girls with neurogenic precocity, especially those who have had cranial irradiation, are at risk of paradoxically having GH deficiency.[484] Coexistent GH deficiency masks the seriousness of the precocity. The growth rate is normal (not accelerated) and breast development is attenuated. However, the disparity between bone age and height age is extreme.

The laboratory investigation of premature pubertal development requires determinations of sex steroids, LH, and FSH by high sensitivity-specificity "pediatric" assays of high sensitivity and specificity in laboratories with well-established normal ranges for children. These assays should have a sensitivity of at least 10 pg/ml for estradiol, 10 ng/dl for testosterone, and 0.2 U/L for LH and FSH. Measurement of serum thyroxine and prolactin is indicated if the sexual precocity is accompanied by growth arrest and/or galactorrhea. Day time plasma estradiol concentration is usually pubertal, typically 10 pg/mL (37 pmol/L) or greater in true isosexual precocity.[558] An estradiol level at the upper end of the premenarcheal normal range (75 pg/mL) or greater is atypical and necessitates a prompt workup to distinguish ovarian or adrenal tumor from true isosexual precocity.[559]

Weekly determinations of estradiol may be necessary to determine whether the level is fluctuating in the normal cyclic fashion of true precocious puberty or is persistently elevated. Because of the episodic and cyclic nature of sex hormone secretion, examination of the vaginal mucosa for estrogen effect is a more accurate indicator of the presence of early puberty than is the estradiol blood level because the vaginal cytology represents the integrated effect of estrogen over the preceeding few weeks (Figure 14-11). Uterine size (e.g., uterine width >1.5 cm) is an objective indicator of overall estrogen effect.[78] Androgen levels are appropriate for the stage of pubarche in true precocity.

Third-generation monoclonal-antibody-based immunoassays for gonadotropins are important to the differential diagnosis. Daytime basal and GnRH-stimulated peak LH levels exceeding 0.6 and 6.9 U/L in girls have been found to be respectively 70 and 92% sensitive for the diagnosis of central precocious puberty.[468] FSH levels are not as helpful diagnostically. A GnRH agonist test yields similar diagnostic information and permits assessment of the ovarian secretory capacity. In response to these tests, children with unsustained pseudopuberty as variants of normal will have a minimal gonadotropin response— whereas children with gonadotropin-independent precocity will have suppressed responses.[81,82,560] Demonstration of a sleep-related rise of plasma LH is an alternative diagnostic procedure. Table 14-6 gives criteria for the diagnosis of the rapidly progressive type of complete sexual precocity that requires treatment.[561,562]

Determination of the plasma androgen pattern is useful in discriminating among the causes of premature pubarche and virilization. Androgen determinations are most accurately performed by a specialty laboratory.[339] Premature adrenarche is characterized by a pubertal level of DHEAS, whereas plasma testosterone and androstenedione are at most marginally elevated above the prepubertal range. A greatly elevated level of DHEAS is characteristic of adrenal tumors. Androstenedione and 17-hydroxyprogesterone levels are disproportionately elevated compared to testosterone or DHEAS levels in congenital adrenal hyperplasia and many ovarian tumors. Dexamethasone suppression testing and other means of determining the source of androgen excess are discussed in the section on hyperandrogenemia.

Ultrasonography is indicated to rule out abdominal or pelvic masses when feminizing or virilizing disorders are suspected. The ovaries of girls with true sexual precocity resemble those of normal pubertal girls.[75,562] A cyst of 10 mm or more in diameter is usually due to a transient preovulatory follicle. However, the differential diagnosis of a persistant cyst or of multicystic ovaries includes McCune-Albright syndrome,[534] tumor,[563] and premature ovarian failure.[564] Magnetic resonance imaging (MRI) of the hypothalamic-pituitary area is indicated in rapidly progressive true sexual precocity, especially for those less than 6 years old or those at risk of organic causes by virtue of their underlyng condition or neurologic symptoms and signs.[558,565]

The situation of a girl presenting with the onset of breast development or pubic hair between 6 and 8 years of age warrants special consideration. Breast and pubic hair development have been reported in 15 to 20% of U.S. black girls in office practice, in contrast to less than 5% of white girls.[483] Subsequent studies have indicated that breast development between 7 and 8 years of age may be normal in blacks and Hispanics, whereas sexual pubic hair is not (Table 14-4). However, pubertal development in girls in the 6- to 8–year-old age range may be associated with pathology—with excessive adiposity an important factor in many.[204,205,464,566] Those with rapidly progressive precocity benefit from GnRHag therapy.[567-569]

On the other hand, many girls in this age range have slowly progressive precocity—with a normal timing of menarche—and are not at risk of short adult stature. Such girls achieve no increase in stature from GnRHag therapy.[503,569,570] We conclude that a less comprehensive investigation may be warranted in selected girls presenting with thelarche between 6 and 8 years of age. For most such girls, a complete history and physical exam (including obesity evaluation and a bone age determination) may be all that is needed—along with careful longitudinal follow-up.[472,503,570] However, 6- to 8-year-old girls with a suggestion of rapidly progressive or excessive androgenization or feminization, neurologic symptoms, linear growth acceleration, or significant bone age advancement should be more completely evaluated (as outlined previously).

Management

The guidelines for management are to rule out an organic disorder that requires treatment in and of itself and to ascertain whether sexual precocity is either rapidly compromising height potential or resulting in important secondary emotional disturbances in the child. Intracranial lesions must be treated by appropriate measures, such as neurosurgery or irradiation. Shunting for hydrocephalus may stop the precocity. Granulosa cell tumors confined to the ovary have a good prognosis for cure by unilateral oophorectomy. Recurrence of tumor may occur up to 20 years after the initial operation, however. Biopsy of the opposite ovary is indicated in unilateral ovarian neoplasms. Compensatory ovarian hypertrophy can be expected at any age after removal of a single ovary.[571]

The only permanent physical complication of true isosexual precocity, all else being normal, is short adult height. Excessive sex hormone production in the first decade of life causes early maturation of the epiphyses, resulting in their premature closure. About half the girls with this disorder reach an adult height of 53 to 59 inches, and the remainder are more than 60 inches tall.[484,503] The mismatch between physical, hormonal, and psychological development may cause behavior changes ranging from social withdrawal to aggression or sexuality. However, frank behavioral problems are unusual in girls and are therefore by themselves seldom indications for treatment.

TABLE 14-6

Laboratory Criteria for Rapidly Progressive Complete Precocious Puberty

- Sex hormone level pubertal (diurnal early)
  - Estrogen (girls, cyclical): $E_2 > 9$ pg/mL, vaginal cornification
  - Testosterone (boys): 20–1200 ng/dL
  - DHEAS normal for age > height age >
- Sex hormone excess is sustained:
  - Bone age > height age > chronologic age
- LH and FSH pubertal
  - Sleep-associated LH rise initiates puberty
  - Basal: LH.0.6 and FSH.2.0 IU/L or more (monoclonal RIA)[a]
  - Post-GnRH LH>4.2 IU/L[a]
- Exclude: tumor, hypothyroidism, gonadotropin-independent precocity

---

[a]. Exact values vary among laboratories.
DHEAS, dehydroepiandrosterone sulfate; E2, estradiol; FSH, follicle-stimulating hormone; GnRH, gonadotropin-releasing hormone; LH, luteinizing hormone; and RIA, radioimmunoassay.

When true sexual precocity is rapidly progressive to the point of significantly compromising height potential and its cause cannot be directly alleviated, the best mode of treatment is with GnRH agonists. The down-regulating effect of these agents on pituitary gonadotropin release inhibits gonadotropin secretion. Suggested criteria for the use of these drugs are presented in Table 14-7.[561] The most widely used agents in the United States are leuprolide acetate (ordinarily given as Lupron depot/ped 7.5–15 mg/mo IM) and nafarelin acetate (Synarel 800 μg bid IN). A long-acting histrelin implant was recently introduced.[571a] These doses are larger than the usual adult dosage in order to avoid worsening the status by an agonist effect. Dosage can be adjusted later as necessary. It is unclear whether the longer-acting depot forms of leuprolide are as effective.[572]

Treatment is adequate if the estradiol level becomes prepubertal[573] or LH is below 6.6 U/L 2 hours after GnRH agonist[574] 1 month after institution of therapy. A withdrawal period may occur at that time, but none should be expected thereafter. Puberty and the pubertal growth spurt are arrested. Concomitantly, epiphyseal closure is delayed and adult height potential is improved because a type of catch-up growth occurs in which height age catches up to bone age. Adult height is greatest when treatment is started soon after onset at an early age, yielding an average height gain above pretreatment height prediction of about 1.4 cm for each year of therapy.[503, 568,569] Prolonging treatment beyond a chronological or bone age of 12.0-12.5 years of age generally leads to little further increase in adult height potential, regardless of the prediction of residual height potential from bone age.

Coincident GH-deficiency must be treated for optimal growth.[575] GH-sufficient patients with central precocity who are started on treatment relatively late and whose height velocity falls below the prepubertal normal range after 2 to 3 years appear to gain an average of 2 cm per year when GH therapy is added.[576] Treatment is ordinarily continued until the normal age for puberty to begin.[568]

TABLE 14-7

Suggested Indications for Gonadotropin-Releasing Hormone Agonist Therapy of Precocious Puberty

Complete precocious puberty
Pubertal sex hormone levels (in sensitive assays)
plus
    Abnormal height potential
    (predicted adult height falling significantly or below 5th
       percentile)
or
    Psychosocial considerations, individualized
    Menses in the mentally or emotionally immature
    Other (e.g., behavioral or emotional disturbance)

Modified from Rosenfield RL (1994). Selection of children with precocious puberty for treatment with gonadotropin releasing hormone analogs. J Pediatr 124:989.

Use of the depot form of GnRH agonist is complicated by sterile abscesses at injection sites in about 5% of cases. Anaphylaxis is a rare complication.[577] No other serious side effects have come to light, but long-term safety remains to be established. The potential risk of bone demineralization has not proven to materialize after GnRH agonist therapy of precocious puberty.[504]

Girls with slowly progressive idiopathic puberty of onset between 6 and 8 years of age or early fast puberty between 8 and 9 years of age tend to be tall at the onset of puberty, follow an advanced growth pattern, and reach their target height without GnRH agonist therapy.[503,570,579-581] Therefore, this treatment is only indicated if there are other compelling reasons to slow the pace of puberty. Those who are obese may have slower pace of puberty if insulin resistance is ameliorated.[581a]

Medroxyprogesterone acetate (Depo-Provera) is useful for stopping menses and as a contraceptive in mentally retarded girls in whom preservation of height potential is not important. It is begun in a dosage commencing at 50 mg/month intramuscularly. Doses as high as 400 mg/month have been used, although Cushingoid side effects may be observed at this level.[582] Although this treatment reverses some of the physical changes of premature puberty, it does not reverse the inordinately rapid maturation of the skeleton—possibly because of its inherently weak androgenicity. In addition, use of medroxyprogesterone acetate is associated with a loss of bone mineral density—which must be considered if long-term use is being contemplated.[583]

A variety of drugs have been used off-label to treat gonadotropin-independent precocity. Antiestrogen and aromatase treatment for McCune-Albright syndrome has met with varying degrees of success.[584,585] Ketoconazole, an antifungal agent that inhibits 17,20-lyase activity and other steroidogenic enzymes, has been used to treat a similar condition in boys[586] and might be useful in girls as well. Gonadotropin-releasing hormone agonist treatment may be necessary for those in whom true puberty becomes superimposed because the bone age has reached a pubertal level.[194,195,587] The fibrous dysplasia of McCune-Albright syndrome may be amenable to treatment with bisphosphonates,[588,589] although this is not a suitable long-term treatment in childhood.[590]

Patients with premature thelarche or pubarche as variations of normal are counseled as follows. The child's early development seems to be a matter of a normal stage of puberty occurring early. It is due to an incomplete slow type of puberty or to increased sensitivity to the trace levels of hormones normally present in childhood. Feminization with breast development and eventual menstruation can be expected to occur at an appropriate age. No treatment is indicated. To exclude subtle sex hormone excess or eventual anovulatory syndromes, long-term follow-up is advisable.

In addition to dealing with the physical consequences of true isosexual precocity, the physician must be ready to help the family and child cope with the psychological problems that come with early physical maturation. The doctor can help the family by explaining that even though their child looks older and more mature than other children of the same age the child will not behave more maturely. The libido of young children with precocity is not increased. The family should be advised to take some precautions to downplay their child's development (for example, in the choice of clothing and swimsuits). Friendships with children a bit older will help shorten the time affected children spend in social limbo. This may be more easily said than done, however, because the intellectual and social maturity of these patients is not advanced. Early on, any children with these disorders tend to be withdrawn because they feel that they are different from their peers. Later on, they tend to enter into romantic relationships early. It is important to remind the family and child that in a few years the child will not be unique from the standpoint of sexual development.[484] The following books may be helpful in explaining precocious puberty: for children, *What's Happening to Me?*, by Peter Mayle (Lyle Stuart, Inc., Secaucus, NJ, 1973); for parents, *Sex Errors of the Body, Second Edition*, by John Money (Paul H. Brookes Publishing Co., Inc., Baltimore, MD, 1994).

HYPOGONADISM

Causes

If hypogonadism is complete and present prepubertally, it causes sexual infantilism in females or disorders of sexual differentiation in genetic males. If it is slightly less severe or of onset in the early teenage years, it may permit too limited a degree of feminization to permit the onset of menses at a normal age (primary amenorrhea). Milder, partial, or incomplete forms of hypogonadism may cause secondary amenorrhea or oligomenorrhea.[489a]

At its mildest, hypogonadism may present with the anovulatory symptoms of dysfunctional uterine bleeding or with excessively frequent periods due to short luteal phase. Consequently, disorders causing hypogonadism appear in the differential diagnosis of disorders of sexual differentiation, sexual infantilism, failure of pubertal progression, and menstrual irregularity. The causes of hypogonadism are listed in the differential diagnosis of amenorrhea in Table 14-8.

Primary Ovarian Failure. Primary ovarian failure is characterized by high levels of gonadotropins, particularly FSH. Two exceptions exist to this rule. First, the gonadotropins may not be elevated until CNS maturation has reached a pubertal stage—as indicated by a bone age of approximately 10 to 11 years (Table 14-9).[591] Second, patients with partial ovarian failure (as is frequent in women during the menopausal transition) do not have high baseline gonadotropin levels.[592-594] FSH may hyperrespond to GnRH and estrogen may hyporespond to GnRH agonist challenge. It seems as if relatively few ovarian follicles (too few to permit the cyclic emergence of preovulatory follicles) suffice to prevent the characteristic rise in basal FSH levels.

Primary ovarian failure may occur before or during puberty (causing primary amenorrhea) or after puberty has occurred, causing secondary amenorrhea. The latter is termed *premature ovarian failure* and resembles premature menopause except that about half of cases sometimes ovulate.[595,596]

TABLE 14-8

Differential Diagnosis of Amenorrhea

Abnormal Genital Structure
- Ambiguous genitalia
  - Intersex
  - Pseudointersex
- Aplasia[α]
  - Hymenal
  - Vaginal
  - Müllerian
  - Intersex
- Endometrial atrophy

Anovulatory Disorders
Hypoestrogenism, FSH Elevated
- Primary ovarian failure
  - Congenital
    - Gonadal dysgenesis
    - Steroidogenic blocks
    - Resistant ovaries
  - Acquired
    - Oophorectomy
    - Oophoritis
    - Radiotherapy or chemotherapy
- Bioinactive gonadotropin

Hypoestrogenism, FSH Not Elevated
- Primary ovarian failure
  - Complete if BA <11 yr[α]
  - Incomplete if BA >11 yr
- Delayed puberty
  - Constitutional delay[α]
  - Growth-retarding disease
- Hypogonadotropic hypogonadism
  - Congenital
  - Acquired
    - Organic
    - Functional
  - Virilization

Estrogenized, FSH Not Elevated
- Hypothalamic anovulation
  - Hypothalamic amenorrhea
  - Athletic/psychogenic amenorrhea
  - Post-pill amenorrhea
- Nonhypothalamic extraovarian disorders
  - Pregnancy
  - Obesity or undernutrition
  - Cushing syndrome
  - Hypothyroidism
  - Hyperprolactinemia
  - Ectopic gonadotropin secretion
- Hyperandrogenism

---

[a]. Cause only primary amenorrhea.
BA, bone age; and FSH, follicle-stimulating hormone.

Gonadal dysgenesis due to deficiency of genes on the X-chromosome is the most common cause of primary ovarian failure. It is usually due to a relatively large scale deletion of X-chromosomal material, which is associated with a characteristic, but variable, phenotype and is termed Turner syndrome (see Chapter 15). Fetuses with a 45,X karyotype have a normal number of oocytes in the ovary at mid-gestation, but a drastic reduction in the number of follicles,[30] which appears to cause gonadal

TABLE 14-9

Bone Age in Workup of Sexually Infantile Girls with Normal Follicle-Stimulating Hormone Level

	Bone Age (Years)		
	<11	11–13	>13
Primary hypogonadism	Yes		
Delayed puberty	Yes	Yes	
Gonadotropin deficiency	Yes	Yes	Yes

Based on Rosenfield RL, Barnes RB (1993). Menstrual disorders in adolescence. Endocrinol Metab Clin North Am 22:491.

streaks via an accelerated rate of apoptosis. However, the gonadal dysgenesis (like other features of the syndrome) is often incompletely expressed.[596] Thus, Turner syndrome should be considered in all girls with primary hypogonadism or secondary amenorrhea whether or not they have the typical stigmata of Turner syndrome

Specific loci on the X-chromosome are associated with primary ovarian failure. Xp11.2 harbors BMP15, a specific ovarian differentiation factor, a heterozygous mutation of which is a rare cause of gonadal dysgenesis. Xq harbors two independent loci in addition to the fragile X premutation, which is associated with about 7-14% of primary ovarian failure.[595,596] Other genes have been incriminated in the ovarian failure of mouse models.[597]

Gonadal dysgenesis also results from 46, XY complete gonadal dysgenesis and certain forms of autosomal aneuploidy.[432,595,598] A variable degree of ovarian dysgenesis occurs in autosomal trisomy 21. Delayed menarche, anovulatory cycles, and primary gonadal failure are occasionally seen.[599] However, pregnancy has been reported. Trisomic offspring are common.[600] Oocytes are virtually absent in trisomies 13 and 18. Ovarian dysgenesis also occasionally occurs as part of the Denys-Drash syndrome due to a WT-1 mutation.[601] There are associations of primary ovarian failure with cerebellar ataxia.[602,26] Other autosomal genetic disorders causing premature ovarian failure include blepharophimosis, galactosemia, leukodystrophies, and myotonia dystrophica.[597,604]

Physical or medical destructive injury to the ovary is a common cause of primary ovarian failure. *Irradiation and chemotherapy* for childhood neoplasia are becoming increasingly frequent causes of primary ovarian failure now that life is effectively prolonged.[604,605] Ionizing radiation and alkylating agents damage DNA whether or not a cell is replicating.[606] A radiation dose of 20 Gy or more to the ovaries causes acute ovarian failure in about 85% of children and adolescents.[607] A cumulative cyclophosphamide dose of about 100 mg/kg causes equivalent damage. Fertility is even more rare when these modalities are combined. Prepubertal girls are about half as sensitive to these therapies as postpubertal females: among girls who receive 1-10 Gy, acute ovarian failure develops in about 10% of girls under 13 years, but in 25% of those ≥13. After prepubertal chemotherapy and radiotherapy for leukemia, half of patients can be anticipated to enter puberty and menstruate regularly, and one-quarter to have normal pituitary-ovarian function 7 years later.[608] Some with early

hypergonadotropinism will experience ovarian recovery. However, all will develop premature menopause because of the reduced number of oocytes. Several non-alkylating chemotherapies are also gonadotoxic.[609,610] However, data are scarce and the interactions among various classes of chemotherapeutic agents is poorly understood. As a consequence of gonadotropin elevation when gonadal failure begins, puberty may progress rapidly.[516]

Sterilization by irradiation can be obviated by transposing the ovaries out of the irradiation field if possible. Administration of a GnRH agonist prior to cyclophosphamide administration may decrease ovarian injury.[606] Mumps oophoritis is a classic but rare cause of ovarian failure.

Functional ovarian failure can arise from autosomal-recessive ovarian mutations of the LH or FSH receptor.[595,603,611,612] These have been associated with a spectrum of defects ranging from primary amenorrhea to oligomenorrhea. Ovarian histology in typical resistance to gonadotropin action (Savage syndrome) shows a normal number of primordial follicles but a paucity of growing follicles. Partial gonadotropin resistance is common in the Albright osteodystrophy form of pseudohypoparathyroidism, in association with the generalized defect in G-protein signal transduction.[613] The carbohydrate-deficient glycoprotein syndrome reduces gonadotropin bioactivity and causes hypergonadotropic hypogonadism.[614]

Autoimmune oophoritis is the basis of approximately half of spontaneous premature ovarian failure,[618] *though estimates* vary from 5-85% in *various series*.[595,615,616] It is diagnosed by its association with any of a variety of autoimmune endocrine or nonendocrine disorders, manifest or subclinical, that have in common defects in T cell suppressor function. Autoimmunity may be directed against the granulose cell, oocyte, or theca cell. The clinical picture may resemble relatively selective resistance to FSH or, less frequently, to LH.[617] The latter results from lymphocytic infiltration of theca with sparing of primordial follicles. These patients have autoantibodies to steroidogenic cells and have or are at risk for adrenal failure. Usually these antibodies are directed against 21-hydroxylase, less frequently to side chain cleavage or 17-hydroxylase, seldom to 3β-hydroxysteroid dehydrogenase. Replacement glucocorticoid therapy may temporarily ameliorate the immune oophoritis in such cases.[618] A case with autoantibodies to testosterone has been reported.[619] Autoimmune gene regulator (AIRE) gene mutations have been identified as causative of type 1 polyendocrine failure. Ultrasonographic and histologic findings are variable in premature ovarian failure and include large or small ovaries, inactive or polyfollicular ovaries, loss or preservation of primordial follicles, and infiltration by lymphocytes or plasma cells.

Functional gonadal failure can also result from specific autosomal-recessive defects in the biosynthesis of androgens and estrogens (or aromatase deficiency, a virilizing disorder). Enzyme blocks can cause gonadal insufficiency in genetic males who are phenotypic females. This occurs in lipoid congenital adrenal hyperplasia (StAR and side chain cleavage mutations, Figure 14-23), 17α-hydroxylase deficiency, 17,20-lyase deficiency, 3β-HSI deficiency, and

17β-HSD3 deficiency. All but the latter are associated with congenital adrenal hyperplasia. Congenital lipoid adrenal hyperplasia is unique in that underlying StAR deficiency has too little direct impact on ovarian function to interfere with the early phases of puberty. However, the gradual buildup of intraovarian lipid deposits resulting from enzyme deficiency (a "second hit") causes ovarian damage with anovulation and late ovarian failure.[620,621]

Gonadotropin Deficiency. Congenital gonadotropin deficiency can occur in association with cerebral, hypothalamic, or pituitary dysfunction or as an isolated defect.[622] Congenital defects in hypothalamic-hypophyseal formation may be associated with midline facial defects. Congenital hypothalamic dysfunction may be associated with other neurologic or endocrine dysfunction, such as in the Prader-Willi syndrome (congenital hypotonia and neonatal failure to thrive followed by hypothalamic obesity, sometimes with hypopituitarism) or the Laurence-Moon-Biedl syndrome (retinitis pigmentosa, obesity, mental deficiency). The autosomal-recessive form of congenital combined pituitary hormone deficiency due to PROP1 mutation is associated with gonadotropin deficiency. Leptin- and leptin-receptor-inactivating mutations cause gonadotropin deficiency in combination with extreme obesity.

Gonadotropin deficiency may be associated with anosmia (olfactory-genital dysplasia or Kallmann syndrome).[182] This syndrome is one-fifth as frequent in females as in males.[623] Mutations in the KAL-1 gene on the pseudoautosomal region of the X-chromosome cause the X-linked form, are highly penetrant, and account for 10% of cases. This mutation causes deficiency of anosmin-1. Inactivating mutation of the fibroblast growth factor receptor-1c isoform accounts for another 10% of cases, and these are inherited as an autosomal-dominant trait with variable penetrance and occasional association with cleft palate and facial defects. FGFR-1c signaling has been hypothesized to occur at least in part through anosmin-1.

Isolated gonadotropin deficiency arises from GnRH receptor mutations in about half of autosomal recessively inherited cases.[624] Partial gonadotropin deficiency can rarely result from mutation of the G-protein–coupled receptor GPR54.[186] The degree of hypogonadism is variable, even within a family, with delayed puberty and delayed menarche as one presentation.[625-627] Isolated hypogonadotropic hypogonadism has also been reported in a woman homozygous for a nonsense mutation of the X-linked DAX1 gene, which was associated with adrenal insufficiency in her brothers.[628] Isolated FSH deficiency due to mutation in the β-subunit has been reported to cause primary amenorrhea in association with a unique test panel of low FSH, elevated LH, and low testosterone levels.

Acquired gonadotropin deficiency can be a consequence of tumors, trauma, autoimmune hypophysitis,[629,630] degenerative disorders involving the hypothalamus and pituitary,[631] irradiation,[632] or chronic illness.[633] Pituitary adenoma, craniopharyngioma, and dysgerminoma are the most common neuroendocrine neoplasms responsible in children. Most "nonfunctioning" pituitary adenomas are gonadotrope adenomas that secrete gonadotropin subunits in response to thyrotropin-releasing hormone.[634] A case of hypothalamic tumor is presented

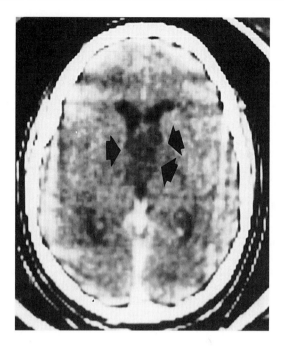

Figure 14-39 Computed tomography of the brain of a 16-year-old girl with hypothalamic astrocytoma. The low-density tumor mass (arrows) extends superiorly from the hypothalamus, obliterates the third ventricle, and partially compresses the frontal horns of the lateral ventricles (particularly the right). This patient presented with secondary amenorrhea. Menarche had occurred at age 13, and menses were normal until 15.3 years. The patient then became amenorrheic in association with ethargy, episodic headaches, polyuria, and weight gain—despite little change in appetite. Physical examination was negative. The skull radiograph, electroencephalogram, visual fields, and serum prolactin and thyroxine levels were normal—and urine-specific gravity was 1.016. After biopsy of the cyst wall, studies revealed her to have gonadotropin, growth hormone, and partial antidiuretic hormone deficiencies.

with Figure 14-39. Pinealomas most commonly cause sexual infantilism. They may act by secreting an inhibitory substance, rather than by compressing key areas of the hypothalamus.[514]

Anorexia nervosa is the prototypic form of eating disorder, a common cause of hypogonadotropinism in teenagers. It is a syndrome of undernutrition due to voluntary starvation with a particular psychological dysfunction that results in amenorrhea.[635-637] Patients uniformly consider themselves too fat in the face of objective evidence that they are underweight. The psychiatric criteria that distinguish this disorder from food faddism and fear of obesity consist of refusal to gain or maintain body weight to a minimally normal level for height and age (less than the 15th percentile; body mass index ≤ 17.5 for postmenarcheal cases) with all of the following being present: intense fear of gaining weight or becoming fat, even though underweight; an inaccurate perception of body weight, such that they have a disturbance in the way that body weight, size, or shape is experienced; undue influence of body shape and weight on self-evaluation or denial of the seriousness of current low body weight; and amenorrhea for 3 or more months in postmenarcheal females.

Bulimia nervosa, the binge-eating/purging variant eating disorder, is similar in the overevaluation of body shape and weight and the use of extreme weight control behaviors. Physical activity tends to be high. These disorders may be manifest at an early stage as atypical eating disorders, before weight or amenorrhea criteria are met or when the binge is subjective. The cognitive defect that weight can serve as the predominant value in judging self-worth is central to anorexia nervosa. In contrast to other depressive individuals, these patients are generally content with themselves in the areas of intellectual and vocational achievement.

The pathogenesis is multifactorial. It involves a genetic predisposition. Concordance rates for the anorexic type are about 50% for monozygous twins, compared with about 5% for dizygotic twins. Many other risk factors have been implicated. Familial factors also include eating disorders of any type, depression, substance abuse, and adverse family interactions. Premorbid experiences (such as sexual abuse or social pressures) or premorbid characteristics (such as low self-esteem, compulsiveness, and perfectionism) are also important. Dieting meets a need for approval in our culture, with its emphasis on dietary restriction and thinness as goals for women. Anorexia is often precipitated in vulnerable children by a new experience (such as puberty, leaving home, or beginning college) or by adverse life events. The disorder is perpetuated by the complications of starvation, such as depression and reduced gastric emptying.

The onset tends to be at 12 years of age or later. Earlier onset is associated with growth arrest, delay of puberty, and primary amenorrhea.[638] GH deficiency is common.[639,640] The medical complications of anorexia nervosa are serious. The risk of death is approximately tenfold increased. Electrolyte imbalance, hypoglycemia, cardiovascular instability, bone marrow hypocellularity predisposing to silent infection, and renal failure account for about half of the mortality. Suicide accounts for the rest.

The weight changes leading to cessation or restoration of menstrual cycles are in the range of 10% to 15% of body weight. Recovery is associated with achieving a critical level of body fat stores above the 10th percentile (>20% body fat) (Figure 14-40) at a BMI averaging 20.[641,642] There is an inverse relationship between body

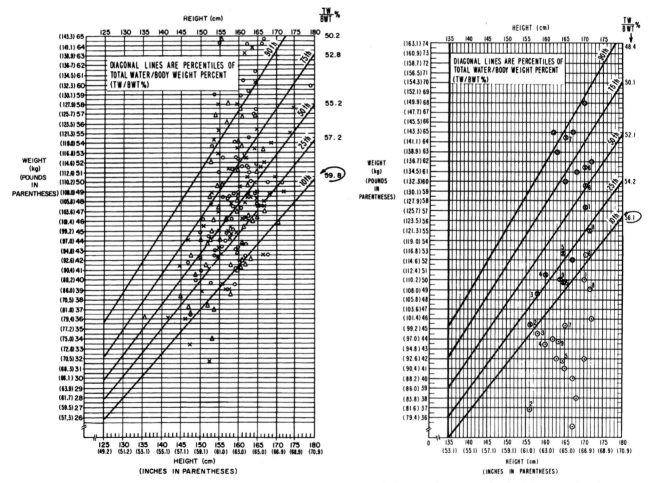

Figure 14-40 Percentiles of fatness (diagonal lines) for white girls at menarche (left) and after menarche (right) equated with computed percentiles of total water as a percentage of total body weight. The minimal weight necessary at a particular height for the onset or maintenance of menses is very close to the 10th percentile of fatness on these respective charts. Data for anorexia nervosa cases are shown on the right-hand chart: • at presentation; x at resumption of menses. [From Frisch RE, McArthur JW (1974). Menstrual cycles: Fatness as a determinant of minimum weight for height necessary for their maintenance or onset. Science 185:949. Copyright © by the American Association for the Advancement of Science.]

weight and the maturity of gonadotropin release in these patients. The 24-hour pattern of gonadotropin release tends to be immature (prepubertal or pubertal), and the diurnal LH pattern becomes mature upon recovery from undernutrition.[643] Luteinizing hormone pulsatility is low, and may be restored by opiate antagonists.[88] The gonadotropin response to GnRH and ovulatory response to clomiphene citrate are blunted in the malnourished state and become normal with weight gain to about 80% of ideal.[644,645] Leptin levels are significantly decreased and are a major contributor to the gonadotropin deficiency and to changes in the thyroid and GH axes.[646]

Mild hypercortisolism is frequent and may contribute to the anovulation by mechanisms discussed further under the section on hypothalamic anovulation.[647] Afternoon ACTH and cortisol levels are significantly higher than normal, and the response to CRH is significantly lower than normal. In contrast to Cushing syndrome, DHEAS levels tend to be blunted as a consequence of undernutrition.[648]

A fundamental neuropsychological flaw or hypothalamic disturbance[649] seems necessary to explain the high incidence of GH deficiency, why some patients become amenorrheic before losing weight, and why about half of the cases remain amenorrheic after treatment. The serotonergic systems implicated in the regulation of feeding and mood seem to remain altered even after weight restoration. The authors favor the concept that these psychological problems lead to amenorrhea only in women predisposed to it by a unique preexisting hypothalamic dysfunction. Evidence has recently been obtained for marked individual differences in reactivity of the neuroendocrine system to stress.[650]

A number of features attributed to hypothalamic dysfunction, such as cold intolerance, may be due to the subtle hypothyroid state secondary to the malnutrition.[647] Serum triiodothyronine levels are consistently low, serum thyroxine levels tend to be lower than average (although usually within normal limits), the pattern of TSH release indicates TRH deficiency, and the state of deep tendon reflexes and metabolism is consistent with hypothyroidism. Hypothyroidism may in part complicate malnutrition as a consequence of the interference with IGF-1 generation. Low IGF-I initiates GH excess, compensatory somatostatin release, and subsequent inhibition of the thyrotropin response to thyrotropin-releasing hormone. Undernutrition also diverts the generation of thyroxine metabolites away from triiodothyronine toward reverse triiodothyronine.

Hyperprolactinemia can cause functional gonadotropin deficiency.[651] Galactorrhea is present in about half of the patients, particularly those with residual estrogen production. The causes of hyperprolactinemia are diverse, including hypothalamic or pituitary disorders, drugs, hypothyroidism, renal or liver failure, peripheral neuropathy, stress, autoimmunity, macroprolactinemia, and idiopathology.[652-654] Elevated serum prolactin levels occur with a variety of tumors that cause functional or anatomic pituitary stalk section, thereby preventing inhibitory pituitary control. About a third of hyperprolactinemic women have an identifiable pituitary adenoma. Prolactinomas less than 1 cm in diameter (microadenomas) cause no problems due to local extension. Prolactinoma may be associated with multiple endocrine neoplasia type 1.[655] In about a quarter of adult cases, the malfunction is due to the ingestion of drugs such as phenothiazines, estrogen, or cocaine.[656] Considerable hyperprolactinemia is idiopathic. Decreased sensitivity to dopaminergic inhibition may underlie such cases.[657]

Macroprolactinemia is due to a variant molecule or autoantibody formation. In this situation, direct immunoassay indicates elevated levels of prolactin. However, the biologically available or active prolactin level is normal. Thus, there is no physiologic consequence to the macroprolactinemia.

Hyperprolactinemia results in luteinizing hormone pulses that tend to be infrequent and LH secretion that is variable in response to GnRH.[658] Selective prolactin excess causes variable degrees of gonadotropin deficiency, ranging from severe to partial (hypothalamic amenorrhea). Adrenal hyperandrogenism, hirsutism, and seborrhea are common.[266] Frank virilization as a result of very high androgen levels suppresses gonadotropin levels and thus causes defeminization. However, the more common moderately hyperandrogenic disorders discussed in material following are associated with normal estrogenization.

Differential Diagnosis

The differential diagnosis of hypogonadism is included in Table 14-8. Investigation should be begun for hypogonadism when the onset of puberty has not begun by the chronologic or bone age of 13 years, if puberty has not progressed as indicated by failure of menses to occur within 4.5 years of the onset of puberty, or if secondary amenorrhea or oligomenorrhea has persisted for 2 years. A family history of delayed puberty is compatible with the delay being constitutional rather than having an organic basis. The history should include a thorough past medical history and systemic review, including systemic, intracranial, visual, olfactory, emotional, abdominal, and pelvic symptoms. It should be kept in mind that chronic endocine, metabolic, or systemic disease of almost any type can lead to delayed puberty.

Upon examining the patient, the height and weight should be carefully measured and growth rate and appropriateness of weight for height determined (Figure 14-40). Careful categorization of the stage of breast and sexual hair development are essential. Examination of the mature breast should include an attempt to express milk from the ducts to the nipple. The finding of a structural genital abnormality may indicate that amenorrhea is due to abnormal genital tract development, whereas clitoromegaly[659] is a clue to a virilizing disorder. Neurologic examination should include evaluation of eye movements, visual fields, and optic fundi—as well as a search for anosmia and midline defects.

An algorithmic approach to the workup of patients with menstrual disorders is shown in Figures 14-41 through 14-43.[660] The laboratory workup depends on the degree of estrogenization, as initially assessed from the stage of breast development. It includes a bone age radiograph in adolescents who are not sexually mature

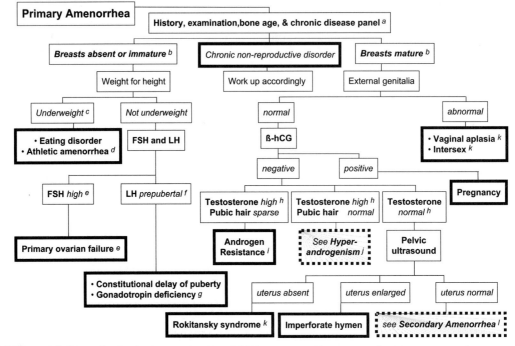

Figure 14-41 Differential diagnosis of primary amenorrhea. (*a*) Prime among the causes of primary amenorrhea are growth-retarding or -attenuating disorders. In the absence of specific symptoms or signs to direct the workup, laboratory assessment for chronic disease typically includes bone age radiograph if the adolescent is not sexually mature and a chronic disease panel (complete blood count and differential, sedimentation rate, comprehensive metabolic panel, celiac panel, thyroid panel, cortisol and insulin-like growth factor-I levels, and urinalysis). (*b*) Breast development ordinarily signifies the onset of pubertal feminization. However, mature breast development does not ensure ongoing pubertal estrogen secretion (see Figure 14-42 and 14-43). (*c*) Underweight is defined as body fat 20% or less of body mass. Although this generally corresponds to BMI < 10th percentile, BMI may not accurately reflect body fat in serious athletes (who have a disproportionately greater muscle mass) or bulimia nervosa. (*d*) Low body fat is associated with amenorrhea in girls underweight (e.g., anorexia nervosa, a symptom complex consisting of amenorrhea, voluntary starvation, and a self-delusional disturbance in the perception of body fatness), not necessarily underweight (bulimia), and from athletic activity out of proportion to caloric intake (serious athletes). (*e*) FSH is preferentially elevated over LH in primary ovarian failure. The most common cause of primary amenorrhea due to primary ovarian failure is gonadal dysgenesis due to Turner syndrome, but acquired causes must be considered (such as cytotoxic therapy). The workup of primary ovarian failure is considered in detail in the next algorithm (Figure 14-42, secondary amenorrhea and oligomenorrhea). Lack of FSH elevation virtually rules out primary ovarian failure only when the bone age is appropriate for puberty (11 years or more). (*f*) A low LH level is more characteristic of delayed puberty and gonadotropin deficiency than a low FSH level. Congenital gonadotropin deficiency is closely mimicked by the more common extreme variation of normal, constitutional delay of puberty (Table 14-10). (*g*) History and examination may yield clues to the cause of hypogonadotropic hypogonadism, such as evidence of hypopituitarism (midline facial defect, extreme short stature) or anosmia (Kallmann's syndrome). Random LH levels in hypogonadotropic patients are typically below 0.15 IU/L, but often overlap those of normal pre- and mid-pubertal children. The GnRH test, measuring the gonadotropin response to a 50- to 100-μg bolus, in the premenarchial teenager strongly suggests gonadotropin deficiency if the LH peak is less than 7.0 IU/L by monoclonal assay. However, the GnRH test has limitations because of overlap between hypogonadotropic and normal teenager responses. GnRH agonist testing (e.g., leuprolide acetate injection 10 μg/kg SC) may discriminate better. It may not be possible to definitively establish the diagnosis of gonadotropin deficiency until puberty fails to begin by 16 years of age. (*h*) Plasma total testosterone is normally about 20 to 60 ng/dL (0.7–2.1 nM), but varies somewhat among laboratories. (*i*) Androgen resistance is characterized by a male plasma testosterone level (when sexual maturation is complete), male karyotype (46, XY), and absent uterus. External genitalia may be ambiguous (partial form) or normal female (complete form). (*j*) The differential diagnosis of hyperandrogenism is shown in Figure 14-46. (*k*) Vaginal aplasia in a girl with normal ovaries may be associated with uterine aplasia (Rokitansky-Kustner-Hauser syndrome). When the vagina is blind and the uterus aplastic, this disorder must be distinguished from androgen resistance. If the external genitalia are ambiguous, it must be distinguished from other disorders of sexual differentiation (intersex). (*l*) Secondary amenorrhea differential diagnosis is presented in Figure 14-42. [Modified with permission from Rosenfield RL (2003). Menstrual disorders and hyperandrogenism in adolescence. In Radovick S, MacGillivray MH (eds.), *Pediatric endocrinology: A practical clinical guide*. Totowa, NJ: Humana Press 451–478.]

and generally begins with a chronic disease panel and determining gonadotropins, estradiol, and testosterone level. A pregnancy test is indicated in a sexually mature adolescent. The diagnostic considerations differ in the anovulatory girl without FSH elevation, depending on whether she is hypoestrogenic or well estrogenized (Table 14-8) (Figures 14-41 and 14-42).

FSH elevation indicates primary ovarian failure (Figures 14-41 and 14-42). Chromosome abnormalities are ordinarily the first consideration because the most common cause is Turner syndrome and its variants. Those individuals with primary ovarian failure that is not due to Turner syndrome and its variants should be investigated for the fragile X premutation.

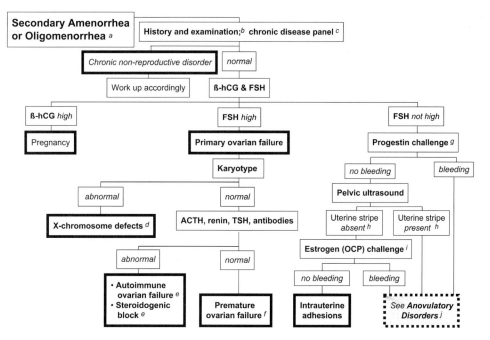

Figure 14-42 Differential diagnosis of secondary amenorrhea or oligomenorrhea. (*a*) Mature secondary sex characteristics are characteristic because the occurrence of menarche indicates a substantial degree of development of the reproductive system. (*b*) Diverse disorders of many systems cause anovulation. The history may reveal excessive exercise, symptoms of depression, gastrointestinal symptoms, radiotherapy to the brain or pelvis, or rapid virilization. Physical findings may include hypertension (forms of congenital adrenal hyperplasia, chronic renal failure), short stature (hypopituitarism, Turner syndrome, pseudohypoparathyroidism), abnormal weight for height (anorexia nervosa, obesity), decreased sense of smell (Kallmann's syndrome), optic disc or visual field abnormality (pituitary tumor), cutaneous abnormalities (neurofibromatosis, lupus), goiter, galactorrhea, hirsutism, or abdominal mass. (*c*) In the absence of specific symptoms or signs to direct the workup, evaluation for chronic disease in a sexually mature adolescent typically includes complete blood count and differential, sedimentation rate, comprehensive metabolic panel, celiac panel, thyroid panel, cortisol and insulin-like growth factor-I levels, and urinalysis. (*d*) Patients missing only a small portion of an X-chromosome may not have the Turner syndrome phenotype. Indeed, among 45,X patients the classic Turner syndrome phenotype is found in less than one-third (with the exception of short stature in 99%). Ovarian function is sufficient for about 10% to undergo some spontaneous pubertal development and for 5% to experience menarche. If chromosomal studies are normal and there is no obvious explanation for the hypogonadism, special studies for fragile X premutation and autoimmune oophoritis should be considered. (*e*) Autoimmune ovarian failure may be associated with tissue-specific antibodies and autoimmune endocrinopathies such as chronic autoimmune throiditis, diabetes, adrenal insufficiency, and hypoparathyroidism. Nonendocrine autoimmune disorders may occur, such as mucocutaneous candidiasis, celiac disease, and chronic hepatitis. Rare gene mutations causing ovarian insufficiency include steroidogenic defects that affect mineralocorticoid status (17-hydroxylase deficiency is associated with mineralocorticoid excess and lipoid adrenal hyperplasia with mineralocorticoid deficiency) and mutations of the gonadotropins or their receptors. Ovarian biopsy is of no prognostic or therapeutic significance. (*f*) The history may provide a diagnosis (e.g., cancer chemotherapy or radiotherapy). Other acquired causes include surgery and autoimmunity. Chromosomal causes of premature ovarian failure include X-chromosome fragile site and point mutations. Other genetic causes include gonadotropin-resistance syndromes such as LH or FSH receptor mutation and pseudohypoparathyroidism. A pelvic ultrasound that shows preservation of ovarian follicles carries some hope for fertility. (*g*) Withdrawal bleeding in response to a 5- to 10-day course of progestin (e.g., medroxyprogesterone acetate 10 mg HS) suggests an overall estradiol level greatert than 40 pg/mL. However, this is not entirely reliable and thus in the interest of making a timely diagnosis it is often worthwhile to proceed to further studies. (*h*) A thin uterine stripe suggests hypoestrogenism. A thick one suggests endometrial hyperplasia, as may occur in polycystic ovary syndrome. (*i*) A single cycle of an OCP containing 30 to 35 μg ethinyl estradiol generally suffices to induce withdrawal bleeding if the endometrial lining is intact. (*j*) The differential diagnosis of other anovulatory disorders continues in Figure 14-43. [Modified with permission from Rosenfield RL (2003). Menstrual disorders and hyperandrogenism in adolescence. In Radovick S, MacGillivray MH (eds.), *Pediatric endocrinology: A practical clinical guide*. Totowa, NJ: Humana Press 451–478.]

Lack of FSH elevation in a prepubertal patient does not rule out primary ovarian failure if bone age is below 11 years because neuroendocrine puberty may not have occurred, in which case primary ovarian failure is not hypergonadotropic (Table 14-9).[591] If gonadotropins are not elevated and bone age has reached 11 years, in a prepubertal girl without a growth-attenuating or growth-retarding disorder one is dealing with constitutional delay of puberty or isolated gonadotropin deficiency (Figure 14-41). "Constitutional" delay of puberty is the most likely diagnosis until the bone age reaches 11 to 13 years

(Table 14-9).[591] Its distinction from isolated gonadotropin deficiency may be difficult.

The features that help to distinguish it from isolated gonadotropin deficiency are listed in Table 14-10 and discussed in the footnotes to Figure 14-41. The single most useful test is the LH level in response to GnRH testing because random LH levels in hypogonadotropic patients often overlap those of pre- and midpubertal normal children.[95] GnRH agonist testing may discriminate between these disorders better[81] and adds the dimension of assessing the gonadal secretory response to the secreted

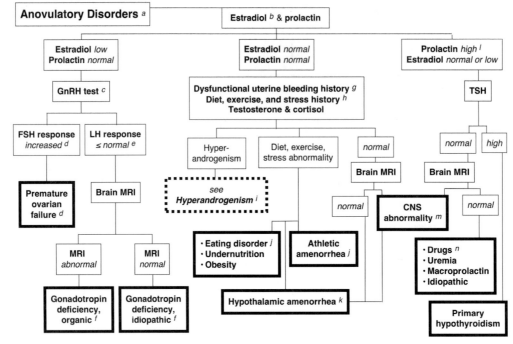

Figure 14-43 Differential diagnosis of anovulatory disorders. (*a*) Anovulatory disorders should be considered in any girl with unexplained amenorrhea or oligomenorrhea, irregular menstrual bleeding, short cycles, or excessive menstrual bleeding. The workup should be initiated as indicated in Figure 14-42, including history and examination, a chronic disease panel, pregnancy test, and gonadotropin levels. (*b*) Once breast development has matured, the breast contour does not substantially regress when hypoestrogenism develops. Hypoestrogenism is suggested if plasma estradiol is persistently <40 pg/mL in an assay sensitive to <10 pg/mL. However, a single estradiol level may be misleading because of cyclic or episodic variations. (*c*) Baseline gonadotropin levels may not be low in gonadotropin-deficient patients, especially according to polyclonal antibody-based assays. Gonadotropin-releasing hormone (GnRH) testing is usually performed by assaying LH and FSH before and 0.5 hour after the administration of 1 mcg/kg GnRH intravenously. GnRH agonist testing may alternatively be performed by administering 10 mcg/kg leuprolide acetate subcutaneously and assaying LH and FSH at 4 hours to assess gonadotropin reserve and at 24 hours to assess the ovarian steroid response to endogenous gonadotropin release. (*d*) Baseline gonadotropin levels may be normal as the ovary begins to fail, as in menopause, but an exaggerated FSH response to GnRH and subnormal E2 response to the gonadotropin elevation induced by acute GnRH agonist challenge are characteristic. The further workup is shown in Figure 14-42. (*e*) Responses to GnRH may vary from nil to normal in gonadotropin deficiency. Normal LH and FSH responses in the presence of hypoestrogenism indicate inadequate compensatory hypothalamic GnRH secretion. (*f*) Gonadotropin deficiency may be congenital or acquired, organic or functional. Congenital causes include midline brain malformations or specific genetic disorders such as Prader-Willi syndrome, Laurence-Moon-Biedl syndrome, or Kallmann syndrome. Kallmann's, the association of anosmia with gonadotropin deficiency, occurs in both the X-linked and autosomal-recessive forms. Special MRI views often demonstrate absence of the olfactory tracts. Acquired gonadotropin deficiency may be secondary to a variety of organic CNS disorders, varying from hypothalamic-pituitary tumor to radiation damage to empty sella syndrome. Autoimmune hypophysitis is a rare disorder, sometimes accompanying a polyendocrine deficiency syndrome. The prototypic form of functional gonadotropin deficiency is anorexia nervosa. Idiopathic hypogonadotropic deficiency may sometimes occur in families with anosmia, suggesting a relationship to Kallmann's syndrome. (*g*) Dysfunctional uterine bleeding or menorrhagia not controlled by progestin or OCP therapy additionally requires a pelvic ultrasound examination (for genital tract tumor or feminizing tumor), coagulation workup (which includes platelet count, prothrombin time, thromboplastin generation test, and bleeding time), and consideration of the possibility of sexual abuse. (*h*) The equivalent of 4 miles per day or more is generally required before body fat stores fall to the point where amenorrhea occurs. Physical or psychosocial stress may cause amenorrhea. (*i*) Hyperandrogenism differential diagnosis is outlined in Figure 14-46. (*j*) Mild forms of stress disorders associated with low body fat (anorexia nervosa, bulimia nervosa, and athletic amenorrhea) may cause acquired hypothalamic amenorrhea rather than frank gonadotropin deficiency. The low body fat content of athletic amenorrhea may not be reflected by weight for height because of high muscularity. Dual-photon absorptiometry scan may be useful in documenting body fat below 20%. Patients with anorexia nervosa may become amenorrheic before or when weight loss begins, indicating an important psychological component to the etiology. Obesity is also associated with anovulatory cycles. (*k*) Hypothalamic amenorrhea is a diagnosis of exclusion. It is a form of partial gonadotropin deficiency in which baseline estrogen secretion is normal but a preovulatory LH surge cannot be generated. It may result from organic CNS disorders. Functional hypothalamic amenorrhea may be stress or undernutrition related or idiopathic. It may be secondary to chronic illness or result from obesity or diverse types of endocrine dysfunction. Research studies show subnormal LH pulsatility or estrogen induceability of the LH surge. (*l*) Hyperprolactinemia is heterogeneous in its presentation. Galactorrhea is found in half of patients. Some have normoestrogenic anovulation, which may be manifest as hypothalamic anovulation, hyperandrogenism, dysfunctional uterine bleeding, or short luteal phase. On the other hand, some are hypoestrogenic. These do not have galactorrhea. (*m*) Hyperprolactinemia may be caused by prolactinomas, which secrete excess prolactin, or may be secondary to interruption of the pituitary stalk by large hypothalamic-pituitary tumors or other types of CNS injury. The latter cause variable pituitary dysfunction, which may include complete gonadotropin deficiency and various manifestations of hypopituitarism (including secondary hypothyroidism). (*n*) Drugs, particularly neuroleptics of the phenothiazone or tricyclic type, may induce hyperprolactinemia. [Modified with permission from Rosenfield RL (2003). Menstrual disorders and hyperandrogenism in adolescence. In Radovick S, MacGillivray MH (eds.), *Pediatric endocrinology: A practical clinical guide.* Totowa, NJ: Humana Press 451–478.]

TABLE 14-10

Features That Distinguish Gonadotropin Deficiency from Constitutional Delay of Puberty

In a healthy delayed prepubertal girl with BA >11 yr and prepubertal FSH, gonadotropin deficiency is:

- Possible if:
  - Weight loss greater than 5% to 8% (BMI <10th to15th percentile for height age)
  - Midline facial defect
  - CNS dysfunction
  - CT or MRI brain scan abnormal
- Probable if:
  - BA >13 yr and LH <0.15 U/L in early daytime
  - Anosmia or panhypopituitarism
- Diagnostic if:
  - Sleep-associated increase in LH lacking
  - GnRH (agonist) test → flat response
  - Chronologic age >16 yr

Reproduced with permission from Rosenfield RL, Barnes RB (1993). Menstrual disorders in adolescence. Endocrinol Metab Clin N Am 22:491–505.

gonadotropins.[594] Gonadotropin profiles during sleep have not proven to necessarily distinguish hypothalamic dysfunction from constitutional delay of puberty.[661]

The assessment of an adolescent's degree of estrogenization is often difficult. Breast development indicates that there has been estrogen exposure but does not mean that it is current. Determination of plasma estradiol is the simplest test, but diurnal and cyclic variations must be taken into account. Determination of hormonal effects on vaginal cytology is the most indicative of overall estrogen exposure (Figure 14-29), but is less well accepted by patients. A progestin withdrawal test is often helpful. A female who does not experience progestin withdrawal bleeding (Figure 14-42) probably has an ambient estradiol level of less than about 40 pg/mL.[662] If bleeding does not occur in response to this maneuver, the integrity of the uterus can be tested by the response to a 3-week course of estrogen-progestin—most conveniently administered in the form of birth control pills.

A prolactin level is indicated in the initial workup of normogonadotropic patients, regardless of their estrogen status. The prolactin level correlates with the size of prolactinomas, and a level greater than 200 ng/mL is typical of a macroprolactinoma. A prolactin level that does not correlate with the size of a large pituitary tumor suggests that the tumor is not a prolactinoma and is causing a functional pituitary stalk section or that the tumor is a macroprolactinoma elaborating such high levels of prolactin as to artefactually lower the immunoassayable prolactin level by a "hook effect."[663] Very high blood or cerebrospinal fluid prolactin levels suggest invasiveness. The workup for this should include formal testing of visual fields (Goldman perimetry or evoked response).

Pituitary microadenomas may be "incidentalomas" of no clinical significance, judging from an approximate 10% incidence in autopsy material.[664] However, they require careful assessment of pituitary function and follow-up.[665] Macroprolactinemia should be considered in the absence of clearly related symptoms, and when MRI is negative or in the setting of autoimmune disease.[653,654] Macroprolactinemia is confirmed when the prolactin level measured after precipitation of serum using polyethylene glycol is normal (or substantially reduced compared to the level measured in untreated serum.)

Imaging studies are important ancillary measures. Pelvic ultrasound may demonstrate hypoplastic ovaries, endometrial hypoplasia or disorders, and multicystic or polycystic ovaries. MRI of the hypothalamic-pituitary area is important in the workup of gonadotropin deficiency, hyperprolactinemia, and hypothalamic anovulation. Anorexic patients require psychiatric evaluation and consideration of brain tumor and partial bowel obstruction. Diet faddism and athletic addiction may be difficult to distinguish from anorexia nervosa. Constitutional thinness is a variant of normal with normal menses and a distinct hormonal profile.[666] It is unclear whether the superior mesenteric artery syndrome is a primary disorder that mimics anorexia nervosa or is a complication of it.[667]

Management

Underlying disorders must be treated appropriately. For example, tumors require surgery and/or radiotherapy. For prolactinoma, dopaminergic treatment is the initial treatment of choice unless the patient's conditon or eyesight is critical.[668] Hyperprolactinemia will be maximally suppressed within 1 month, and the menstrual cycle normalized within 3 months, by an effective dopaminergic agonist regimen. Cabergoline 0.5 to 1.0 mg once or twice weekly will usually control galactorrhea and shrink prolatinomas.[652,669] To minimize nausea, it is best to start with a low dose at bedtime.

Recent data implicate cabergoline as increasing the risk of cardiac valve regurgitation about fivefold in the elderly, albeit at generally tenfold or higher doses than used to treat hyperprolactinemia.[670,671] Bromocriptine does not activate the serotonin 5-HT(2B) receptor, the proposed mechanism through which cabergoline is thought to stimulate valve hypertrophy, and thus bromocriptine should not be associated with an increased risk of cardiac valve regurgitation and may be considered an alternative to cabergoline treatment—albeit a less effective one. The usual bromocriptine maintenance dose is 0.25 to 0.5 mg twice daily.

Anorexia nervosa is best managed by an experienced multidisciplinary team. Refeeding is the first priority, and once steady weight gain is evident the psychodynamic issues can be dealt with.[672] Family therapy, given on an outpatient basis, for medically uncomplicated cases of anorexia nervosa generally yields the best results—with good improvement in over half of patients. Inpatient intervention for rehydration and metabolic stabilization or failure of weight gain with ongoing cachexia may be required at any time. Menses resume when psychotherapy is effective and body fat is restored to normal (Figure 14-40). The induction of menses by estrogen-progestin replacement is usually injudicious because it provides a false sense of recovery and does not yield the recovery of bone loss that occurs with weight gain.[673] Although the acute episode can usually be successfully treated, there is a high rate of ongoing psychiatric disability and medical complications. Anorexia nervosa "by proxy" has been described in the offspring of former patients.[674]

There are two aspects of therapy that are uniformly involved in managing hypogonadism: psychological support and hormone administration. Patients with delayed development that is a variation of normal should be reassured that there is nothing wrong. They are simply among those who are experiencing a delay in timing of the onset of puberty. The wide normal variation in the pattern and time of the pubertal growth spurt should be explained in detail and the girl should be informed of her predicted eventual height. The majority of children with delayed puberty do not have overt psychological symptoms. Complex compensations and sublimations obviously occur. However, peer group pressures may make adjustment to sexual infantilism especially difficult when the age of 13 is approached[675]—and a poor self-image may lead to social withdrawal and feelings of hopelessness. Physical immaturity may prolong psychological immaturity.

A short course of physiologic sex hormone therapy at this time may help alleviate these anxieties. The physician should discuss the fact, when the evidence favors it, that the odds are overwhelmingly in favor of the "timer in the subconscious area of the brain" eventually turning on. When this will happen can be approximated from the skeletal age. One should not hesitate to advise more intensive psychological counseling if it becomes apparent that the concern about puberty is but one aspect of a more general maladjustment. Ultimately, the decision as to whether to undertake treatment for delayed puberty is up to the patient and her family.

It is important to assure the teenager with an organic basis for hypoestrogenism that feminization will occur, although in response to appropriate hormone treatment. It should be kept in mind that attainment of normal breast development in the girl with panhypopituitarism requires replacement of GH and cortisol deficits. It is difficult, however, to induce secondary sex characteristics in some patients with systemic chronic inflammatory disease such as lupus erythematosus.

In patients in whom short stature is a major concern, as in Turner syndrome, growth potential must be considered before undertaking estrogen replacement. GH therapy improves the adult height potential of patients with Turner syndrome, especially when started as soon as growth failure becomes apparent.[676] GH therapy in the United States is generally initiated at the FDA-approved dose of 0.375 mg/kg per week. In older girls, or those with extreme short stature, therapy with oxandrolone [2-oxo-17α-methyldihydrotestosterone (Anavar)] 0.05 mg/kg/day (which augments GH action) can be considered.[677] Clitoromegaly is ordinarily negligble on this dosage. Liver function should be monitored.

Estrogen replacement therapy starting at about one-tenth of the adult dose does not seem to interfere with the positive effect that GH has on adult height.[676,678] A physiologic form of treatment is to begin with intramuscular depot E2 0.2 mg/month and to increase the dose by 0.2 mg every 6 months until a midpubertal dose is reached, at which time it can be increased by 0.5 mg every 6 months. Midpubertal sex hormone production is approximated by delivering 1.0 to 1.5 mg of depot E2 per month, which alone permits achievement of height potential and typically induces menarche within 1 year. An equivalent starting dose of transdermal E2 appears to be 6.25 µg daily, which requires intermittent or fractionated delivery of the lowest-dose patches currently available. A reasonable alternative regimen begins with 0.25 mg micronized E2 by mouth daily. Adult replacement doses are 100 µg transdermal or 2 to 4 mg oral E2 daily.

Progestin should be added to estrogenic regimens after 2 years of estrogen replacement treatment or after withdrawal bleeding occurs. A physiologic replacement regimen consists of micronized progesterone 200 mg daily for 10 days monthly. We typically begin with half of this dose to minimize premenstrual symptoms, but full replacement appears necessary to lower the risk of endometrial hyperplasia and endometrial carcinoma.[679,680] Once optimal height is achieved, most patients prefer to switch to birth control pills as a convenient form of estrogen-progestin therapy. The pills containing the lowest dose of estrogen that will result in normal menstrual cycles are advisable. The lowest estrogen dosages currently available in combination contraceptive pills in the United States contain 20 µg (Mircette) to 30 µg (Yasmin) ethinyl estradiol.

Hypogonadotropic patients can achieve ovulation with gonadotropin therapy. There has been considerable success in treating those patients with hypothalamic GnRH deficiency by pulsatile GnRH.[88,661] Fertility has been achieved by this means. Induction of ovulation is best carried out by a gynecologist specializing in reproductive endocrinology. Patients with primary ovarian failure can successfully achieve pregnancy after oocyte donation and in vitro fertilization.[681]

Turner syndrome patients are at high risk for obstetrical complications in the areas of uterine anomalies, carbohydrate intolerance, and cardiovascular complications. Oocyte cryopreservation and ovarian tissue cryopreservation and transplantation have been explored to preserve fertility in patients with gonadal dysgenesis and disorders requiring cytotoxic chemotherapy or gonadectomy.[682-684] Data are limited, but the modest success with the former outstrips the rare success with the latter. Each technique has limitations and risks. These procedures should currently be considered experimental until greater evidence for efficacy and safety is available.

NORMOESTROGENIC MENSTRUAL DISTURBANCES

Hypothalamic Anovulation

Hypothalamic anovulation causes menstrual disturbances in sexually mature well-estrogenized women through a deficiency in GnRH secretion too subtle to cause frank hypoestrogenism. The neuroendocrine system stimulates ovarian estrogen secretion to a level normal for an early- or mid-follicular-phase female, but follicular development is inadequate for a normal dominant follicle to emerge. Amenorrhea or oligomenorrhea may result.

However, in some patients sufficient estrogenization occurs to cause dysfunctional uterine bleeding (discussed in the next section).

Reduced LH pulsatility occurs in the great majority[685]—failure to generate a midcycle LH surge in the remainder.[686,687] The pathophysiology seems to involve varying degrees of undernutrition and/or CRH excess. Negative energy balance may be present even in patients of normal, but lower than average, weight and fat stores.[371,646] Leptin deficiency is an important determinant of the decreased LH pulsatility. The anovulation of psychic or physical stress may involve CRH excess.[647] In the brain, CRH releases β-endorphin from proopiomelanocortin. This endorphin in turn inhibits GnRH release. This seems to be the major mechanism of anovulation because naloxone blockade of opioid action normalizes gonadotropin secretion.[88]

In the pituitary, CRH increases the set-point for ACTH release. This brings about a new steady state of increased cortisol secretion. Further ACTH response to CRH is blunted by the negative feedback of this cortisol excess. The result is a mildly Cushingoid cortisol rhythm. Cortisol excess itself can contribute to the amenorrhea by inhibiting the response to GnRH,[688] as well as by antagonizing some sex hormone actions. Adrenal androgens are elevated in competitive athletes who maintain body fat stores.[689]

Causes. *Functional hypothalamic amenorrhea* is a term commonly used to describe unexplained hypothalamic anovulation. The endocrine features of these patients resemble those of patients with the athletic or psychogenic types of hypothalamic anovulation. A primate model indicates that hypothalamic anovulation develops in stress-sensitive individuals from an innocuous combination of mild stress and mild caloric restriction.[689a] *Athletic amenorrhea* is the term used for the hypothalamic anovulation associated with excessive exercise and with low body fat stores. The female athletic triad consists of menstrual disturbance, eating disorder, and osteoporosis.[690] Primary or secondary amenorrhea, oligomenorrhea, or short luteal phase are common in athletes.[691] Ovarian function decreases approximately in proportion to the amount of physical activity and dietary restriction. Weight-bearing exercise is only partly protective of the effects of hypoestrogenism on weight-bearing bone.

There is concern that amenorrheic athletes may be left with a pemanent deficit in bone mass.[692] Weight loss to 10% below ideal body weight and body fat less than 10% are risk factors for amenorrhea. Body mass index does not accurately reflect body fat stores in athletes.[693] Energy balance seems to be more critical than low body fat stores in mediating the anovulation.[691,694] Menarche may occur or menses resume when the athlete's activity level suddenly decreases and before weight gain occurs. Other factors contribute to cause amenorrhea. Nutritional deficiencies may coexist. Chronic undernutriton may suppress thyroid function, as in anorexia nervosa.[647] Delayed menarche may preexist, possibly indicating genetic susceptibility. Athletic amenorrhea resembles anorexia nervosa in patients' obsession with weight control.[691,695]

Psychogenic amenorrhea from severe psychic stress has long been known (e.g., "boarding-school amenorrhea").[696] The onset of psychogenic amenorrhea may be identified as being associated with a discrete event, but the ovarian dysfunction tends to be long lasting. Subtle nutritional deficits contribute.[371] Pseudocyesis is an extremely rare form of psychogenic amenorrhea that is due to persistence of the corpus luteum. This syndrome tends to occur in infertile women with an overwhelming desire for pregnancy and conversion hysteria. Prolactin and LH excess appear to mediate this rare syndrome.[697]

Post-pill amenorrhea has been a term applied to the amenorrhea that sometimes follows the long-term use of hormonal contraceptives. This in the past was attributed to oversuppression, but oversuppression should not be expected to be the case with the current generation of oral contraceptives.[242] About a third of patients with secondary amenorrhea after discontinuation of estrogen- and progestin-containing pills have a history of previous menstrual disturbance and ongoing menstrual problems.[698] Another third can expect spontaneous remission of the amenorrhea. About half of the remainder of cases will have resolution of their menstrual disturbance after induced pregnancy.

The most common cause of post-pill amenorrhea is probably hyperprolactinemia because more than 20% of such cases have galactorrhea. How often this antedates ingestion of the contraceptive pill is unknown. Menses may be restored in normoprolactinemic cases by dopaminergic treatment, which suggests that in such cases there is excessive pituitary prolactin secretion that is too subtle to be detected by measurement of plasma levels.[699] The anovulation resulting from depot-medroxyprogesterone acetate contraception is related to the extremely slow rate of absorption and metabolism of this steroid. Menses return when the blood levels of this progestin fall below the threshold for suppression of the LH surge,[700] and only rarely has it been associated with disturbed prolactin secretion.[701]

Differential Diagnosis. Disorders outside the neuroendocrine-gonadal axis may mimic hypothalamic anovulation. These include pregnancy, nutritional disturbance, glucocorticoid excess, disturbed thyroid function, drug abuse, chronic illness, hyperprolactinemia, and ectopic LH secretion. Pregnancy must be excluded in all sexually mature adolescents wtih amenorrhea. An elevation of the plasma β-hCG level is the earliest laboratory sign.[702] Constant overproduction of estrogens and progestins by the hCG-driven corpus luteum of pregnancy and the fetoplacental unit leads to the suppression of endogenous pituitary gonadotropin release that underlies the amenorrhea.

Overnutrition or undernutrition may cause hypothalamic amenorrhea. Overproduction of estrogen from plasma precursors in adipose tissue appears to mediate the effect of obesity.[334] The effect of undernutrition seems to be mediated by factors related to energy balance, as discussed previously. Cushing syndrome (glucocorticoid excess) seems to cause menstrual irregularity by mechanisms discussed earlier in this section. Thyroid hormone deficiency interferes with gonadotropin action on the ovary,[703] and may interfere with endometrial function by actions on steroid metabolism[704] and action.[705] Hypothalamic anovulation may be caused by drug abuse with tetrahydrocannabinol, ethanol, or opiates.[706,707]

Cocaine causes menstrual irregularity by suppressing gonadotropin secretion through mechanisms that include depletion of dopaminergic stores (resulting in hyperprolactinemia) and stimulation of CRH release.[656,708] Inflammatory illness acutely disrupts the estradiol-induced LH surge[709] and chronically causes gonadotropin deficiency, which may be mediated partly by undernutrition and partly by cytokines.[633] Disorders as diverse as diabetes mellitus and iron overload all impact GnRH secretion.[710,711] Chronic renal failure causes complex dysfunction of the reproductive system, including poor clearance of gonadotropins and prolactin in the presence of inhibition of gonadotropins by a nondialyzable factor.[712]

Hyperprolactinemia occasionally causes secondary amenorrhea without frank hypoestrogenism.[713] This situation probably results from a diminution in FSH secretion that is so marginal as to only inhibit the emergence of a dominant follicle. Ectopic LH or hCG secretion by a tumor can cause normoestrogenic anovulation.[714] Sex steroid levels are normal due to ovarian desensitization to LH. Hypothalamic anovulation is ordinarily a diagnosis of exclusion. The medical evaluation should be performed as discussed in the preceding section, with particular attention to the possibilities of emotional disturbances, excessive exercise, the use of birth control pills or other drugs, and state of health.

The physical examination should be particularly directed to the state of nutrition, the possibilities of intracranial or systemic disease, galactorrhea, thyroid dysfunction, glucocorticoid excess, hirsutism, and obesity. If this workup is negative, an MRI of the hypothalamic-pituitary area is indicated. The response to a GnRH test may be immature, but it is not necessarily helpful. Hypothalamic anovulation may be documented by demonstrating subnormal LH pulse frequency, but this is not generally practical. Leptin levels tend to be low but nondiagnostic.[646] Dysfunctional uterine bleeding from hypothalamic anovulation must be distinguished from that due to other causes (see next section).

Management. Many patients with hypothalamic anovulation will benefit from nutritional counseling. Diet faddists and athletes should be advised about the necessity of optimal body energy reserves for the maintenance of normal menstrual cycles (see Figure 14-40). The teleologic significance of this may be pointed out; namely, that inherent in the evolutionary process is the inhibition of pregnancy in times of inadequate food supplies. Ongoing psychological counseling is advisable for patients who cannot change their dietary or exercise patterns because of an abnormal body image. Mature athletes who are hypoestrogenic may benefit from estrogen replacement. Obese girls should be advised that there is a substantial possibility that reduction to a normal weight will result in restoration of menses and improved probability of fertility.

Mature teenagers whose amenorrhea is unexplained should be assured that they have a high likelihood of fertility with appropriate endocrinologic treatment. However, such treatment is unlikely to be of any benefit to them until such time as they desire to become pregnant. In the meanwhile, the main objective of therapy is to normalize the endometrial cycle by periodic progestin administration. For this purpose, medroxyprogesterone acetate (up to 10 mg at bedtime for 14 consecutive days) is usually effective in inducing withdrawal periods. During the first few years after menarche, it is reasonable to administer this treatment on alternate months to allow detection of late maturation of a regular menstrual cycle.

Induction of an ovulatory cycle has been reported to occasionally result in resumption of spontaneous normal menses.[698] An ovulatory cycle can normally be induced by the administration of clomiphene citrate once nightly for five doses. If treatment is successful, bleeding generally occurs about 1 month from commencement of the treatment. One should start with the 50-mg dose because larger doses may cause hyperstimulation of the ovaries with the development of ovarian cysts. For this reason, one should perform an ultrasound examination to rule out cystic ovaries before going successively to 100- to 150-mg dosage. This treatment is not generally recommended in the teenage years, however. Dopaminergic therapy has been reported to be successful in causing the resumption of ovulation in post-pill amenorrhea, modest undernutrition, and other unexplained cases of secondary amenorrhea. Otherwise, induction of ovulation is best left to the endocrinologic gynecologist to supervise at such time as the woman wishes to conceive. The vast majority of patients with no obvious cause for their secondary amenorrhea will become pregnant after appropriate treatment with estrogen, clomiphene, dopaminergic agonist, human menopausal gonadotropins, or pulsatile GnRH therapy.

Dysfunctional Uterine Bleeding

Causes. Dysfunctional uterine bleeding (anovulatory bleeding that is too frequent or excessive) is a manifestation of anovulatory cycles in which there is overall excessive estrogen production.[591] It is most often a manifestation of physiologic adolescent anovulation. Hyperandrogenism, particularly polycystic ovary syndrome and its variants, is a common cause of dysfunctional bleeding. In some cases it arises from hypothalamic anovulation (discussed previously). Less common are estrogen-producing cysts or tumors, hypothyroidism, hyperprolactinemia, and incipient premature ovarian failure. The workup should therefore include measurement of androgens, prolactin, thyroid function, and FSH blood levels.

Corpus luteum insufficiency presents as short (less than 22 days) ovulatory cycles, and thus excessively frequent menses. The immediate cause of an inadequate luteal phase is insufficent progesterone production to sustain a pregnancy.[715,716] This in turn may arise from subtle deficiency of FSH during the follicular phase, resultant incomplete emergence of a dominant follicle, and the subsequent formation of an inadequate corpus luteum. Alternatively, the corpus luteum may not be responsive to LH.[717] Luteal insufficiency may be the result of hyperprolactinemia,[718] obesity, or hyperandrogenism.

Differential Diagnosis. Dysfunctional uterine bleeding must be distinguished from the other causes of abnormal genital bleeding listed in Table 14-11.[591,719] The possibility that it is pregnancy related must be considered and a pregnancy test performed in a sexually active teenager. Sexual

TABLE 14-11

Differential Diagnosis of Abnormal Genital Bleeding

- Dysfunctional uterine bleeding (anovulation)
  - Physiologic anovulation (perimenarcheal)
  - Hyperandrogenism
    - Polycystic ovary syndrome
  - Hyperestrogenism
  - Hypothyroidism
  - Hypothalamic anovulation
    - Hyperprolactinemia
  - Chronic disease
  - Incipient premature ovarian failure
- Luteal phase defects
- Pregnancy-related bleeding
  - Threatened, missed, or incomplete abortion
  - Molar pregnancy
  - Ectopic pregnancy
- Vaginal bleeding
  - Trauma
  - Tumor
- Menorrhagia
  - Essential menorrhagia
  - Bleeding diathesis
  - Uterine tumor, polyp, adenomyosis, intrauterine device

Based on Rosenfield RL, Barnes RB (1993). Menstrual disorders in adolescence. Endocrinol Metab Clin North Am 22:491.

abuse is a prime consideration in recurrant vaginal bleeding. Genital tract or feminizing tumors characteristically cause bleeding that cannot be controlled with cyclic progestin or estrogen-progestin therapy. Menorrhagia can be pragmatically considered to exist if prolonged or excessive menses is associated with iron deficiency anemia.

Essential or idiopathic menorrhagia is the single most common cause in adolescents. It is theorized to result from imbalance of vasodilating and vasocontricting prostanoid action on the endometrium.[720] However, pathologic causes must be considered because bleeding disorders are present in about 20% of adolescents with menorrhagia requiring hospitalization and in 50% of those presenting at menarche.

Patients requiring hospitalization for abnormal bleeding should have a platelet count, prothrombin time, partial thromboplastin time, and bleeding time performed. Transvaginal ultrasound, which is not often feasible in the virginal adolescent, is as reliable as hysteroscopy in determining whether or not the endometrial cavity is normal. Failure of serum progesterone to rise above 500 ng/dL during the luteal phase is diagnostic of corpus luteum insufficiency. However, a higher progesterone level may be compatible with inadequacy if not sustained.

Management. Estrogen is required to stop an acute episode of dysfunctional bleeding. It can be given together with a progestin as a low-dose oral contraceptive pill, one tablet four times daily for 7 days. Treatment is then stopped for 5 days, and the patient warned that heavy withdrawal bleeding with cramps may occur. Therapy with a low-dose pill, given as for contraception, is then begun to prevent recurrence of dysfunctional bleeding and is continued for about three cycles. If the patient is sexually active, oral contraceptive therapy can be continued indefinitely as necessary.

A progestin can be used as an alternative to the oral contraceptive pill to prevent recurrent dysfunctional bleeding in a patient who is not sexually active. Medroxyprogesterone acetate 10 mg/day for 1 week is given at 3- to 4-week intervals. After the third month, therapy is stopped and the patient is observed for 1 to 2 months for spontaneous bleeding. If none occurs, the progestin can be given every other month in a dosage of 5 to 10 mg for 7 to 14 days to prevent recurrent dysfunctional bleeding. If in the progestin-free month spontaneous bleeding occurs, progestins are withheld in the subsequent month to determine if the patient has developed regular ovulatory cycles.

A patient who is hypovolemic because of rapid and heavy dysfunctional bleeding should be hospitalized and treated with intravenous fluids and blood products as necessary. Premarin can be administered in a dose of 25 mg intravenously every 3 to 4 hours for three to four doses. When medical management fails, a bleeding diathesis or uterine structural abnormality should be considered (see material following). If heavy bleeding persists, curettage should be performed by a gynecologist.

Unexplained ("essential") menorrhagia is treated much the same way as dysmenorrhea. The oral contraceptive pill will decrease menstrual blood loss by about 50% in women with essential menorrhagia. Antiprostaglandins, such as naproxen 500 mg twice a day, decrease blood loss nearly as effectively.

Perimenstrual Symptoms

Dysmenorrhea. Pain with menses becomes a source of morbidity in 14% of adolescents.[721] When pain is acute and qualitatively different from the usual menstrual pain, ectopic pregnancy must be considered.[702,722] An ectopic pregnancy often causes vaginal bleeding that occurs 2.5 weeks later than the time of the expected next menstrual period and is typically light. However, the bleeding may be heavy and thus resemble an episode of dysfunctional uterine bleeding. Ectopic pregnancy is usually diagnosable by a combination of ultrasonography, a serum β-hCG level >1,000 IU/L, and a progesterone level of <2,500 ng/dL.

In patients with chronic pelvic pain unresponsive to antiprostaglandins or the oral contraceptive pill, psychological overlay is possible. However, attention should be directed to the possibility of endometriosis, uterine outlet obstruction, or gynecologic tract masses. Ultrasonography and laparoscopy may be indicated to further evaluate these patients. Endometriosis accounts for approximately half of the cases of chronic pelvic pain in teenagers.[723] Genetic factors and congenital obstruction of the genital tract predispose to endometriosis, and aberrant estradiol formation in endometrial stroma[724] has been incriminated in the pathogenesis. Lack of expression of the cell adhesion molecule integrin in the luteal phase endometrium is associated with a form of endometriosis that is mild but accompanied by infertility.[725]

Dysmenorrhea may be ameliorated by antiprostaglandin therapy. Naproxen (275 mg qid after a 550-mg loading dose) has been shown to be superior to aspirin

(650 mg qid) or placebo when begun 2 days before the anticipated onset of menses.[726] The oral contraceptive pill is an alternative that will relieve dysmenorrhea in about 90% of cases, presumably by reducing endometrial mass.[591] Because smoking, alcohol intake, and excessive weight are risk factors, lifestyle counselling is advisable.

Premenstrual Syndrome. *Premenstrual syndrome* is the term applied when cylic mood changes confined to the second half of the menstrual cycle become debilitating.[727] It is often disruptive to women's personal, social, and occupational function. If symptoms of marked mood swings, depressed mood, anxiety, and irritability occur, it is classified as premenstrual dysphoric disorder.[728] Neuropsychiatric symptoms may include epilepsy[729] and bizarre behavior.[730] These seem to represent aberrant responses to normal cyclic hormonal changes.[731] Subnormal activation of the hypothalamic-pituitary-adrenal axis in response to progesterone has been found.[732]

Some evidence indicates that variation in the degree of progesterone metabolism to neuroactive steroids affects the severity of symptomatology.[733] Oral contraceptive therapy with the antimineralocorticoid progestin drospirenone is indicated if psychotropic therapy is unsuccessful. Down-regulation of pituitary gonadotropin secretion by GnRH agonist therapy is efficacious, but its usefulness is limited by the side effects of estrogen deficiency. The relationship of premenstrual syndrome to other luteal phase symptomatology, such as recurrent fever and autoimmune symptoms, is unclear.[734,735]

HYPERANDROGENISM IN ADOLESCENCE

Hyperandrogenism of a mild to moderate degree is the most common cause of normoestrogenic menstrual disturbances. It arises from ovarian or adrenal dysfunction in the vast majority of cases, and abnormal peripheral formation of androgen in most others (Table 14-12).[339,736,737] Virilizing tumors are rare (accounting for about 0.2% of hyperandrogenism). These are discussed in the section on precocious puberty.

Causes

Polycystic Ovary Syndrome. Polycystic ovary syndrome (PCOS) is the most common cause of hyperandrogenism presenting at or after the onset of puberty. It is a heterogeneous syndrome of unexplained chronic hyperandrogenism and oligo-anovulation, with a polycystic ovary being an alternative diagnostic criterion (Table 14-13).[268,736-738] Whether the syndrome can be diagnosed in the absence of hyperandrogenism is controversial. Insulin resistance and LH excess contribute to the pathogenesis of the syndrome, but neither is a criterion for diagnosis. The syndrome is variable both clinically and endocrinologically (Figure 14-44).[736] The syndrome in adolescents resembles that in adults. The cardinal symptoms typically begin in the perimenarcheal stage, and it has been documented in children as young as 10 years of age. Adolescents with classic PCOS develop higher LH levels and greater insulin resistance than normal.

The classic Stein-Leventhal form of PCOS is characterized clinically by menstrual irregularity, hirsutism (or

---

TABLE 14-12

Causes of Adolescent Hyperandrogenism

Functional Gonadal Hyperandrogenism
- Primary (dysregulational) functional ovarian hyperandrogenism*
- Secondary polycystic ovary syndrome
  - Poorly controlled classic congenital adrenal hyperplasia
  - Ovarian steroidogenic blocks
  - Syndromes of severe insulin resistance
  - Portohepatic shunting
  - Epilepsy or valproic acid therapy
- Adrenal rests
- Ovotesticular disorder of sexual differentiation
- Chorionic gonadotropin related

Functional Adrenal Hyperandrogenism
- Primary (dysregulational) functional adrenal hyperandrogenism**
- Congenital adrenal hyperplasia
- Prolactin or growth hormone excess
- Dexamethasone-resistant functional adrenal hyperandrogenism
  - Cushing syndrome
  - Cortisol resistance
  - Apparent cortisone reductase deficiency

Peripheral Androgen Overproduction
- Obesity
- Idiopathic hyperandrogenism

Tumoral Hyperandrogenism
Androgenic Drugs

* Common form of PCOS.
** Uncommon form of PCOS.
Modified with permission from Buggs C, Rosenfield RL (2005). Polycystic ovary syndrome in adolescence. Endocrinol Metab Clin North Am 34:677–705.

TABLE 14-13

Diagnostic Criteria for Polycystic Ovary Syndrome

National Institutes of Health (NIH) Criteria
- Clinical and/or biochemical signs of hyperandrogenism
- Anovulatory symptoms

Rotterdam criteria
- NIH criteria
- Ultrasonographic evidence of a polycystic ovary as an alternative to either specific NIH criterion

Modified with permission from Buggs C, Rosenfield RL (2005). Polycystic ovary syndrome in adolescence. Endocrinol Metab Clin North Am 34:677–705.

---

hirsutism equivalents such as seborrhea, acne, and alopecia), and obesity (often with acanthosis nigricans). Endocrinologically, they are characterized by hyperandrogenemia and by polycystic ovaries or about twofold elevation of serum LH—although the more obese the patient the less likely serum LH is to be elevated.[739,740] However, half the cases are nonclassic or atypical. Nonclassic PCOS patients are hyperandrogenic and have anovulatory symptoms, but lack a polycystic ovary (meeting NIH criteria) or have normal menses yet a polycystic ovary (meeting Rotterdam criteria) (Table 14-13). The broad

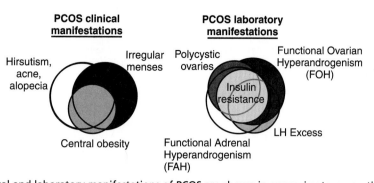

Figure 14-44 The major clinical and laboratory manifestations of PCOS are shown in approximate proportion to their relative incidence and coincidence. [Modified with permission from Buggs C, Rosenfield RL (2005). Polycystic ovary syndrome in adolescence. Endocrinol Metab Clin North Am 34:677–705.]

spectrum of the disorder includes atypical hyperandrogenemic cases with cutaneous manifestations or central obesity that do not fit current diagnostic criteria because they lack clinical or ultrasonographic evidence of ovarian dysfunction, although they have the typical endocrine dysfunction of the ovaries or adrenal glands.

Functional ovarian hyperandrogenism (FOH) is the source of the androgen excess in about 80% of cases. It is characterized by 17-hydroxyprogesterone (17PROG) hyperresponsiveness to the gonadotropin stimulation of GnRH agonist (GnRHag) or human chorionic gonadotropin testing and subnormal suppressibility of plasma testosterone upon adrenal suppression by glucocorticoid. About 60% of cases have a typical form of dexamethasone-suppressible functional adrenal hyperandrogenism (FAH) that is characterized by moderate 17-hydroxypregnenolone or DHEA hyperresponsiveness to ACTH. FAH accompanies FOH about half the time, but in atypical PCOS it may be the sole source of androgen excess.

Pathogenesis. The central abnormality in primary FOH usually seems to be intraovarian androgen excess (Figure 14-45). The hyperandrogenemia results in the pilosebaceous manifestations. The disproportionately high intraovarian androgen concentration arising from FOH seems to recruit excessive growth of small follicles while hindering the follicular maturation involved in the emergence of a dominant follicle, as well as causing thecal and stromal hyperplasia.

Dysregulation of steroidogenesis appears to account for primary FOH and primary FAH. Dysregulation is postulated to result from imbalance among the various intrinsic and extrinsic factors involved in the modulation of trophic hormone action. Within the ovary, there appear to be flaws in the processes that normally coordinate androgen and estrogen secretion (Figure 14-20). This causes the ovaries to hyperrespond to LH, rather than undergoing down-regulation in response to LH stimulation. The majority of cases appear to have an intrinsic theca cell defect that causes widespread overexpression of steroidogenic enzymes, particularly 17-hydroxylase and 17,20-lyase (both properties of P450c17, which are the rate-limiting steps in the biosynthesis of testosterone precursors).

As in the ovary, dysregulation of local steroidogenic regulatory processes within the adrenal cortex appears to cause excessive 17-ketosteroid formation as by-products of cortisol secretion. Granulosa cells also exhibit ste-

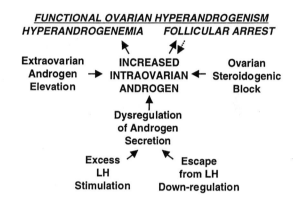

Figure 14-45 Model of the pathogenesis of functional ovarian hyperandrogenism. Increased intraovarian androgen concentration is central and causes hyperandrogenemia and follicular maturation arrest. It can also result from follicular atresia. Additional causes of increased intraovarian androgen levels include extraovarian androgen excess, ovarian steroidogenic blocks, and dysregulation of androgen secretion. The latter may result from luteinizing hormone (LH) excess or from escape from desensitization to LH action by insulin, insulin-like growth factors, or other peptides. [Modified from Ehrmann DA, et al. (1995). Polycystic ovary syndrome as functional ovarian hyperandrogenism as dysregulation of androgen secretion. Endocr Rev 16:322. Copyright © 1995 The Endocrine Society.]

roidogenic dysregulation. They are excessively responsive to FSH, particularly at high dosage. This accounts for the tendency of PCOS women to develop the dangerous ovarian hyperstimulation syndrome during fertility treatment. It may also aggravate thecal androgen secretion via a paracrine action.[129] The fundamental defect may be a generalized disorder involving specific transcriptional coregulators also involved in the regulation of glucose and fat metabolism.

Insulin excess appears to be an important extrinsic factor in dysregulation. As a group, PCOS patients are significantly hyperinsulinemic in association with a state of insulin resistance—and treatments that lower insulin levels reduce the androgen excess moderately. The insulin/IGF system seems to act in synergism with trophic hormones to cause ovarian or adrenal androgen excess. The ovaries and adrenal glands function as if responding to the hyperinsulinemic state in spite of the resistance to the effects of insulin on skeletal glucose metabolism. This paradox remains to be resolved.

Excessive LH secretion, found in 50% to 75% of cases, was once thought to be central to the pathogenesis of PCOS due to a complex cycle of events in which peripheral conversion of adrenal androstenedione to estrone-sensitized gonadotropes to GnRH.[741] However, evidence is accumulating that it results from hyperandrogenemia interfering with progesterone negative feedback effect on LH secretion.[55,252,253] Nevertheless, the possibility of a primary role for LH excess remains—particularly in the PCOS that is secondary to congenital virilizing disorders.

Etiology. Increasing evidence suggests that PCOS arises as a complex trait with contributions from both heritable and nonheritable factors. Polygenic influences appear to account for about 70% of the variance in pathogenesis. Hyperandrogenemia and polycystic ovaries each appear to be inherited as independent autosomal-dominant traits. Nearly half of sisters of women with PCOS have an elevated plasma testosterone level, although only half of them are symptomatic. Asymptomatic polycystic ovaries are found in about 10% of women, but they are often accompanied by a subclinical PCOS-type of ovarian dysfunction.

Central obesity and insulin resistance seem to play important roles in PCOS, perhaps by accentuating steroidogenic dysregulation—but perhaps more fundamentally because PCOS is closely related to metabolic syndrome in parents. Gestational factors have also been incriminated. The syndrome has been associated with high and low birth weight, and it can develop secondary to fetal virilization. Thus, the syndrome seems to arise from an intrinsic genetic trait that becomes manifest only when interacting with other congenital or environmental factors, excessive adiposity being the most common precipitant.

Other Causes of Functional Ovarian Hyperandrogenism. Secondary PCOS can result from several disorders (Table 14-12).[742] Extraovarian androgen excess (as in poorly controlled congenital adrenal hyperplasia) and ovarian steroidogenic blocks (such as 3β-hydroxysteroid dehydrogenase, 17β-hydroxysteroid dehydrogenase, and aromatase deficiency) are causes. Excessive stimulation of the LH receptor appears to mediate the hyperandrogenism reported in chorionic gonadotropin-related ovarian dysfunction during pregnancy, and appears to have played a role in a case of FSH-resistant ovarian follicles.[743]

All known forms of extreme insulin resistance (including hereditary cases of insulin receptor mutations, as well as acromegaly) are accompanied by PCOS, possibly by acting through the IGF-I signal transduction pathway to cause escape from desensitization to LH. Functional ovarian hyperandrogenism may also result from adrenal rests of the ovaries in congenital adrenal hyperplasia and from true hermaphroditism. PCOS has also been reported as a complication of portasystemic shunting. Impaired steroid metabolism has been postulated as the mechanism.

Other Causes of Functional Adrenal Hyperandrogenism. The PCOS type of primary (dysregulational) FAH occurs as an isolated entity, not associated with FOH, in about 25% of hyperandrogenic women. This may sometimes be an outcome of exaggerated adrenarche. This type of adrenal dysfunction was previously mistaken for nonclassic 3β-hydroxysteroid dehydrogenase deficiency, which is now known to be a rare disorder.[744] Less than

10% of adrenal hyperandrogenism can be attributed to the more well-understood disorders listed in Table 14-11. Most are due to nonclassic congenital adrenal hyperplasia, which accounts for less than 5% of hyperandrogenism in the general U.S. population, and to the various hyperandrogenic forms of Cushing syndrome. Prolactin excess causes adrenal hyperandrogenism, sometimes in association with polycystic ovaries. Adrenal hyperandrogenism can on rare occasions arise from cortisol resistance or apparent cortisone reductase deficiency.

Peripheral Androgen Overproduction. In nearly 10% of hyperandrogenic patients, an ovarian or adrenal source cannot be ascertained by thorough testing. This is idiopathic hyperandrogenemia. Obesity seems to explain some of these cases because adipose tissue has the capacity to form testosterone from androstenedione. Obesity may simulate PCOS by causing amenorrhea, acanthosis nigricans, and hyperandrogenemia. Other idiopathic cases may be due to hereditary quirks in peripheral metabolism of steroids.

Differential Diagnosis

Hyperandrogenism should be considered in any girl who presents with hirsutism or cutaneous hirsutism equivalents, menstrual disturbance, or central obesity during puberty. PCOS is by far the most common cause, and its manifestations are variable (Figure 14-44). Hirsutism, acne, and alopecia are inconsistently expressed manifestations of androgen excess. If acne vulgaris is unusually early in its age of onset, if severe acne is persistent, or if Accutane treatment is being considered, the possibility of hyperandrogenemia should be investigated. Androgenetic alopecia is manifest as a diffuse pattern in females.

Hyperhidrosis or hidradenitis suppurativa may be the only dermatologic manifestation. On the other hand, some of the cardinal symptoms or signs of androgen excess may not be present. Many cases of hyperandrogenemia are entirely cryptic. Menstrual irregularity of any sort (i.e., ranging from amenorrhea to dysfunctional uterine bleeding) that persists for 2 years has a two-thirds probability of being persistent and thus is an indication for workup for androgen excess. Conversely, a history of normal menstrual cyclicity does not necessarily indicate ovulatory cycles—and some cases are not diagnosed until they present as adults with unexplained infertility[745] or with recurrent miscarriages.[746]

Intractable obesity, large waist circumference (>88 cm), or acanthosis nigricans should raise concern for PCOS. The possibility of PCOS is heightened if the previously cited symptoms are associated with a history of prepubertal risk factors for PCOS, including congenital virilizing disorders; premature adrenarche, particularly exaggerated adrenarche; atypical sexual precocity; and intractable prepubertal obesity, particularly if associated with pseudo-Cushing syndrome, pseudo-acromegaly, or a family history of metabolic syndrome.

Most hyperandrogenic girls present when sexually mature and normoestrogenic. However, if there is any doubt about whether feminization is adequate and ongoing (as when the presenting symptom is primary amenorrhea) the evaluation should include bone age, estradiol, and gonadotropin levels as outlined previously (Figure 14-41).

Hirsutism must be differentiated from hypertrichosis, the situation in which vellus hair predominates on "nonsexual" areas of the body. Hypertrichosis is not caused by sex hormone imbalance but appears with heredity, glucocorticoid excess, starvation, and medications such as phenytoins, cyclosporine, and valproic acid.[339]

The history and examination should also address risk factors for androgenic medications, other endocrinopathies (the most common of which are nonclassic congenital adrenal hyperplasia, Cushing syndrome, hyperprolactinemia, and thyroid dysfunction), and virilizing disorders. A rapid pace of development or progression of hirsutism, evidence of virilization (such as clitoromegaly, genital ambiguity, or increasing muscularity), or an abdominal mass would raise concern for an androgen-secreting neoplasm. However, tumors producing moderately excessive androgen can have indolent presentations.

The goals of the laboratory evaluation for PCOS are to attempt to document hyperandrogenism, to determine the specific etiology, and to provide a baseline in case it becomes necessary to reassess because of progression of the disorder. The diagnosis is on the firmest grounds if hyperandrogenism is demonstrated biochemically, rather than relying on hirsutism as a surrogate for it—although documentation of hyperandrogenemia can be problematic.

An approach to the workup that depends on assessing the degree of hirsutism and elucidating risk factors for virilizing disorders, androgenic medications, PCOS, and other endocrinopathies is suggested (Figure 14-46).[339] If hirsutism is mild and menses are regular with no evidence of risk factors that would suggest a secondary cause, it is reasonable not to pursue laboratory evaluation—given the high likelihood of idiopathic hirsutism (a cutaneous rather than endocrine disorder)—unless the patient is of Asian ethnicity. If hirsutism is moderate or severe or there are features to suggest an underlying disorder, excess androgen production should be ruled out. Risk factor assessment includes follow-up to evaluate response to therapy.

Plasma testosterone is the single most important androgen to evaluate. Plasma free testosterone is about 50% more sensitive in detecting excessive androgen production because hyperandrogenic women have a relatively low level of SHBG. Many commercial total and free testosterone assays are not suitable for the evaluation of women and children. Therefore, these assays are best performed by a specialty laboratory that has extensively validated them. Although other androgens are present in blood, their assessment makes little difference in management if plasma free testosterone is normal. However, the variation in androgen levels may miss an occasional case of nonclassic congenital adrenal hyperplasia and therefore further studies are indicated in patients at high risk by virtue of family history or ethnicity. These tests are most clearly interpreted when samples are drawn in the early morning of the mid-follicular (or anovulatory) phase of a menstrual cycle.

If androgen elevation is found, the next step in the differential diagnosis is ordinarily to obtain an ultrasound examination of the pelvis. A polycystic ovary is specifically defined as one that exceeds a critical volume (>10.8 cc in adolescents) or is polyfollicular (containing 10 or more follicles in the maximum plane).[463] The volume criterion assumes the absence of a dominant follicle (>10 mm in diameter) or a corpus luteum. Ovarian enlargement is the most solid criterion because multifollicular ovaries, normal in adolescence and present in other anovulatory states, are distinguishable from polycystic ovaries primarily on the basis of whether volume is normal or abnormal (which can be problematic).

These findings are not completely specific to PCOS and require excluding disorders that may secondarily cause PCOS. On the other hand, a negative ultrasound examination does not exclude nonclassic PCOS. However, it is useful in ruling out tumor and disorders of sexual differentiation as a cause of the androgen excess.[736] Simultaneous ultrasound imaging of the abdomen can be a cost-effective screening test for adrenal neoplasm in the hands of an experienced ultrasonographer.

Additional testing may include tests to exclude pregnancy and hyperprolactinemia. It may also include measurement of DHEAS and early-morning 17-hydroxyprogesterone if adrenal hyperandrogenism is suspected, and assessment for Cushing syndrome, thyroid dysfunction, or acromegaly if clinically indicated. If this evaluation for the most common disorders that mimic polycystic ovary syndrome is negative, the association of testosterone elevation with anovulatory symptoms or a polycystic ovary fulfills standard diagnostic criteria for polycystic ovary syndrome (Table 14-13). However, it does not exclude some fairly rare hyperandrogenic disorders. The approach to further studies to determine the source of hyperandrogenemia varies among subspecialists and with the needs of the individual patient.

Our preference is to use a dexamethasone suppression test to attempt to make a positive diagnosis of the ovarian or adrenal dysfunction of PCOS or to determine whether further workup is necessary for rare forms of CAH or other rare adrenal disorders (Figure 14-47).[736] The degree of suppression of plasma androgens and cortisol in response to a low-dose dexamethasone suppression test segregates patients diagnostically. Total testosterone levels of adrenal tumors fail to suppress more than 40% after a 2-day test.[747] A more prolonged course of low-dose dexamethasone is normally required to lower adrenal androgens below normal levels, and thus we prefer a "dexamethasone androgen-suppression test" (Figure 14-47).

Subnormal androgen suppression with normal adrenocortical suppression indicates a source of androgen other than an ACTH-dependent adrenal one. This is typical of PCOS if tumor or other ovarian pathology has not been found by ultrasound examination. If both cortisol and androgen suppression are subnormal, the androgen excess may be secondary to noncompliance with taking dexamethasone, to Cushing syndrome, or to defective cortisol metabolism or action. If androgen suppression is normal, ACTH (cosyntropin) stimulation testing to assess 17-hydroxyprogesterone and other steroid intermediates is recommended.

Further extensive diagnostic studies are seldom indicated unless there is reason to suspect a virilizing tumor

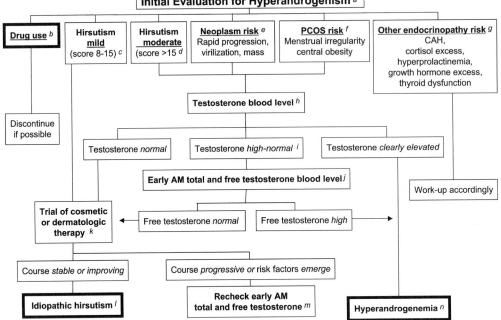

Figure 14-46 Differential diagnosis of hyperandrogenism and hirsutism. (*A*) Risk assessment includes assessment for the degree of hirsutism, menstrual irregularity, central obesity, and the other risk factors shown. Acne vulgaris, seborrhea, pattern alopecia, hyperhidrosis, and hidradenitis suppurativa are "cutaneous hirsutism equivalents" and may be alternative signs of hyperandrogenism. A small amount of sexual hair growth is normal (Ferriman-Gallwey score <8). However, if other risk factors are present (even in the absence of hirsutism) androgen excess should be considered. (*B*) Medications that cause hirsutism include anabolic or androgenic steroids (consider in athletes and patients with endometriosis or sexual dysfunction). Valproic acid, an antiepileptic drug, raises testosterone levels. (*C*) Mild hirsutism in the absence of the risk factors shown is likely to be idiopathic and to respond to cosmetic or dermatologic therapy. Therefore, it is reasonable to embark on these treatments without an endocrine evaluation. (*D*) Acne vulgaris of early onset or unresponsive to ordinary dermatologic measures, including antibiotic therapy, and pattern balding are similarly risk factors for hyperandrogenism. (*E*) Neoplasm risk is suggested by sudden onset, rapid progression, virilization, or an abdominal or pelvic mass. (*F*) In some hyperandrogenic cases, there is no cutaneous symptomatology ("cryptic hyperandrogenism") and androgen excess is suspected only because of menstrual irregularity, central obesity, or acanthosis nigricans. (*G*) The most common hyperandrogenic endocrine disorder other than PCOS in adolescents is nonclassic congenital adrenal hyperplasia (CAH). Risk is increased if family history is positive or in certain ethnic groups, such as Ashkenazi Jews (prevalence 1:27), Hispanics (1:40), and Slavics (1:50). (*H*) A random sample for plasma total testosterone is a reasonable screening test if reliable assessment of free testosterone is not available. At 8:00 a.m. during the mid-follicular phase of the menstrual cycle (days 4–10), the normal upper limit for plasma total testosterone is typically about 60 ng/dL (2.1 nM) for postmenarcheal adolescents when determined by a specialty laboratory. The upper limit of normal for plasma free testosterone under these conditions is 9 pg/mL (32 pM) in our laboratory. Unfortunately, the methodology for plasma free or bioavailable testosterone yields method-specific norms. (*I*) A high-normal testosterone level may not reflect a hyperandrogenic state if drawn after the early morning because of diurnal variation—or if only the total testosterone is initially assayed because the plasma free testosterone can be high when total testosterone is normal in that sex hormone binding globulin (SHBG), the major determinant of the bioavailable testosterone, is commonly low in hyperandrogenic women. (*J*) An early-morning plasma free testosterone determined by a specialty laboratory is indicated on days 4 through 10 of the menstrual cycle or during a period of amenorrhea, when the plasma testosterone is high-normal in patients with moderate or severe hirsutism, if features suggestive of other disorders are present or emerge, or if the response to cosmetic-dermatologic therapy is unsatisfactory. Simultaneous assay of 17-hydroxyprogesterone is indicated in subjects at high risk for CAH, which is suggested by a level greater than 150 ng/dL (4.5 nM)—and is virtually assured by a level greater than 1,200 ng/dL (36 nM). (*K*) Cosmetic therapies include bleaching, shaving, and waxing. Dermatologic therapies include topical eflornithine and laser treatment. OCP treatment is a useful and effective adjunct if hirsutism is more than minimal. (*L*) Idiopathic hirsutism may be mimicked by otherwise asymptomatic idiopathic hyperandrogenism, which may be due to atypical polycystic ovary syndrome or abnormal peripheral metabolism of prohormones. (*M*) Because testosterone undergoes episodic and cyclic changes in addition to diurnal ones, recheck is indicated if the course is progressive or risk factors emerge. (*N*) Hyperandrogenism with a polycystic ovary or menstrual irregularity in the absence of drug use, neoplasm, or other endocrinopathy meets standard criteria for the diagnosis of PCOS. Therefore, ultrasonic imaging of the ovaries and adrenal glands is usually advisable. See Figure 14-47 for potential further workup to determine the source of androgen excess. [Modified with permission from Rosenfield RL (2005). Clinical practice: Hirsutism. N Engl J Med 353:2578–2588.]

or a disorder of sexual differentiation. Further or alternative workup may include computed tomography for adrenal tumor, acute gonadotropin-releasing hormone agonist administration, or assessment of the response to hormonal suppression treatment to determine the source of androgen.

Management

Management is individualized according to symptoms and patient goals (e.g., hirsutism, acne, and alopecia; menstrual irregularity; obesity and insulin resistance) and the source of androgen excess.[339,736,737] Because PCOS is

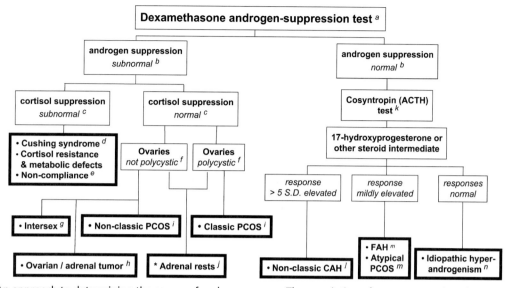

Figure 14-47 An approach to determining the source of androgen excess. The association of testosterone elevation with otherwise unexplained anovulatory symptoms (see Figures 14-42 and 14-43) or a polycystic ovary fulfills standard diagnostic criteria for PCOS, which in its various forms accounts for about 80 to 90% of adolescent hyperandrogenism. Determination of the source of excess androgen often permits a positive diagnosis of the characteristic FOH or FAH and rules out rare disorders that mimic PCOS. (A) Our standard dexamethasone androgen suppression test dose is 1 mg/m² in four divided doses (0.5 mg qid in adult) for 4 days, and plasma cortisol, free testosterone, 17-OHP, and DHEAS are measured on the morning of the fifth day after the final dexamethasone dose. For individuals weighing 100 kg or more, dexamethasone is given for 7 days. (B) Dexamethasone suppression of ACTH-dependent adrenal function normally causes plasma total testosterone to fall below 35 ng/dL (1.2 nM), free testosterone to below 8 pg/mL (28 pM), DHEAS by 75% to below 80 μg/dL (2.1 μM), and 17-OHP to less than 50 ng/dL (1.5 nM). Total testosterone is not as discriminating a criterion as the free testosterone (unfortunately, a method-dependent criterion) or 17-OHP criteria. Subnormal androgen suppression with normal adrenocortical suppression indicates a source of androgen other than an ACTH-dependent adrenal one. (C) Normally, cortisol falls below 1.5 mcg/dL (45 nM). (D) Cushing syndrome is an infrequent cause of hyperandrogenism and requires a more definitive workup. Hyperandrogenism has been reported in the rare conditions of cortisol resistance and cortisone reductase deficiency. (E) Subnormal cortisol suppression is most often due to noncompliance with taking dexamethasone tablets. (F) Ultrasonographic visualization of the ovaries by the vaginal route yields better definition than by the abdominal route, but this is not a generally acceptible technique in the virginal child. An adolescent polycystic ovary is defined as one with a volume greater than 10.8 cc or maximal area greater than 5.5 cm² or with 10 or more follicles in the maxmum plane. (G) Ovo-testicular DSD patients may only have a clearly elevated plasma testosterone level in response to a midcycle LH surge, hCG, or GnRH agonist test. (H) The baseline pattern of plasma androgens may yield a clue to the type of tumor. A DHEAS level greater than 700 mcg/dL (19 μmol/L) is suspicious for adrenal tumor. In the absence of a high DHEAS, disproportionate elevation of plasma androstenedione relative to testosterone or elevated 17-hydroxyprogesterone is typical of a virilizing tumor. Poor dexamethasone suppressibility of testosterone and/or DHEAS is very suggestive of adrenal tumor. CT scan of the abdomen may be indicated in such cases. (I) Polycystic ovary syndrome (PCOS) is a symptom complex with various combinations of hirsutism or its cutaneous equivalents anovulation and central obesity. A polycystic ovary is a classic diagnostic criterion, but is not necessary or specific for the diagnosis. Nonclassic PCOS includes anovulatory hyperandrogenic girls who lack a polycystic ovary. Most have the typical PCOS-type of functional ovarian hyperandrogenism on dexamethasone suppression or GnRH agonist testing. (J) Virilizing adrenal rests of the ovaries may complicate congenital adrenal hyperplasia. They may resemble a polycystic ovary. (K) The standard ACTH test is performed by infusing 250 mcg ACTH1-24 intravenously over a period of 1 minute and obtaining a blood sample before injection 1 hour later. (L) Congenital adrenal hyperplasia (CAH) cannot be confirmed upon mutation analysis unless the steroid intermediates immediately prior to the enzyme block rise 5 standard deviations above average in response to ACTH. For 17-OHP, this is greater than 1,200 ng/dL (36.5 nmol/L). For DHEA, this is greater than 3,000 ng/dL (104 nmol/L) in adolescents. (M) *Primary functional adrenal hyperandrogenism* (FAH) is a term for idiopathic ACTH-dependent (dexamethasone-suppresible) adrenal hyperandrogenism in which modest rises in DHEA, 17-OHP, and so on do not meet the criteria for the diagnosis of congenital adrenal hyperplasia. It is often found in atypical PCOS. (N) Idiopathic hyperandrogenemia is distinguished from idiopathic hirsutism. About 8% of chronic hyperandrogenemia remains unexplained after intensive investigation, which includes GnRH agonist testing to detect the occasional case of ovarian hyperandrogenism not detected by the dexamethasone test. [Modified with permission from Buggs C, Rosenfield RL (2005). Polycystic ovary syndrome in adolescence. Endocrinol Metab Clin North Am 34:677–705.]

associated with metabolic syndrome, a fasting lipid panel and oral glucose tolerance test are recommended in patients with central obesity or hypertension.[748] The two-hour blood sugar during an oral glucose tolerance test deteriorates at an average rate of 9 mg/dL/year.[749] Because PCOS is closely related to parental metabolic syndrome, we recommend a similar evaluation of primary relatives.

Cosmetic measures are the cornerstone of care for hirsutism. Bleaching and shaving suffice for many. Depilat-

ing agents and waxing treatments are useful but are prone to causing skin irritation. Eflornithine hydrochloride cream brings about marked improvement of hirsutism in about a third of patients, with the maximal effect by 2 to 6 months. The FDA has permitted marketing of many laser devices, and equivalents such as diode and flashlamp, as effective for permanent hair reduction—for which the criterion is persistant reduction in hair density by 30% or more after three to four treatments of a site.

Wavelengths between 694 and 1064 nm damage hair follicles by combining relatively selective absorption of heat by dark hairs with penetration into the dermis. Light-skinned individuals are the best candidates, requiring the lower energy pulses. Those with heavily tanned or darker skin require the use of cooling procedures and adjustment of energy levels to minimize the risk of skin side effects. Laser treatment is coming to be preferred to electrolysis, but both types of treatment require trained personnel; are repetitious, expensive, and painful; are practical only for treating limited areas; and may result in local reactions, including burns, dyspigmentation, and scarring. Endocrine therapy is directed at interrupting androgen production or action. This causes the pilosebaceous unit to revert toward the prepubertal vellus type.

Endocrinologic treatment of cutaneous symptoms is indicated before undertaking treatment with laser treatment—using Accutane or Rogane if standard cosmetic or topical dermatologic measures are inadequate. The maximal effect on the sebaceous gland occurs within 3 months, but that on sexual hairs requires 9 to 12 months of treatment because of the long duration of the hair growth cycle. All are effective only as long as the patient wishes to maintain her improvement in hirsutism.

Combination oral contraceptive pills (OCPs) are the first-line endocrine treatment for women with the dermatologic or menstrual abnormalities of PCOS. They act by suppressing plasma androgens, particularly free testosterone, mainly by inhibiting ovarian function. They also raise SHBG and modestly lower DHEA sulfate levels. They normalize androgen levels within the first month of therapy.

All estrogen-progestin combinations generally suffice for women with acne or mild hirsutism, in combination with cosmetic measures. Those with nonandrogenic progestins, such as norgestimate or ethynodiol diacetate combined with 35 μg ethiny E2, have generally favorable risk-benefit ratios and optimize lipid profiles. Those with antiandrogenic progestins in low dose may confer an additional benefit. Drospirenone is available in the United States (with 30 μg ethinyl E2) and in Canada, Mexico, and abroad (with cyproterone acetate 2 mg with 35 μg ethinyl E2). The larger estrogen doses may be necessary in larger girls to provide menstrual regularity.

OCPs are also effective in management of menstrual irregularity, which requires treatment because chronic anovulation is associated with increased risk of developing endometrial hyperplasia and carcinoma. There are, however, several potential disadvantages to the use of OCPs in the management of PCOS in adolescents. They will bring growth to end in perimenarcheal girls. OCPs, particularly some third-generation OCPs, may be contraindicated in patients who are at risk for venous thrombosis. In patients with migraine headaches, OCPs should be used with caution and in the lowest estrogen dose possible. Patients may use OCPs as an excuse for not losing weight. The patient may believe that the treatment is curative and defer a definitive diagnostic workup. OCPs do not permit conception if and when it is desired. The long-term consequences of these agents on fertility are unknown. There is the theoretic possibility of post-pill amenorrhea because high-dose estrogen begun in early adolescence may increase the risk of infertility.[750]

It is advisable to recheck patients after 3 months of therapy to assess the efficacy of treatment and normalization of androgen levels. As a general rule, OCP treatment should be continued until the patient is gynecologically mature (5 years postmenarcheal) or has lost a substantial amount of excess weight. At that point, withholding treatment for a few months to allow recovery of suppression of pituitary-gonadal function and to ascertain whether the menstrual abnormality persists is usually advisable. In doing so, however, one must keep in mind that the anovulatory cycles of PCOS lead to relative infertility (not absolute infertility). The need for continued use of OCP for contraceptive purposes must be considered.

Progestin monotherapy is an alternative to OCPs for the control of menstrual irregularities. Micronized progesterone (Prometrium) 100 to 200 mg daily at bedtime for 7 to 10 days induces withdrawal bleeding in the majority of patients, but some do not respond—apparently because of an antiestrogenic effect of androgen excess on the endometrium. Breakthough bleeding is more likely with progesterone than with OCPs. Progestin therapy has the appeal of permitting the detection of the emergence of normal menstrual cyclicity. However, it does not normalize androgen levels and is not an adequate treatment if hirsutism or hirsutism equivalents are a problem. The perimenarcheal girl who responds well to progestin therapy can be maintained at approximately 6-week cycles to permit the detection of spontaneous menses. Side effects of progestin include mood symptoms (depression), bloating, and breast soreness. Patients must be informed that oral progestin dosed in this way is not a means of contraception.

Antiandrogens generally yield improvement in hirsutism beyond that attainable with OCPs. They can be expected to reduce the Ferriman-Gallwey score by 15% to 40%, although there is considerable variation among individuals. Antiandrogen use for this purpose is off-label because all carry the risk of causing pseudohermaphroditism of the male fetus. Therefore, all antiandrogens should be prescribed with a contraceptive—preferably an OCP. They may have a modest effect on the metabolic abnormalities associated with PCOS.[751]

Spironolactone in high dosage is the safest potent antiandrogen in the United States. We recommend starting with 100 mg twice a day until the maximal effect has been achieved, and then attempting to reduce the dose to 50 mg twice a day for maintenance therapy. Spironolactone is usually well tolerated, but it is contraindicated in patients with adrenal, hepatic, or renal insufficiency. Women are at risk of hyperkalemia if on potassium-sparing diuretics, potassium supplements, daily nonsteroidal anti-inflammatory drugs, angiotensin-converting enzyme inhibitors, heparin, or such drugs. Therefore, electrolytes should be monitored. Alone, spironolactone tends to cause irregular bleeding.

Other antiandrogens used to treat hirsutism and hirsutism equivalents include cyproterone acetate, flutamide, and finasteride. Cyproterone acetate is a potent progestational antiandrogen used with estrogen in a reverse sequential regimen: 50 to 100 mg is given during days 1 to

10 of cycles in which estrogen is given from days 1 to 21. Flutamide is a more specific antiandrogen with efficacy similar to that of cyproterone and spironolactone, but it is more expensive and rarely causes fatal hepatic failure. Finasteride, a type-1 5-alpha-reductase inhibitor, seems less effective than other antiandrogens in the treatment of hirsutism and less effective in pattern hair loss in females than in males.

Although topical minoxidil is the only medication approved for alopecia treatment, antiandrogen-OCP therapy may be superior in those with PCOS. Insulin-lowering treatments, from weight loss to drug treatment, have about a 50% probability of improving menstrual cyclicity and ovulatory status—which seems greater than explicable by the modest reduction in androgen levels that they bring about.[268] The effect on hirsutism is neglible. Although weight reduction is indicated in obese PCOS patients, it is typically difficult to achieve.

Metformin appears to have more utility than thiazolidines in the management of adolescents because it suppresses appetite and enhances weight loss, albeit to a modest degree. It is most effective in combination with a behavioral weight-reduction program.[751] Therapy should start with 500 mg daily of the extended release form before the evening meal, with an increase in the dose by 500 mg per week to a maximal dose of 2,000 mg daily as tolerated. The larger doses are often better tolerated when divided into two daily doses. It is advisable to obtain a comprehensive metabolic panel at baseline and every 3 to 6 months, or as necessary, because of the rare complication of lactic acidosis.

Other hormonal manipulations may be useful in specific unusual situations. Prednisone therapy has little utility in the management of the hirsutism or menstrual irregularity of PCOS, although it may potentially be worth a trial in the atypical nonobese hirsute patient with isolated FAH as a single 5% to 7.5-mg bedtime dose. Gonadotropin-releasing hormone agonists are an oral contraceptive alternative when OCPs are contraindicated. They should be used with estradiol replacement therapy.

Future Directions

Tremendous advances continue to occur in our understanding of puberty. The identification of genes involved in ovarian differentiation, the discovery of new hormones and hormone receptors, new insights into the regulation of gene transcription and signal transduction, further identification of the role of genetic factors and prenatal imprinting on pubertal disorders, and advances in the application of mass spectrometry to steroid assays can also be anticipated to occur in the next 5 years.

We are in the midst of an explosion of information in the biological sciences. It is becoming clear that the body puts a wide but finite repertoire of hormones and growth factors to myriad and unexpected uses. Many concepts we hold dear at this moment are at the best likely to be shown to be oversimplifications; at worst, wrong. New information comes to light faster than we can assimilate it. The understanding of the interactions of the human genome with environmental factors can be expected to yield new insights into our understanding of puberty and its disorders.

ACKNOWLEDGMENTS

The authors' studies were supported in part by USPHS grants U54-041859 (RLR, SR) and RR-00055 (RLR).

REFERENCES

1. Donovan B, van der Werff ten Bosch J (1965). *Physiology of puberty.* London: Edward Arnold.
2. Wilkins L (1965). The Diagnosis and Treatment of Endocrine Disorders in Childhood and Adolescence. In Thomas C Springfield: MO.
3. Ramirez D, McCann S (1963). Comparison of the regulation of luteinizing hormone (LH) secretion in immature and adult rats. Endocrinology 72:452.
4. Mills I, Brooks R, Prunty F (1962). The relationship between the production of cortisol and androgen by the human adrenal. In Currie A, Symington T, Grant J (eds.), *The human adrenal cortex.* Baltimore: Williams & Wilkins.
5. Krsmanovic LZ, Stojilkovic SS, Catt KJ (1996). Pulsatile gonadotropin-releasing hormone release and its regulation. Trends Endocrinol Metab 7:56–59.
6. Grumbach M, Roth J, Kaplan S, Kelch R (1974). Hypothalamic-pituitary regulation of puberty in man: Evidence and concepts derived from clinical research. In Grumbach M, Grave C, Mayer F (eds.), *The control of the onset of puberty.* New York: John Wiley & Sons 115–207.
7. Winter J, Faiman C, Hobson W, Prasad A, Reyes F (1975). Pituitary-gonadal relations in infancy: I. Patterns of serum gonadotropin concentrations from birth to four years of age in man and chimpanzee. J Clin Endocrinol Metab 40:545.
8. Arey L (1974). Development of the female reproductive system. In, *Developmental anatomy.* Philadelphia: WB Saunders.
9. Schwanzel-Fukuda M, Jorgenson K, Bergen H, Weesner G, Pfaff D (1992). Biology of normal luteinizing hormone-releasing hormone neurons during and after their migration from olfactory placode. Endocr Rev 13:623.
10. Clements J, Reyes F, Winter J, et al. (1980). Ontogenesis of gonadotropin-releasing hormone in the human fetal hypothalamus. Proc Soc Exp Biol Med 163:437.
11. Kaplan S, Grumbach M, Aubert M (1976). The ontogenesis of pituitary hormones and hypothalamic factors in the human fetus. Recent Prog Horm Res 32:161.
12. Tapanainen J, Koivisto M, Vihko R, Huhtaniemi I (1981). Enhanced activity of the pituitary-gonadal axis in premature human infants. J Clin Endocrinol Metab 52:235–238.
13. King J, Gerall A (1976). Localization of luteinizing hormone-releasing hormone. J Histochem Cytochem 24:829.
14. Raisman G, Field P (1973). Sexual dimorphism in the neuropil of the preoptic area of the rat and its dependence on neonatal androgen. Brain Res 54:1.
15. Gorski R (1985). Sexual differentiation of the brain: possible mechanisms and implications. Can J Physiol Pharmacol 63:577–594.
16. Sarma HN, Manikkam M, Herkimer C, et al. (2005). Fetal programming: excess prenatal testosterone reduces postnatal luteinizing hormone, but not follicle-stimulating hormone responsiveness, to estradiol negative feedback in the female. Endocrinology 146:4281–4291.
17. Gulyas B, Hodgen G, Tullner W, et al. (1977). Effects of fetal or maternal hypophysectomy on endocrine organs and body weight in infant rhesus monkeys (Macaca mulatto): With particular emphasis on oogenesis. Biol Reprod 16:216.
18. Merrill J (1959). Ovarian hilus cells. Am J Obstet Gynecol 78:1258.
19. Carney JA (1987). Unusual tumefactive spindle-cell lesions in the adrenal gland. Hum Pathol 18:980–985.
20. Lim HN, Hawkins JR (1998). Genetic control of gonadal differentiation. Baillière's Clin Endocrinol Metab 12:1–16.
21. Rabinovici J, Jaffe R (1990). Development and regulation of growth and differentiated function in human and subhuman primate fetal gonads. Endocr Rev 11:532.

22. Vainio S, Heikkila M, Kispert A, Chin N, McMahon AP (1999). Female development in mammals is regulated by Wnt-4 signalling. Nature 397:405–409.

23. Yao HH, Matzuk MM, Jorgez CJ, et al. (2004). Follistatin operates downstream of Wnt4 in mammalian ovary organogenesis. Dev Dyn 230:210-215

24. Peters H (1970). Migration of gonocytes into the mammalian gonad and their differentiation. Philos Trans R Soc Lond [Biol] 259:91.

25. Baker T (1963). A quantitative and cytological study of germ cells in human ovaries. Proc R Soc Lond B Biol Sci 158:417–433.

26. Peters H, Byskov A, Grinsted J (1978). Follicular growth in fetal and prepubertal ovaries of humans and other primates. Clin Endocrinol Metab 7:469.

27. Ross GT, Schreiber JR (1978). The ovary. In Yen SSC, Jaffe R (eds.), Reproductive endocrinology. Philadelphia: WB Saunders.

28. Peters H (1979). The human ovary in childhood and early maturity. Eur J Obstet Gynecol Reprod Biol 9:137.

29. Gougeon A (1996). Regulation of ovarian follicular development in primates: Facts and hypotheses. Endocrin Rev 17:121–155.

30. Carr D, Naggar R, Hart A (1968). Germ cells in the ovaries of XO female infants. Am J Clin Pathol 19:521.

31. Block E (1953). A quantitative morphological investigation of the follicular system in newborn female infants. Acta Anat 17:201–206.

32. Richardson S, Senikas V, Nelson J (1987). Follicular depletion during the menopausal transition: Evidence for accelerated loss and ultimate exhaustion. J Clin Endocrinol Metab 65:1231.

33. Gartler S, Andina R, Cant N (1975). Ontogeny of X chromosome inactivation in the female germ line. Exp Cell Res 91:454.

34. Zinn AR (2000). The X chromosome and the ovary. J Soc Gynecol Investig 8:S34–S36.

35. McGee E, Hsueh A (2000). Initial and cyclic recruitment of ovarian follicles. Endocrine Reviews 21:200–214.

36. Yamamoto N, Christenson LK, McAllister JM, Strauss JF III (2002). Growth differentiation factor-9 inhibits 3'5'-adenosine monophosphate-stimulated steroidogenesis in human granulosa and theca cells. J Clin Endocrinol Metab 87:2849–2856.

37. Knight PG, Glister C (2006). TGF-beta superfamily members and ovarian follicle development. Reproduction 132:191-206.

38. Richards JS (2001). Perspective: the ovarian follicle--a perspective in 2001. Endocrinology 142:2184-2193.

39. Dissen GA, Romero C, Hirshfield AN, Ojeda SR (2001). Nerve growth factor is required for early follicular development in the mammalian ovary. Endocrinology 142:2078–2086.

40. Pru JK, Tilly JL (2001). Programmed cell death in the ovary: insights and future prospects using genetic technologies. Mol Endocrinol 15:845–853.

41. Robles R, Morita Y, Mann KK, et al. (2000). The aryl hydrocarbon receptor, a basic helix-loop-helix transcription factor of the PAS gene family, is required for normal ovarian germ cell dynamics in the mouse. Endocrinology 141:450–453.

42. Besedovsky H, Sorkin E (1974). Thymus involvement in female sexual maturation. Nature 249:356.

43. de Bruin JP, Dorland M, Bruinse HW, Spliet W, Nikkels PG, Te Velde ER (1998). Fetal growth retardation as a cause of impaired ovarian development. Early Hum Dev 51:39–46.

44. Gagnon R (1998). Fetal endocrine adaptation to placental insufficiency. The Endocrinologist 8:436–442.

45. Cole B, Hensinger K, Maciel GA, Chang RJ, Erickson GF (2006). Human fetal ovary development involves the spatiotemporal expression of p450c17 protein. J Clin Endocrinol Metab 91:3654–3661.

46. Terasawa E, Fernandez DL (2001). Neurobiological mechanisms of the onset of puberty in primates. Endocr Rev 22:111–151.

47. Shahab M, Mastronardi C, Seminara SB, Crowley WF, Ojeda SR, Plant TM (2005). Increased hypothalamic GPR54 signaling: A potential mechanism for initiation of puberty in primates. Proc Natl Acad Sci USA 102:2129–2134.

48. Ojeda SR, Lomniczi A, Mastronardi C, et al. (2006). The neuroendocrine regulation of puberty: Is the time ripe for a systems biology approach? Endocrinology 147:1166–1174.

49. Plant TM, Witchel SF (2006). Puberty in non-human primates and humans. In Challis JRG, de Kretser DM, Neill JD, et al. (eds.), Knobil and Neill's physiology of reproduction. New York: Elsevier 2177–2230.

50. Hughes IA, Kumanan M (2006). A wider perspective on puberty. Mol Cell Endocrinol 254:1–7.

51. Winter J, Faiman C (1973). Pituitary-gonadal relations in female children and adolescents. Pediatr Res 7:948.

52. Winter JSD, Hughes IA, Reyes Fl, Faiman C (1976). Pituitary-gonadal relations in infancy: 2. Patterns of serum gonadal steroid concentrations in man from birth to two years of age. J Clin Endocrinol Metab 42:679.

53. Danon M, Velez O, Ostrea T, Crawford JD, Beitins IZ (1988). Dynamics of bioactive luteinizing hormone-human chorionic gonadotropin during the first 7 days of life. Pediatr Res 23:530–533.

54. Bangham DR, Berryman I, Burger H, et al. (1973). An international collaborative study of 69-104, a reference preparation of human pituitary FSH and LH. J Clin Endocrinol Metab 36:647–660.

55. Bouvattier C, Carel JC, Lecointre C, et al. (2002). Postnatal changes of T, LH, and FSH in 46,XY infants with mutations in the AR gene. J Clin Endocrinol Metab 87:29–32.

56. Sullivan SD, Moenter SM (2004). Prenatal androgens alter GABAergic drive to gonadotropin-releasing hormone neurons: Implications for a common fertility disorder. Proc Natl Acad Sci USA 101:7129–7134.

57. Bidlingmaier F, Kiiorr D (1978). Oestrogens: Physiological and clinical aspects. Pediatr Adolesc Endocrinol 4:43.

58. Betend B, Claustrat B, Bizollon C, Ehre C, Francois R (1975). Etude de la fonction gonadotrope hypophysaire par le test a la LH-RH pendant la premiere année de la vie. Ann Endocrinol (Paris) 36:325.

59. Rosenfield RL, Burstein S, Cuttler L, et al. (1989). Use of nafarelin for testing pituitary-ovarian function. J Reprod Med 34:1044–1150.

60. Chellakooty M, Schmidt IM, Haavisto AM, et al. (2003). Inhibin A, inhibin B, follicle-stimulating hormone, luteinizing hormone, estradiol, and sex hormone-binding globulin levels in 473 healthy infant girls. J Clin Endocrinol Metab 88:3515–3520.

61. Conte F, Grumbach M, Kaplan S, et al. (1980). Correlation of luteinizing hormone-releasing factor-induced luteinizing hormone and follicle-stimulating hormone release from infancy to 19 years with the changing pattern of gonadotropin secretion in agonadal patients: Relation to the restraint of puberty. J Clin Endocrinol Metab 50:163.

61a. Sedin G, Bergquist C, Lindgren PG (1985). Ovarian hyperstimulation syndrome in preterm infants. Pediatr Res 19:548-552.

62. Penny R, Olambiwonnu N, Frasier S (1974). Serum gonadotropin concentrations during the first four years of life. J Clin Endocrinol Metab 38:320.

63. Elsholz DD, Padmanabhan V, Rosenfield RL, Olton PR, Phillips DJ, Foster CM (2004). GnRH agonist stimulation of the pituitary-gonadal axis in children: Age and sex differences in circulating inhibin-B and activin-A. Hum Reprod 19:2748–2758.

64. Bourguignon J-P, Hoyoux C, Reuter A, et al. (1979). Urinary excretion of immunoreactive luteinizing hormone-releasing hormone-like material and gonadotropins at different stages of life. J Clin Endocrinol Metab 48:78.

65. Rosenfield RL (1977). Hormonal events and disorders of puberty. In Givens J (ed.), Gynecologic endocrinology. Chicago: Year Book Medical Publishers 1–19.

66. Attardi B, Ohno S. Androgen and estrogen receptors in the developing mouse brain. Endocrinology 1976;99:1279.

67. Rifkind A, Kulin H, Ross G (1967). Follicle stimulating hormone (FSH) and luteinizing hormone (LH) in the urine of prepubertal children. J Clin Invest 46:1925.

68. Maesaka H, Tachibana K, Adachi M, Okada T (1996). Monthly urinary gonadotropin and ovarian hormone excretory patterns in normal girls and female patients with idiopathic precocious puberty. Pediatr Res 40:853–860.

69. Apter D, Butzow TL, Laughlin GA, Yen SS (1993). Gonadotropin-releasing hormone pulse generator activity during pubertal transition in girls: Pulsatile and diurnal patterns of circulating gonadotropins. J Clin Endocrinol Metab 76:940–949.

70. Wilson ME, Fisher J, Chikazawa K (2004). Estradiol negative feedback regulates nocturnal luteinizing hormone and follicle-stimulating hormone secretion in prepubertal female rhesus monkeys. J Clin Endocrinol Metab 89:3973–3978.

71. Mitamura R, Yano K, Suzuki N, Ito Y, Makita Y, Okuno A (2000). Diurnal rhythms of luteinizing hormone, follicle-stimulating hormone, testosterone, and estradiol secretion before the onset of female puberty in short children. J Clin Endocrinol Metab 85:1074–1080.

72. Gruijters MJ, Visser JA, Durlinger AL, Themmen AP (2003). Anti-Mullerian hormone and its role in ovarian function. Mol Cell Endocrinol 211:85-90.

73. Merrill J (1963). The morphology of the prepubertal ovary: Relationship to the polycystic ovary syndrome. Southern Medical Journal 225–231.

74. Kraus F, Neubecker R (1962). Luteinization of the ovarian theca in infants and children. Am J Clin Pathol 37:389–397.

75. Stanhope R, Adams J, Jacobs H, Brook C (1985). Ovarian ultrasound assessment in normal children, idiopathic precocious puberty, and during low dose pulsatile gonadotrophin releasing hormone treatment of hypogonadotrophic hypogonadism. Arch Dis Child 60:116.

76. Bridges NA, Cooke A, Healy MJR, Hindmarsh PC, Brook CGD (1993). Standards for ovarian volume in childhood and puberty. Fertil Steril 60:456–460.

77. Buzi F, Pilotta A, Dordoni D, Lombardi A, Zaglio S, Adlard P (1998). Pelvic ultrasonography in normal girls and in girls with pubertal precocity. Acta Paediatr 87:1138–1145.

78. de Vries L, Horev G, Schwartz M, Phillip M (2006). Ultrasonographic and clinical parameters for early differentiation between precocious puberty and premature thelarche. Eur J Endocrinol 154:891–898.

79. Klein KL, Mericq V, Brown-Dawson JM, Larmore KA, Cabezas P, Cortinez A (1999). Estrogen levels in girls with premature thelarche compared with normal prepubertal girls as determined by an ultrasensitive recombinant cell bioassay. J Pediatr 134: 190–192.

80. Collett-Solberg P, Grumbach M (1965). A simplified procedure for evaluating estrogenic effects and the sex chromatin pattern in exfoliated cells in urine: Studies in premature thelarche and gynecomastia of adolescence. J Pediatr 66:883.

81. Goodpasture J, Ghai K, Cara J, Rosenfield R (1993). Potential of gonadotropin-releasing hormone agonists in the diagnosis of pubertal disorders in girls. Clin Obstet Gynecol 36:773–785.

82. Ibañez L, Potau N, Zampolli M, et al. (1994). Use of leuprolide acetate response patterns in the early diagnosis of pubertal disorders: Comparison with the gonadotropin-releasing hormone test. J Clin Endocrinol Metab 78:30–35.

83. Norjavaara E, Ankargerg C, AAlbertsson-Wikland K (1996). Diurnal rhythm of 17ß-estradiol secretion throughout pubertal development in healthy girls: Evaluation by a sensitive radioimmunoassay. J Clin Endocrinol Metab 81:4095–4102.

84. Dickerman Z, Prager-Lewin R, Laron Z (1976). Response of plasma LH and FSH to synthetic LHRH in children at various pubertal stages. Am J Dis Child 130:634–638.

85. Rettig K, Duckett CE, Sweetland M, Reiter EO, Root AW (1981). Urinary excretion of immunoreactive luteinizing hormone-releasing hormone-like material in children: Correlation with pubertal development. J Clin Endocrinol Metab 52:1150.

86. Barnea A, Cho C, Porter J (1979). A role for the ovaries in maturational processes of hypothalamic neurons containing luteinizing hormone-releasing hormone. Endocrinology 105:1303.

87. Knobil E (1980). The neuroendocrine control of the menstrual cycle. Recent Prog Horm Res 36:53.

88. Marshall J, Kelch R (1986). Gonadotropin-releasing hormone: Role of pulsatile secretion in the regulation of reproduction. N Engl J Med 315:1459.

89. Crowley WF Jr., Filicori M, Santoro NF (1987). GnRH secretion across the normal menstrual cycle. In Crowley WJ, Hofler J (eds.), *The episodic secretion of hormones*. New York: John Wiley/Churchill Livingstone 219–231.

90. Kulin H, Reiter E (1973). Gonadotropins during childhood and adolescence: A review. Pediatrics 51:260.

91. Hansen J, Hoffman H, Ross C (1975). Monthly gonadotropin cycles in premenarcheal girls. Science 190:161.

92. Weitzman E, Perlow M, Boyar R, Hellman L (1972). Light and luteinizing hormone. N Engl J Med 286:932.

93. Boyar RM, Wu RHK, Roffwarg H, et al. (1976). Human puberty: 24-Hour estradiol patterns in pubertal girls. J Clin Endocrinol Metab 43:1418.

94. Lucky AW, Rich BH, Rosenfield RL, Fang VS, Roche-Bender N (1980). LH bioactivity increases more than immunoreactivity during puberty. J Pediatr 97:205.

95. Rosenfield RL, Helke J (1992). Is an immunoassay available for the measurement of bioactive LH in serum? J Androl 13:1–10.

96. Beitins I, Padmanabhan V (1991). Bioactivity of gonadotropins. Endocrinol Metab Clin N Am 20:85–120.

97. Legro RS, Lin HM, Demers LM, Lloyd T (2000). Rapid maturation of the reproductive axis during perimenarche independent of body composition. J Clin Endocrinol Metab 85:1021–1025.

98. Elkind-Hirsch K, Ravnikar V, Schiff I, Tulchinsky D, Ryan K (1982). Determinations of endogenous immunoreactive luteinizing hormone-releasing hormone in human plasma. J Clin Endocrinol Metab 54:602.

99. Xia L, Van Vugt D, Alston E, Luckhaus J, Ferin M (1992). A surge of gonadotropin-releasing hormone accompanies the estradiol-induced gonadotropin surge in the Rhesus monkey. Endocrinol 131:2812–2820.

100. McCartney CR, Blank SK, Marshall JC (2007). Progesterone acutely increases LH pulse amplitude but does not acutely influence nocturnal LH pulse frequency slowing during the late follicular phase in women. Am J Physiol Endocrinol Metab 292:E900-E906.

101. Lin W, Ramirez V (1988). Effect of pulsatile infusion of progesterone on the in vivo activity of the luteinizing hormone-releasing hormone neural apparatus of awake unrestrained female and male rabbits. Endocrinology 122:868.

102. Moll GW Jr., Rosenfield RL (1984). Direct inhibitory effect of estradiol on pituitary luteinizing hormone responsiveness to luteinizing hormone releasing hormone is specific and of rapid onset. Biol Reprod 30:59.

103. Young J, Jaffe R (1976). Strength-duration characteristics of estrogen effects on gonadotropin response to gonadotropin-releasing hormone in women: II. J Clin Endocrinol Metab 42:432.

104. March CM, Goebelsmann U, Nakamura RM, Mishell DR Jr. (1979). Roles of estradiol and progesterone in eliciting the midcycle luteinizing hormone and follicle-stimulating hormone surges. J Clin Endocrinol Metab 49:507.

105. Chang R, Jaffe R (1978). Progesterone effects on gonadotropin release in women pretreated with estradiol. J Clin Endocrinol Metab 47:119.

106. Advis J, cause J, McKelvy J (1983). Evidence that endopeptidase-catalyzed luteinizing hormone releasing hormone cleavage contributes to the regulation of median eminence LHRH levels during positive steroid feedback. Endocrinology 11:1147.

107. Harlow C, Shaw N, Hillier S, Hodges J (1988). Factors influencing follicle-stimulating hormone-responsive steroidogenesis in marmoset granulosa cells: Effects of androgens and the stage of follicular maturity. Endocrinology 122:2780.

108. Richards J, Bogovich K (1982). Effects of human chorionic gonadotropin and progesterone on follicular development in the immature rat. Endocrinol 111:1429–1438.

109. Jia X-C, Kessel B, Welsh TN J, Hsueh A (1985). Androgen inhibition of follicle-stimulating hormone-stimulated luteinizing hormone receptor formation in cultured rat granulosa cells. Endocrinology 117:13.

110. Hsueh AJW, Adashi EY, Jones PBC, Welsh TNJ (1984). Hormonal regulation of the differentiation of cultured ovarian granulosa cells. Endocrinol Rev 5:76.

111. Findlay J (1994). Peripheral and local regulators of folliculogenesis. Reprod Fertil Dev 6:1–13.

112. White SS, Ojeda SR (1981). Changes in ovarian LHRH receptor content during the onset of puberty in the female rat. Endocrinology 108:347.

113. Eckstein B, Shani J, Ravid R, Goldhaber G (1981). Effect of androstanediol sulfates on luteinizing hormone release in ovariectomized rats. Endocrinology 108:500.

114. Polhemus D (1953). Ovarian maturation and cyst formation in children. Pediatr 11:588–593.

115. Brook C, Jacobs H, Stanhope R (1988). Polycystic ovaries in childhood. Br Med J 296:878.

116. Adams J, Franks S, Polson DW, et al. (1985). Multifollicular ovaries: clinical and endocrine features and response to pulsatile gonadotrophin releasing hormone. Lancet 2:1375–1378.

116a. van Hooff MH, Voorhorst FJ, Kaptein MB, et al (2000). Polycystic ovaries in adolescents and the relationship with menstrual cycle patterns, luteinizing hormone, androgens, and insulin. Fertil Steril 74:49-58.

117. Venturoli S, Porcu E, Fabbri R, et al. (1995). Longitudinal change of sonographic ovarian aspects and endocrine parameters in irregular cycles of adolescence. Pediatr Res 38:974–980.

118. Abraham G (1974). Ovarian and adrenal contributions to peripheral androgens during the menstrual cycle. J Clin Endocrinol Metab 39:340.

119. Ross GT, Cargille CM, Lipsett MB, et al. (1970). Pituitary and gonadal hormones in women during spontaneous and induced ovulatory cycles. Recent Prog Horm Res 26:1.

120. McCartney CR, Gingrich MB, Hu Y, Evans WS, Marshall JC (2002). Hypothalamic regulation of cyclic ovulation: evidence that the increase in gonadotropin-releasing hormone pulse frequency during the follicular phase reflects the gradual loss of the restraining effects of progesterone. J Clin Endocrinol Metab 87:2194–2200.

121. Johnson D, Naqvi R (1969). A positive feedback action of androgen on pituitary follicle stimulating hormone: Induction of a cyclic phenomenon. Endocrinology 85:881.

122. Melrose P, Gross R (1987). Steroid effects on the secretory modalities of gonadotropin-releasing hormone release. Endocrinology 121:190.

123. Erickson GF, Magoffin DA, Dyer CA, Hofeditz C (1985). The ovarian androgen producing cells: A review of structure/function relationships. Endocrin Rev 6:371–399.

124. Richards J (1994). Hormonal control of gene expression in the ovary. Endocrine Rev 15:725.

125. Castrillon DH, Miao L, Kollipara R, Horner JW, DePinho RA (2003). Suppression of ovarian follicle activation in mice by the transcription factor Foxo3a. Science 301:215–218.

126. Ibañez L, Valls C, Cols M, Ferrer A, Marcos MV, De Zegher F (1988). Hypersecretion of FSH in infant boys and girls born small for gestational age. J Clin Endocrinol Metab 87:1986–1988.

127. Ross C (1974). Gonadotropins and preantral follicular maturation in women. Fertil Steril 25:52.

128. Kumar TR, Wang Y, Lu N, Matzuk MM (1997). Follicle stimulating hormone is required for ovarian follicle maturation but not male fertility. Nat Genet 15:201–204.

129. Barnes RB, Namnoum AB, Rosenfield RL, Layman LC (2002). The role of LH and FSH in ovarian androgen secretion and ovarian follicular development: Clinical studies in a patient with isolated FSH deficiency and multicystic ovaries, Case report. Hum Reprod 17:88–91.

130. Weil S, Vendola K, Zhou J, Bondy CA (1999). Androgen and follicle-stimulating hormone interactions in primate ovarian follicle development. J Clin Endocrinol Metab 84:2951–2956.

131. Vendola KA, Zhou J, Adesanya OO, Weil SJ, Bondy CA (1998). Androgens stimulate early stages of follicular growth in the primate ovary. J Clin Invest 15:2622–2629.

132. Shiina H, Matsumoto T, Sato T, et al. (2006). Premature ovarian failure in androgen receptor-deficient mice. Proc Natl Acad Sci USA 103:224–229.

133. Voutilainen R, Tapanainen J, Chung B, Matteson K, Miller W (1986). Hormonal regulation of P450scc (20,22-desmolase) and P450c17 (17α-hydroxylase/17,20-lyase) in cultured human granulosa cells. J Clin Endocrinol Metab 63:202–207.

134. Inkster S, Brodie A (1991). Expression of aromatase cytochrome P-450 in premenopausal and postmenopausal human ovaries: An immunocytochemical study. J Clin Endocrinol Metab 73:717–726.

135. McNatty KP, Makris A, Reinhold VN (1979). Metabolism of androstenedione by human ovarian tissues in vitro with particular reference to reductase and aromatase activity. Steroids 34:429.

136. McNatty KP, Smith DM, Makris A, Osathanondh R, Ryan KJ (1979). The microenvironment of the human antral follicle: Interrelationships among the steroid levels in antral fluid, the population of granulosa cells, and the status of the oocyte in vivo and in vitro. J Clin Endocrinol Metab 49:851.

137. Erickson GF, Hsueh AJ, Quigley ME, Rebar RW, Yen SS (1979). Functional studies of aromatase activity in human granulosa cells from normal and polycystic ovaries. J Clin Endocrinol Metab 49:514.

138. Tsang B, Armstrong D, Whitfield J (1980). Steroid biosynthesis by isolated human ovarian follicular cells in vitro. J Clin Endocrinol Metab 51:1407–1411.

139. Mason HD, Willis DS, Beard RW, Winston RM, Margara R, Franks S (1994). Estradiol production by granulosa cells of normal and polycystic ovaries: Relationship to menstrual cycle history and concentrations of gonadotropins and sex steroids in follicular fluid. J Clin Endocrinol Metab 79:1355–1360.

140. Haning Jr R, Hackett R, Flood C, Loughlin J, Zhao Q, Longcope C (1993). Testosterone, a follicular regulator: Key to anovulation. J Clin Endocrinol Metab 77:710–715.

141. Karnitis V, Townson D, Friedman C, Danforth D (1994). Recombinant human follicle-stimulating hormone stimulates multiple follicular growth, but minimal estrogen production in gonadotropin-

142. Meduri G, Touraine P, Beau I, et al. (2003). Delayed puberty and primary amenorrhea associated with a novel mutation of the human follicle-stimulating hormone receptor: Clinical, histological, and molecular studies. J Clin Endocrinol Metab 88:3491–3498.

143. Zhou J, Kumar R, Matzuk MM, Bondy C (1997). Insulin-like growth factor I regulates gonadotropin responsiveness in the murine ovary. Molec Endocrinol 11:1924–1933.

144. McNatty KP, Hunter WM, MacNeilly AS, Sawers RS (1975). Changes in the concentration of pituitary and steroid hormones in the follicular fluid of human Graafian follicles throughout the menstrual cycle. J Endocrinol 64:555.

145. McNatty KP, Makris A, De Grazia C, Osathanondh R, Ryan KJ (1980). Steroidogenesis by recombined follicular cells from the human ovary in vitro. J Clin Endocrinol Metab 51:1286.

146. Couse JF, Hewitt SC, Bunch DO, et al. (1999). Postnatal sex reversal of the ovaries in mice lacking estrogen receptors alpha and beta. Science 286:2328-31.

146a. Lofrano-Porto A, Barra GB, Giacomini LA, et al (2007). Luteinizing hormone beta mutation and hypogonadism in men and women. N Engl J Med 357:897-904.

147. Richards JS, Russell DL, Ochsner S, et al. (2002). Novel signaling pathways that control ovarian follicular development, ovulation, and luteinization. Recent Prog Horm Res 57:195–220.

148. Jonassen J, Bose K, Richards J (1982). Enhancement and desensitization of hormone-responsive adenylate cyclase in granulosa cells of preantral and antral ovarian follicles: Effects of estradiol and follicle-stimulating hormone. Endocrinology 111:74.

149. Masciarelli S, Horner K, Liu C, et al. (2004). Cyclic nucleotide phosphodiesterase 3A-deficient mice as a model of female infertility. J Clin Invest 114:196–205.

150. Lindner HR, Tsafriri A, Lieberman ME, et al. (1974). Gonadotropin action on cultured Graafian follicles: Induction of maturation division of the mammalian oocyte and differentiation of the luteal cell. Recent Prog Horm Res 30:79.

151. Hillier S, Ross C (1979). Effects of exogenous testosterone on ovarian weight, follicular morphology and intraovarian progesterone concentration in estrogen-primed hypophysectomized immature female rats. Biol Reprod 20:261.

152. Poland M, Seu D, Tarlatzis B (1986). Human chorionic gonadotropin stimulation of estradiol production and androgen antagonism of gonadotropin-stimulated responses in cultured human granulosa luteal cells. J Clin Endocrinol Metab 62:628.

153. Chaffkin L, Luciano A, Peluso J (1993). The role of progesterone in regulating human granulosa cell proliferation and differentiation in vitro. J Clin Endocrinol Metab 76:696–700.

154. Schreiber J, Nakamura K, Truscella A, Erickson G (1982). Progestins inhibit FSH-induced functional LH receptors in cultured rat granulosa cells. Molec Cell Endocrinol 25:113.

155. Fauser BC, Van Heusden AM (1997). Manipulation of human ovarian function: physiological concepts and clinical consequences. Endocr Rev 18:71–106.

156. Couse JF, Korach KS (1999). Estrogen receptor null mice: What have we learned and where will they lead us? [published erratum appears in Endocr Rev 20(4):459, 1999]. Endocr Rev 20:358–417.

157. Couse JF, Bunch DO, Lindzey J, Schomberg DW, Korach KS (1999). Prevention of the polycystic ovarian phenotype and characterization of ovulatory capacity in the estrogen receptor-alpha knockout mouse. Endocrinology 140:5855–5865.

158. Cheng G, Weihua Z, Makinen S, et al. (2002). A role for the androgen receptor in follicular atresia of estrogen receptor beta knockout mouse ovary. Biol Reprod 66:77–84.

159. Lyet L, Louis F, Forest MG, Josso N, Behringer RR, Vigier B (1995). Ontogeny of reproductive abnormalities induced by deregulation of anti-mullerian hormone expression in transgenic mice. Biol Reprod 52:444–454.

160. Carlsson IB, Scott JE, Visser JA, et al. (2006). Anti-Mullerian hormone inhibits initiation of growth of human primordial ovarian follicles in vitro. Hum Reprod 21:2223-2227.

161. Catteau-Jonard S, Pigny P, Reyss AC, et al. (2007). Changes in serum anti-Mullerian hormone level during low-dose recombinant follicular-stimulating hormone therapy for anovulation in polycystic ovary syndrome. J Clin Endocrinol Metab 92:4138-143.

162. Burger HG, Groome NP, Robertson DM (1998). Both inhibin A and B respond to exogenous follicle-stimulating hormone in the follicular phase of the human menstrual cycle. J Clin Endocrinol Metab 83:4167–4169.

163. Welt CK, Smith ZA, Pauler DK, Hall JE (2001). Differential regulation of inhibin A and inhibin B by luteinizing hormone, follicle-stimulating hormone, and stage of follicle development. J Clin Endocrinol Metab 86:2531–2537.

164. Richards J, Hegin L, Caston L (1986). Differentiation of rat ovarian thecal cells: Evidence for functional luteinization. Endocrinol 118:1660–1668.

165. Auletta F, Flint A (1988). Mechanisms controlling corpus luteum function in sheep, cows, nonhuman primates, and women especially in relation to the time of luteolysis. Endocr Rev 9:88.

166. Vande Wiele RL, Bogumil J, Dyrenfurth I, et al. (1970). Mechanisms regulating the menstrual cycle in women. Recent Prog Horm Res ;26:63.

167. Stouffer R, Hodgen C, Ottobre A, Christina C (1984). Follicular fluid treatment during the follicular versus luteal phase of the menstrual cycle: Effects on corpus luteum function. J Clin Endocrinol Metab 58:1027.

168. Parent AS, Teilmann G, Juul A, Skakkebaek NE, Toppari J, Bourguignon JP (2003). The timing of normal puberty and the age limits of sexual precocity: Variations around the world, secular trends, and changes after migration. Endocr Rev 24:668–693.

169. Fischbein S (1977). Intra-pair similarity in physical growth of monozygotic and of dizygotic twins during puberty. Ann Hum Biol 4:417–430.

170. Garn SM, Bailey SM (1978). Genetics and maturational processes. In Falkner F, Tanner JM (eds.), Human growth 1: Principles and prenatal growth. New York: Plenum Press 307–330.

171. Sharma JC (1983). The genetic contribution to pubertal growth and development studied by longitudinal growth data on twins. Ann Hum Biol 10:163–171.

172. Kaprio J, Rimpela A, Winter T, Viken RJ, Rimpela M, Rose RJ (1995). Common genetic influences on BMI and age at menarche. Hum Biol 67:739–753.

173. Sun SS, Schubert CM, Chumlea WC, et al. (2002). National estimates of the timing of sexual maturation and racial differences among U.S. children. Pediatrics 110:911–919.

174. Chumlea WC, Schubert CM, Roche AF, et al. (2003). Age at menarche and racial comparisons in US girls. Pediatrics 111:110–113.

175. Sedlmeyer IL, Hirschhorn JN, Palmert MR (2002). Pedigree analysis of constitutional delay of growth and maturation: determination of familial aggregation and inheritance patterns. J Clin Endocrinol Metab 87:5581–5586.

176. Sedlmeyer IL, Palmert MR (2002). Delayed puberty: analysis of a large case series from an academic center. J Clin Endocrinol Metab 87:1613–1620.

177. Eaves L, Silberg J, Foley D, et al. (2004). Genetic and environmental influences on the relative timing of pubertal change. Twin Res 7:471–481.

178. Herman-Giddens ME, Kaplowitz PB, Wasserman R (2004). Navigating the recent articles on girls' puberty in Pediatrics: What do we know and where do we go from here? Pediatrics 113:911–917.

179. Nathan BM, Hodges CA, Palmert MR (2006). The use of mouse chromosome substitution strains to investigate the genetic regulation of pubertal timing. Mol Cell Endocrinol 254/255:103–108.

180. Franco B, Guioli S, Pragliola A, et al. (1991). A gene deleted in Kallmann's syndrome shares homology with neural cell adhesion and axonal path-finding molecules. Nature 353:529–536.

181. Seminara SB (2006). Mechanisms of disease: The first kiss-a crucial role for kisspeptin-1 and its receptor, G-protein-coupled receptor 54, in puberty and reproduction. Nat Clin Pract Endocrinol Metab 2:328–334.

182. Pitteloud N, Meysing A, Quinton R, et al. (2006). Mutations in fibroblast growth factor receptor 1 cause Kallmann syndrome with a wide spectrum of reproductive phenotypes. Mol Cell Endocrinol 254-255:60-69.

182a. Pfaeffle RW, Savage JJ, Hunter CS, et al. (2007). Four novel mutations of the LHX3 gene cause combined pituitary hormone deficiencies with or without limited neck rotation. J Clin Endocrinol Metab 92:1909-1919.

183. Sedlmeyer IL, Pearce CL, Trueman JA, et al. (2005). Determination of sequence variation and haplotype structure for the gonadotropin-releasing hormone (GnRH) and GnRH receptor genes: Investigation of role in pubertal timing. J Clin Endocrinol Metab 90:1091–1099.

184. Plant TM, Barker-Gibb ML (2004). Neurobiological mechanisms of puberty in higher primates. Hum Reprod Update 10:67–77.

185. Ojeda SR, Urbanski HF (1994). Puberty in the rat. In Knobil E, Neill JD (eds.), The physiology of reproduction. New York: Raven Press 363–407.

186. Seminara SB, Messager S, Chatzidaki EE, et al. (2003). The GPR54 gene as a regulator of puberty. N Engl J Med 349:1614–1627.

187. Semple RK, Achermann JC, Ellery J, et al. (2005). Two novel missense mutations in g protein-coupled receptor 54 in a patient with hypogonadotropic hypogonadism. J Clin Endocrinol Metab 90:1849–1855.

188. Lanfranco F, Gromoll J, von Eckardstein S, Herding EM, Nieschlag E, Simoni M (2005). Role of sequence variations of the GnRH receptor and G protein-coupled receptor 54 gene in male idiopathic hypogonadotropic hypogonadism. Eur J Endocrinol 153:845–852.

189. Navarro VM, Fernandez-Fernandez R, Castellano JM, et al. (2004). Advanced vaginal opening and precocious activation of the reproductive axis by KiSS-1 peptide, the endogenous ligand of GPR54. J Physiol 561:379–386.

190. Castellano JM, Navarro VM, Fernandez-Fernandez R, et al. (2005). Changes in hypothalamic KiSS-1 system and restoration of pubertal activation of the reproductive axis by kisspeptin in undernutrition. Endocrinology 146:3917–3925.

191. Han SK, Gottsch ML, Lee KJ, et al. (2005). Activation of gonadotropin-releasing hormone neurons by kisspeptin as a neuroendocrine switch for the onset of puberty. J Neurosci 25:11349–11356.

192. Partsch CJ, Dreyer G, Gosch A, et al. (1999). Longitudinal evaluation of growth, puberty, and bone maturation in children with Williams syndrome. J Pediatr 134:82–89.

193. Terasawa E, Noonan J, Nass T, Loose M (1984). Posterior hypothalamic lesions advance the onset of puberty in the female rhesus monkey. Endocrinology 115:2241.

194. Pescovitz OH, Comite F, Cassorla F, et al. (1984). True precocious puberty complicating congenital adrenal hyperplasia: Treatment with a luteinizing hormone-releasing hormone analog. J Clin Endocrinol Metab 58:857.

195. Foster C, Comite F, Pescovitz O, Ross J, Loriaux D, Cutler CJ (1984). Variable response to a long-acting agonist of luteinizing hormone-releasing hormone in girls with McCune-Albright syndrome. J Clin Endocrinol Metab 59:801.

196. Wilson ME, Tanner JM (1994). Somatostatin analog treatment slows growth and the tempo of reproductive maturation in female rhesus monkeys. J Clin Endocrinol Metab 79:495–501.

197. Hiney JK, Srivastava V, Nyberg CL, Ojeda SR, Dees WL (1996). Insulin-like growth factor I of peripheral origin acts centrally to accelerate the initiation of female puberty. Endocrinol 137:3717–3728.

198. Childs GV (2000). Growth hormone cells as co-gonadotropes: partners in the regulation of the reproductive system. Trends Endocrinol Metab 11:168–175.

199. Marshall W (1974). Interrelationships of skeletal maturation, sexual development and somatic growth in man. Ann Human Biol 1:29.

200. Simmons K, Greulich W (1943). Menarcheal age and the height, weight, and skeletal age of girls age 7 to 17 years. J Pediatr 22:518.

201. Boyar R, Finkelstein J, David R, et al. (1973). Twenty-four hour patterns of plasma luteinizing hormone and follicle-stimulating hormone in sexual precocity. N Engl J Med 289:282.

202. Tanner J, Whitehouse R (1975). A note on the bone age at which patients with true isolated growth hormone deficiency enter puberty. J Clin Endocrinol Metab 41:788.

203. Frisch R (1984). Body fat, puberty, and fertility. Biol Rev 5:161–188.

204. Kaplowitz PB, Slora EJ, Wasserman RC, Pedlow SE, Herman-Giddens ME (2001). Earlier onset of puberty in girls: Relation to increased body mass index and race. Pediatrics 108:347–353.

205. Wang Y (2002). Is obesity associated with early sexual maturation? A comparison of the association in American boys versus girls. Pediatrics 110:903–910.

206. Rosenbaum M, Leibel RL (1999). The role of leptin in human physiology [editorial; comment]. N Engl J Med 341:913–915.

207. Ahima RS, Kelly J, Elmquist JK, Flier JS (1999). Distinct physiologic and neuronal responses to decreased leptin and mild hyperleptinemia. Endocrinology 140:4923–4931.

208. Yura S, Ogawa Y, Sagawa N, et al. (2000). Accelerated puberty and late-onset hypothalamic hypogonadism in female transgenic skinny mice overexpressing leptin. J Clin Invest 105:749–755.

209. Schwartz J, Cherny R (1992). Intercellular communication within the anterior pituitary influencing the secretion of hypophysial hormones. Endocr Rev 13:453.

210. Mann DR, Johnson AO, Gimpel T, Castracane VD (2003). Changes in circulating leptin, leptin receptor, and gonadal hormones from infancy until advanced age in humans. J Clin Endocrinol Metab 88:3339–3345.

211. Loucks AB, Thuma JR (2003). Luteinizing hormone pulsatility is disrupted at a threshold of energy availability in regularly menstruating women. J Clin Endocrinol Metab 88:297–311.

212. Garcia MC, Lopez M, Alvarez CV, et al. (2007). Role of ghrelin in reproduction. Reproduction 133:531-540.

213. Bruning JC, Gautam D, Burks DJ, et al. (2000). Role of brain insulin receptor in control of body weight and reproduction. Science 289:2122–2125.

214. Reiter R (1980). The pineal and its hormones in the control of reproduction in mammals. Endocrinology 1:109.

215. Brzezinski A (1997). Melatonin in humans. N Engl J Med 336:186–195.

216. Reiter E, Kulin H, Hamwood S (1974). The absence of positive feedback between estrogen and luteinizing hormone in sexually immature girls. Pediatr Res 8:740.

217. Rosenfield RL, Fang VS (1974). The effects of prolonged physiologic estradiol therapy on the maturation of hypogonadal teenagers. J Pediatr 85:830–837.

218. Bogumil R, Ferlin M, Rootenberg J, et al. (1972). Mathematical studies of the human menstrual cycle. l. Formation of a mathematical model. J Clin Endocrinol Metab 35:126.

219. Levine JE (1999). Pulsatility in primates: A perspective from the placode. Endocrinol 140:1033–1035.

220. Wuttke W, Leonhardt S, Jarry H, Lopez P, Hirsch B (1992). Involvement of catecholamines and amino acid neurotransmitters in the generation of GnRH pulses. In Rosmanith W, Scherbaum W (eds.), *New developments in biosciences 6: Neuroendocrinology of sex steroids, Basic knowledge and clinical implications.* Berlin: de Gruyter 109–123.

221. Favit A, Wetsel W, Negro-Vilar A (1993). Differential expression of γ-aminobutyric acid receptors in immortalized luteinizing hormone-releasing hormone neurons. Endocrinol 133:1983–1989.

222. Chappell PE, Lee J, Levine JE (2000). Stimulation of gonadotropin-releasing hormone surges by estrogen: II. Role of cyclic adenosine 3′,5′-monophosphate. Endocrinol 141:1486–1492.

223. Radovick S, Ticknor CM, Nakayama Y, et al. (1991). Evidence for direct estrogen regulation of the human gonadotropin- releasing hormone gene. J Clin Invest 88:1649–1655.

224. Roy D, Angelini NL, Belsham DD (1999). Estrogen directly represses gonadotropin-releasing hormone (GnRH) gene expression in estrogen receptor-a (ERα)- and ERβ-expressing GT1-7 GnRH neurons. Endocrinol 140:5045–5053.

225. Kepa JK, Jacobsen BM, Boen EA, et al. (1996). Direct binding of progesterone receptor to nonconsensus DNA sequences represses rat GnRH. Mol Cell Endocrinol 117:27–39.

226. Couzinet B, Young J, Kujas M, et al. (1999). The antigonadotropic activity of a 19-nor-progesterone derivative is exerted both at the hypothalamic and pituitary levels in women. J Clin Endocrinol Metab 84:4191-196.

227. Garcia A, Herbon L, Barkan A, Papavasiliou S, Marshall J (1985). Hyperprolactinemia inhibits gonadotropin-releasing hormone (GnRH) stimulation of the number of pituitary GnRH receptors. Endocrinology 117:954.

228. Milenkovic L, D'Angelo G, Kelly PA, Weiner RI (1994). Inhibition of gonadotropin hormone-releasing hormone release by prolactin from GT1 neuronal cell lines through prolactin receptors. Proc Natl Acad Sci USA 91:1244–1247.

229. Petraglia F, Sutton S, Vale W, et al. (1987). Corticotropin-releasing factor decreases plasma luteinizing hormone levels in female rats by inhibiting gonadotropin-releasing hormone release into hypophysial-portal circulation. Endocrinol 120:1083.

230. Rivest S, Lee S, Attardi B, Rivier C (1993). The chronic intracerebroventricular infusion of interleukin-1ß alters the activity of the hypothalamic-pituitary-gonadal axis of cycling rats: I. Effect on LHRH and gonadotropin biosynthesis and secretion. Endocrinol 133:2424–2430.

231. Evans JJ (1999). Modulation of gonadotropin levels by peptides acting at the anterior pituitary gland. Endocr Rev 20:46–67.

232. Campbell RE, ffrench-Mullen JM, Cowley MA, Smith MS, Grove KL (2001). Hypothalamic circuitry of neuropeptide Y regulation of neuroendocrine function and food intake via the Y5 receptor subtype. Neuroendocrinology 74:106–119.

233. Vitale M, Chiocchio S (1993). Serotonin, a neurotransmitter involved in the regulation of luteinizing hormone release. Endocr Rev 14:480.

234. Conn P, Crowley WJ (1991). Gonadotropin-releasing hormone and its analogues. New Engl J Med 324:93–103.

235. Norwitz ER, Jeong KH, Chin WW (1999). Molecular mechanisms of gonadotropin-releasing hormone receptor gene regulation. J Soc Gynecol Investig 6:169–178.

236. Hirono M, lgarashi M, Matsumoto S (1971). Short- and auto-feedback mechanism of LH. Endocrinology 18:175.

237. Patritti-Laborde N, Wolfsen A, Odell W (1981). Short loop feedback system for the control of follicle-stimulating hormone in the rabbit. Endocrinology 108:72.

238. Kirk S, Dalkin A, Yasin M, Haisenleder D, Marshall J (1994). Gonadotropin-releasing hormone pulse frequency regulates expression of pituitary follistatin messenger ribonucleic acid: A mechanism for differential gonadotrope function. Endocrinol 13:876–880.

239. McArdle C (1994). Pituitary adenylate cyclase-activating polypeptide: A key player in reproduction? Endocrinol 135:815–816.

240. Drouin J, Labrie F (1981). Interactions between 17ß-estradiol and progesterone in the control of luteinizing hormone and follicle-stimulating hormone release in rat anterior pituitary cells in culture. Endocrinology 108:52.

241. Turgeon JL, Waring DW (1999). Androgen modulation of luteinizing hormone secretion by female rat gonadotropes. Endocrinology 140:1767-1774.

242. Hemrika D, Slaats E, Kennedy J, et al. (1993). Pulsatile luteinizing hormone patterns in long term oral contraceptive users. J Clin Endocrinol Metab 77:420.

243. Wildt L, Hutchison J, Marshall C, et al. (1981). On the site of action of progesterone in the blockade of the estradiol-induced gonadotropin discharge in the rhesus monkey. Endocrinology 109:1293.

244. Couse JF, Yates MM, Walker VR, Korach KS (2003). Characterization of the hypothalamic-pituitary-gonadal axis in estrogen receptor (ER) Null mice reveals hypergonadism and endocrine sex reversal in females lacking ERalpha but not ERbeta. Mol Endocrinol 17:1039–1053.

245. Griffin LD, Mellon SH (2001). Biosynthesis of the neurosteroid 3alpha-hydroxy-4-pregnen-20-one (3alphahp), a specific inhibitor of fsh release. Endocrinology 142:4617–4622.

246. Groome N, Illingworth P, O'Brien M, et al. (1996). Measurement of dimeric inhibin B throughout the human menstrual cycle. J Clin Endocrinol Metab 81:1401–1405.

247. Hayes FJ, Hall JE, Boepple PA, Crowley WF Jr. (19989). Clinical review 96: Differential control of gonadotropin secretion in the human: endocrine role of inhibin. J Clin Endocrinol Metab 83:1835–1841.

248. Lumpkin M, Negro-Vilar A, Franchimont P, et al. (1981). Evidence for a hypothalamic site of action of inhibin to suppress FSH release. Endocrinology 108:1101.

249. Bilezikjian LM, Blount AL, Donaldson CJ, Vale WW (2006). Pituitary actions of ligands of the TGF-beta family: Activins and inhibins. Reproduction 132:207–215.

250. Fraser H, Lunn S (1993). Does inhibin have an endocrine function during the menstrual cycle? TEM 4:187–194.

251. Meriggiola M, Dahl K, Mather J, Bremner W (1967). Follistatin decreases activin-stimulated FSH secretion with no effect on GnRH-stimulated FSH secretion in prepubertal male monkeys. Endocrinol 134:1967.

252. Eagleson CA, Gingrich MB, Pastor CL, et al. (2000). Polycystic ovarian syndrome: Evidence that flutamide restores sensitivity of the gonadotropin-releasing hormone pulse generator to inhibition by estradiol and progesterone. J Clin Endocrinol Metab 85:4047–4052.

253. Pielecka J, Quaynor SD, Moenter SM (2006). Androgens increase gonadotropin-releasing hormone neuron firing activity in females and interfere with progesterone negative feedback. Endocrinology 147:1474–1479.

254. Rosenfield RL (1999). Ovarian and adrenal function in polycystic ovary syndrome. Endocrinol Metab Clin N Am 28:265–293.

255. Ehrmann DA, Barnes RB, Rosenfield RL (1995). Polycystic ovary syndrome as a form of functional ovarian hyperandrogenism due to dysregulation of androgen secretion. Endocrin Rev 16:322–353.

256. Udoff LC, Adashi EY (1999). Autocrine/paracrine regulation of the ovarian follicle. The Endocrinologist 9:99–106.

257. Yoshimura Y, Washita M, Karube M, et al. (1994). Growth hormone stimulates follicular development by stimulating ovarian production of insulin-like growth factor-I. Endocrinol 135:887–894.

258. Mason HD, Margara R, Winston RML, Beard RW, Reed MJ, Franks S (1990). Inhibition of oestradiol production by epidermal growth factor in human granulosa cells of normal and polycystic ovaries. Clin Endocrinol 33:511–517.

259. Mayerhofer A, Hemmings HC Jr., Snyder GL, et al. (1999). Functional dopamine-1 receptors and DARPP-32 are expressed in human ovary and granulosa luteal cells in vitro. J Clin Endocrinol Metab 84:257–264.

260. Agarwal SK, Vogel K, Weitsman SR, Magoffin DA (1999). Leptin antagonizes the insulin-like growth factor-I augmentation of steroidogenesis in granulosa and theca cells of the human ovary. J Clin Endocrinol Metab 84:1072–1076.

261. Feng P, Catt K, Knecht M (1988). Transforming growth factor-ß stimulates meiotic maturation of the rat oocyte. Endocrinology 122:181.

262. Aten R, Poland M, Bayless R, Behrman H (1987). A gonadotropin-releasing hormone (GnRH)-like protein in human ovaries: Similarity to the GnRH-like ovarian protein of the rat. J Clin Endocrinol Metab 64:1288.

263. Barnes RB, Scommegna A, Schreiber JR (1987). Decreased ovarian response to human menopausal gonadotropin caused by subcutaneously administered gonadotropin-releasing hormone agonist. Fertil Steril 47:512.

264. Advis J, Richards J, Ojeda S (1981). Hyperprolactinemia-induced precocious puberty: Studies on the intraovarian mechanism(s) by which PRL enhances ovarian responsiveness to gonadotropins in prepubertal rats. J Clin Endocrinol Metab 108:1333.

265. Demura R, Ono M, Demura H, Shizume K, Oouch H (1982). Prolactin directly inhibits basal as well as gonadotropin-stimulated secretion of progesterone and 17ß-estradiol in the human ovary. J Clin Endocrinol Metab 54:1246.

266. Glickman SP, Rosenfield RL, Bergenstal RM, Helke J (1982). Multiple androgenic abnormalities, including elevated free testosterone, in hyperprolactinemic women. J Clin Endocrinol Metab 55:251–257.

267. Rosenfield RL, Qin K (2006). Normal adrenarche. In Rose BD (ed.), UpToDate.Wellesley, MA: UpToDate.

268. Rosenfield RL (2007). Identifying children at risk of polycystic ovary syndrome. J Clin Endocrinmol Metab [in press].

269. Rittmaster R, Givner M (1988). Effect of daily and alternate day low dose prednisone on serum cortisol and adrenal androgens in hirsute women. J Clin Endocrinol Metab 67:400–403.

270. Cutler GJ, Davis S, Johnsonbaugh R, Loriaux L (1979). Dissociation of cortisol and adrenal androgen secretion in patients with secondary adrenal insufficiency. J Clin Endocrinol Metab 49:604.

271. Auchus RJ, Rainey WE (2004). Adrenarche: - pPhysiology, biochemistry and human disease. Clin Endocrinol (Oxford) 60:288–296.

272. Taha D, Mullis PE, Ibanez L, de Zegher F (2005). Absent or delayed adrenarche in Pit-1/POU1F1 deficiency. Horm Res 64:175–179.

273. Biason-Lauber A, Zachmann M, Schoenle EJ (2000). Effect of leptin on CYP17 enzymatic activities in human adrenal cells: New insight in the onset of adrenarche. Endocrinology 141:1446–1454.

274. Ehrhart-Bornstein M, Hinson J, Bornstein S, Scherbaum W, Vinson G (1998). Intraadrenal interactions in the regulation of adrenocortical steroidogenesis. Endocr Rev 19:101–143.

275. Martin DD, Schweizer R, Schwarze CP, Elmlinger MW, Ranke MB, Binder G (2004). The early dehydroepiandrosterone sulfate rise of adrenarche and the delay of pubarche indicate primary ovarian failure in Turner syndrome. J Clin Endocrinol Metab 89:1164–1168.

276. Cumming D, Rebar R, Hopper B, Yen S (1982). Evidence for an influence of the ovary on circulating dehydroepiandrosterone sulfate levels. J Clin Endocrinol Metab 54:1069.

277. Paul S, Purdy R (1992). Neuroactive steroids. FASEB J 6:2311–2322.

278. Remer T, Boye KR, Hartmann M, et al. (2003). Adrenarche and bone modeling and remodeling at the proximal radius: Weak androgens make stronger cortical bone in healthy children. J Bone Miner Res 18:1539–1546.

279. Remer T, Manz F (2001). The midgrowth spurt in healthy children is not caused by adrenarche. J Clin Endocrinol Metab 86:4183–4186.

280. Nair KS, Rizza RA, O'Brien P, et al. (2006). DHEA in elderly women and DHEA or testosterone in elderly men. N Engl J Med 355:1647–1659.

281. Brooke AM, Kalingag LA, Miraki-Moud F, et al. (2006). Dehydroepiandrosterone improves psychological well-being in male and female hypopituitary patients on maintenance growth hormone replacement. J Clin Endocrinol Metab 91:3773–3779.

282. Apaja PM, Aatsinki JT, Rajaniemi HJ, Petaja-Repo UE (2005). Expression of the mature luteinizing hormone receptor in rodent urogenital and adrenal tissues is developmentally regulated at a posttranslational level. Endocrinology 146:3224–3232.

283. Spiegel A, Shenker A, Weinstein L (1992). Receptor-effector coupling by G proteins: implications for normal and abnormal signal transduction. Endocrine Rev 13:536.

284. Carvalho CR, Carvalheira JB, Lima MH, et al. (2003). Novel signal transduction pathway for luteinizing hormone and its interaction with insulin: activation of Janus kinase/signal transducer and activator of transcription and phosphoinositol 3-kinase/Akt pathways. Endocrinology 144:638–647.

285. Orly J, Rei Z, Greenberg N, Richards J (1994). Tyrosine kinase inhibitor AG18 arrests follicle-stimulating hormone-induced granulosa cell differentiation: use of reverse transcriptase-polymerase chain reaction assay for multiple messenger ribonucleic acids. Endocrinol 134:2336–2346.

286. Adelman J, Mason A, Hayflick J, Seeburg P (1986). Isolation of the gene and hypothalamic cDNA for the common precursor of gonadotropin-releasing hormone and prolactin release-inhibiting factor in human and rat. Proc Natl Acad Sci (USA) 83:179.

287. Redding TW, Schally AV, Arimura A, Matsuo H (1972). Stimulation of release and synthesis of luteinizing hormone (LH) and follicle stimulating hormone (FSH) in tissue cultures of rat pituitaries in response to natural and synthetic LH and FSH releasing hormone. Endocrinology 90:764.

288. Kauffman AS, Rissman EF (2004). A critical role for the evolutionarily conserved gonadotropin-releasing hormone II: Mediation of energy status and female sexual behavior. Endocrinology 145:3639–3646.

289. Millar R, Lowe S, Conklin D, et al. (2001). A novel mammalian receptor for the evolutionarily conserved type II GnRH. Proc Natl Acad Sci (USA) 98:9636–9641.

290. Phifer R, Midgley A, Spicer S (1973). Immunohistologic and histologic evidence that follicle-stimulating hormone and luteinizing hormone are present in the same cell type in the human pars distalis. J Clin Endocrinol Metab 36:125.

291. Hammond E, Griffin J, Odell W (1991). A chorionic gonadotropin-secreting human pituitary cell. J Clin Endocrinol Metab 72:747–754.

292. Combarnous Y (1992). Moecular basis of the specificity of binding of glycoprotein hormones to their receptors. Endocr Rev 13:670–685.

293. Dahl K, Stone M (1992). FSH isoforms, radioimmunoassays, bioassays, and their significance. J Andrology 13:11–12.

294. Arey BJ, Stevis PE, Deecher DC, et al. (1997). Induction of promiscuous G protein coupling of the follicle-stimulating hormone (FSH) receptor: A novel mechanism for transducing pleiotropic actions of FSH isoforms. Mol Endocrinol 11:517–526.

295. West CR, Carlson NE, Lee JS, et al. (2002). Acidic mix of FSH isoforms are better facilitators of ovarian follicular maturation and E2 production than the less acidic. Endocrinology 143:107–116.

296. Themmen APN, Huhtaniemi IT (2000). Mutations of gonadotropins and gonadotropin receptors: Elucidating the physiology and pathophysiology of pituitary-gonadal function. Endocr Rev 21:551–583.

297. Weiss J, Axelrod L, Whitcomb R, Harris P, Crowley W, Jameson J (1992). Hypogonadism caused by a single amino acid substitution in the ß subunit of luteinizing hormone. New Engl J Med 326:179–184.

298. Pettersson K, Ding Y-Q, Huhtaniemi I (1992). An immunologically anomalous luteinizing hormone variant in a healthy woman. J Clin Endocrinol Metab 74:164–171.

299. Tapanainen JS, Koivunen R, Fauser BC, et al. (1999). A new contributing factor to polycystic ovary syndrome: The genetic variant of luteinizing hormone. J Clin Endocrinol Metab 84:1711–1715.

300. Solano A, Garcia-Vela A, Catt K, et al. (1980). Modulation of serum and pituitary luteinizing hormone bioactivity by androgen in the rat. Endocrinology 106:1941.

301. Lucky AW, Rebar RW, Rosenfield RL, Roche-Bender N, Helke J (1979). Estrogen reduces the potency of luteinizing hormone. N Engl J Med 3030:1034.

302. Dahl K, Bicxak T, Hsueh A (1988). Naturally occurring antihormones: Secretion of FSH antagonists by women treated with a GnRH analog. Science 239:72.

303. Tilly J, Aihara T, Nishimori K, et al. (1992). Expression of recombinant human follicle-stimulating hormone receptor: Species-specific ligand binding, signal transduction, and identification of multiple ovarian messenger ribonucleic acid transcripts. Endocrinol 131:799–806.

304. Taylor A, Khoury R, Crowley WJ (1994). A comparison of 13 different immunometric assay kits for gonadotropins: implications for clinical investigation. J Clin Endocrinol Metab 79:240–247.

305. Yen S, Llerena O, Little B, et al. (1968). Disappearance rates of endogenous luteinizing hormone and chorionic gonadotropin in man. J Clin Endocrinol Metab 28:1763.

306. Yen S, Vela P, Rankin J (1970). Inappropriate secretion of follicle-stimulating hormone and luteinizing hormone in polycystic ovarian disease. J Clin Endocrinol Metab 30:435–442.

307. Veldhuis J, Johnson M (1988). In vivo dynamics of luteinizing hormone secretion and clearance in man: Assessment by deconvolution mechanics. J Clin Endocrinol Metab 66:1291.

308. Raiti S, Foley TJ, Penny R, et al. (1975). Measurement of the production rate of human luteinizing hormone using the urinary excretion technique. Metabolism 24:937.

309. Prentice L, Ryan R (1975). LH and its subunits in human pituitary, serum and urine. J Clin Endocrinol Metab 40:303.

310. Kohler P, Ross C, Odell W (1968). Metabolic clearance and production rates of human luteinizing hormone in pre- and postmenopausal women. J Clin Invest 47:38.

311. Coble YD, Jr., Kohler PO, Cargille CM, Ross GT (1969). Production rates and metabolic clearance rates of human follicle-stimulating hormone in premenopausal and postmenopausal women. J Clin Invest 48:359.

312. Rosenfield RL (1972). Role of androgens in growth and development of the fetus, child, and adolescent. Adv Pediatr 19:171–213.

313. Baulieu E, Corpechot C, Dray F, et al. (1965). An adrenal-secreted "androgen": Dehydroisoandrosterone sulfate. Recent Prog Horm Res 21:411.

314. Sandberg E, Gurpide E, Lieberman S (1964). Quantitative studies on the metabolism of dehydroisoandrosterone sulfate. Biochemistry 3:1256.

315. Longcope C, Pratt J (1977). Blood production rates of estrogens in women with differing ratios of urinary estrogen conjugates. Steroids 29:483–492.

316. Strott C, Hoshimi T, Lipsett M (1989). Plasma progesterone and 17-hydroxyprogesterone in normal men and children with congenital adrenal hyperplasia. J Clin Invest 48:930–939.

317. Lin TJ, Billiar RB, Little B (1972). Metabolic clearance of progesterone in the menstrual cycle. J Clin Endocrinol Metab 35:879–886.

318. Sinha Y (1992). Prolactin variants. Trends Endocrinol Metab 3:100–106.

319. Frawley L. Role of the hypophyseal neurointermediate lobe in the dynamic release of prolactin. Trends Endocrinol Metab 1994;5:107–112.

320. Pangas SA, Rademaker AW, Fishman DA, Woodruff TK (2002). Localization of the activin signal transduction components in normal human ovarian follicles: Implications for autocrine and paracrine signaling in the ovary. J Clin Endocrinol Metab 87:2644–2657.

321. Rosenfield RL, Lucky AW, Allen TD (1980). The diagnosis and management of intersex. Curr Probl Pediatr 10:1–66.

322. Wu Q, Sucheta S, Azhar S, Menon KM (2003). Lipoprotein enhancement of ovarian theca-interstitial cell steroidogenesis: relative contribution of scavenger receptor class B (type I) and adenosine 5'-triphosphate- binding cassette (type A1) transporter in high-density lipoprotein-cholesterol transport and androgen synthesis. Endocrinology 144:2437–2445.

323. Scott RR, Gomes LG, Huang N, et al. (2007). Apparent manifesting heterozygosity in P450 oxidoreductase deficiency and its effect on coexisting 21-hydroxylase deficiency. J Clin Endocrinol Metab 92:2318-2322.

324. Rheaume E, Lachance Y, Zhao HF, et al. (1991). Structure and expression of a new complementary DNA encoding the almost exclusive 3ß-hydroxysteroid dehydrogenase/Δ5-Δ4-isomerase in human adrenals and gonads. Molec Endocrinol 5:1147–1157.

325. Qin K, Rosenfield RL (1998). Role of cytochrome P450c17 in polycystic ovary syndrome. Molec Cell Endocrinol 145:111–121.

326. Nelson VL, Qin Kn K, Rosenfield RL, et al. (2001). The biochemical basis for increased testosterone production in theca cells propagated from patients with polycystic ovary syndrome. J Clin Endocrinol Metab 86:5925–5933.

327. Simpson E, Mahendroo M, Means G, et al. (1994). Aromatase cytochrome P450, the enzyme responsible for estrogen biosynthesis. Endocr Rev 15:342.

328. Rosenfield RL (1973). Relationship of androgens to female hirsutism and infertility. J Reprod Med 11:87–95.

329. Alonso LC, Rosenfield RL (2002). Oestrogens and puberty. Best Pract Res Clin Endocrinol Metab 16:13–30.

330. Siiteri P, MacDonald P (1973). Role of extraglandular estrogen in human endocrinology. In Greep R, Astwood E (eds.), *Handbook of physiology*. Washington, D.C.: American Physiology Society 615.

331. Morimoto I, Edmiston A, Hawks D, Horton R (1981). Studies of the origin of androstanediol and androstanediol glucuronide in young and elderly men. J Clin Endocrinol Metab 52:772.

332. Heinrichs WL, Tabei T, Kuwabara Y, et al. (1979). Differentiation and regulation of peripheral androgen metabolism in rats and rhesus monkeys. Am J Obstet Gyn 135:974.

333. Mode A, Norstedt G, Eneroth H, Gustafsson J-A (1983). Purification of liver feminizing factor from rat pituitaries and demonstration of its identity with growth hormone. Endocrinol 113:1250–1260.

334. Edman CD, MacDonald PC (1978). Effect of obesity on conversion of plasma androstenedione to estrone in ovulatory and anovulatory young women. Am J Obstet Gynecol 130:456–461.

335. Kadlubar FF, Berkowitz GS, Delongchamp RR, et al. (2003). The CYP3A4*1B variant is related to the onset of puberty, a known risk factor for the development of breast cancer. Cancer Epidemiol Biomarkers Prev 12:327–331.

336. Harris RM, Wood DM, Bottomley L, et al. (2004). Phytoestrogens are potent inhibitors of estrogen sulfation: Implications for breast cancer risk and treatment. J Clin Endocrinol Metab 89:1779–1787.

337. Giorgi E, Stein W (1981). The transport of steroids into animal cells in culture. Endocrinology 108:688.

338. Martin K, Chang R, Ehrmann D, et al. (2008). Evaluation and treatment of hirsutism in premenopausal women: an Endocrine Society Clinical Practice Guideline. J Clin Endocrin Metab [E-pub ahead of print] doi:10.1210/jc.2007-2437.

339. Rosenfield RL (2005). Clinical practice: Hirsutism. N Engl J Med 353:2578–2588.

340. Rosenfield RL (1975). Studies of the relation of plasma androgen levels to androgen action in women. J Steroid Biochem 6:695–702.

341. Kahn SM, Hryb DJ, Nakhla AM, et al. (2002). Sex hormone-binding globulin is synthesized in target cells. J Endocrinol 175:113-120.

342. Hammes A, Andreassen TK, Spoelgen R, et al. (2005). Role of endocytosis in cellular uptake of sex steroids [Comments in: Cell. 2005 Sep 9;122(5):647-9;Cell. 2006 Feb 10;124(3):455-6; author reply 456-7]. Cell 2005;122:751-762.

343. Nestler J, Powers L, Matt D, et al. (1991). A direct effect of hyperinsulinemia on serum sex-hormone binding globulin levels in obese women with the polycystic ovary syndrome. J Clin Endocrinol Metab 72:83–89.

344. Nimrod A, Rosenfield RL, Otto P (1980). Relationship of androgen action to androgen metabolism in isolated rat granulosa cells. J Steroid Biochem 13:1015.

345. Yang S, Fang Z, Gurates B, et al. (2001). Stromal PRs mediate induction of 17beta-hydroxysteroid dehydrogenase type 2 expression in human endometrial epithelium: A paracrine mechanism for inactivation Of E2. Mol Endocrinol 15:2093–2105.

346. Wilson JD, Griffin JE, Russell DW (1993). Steroid 5 alpha-reductase 2 deficiency. Endocr Rev 14:577–593.

347. Hochberg RB (1998). Biological esterification of steroids. Endocr Rev 19:331–348.

348. Baracat E, Haidar M, Lopez FJ, Pickar J, Dey M, Negro-Vilar A (1999). Estrogen activity and novel tissue selectivity of delta8,9-dehydroestrone sulfate in postmenopausal women. J Clin Endocrinol Metab 84:2020–2027.

349. Katzenellenbogen BS, Montano MM, Ediger TR, et al. (2000). Estrogen receptors: Selective ligands, partners, and distinctive pharmacology. Recent Prog Horm Res 55:163–193; discussion 194–195.

350. O'Malley BW (2005). A life-long search for the molecular pathways of steroid hormone action. Mol Endocrinol 19:1402–1411.

351. Chen H, Hu B, Huang GH, Trainor AG, Abbott DH, Adams JS (2003). Purification and characterization of a novel intracellular 17 beta-estradiol binding protein in estrogen-resistant New World primate cells. J Clin Endocrinol Metab 88:501–504.

352. Cheung J, Smith DF (2000). Molecular chaperone interactions with steroid receptors: An update. Molec Endocrinol 14:939–946.

353. Alarid ET, Bakopoulos N, Solodin N (1999). Proteasome-mediated proteolysis of estrogen receptor: A novel component in autologous down-regulation. Mol Endocrinol 13:1522–1534.

354. Korenman S (1968). Radio-ligand binding assay of specific estrogens using a soluble uterine macromolecule. J Clin Endocrinol Metab 28:127.

355. French FS, Lubahn DB, Brown TR, et al. (1990). Molecular basis of androgen insensitivity. Rec Prog Horm Res 46:1.

356. Connor CE, Norris JD, Broadwater G, et al. (2001). Circumventing tamoxifen resistance in breast cancers using antiestrogens that induce unique conformational changes in the estrogen receptor. Cancer Res 61:2917–2922.

357. Melamed M, Castano E, Notides AC, Sasson S (1997). Molecular and kinetic basis for the mixed agonist-antagonist activity of estriol. Molec Endocrinol 11:1868–1878.

358. Kemppainen JA, Langley E, Wong CI, Bobseine K, Kelce WR, Wilson EM (1999). Distinguishing androgen receptor agonists and antagonists: Distinct mechanisms of activation by medroxyprogesterone acetate and dihydrotestosterone. Mol Endocrinol 13:440–454.

359. Negro-Vilar A (1999). Selective androgen receptor modulators (SARMs): A novel approach to androgen therapy for the new millennium. J Clin Endocrinol Metab 84:3459–3462.

360. McDonnell DP (2000). Selective estrogen receptor modulators (SERMs): A first step in the development of perfect hormone replacement therapy regimen. J Soc Gynecol Investig 7: S10–S15.

361. Yang NN, Venugopalan M, Hardikar S, Glasebrook A (1996). Identification of an estrogen response element activated by metabolites of 17beta-estradiol and raloxifene [published erratum appears in Science 275(5304):1249, 1997]. Science 273:1222–1225.

362. Dowsett M, Ashworth A (2003). New biology of the oestrogen receptor. Lancet 362:260–262.

363. Smid-Koopman E, Blok LJ, Kuhne LC, et al. (2003). Distinct functional differences of human progesterone receptors A and B on gene expression and growth regulation in two endometrial carcinoma cell lines. J Soc Gynecol Investig 10:49–57.

364. McPhaul MJ, Young M (2001). Complexities of androgen action. J Am Acad Dermatol 45:S87–S94.

365. Lindberg MK, Moverare S, Skrtic S, et al. (2003). Estrogen receptor (ER)-beta reduces ERalpha-regulated gene transcription, supporting a "ying yang"relationship between ERalpha and ERbeta in mice. Mol Endocrinol 17:203–208.

366. Smith EP, Boyd J, Frank GR, et al. (1994). Estrogen resistance caused by a mutation in the estrogen-receptor gene in a man. N Engl J Med 331:1056–1061.

367. Nilsson S, Kuiper G, Gustafsson J-A (1998). ERß: A novel estrogen receptor offers the potential for new drug development. Trends Endocrinol Metab 9:387–395.

368. Conneely OM, Lydon JP, De Mayo F, O'Malley BW (2000). Reproductive functions of the progesterone receptor. J Soc Gynecol Investig 7:S25–S32.

369. Barbulescu K, Geserick C, Schuttke I, Schleuning WD, Haendler B (2001). New androgen response elements in the murine pem promoter mediate selective transactivation. Mol Endocrinol 15:1803–1816.

370. McKenna NJ, Lanz RB, O'Malley BW (1999). Nuclear receptor coregulators: Cellular and molecular biology. Endocr Rev 20: 321–344.

371. Laughlin GA, Dominguez CE, Yen SS (1998). Nutritional and endocrine-metabolic aberrations in women with functional hypothalamic amenorrhea. J Clin Endocrinol Metab 83:25–32.

372. Lu S, Jenster G, Epner DE (2000). Androgen induction of cyclin-dependent kinase inhibitor p21 gene: Role of androgen receptor and transcription factor Sp1 complex. Mol Endocrinol 14:753–760.

373. Kousteni S, Bellido T, Plotkin LI, et al. (2001). Nongenotropic, sex-nonspecific signaling through the estrogen or androgen receptors: Dissociation from transcriptional activity. Cell 104:719–730.

374. Nilsson O, Falk J, Ritzen EM, Baron J, Savendahl L (2003). Raloxifene acts as an estrogen agonist on the rabbit growth plate. Endocrinology 144:1481–1485.

375. Cranney A, Adachi JD (2005). Benefit-risk assessment of raloxifene in postmenopausal osteoporosis. Drug Saf 28:721–730.

376. Emlet DR, Schwartz R, Brown KA, Pollice AA, Smith CA, Shackney SE (2006). HER2 expression as a potential marker for response to therapy targeted to the EGFR. Br J Cancer 94:1144–1153.

377. Cenni B, Picard D (1999). Ligand-independent activation of steroid receptors: New roles for old players. Trends Endocrinol Metab 10:41–46.

378. Apostolakis EM, Garai J, Lohmann JE, Clark JH, O'Malley, BW (2000). Epidermal growth factor activates reproductive behavior independent of ovarian steroids in female rodents. Molec Endocrinol 14:1086–1098.

379. Platet N, Cunat S, Chalbos D, Rochefort H, Garcia M (2000). Unliganded and liganded estrogen receptors protect against cancer invasion via different mechanisms. Molec Endocrinol 14:999–1009.

380. Song RX, McPherson RA, Adam L, et al. (2002). Linkage of rapid estrogen action to MAPK activation by ERalpha-Shc association and Shc pathway activation. Mol Endocrinol 16:116-27.

381. Razandi M, Pedram A, Park ST, Levin ER (2003). Proximal events in signaling by plasma membrane estrogen receptors. J Biol Chem 278:2701–2712.

382. Lu ML, Schneider MC, Zheng Y, Zhang X, Richie JP (2001). Caveolin-1 interacts with androgen receptor: A positive modulator of androgen receptor mediated transactivation. J Biol Chem 276:13442–13451.

383. Lutz LB, Cole LM, Gupta MK, Kwist KW, Auchus RJ, Hammes SR (2001). Evidence that androgens are the primary steroids produced by Xenopus laevis ovaries and may signal through the classical androgen receptor to promote oocyte maturation. Proc Natl Acad Sci (USA) 98:13728–13733.

384. Boonyaratanakornkit V, Scott MP, Ribon V, et al. (2001). Progesterone receptor contains a proline-rich motif that directly interacts with SH3 domains and activates c-Src family tyrosine kinases. Mol Cell 8:269–280.

385. Ashley RL, Clay CM, Farmerie TA, et al. (2006). Cloning and characterization of an ovine intracellular seven transmembrane receptor for progesterone that mediates calcium mobilization. Endocrinology 147:4151-4159.

385a.Chagin AS, Savendahl L (2007). GPR30 estrogen receptor expression in the growth plate declines as puberty progresses. J Clin Endocrinol Metab 92:4873-877.

386. Mellon S (1994). Neurosteroids: Biochemistry, modes of action. and clinical relevance. J Clin Endocrinol Metab 78:1003–1008.

387. Baulieu EE (1999). Neuroactive neurosteroids: Dehydroepiandrosterone (DHEA) and DHEA sulphate. Acta Paediatr Suppl 88:78–80.

388. Zwain IH, Yen SS (1999). Neurosteroidogenesis in astrocytes, oligodendrocytes, and neurons of cerebral cortex of rat brain. Endocrinology 140:3843–3852.

389. Ramirez VD, Zheng J (1996). Membrane sex-steroid receptors in the brain. Front Neuroendocrinol 17:402–439.

390. Wetzel CH, Hermann B, Behl C, et al. (1998). Functional antagonism of gonadal steroids at the 5-hydroxytryptamine type 3 receptor. Mol Endocrinol 12:1441–1451.

391. McEwen BS (1999). Clinical review 108: The molecular and neuroanatomical basis for estrogen effects in the central nervous system. J Clin Endocrinol Metab 84:1790–1797.

392. MacLusky N, McEwen B (1980). Progestin receptors in rat brain: Distribution and properties of cytoplasmic progestin-binding sites. Endocrinology 106:192.

393. Attardi B (1981). Facilitation and inhibition of the estrogen-induced luteinizing hormone surge in the rat by progesterone: Effects on cytoplasmic and nuclear estrogen receptors in the hypothalamic-preoptic area, pituitary, and uterus. Endocrinology 108:1487.

394. Pacifici R (1998). Cytokines, estrogen, and postmenopausal osteoporosis: The second decade. Endocrinology 139:2659–2661.

395. Gupta C, Goldman A (1986). The arachidonic acid cascade is involved in the masculinizing action of testosterone on embryonic external genitalia in mice. Develop Biol 83:4346–4349.

396. Rosenfield RL, Kentsis A, Deplewski D, Ciletti N (1999). Rat preputial sebocyte differentiation involves peroxisome proliferator-activated receptors. J Invest Dermatol 112:226–232.

397. Maor G, Segev Y, Phillip M (1999). Testosterone stimulates insulin-like growth factor-I and insulin-like growth factor-I-receptor gene expression in the mandibular condyle: A model of endochondral ossification. Endocrinology 140:1901–1910.

398. Greco T, Duello T, Gorski J (1993). Estrogen receptors, estradiol, and diethylstilbestrol in early development: The mouse as a model for the study of estrogen receptors and estrogen sensitivity in embryonic development of male and female reproductive tracts. Endocr Rev 14:59.

399. Kalloo N, Gearhart J, Barrack E (1993). Sexually dimorphic expression of estrogen receptors, but not of androgen receptors in human fetal external genitalia. J Clin Endocrinol Metab 77:692–698.

400. Ammini A, Vijyaraghavan M, Sabherwal U (1994). Human female phenotypic development: role of fetal ovaries. J Clin Endocrinol Metab 79:604–608.

401. Tewari K, Bonebrake R, Asrat T, Shanberg A (1997). Ambiguous genitalia in infant exposed to tamoxifen in utero. Lancet 350:183.

402. Futterweit W, Deligdisch L (1986). Histopathological effects of exogenously administered testosterone in 19 female to male transsexuals. J Clin Endocrinol Metab 62:16–21.

403. Glasier A (1997). Emergency postcoital contraception. N Engl J Med 337:1058–1064.

404. Westhoff C (2003). Clinical practice. Emergency contraception. N Engl J Med 349:1830–1835.

405. Rochwerger L, Buchwald M (1993). Stimulation of the cystic fibrosis transmembrane regulator expression by estrogen in vivo. Endocrinol 133:921–930.

406. Paek SC, Merritt DF, Mallory SB (2001). Pruritus vulvae in prepubertal children. J Am Acad Dermatol 44:795–802.

407. Wied C, Bibbo M (1975). Evaluation of endocrinologic condition by exfoliative cytology. In Cold J (ed.), *Gynecologic endocrinology.* New York: Harper & Row.

408. Rosenfield RL, Fang VS, Dupon C, Kim MH, Refetoff S (1973). The effects of low doses of depot estradiol and testosterone in teenagers with ovarian failure and Turner's syndrome. J Clin Endocrinol Metab 37:574–580.

409. Berenson A, Heger A, Hayes J, Bailey R, Emans S (1992). Appearance of the hymen in prepubertal girls. Pediatr 89:387–394.

410. Gardner J (1992). Descriptive study of genital variation in healthy, nonabused premenarcheal girls. J Pediatr 120:251–257.

411. Robbins S, Cotran R (1979). The breast. In Kumar V (ed.), *Pathologic basis of disease.* Philadelphia: WB Saunders 1165–1191.

412. Rilemma J (1994). Development of the mammary gland and lactation. Trends Endocrinol Metab 5:149–154.

413. Lyons W (1958). Hormonal synergism in mammary growth. Proc Roy Soc Lond [Biol] 149:303.

414. Bole-Feysot C, Goffin V, Edery M, Binart N, Kelly PA (1998). Prolactin (PRL) and its receptor: Actions, signal transduction pathways and phenotypes observed in PRL receptor knockout mice. Endocr Rev 19:225–268.

415. Ma Y, Katiyar P, Jones LP, et al. (2006). The breast cancer susceptibility gene BRCA1 regulates progesterone receptor signaling in mammary epithelial cells. Mol Endocrinol 20:14–34.

416. Deplewski D, Rosenfield RL (2000). Role of hormones in pilosebaceous unit development. Endocr Rev 21:363–392.

417. Daughaday WH, Rotwein P (1989). Insulin-like growth factors I and II: Peptide, messenger ribonucleic acid and gene structures, serum, and tissue concentrations. Endocr Rev 10:68–91.

418. Abu AO, Horner A, Kusec V, Triffitt JT, Compston JE (1997). The localization of androgen receptors in human bone. J Clin Endocrinol Metab 82:3493–3497.

419. Bachrach BE, Smith EP (1996). The role of sex steroids in bone growth and development: Evolving new concepts. The Endocrinol 6:362–368.

420. Seeman E (2003). The structural and biomechanical basis of the gain and loss of bone strength in women and men. Endocrinol Metab Clin North Am 32:25–38.

421. Mora S, Gilsanz V (2003). Establishment of peak bone mass. Endocrinol Metab Clin North Am 32:39–63.

422. Migliaccio S, Newbold RR, Bullock BC, et al. (1996). Alterations of maternal estrogen levels during gestation affect the skeleton of female offspring. Endocrinology 137:2118–2125.

423. Eastell R (2005). Role of oestrogen in the regulation of bone turnover at the menarche. J Endocrinol 185:223–234.

424. Price TM, O'Brien SN, Welter BH, George R, Anandjiwala J, Kilgore M (1998). Estrogen regulation of adipose tissue lipoprotein lipase: Possible mechanism of body fat distribution. Am J Obstet Gynecol 178:101–107.

425. Machinal F, Dieudonne MN, Leneveu MC, Pecquery R, Giudicelli Y (1999). In vivo and in vitro ob gene expression and leptin secretion in rat adipocytes: Evidence for a regional specific regulation by sex steroid hormones. Endocrinology 140:1567–1574.

426. Wajchenberg BL (2000). Subcutaneous and visceral adipose tissue: their relation to the metabolic syndrome. Endocr Rev 21:697–738.

427. Veldhuis JD, Roemmich JN, Richmond EJ, et al. (2005). Endocrine control of body composition in infancy, childhood, and puberty. Endocr Rev 26:114–146.

428. Bottner A, Kratzsch J, Muller G, et al. (2004). Gender differences of adiponectin levels develop during the progression of puberty and are related to serum androgen levels. J Clin Endocrinol Metab 89:4053–4061.

429. Perseghin G, Scifo P, Pagliato E, et al. (2001). Gender factors affect fatty acids-induced insulin resistance in nonobese humans: Effects of oral steroidal contraception. J Clin Endocrinol Metab 86:3188–3196.

430. Sherwin BB (2003). Estrogen and cognitive functioning in women. Endocr Rev 24:133-51.

431. Wilson JD (2001). Androgens, androgen receptors, and male gender role behavior. Horm Behav 40:358–366.

432. Hughes IA, Houk C, Ahmed SF, Lee PA (2006). Consensus statement on management of intersex disorders. Arch Dis Child 91:554–563.

433. Swaab DF, Hofman MA (1995). Sexual differentiation of the human hypothalamus in relation to gender and sexual orientation. Trends Neurosci 18:264–270.

434. Cosgrove KP, Mazure CM, Staley JK (2007). Evolving knowledge of sex differences in brain structure, function, and chemistry. Biol Psychiatry 62:847-855.

435. Abdelgadir S, Resko J, Ojeda S, Lephart E, McPhaul M, Roselli C (1994). Androgens regulate aromatase cytochrome P450 messenger ribonucleic acid in rat brain. Endocrinol 135:395–401.

436. Beyer C, Green S, Hutchison J (1994). Androgens influence sexual differentiation of embryonic mouse hypothalamic aromatase neurons in vitro. Endocrinol 135:1220–1226.

437. Ogawa S, Eng V, Taylor J, Lubahn DB, Korach KS, Pfaff DW (1998). Roles of estrogen receptor-alpha gene expression in reproduction-related behaviors in female mice. Endocrinology 139:5070–5081.

438. Gladue B, Clemens L (1980). Flutamide inhibits testosterone-induced masculine sexual behavior in male and female rats. Endocrinology 106:1917–1922.

439. Poletti A, Negri-Cesi P, Rabuffetti M, Colciago A, Celotti F, Martini L (1998). Transient expression of the 5alpha-reductase type 2 isozyme in the rat brain in late fetal and early postnatal life. Endocrinology 139:2171–2178.

440. Roselli CE, Klosterman SA (1998). Sexual differentiation of aromatase activity in the rat brain: effects of perinatal steroid exposure. Endocrinology 139:3193–201.

441. Shughrue P, Stumpf W, Elger W, Schulze P-E, Sar M (1991). Progestin receptor cells in the 8-day-old male and female mouse cerebral cortex: Autoradiographic evidence for a sexual dimorphism in target cell number. Endocrinol 128:87–95.

442. Mani S, Blaustein J, Allen J, Law S, O'Malley B, Clark J (1994). Inhibition of rat sexual behavior by antisense oligonucleotides to the progesterone receptor. Endocrinol 135:1409–1414.

443. Cooke BM, Woolley CS (2005). Gonadal hormone modulation of dendrites in the mammalian CNS J Neurobiol 64:34-46.

444. Naftolin F, Garcia-Segura LM, Horvath TL, et al. (2007). Estrogen-induced hypothalamic synaptic plasticity and pituitary sensitization in the control of the estrogen-induced gonadotrophin surge. Reproductive Sciences 14:101-116.

445. Lu SF, McKenna SE, Cologer-Clifford A, Nau EA, Simon NG (1998). Androgen receptor in mouse brain: Sex differences and similarities in autoregulation. Endocrinology 139:1594–1601.

446. Cooke BM, Tabibnia G, Breedlove SM (1999). A brain sexual dimorphism controlled by adult circulating androgens. Proc Natl Acad Sci (USA) 96:7538–7540.

447. Levy J, Heller W (1992). Gender differences in human neuropsychological function. In Gerall AA, Moltz H, Ward I (eds.), *Sexual differentiation: A lifespan approach, Handbook of behavioral neurobiology* (vol. 11). New York: Plenum Press 245–274.

448. Levine SC, Huttenlocher J, Taylor A, Langrock A (1999). Early sex differences in spatial skill. Dev Psychol 35:940–949.

449. Schoentjes E, Deboutte D, Friedrich W (1999). Child sexual behavior inventory: A Dutch-speaking normative sample. Pediatrics 104:885–893.

450. McClintock M, Herdt G (1996). Rethinking puberty: The development of sexual attraction. Cur Direct Psychol Sci 5:178–183.

451. Finkelstein JW, Susman EJ, Chinchilli VM, et al. (1997). Estrogen or testosterone increases self-reported aggressive behaviors in hypogonadal adolescents. J Clin Endocrinol Metab 82:2433–2438.

452. Finkelstein JW, Susman EJ, Chinchilli VM, et al. (1998). Effects of estrogen or testosterone on self-reported sexual responses and behaviors in hypogonadal adolescents. J Clin Endocrinol Metab 83:2281–2285.

453. LeVay S (1991). A difference in hypothalamic structure between heterosexual and homosexual men. Science 253:1034–1037.

454. Allen LS, Gorski RA (1992). Sexual orientation and the size of the anterior commissure in the human brain. Proc Natl Acad Sci (USA) 89:7199–7202.

455. Zhou Z-X, Lane M, Kemppainen J, French F, Wilson E (1995). Specificity of ligand-dependent androgen receptor stabilization: Receptor domain interactions influence ligand dissociation and receptor stability. Molec Endocrinol 9:208–218.

456. Berglund H, Lindstrom P, Savic I (20060. Brain response to putative pheromones in lesbian women. Proc Natl Acad Sci (USA) 103:8269–8274.

457. Yoon H, Enquist LW, Dulac C (2005). Olfactory inputs to hypothalamic neurons controlling reproduction and fertility. Cell 123:669–682.

458. Papanicolaou DA, Vgontzas AN (2000). Interleukin-6: The endocrine cytokine. J Clin Endocrinol Metab 85:1331–1333.

459. Rosing J, Middeldorp S, Curvers J, et al. (1999). Low-dose oral contraceptives and acquired resistance to activated protein C: A randomised cross-over study. Lancet 354:2036–2040.

460. Knauthe R, Diel P, Hegele-Hartung C, Engelhaupt A, Fritzemeier KH (1996). Sexual dimorphism of steroid hormone receptor messenger ribonucleic acid expression and hormonal regulation in rat vascular tissue. Endocrinology 137:3220–3227.

461. Drobac S, Rubin K, Rogol AD, Rosenfield RL (2006). A workshop on pubertal hormone replacement options in the United States. J Pediatr Endocrinol Metab 19:55–64.

462. Grodstein F, Manson JE, Stampfer MJ (2006). Hormone therapy and coronary heart disease: The role of time since menopause and age at hormone initiation. J Womens Health (Larchmt) 15:35–44.

463. Mortensen M, Rosenfield RL, Littlejohn E (2006). Functional significance of polycystic-size ovaries in healthy adolescents. J Clin Endocrinol Metab 91:3786–3790.

464. Bordini BD, Littlejohn EE, Rosenfeld RL (2007). Blunted sleep-related LH increase in early pubertal overweight healthy girls. Pediatric Academic Society Annual Meeting,Toronto, Canada, May 3-8, 2007; E-PAS2007:61:7515.2. (http://www.pas-meeting.org/2008%20Honolulu/abstract_archives.asp)

465. Forest M (1979). Function of the ovary in the neonate and infant. Eur J Obstet Gynecol Reprod Biol 9:145-160.

466. Solomon LM, Esterly NB (1970). Neonatal dermatology: I. The newborn skin. J Pediatr 77:888–894.

467. Rosenfield RL (1994). Normal and almost normal variants of precocious puberty: Premature pubarche and premature thelarche revisited. Horm Res 41:7–13.

468. Brito VN, Batista MC, Borges MF, et al. (1999). Diagnostic value of fluorometric assays in the evaluation of precocious puberty. J Clin Endocrinol Metab 84:3539–3544.

468a.Resende EA, Lara BH, Reis JD, et al. (2007). Assessment of basal and gonadotropin-releasing hormone-stimulated gonadotropins by immunochemiluminometric and immunofluorometric assays in normal children. J Clin Endocrinol Metab 92:1424-1429.

469. Ehara Y, Yen S, Siler T (1975). Serum prolactin levels during puberty. Am J Obstet Gynecol 121:995.

470. Marshall W, Tanner J (1969). Variations in pattern of pubertal changes in girls. Arch Dis Child 44:291.

471. Ross GT, Vande Wiele R (1974). The ovary. In Williams R (ed.), Textbook of endocrinology. Philadelphia: WB Saunders.

472. Rosenfield RL, Bachrach LK, Chernausek SD, et al. (2000). Current age of onset of puberty. Pediatrics 106:622.

473. Frontini MG, Srinivasan SR, Berenson GS (2003). Longitudinal changes in risk variables underlying metabolic Syndrome X from childhood to young adulthood in female subjects with a history of early menarche: The Bogalusa Heart Study. Int J Obes Relat Metab Disord 27:1398–1404.

474. Rosenfield RL, Lipton RB, Drum ML (2007). Pubertal milestone attainment in normal-weight girls. E-PAS2007; 7914.11.

475. Freedman DS, Khan LK, Serdula MK, Dietz WH, Srinivasan SR, Berenson GS (2002). Relation of age at menarche to race, time period, and anthropometric dimensions: The Bogalusa Heart Study. Pediatrics 110:e43.

476. Demerath EW, Towne B, Chumlea WC, et al. (2004). Recent decline in age at menarche: The Fels Longitudinal Study. Am J Hum Biol 16:453–457.

477. de Ridder C, Thijssen J, Bruning P, Van den Brande J, Zonderland M, Erich W (1992). Body fat mass, body fat distribution, and pubertal development: A longitudinal study of physical and hormonal sexual maturation of girls. J Clin Endocrinol Metab 75:442–446.

478. Marti-Henneberg C, Vizmanos B (1997). The duration of puberty in girls is related to the timing of its onset. J Pediatr 131:618–621.

479. Biro FM, Huang B, Crawford PB, et al. (2006). Pubertal correlates in black and white girls. J Pediatr 148:234-240.

479a.Lee JM, Appugliese D, Kaciroti N, et al. (2007). Weight status in young girls and the onset of puberty. Pediatrics 119:e624-e630.

480. Ibañez L, Jimenez R, de Zegher F (2006). Early puberty-menarche after precocious pubarche: Relation to prenatal growth. Pediatrics 117:117–121.

481. Tanner JM, Davies PS (1985). Clinical longitudinal standards for height and height velocity for North American children. J Pediatr 107:317–329.

482. Bennett D, Ward M, Daniel WJ (1976). The relationship of serum alkaline phosphatase concentrations to sex maturity ratings in adolescents. J Pediatr 88:633.

483. Herman-Giddens ME, Slora EJ, Wasserman RC, et al. (1997). Secondary sexual characteristics and menses in young girls seen in office practice: A study from the Pediatric Research in Office Settings network. Pediatrics 99:505–512.

484. Kreiter M, Cara J, Rosenfield R (1993). Modifying the outcome of complete precocious puberty. To treat or not to treat. In Grave G, Cutler G (eds.), Sexual precocity: Etiology, diagnosis, and management. New York: Raven Press 109–120.

485. Roman R, Johnson MC, Codner E, Boric MA, aVila A, Cassorla F (2004). Activating GNAS1 gene mutations in patients with premature thelarche. J Pediatr 145:218–222.

486. Witchel SF, Lee PA, Suda-Hartman M, Hoffman EP (1997). Hyperandrogenism and manifesting heterozygotes for 21-hydroxylase deficiency. Biochem Mol Med 62:151–158.

487. Nayak S, Lee PA, Witchel SF (1998). Variants of the type II 3beta-hydroxysteroid dehydrogenase gene in children with premature pubic hair and hyperandrogenic adolescents. Mol Genet Metab 64:184–192.

488. Apter D, Vihko R (1977). Serum pregnenolone, progesterone, 17-hydroxyprogesterone, testosterone, and 5α-dihydrotestosterone during female puberty. J Clin Endocrinol Metab 45:1039.

489. Treloar A, Boynton R, Benn B, Brown B (1967). Variation of human menstrual cycle through reproductive life. Int J Fertil 12:77–84.

489a.Diaz A, Laufer MR, Breech LL (2006). Menstruation in girls and adolescents: using the menstrual cycle as a vital sign. Pediatrics 118:2245-2250.

490. Siegberg R, Nilsson CG, Stenman UH, Widholm O (1986). Endocrinologic features of oligomenorrheic adolescent girls. Fertil Steril 46:852–857.

491. Venturoli S, Porcu E, Fabbri R, et al. (1986). Menstrual irregularities in adolescents: Hormonal pattern and ovarian morphology. Hormone Res 24:269–279.

492. Ardaens Y, Robert Y, Lemaitre L, Fossati P, Dewailly D (1991). Polycystic ovarian disease: contribution of vaginal endosonoggraphy and reassessment of ultrasonic diagnosis. Fertil Steril 55:1062–1068.

493. Apter D, Bützow T, Laughlin G (1993). Hyperandrogenism during puberty and adolescence, and its relationship to reproductive function in the adult female. In Frajese G, Steinberger E, Rodriguez-Rigau L (eds.), Reproductive medicine. New York: Raven Press 265–275.

494. Southam A, Richart E (1966). The prognosis for adolescents with menstrual abnormalities. Am J Obstet Gynecol 94:637.

495. Lucky AW, Biro FM, Huster GA, Leach AD, Morrison JA, Ratterman J (1994). Acne vulgaris in premenarchal girls. Arch Dermatol 130:308–314.

496. McClintock M (1971). Menstrual synchrony and suppression. Nature 229:244.

497. Rosenfield RL (1979). Plasma free androgen patterns in hirsute women and their diagnostic implications. Am J Med 66:417.

498. Vekemans M, Delvoye P, L'Hermite M, Robyn C (1977). Serum prolactin levels during the menstrual cycle. J Clin Endocrinol Metab 44:989.

499. Kolodny R, Jacobs L, Daughaday W (1972). Mammary stimulation causes prolactin secretion in non-lactating women. Nature 238:284.

500. Stern K, McClintock MK (1998). Regulation of ovulation by human pheromones. Nature 392:177–179.

501. Jacob S, McClintock MK (2000). Psychological state and mood effects of steroidal chemosignals in women and men. Horm Behav 37:57–78.

502. Golan A, Langer R, Bukovsky I, Caspi E (1989). Congenital anomalies of the Müllerian system. Fertil Steril 51:747–754.

502a. Biason-Lauber A, De Filippo G, Konrad D, et al. (2007). WNT4 deficiency--a clinical phenotype distinct from the classic Mayer-Rokitansky-Kuster-Hauser syndrome: a case report. Hum Reprod 22:224-229.

503. Brauner R, Adan L, Malandry A, Zantleifer D (1994). Adult height in girls with idiopathic true precocious puberty. J Clin Endocrinol Metab 79:415–420.

504. Pasquino AM, Pucarelli I, Accardo F, et al. (2008). Long-term observation of 87 girls with idiopathic central precocious puberty treated with GnRH analogues: impact on adult height, body mass index, bone mineral content and reproductive function. J Clin Endocrinol Metab 93:190-195.

505. Fokstuen S, Ginsburg C, Zachmann M, Schinzel A (1999). Maternal uniparental disomy 14 as a cause of intrauterine growth retardation and early onset of puberty. J Pediatr 134:689–695.

506. Bourguignon JP, Jaeken J, Gerard A, de Zegher F (1997). Amino acid neurotransmission and initiation of puberty: Evidence from nonketotic hyperglycinemia in a female infant and gonadotropin-releasing hormone secretion by rat hypothalamic explants. J Clin Endocrinol Metab 82:1899–1903.

507. Junier M-P, Wolff A, Hoffman G, Ma Y, Ojeda S (1992). Effect of hypothalamic lesions that induce precocious puberty on the morphological and functional maturation of the luteinizing hormone-releasing hormone neuronal system. Endocrinol 131:787–798.

508. Cacciari E, Zucchini S, Ambrosetto P, et al. (1994). Empty sella in children and adolescents iwth possible hypothalamic-pituitary disorders. J Clin Endocrinol Metab 78:767–771.

509. Laue I, Comite F, Hench K, Loriaux D, Cutler CJ, Pescovitz O (1985). Precocious puberty associated with neurofibromatosis and optic gliomas. Am J Dis Child 139:1097.

510. Zacharin M (1997). Precocious puberty in two children with neurofibromatosis type I in the absence of optic chiasmal glioma. J Pediatr 130:155–157.

511. Mahachoklertwattana P, Kaplan S, Grumbach M (1993). The luteinizing hormone-releasing hormone-secreting hypothalamic hamartoma is a congenital malformation: Natural history. J Clin Endocrinol Metab 77:118–124.

512. Jung H, Carmel P, Schwartz MS, et al. (1999). Some hypothalamic hamartomas contain transforming growth factor alpha, a puberty-inducing growth factor, but not luteinizing hormone-releasing hormone neurons. J Clin Endocrinol Metab 84:4695–4701.

513. Kitay J, Altschule M (1964). *The pineal gland.* Cambridge, MA: Harvard Univ Press.

514. Cohen R, Wurtman R, Axelrod J, et al. (1964). Some clinical, biochemical, and physiological actions of the pineal gland. Ann Intern Med 61:1144.

515. Baer K (1977). Premature ovarian failure and precocious puberty. Obstet Gynecol 49:15s.

516. Quigley C, Cowell C, Jimenez M, et al. (1989). Normal or early development of puberty despite gonadal damage in children treated for acute lymphoblastic leukemia. N Engl J Med 321:143–151.

517. Root AW, Moshang T Jr. (1984). Evolution of the hyperandrogenism-polycystic ovary syndrome from isosexual precocious puberty: report of two cases. Am J Obstet Gynecol 149:763–767.

518. Cisternino M, Dondi E, Martinetti M, et al. (1998). Exaggerated 17-hydroxyprogesterone response to short-term adrenal stimulation and evidence for CYP21B gene point mutations in true precocious puberty. Clin Endocrinol (Oxford) 48:555–560.

519. Jensen AM, Brocks V, Holm K, Laursen EM, Muller J (1998). Central precocious puberty in girls: Internal genitalia before, during,

and after treatment with long-acting gonadotropin-releasing hormone analogues. J Pediatr 132:105–108.

520. Blanco-Garcia M, Evain-Brion D, Roger M, Job M (1985). Isolated menses in prepubertal girls. Pediatrics 76:43.

521. Sklar C, Conte F, Kaplan S, Grumbach M (1981). Human chorionic gonadotropin-secreting pineal tumor: Relation to pathogenesis and sex limitation of sexual precocity. J Clin Endocrinol Metab 53:656–660.

522. Hibi I, Fujiwara K (1987). Precocious puberty of cerebral origin: A cooperative study in Japan. Prog Exp Tumor Res 30:224–238.

523. Starzyk J, Starzyk B, Bartnik-Mikuta A, Urbanowicz W, Dziatkowiak H (2001). Gonadotropin releasing hormone-independent precocious puberty in a 5 year-old girl with suprasellar germ cell tumor secreting beta-hCG and alpha-fetoprotein. J Pediatr Endocrinol Metab 14:789–796.

524. O'Marcaigh AS, Ledger GA, Roche PC, Parisi JE, Zimmerman D (1995). Aromatase expression in human germinomas with possible biological effects. J Clin Endocrinol Metab 80:3763–3766.

525. Rosenfeld R, Reitz R, King A, Hintz R (1980). Familial precocious puberty associated with isolated elevation of luteinizing hormone. N Engl J Med 303:859.

526. Van Wyk J, Grumbach M (1960). Syndrome of precocious menstruation and galactorrhea in juvenile hypothyroidism: An example of hormonal overlap in pituitary feedback. J Pediatr 57:416.

527. Lindsay A, Voorhess M, MacGillivray M (1980). Multicystic ovaries detected by sonography in children with hypothyroidism. Am J Dis Child 134:588.

528. Lee P, Blizzard R (1974). Serum gonadotropins in hypothyroid girls with and without sexual precocity. Johns Hopkins Med J 135:55.

529. Beitins I, Bode H (1980). Hypothyroidism with elevated gonadotropin secretion. Pediatr Res 14:475.

530. Ryan GL, Feng X, d'Alva CB, et al. (2007). Evaluating the roles of follicle-stimulating hormone receptor polymorphisms in gonadal hyperstimulation associated with severe juvenile primary hypothyroidism. J Clin Endocrinol Metab 92:2312-2317.

531. De Leener A, Montanelli L, Van Durme J, et al. (2006). Presence and absence of follicle-stimulating hormone receptor mutations provide some insights into spontaneous ovarian hyperstimulation syndrome physiopathology. J Clin Endocrinol Metab 91:555–562.

532. Copmann T, Adams W (1981). Relationship of polycystic ovary induction to prolactin secretion: Prevention of cyst formation by bromocriptine in the rat. Endocrinology 108:1095.

533. Shenker A, Weinstein L, Moran A, et al. (1993). Severe endocrine and nonendocrine manifestations of the McCune-Albright syndrome associated with activating mutations of stimulatory G protein Gs. J Pediatr 123:509–518.

534. Frisch L, Copeland K, Boepple P (1992). Recurrent ovarian cysts in childhood: Diagnosis of McCune-Albright syndrome by bone scan. Pediatr 90:102–104.

535. Scanlon E, Burkett F, Sener S, et al. (1974). Breast carcinoma in an 11-year-old girl with Albright's syndrome. Breast 6:5.

536. Lumbroso S, Paris F, Sultan C (2004). Activating Gsalpha mutations: Analysis of 113 patients with signs of McCune-Albright syndrome, a European Collaborative Study. J Clin Endocrinol Metab 89:2107–2113.

537. Kalter-Leibovici O, Dickerman Z, Zamir R, Weiss I, Kaufman H, Laron Z (1989). Late onset 21-hydroxylase deficiency in a girl mimicking true sexual precocity. J Pediat Endocrinol 3:121–124.

538. Uli N, Chin D, David R, et al. (1997). Menstrual bleeding in a female infant with congenital adrenal hyperplasia: Altered maturation of the hypothalamic-pituitary-ovarian axis. J Clin Endocrinol Metab 82:3298–3302.

539. Boepple P (1989). Case records of the Massachusetts General Hospital. N Engl J Med 321:1463.

540. Schneider DT, Calaminus G, Wessalowski R, et al. (2003). Ovarian sex cord-stromal tumors in children and adolescents. J Clin Oncol 21:2357-2363.

541. Gallion H, van Nagell J, Donaldson E, Powell D (1988). Ovarian dysgerminoma: Report of seven cases and review of the literature. Am J Obstet Gynecol 158:591.

542. Silverman LA, Gitelman SE (1996). Immunoreactive inhibin, mullerian inhibitory substance, and activin as biochemical markers for juvenile granulosa cell tumors. J Pediatr 129:918–921.

543. Vaz R, Turner C (1986). Ollier disease (enchondromatosis) associated with ovarian juvenile granulosa cell tumor and precocious pseudopuberty. J Pediatr 108:945.

544. Orselli RC, Bassler TJ (1973). Theca granulosa cell tumor arising in adrenal. Cancer 31:474–477.

544. Gustafson M, Lee M, Scully R, et al. (1992). Müllerian inhibiting substance as a marker for ovarian sex-cord tumor. New Engl J Med 326:466–467.

545. Mehenni H, Blouin JL, Radhakrishna U, et al. (1997). Peutz-Jeghers syndrome: Confirmation of linkage to chromosome 19p13.3 and identification of a potential second locus, on 19q13.4. Am J Hum Genet 61:1327–1334.

546. Fragoso MC, Latronico AC, Carvalho FM, et al. (1998). Activating mutation of the stimulatory G protein (gsp) as a putative cause of ovarian and testicular human stromal Leydig cell tumors. J Clin Endocrinol Metab 83:2074–2078.

547. Mandel FP, Voet RL, Weiland AJ, Judd HL (1981). Steroid secretion by masculinizing and "feminizing" hilus cell tumors. J Clin Endocrinol Metab 52:779.

548. Rosenfield RL, Cohen RM, Talerman A (1987). Lipid cell tumor of the ovary in reference to adult-onset congenital adrenal hyperplasia and polycystic ovary syndrome. J Reprod Med 32:363.

549. Lin CJ, Jorge AA, Latronico AC, et al. (2000). Origin of an ovarian steroid cell tumor causing isosexual pseudoprecocious puberty demonstrated by the expression of adrenal steroidogenic enzymes and adrenocorticotropin receptor. J Clin Endocrinol Metab 85:1211–1214.

550. Phornphutkul C, Okubo T, Wu K, et al. (2001). Aromatase p450 expression in a feminizing adrenal adenoma presenting as isosexual precocious puberty. J Clin Endocrinol Metab 86:649–652.

551. Wilkin F, Gagne N, Paquette J, Oligny LL, Deal C (2000). Pediatric adrenocortical tumors: Molecular events leading to insulin-like growth factor II gene overexpression. J Clin Endocrinol Metab 85:2048–2056.

552. Saenz de Rodriguez CA, Bongiovanni AM, Conde de Borrego L (1985). An epidemic of precocious development in Puerto Rican children. J Pediatr 107:393–396.

553. Setchell KD, Zimmer-Nechemias L, Cai J, Heubi JE (1997). Exposure of infants to phyto-oestrogens from soy-based infant formula. Lancet 350:23–27.

554. Zava DT, Dollbaum CM, Blen M. Estrogen and progestin bioactivity of foods, herbs, and spices. Proc Soc Exp Biol Med 1998;217:369–378.

554a. Henley DV, Lipson N, Korach KS, Bloch CA (2007). Prepubertal gynecomastia linked to lavender and tea tree oils. N Engl J Med 356:479–485.

555. Kunz GJ, Klein KO, Clemons RD, Gottschalk ME, Jones KL (2004). Virilization of young children after topical androgen use by their parents. Pediatrics 114:282–284.

556. Stratakis CA, Vottero A, Brodie A, et al. (1998). The aromatase excess syndrome is associated with feminization of both sexes and autosomal dominant transmission of aberrant P450 aromatase gene transcription. J Clin Endocrinol Metab 83:1348–1357.

557. Balducci R, Boscherini B, Mangiantini A, Morellini M, Toscanii V (1994). Isolated precocious pubarche: An approach. J Clin Endocrinol Metab 79:582–589.

558. Trivin C, Couto-Silva AC, Sainte-Rose C, et al. (2006). Presentation and evolution of organic central precocious puberty according to the type of CNS lesion. Clin Endocrinol (Oxford) 65:239–245.

559. Bidlingmaier F, Butenandt O, Knorr D (1977). Plasma gonadotropins and estrogens in girls with idiopathic precocious puberty. Pediatr Res 11:91.

560. Rosenthal I, Refetoff S, Rich B, et al. (1996). Response to challenge with gonadotropin-releasing hormone agonist in a mother and her two sons with a constitutively activating mutation of the luteinizing hormone receptor: A clinical research center study. J Clin Endocrinol Metab 81:3802–3806.

561. Rosenfield RL (1994). Selection of children with precocious puberty for treatment with gonadotropin releasing hormone analogs. J Pediatr 124:989–991.

562. Klein KO (1999). Precocious puberty: who has it? Who should be treated? J Clin Endocrinol Metab 84:411–414.

563. Stratakis CA, Papageorgiou T, Premkumar A, et al. (2000). Ovarian lesions in Carney complex: Clinical genetics and possible predisposition to malignancy. J Clin Endocrinol Metab 85:4359–4366.

564. Lonsdale RN, Roberts PF, Trowell JE (1991). Autoimmune oophoritis associated with polycystic ovaries. Histopathology 19:77–81.

565. Grunt JA, Midyett LK, Simon SD, Lowe L (2004). When should cranial magnetic resonance imaging be used in girls with early sexual development? J Pediatr Endocrinol Metab 17:775–780.

566. Midyett LK, Moore WV, Jacobson JD (2003). Are pubertal changes in girls before age 8 benign? Pediatrics 111:47–51.

567. Heger S, Partsch CJ, Sippell WG (1999). Long-term outcome after depot gonadotropin-releasing hormone agonist treatment of central precocious puberty: Final height, body proportions, body composition, bone mineral density, and reproductive function. J Clin Endocrinol Metab 84:4583–4590.

568. Klein KO, Barnes KM, Jones JV, et al. (2001). Increased final height in precocious puberty after long-term treatment with LHRH agonists: the National Institutes of Health experience. J Clin Endocrinol Metab 86:4711-4716.

569. Lazar L, Padoa A, Phillip M (2007). Growth pattern and final height after cessation of gonadotropin-suppressive therapy in girls with central sexual precocity. J Clin Endocrinol Metab 92:3483-3489.

570. Palmert MR, Malin HV, Boepple PA (1999). Unsustained or slowly progressive puberty in young girls: initial presentation and long-term follow-up of 20 untreated patients. J Clin Endocrinol Metab 84:415-423.

571. Alvarez R, Grizzle W, Smith L, Miller D (1989). Compensatory ovarian hypertrophy occurs by a mechanism distinct from compensatory growth in the regenerating liver. Am J Obstet Gynecol 161:1653–1657.

571a. Eugster EA, Clarke W, Kletter GB, et al. (2007). Efficacy and safety of histrelin subdermal implant in children with central precocious puberty: a multicenter trial. J Clin Endocrinol Metab 92:1697-704.

572. Badaru A, Wilson DM, Bachrach LK, et al. (2006). Sequential comparisons of one-month and three-month depot leuprolide regimens in central precocious puberty. J Clin Endocrinol Metab 91:1862–1867.

573. Klein KO, Baron J, Barnes KM, Pescovitz OH, Cutler GB Jr. (1998). Use of an ultrasensitive recombinant cell bioassay to determine estrogen levels in girls with precocious puberty treated with a luteinizing hormone-releasing hormone agonist. J Clin Endocrinol Metab 83:2387–2389.

574. Brito VN, Latronico AC, Arnhold IJ, Mendonca BB (2004). A single luteinizing hormone determination 2 hours after depot leuprolide is useful for therapy monitoring of gonadotropin-dependent precocious puberty in girls. J Clin Endocrinol Metab 89:4338–4342.

575. Adan L, Souberbielle JC, Zucker JM (1997). Adult height in 24 patients treated for growth hormone deficiency and early puberty. J Clin Endocrinol Metab 82:229–233.

576. Pasquino AM, Pucarelli I, Segni M, Matrunola M, Cerroni F, Cerrone F (1999). Adult height in girls with central precocious puberty treated with gonadotropin-releasing hormone analogues and growth hormone [published erratum appears in J Clin Endocrinol Metab 84(6):1978, 1999]. J Clin Endocrinol Metab 84:449–452.

577. Letterie GS, Stevenson D, Shah A (1991). Recurrent anaphylaxis to a depot form of GnRH analogue. Obstet Gynecol 78:943–946.

578. Antoniazzi F, Zamboni G, Bertoldo F, et al. (2003). Bone mass at final height in precocious puberty after gonadotropin-releasing hormone agonist with and without calcium supplementation. J Clin Endocrinol Metab 88:1096–1101.

579. Rosenfield RL (1996). Essentials of growth diagnosis. Endocrinol Metab Clin N Am 25:743–758.

580. Papadimitriou A, Beri D, Tsialla A, Fretzayas A, Psychou F, Nicolaidou P (2006). Early growth acceleration in girls with idiopathic precocious puberty. J Pediatr 149:43–46.

581. Lazar L, Kauli R, Pertzelan A, Phillip M (2002). Gonadotropin-suppressive therapy in girls with early and fast puberty affects the pace of puberty but not total pubertal growth or final height. J Clin Endocrinol Metab 87:2090–2094.

582. Richman RA, Underwood LE, French FS, Van Wyk JJ (1971). Adverse effects of large doses of medroxyprogesterone (MPA) in idiopathic isosexual precocity. J Pediatr 79:963.

583. Lopez LM, Grimes DA, Schulz KF, Curtis KM (2006). Steroidal contraceptives: Effect on bone fractures in women. Cochrane Database Syst Rev CD006033.

584. Eugster EA, Rubin SD, Reiter EO, Plourde P, Jou HC, Pescovitz OH (2003). Tamoxifen treatment for precocious puberty in McCune-Albright syndrome: A multicenter trial. J Pediatr 143:60–66.

585. Feuillan P, Calis K, Hill S, et al. (2007). Letrozole treatment of precocious puberty in girls with the McCune-Albright syndrome: a pilot study. J Clin Endocrinol Metab 92:2100-2106.

586. Holland F, Kirsch S, Selby R (1987). Gonadotropin-independent precocious puberty ("testotoxicosis"): Influence of maturational status on response to ketoconazole. J Clin Endocrinol Metab 64:328–333.

587. Laven JS, Lumbroso S, Sultan C, Fauser BC (2001). Dynamics of ovarian function in an adult woman with McCune-Albright syndrome. J Clin Endocrinol Metab 86:2625–2630.

588. Chapurlat RD, Meunier PJ (2000). Fibrous dysplasia of bone. Baillieres Best Pract Res Clin Rheumatol 14:385–398.

589. Lala R, Matarazzo P, Bertelloni S, Buzi F, Rigon F, de Sanctis C (2000). Pamidronate treatment of bone fibrous dysplasia in nine children with McCune-Albright syndrome. Acta Paediatr 89:188–193.

590. Whyte MP, Wenkert D, Clements KL, McAlister WH, Mumm S (2003). Bisphosphonate-induced osteopetrosis. N Engl J Med 349:457–463.

591. Rosenfield RL, Barnes RB (1993). Menstrual disorders in adolescence. Endocrinol Metab Clin N Am 22:491–505.

592. Razdan A, Rosenfield R, Kim M (1976). Endocrinologic characteristics of partial ovarian failure. J Clin Endocrinol Metab 43:449.

593. Page L, Beauregard L, Bode H, Beitins I (1990). Hypothalamic-pituitary-ovarian function in menstruating women with Turner syndrome (45,X). Pediatr Res 28:514–517.

594. Winslow KL, Toner JP, Brzyski RG, Oehninger SC, Acosta AA, Muasher SJ (1991). The gonadotropin-releasing hormone agonist stimulation test: A sensitive predictor of performance in the flare-up in vitro fertilization cycle. Fertil Steril 56:711–717.

595. Goswami D, Conway GS (2005). Premature ovarian failure. Hum Reprod Update 11:391-410.

596. Welt CK, Hall JE, Adams JM, Taylor AE (2005). Relationship of estradiol and inhibin to the follicle-stimulating hormone variability in hypergonadotropic hypogonadism or premature ovarian failure. J Clin Endocrinol Metab 90:826-830.

597. Mazzanti L, Cacciari E, Bergamaschi R, et al. (1997). Pelvic ultrasonography in patients with Turner syndrome: Age-related findings in different karyotypes. J Pediatr 131:135–140.

598. Cunniff C, Jones K, Benirschke K (1990). Ovarian dysgenesis in individuals with chromosomal abnormalities. Hum Genet 86:552–556.

599. Hansen J, Boyar R, Shapiro L (1980). Gonadal function in trisomy 21. Horm Res 12:345.

600. Bovicelli L, Orsini LF, Rizzo N, Montacuti V, Bacchetta M (1982). Reproduction in Down syndrome. Obstet Gynecol 59:13S–17S.

601. Pelletier J, Bruening W, Kashtan C, et al. (1991). Germline mutations in the Wilms' tumor suppressor gene are associated with abnormal urogenital development in Denys-Drash syndrome. Cell 67:437–447.

602. Skre H, Bassoe HH, Berg K, Frovig AG (1976). Cerebellar ataxia and hypergonadotrophis hypogonadism in two kindreds: Chance concurrence, pleiotropism or linkage. Clin Genet 9:234.

603. McDonough PG (2003). Selected enquiries into the causation of premature ovarian failure. Hum Fertil (Camb) 6:130-136.

604. Goldman S, Johnson F (1993). Effects of chemotherapy and irradiation on the gonads. Endocrinol Metab Clin N Am 22:617–629.

605. Cohen LE (2005). Endocrine late effects of cancer treatment. Endocrinol Metab Clin North Am 34:769-789.

606. Oktay K, Sonmezer M, Oktem O, et al. (2007). Absence of conclusive evidence for the safety and efficacy of gonadotropin-releasing hormone analogue treatment in protecting against chemotherapy-induced gonadal injury. Oncologist 12:1055-1066.

607. Chemaitilly W, Mertens AC, Mitby P, et al. (2006). Acute ovarian failure in the childhood cancer survivor study. J Clin Endocrinol Metab 91:1723-1728.

608. Sarafoglou K, Boulad F, Gillio A, Sklar C (1997). Gonadal function after bone marrow transplantation for acute leukemia during childhood. J Pediatr 130:210–216.

609. Yeung SC, Chiu AC, Vassilopoulou-Sellin R, Gagel RF (1998). The endocrine effects of nonhormonal antineoplastic therapy. Endocr Rev 19:144–172.

610. Larsen EC, Muller J, Schmiegelow K, et al. (2003). Reduced ovarian function in long-term survivors of radiation- and chemotherapy-treated childhood cancer. J Clin Endocrinol Metab 88:5307-5314.

611. Toledo S, Brunner H, Kraaij R, et al. (1996). An inactivating mutation of the luteinizing hormone receptor causes amenorrhea in a 46,XX female. J Clin Endocrinol Metab 81:3850–3854.

612. Layman LC, McDonough PG (2000). Mutations of follicle stimulating hormone-beta and its receptor in human and mouse: Genotype/phenotype. Mol Cell Endocrinol 161:9–17.

613. Namnoum AB, Merriam GR, Moses AM, Levine MA (1998). Reproductive dysfunction in women with Albright's hereditary osteodystrophy. J Clin Endocrinol Metab 83:824–829.

614. de Zegher F, Jaeken J (1995). Endocrinology of the carbohydrate-deficient glycoprotein syndrome type 1 from birth through adolescence. Pediatr Res 37:395.

615. Betterle C, Dal Pra C, Mantero F, Zanchetta R (2002). Autoimmune adrenal insufficiency and autoimmune polyendocrine syndromes: Autoantibodies, autoantigens, and their applicability in diagnosis and disease prediction. Endocr Rev 23:327–364.

616. Bakalov VK, Anasti JN, Calis KA, et al. (2005). Autoimmune oophoritis as a mechanism of follicular dysfunction in women with 46,XX spontaneous premature ovarian failure. Fertil Steril 84:958-965.

617. Welt CK, Falorni A, Taylor AE, et al. (2005). Selective theca cell dysfunction in autoimmune oophoritis results in multifollicular development, decreased estradiol, and elevated inhibin B levels. J Clin Endocrinol Metab 90:3069-3076.

618. Lucky AW, Rebar RW, Blizzard RM, Goren EM (1977). Pubertal progression in the presence of elevated serum gonadotropins in girls with multiple endocrine deficiencies. J Clin Endocrinol Metab 45:673-678.

619. Kuwahara A, Kamada M, Irahara M, Naka O, Yamashita T, Aono T (1998). Autoantibody against testosterone in a woman with hypergonadotropic hypogonadism. J Clin Endocrinol Metab 83:14–16.

620. Bose HS, Pescovitz OH, Miller WL (1997). Spontaneous feminization in a 46,XX female patient with congenital lipoid adrenal hyperplasia due to a homozygous frameshift mutation in the steroidogenic acute regulatory protein. J Clin Endocrinol Metab 82:1511–1515.

621. Tanae A, Katsumata N, Sato N, Horikawa R, Tanaka T (2000). Genetic and endocrinological evaluations of three 46,XX patients with congenital lipoid adrenal hyperplasia previously reported as having presented spontaneous puberty. Endocr J 47:629–634.

622. Layman LC (1999). Genetics of human hypogonadotropic hypogonadism. Am J Med Genet 89:240–248.

623. Jones J, Kemmann E (1976). Olfacto-genital dysplasia in the female. Obstet Gynecol Ann 5:443–466.

624. Beranova M, Oliveira LM, Bedecarrats GY, et al. (2001). Prevalence, phenotypic spectrum, and modes of inheritance of gonadotropin-releasing hormone receptor mutations in idiopathic hypogonadotropic hypogonadism. J Clin Endocrinol Metab 86:1580–1588.

625. de Roux N, Young J, Misrahi M, et al. (1997). A family with hypogonadotropic hypogonadism and mutations in the gonadotropin-releasing hormone receptor. New Engl J Med 337:1597–1602.

626. de Roux N, Young J, Brailley-Tabard S, Misrahi M, Milgrom E, Schaison G (1999). The same molecular defects of the gonadotropin-releasing hormone receptor determine a variable degree of hypogonadism in affected kindred. J Clin Endocrinol Metab 84:567–572.

627. Seminara SB, Beranova M, Oliveira LMB, Martin KA, Crowley WFJ, Hall JE (2000). Successful use of pulsatile gonadotropin-releasing hormone (GnRH) for ovulation induction and pregnancy in a patient with GnRH receptor mutations. J Clin Endocrinol Metab 85:556–562.

628. Merke DP, Tajima T, Baron J, Cutler GB Jr. (1999). Hypogonadotropic hypogonadism in a female caused by an X-linked recessive mutation in the DAX1 gene. N Engl J Med 340:1248–1252.

629. Barkan A, Kelch R, Marshall J (1985). Isolated gonadotrope failure in the polyglandular autoimmune syndrome. N Engl J Med 312:1535.

630. Komatsu M, Kondo T, Yamauchi K, et al. (1988). Antipituitary antibodies in patients with the primary empty sella syndrome. J Clin Endocrinol Metab 67:633.

631. Hendricks SA, Lippe BM, Kaplan SA, Bentson JR (1981). Hypothalamic atrophy with progressive hypopituitarism in an adolescent girl. J Clin Endocrinol Metab 52:562.

632. Rappaport R, Brauner R, Czernichow P, et al. (1982). Effect of hypothalamic and pituitary irradiation on pubertal development in children with cranial tumors. J Clin Endocrinol Metab 54:1164.

633. Van den Berghe G, de Zegher F, Bouillon R (1998). Clinical review 95: Acute and prolonged critical illness as different neuroendocrine paradigms. J Clin Endocrinol Metab 83:1827–1834.

634. Molitch M (1991). Gonadotroph-cell pituitary adenomas. N Engl J Med 324:626–627.

635. Fairburn CG, Harrison PJ (2003). Eating disorders. Lancet 361: 407–416.
636. American Academy of Pediatrics Policy Statement (2003). Identifying and treating eating disorders. Pediatrics 111:204–211.
637. Yager J, Andersen AE (2005). Clinical practice: Anorexia nervosa. N Engl J Med 353:1481–1488.
638. Pugliese M, Lifshitz F, Grad C, Fort P, Marks-Katz M (1983). Fear of obesity: A cause of short stature and delayed puberty. N Engl J Med 309:513.
639. Golden N, Kreitzer P, Jacobson M, et al. (1994). Disturbances in growth hormone secretion and action in adolescents with anorexia nervosa. J Pediatr 125:655–660.
640. Newman M, Halmi K (1988). The endocrinology of anorexia nervosa and bulimia nervosa. Endocrinol Metab Clin N Am 17:195.
641. Frisch R, McArthur J (1974). Menstrual cycles: Fatness as a determinant of minimum weight for height necessary for their maintenance or onset. Science 185:949.
642. Misra M, Prabhakaran R, Miller KK, et al. (2006). Role of cortisol in menstrual recovery in adolescent girls with anorexia nervosa. Pediatr Res 59:598–603.
643. Boyar RM, Katz J, Finkelstein JW, et al. (1974). Anorexia nervosa: Immaturity of the 24-hour luteinizing hormone secretory pattern. N Engl J Med 291:861.
644. Beumont PJ, George GC, Pimstone BL, Vinik AI (1976). Body weight and the pituitary response to hypothalamic releasing hormones in patients with anorexia nervosa. J Clin Endocrinol Metab 43:487.
645. Marshall J, Fraser T (1971). Amenorrhoea in anorexia nervosa: Assessment and treatment with clomiphene citrate. Br Med J 4:590.
646. Welt CK, Chan JL, Bullen J, et al. (2004). Recombinant human leptin in women with hypothalamic amenorrhea. N Engl J Med 351:987–997.
647. Chrousos G, Gold P (1992). The concepts of stress and stress system disorders: Overview of physical and behavioral homeostasis. JAMA 267:1244–1252.
648. Winterer J, Gwirtsman HE, George DT, Kaye WH, Loriaux DL, Cutler GB Jr. (1985). Adrenocorticotropin-stimulated adrenal androgen secretion in anorexia nervosa: Impaired secretion at low weight with normalization after long-term weight recovery. J Clin Endocrinol Metab 61:693.
649. Mecklenburg RS, Loriaux DL, Thompson RH, Andersen AE, Lipsett MB (1974). Hypothalamic dysfunction in patients with anorexia nervosa. Medicine 53:147.
650. Petrides J, Mueller G, Kalogeras K, Chrousos G, Gold P, Deuster P (1994). Exercise-induced activation of the hypothalamic-pituitary-adrenal axis: Marked differences in the sensitivity to glucocorticoid suppression. J Clin Endocrinol Metab 79:377–383.
651. Molitch M (1992). Pathologic hyperprolactinemia. Endocrinol Metab Clin N Am 21:877–901.
652. Colao A, Loche S, Cappa M, et al. (1998). Prolactinomas in children and adolescents: Clinical presentation and long-term follow-up. J Clin Endocrinol Metab 83:2777–2780.
653. Blanco-Favela F, Quintal Ma G, Chavez-Rueda AK, et al. (2001). Anti-prolactin autoantibodies in paediatric systemic lupus erythematosus patients. Lupus 10:803–808.
654. Schlechte JA (2002). The macroprolactin problem. J Clin Endocrinol Metab 87:5408–5409.
655. Greenberg LW, Badosa F, Niakosari A, Schneider A, Zaeri N, Schindler AM (2000). Clinicopathologic exercise: Hypoglycemia in a young woman with amenorrhea. J Pediatr 136:818–822.
656. Mendelson J, Mello N, Teoh S, Ellingboe J, Cochin J (1989). Cocaine effects on pulsatile secretion of anterior pituitary, gonadal, and adrenal hormones. J Clin Endocrinmol Metab 69:1256.
657. Tallo D, Malarkey W (1985). Physiologic concentrations of dopamine fail to suppress prolactin secretion in patients with idiopathic hyperprolactinemia or prolactinomas. Am J Obstet Gynecol 151:651.
658. Sauder S, Frager M, Case C, Kelch R, Marshall J (1984). Abnormal patterns of pulsatile luteinizing hormone secretion in women with hyperprolactinemia and amenorrhea: Responses to bromocriptine. J Clin Endocrinol Metab 59:941.
659. Sane K, Pescovitz O (1992). The clitoral index: A determination of clitoral size in normal girls and in girls with abnormal sexual development. J Pediatr 120:264–266.
660. Rosenfeld RL (2003). Menstrual disorders and hyperandrogenism in adolescence. In Radovick S, MacGillivray MH (eds.), *Pediatric*

endocrinology: A practical clinical guide. Totowa, NJ: Humana Press 451–478.
661. Stanhope R, Pringle P, Brook C, Adams J, Jacobs N (1987). Induction of puberty by pulsatile gonadotropin releasing hormone. Lancet 2:552.
662. Rebar R, Connolly H (1990). Clinical features of young women with hypergonadotropic amenorrhea. Fertil Steril 53:804–810.
663. Petakov MS, Damjanovic SS, Nikolic-Durovic MM, et al. (1998). Pituitary adenomas secreting large amounts of prolactin may give false low values in immunoradiometric assays: The hook effect. J Endocrinol Invest 21:184–188.
664. Kovacs K, Horvath E (1983). Tumors of the pituitary gland. In Hartmann W, Sobin L (eds.), *Atlas of tumor pathology*. Washington, DC: Armed Forces Inst of Pathology 205–209.
665. Schroeder I, Johnson J, Malarkey W (1976). Cerebrospinal fluid prolactin: A reflection of abnormal prolactin secretion in patients with pituitary tumors. J Clin Endocrinol Metab 43:1255.
666. Germain N, Galusca B, Le Roux CW, et al. (2007). Constitutional thinness and lean anorexia nervosa display opposite concentrations of peptide YY, glucagon-like peptide 1, ghrelin, and leptin. Am J Clin Nutr 85:967-971.
667. Gardner D (1993). Pathogenesis of anorexia nervosa. Lancet 341:1631–1634.
668. Molitch ME, Thorner MO, Wilson C (1997). Management of prolactinomas. J Clin Endocrinol Metab 82:996–1000.
669. Colao A, Di Sarno A, Landi ML, et al. (2000). Macroprolactinoma shrinkage during cabergoline treatment is greater in naive patients than in patients pretreated with other dopamine agonists: A prospective study in 110 patients. J Clin Endocrinol Metab 85:2247–2252.
670. Schade R, Andersohn F, Suissa S, Haverkamp W, Garbe E (2007). Dopamine agonists and the risk of cardiac-valve regurgitation. N Engl J Med 356:29–38.
671. Zanettini R, Antonini A, Gatto G, Gentile R, Tesei S, Pezzoli G (2007). Valvular heart disease and the use of dopamine agonists for Parkinson's disease. N Engl J Med 356:39–46.
672. Lock J, le Grange D, Agras WS, Dare C (2001). *Treatment manual for anorexia nervosa*. New York: Guilford.
673. Misra M, Klibanski A (2006). Anorexia nervosa and osteoporosis. Rev Endocr Metab Disord :91-99.
674. Katz R, Mazer C, Litt I (1985). Anorexia nervosa by proxy. J Pediatr 107:247.
675. Rothchild E, Owens R (1972). Adolescent girls who lack functioning ovaries. J Am Acad Child Psychiatry 11:88.
676. Bondy CA, for the Turner Syndrome Consensus Study Group (2007). Care of girls and women with Turner syndrome: A guideline of the Turner syndrome study group. J Clin Endocrinol Metab 92:10–25.
677. Rosenfeld RG, Frane J, Attie KM, et al. (1992). Six-year results of a randomized prospective trial of human growth hormone and oxandrolone in Turner syndrome. J Pediatr 121:49–55.
678. Rosenfield R, Kiess W, Keizer-Schrama S (2006). Physiologic induction of puberty in Turner syndrome with very low-dose estradiol. In Gravholt C, Bondy C (eds.), *Wellness for girls and women with Turner syndrome*. Amsterdam: Elsevier Science 71–79.
679. Woodruff J, Pickar J (1994). Incidence of endometrial hyperplasia in postmenopausal women taking conjugated estrogens (Premarin) with medroxyprogesterone acetate or conjugated estrogens alone. Am J Obstet Gynecol 170:1213–1223.
680. Voight L, Weiss N, Chu J, Daling J, McKnight B, Van Belle G (1991). Progestagen supplementation of exogenous oestrogens and risk of endometrial cancer. Lancet 338:274.
681. Devroey P, Camus M, Palermo G, et al. (1990). Placental production of estradiol and progesterone after oocyte donation in patients with primary ovarian failure. Am J Obstet Gynecol 162:66–70.
682. Silber SJ, Lenahan KM, Levine DJ, et al. (2005). Ovarian transplantation between monozygotic twins discordant for premature ovarian failure. N Engl J Med 353:58–63.
683. Shamonki MI, Oktay K (2005). Oocyte and ovarian tissue cryopreservation: indications, techniques, and applications. Semin Reprod Med 23:266-276.
684. Jahnukainen K, Ehmcke J, Soder O, Schlatt S (2006). Clinical potential and putative risks of fertility preservation in children utilizing gonadal tissue or germline stem cells. Pediatr Res 59:40R–47R.
685. Perkins RB, Hall JE, Martin KA (1999). Neuroendocrine abnormalities in hypothalamic amenorrhea: Spectrum, stability, and response to neurotransmitter modulation. J Clin Endocrinol Metab 84:1905–1911.

686. Shaw R (1979). Differential response to LHRH following oestrogen therapy in women with amenorrhoea. Br Obstet Gynaecol 86:69–75.

687. Weiss C, Nachtigall L, Ganguly M (1976). Induction of an LH surge with estradiol benzoate. Obstet Gynecol 47:415–418.

688. Lado-Abeal J, Rodriguez-Arnao J, Newell-Price JDC, et al. (1998). Menstrual abnormalities in women with Cushing's disease are correlated with hypercortisolemia rather than raised circulating androgen levels. J Clin Endocrinol Metab 83:3083–3088.

689a.Centeno ML, Sanchez RL, Cameron JL, Bethea CL (2007). Hypothalamic expression of serotonin 1A, 2A and 2C receptor and GAD67 mRNA in female cynomolgus monkeys with different sensitivity to stress. Brain Res 1142:1-12.

689. Constantini N, Warren M (1995). Menstrual dysfunction in swimmers: A distinct entity. J Clin Endocrinol Metab 80:2740.

690. Tofler IR, Stryer BK, Micheli LJ, Herman LR (1996). Physical and emotional problems of elite female gymnasts. N Engl J Med 335:281–283.

691. Warren M (1992). Amenorrhea in endurance runners. J Clin Endocrinol Metab 75:1393-1397.

692. Drinkwater B, Bruemner B, Chestnut CI (1990). Menstrual history as a determinant of current bone density in young athletes. JAMA 263:545–548.

693. Frisch R, Snow R, Johnson L, Gerard B, Barbieri R, Rosen B (1993). Magnetic resonance imaging of overall and regional body fat, estrogen metabolism, and ovulation of athletes compared to controls. J Clin Endocrinol Metab 77:471–477.

694. Weltman E, Stern R, Doershuk C, Moir R, Palmer K, Jaffe A (1990). Weight and menstrual function in patients with eating disorders and cystic fibrosis. Pediatr 85:282–287.

695. Frisch R, Wyshak G, Vincent I (1980). Delayed menarche and amenorrhea in ballet dancers. N Engl J Med 303:17.

696. Rakoff A (1962). Psychogenic factors in anovulatory women. Fertil Steril 13:1.

697. Yen SSC (1978). Chronic anovulation due to CNS-hypothalamic-pituitary dysfunction. In Yen Y, Jaffe R (eds.), *Reproductive endocrinology*. Philadelphia: WB Saunders.

698. Shearman R (1974). Secondary amenorrhoea after oral contraceptives: Treatment and follow-up. Contraception 11:123.

699. van der Steeg N, Bennink H (1977). Bromocriptine for induction of ovulation in normoprolactinaemic post-pill anovulation. Lancet 1:502.

700. Ortiz A, Hirol M, Stanczyk FZ, Goebelsmann U, Mishell DR Jr. (1977). Serum medroxy-progesterone acetate (MPA) concentrations and ovarian function following intramuscular injection of depo-MPA. J Clin Endocrinol Metab 44:32.

701. Bolognese R, Piver S, Feldman J (1967). Galactorrhea and abnormal menses associated with a long-acting progesterone. JAMA 199:100.

702. Carson S, Buster J (1993). Ectopic pregnancy. New Engl J Med 16:1174.

703. Maruo T, Nayashi M, Matsuo H, Yamamoto T, Okada H, Mochizuki M (1987). The role of thyroid hormone as a biological amplifier of the actions of follicle-stimulating hormone in the functional differentiation of cultured porcine granulosa cells. Endocrinology 121:1233.

704. Boyar RM, Hellman LD, Roffwarg H, et al. (1977). Cortisol secretion and metabolism in anorexia nervosa. N Engl J Med 296:190–193.

705. Winters SJ, Berga SL (1997). Gonadal dysfunction in patients with thyroid disorders. The Endocrinologist 7:167–173.

706. Asch RH, Smith CG, Siler-Khodr TM, Pauerstein CJ (1981). Effects of Δ5-tetrahydrocannabinol during the follicular phase of the rhesus monkey (Mocaca mulatto). J Clin Endocrinol Metab 52:50.

707. Dees WL, Dissen GA, Hiney JK, Lara F, Ojeda SR (2000). Alcohol ingestion inhibits the increased secretion of puberty-related hormones in the developing female rhesus monkey. Endocrinology 141:1325–1331.

708. Chen EC, Samuels MH, Luther MF, et al. (1998). Cocaine impairs follicular phase pulsatile gonadotropin secretion in rhesus monkeys. J Soc Gynecol Investig 5:311–316.

709. Battaglia DF, Beaver AB, Harris TG, Tanhehco E, Viguie C, Karsch FJ (1999). Endotoxin disrupts the estradiol-induced luteinizing hormone surge: Interference with estradiol signal reading, not surge release. Endocrinology 140:2471–2479.

710. Oerter K, Kampf G, Munson P, Nienhuis A, Cassorla F, Manasco P (1993). Multiple hormone deficiencies in children with hemochromatosis. J Clin Endocrinol Metab 76:357–361.

711. South S, Asplin C, Carlsen E, et al. (1993). Alterations in luteinizing hormone secretory activity in women with insulin-dependent diabetes mellitus and secondary amenorrhea. J Clin Endocrinol Metab 76:1048–1053.

712. Lim V, Kathpalia S, Henriquez C (1978). Endocrine abnormalities associated with chronic renal failure. Med Clin N Am 62:1341.

713. Boyar RM, Kapen S, Weitzman ED, Hellman L (1976). Pituitary microadenoma and hyperprolactinemia. N Engl J Med 294:263.

714. Hirshberg B, Conn PM, Uwaifo GI, Blauer KL, Clark BD, Nieman LK (2003). Ectopic luteinizing hormone secretion and anovulation. N Engl J Med 348:312–317.

715. Soules M, McLachlan R, Ek M, Dahl K, Cohen N, Bremner W (1989). Luteal phase deficiency: characterization of reproductive hormones over the menstrual cycle. J Clin Endocrinol Metab 69:804.

716. Daya S (1989). Optimal time in the menstrual cycle for serum progesterone measurement to diagnose luteal phase defects. Am J Obstet Gynecol 161:1009–1011.

717. Hinney B, Henze C, Kuhn W, Wuttke W (1996). The corpus luteum insufficiency: A multifactorial disease. J Clin Endocrinol Metab 81:565–570.

718. Seppala M, Nirvonen E, Ranta T (1976). Hyperprolactinaemia and luteal insufficiency. Lancet 1:229.

719. Wathen PI, Henderson MC, Witz CA (1995). Abnormal uterine bleeding. Med Clin North Am 79:329–344.

720. Carlson KJ, Schiff I (1996). Alternatives to hysterectomy for menorrhagia. New Engl J Med 335:198–199.

721. Kennedy S (1997). Primary dysmenorrhoea. Lancet 349:1116.

722. Ammeman S, Shafer M-A, Snyder D (1990). Ectopic pregnancy in adolescents: A clinical review for pediatricians. J Pediatr 117:677–684.

723. Olive D, Schwartz L (1993). Endometriosis. New Engl J Med 328:1759–1768.

724. Zeitoun K, Takayama K, Sasano H, et al. (1998). Deficient 17ß-hydroxysteroid dehydrogenase type 2 expression in endometriosis: Failure to metabolize 17ß-estradiol. J Clin Endocrinol Metab 83:4474–4480.

725. Lessey B, Castelbaum A, Sawin S, et al. (1994). Aberrant integrin expression in the endometrium of women with endometriosis. J Clin Endocrinol Metab 79:643–649.

726. Rosenwaks Z, Jones GS, Henzl MR, Dubin NH, Ghodgaonkar RB, Hoffman S (1981). Naproxin sodium, aspirin, and placebo in primary dysmenorrhea. Am J Obstet Gynecol 140:592.

727. DeVane G (1991). Premenstrual syndrome. J Clin Endocrinol Metab 72:250.

728. Grady-Weliky TA (2003). Clinical practice: Premenstrual dysphoric disorder. N Engl J Med 348:433–438.

729. Schachter SC (1988). Hormonal considerations in women with seizures. Arch Neurol 45:1267–1270.

730. Dalton K (1980). Cyclical criminal acts in premenstrual syndrome. Lancet 2:1070.

731. Schmidt PJ, Nieman LK, Danaceau MA, Adams LF, Rubinow DR (1998). Differential behavioral effects of gonadal steroids in women with and in those without premenstrual syndrome. N Engl J Med 338:209–216.

732. Roca CA, Schmidt PJ, Altemus M, et al. (2003). Differential menstrual cycle regulation of hypothalamic-pituitary-adrenal axis in women with premenstrual syndrome and controls. J Clin Endocrinol Metab 88:3057–3063.

733. Wang M, Seippel L, Purdy RH, Backstrom T (1996). Relationship between symptom severity and steroid variation in women with premenstrual syndrome: Study on serum pregnenolone, pregnenolone sulfate, 5 alpha-pregnane-3,20-dione and 3 alpha-hydroxy-5 alpha-pregnan-20-one. J Clin Endocrinol Metab 81:1076–1082.

734. Rutanen E-M, Teppo A-M, Stenman U-H, Tiitinen A, Fyhrquist F, Ylikorkala O (1993). Recurrent fever associated with progesterone action and persistently elevated serum levels of immunoreactive tumor necrosis factor-α and interleukin-6. J Clin Endocrinol Metab 76:1594–1598.

735. Cannon JG, Angel JB, Abad LW, et al. (1997). Interleukin-1 beta, interleukin-1 receptor antagonist, and soluble interleukin-1 receptor type II secretion in chronic fatigue syndrome. J Clin Immunol 17:253–261.

736. Buggs C, Rosenfield RL (2005). Polycystic ovary syndrome in adolescence. Endocrinol Metab Clin North Am 34:677–705.

737. Rosenfield RL (2006). Polycystic ovary syndrome in adolescents. In Rose BD (ed.), *UpToDate.*Wellesley, MA: UpToDate.

738. Azziz R, Carmina E, Dewailly D, et al. (2006). Criteria for defining polycystic ovary syndrome as a predominantly hyperandrogenic syndrome: An androgen excess society guideline. J Clin Endocrinol Metab 91:4237–4245.

739. Taylor AE, McCourt B, Martin KA, et al. (1997). Determinants of abnormal gonadotropin secretion in clinically defined women with polycystic ovary syndrome. J Clin Endocrinol Metab 82:2248–2256.

740. Arroyo A, Laughlin GA, Morales AJ, Yen SSC (1997). Inappropriate gonadotropin secretion in polycystic ovary syndrome: Influence of adiposity. J Clin Endocrinol Metab 82:3728–3733.

741. McKenna T (1988). Pathogenesis and treatment of polycystic ovary syndrome. N Engl J Med 318:558.

742. Rosenfield R (1997). Current concepts of polycystic ovary syndrome. Baillière's Clin Obstet Gynaecol 11:307–333.

743. Meldrum D, Frumar A, Shamonki I, et al. (1980). Ovarian and adrenal steroidogenesis in a virilized patient with gonadotropin-resistant ovaries and hilus cell hyperplasia. Obstet Gynecol 56:216.

744. Carbunaru G, Prasad P, Scoccia B, et al. (2004). The hormonal phenotype of Nonclassic 3 beta-hydroxysteroid dehydrogenase (HSD3B) deficiency in hyperandrogenic females is associated with insulin-resistant polycystic ovary syndrome and is not a variant of inherited HSD3B2 deficiency. J Clin Endocrinol Metab 89:783–794.

745. Suikkari A-M, MacLachlan V, Montalto J, Calderon I, Healy D, McLachlan R (1995). Ultrasonographic appearance of polycystic ovaries is associated with exaggerated ovarian androgen and oestradiol responses to gonadotropin-releasing hormone agonist in women undergoing assisted reproduction treatment. Hum Reprod 10:513–519.

746. Okon MA, Laird SM, Tuckerman EM, Li TC (1998). Serum androgen levels in women who have recurrent miscarriages and their correlation with markers of endometrial function. Fertil Steril 69:682–690.

747. Kaltsas GA, Isidori AM, Kola BP, et al. (2003). The value of the low-dose dexamethasone suppression test in the differential diagnosis of hyperandrogenism in women. J Clin Endocrinol Metab 88:2634–2643.

748. Leibel NI, Baumann EE, Kocherginsky M, Rosenfield RL (2006). Relationship of adolescent polycystic ovary syndrome to parental metabolic syndrome. J Clin Endocrinol Metab 91:1275–1283.

749. Ehrmann DA, Barnes RB, Rosenfield RL, Cavaghan MK, Imperial J (1999). Prevalence of impaired glucose tolerance and diabetes in women with polycystic ovary syndrome. Diabetes Care 22:141–146.

750. Venn A, Bruinsma F, Werther G, et al. (2004). Oestrogen treatment to reduce the adult height of tall girls: Long-term effects on fertility. Lancet 364:1513–1518.

751. Gambineri A, Patton L, Vaccina A, et al. (2006). Treatment with flutamide, metformin, and their combination added to a hypocaloric diet in overweight-obese women with polycystic ovary syndrome: A randomized, 12-month, placebo-controlled study. J Clin Endocrinol Metab 91:3970–3980.

Turner Syndrome

PAUL SAENGER, MD

Introduction

It has been more than 60 years since Henry Turner, an internist, reported the clinical characteristics of the seven patients whose phenotype now bears his name.[1] Six of these women are shown in Figure 15-1. These women had short stature in association with sexual infantilism, webbing of the neck, low posterior hairline, and increased carrying angle of the elbows (cubitus valgus). In 1930, Ullrich described an 8-year-old girl with short stature; lymphedema of the neck, hands, and feet; subsequent neck webbing, cubitus valgus, and other phenotypic abnormalities (including a high arched palate, ptosis, low-set auricles, and small upwardly curved

nails); and several other features that are now associated with Turner syndrome. This gave rise to the less common but more appropriate eponym *Ullrich-Turner syndrome.*

Ullrich later recognized that his patients and those of Turner appeared to have the same condition.[2] He also called attention to the work of Bonnevie, who described a group of congenital anomalies in mice consisting of distention of the neck and malformations of the ears, face, and limb buds—all secondary to dissection of the subcutaneous tissues by fluid. This "bleb" mechanism for producing multiple anomalies was suggested by Ullrich as being responsible for the cervical lymphangiectasia noted in some human female abortuses that appeared to produce a scarred webbed neck (pterygium colli). Ullrich

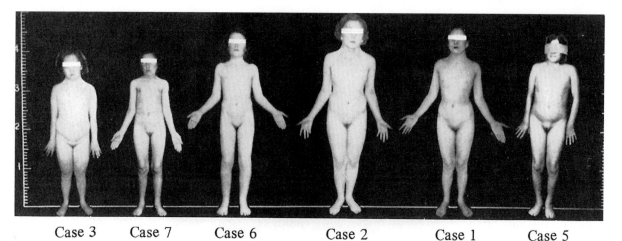

Figure 15-1 Patients exhibiting the syndrome of infantilism, webbed neck, and cubitus valgus. Note the height marker at the left indicating the short stature. [From Turner HH (1938). A syndrome of infantilism, congenital webbed neck and cubitus valgus. Endocrinology 23:566.]

proposed the eponym *status Bonnevie-Ullrich* to describe the set of specific anomalies arising from a single mechanism (lymphangiectasia) and resulting in the phenotype of Turner syndrome.

The links among these phenotypic descriptions, the pathologic evidence of streak ovaries, and the abnormal X chromosomes came with the introduction of the technique for sex chromatin identification by Barr and the demonstration that most patients with Turner syndrome lacked the sex chromatin material.[3] Initially, this absence of sex chromatin (or lack of a Barr body) was associated with "maleness" because a similar pattern was found in normal phenotypic males. Only after it was demonstrated that it was the second X chromosome that in the inactivated state constituted the Barr body was it clear that the 45,X karyotype would result in a chromatin pattern similar to the normal 46,XY karyotype.

It was not until 1961 that techniques became available for the analysis of the chromosomal constitution and the sex chromosome constitution was shown in a 14-year-old phenotypic female with Turner syndrome to be indeed 45,X.[4] Thus, Turner syndrome patients were not XY males but in most cases 45,X females. The original patient of Ullrich was studied in the 1960s and found to have a 45,X karyotype (D. Knorr, personal communication to the author). One of the original seven patients Turner described was also reinvestigated and found to have a 45,X chromosomal karyotype.[4]

The X Chromosome and the Chromosomal Karyotype

A chromosomal karyotype (prepared from peripheral leukocytes, skin fibroblasts, bone marrow elements, or tissue samples) should always be used in making the definitive diagnosis of Turner syndrome. The normal karyotype consists of 22 pairs of homologous autosomes and 1 pair of sex chromosomes. The chromosomes were classified originally into seven groups, A through G, according to the length of the chromosome and the posi-

tion of the centromere. By convention, the short arms were designated by lowercase p (petit), whereas the long arms were assigned the next letter in the alphabet (lowercase q). The X chromosome has the characteristic of a C-group chromosome. It is similar in size and has a metacentric centromere. The Y chromosome, on the other hand, is a small structure—similar in configuration to the G-group chromosomes.[5]

If part of the short arm of one of the X chromosomes were missing, the karyotype would be reported as 46,XXp2. Similarly, if part of the long arm were deleted this would be designated 46,XXq2. Should a ring (r) chromosome be identified, composed of material with X-like staining patterns of both the short and long arms, it would be designated 46,X,r(X). In some cases, the ring X chromosome is tiny. Those patients with a small ring X may be much more severely affected than those with a nonmosaic 45,X karyotype. They may have severe mental retardation, developmental delay, profound growth retardation at birth, and multiple congenital anomalies—including dysmorphism (coarse facial features), epicanthal folds, upturned nares, long philtrum, hypertelorism, strabismus, soft-tissue syndactyly of upper and lower limbs, and increased frequency of heart defects (particularly ventricular septal defects and mitral valve stenosis).[6-8]

Small ring X chromosomes are more detrimental than large ones because they are unable to inactivate, and therefore some genes (those within the ring) are expressed from both the X ring and the normal X chromosome. It has also been shown that the X inactivation specific transcript (XIST) locus on the X chromosome is uniquely transcribed on the inactive X chromosome. It has been proposed that this locus is required for a chromosome to become inactive. Failure of X inactivation has been observed to result from deletion of the XIST gene or deficient transcription of XIST. Ring chromosomes may have a functional disomy for genes present on the ring, leading to the more severe phenotype. The XIST locus is expressed only from the inactive X chromosome residing at the putative X inactivation center. In patients with tiny ring X chromosome XIST, transcription is therefore absent and the inability of these rings to be inactive is responsible for the severe clinical phenotype often associated with severe mental retardation.[9,10]

Another recognized rearrangement is when the entire X chromosome appears to consist of almost two complete long arms with little short-arm material or two short arms with little or no long-arm material. These structurally abnormal chromosomes are called isochromosomes, and the most common one is for the long arm [X,i(Xq)]. Banding and other molecular marker techniques have been used to number all regions of the chromosome, and very specific deletions, translocations, and rearrangements are designated by their numerical region on the short arm or on the long arm.

X CHROMOSOME GENES

Concurrent with the development of techniques for chromosome identification, cytogenetic, clinical, and experimental investigations were carried out to attempt to localize specific genes to the X chromosome and to characterize which regions of the chromosome are responsible for the genotypic and phenotypic abnormalities that occur in women with X chromosome disorders. It is beyond the scope of this discussion to review the historical data localizing the genes for such factors as the Xga blood group antigens and the genes for enzymes such as phosphoglycerate kinase and α-galactosidase to the X chromosome, except to mention that genetic studies of families often use the measurement of these gene products in linkage analysis.

Similarly, although a complete review of X-linked disorders (such as hemophilia A,[11] red-green color blindness, ocular albinism, muscular dystrophy, and ichthyosis) is not feasible here, it is noteworthy that full expression of these disorders has been reported in females with Turner syndrome. Genetic determinants for thyroxine-binding globulin is X linked as well, and thyroxine-binding globulin deficiency has been reported in a 45,X member of an affected kindred.[12]

With the introduction of molecular techniques for the exploration of the human genome, the X chromosome is being mapped at a rapidly expanding pace. The techniques include classic Southern blot analysis of DNA with X- or Y-specific probes, fluorescence in situ hybridization,[13] bivariate flow karyotyping,[14] and polymerase chain reaction amplification. Parenthetically, the fluorescence in situ hybridization technique (with both X and Y probes) can be applied to entire cells and tissues—not unlike a molecular version of the historical buccal smear—and is especially useful in identifying low-frequency cell lines and unknown markers.[15]

Numerous studies have examined the relationship between the chromosomal karyotype and the phenotypic characteristics that appear in Turner syndrome. In a classic article by Ferguson-Smith,[16] the karyotypes of 307 patients with various forms of gonadal dysgenesis were correlated with their clinical findings. He noted that short stature was the only clinical finding invariably associated with the 45,X karyotype. Complete gonadal insufficiency was not always present because seven patients with a 45,X karyotype demonstrated evidence of spontaneous puberty. He also noted that as a whole patients with mosaic karyotypes, including one normal XX line (i.e., 45,X/46,XX), tended to have fewer phenotypic abnormalities.

Save for a very few mosaic patients who were not short, however, on physical examination individual patients with mosaicism could not be readily distinguished from patients with the monosomic karyotype. Finally, he proposed that the area of the X chromosome responsible for the disturbance in growth was localized to the short arm of the X chromosome. Although banding studies were not yet available at the time of this study, the majority of these observations are still valid. A subsequent study of a large group of patients, which included banding,[17] confirmed that short stature is the only characteristic present in virtually 100% of patients.

Phenotypic abnormalities are most easily understood as resulting from altered dosage of certain genes.[18] Genes expected to have an altered dose in Turner individuals are those that escape the process of X inactivation and that have functional homologues on the Y chromosome. Molecular studies to further correlate critical regions with phenotype have tended to confirm the distal pseudoautosomal region (the region that participates in X-Y meiotic pairing and in which recombination takes place) of the short arm as the putative site of at least one stature gene.[19]

Although this idea was proposed in the pathogenesis of Turner syndrome for many years, only in the past several years have strong candidate genes emerged (Figure 15-2). Zinn et al.[20] have argued that there is locus in the interval Xp11.1-p22 encoding for the gene (or genes) pertinent to stature, and have proposed that the transcriuption factor ZFX is the likely candidate gene. To date, there are no genetic data available that would explain the soft tissue and visceral stigmata (such as lymphedema, webbing of the neck, and congenital heart failure) in Turner syndrome… It has been proposed that in primary lymphatic hypoplasia tissues and organs in the vicinity of the affected lymphatic system are secondarily affected.[21,22] In analogy to genes affecting skeletal and statural growth, it is inferred that a lymphogenic gene escaping X inactivation is present on the sex chromosomes. It has been suggested that genes residing in the vicinity of Xp11.3 are relevant to this issue.

USP9X (DFRX) is a second candidate for the Turner syndrome gonadal dysgenesis gene. DFRX (drosophila fat facets related X) is the human homologue of a fruit fly gene involved in oogenesis and eye development. DFRX escapes X inactivation and maps to Xp11.4, a region of proximal Xp implicated in ovarian failure. Two other candidate genes have been described on Xq. RPS4X encodes an isoform of ribosomal protein S4, which lies within a critical region for the lymphedema-related Turner syndrome phenotype and may also relate to poor viability in utero. Evidence against such a role has been reported.[20,21] DIAPH2 is the second gene and is the human homologue of the drosophila diphanous (DIA) gene. DIAPH2 is required for normal ovarian function.[2,22]

The prototypes of genes that would escape X inactivation and show expression from the Y chromosome are

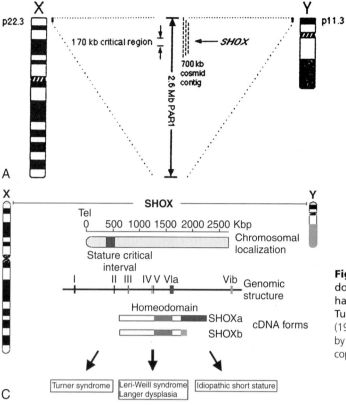

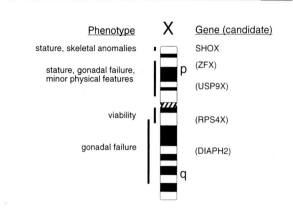

Figure 15-2 (*A*) X and Y chromosomes showing the terminal pseudoautosomal regions (Xp22.3 and Yp11.3) where the SHOX gene has been identified and cloned. (*B*) The X chromosome with the Turner syndrome critical region and (candidate) genes. [From Zinn AR (1997). Growing interest in Turner syndrome. Nat Genet 16:3.] Reprinted by permission from Macmillan Publisher Ltd: Nature Genetics (16(1): 3-4), copyright (1997)

genes in the pseudoautosomal region (PAR) of the X and Y chromosomes located at the distal ends of the short and long arms. In 1997, two groups[18,24] described independently a pseudoautosomal gene—both using a positional cloning strategy. The gene is 500 kb from the telomere of the sex chromosomes (Figure 15-2). It is located in the pseudoautosmal region 1 (PAR 1) on the distal end of the X and Y chromosomes at Xp22.3 and Yp11.3. Because genes in PAR 1 do not undergo X inactivation, healthy individuals express two copies of the SHOX gene: one from each of the sex chromosomes in 46,XX and 46,XY individuals. Because this gene contained a homeobox, it was named SHOX for "short stature homeobox-containing" gene.

There are two isoforms, SHOX A and SHOX B. Both forms were shown to be expressed from the active as well as the inactive X chromosome, with the highest expression levels in bone marrow fibroblasts. The SHOX gene covers a genomic region of approximately 40 kb, consists of seven exons, and encodes two transcripts generated by alternative splicing of its 39 prime exons. It is expressed highly in bone morphogenetic tissues. SHOX mutations have also been described in Leri-Weill dyschondrosteosis, a pseudoautosomal-dominant condition with greater penetrance in females than in males. These patients have shortening and bowing of the radius (with a dorsal subluxation) of the distal ulna, resulting in a dinner-fork-like twist (Madelung deformity) and with distal hypoplasia of the ulna and proximal hypoplasia to aplasia of the fibula (mesial segments). Haploinsufficiency of SHOX is thus the cause of Leri-Weill dyschondrosteosis deformity and probably part of the cause for the short stature seen in Turner syndrome.[25]

The rare homozygous (or compound heterozygous) form of SHOX deficiency is referred to as Langer mesomelic dysplasia. It is characterized by extreme dwarfism, profound mesomelia, and severe limb deformity. The elucidation of the role of SHOX in the growth failure of Leri-Weill dyschondrosteosis and Turner syndrome adds to our understanding of the multifactorial nature of growth.[26] SHOX is so far the only molecularly characterized growth gene on the X chromosome. Further evidence for SHOX as the short stature gene in Turner syndrome comes from XY females with interstitial Yp deletions and from 45,X/46,X,der (X) patients. These patients have Turner stigmata but are of normal size.

The Turner growth gene in the pseudoautosomal region is present in double dosage in these females.[22,27] Could SHOX haploinsufficiency also account for additional somatic features in Turner syndrome? SHOX expression also occurs in the first and second pharyngeal arches, ulna, radius, elbow, wrist, and equivalent bones of the leg. This suggests an involvement of SHOX-related growth impairment in the expression of additional somatic Turner syndrome stigmata such as high arched palate, abnormal auricular development, cubitus valgus, genu valgum, and appearance of the carpal bones (including the characteristic short fourth metacarpals).

The protein is specifically expressed in the growth plate in hypertrophic chondrocytes undergoing apoptosis, and appears likely to play an important role in regulating chondrocyte differentiation and proliferation.[28-31] The state of SHOX haplonsufficency appears to be substantially responsible for the average 20-cm height deficit in untreated women with Turner syndrome. These studies have led to the concept of SHOX haploinsufficiency as a common underlying mechanism in the short stature of Turner syndrome, Leri-Weill dyschondrosteosis, and 2% to 15% of children with idiopathic short stature.[25,30]

Variations in the expression level of the remaining (intact) SHOX gene copy help to explain the variable severity in the manifestations of SHOX mutations. Alternatively, the cause for phenotypic variability might reside in chemical properties of the SHOX encoded transcription factor. An additional area that requires further study is the association of features of Turner syndrome with karyotypes that have no apparent X chromosome abnormality. One group of patients consists of those in whom the phenotype of webbed neck and short stature is associated with normal chromosomes in XX females and XY males. A group of these patients was described by Noonan,[32] who noted the frequent occurrence of pulmonic valvular heart disease. The eponym *Noonan syndrome* is applied to these patients.

This syndrome is often confused with Turner syndrome, and when it occurs in males it has been referred to as the male Turner syndrome phenotype. The chromosomes are normal in 46,XX females and 46,XY males who bear this phenotype, however. No point mutations in the SHOX gene have been described in patients with Noonan syndrome.[33] Their growth failure must have other causes, and a gene PTPN 11 encoding a tyrosine phosphatase SHP-2 as one of the causes of Noonan syndrome has been identified.[34]

Noonan syndrome patients with short stature (approximately 50%) respond poorly to growth hormone and may have some form of growth hormone resistance The gonads of the females do not show the early follicular loss or fibrosis characteristic of X chromosome abnormalities, nor is there a chromosomal abnormality in those males in whom cryptorchidism occurs. Therefore, Noonan syndrome in both males and females should be clearly separated from Turner syndrome. The nomenclature, evaluation, genetic counseling, and endocrine management that are appropriate to the female with Turner syndrome do not apply to patients with Noonan syndrome.

Another area of confusion arises from the demonstration of gonadal dysgenesis or aplasia in 46,XX females without demonstrable chromosomal abnormalities. In this condition, often called "pure gonadal dysgenesis," most of these patients tend to have normal phenotypes and normal stature—and some have similarly affected siblings, which is consistent with an autosomal-recessive pattern of inheritance. Finally, there is a group of phenotypic female patients with gonadal dysgenesis and a 46,XY karyotype. These patients (who should not be confused with those with testicular feminization) also have a genetic disorder affecting testicular induction such that gonads do not form. Thus, the concept of gonadal dysgenesis (elegantly reviewed by Opitz and Pallister[35]) includes a large number of disorders. For the purpose of this chapter, Turner syndrome will be used to describe the patient with an abnormality of the chromosomal karyotype involving loss of part or all of the X chromosome associated with phenotypic abnormalities that include short stature and the potential for or the presence of ovarian failure.

GENOMIC IMPRINTING

The selective silencing of certain alleles depending on the parent of origin is known as genomic imprinting. The putatively imprinted traits in Turner syndrome reflect typical differences between eukaryotic males and females. So far there are three areas in which X-imprinting effects have been found: cognitive function, statural growth, and possible visceral adiposity and lipid metabolism. They are at present rather preliminary and require independent confirmation as well as further work to define the genetic and epigenetic mechanisms.[36]

MULTIPLE X CHROMOSOMES

When there is an excessive rather than deficient number of X chromosomes, ovarian function may also be impaired. The incidence of the 47,XXX (triplo-X) karyotype in newborn phenotypic female infants is approximately 1:1,000.[37] The majority of these patients do not have obvious phenotypic or developmental abnormalities and would be unrecognized except for the research-based chromosome screening programs that identified them. When prospective studies are performed on women with the 47,XXX karyotype, however, infertility and gonadal failure are noted more frequently than in the normal population.[38]

Gonadotropins are increased in the plasma, indicating that the hypogonadism is caused by primary gonadal failure. Histologic data are scanty, but the mechanism of ovarian failure is presumed to be accelerated follicular atresia. Therefore, the manner in which this diagnosis is established is somewhat similar to that of the phenotypically normal patient with Turner syndrome. Primary gonadal failure per se, whether short stature is present or not, necessitates a complete chromosomal karyotype. Should the triplo-X karyotype be identified in a girl before pubertal development, however, assurance may be given that the majority of the patients are fertile. They appear to have a spectrum of neurodevelopmental disorders characterized by gross and fine motor dysfunction,[39] speech and language deficiencies, and a high incidence of psychiatric disturbances.[40] There is also a low incidence of chromosomal aneuploidy among their offspring.[41] Although amniocentesis might be performed during pregnancy, the value of this procedure in prenatal counseling is debatable.

The 48,XXXX karyotype is exceedingly rare,[42] with fewer than 50 cases reported. These patients are also phenotypic females, but they tend to have more phenotypic abnormalities—including skeletal dysplasias, intellectual impairment, and speech dysfunctions.[43] The skeletal abnormalities, including those of carrying-angle varus disturbances and radioulnar synostosis, are similar to those in Klinefelter syndrome. Thus, in contrast to the increased carrying angle of the 45,X patient or the normal angle of the 46,XX patient the angle of the 48,XXXX patient may be decreased to an extent indistinguishable from that of the 47,XXY or 48,XXXY male.

In these so-called tetra-X women fertility appears to be decreased to an extent even greater than in triplo-X patients. Again, primary gonadal failure is responsible.

Plasma gonadotropin concentrations in adolescence are helpful in predicting whether ovarian function and fertility will be normal. We reported one such patient in whom ovarian development was virtually absent. This case represents one extreme within the spectrum of the abnormality.[42] The penta-X karyotype 49,XXXXX has also been reported.[44,45] It is extremely rare, and the principal phenotypic features are those associated with microcephaly, postnatal growth failure, cardiac defects, and skeletal dysplasia (including radioulnar synostosis). The frequency with which gonadal function is impaired, however, is less well documented because the oldest patient was only 16 years old when reported.

This patient was still not fully pubertal, and this suggests that she had ovarian dysfunction. Thus, the evidence confirms that ovarian function may be adversely affected by the presence of multiple X chromosomes. The mechanism is unknown because the precise effect of aneuploidy, be it autosomal or X chromosomal, is unclear. The presence of an additional X chromosome or multiple X chromosomes, however, appears to accelerate the rate of follicular atresia in most patients. In some patients, such as our patient with apparent ovarian agenesis, normal induction of the ovaries may be impaired in the fetus. A possible mechanism for the ovarian failure could be impaired migration of the abnormally constituted germ cells. In no cases without demonstrable or presumptive Y chromosomal material has ovarian neoplasia been documented, and surgical intervention is therefore not indicated.

Turner Syndrome

INCIDENCE AND ETIOLOGY

The incidence of abnormalities in the sex chromosomal karyotype resulting in the loss of all or part of an X chromosome has been variously reported as 1:2,000 to 1:5,000 in live-born phenotypic females.[46,47] Population screenings by Barr body assessment were likely to have underestimated the incidence because mosaic or structural X abnormalities may have been missed. Studies with lymphocyte chromosomal analysis would have detected some mosaic karyotypes such as 45,X/46,XX [as well as some nonmosaic karyotypes such as 46,X,r(X)], but may have missed deletions and rearrangements. Finally, studies with banding techniques applied to the lymphocyte karyotype analysis would tend to detect minor changes in the architecture of the X chromosome (such as partial deletions or an X isochromosome) and should yield a higher incidence.

A standard 30-cell karyotype is recommended by the American College of Medical Genetics. This karyotype identifies at least 10% of mosaicism with 95% confidence, although additional metaphases may be counted or fluorescent in situ hybridization (FISH) studies performed if there is suspicion of undetected mosaicism. In rare instances, additional tissues (such as skin) need to be examined if there is strong clinical suspicion of Turner syndrome.[48]

Although clinical series using these techniques report a distribution of karyotypes with 45,X approximating 50%,[49,50] prospective newborn series might differ. In one prospective study of 34,910 newborn children (17,038 girls) born in Arhus, Denmark,[30] cytogenetic analysis detected nine karyotypes consistent with Turner syndrome for an incidence of 1:1,893 live female births. Of note is that only one of the nine had a 45,X karyotype. The other eight were mosaic and included a wide range of abnormalities. A compilation of studies of newborns from centers throughout the world suggests not only that the prevalence might differ in different populations but that within the same center the distribution of karyotypes is shifting toward much higher rates of mosaicism.[51] Whether this represents increased technical sophistication in detection or some biologic variable remains to be determined.

Our data for a group of 205 patients are shown in Table 15-1. The 45,X karyotype was found in 54.6%, which is consistent with the distribution reported in retrospective clinical series. This percentage, coupled with the prospective incidence data from Aarhus (including the low percentage of 45,X in that series), supports the calculation that the incidence of Turner syndrome in liveborn females is at least 1:2,000. All series, including our own, include a small percentage of patients with cytogenetic evidence of a cell line containing a Y chromosome. For the most part, when those patients are examined they show no evidence of virilization. The same is true for the patients in whom a small marker chromosome, which could be derived from the Y chromosome, is present. The use of molecular techniques has improved the ability to detect Y-specific sequences. Thus, the DNA from Turner syndrome patients can be examined to determine whether the marker chromosome is of Y origin and to detect putative Y sequences in patients with no cytogenetically detectable Y material.

The significance of the detection of occult Y chromosomal material is twofold: the association with the risk of gonadoblastoma (see later section on gonadoblastoma for a clinical discussion) and the issue of mosaicism as it relates to fetal survival. With regard to the risk of gonadoblastoma, in one study polymerase chain reaction was used to amplify the gene for the sex-determining region of the Y chromosome (SRY) in a group of 40 patients with Turner syndrome.[52]

Although the authors detected a very low frequency (1:40) of unrecognized Y material (in an adolescent who had clinical evidence of androgen excess), they suggested that this test may be useful in screening all patients regardless of phenotype. Others,[53,54] who reported an even higher frequency of apparent SRY positivity with variable centromeric data, have made the same recommendation.

There is no evidence that the SRY gene confers a risk for gonadoblastoma. In fact, there is evidence to the contrary. Deletion analysis of genomic material from numerous patients with gonadoblastoma suggests that the putative gonadoblastoma gene (GBY) is located near the centromere, not on distal Yp.[55] A putative candidate gene, TSPY, has been identified by one group.[56] In addition, in a report of a girl with Turner syndrome, a gonadoblastoma,[57] and a small Y fragment that contained

TABLE 15-1

Summary of the Cytogenetic Findings in 207 Patients with Turner Syndrome

No.	%	Karyotype	
112	54.6	45,X	
34	16.6	46,X,i(Xq)	22: 45,X/46,X,i(Xq)
			11: 46,X,i(Xq)
			1: 45,X/46,X,i(Xq)/
			46,XXp2
26	12.6	45,X/46,XX	24: 45,X/46,XX
			1: 45,X/46,XX1mar*
			1: 45,X/45,X1mar†
11	5.3	46,X,r(X)	All: 45,X/46,X,r(X)
10	4.9	45,X/46,XY‡	
5	2.4	46,XXq2	2: 45,X/46,XXq2
			3: 46,XXq2
4	1.9	46,XXp2	2: 46,XXp2
			1: 45,X/46,XXp2
			1: 45,X/46,XXp2/
			46,X1mar
4	1.4	45,X/47,XXX	
1	0.5	46,X,t(X;15)	(q22.1;q24)

* DNA was examined with Y chromosome–specific probes and found to contain Y sequences. Gonadal streaks were removed, and an in situ gonadoblastoma was found.

† Leukocytes examined by fluorescent in situ hybridization with X- and Y-specific pericentromeric probes showed presence of one cell line positive only for X probe and one cell line positive for both probes. Gonadal streaks were removed and were tumor free.

‡ Eight patients had removal of gonadal streaks. One macroscopic calcified gonadoblastoma and three in situ gonadoblastomas were found. Two patients who did not have surgery were lost to follow-up.

pericentromeric material SRY analysis was negative. This supports the assertion of Page[58] that in the absence of the centromere the presence or absence of SRY probably has little bearing on the risk of gonadoblastoma.

Conversely, if there is a clinical reason to test for occult Y material to assess gonadoblastoma risk, fluorescence in situ hybridization technology with Y-specific centromeric probes may be the applicable method.[59] Finally, in one population study of 114 Turner women there were no gonadoblastomas identified among 7 women with occult Y chromosomal material identified only by polymerase chain reaction, and only one gonadoblastoma identified among the 7 women with a karyotypic Y chromosome.[60] Thus, in the absence of a demonstrable marker chromosome or clinical evidence of virilization screening of all patients with Turner syndrome for Y sequences is not recommended by the authors at this time.[61]

Testing for Y chromosome material should, however, be performed in any Turner syndrome patient with a marker[61] chromosome. It should be stressed that the prevalence and clinical significance of cryptic Y material detected only by FISH or DNA analysis in patients without virilization or a marker chromosome need additional investigation. False positives may be a problem with highly sensitive PCR-based Y detection methods.[62] According to recent analysis of pooled data, true presence of Y chromosome material is associated with an approximately 12% risk of gonadoblastoma.[63] The current

recommendation is for laparascopic prophylactic gonadectomy. It is often assumed that gonads in Turner patients with Y chromosome mosaicism have no reproductive potential, but spontaneous pregnancies in such women have been reported. Thus, preservation of follicles or oocytes may be a future option for some patients undergoing gonadectomy.[64,65]

The presence of occult chromosomal mosaicism, whether a second cell line contains a second X or Y chromosome, may relate to fetal survival. It is known that the number of affected live births reflects only a small proportion of total conceptuses with X chromosome abnormalities. It is estimated that 99.9% of 45,X conceptuses do not survive beyond 28 weeks' gestation and that the 45,X karyotype occurs in 1 of 15 spontaneous abortions.

It is believed that mosaicism accounts for some of the survival of apparent 45,X fetuses owing to a fetoprotective effect of more than one dose of some loci on the long arm of the X. One piece of evidence to support this hypothesis is that live-born infants with the X,i(Xq) karyotype constitute an unusually large percentage of Turner syndrome individuals compared to the proportion of this karyotype found in early abortuses.[46,47] In a cytogenetic and molecular study of 91 patients, low-level mosaicism—attributable to a second cell line (containing small marker chromosomes or small ring chromosomes)—was detected in cell culture of fibroblasts and lymphocytes from a high proportion of individuals originally diagnosed as having 45,X.[66] Finally, the expanded use of prenatal chromosomal analysis obtained by chorionic villus sampling or amniocentesis may document mosaicism that is not present at birth. Chorionic villus sampling demonstrates 45,X monosomy at a frequency of 1% compared to 0.08% at amniocentesis.

Although part of the discrepancy can be explained by failure of some 45,X pregnancies to survive or a tendency of monosomic cell lines to die out,[67] a proportion may be caused by anaphase lag during development of the cytotrophoblast but not the mesenchymal core of the villus.[68] Some discrepancies have also been reported between mosaicism detected on amniocentesis and results of postnatal karyotype analysis.[69] The significance of mosaicism and the differences between prenatal and postnatal karyotype go beyond issues of mechanism to create a significant genetic counseling dilemma. Termination of pregnancy for false positive 45,X results on chorionic villus sampling has been pointed out as a danger of this method.[70] In addition, all infants who have been diagnosed prenatally with Turner syndrome merit a repeat karyotype on delivery because maternal cell contamination, placental mosaicism, and other factors could result in differences between the prenatal and postnatal karyotype.

The 45,X/46,XY karyotype present in multiple cultures of amniotic fluid cells presents a different problem because this may be associated with a spectrum of phenotypes from normal female to normal male to genital abnormalities, including the phenotype of mixed gonadal dysgenesis. In a large collaborative international survey of more than 730 cytogenetic laboratories, 92 cases of the 45,X/46,XY mosaicism were identified.[71] Seventy-six patients had physical examinations either at birth or at termination of pregnancy. Ninety-five percent had normal male genitalia, and only 5% had genital ambiguity or female genitalia with features of Turner syndrome. There was no association between phenotype and the degree of mosaicism. Ultimate gonadal function, stature, and tumor risk remain to be studied. Similar data were reported by Hsu. In her series of some 80 prenatally diagnosed patients, 74 (92%) had normal male external genitalia.[72] The role of prenatal ultrasonography as an adjunct in counseling was not evaluated in the series but is advocated by Hsu. These data contrast with a large series of postnatally reported patients with this mosaicism.[73]

In this series, there was a wide spectrum of abnormal phenotypes that could not be correlated with the degree of mosaicism found in blood. Therefore, with prenatally diagnosed 45,X/46,XY mosaicism the majority of patients will have normally appearing male genitalia at birth. Only determination by physical examination, starting in utero and completed postnatally (not by karyotype), can distinguish patients in whom male gonadal function is sufficient for complete masculinization of external genital development from those with genital ambiguity or normal female genitalia and a Turner phenotype.

The high incidence of X chromosome monosomy raises multiple questions about etiology. In abortuses, there is an inverse correlation with maternal age for the 45,X karyotype but not for mosaic or structural X abnormalities.[74] There is no correlation with maternal age for viable 45,X infants, however. Thus, young women do not have an increased risk for having a term infant with Turner syndrome—only for having the abnormality in a fetus spontaneously aborted. There are no data to support a positive or negative correlation between the 45,X karyotype in aborted or term pregnancies and paternal age. There is a suggestion that the mechanism responsible for the 45,X conceptus may be different from that responsible for structural X chromosome rearrangements. There is evidence, for example, that the X,i(Xq) karyotype is associated with advanced paternal age.[75]

If the mechanisms responsible for the loss of the X chromosome are not directly age dependent, the question arises whether there is a relationship between which chromosomes are lost and which are retained. Early studies of the parental origin of the retained X chromosome were performed with Xg blood group linkage but were often uninformative. The introduction of molecular techniques has made it possible to assign parental origin of the single X in almost all affected individuals. With this technique, Mathur et al. and others[76-79] have determined that there is no significant parental age effect between the groups retaining the maternal X or the paternal X. In addition, the ratio of maternal X to paternal X is just over 2-3:1, which is consistent with the expected proportion of meiotic or mitotic products—with equal loss at each step, given the nonviability of 45,Y.

Finally, Tsezou et al. and others[80,81] were unable to find significant differences in physical phenotype between the two groups—providing no evidence for a parental X-imprinting effect. This lack of X imprinting on physical phenotype is also suggested by the finding that there are no significant clinical differences in patients with Klinefelter syndrome between those with two maternal X chromosomes and those with one,[82] and by the report of mild stigmata of Turner syndrome without any other significant phenotypic disturbances in a patient with 45,X/46,XX mosaicism in whom all X chromosomes are of paternal origin.[83] Conversely, there are data to suggest that X-linked imprinted loci may have a subtle effect on neuropsychological function.

Skuse and co-workers[84] found evidence of an X-linked imprinted locus by comparing females with Turner syndrome who had retained the maternal X (Xm) to those who had retained the paternal X (Xp). In 80 45,X females these authors found 25 to be 45,Xp and 55 to be 45,Xm. Females with a single paternal X chromosome possessed superior social-communicative skills and high-order executive function skills compared with those whose single X was maternal in origin. Neuropsychological and molecular investigation of eight females with partial deletion of the short arm of the X chromosome indicated that the putative imprinted locus escapes X inactivation and probably lies on Xq or close to the centromere on Xp. These preliminary findings, which await confirmation, provide evidence for the evolution of an imprinted X-linked locus that underlies the development of sexual dimorphism in social behavior.

The association of a seasonal incidence with a birth abnormality such as Turner syndrome would implicate an environmental cause or an environmental effect on preservation of prenatal viability. When such associations are sought in Turner syndrome, the results are somewhat conflicting. However, when all of the series are reviewed significant peaks do not appear to emerge.

Other etiologic factors examined previously include birth order and sibling sex (for which there were no apparent associations) and twinning. In the latter, there appears to be a slightly higher occurrence rate for the 45,X[85] and X,i(Xq) karyotypes, although not at a level of statistical significance. At least three cases of Turner syndrome resulting from artificial insemination have been reported.[86] In two, studies of blood group antigens suggest that the lost chromosome was of paternal origin. In our series, one patient was the offspring from pregnancy by artificial insemination.

The issue of the relationship between autoimmune disorders and chromosomal defects is unresolved. It has been well documented that autoimmune phenomena occur with increased frequency, not only in Turner syndrome but in trisomy 21 and Klinefelter syndrome.[87] It has also been suggested that autoimmune disorders occur with increased frequency in first-degree relatives of affected individuals. Preliminary studies of the human leukocyte antigens (HLAs) of Turner syndrome patients and their families failed to show any preponderance of those specific types most commonly associated with autoimmune disorders (HLA B8 and Bw15).[88]

The role of environmental factors (such as maternal or paternal drug abuse or ethanol consumption, therapeutic medications, cigarette smoking, and so on) in the pathogenesis of Turner syndrome has not been systematically investigated or reported. The lack of evidence for any etiologic mechanisms responsible for the occurrence of Turner syndrome applies equally to the occurrence of the Turner-Down polysomy, or double aneuploidy syndrome.

In this condition, trisomy 21 is associated with a 45,X karyotype or mosaic cell lines for the X chromosome. Although this is a rare occurrence, its frequency is estimated to be greater than that caused by chance alone.[89] Similarly, the double aneuploidy for Down syndrome and Klinefelter syndrome occurs with a frequency greater than that expected from chance alone.

There does not appear to be an increased risk for the recurrence of the 45,X karyotype in families. X chromosome structural abnormalities may have an increased risk of recurrence because some deletions, for example, may be transmitted by the carrier of a balanced translocation[90] and others may be transmitted on the X by a mother with the Turner phenotype but preserved fertility.[91] There also are reports in the literature of trisomy 21 and Turner syndrome occurring in the same sibship.[92] We have two such sibships in our series. Taken in conjunction with the evidence that there appears to be an increased risk of a second defect occurring in most other chromosomal disorders, one would have to counsel parents accordingly. In the absence of significantly increased parental age, assignment of a risk figure of 1% may be reasonable.

PRENATAL DIAGNOSIS

The use of multiple modalities for prenatal diagnosis and pregnancy monitoring (including chorionic villus sampling, amniocentesis, maternal serum screening, and fetal ultrasound) has increased the number of conditions diagnosed prenatally, including that of Turner syndrome. Although the pitfalls of trying to correlate phenotype with prenatal genotype have been discussed in the previous section, the methodologies that increase the ascertainment of a Turner pregnancy and the issues of outcome based on the diagnosis merit discussion.

The measurement of concentrations of human chorionic gonadotropin (hCG), a-fetoprotein (AFP), and unconjugated estriol (uE3) in maternal serum in conjunction with maternal age has been used as a prenatal screen for Down syndrome and trisomy 18. The basis for the utility of this screen is that in fetal trisomy 21 the average hCG is higher than normal and the AFP and uE3 are lower than normal in the presence of fetal trisomy 21. As the screening programs progressed, it was noted that fetuses affected with Turner syndrome were detected among the pregnancies identified at risk for Down syndrome or trisomy 18. In these pregnancies, the abnormality in the screen was most consistently that of high hCG—especially in those with hydropic pregnancies, with more variable findings of normal or low AFP and uE3.[93]

Subsequent studies of the association of fetal hydrops and increased hCG have concluded that the morphologic defect of hydrops rather than the chromosomal aneuploidy per se may be the reason for the positive detection of the Turner fetus by maternal screening. In addition, second-trimester maternal serum progesterone levels and inhibin A are also elevated in the presence of Turner syndrome with hydrops—further supporting the concept that placental hypersecretion may be a consequence of hydrops rather than aneuploidy.[94]

Because cystic hygroma, increased nuchal translucency, and overt hydrops can also be detected by ultrasound—and ultrasound has detected these abnormalities in some pregnancies identified as at risk for Down syndrome and Turner syndrome by maternal fetal screening—the utility of fetal nuchal translucency as a primary screen for chromosomal abnormalities was evaluated.[95] In an unselected population of pregnant adolescents and women, Taipale and co-workers found a 0.8% incidence of nuchal translucency or cystic hygroma. Of the detected fetuses, 24% had an abnormal karyotype and 28% of these had Turner syndrome.

All of the fetuses with Turner syndrome had nuchal translucency consistent with hygromas. When fetuses with cystic hygroma are classified by gestational age, autosomal trisomies with cystic hygromas are more often seen in the first trimester and those with Turner syndrome in the second trimester and the fetuses that already demonstrate hygroma in the first trimester are more likely to spontaneously abort.[96] A characteristic ultrasound of a 14-week-old Turner fetus with a cystic hygroma is shown in Figure 15-3a and b, compared with a normal fetus in Figure 15-3c. Ultrasound and maternal serum screening are not diagnostic, and to make a prenatal diagnosis of Turner syndrome karyotype confirmation is necessary. Chromosomes should be reevaluated postnatally in all cases. The degree of mosaicism detected prenatally is not generally predictive of the severity of the Turner syndrome phenotype.[97]

The issue of fetal outcome is affected not only by karyotype and phenotype (hydrops and cardiac abnormalities, in which more 45,X fetuses and those with abnormal phenotypes will spontaneously abort than those with mosaic karyotype) but by decision for elective termination. Buckway and colleagues have reviewed a summary of a series of 24 published studies that reported that only 25% of prenatally diagnosed Turner syndrome pregnancies were continued after counseling, whereas in specific instances in a center with a long-standing developmental focus more than 50% of 45,X pregnancies and more than 80% of mosaic pregnancies were continued.[98] They also note that even the hydropic 45,X fetus does not spontaneously abort 100% of the time. Therefore, karyotype and phenotype are not necessarily always a predictor of a poor outcome—and knowledge of the heterogeneity of the phenotype is essential to informed counseling.

INDICATIONS FOR KARYOTYPE

The diagnosis of Turner syndrome should be considered in any female with unexplained growth failure or pubertal delay or any constellation of the following clinical findings: edema of the hands and feet, nuchal folds, left-sided cardiac anomalies, low hairline, low-set ears, small mandible, short stature, markedly elevated FSH levels, cubitus valgus, nail hypoplasia, hyperconvex uplifted nails, multiple nevi, characteristic facies, short fourth metacarpal, high-arched palate, and chronic otitis media.[61] Newborn screening underdiagnosis and delayed diagnosis remain a problem.[99] PCR-based screening methods to detect sex chromosome aneuploidy are feasible but have not been validated on a newborn population sample.

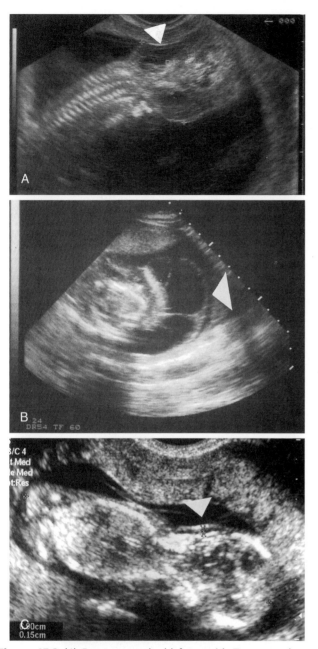

Figure 15-3 (A) Fourteen-week-old fetus with Turner syndrome and a cystic hygroma (arrow). (B) A 13-week-old fetus with a normal karyotype and normal nuchal translucency of 1.5 mm (arrow). (C) Same fetus as in view A in transverse plane. Large septated cystic hygroma (arrow) can be seen around the fetal neck. [Courtesy of Pekka Taipale, MD, PhD, Kuppio University Hospital, Finland.]

Again, positive findings will require karyotype confirmation. Screening using FSH levels at 1 to 2 years of age may also be useful.[100] Although upholding personal choice about reproduction is a widely embraced ethical principle, decisions to terminate a fetus with Turner syndrome should never be based on misunderstood or unbalanced information.[101-103] Outcomes of incidentally detected 45,X/46, XX mosaicism detected by screening on the basis of advanced maternal age, which incidentally is not associated with an increased incidence of Turner syndrome, often tend to be less affected than those diagnosed postnatally on clinical grounds.[97,104,105]

Clinical Findings

Since the original description of Turner, it has been recognized that there are a multiplicity of findings in patients with Turner syndrome—occurring with varying frequencies. More significantly, it has been recognized that the multiple findings may reflect a smaller number of fundamental events. In Table 15-2 and in the following discussion, the common features illustrated by the patients in our series are described—and when possible categorized according to the developmental defects proposed to be fundamentally responsible. What cannot be illustrated are the multiple combinations of findings that occur in any one patient. Thus, it is difficult to appreciate from Table 15-2 that in fact one patient may have only one of the many features described (whereas others may have multiple features).

Physical Features

SKELETAL GROWTH DISTURBANCES

The most common physical abnormality associated with Turner syndrome is short stature. The impairment is most pronounced along the longitudinal body axis (the entire problem of the growth disturbance in Turner syndrome is discussed in a subsequent section).[106] This gives affected individuals the visual appearance of being stocky or squarely shaped and accounts for the predominantly illusory finding of widely spaced nipples[107] and a shieldlike chest. In fact, when chest width and internipple distances are measured and ratios are calculated, the majority of patients do not differ from normal subjects of the same age. What differs is their overall height and the relative width to height of the thorax. Thus, the impaired longitudinal osseous growth is the primary defect.

Conversely, the short neck is not illusory but secondary in many cases to hypoplasia of one or more of the cervical vertebrae.[108] The osseous abnormalities responsible for the short stature are not limited to the cervical vertebrae. Our own data, and those of others, confirm that long bone growth may be impaired even to a greater degree than vertebral growth. Thus, there is disproportion in the axial segmental measurements resulting in short-leggedness and an abnormal upper-to-lower segment ratio.[109] The limbs themselves do not have the radiologic or histologic appearance of a true skeletal dysplasia, however. The low hairline, on the other hand, is secondary to the short neck and to the intrauterine mechanism responsible for the neck webbing (see "Lymphatic Obstruction").

Individual bones appear to be affected to varying degrees. For example, cubitus valgus is commonly appreciated. What this reflects is an increase in the carrying angle. Clinically, this can be measured as the angle of intersection of the long axis of the upper arm with the long axis of the supinated forearm when the elbow is fully extended. In radiographs, it is measured as the acute angle formed between the humerus and the ulna. Normally, in adult women this angle is approximately

TABLE 15-2

Clinical Findings Commonly Described in Patients with Turner Syndrome

Primary Defects	Secondary Features	Incidence (%)
Physical Features		
Skeletal growth disturbances	Short stature	100
	Short neck	40
	Abnormal upper-to-lower segment ratio	97
	Cubitus valgus	47
	Short metacarpals	37
	Madelung deformity	7.5
	Scoliosis	12.5
	Genu valgum	35
	Characteristic facies with micrognathia	60
Lymphatic obstruction	Webbed neck	25
	Low posterior hairline	42
	Rotated ears	Common
	Edema of hands/feet	22
	Severe nail dysplasia	13
	Characteristic ermatoglyphics	35
Unknown factors	Strabismus	17.5
	Ptosis	11
	Multiple pigmented nevi	26
Physiologic Features		
Skeletal growth disturbances	Growth failure	100
	Otitis media	73
Germ cell chromosomal defects	Gonadal failure	90
	Infertility	95
Unknown factors—embryogenic	Cardiovascular anomalies	55
	Hypertension	7
Unknown factors	Strabismus	17.5
	Renal and renovascular anomalies	39
Unknown factors—metabolic	Hashimoto thyroiditis	34
	Hyperthyroidism	10
	Alopecia	2
	Vitiligo	2
	Gastrointestinal disorders	2.5
	Carbohydrate intolerance	40

12 degrees—whereas in adult men it is approximately 6 degrees.[110] The major determinant of the angle is the depth of the inner lip of the trochlea of the ulna relative to the outer lip.

When this relationship is disturbed, abnormalities occur. In many patients with Turner syndrome the angle will be between 15 and 30 degrees (Figure 15-4) as a consequence of developmental abnormalities of the trochlear head. Thus, it is a skeletal abnormality responsible for a physical finding. That the development of the head of the ulna appears to be regulated by the sex chromosomes (and not, as has been previously inferred, primarily by sex hormones during puberty) is suggested by the abnormalities in Turner syndrome as well as by those in other disorders. The carrying angle is most pronounced with the 45,X karyotype, and the angle decreases progressively in association with XX and XY karyotypes. The angle further decreases, approaching cubitus rectus, in patients with an extra X or Y—and frank radioulnar synostosis and radial head

dislocation occur in many patients with multiple extra sex chromosomes.[111]

The knuckle sign, a depression caused by diminished prominence of the head of the fourth metacarpal so that a straight edge can be placed between the third and fifth metacarpals, is another physical finding that occurs in a large number of patients. It, as well as the so-called knuckle-knuckle-dimple-dimple sign (reflecting a depression of both the fourth and fifth knuckles), is a consequence of abnormally small metacarpals. These signs may be seen on a bone age radiograph and are often clues to the possible diagnosis (Figure 15-5A). Short toes, owing to shortening of the metatarsals, may also be found.

Other deformities of the hand and wrist occur commonly. The carpal bones of the first line are frequently arched together abnormally. Superimposed on this is a further deformity (originally described by Madelung in 1898) occurring in 7.5% of our patients. This so-called bayonet deformity is caused by lateral and dorsal bowing

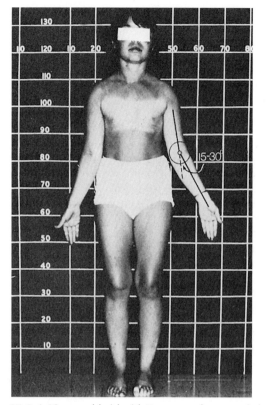

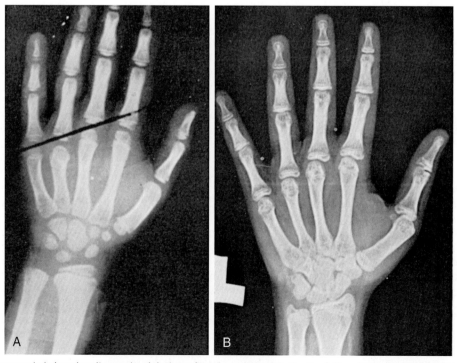

of the radius, coupled with the carpal crowding and dorsal dislocation or subluxation of the distal ulna (Figure 15-6).[112] It also occurs as part of the autosomal-dominant mesomelic chondrodystrophy, dyschondrosteosis, or Leri-Weill syndrome. We have discussed, in the section on the X chromosome, the SHOX gene on the short arm pseudoautosomal region (PAR 1) of the sex chromosomes.

Through other workers identifying the same gene simultaneously, the term *PHOG* (pseudoautosomal homeobox-containing osteogenic gene) was also introduced. Haploinsufficiency of SHOX has been shown to cause Leri-Weill dyschondrosteosis, as well as other limb skeletal anomalies—such as short fourth metacarpals and cubitus valgus. SHOX deletions or insertions accounted for all Leri-Weill syndrome cases in a recent review.[113] Thus, SHOX haploinsufficiency is common to Turner syndrome and Leri-Weill syndrome and accounts for the difficulty in the differential diagnosis. Although gonadal dysgenesis is not a feature of Leri-Weill syndrome, chromosomal analysis may be necessary to distinguish the two—especially in the prepubertal girl without an obviously affected parent. Conversely, gonadal estrogens may play a role in the development of skeletal lesions (in particular, the Madelung deformity) in both conditions.[114]

The mechanism may be that estrogens exert a maturational effect on skeletal tissues that are susceptible to premature fusion of growth plates because of haploinsufficiency of SHOX, thereby accelerating the development of skeletal lesions such as short fourth metacarpals and Madelung deformity. Both skeletal lesions are associated with premature fusion of epiphyses and may thus become evident in the peripubertal period. This may account for the more pronounced lesions in the girl with

Figure 15-4 A 16-year-old girl with Turner syndrome and absence of puberty. Note absence of most characteristic stigmata save short stature and an increased carrying angle.

Figure 15-5 Two characteristic hand radiographs. (*A*) Short fourth metacarpal, the tip falling below a straight line drawn between the third and fifth metacarpals. (*B*) Generalized lacy ("fish net") appearance of the carpals and tufting of the distal phalanges, characteristic of the osteoporotic appearance of the bones of patients with Turner syndrome.

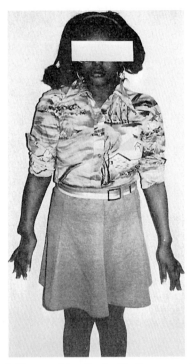

Figure 15-6 A 19-year-old-patient with Turner syndrome and bilateral bayonet-like Madelung deformities of the wrists.

Leri-Weill dyschondrosteosis compared to the girl with Turner syndrome and for the failure of late estrogen therapy in the girl with Turner syndrome to induce Madelung deformity.

Scoliosis is reported in a significant number of patients. In our own series, 12.5% had a deformity. The cause was demonstrated radiologically to be secondary to obvious hemivertebrae in three patients and secondary to documented leg-length inequality, with a functional scoliosis occurring secondarily in two patients. In the remaining patients, no obvious bony deformities were noted—and the scoliosis was classified as idiopathic. That severity sufficient to warrant surgical correction has not been reported may be related to the lack of a pubertal growth spurt. As we begin to use more aggressive programs of hormonal treatment for growth acceleration, we may find an increase in clinically significant scoliosis—and appropriate measures should be taken to ensure its early detection.

The knock-kneed appearance of many patients described in the literature is caused by abnormalities in the medial tibial and femoral condyles. The medial tibial condyles are enlarged and project medially, the medial femoral condyles are enlarged and project downward below the levels of the lateral condyles, and the epiphyseal plates are deformed and displaced.[115]

The development of the face is also affected by a number of osseous malformations, contributing in part to the characteristic facies. The high incidences of micrognathia, antimongoloid palpebral fissures, downward droop of the outer corners of the eyes, and epicanthal folds are also consequences of defective facial morphogenesis. The palate is frequently abnormally arched, and when examined using maxillary casts exhibits deformi-

ties that differ from the more typical gothic or inverted V shape of other syndromes. Instead, an inverted U shape form and a form with a narrow vault and bulges of the lateral alveolar ridges have been described.[116]

Not manifest clinically but present radiologically is the osteoporotic appearance of the bones. Examination of the hand and wrist for bone age, a procedure frequently performed even before the diagnosis of Turner syndrome is established, often reveals this osteoporotic appearance. In some patients, the carpal bones may be so characteristically affected that the appearance (which we describe as fish net) has been reported as a clue to the diagnosis.[117] Others find that ballooning of the tips of the terminal phalanges is a most consistent finding.[118] Both findings are illustrated in Figure 15-5B.

That this osteoporotic appearance is observed in childhood suggests it may be more related to the developmental localization of SHOX than to primary estrogen deficiency. Both a primary skeletal disorder and estrogen deficiency could compromise bone mass, however. Bone mineral content and bone mineral density are reduced for age in children and adults with Turner syndrome, but these deficits are reduced or diminished when adjustments are made for small bone size and delayed bone maturation.[119-121] When looked at in a longitudinal fashion and when compared with control data related to body weight and pubertal status, no advantage was found with early estrogen replacement or growth hormone (GH) therapy in optimizing bone mineralization.[119,120]

Shaw and associates demonstrated normal bone density in children and adolescents with Turner syndrome using dual-energy x-ray absorptiometry.[122] In older adolescents and adults, a normal femoral neck bone mass is not achieved. This may be because of the low-dose estrogen therapy used by some (20 to 30 mg of ethinyl estradiol), which may simply not be enough. Thus, the risk of osteoporosis and fracture appear to be increased—particularly after age 45.[123-124] After adolescence, estrogen therapy seems to be the single most important factor in maintaining peak bone mass. In summary, the cause of the apparent early and true late osteopenia in Turner syndrome remains controversial. However, it is most likely the result of an intrinsic bone matrix defect combined with estrogen deficiency or inadequate estrogen replacement.[125]

LYMPHATIC OBSTRUCTION

The appearance of the 45,X fetus illustrated in Figure 15-7 dramatically shows the fetal edema that occurs in many concept uses with Turner syndrome. The edema appears to result from lymphatic malformations and obstruction.[126] This type of obstruction may result from a lag in the formation of a communication between the developing jugular lymph sac and the internal jugular vein. This communication normally develops between the fifth and sixth weeks of gestation, and failure to establish it appropriately results in lymphatic distention.[127] The search for the gene or genes on the X chromosome responsible for this developmental abnormality is underway.

The maldevelopment occurs most often in the nuchal region, with the dilatation of at least two cavities separated

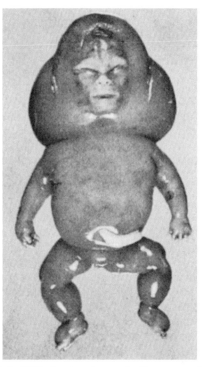

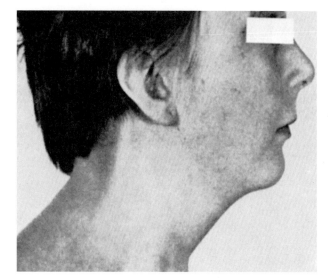

Figure 15-8 Lateral view of the face of a girl with Turner syndrome, demonstrating low posterior hairline, residual webbing, and micrognathia.

Figure 15-7 A 45,X abortus demonstrating generalized lymphedema. Note the distended cervical region. With resolution of the edema, the redundant skin may cicatrize—resulting in a webbed neck. The edema of the hands and feet may persist and be present at birth. [From Gellis SS, Feingold M (1978). Picture of the month. Am J Dis Child 132:417. Copyright © 1978, American Medical Association.)

by the nuchal ligament. In many cases, each cavity is subdivided by incomplete septa. The cavities extend from the upper part of the occipital bone caudad to the scapular region and medially to beneath the sternocleidomastoid muscle. If the blockage persists, the increased pressure within the lymphatics may alter their development and result in the more generalized malformations of peripheral lymphatics. Peripheral lymphatic hypoplasia or aplasia has also been demonstrated using lymphangiography in adult patients with Turner syndrome.[21] Thus, as in the case of the mice with subcutaneous blebs described by Bonnevie a single process may be responsible for a host of the apparently varied physical findings in this syndrome.

Webbed neck, or pterygium colli, is perhaps the most obvious consequence of lymphatic obstruction. It results from a scarring process that affects the distended loose skin over the large cystic hygromas that were present in the nuchal region. Some patients may, therefore, have a severe anomaly. Others, however, who never had significant distention or in whom the obstruction was minimal or in whom rupture and decompression occurred early do not have a webbed neck. In fact, in some patients in whom neither webbing nor abnormalities of the cervical vertebrae exist the neck will appear long in proportion to the stature (Figure 15-4). Thus, webbing per se is not a primary anomaly. In our series, only 25% of patients had any webbing at all.

The dilatation of the nuchal region is also believed to be responsible for mechanical effects on the pattern of hair direction, resulting in the lower position of the posterior hairline (Figure 15-8). This may also be responsible for the heavy extended growth of the eyebrow. Similarly, the dilatation may result in rotation of the axis of the auricle posteriorly and elevation of the lower pinna—resulting in the prominent and low-set appearance of the ears.[128]

Edema of the dorsum of the hands and feet at birth is an obvious consequence of the incompletely resolved process if it involved peripheral lymphatics. Postnatally, the lymphedema usually resolves—although some patients demonstrate residual involvement. Others may complain of intermittent or recurrent edema, often after institution of estrogen replacement therapy. Less obvious are the mechanical effects the lymphedema may have had on the developing extremities. It is probable that the abnormalities in the nails described in many patients (deeply set into the nail bed with lateral hyperconvexity) are secondary to mechanical distortion of the developing nail bed.[129] Severely dysplastic or even absent nails are noted at birth in some patients as a more obvious consequence. The result on the fingertip pads is a predominance of dermal ridge whorl patterning, a characteristic dermatoglyphic feature.[129] A compressive or restrictive effect on the developing ossification centers resulting in some of what has been categorized as skeletal defects is also possible.

UNKNOWN FACTORS: EYE, EAR, SKIN

The factors responsible for several other common physical features are less clear. Strabismus and unilateral or bilateral ptosis occur more commonly than normal, contributing other features to the characteristic facies.

Multiple pigmented nevi, in excess of that expected from familial patterns, occur frequently and were noted in 26% of our patients. Several had surgical excisions of one or more lesions that had been subjected to trauma, and histologic examination did not show evidence of

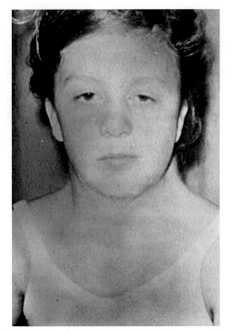

Figure 15-9 Unilateral ptosis in a girl with Turner syndrome. Note also significant webbing of the neck on the affected side.

malignant degeneration. The mechanism responsible for the excessive presence of these lesions, especially on the face and arms, is unknown. Because migration of melanocytes into the skin begins at a relatively early stage (10 weeks), it is unlikely that this process is affected by the lymphedema.[130]

Physiologic Features

SKELETAL GROWTH FAILURE

Short stature appears to be the most common phenotypic feature of children and adults with Turner syndrome and has been noted in almost all articles and reviews since Turner's report in 1938. The first comprehensive assessment of cross-sectional and longitudinal growth and final height did not appear until the report of Ranke and colleagues in 1983.[131] Patterns of growth are illustrated in Figure 15-10, which shows cross-sectional height and velocity data from a series of 150 Turner children who had not received therapy for growth promotion.

These patterns described by Ranke and colleagues are distinguished by four components: intrauterine growth retardation [with mean birth length 1 standard deviation (SD) below the mean or an average reduction of 2.8 cm] and mean birth weight (not shown in the figure) of 2.18 kg, which is also 1 SD below the mean; a period of what initially appeared to be near-normal growth velocity for 2 to 3 years, which has now been characterized by growth deceleration to a mean of −2.18 SD at 1.5 years[132] and a further loss by age 3 years[133]; after age 3, continued deceleration, so that between ages 3 and 13 years the Turner syndrome girls fall farther and farther away from the normal height curves; and if untreated failure to experience a pubertal growth spurt but continued growth at a slow rate for several more years.

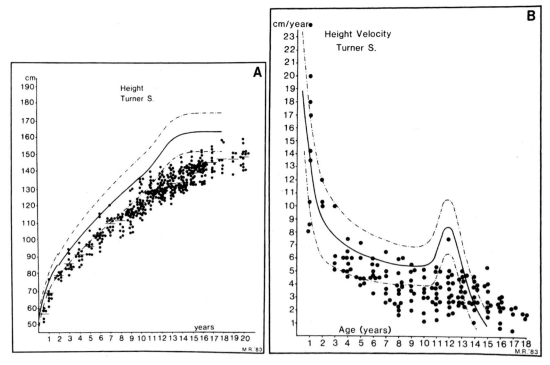

Figure 15-10 Height and height velocity in Turner syndrome. (*A*) Three hundred eighty-four single measurements of height for 150 children with Turner syndrome. (*B*) Height velocity from a total of 159 measurements. The normal ranges are shown by the heavy and dashed lines. [From Tanner JM, Whitehouse RH, Takaishi M (1965). Standards from birth to maturity for height, weight, height velocity and weight velocity: British children. Arch Dis Child 41:454, 613; and from Ranke MD, Pfluger H, Rosendahl W, et al. (1983). Turner syndrome: Spontaneous growth in 150 cases and review of the literature. Eur J Paediatr 141:81.]

A positive correlation is found among height at diagnosis,[134] ultimate height achieved, and midparental height.[135] The final height deficit, using comparative data on adult heights in patients with different ethnic backgrounds, is approximately 20 cm.[136] These authors concluded that the short stature was primarily the result of a generalized abnormality in the growth response of the skeleton but that other genetic factors such as a prolongation of cell generation time associated with the chromosomal disturbance per se[137] may also play a part.

Lippe et al.[138] have shown that disproportionate growth of the lower extremities appears to contribute, in some degree, to the short stature in Turner syndrome. In a group of 16 adult Turner syndrome patients not treated with growth hormone, the mean height was 144.2.0 cm, the sitting height was 79.6 cm, and the sitting height-to-height ratio was 0.55. This observation of a short lower segment has been confirmed by some,[139] but not all,[140] observers. In addition we found a significant negative correlation between the ratio of sitting height to lower segment and height, indicating that the patients with the greatest proportional reduction in the length of their legs were the shortest. The description of the SHOX gene and its role in statural growth, including mesomelic short stature, may explain the major component of the statural deficit (as discussed previously).

After the report of Ranke and colleagues,[131] Lyon and associates[141] used the data from that report and from three other European centers to synthesize a series of growth curves for Turner syndrome. The curves provided mean height and SD values for age. The mean adult height from these series was 143.1 cm. In the United States, we obtained 3,460 cross-sectional and longitudinal height determinations from 1,363 individuals to validate the applicability of these Western European–derived growth curves to U.S. girls with Turner syndrome.[142]

Our data (Figure 15-11, left) demonstrate that U.S. girls with Turner syndrome fit almost exactly the Lyon-Turner curve, with a final height of 144.3 cm, in 584 patients untreated with growth-promoting agents or estrogen before age 18 years. When the smoothed mean values (splines) are compared (right), there is a small but significant increase in the heights of U.S. girls between ages 12 and 16 that might represent the so-called spontaneous growth spurt that has been described by other groups with mathematical models.[143,144]

With their longitudinal patient data, Lyon and colleagues also noted a very strong correlation (0.95) between the initial height SD on these Turner curves and the adult height SD achieved regardless of whether the patient had received late estrogen replacement therapy and essentially independent of bone age at the time of the first height. Thus, they concluded that one could actually predict, or project, the adult height of a girl with Turner syndrome based on her height at an earlier age. In our study, we validated this projection method with a longitudinal assessment of 56 patients who had not received growth-promoting therapy and for whom we had both childhood heights and heights after the age of 18 years. The results showed a mean difference of less than 1 cm between the projection and the final height achieved. Data such as these have proved invaluable in assessing the efficacy of growth-promoting therapy.

Growth-Promoting Therapy

Early studies on the use of growth hormone (GH), dating back to the 1960s, yielded conflicting and inconclusive results.[145] Some studies were very short term, others did not use comparable doses of GH—and few patients were followed to adult height. This failure to confirm or preclude a role for GH was confounded by the debate

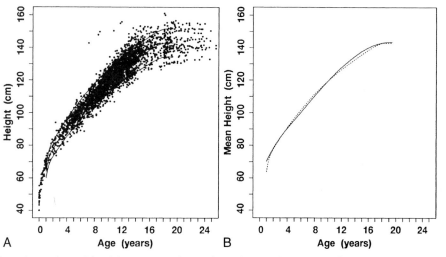

Figure 15-11 (*A*) Heights of American girls with Turner syndrome (superimposed on curves of Lyon and associates) representing the 10th, 50th, and 90th percentiles. (*B*) Spline fit to the American heights (solid curve) together with a dashed curve showing spline fit of Lyon European data. [From Lippe B, Plotnick L, Attie K, et al. (1993). Growth in Turner syndrome: Updating the United States experience. In Hibi I, Takano K (eds.), *Basic and clinical approach to Turner syndrome*. Amsterdam: Elsevier Science.]

over the status of GH secretion in Turner syndrome. Although it is clear that girls with Turner syndrome as a group do not have classic GH deficiency, there is no consensus on the nature of their secretory dynamics. In an international workshop on Turner syndrome, four groups reported differing data with regard to spontaneous GH secretion.[146-149] These differences in data persist even when age-matched groups are compared. For example, several groups found normal GH secretion in younger girls with Turner syndrome compared with their peers but not in older girls compared with normal adolescents.[150-151]

Although this might be expected because girls with Turner syndrome do not for the most part experience an estrogen increase with puberty, other groups have not found this difference at puberty.[152] In addition, when studied in a longitudinal manner ethinyl estradiol treatment resulted in increased GH pulse amplitude. However, in a cross-sectional study there was no difference in GH secretion between Turner syndrome girls with or without spontaneous breast development or with or without estrogen therapy.[153] These data are further confounded by methodologic differences in assessment,[154] assay differences,[155-156] and biologic variables such as body weight differences[157] between Turner syndrome girls and normal girls. Because the consensus is that there is no GH deficiency, however, provocative GH testing is obsolete and need not be performed unless growth velocity is abnormal relative to that expected for Turner syndrome.

The use of anabolic steroids in Turner syndrome also dates back to the 1960s,[158] but their efficacy in increasing final adult height is still being debated. Some studies indicate that augmented growth velocity may not be accompanied by a concomitant bone age increase and suggest that ultimate height is increased.[159-161] Others either found no differences in adult height between androgen- and estrogen-treated girls[162] or pointed out that over time changes in stature could make the results difficult to interpret if treated patients were compared with untreated controls of previous years.[163]

Of the more recent studies, two conclude that androgens alone do have a positive effect on final height[165-166] and two conclude that they do not.[166-167] Our retrospective analysis of growth data failed to demonstrate that anabolic steroids promoted a statistically significant increase in final adult height. We and others,[169,170] however, have confirmed that they do promote marked growth acceleration in the first year or more of therapy—which was perceived as highly beneficial by the patients and their families.

The use of a combination of androgen and GH was first reported in 1980, and it was suggested that short-term combination therapy might promote more rapid growth than either agent alone.[170,171] The availability of unlimited recombinant human GH has made it possible to conduct carefully designed studies and to evaluate the growth response to GH and the combination of GH with androgens and/or estrogens. This forms the basis for a large U.S. multicenter study that has now been completed.[171] In 1983, this multicenter prospective randomized trial of recombinant human GH alone and in combination with oxandrolone was initiated.

The mean adult height for the 17 recipients of GH alone was 150.5 cm, which was 8.5 cm above their projected adult heights. For the 43 subjects treated with a combination of GH and oxandrolone, the mean adult height was 152.2 cm—10.4 cm taller than their projected adult heights. Fifty-eight of the 62 GH-treated subjects (94%) attained an adult height greater than their projected adult heights. The mean adult height attained by a retrospective control group as part of this study was 144.3 cm (Figure 15-12). These results compare favorably not only with the matched American control group but with previous reports of final heights in girls with untreated Turner syndrome from the United States and many other countries.[131,142,147,172-176]

The increment in final height, above the projected adult height, of the group receiving combination therapy was modestly but significantly greater than that in the group receiving GH alone (2.9 + 0.5 cm). This improved growth response was attained despite the fact that GH administration in the combination group was 1.5 years briefer than in the group receiving GH alone.

Combination therapy appears to offer certain advantages over GH alone: increased growth over the first 6 years of treatment (37.3 cm for the combination group versus 31.2 for GH alone), thereby allowing for better normalization of height during childhood; potential for earlier initiation of estrogen replacement because girls will have attained greater heights by adolescence with

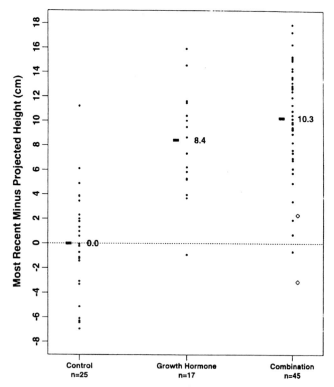

Figure 15-12 Most recent height of each subject (or American historical control subject) relative to each subject's projected adult height (indicated by dotted zero line). Mean increment in height (in centimeters) relative to projected adult height is indicated. Diamond symbols in the combination group indicate the two subjects who discontinued treatment early. [From Rosenfeld RG, Attie KM, Frane J, et al. (1998). Growth hormone therapy of Turner's syndrome: Beneficial effect on adult height. J Pediatr 132:319.]

combination treatment; and a briefer requirement for GH. Side effects associated with oxandrolone, 0.0625 mg/kg/ day, were minimal—and skeletal maturation averaged only 1.04 years per year of treatment. Experience with oxandrolone in young girls with Turner syndrome (6 years old) is limited, however, and it remains unclear whether it is better in young patients to initiate therapy with GH alone or in combination with oxandrolone.[170] In several other studies in which older Turner syndrome patients were treated with lower doses of GH, improvement of height was not as satisfactory.[176]

The results of the U.S. study also compare favorably to preliminary data from a second U.S. study[177] looking both at the role of GH and at the role of early versus late estrogen therapy. Twenty-nine girls receiving GH alone (plus estrogen replacement at 15 years of age) achieved a mean height of 150.5 cm, which was 8.5 cm above their projected adult heights. This is almost identical to the results of the first U.S. study. The 26 patients in whom estrogen therapy was initiated at age 12 gained only 5.1 cm on average beyond their projected height and achieved a final height of 147.1 cm (Figure 15-13).

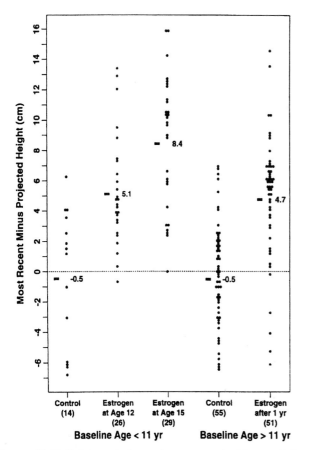

Figure 15-13 Height gain for patients treated with growth hormone compared with controls. Data are plotted for individual patients, with the most recent height minus the pretreatment projected height determined as indicated in the text. The mean values for each group are indicated by a dash. Control patients were matched from a historical database (as described in the text). [From Chernausek S, Attie KM, Cara JF, et al. (2000). Growth hormone therapy of Turner syndrome: The impact of age of estrogen replacement on final height. J Clin Endocrinol Metab 85:2439.]

A multivariate analysis was used to examine several factors that might influence the gain in stature. The number of years of GH therapy before estrogen treatment was a strong predictor. These data show that the early introduction of estrogen has a significant negative impact on adult height. Several published studies have reported that GH therapy results in an average height gain of 5 to 10 cm, a range that represents a surprising variability in outcome.[171-182] It appears that at least some of this variability may be caused by differences in the ages in which estrogen therapy was begun in these patients. Some of the reports showed that patients who had more modest apparent gains in final height also had relatively short periods of GH administration before the introduction of estrogen therapy.[180,182]

The method used to estimate what the adult height would have been without treatment with GH will affect the observed gain in height. Attie and Frane[183] compared five methods of predicting adult height in patients with Turner syndrome, using data from patients with Turner syndrome in the United States who had not been given growth-promoting drugs. They found that the Lyon projection method,[141] used in the two U.S. studies previously discussed,[171,177] was one of the most reliable means of predicting adult height—with the mean error of overprediction being only 0.3 cm.

Several studies that did not achieve such reassuring gains in final height[180,182] were also utilizing lower GH doses than the U.S. study groups.[171,177] This became particularly apparent in elegant studies carried out by the Dutch Advisory Group on GH.[184] Their final assessment of 7-year data clearly shows that in a carefully conducted dose-response study the increased dose of GH led to impressive increases in final height exceeding even the data seen in the U.S. studies. These investigators treated 68 patients with chronologic ages between 2 and 11 years and heights below the 50th percentile for healthy Dutch girls. The dosages employed were from 1.3 mg/m^2/day (0.23 mg/kg/week) to as high as 2.7 mg/m^2/day (0.63 mg/kg/week). It is clear from this study that there is a dose-response curve and that patients with the higher GH dose grew significantly better.

The patients were divided into three groups. In the first year, all three groups received GH at the starting dose of 1.3 mg/m^2/day. In the second year, two groups were switched to doses of 2 mg/m^2/day. In the third year, one of these two groups was switched to 2.7 mg/m^2/day. All were then treated at these doses for the remainder of the study period. After 7 years of GH treatment, mean final heights were 159.1, 161.8, and 162.7, respectively, for the three groups. These investigators concluded that after 7 years of GH treatment most girls with Turner syndrome are growing within the height range for healthy normal girls (Table 15-3, Figure 15-14). In fact, adult height was above 170 cm in 5 girls and above 160 cm in 17 girls. Growth-promoting therapy in these patients was not marked by any major clinical or metabolic side effects (see "Safety of Growth-Promoting Therapy"). Concerns about elevation of IGF-1 levels during GH therapy in Turner syndrome would suggest that inappropriate elevation of IGF-1 levels in the long term should be avoided.[185]

TABLE 15-3

Final Height in Turner Syndrome

	Dose	Final Height (CM)	Gain (CM)	Duration of Treatment (YR)
U.S. study (Genentech)* GH (n517)	0.375 (mg/kg/wk)	150.465.5	8.464.5	7.662.2
GH1oxandrolone (n543)	0.3751 oxandrolone 50.0625 (mg/kg/day)	152.165.9	10.364.5	6.161.9
U.S. study (NCGS)† (n5622)	0.35 (mg/kg/wk)	148.365.6	6.464.9	3.761.9
Dutch study (dose response)‡ (n568)	0.23 to 0.63 (mg/kg/wk) to 162.3 (154.3-170.3)	158.8 (148.3–172.4) to 16.0 (10.0-24.8)	12.5 (7.8–15.7)	7

* Data from van Es A, Massarano AA, Wit JM, et al. (1991). 24-hour growth hormone secretion in Turner syndrome. In Ranke MB, Rosenfeld RG (eds.), *Turner syndrome: Growth promoting therapies.* Amsterdam: Elsevier Science 29–33.
† Data from Urban MD, Lee PA, Dorst JP, et al. (1979). Oxandrolone therapy in patients with Turner syndrome. J Pediatr 94:823.
‡ Data from Rosenbloom AL, Frias JL (1973). Oxandrolone for growth promotion in Turner syndrome. Am J Dis Child 125:385.
GH, growth hormone; and NCGS, Genentech's National Cooperative Growth Study.

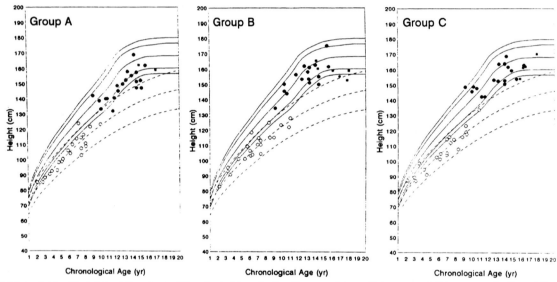

Figure 15-14 Individual heights at the start of the study (s) and after 7 years of growth hormone (d) in groups A, B, and C, respectively. Twelve girls had completed the trial during the 7-year study period (j). Reference curves for healthy Dutch girls (3rd, 10th, 50th, 90th, and 97th percentiles) and for untreated girls with Turner syndrome (North European references for 3rd, 50th, and 97th percentiles) are given. [From Sas TCJ, de Munick Keizer-Schrama SMPF, Stijnen T, et al. (1999). Normalization of height in girls with Turner syndrome after long-term growth hormone treatment: Results of a randomized dose-response trial. J Clin Endocrinol Metab 84:4607.]

In summary, it should be pointed out that final height data reported by many groups in different countries using different study protocols are most likely conservative estimates of the effect of therapeutic intervention with GH on height potential in patients with Turner syndrome. Many of these patients were enrolled at older ages, thus limiting the duration of GH therapy. Doses of GH employed were often well below the mean dose of 0.33 mg/kg/week used in the United States.[186] Some investigators began estrogen replacement in patients as early as age 12 years and used relatively high dosages of estrogen. This will only hasten epiphyseal fusion and thus compromise height potential.

In general, one can expect only 18 to 24 months continued growth after the initiation of estrogens. If there is still a large height deficit at 12 to 13 years of age, estrogen therapy should be delayed. There is no evidence that low-dose estrogen given at any age in growth-promoting dosages before it is used for induction of puberty is advantageous, and it may even curtail final height[187] (although spontaneous puberty per se does not appear to reduce final height).[188] However, the magnitude of the benefit has varied greatly depending on study designs and treatment parameters. Factors predictive of taller adult stature include a relatively tall height at initiation of therapy, tall parents, young age at initiation of therapy, a long duration of therapy, and a high GH dose.[61,189]

Therapeutic regimens aiming at early GH treatment initiation and optimizing the dose of GH may well allow for normalization of height during school-age years and thus earlier introduction of estrogens.[170,177,189] The recently

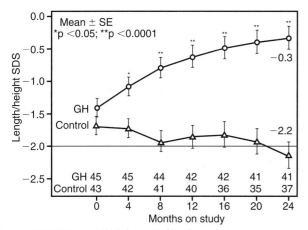

Figure 15-15 Length/height SDS for the nontreatment control group (open symbols) and the growth hormone treatment group (filled symbols) of toddlers with Turner syndrome during the 2-year study. Between-group difference at endpoint was 1.6 + 0.6 SDS (p <0.0001). Mean age at baseline was 24 + 12.1 months. Published with permission from Davenport ML, Crowe BJ, Travers SH, et al. (2007). Grwoth Hormone Treatment of Early Growth Failure in Toddlers with Turner Syndrome: A Randomized, Controlled, Multicenter Trial. JCEM 93(9): 3406-3416.

completed toddler Turner study in the United States began GH treatment between 9 months and 4 years in 88 girls. GH therapy is effective as early as 9 months of age. Treatment with GH should be considered as soon as growth failure (decreasing height percentiles on the normal curve) is demonstrated and its potential risks and benefits have been discussed with the family[81] (Figure 15-15).

SAFETY OF GROWTH-PROMOTING THERAPY

Human recombinant growth hormone (hrGH) was introduced into the United States in 1985, and worldwide shortly thereafter. Its introduction followed on the heels of the recognition that Creutzfeldt-Jacob disease had been transmitted to patients from some batches of human pituitary-derived GH.[190] This serious safety issue, coupled with the fact that hrGH was the first recombinant protein available as a pharmaceutical, has resulted in extensive worldwide scrutiny of this drug. Because it is beyond the scope of this chapter to discuss GH safety in its entirety, we will focus on several specific clinical and metabolic issues related to GH therapy in Turner syndrome.

The issue of whether GH alters the body proportions of girls with Turner syndrome has been of interest since the early studies of GH use.[191] The report by Sas and associates[192] of more than 60 girls observed for up to 7 years on increasingly high doses of GH addresses this issue in depth. Height, sitting height, hand and foot length, and biacromial and bi-iliacal diameters were measured. They note that at the outset Turner syndrome girls have relatively large trunks, hands, and feet and broad shoulders and pelvis compared with height. This is in concert with the reference data,[193] illustrating the relative disproportion that these girls have before GH is initiated.

Long-term GH therapy tends to normalize height, improve the disproportion between height and sitting height, and have little effect on hand length or shoulder or pelvic proportions. Foot length increases disproportionately in a dose-dependent fashion and in their series played a role in the decision of some patients to discontinue GH therapy in the last phases of growth. Scoliosis was not specifically addressed in this paper. The incidence of scoliosis is as high as 35% (Table 15-2) in untreated patients with Turner syndrome. Although it is also reported to be increased after GH treatment compared with GH-deficient patients so treated, it may not be increased compared with untreated patients. In addition, progression to surgical intervention is rare in both the treated and the untreated patient.

Sas and associates also evaluated the effect of GH on cardiac left ventricular dimensions and blood pressure in this cohort.[193] They found that the growth of the left ventricle was comparable to that of healthy girls, confirming the earlier findings of Saenger and colleagues.[192] Sas and associates[194] also found that whereas blood pressure in these girls was within the normal range for age at the start of therapy it was significantly higher than in healthy control subjects. Seven years of GH therapy had no significant effect on systolic blood pressure and had a small lowering effect on diastolic blood pressure. Finally, during the course of this 7-year GH trial there was no significant dilation of the aortic root (S.M.P.F. de Muinck Keizer-Schrama, MD, personal communication).

Two studies have looked at long-term effects on plasma lipids. van Teunenbroek and co-workers evaluated the effects of GH in two different study groups over time and found that in one group the atherogenic index improved with long-term treatment, whereas in the other it remained the same.[196] Querfeld and co-workers evaluated the effect of GH on lipoprotein(a) and found no effect, either alone or in combination with oxandrolone, on lipoprotein(a) levels after a median of 27 months of therapy.[197] Lanes and colleagues found normal lipoproteins in the untreated state and a decrease in total and low-density lipoprotein cholesterol during treatment.[198] Thus, long-term GH therapy does not appear to have a deleterious effect on cardiac structure or on cardiovascular risk factors and in a high-dose study led to a cardioprotective profile.

Other aspects of the safety assessment of GH therapy in these clinical trials showed there were no adverse effects of GH treatment on carbohydrate metabolism. Hgb A1c levels did not change, and glucose levels remained normal. In most studies, fasting and postprandial insulin levels increase during GH therapy but return to normal after GH treatment is stopped.[199,200] Liver abnormalities, characterized by transient increases in transaminase and/or g-glutamyl transpeptidase concentrations, have been occasionally reported in GH-deficient and Turner syndrome 2 children during GH therapy.[201,202] Spontaneous resolution usually takes place within 3 to 6 months of identification.

In Turner syndrome specifically, treatment with estrogens or androgens or the presence of autoimmune liver disease was more commonly associated with the increase in liver enzymes than was GH treatment.[201] Conversely, in adult women with Turner syndrome hepatic enzyme levels are higher than in normal women but have been found to decrease with estrogen therapy.[203] Thus, the tendency of liver enzymes to be increased in both girls and women with Turner syndrome appears to reflect both intrinsic and exogenous mechanisms but rarely reflects active dysfunction or disease. Finally, what appears to be hepatic enzymes may be confounded by transient increases in muscle creatine phosphokinase (CK) that has been reported after GH therapy.[204]

In 1993, Bourguignon and colleagues[205] reported that melanocytic nevi may grow more rapidly during GH therapy based on clinical observation and immunoantibody staining for actively growing melanocytes. Subsequently, the issue has been of concern—albeit there are no reports of increased melanoma frequency in patients with acromegaly. Zvulunov and associates evaluated this question in two studies,[206,207] concluding that whereas the number of nevi are increased in Turner syndrome GH therapy in GH deficiency is not associated with an increased count or density of nevi (both factors in increasing melanoma risk) and is therefore unlikely to potentiate the risk for melanoma in Turner syndrome. To date, this conclusion is supported by a lack of reports indicating an increased incidence of melanoma in Turner syndrome patients treated with GH.

The role of GH as an immunoregulator has been reviewed.[208] Although there are data that suggest that GH replacement therapy has a transient effect on B cells,[209] clinically significant effects of GH on immune function have not been described. Because Turner syndrome patients are known to have a high incidence of autoimmune thyroiditis, the effect of GH therapy on the incidence of thyroid antibodies was studied.[210] No increase in the prevalence of thyroid antibodies was observed.

Among adverse events related to GH reported in the Pharmacia International Growth Study database (KIGS), the incidence of pseudotumor cerebri appears to be higher in Turner syndrome patients (and in patients with chronic renal failure and organic GH deficiency) than in other subgroups of patients treated with GH. Scoliosis is also higher in Turner syndrome and in Prader-Willi syndrome patients, conditions known to be associated with scoliosis in the untreated state. Malignancy rates are not increased in Turner syndrome during GH therapy.[211]

OTITIS AND HEARING LOSS

Perhaps the most common medical problem reported by patients with Turner syndrome is bilateral otitis media. In a series of 76 patients, Anderson and co-workers[212] recorded medically significant middle ear infection in 68%—with more than one half of these patients reporting not only recurrent episodes but spontaneous perforations, the need for surgical treatment, or both. Hearing problems and ear malformations correlate with karyotype.[213-215] In Figure 15-16, the audiogram shows the typical dip in sensorineural hearing paricularly prevalent in higher frequencies.

In our series, complete system reviews were recorded for more than 80% of patients. Of these, almost 75% had undergone tonsillectomy and adenoidectomy because of recurrent otitis or had had polyethylene tubes placed for the drainage of serous otitis media or had both procedures performed. Of these, five patients had also under-

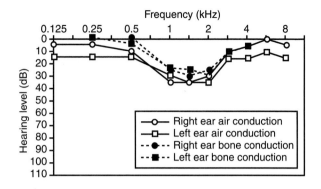

Figure 15-16 Audiogram showing the typical dip with the peak of 35 dB in the 1.5-kHz frequency region in a 12-year-old girl with Turner's syndrome (karyotype 45,X). This girl has no subjective hearing problems.[From Stenberg AE, et al. (1998). Otological problems in children with Turner syndrome. Hearing Research 124:85–90.]

gone mastoid surgery. The cause of otitis does not appear to be related to a specific or generalized immunologic dysfunction. Other infections, as well as other disorders of the mucous membranes, are not reported to occur with increased frequency in Turner syndrome.

Although levels of secretory immunoglobulins have not been reported, serum concentrations are not abnormal. IgG and IgA concentrations, however, appear to be in the adult male range—which is significantly lower than the adult female range.[216] Instead, frequent occurrence of otitis may be the consequence of abnormalities in growth of the cranial base in Turner syndrome. Cephalometry[212,217] has demonstrated that both structural growth of the temporal bone and growth of the condylar cartilage and spheno-occipital synchondrosis are abnormal. The result is that the final development of the facial skeleton reaches a level only corresponding to that of an 11-year-old girl, whereas that of the posterior portion of the cranial base is even less advanced. As a consequence, not only is the position of the external auditory meatus abnormal (giving the appearance of low-set ears) but the relationship of the middle ear to the eustachian tube is disturbed. These factors, coupled with abnormalities in the shape of the palate, create a predisposition to fluid collection and secondary infection. Marked hypocellularity of the mastoid air cells may also be found, further predisposing the individual to acute and chronic suppurative disease.[218]

The relationship of chronic otitis media to hearing deficit was also explored by Anderson and colleagues.[188] Their data suggest that a component of the hearing loss reported to be a common occurrence in Turner syndrome is conductive in nature. A high incidence of eardrum disease and conductive hearing loss (43%) was also reported more recently.[219] True sensorineural hearing impairment was also documented in both series. This was generally bilateral and characterized by symmetrical sensorineural dips in the audiogram in the midfrequency range. Audiologic manipulations tended to identify the defect as one of recruitment and specifically localized the defect to the outer hair cells of the organ of Corti.

When older patients were compared with children younger than the age of 10, conductive losses were more frequently found in the children and sensorineural losses were more frequently found in the adults. Thus, the sensorineural losses appear to develop with age and represent a degenerative rather than a congenital abnormality. In addition to the findings reported previously, high-frequency audiometry also reveals a high prevalence of hearing loss that may precede the mid-frequency dip.[220] A relationship between auricular abnormalities and hearing loss and those karyotypes with complete loss of the X or Xp2 is suggested and may confirm the hypothesis that growth dysregulation of the cranial base owing to loss of the growth-regulating genes such as SHOX is in part responsible for the findings.[221]

Alternatively, growth dysregulation of the cranial base may be secondary to delayed cell cycle caused by chromosomal aberrations per se and not only genes deleted on the X chromosome.[222] In older girls and women with Turner syndrome with no history of hearing loss, audiologic surveillance is warranted every 2 to 3 years. The assiduous treatment of ENT problems in childhood and avoiding potential injuries to the inner ear may reduce the risk of hearing loss.[61] Removal of the adenoids may exacerbate palatal dysfunction and negatively influence quality of speech, factors that must taken into consideration prior to surgery.

GERM CELL CHROMOSOMAL DEFECTS

Gonadal Failure

Histologic evidence suggests that the ovary of the fetus with a 45,X karyotype (and presumably the ovary of the fetus with karyotypes with X chromosome deletions, rings, or mosaicism) undergoes an initial phase of differentiation that is the same as that in the 46,XX fetus. If the ovary is examined at 14 to 18 weeks of gestation, no abnormalities are seen. Subsequently, however, when there is a chromosomal defect in the germ cells the process of oocyte loss appears to be accelerated—with a concomitant acceleration of stromal fibrosis. Thus, what is considered the normal process of oocyte loss (beginning prenatally and continuing over 30 to 50 years of postnatal life in normal females) occurs entirely prenatally or in the first few months or years of postnatal life in most females with Turner syndrome.[223,224]

The triggering mechanism for this premature follicular atresia is postulated to be in part secondary to meiotic pairing anomalies in prophase,[225] and may be seen in other chromosomal abnormalities (such as trisomy 13 and trisomy 18).[226] The molecular mechanisms presumably involve the acceleration of an oocyte-intrinsic apoptosis defect regulated by members of the Bcl-2 gene family[198] and the caspase family of proteases.[227] The processes of oocyte loss and fibrosis are, however, neither absolute nor inevitable. Whereas the older literature documents both spontaneous puberty and menarche in a small number of patients with Turner syndrome,[228-231] the low percentages reported may be the result of ascertainment of only the most phenotypically obvious Turner syndrome patients.

The report of Pasquino and co-workers,[188] which includes more than 500 patients older than the age of 12 years, documents a high rate of spontaneous puberty—with an incidence of 14% in monosomic X patients and 32% in patients with cell lines with more than one X. In the series of Lippe et al.[232] of 141 girls who were in the pubertal age range, 29 (21%) had the onset of breast development to Tanner III or more—with menses occurring at least once in 25 and menses persisting into at least young adulthood in 15 (50% of those with initial ovarian function, or 11% of the entire pubertal age group).

Seven of the 29 with some degree of ovarian function had a 45,X karyotype. Of note is that although these 7 girls had some phenotypic features of Turner syndrome they did not have the webbed neck phenotype we associate with the presence of fetal lymphedema. The remaining 22 patients had mosaicism or structural abnormalities, with the highest number of girls with menses in the 45,X/46,XX group. Again, these girls lacked the webbed neck phenotype. Thus, maintenance of some degree of ovarian function can occur in Turner syndrome patients regardless of karyotype—although it is more common in those with cell lines with more than one X, and clearly more common in those who lack the webbed neck phenotype.

Pregnancy has been reported in more than 60 patients with Turner syndrome, including those with a 45,X karyotype on multiple tissues.[234-238] Although these latter cases remain rare enough to continue to merit individual reports, they illustrate the spectrum of ovarian function in this condition. Counseling about the expectations and future management of the patient with Turner syndrome diagnosed before puberty needs to include the probability of gonadal failure and infertility but not its inevitable occurrence. Even in those instances in which fertility does occur, however, reproductive failure is high and the risk of an abnormal offspring (notably one with trisomy 21) appears significant.[237-239]

In the series of Pasquino and co-workers,[188] there were three patients with spontaneous pregnancies (3.6%). One patient had two pregnancies, one with a normal male karyotype and one female with the same structurally abnormal X as the mother (i.e., Turner syndrome). One patient had twins with normal karyotype but severe cleft palate, and one patient had a normal infant. Ultimately, morethan 90% of indianals with Turner syndrome will have gonadal failure.[61] Physiologic evidence for gonadal failure in Turner syndrome is provided by the response of the hypothalamic-pituitary axis to functional agonadism.

It has long been recognized that the negative feedback loop between the gonad and the hypothalamic-pituitary axis is operative in the fetus and demonstrable at birth. In normal infants, follicle-stimulating hormone (FSH) and luteinizing hormone (LH) rise after birth. In the male, the gonadotropin rise is accompanied by a significant surge in plasma testosterone in the first months of life. Gonadotropin and testosterone then gradually decline to prepubertal concentrations by the end of the first year. In the female, although the gonadotropin rise does not appear to be accompanied by as striking a response in estradiol secretion from the ovary the plasma FSH remains slightly elevated for a period of several years.

In Turner syndrome, a markedly exaggerated rise in both plasma gonadotropins (but especially in FSH) has been demonstrated as early as 5 days of age in one study.[240] In a more recent study, however, with the blood spot obtained used for neonatal screening[241] a clear-cut elevation of FSH could not be demonstrated in patients with known karyotype abnormalities consistent with Turner syndrome—suggesting that FSH cannot be used for neonatal screening for Turner syndrome. In the series by Lippe et al.,[232] the investigators evaluated 14 patients with karyotypes consistent with Turner syndrome at 2 weeks of age or later in the first year of life. Of those who presented with lymphedema at birth, all had FSH determinations of more than 40 mIU/mL.

Conversely, of the patients who had the diagnosis of an X chromosome abnormality made by amniocentesis only 50% had evidence of castrate levels of FSH. Thus, although an abnormally high FSH in the neonatal or infancy period is useful to detect gonadal failure a normal level does not preclude the diagnosis of Turner syndrome. Whether the girls with normal FSH levels in infancy will go on to have gonadal failure at adolescence or will turn out to be the 10% to 30% who have some gonadal function remains to be determined. Pelvic ultrasound may have prognostic value in predicting the future sexual development of patients with normal gonadotropins. Data of Mazzanti and associates[242] suggest that detection of ovaries bilaterally in patients without castrate levels of gonadotropins and mosaic karyotypes correlated best with preservation of some ovarian function at puberty.

When abnormally elevated in infancy, the gonadotropin levels decline again after the first 2 years—although to mean concentrations significantly higher than those in gonadally competent female children. Between ages 4 and 10 to 11 years, a trough is noted, which is followed by the gradual rise of gonadotropins in normal children and a more rapid and exaggerated rise in most children with Turner syndrome. This diphasic pattern of FSH, determined on a large number of patients with gonadal dysgenesis, is illustrated in Figure 15-17A. In Figure 15-17B, serial determinations graphically demonstrate the fall that occurs in the first years of life and the abrupt rise that occurs in early adolescence. The range of values considered normal for a female varies with the assay method and the standard used, and thus the values in the figure are illustrative but will not be normative for most current commercial assays.

The mechanisms responsible for the feedback suppression of gonadotropin secretion in the normal child and the similar pattern, although at a higher set point, in the child with gonadal dysgenesis are unclear. It has been presumed that increased sensitivity to circulating steroids of gonadal and adrenal origin results in decreased hypothalamic gonadotropin-releasing hormone (GnRH) release in the prepubertal subject. Studies in primate species suggest that one component of the feedback inhibition may be at the level of the pituitary and that another may be at the hypothalamic level. There may also be significant central neuronal inhibition that is not affected by gonadal steroids.

Plasma gonadotropin concentrations can be assessed at the time of diagnosis and again in early adolescence before the institution of steroid hormone therapy and counseling

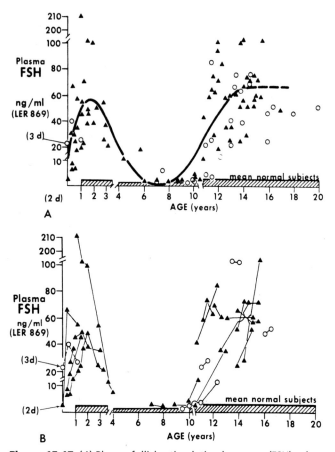

Figure 15-17 (*A*) Plasma follicle-stimulating hormone (FSH) values in patients with Turner syndrome. Triangles (m) indicate patients with 45,X karyotype, and circles (s) denote those with X chromosome mosaicism or structural abnormalities of the X. The curve is a polynomial regression plot. The hatched lines indicate mean plasma FSH values in normal females. Note the very high levels in infancy and adolescence, with lower levels in the mid first decade. FSH is expressed as nanograms per milliliter of standard LER-869. To convert these values to milli-International Units per milliliter of the second IRP, multiply by 3.5. (*B*) Symbols indicating that serial plasma FSH values in several individuals are connected by straight lines. Note the rise and fall in infancy and the dramatic and abrupt rises in adolescence. [From Conte FA, Grumbach MM, Kaplan SL (1975). A diphasic pattern of gonadotropin secretion in patients with the syndrome of gonadal dysgenesis. J Clin Endocrinol Metab 40:670.]

about ultimate fertility. When GnRH is administered to assess the function of the hypothalamic-pituitary axis, the responses of patients with Turner syndrome with gonadal failure are exaggerated compared with normal subjects.[243] This procedure may be used to provide a second test for gonadal integrity in some patients. In one study of two 45,X menstruating adolescents with both documented anovulatory cycles and ovulatory cycles with a prolonged follicular phase and short luteal phases, however, GnRH testing did not show exaggerated responses.[244]

Nevertheless, in most adolescent patients a single determination of plasma FSH and LH is sufficient to document gonadal failure. In the absence of estrogen replacement therapy, gonadotropin secretion will continue unabated and unmodulated. Although no systemic manifestations are known to result from these excessive concentrations of

FSH and LH, reactive pituitary abnormalities have been reported in some patients.[245] Skull radiographs may show enlargement of the pituitary fossa, which is suggestive of pituitary hyperplasia or microadenoma formation. Although enlargement sufficient to result in organic dysfunction has not yet been reported, the recognition of this phenomenon is important so that the gonadal dysgenesis is not misdiagnosed as being secondary to a pituitary tumor. The potential for progressive pituitary enlargement is an additional reason for instituting estrogen replacement therapy.

Gonadoblastoma

Gonadoblastomas are distinctive tumors composed of at least two different cell types. The large cells have the appearance and ultrastructure of oogonial germ cells, and the small cells are ovarian stromal cells that are not clearly differentiated.[246] The small cells most closely resemble primitive sex-cord mesenchymal cells and are termed *granulosa-Sertoli cells*. The tumor arises in a gonad that is dysgenetic; that is, a gonad that has not completely differentiated into a normal ovary or normal testis or that does not behave like a normal ovary or normal testis. The dysgenesis that leads to gonadoblastoma formation almost invariably occurs in patients with Y chromosome material in their karyotype. In the case of Turner syndrome, most karyotypes do not contain a Y. The ovary is induced normally and then usually rapidly degenerates into fibrous streaks with loss of oogonial germ cells. These ovaries are not believed to be at risk for gonadoblastoma formation.

There is a small percentage of patients (between 2 and 5% in most series and 5% in our series), however, who fit all of the criteria for Turner syndrome and in whom the karyotype contains a Y chromosome. There is an even smaller percentage with a marker chromosome. Most often, the karyotype is the mosaic 45,X/46,XY. More complex karyotypes (including 46,XX/45,X/46,XY and even 46,XY), however, have been associated with Turner syndrome. Thus, the karyotype per se does not determine the phenotype.

What defines these patients as having Turner syndrome (rather than being hermaphrodites or having mixed gonadal dysgenesis) is their short stature, their symmetrical female external genitalia, and their normal female internal genitalia (bilateral fallopian tubes, uterus, and vagina). The only expression of the Y may be its effect on gonadal ridge induction, with the result that a number of cells no longer resemble differentiated ovarian stroma. In this case, all of the oogonial germ cells that develop in these dysgenetic ridges do not necessarily undergo atresia as rapidly as they do in typical Turner syndrome. Instead, some may persist, continue to divide, and develop into a gonadoblastoma.

In some patients with a Y in their karyotype, the granulosa/Sertoli cell stroma more closely resembles a testis and produces some androgen. This may occur regardless of whether a gonadoblastoma will eventually develop. These patients, although still having the Turner phenotype, may show some evidence of virilization—including clitoromegaly or partial fusion of the posterior labia. Virilization is in itself an indication for gonadectomy, whether a gonadoblastoma is present or not. Because many patients bearing the Y will not virilize, however, these findings are not necessarily helpful in deciding which Turner syndrome patient may be at risk for gonadoblastoma. For this reason, it is essential to obtain a complete chromosomal karyotype even in the most obvious of Turner syndrome patients. If a marker or fragment chromosome is detected that cannot be assigned to a specific chromosome, more specific studies can be performed (see "Incidence and Etiology" for a discussion of the role of Y chromosome-derived genes in gonadoblastoma formation).

The risk for the development of the tumor, unilaterally or bilaterally, in the patients with the Y-bearing dysgenetic gonad has been estimated to be as high as 15% to 25%[247]—although in the recent population study from Denmark by Gravholt and co-workers the risk appears to be much lower.[60] In the series by Lippe et al.,[232] four of the eight patients with an intact Y chromosome and one of the two with a Y-derived marker had histologic gonadoblastomas. As discussed previously, these data do not pertain to use of molecular markers for any Y-derived genetic material and should not be extrapolated to imply that patients should be screened with molecular markers to detect Y material to monitor them for gonadoblastoma or perform gonadectomy.

Although gonadoblastomas usually do not metastasize, local invasion of the surrounding stroma to form microscopic or gross germinomas is seen in about half of cases.[248] Gonadoblastomas may also be found in conjunction with malignant germinomas, although these latter tumors tend to occur in conditions other than Turner syndrome. The age at which these tumors are detected varies, but a number have been reported in early childhood.[249,250] In some patients, calcification is present— which assists in detection. In others, a tumor mass may be demonstrated with ultrasound, magnetic resonance imaging (MRI), or computed tomography. In many, however, the disease is microscopic.

Recommendations for dealing with the problem vary from prophylactic removal of the gonadal ridge streaks in all Turner syndrome patients with an intact Y or marker chromosome in their karyotype to prospective monitoring of the patient at risk with some visualization technique such as ultrasonography. Until the gonadoblastoma gene locus is identified, we do not recommend removal of gonadal streaks based on molecular marker testing in the absence of a cytogenetic Y but do recommend prophylactic removal if a cytogenetic Y or marker chromosome or virilization is present. Gravholt's data might indicate that even this is too aggressive in all cases, however, and monitoring alone may be sufficient in some. Examples of ultrasonographic studies in a normal pubertal female, a girl with Turner syndrome, and a girl with Turner syndrome and a gonadoblastoma are shown in Figure 15-18.

CARDIOVASCULAR ABNORMALITIES

The association of cardiovascular abnormalities, notably coarctation of the aorta, with Turner syndrome has been well documented.[16,251-254] The haploinsufficiency of the X

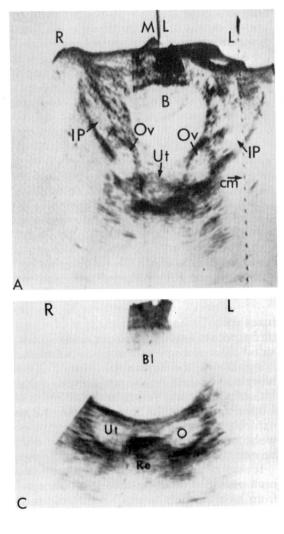

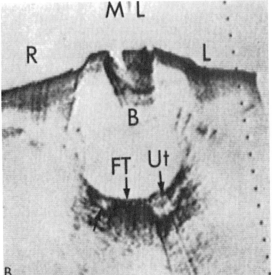

Figure 15-18 Examples of pelvic ultrasound studies. (*A*) Normal pubertal female demonstrating ovaries of adult size. (*B*) Patient with Turner syndrome. The corpus of the uterus is seen slightly to the left of the midline. The fallopian tube can be followed into the right adnexa and observed to terminate in a small structure (arrow) believed to be the fimbriated end of the tube. No ovaries are identified. (*C*) Patient with 45,X/46,XY Turner syndrome previously treated with estrogen. The corpus of the uterus is enlarged to adult size. In the left adnexa, a large gonadal mass (O) is seen. Histologically, this was identified as a gonadoblastoma. The images are transverse, oriented right (R) and left (L) of the midline (ML). The dotted scales are in centimeters. B, BL, bladder; FT, fallopian tube; IP, iliopsoas; O, gonadoblastoma; OV, ovary; Re, rectum; and Ut, uterus.

chromosome causes the most serious life-threatening consequences involving the cardiovascular system. The determination of its frequency, however [as well as the clarification of the conflicting reports of occurrence of other major structural cardiovascular malformations (CVMs)], was impaired by the lack of chromosomal karyotyping in early series.

One of the major sources of confusion was the inclusion of patients with normal chromosomes but phenotypic abnormalities, of whom a large number may have had Noonan syndrome.[254,255] CVMs occur in approximately 75% of spontaneously aborted Turner fetuses and 30% of living patients. Obstructive lesions of the left side of the heart predominate, ranging in severity from nonstenotic bicuspid aortic valve to aortic stenosis, coarctation of the aorta, and mitral valve anomalies (Table 15-4).[256-264] The most severe form of left-sided hypoplasia (hypoplastic left heart syndrome) also occurs, although it is uncommon.[265,266] The association of Turner syndrome and the entire spectrum of left-sided cardiovascular malformation is distinctive among malformation syndromes.

Only Williams syndrome, commonly associated with supravalvar aortic stenosis, shares this left-sided association. The largest series of patients comes from Italy, where Mazzanti and colleagues[259] analyzed the cardiac

evaluation of 594 Turner syndrome patients ranging from 1 month to 24 years of age. In addition, various other authors[260,262] have over the past years published type and frequency of cardiovascular malformations (Table 15-4). The prevalence of congenital heart disease and the relative risk in Turner syndrome patients compared to the general population are shown in Table 15-5.

Coarctation per se (especially the preductal adult-type coarctation most characteristic of this condition) is not likely to result from the same mechanisms as other congenital heart defects. Although the final structure of the four chambers of the heart and the orientation of the great vessels are established by 6 to 7 weeks after fertilization, the preductal area of the aorta subject to coarctation may be affected at any time. Moreover, coarctation occurring in this isthmus region has been considered in some cases to be a result of the differential flows through the two fetal circulatory systems that interface at this point (the ductal-placental flow and the systemic-cardiac-pulmonary flow).

Clark[267] elegantly reviewed the embryology of lymphatic sac drainage into the venous system and noted that in the chick disordered drainage implicates a mechanism that distends the cardiac lymphatics. He proposed that this would encroach on the ascending aorta and alter

TABLE 15-4

Cardiovascular Malformation in Turner Syndrome

	Gotzsche et al.[232]	Sybert[234]	Lin et al.[233]	Mazzanti et al.[231]
Year	1994			
No. of patients	179			
Type and frequency (rounded)				
All types	25%			
Among fetuses: 75%				
Left-sided obstruction, total	95%	75%	70%	100%
BAV 6 CVM	45%	25%	25%	55%
COA 6 other CVM	30%	30%	30%	30%
COA/BAV	10%	5%	10%	
Aortic stenosis, without BAV	10%	10%	5%	15%
Mitral stenosis, hypoplasia				
Hypoplastic left heart syndrome		5%		
Other, total		15%-20%	25%-30%	15%-20%
Membranous VSD		5%	.5%	.5%
ASD2		5%	.5%	.5%
PAPVR		.5%	.5%	10%
Mitral valve prolapse		5%	15%	10%

ASD2, atrial septal defect, secundum type; BAV, bicuspid aortic valve; COA, coarctation; CVM, cardiovascular malformation; PAPVR, partial anomalous venous return; and VSD, ventricular septal defect.
From Lin AE (2000). Management of cardiac problems. In Saenger P, Pasquino AM (eds.), *Optimizing health care for Turner patients in the 21st century: Proceedings of the 5th International Symposium on Turner Syndrome, Naples, Italy.* Amsterdam: Elsevier Science 115–123.

TABLE 15-5

Prevalence of Congenital Heart Disease and Relative Risk in Turner Patients and in the General Population

	Turner Patients (%)	General Population (%)	Relative Risk
Congenital heart disease	22.9 (136)	2	11.4
Bicuspid aortic valve	12.5 (74)	1.28	9.8
Coarctation of the aorta	6.9 (41)	0.043	160.5
Aortic valve disease	3.2 (19	0.035	91.4
Partial anomalous pulmonary discharge	2.9 (17)	0.009	320
Ostium secundum atrial septal defect	2.2 (13)	0.064	34.4
Ventricular septal defect	0.5 (3)	0.188	2.7
Atrioventricular septal defect	0.2 (1)		

From Mazzanti L, et al. (2000). Italian Turner syndrome study: Cardiac function and complications. In Saenger PH, Pasquino AM (eds.), *Optimizing health care for Turner patients in the 21st century: Proceedings of the 5th International Symposium on Turner Syndrome, Naples, Italy.* Amsterdam: Elsevier Science 125–136.

intracardiac blood flow. A more recent pathologic examination of 12 fetuses with Turner phenotype of nuchal cystic hygromas found that 75% had left-sided flow defects and aberrations of the lymphatics at the base of the heart.[268]

These cystic hygromas resolve as lymphatic ducts open in later gestation but often result in residual webbing of the neck. Finally, Miyabara and co-workers[269] analyzed 13 fetuses with 45,X karyotypes with cystic hygroma and documented that almost all had bicuspid aortic valves and many tubular hypoplasias of the aortic arch. They postulated that a homeobox gene or genes,

not SHOX, could be responsible for what appears to be a generalized hypoplasia of tissues of the fourth branchial arch. This further confirms a relationship between the nuchal hygroma/webbed neck phenotype and the cardiac defects found clinically in the 45,X karyotype.

Mazzanti and co-workers[259] showed that a 45,X karyotype is more likely to be associated with webbing, more severe CVMs, and in particular coarctation and partial anomalous pulmonary venous return. We and others also showed a similar association between the webbed neck phenotype and coarctation.[253,269] In contrast, X-structural abnormalities are more likely to be associated with bicuspid aortic valve and aortic valve disease. Less frequent than a left-sided obstruction, CVMs are membranous ventricular septal defects, secundum-type atrial septal defects, partial anomalous pulmonary venous return, and mitral valve prolapse.[259-262,268]

Another cardiovascular abnormality that occurs in Turner syndrome is aortic dilation, dissection, or rupture. Approximately 90% of the cases of dissection or rupture had an associated cardiac malformation, including previous coarctation, "pseudocoarctation," bicuspid aortic valve, or some degree of hypertension.[271] Other large series of Turner syndrome patients have also provided data on aortic root dilation, although the prevalence and natural history remain incomplete.[259,260,262] One large series of 244 patients followed in a Turner syndrome clinic in Seattle, Washington, provided both cross-sectional and longitudinal data about cardiac anomalies.[262] The frequency of aortic dilation was not reported, but aortic dissection occurred in three patients (1%): one with chest trauma, one with previous coarctation repair, and one with chronic hypertension and obesity.

We also analyzed the responses of 245 of 1,000 members of the Turner's Syndrome Society of the United States.[261] Confirmation of karyotype, however, was not obtained. Thirty-five percent were 10 years of age or younger, and a substantial 14% were 41 years or older. Among all respondents, 15 (6%) reported aortic dilation (8% of those who had specifically been evaluated). Of those reporting dilation, 80% reported having a CVM— usually bicuspid aortic valve, aortic valve stenosis, or coarctation (alone or in combination).

About two-thirds of the patients with aortic dilation were younger than 21 years of age, and most had an associated CVM. However, two of the three patients who had aortic dilation without a CVM or other risk factor were also in this younger age group. Despite the limitations of a self-reporting survey, the study provided a conservative estimate of the frequency of aortic dilation. The vast majority of Turner syndrome patients in this survey and the literature have an associated risk factor for aortic dilation. Nevertheless, of concern to patients and health care professionals are the small number in whom there is no risk factor.[272,273]

Figure 15-19 and Figure 15-20 demonstrates the utility of echocardiography in assessment of the aortic root, as well as of MRI in the imaging of the entire aorta. A prospective study of thoracic cardiovascular MRI of 40 girls with Turner syndrome revealed an overall frequency of anomalies of more than 45%.[274] These included not only bicuspid aortic valve (17.5%) and aortic coarctation

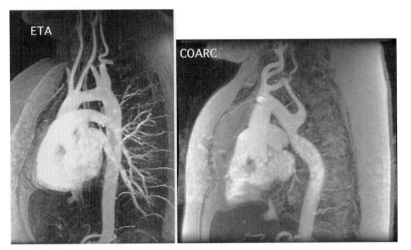

Figure 15-19 Cardiac imaging in Turner syndrome. In older children, MRI is the preferred study because it gives better resolution. In younger children, ultrasonography is still the method of choice. This panel shows coarctation of the aorta (R) and elongated transverse aortic arch (ETA) (L), which my lead to coarctation. Courtesy of C. Bonoly.

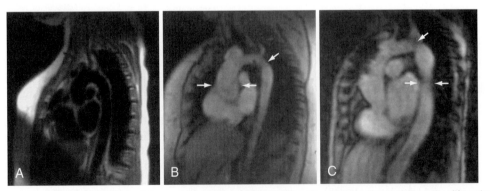

Figure 15-20 Three examples of coarctation of the aorta as seen on MRI studies. Please note the poststenotic dilatation, seen especially in panels B and C. Courtesy of G. Conway.

(12.5%) but dilated ascending aorta (12.5%). Aortic coarctation and bicuspid aortic valve are each almost fourfold more frequent in patients with webbed necks (e.g., 37% of patients with neck webbing have a BAV, compared to 12% in those without webbing).[275]

The authors point out that three of five aortic coarctations and four of five ascending aortic dilations were solely detected with MRI and were not evident on echocardiographic examination. Thus, these findings and other series[276,278] suggest an MRI is a valuable adjunct in the cardiovascular evaluation of girls with Turner syndrome. In fact, MRI may dectect coarcation missed by echocardiography in infancy.[279-281] The risks associated with BAV in Turner syndrome are probably similar to those for nonsyndromic cases. The abnormal valve is at risk for infective endocarditis, and over time it may deteriorate—leading to clinically significant aortic stenosis or regurgitation. BAV can also be associated with aortic wall abnormalirties, including ascending aortic diltation, aneurysm formation, and aortic dissection.[282]

Recent studies suggest a broader spectrum of CVM than previously recognized. Magnetic resonance angiographic (MRA) screening studies of asymptomatic inviduals with Turner syndrome have identified a high prevalence of vascular anomalies of uncertain clinical significance. Almost 50 have an unusual elongation and angulation of the aortic arch termed *elongated transverse arch* (ETA) by Ho et al.[280] This may reflect an abnormal aortic wall prone to dilation. Additional anomalies are partial anomalous pulmonary connection (PAPVC) and persistent left superior vena cava, affecting 13 versus <1% b in the general population. Whether this defect is clinically significant depends on the degree of the left to right shunt.[283-285] There seems to be a generalized dilation of major vessels in women with Turner syndrome, including the brachial and carotid arteries as well as the aorta. The distal extent of this vasculopathy is unknown. Estrogen deficiency contributes to greater intima medial thickness and altered arterial wall dynamics but not the increased caliber of the vessels[286-287] (Figure 15-19).

The data from this group and another using echocardiography suggest that aortic root diameters are greater in 45,X patients than in matched controls.[288] Whereas both studies compared aortic root dimensions to body surface area, which in a condition of short stature may not be the appropriate control group (may be more appropriate to match for age),[271] the findings suggest a degree of intrinsic primary abnormality. Pathologic evidence of cystic medial necrosis is reported in some cases of dissection and suggests that the intrinsic disorder might represent an example of a mesenchymal defect in Turner syndrome. This may explain the increased incidence of mitral valve prolapse as well.

Alternatively, the tendency toward significant aortic root dilation may be related to the intrauterine hemodynamic events that are a consequence of the lymphatic disorder. The longitudinal survey report that 25% of normal patients had increased aortic root diameters 2 years after the first study[277] (coupled with a report that death from aortic dissection was greatly in excess of that expected in a large prospective study of Turner syndrome patients registered with a karyotype registry[289]) prompted

us to adopt an aggressive approach to diagnosis, follow-up, and risk factor management in these patients. Data at present are not adequate to recommend routine prophylaxis with beta-blocking drugs, although this therapy may be appropriate for those with significant aortic root dilation (e.g., Marfan syndrome)—especially those with bicuspid aortic valve.[290]

Of particular importance is the increased risk of aortic dissection in pregnancy among Turner syndrome women.[291] As more Turner syndrome women contemplate pregnancy, it seems prudent to identify those with aortic root dilation before the pregnancy. Those with a previous risk factor (bicuspid aortic valve, coarctation, hypertension) should be monitored very closely. Those women without abnormal risk factors also require close attention.[236,291-296]

It is also clear from reports of a high incidence of unclassified murmurs and from early patient series[297] that the incidence of aortic valvular abnormalities is also increased in Turner syndrome. With the introduction of echocardiography, we were able to undertake a study of the frequency of this association.[256] Of 67 patients without coarctation studied with two-dimensional or M-mode echocardiography (or both), 20 (almost 30%) have findings characteristic of bicuspid aortic valve. Some of these valves are anatomically tricuspid but have eccentric closure and are functionally bicuspid, whereas the majority are actually bicuspid.

Our data, and the more recent confirmatory data from Mazzanti and co-workers,[259] indicate that the percentage distribution of patients with isolated bicuspid valve does not appear to be confined to any karyotype—nor does there appear to be a preponderance of the webbed neck phenotype. Thus, bicuspid aortic valve not only may be more common than coarctation but may represent a more fundamental manifestation of an X chromosome defect in Turner syndrome. We also diagnosed six patients as having mitral valve prolapse (Barlow syndrome), a finding confirmed by a second group.[257] The frequency, 10% to 15%, is in excess of that believed to be the occurrence rate in the population at large.[298]

Mazzanti and co-workers also found a significant number of patients with partial anomalous pulmonary venous return, a rare malformation, and thus the malformation with the highest relative risk of occurrence compared with normals[259] (Table 15-5). In a follow-up study of adult Turner women, only 11 of 25 adult women with Turner syndrome had normal cardiac findings using a combined echocardiography and MRI screen of the aorta. Twelve had aortic root dilation, three had bicuspid aortic valve, and five had pseudocoarctation of the aorta.[299] Finally, hypoplastic left heart syndrome has been described during prenatal echocardiography[266]—and four Turner syndrome infants are described in a large outcome study, with limited survival in two.[267]

Adults with Turner syndrome have a high prevalence of electrcardiographic conduction and repolarization abnormalities, as well as prolonged QT intervals. Therefore, monitoring of echocardiograms (ECGs) in Turner syndrome appears warranted.[300] In addition to congenital structural anomalies, there are several acquired cardiac problems that have been noted in Turner syndrome women—although their prevalence is not well established. In some series, hypertension occurs in about 15% to 25% of girls (and in a larger percentage of adults with Turner syndrome).[259,262,301,302] A threefold relative risk for high blood pressure was noted in Denmark, but patients with repaired coarctation had not been removed from the sample.[303]

Stratification by age and weight has not been performed. Several large series from different countries also support an increased prevalence of hypertension. These analyses did not consistently analyze patients based on age, weight, and coarctation repair. Nevertheless, in the Danish study of morbidity in Turner syndrome women along with hypertension there were also marked increases in ischemic heart disease and stroke.[303] In a Swedish morbidity study, cardiac anomalies and hypertension were common but plasma lipid levels did not differ from those of normal subjects.[304]

Although a renovascular abnormality is considered the most likely mechanism for development of hypertension, especially in younger patients, obvious structural renal lesions are not always present. Similarly, a history of infectious nephritis or even urinary tract infection is usually absent. Thus, in the majority of patients the cause of the hypertension is unknown. In our series, nine patients with hypertension were identified and in only one did it appear to be of renovascular origin (Figure 15-21). One of the earliest abnormalities in blood pressure regulation is the disappearance of the physiologic nighttime dipping in blood pressure as prodromal state of hypertension[61] (Table 15-6). Systemic hypertension is an important risk factor for aortic dilation and dissection. Therefore, blood pressure should be monitored frequently and treated vigorously in all patients with Turner syndrome.

If the baseline ECG reveals a significantly prolonged QTc, medications that might further prolong the QT should be avoided.[61] There was no apparent relationship to any particular karyotype or phenotype. Other infrequent abnormalities include endocardial fibroelastosis[258] and cardiomyopathy.[305] In two studies of Turner syndrome girls without major cardiac abnormalities who received GH treatment there was no evidence of left ventricular hypertrophy or hypertension.[194,195] In one, after 7 years there was no significant dilation of the aorta (S.M.P.F. de Muinck Keizer-Schrama, MD, personal communication).

TABLE 15-6

Cardiovascular Screening and Monitoring Algorithm for Girls and Women with Turner Syndrome

Screening (All Patients at Time of Diagnosis)
- Evaluation by cardiologist with expertise in congenital heart disease.
- Comprehensive exam, including blood pressure in all extremities.
- All require clear imaging of heart, aortic valve, aortic arch, and pulmonary veins.
- Echocardiography is usually adequate for infants and young girls.
- MRI and echo for older girls and adults.
- ECG.

Monitoring (Follow-up Depends on Clinical Situation)
- For patients with apparently normal cardiovascular system and age-appropriate blood pressure.
  - Reevaluation with imaging at timely occasions (e.g., at transition to adult clinic), before attempting pregnancy, or with appearance of hypertension. Girls that have only had echocardiography should undergo MRI when old enough to cooperate with the procedure.
  - Otherwise, imaging about every 5 to 10 years.
- For patients with cardiovascular pathology, treatment and monitoring determined by cardiologist.

From Bondy CA for the Turner Syndrome Study Group (2007). Care of girls and women with Turner syndrome. *J Clin Endocrinol and Metab* 92(1):10–25.

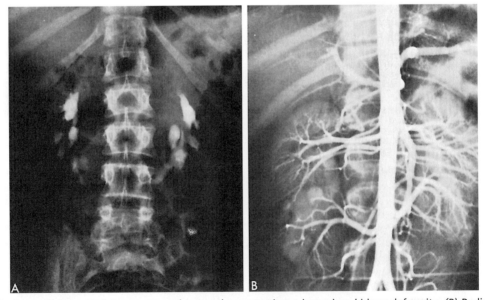

Figure 15-21 *(A)* Radiograph from an intravenous pyelogram demonstrating a horseshoe kidney deformity. *(B)* Radiograph after an aortic injection, illustrating multiple renal arteries in a patient with Turner syndrome and hypertension.

Ongoing Cardiac Care

For the patient with no identified cardiovascular defects, routine pediatric care is advised with continued monitoring of blood pressure. It seems also prudent to reevaluate aortic dimension at 5- to 10-year intervals. Patients with significant cardiovascular defects need continued monotoring by a cardiologist, with frequency of monitoring determined by circumstances. Children considered at increased risk for hypertension should be educated about this risk, the need for compliance with medical monitoring and treatment, and the possible presenting symptoms (e.g., chest or back pain). Patients with multiple risk factors (BAV, dilated aortic root, hypertension) that put them at high risk for aortic deterioration might want to consider carrrying a medical ID bracelet. They also need to be informed that prophylactic antibiotics should be given before dental procedures or surgery.

MONITORING FOR AORTIC DILATION

All measurements of the aorta should be done at end systole. The ascending aorta should be measured at the level of the annulus at the hinge points of the valve, at the level of the sinuses of valsalva perpendicular to the ascending aorta long axis, and at the ascending aorta 10 mm above the sinotubular junction. Normative data for aortic diameters as a function of body surface area are available.[282,286,306] Review of available data suggests that unadjusted values greater than 28 to 32 mm will identify patients with diameters greater than 95% of controls, which would clearly be abnormal for women with Turner syndrome who are generally smaller. When aortic root enlargement is found, medical therapy and detailed imaging is recommended.

In hypertensive patients with aortic root enlargement who also have resting tachycardia, beta adrenergic receptor blockade is an excellent therapeutic option. Beta-blockers have been shown to reduce the rate of aortic dilation and dissection in Marfan syndrome,[307] although efficacy in treating aortic dilation in Turner syndrome has not yet been investigated.

Heart-healthy exercise with moderate aerobic exercise is emphasized and should be encouraged. Eligibility for competitive sports for all those with Turner syndrome should be determined by a cardiologist after a comprehensive evaluation that includes an MRI of the aorta. Experts polled on this issue at the most recent Turner syndrome guidelines meeting agreed that aortic enlargement in Turner syndrome may be defined as an aortic sinus of valsalva or ascending aorta, body size adjusted Z score >2 plus evidence of increasing Z score on a subsequent imaging study of the aorta or a single Z score >3. In those cases, participation in competitive sports is contraindicated.[308]

PREGNANCY AND CARDIAC CARE

Spontaneous or assisted pregnancy in Turner syndrome should be undertaken only after thorough cardiac evaluation. Alarming reports of fatal aortic dissection during pregnancy and the postpartum period have raised concern about the safety of pregnancy in Turner syndrome. If pregnancy is being considered, preconception assessment must include cardiology evaluation with imaging of the aorta. A history of surgically repaired cardiovascular defect, the presence of BAV, or current evidence of aortic dilation or systemic hypertension should probably be considered as relative contraindications to pregnancy.[309]

GROWTH HORMONE TREATMENT AND THE CARDIOVASCULAR SYSTEM

Several echocardiographic studies reported normal left ventricular and septal morphology and function in GH-treated girls with Turner syndrome,[310] and two recent MR studies found no deleterious effect of GH treatment on aortic diameter[311] or compliance.[312] It is particularly reassuring that when adult Dutch Turner women were examined for aortic distensibility and the effects of growth hormone on aortic dimensions the patients who had received the higher growth hormones doses (47 mg/kg/week) had better cardiac health based on the parameters measured.[312]

In regard to the lymphatic system, abnormalities of cardiovascular and lymphatic development are found in most TS fetuses that fail to survive the first trimester.[21,269,313] For those girls who survive, the residua of the fetal lymphedema and cystic hygromas are peripheral lymphedema and webbed neck. Often the newborn lymphedema resolves by 2 years of age without therapy. It may recur at any age and may be associated with initiation of GH or estrogen therapy. Some children and adolescents may require support stockings. Complete decongestive physiotherapy (a four-step process involving skin and nail care, massage for manual lymph drainage, compression bandaging, and a subsequent remedial exercise regimen) is recommended for those with more significant lymphedema.[314] Long-term diuretic use should be avoided, as should vascular surgery. Families should be directed to the National Lymphedema Network (*http://www.lymphnet.org*) for more information.[61]

RENAL AND RENOVASCULAR ABNORMALITIES

Renal and renovascular abnormalities occur in Turner syndrome with greatly increased frequency. Although the incidence varies from 25% to 70% among different series reported,[315-319] the abnormalities tend to be of three specific types: those that primarily involve the pelvocaliceal collecting system, such as complete or partial duplication; those associated with the position and alignment of the organ, such as horseshoe kidney and retrocaval ureter; and those associated with abnormal vascular supply. In a recent study,[320] no patient with a normal baseline ultrasound developed renal disease during a follow-up period averaging 6 years. However, some of those with malformations developed hypertension and urinary tract infections.

The development of the collecting system begins with the formation of the ureteric bud, its dorsocranial migration, and its penetration of the metanephric blastema. At about 5 weeks of gestation it dilates into a primitive pelvis and simultaneously splits into cranial and caudal portions—forming the future major calyces. Thus, duplications of the collecting system are caused by abnormal or early splitting of the ureteric bud at or before 5 fetal weeks and are therefore primary malformations of organogenesis. Conversely, the upward migration of the already preformed kidney from its position in the pelvis to the lumbar region is a somewhat later event. The kidney must pass through the arterial fork formed by the umbilical arteries, and if there are disturbances in either the anatomy of these vessels or the path of migration secondary positional malformations occur. If one kidney fails to traverse the arterial fork, it will remain ectopically in the pelvis. If there is a partial mechanical effect on the kidney during migration, rotational abnormalities may result.

The vascular supply of the kidneys may be anomalous (Figure 15-20B), secondary to the multiple budding segments of the kidney, the final positioning, or the presence of an aberrant vessel crossing the upper renal pole. Finally, the horseshoe kidney [which occurs with increased frequency (Figure 15-20A)] may represent a primary defect in embryogenesis resulting in the union of the two metanephric blastemas or a secondary defect caused by malposition of the umbilical arteries.

In the experience of Lippe et al.[142] patients studied with intravenous pyelography, with contrast medium enhancement at the time of cardiac catheterization, or with ultrasonography we found that 47 patients (33%) had some structural. The lesions we detected covered the spectrum of defects described previously, except that we did not have a case of retrocaval ureter.[321,322] Ultrasound, as the initial screening method in recent years, was effective in demonstrating all anomalies previously seen with intravenous pyelography except for mild clinically insignificant rotational abnormalities.

Although the overall morbidity of the renal lesions is relatively low (with only four patients requiring surgery, one requiring long-term antibiotic therapy, and four having an absent kidney), the potential for caliceal obstruction, parenchymal infection, and secondary renal impairment is real—and we therefore suggest that all patients should undergo an ultrasound imaging study. The high percentage of horseshoe kidneys (up to 7%[320]) merits further comment because there may be an increased incidence of Wilms' tumor in the horseshoe kidney.[322]

If the increased incidence of Wilms' tumor results from an abnormal proliferation of the metanephric blastema and if that were the mechanism in Turner syndrome, these patients would be at the same risk as other patients with a horseshoe kidney—and the incidence of Wilms' tumor in Turner syndrome should be high. Alternatively, if the mechanism in Turner syndrome is vascular these patients should be at no greater risk for Wilms' tumor than the general population. At present, only one patient with both Wilms' tumor and Turner syndrome has been reported—suggesting that the latter hypothesis is correct. In a recent paper by Sagi et al.,[316] kidney malformations were exclusively found in those patients who had retained the maternal X chromosome.

UNKNOWN METABOLIC FACTORS

Autoimmune Disorders

An apparent increased frequency of autoimmune disorders has been noted in patients with Turner syndrome. The reason for this increase is unknown, but it has been theorized that families with a high frequency of autoimmune diseases may be prone to nondisjunctional events. This hypothesis is based on the observations that there is also an increased frequency of autoimmune disorders in other nondisjunctional chromosomal disorders, such as Down and Klinefelter syndromes, and that when the families of patients with Turner and Down syndromes are investigated autoimmune disease appears to be reported or diagnosed frequently. It should be noted, however, that these studies were retrospective and did not test the parents for antibodies at the time of delivery.

A recent prospective study of thyroid antibody positivity as a risk factor for nondisjunction failed to show an association.[323] A second theory that autoimmune diseases might result from, or be associated with, genes or gene mutations on the X chromosome is supported by the increased incidence of these disorders in X chromosomal disorders as well as by their increased incidence in women. A third theory, that familial (maternal) autoimmunity may lead to the preferential survival of a fetus with chromosomal aneuploidy (albeit a general risk for pregnancy loss),[324] remains to be investigated.

The most prevalent autoimmune disorder in Turner syndrome appears to be Hashimoto lymphocytic thyroiditis. Depending on the series reported and on the methods used to measure the antibodies, the prevalence of significant titers may be as high as 50%.[210] Although originally described in association with structurally abnormal X chromosomes, notably the isoX,[325] increased titers of antithyroid antibodies with or without thyroid failure have been reported in 45,X individuals as well as in patients with mosaic karyotypes without a structurally abnormal X (i.e., 45,X/46,XX).[326-328]

In our series, approximately 30% of patients have positive antithyroid antibodies at the time of first testing. Of six patients who were overtly hypothyroid, however, two did not have abnormal antibody titers at the time of diagnosis. This is not unexpected because it is well known that children with biopsy-proven Hashimoto thyroiditis often do not have abnormal titers of circulating antithyroid antibodies.[329] The clinical picture of overt hypothyroidism in Turner syndrome may be different from the normal population because it has been reported that even severely affected individuals may not show any signs or symptoms of the disease.[330] This, coupled with the high frequency, mandates periodic screening of all Turner syndrome patients.

There are reports that indicate that Grave's hyperthyroidism[331] may also occur more commonly than previously recognized in girls with Turner syndrome, and we have one affected girl in our series. One report notes that in one patient during the hyperthyroid phase there was a marked increase in growth velocity.[332] Final height, however, did not appear to be adversely or positively influenced. In a recent study, 24% of 84 children (0–19 years old) with Turner syndrome who were followed (longitudinally mean duration = 8 years) developd hypothyroidism (and 2.5% developd hyperthyroidism).[333] Thyroid disease has been reported as early as 4 years.[334] Therefore, all patients with Turner syndrome should be screened annually for autoimmune thyroid disease with a TSH and a free T4 level from 4 years of age onward.

We also have two patients with vitiligo and three with alopecia. Other forms of polyglandular autoimmunity (such as Addison disease, hypoparathyroidism, and pernicious anemia) have not been noted to be increased in frequency in Turner syndrome patients. The association of juvenile rheumatoid arthritis and Turner syndrome had only been reported in single case reports until the study of Zulian and colleagues.[335]

The authors conducted a survey of 28 pediatric rheumatology centers (15 U.S., 10 European, 3 Canadian) comprising an aggregate patient population of some 15,000 patients. Eighteen cases of juvenile rheumatoid arthritis were found in patients with Turner syndrome, of which 7 were polyarticular and 11 monoarticular. The authors calculated that this represented a sixfold increase over what would be expected, thus strongly suggesting an association between Turner syndrome and the occurrence of juvenile rheumatoid arthritis. The karyotypes of the affected individuals varied, but there appeared to be a predominance of 45,X patients with the more severe polyarticular form.

Gastrointestinal Disorders

A number of reports have called attention to gastrointestinal bleeding, often massive, occurring in patients with Turner syndrome.[336,337] The bleeding has been ascribed to intestinal telangiectasia, hemangiomatoses, phlebectasia, or dilated veins and venules. These vascular malformations occur without evidence of mesenteric, portal, or hepatic vascular abnormalities—which suggests a developmental rather than acquired cause. They do not appear to be associated with cutaneous hemangiomas reported in some Turner syndrome patients, however.[338] It is not known which patients may be at risk for development of vascular bleeding. Whether these vascular abnormalities are a consequence of the same obstructive processes that result in the lymphedema is not known.

Because large segments of bowel may be involved, we recommend conservative management when possible to avoid massive resections. If the patient has discontinued estrogen-progesterone replacement therapy, we recommend that it be reinstituted because this therapy appears to be efficacious in treating the bleeding of severe gastrointestinal vascular malformations[339] and was reported as appearing to help one affected patient with Turner syndrome.[340]

A second cause of gastrointestinal bleeding and dysfunction appears to be inflammatory bowel disease. Several reports suggest an increased incidence of Crohn disease and ulcerative colitis in infants and children with Turner syndrome.[341-345] Whether this increase may represent another autoimmune phenomenon or is associated with a particular genetic haplotype (HLA type) that may also prove to be increased in Turner syndrome remains

to be established. Similarly, there is no conclusive evidence for a genetic or familial predisposition to ulcerative colitis in these patients. Because growth retardation and delayed sexual maturation are characteristic manifestations of inflammatory bowel disease and of Turner syndrome, careful attention must be paid to the review of systems in these patients. Conversely, short girls with inflammatory bowel disease and growth and pubertal delay may need assessment of gonadal function (measurement of gonadotropins) before their sexual delay is ascribed to their bowel disease alone.

Celiac disease is also being detected in Turner syndrome patients in frequencies that may exceed ethnic population norms.[346-348] There is also a suggestion that this may occur in association with immunoglobulin A deficiency, a known risk factor for the development of celiac disease.[337] Considering that growth failure and pubertal delay can be manifestations of celiac disease and Turner syndrome, consideration has to be given to testing short girls with celiac disease with or without pubertal delay (especially if they are on dietary management and have not had catch-up growth) for Turner syndrome. In addition, the issue is raised whether screening girls with Turner syndrome for celiac disease is warranted in the absence of clinical symptoms.

Based on recent data, the risk of celiac disease is increased in Turner syndrome (up to 6% of individuals are affected). Turner syndrome girls should be screened by measurement of tissue tranglutaminase IgA antibodies. Periodic screening is best begun at age 4, and should be repeated every 2 to 5 years.[349,350] Whereas hepatic abnormalities have not in the past been reported to be a typical finding in Turner syndrome individuals, a report by Salerno and co-workers[201] references 10 papers that describe a range of hepatic disorders/dysfunction in children and adults with Turner syndrome. A second paper[351] describes three additional adult patients with varying forms of hepatic disease. In the pediatric age group, Salerno's group followed some 70 girls prospectively for a mean of 7.6 years for the development of increased hepatic serum enzymes. They found a significant increase in liver enzymes in 20% over time. The majority appeared to be associated with the institution of oral androgen therapy for growth promotion or oral estrogen therapy for feminization, which were reversed with cessation of drug therapy.

That the association was with the estrogen and not the progestational agent is supported by a previous report.[352] As previously discussed, GH replacement does not appear to be associated with this finding. Among Salerno's patients,[201] however, were several who were thought to have autoimmune disease (one associated with celiac disease and one with hypergammaglobulinemia and a biopsy consistent with autoimmune hepatitis). In addition, two patients had mild steatofibrosis of unknown cause. Thus, there may be an increase (starting in childhood) in evidence of mild hepatic dysfunction from a variety of causes.

Steatosis, steatofibrosis, and steatohepatitis are frequently seen.[353] In a review of the Danish Cytogenetic Central Registry, a cohort of more than 500 adult patients with Turner syndrome was identified.[303] These were cross referenced against the Danish National Registry of Patients to obtain data on first hospitalization diagnoses for these patients. Statistical analysis was done by comparing the patients with population controls to determine the relative risks for the diagnoses given.

The relative risk for a diagnosis of cirrhosis of the liver was 5.69 (1.55 to 14.56). Therefore, adult Turner syndrome individuals appear to be at risk for progressive hepatic disease. Regular monitoring of hepatic enzymes, at least in adults, may be indicated. Consideration can be given to using transdermal estrogen therapy rather than oral therapy in girls and women who appear to show liver abnormalities because the transdermal route results in fewer effects on hepatic metabolism than does the oral route.[354] Conversely, a study of transdermal estrogen replacement therapy in young healthy women with Turner syndrome showed mildly elevated liver enzymes at the time of estrogen washout—which normalized with oral estrogen replacement.[355] Thus, multiple mechanisms for the liver enzyme abnormalities appear to be operative.

CARBOHYDRATE TOLERANCE

The high incidence of carbohydrate intolerance, including frank diabetes in patients with Turner syndrome, has been documented over the past 40 years.[356-359] In our series, 40% of patients tested with oral glucose tolerance tests showed abnormal responses.[360] The clinical features are those of type 2 diabetes mellitus. Patients are non insulin dependent and are not ketosis prone. The abnormality may be reflected in a hyperglycemic response to oral glucose or to a meal, or it may progress to fasting hyperglycemia and polyuria. Insulin levels in the serum may be elevated, in the normal range, or low.

Some genetic evidence suggests that the diabetes is the familial type 2 variety because abnormal or borderline glucose tolerance tests have been demonstrated in 51% of parents of patients.[360] In that series, however, only one parent had clinical diabetes—which is far fewer than the usual clinical expression in type 2 families. Type 1 diabetes mellitus is infrequent, and in children most reports indicate that it is not in excess of that seen in the childhood population. There are no data on islet cell antibodies or glutamic acid decarboxylase antibodies available in Turner syndrome patients.

The metabolic/endocrine abnormality most frequently reported in children and adolescents with Turner syndrome not receiving GH replacement therapy is a greater glucose response to an oral glucose challenge than that noted in age-matched control subjects.[361,362] Insulin responses vary from series to series, and when increased in young patients may be related to concomitant androgen or estrogen therapy. Particularly, oxandrolone has been shown to be causing higher insulin levels in glucose tolerance tests than GH alone.[363,364]

When the metabolic defect was studied with a euglycemic insulin clamp technique to evaluate insulin sensitivity, and with indirect calorimetry to study whole-body glucose and lipid oxidation, insulin resistance was documented.[365] The defect appeared to be restricted to nonoxidative pathways of intracellular glucose metabolism and was present in a group of young girls who had never received any form of hormone therapy. The authors concluded that the defect is similar to that found in type 2 diabetes mellitus. These data suggest that in naive patients with Turner syndrome insulin resistance is a very early metabolic defect. Other groups have not found this abnormality, however. A possible explanation may be the fact that the clamp studies were methodologically different, employing differing insulin levels.[366]

A number of physiologic factors are known to be associated with this form of diabetes. Their role in contributing to the insulin resistance of Turner syndrome has not been clearly documented. Obesity per se could be a factor, but when assessed by measurements of skin-fold thickness the majority of the patients are not obese.[367] When this method was used in conjunction with standards for ideal body weight appropriate for height and age, we found that the degree of fat or percentage of ideal body weight did nor correlate with their carbohydrate intolerance.[360] In the study by Caprio and colleagues,[365] body mass index alone was used and there was no correlation between body mass index and insulin-stimulated glucose metabolism.

Estrogen-progesterone replacement therapy is known to be associated with changes in carbohydrate tolerance. Data now suggest that it is the chemical structure of the progestins used in oral contraceptives that contributes most to the defect.[367] In Turner syndrome, the use of estrogen replacement is probably not an important factor in pathogenesis or progression of insulin resistance. In a 6-month intervention study in adult Turner syndrome patients, a deterioration took place in the glycemic response during treatment with sex hormones (without a change in insulin sensitivity)—although a significant reduction in the level of fasting insulin was seen.[368] Others have found a slight improvement in glycemia and insulin when formally testing insulin sensitivity.[369] Longer-term treatment with sex hormones may show an improvement in the indices of carbohydrate metabolism, perhaps partly through the expedient effects of sex hormone replacement on physical fitness, body composition, and blood pressure. Hormone replacement therapy did have a beneficial effect on aortic stiffness and cholesterol levels.[370]

The use of GH alone or in combination with anabolic steroids has prompted a reassessment of the carbohydrate status of girls with Turner syndrome, with specific focus on the effects of these agents. In a study of 71 girls enrolled in the previously discussed GH/oxandrolone protocol of Rosenfeld and colleagues,[146] glucose tolerance status was evaluated acutely (before and after 5 days) and after longer-term (2 and 12 months) administration of GH alone, oxandrolone alone, or combination therapy. Pretreatment fasting glucose concentrations were normal in the Turner syndrome patients, but their glucose responses to an oral glucose challenge were higher than in control subjects—with 15% classified as having impaired glucose tolerance. Insulin responses were so varied as to be impossible, as a group, to distinguish from normal. After acute or chronic GH therapy, carbohydrate tolerance as measured by integrated insulin or glucose responses did not change in the GH group.[371]

In the Dutch Turner syndrome study, in which there was a higher than conventional GH treatment group, Hgb

A1c levels did not change from baseline yet decreased after discontinuation of GH treatment.[200] Although there was clearly a trend toward higher fasting insulin levels with the higher GH doses after 4 years of treatment, no significant differences in the change of fasting insulin level or area under the curve for insulin between the GH dosage groups were found. After a mean period of 7.3 years of treatment, insulin levels decreased to values close to or equal to pretreatment values after discontinuation of GH treatment. Long-term results of the effect of GH treatment on lipid metabolism showed no abnormal effects.[196]

In another analysis of U.S. patients treated with GH, mean Hgb A1c levels also remained within the low to middle end of the normal range. Fasting insulin levels remained unchanged, whereas postprandial insulin levels rose and yet remained within the normal range at the 5-year mark.[372] In a few patients, insulin responses were studied after GH was discontinued. Levels returned to normal except in those patients markedly obese (P.H. Saenger, unpublished data). Although the reversibility of the effects of long-term GH is reassuring, the consequences of hyperinsulinism lasting for several years during GH therapy are still unknown.

In summary, glucose-stimulated insulin responses may be increased in children with Turner syndrome whether or not they are treated with GH, but these alterations may be further exaggerated by GH treatment[373,374]—with hyperinsulinemic responses appearing to compensate for reductions in insulin sensitivity.

Data on disease prevalence in adult patients with Turner syndrome suggest an increased incidence of both type 2 and type 1 diabetes mellitus, suggesting an influence of haploinsufficiency of genes on the X chromosome. In adults, the relative risk of type 2 diabetes mellitus was 11.56%. The relative risk of type 1 diabetes mellitus was 4.38%. Because these data are from a medical registry, the risk of misclassification between type 2 diabetes mellitus and type 1 diabetes mellitus cannot be ruled out. The relative risk of diabetes certainly does not seem to be below 2, however. The increased risk for type 2 diabetes mellitus may be secondary to the increased prevalence of obesity in adult women with Turner syndrome.[303,368,369] The data on lipid metabolism are more heterogenous and more studies are needed to determine whether or not lipid metabolism is really altrered in Turner syndrome.[370]

Neuropsychological Features

The consensus regarding the currently available evidence is that the intelligence of persons with Turner syndrome is normal. There does not appear to be an increased incidence of moderate or severe mental retardation, nor do the individuals differ from their siblings in overall intelligence.[375] The only clearly documented association among karyotype, phenotype, and the occurrence of mental retardation is the presence of a small ring X chromosome.[6-10] In these patients, the high risk of mental retardation is most likely caused by the lack of lyonization of the ring X from loss of the X inactivation center—thus creating disomy for some X genes (see section on X chromosome genes).

Of note is a report from 1973 of two severely retarded institutionalized patients with the Turner syndrome phenotype. In these patients, in addition to the 45,X karyotype extrachromosomal material (believed to be of chromosome 21 in origin) was described.[316] Thus, some of the earlier reports of mental retardation[16] may be the result of a small ring X or unrecognized coexistent autosomal aneuploidy—a condition recognized to occur in association with Turner syndrome. We have also found a potential physiologic or genetic correlate with IQ. In a group of 33 Turner syndrome patients who underwent neuropsychological testing, we also tested for thyroid autoimmunity.[377]

The group of 9 girls who had positive antithyroid microsomal antibodies had significantly lower verbal and full-scale IQ scores than the 24 patients in the antibody negative group and the 24 control children. Although overt hypothyroidism was not the mechanism, subclinical or variably transient periods of hypothyroidism could not be ruled out. Alternatively, because thyroid autoimmunity may be familial two other explanations are tenable. One is that the mothers of these patients had subclinical hypothyroidism, a mechanism now documented to account for statistically lower IQ scores in their offspring.[378] A second is that there may be a genetic linkage of autoimmunity and learning disability. At this time, we consider that thyroid autoimmunity may be a marker of cognitive impairment in Turner syndrome and recommend early screening; periodic follow-up of thyroid function, including autoantibodies; and careful developmental assessment.

Whereas individuals with Turner syndrome have normal intelligence and are characterized by normal verbal skills, they have selective impairments in nonverbal skills—including visual-spatial information processing, arithmetic skills, and the coordination of motor and visual-perceptual skills[379-381] (coupled in some with a degree of hyperactivity).[382] Studies suggest that these individuals also have an associated movement (motor) problem in daily life that cannot be directly attributed to cognitive dysfunction.[383,384] As a group, Turner syndrome children also exhibit delayed emotional maturity, poor relations with peers, timidity, and negative body image.[385]

This negative body image may also be secondary to the fact that their short stature could negatively affect psychosocial function and self-esteem, although the severity of psychosocial problems associated with short stature is quite variable.[386] Although Rovet and Holland reported a positive correlation between height and social competence in patients with Turner syndrome,[387] in a more recent study no significant changes in psychosocial function were seen during GH therapy of 2 years.[386]

Although almost all investigators concur that specific cognitive deficits are present, the areas of presumed cognitive dysfunction differ in different reports—and interpretation of the results depends on numerous variables relating to the testing instrument and data analysis. The discrepancy between verbal and performance IQ appears to be, however, confirmed by many studies and may range between 10 and 15 points—with verbal being higher than performance.[379-381,388-390]

In a study dividing patients by karyotype, the 45,X group showed the greatest discrepancy compared with patients with the mosaic or the structurally abnormal X group.[388] The performance task was clearly affected and involved mental rotation tasks, particularly of the block design and object assembly type.[320,388] Turner syndrome girls are also described as exhibiting deficits in tasks of left/right discrimination, road map skills, mental rotation, line orientation rotation, and integration of motor and visual-perceptual skills.[382,389]

Abnormalities in the cognitive and psychosocial abilities in persons with Turner syndrome likely reflect underlying atypical brain development and function.[391] Therefore, investigators have attempted to use specific tests of brain function in an attempt to more clearly elucidate the neuropathologic basis for these performance differences as well as to examine the more general question of the role of the sex chromosomes and/or gonadal hormones in brain development and hemispheric specialization. Qualitative and quantitative analyses of electroencephalographic background data suggested transiently appearing hypofunction at the parietal, temporal, and occipital areas.[392] Lateralization, however, was inconsistent. Electrical activity, measured as event-related brain potential and reaction time to auditory stimuli, was assessed in groups of young and older Turner syndrome girls.[393]

Their event-related brain potential data suggested a slower than normal maturational change, whereas their reaction time responses were less than those of control subjects in both age groups. In one study of a pair of prepubertal monozygotic twins discordant for X monosomy, extensive neurobehavioral and anatomic (MRI) data are presented.[394] The data demonstrate that although both sisters scored in the superior range of intelligence the affected twin had a wide discrepancy in her performance compared with her verbal scores, which was not present in the unaffected twin. The neuroanatomic findings for both sisters fell in the range of normal, but there were significant differences between the twins—the relevance of which is unknown.

In a more extensive MRI study comparing 18 adult women with Turner syndrome and appropriate controls, the subjects had significantly smaller values than the control subjects in MRI-measured volumes of multiple nuclei as well as in bilateral parieto-occipital brain matter.[395] The authors postulate that the X chromosome modulates development of gray matter in striatum, diencephalon, and cerebral hemispheres. Others,[396] including the group of Lippe et al.,[397] have used positron emission tomography in an attempt to correlate regional abnormalities in cerebral metabolic rates with neuropsychological profiles.

These initial studies suggest that hypometabolism in the parietal and occipital lobes may be common among Turner syndrome girls with learning disabilities and also may help explain the impaired visual-spatial information processing. In addition, preliminary studies using functional MRI show activation deficits, particularly in the dorsal lateral prefrontal area of the cortex. This area may be related to executive function, another area of deficit observed in women with Turner syndrome,[398] and to-

gether with the other findings may account for the neurobehavioral phenotype in this condition.

Recently published results of neurogenetic research have stimulated interest and controversy. Thus, the differential gene expression known to depend on the parental origin of chromosomes (genomic imprinting) is now being associated with the possibility that in Turner syndrome genes may be differentially expressed according to the origin of the X chromosome present. It is known that in 45,X Turner syndrome the X chromosome is of maternal origin in about 70% to 80.5% of cases.[76-78] Skuse and associates investigated 80 females with Turner syndrome, of whom 25 (the expected proportion) had an X chromosome of paternal origin (Xp). These girls showed satisfactory social adjustment and had higher verbal and executive functional skills than the larger group of girls with the retained X chromosome of maternal origin (Xm).[84]

In an extension of these studies, the Skuse group investigated the relationship of verbal and nonverbal memory with origin of the X chromosome.[399] They observed that 45,Xp Turner females matched controls in verbal memory, whereas this was not the case in the 45,Xm females. In contrast, the results of 45,Xm patients matched those of controls in visual-spatial memory tests but the 45,Xp group did not. The authors conclude that these data indicate an imprinted locus for social cognition on the X chromosome that is not expressed (silenced) on the maternally derived X (putting males and Xm Turner females at risk for developmental disorders of language and social cognition but protecting girls and Xp Turner females). This defect in social cognition may translate into difficulties or lack of understanding of social and nonverbal cues. For example, a young sibling of an adolescent Turner syndrome patient commented about her sister, "She just doesn't get the point and that isolates her"—and a mother commented that her daughter "was not street wise." Many of the girls and women tend not to "read" sarcastic facial expressions or understand double entendres.

The differences in cognition associated with parental X chromosome origin, however, have not been reported by all investigators and need to be corroborated by other groups. For example, Haverkamp and co-workers also examined parental origin of the X chromosome in relation to cognition and came to the conclusion that age and familial covariance also influence cognitive function in Turner syndrome patients.[400] These factors may not have been controlled for in the previous studies. In other words, social cognition and visual-spatial abilities change with age—and differences were no longer apparent in the Haverkamp cohort of adolescent Turner syndrome patients when compared with the normal population.

The role of estrogen deficiency and estrogen replacement therapy also needs to be considered in the context of organic causes for the cognitive, social, and functional profiles of girls and women with Turner syndrome. Indeed, estrogen replacement has been suggested as an explanation for improved motor speed, nonverbal processing, and memory in estrogen-treated Turner syndrome patients compared with placebo-treated patients.[401,402] Whether these findings will influence the quality of life of females with Turner syndrome is not yet known, although the positive effect on motor function could mitigate the findings of motor impairment described in prepubertal girls.

Some of these deficits may be improved by hormonal therapy at puberty.[402,403] Difficulties in visual-spatial organization, social cognition, and problem solving (mathematics) and motor deficits describe specific neuropsychological deficits that do not improve with time or estrogens.[404-408] As a group, girls and women with Turner syndrome excel at verbal skills, and many adults with Turner syndrome have university level education.[408-409] Recent studies do not support the influence of height as influential on dating and initiation of sexual activities, but the role of physical abnormalities is unclear.[410-412] The developmental process is likely affected by treatment with GH and estrogen that potentially may influence the child's perception of herself.[61] In open-ended interviews, women with Turner syndrome reported that dealing with premature ovarian failure and loss of fertility was the most difficult part of having the condition.[413]

Psychiatric disorders have not previously been reported to be increased in Turner syndrome, but there have been a number of reports describing the occurrence of anorexia nervosa in patients with Turner syndrome.[414] It is presently unclear whether this is increased in comparison with normal girls. Kron and colleagues[414] have pointed out the danger of overlooking an X chromosomal disorder in a patient in whom growth arrest and pubertal delay are attributed to excessive weight loss alone. This is especially relevant because gonadotropins may revert to prepubertal levels.[415] One report, in which the literature was reviewed as well as reporting two patients, suggests that schizophrenia may be increased in women with a mosaic chromosomal karyotype[416] (but again this remains to be confirmed).

Finally, Skuse and co-workers have reported what appears to be a significantly increased risk of autism among Turner syndrome individuals.[417] They noted that this appeared to be in excess in those girls who had retained the maternal X chromosome (Xm) and had either a missing or a structurally abnormal second X. A report of a Turner individual with autism and an Xm genotype[418] is supportive but not confirmatory of this hypothesis because the majority of patients with Turner syndrome are Xm. The hypothesis of Skuse and co-workers that unmaking of a familial predisposition toward autism may occur by the deletion of the protective paternal X chromosome remains to be tested.[419]

A final aspect of the neuropsychological profile of girls and women with Turner syndrome might be called personality. The first systematic investigation of the personality of girls and women with Turner syndrome was conducted in the 1970s.[420] This study and subsequent studies indicate that some personality traits are common to the majority of women and that Turner syndrome individuals had a high stress tolerance, a tendency toward overcompliance, and a higher degree of dependence and limitations in emotional competence.[382,421,422] They also may have an impairment of self-esteem.[423]

The role of the previously described cognitive differences in affecting adaptive personality traits needs to be investigated. Studies indicate that women with Turner syndrome have a typically female pattern of development with unambiguous female gender identification.[424] The scant data available indicate that heterosexual romantic fantasies are common but that dating and initiation of sexual activities may be somewhat delayed or infrequent and that they leave home later than their siblings. A Swedish psychosocial report from 22 middle-aged women with Turner syndrome notes adequate adjustment as adults but a prolonged and isolated adolescence, concerns about infertility, and poor compliance with hormone replacement therapy.[425]

Another report from Israel, however, notes a high degree of adjustment that may relate to the more structured environment.[426] In the context of psychosexual adaptation, attention should be paid to sex education and orientation in adult sexuality. Because some of these girls mature more slowly than their peers, they may not be ready for or interested in sex education when it is given at school. They may also be more self-conscious in relation to beginning a sexual relationship because of being "different." More attention to sex education and sex therapy may be necessary to address this area. Information about assisted reproductive techniques should also be provided.

RECOMMENDATIONS

Whether this complex psychosocial behavior is endogenous or adaptive, as more aggressive and innovative endocrine therapies begin to alter the outlook for stature, timing of feminization, and fertility attention should still be paid to assessment of psychosocial adaptation. Because the factors that affect the quality of life are the same as those that affect the rest of society, psychological care should be provided within the context of helping to prevent difficulties and normalizing the developmental process rather than operating from an illness model. Plans for both medical and psychological intervention should be developed so as to reinforce and support the individual's self-esteem and to ensure that individuals with Turner syndrome remain in the mainstream of social, educational, and employment activities.

A comprehensive psycho-educational evaluation is recommended preceding school entry. Children with Turner syndrome may have other conditions (e.g., dyslexia or attention deficit) that need to be addressed. In view of slower processing speed, untimed testing may be appropriate. Age-appropriate pubertal induction is recommended. It is important to address all issues surrounding sexuality, infertility, and reproductive options in an honest and open manner because "secret-keeping" may have unintended negative consequences and actually amplify the problems.[61,427]

Many of these issues are discussed in patient-oriented material available through the Turner's Syndrome Society of the United States web site (*www.turner-syndrome-us. org*). Similar web sites exist for other national Turner syndrome organizations. Patients with Turner syndrome and their parents need to be well informed about the learning problems associated with Turner syndrome because most individuals are affected by these difficulties, if only to a mild degree. They need to understand that even with intervention some of these learning difficulties do not disappear with age but persist throughout adult life. Learning disabilities can be a major impediment to emancipation from family and to career enhancement, although many women with Turner syndrome do achieve high professional status.[428]

Management: Pediatric And Adult

EVALUATION

The clinical aspects of which child should be evaluated for Turner syndrome, and at what age, have been addressed in part in this chapter and in the previous chapter on disorders of puberty. Nevertheless, certain clinical aspects warrant review. It is obvious that the female neonate with a webbed neck or edema of the hands and feet merits further investigation. Similarly, the girl with multiple physical stigmata, the girl with coarctation of the aorta, or the girl with radiologic evidence of abnormalities in the urinary collecting system or a horseshoe kidney should also be considered for evaluation. What is less obvious is which girl without obvious stigmata or highly suggestive organic defects should be evaluated (Tables 15-7 and 15-8).

Many girls with Turner syndrome do not have obvious physical stigmata, and it is necessary to recognize that the diagnosis may be difficult in such cases. We reviewed the records of 144 of our patients and found that only 41 had been diagnosed as neonates or toddlers because of obvious physical stigmata. The remaining 103 (71%) presented with short stature or short stature and pubertal delay.[424] In a report of 100 patients, a similar finding was noted.[111] Only 15% were diagnosed at birth. The remaining patients were diagnosed often only after 12 years of age.[134]

The incidence of Turner syndrome is about 1:2,000 live female births, but the statistics change as one considers stature. For example, among 2,000 girls in childhood only 60 are at or below the third percentile—leaving most of the group at risk (excluding infancy and early childhood, and even if no stigmata are present) much smaller. Given other genetic causes for short stature among this group (as well as other acquired causes, and the possible presence of one or more clinical features), the number of girls who might need evaluation becomes less than 1 in 60. Thus, the rationale for considering performing a complete chromosomal karyotype on a girl with short stature becomes even more obvious. The role and utility of SHOX gene testing as part of a short stature evaluation remains to be evaluated.

Once the diagnosis of Turner syndrome has been established and a chromosome analysis has been carried out, additional diagnostic procedures are indicated. These diagnosis and management strategies have been published as recommendations from a consensus workshop. As participants in that workshop, our recommendations tend to be consistent with these recommendations.[61,428]

TABLE 15-7
Screening at Diagnosis of Turner Syndrome in Children and Adults

All Patients
- Cardiovascular evaluation by specialist[a]
- Renal ultrasound
- Hearing evaluation by an audiologist
- Evaluation for scoliosis/kyphosis
- Evaluation for knowledge of Turner syndrome; referral to support groups
- Evaluation for growth and pubertal development

Ages 0-4 Years
- Evaluation for hip dislocation
- Eye exam by pediatric ophthalmologist (if age ≥ 1)

Ages 4-10 Years
- Thyroid function tests (T_4, TSH) and celiac screen (TTG Ab)
- Educational/psychosocial evaluation
- Orthodontic evaluation (if age ≥ 7)

Ages $\geq$ 10 Years
- Thyroid function tests (T_4, TSH) and celiac screen (TTG Ab)
- Educational and psychosocial evaluations
- Orthodontic evaluation
- Evaluation of ovarian function/estrogen replacement
- LFTs, FBG, lipids, CBC, Cr, BUN
- BMD (if age 18)

BUN, blood urea nitrogen; CBC, complete blood count; Cr, creatinine; FBG, fasting blood glucose; and LFTs, liver function tests.

[a] See Table 15-6.

From Bondy CA for the Turner Syndrome Study Group (2007). Care of girls and women with Turner syndrome. J Clin Endocrinol and Metab 92(1):10–25.

TABLE 15-8
Ongoing Monitoring in Turner Syndrome

All Ages
- Cardiological evaluation as indicated[a]
- Blood pressure annually
- ENT and audiology every 1-5 years

Girls <5 Years
- Social skills at age 4-5 years

School Age
- Liver and thyroid screening annually
- Celiac screen every 2-5 years
- Educational and social progress annually
- Dental and orthodontic as needed

Older Girls and Adults
- Fasting lipids and blood sugar annually
- Liver and thyroid screening annually
- Celiac screen as indicated
- Age-appropriate evaluation of pubertal development and psychosexual adjustment

[a]See Table 15-6.

From Bondy CA for the Turner Syndrome Study Group (2007). Care of girls and women with Turner syndrome. J Clin Endocrinol and Metab 92(1):10–25.

Initial and Follow-up Studies in Adolescence and Adulthood

Because the clinical manifestations of gradually developing thyroid failure can be subtle and easily overlooked in a short child, routine serum thyroid function tests (including thyroxine, thyroid-stimulating hormone, and antithyroid antibodies) are indicated. Subsequently, thyroxine and thyroid-stimulating hormone or thyroid-stimulating hormone alone should be determined at 1- to 2-year intervals in all patients regardless of whether significant titers of antithyroid antibodies were detected initially. This follow-up should be continued as an adult. Routine testing for other autoimmune glandular failures does not appear necessary unless other evidence of autoimmune disease develops, such as alopecia, vitiligo, or a glandular failure (other than the ovary).

Routine renal ultrasound may detect structural abnormalities in renal architecture or collecting system anatomy. If no abnormalities are present, follow-up studies are not routinely indicated. If significant abnormalities are detected, follow-up evaluation and therapy may be indicated and long-term screening for urinary tract infection may be necessary.

Infants with Turner syndrome may have an increased risk of congenital hip dislocation,[428] and care should be taken to evaluate the infant. Poor management in childhood can result in serious morbidity in the adult woman. Although the other osseous abnormalities of Turner syndrome may be multiple, unless they cause significant morbidity radiologic survey of the entire skeleton is not routinely recommended. Once a skeletal deformity is noted, however, orthopedic consultation may be indicated. In addition, the practical effects of having an increased carrying angle (e.g., interference with activities such as swimming using a backstroke) need to be recognized and discussed.

Abnormalities of the fingernails and toenails are usually only of mild cosmetic interest. A report of cellulitis and infection secondary to ingrown toenails warrants calling attention to the toenail deformity (if present) and its predisposing conditions (including intermittent lymphedema) and taking care to prevent the ingrown condition.[430] This issue may continue into adulthood. Scoliosis is common but usually does not progress rapidly and can most often be managed conservatively. If growth-promoting regimens are used, careful attention should be paid to detecting progressive scoliosis.

If noted, its cause should be determined radiographically. We have observed two patients in whom it was caused by leg-length inequality. Madelung deformity requires recognition so as to exclude other causes of this bony malposition, but it does not require orthopedic correction. It is actually rather infrequent in Turner syndrome.[431] Girls with Turner syndrome have higher risks for scoliosis and kyphosis than the general population. Ten to twenty percent of girls with Turner syndrome develop scoliosis and kyphosis. Vertebral wedging also appears to be more common.[432,433] Both problems can be accentuated with rapid growth. Phalangeal bone density has been reported to be normal during childhood.[434]

Plasma FSH and LH concentrations at the time of diagnosis may or may not be elevated. They could serve as an indication of future gonadal function but should not be used to screen for the diagnosis of Turner syndrome. In addition, we observed two girls with significantly elevated FSH levels in early childhood who went on to spontaneous onset of puberty (although subsequent ovarian failure). Therefore, predictions of gonadal failure based on high infant/childhood FSH may be given, but with care. Pelvic visualization techniques, including ultrasound and MRI, appear to be clinically indicated only in those situations in which there is a question of gonadal anatomy or potential pubertal function.

The absolute indication is the patient with a Y chromosome or marker chromosome in the karyotype because she is at risk for the development of gonadoblastoma. The ultrasound may demonstrate an adnexal mass in the patient with the Y chromosome in comparison with the normal female (Figure 15-18). Surgical removal of the bilateral adnexal structures is then indicated. The recommendation for concomitant hysterectomy as a prophylactic measure against endometrial carcinoma in an agonadal individual who will be on long-term estrogen replacement therapy is controversial.

Some physicians believe that because it lends little extra morbidity to the indicated pelvic surgery it is a warranted consideration. Others believe that the psychological benefit of monthly menstruation, independent of the artificiality of its method of production and its irrelevance to fertility, precludes the procedure unless there is evidence of local spread of the gonadoblastoma. Finally, oocyte donation, in vitro fertilization, and embryo transfer are being performed successfully in agonadal women—including women with Turner syndrome who have an intact uterus.[435-437] Thus, the issue bears complete discussion with the individual patient and physicians involved—as well as informed patient consent.

A more difficult management decision concerns the method of follow-up of the patient with a cytogenetically documented Y chromosome or molecularly detected Y-derived marker chromosome in the karyotype in whom the initial radiographic studies are normal. The question of whether prophylactic removal of the adnexal streaks should be performed electively or delayed until the ultrasound or MRI suggests a mass has not been entirely resolved. Data indicating that tumor formation may be present microscopically at a very young age are a strong argument for elective surgery, however, even in the absence of a demonstrable mass.[228] However, data from the Danish cancer registry failed to show the presence of gonadoblastoma or dysgerminoma in 29 women with a Y chromosome—suggesting that the risk may be overestimated.[60]

Pelvic visualization techniques may also be useful in patients with evidence of some gonadal function at puberty.[438] In such patients, unilateral or bilateral ovarian structures indistinguishable from normal may be demonstrable. The anatomic findings would lend supportive evidence to the clinical or gonadotropin data and might deter the physician from the institution of hormonal replacement therapy. It is important to point out that spontaneous puberty, even with menses that appear cyclic, does not always mean that normal ovulatory cycles are occurring or will continue to occur normally in these patients.[232,244] Anovulatory cycles do not result in normal endometrial histology and could impair the capacity for successful ovum implantation and predispose to endometrial hyperplasia or cancer. Although it is clinically impractical to study a complete cycle, efforts should be made to ensure that most cycles are ovulatory. If not, the patient should be either cycled artificially or given periodic courses of progesterone for withdrawal.

Otologic abnormalities are very frequent. Deformation of the pinna is most frequent in patients with the lymphedema phenotype. Otitis media is extremely common and should be treated immediately. The high prevalence of hearing loss, either primary or secondary to residual serous otitis media, suggests that otorhinolaryngologic evaluation with audiometry may be indicated in a large number of patients. In infancy, feeding techniques such as those used for cleft palate patients may also be indicated. We have the clinical impression that mild abnormalities in phonation, independent of hearing impairment, are present in a number of our older patients.

Because these abnormalities in speech may be a consequence of a palatal deformity, speech evaluation may also be indicated. Myringotomy and polyethylene tube placement are considered the primary modes of therapy for serous otitis media in Turner syndrome, and tonsillectomy or adenoidectomy or both should be avoided if possible. Removal of the tonsils and adenoids may not be advisable because of its dubious value for the treatment of serous otitis media and because the pharyngeal tissue often serves as an anatomic prosthesis for pharyngeal competence.

Ophthalmologic abnormalities are common, and an appropriate examination should be performed.[130] Ptosis, hypertelorism epicanthal folds, and upward slanting palpebral fissures are common in Turner syndrome. Red-green color deficiency is present in 8% of the population, a percentage similar to that found in most males. Strabismus and hyperopia occur in 25% to 35% of these children, putting them at high risk for amblyopia. To promote early detection and treatment and to prevent visual loss, children with Turner syndrome should be evaluated by a pediatric ophthalmologist at 12 to 18 months of age.[61]

Hypertension is common in Turner syndrome, and blood pressure should be measured at each visit. Renal arteriography, selective venous catheterization, or both may be indicated in some patients with hypertension. Although the evidence of multiple arterial and venous abnormalities in Turner syndrome suggests that gross or segmental renal vascular disease may be responsible for the hypertension, the disordered anatomy may also render detection of treatable lesions difficult. An example of a study performed in an 11-year-old patient with significant hypertension is shown in Figure 15-20B.

Multiple renal arteries and veins were noted, and selective catheterization was virtually impossible. Nevertheless, in some patients surgically treatable lesions may be apparent. The risk of hypertension continues into adulthood and is a major risk factor for aortic dilation. Adult women with Turner syndrome are also at risk for cardiovascular disease. Therefore, when hypertension is detected in the child or in the adult it should be treated aggressively to minimize the risk of cardiovascular disease as well as of progressive dilation and aortic dissection.[439]

Because the detection of cardiovascular abnormalities requires specialized diagnostic and clinical evaluation, and because their presence may indicate the need for cardiac surgery or lifelong antibiotic therapy for subacute bacterial endocarditis prophylaxis, a cardiologic consultation should be obtained for all patients and should include an ECG. A prenatal ECG does not obviate the need for a postnatal examination because bicuspid aortic valve and coarctation may not be detected in utero. A cardiologist skilled in the assessment of congenital heart disease should interpret the ECG.

If no abnormalities are detected in childhood, a repeat cardiovascular examination and ECG should be conducted during adolescence because aortic dilation may occur without any other risk factors. If bicuspid aortic valve or mitral valve prolapse is detected, subacute bacterial endocarditis prophylaxis is recommended and follow-up should be more frequent. If aortic root dilation is found, the cardiologist should obtain follow-up ECGs at a frequency based on the severity of the dilation present and the presence or absence of other risk factors for dilation (such as hypertension, bicuspid aortic valve, and previously repaired coarctation).

Although we consider the potential morbidity and mortality of this condition (when present) to be similar to that of Marfan syndrome, there are no outcome data to absolutely recommend Marfan management strategies. The role of long-term prophylactic β-adrenergic blockade to slow the rate of dilation and lessen the development of aortic complications in some patients needs to be assessed.[420] Prophylactic aortic root repair may have to be considered for the patient with marked and progressive dilation, however. If unexplained chest pain occurs, even with initially normal studies, the diagnosis of aneurysm or dissection must always be considered.

Coarctation of the aorta is treated surgically in most cases. Although the postoperative risk of the development of mesenteric arteritis is higher in males than in females,[441] we have observed this syndrome in a patient with Turner syndrome. Long-term prognosis is generally good, with few reports of recurrence or complications. However, asymptomatic poststenotic aneurysmal dilation of the aorta may be detectable on screening chest radiography or cardiac MRI (Figure 15-19B and C) and should be followed carefully to prevent dissection or rupture.

The decision to seek consultation for plastic surgery to correct the webbed neck deformity or the forwardly displaced ears is individual. It must be pointed out to the patient and family that in addition to the webbing the neck may also be short. Therefore, cosmetic surgery may be somewhat disappointing. In some cases, however, satisfactory results are achieved. The apparent predisposition toward the development of keloids in these patients must also be taken into account. There is some evidence to suggest that early surgery may have a better cosmetic result.[442] Keloids have also been seen in conjunction with ear piercing, suggesting that this procedure should be avoided or performed with great care.

If, or when, psychometric testing should be performed is an individual family decision. Nevertheless, a preschool evaluation to rule out major areas of cognitive dysfunction might be advisable. In light of the previous discussion, school performance should be monitored—and specific problems should be attended to with skilled cognitive specialists.

Endocrinologic Management

The data show that GH safely increases growth velocity and final adult height in Turner syndrome and have led to regulatory approval for the use of GH in many countries. The criteria for which girls are potential candidates for GH vary. The previously cited guidelines suggest GH should be initiated when the Turner syndrome girl drops below the 5th percentile of the normal curve. This may delay therapy, however, in some girls who could benefit from early therapy and earlier initiation of estrogen replacement (see Turner Toddler study[81]). It also fails to consider genetic midparental target height.

An alternative is to use Lyon curves for Turner syndrome patients as previously described, project their final height if untreated, and initiate therapy if this falls below the 5th through 10th percentiles for normal girls or −1 to −2 SDs below their genetic target midparental height if they are from tall families. A target goal should be set after discussion with the family or with the patient and family, with the emphasis that therapy will be a long process and will not necessarily result in complete normalization of target midparental height.

There are data to document that the response to GH in Turner syndrome does not differ between patients with normal GH responses to pharmacologic stimuli and those with insufficient responses.[443,444] Therefore, GH-provocative testing is neither required by regulatory agencies for GH use nor recommended unless the patient's growth velocity is significantly below the Turner velocity for age (suggesting the presence of hypothalamic-pituitary disease). When GH is started in young girls, concomitant anabolic steroids may not be needed—and there might be some theoretical reasons to avoid years of anabolic steroid therapy.

In older girls (9 to 12 years) or in girls older than 8 in whom therapy is started at a significant height deficit, consideration should be given to starting combined therapy with GH and a nonaromatizable androgen such as oxandrolone because it is aromatization to estrogen that promotes epiphyseal fusion. The recommended dose of oxandrolone should not be above 0.05 mg/kg/day, significantly lower than that used as the initial dose, and slightly lower than that finally used in an often cited study.[171]

Dosing with GH has been previously discussed in the section on growth-promoting therapy. The starting dose is 0.05 mg/kg/day. Individualization of dose can be considered, depending on the patient's growth response. Prediction models may help in this respect.[445] GH should be continued until the final target height previously agreed on with the family (or patient and family) is achieved or until near epiphyseal fusion precludes a significant effect. If androgen is being used, it should be discontinued when the decision is made to begin estrogen therapy.

The issue of when to begin estrogen therapy in this paradigm of GH treatment is less clear. The earlier discussion in this chapter reviews data that suggest that estrogen alone is not useful for augmentation of final height. There are also data that suggest that epiphyseal fusion progresses significantly after 12 to 18 months of estrogen therapy. In addition, when estrogen is used for feminization in conjunction with ongoing GH therapy further growth augmentation may not occur.[446] Finally, in one paper it was documented that the longer the estrogen-free years of GH therapy the taller the final height.

The data in this report also showed that if GH is begun early, however, estrogen treatment could be begun at a younger more appropriate age and still have a greater gain in projected final height.[447] Thus, in aggregate the data suggest that estrogen therapy for feminization should not begin until the patient has reached the estimated height at which she will require only 1 to 2 more years of GH therapy. With the early initiation of GH therapy, that age is likely to be one that is socially acceptable and physiologically normal.

In a recent report,[448] Quigley et al. report positive data of the synergistic effect of early low-dose estrogen (ethinyl estradiol 25 ng/kg/day from age 5 years on) and growth hormoone on adult height. An additional management issue has developed with respect to girls with spontaneous ovarian function. Although studies done before GH treatment suggest that final height does not appear to differ between those girls with spontaneous and induced puberty,[231] there are few data that are applicable to the GH-treated girl.

In one study,[449] four girls developed spontaneous puberty during the first year of GH treatment. They appeared to have an augmented growth velocity compared with the prepubertal girls that persisted into the second year of therapy. Final height data are not available, however. In the study of Reiter and associates, the relationship to estrogen-free years held whether the estrogen was exogenous or endogenous.[447] Thus, if a girl has been treated for several years with GH and has achieved significant height augmentation spontaneous puberty may be of no concern with respect to final height. If it occurs in a girl who is just beginning therapy, however, the initial augmentation could be offset by subsequent epiphyseal closure. Therefore, in a very short girl in whom a significant height augmentation has not yet been achieved and puberty occurs relatively early some consideration may be in order to inhibit puberty with long-acting GnRH analogues.

If GH therapy is not available or otherwise contraindicated, consideration of the use of anabolic steroids as a growth promoter before estrogen therapy in girls 10 to 13 years old who have no clinical or hormonal evidence of ovarian function might be appropriate. The rationale for this, recognizing that it may not increase final adult height, is that it could provide a growth spurt so that when feminization is induced the patient is at a height somewhat closer to that which appears appropriate for obvious signs of puberty. Oxandrolone, 0.05 mg/kg/day, could be used—with side effects (including clitoromegaly and facial hair) monitored.

If the growth velocity begins to decline (usually after 12 months) and if epiphyseal fusion has not taken place, the steroid dose could be increased (0.075 to 0.1 mg/kg/day) to see whether a second spurt can be induced. After that, the medication is discontinued, gonadal status is reassessed, and estrogen therapy is initiated. Finally, some have considered orthopedic leg lengthening as an alternative approach for correction of short stature in Turner syndrome. Experience with this procedure in this condition is still very limited, however.

Although there is controversy over the risks and benefits of hormone replacement therapy in the postmenopausal woman,[450,451] the psychological needs for estrogen in the induction and maintenance of secondary sexual characteristics in young women—and the physiologic needs, among others, for induction of peak bone mass and mineral maintenance and metabolism—are well accepted. Compared with the emphasis on developing optimal regimens for postmenopausal hormonal replacement therapy,[450-455] however, there are few reviews of the optimum preparation and dose schedule for long-term use in younger agonadal women.

With regard to maintenance of bone mineral, the issue is further confounded in Turner syndrome by the difficulty in deciding what standards to apply to the measurements of bone mineral density,[121] the presence of an intrinsic appearance of osteopenia,[456] and the role GH therapy might have in altering bone mineral content.[457] Nevertheless, extrapolation from previous clinical practice and the newer data allow clinicians to develop a rational approach to the principles of therapy. These include long-term cyclic therapy to prevent estrogen-related uterine neoplasia and adequate estrogen to achieve and maintain bone mineral content and preserve the cardioprotective effects on plasma lipids and lipoproteins.

Cyclic therapy is recommended, not only for its positive psychological effect in the adolescent but for its uterine protective effect.[429,458] Data on steroid receptors in hormone-dependent target tissues suggest that progesterone down-regulates or blocks the estrogen receptors,[459] and that when given in conjunction with estrogen may be protective against estrogen-induced neoplasia. Progestins also act to attenuate the action of estrogen by increasing the activities of enzymes that convert estrogen into biologically less active estrone and inactive estrogen sulfate.

When endometrial responses were prospectively evaluated in Turner syndrome patients receiving long-term replacement therapy, hyperplastic changes were noted in only a small percentage of those receiving combined therapy compared with those receiving cyclic estrogen alone.[460] The goal is the complete conversion of the endometrium from a proliferative to a wholly or predominantly secretory state. The dose of progesterone should be minimized to prevent an adverse effect on carbohydrate tolerance[461] and lipid metabolism.[462,463] Therefore, the use of traditional-dose oral contraceptives as long-term therapy is not ideal—given that their progesterone content may be higher than is necessary or optimal.

The estrogen dose needed to achieve maximum bone mineral and to prevent bone mineral loss in Turner syndrome is not known. There are data in adult women with Turner syndrome, however, to show that there is a positive correlation between bone mineral content and the duration of estrogen treatment.[464] A short-term study compared the metabolic effects of low-dose oral conjugated estrogen (0.625 mg) with relatively high-dose ethinyl estradiol (30 ug) combined with progesterone in young women with Turner syndrome.[465] Whereas both regimens normalized the hypotrophic endometria and suppressed hyperinsulinemia, only the higher dose normalized FSH. Neither agent completely normalized the bone metabolic profile, although the higher-dose ethinyl estradiol regimen was more effective in normalizing bone turnover markers. Future investigations of selective estrogen receptor modulators, as well as calcium and vitamin D, were suggested.

Thus, the recommendations for postmenopausal women (0.625 mg of conjugated equine estrogen or its equivalent)—which approximates 60 pg/mL estradiol—may not be adequate long-term replacement for the agonadal woman. Therefore, although this was our previous recommendation for the patient with Turner syndrome it is unlikely that it represents sufficient physiologic long-term replacement. Somewhat higher doses (to achieve the equivalence of 90 to 120 pg/mL) would appear to be more logical. A dose of 2 mg of micronized 17b-estradiol, which is relatively equal to 1.25 mg conjugated estrogen (Premarin), has been shown to have a greater effect in increasing spinal trabecular bone density in postmenopausal women than did the more commonly used 1-mg dose.[465] These estrogen doses are still lower than those in most oral contraceptives.

As most girls are treated from infancy or early childhood on with GH, they are at a better height percentile by age 12 to 13 years. Based on these considerations, hormone replacement therapy may begin sooner (Table 15-9). To initiate feminization, one can begin with 0.3 to 0.625 mg conjugated estrogen daily for 6 to 12 months. After initiation and progression of breast development and uterine growth, the estrogen may be increased to 0.9 to 1.25 mg and cyclic therapy with progesterone [e.g., 10 mg medroxyprogesterone (Provera)] begun. Alternatively, progressive doses of 17β-estradiol can be used (if available), culminating in a final maintenance dose of 2 mg. A calendar month can be used for convenience, beginning with estrogen on day 1 and continuing it through day 23.

Progesterone is started on day 10 and continued through day 23. No medication is ingested for the remainder of the calendar month, when withdrawal menses usually ensue. Estrogen is then restarted on day 1 of the next calendar month, and the cycles are repeated. Follow-up includes monthly breast self-examination. Pelvic examinations and Papanicolaou smears should commence yearly if the patient is sexually active. Otherwise, frequency of these examinations can be determined by the gynecologist to whom the patient is referred as an adult. Cyclic therapy, and maintaining a normal adult uterine endometrium, also enhances the potential for success for reproductive options such as in vitro fertilization.

In addition, for those girls with some residual ovarian function advances are now being made in the area of oocyte cryopreservation coupled with later intracytoplasmic sperm injection.[189] This potential option also enhances the reasons for preservation of the uterus. When

Turner women are older, the issue of whether cyclic therapy should be converted to continuous therapy to prevent menopausal symptoms in the "off week" needs to be considered. This can be achieved safely if the progesterone dose is sufficient to prevent hyperplasia.

The use of other preparations of estrogen and progesterone should also be assessed for long-term use as replacement therapy. These include oral synthetic ethinyl estradiol, transdermal estradiol-17β, and transvaginal suppositories of estrogen and progesterone. The issues that need to be considered are the route of administration and effects of different preparations on systems (such as the hepatic enzymes) that contribute to the potential adverse affects of estrogen on blood pressure, clotting, and gallstone formation. Transdermal estrogen, for example (unlike oral estrogens), avoids the first-pass effect on the liver and may therefore obviate adverse effects on hepatic proteins.[466]

Our initial experience with transdermal estradiol was in a Turner syndrome patient who had recurrence of pedal lymphedema with the institution of oral estrogen replacement. She experienced less swelling with the transdermal preparation. Other patients were started on oral estrogen and then switched to patch estrogen with oral progesterone. For this form of therapy, one can use a 100-mg patch—which appears to be similar in potency to 1.25 mg of conjugated estrogen or 2 mg of estradiol. The patient changes the patch after 3.5 days (two per week) for the first 21 days (3 weeks) of the calendar month. Progesterone is taken from days 10 through 21, and no patch or progesterone is used after day 21 until the next month. Follow-up is the same as for oral estrogen therapy.

An additional comment should be made about breast development in response to estrogen replacement in Turner syndrome. We have observed that the final size of the breast appears to be more consistent with genetic predisposition than with the dose of estrogen or the time it was initiated. The only clear exception appears to be in the girl in whom there are marked clinical signs of extensive fetal edema of the upper body. This includes severe webbing and/or marked nipple hypoplasia at birth. It appears that some of these girls develop very little breast tissue in response to estrogen and that this may be caused by mechanical damage to the breast primordium in utero. In such patients, breast augmentation in late adolescence may be necessary (if the patient is so inclined and if she has not had a problem with keloid formation).

Finally, it must be emphasized that repeated discussion of important issues must take place among family, patient, and clinician. After years of follow-up, one tends to overlook the fact that the patient is no longer a child—and reeducation and new lines of communication need to be established with the patient as an emerging adult.

Transition Management

The transition from pediatric to adult health care should occur at the completion of growth and puberty during late-stage adolescence (usually by 18 to 21 years). However, transition should be initiated as a staged process.

Beginning at approximately 12 years of age, the center of care should be shifted incrementally from the parent to the adolescent with Turner syndrome. The health care focus also shifts from maximizing height to including feminization, counseling the adolescent with Turner syndrome about the evolving impact of her condition into adulthood, and promoting the development of independent self-care behaviors.[61,467]

The Adult with Turner Syndrome

The number of recent excellent papers and reports that now deal with adult women with Turner syndrome strengthens the fact that awareness is growing that this is a large segment of the adult population and that a comprehensive approach to care is needed.[299,425,441,469,470] Most importantly, it needs to be stressed that cardiac care continues. It also must be stressed that women with Turner syndrome receive cylical estrogen and progestin and discontinuation should occur at the age of normal menopause and not before.

Recent studies show that women with Turner syndrome become pregnant as easily as other women with other types of infertility and carry their pregnancies to term without an increased miscarriage rate.[470,471] Because of their small size and and the narrow android pelvis, most women with Turner syndrome need to deliver by Cesarean section. Most critically, the risk for dilatation and dissection of the aorta appears to increase during pregnancy.[471] New data have emerged showing that adolescents with only few signs of spontaneous puberty may still have ovaries with functioning follicles.[472] The possibility of using cryopreserved ovarian tissue and immature oocytes, obtained before regression of follicles occurs, is currently under intense investigation and results seem promising.[61]

With unpredictable changes occurring in health care delivery, however, it is of concern that patients who require a long-term multidisciplinary approach to management may be lost in the medical system. We attempted to reach a consensus in the recently published *Guidelines for the Care of Girls and Women with Turner Syndrome*,[61] which together with previous recommendations[430] reflects our desire to make these guidelines for pediatricians and internists more broadly known.

The consensus document suggests that puberty should be induced at a physiologically appropriate age to optimize self-esteem, social adjustment, and the potential for initiation of sexual relationships. With the quest for earlier diagnosis and hence earlier introduction of growth-promoting therapy, these recommendations (based on a French survey of 566 Turner women aged 18 to 31 years) should guide the clinician in future therapy.[411]

Because the parental origin of the missing X chromosome appears to have an impact on renal development and on ocular features, weight, and academic achievement, it may be appropriate to determine parental origin of the X chromosome using polymorphic microsatellite markers on the X and Y chromosomes.[317,473] It is clear, however, that the pediatric health care provider will be the major resource for translating the ideas expressed into a future management plan for these patients. The strongest ally the practitioner has may be the patient herself. A well-informed and educated patient will become her own best advocate. Information and materials are available from the Turner's Syndrome Society of the United States (*www.turner-syndrome-us.org*), regional affiliates, and international societies. With the intervention strategies described, girls and women with Turner syndrome now—more than ever—have the capability of achieving their full potential.

REFERENCES

1. Turner HH (1938). A syndrome of infantilism, congenital webbed neck and cubitus valgus. Endocrinology 23:566.
2. Ullrich O (1949). Turner's syndrome and status Bonnevie-Ullrich. Am J Hum Genet 1:179.
3. Barr ML, Bertram EG (1949). A morphological distinction between neurones of the male and female and the behavior of the nucleolar satellite during accelerated nucleo-protein synthesis. Nature 163:676.
4. Males JL, Seely JR (1978). Turner's syndrome: Index case after 44 years (a tribute to Dr. Henry H. Turner). J Clin Endocrinol Metab 46:163.
5. deGrouchy J, Turleau C (1977). *Clinical atlas of human chromosomes.* New York: John Wiley & Sons 222.
6. Van Dyke DL, Wiktor A, Roberson JR, et al. (1991). Mental retardation in Turner syndrome. J Pediatr 118:415.
7. Grompe M, Rao N, Elder FFB, et al. (1992). 45,X/46,X,1r(X) can have a distinct phenotype different from Ullrich-Turner syndrome. Am J Hum Genet 42:39.
8. Van Dyke DL, Wiktor A, Palmer CG, et al. (1992). Ullrich-Turner syndrome with a small ring X chromosome and presence of mental retardation. Am J Hum Genet 43:996.
9. Migeon BR, Luo S, Jani M, Jeppesen P (1994). The severe phenotype of females with tiny ring X chromosomes is associated with inability of these chromosomes to undergo X inactivation. Am J Hum Genet 55:497.
10. Jani MM, Torchi BS, Pai GS, Migeon BR (1995). Molecular characterization of tiny ring X chromosomes from females with functional X chromosome disomy and lack of cis X inactivation. Genomics 27:182.
11. Gilchrist GS, Hammond D, Melnyk J (1965). Hemophilia A in a phenotypically normal female with XX/XO mosaicism. N Engl J Med 273:1403.
12. Refetoff S, Selenkow HA (1968). Familial thyroxine-binding globulin deficiency in a patient with Turner's syndrome (XO): Genetic study of a kindred. N Engl J Med 278:1081.
13. Trask BJ, Massa H, Kenwrick S, et al. (1991). Mapping of human chromosome Xq28 by two-color fluorescence in situ hybridization of DNA sequences to interphase cell nuclei. Am J Hum Genet 48:1.
14. McCabe ERB, Towbin JA, van den Engh G, et al. (1992). Xp21 contiguous gene syndromes: Deletion quantitation with bivariate flow karyotyping allows mapping of patient breakpoints. Am J Hum Genet 51:1277.
15. Abulhasan SJ, Tayel SM, Al-Awadi SA (1999). Mosaic Turner syndrome: Cytogenetics versus FISH. Ann Hum Genet 63:199.
16. Ferguson-Smith MA (1965). Karyotype-phenotype correlations in gonadal dysgenesis and their bearing on the pathogenesis of malformations. J Med Genet 2:142.
17. Palmer CG, Reichman A (1976). Chromosomal and clinical findings in 110 females with Turner syndrome. Hum Genet 35:35.
18. Ellison JW, Wardak Z, Young MF, et al. (1997). PHOG: A candidate gene for involvement in the short stature of Turner syndrome. Hum Mol Genet 6:1341.
19. Ballabio A, Bardoni B, Carrozzo R, et al. (1989). Contiguous gene syndromes due to deletions in the distal short arm of the human X chromosome. Proc Natl Acad Sci USA 86:10001.
20. Zinn AR, Ross JL (2000). Critical regions for Turner syndrome phenotype on the X chromosome. In Saenger PH and Pasquino AM (eds.), *Optimizing health care for Turner patients in the 21st Century: Proceedings of the 5th International Symposium on Turner Syndrome, Naples, Italy.* Amsterdam: Elsevier Science 19–28.
21. Vittay P, Bosze P, Gaal M, Laszlo J (year). Lymph vessel defects in patients with oovarian dysgenesis. Clin Genet 180(18):387–391.
22. Watanabe M, Zinn AR, Page DC, Nishimoto T (1993). Functional equivalence of human X- and Y-encoded isoforms of ribosomal protein S4 consistent with a role in Turner syndrome. Nat Genet 4:268.
23. Geerkens C, Just W, Held KR, Vogel W (1996). Ullrich-Turner syndrome is not caused by haploinsufficiency of PRS4X. Hum Genet 97:39.
24. Rao E, Weiss B, Fukami M, et al. (1977). Pseudoautosomal deletions encompassing a novel homeobox gene cause growth failure in idiopathic short stature and Turner syndrome. Nat Genet 16:54.
25. Blaschke RJ, Rappold GA (2000). SHOX: Growth, Leri-Weill and Turner syndrome. Trends Endocrinol Metab 11:227.
26. Rosenfeld RG (2000). A SHOX to the system. J Clin Endocrinol Metab 86:5672.
27. Ogata T, Kosho T, Wakui K, et al. (2000). Short stature homeobox-containing gene duplication on the der (X) chromosome in a female with 45,X/46,X,der (X), gonadal dysgenesis, and tall stature. J Clin Endocrinol Metab 85:2927.
28. Marchini A, Marttila T, Winter A, Caldeira S, et al. (2004). The Short Stature Homeodomain Protein SHOX induces cellulate growth arrest and apoptosis and is expressed in human growth plate chondrocytes. J Biol Chem 279:37103–4135.
29. Munns CJF, Haase HR, Crowther LM, Hayes MT, et al. (2004). Expression of SHOX in human fetal and childhood growth plate C. Clin Endocrinol Metab 89:4130–4135.
30. Blum WF, Crowe B, Quigley C, Jung H, et al. (2007). Growth hormone is effective in treatment of short stature associated with SHOX deficiency: Results of a randomized, controlled multicenter trial. J Clin Endocrinol Metab (in press).
31. Rappold G, Shanske AI, Saenger P (2005). All shook up about SHOX deficiency. J Ped 147:422–424.
32. Noonan JA (1968). Hypertelorism with Turner phenotype: A new syndrome with associated congenital heart disease. Am J Dis Child 116:373.
33. Souza SCAL, Jorge AL, Nishi MY, et al. (2000). Absence of point mutations in exons 3 and 4 of SHOX gene in patients with Noonan syndrome. In [editor(s)], *Proceedings of the 82nd annual meeting of the Endocrine Society, Toronto.* Bethesda MD: The Endocrine Society Press, abstract 2111.
34. Tartaglia M, Mehler EL, Goldberg R, et al. (2001). Mutations in PTPN11, encoding the protein tyrosine phosphatase SHP-2, cause Noonan syndrome. Nat Genet 29:465.
35. Opitz JM, Pallister PD (1979). Brief historical note: The concept of "gonadal dysgenesis." Am J Med Genet 4:333.
36. Bondy CA (2007). Genomic imprinting in Turner syndrome. In CH Gravholt, CA Bondy (eds.), *Wellness for girls and women with Turner syndrome.* International Congress Series 1298, Amsterdam: Elsevier.
37. Nielsen J, Wohlert M (1991). Chromosome abnormalities found among 34,910 newborn children: Results from a 13-year incidence study in Arhus, Denmark. Hum Genet 87:81.
38. Smith HC, Seale JP, Posen S (1974). Premature ovarian failure in a triple X female. J Obstet Gynecol Br Commonw 81:405.
39. Salbenblatt JA, Meyers DC, Bender BG, et al. (1989). Gross and fine motor development in 45,X and 47,XXX girls. Pediatrics 84:678.
40. Linden MG, Bender BG, Harmon RJ, et al. (1988). 47,XXX: What is the prognosis? Pediatrics 82:619.
41. Neri G (1984). A possible explanation for the low incidence of gonosomal aneuploidy among the offspring of Triplo-X individuals. Am J Med Genet 18:357.
42. Collen RJ, Falk RE, Lippe BM, Kaplan SA (1980). A 48,XXXX female with absence of ovaries. Am J Med Genet 6:275.
43. Gardner RJM, Veale AMO, Sands VE, et al. (1973). XXXX syndrome: Case report, and a note on genetic counseling and fertility. Hum Genet 17:323.
44. Monheit A, Francke U, Saunders B, et al. (1980). The penta-X syndrome. J Med Genet 17:392.
45. Zerres K, Schuler H, Kautza M, et al. (1997). Penta-X syndrome: Report on four new cases and further delineation of a rare syndrome. Acta Med Auxol 29:111.
46. Hook EB, Hamerton JL (1977). The frequency of chromosome abnormalities detected in consecutive newborn studies. Differences between studies: Results by sex and severity of phenotypic involvement. In Hooke B, Porter IH (eds.), *Population cytogenetics.* New York: Academic Press 63–79.

47. Hook EB, Warburton D (1983). The distribution of chromosomal genotypes associated with Turner's syndrome: Live-birth prevalence rates and evidence for diminished fetal mortality and severity in genotypes associated with structural X abnormalities or mosaicism. Hum Genet 64:24.

49. Jacobs PA, Betts PR, Cockwell AE, et al. (1990). A cytogenetic and molecular reappraisal of a series of patients with Turner's syndrome. Ann Hum Genet 54:209.

48. Hook EB (1977). Exclusion of chromosomal mosaicism: Tables of 90%, 95% and 99% confidence limits and comments on use. Am J Hum Genet 29:94–97.

50. Hall JG, Sybert VP, Williamson RA, et al. (1982). Turner's syndrome. West J Med 137:32.

51. Imaizumi K, Kuroki Y (1993). Prevalence of Turner syndrome in Japan. In Hibi I, Takano K (eds.), *Basic and clinical approach to Turner Syndrome: Proceedings of the 3rd International Symposium on Turner Syndrome, Chiba, Japan.* Amsterdam: Elsevier Science 3–6.

52. Medlej R, Lobaccaro JM, Berta P, et al. (1992). Screening for Y-derived sex determining gene SRY in 40 patients with Turner syndrome. J Clin Endocrinol Metab 75:1289.

53. Kocova M, Siegel SF, Wenger SL, et al. (1993). Detection of Y chromosome sequences in Turner's syndrome by Southern blot analysis of amplified DNA. Lancet 342:140.

54. Kocova M, Trucco M (1994). Centromere of Y chromosome in Turner's syndrome. Lancet 343:925.

55. Tsuchiya K, Reijo R, Page DC, Disteche CM (1995). Gonadoblastoma: Molecular definition of the susceptibility region on the Y chromosome. Am J Hum Genet 57:1400.

56. Lau Y-FC (1999). Gonadoblastoma, testicular and prostate cancers, and the TSPY gene. Am J Hum Genet 64:921.

57. Petrovic V, Nasioulas S, Chow CW, et al. (1992). Minute Y chromosome derived marker in a child with gonadoblastoma: Cytogenetic and DNA studies. J Med Genet 29:542.

58. Page DC (1994). Y chromosome sequences in Turner's syndrome and risk of gonadoblastoma or virilisation. Lancet 343:240.

59. Held KR (1993). Turner's syndrome and chromosome Y. Lancet 342:128.

60. Gravholt CH, Fedder J, Naeraa RW, Muller J (2000). Occurrence of gonadoblastoma in females with Turner syndrome and Y chromosome material: A population study. J Clin Endocrinol Metab 85:3199.

61. Bondy C for the Turner Syndrome Consensus Study Group (2007). Guidelines for the care of girls and women with Turner Syndrome. J Clin Endocrinol Metab [volume].

62. Nishi MY, Domenice S, Medeiros MA, et al. (2002). Detection of Y-specific sequences in 122 patients with Turner syndrome: Nested PCR is not a reliable method. Am J Hum Genet 107:299–305.

63. Cools M, Drop SLS, Wolffenbuttel KG, et al. (2006). Germ cell tumours in the intersex gonad: Old paths, new directions, moving frontiers. Endocr Rev [volume/pages].

64. Wei F, Cheng S, Badie N, et al. (2001). A man who inherited his SRY gene and Leri-Weill dyschondrosteosis from his mother and neurofibromatosis type 1 from his father. Am J Med Genet 102:353–358.

65. Landin-Wilhelmsen K, Bryman I, Hanson C, et al. (2004). Spontaneous pregnancies in a Turner syndrome women with Y-chromosome mosaicism. J Assist Reprod Genet 21:229–230.

66. Held KR, Kerber S, Kaminsky E, et al. (1992). Mosaicism in 45,X Turner syndrome: Does survival in early pregnancy depend on the presence of two sex chromosomes? Hum Genet 88:288.

67. Rubin CH, Williams J, Wang BBT (1993). Discrepancy in mosaic findings between chorionic villi and amniocytes: A diagnostic dilemma involving 45,X, 46,XY, and 47,XYY cell lines. Am J Med Genet 46:457.

68. Qumsiyeh MB, Tharapel AT, Shulman LP, et al. (1990). Anaphase lag as the most likely mechanism for monosomy X in direct cytotrophoblasts but not in mesenchymal core cells from the same villi. J Med Genet 27:780.

69. Kelly TE, Ferguson JE, Golden W (1992). Survival of fetuses with 45,X: An instructive case and an hypothesis. Am J Med Genet 42:825.

70. MRC Working Party on the Evaluation of Chorion Villus Sampling (1991). Medical Research Council European Trial of Chorion Villus Sampling. Lancet 337:1491.

71. Chang HJ, Clark RD, Bachman H (1990). The phenotype of 45,X/46,XY mosaicism: An analysis of 92 prenatally diagnosed cases. Am J Hum Genet 46:156.

72. Hsu LYF (2000). Prenatal diagnosis of sex chromosome abnormalities. In Saenger PH, Pasquino AM (eds.), *Optimizing health care for Turner patients in the 21st century: Proceedings of the 5th International Symposium on Turner Syndrome, Naples, Italy.* Amsterdam: Elsevier Science 47–59.

73. Telvi L, Lebbar A, Del Pino O, et al. (1999). 45,X/46,XY mosaicism: Report of 27 cases. Pediatrics 104:304.

74. Kajii T, Ohama K (1980). Inverse maternal age effect in monosomy X. Hum Genet 51:147.

75. Carothers AD, Frackiewicz A, DeMey R, et al. (1980). A collaborative study of the aetiology of Turner syndrome. Ann Hum Genet 43:355.

76. Mathur A, Stekol L, Schatz D, et al. (1991). The parental origin of the single X chromosome in Turner syndrome: Lack of correlation with parental age or clinical phenotype. Am J Hum Genet 48:682.

77. Hassold T, Pettay D, Robinson A, et al. (1992). Molecular studies of parental origin and mosaicism in 45,X conceptuses. Hum Genet 89:647.

78. Lorda-Sanchez I, Binkert F, Maechler M, et al. (1992). Molecular study of 45,X conceptuses: Correlation with clinical findings. Am J Med Genet 42:487.

79. Jacobs P, Dalton P, James R, et al. (1997). Turner syndrome: A cytogenetic and molecular study. Ann Hum Genet 61:471.

80. Tsezou A, Hadjiathanasiou C, Gourgiotis D, et al. (1999). Molecular genetics of Turner syndrome: Correlation with clinical phenotype and response to growth hormone therapy. Clin Genet 56:441.

81. Davenport ML, Crowe BJ, Travers SH, et al. (2007). Growth hormone Growth hormone treatment of early growth failure in toddlers with Turner syndrome: a randomized, controlled, multicenter trial. J Clin Endocrinol Metab 92:3406-3416.

82. Lorda-Sanchez I, Binkert F, Maechler M, et al. (1992). Reduced recombination and paternal age effect in Klinefelter syndrome. Hum Genet 89:524.

83. Schinzel AA, Robinson WP, Binkert F, et al. (1993). Exclusively paternal X chromosomes in a girl with short stature. Hum Genet 92:175.

84. Skuse DH, James RS, Bishop DVM, Coppin B, et al. (1997). Evidence from Turner's syndrome of an imprinted X-linked locus affecting cognitive function. Nature 387:705.

85. Pescia G, Ferrier PE, Wyss-Hutin D, et al. (1975). 45,X Turner's syndrome in monozygotic twin sisters. J Med Genet 12:390.

86. King CR, Magenis E (1978). Turner syndrome in the offspring of artificially inseminated pregnancies. Fertil Steril 30:604.

87. Salmon MA, Ashworth M (1970). Association of autoimmune disorders and sex chromosome anomalies. Lancet 2:1085.

88. Cassidy SB, Niblack GD, Lorber CA, et al. (1978). HLA frequencies, diabetes mellitus and autoimmunity in Turner's patients and their relatives. Ann Genet 21:203.

89. Villaverde MM, DaSilva JA (1975). Turner-mongolism polysyndrome: Review of the first eight known cases. JAMA 234:844.

90. Leichtman DA, Schmickel RD, Gelehrter TD, et al. (1978). Familial Turner syndrome. Ann Intern Med 89:473.

91. Massa G, Vanderschueren-Lodeweyckx M, Fryns J-P (1992). Deletion of the short arm of the X chromosome: A hereditary form of Turner syndrome. Eur J Pediatr 151:893.

92. Casteels-Van Daele M, Proesmans W, Van den Berghe H, et al. (1970). Down's anomaly (21 trisomy) and Turner's syndrome (46,XXqi) in the same sibship. Helv Paediatr Acta 25:412.

93. Ruiz C, Lamm F, Hart PS (1999). Turner syndrome and multiple-marker screening. Clin Chem 45:12.

94. Lambert-Messerlian GM, Saller DN Jr., Tumber MB, et al. (1999). Second-trimester maternal serum progesterone levels in Turner syndrome with and without hydrops and in trisomy 18. Prenat Diagn 19:476.

95. Taipale P, Hiilesmaa V, Salonen R, Ylostalo P (1997). Increased nuchal translucency as a marker for fetal chromosomal defects. N Engl J Med 337:1654.

96. Taipale P (2000). Prenatal nuchal studies in Turner syndrome. In Saenger PH, Pasquino AM (eds.), *Optimizing health care for Turner patients in the 21st century: Proceedings of the 5th International Symposium on Turner Syndrome, Naples, Italy.* Amsterdam: Elsevier Science 61–67.

97. Gunther DF, Eugster E, Zagar AJ, et al. (2004). Ascertainment bias in Turner syndrome : New insights from girls were diagnosed incidentally in prenatal life. Pediatrics 114:640–644.

98. Buckway CK, Magenis RE, Bissonnette JM, et al. (2000). Prenatal diagnosis of Turner syndrome: The Portland experience. In Saenger PH, Pasquino AM (eds.), *Optimizing health care for Turner patients in the 21st century: Proceedings of the 5th International Symposium on Turner Syndrome, Naples, Italy.* Amsterdam: Elsevier Science 69–76.

99. Gravholt CH, Juul S, Naeraa RW, et al. (1996). Prenatal and postnatal prevalence of Turner's syndrome: A registry study. BMJ 312:16–21.

100. Fechner PY, Davenport ML, Qualy RL, et al. (2006). Differences in FSH secretion between 45,X monosomy Turner syndrome and 45,X?46,XX mosaicism are evident at an early age. J Clin Endocrinol Metab 91:4896–4902.

101. Baena N, De Vigan C, Cariati E, et al. (2004). Turner syndrome: Evaluation of prenatal diagnosis in 19 European registries. Am J Med Genet A 129:16–20.

102. Hamamy HA, Dahoun S (2004). Parental decisions following the prenatal diagnosis of sex chromosome abnormalities. European J Obstetrics and Gynecology and Reproductive Biology 116:58–62.

103. Hall S, Abramsky L, Marteau TM (2003). Health professionals' report of information given to parents following the prenatal diagnosis of sex chromosome anomalies and outcomes of pregnancies: A pilot study. Prenat Diag 23:535–538.

104. Koeberl DD, McGillivray B, Sybert VP (1995). Prenatal diagnosis of 45,X/46,XX mosaicism and 45,X: Implications for postnatal outcome. Am J Hum Genet 57:661–666.

105. Warburton D, Kline J, Stein Z, Susser M (1980). Monosomy X: A chromosomal anomaly associated with young maternal age. Lancet 1:167–169.

106. Park E (1977). Body shape in Turner's syndrome. Hum Biol 49:215.

107. Collins E (1973). The illusion of widely spaced nipples in the Noonan and the Turner syndromes. J Pediatr 83:557.

108. Felix A, Capek V, Pashayan M (1974). The neck in the XO and XX/XO mosaic Turner's syndrome. Clin Genet 5:77.

109. Neufeld ND, Lippe BM, Kaplan SA (1978). Disproportionate growth of the lower extremities: A major determinant of short stature in Turner's syndrome. Am J Dis Child 132:296.

110. Beals RK (1974). Orthopedic aspects of the XO (Turner's) syndrome. Clin Orthop 97:19.

111. Baughman FA, Higgins JV, Wadsworth TG, et al. (1974). The carrying angle in sex chromosome anomalies. JAMA 230:718.

112. Kaitila II, Leisti JT, Rimoin DL (2001). Mesomelic skeletal dysplasias. Clin Orthop 114:94.

113. Ross JL, Scott C Jr, Marttila P, et al. (2001). Phenotypes associated with SHOX deficiency. J Clin Endocrinol Metab 86:5674.

114. Kosho T, Muroya K, Nagai T, et al. (1999). Skeletal features and growth patterns in 14 patients with haploinsufficiency of SHOX: Implications for the development of Turner syndrome. J Clin Endocrinol Metab 84:4613.

115. Levin B (1962). Gonadal dysgenesis: Clinical and roentgenologic manifestations. Am J Roentgenol Rad Ther Nucl Med 87:1116.

116. Horowitz SL, Morishima A (1974). Palatal abnormalities in the syndrome of gonadal dysgenesis and its variants and in Noonan's syndrome. Oral Surg 38:839.

117. Bercu BB, Kramer SS, Bode HH (1976). A useful radiologic sign for the diagnosis of Turner's syndrome. Pediatrics 48:737.

118. Necic S, Grant DB (1978). Diagnostic value of hand X-rays in Turner's syndrome. Acta Paediatr Scand 67:309.

119. Neely EK, Marcus R, Rosenfeld RG, Bachrach LK (1993). Turner syndrome in adolescents receiving growth hormone are not osteopenic. J Clin Endocrinol Metab 76:861.

120. Bachrach LK (2000). Routine monitoring of bone mineral density is not warranted in patients with Turner syndrome. In Saenger P, Pasquino AM (eds.), *Optimizing health care for Turner patients in the 21st century.* Amsterdam: Elsevier Science 267–273.

121. Ross JL, Long LM, Feuillan P, et al. (1991). Normal bone density of the wrist and spine and increased wrist fractures in girls with Turner's syndrome. J Clin Endocrinol Metab 73:335.

122. Shaw NJ, Rehan VK, Husain S, et al. (1997). Bone mineral density in Turner's syndrome: A longitudinal study. Clin Endocrinol 47:367.

123. Masters KC (1996). Treatment of Turner syndrome: A concept. Lancet 348:681.

124. Landin-Wilhelmsen K, Bryman I, Windh M, Wilhelmsen L (1999). Osteoporosis and fractures in Turner syndrome-importance of growth promoting and estrogen therapy. Clin Endocrinol 51:497.

125. Emans SJ, Grace E, Hoffer FA, et al. (1990). Estrogen deficiency in adolescents and young adults: Impact on bone mineral content and effects of estrogen replacement therapy. Obstet Gynecol 76:585.

126. van der Putte SCJ (1977). Lymphatic malformation in human fetuses: A study of fetuses with Turner's syndrome or status Bonnevie-Ullrich. Virchows Arch Hum Pathol Anat Histol 376:233.

127. Smith DW (1981). *Recognizable patterns of human deformation.* Philadelphia: WB Saunders 119–120.

128. Horowitz SL, Morishima A, Vinkk A (1976). The position of the external ear in Turner's Syndrome. Clin Genet 9:333.

129. Reed T, Reichmann A, Palmer CG (1977). Dermatoglyphic differences between 45,X and other chromosomal abnormalities of Turner syndrome. Hum Genet 36:13.

130. Denniston A (2001). Turner's syndrome. Lancet 358:2169.

131. Ranke MB, Pfluger H, Rosendahl W, et al. (1983). Turner syndrome: Spontaneous growth in 150 cases and review of the literature. Eur J Paediatr 141:81.

132. Davenport ML, Punyasavatsut N, Gunther D, et al. (1999). Turner syndrome: A pattern of early growth failure. Acta Paediatr Suppl 433:118.

133. Even L, Cohen A, Marbach N, et al. (2000). Longitudinal analysis of growth over the first 3 years of life in Turner's syndrome. J Pediatr 137:460.

134. Massa GG, Vanderschueren-Lodeweyckx M (1991). Age and height at diagnosis in Turner syndrome: Influence of parental height. Pediatrics 88:1148.

135. Brook CGD, Murset G, Zachmann M, et al. (1974). Growth in children with 45,XO Turner's syndrome. Arch Dis Child 49:789.

136. Ranke MB (1999). Turner syndrome. Eur J Endocrinol 141:216.

137. Verp MS, Rosinsky B, Le Beau MM, et al. (1988). Growth disadvantage of 45,X and 46,X,del (Xp11) fibroblasts. Clin Genet 33:277.

138. Neufeld ND, Lippe BM, Kaplan SA (1978). Disproportionate growth of the lower extremities: A major determinant of short stature in Turner's syndrome. Am J Dis Child 132:296.

139. Ikeda Y, Higurashi M, Egi S, et al. (1982). An anthropometric study of girls with Ullrich-Turner syndrome. Am J Med Genet 12:271.

140. Varrela J, Vinkka H, Alvesalo L (1984). The phenotype of 45,X females: An anthropometric quantification. Ann Hum Biol 11:53.

141. Lyon AJ, Preece MA, Grant DB (1985). Growth curve for girls with Turner syndrome. Arch Dis Child 60:932.

142. Lippe B, Plotnick L, Attie K, et al. (1993). Growth in Turner syndrome: Updating the United States experience. In Hibi I, Takano K (eds.), *Basic and clinical approach to Turner syndrome: Proceedings of the 3rd International Symposium on Turner Syndrome, Chiba, Japan.* Amsterdam: Elsevier Science 77–82.

143. Pelz L, Sager G, Hinkel GK, et al. (1991). Delayed spontaneous pubertal growth spurt in girls with Ullrich-Turner syndrome. Am J Med Genet 40:401.

144. Haeusler G, Schemper M, Frisch H, et al. (1992). Spontaneous growth in Turner syndrome: Evidence for a minor pubertal growth spurt. Eur J Pediatr 151:283.

145. Wilton P (1987). Growth hormone treatment in girls with Turner's syndrome: A review of the literature. Acta Paediatr Scand 76:193.

146. Albertsson-Wikland K, Rosberg S (1991). Pattern of spontaneous growth hormone secretion in Turner syndrome. In Ranke MB, Rosenfeld RG (eds.), *Turner syndrome: Growth promoting therapies.* Amsterdam: Elsevier Science 23–28.

147. van Es A, Massarano AA, Wit JM, et al. (1991). 24-hour growth hormone secretion in Turner syndrome. In Ranke MB, Rosenfeld RG (eds.), *Turner syndrome: Growth promoting therapies.* Amsterdam: Elsevier Science 29–33.

148. Frisch H, Haeusler G, Blumel P, et al. (1991). Relation of spontaneous nocturnal GH secretion to GH stimulation and the influence of estrogen pretreatment in Turner syndrome. In Ranke MB, Rosenfeld RG (eds.), *Turner syndrome: Growth promoting therapies.* Amsterdam: Elsevier Science 35–40.

149. Tanaka T, Hibi I, Shizume K (1991). GH secretion capacity in Turner syndrome and its influence on the effect of GH treatment. In Ranke MB, Rosenfeld RG (eds.), *Turner syndrome: Growth promoting therapies.* Amsterdam: Elsevier Science 41–45.

150. Zadik Z, Landau H, Chen M, et al. (1992). Assessment of growth hormone (GH) axis in Turner's syndrome using 24-hour integrated

concentrations of GH, insulin-like growth factor-I, plasma GH-binding activity, GH binding to IM9 cells, and GH response to pharmacological stimulation. J Clin Endocrinol Metab 75:412.

151. Ross JL, Long LM, Loriaux DL, Cutler GB (1985). Growth hormone secretory dynamics in Turner syndrome. J Pediatr 106:202.

152. Lanes R, Brito S, Suniaga M, et al. (1990). Growth hormone secretion in pubertal age patients with Turner's syndrome. J Clin Endocrinol Metab 71:770.

153. Wit JM, Massarano AA, Kamp GA, et al. (1992). Growth hormone secretion in patients with Turner's syndrome as determined by time series analysis. Acta Endocrinol 127:7.

154. Veldhuis JD, Sotos JF, Sherman BM (1991). Decreased metabolic clearance of endogenous growth hormone and specific alterations in the pulsatile mode of growth hormone secretion occur in prepubertal girls with Turner's syndrome. J Clin Endocrinol Metab 73:1073.

155. Blethen SL, Albertsson-Wikland K, Faklis EJ, et al. (1994). Circulating growth hormone isoforms in girls with Turner's syndrome. J Clin Endocrinol Metab 78:1439.

156. Foster CM, Borondy M, Markovs ME, et al. (1994). Growth hormone bioactivity in girls with Turner's syndrome: Correlation with insulin-like growth factor I. Pediatr Res 35:218.

157. Lu PW, Cowell CT, Jimenez M, et al. (1991). Effect of obesity on endogenous secretion of growth hormone in Turner's syndrome. Arch Dis Child 66:1184.

158. Whitelaw MJ, Thomas SF, Graham W, et al. (1962). Growth response in gonadal dysgenesis to the anabolic steroid norethandrolone. Am J Obstet Gynecol 84:501.

159. Johanson AJ, Brasel JA, Blizzard RM (1969). Growth in patients with gonadal dysgenesis receiving fluoxymesterone. J Pediatr 75:1015.

160. Rosenbloom AL, Frias JL (1973). Oxandrolone for growth promotion in Turner syndrome. Am J Dis Child 125:385.

161. Urban MD, Lee PA, Dorst JP, et al. (1979). Oxandrolone therapy in patients with Turner syndrome. J Pediatr 94:823.

162. Lev Ran A (1977). Androgens, estrogens, and the ultimate height in XO gonadal dysgenesis. Am J Dis Child 131:648.

163. Snider ME, Solomon IL (1974). Ultimate height in chromosomal gonadal dysgenesis without androgen therapy. Am J Dis Child 127:673.

164. Joss E, Zuppinger K (1984). Oxandrolone in girls with Turner's syndrome: A pair-matched controlled study up to final height. Acta Paediatr Scand 73:674.

165. Stahnke N, Lingstaedt K, Willig RP (1985). Oxandrolone increased final height in Turner's syndrome. Pediatr Res 19:620.

166. Sybert VP (1984). Adult height in Turner syndrome with and without androgen therapy. J Pediatr 104:365.

167. Lenko HL, Soderholm A, Perheentupa J (1988). Turner syndrome: Effect of hormone therapies on height velocity and adult height. Acta Paediatr Scand 77:699.

168. Moore DC, Tattoni DS, Ruvalcaba RHA, et al. (1977). Studies of anabolic steroids: VI. Effect of prolonged administration of oxandrolone on growth in children and adolescents with gonadal dysgenesis. J Pediatr 90:462.

169. Rudman D, Goldsmith M, Kutner M, Blackston D (1980). Effect of growth hormone and oxandrolone singly and together on growth rate in girls with X chromosome abnormalities. J Pediatr 96:132.

170. Saenger P (1996). Turner's syndrome. N Engl J Med 335:1749.

171. Rosenfeld RG, Attie KM, Frane J, et al. (1998). Growth hormone therapy of Turner's syndrome: Beneficial effect on adult height. J Pediatr 132:319.

172. Bernasconi S, Giovanelli G, Volta C, et al. (1991). Spontaneous growth in Turner syndrome: Preliminary results of an Italian multicenter study. In Ranke MB, Rosenfeld R (eds.), Turner's syndrome: Growth promoting therapies. Amsterdam: Elsevier Science 53–57.

173. Hausler G, Schemper M, Frisch H, et al. (1991). Spontaneous growth in Turner syndrome: Evidence for a minor pubertal growth spurt. In Ranke MB, Rosenfeld R (eds.), Turner's syndrome: Growth promoting therapies. Amsterdam: Elsevier Science 67–73.

174. Hibi I, Tanae A, Tanaka T, et al. (1991). Spontaneous puberty in Turner syndrome: Its incidence, influence on final height and endocrinological features. In Ranke MB, Rosenfeld R (eds.), Turner's syndrome: Growth promoting therapies. Amsterdam: Elsevier Science 75–81.

175. Naeraa RW, Nielsen J (1990). Standards for growth and final height in Turner's syndrome. Acta Paediatr Scand 79:182.

176. Donaldson MDC (1997). Growth hormone therapy in Turner syndrome-current uncertainties and future strategies. Horm Res 47(5):35.

177. Chernausek SD, Attie KM, Cara JF, et al. (2000). Growth hormone therapy of Turner syndrome: The impact of age of estrogen replacement on final height. J Clin Endocrinol Metab 85:2439.

178. Attanasio A, James D, Reinhardt R, Rekers-Mombarg L (1995). Final height and long-term outcome after growth hormone therapy in Turner syndrome: Results of a German multicentre trial. Horm Res 43:147.

179. Nilsson KO, Albertsson-Wikland K, Alm J, et al. (1996). Improved final height in girls with Turner's syndrome treated with growth hormone and oxandrolone. J Clin Endocrinol Metab 81:635.

180. Taback SP, Collu R, Deal CL, et al. (1996). Does growth hormone supplementation affect adult height in Turner's syndrome? Lancet 34:25.

181. Takano K, Shizume K, Hibi I, and the Committee for the Treatment of Turner Syndrome (1995). Long-term effects of growth hormone on height in Turner syndrome: Results of a six year multicentre study in Japan. Horm Res 43:141.

182. Van den Broeck J, Massa GG, Attanasio A, et al. (1995). Final height after long-term growth hormone treatment in Turner syndrome. J Pediatr 125:729.

183. Attie KM, Frane JW (1997). Accuracy of adult height prediction methods for Turner syndrome using US untreated control data. Horm Res 48(1):60.

184. Sas TCJ, de Muinck Keizer-Schrama SM, Stijnen T, et al. (1999). Normalization of height in girls with Turner syndrome after long-term growth hormone treatment: Results of a randomized dose-response trial. J Clin Endocrinol Metab 84:4607.

185. Park P, Cohen P (2004). The role of insulin-like growth factor I monitoring in growth hormone-treated children. Horm Res 62: 59–65.

186. Plotnick L, Attie KM, Blethen SL, Sy JP (1998). Growth hormone treatment of girls with Turner syndrome: The National Cooperative Growth Study Experience. Pediatrics 102:479.

187. Johnston DI, Betts P, Dunger D, et al. (2001). A multicentre trial of recombinant growth hormone and low dose oestrogen in Turner syndrome: Near final height analysis. Arch Dis Child 84:76.

188. Pasquino AM, Passeri F, Pucarelli I, et al. (1997). Spontaneous pubertal development in Turner's syndrome. J Clin Endocrinol Metab 82:1810.

189. Saenger P (1993). The current status of diagnosis and therapeutic intervention in Turner's syndrome. J Clin Endocrinol Metab 77:297.

190. Brown P, Gajdusek DC, Gibbs CJ Jr., Asher DM (1985). Potential epidemic of Creutzfeldt-Jakob disease from human growth hormone therapy. N Engl J Med 313:728.

191. Gerver WJM, Drayer NM, Van EA (1992). Does growth hormone treatment of patients with Turner's syndrome cause an abnormal body shape? Acta Paediatr 81:691.

192. Sas TCJ, Gerver W-JM, De Bruin R, et al. (1999). Body proportions during long-term growth hormone treatment in girls with Turner syndrome participating in a randomized dose-response trial. J Clin Endocrinol Metab 84:4622.

193. Gravholt CH, Naeraa RW (1997). Reference values for body proportions and body composition in adult women with Ullrich-Turner syndrome. Am J Med Genet 72:403.

194. Sas TC, Cromme-Dijkhuis AH, de Muinck Keizer-Schrama SM, et al. (1999). The effects of long-term growth hormone treatment on cardiac left ventricular dimensions and blood pressure in girls with Turner's syndrome. J Pediatr 135:470.

195. Saenger P, Wesoly S, Glickstein J, et al. (1995). No evidence for ventricular hypertrophy in Turner syndrome after growth hormone therapy. In Albertsson-Wikland K, Ranke MB (eds.), Turner syndrome in a life span perspective: Research and clinical aspects, Proceedings of the 4th International Symposium on Turner Syndrome, Gothenburg. Amsterdam: Elsevier Science 259–262.

196. van Teunenbroek A, de Muinck Keizer-Schrama SMPF, Aanstoot HJ, et al. (1999). Carbohydrate and lipid metabolism during various growth hormone dosing regimens in girls with Turner syndrome. Metabolism 48:7.

197. Querfeld U, Döpper S, Gradehand A, et al. (1999). Long-term treatment with growth hormone has no persisting effect on lipoprotein(a)

in patients with Turner's syndrome. J Clin Endocrinol Metab 84:967.

198. Lanes R, Gunczler P, Palacios A, Villaroel O (1997). Serum lipids, lipoprotein Ip(a), and plasminogen activator inhibitor-1 in patients with Turner's syndrome before and during growth hormone and estrogen therapy. Fertil Steril 68:473.

199. Saenger P, Wesoly S, Wasserman EJ, et al. (1996). Safety aspects of growth hormone therapy in Turner syndrome (TS): No evidence for ventricular hypertrophy (VH) and normalization of insulin levels after discontinuation of growth hormone. Pediatr Res 39(4/2):98A.

200. Sas TCJ, de Muinck Keizer-Schrama SMPF, Stijnen T, et al. (2000). Carbohydrate metabolism during long-term growth hormone (GH) treatment and after discontinuation of GH treatment in girls with Turner syndrome participating in a randomized dose-response study. J Clin Endocrinol Metab 141:769.

201. Salerno M, Di Maio S, Gasparini N, et al. (1999). Liver abnormalities in Turner syndrome. Eur J Pediatr 158:618.

202. Salerno M, Di Maio S, Ferri P, et al. (2000). Liver abnormalities during growth hormone treatment. J Pediatr Gastroenterol Nutr 31:149.

203. Gravholt CH (2000). Morbidity in Turner syndrome. In Saenger PH, Pasquino AM (eds.), *Optimizing health care for Turner patients in the 21st century: Proceedings of the 5th International Symposium on Turner Syndrome, Naples, Italy.* Amsterdam: Elsevier Science 285–294.

204. Momoi T, Yamanaka C, Tanaka R, et al. (1995). Elevation of serum creatine phosphokinase during growth hormone treatment in patients with multiple pituitary hormone deficiency. Eur J Pediatr 154:886.

205. Bourguignon JP, Pierard GE, Ernould C, et al. (1993). Effects of human growth hormone therapy on melanocytic naevi. Lancet 341:1505.

206. Zvulunov A, Wyatt DT, Laud PW, Esterly NB (1998). Influence of genetic and environmental factors on melanocytic naevi: A lesson from Turner's syndrome. Br J Dermatol 138:993.

207. Zvulunov A, Wyatt DT, Laud PW, Esterly NB (1997). Lack of effect of growth hormone therapy on the count and density of melanocytic naevi in children. Br J Dermatol 137:545.

208. Dorshkind K, Horseman ND (2000). The roles of prolactin, growth hormone, insulin-like growth factor-I, and thyroid hormones in lymphocyte development and function: Insights from genetic models of hormone and hormone receptor deficiency. Endocr Rev 21:292.

209. Rapaport R, Oleske J, Ahdieh H, et al. (1986). Suppression of immune function in growth hormone-deficient children during treatment with human growth hormone. J Pediatr 109:434.

210. Ivarsson S-A, Ericsson U-B, Nilsson KO, et al. (1995). Thyroid autoantibodies, Turner's syndrome and growth hormone therapy. Acta Paediatr 84:63.

211. Wilton P (1999). Adverse events during GH treatment: 10 years' experience in KIGS, a pharmacoepidemiological survey. In Ranke MB, Wilton P (eds.), *Growth hormone therapy in KIGS: 10 years' experience.* Heidelberg: Johann Ambrosius Barth Verlag.

212. Anderson H, Filipsson R, Fluur E, et al. (1969). Hearing impairment in Turner's syndrome. Acta Otolaryngol Suppl 247:1.

213. Barrenaes M, Landin-Wilhelmsen K, Hanson C (2000). Ear and hearing in relation to genotype and growth in Turner syndrome. Hear Res 144:21–28.

214. Dhooge IJ, De Vel E, Verhoye C, et al. (2005). Otologic disease in Turner's syndrome. Otol Neurotol 26:145–150.

215. Saenger P, Nussbaum, Lippe B (2007). Ophthalmological and otological problems in Turner syndrome. In Gravholt CH, Bondy CA (eds.), *Wellness for girls and women with Turner syndrome.* Elsevier International Congress Series 1298, Amsterdam: Elsevier 49–57.

216. Jensen K, Petersen PH, Nielsen EL, et al. (1976). Serum immunoglobulin M, G, and A concentration levels in Turner's syndrome compared with normal women and men. Hum Genet 31:329.

217. Filipsson R, Lindsten J, Almquist S (1965). Time of eruption of the permanent teeth, cephalometric and tooth measurement and sulphation factor activity in 45 patients with Turner's syndrome with different types of X chromosome aberrations. Acta Endocrinol 48:91.

218. Szpunar J (1968). Middle ear disease in Turner's syndrome. Arch Otolaryngol 87:34.

219. Stenberg AE, Nylen O, Windh M, Hultcrantz M (1998). Otological problems in children with Turner's syndrome. Hear Res 124:85.

220. Güngör N, Böke B, Belgin E, Tunçbilek E (2000). High frequency hearing loss in Ullrich-Turner syndrome. Eur J Pediatr 159:740.

221. Barrenäs M-L, Nylén O, Hanson C (1999). The influence of karyotype on the auricle, otitis media and hearing in Turner syndrome. Hear Res 138:163.

222. Barrenas M-L, Landin-Wilhelmsen K, Hanson C (2000). Ear and hearing in relation to genotype and growth in Turner syndrome. Hear Res 144:21.

223. Weiss L (1971). Additional evidence of gradual loss of germ cells in the pathogenesis of streak ovaries in Turner's syndrome. J Med Genet 8:540.

224. Singh RP, Carr DH (1965). The anatomy and histology of XO human embryos and fetuses. Anat Rec 155:369.

225. Speed RM (1988). The possible role of meiotic pairing anomalies in the atresia of human fetal oocytes. Hum Genet 78:260.

226. Morita Y, Perez GI, Maravei DV, et al. (1999). Targeted expression of Bcl-2 in mouse oocytes inhibits ovarian follicle atresia and prevents spontaneous and chemotherapy-induced oocyte apoptosis in vitro. Mol Endo 13:841.

227. Bergeron L, Perez GI, Macdonald G, et al. (1998). Defects in regulation of apoptosis in caspase-2-deficient mice. Gene Dev 12:1304.

228. McDonough PG, Byrd RJ, Tho PT, et al. (1977). Phenotypic and cytogenetic findings in eighty-two patients with ovarian failure: Changing trends. Fertil Steril 28:638.

229. Rosenfield RL (1990). Spontaneous puberty and fertility in Turner syndrome. In Rosenfield RG, Grumbach MM (eds.), *Turner syndrome.* New York: Marcel Dekker 131–144.

230. Page LA (1993). Final heights in 45,X Turner's syndrome with spontaneous sexual development: Review of European and American reports. J Pediatr Endocrinol 6:153.

231. Massa G, Vanderschueren-Lodeweyckx M, Malvaux P (1990). Linear growth in patients with Turner syndrome: Influence of spontaneous puberty and parental height. Eur J Pediatr 149:246.

232. Lippe B, Westra SJ, Boechat MI (1993). Ovarian function in Turner syndrome: Recognizing the spectrum. In Hibi I, Takano K (eds.), *Basic and clinical approach to Turner syndrome: Proceedings of the 3rd International Symposium on Turner Syndrome, Chiba, Japan.* Amsterdam: Elsevier Science 117–122.

233. King CR, Magenis E, Bennett S (1978). Pregnancy and the Turner syndrome. Obstet Gynecol 52:617.

234. Reyes FI, Koh KS, Faiman C (1976). Fertility in women with gonadal dysgenesis. Am J Obstet Gynecol 126:668.

235. Philip J, Sele V (1976). 45,XO Turner's syndrome without evidence of mosaicism in a patient with two pregnancies. Acta Obstet Gynecol Scand 55:283.

236. Swapp GH, Johnston AW, Watt JL, et al. (1989). A fertile woman with non-mosaic Turner's syndrome: Case report and review of the literature. Br J Obstet Gynaecol 96:876.

237. Kaneko N, Kawagoe S, Hiroi M (1990). Turner's syndrome: Review of the literature with reference to a successful pregnancy outcome. Gynecol Obstet Invest 29:81.

238. Dewhurst J (1977). Fertility in 47,XXX and 45,X patients. J Med Genet 15:132.

239. King CR, Magenis E (1977). Fetal wastage and chromosome anomalies in offspring of patients with Turner syndrome. Lancet 2:928.

240. Conte FA, Grumbach MM, Kaplan SL (1975). A diphasic pattern of gonadotropin secretion in patients with the syndrome of gonadal dysgenesis. J Clin Endocrinol Metab 40:670.

241. Heinrichs C, Bourdoux P, Saussez C, et al. (1994). Blood spot follicle stimulating hormone during early postnatal life in normal girls and Turner syndrome. J Clin Endocrinol Metab 78:978.

242. Mazzanti L, Cacciari E, Bergamaschi R, et al. (1997). Pelvic ultrasonography in patients with Turner syndrome: Age-related findings in different karyotypes. J Pediatr 131:135.

243. Illig R, Tolksdorf M, Murset G, et al. (1975). LH and FSH response to synthetic LH-RH in children and adolescents with Turner's and Klinefelter's syndrome. Helv Paediatr Acta 30:221.

244. Page LA, Beauregard LJ, Bode HH, et al. (1990). Hypothalamic-pituitary ovarian function in menstruating women with Turner syndrome (45,X). Pediatr Res 28:514.

245. Samaan NA, Stepanas AV, Danziger J, et al. (1979). Reactive pituitary abnormalities in patients with Klinefelter's and Turner's syndrome. Arch Intern Med 139:198.

246. Hou-Jensen K, Kempson RL (1974). The ultrastructure of gonadoblastoma and dysgerminoma. Hum Pathol 5:79.

247. Mulvihill JJ, Wade WM, Miller RW (1975). Gonadoblastoma in dysgenetic gonads with a Y chromosome. Lancet 1:863.

248. Scully RE (1970). Gonadoblastoma: A review of 74 cases. Cancer 25:1340.

249. Cuseen LJ, MacMahon RA (1979). Germ cells and ova in dysgenetic gonads of a 46-XY female dizygotic twin. Am J Dis Child 133:373.

250. Khodr GS, Cadena GD, Ong TC, et al. (1979). Y-autosome translocation, gonadal dysgenesis, and gonadoblastoma. Am J Dis Child 133:277.

251. Haddad HM, Wilkins L (1959). Congenital anomalies associated with gonadal aplasia: Review of 55 cases. Pediatrics 23:885.

252. Goldberg MB, Scully AL, Solomon IL, et al. (1968). Gonadal dysgenesis in phenotypic female subjects: A review of eighty-seven cases, with cytogenetic studies in fifty-three. Am J Med 45:529.

253. Engel E, Forbes AP (1965). Cytogenetic and clinical findings in 48 patients with congenitally defective or absent ovaries. Medicine 44:135.

254. Nora JJ, Torres FG, Sinha AK, et al. (1970). Characteristic cardiovascular anomalies of XO Turner syndrome, XX and XY phenotype and XO/XX Turner mosaic. Am J Cardiol 25:639.

255. Rainier-Pope CR, Cunningham RD, Nadas AS, et al. (1964). Cardiovascular malformations in Turner's syndrome. Pediatrics 33:919.

256. Miller MJ, Geffner ME, Lippe BM, et al. (1983). Echocardiography reveals a high incidence of bicuspid aortic valve in Turner syndrome. J Pediatr 102:47.

257. Bastianon V, Pasquino AM, Giglioni E, et al. (1989). Mitral valve prolapse in Turner syndrome. Eur J Pediatr 148:533.

258. Lin AE, Lippe BM, Geffner ME, et al. (1986). Aortic dilation, dissection, and rupture in patients with Turner syndrome. J Pediatr 109:820.

259. Mazzanti L, Cacciari E, and the Italian Study Group for Turner Syndrome (1998). Congenital heart disease in patients with Turner's syndrome. J Pediatr 133:688.

260. Goetzsche CO, Krag-Olsen B, Nielsen J, et al. (1994). Prevalence of cardiovascular malformations and association with karyotypes in Turner's syndrome. Arch Dis Child 71:433.

261. Lin AE, Lippe B, Rosenfeld RG (1998). Further delineation of aortic dilation, dissection, and rupture in patients with Turner syndrome. Pediatrics 102:e12 (http://www.pediatrics.org/cgi/content/full/102/1/e12).

262. Sybert VP (1998). Cardiovascular malformations and complications in Turner syndrome. Pediatrics 101:e11 (http://www.pediatrics.org/cgi/content/full/101/1/e11).

263. Lin AE (1994). Congenital heart defects in chromosome abnormality syndromes. In Emmanoulides GC, Reimenschneider TA, Allen HD, Gutgesell HP (eds.), Moss and Adams' heart disease in infants, children and adolescents, including the fetus and young adult, Fifth edition. Baltimore: Williams & Wilkins 633–643.

264. Prandstraller D, Mazzanti L, Picchio FM, et al. (1999). Turner's syndrome: Cardiologic profile according to the different chromosomal patterns and long-term clinical follow-up of 136 nonpreselected patients. Pediatr Cardiol 20:108.

265. Reis PM, Punch MR, Bove EL, Van de Ven CJM (1999). Outcome of infants with hypoplastic left heart and Turner syndromes. Obstet Gynecol 93:532.

266. Brackley KJ, Kilby MD, Wright JG, et al. (2000). Outcome after prenatal diagnosis of hypoplastic left-heart syndrome: A case series. Lancet 356:1143.

267. Clark EB (1984). Neck web and congenital heart defects: A pathogenic association in 45 X-O Turner syndrome? Teratology 29:355.

268. Larco RV, Jones KL, Bernirschke K (1988). Coarctation of the aorta in Turner syndrome: A pathologic study of fetuses with nuchal cystic hygromas, hydrops fetalis, and female genitalia. Pediatrics 81:445.

269. Miyabara S, Nakayama M, Suzumori K, et al. (1997). Developmental analysis of cardiovascular system of 45,X fetuses with cystic hygroma. Am J Med Genet 68:135.

270. Lippe BM, Saenger P (2002). Turner syndrome. In Sperling MA (ed.), Pediatric endocrinology, Second edition. Philadelphia: WB Saunders 387–421.

271. Lin AE (2000). Management of cardiac problems. In Saenger PH, Pasquino AM (eds.), Optimizing health care for Turner patients in the 21st century: Proceedings of the 5th International Symposium on Turner Syndrome, Naples, Italy. Amsterdam: Elsevier Science 115–123.

272. Rubin K (1993). Aortic dissection and rupture in Turner syndrome. J Pediatr 122:670.

273. Lippe B (1993). Letter to the editor. J Pediatr 122:670.

274. Dawson-Falk KL, Wright AM, Bakker B, et al. (1992). Cardiovascular evaluation in Turner syndrome: Utility of MR imaging. Australas Radiol 36:204.

275. Loscalco ML, Van Pl, Ho VB, et al. (2005). Association between fetal lymphedema and congenital cardiovascular defects in Turner syndrome. Pediatrics 115:732–735.

276. Ostberg JM, Conway GS (2000). A comparison of echocardiography and magnetic resonance imaging of the aorta in women with Turner syndrome. In Saenger PH, Pasquino AM (eds.), Optimizing health care for Turner patients in the 21st century: Proceedings of the 5th International Symposium on Turner Syndrome, Naples, Italy. Amsterdam: Elsevier Science 331.

277. Sykes KS, Neely EK, Pitlick P, Wilson DM (1998). A longitudinal study of aortic diameter in Turner syndrome. Pediatr Res 43:84A.

278. Chalard F, Ferey S, Teinturier C, et al. (2005). Aortic dilatation in Turner syndrome: The role of MRI in early recognition. Pediatr Radiol 35:323–326.

279. Castro AV, Okoshi K, Ribeiro SM, et al. (2002). Cardiovascular assessment of patients with Ulrich-Turner syndrome on Doppler echocardiography and magnetic resonance imaging. Arq Bras Cardiol 78:51–58.

280. Ho VB, Bakalov VK, Cooley M, et al. (2004). Major vascular anomalies in Turner syndrome: Prevalence and magnetic resonance angiographic features. Circulation 110:1694–1700.

281. Ostberg JE, Brookes JAS, McCarthy C, et al. (2004). A comparison of echocardiographic and magnetic resonance imaging in cardiovascular screening of adults with Turner syndrome. J Clin Endocrinol Metab 89:5966–5971.

282. Elsheihk M, Casadei B, Conway GS, et al. (2001). Hypertension is a major risk factor for aortic root dilatation in women with Turner's syndrome Clin Endocrinol (Oxford) 54:69–73.

283. Bechtold SM, Dalla Pozza R, Becker A, et al. (2004). Partial anomalous pulmonary vein connection: An underestimated cardiovascular defect in Ullrich-Turner syndrome. Eur J Pediatr 163:158–162.

284. Shiroma K, Ebine K, Tamura S, et al. (1997). A case of Turner's syndrome associated with partial anomalous pulmonary venous return complicated by dissecting aortic aneurysm and aortic regurgitation. J Cardiovasc Surg (Torino) 38:257–259.

285. Van Wasenaer AG, Lubbers LJ, Losekoit G (1988). Partial abnormal pulmonary venous return in Turner syndrome. Eur J Pediatr 148:101–103.

286. Ostberg JE, Donald AE, Halcox JPJ, et al. (2005). Vasculopathy in Turner syndrome: Arterial dilatation and intimal thickening without endothelial dysfunction. J Clin Endocrinol Metab 90:5161–5166.

287. Baguet JP, Douchin S, Pierre H, et al. (2005). Structural and functional abnormalities of large arteries in Turner syndrome. Heart 048371.

288. Allen DB, Hendricks SA, Levy JM (1986). Aortic dilation in Turner syndrome. J Pediatr 109:302.

289. Price WH, Clayton JF, Collyer S, et al. (1986). Mortality ratios, life expectancy, and causes of death in patients with Turner's syndrome. J Epidemiol Community Health 40:97.

290. Silberbach M (2000). Dissection of the aorta: Lessons learned from Marfan syndrome. In Saenger PH, Pasquino AM (eds.), Optimizing health care for Turner patients in the 21st century: Proceedings of the 5th International Symposium on Turner Syndrome, Naples, Italy. Amsterdam: Elsevier Science 145–152.

291. Larson EW, Edwards WD (1984). Risk factors for aortic dissection: A necropsy study of 161 cases. Am J Cardiol 53:849.

292. Garvey P, Elovitz M, Landsberger EJ (1998). Aortic dissection and myocardial infarction in a pregnant patient with Turner syndrome. Obstet Gynecol 91:864.

293. Nagel TC, Tesch LG (1997). ART and high risk patients. Fertil Steril 68:748.

294. Birdsall M, Kenny S (1996). The risk of aortic dissection in women with Turner syndrome. Hum Reprod 11:587.

295. Lipscomb KJ, Smith JC, Clarke B, et al. (1997). Outcome of pregnancy in women with Marfan's syndrome. Br J Obstet Gynaecol 104:201.

296. Hahn RT, Roman MJ, Mogtader AH, Devereux RB (1992). Association of aortic dilation with regurgitant, stenotic and functionally normal bicuspid aortic valves. J Am Coll Cardiol 19:283.

297. Gunning JF, Oakley CM (1970). Aortic-valve disease in Turner's syndrome. Lancet 1:389.

298. Bisset GS, Schwartz DC, Meyer RA, et al. (1980). Clinical spectrum and long-term follow-up of isolated mitral valve prolapse in 119 children. Circulation 62:423.

299. Conway GS, Elsheikh M, Cadge B, Ostberg J (2000). Adult Turner follow-up-the Middlesex Experience. In Saenger PH, Pasquino AM (eds.), Optimizing health care for Turner patients in the 21st century. Proceedings of the 5th International Symposium on Turner Syndrome, Naples, Italy. Amsterdam: Elsevier Science 295–306.

300. Bondy CA, Van PL, Bakalov VK, et al. (2006). Prolongation of cardiac QTc interval in Turner syndrome. Medicine 85:75–81.

301. Nathwani NC, Unwin R, Brook CG, et al. (2000). The influence of renal and cardiovascular abnormalities on blood pressure in Turner syndrome. Clin Endocrinol (Oxford) 52:371–377.

302. Gravholt CH, Naeraa RW, Nyholm B, et al. (1998). Glucose metabolism, lipid metabolism, and cardiovascular risk factors in adult Turner's syndrome: The impact of sex hormone replacement. Diabetes Care 21:1062–1070.

303. Gravholt CH, Juul S, Naeraa RW, Hansen J (1998). Morbidity in Turner syndrome. J Clin Epidemiol 51:147.

304. Landin-Wilhelmsen K, Sylven L, Berntorp K, et al. (2000). Swedish cardiac morbidity study in Turner syndrome. In Saenger PH, Pasquino AM (eds.), Optimizing health care for Turner patients in the 21st century: Proceedings of the 5th International Symposium on Turner Syndrome, Naples, Italy. Amsterdam: Elsevier Science 137–144.

305. Skemp AM, Pierpont MEM (1998). Cardiomyopathy, conduction abnormalities and aortic dilation in Turner syndrome. Int Pediatr 13:27.

306. Roman MJ, Devereux RB, Kramer-Fix R, et al. (1989). Two-dimensional echocardiographic aortic root dimensions in normal children and adults Amer J Cardiol 63:507–512.

307. Shores J, Berger KR, Murphy EA, et al. (1994). Progression of aortic dilatation and the benefit of long-term beta adrenergic blockade in Marfan's syndrome. N Engl J Med 330:1335–1341.

308. Fletcher GF (1997). How to implement physical activity in primary and secondary prevention. Circulation 96:355–357.

309. Karnis MF, Zimon AE, Lalwani SI, et al. (2003). Risk of death in pregnancy achieved through oocyte donation in patients with Turner syndrome: A national survey. Fertility and Sterility 80:498–501.

310. Radetti G, Crepaz R, Milanesi O, et al. (2001). Cardiac performance in Turners syndrome patients on growth hormone therapy. Horm Res 55:240–244.

311. Bondy CA, Van PL, Bakalov VK, et al. (2006). Growth hormone treatment and aortic dimensions in Turner syndrome. J Clin Endocrinol Metab 91:1785–1788.

312. Van den Berg J, Bannink EM, Wielopolski PA, et al. (2006). Aortic distensibility and dimensions and the effects of growth hormone treatment in the Turner syndrome. Amer J Cardiology 97:1644–1649.

313. H Surerus E, Huggon IC, Allan LD (2003). Turner syndrome in fetal life. Ultrasound Obstetr Gynecol 22:264–267.

314. Bernas MJ, Witte CL, Witte MH (2001). The diagnosis and treatment of peripheral lymphedema: 1995 consensus document revision. Lymphology 38:84–91.

315. Reveno JS, Palubinskas AJ (1966). Congenital renal abnormalities in gonadal dysgenesis. Radiology 86:49.

316. Sagi L, Zuckerman-Levin N, Gawlik A, et al. (2006). Clinical signific`ance of the parental origin of the X chromosome in Turner syndrome. J Clin Endocrinol Metab 92:848.

317. Litvak AS, Rousseau TG, Wrede LD, et al. (1978). The association of significant renal anomalies with Turner's syndrome. J Urol 120:671.

318. Flynn MT, Ekstrom L, De Arce M, et al. (1996). Prevalence of renal malformation in Turner syndrome. Pediatr Nephrol 10:498.

319. Mazzanti L, Bergamaschi R, Scarano E, et al. (1999). Renal malformations in patients with Turner's syndrome. Horm Res 51(2):59.

320. Bilge I, Kayserili H, Emre S, et al. (2000). Frequency of renal malformations in Turner syndrome: Analysis of 82 Turkish children. Pediatr Nephrol 14:1111–1114.

321. Cleeve DM, Older RA, Cleeve LK, et al. (1979). Retrocaval ureter in Turner syndrome. Urology 8:544.

322. Mesrobian H-GJ, Kelalis PP, Hrabovsky E, et al. (1985). Wilms tumor in horseshoe kidneys: A report from the National Wilms Tumor Study. J Urol 133:1002.

323. Torfs CP, van den Berg BJ, Oechsli FW, et al. (1990). Thyroid antibodies as a risk factor for Down syndrome and other trisomies. Am J Hum Genet 47:727.

324. Stagnaro-Green A, Roman SH, Cobin RH, et al. (1990). Detection of at-risk pregnancy by means of highly sensitive assays for thyroid autoantibodies. JAMA 264:1422.

325. Sparkes RS, Motulsky AB (1963). Hashimoto's disease in Turner's syndrome with isochromosome X. Lancet 1:947.

326. Pai GS, Leach DC, Weiss L, et al. (1977). Thyroid abnormalities in 20 children with Turner's syndrome. J Pediatr 91:267.

327. Germain EL, Plotnick LP (1986). Age-related anti-thyroid antibodies and thyroid abnormalities in Turner syndrome. Acta Paediatr Scand 75:750.

328. Fleming S, Cowell C, Bailey J, et al. (1988). Hashimoto's disease in Turner's syndrome. Clin Invest Med 11:243.

329. Ling SM, Kaplan SA, Weitzmann JJ, et al. (1969). Euthyroid goiters in children: Correlation of needle biopsy with other clinical and laboratory findings in chronic lymphocytic thyroiditis and simple goiter. Pediatrics 44:695.

330. Radetti G, Mazzanti L, Paganini C, et al. (1995). Frequency, clinical and laboratory features of thyroiditis in girls with Turner's syndrome. Acta Paediatr 84:909.

331. Brooks WH, Meek JC, Schimke RN (1977). Gonadal dysgenesis with Graves' disease. J Med Genet 14:128.

332. Massa G, de Zegher F, Dooms L, et al. (1992). Hyperthyroidism accelerates growth in Turner's syndrome. Acta Paediatr 81:362.

333. El Mansoury M, Bryman I, Berntorp K, et al. (2002). Hypothyroidism is common in Turner syndrome: Results of a five year follow up. J Clin Endocrinol Metab 90:2131–2135.

334. Livada S, Xekouki P, Fouka F, et al. (2005). Prevalence of thyroid dysfunction in Turner syndrome. Thyroid 15:1061–1066.

335. Zulian F, Schumacher HR, Calore A, et al. (1998). Juvenile arthritis in Turner's syndrome: A multicenter study. Clin Exp Rheumatol 16:489.

336. Rosen KM, Sirota DK, Marinoff SC (1967). Gastrointestinal bleeding in Turner's syndrome. Ann Intern Med 67:145.

337. Salomonowitz E, Staffen A, Potzi R, et al. (1983). Angiographic demonstration of phlebectasia in a case of Turner's syndrome. Gastrointest Radiol 8:279.

338. Weiss SW (1988). Pedal hemangioma (venous malformation) occurring in Turner's syndrome: An additional manifestation of the syndrome. Hum Pathol 9:1015.

339. van Cutsem E, Rutgeerts P, Vantrappen G (1990). Treatment of bleeding gastrointestinal vascular malformations with oestrogen-progesterone. Lancet 335:953.

340. O'Hare JP, Hamilton M, Davies JD, et al. (1986). Oestrogen deficiency and bleeding from large bowel telangiectasia in Turner's syndrome. J R Soc Med 79:746.

341. Arulanantham K, Kramer MS, Gryboski JD (1980). The association of inflammatory bowel disease and X chromosomal abnormality. Pediatrics 66:63.

342. Price WH (1979). A high incidence of chronic inflammatory bowel disease in patients with Turner's syndrome. J Med Genet 16:263.

343. Knudtzon J, Svane S (1988). Turner's syndrome associated with chronic inflammatory bowel disease: A case report and review of the literature. Acta Med Scand 223:375.

344. Manzione NC, Kram M, Kram E, et al. (1988). Turner's syndrome and inflammatory bowel disease: A case report with immunologic studies. Am J Gastroenterol 83:1294.

345. Hayward PAR, Satsangi J, Jewell DP (1996). Inflammatory bowel disease and the X chromosome. QJM 89:713.

346. Bonamico M, Bottaro G, Pasquino AM, et al. (1998). Celiac disease and Turner syndrome. J Pediatr Gastroenterol Nutr 26:496.

347. Ivarsson S-A, Carlsson A, Bredberg A, et al. (1999). Prevalence of coeliac disease in Turner syndrome. Acta Paediatr 88:933.

348. Schewior S, Brand M, Santer R (1999). Celiac disease and selective IgA deficiency in a girl with atypical Turner syndrome. J Pediatr Gastroenterol Nutr 28:353.

349. Bonamico M, Pasquino AM, Mariani P, et al. (2002). Prevalence and clinical picture of celiac disease in Turner syndrome. J Clin Endocrinol Metab 87:5495–5498.

350. Hill ID, Dirks MH, Liptak GS, et al. (2005). Guideline for the diagnosis and treatment of celiac disease in children. J Pediatr Gastroenterology 40:1–19.

351. Floreani A, Molaro M, Baragiota A, Naccarato R (1999). Chronic cholestasis associated with Turner's syndrome. Digestion 60:587.

352. Wemme H, Pohlenz J, Schonberger W (1995). Effect of oestrogen/gestagen replacement therapy on liver enzymes in patients with Ullrich-Turner syndrome. Eur J Pediatr 154:807.

353. Roulot D, Valla D (2007). Hepatic disease in Turner syndrome. In [editor(s)], *Wellness for girls and women with Turner syndrome.* Elsevier International Congress Series 1298. Amsterdam: Elsevier 146–151.

354. Jospe N, Orlowski CC, Furlanetto R (1995). Comparison of transdermal and oral estrogen therapy in girls with Turner's syndrome. J Pediatr Endocrinol Metab 8:111.

355. Guttmann H, Weiner Z, Nikolski E, et al. (2001). Choosing an oestrogen replacement therapy in young adult women with Turner syndrome. Clin Endocrinol 54:159.

356. Forbes AP, Engel E (1963). The high incidence of diabetes mellitus in 41 patients with gonadal dysgenesis, and their close relatives. Metabolism 12:428.

357. Nielsen J, Johansen K, Yde H (1969). The frequency of diabetes mellitus in patients with Turner's syndrome and pure gonadal dysgenesis. Acta Endocrinol 62:251.

358. Costin G, Kogut MD (1985). Carbohydrate intolerance in gonadal dysgenesis: Evidence for insulin resistance and hyperglucagonemia. Horm Res 22:260.

359. Rimoin DL, Harder E, Whitehead B, et al. (1970). Abnormal glucose tolerance in patients with gonadal dysgenesis and their parents. Clin Res 18:395.

360. Neufeld ND, Lippe B, Sperling MA (1980). Carbohydrate (CHO) intolerance in gonadal dysgenesis: A new model of insulin resistance. Diabetes 25:379.

361. Karp M, Snir A, Doron M, et al. (1975). Glucose tolerance tests and insulin response in juvenile patients with gonadal dysgenesis. Mod Probl Paediatr 12:251.

362. Cicognani A, Mazzanti L, Tassinari D, et al. (1988). Differences in carbohydrate tolerance in Turner syndrome depending on age and karyotype. Eur J Pediatr 148:64.

363. Stahnke N, Stubbe P, Keller E (1992). Recombinant human growth hormone and oxandrolone in treatment of short stature in girls with Turner syndrome. Horm Res 37(2):37.

364. Almaguer M, Saenger P, Frane J, et al. (1993). Six year data of carbohydrate tolerance in Turner syndrome treated with growth hormone and oxandrolone. Pediatr Res 33:S67.

365. Caprio S, Boulware S, Diamond M, et al. (1991). Insulin resistance: An early metabolic defect of Turner's syndrome. J Clin Endocrinol Metab 72:832.

366. Monti LD, Brambilla P, Caumo A, et al. (1997). Glucose turnover and insulin clearance after growth hormone treatment in girls with Turner's syndrome. Metabolism 46:1482.

367. Harvengt C (1992). Effect of oral contraceptive use on the incidence of impaired glucose tolerance and diabetes mellitus. Diabetes Metab 18:71.

368. Gravholt CH, Naeraa RW, Nyholm B, et al. (1998). Glucose metabolism, lipid metabolism, and cardiovascular risk factors in adult Turner's syndrome: The impact of sex hormone replacement. Diabet Care 21:1062.

369. Elsheikh M, Bird R, Casadei B, et al. (2000). The effect of hormone replacement therapy on cardiovascular hemodynamics in women with Turner's syndrome. J Clin Endocrinol Metab 85:614.

370. Hjerrild BE, Gravholt CH (2007). Diabetes and lipid disorders. In [editor(s)] (eds.), *Wellness for girls and women with Turner syndrome.* International Congress Series 1298, [city]: Elsevier 152–159.

371. Wilson DM, Frane JW, Sherman B, et al. (1988). Carbohydrate and lipid metabolism in Turner syndrome: Effect of therapy with growth hormone, oxandrolone, and a combination of both. J Pediatr 112:210.

372. Saenger P, Attie KM, DiMartino-Nardi J, Fine RN (1996). Carbohydrate metabolism in children receiving growth hormone for 5 years: Chronic renal insufficiency compared with growth hormone deficiency, Turner syndrome, and idiopathic short stature. Pediatr Nephrol 10:261.

373. Caprio S, Boulware S, Press M, et al. (1992). Effect of growth hormone treatment on hyperinsulinemia associated with Turner syndrome. J Pediatr 120:238.

374. Caprio S (2000). Lipoproteins and carbohydrate metabolism in Turner syndrome. In Saenger PH, Pasquino AM (eds.), *Optimizing health care for Turner patients in the 21st century: Proceedings of the 5th International Symposium on Turner Syndrome, Naples, Italy.* Amsterdam: Elsevier Science 257–260.

375. Garron DC (1977). Intelligence among persons with Turner's syndrome. Behav Genet 7:105.

376. Nielsen J, Fischer M, Friedrich U (1973). Mental retardation in Turner's syndrome. J Ment Defic Res 17:227.

377. Watkins JM, Elliott TE, Neely EK, et al. (1993). Thyroid autoimmunity is associated with cognitive impairment in Turner syndrome. Pediatr Res 33:S94.

378. Haddow JE, Palomaki GE, Allan WC, et al. (1999). Maternal thyroid deficiency during pregnancy and subsequent neuropsychological development of the child. N Engl J Med 341:549.

379. Silbert A, Wolff PH, Lilienthal J (1977). Spatial and temporal processing in patients with Turner's syndrome. Behav Genet 7:11.

380. Nyborg H, Nielsen J (1977). Sex chromosome abnormalities and cognitive performance: III. Field dependence, frame dependence, and failing development of perceptual stability in girls with Turner's syndrome. J Psychol 96:205.

381. Waber DP (1979). Neuropsychological aspects of Turner's syndrome. Dev Med Child Neurol 21:58.

382. McCauley E, Kay T, Ito J, Treder R (1987). The Turner syndrome: Cognitive deficits, affective discrimination, and behavior problems. Child Dev 58:464.

383. Ross JL, Kushner H, Roeltgen DP (1996). Developmental changes in motor function in girls with Turner syndrome. Pediatr Neurol 15:317.

384. Nijhuis-van der Sanden RWG, Smits-Engelsman BCM, Eling PATM (2000). Motor performance in girls with Turner syndrome. Dev Med Child Neurol 42:685.

385. McCauley E, Ross JL, Kushner H, Cutler G (1995). Self-esteem and behavior in girls with Turner syndrome. J Dev Behav Pediatr 16:82.

386. Lagrou K, Xhrouet-Heinrichs D, Heinrichs C, et al. (1998). Age-related perception of stature, acceptance of therapy, and psychosocial functioning in human growth hormone-treated girls with Turner's syndrome. J Clin Endocrinol Metab 83:1494.

387. Rovet J, Holland J (1993). Psychological aspects of the Canadian randomized control trial of human growth hormone and low dose ethinyl oestradiol in children with Turner syndrome. Horm Res 39:60.

388. Rovet J, Netley C (1982). Processing deficits in Turner's syndrome. Dev Psychol 18:77.

389. Temple CM, Carney RA (1993). Intellectual functioning of children with Turner syndrome: A comparison of behavioural phenotypes. Dev Med Child Neurol 35:691.

390. Ross JL, Stefanatos G, Roeltgen D, et al. (1995). Ullrich-Turner syndrome: Neurodevelopmental changes from childhood through adolescence. Am J Med Genet 58:74.

391. Zinn AR, Ross JL (2000). Critical regions for Turner syndrome phenotypes on the X chromosome. In Saenger PH, Pasquino AM (eds.), *Optimizing health care for Turner patients in the 21st century: Proceedings of the 5th International Symposium on Turner Syndrome, Naples, Italy.* Amsterdam: Elsevier Science 19–28.

392. Tsuboi T, Nielsen J, Nagayama I (1988). Turner's syndrome: A qualitative and quantitative analysis of EEG background activity. Hum Genet 78:206.

393. Johnson R, Rohrbaugh JW, Ross JL (1993). Altered brain development in Turner's syndrome: An event-related potential study. Neurology 43:801.

394. Reiss AL, Freund L, Plotnick L, et al. (1993). The effect of X monosomy on brain development: Monozygotic twins discordant for Turner's syndrome. Ann Neurol 34:95.

395. Murphy DGM, DeCarli C, Daly E, et al. (1993). X-chromosome effects on female brain: A magnetic resonance imaging study of Turner's syndrome. Lancet 342:1197.

396. Clark C, Klonoff H, Hayden M (1990). Regional cerebral glucose metabolism in Turner syndrome. Can J Neurol Sci 17:140.

397. Watkins JM, Chugani HT, Elliott TK, et al. (1991). Positron emission tomography and neuropsychological correlations in Turner syndrome. Ann Neurol 30:454.

398. Haberecht M, Menon V, Warofsky I, et al. (2000). Neurocognitive function in Turner syndrome: A review of neuroimaging and behavioral studies. In Saenger PH, Pasquino AM (eds.), *Optimizing health care for Turner patients in the 21st century: Proceedings of*

the 5th International Symposium on Turner Syndrome, Naples, Italy. Amsterdam: Elsevier Science 79–84.

399. Bishop DV, Canning E, Elgar K, et al. (2000). Distinctive patterns of memory function in subgroups of females with Turner syndrome: Evidence for imprinted loci on the X-chromosome affecting neurodevelopment. Neuropsychologia 38:712.

400. Haverkamp F, Keuker T, Kaiser G, et al. (2000). Social cognition in relation to different visuospatial cognitive styles in Ullrich-Turner syndrome: Evidence for a selective deficit in social context dependent visual integration. In Saenger PH, Pasquino AM (eds.), *Optimizing health care for Turner patients in the 21st century: Proceedings of the 5th International Symposium on Turner Syndrome, Naples, Italy.* Amsterdam: Elsevier Science 97–103.

401. Ross JL, Roeltgen D, Feuillan P, et al. (1998). Effects of estrogen on nonverbal processing speed and motor function in girls with Turner's syndrome. J Clin Endocrinol Metab 83:3198.

402. Ross JL, Roeltgen D, Feuillan P, et al. (2000). Use of estrogen in young girls with Turner syndrome: Effects on memory. Neurology 54:164.

403. Romans SM, Stefanatos G, Roeltgen DP, et al. (1998). Transition to young adulthood in Ullrich-Turner syndrome: Neurodevelopmental changes. Am J Med Genet 79:140.

404. Rovet JF (1993). The psychoeducational characteristics of children with Turner syndrome. J Learn Disabil 26:333–341.

405. Mazzocco MM, Singh Bhatia N, Lesniak-Karpiak K (2006). Visuispatial skills and their association with math performance in girls with fragile X or Turner syndrome. Child Neuropsychol 12:87–110.

406. Ross, JL, Zinn A, McCauley E (2000). Neurodevelopmental and psychosocial aspects of Turner syndrome. Ment Retard Dev Disabil Res Rev 6:135–141.

407. Verlinde F, Massa G, Lagrou K, et al. (2004). Health and psychosocial status of patients with Turner syndrome after transition to adulthood. Horm Res 62:161–167.

408. Hanton L, Axelrod L, Bakalov V, et al. (2003). The importance of estrogen replacement in young women with Turner syndrome. J Womens Health (Larchmt) 12:971–977.

409. Okada Y (1994). The quality of life of Turner women in comparison with grown-uo Gh-deficient women. Endocr J 41:345–354.

410. Pavlidis K, McCauley E, Sybert VP (1995). Psychosocial and sexual functioning in women with Turner syndrome. Clin Genet 47:85–89.

411. Carel JC, Elie C, Ecosse E, et al. (2006). Self-esteem and social adjustment in young women with Turner syndrome: Influence of pubertal management and sexuality, population-based cohort study. J Clin Endocrinol Metab 91:2972–2979.

412. Schmidt PJ, Cardoso GMP, Ross JL, et al. (2002). Shyness, social anxiety and impaired self-esteem in Turner syndrome and premature ovarian failure. JAMA 295:1374–1376.

413. Sutton EJ, McInerney-Leo A, Bondy CA, et al. (2005). Turner syndrome: Four challenges across the life span. Am J Med Genet 139:57–66.

414. Kron L, Katz JL, Gorzynski G, et al. (1977). Anorexia nervosa and gonadal dysgenesis: Further evidence of a relationship. Arch Gen Psychiatry 34:332.

415. Kauli R, Gurewitz R, Galazer A, et al. (1982). Effect of anorexia nervosa on gonadotropin secretion in a patient with gonadal dysgenesis. Acta Endocrinol 100:363.

416. Prior TI, Chue PS, Tibbo P (2000). Investigation of Turner syndrome in schizophrenia. Am J Med Genet (Neuropsychiatr Genet) 96:373.

417. Creswell CS, Skuse DH (1999). Autism in association with Turner syndrome: Genetic implications for male vulnerability to pervasive developmental disorders. Neurocase 5:101.

418. Donnelly SL, Wolpert CM, Menold MM, et al. (2000). Female with autistic disorder and monosomy X (Turner syndrome): Parent-oforigin effect of the X chromosome. Am J Med Genet (Neuropsychiatr Genet) 96:312.

419. Skuse D, Kuntsi J, Elgar K (2000). Evidence that X-linked genes of maternal and paternal origin differentially contribute to the development of cognitive brain systems. In Saenger PH, Pasquino AM (eds.), *Optimizing health care for Turner patients in the 21st century: Proceedings of the 5th International Symposium on Turner Syndrome, Naples, Italy.* Amsterdam: Elsevier Science 85–95.

420. Money J, Mittenthal S (1970). Lack of personality pathology in Turner's syndrome: Relation to cytogenetics, hormones, and physique. Behav Genet 1:43.

421. Downey J, Ehrhardt AA, Gruen R, et al. (1989). Psychopathology and social functioning in women with Turner syndrome. J Nerv Ment Dis 177:191.

422. McCauley E, Sybert V, Ehrhardt AA (1986). Psychosocial adjustment of adult women with Turner syndrome. Clin Genet 29:284.

423. McCauley E, Ito J, Kay T (1986). Psychosocial functioning in girls with Turner's syndrome and short stature: Social skills, behavior problems, and self-concept. J Am Acad Child Psychiatry 25:105.

424. Garron DC, Van der Stoep LP (1969). Personality and intelligence in Turner's syndrome. Arch Gen Psychiatry 21:339.

425. Sylven L, Magnusson C, Hagenfeldt K, et al. (1993). Life with Turner's syndrome: A psychosocial report from 22 middle-aged women. Acta Endocrinol 129:188.

426. Aran O, Galatzer A, Kauli R, et al. (1992). Social, educational and vocational status of 48 young adult females with gonadal dysgenesis. Clin Endocrinol 36:405.

427. Sutton EJ, Young J, McInerney-Leo A, Bondy CA (2006). Truthtelling and Turner syndrome: The importance of diagnostic disclosure. J Ped 148:102–107.

428. Saenger P, Wikland KA, Conway GS, et al. (2001). Recommendations for the diagnosis and management of Turner syndrome. J Clin Endocrinol Metab 86:3061.

429. Gottschalk M, Lippe BM, Frane JW (1989). Turner syndrome: Delayed diagnosis when short stature is the predominant finding. Clin Res 37:184A.

430. Findlay CA, Donaldson MDC, Watt G (2001). Foot problems in Turner's syndrome. J Pediatr 138:775.

431. Binder G, Fritsch H, Schweizer R, et al. (2001). Radiological signs of Leri-Weill dyschondrosteosis in Turner syndrome. Horm Res 55:71–76.

432. Elder DA, Roper MG, Henderson RC, et al. (2002). Kyphosis in a Turner syndrome population. Pediatrics 109:e93.

433. Kim JY, Rosenfeld SR, Keyak JH (2001). Increased prevalence of scoliosis in Turner syndrome. J Pediatr Orthop 21:765–766.

434. Sas TC, Munick Keizer-Schrama SM, Stijnen T, et al. (2000). A longitudinal study on bone mineral density until adulthood in girls with Turner's syndrome participating in a growth hormone injection frequency-response trial. Clin Endocrinol (Oxford) 52:531–536.

435. Navot D, Laufer N, Kopolovic J, et al. (1986). Artificially induced endometrial cycles and establishment of pregnancies in the absence of ovaries. N Engl J Med 314:806.

436. Rogers PAW, Murphy CR, Leeton J, et al. (1992). Turner's syndrome patients lack tight junctions between uterine epithelial cells. Hum Reprod 7:883.

437. Hovatta O (1999). Pregnancies in women with Turner's syndrome. Ann Med 31:106.

438. Massarano AA, Adams JA, Preece MA, et al. (1989). Ovarian ultrasound appearances in Turner syndrome. J Pediatr 114:568.

439. Elsheikh M, Casade B, Conway GS, Wass JAH (2001). Hypertension is a major risk factor for aortic root dilatation in women with Turner's syndrome. Clin Endocrinol 54:69.

440. Shores J, Berger KR, Murphy EA, et al. (1994). Progression of aortic dila-tation and the benefit of long-term b-adrenergic blockade in Marfan's syndrome. N Engl J Med 330:1335.

441. Ho ECK, Moss AJ (1972). The syndrome of "mesenteric arteritis" following surgical repair of aortic coarctation: Report of nine cases and review of the literature. Pediatrics 49:40.

442. Crawford JD (1979). Management of children with Turner's syndrome. In [editor(s)] (ed.), *The management of genetic disorders.* New York: Alan R. Liss 97–109.

443. Massa G, Vanderschueren-Lodeweyckx M, Craen M, et al. (1991). Growth hormone treatment of Turner syndrome patients with insufficient growth hormone response to pharmacological stimulation tests. Eur J Pediatr 150:460.

444. Pasquino AM, Bernardini S, Cianfarani S, et al. (1992). GH assessment and three years' hGH therapy in girls with Turner syndrome. Horm Res 38:120.

445. Ranke MB, Lindberg A, Chatelain P, et al. (2000). Prediction of long-term response to recombinant human growth hormone (GH) in Turner syndrome: Development and validation of mathematical models. J Clin Endocrinol Metab 85:4212.

446. Neely EK, Rosenfeld RG (1993). First year results of a randomized, placebo controlled trial of low dose ethinyl estradiol for feminization during growth hormone therapy for Turner syndrome. Pediatr Res 33:S89.

447. Reiter EO, Blethen SL, Baptista J, Price L (2001). Early initiation of growth hormone treatment allows age-appropriate estrogen use in Turner's syndrome. J Clin Endocrinol Metab 86:1936.

448. Ross Jl, Quigley CA, Dachuang C, et al. (2007). *Synergistic effect of GH and early low dose estrogen on adult height in Turner syndrome: Results of a randomised, double-blind, placebo-controlled trial.* [city]: The Endocrine Society 34.

449. Massa G, Maes M, Heinrichs C, et al. (1993). Influence of spontaneous or induced puberty on the growth promoting effect of treatment with growth hormone in girls with Turner's syndrome. Clin Endocrinol 38:253.

450. Santoro NF, Col NF, Eckman MH, et al. (1999). Therapeutic controversy: Hormone replacement therapy-where are we going? J Clin Endocrinol Metab 84:1798.

451. Greendale GA, Lee NP, Arriola ER (1999). The menopause. Lancet 353:571.

452. Voigt LF, Weiss NS, Chu J, et al. (1991). Progestagen supplementation of exogenous oestrogens and risk of endometrial cancer. Lancet 338:274.

453. Lobo RA (1991). Clinical Review 27: Effects of hormonal replacement on lipids and lipoproteins in postmenopausal women. J Clin Endocrinol Metab 73:925.

454. Whitcroft SIJ, Stevenson JC (1992). Hormone replacement therapy: Risks and benefits. Clin Endocrinol 36:15.

455. Belchetz PE (1994). Hormonal treatment of postmenopausal women. N Engl J Med 330:1062.

456. Rubin KR (1988). Osteoporosis in Turner syndrome. In Rosenfeld RG, Grumbach MM (eds.), *Turner syndrome.* New York: Marcel Dekker 301–317.

457. Neely EK, Marcus R, Rosenfeld RG, et al. (1993). Turner syndrome adolescents receiving growth hormone are not osteopenic. J Clin Endocrinol Metab 76:861.

458. Dewhurst CJ, DeKoos EB, Haines RM (1975). Replacement hormone therapy in gonadal dysgenesis. Br J Obstet Gynaecol 82:412.

459. Chan L, O'Malley BW (1976). Mechanism of action of the sex steroid hormones. N Engl J Med 294:1430.

460. Benjamin I, Block RE (1977). Endometrial response to estrogen and progesterone therapy in patients with gonadal dysgenesis. Obstet Gynecol 50:137.

461. Padwick ML, Pryse-Davies J, Whitehead MI (1986). A simple method for determining the optimal dosage of progestin in postmenopausal women receiving estrogens. N Engl J Med 315:930.

462. Elkind-Hirsch KE, Sherman LD, Malinak R (1993). Hormone replacement therapy alters insulin sensitivity in young women with premature ovarian failure. J Clin Endocrinol Metab 76:472.

463. Godsland IF, Crook D, Simpson R, et al. (1990). The effects of different formulations of oral contraceptive agents on lipid and carbohydrate metabolism. N Engl J Med 323:1375.

464. Naeraa RW, Brixen K, Hansen RM, et al. (1991). Skeletal size and bone mineral content in Turner's syndrome: Relation to karyotype, estrogen treatment, physical fitness, and bone turnover. Calcif Tissue Int 49:77.

465. Ettinger B, Genant HK, Steiger P, et al. (1992). Low-dosage micronized 17b-estradiol prevents bone loss in postmenopausal women. Am J Obstet Gynecol 166:479.

466. Porcu E, Fabbri R, Damiano G, et al. (2000). Clinical experience and applications of oocyte cryopreservation. Mol Cell Endocrinol 169:33.

467. Lufkin EG, Ory SJ (1994). Relative value of transdermal and oral estrogen therapy in various clinical situations. Mayo Clin Proc 69:131.

468. Elsheikh M, Conway GS, Wass JAH (1999). Medical problems in adult women with Turner syndrome: Trends in medical practice. Ann Med 31:99.

469. Gravholt CH, Bondy CA (2007). *Wellness for girls and women with Turner syndrome.* International Congress Series 1298, Amsterdam: Elsevier.

470. Foudila T, Soderstrom-Antitila V, Hovatta O (1999). Turner syndrome and pregnancies after oocyte donation. Hum Reprod 14:532–535.

471. Bodri D, Vernaeve V, Figueras F, et al. (2006). Oocyte donation in patients with Turner syndrome: A successful technique but with an accompanying risk of hypertensive disorders during pregnancy. Hum Reprod 21: 829–832.

472. Hreinsson JG, Otala M, Fridstrom M, et al. (2005). Follicles are found in the ovaries of adolescent girls with Turner syndrome. J Clin Endocrinol Metab 87:3618–3623.

473. Ferraz de Souza B, Lin L, Woodruff TK, Achermann JC (2007). Reproductive endocrinology. In Carel JC, Hochberg Z (eds.), *Yearbook of peditaric endocrinology.* Basel: Karger 71–86.

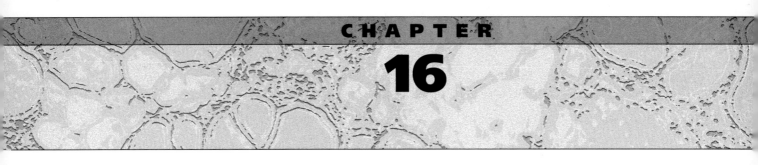

The Testes: Disorders of Sexual Differentiation and Puberty in the Male

IEUAN A. HUGHES, MD, FRCP

Introduction

Development of the testes is essential for three key components of male reproductive function: sex determination and differentiation, stimulating the somatic components of male puberty, and development of spermatogenesis and acquisition of reproductive capacity. A trio of cells orchestrates these developments: Leydig cells, Sertoli cells, and germ cells. This chapter focuses on the genetic and hormonal factors that enable a testis to develop, the production of testicular androgens and their mode of action, and how disturbances in these pathways result in disorders seen in pediatric endocrine practice. Endocrine disorders are confined to those resulting from an intrinsic abnormality in testicular function, including a section on testicular tumors. Disorders of male puberty are also covered in this chapter

Fetal Male Development

EMBRYOLOGY

Sex development comprises the dual components of sex determination (the process whereby the bipotential gonad develops as a testis or as an ovary) and sex differentiation (the phenotypic expression of the action of testicular hormones). The summation and amplification of these processes postnatally is manifest at puberty and followed by the acquisition of reproductive capacity. The entire process, extending from fetal life to adulthood, is a dynamic process dependent on the appropriate and timely interaction of a multitude of genes, proteins, signaling molecules, paracrine factors, and endocrine stimuli.[1-4]

The bipotential primitive gonad arises from a condensation of the mesoderm at the medioventral region of the urogenital ridge (Figure 16-1). This process begins at about 4 to 5 weeks of gestation in humans. The urogenital region is the site of development of the kidney, gonad, and adrenals. Consequently, when disrupted in mice genes (such as WT1 and SF1) that are key to urogenital development result in absent kidney/gonad and adrenal/gonad development (respectively). Inactivating mutations of these genes in humans lead to syndromes [such as Denys-Drash and Frasier (WT1)] and to XY sex reversal with adrenal failure (SF1).[5,6]

Once the urogenital ridge is formed, the mesonephros becomes essential to the development of the testis as a source of somatic cells—which migrate to encompass the primordial germ cells that have also migrated to this site from the yolk sac. The testis and ovary are morphologically indistinguishable until about 6 weeks of gestation. Then, the appearance of Sertoli cells and seminiferous cords developing adjacent to a prominent coelomic blood vessel are the hallmarks of the developing testis. No such morphologic differentiation occurs in the developing ovary until weeks later. Later, interstitial cells differentiate in the testis into Leydig cells and start producing testosterone for the next stage in development: sex differentiation.

The adrenal primordium separates from the developing gonad at about 8 weeks of gestation. However, when the testis later migrates trans-abdominally to reach its scrotal position a nidus of adrenal cell rests may also be sited in this position. It is estimated that adrenal rests are found within, or adjacent to, the testis in up to 15% of neonates.[7] These rests usually regress in later infancy, although they may persist and form testicular "tumors" in males with congenital adrenal hyperplasia.[8] This tissue has characteristics of adrenocortical tissue, such as the production of adrenal-specific steroids and expression of adrenal-specific steroidogenic enzymes.

The internal genitalia are also bipotential, with the anlage for development of the male and female internal genital ducts initially present in both sexes. In the male, regression of the Mullerian ducts (destined to form the uterus and fallopian tubes) and stabilization of the Wolffian ducts (destined to form the vas deferens, epididymis, and seminal vesicles) are prerequisites of normal development. This is mediated by the anti-Mullerian hormone (AMH) acting on its type II AMH receptor expressed in the Mullerian mesenchyme.[9] Maximum sensitivity to AMH action occurs in a window of 9 to 12 weeks of gestation. Wolffian duct stabilization and differentiation is mediated by testosterone produced in large concentrations by the ipsilateral testis and acting predominantly in a paracrine manner.[10]

The external genitalia develop from a common anlage, with androgens playing a trophic role to enable the external genitalia to become sexually dimorphic. Thus, under the influence of androgens the genital tubercle differentiates and enlarges to become a penis, the urethral folds form the penile urethra, and labioscrotal swellings fuse to form the scrotum. The 5α-reduced metabolite of testosterone, dihydrotestosterone (DHT), appears to be essential to this component of sex differentiation based on the anatomic consequences of the human syndrome of 5α-reductase deficiency.[11]

The final step in fetal male development is descent of the testis in two stages: trans-abdominal and transinguinal. The

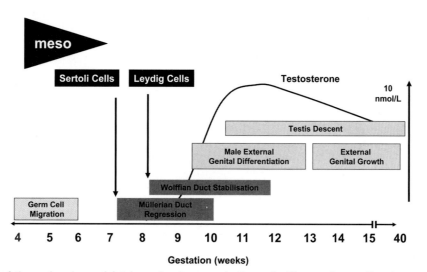

Figure 16-1 Schematic of the embryology of fetal sex development in the male. The continuous line denotes the rise in fetal serum testosterone during the period of sex differentiation.

first stage, which begins at about 12 weeks of gestation and is completed by the middle of the second trimester, involves contraction and thickening of the gubernacular ligament.[12] This phase of descent appears to be controlled by a Leydig cell product [insulin-like 3 (INSL3)] binding to its G-protein–coupled receptor [GREAT, also known as leucine-rich repeat-containing G-protein–coupled receptor 8 (LGR-8) and as GPR106].[13] The phase of transinguinal descent is predominantly androgen dependent.

GENETIC AND HORMONAL CONTROL

A panoply of genes is involved in fetal sex determination and sex differentiation. Much of the knowledge gained, particularly in relation to the genetic control of urogenital development and testis determination, has arisen from mouse models of targeted disruption of candidate genes. However, several of these genes (such as Lim1, Emx2, Pdgfrα, testatin, and SOX3) have not yet been shown to be key components in human sex development based on the effects of inactivating mutations. Figure 16-2 shows a simplified outline of those genes relevant to human fetal sex development. The SRY gene remains the key orchestrator of testis determination, with the most profound evidence illustrated by its expression in more than 90% of phenotypic human males with an XX karyotype[14] and the induction of an XX male mouse by transgenesis.[15]

Inactivating mutations in SRY are found in only 10% to 15% of sex-reversed females with complete XY gonadal dysgenesis. Consequently, genes additional to SRY are required for testis determination. Although SRY is a known transcription factor, little is known of the nature of downstream genes controlled by SRY. It is linked to SOX9, another member of the high-mobility group (HMG) box family of proteins to which SRY belongs, and it is possible that SRY acts by disrupting the binding and function of a repressor—thus allowing activation of downstream genes (such as SOX9).[16] The genes involved in mediating sex differentiation are well characterised and are predominantly those that encode for peptide hormones, such as AMH, and for the steroidogenic enzymes required for androgen biosynthesis. For androgen signaling, the ligand-activated nuclear androgen receptor (AR) is a crucial element in the pathway of male sex development.

The pathway of fetal testicular steroidogenesis is shown in Figure 16-3. The production of androgens by fetal Leydig cells occurs as early as 8 to 9 weeks of gestation and is initially autonomous, before becoming dependent on placental hCG secretion.[17] Fetal serum testosterone concentrations increase between 10 and 16 weeks of gestation to levels approaching the adult male range. The pathways shown in Figure 16-3 highlight the importance of CYP17 and the POR gene as regulators of androgen biosynthesis. It is possible that the cytochrome P450 oxidoreductase (POR) enzyme is used preferentially to synthesise DHT by an alternative pathway specific to the fetal testis.[18]

All androgens bind intracellularly with high affinity to a single nuclear AR to mediate androgenic effects, including sex differentiation. The AR is a transcription factor encoded by a gene on chromosome Xq11-q12. The receptor, in common with other members of the large nuclear receptor family, comprises an N-terminal domain (involved in transcriptional activity), a central DNA-binding domain, and a C-terminal domain involved in hormone binding.[19] Subdomains are involved in intramolecular interactions, as well as binding to a number of co-regulators that bridge the AR to the general transcriptional machinery.[20] The AR is ubiquitously expressed, including the fetal reproductive tract.

Disorders of Sex Development

Normal testis development and production of its hormones in an optimal concentration and time-dependent manner is crucial to enable male development to occur against a constitutive background of female fetal development. Consequently, an abnormality of testis function may manifest as a disorder of sex development (DSD). Indeed, it ranks second only to congenital adrenal hyperplasia as the most common cause of ambiguous genitalia of the newborn. This clinical disorder is discussed further in Chapters 4 and 12. The recent changes in terminology and classification of DSD[21,22] (which provide a more rational approach to considering causation related to testicular disease) are outlined in Tables 16-1 and 16-2. From an endocrine perspective, the broad categories of causation are threefold: testicular dysgenesis (a defect in testis determination), a defect in testicular hormone production, and a defect in testicular hormone signaling or action.

Defect in Testis Determination

SEX CHROMOSOME ANOMALIES

Klinefelter syndrome is the male exemplar of the gonadal manifestation of an abnormality in sex chromosomes. This is the most frequent form of sex chromosome aneuploidy. An incidence of about 1 in 600 live births is approximately quadruple the figure obtained in adulthood based on karyotype analysis.[23] This mismatch, indicating a significant rate of underdiagnosis, is presumably the result of not recognizing the pathognomonic sign of small firm testes. Not surprisingly, less than 10% of cases are recognized before puberty. The classic 47,XXY karyotype

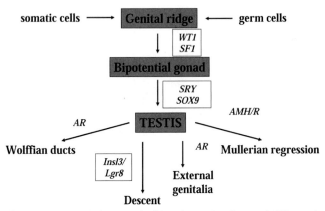

Figure 16-2 Genetic control of sex determination and differentiation in the male related to morphogenetic events.

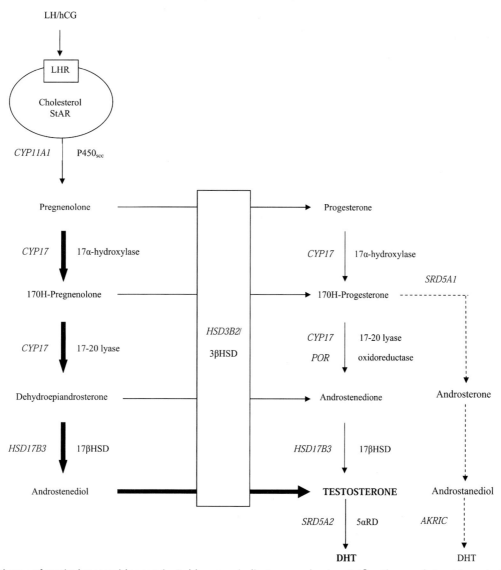

Figure 16-3 Pathway of testicular steroidogenesis. Bold arrows indicate a predominant Δ^5 pathway of steroid production. The dotted lines denote a "backdoor" pathway to DHT synthesis postulated to be specific to the fetus. The steroidogenic enzymes and their cognate genes are shown.

is the result of meiotic non-disjunction during gametogenesis, of which 60% occur during oogenesis.

About 10% of cases are mosaic (46,XY/47,XXY) and tend to have a milder phenotype. Typically, the external genitalia are normal at birth—although there may be anomalies such as hypospadias, micropenis, and undescended testes.[24] The reduced testis size in Klinefelter syndrome is the result of degeneration of the seminiferous tubules. The process has its onset in the fetus, progresses through infancy, and accelerates at puberty.[25] Although the number of germ cells is reduced, there is preservation of Leydig cell development—which is reflected in spontaneous onset of puberty in the majority of boys with Klinefelter syndrome.[26]

Seldom is it necessary to induce puberty with androgens, although supplementary testosterone may be required in adulthood. Fertility has occurred in association with the mosaic forms of Klinefelter syndrome, but with the use of testicular sperm extraction and intracytoplasmic

sperm injection (ICSI) a significant number of pregnancies can now be attained in men with the 47,XXY karyotype.[27] Other variants of Klinefelter syndrome can be associated with 46,XY/47,XXY mosaicism and karyotypes as diverse as 48,XXYY, 48,XXXY, 49,XXXYY, and 49,XXXXY. All have in common small testes, tall stature, some genital anomalies, and varying degrees of abnormal cognitive performance.

The XX male syndrome is also similar in nature to Klinefelter syndrome, as characterized by small testes but with some features that differ. The testes are more likely to be undescended, and the incidence of genital anomalies is higher. Adult XX males are shorter, and gynecomastia is more common.[28,29] Azoospermia is universal so that infertility is absolute. The incidence is about 1 in 20,000 phenotypic males. About 10% of XX males lack translocation of the Y-chromosomal SRY gene. They have a higher incidence of genital anomalies such as micropenis, hypospadias, and undescended testes.

TABLE 16-1

Nomenclature Relating to Disorders of Sex Development

Previous	Proposed
Intersex	Disorders of sex development (DSD)
Male pseudohermaphrodite Undervirilization of an XY male Undermasculinization of an XY male	46,XY DSD
Female pseudohermaphrodite Overvirilization of an XX female Masculinization of an XX female	46,XX DSD
True hermaphrodite	Ovotesticular DSD
XX male or XX sex reversal	46,XX testicular DSD
XY sex reversal	46,XY complete gonadal dysgenesis

It is also possible that XX ovotesticular DSD (true hermaphroditism) is part of this subgroup etiologically, subject to ovarian-tissue-containing follicles having been confirmed in an affected individual. There is yet no molecular explanation for male development in the absence of Y-chromosomal material. Proposals include a loss-of-function mutation in a gene that normally inhibits testis formation in the XX female, a gain-of-function mutation in a gene downstream of the SRY transcription factor, and mosaicism for a Y-bearing cell line expressed in the gonads.[30,31] These unidentified genes could be autosomal or X-linked.

GONADAL DYSGENESIS

The term *dysgenesis* should only strictly be used where the definition is based on histology of the gonad. In relation to the testis and disorders of sex development, the appearances on histology accepted to define dysgenesis include carcinoma in situ, immature tubules with undifferentiated Sertoli cells, the presence of microliths (sometimes visible on testicular ultrasound), and a Sertoli cell-only pattern.[32,33]

TABLE 16-2

A Proposed Classification of Causes of DSD

Sex Chromosome DSD	46,XY DSD	46,XX DSD
A: 47,XXY (Klinefelter syndrome and variants)	A: Disorders of gonadal (testicular) development 1. Complete or partial gonadal dysgenesis (e.g., SRY, SOX9, SF1, WT1, DHH, etc.) 2. Ovotesticular DSD 3. Testis regression	A: Disorders of gonadal (ovarian) development 1. Gonadal dysgenesis 2. Ovotesticular DSD 3. Testicular DSD (e.g., SRY+, dup SOX9, RSP01)
B: 45,X (Turner syndrome and variants)	B: Disorders in androgen synthesis or action 1. Disorders of androgen synthesis LH receptor mutations Smith-Lemli-Opitz syndrome Steroidogenic acute regulatory protein mutations Cholesterol side-chain cleavage (CYP11A1) 3β-hydroxysteroid dehydrogenase (HSD3B2) 17α hydroxylase/17,20-lyase (CYP17) P450 oxidoreductase (POR) 17β-hydroxysteroid dehydrogenase (HSD17B3) 5α-reductase (SRD5A2)	B: Androgen excess 1. Fetal 3β-hydroxysteroid dehydrogenase 2HSD3B2 21-hydroxylase (CYP21A2) P450 oxidoreductase (POR) 11β-hydroxylase (CYP11B1) Glucocorticoid receptor mutations 2. Fetoplacental Aromatase (CYP19) deficiency Oxidoreductase (POR) deficiency 3. Maternal Maternal virilizing tumors (e.g., luteomas) Androgenic drugs
C: 45,X/46,XY (mixed gonadal dysgenesis)	2. Disorders of androgen action Androgen insensitivity syndrome Drugs and environmental modulators	
D: 46,XX/46,XY (chimerism)	C: Other 1. Syndromic associations of male genital development (e.g., cloacal anomalies, Robinow, Aarskog, hand-foot-genital, popliteal pterygium) 2. Persistent Mullerian duct syndrome 3. Vanishing testis syndrome 4. Isolated hypospadias (CXorf6) 5. Congenital hypogonadotropic hypogonadism 6. Cryptorchidism (INSL3, GREAT) 7. Environmental influences	C: Other 1. Syndromic associations (e.g., cloacal anomalies) 2. Mullerian agenesis/hypoplasia (e.g., MURCS) 3. Uterine abnormalities (e.g., MODY5) 4. Vaginal atresia (e.g., KcKusick-Kaufman) 5. Labial adhesions

Gonadal dysgenesis as applied to the testis arises from a defect in sex determination during embryogenesis, which may be associated with a sex chromosome anomaly (as in Klinefelter syndrome) or due to inactivation of a testis-determining gene such as SRY or SF1.

The term *gonadal dysgenesis* is also used more loosely in association with indirect evidence of gonadal dysfunction such as elevated gonadotrophin and decreased testosterone levels in an XY subject with failure of Mullerian duct regression. A wide range of genital anomalies occurs with gonadal dysgenesis, and some classification systems are all embracing—including Turner syndrome. In the context of this chapter on the testis, Table 16-2 lists the disorders that need to be considered.

Complete or pure XY gonadal dysgenesis is also known as Swyer syndrome, and is characterized by complete phenotypic sex reversal in an XY female. There are normal female genitalia at birth, but breast development is delayed at puberty. The uterus and fallopian tubes are present, but Wolffian duct remnants are not found. Gonadotrophin levels are characteristically markedly elevated by the time of puberty. Histology shows "streak" gonads indicating no morphological definition of testis development. There is a high risk of tumor development. The incomplete form is defined by any evidence of some masculinizing effects such as ambiguity of the genitalia at birth or virilization at puberty in the form of clitoromegaly, hirsutism, and deepening of the voice.

Histology may reveal some evidence of testis development, but dysgenetic in nature. The molecular pathogenesis of XY gonadal dysgenesis should be explained by a mutation in one of a number of genes involved in testis determination, but only 10% to 15% of individuals with the complete form have a mutation of the SRY gene.[34,35] SRY mutations are rarely found in partial XY gonadal dysgenesis. The first reports of SF1 mutations in humans described the expected phenotype of gonadal dysgenesis and primary adrenal failure.[36] Now, there are examples identified in which adrenal failure does not appear to be a concomitant component of the syndrome of SF1 deficiency.[37] This implies that the yield for identifying mutations in cases of gonadal dysgenesis may be higher if clinicians are more aware of expanded phenotypic spectra associated with testis-determining gene mutations.

MIXED GONADAL DYSGENESIS

This form of gonadal dysgenesis is typically associated with a mosaic 45,X/46,XY karyotype, although additional karyotypes include 45,X/47,XXY and 45,X/46,XY/47,XYY. The phenotype is highly variable. There is a referral bias toward the spectrum of ambiguous genitalia manifest generally as micropenis, severe hypospadias, and bifid scrotum. Such a clinical presentation can be seen with so many causes of DSD. The clinical phenotype in mixed gonadal dysgenesis may range from almost normal female external genitalia with mild clitoromegaly, through ambiguous genitalia, to isolated hypospadias or normal male external genitalia. Indeed, when a 45,X/46,XY karyotype has been found seren-

dipitously on prenatal testing most infants have normal male external genitalia at birth.[38]

There is no information on the longer-term follow-up of these infants with respect to growth, pubertal development, fertility, and risk of gonadal tumors. It is clear that there are normal men in whom this mosaic karyotype is present but unknown, as rarely this sex chromosome anomaly is identified in an infertility clinic setting. The internal genital ducts in mixed gonadal dysgenesis align in general with the nature of the ipsilateral gonad, with retention of a fallopian tube on the side adjacent to a severely dysgenetic streak gonad. The presence of a 45,X line may manifest with Turner-like somatic features of nuchal folds and low-set hairline, associated cardiac and renal anomalies, and short stature.

The gonads in this disorder are generally a combination of a well-formed testis on one side and a streak dysgenetic gonad on the contralateral side. Their positions are usually inguinal/scrotal and intra-abdominal, respectively. The assignment of gender in the biased referred population can be difficult and depends on several factors. Many are now assigned male and will require careful long-term monitoring at puberty and beyond with respect to malignancy risk. The streak gonad is usually removed during early childhood. Infants with female or only mild clitoromegaly are assigned female. The presence of Mullerian remnants in the form of a uterus or hemi-uterus provides an option later for pregnancy by ovum donation. It is essential to remove dysgenetic/streak gonadal material. Mutations in testis-determining genes such as SRY are not generally found in this condition.[39]

Ovotesticular DSD (also previously termed *true hermaphroditism*) can only be defined on histologic criteria according to the presence of ovarian tissues (containing follicles) and testicular tissue present in the same gonad (ovotestis) or as the morphologic appearance of the contralateral gonad. Often, the internal gonads may be in the form of bilateral ovotestes. The most common karyotype is 46,XX, with about 10% of cases having a 46,XY karyotype. An ovotestis is the most frequent gonad, and about a third of 46,XX cases are SRY positive.[40]

Rarely, an SRY mutation may be identified in XY ovotesticular DSD.[41] The phenotype in ovotesticular DSD is variable, although the predominant presentation is ambiguous genitalia or severe hypospadias. In 46,XX cases with an ovotestis and contralateral ovary, sex assignment is generally female with spontaneous onset of breast development and menses at puberty. All testicular tissue should be removed as completely as possible, and remnants monitored by serum AMH levels and the testosterone response to HCG stimulation. Pregnancies are reported in ovotesticular DSD.[42,43] Those raised male will generally require hypospadias repair, orchidopexy, and removal of Mullerian remnants. Any ovarian tissue must be removed before puberty to avoid the risk of breast development. Scrotally sited testicular tissue can be monitored for tumor development, a rare occurrence in this type of DSD. Fertility is uncommon.[44]

Disorders of Androgen Synthesis

GENERAL

The pathway of testicular steroidogenesis is outlined in Figure 16-3. A number of defects in the more proximal intratesticular pathway of steroidogenesis are also manifest as defects in adrenal steroidogenesis (see Chapter 12). These include StAR protein defect (lipoid congenital adrenal hyperplasia), P450 side-chain cleavage deficiency (CYP11A1), 3β-hydroxysteroid dehydrogenase deficiency, 17α-hydroxylase/17,20-lyase deficiency (CYP17), and P450 oxidoreductase (POR) deficiency. The predominant mode of presentation is generally adrenal failure with associated varying degrees of genital anomalies. In contrast, the classic presentation of combined CYP17 deficiency is absent puberty in a phenotypic XY female with low renin hypertension and hypokalemic alkalosis.

Allied to this enzyme, central to androgen production is the co-enzyme P450 oxidoreductase—which is a key participant in the transfer of electrons to P450 enzymes, including the 17,20-lyase reaction of the CYP17 enzyme.[45] Uniquely, deficiency of this enzyme can lead on the one hand to virilization of an affected female (XX, DSD) and on the other to undermasculinization of an affected male (XY,DSD). The underlying mechanism is explained by an apparent combined deficiency of two P450 enzymes (CYP17 and CYP21) and a hitherto unrecognized alternative pathway of androgen biosynthesis specific to the fetus.[46]

P450-oxidoreductase deficiency is also a feature of a subset of cases of Antley-Bixler syndrome.[47] This is characterized by ambiguous genitalia and skeletal dysplasia, the latter comprising craniosynostosis, brachycephaly, midfacial hypoplasia, synostosis of the radioulnar or radiohumeral joints, bowing of the femora, and arachnodactyly. The syndrome also manifests in the absence of a defect in steroidogenesis. This is caused by mutations in the FGFR2 gene (fibroblast growth factor receptor) and is autosomal dominant. The defects in androgen synthesis confined solely to the production and testicular androgens include Leydig cell hypoplasia and deficiencies of the 17β-hydroxysteroid dehydrogenase and 5α-reductase enzymes.

LEYDIG CELL HYPOPLASIA

Placental HCG during early gestation and pituitary LH thereafter in late fetal and postnatal development stimulate testicular androgen synthesis through binding to the LH receptor expressed in Leydig cells. Both ligands bind with similar affinity. The LH receptor is a glycoprotein hormone receptor and a member of the large group of G-protein–coupled receptors. These receptors are characterized by a large extracellular domain of about 400 amino acids and a transmembrane domain comprising a 7-transmembrane serpentine structure.[48] If the receptor is inactivated, the result is a spectrum of undermasculinization in affected males ranging from a complete female phenotype to isolated micropenis. Inactivating mutations of the LH receptor are rare, and usually present with genital anomalies such as severe hypospadias and cryptorchidism.

More than 30 loss-of-function homozygous or heterozygous mutations of the LH receptor gene (residing on chromosome 2p21) are now described.[49,50] Complete resistance may present with primary amenorrhoea and lack of breast development in a phenotypic female who has XY chromosomes. The lack of breast development is a distinguishing clinical feature from the complete androgen insensitivity syndrome. The endocrine profile is as expected: elevated serum LH but normal FSH and low testosterone, which does not respond to HCG stimulation.

Mullerian structures are absent, indicative of normal testicular AMH function. However, the epididymis and vas deferens may be present. It is not clear how Wolffian ducts are stabilized in the absence of fetal androgens. Inactivating LH receptor mutations manifest differently in affected females, who develop puberty normally but thereafter have ovarian dysfunction. There is a tendency for partial loss-of-function mutations that result in mild hypospadias or isolated micropenis to localize in the seventh transmembrane domain. Histology of the gonads shows decreased or absent Leydig cells after puberty. These appearances are less definitive in the prepubertal testis.

17β-HYDROXYSTEROID DEHYDROGENASE DEFICIENCY

The 17β-hydroxysteroid dehydrogenase reaction is mediated by six isoenzymes in humans that convert androstenedione to testosterone, dehydroepiandrosterone to androstenediol, and estrone to estradiol (Figure 16-3). The type 3 enzyme encoded by HSD17B3 located on chromosome 9q22 is testis specific and is key to converting the weak androgen androstenedione to the potent major androgen testosterone.

17β-HSD deficiency (also termed *17β-hydroxysteroid oxidoreductase* or *17-ketosteroid reductase*) is now a well-characterized cause of 46,XY DSD.[51-53] Most affected males have female external genitalia at birth but may present with inguinal swellings similar to infants with complete androgen insensitivity syndrome. Alternatively, the presentation is at puberty when an affected individual (whose sex is assigned female at birth) becomes profoundly virilized—with deepening of the voice, hirsutism, muscle development, and clitoromegaly. Why such virilization should occur at puberty and yet the fetus not masculinized in utero is not adequately explained.

The gonadotrophin rise at puberty increases androstenedione substrate, which can be metabolized to testosterone by extraglandular conversion via alternative 17βHSD isoenzymes (such as the aldoreductase type 5 17β-HSD isoenzyme AKRIC3).[54] The development of gynecomastia occurs by converson of androstenedione by aromatase enzyme in extraglandular tissues and the action of type 1 or type 2 17β-HSD isoenzymes. The virilization that occurs at puberty is occasionally followed by gender role reassignment from female to male, similar to that observed in 5α-reductase deficiency. If the gender remains female, urgent gonadectomy is required—with clitoroplasty and usually vaginoplasty. The deepening of the voice is seldom completely reversible.

More than 20 mutations in the HSD17B3 gene have now been described.[4] Most are missense mutations, with some patients displaying compound heterozygosity. Functional studies of mutant enzymes expressed in vitro generally show complete lack of ability to convert androstenedione to testosterone. Consequently, these studies bear little relationship to predicting the degree of virilization expected at puberty. An inbred population in Gaza has the more frequent mutation causing 17β-HSD deficiency, resulting from conversion of arginine to glutamine (R80Q) at codon 80.[55] This population also serves to illustrate that deficiency of this enzyme in females has no functional consequences because females homozygous for the mutation were normal.

5α-REDUCTASE DEFICIENCY

This cause of XY DSD is also characterized by profound virilization at puberty in an affected individual/raised female. The condition came to prominence through the reporting of a genetic isolate in the Dominican Republic, where gender role changes at puberty are not uncommon.[56,57] However, unlike 17β-hydroxysteroid dehydrogenase deficiency the external genitalia are more ambiguous at birth—with severe hypospadias, micropenis, bifid scrotum/labioscrotal folds, and a urogenital sinus.

The testes transcend the abdomen to lie in the inguinal canals or within the bifid/labioscrotal folds. There are no Mullerian structures, and the Wolffian ducts are normally stabilized to form the epididymis, vas deferens, and seminal vesicle. The prostate gland remains hypoplastic at puberty, indicating the specific dependence of this structure on DHT. Furthermore, adult males do not develop acne or temporal hair recession. Fertility is reduced probably as a result of the mal-positioned testes. However, there are reports of fertility—spontaneous and by artificial reproductive techniques.[58,59]

The enzyme deficiency is caused by mutations in the SRD5A2 gene located on chromosome 2p23. More than 40 mutations have been identified, the majority being missense mutations.[4] A genetic isolate affecting the New Guinea population is due to a complete gene deletion. Females homozygous for 5α-reductase deficiency have normal fertility.[60] The biochemical diagnosis centers on demonstrating an elevated ratio of testosterone to dihydrotestosterone (DHT) in serum (following HCG stimulation in prepubertal patients) and a diminished ratio of urinary 5α to 5α-reduced C_{19} and C_{21} steroids. Even after gonadectomy, a biochemical diagnosis can still be ascertained because of the role of 5α-reductase in metabolism of glucocorticoids.

Disorders of Androgen Action

GENERAL

The key role of androgens in male sex differentiation is vividly illustrated by the consequence of a total lack of response to androgens in target tissues—a complete female phenotype in a 46,XY individual with normally formed testes producing age-appropriate testosterone levels. This is the paradigm of a hormone resistance syndrome. Formerly called the testicular feminization syndrome, the favored terminology is now *androgen insensitivity syndrome* (AIS)—subclassified into complete (CAIS) and partial (PAIS) forms.[61,62]

Male sex differentiation and the subsequent acquisition of secondary sex characteristics at puberty, and the onset of spermatogenesis, are all mediated by androgens binding to a single intracellular androgen receptor (AR) ubiquitously expressed in target tissue. The AR is one of a quartet of nuclear receptors (glucocorticoid, mineralocorticoid, progesterone, and androgen) closely related within a large superfamily. It can activate gene transcription via a common hormone response element. The single-copy gene encoding the AR is located on Xq11-q12 and is made up of 8 exons that encode a protein of 919 amino acid residues. The major functional domains comprise an N-terminal transactivation domain (NTD), a central highly conserved DNA-binding domain (DBD), and a hinge region that connects the DBD to the C-terminal ligand-binding domain (LBD) (Figure 16-4).

The DBD contains cysteine residues that coordinate zinc atoms to form the zinc fingers characteristic of all nuclear receptors and many other transcription factors. The main domains comprise subsidiary functions that include dimerization, binding to co-regulator proteins, interaction with heat shock proteins, and transcriptional regulation.[63] The two subdomains most involved in activation of transcription are the motif activation function-1 (AF1) in the NTD and the motif activation function-2 (AF2) in the LBD. AF2 also interacts with steroid receptor coactivators such as SRC1, SRC2/TIF2, and SRC3 via their LXXLL motifs—where L is a leucine and X is any amino acid.[64] This interaction is weaker in the case of the androgen receptor AF2 subdomain, which uniquely interacts in an intramolecular manner with its cognate AF1 subdomain in the NTD.[64] N- and C-terminal interaction stabilizes the AR and slows down the dissociation of the ligand from its receptor.

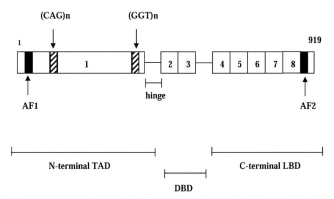

Figure 16-4 A schematic of the functional domains of the androgen receptor. Numbers inside boxes refer to exons 1 through 8. AF1 is activation function 1. AF2 is activation function 2. (CAG)n encodes for a polyglutamine stretch. (GGT)n encodes for a polyglycine stretch. The three main domains are TAD (transactivation domain), DBD (DNA-binding domain), and LBD (ligand-binding domain).

A sequence of CAG repeats in exon 1 of the AR gene encodes for a homopolymeric stretch of glutamines, which ranges from 11 to 31 repeats in the general population. Another repeat of glycines ranges from 10 to 25. In vitro studies show that the length of the CAG repeat is inversely proportional to the activity of the AR as a transcription factor.[65]

Figure 16-5 shows a schematic of how androgens interact with the AR on entering target cells. The figure also shows subsequent activation of target genes. A single receptor binds testosterone and DHT, the latter being a biologically more potent androgen because of dissociating from the AR at a slower rate. The AR in the unliganded state is located in the cytoplasm complexed to heat shock proteins (HSPs) such as HSP70 and HSP90. These in turn are also complexed to co-chaperone proteins such as FKBP52.[66] Ligand binding initiates dissociation to allow translocation of the AR to the nucleus, where it binds as a homodimer to DNA hormone response elements. The action of the AR is further modulated by interaction with co-regulatory proteins, which function either as coactivators or co-repressors. These proteins act as a physical bridge connecting the receptor to the basal transcription machinery. Coactivators ARA24, ARA55, and ARA70 are AR specific.

The three-dimensional structure of a nuclear receptor LBD comprises 12α helices associated with anti-parallel β sheets arranged in the form of a tripartite sandwich. A hydrophobic pocket is formed by helixes, 4, 5, 7, 11, and 12—to which the ligand is bound on contact with its cognate receptor. Helix 12 is the outermost α-helix, which folds back on top of the ligand hydrophobic pocket like a lid closing on a box. This has been referred to as the "mousetrap effect" to capture the ligand and retain it by slowing the rate of ligand-receptor dissociation. This trapping effect by helix 12 also permits interaction between the LBD and AF2 subdomain and the LXXLL motif in associated co-regulator proteins. Much information about the structural and functional aspects of the AR has been obtained through studying the functional effects of AR mutations that lead to AIS.

The phenotype of CAIS is that of a normal female, with a prevalence for this X-linked recessive disorder ranging from 1 in 20,400 genetic males to 1 in 99,000 genetic males.[67,68] The typical presentation is primary amenorrhoea in an otherwise normally developed adolescent female. The uterus is absent as a result of normal AMH action. The Wolffian ducts are surprisingly stabilized in many patients.[69] The main differential at this age is XY complete gonadal dysgenesis (Swyer syndrome), which is distinguished by poor breast development and a shorter stature. The other typical presentation in early life for CAIS is with bilateral inguinal or labial swellings. This can also occur in 17β-HSD deficiency.

Bilateral inguinal herniae are rare in girls, and it has been estimated that 1% to 2% of such cases have CAIS. Consequently, it is now generally recommended that a CAIS diagnosis be considered in all girls with this type of hernia and the presence of a Y chromosome be checked by FISH analysis and a full karyotype. If the content of the

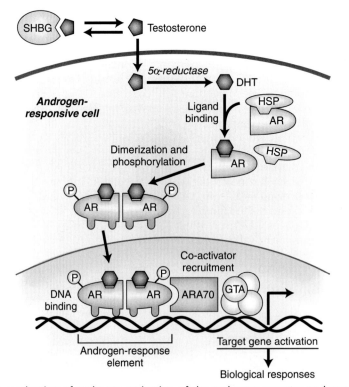

Figure 16-5 A schematic of the mechanism of androgen activation of the androgen receptor and gene transcription. HSP, heat shock proteins; ARA70, an androgen receptor-specific coactivator; and GTA, general transcriptional apparatus. [From Feldman BJ, Feldman D (2001). The development of androgen-independent prostate cancer. Nature Rev Cancer 1:34–45. Copyright © of and adapted by permission from Macmillan Publishers Ltd.]

hernial sac contain gonads, a biopsy should be taken in concert with the cytogenetic studies.[70] A family history of an older female sibling having had an inguinal hernia repair in infancy but with the diagnosis of CAIS missed is not unusual. Another mode of presentation is mismatch between a prenatal XY karyotype and a female phenotype at birth.

The syndrome of PAIS occurs when there is some biologic response to androgens. The external genitalia may be ambiguous at birth, but the prototypic phenotype for PAIS is perineoscrotal hypospadias, micropenis, bifid scrotum, and undescended testes. The more severe form of PAIS presenting as isolated clitoromegaly is only marginally different from CAIS. At the other end of the phenotypic spectrum there may be just isolated hypospadias or even normal male development at birth but gynaecomastia and infertility presenting in adulthood. Surveys of male factor infertility characterized by elevated LH and testosterone levels have revealed a minority to have a mutation in the AR gene.[71] High doses of androgens may lead to fertility.[72] The list of disorders to consider within the 46,XY DSD category is much larger with the PAIS phenotype. They can be broadly classified as partial gonadal dysgenesis, a defect in androgen biosynthesis (LH receptor, SF1, 17β-HSD and 5α-RD deficiencies), and mixed gonadal dysgenesis in association with 45,X/46,XY mosaicism.

The hormone profile in AIS shows an increased age-related testosterone level, increased LH, and only a slightly elevated FSH level. Serum estradiol is increased at puberty from aromatization of testosterone. Concentrations of sex hormone binding globulin (SHBG), a protein produced by the liver, are sexually dimorphic—with levels in CAIS similar to those found in normal females. This hepatic resistance to the action of androgens has been proposed as a biologic marker of androgen responsiveness in AIS.[73] Stanazolol, a synthetic nonaromatizable androgen, is administered orally—and the decrement in serum SHBG levels measured. There is normally a 50% reduction, but the change is insignificant in CAIS. There is a moderate response in PAIS, but overlapping with normals.

A further biochemical test, available only in research laboratories, used in the investigation of androgen resistance is measurement of androgen binding in genital skin fibroblasts. The AR is ubiquitously expressed, and in greater quantities in genital versus nongenital skin. A small genital skin biopsy collected at genitoplasty or during an examination under anesthetic can be used to generate a cell line to perform a binding assay using radiolabeled androgens. A quantitative and qualitative measure of binding can be determined from a Scatchard plot analysis. Typically, there is absent binding when a nonsense mutation results in a truncated AR. Such a mutation is sufficiently pathogenic to lead to a CAIS phenotype. Alternatively, there may be binding of androgens to the AR—but with lower affinity. A missense mutation is generally associated with such findings, resulting usually in a PAIS phenotype. The cell line is also a source of RNA, which can be analyzed for length if a mutation is suspected to be residing in the noncoding region of the AR gene.

MOLECULAR PATHOGENESIS OF ANDROGEN INSENSITIVITY SYNDROMES

Information about the various mutations that affect the AR and give rise to clinical disease is recorded on an International Mutation Database at McGill University (*http://www.androgendb.mcgill.ca*). The majority of mutations relate to syndromes of androgen insensitivity, but in addition somatic mutations identified in prostate carcinoma are listed. The database records more than 300 different mutations that can cause AIS. These are distributed throughout the gene, with no specific "hot spot" of mutations but about two-thirds are located in the LBD.

The range of mutations identified through the Cambridge DSD database is shown in Figure 16-6. Identifying a mutation, particularly if missense, does not necessarily imply pathogenicity. If the mutation is novel, it is advisable to recreate the mutant AR for functional studies using a reporter gene assay. It is also possible to undertake structure-guided modeling of the mutant protein to provide insight into AR dysfunction.[74] There is considerable heterogeneity in the phenotypic expression of a particular mutation, sometimes even within families. For example, a missense mutation at codon 703 in exon 4 of the LBD (which changes a serine to a glycine) is reported in four separate individuals on the McGill database. One patient had a normal female phenotype, whereas the other three cases all had ambiguous genitalia consistent with PAIS. However, the degree of androgenization of the external genitalia was sufficiently variable that two were raised male and the other female.[75,76] Rarely, two affected members in the same family can be respectively phenotypically CAIS and PAIS.

X-linked disorders are associated with a high rate of mutations that are de novo. The rate in AIS is about 30%. Such mutations arise as a single mutational event in a parental germ cell (maternal in the case of AIS) or as a germ cell mosaicism in the maternal gonad. Somatic mosaicism occurs when the mutation arises at the post-zygotic stage. Consequently, there is expression of both mutant and wild-type AR in different target tissues, including the external genitalia. About a third of de novo mutations in AIS arise at the post-zygotic stage, thereby explaining some of the variable phenotype in PAIS.[77] Other modulatory factors may include differences in 5α-RD 2 expression and reduced AR transcription and translation.[78,79]

No AR gene mutation is found in a minority of cases of CAIS or in a significant number of cases of PAIS. Nevertheless, it appears that there is clinical and biochemical evidence of androgen resistance. It is possible that patients with CAIS or PAIS in whom no mutation has been found in the AR gene may have a mutant coactivator protein to explain the androgen resistance. There is increasing evidence that nuclear receptor co-regulators play a role in the formation of mammalian phenotypes and perhaps in human disease.[20,81] In a study of the two AR-related coactivators, ARA24 and ARA 70, no substantive variations were found in amino acid residues in a series of patients with PAIS and a normal AR.[81,82]

Disruption of the steroid receptor coactivator-3 (SRC) in mice results in a phenotype of general hormone resistance, including features consistent with PAIS.[83] The SRC3

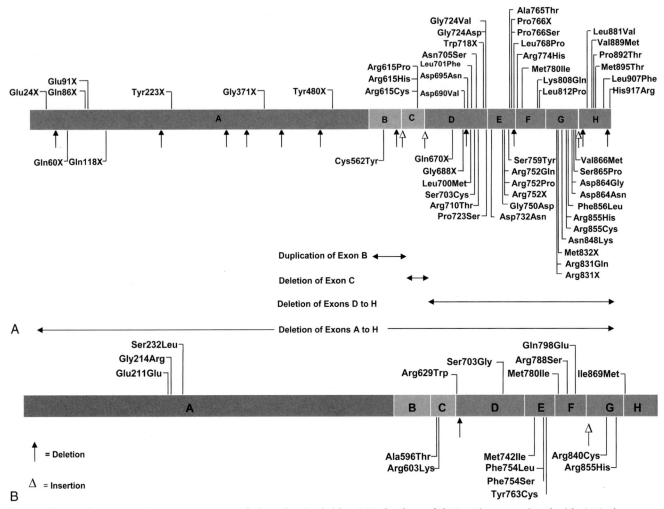

Figure 16-6 Androgen receptor mutations recorded on the Cambridge DSD database. *(A)* Mutations associated with CAIS phenotype. *(B)* Mutations associated with PAIS phenotype.

gene contains a variable track of CAG/CAA triplets that encode a polyglutamine repeat. The lengths of glutamine repeats were found to be shorter in PAIS subjects compared with controls.[84] The large number of co-regulator proteins (more than 300), their array of mechanisms to modulate transcription, and promiscuous binding to nuclear receptors in general makes it unlikely that a single mutant protein in this family would explain the mechanism of androgen resistance in CAIS or PAIS patients who have a normal AR. One patient with CAIS with a normal AR, in whom a subdomain of the AR failed to stimulate transcription of AR target genes, was suggested as evidence for a defect in an AR-specific coactivator.[85,86]

The polymorphic region in the N-terminal domain of the AR of glutamine repeats has biologic relevance to human disease. A toxic gain-of-function from hyperexpansion (>40 repeats) is found in Kennedy's disease and in spinal and bulbar muscular atrophy (SBMA).[87] Affected males have testicular atrophy, decreased spermatogenesis, and gynaecomastia despite elevated androgen levels (in keeping with a degree of androgen resistance). Variations in the length of the polyglutamine tract within the normal range are reported in association with disorders such as hypospadias,[88] reduced spermatogenesis,[89] and the phenotype of Klinefelter syndrome.[90]

Shorter glutamine repeats and relative hyperandrogenic states are reported in prostate cancer[91] androgenetic alopecia and acne,[92] and ovarian hyperandrogenism.[93] The polymorphic stretch of glycines is also significantly longer in patients with cryptorchidism and in a separate group with hypospadias compared with controls.[94] When CAG (glutamine) and GGN (glycine) lengths are analyzed together in the context of a missense mutation in the AR gene causing AIS, the combined effects appear to modulate the phenotypic expression of a given AR mutant in different affected individuals.[95]

Disorder of AMH

PERSISTENT MULLERIAN DUCT SYNDROME

Anti-Mullerian hormone (AMH) is a Sertoli-cell-produced glycoprotein homodimer encoded by a 2.75-kb gene on chromosome 19p13.3. The AMH type II receptor is a serine/threonine kinase with a single transmembrane domain encoded by a gene located on 12q13.[96] Persistent Mullerian duct syndrome (PMDS, *herniae uteri inguinale*) is a condition affecting males who have normally developed testes, internal male ducts, and external genitalia but persistent Mullerian duct derivatives. The diagnosis is often made when a fallopian tube and uterus are found during an inguinal hernia repair or an orchidopexy procedure. The hernia contains a partially descended or scrotal testis, as well as an ipsilateral tube and uterus. Sometimes the contralateral testis is also present in the hernial sac. Such transverse testicular ectopia is virtually pathognomonic of PMDS.

PMDS in normally differentiated males may result from failure of the Sertoli cells to synthesize AMH or from resistance to the action of AMH because of an AMH type II receptor defect. There is an even distribution of genetically proven cases of PMDS being the result of AMH or AMH type II receptor gene mutations.[97] AMH gene mutations are most common in Mediterranean, Northern African, and Middle Eastern countries and are usually familial homozygous mutations.[98] In contrast, mutations in the AMH type II receptor gene are more common in France and Northern Europe and are often compound heterozygous in nature.[99] Serum AMH measurement is a useful marker of the likely gene affected. Thus, low or undetectable levels are indicative of a mutation in the AMH gene—whereas a normal or increased serum concentration of AMH points to a defect in the AMH type II receptor gene.

Other Testis-Related Disorders

ANORCHIA AND CRYPTORCHIDISM

The term *vanishing testis syndrome* was coined for the phenotype of bilateral anorchia in an otherwise normally developed male infant. It recognizes the presence of normal testes in early gestation functioning to induce Mullerian duct regression, stabilize Wolffian duct development, and differentiate male external genitalia. Any ambiguity of the external genitalia suggests a variant of the syndrome related to some form of XY gonadal dysgenesis. Bilateral anorchia with normal differentiated but small phallus (micropenis) is also a recognized variant of the syndrome.[100]

A rare finding in such cases is a heterozygous partial loss-of-function mutation in SF1.[101] Otherwise, the cause is unknown other than invoking an interruption to the testis blood supply from a torsion or vascular occlusion event in utero. Surgical exploration and histologic findings typically show nubbins of fibrous tissue as remnants of gonads, associated with a vas deferens in the majority and some epididymal tissue.[102,103] The presence of hemosiderin-laden macrophages and dystrophic calcification is in keeping with the vascular accident hypothesis.

Establishing complete anorchia is based on a combination of biochemical tests, imaging studies, and surgical exploration.[104] An undetectable serum AMH level is a reliable marker when evaluating infants with nonpalpable gonads.[105] This, coupled with elevated serum gonadotrophins and an absent testosterone response to hCG stimulation, is predictive of the absence of testes. A low inhibin B level is also confirmatory. Imaging with CT or MRI may be useful prior to laparoscopy. Most centers would currently still undertake surgical exploration to remove testicular remnants, even though there is usually no evidence of malignancy found. Such a procedure could be deferred until the time of insertion of testicular prostheses.

Testes that have not descended at birth (cryptorchidism) is the most common congenital abnormality in boys, affecting 2% to 9% male live births.[106] The strong association with low birth weight is well recognized, as are disorders of the pituitary-gonadal axis [such as hypogonadotrophic hypogonadism (HH) and the androgen insensitivity syndrome]. The association with disorders of androgen production or action is in keeping with the role of androgens in the inguinoscrotal phase of testis descent. Mutations in INSL3 and GREAT (also known as LGR8) are reported in a minority of boys with cryptorchidism.[107-109]

Greater exposure to pesticides has been reported in cryptorchid boys based on analyses of breast milk samples as a proxy for fetal exposure.[110] Epidemiologic evidence for secular trends in the prevalence of cryptorchidism, and geographic variations in birth prevalence, point to environmental chemicals having an adverse effect on the genetic and hormonal control of testis descent.[111-115] Cryptorchidism may be associated with hypospadias. In turn, both are coupled to an increased risk for abnormal spermatogenesis and testicular cancer—two male reproductive tract disorders also increasing in prevalence.[116,117] This quartet of disorders constitutes a testicular dysgenesis syndrome (TDS) postulated to be of fetal origin and triggered by environmental chemicals disrupting an androgen/estrogen balance critical to normal sex development.[118]

The clearest evidence that certain chemicals (such as herbicides, fungicides, bisphenol A, and phthalates) can act as endocrine disruptors is derived from observations of wildlife and laboratory animal experiments. It remains uncertain whether there is also a new and emerging public health problem.[119] Direct evidence of toxic effects in humans has yet to be established. The previous practice of using diethyl stilbestrol (DES) to prevent recurrent miscarriages has resulted in transgenerational effects in the form of urogenital anomalies, including cryptorchidism in male offspring.[120] Sons of agricultural workers have an increased risk of cryptorchidism, which is related to levels of pesticide exposure.[121] The anogenital distance is a measurement used by reproductive toxicologists as a sensitive marker of prenatal exposure to androgen action in rodent studies.[122] In a human study, there was an inverse relationship between the anogenital distance in male infants and the levels of several phthalates measured in maternal urine.[123] Furthermore, the anogenital distance was shorter in boys with cryptorchidism.

HYPOSPADIAS

Hypospadias is incomplete fusion of the penile urethra defined by an arrest in development of the urethral spongiosum and ventral prepuce.[124] The normal embryologic correction of penile curvature is also interrupted. It is a common congenital anomaly, with birth prevalence estimated at about 3 to 4 per 1,000 live births. Despite extensive effort at investigation, the cause is unknown in the majority of cases.[125,126] An occasional case of isolated hypospadias has been identified with a mutation in WT1, SF1, LHR, CYP17, or the AR gene. The CXorf6 gene on chromosome Xq28 has been found to be mutated in some cases of hypospadias.[127] The mouse homologue is expressed in Leydig and Sertoli cells coincident with the period of sex differentiation (E12.5-E14.5).

Because expression of this gene is insignificant in the external genital anlagen, this suggests a transient Leydig cell dysfunction as an explanation for hypospadias in these cases. A mutation screen of BMP4, BMP7, HOXA4, and HOXB6 identified mutations in 14 of 90 cases of hypospadias in a Chinese population (all in the heterozygous state).[128] Mutations in HOXA13 are found in the hand-foot-genital syndrome, which includes hypospadias.[129] There is generally a familial clustering of cases in hypospadias, with a 7% incidence of one or more additional affected family members.[130] Furthermore, the twinning rate is higher than in the general population—of which two-thirds are monozygotic.

Associations observed in hypospadias include increased maternal age, mother exposed to DES in utero, paternal subfertility, maternal vegetarian diet, maternal smoking, assisted reproductive techniques, paternal exposure to pesticides, and fetal growth restriction.[131] The association with low birth weight suggests a link between factors operating to cause fetal growth restriction and the process of completing fusion of the urethral folds by the early second trimester. Gene expression profiles during urethral development in the mouse indicate that a number of signaling pathways are involved.[132]

Testis Tumors

GENERAL

Testis cancer is rare and has the highest prevalence in young men in the third and fourth decades of life.[133] The majority are germ cell in origin, manifesting as seminoma or nonseminoma tumors. The World Health Organization (WHO) classification system is the basis on which histologic typing of testis tumors is practiced.[134-136]

Tumors arise from the three principal cell types that comprise the formation of the testis: germ cells derived from primitive gonocytes, the supporting cells that differentiate as Sertoli cells, and the stromal interstitial cells that differentiate as Leydig cells. Rarely, tumors can arise from nonspecific testis tissue such as muscle (rhabdomyosarcoma), blood vessels (hemangioma), fibrous tissue (fibroma), and as a result of infiltration (leukemias, lymphoma). Germ cell tumors account for the vast majority, some of which manifest in early life. Leydig cell tumors also occur in childhood.

GERM CELL TUMORS

There are five categories of germ cell tumors described, of which types I through III involve the testis.[137] The WHO histologic classification of germ cell tumors is shown in

Table 16-3. The teratoma/yolk sac tumor presents in infancy and childhood and is not confined to the testis. Other sites include the mediastinum, retroperitoneum, sacral region, and midline brain. Yolk sac tumor is the most common testis tumor occurring before puberty, followed by embryonal carcinoma.[138] Type II tumors (comprising seminoma, nonseminoma, and dysgerminoma) originate from primordial germ cells or gonocytes.

A premalignant lesion develops initially, termed *intratubular germ cell neoplasia unclassified* (IGCNU) or *carcinoma in situ* (CIS). When the gonad is dysgenetic in nature, the premalignant condition is in the form of a gonadoblastoma. They progress to an invasive tumor manifest as a seminoma or nonseminoma and as a dysgerminoma in a dysgenetic gonad or an ovary.[139] The existence of a locus on the Y chromosome predisposes a gonadoblastoma to form in dysgenetic gonads. The TSPY (testis-specific protein Y-encoded) gene located on the short arm of the Y chromosome is one such oncogene that is abundantly expressed in the germ cells of XY individuals with DSD.

Gonocytes and CIS cells share similarities in morphology and in the expression of certain fetal proteins.[140] It is hypothesized that CIS represents delayed maturation of germ cells, which gives rise to an increased risk of germ cell tumors. This is found not only in XY DSDs but in trisomy 21, where there is a fiftyfold higher incidence of seminoma.[141] CIS is generally associated with germ cells developing in a depleted androgen environment, whether it be the result of insufficient androgen production or resistance to the action of androgen (as in syndromes of androgen insensitivity).

The propensity for gonadoblastomas to develop in gonadal dysgenesis (92%, as opposed to only 8% incidence of CIS) may be explained by the undifferentiated state of dysgenetic gonadal tissue. Invasive germ cell tumors are

TABLE 16-3

Classification of Germ Cell Tumors

Type	Site	Phenotype	Age
I	Testis/ovary/ retroperitoneum Mediastnum/ midline brain	Teratoma/ yolk sac tumor	Neonates Children
II	Testis	Seminoma/ non-seminoma	Young adult
	Ovary	Dysgerminoma	Childhood → young adult
	Dysgenetic gonad	Dysgerminoma/ non-seminoma	congenital
III	Testis	Spermatocytic seminoma	>50 yr
IV	Ovary	Dermoid cysts	Children/young adults
V	Placenta/uterus	Hydatidiform mole	Fetal life

Adapted from Cools M, Drop SLS, Wolffenbuttel KP, Oosterhuis JW, Looijenga LHJ (2006). Germ cell tumors in the intersex gonad: Old paths, new directions, moving frontiers. Endocr Rev 27:468-484.

rare before puberty in CAIS. Thereafter, with the rise of estrogens at puberty there may be estrogen-stimulated induction of the c-kit ligand—which can stimulate primordial germ cell growth.[142] In contrast, germ cell tumors occur at an earlier age in gonadal dysgenesis as a result of progressive genetic instability.[137,140,143]

A number of tumor markers can be used for immunohistochemical analysis to identify a premalignant state. These include placental-like alkaline phosphatase (PLAP), KIT (a membrane tyrosine kinase receptor for stem cell factor), AP2 gamma (activator protein-2 gamma), and OCT ¾.[139] These protein markers are normally expressed by fetal germ cells (and occasionally in postnatal life) until about 12 months of age. Thereafter, any expression in germ cells is abnormal and indicative of CIS or IGCNU. These tumor markers are not detected in serum, but have been identified in semen samples.[144] The risk of gonadal tumor in various causes of DSD can now be quantified reasonably well, particularly for gonadal dysgenesis and AIS (Table 16-4).

NON GERM CELL (SEX CORD STROMAL) TUMORS

Other tumors of the testis of relevance to infancy and childhood include Sertoli cell, Leydig cell, and adrenal rest tumors—which are stromal in origin and generally benign. Sertoli cell tumors can be bilateral, large and calcified, and associated with syndrome complexes such as the Peutz-Jeghers syndrome[145] and the Carney complex.[146] A feature of such tumors is associated breast development from increased estrogen production. Inhibin B, a product of the Sertoli cell, may be elevated in serum as a marker of Sertoli cell tumors.[147]

Leydig cell tumors are rare and comprise only 1 to 3% of testis tumors.[148] They are most common in the prepubertal age group, where they are always benign. In adults, 10% of cases are malignant. Leydig cell tumors are characterized clinically by the manifestations of their increased steroid production, which is generally androgenic. Consequently, precocious puberty is the hallmark in childhood. Estrogens can also be produced, either directly by the tumor or via peripheral aromatization. A testicular mass may be palpable, but the tumor can be occult and only visible on ultrasound examination. Characteristic histologic features include abundant cytoplasmic lipofuscin pigment and Reinke crystals.[149] Immunohistochemical markers specific for Leydig cell tumors include α-inhibin (particularly useful to distinguish from germ cell tumors), calretinin, and Melan-A.

Aberrant adrenal "tumors" may develop from the rest cells found within the testis in up to 15% of neonates.[7] The aberrant cells remain ACTH responsive and express adrenal-specific steroidogenic enzymes.[150] Consequently, the cells can become hyperplastic to form testicular adrenal rest tumors (TARTs) under states of ACTH hypersecretion in congenital adrenal hyperplasia (CAH), Addison's disease, and Nelson's syndrome.[151-153] There is almost uniform prevalence of TART in adult male patients with CAH when screened routinely by testicular ultrasound examination.[151] Even in male children with CAH, the prevalence is 24%.[154] The tumors are usually bilateral and benign. Histologically, they are sometimes difficult to separate from Leydig cell tumors—although the absence of Reinke crystals is a distinguishing feature.[155] The tumors are sited adjacent to the mediastinum testis, which can cause obstruction of the seminiferous tubules. This is invoked as one possible reason for gonadal dysfunction and infertility associated with TART.[156]

An endocrine explanation of infertility centers on the inhibitory role elevated endogenous levels of adrenal steroids may have on gonadotrophin secretion in males with inadequately treated CAH.[157,158] Fertility may be restored with improved medical control.[159] Testis-sparing surgery by tumor enucleation does not appear to improve pituitary-gonadal function.[160] Due recognition must be given to a testicular mass in males with CAH as most likely being a TART. Orchidectomy is not the preferred treatment.

There are other causes of testis enlargement that are not tumor related. Macro-orchia is a feature of the fragile

---

TABLE 16-4

Estimated Risks of Gonadal Tumors in Various Forms of DSD

Risk Group	Disorder	Malignancy Risk (%)	Recommended Action	Numbers: Studies (n)	Numbers: Patients (n)
High	GD (+Y) intra-abd.	15-35	gonadectomy	12	>350
	PAIS non-scrotal	50	gonadectomy	2	24
	Frasier	60	gonadectomy	1	15
	Denys-Drash (+Y)	40	gonadectomy	1	5
Intermediate	Turner (+Y)	12	gonadectomy	11	43
	17β-HSD	28	monitor	2	7
	GD (+Y) scrotal	unknown	biopsy and irrad.	0	0
	PAIS scrotal gonad	unknown	biopsy and irrad.	0	0
Low	CAIS	2	biopsy and testis	2	55
	ovotest. DSD	3	tissue removal	3	426
	Turner (−Y)	1	None	11	557
No	5α-reductase	0	unresolved	1	3
	Leydig cell hypoplasia	0	unresolved	2	

X syndrome, which is associated with mental retardation.[161] The cytogenetic fragile site on Xq27.3 harbors the FMRI gene, which has a tandem repeat of CGG trinucleotides in its 5' untranslated region. Expansion of this repeat is responsible for the syndrome, with its onset occurring before germ line segregation based on analysis of allele expansions in early fetal ovaries and testes.[162] The FMRP protein is widely expressed and is predominant in the brain and testes (mainly Sertoli cells), consistent with the key clinical features of the syndrome.

Macro-orchidism is most obvious after puberty, with testicular volume greater than 30 mL characteristically present. However, anthropometric measurements of males with fragile X syndrome from birth to adulthood shows an increase in testicular volume already in childhood—with the 50th percentile equivalent to the normal 95th percentile by 6 years of age.[163] Indeed, macro-orchidism has been documented as early as 5 months of age postnatally[164]—and in the fetus by 24 weeks of gestation.[165] Information on testicular histology is scanty. The mass of Sertoli cells is the primary determinant of testis volume. Biopsy studies of macro-orchid adult testes showed interstitial edema, increased lysosomal inclusions in Sertoli cells, and abnormal spermatogenesis.[166] In the male Fmr1 mouse knockout model, the rate of Sertoli cell proliferation is increased and is independent of any change in FSH signaling.[167]

The dominance of Sertoli cells in constituting testis volume is further illustrated by the observation of testis enlargement in males with the McCune-Albright syndrome.[168,169] In contrast to affected females, however, precocious signs of hyperandrogenism are often absent. The Gs-alpha-activating mutation, the cause of this syndrome, is manifest in somatic cells and occurs early in development.[170] The prevalence of this apparent sex dimorphism in sexual precocity is explained by the observation that in one affected patient of the typical Gs-alpha mutation (Arg201His) the GNAS1 allele was present only in Sertoli cells—explaining the lack of Leydig cell hyperfunction.[171]

Macro-orchidism may occur without any known cause, including the exclusion of activating mutations in the FSH receptor gene.[172] Severe hypothyroidism of long standing can paradoxically result in precocious puberty, particularly in girls (VanWyk-Grumbach syndrome). The manifestation when it occurs in boys is with macro-orchidism.[173,174] It has been postulated that the markedly elevated TSH levels have additional gonadotrophin-stimulating effects by binding promiscuously to the FSH receptor.[175] Restoring a euthyroid state with thyroxine replacement leads to resolution of the early signs of puberty. There is no evidence to indicate that early puberty in primary hypothyroidism is due to activating mutations in the FSH receptor gene.[176]

Puberty and the Testis

GENERAL

The testis is clearly an essential conduit in producing the sex steroid endpoint for translating activation of the GnRH pulse generator into the somatic features characteristic of male puberty. Although most pubertal disorders are not the result of a primary testis dysfunction, an overview of puberty and its disorders in the male is briefly provided in this chapter. The control of the onset of puberty remains an enigma because the primary mechanism that awakens the dormant neuroendocrine machinery remains unclear.[177] The physiologic paradigm of puberty centers on a period of "restraint" on gonadotrophin secretion during childhood that when released via genetic and extrinsic mechanisms allows puberty to be reactivated. This is based on evidence of prior increased gonadotrophin activity during fetal life and early infancy.

Placental gonadotrophin (HCG) and fetal pituitary gonadotrophins (FSH/LH) secretion are essential to sufficient production of testosterone for male genital differentiation and descent of the testes. Placental HCG secretion rises abruptly after 6 weeks, reaching a peak at about 12 weeks of fetal life and then declining to low levels by 18 to 20 weeks of gestation. The rise in fetal HCG is mirrored by a sharp rise in fetal circulating testosterone, essential to the normal development of the internal and external male genitalia. The second half of gestation is characterized by increasing FSH and LH secretion, which stimulate testicular size, descent, and penile growth. At birth, after separation of the umbilical cord there is a rapid rise in testosterone—reaching levels as high as 400 ng/dL in the first day of life.

Testosterone levels then decline rapidly during the first week to levels of 20 to 50 ng/dL but then increase again to levels between 60 and 400 ng/dL between 20 and 60 days of life. Thereafter, levels decline to the prepubertal range of less than 10 ng/dL by the end of the first year of life. These surges in testosterone are induced by gonadotrophins. A GnRH stimulation test evokes a greater rise in FSH than LH at these times. What purpose is served by the gonadotrophin-induced surge in testosterone in the first hours and days of neonatal life is less clear. Penile length increases during infancy, particularly during the first 3 months, and is positively correlated with serum concentrations of testosterone.[178] Inhibin B, a marker of Sertoli cell mass, is also elevated at 3 months of age and remains so for about another year.[179] Sertoli cell numbers proliferate during fetal and early postnatal life, the total number ultimately being a determinant of sperm quantity in adulthood.[180]

That these changes are FSH dependent is suggested by the observation of larger testis volume at 3 months of age in normal Finnish versus Danish male infants, and related to higher FSH and inhibin levels.[181] Furthermore, boys with cryptorchidism have higher FSH levels compared with controls.[182] Collectively, these observations indicate that the testis is responsive to a surge in gonadotrophin secretion during infancy. However, FSH and LH secretion abate (and serum levels are quite low) in the prepubertal years. Puberty is heralded by the appearance of nocturnal-sleep-related FSH and LH pulses, a reflection of the reawakening of the GnRH pulse generator (which has been "restrained" by an as yet unidentified mechanism).

If puberty is indeed the result of removing a restraint mechanism, it is not initiated by the gonads because a rise in gonadotrophins occurs at the expected time of puberty in girls with Turner syndrome, boys with Klinefelter syndrome, and boys with anorchia.[183] Studies in agonadal nonhuman primates show similar findings.[184] In addition, severe head injuries and irradiation of the skull may be associated with precocious puberty (Table 16-5)—implying damage to the region that regulates the restraint of puberty. Thus, the restraint of puberty is orchestrated in the brain (not the gonad).[185-186]

The first sign of puberty in boys is an increase in testis volume from a prepubertal value of 3 to 4 mL. This occurs on average between 11 and 11.5 years of age. The timing and tempo of puberty are related to a host of interacting factors comprising GnRH, neuropeptide-Y,

gamma aminobutyric acid (GABA), leptin, and transforming growth factor-alpha (TGFα). A recent addition to this list is a G-protein–coupled receptor (GPR54) and its ligand (kisspeptin 54), which act upstream of the GnRH pulse generator (Figure 16-7). The kisspeptins appear to be a gatekeeper to puberty and to play a key role in the negative and positive feedback control of gonadotrophin secretion by sex steroids.[187,188] Mutations in the GPR54 gene in humans results in delayed puberty due to HH.[189,190] Treatment with exogenous kisspeptin induces a rapid increase in LH and FSH levels in humans and can induce puberty in primates.[184,191,192]

DISORDERS OF PUBERTY

It is generally accepted that the age boundaries for the first sign of puberty (Tanner stage G2) in normal males extends from 9 years to 13.5 years. Thus, a boy starting puberty before 9 years of age is deemed precocious in development—whereas delayed puberty warrants investigation if G2 is not reached by 13 to 14 years of age. By far the most common clinical scenario to investigate is constitutional delay in pubertal development, a condition that implies normal but delayed onset of puberty in otherwise healthy boys. There is often a positive family history of similar delay in pubertal onset in the mother or father, suggesting a genetically regulated timing in the awakening of the GnRH pulse generator.

This is not a disorder per se, but can cause significant problems relating to self-esteem. It should be distinguished from HH, but this distinction is not easy because low basal FSH and LH levels with a prepubertal low response to a pulse of GnRH will occur in both. Some advocate a short course of exogenous testosterone (100-200 mg IM monthly for 4 to 6 injections). Such treatment improves self-image, promotes linear growth without impairing final adult height, and may result in the initiation of puberty—reflected in part by growth of the testis, which occurs in constitutional delay but not in disorders of HH.[193]

Because the disorders of puberty are primarily extratesticular in origin, reference to Tables 16-5 and 16-6 will suffice to summarize a general classification for disorders

TABLE 16-5

General Classification of Causes of Precocious and Delayed Puberty in the Male

Precocious Puberty

Gonadotrophin-Dependent
- Idiopathic central precocious puberty
- Organic central precocious puberty
  - Hypothalamic hamartoma
  - Post head trauma
  - Post cranial radiotherapy
  - Neurofibromatosis
  - HCG-secreting germ cell tumor

Gonadotrophin-Independent
- Activating LH receptor mutation (*testotoxicosis*)
- McCune-Albright syndrome
- Leydig cell tumor
- Extratesticular hyperandrogenism
  - Congenital adrenal hyperplasia
  - Adrenal tumor

Delayed Puberty

Hypogonadotrophic Hypogonadism
- Genetic
  - KAL1, FGFR1, GnR, GPR54, SF1, DAX1, Leptin R, STAT5b
- Organic
  - Craniopharyngioma
  - Post head trauma
  - Cranial irradiation
  - Multiple pituitary hormone deficiency
  - Isolated gonadotrophin deficiency
- Syndromal
  - Prader-Willi syndrome
  - Lawrence-Moon-Biedl syndrome
  - Kallmann syndrome
- Chronic disorders
  - Inflammatory bowel disease
  - Renal failure
  - Thalassemia
  - Emotional deprivation
  - Cystic fibrosis

Hypergonadotrophic Hypogonadism
- Syndromal
  - Klinefelter syndrome
  - XX male
  - Noonan syndrome
  - Frasier syndrome
- Primary testicular
  - Gonadal dysgenesis
  - Androgen biosynthetic defects
  - Anorchia/cryptorchidism
  - Chemotherapy

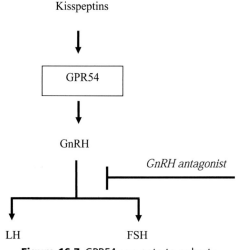

Figure 16-7 GPR54 as a gate to puberty.

of precocious and delayed puberty. Precocious puberty involves the gonads (gonadarche) and must not be equated with premature adrenarche, a condition in which adrenal androgens induce premature pubic hair development without virilization or advanced bone age (as discussed in detail in Chapters 4 and 12). It is logical and practical to base classification on the status of gonadotrophin secretion, the prime driver of normal puberty. Some testis-specific disorders are mentioned in further detail.

Constitutive activation of mutant LH receptors leads to precocious puberty. This condition is limited to males (testotoxicosis) and is familial in a heterozygous (autosomal-dominant) manner.[50] Puberty occurs in early childhood and is characterized by elevated serum testosterone and suppressed serum LH levels. Missense mutations are confined to exon 11 of the LH receptor gene, which encodes for the signal-transducing transmembrane domain of the receptor. This contrasts with inactivating LH receptor mutations causing DSD, which are distributed throughout the gene.

Mutant LH receptors causing testotoxicosis, when expressed in vitro, show basal constitutive activation of the cAMP signaling pathway in transfected cells in the absence of agonist compared with wild-type receptor. Mutant receptors also demonstrate a dose-response relationship with added LH or HCG.[194] It is a curious observation that females heterozygous for LH receptor mutations do not develop early puberty. The explanation lies with the observation that LH receptor expression in the ovary is dependent on FSH levels. Because FSH levels are low in childhood, ovarian follicles do not differentiate and hence LH receptor expression is also not enacted at this time. However, it is not clear why mothers of sons with LH-receptor-activating mutations have no discernible phenotype.

There is a relative hot spot of mutations at codon 578 in the sixth transmembrane helix, where aspartic acid (Asp) can be changed to glycine, tyrosine, or glutamic acid. A mutation at this codon (Asp578His) is found in somatic form only, and results in precocious puberty due to a Leydig cell adenoma.[195,196] This particular mutation is highly active basally when expressed in transfected cells but does not respond to LH or HCG. Furthermore, the mutant LH receptor constitutively activates an alternative signal transduction pathway involving the phospholipase C pathway.[197] The management of precocious puberty due to germline-activating mutations of the LH receptor is a challenge because the conventional approach of using a GnRH analogue to desensitise the gonadotrophes is not applicable.

The mainstay of current treatment is to use a combination of an antiandrogen to block the direct biologic effects of androgens and an aromatase inhibitor to reduce the accelerating effects on growth plate closure from estrogens produced from aromatization of increased androgens. An effective combination appears to be bicalutamide (a nonsteroidal antiandrogen) and anastrozole, a third-generation aromatase inhibitor.[198] This combination has produced a reversal of signs of hyperandrogenism, as well as reduction in growth velocity and rate of skeletal maturation.

A similar gonadotrophin-independent increased sex steroid secretion is the cause of precocious puberty in the McCune-Albright syndrome.[170] In this case, the pathophysiology relates to an activating mutation in the ubiquitously expressed G-protein α-subunit (Gsα), a major product of the GNAS gene.[199] The classic features of the syndrome comprise gonadotrophin-independent precocious puberty, café-au-lait lesions of the skin of a specific distribution, and polyostotic fibrous dysplasia. The pubertal manifestation occurs mainly in affected females. When it occurs in males, there is asymmetric enlargement of the testes. The Gsα mutation is somatic and is invariably a substitution of glycine for arginine at codon 201. Treatment for pubertal precocity associated with the McCune-Albright syndrome is similar to that used for LH-receptor-activating mutations.

Treatment of central precocious puberty relies primarily on the use of long-acting GnRH agonists that suppress the ability of endogenous GnRH to bind to its cognate receptor and evoke an appropriate increase in FSH and LH. It is based on the discovery that a single pulse of GnRH evokes an appropriate gonadotrophin response, whereas continuous infusion of GnRH down-regulates and abrogates the response.[200] Until recently, such GnRH long-acting agonists were administered by monthly IM injections—adjusting the dose to ensure suppression of response to exogenous GnRH.

A long-acting form of GnRH that can be implanted subcutaneously and last for 1 year has recently been introduced.[201] In addition to suppressing GnRH secretion, a form of reversible "medical castration," a primary underlying cause must be excluded by appropriate investigation—including cranial imaging. "Idiopathic" precocious puberty is more common in girls than in boys. The causes of delayed puberty can also be classified according to the status of gonadotrophin secretion. Table 16-6 outlines a general classification of causes in males.

GENETIC CAUSES OF HYPOGONADOTROPHIC HYPOGONADISM

The genetic causes of HH have been the subject of interest and investigation, resulting in the discovery of novel genes involved in the regulation of puberty via the hypothalamic-pituitary-gonadal axis. Kallmann syndrome consists of isolated HH plus anosmia. An X-linked form and several variants encoded by autosomal genes are described. The gene for the X-linked form KAL1 encodes the protein anosmin, which is a major regulator of the migration of GnRH neurones and olfactory nerves from the olfactory placode to the hypothalamus.

Males with this condition have agenesis of the olfactory lobes, which may be detected on MRI imaging, as well as hypogonadism secondary to deficiency of hypothalamic GnRH. Transmitting females may have partial or complete anosmia. Renal agenesis, high-arched palate, cerebellar ataxia, and mirror movements of the hands (synkinesia) have been described. The X-linked form due to KAL1 is listed as Kallmann syndrome 1 in the Online Mendelian Inheritance in Man (OMIM) database (*www.ncbi.nlm.nih.gov*). Kallman syndrome 2, KAL2, is an autosomal-recessive form due to a mutation in the gene encoding fibroblast growth factor receptor-1 (FGFR-1) and is associated with cleft lip or palate plus tooth agenesis in addition to the anosmia and hypogonadism. KAL 3 is caused by a mutation in the PROKR2 gene, and KAL 4 is caused by a mutation in PROK 2.

Together, these gene abnormalities account for about a third of all cases of Kallmann syndrome. Treatment with GnRH injected subcutaneously as pulses via a programmable pump can restore normal gonadal development and function. In some, the treatment can be discontinued while the patient retains normal gonadal function.[202] The role of Kisspeptin and its cognate receptor in regulating GnRH secretion and hence puberty has been described.[189,191,192] The DAX1 and SF1 genes interact in a complex manner in the formation of the GnRH region of the hypothalamus, as well as the formation of the adrenal gland. They are discussed in detail in Chapter 12.

Leptin secreted by fat tissue also regulates gonadotrophin secretion. Inactivating mutations in the genes for leptin or its receptor lead to obesity.[203,204] Leptin may be a signal in the initiation of puberty, indicating a link between nutritional status and reproductive capacity and the secular trend of pubertal onset in well-nourished societies. That leptin may be regarded as a metabolic gate to puberty is illustrated by the effect of leptin facilitating appropriately timed puberty when administered to children with congenital leptin deficiency.[205] Leptin signaling may play an important role in the HH of chronic wasting illnesses, including anorexia nervosa and the chronic disorders listed in Table 16-6.

The Prader-Willi syndrome is typically characterized by hypotonia, developmental delay, hypogonadism, and obesity. Stereotypic behavioral abnormalities also occur. The defect is encoded by a gene or genes on the paternal short arm of chromosome 15. Most disorders primarily testicular in nature have been discussed. Management of delayed puberty in the male is dependent on the underlying etiology. The overriding practical issue is to induce somatic signs of puberty in the event of this not occurring spontaneously from endogenous androgen production.

A commonly used treatment is Sustanon, a mixture of testosterone esters, given by monthly intramuscular injections at a starting dose of 25 mg and thereafter increasing to adult doses of 250 mg monthly. A wide variety of injectable, oral, implantable, cutaneous patch, and gel preparations of androgens are available.[206,207] Although the low-dose Sustanon modality is suited to replicate pubertal changes in a slow and timely fashion, regular hormone replacement in adulthood for persistent hypogonadism is increasingly employing topical delivery systems that appear to provide serum testosterone and DHT profiles similar to those found in normal males.[208,209]

Investigating Testis Function

GENERAL

There is no algorithmic-based panacea on how to investigate testis function. The choice of tests should be dictated by the clinical problem to be addressed and the nature of the questions posed. A number of sources provide recipes for investigation of the endocrine system.[210-212]

TABLE 16-6
General Classification of Causes of Delayed Puberty in the Male

Hypogonadotrophic Hypogonadism[229,230]
  Genetic
    KAL1, FGFR1, GnRH, GPR54, SF1, DAX1, Leptin R, STAT5b
  Organic
    craniopharyngioma
    post-head trauma
    cranial irradiation
    multiple pituitary hormone deficiency
    isolated gonadotrophin deficiency
  Syndromal
    Prader-Willi syndrome[231]
    Lawrence-Moon-Biedl syndrome[232]
    Kallmann syndrome[233]
  Chronic disorders
    inflammatory bowel disease
    renal failure
    thalassaemia
    emotional deprivation
    cystic fibrosis

Hypergonadotrophic Hypogonadism
  Syndromal
    Klinefelter syndrome[234]
    XX male
    Noonan syndrome[235]
    Frasier syndrome[236]
  Primary testicular
    gonadal dysgenesis
    androgen biosynthetic defects
    anorchia/cryptorchidism
    chemotherapy[237]

AMBIGUOUS GENITALIA (also see Chapter 14)

The approach to the investigation of a newborn infant with ambiguous genitalia requires a two-tiered approach to the choice of tests (Table 16-7). Establishing the karyotype, together with confirming or excluding CAH (the most common cause of ambiguous genitalia of the newborn), is the first task to be undertaken. The clear presence of a uterus/cervix on ultrasound and a markedly elevated serum 17OH-progesterone level in a full-term infant with a 46,XX karyotype confirms a diagnosis of CAH due to 21-hydroxylase deficiency.

If the karyotype is 46,XY (or 45X/46,XY), one determines whether testes are present—and if present whether they produce normal age-related amounts of testosterone. Table 16-7 does not contain an exhaustive list for this second-tier level of investigation but should allow resolution of the determinations cited. An understanding of the DSD classification shown in Table 16-2 is a guide to a logical pathophysiologic approach to investigation.

The HCG stimulation test is the bedrock of investigation for the XY DSD infant. The protocol and timing for this test varies considerably among centers.[213] The author's center uses as a standard three daily injections of HCG (1,500 units by intramuscular injection). A post-HCG

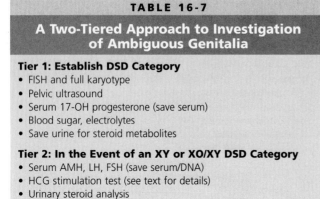

TABLE 16-7

A Two-Tiered Approach to Investigation of Ambiguous Genitalia

Tier 1: Establish DSD Category
- FISH and full karyotype
- Pelvic ultrasound
- Serum 17-OH progesterone (save serum)
- Blood sugar, electrolytes
- Save urine for steroid metabolites

Tier 2: In the Event of an XY or XO/XY DSD Category
- Serum AMH, LH, FSH (save serum/DNA)
- HCG stimulation test (see text for details)
- Urinary steroid analysis
- Imaging (MRI)
- Laparoscopy/gonadal biopsy

blood sample is collected 24 hours after the last injection for analysis of testosterone (coupled with androstenedione and DHT tests if indicated). An acute LHRH stimulation test may also be undertaken just prior to the first HCG injection. Occasionally, the HCG stimulation test is extended over 3 weeks (twice-weekly injections).

This protocol has the potential for coupling investigation and management where the clinical problem is testis maldescent.[214] The timing of an HCG test should be planned to coincide with the endogenous LH-induced rise in testosterone production at about 4 to 8 weeks of postnatal age, but local circumstances may dictate that the test be performed shortly after birth. This may create difficulties with the interpretation of neonatal serum steroid levels if nonextraction or non-chromatographic assays are performed.[215] Analysis of urinary steroid metabolites by sensitive highly specific chromatographic techniques may delineate defects in androgen biosynthesis such as P450-oxidoreductase deficiency and 5α-reductase deficiency.

ABSENT TESTES

When testes are not palpable at birth in an otherwise normal male infant, a karyotype is still mandatory. The phenotype may be the result of a fully virilized 46,XX infant with CAH. The main question asked of an endocrine investigation of a 46,XY infant with nonpalpable testes is whether testes are present. The HCG stimulation test and baseline LH and FSH measurements will generally answer the question. In addition, serum AMH is proving to be a reliable additional test—measuring levels otherwise almost undetectable in the case of anorchia.[216-219] Measurement of serum inhibin B levels appears to be equally effective as a marker of loss of Sertoli cells.

Undetectable levels of testosterone after HCG stimulation, elevated gonadotrophins (particularly FSH), and very low or undetectable levels of AMH are strongly suggestive of absent testicular tissue. However, efforts are usually made to locate testicular tissue and imaging is not sufficiently reliable for this purpose. Laparoscopic exploration generally reveals just nubbins of fibrous tissue at the end of a vas deferens.[102,103] If the genitalia are not otherwise completely normal (for example, an associated micropenis), the anorchia may be a form of gonadal dysgenesis in which there is occasionally a mutation in the SF1 gene.[220]

TESTIS TUMORS

Imaging, together with histology and immunohistochemical analysis of a testicular biopsy, is the key investigation for a testis mass. The relevant tumor markers have been listed previously. Ultrasound distinguishes among cystic, solid, or complex scrotal masses and is useful in longitudinal screening of patients with testicular microlithiasis.[221] However, microlithiasis is present in 5.6% of the young adult male population—and most men with such an isolated finding do not develop testis cancer.[222] Regular self-examination of the testes is the recommended surveillance procedure.

PUBERTAL DISORDERS

A basal and acute LHRH-stimulated LH and FSH level, with interpretation of age-appropriate serum testosterone measurements, is the mainstay of the investigation of puberty-related testis disorders. The original term, *testotoxicosis*, for the clinical syndrome due to LH-receptor-activating mutations is affirmation that elevated testosterone with totally suppressed LH levels is akin to the TSH/FT4 profile in thyrotoxicosis (Grave's disease). Assessment of LH/FSH levels provides the division between hyper-/hypogonadotrophic states and gonadotrophin dependency, as outlined in Tables 16-4 and 16-5. In pituitary-gonadal interrelationships, the negative feedback effect appears to be more profound on FSH levels than on LH levels.

In gonadal dysgenesis, for example, basal FSH levels are usually more elevated than LH levels. Primary hypogonadism may be the result of chemotherapy for cancer in childhood. The germ cells are more susceptible to damage than Leydig cells, and thus boys often develop puberty spontaneously. Fertility is a later problem, with lower than normal testosterone levels for young adulthood subsequently found.[223] Whereas the basal FSH level is usually a reliable indicator of germ cell damage and is a predictor of abnormal spermatogenesis, the basal LH is not as predictive of androgen deficiency.

It is generally not appropriate to undertake seminal fluid analysis in pubertal boys as a measure of testis function, although obtaining a semen sample for cryopreservation is offered to pubertal boys undergoing cancer treatment.[224] Inhibin B levels increase markedly at puberty and correlate with measurements of testis volume and testosterone, LH, and FSH levels.[225] The level of inhibin is inversely correlated with FSH levels at mid-puberty (G3-G4), when spermatogenesis is becoming established. This concurs with the results of indirect semen analysis using the observation that spermatozoa can be identified in early-morning urine samples from pubertal boys.[226]

Spermaturia as an index of the onset of spermatogenesis (spermarche) is possible at a median age of 13.4 years, although there is a large variation between boys of the same pubertal stage.[227] Nevertheless, this minimally invasive method of assessing developing germ cell function in adolescent boys has applicability in epidemiologic studies—including the effects of changes in the environment on male reproductive function. Thus, the effects of exposure to toxic chemicals before birth may be measurable by spermaturia analysis at puberty.[228] The assessment of testis function needs to be designed not only to determine the cause of intrinsic disorders related to the pituitary-gonadal interplay but to account for the increasing evidence that disorders of the testis may have a causation in part environmental in origin.

REFERENCES

1. Brennan J, Capel B (2004). One tissue, two fates: Molecular genetic events that underlie testis versus ovary development. Nat Rev Genet 5:509–521.
2. Park SY, Jameson JL (2005). Transcriptional regulation of gonadal development and differentiation. Endocrinol 146:1035–1042.
3. Wilhelm D, Koopman P (2006). The makings of maleness: Towards an integrated view of male sexual development. Nat Rev Genet 7:620–632.
4. Achermann JC, Hughes IA (2007). Disorders of sex differentiation. In Larsen PR, Kronenberg HM, Melmed S, Polonsky KS (eds.), Williams' textbook of endocrinology, Eleventh edition. Philadelphia: WB Saunders pp 783-848.
5. Koziell A, Charmandari E, Hindmarsh PC, Rees L, Scambler P, Brook CG (2000). Frasier syndrome, part of the Denys-Drash continuum or simply a WT1 gene associated disorder of intersex and nephropathy? Clin Endocrinol 52:519–524.
6. Ozisik G, Achermann JC, Meeks JJ, Jameson JL (2003). SF1 in the development of the adrenal gland and gonads. Horm Res 59(1):94–98.
7. Sullivan JG, Gohel M, Kinder RB (2005). Ectopic adrenocortical tissue found at groin exploration in children: Incidence in relation to diagnosis, age and sex. BJU Int 95:407–410.
8. Claahsen-van der Grinten HL, Otten BJ, Sweep FC, et al. (2007). Testicular tumors in patients with congenital adrenal hyperplasia due to 21-hydroxylase deficiency show functional features of adrenocortical tissue. J Clin Endocrinol Metab 92:3674–3680.
9. Josso N, Clemente N (2003). Transduction pathway of anti-Müllerian hormone, a sex-specific member of the TGF-beta family. Trends Endocrinol Metab 14:91–97.
10. Hannema SE, Hughes IA (2007). Regulation of Wolffian duct development. Horm Res 67:142–151.
11. Wilson JD, Griffin JE, Russell DW (1993). Steroid 5α-reductase 2 deficiency. Endocr Rev 14:577–593.
12. Hutson JM, Hasthorpe S (2004). Testicular descent and cryptorchidism: The state of the art in 2004. J Pediatr Surg 40:297–302.
13. Zimmermann S, Steding G, Emmen JMA, et al. (1999). Targeted disruption of the Insl3 gene causes bilateral cryptorchidism. Mol Endocrinol 13:681–691.
14. Boucekkine C, Toublanc JE, Abbas N, et al. (1994). Clinical and anatomical spectrum in XX sex reversed patients: Relationship to the presence of Y specific DNA-sequences. Clin Endocrinol 40:733–742.
15. Koopman P, Gubbay J, Vivian N, Goodfellow P, Lovell-Badge R (1991). Male development of chromosomally female mice transgenic for Sry. Nature 351:117–121.
16. McElreavey K, Vilain E, Abbas N, Herskowitz I, Fellous M (1993). A regulatory cascade hypothesis for mammalian sex determination: SRY represses a negative regulator of male development. Proc Natl Acad Sci USA 90:3368–3372.
17. O'Shaughnessy PJ, Baker PJ, Johnston H (2006). The foetal Leydig cell: Differentiation, function and regulation. Int J Androl 29:90–95.
18. Auchus RJ (2004). The backdoor pathway to dihydrotestosterone. Trends Endocrinol Metab 15:432–438.
19. Hughes IA, Deeb A (2006). Androgen resistance. Best Pract Res Clin Endocrinol Metab 20:577–598.
20. Lonard DM, O'Malley BW (2007). Nuclear receptor coregulators: Judges, juries, and executioners of cellular regulation. Mol Cell 27:691–700.
21. Hughes IA, Houk C, Ahmed SF, Lee PA (2006). Consensus statement on management of intersex disorders. Arch Dis Child 91:554–563.
22. Houk CP, Hughes IA, Ahmed SF, Lee PA for the Writing Committee for the International Consensus Conference Participants (2006). Summary of consensus statement on intersex disorders and their management. Pediatrics 118:753–757.
23. Bojesen A, Juul, S, Gravholt CH (2003). Prenatal and postnatal prevalence of Klinefelter syndrome: A national registry study. J Clin Endocrinol Metab 88:622–626.
24. Lee YS, Cheng AW, Ahmed SF, Shaw NJ, Hughes IA (2007). Genital anomalies in Klinefelter's syndrome. Horm Res 68:150–155.
25. Aksglaede L, Wikström AM, Rajpert-De Meyts E, Dunkel L, Skakkebaek NE, et al. (2006). Natural history of seminiferous tubule degeneration in Klinefelter syndrome. Hum Reprod Update 12:39–48.
26. Wikström AM, Dunkel L, Wickman S, Norjavaara E, Ankarberg-Lindgren C, Raivio T (2006). Are adolescent boys with Klinefelter syndrome androgen deficient?: A longitudinal study of Finnish 47,XXY boys. Pediatr Res 59:854–859.
27. Schiff JD, Palermo GD, Veeck LL, Goldstein M, Rosenwaks Z, Schlegel PN (2005). Success of testicular sperm extraction (corrected) and intracytoplasmic sperm injection in men with Klinefelter syndrome. J Clin Endocrinol Metab 90:6263–6267.
28. de la Chapelle A (1981). The etiology of maleness in XX men. Hum Genet 58:105–116.
29. Vorona E, Zitzmann M, Gromoll J, Schüring AN, Nieschlag E (2007). Clinical, endocrinological, and epigenetic features of the 46,XX male syndrome, compared with 47,XXY Klinefelter patients. J Clin Endocrinol Metab 92:3458–3465.
30. Abusheikha N, Lass A, Brinsden P (2001). XX males without SRY gene and with infertility. Hum Reprod 16:717–718.
31. Rajender S, Rajani V, Gupta NJ, Chakravarty B, Singh L, Thangaraj K (2006). SRY-negative 46,XX male with normal genitals, complete masculinisation and infertility. Mol Hum Reprod 12:341–346.
32. Hoei-Hansen CE, Holm M, Rajpert-De Meyts E, Skakkebaek NE (2003). Histological evidence of testicular dysgenesis in contralateral biopsies from 218 patients with testicular germ cell cancer. J Pathol 200:370–374.
33. Chemes HE, Muzulin PM, Venara MC, Mulhmann Mdel C, Martinez M, Gamboni M (2003). Early manifestations of testicular dysgenesis in children: pathological phenotypes, karyotype correlations and precursor stages of tumor development. APMIS 111:12–24.
34. Cameron FJ, Sinclair AH (1997). Mutations in SRY and SOX9: Testis determining genes. Hum Mut 9:388–395.
35. Gimelli G, Gimelli S, Dimasi N, et al. (2007). Identification and molecular modelling of a novel familial mutation in the SRY gene implicated in pure gonadal dysgenesis. Eur J Hum Genet 15:76–80.
36. Achermann JC, Ozisik G, Ito M, et al. (2002). Gonadal determination and adrenal development are regulated by the orphan nuclear receptor steroidogenic factor-1, in a dose-dependent manner. J Clin Endocrinol Metab 87:1829–1833.
37. Lin L, Philbert P, Ferraz-de-Souza B, et al. (2007). Heterozygous missense mutations in steroidogenic factor 1 (SF1/Ad4BP, NR5A1) are associated with 46,XY disorders of sex development with normal adrenal function. J Clin Endocrinol Metab 92:991–999.
38. Chang HJ, Clark RD, Bachman H (1990). The phenotype of 45,X/46,XY mosaicism: An analysis of 92 prenatally diagnosed cases. Am J Hum Genet 45:156–167.
39. Alvarez-Nava F, Soto M, Borjas L, et al. (2001). Molecular analysis of SRY gene in patients with mixed gonadal dysgenesis. Ann Genet 44:155–159.
40. Verkauskas G, Jambert F, Lortat-Jacob S, Malan V, Thibaud E, Nihoul-Fékété C (2007). The long-term follow up of 33 cases of true hermaphroditism: A 40-year experience with conservative gonadal surgery. J Urol 177:726–731.
41. Maier EM, Leitner C, Löhrs U, Kuhnle U (2003). True hermaphroditism in an XY individual due to a familial point mutation of the SRY gene. J Pediatr Endocrinol Metab 16:575–580.
42. Talerman A, Verp MS, Senekjian E, Gilewski T, Vogelzang N (1990). True hermaphrodite with bilateral ovotestes, bilateral gonadoblastomas and dysgerminomas, 46,XX/46,XY karyotype, and a successful pregnancy. Cancer 66:2668–2672.
43. Williamson HO, Phansey SA, Mathur RS (1981). True hermaphroditism with term vaginal delivery and a review. Am J Obstet Gynecol 141:262–265.
44. Krob G, Braun A, Kuhnle U (2005). True hermaphroditism: geographical distribution, clinical findings, chromosomes and gonadal histology. J Obstet Gynaecol 25:401–403.
45. Krone N, Dhir V, Ivison HE, Arlt W (2007). Congenital adrenal hyperplasia and P450 oxidoreductase deficiency. Clin Endocrinol 66:162–172.

46. Arlt W, Walker EA, Draper N, et al. (2004). Congenital adrenal hyperplasia caused by mutant P450 oxidoreductase and human androgen synthesis: Analytical study. Lancet 363:2128–2135.

47. Flück CE, Miller WL (2006). P450 oxidoreductase deficiency: A new form of congenital adrenal hyperplasia. Curr Opin Pediatr 18:435–441.

48. Ascoli M, Fanelli F, Segaloff DL (2002). The lutropin/choriogonadotropin receptor: A 2002 perspective. Endocr Rev 23:141–174.

49. Huhtaniemi I, Alevizaki M (2006). Gonadotrophin resistance. Best Prac Res Clin Endocrinol Metab 20:561–576.

50. Piersma D, Verhoef-Post M, Berns EM, Themmen APN (2007). LH receptor gene mutations and polymorphisms: An overview. Mol Cell Endocrinol 260–262:282–286.

51. Andersson S, Geissler WM, Wu L, et al. (1996). Molecular genetics and pathophysiology of 17 beta-hydroxysteroid dehydrogenase 3 deficiency. J Clin Endocrinol Metab 81:130–136.

52. Boehmer AL, Brinkmann AO, Sandkuijl LA, et al. (1999). 17 beta-hydroxysteroid dehydrogenase-3 deficiency: diagnosis, phenotypic variability, population genetics, and worldwide distribution of ancient and de novo mutations. J Clin Endocrinol Metab 84:4713–4721.

53. Lee YS, Kirk JM, Stanhope RG, et al. (2007) Phenotypic variability in 17beta-hydroxysteroid dehydrogenase-3 deficiency and diagnostic pitfalls. Clin Endocrinol 67:20–28.

54. Qiu W, Zhou M, Labrie F, Lin SX (2004). Crystal structures of the multispecific 17beta-hydroxysteroid dehydrogenase type 5: Critical androgen regulation in human peripheral tissues. Mol Endocrinol 18:1798–1807.

55. Rösler A, Silverstein S, Abeliovich D (1996). A (R80Q) mutation in 17 beta-hydroxysteroid dehydrogenase type 3 gene among Arabs of Israel is associated with pseudohermaphroditism in males and normal asymptomatic females. J Clin Endocrinol Metab 81:1827–1831.

56. Imperato-McGinley J, Guerrero L, Gautier T, Peterson RE (1974). Steroid 5alpha-reductase deficiency in man: An inherited form of male pseudohermaphroditism. Science 186:1213–1215.

57. Wilson JD, Griffin JE, Russell DW (1993). Steroid 5α-reductase 2 deficiency. Endocr Rev 14:577–593.

58. Katz MD, Kligman I, Cai LQ, et al. (1997). Paternity by intrauterine insemination with sperm from a man with 5α-reductase-2 deficiency. N Eng J Med 336:994–997.

59. Nordenskjöld A, Ivarsson SA (1998). Molecular characterization of 5 alpha-reductase type 2 deficiency and fertility in a Swedish family. J Clin Endocrinol Metab 83:3236–3238.

60. Katz MD, Cai LQ, Zhu YS, et al. (1995). The biochemical and phenotypic characterization of females homozygous for 5 alpha-reductase 2 deficiency. J Clin Endocrinol Metab 80:3160–3167.

61. Quigley C, De Bellis A, Marschke KB, et al. (1995). Androgen receptor defects: Historical, clinical and molecular perspectives. Endocr Rev 16:271–321.

62. Ahmed SF, Cheng A, Dovey L, et al. (2000). Phenotypic features, androgen receptor binding, and mutational analysis in 278 clinical cases reported as androgen insensitivity syndrome. J Clin Endocrinol Metab 85:658–665.

63. Jenster G, van der Korput JA, Trapman J, Brinkmann AO (1992). Functional domains of the human androgen receptor. J Steroid Biochem Mol Biol 41:671–675.

64. Heinlein CA, Chang C (2002). Androgen receptor (AR) coregulators: An overview. Endocr Rev 23:175–200.

65. Tut TG, Ghadessy FJ, Trifiro MA, Pinsky L, Yong EL (1997). Long polyglutamine tracts in the androgen receptor are associated with reduced trans-activation, impaired sperm production, and male infertility. J Clin Endocrinol Metab 82:3777–3782.

66. Cheung-Flynn J, Prapapanich V, Cox MB, Riggs DL, Suarez-Quian C, Smith DF (2005). Physiological role for the cochaperone FKBP52 in androgen receptor signalling. Mol Endocrinol 19:1654–1666.

67. Bangsbøll S, Qvist I, Lebech PE, Lewinsky M (1992). Testicular feminization syndrome and associated gonadal tumors in Denmark. Acta Obstet Gynecol Scand 71:63–66.

68. Boehmer AL, Brinkmann AO, Brüggenwirth H, et al. (2001). Genotype versus phenotype in families with androgen insensitivity syndrome. J Clin Endocrinol Metab 86:4151–4160.

69. Hannema SE, Scott IS, Hodapp J, et al. (2004). Residual activity of mutant androgen receptors explains Wolffian duct development in the complete androgen insensitivity syndrome. J Clin Endocrinol Metab 89:5815–5822.

70. Deeb A, Hughes IA (2005). Inguinal hernia in female infants: A cue to check the sex chromosomes? BJU Int 96:401–403.

71. Yong EL, Loy CJ, Sim KS (2003). Androgen receptor gene and male infertility. Hum Reprod Update 9:1–7.

72. Ong YC, Wong HB, Adaikan G, Yong EL (1999). Directed pharmacological therapy of ambiguous genitalia due to an androgen receptor gene mutation. Lancet 354:1444–1445.

73. Sinnecker GH, Hiort O, Nitsche EM, Holterhus PM, Kruse K (1997). Functional assessment and clinical classification of androgen sensitivity in patients with mutations of the androgen receptor gene: German Collaborative Intersex Study Group. Eur J Pediatr 156:7–14.

74. Nagy L, Schwabe JW (2004). Mechanism of the nuclear receptor molecular switch. Trends Biochem Sci 29:317–324.

75. Radmayr C, Culig Z, Glatzl J, Neuschmid-Kaspar F, Bartsch G, Klocker H (1997). Androgen receptor point mutations as the underlying molecular defect in 2 patients with androgen insensitivity syndrome. J Urol 158:1553–1556.

76. Deeb A, Mason C, Lee YS, Hughes IA (2005). Correlation between genotype, phenotype and sex of rearing in 111 patients with partial androgen insensitivity syndrome. Clin Endocrinol 63:56–62.

77. Köhler B, Lumbroso S, Leger J, et al. (2005). Androgen insensitivity syndrome: Somatic mosaicism of the androgen receptor in seven families and consequences for sex assignment and genetic counselling. J Clin Endocrinol Metab 90:106–111.

78. Boehmer AL, Brinkmann AO, Nijman RM, et al. (2001). Phenotypic variation in a family with partial androgen insensitivity syndrome explained by differences in 5alpha dihydrotestosterone availability. J Clin Endocrinol Metab 86:1240–1246.

79. Holterhus PM, Werner R, Hoppe U, et al. (2005). Molecular features and clinical phenotypes in androgen insensitivity syndrome in the absence and presence of androgen receptor gene mutations. J Mol Med 83:1005–1113.

80. Lonard DM, O'Malley BW (2007). Nuclear receptor coregulators and human disease. Endocr Rev 28:575–587.

81. Mongan NP, Lim HN, Hughes IA (2001). Genetic evidence to exclude the androgen receptor-polyglutamine associated coactivator, ARA-24, as a cause of male undermasculinisation. Eur J Endocrinol 145:809–811.

82. Lim HN, Hawkins JR, Hughes IA (2001). Genetic evidence to exclude the androgen receptor co-factor, ARA70 (NCOA4) as a candidate gene for the causation of undermasculinised genitalia. Clin Genet 59:284–286.

83. Xu J, Liao L, Ning G, Yoshida-Komiya H, Deng C, O'Malley BW (2000). The steroid receptor coactivator SRC-3 (p/CIP/RAC3/AIB1/ACTR/TRAM-1) is required for normal growth, puberty, female reproductive function, and mammary gland development. Proc Natl Acad Sci USA 97:6379–6384.

84. Mongan NP, Jääskeläinen J, Bhattacharyya S, Leu RM, Hughes IA (2003). Steroid receptor coactivator-3 glutamine repeat polymorphism and the androgen insensitivity syndrome. Eur J Endocrinol 148:277–279.

85. Adachi M, Takayanagi R, Tomura A, et al. (2000). Androgen-insensitivity syndrome as a possible coactivator disease. N Eng J Med 343:856–862.

86. Hughes IA (2000). A novel explanation for resistance to androgens. N Engl J Med 343:881–882.

87. La Spada AR, Wilson EM, Lubahn DB, Harding AE, Fischbeck KH (1991). Androgen receptor gene mutations in X-linked spinal and bulbar muscular atrophy. Nature 352:77–79.

88. Lim HN, Chen H, McBride S, et al. (2000). Longer polyglutamine tracts in the androgen receptor are associated with moderate to severe undermasculinized genitalia in XY males. Hum Mol Genet 9:829–834.

89. Mengual L, Oriola J, Ascaso C, Ballesca JL, Oliva R (2003). An increased CAG repeat length in the androgen receptor gene in azoospermic ICSI candidates. J Androl 24:279–284.

90. Zinn AR, Ramos P, Elder FF, Kowal K, Samango-Sprouse C, Ross JL (2005). Androgen receptor CAGn repeat length influences phenotype of 47,XXY (Klinefelter) syndrome. J Clin Endocrinol Metab 90:5041–5046.

91. Tsujimoto Y, Takakuwa T, Takayama H, et al. (2004). In situ shortening of CAG repeat length within the androgen receptor gene in prostatic cancer and its possible precursors. Prostate 58:283–290.

92. Zitzmann M, Nieschlag E (2003). The CAG repeat polymorphism within the androgen receptor gene and maleness. Int J Androl 26:76–83.

93. Ibanez L, Ong KK, Mongan N, et al. (2003). Androgen receptor gene CAG repeat polymorphism in the development of ovarian hyperandrogenism. J Clin Endocrinol Metab 88:3333–3338.

94. Aschim EL, Nordenskjold A, Giwercman A, et al. (2004). Linkage between cryptorchidism, hypospadias, and GGN repeat length in the androgen receptor gene. J Clin Endocrinol Metab 89: 5105–5109.

95. Werner R, Holterhus PM, Binder G, et al. (2006). The A645D mutation in the hinge region of the human androgen receptor (AR) gene modulates AR activity, depending on the context of the polymorphic glutamine and glycine repeats. J Clin Endocrinol Metab 91:3515–3520.

96. Visser JA (2003). AMH signaling: from receptor to target gene. Mol Cell Endocrinol 211:65–73.

97. Josso N, Belville C, di Clemente N, Picard JY (2005). AMH and AMH receptor defects in persistent Müllerian duct syndrome. Hum Reprod Update 11:351–356.

98. Imbeaud S, Carré-Eusèbe D, Rey R, Belville C, Josso N, Picard JY (1994). Molecular genetics of the persistent Müllerian duct syndrome: A study of 19 families. Hum Mol Genet 3:125–131.

99. Imbeaud S, Faure E, Lamarre I, et al. (1995). Insensitivity to anti-Müllerian hormone due to a mutation in the human antiMüllerian hormone receptor. Nat Genet 11:382–388.

100. Zenaty D, Dijoud F, Morel Y, et al. (2006). Bilateral anorchia in infancy: Occurrence of micropenis and the effect of testosterone treatment. J Pediatr 149:687–691.

101. Philibert P, Zenaty D, Lin L, et al. (2007). Mutational analysis of steroidogenic factor 1 (NR5a1) in 24 boys with bilateral anorchia: A French collaborative study. Hum Reprod 22:3255-3261.

102. Law H, Mushtaq I, Wingrove K, Malone M, Sebire NJ (2006). Histopathological features of testicular regression syndrome: Relation to patient age and implications for management. Fetal Pediatr Pathol 25:119–129.

103. Emir H, Ayik B, Eliçevik M, et al. (2007). Histological evaluation of the testicular nubbins in patients with nonpalpable testis: Assessment of etiology and surgical approach. Pediatr Surg Int 23:41–44.

104. McEachern R, Houle AM, Garel L, Van Vliet G (2004). Lost and found testes: The importance of the hCG stimulation test and other testicular markers to confirm a surgical declaration of anorchia. Horm Res 62:124–128.

105. Lee MM, Donahoe PK, Silverman BL, et al. (1997). Measurements of serum Müllerian inhibiting substance in the evaluation of children with nonpalpable gonads. N Engl J Med 336:1480–1486.

106. Boisen KA, Chellakooty M, Schmidt IM, et al. (2005). Hypospadias in a cohort of 1072 Danish newborn boys: Prevalence and relationship to placental weight, anthropometrical measurements at birth, and reproductive hormone levels at three months of age. J Clin Endocrinol Metab 90:4041–4046.

107. Gorlov IP, Kamat A, Bogatcheva NV, et al. (2002). Mutations of the GREAT gene cause cryptorchidism. Hum Molec Genet 11:2309–2318.

108. Ferlin A, Simonato M, Bartoloni L, et al. (2003). The INSL3-LGR8/GREAT ligand-receptor pair in human cryptorchidism. J Clin Endocrinol Metab 88:4273–4279.

109. Yamazawa K, Wada Y, Sasagawa I, Aoki K, Ueoka K, Ogata T (2006). Mutation and polymorphism analyses of INSL3 and LGR8/GREAT in 62 Japanese patients with cryptorchidism. Horm Res 67:73–76.

110. Damgaard IN, Skakkebaek NE, Toppari J, et al. (2006). Persistent pesticides in human breast milk and cryptorchidism. Environ Health Perspect 114:1133–1138.

111. John Radcliffe Hospital Cryptorchidism Study Group (1992). Cryptorchidism: A prospective study of 7500 consecutive male births, 1984–1988. Arch Dis Child 67:892–899.

112. Buemann B, Henriksen H, Villumsen AL, Westh A, Zachau-Christiansen B (1961). Incidence of undescended testes in the newborn. Acta Chir Scand 283:289–293.

113. Boisen KA, Kaleva M, Main KM, et al. (2000). Difference in prevalence of congenital cryptorchidism in infants between two Nordic countries. Lancet 363:1264–1269.

114. Abdullah NA, Pearce MS, Parker L, Wilkinson JR, McNally RJQ (2007). Evidence of an environmental contribution to the aetiology of cryptorchidism and hypospadias? Eur J Endocrinol 22:615–620.

115. Sharpe R (2001). Hormones and testis development and the possible adverse effects of environmental chemicals. Toxicol Lett 120:221–232.

116. Jorgensen N, Asklund G, Carlsen E, Skakkebaek NE (2006). Coordinated European investigations of semen quality: Results from studies of Scandinavian young men is a matter of concern. Int J Androl 29:54–61.

117. Skakkebaek NE, Rajpert-De Meyts E, Jorgensen N, et al. (2007). Testicular cancer trends as "whistle blowers" of testicular developmental problems in populations. Int J Androl 30:198–204.

118. Bay K, Asklund C, Skakkebaek NE, Andersson AM (2006). Testicular dysgenesis syndrome: possible role of endocrine disruptors. Best Pract Res Clin Endocrinol Metab 20:77–90.

119. Acerini CL, Hughes IA (2006). Endocrine disrupting chemicals: A new and emerging public health problem? Arch Dis Child 91:633–641.

120. Swan SH (2000). Intrauterine exposure to diethylstilbestrol: Long-term effects in humans. APMIS 108:793–804.

121. Weidner IS, Moller H, Jensen TK, Skakkebaek NE (1998). Cryptorchidism and hypospadias in sons of gardeners and farmers. Environ Health Perspect 106:793–796.

122. Ema M, Myawaki E, Hirose A, Kamata E (2003). Decreased anogenital distance and increased incidence of undescended testes in fetuses of rats given monobenzyl phthalate, a major metabolite of butyl benzyl phthalate. Reprod Toxicol 17:407–412.

123. Swan SH, Main KM, Liu F, et al. (2005). Decrease in anogenital distance among male infants with prenatal phthalate exposure. Environ Health Perspect 113:1056–1061.

124. Baskin LS, Ebbers MB (2006). Hypospadias: Anatomy, etiology, and technique. J Ped Surg 41:463–472.

125. Rey RA, Codner E, Iniguez G, et al. (2005). Low risk of impaired testicular Sertoli and Leydig cell functions in boys with isolated hypospadias. J Clin Endocrinol Metab 90:6035–6040.

126. Holmes NM, Miller WL, Baskin LS (2004). Lack of defects in androgen production in children with hypospadias. J Clin Endocrinol Metab 89:2811–2816.

127. Fukami M, Wada Y, Miyabayashi K, et al. (2006). CXorf6 is a causative gene for hypospadias. Nat Genet 38:1369–1371.

128. Chen T, Li Q, Xu J, et al. (2007). Mutation screening of BMP4, BMP7, HOXA4 and HOXB6 genes in Chinese patients with hypospadias. Eur J Hum Genet 15:23–28.

129. Goodman FR, Bacchelli C, Brady AF, et al. (2000). Novel HOXA13 mutations and the phenotypic spectrum of hand-foot-genital syndrome. Am J Hum Genet 67:197–202.

130. Fredell L, Kockum I, Hansson E, et al. (2002). Heredity of hypospadias and the significance of low birth weight. J Urol 167:1423–1427.

131. Brouwers MM, Feitz WF, Roelofs LA, Kiemeney LA, de Gier RP, Roeleveld N (2007). Risk factors for hypospadias. Eur J Pediatr 166:671–678.

132. Li J, Willingham E, Baskin LS (2006). Gene expression profiles in mouse urethral development. BJU Int 98:880–885.

133. Laguna MP, Pizzocaro G, Klepp O, et al. (2001). EAU guidelines on testicular cancer. Eur Urol 40:102–110.

134. Mostofi FK, Sobin LH (1977). *Histological typing of testicular tumors: International histological classification of tumors.* Geneva: World Health Organization.

135. Eble JN, Sauter G, Epstein JL (eds.) (2004). *World Health Organization classification of tumors: Pathology and genetics of the urinary system and male genital organs.* [city]: IARC Press.

136. Ulbright TM (2005). Germ cell tumors of the gonads: A selective review emphasizing problems in differential diagnosis, newly appreciated, and controversial issues. Mod Pathol 18:S61–S79.

137. Cools M, Drop SLS, Wolffenbuttel KP, Oosterhuis JW, Looijenga LHJ (2006). Germ cell tumors in the intersex gonad: Old paths, new directions, moving frontiers. Endocr Rev 27:468–484.

138. Bahrami A, Ro, JY, Ayala AG (2007). An overview of testicular germ cell tumors. Arch Pathol Lab Med 131:1267–1280.

139. Hannema SE, Hughes IA (2008). Neoplasia and intersex states. In Hay ID, Wass JAH (eds.), *Clinical endocrine oncology, Second edition.* Oxford (UK): Blackwell (in press).

140. Rajpert-De Meyts E, Bartkova J, Sansom M, et al. (2003). The emerging phenotype of the testicular carcinoma in situ germ cell. APMIS 111:267–278.

141. Satgé D, Sascoe AJ, Cure H, Leduc B, Sommelet D, Vekemans MJ (2003). An excess of testicular germ cell tumors in Down's syndrome: Three case reports and a review of the literature. Cancer 80:929–935.

142. Moe-Behrens GHG, Klinger FG, Eskild W, Grotmol T, Haugen TB, De Felici M (2003). Akt/PTEN signaling mediates estrogen-dependent proliferation of primordial germ cells in vitro. Mol Endocrinol 17:2630–2638.

143. Pena-Alonso R, Nieto K, Alvarez R, et al. (2005). Distribution of Y-chromosome bearing cells inn gonadoblastoma and dysgenetic testis in 45,X,/46,XY infants. Mod Pathol 18:439–445.

144. Hoei-Hansen CE, Carlsen E, Jorgensen N, Leffers H, Skakkebaek NE, Rajpert-De Meyts E (2007). Towards a non-invasive method for early detection of testicular neoplasia in semen samples by identification of fetal germ cell-specific markers. Hum Reprod 22:167–173.

145. Lefevre H, Bouvattier C, Lahlou N, Adamsbaum C, Bougnères P, Carel JC (2006). Prepubertal gynaecomastia in Peutz-Jeghers syndrome: Incomplete penetrance in a familial case and management with an aromatase inhibitor. Eur J Endocrinol 154:221–227.

146. Brown B, Ram A, Clayton P, Humphrey G (2007). Conservative management of bilateral Sertoli cell tumors of the testicle in association with the Carney complex: A case report. J Pediatr Surg 42:E13–E15.

147. Toppari J, Kaipia A, Kalevo M, et al. (1998). Inhibin gene expression in a large cell calcifying Sertoli cell tumor and serum inhibin and activin levels. APMIS 106:101–112.

148. Al-Agha OM, Axiotis CA (2007). An in-depth look at Leydig cell tumor of the testis. Arch Pathol Lab Med 131:311–317.

149. Jain M, Aiyer HM, Bajaj P, Dhar S (2001). Intracytoplasmic and intranuclear Reinke's crystals in a testicular Leydig-cell tumor diagnosed by fine-needle aspiration cytology: A case report with review of the literature. Diagn Cytopathol 25:162–164.

150. Val P, Jeays-Ward K, Swain A (2006). Identification of a novel population of adrenal-like cells in the mammalian testis. Dev Biol 299:250–256.

151. Stikkelbroek NM, Otten BJ, Pasic A, et al. (2001). High prevalence of testicular adrenal rest tumors, impaired spermatogenesis, and Leydig cell failure in adolescent and adult males with congenital adrenal hyperplasia. J Clin Endocrinol Metab 86:5721–5728.

152. Seidenwurm D, Smathers RL, Kan P, Hoffman A (1985). Intratesticular adrenal rests diagnosed by ultrasound. Radiology 155:479–481.

153. Johnson RE, Scheithauer B (1982). Massive hyperplasia of testicular adrenal rests in a patient with Nelson's syndrome. Am J Clin Pathol 77:501–507.

154. Claahsen-van der Grinten HL, Sweep FC, Blickman JG, Hermus AR, Otten BJ (2007). Prevalence of testicular adrenal rest tumors in male children with congenital adrenal hyperplasia due to 21-hydroxylase deficiency. Eur J Endocrinol 157:339–344.

155. Knudsen JL, Savage A, Mobb GE (1991). The testicular "tumor" of adrenogenital syndrome: A persistent diagnostic pitfall. Histopathology 19:468–470.

156. Claahsen-van der Grinten HL, Stikkelbroek NM, Sweep CG, Hermus AR, Otten BJ (2006). Fertility in patients with congenital adrenal hyperplasia. J Pediatr Endocrinol Metab 19:677–685.

157. Ogilvie CM, Crouch NS, Rumsby G, Creighton SM, Liao LM, Conway GS (2006). Congenital adrenal hyperplasia in adults: A review of medical, surgical and psychological issues. Clin Endocrinol 64:2–11.

158. Martinez-Aguayo A, Rocha A, Rojas N, et al. (2007). Testicular adrenal rest tumors and Leydig and Sertoli cell function in boys with classical congenital adrenal hyperplasia. J Clin Endocrinol Metab (E-pub ahead of print).

159. Claahsen-van der Grinten HL, Otten BJ, Sweep FC, Hermus AR (2007). Repeated successful induction of fertility after replacing hydrocortisone with dexamethasone in a patient with congenital adrenal hyperplasia and testicular adrenal rest tumors. Fertil Steril 88:705.e5–e8.

160. Claahsen-van der Grinten HL, Otten BJ, Takahashi S, et al. (2007). Testicular adrenal rest tumors in adult males with congenital adrenal hyperplasia: Evaluation of pituitary-gonadal function before and after successful testis-sparing surgery in eight patients. J Clin Endocrinol Metab 92:612–615.

161. Penagarikano O, Mulle JG, Warren ST (2007). The pathophysiology of fragile X syndrome. Annu Rev Genomics Hum Genet 8:109–129.

162. Malter HE, Iber JG, Willemsen R, et al. (1997). Characterization of the full fragile X syndrome in fetal gametes. Nat Genet 15:165–169.

163. Butler MG, Brunschwig A, Miller LK, Hagerman RJ (1992). Standards for selected anthropometric measurements in males with the Fragile X syndrome. Pediatrics 89:1059–1062.

164. Carmi R, Meryash DL, Wood J, Gerald PS (1984). Fragile-X syndrome ascertained by the presence of macro-orchidism in a 5-month-old infant. Pediatrics 74:883–886.

165. Rudelli RD, Jenkins EC, Wisniewski K, Moretz R, Byrne J, Brown WT (1983). Testicular size in fetal fragile X syndrome. Lancet 1:1221–1222.

166. Johannisson R, Rehder H, Wendt V, Schwinger E (1987). Spermatogenesis in two patients with the fragile X syndrome: I. Histology: light and electron microscopy. Hum Genet 76:141–147.

167. Slegtenhorst-Eegdeman KE, De Rooij DG, Verhoef-Post M, et al. (1998). Macroorchidism in FMR1 knockout mice is caused by increased Sertoli cell proliferation during testicular development. Endocrinology 139:156–162.

168. Coutant R, Lumbroso S, Rey R, et al. (2001). Macroorchidism due to autonomous hyperfunction of Sertoli cells and Gsα gene mutation: An unusual expression of McCune-Albright syndrome in a prepubertal boy. J Clin Endocrinol Metab 86:1778–1881.

169. Arrigo T, Pirazzoli P, De Sanctis L, et al. (2006). McCune-Albright syndrome in a boy may present with a monolateral macroorchidism as an early and isolated clinical manifestation. Horm Res 65:114–119.

170. Spiegel AM, Weinstein LS (2004). Inherited diseases involving G proteins and G protein coupled receptors. Annu Rev Med 55:27–39.

171. Rey RA, Venara M, Coutant R, et al. (2006). Unexpected mosaicism of R201H-GNAS1 mutant-bearing cells in the testis underlie macroorchidism without sexual precocity in McCune-Albright syndrome. Hum Mol Genet 15:3538–3543.

172. Velaga MR, Wright G, Crofton PM, et al. (2005). Macro-orchidism in two unrelated prepubertal boys with a normal FSH receptor. Horm Res 64:1–2.

173. Castro-Magana M, Angulo M, Canas A, Sharp A, Fuentes B (1988). Hypothalamic-pituitary gonadal axis in boys with primary hypothyroidism and macroorchidism. J Pediatr 112:397–402.

174. Jannini EA, Ulisse S, D'Armiento M (1995). Macroorchidism in juvenile hypothyroidism. J Clin Endocrinol Metab 80:2543–2544.

175. De Leener A, Montanelli L, Van Durme J, et al. (2006). Presence and absence of follicle-stimulating hormone receptor mutations provide some insights into spontaneous ovarian hyperstimulation syndrome physiopathology. J Clin Endocrinol Metab 91:555–562.

176. Suarez EA, d'Alva CB, Campbell A, et al. (2007). Absence of mutation in the follicle-stimulating hormone receptor gene in severe primary hypothyroidism associated with gonadal hyperstimulation. J Pediatr Endocrinol Metab 20:923–931.

177. Parent AS, Teilmann G, Juul A, Skakkebaek NE, Toppari J, Bourguignon JP (2003). The timing of normal puberty and the age limits of sexual precocity: Variations around the world, secular trends, and changes after migration. Endocr Rev 24:668–693.

178. Boas M, Boisen KA, Virtanen HE, et al. (2006). Postnatal penile length and growth rate correlate to serum testosterone levels: A longitudinal study of 1962 normal boys. Eur J Endocrinol 154:125–129.

179. Andersson AM, Toppari J, Haavisto AM, et al. (1998). Longitudinal reproductive hormone profiles in infants: Peak of inhibin B levels in infant boys exceeds levels in adult men. J Clin Endocrinol Metab 83:675–681.

180. Sharpe RM, McKinnell C, Kivlin G, Fisher JS (2003). Proliferation and functional maturation of Sertoli cells, and their relevance to disorders of testis function in adulthood. Reproduction 125:769–784.

181. Main KM, Toppari J, Suomi AM, et al. (2006). Larger testes and higher inhibin B levels in Finnish than in Danish newborn boys. J Clin Endocrinol Metab 91:2732–2737.

182. Suomi AM, Main KM, Kaleva M, et al. (2006). Hormonal changes in 3-month old cryptorchid boys. J Clin Endocrinol Metab 91:953–958.

183. Conte FA, Grumbach MM, Kaplan SL (1975). A diphasic pattern of gonadotropin secretion in patients with the syndrome of gonadal dysgenesis. J Clin Endocrinol Metab 4:670–674.

184. Plant TM (2006). The male monkey as a model for the study of the neurobiology of puberty onset in man. Mol Cell Endocrinol 254/255:97–102.

185. Acerini CL, Tasker RC (2007). Traumatic brain injury induced hypothalamic-pituitary dysfunction: A paediatric perspective. Pituitary (E-pub ahead of print).

186. Darzy KH, Shalet SM (2005). Hypopituitarism as a consequence of brain tumors and radiotherapy. Pituitary 8:203–211.

187. Seminara SB (2007). Kisspeptin in reproduction. Semin Reprod Med 25:337–343.

188. Kauffman AS, Clifton DK, Steiner RA (2007). Emerging ideas about kisspeptin-GPR54 signalling in the neuroendocrine regulation of reproduction. Trends Neuroscience 30:504–511.

189. Seminara SG, Messager S, Chatzidaki EE, et al. (2003). The GPR54 gene as a regulator of puberty. N Engl J Med 349:1614–1627.

190. Semple RK, Achermann JC, Ellery J, et al. (2005). Two novel missense mutations in G protein-coupled receptor 54 in a patient with hypogonadotrophic hypogonadism. J Clin Endocrinol Metab 90:1849–1855.

191. Dhillo WS, Chaudhri OB, Patterson M, et al. (2005). Kisspeptin-54 stimulates the hypothalamic-pituitary gonadal axis in human males. J Clin Endocrinol Metab 90:6609–6615.

192. Shahab M, Mastronardi C, Seminara SB, Crowley WF, Ojeda SR, Plant TM (2005). Increased hypothalamic GPR54 signalling: A potential mechanism for initiation of puberty in primates. Proc Natl Acad Sci USA 102:2129–2134.

193. Kaplowitz PB (1989). Diagnostic value of testosterone therapy in boys with delayed puberty. Amer J Dis Child 143:116–120.

194. Kosugi S, Van Dop C, Geffner ME, et al. (1995). Characterisation of heterogeneous mutations causing constitutive activation of the luteinising hormone receptor in familial male precocious puberty. Hum Mol Genet 4:183–188.

195. Richter-Unruh A, Wessels HT, Menken U, et al. (2002). Male LH-independent sexual precocity in a 3.5-year old boy caused by a somatic activating mutation of the LH receptor in a Leydig cell tumor. J Clin Endocrinol Metab 87:1052–1056.

196. d'Alva CB, Brito VN, Palhares HMC, et al. (2006). A single somatic activating Asp578His mutation of the luteinising hormone receptor causes Leydig cell tumor in boys with gonadotrophin-independent precocious puberty. Clin Endocrinol 65:408–410.

197. Liu G, Duranteau L, Carel JC, Monroe J, Doyle DA, Shenker A (1999). Leydig-cell tumors caused by an activating mutation of the gene encoding the luteinising hormone receptor. N Engl J Med 341:1731–1736.

198. Kreher NC, Pescovitz OH, Delameter P, Tiulpakov A, Hochberg Z (2006). Treatment of familial male-limited precocious puberty with bicalutamide and anastrozole. J Pediatr 149:416–420.

199. Weinstein LS, Liu J, Sakamoto A, Xie T, Chen M (2004). GNAS: Normal and abnormal functions. Endocrinology 145:5459–5464.

200. Wildt L, Marshall G, Knobil E (1980). Experimental induction of puberty in the infantile female rhesus monkey. Science 207:1373–1375.

201 Eugster EA, Clarke W, Kletter GB, et al. (2007). Efficacy and safety of histrelin subdermal implant in children with central precocious puberty: A multicenter trial. J Clin Endocrinol Metab 92:1697–1704.

202. Ravio T, Falardeau J, Dwyer A, et al. (2007). Reversal of idiopathic hypogonadotropic hypogonadism. N Engl J Med 357:863–873.

203. Farooqi S, O'Rahilly S (2006). Genetics of obesity in humans. Endocr Rev 27:710–718.

204. Farooqi IS, Wangensteen T, Collins S, et al. (2007). Clinical and molecular genetic spectrum of congenital deficiency of the leptin receptor. N Engl J Med 356:237–247.

205. Farooqi IS, Matarese G, Lord GM, et al. (2002). Beneficial effects of leptin on obesity, T cell hyporesponsiveness, and neuroendocrine/metabolic dysfunction of human congenital leptin deficiency. J Clin Invest 110:1093–1103.

206. Richmond EJ, Rogol AD (2007). Male pubertal development and the role of androgen therapy. Nat Clin Pract Endocrinol Metab 3:338–344.

207. Nieschlag E (2006). Testosterone treatment comes of age: New options for hypogonadal men. Clin Endocrinol 65:275–281.

208. Swerdloff RS, Wang C, Cunningham G, et al. (2000). Long-term pharmacokinetics of transdermal testosterone gel in hypogonadal men. J Clin Endocrinol Metab 85:4500–4510.

209. Mazer N, Bell D, Wu J, et al. (2005). Comparison of the steady-state pharmacokinetics, metabolism, and variability of a transdermal testosterone patch versus a transdermal testosterone gel in hypogonadal men. J Sex Med 2:213–226.

210. Ogilvy-Stuart AL, Brian CE (2004). Early assessment of ambiguous genitalia. Arch Dis Child 89:401–407.

211. Ranke MB (2003). *Diagnostic of endocrine function in children and adolescents, Second edition.* Basel: Karger.

212. Hochberg Z (2007). *Practical algorithms in pediatric endocrinology, Second edition.* Basel: Karger.

213. Ng KL, Ahmed SF, Hughes IA (2000). Pituitary-gonadal axis in male undermasculinisation. Arch Dis Child 82:54–58.

214. Dixon J, Wallace AM, O'Toole S, Ahmed SF (2007). Prolonged human chorionic gonadotrophin stimulation as a tool for investigating and managing undescended testes. Clin Endocrinol (E-pub ahead of print).

215. Tomlinson C, Macintyre H, Dorrian CA, Ahmed SF, Wallace AM (2004). Testosterone measurements in early infancy. Arch Dis Child Fetal Neonatal Ed 89:F558–F559.

216. Rey RA, Belville C, Nihoul-Fékété C, et al. (1999). Evaluation of gonadal function in 107 intersex patients by means of serum antimüllerian hormone measurement. J Clin Endocrinol Metab 84:627–631.

217. Lee MM, Misra M, Donohoe PK, MacLaughlin DT (2003). MIS/AMH in the assessment of cryptorchidism and intersex conditions. Mol Cell Endocrinol 211:91–98.

218. Josso N, Picard JY, Rey R, di Clemente N (2006). Testicular anti-Mullerian hormone: History, genetics, regulation and clinical applications. Pediatr Endocrinol Rev 3:347–358.

219. Bergadá I, Milani C, Bedecarrás P, et al. (2006). Time course of the serum gonadotrophin surge, inhibins, and anti-Mullerian hormone in normal newborn males during the first month of life. J Clin Endocrinol Metab 91:4092–4098.

220. Philibert P, Zenaty D, Lin L, et al. (2007). Mutational analysis of steroidogenic factor 1 (NR5a1) in 24 boys with bilateral anorchia: A French collaborative study. Hum Reprod (E-pub ahead of print).

221. Pearl MS, Hill MC (2007). Ultrasound of the scrotum. Semin Ultrasound CT MR 28:225–248.

222. Costabile RA (2007). How worrisome is testicular microlithiasis? Curr Opinion Urol 17:419–423.

223. Greenfield DM, Walters SJ, Coleman RE, et al. (2007). Prevalence and consequences of androgen deficiency in young male cancer survivors in a controlled cross-sectional study. J Clin Endocrinol Metab 92:3476–3482.

224. Müller J, Sønksen J, Sommer P, et al. (2000). Cryopreservation of semen from pubertal boys with cancer. Med Pediatr Oncol 34:191–194.

225. Radicioni AF, Anzuini A, De Marco E, Nofroni I, Castracane VD, Lenzi A (2005). Change in serum inhibin B during normal male puberty. Eur J Endocrinol 152:403–409.

226. Nielsen CT, Skakkebaek NE, Richardson DW, et al. (1986). Onset of the release of spermatozoa (spermarche) in boys in relation to age, testicular growth, pubic hair, and height. J Clin Endocrinol Metab 62:532–535.

227. Pedersen JL, Nysom, K, Jørgensen M, et al. (1993). Spermaturia and puberty. Arch Dis Child 69:384–387.

228. Mol NM, Sørensen N, Weihe P, et al. (2002). Spermaturia and serum hormone concentrations at the age of puberty in boys prenatally exposed to polychlorinated biphenyls. Eur J Endocrinol 146:357–363.

229. Layman LC (2007). Hypogonadotropic hypogonadism. Endocrinol Metab Clin N Am 36:283–296.

230. Trarbach EB, Silveira LG, Latronio AC (2007). Genetic insights into human isolated gonadotropin deficiency. Pituitary (E-pub ahead of print).

231. Burman P, Ritzen EM, Lindgren AC (2001). Endocine dysfunction in Prader-Willi syndrome: A review with special reference to GH. Endocr Rev 22:787–799.

232. Blaque OE, Leroux MR (2006). Bardet-Biedl syndrome: An emerging pathomechanism of intracellular transport. Cell Mol Life Sci 63:2145–2161.

233. Bhagavath B, Layman LC (2007). The genetics of hypogonadotropic hypogonadism. Semin Reprod Med 25:272–286.

234. Lanfranco F, Kamischke A, Zitzmann M (2004). Klinefelter's syndrome. Lancet 364:273–283.

235. Allanson JE (2007). Noonan syndrome. Am J Genet C Semin Med Genet 145:274–279.

236. Melo KF, Martin RM, Costa EM, et al. (2002). An unusual phenotype of Frasier syndrome due to IVS9 +4C>T mutation in the WT1 gene: Predominantly male ambiguous genitalla and absence of gonadal dysgenesis. J Clin Endocrinol Metab 87:2500–2505.

237. Rutter MM, Rose SR (2007). Long-term endocrine sequelae of childhood cancer. Curr Opin Pediatr 19:480–487.

CHAPTER 17

Disorders of Mineral Homeostasis in the Newborn, Infant, Child, and Adolescent

ALLEN W. ROOT, MD • FRANK B. DIAMOND, JR., MD

Introduction

Disorders of calcium, magnesium, and phosphate metabolism (and of bone formation, accrual, and maintenance) during the first two decades of life result from suboptimal ingestion, absorption, or retention of constit-

uent nutrients; abnormal vitamin D metabolism or bioactivity; disorders of parathyroid hormone (PTH) synthesis, secretion, or function; and intrinsic aberrations in cartilage and bone cells. For an integrated overview of calcium, mineral, and skeletal homeostasis, the reader is referred to Chapter 3.

Mineral Homeostasis: Conception Through Adolescence

PREGNANCY AND LACTATION

The fetus is entirely dependent on the mother for its calcium and phosphate requirements for skeletal formation and cell and tissue growth and function. The fetal-placental unit actively extracts calcium from the maternal circulation, as the mother doubles her rate of intestinal calcium absorption.[1-3] During the first trimester of pregnancy, maternal serum concentrations of total calcium decline and remain low through gestation due to a fall in albumin values and expansion of extracellular fluid volume—whereas serum concentrations of ionized calcium (Ca^{2+}_e) and phosphate remain relatively constant (Figure 17-1).

PTH values decline to 10% to 30% of the nonpregnant range in the first trimester of pregnancy, and then rise to mid nonpregnant levels in the latter half of gestation. The secretion of PTH-related peptide (PTHrP) by the placenta, amnion, decidua, umbilical cord, breast, and fetal parathyroid glands increases severalfold beginning early in the first trimester, and maternal levels rise throughout gestation. Maternal calcitonin values also increase during gestation. Serum concentrations of calcidiol do not change, but levels of calcitriol (synthesized primarily by the maternal kidney but also in part by the placenta, decidua, and fetal kidneys) increase more than twofold as pregnancy advances and substantially accelerate the rate (and augment the amount) of calcium absorbed by the maternal small intestine.

Increased renal synthesis of calcitriol is stimulated primarily by PTHrP but also by prolactin, estrogen, and human chorionic somatomammotropin. Maternal urinary calcium excretion rises (+125%), reflecting the increased absorption of ingested calcium.[4] The rate of maternal bone resorption increases in the first trimester of gestation, as determined by histomorphometric analysis of bone biopsies and by the increase in the urinary excretion rates of pyridinoline (Pyr), desoxypyridinoline (Dpd), N-telopeptide (NTx), and hydroxyproline that occur in early gestation and continue to rise through gestation. Markers of osteoblast activity and bone formation (bone-specific alkaline phosphatase, osteocalcin, carboxyl, and amino terminal propeptides of type I collagen) decline during the first trimester but increase in the third trimester.[4,5]

During a normal 40-week gestation, maternal whole-body bone mineral density (BMD) does not change. Cortical BMD increases (arms +2.8%, legs +1.8%), whereas trabecular BMD declines (vertebrae −4.5%, pelvis −3.2%). However, pregnancy does not appear to have any long-term adverse effects on maternal bone mineralization or fracture risk.[3] Maternal serum values of insulin-like growth factor-I (IGF-I) increase 67% by the third trimester of pregnancy, and the increment correlates positively with the increase in markers of bone turnover and inversely with the change in maternal vertebral BMD. Thus, early in gestation the pregnant woman meets fetal demand for calcium by increasing the rate of resorption of stored bone calcium—whereas the calcium requirement of the more mature fetus is met

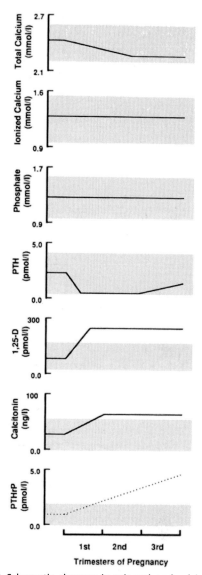

Figure 17-1 Schematic changes in mineral and calciotropic hormone values during pregnancy. The shaded areas represent normal adult ranges. To convert calcium in mmol/L to mg/dL, multiply by 4; to convert phosphate in mmol/L to mg/dL, multiply by 3.097; to convert PTH in pmol/L to pg/mL, multiply by 9.50; and to convert calcitriol in pmol/L to pg/mL, multiply by 0.4166. [Reproduced with permission from Kovacs CS, Kronenberg HM (1997). Maternal-fetal calcium and bone metabolism during pregnancy, puerperium, and lactation. Endocrine Reviews 18:832–872.]

by a substantially increased rate of maternal intestinal calcium absorption.

During lactation, the nursing mother daily transfers to her suckling infant 280 to 400 mg of calcium mobilized from her skeleton in response to PTHrP secreted primarily by the breast.[3] Calcium concentrations are low in colostrum, being approximately 25 mg/dL in breast milk during the first 6 months of lactation and 21 mg/dL during months 6 to 12 of nursing.[6] Maternal total calcium, calcitriol, and calcitonin values are normal, while Ca^{2+}_e, phosphate, and PTHrP levels are increased during lactation.

Urinary levels of markers of bone resorption and serum values of markers of bone formation are elevated during lactation, implying rapid turnover of maternal bone mineral during nursing. Maternal bone mineralization declines 3% to 10% during lactation, only to re-accrue rapidly after weaning.[7] As there is an increasing incidence (or awareness) of vitamin D deficiency in breast-fed infants, supplementation of the breast-fed infant with 400 IU of vitamin D daily and higher than recommended intake (200 IU/day) of vitamin D (up to 2,000 to 4,000 IU/day) have been suggested for pregnant and lactating women.[8-10]

FETUS

During gestation, the fetus accrues 30 to 35 g of calcium. Approximately 80% of calcium accretion occurs in the third trimester.[1,3] At 28 weeks of gestation, calcium is deposited into the fetal skeleton at the rate of approximately 100 mg/day—whereas at 35 weeks calcium is deposited at the rate of approximately 250 mg/day.[2,5,11,12] At birth, whole-body bone mineral content (BMC) is positively related to gestational age, to body length, and most closely to body weight—as are lumbar spine (L1-L4) BMC and BMD (Figures 17-2 and 17-3).[12,13] The fetal skeleton serves two roles: it is a metabolically important source of calcium mobilized by fetal PTH and/or PTHrP acting through the PTH/PTHrP receptor (PTHR1) when the supply of calcium from the mother is limited, and it provides a rigid structural and protective framework for fetal soft tissues.[2]

Fetal serum calcium levels are established independently of, and are not directly related to, maternal calcium concentrations. From at least 15 weeks of gestation, serum concentrations of total calcium (and particularly Ca^{2+}_e) are substantially higher in the human fetus and other mammals (rat, sheep) than in the mother (1.4:1). The physiologic significance of this finding is unknown. In addition, fetal serum concentrations of magnesium and phosphate are greater than maternal values. The parathyroid glands (PTG) are essential to maintenance of normal fetal calcium concentrations. By the tenth week of gestation, they secrete PTH and possibly PTHrP—and both peptides function additively to maintain fetal serum calcium levels. PTH does not stimulate placental calcium transport, but it is secreted by the fetal PTG in response to hypocalcemia. Fetal mice in which the expression of PTH has been ablated (e.g., *Hoxa3* null mice) are hypocalcemic, and their skeletal mineralization is impaired.[1,14]

Maternal hypercalcemia suppresses, and maternal hypocalcemia stimulates, secretion of fetal PTH. Both amino and mid-molecule fragments of PTHrP (e.g., PTHrP[1-86], PTHrP[67-86]) produced by the fetal PTG (possibly), placenta (primarily), amnion, chorion, and umbilical cord maintain high fetal serum calcium concentrations by stimulating active maternal-to-fetal transport of calcium across the placental syncytiotrophoblast against a concentration gradient. This PTHrP effect is mediated in part by receptors that recognize mid-molecule and/or carboxyl terminal fragments of PTHrP, as evidenced in fetal mice in which *Pthr1* has been ablated (placental calcium transport remains active, whereas fetal serum calcium levels are low).

In fetal mice in which the expression of *Pthrp* itself has been impaired, serum calcium levels are lower than control

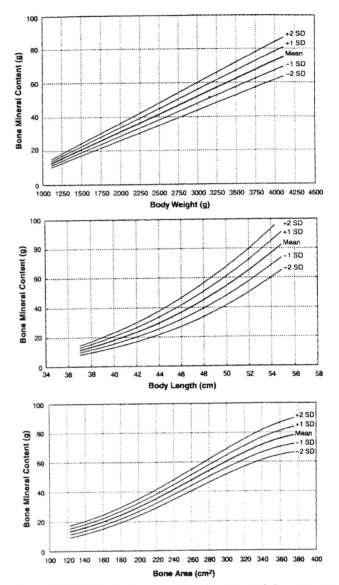

Figure 17-2 Whole-body bone mineral content of the preterm and term neonate relative to body weight, body length, and bone area as determined by dual X-ray absorptiometry near birth. [Reproduced with permission from Rigo J, et al. (2000). Bone mineral metabolism in the micropremie. Clin Perinatol 27:147–170.]

values and are maintained by fetal PTH at values comparable to those of the mother. In *Pthrp* null fetal mice, placental calcium transfer is decreased—and chondrocyte maturation and bone development are abnormal.[1] Although serum concentrations of PTHrP are quite high in the human fetus (term cord blood 2–5 pmol/L), PTH levels are lower than those in maternal serum. *In utero*, calcitonin concentrations are quite high (an appropriate response to the increased serum calcium levels of the fetus)—but this peptide does not have a major impact on fetal calcium homeostasis.[1]

Calcium and magnesium regulate fetal calcium levels through the calcium-sensing receptor (CaSR) that controls the synthesis and secretion of fetal PTH. Thus, in fetal mice in which *Casr* has been knocked out the serum calcium concentration is further elevated—as are values

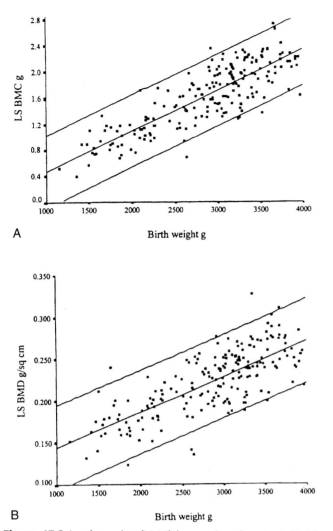

Figure 17-3 Lumbar spine (L1-L4) bone mineral content (BMC). (*A*) Bone mineral density (BMD). (*B*) BMD of preterm and term neonates relative to body weight as determined by dual X-ray absorptiometry near birth. [Reproduced with permission from Koo WWK, Hockman EM (2000). Physiologic predictors of lumbar spine bone mass in neonates. Pediatr Res 48:485–489.]

juxta-articular cells of the long bone regulates the orderly rate of chondrocyte maturation, whereas fetal PTH maintains serum calcium and phosphate values appropriate to bone mineralization. Magnesium is actively transported across the placenta.[19] *In utero* fetal magnesium concentrations exceed maternal values and are inversely related to gestational age, reflecting the third trimester decline in maternal magnesium concentrations.

NEONATE AND INFANT

Calcium levels in cord blood correlate with gestational age and exceed maternal values by 1 to 2 mg/dL as a result of an active placental calcium pump. When the neonate is abruptly removed from the transplacental infusion of maternal calcium, total calcium and Ca^{2+}_e concentrations decline rapidly in the first 6 to 12 hours after delivery to nadir values (from 12 to 9 mg/dL and 1.45 to 1.20 mmol/L, respectively) by 24 to 72 hours of age.[1,2,20] Calcium levels are a bit lower and PTH values higher in neonates delivered by cesarean section than in those delivered vaginally.[21] After birth, PTHrP values decline rapidly. Thus, to maintain mineral homeostasis the neonate becomes dependent on endogenous PTH, exogenous vitamin D, ingested and absorbed calcium, renal tubular reabsorption of calcium, and bone calcium stores for its calcium needs.

In response to the fall in Ca^{2+}_e values, serum levels of PTH begin to increase on the first day of life—resulting in normal calcium values (8.8–11.3 mg/dL) at 48 hours of age, followed by rise in calcitriol concentrations and slow decline (after an initial postnatal rise) in calcitonin values (Figure 17-4).[22] For the first 2 to 4 weeks after birth, there is increased efficiency of intestinal calcium absorption by passive means that are independent of vitamin D—perhaps due to the lactose content of milk, which affects paracellular transport of Ca^{2+}_e (1,2). Later in the neonatal period, vitamin-D-dependent intestinal calcium absorption increases. Renal tubular handling of calcium and the response to PTH mature during the first several weeks of life. Bone calcium accretion continues at the rate of 150 mg/kg/day for several months after birth, a vitamin-D-dependent process.

Due to decreased glomerular filtration and increased tubular reabsorption, serum concentrations of phosphate are maximal in the neonate. After delivery, serum phosphate concentrations increase from cord values of 3.8 to 8.1 mg/dL to levels that range between 4.5 and 9.0 mg/dL during the first week of life and that then stabilize at values between 4.5 and 6.7 mg/dL through the first year of life.[23] In preterm or acutely ill neonates, the fall in calcium values is often exaggerated and more prolonged—and bone mineralization is frequently impaired in very preterm newborns and infants. Maternal hypercalcemia suppresses, and maternal hypocalcemia stimulates, secretion of fetal PTH—effects that may carry over to the neonate for several days. In infants and children, serum magnesium concentrations are quite stable—ranging between 1.5 and 2.2 mg/dL through 4 months of age and between 1.7 and 2.3 mg/dL through 5 years of age.

Human breast milk contains (on average) calcium at 28 mg/dL, phosphate at 13 mg/dL, and vitamin D 15 to

of PTH and calcitriol.[1,15] The CaSR is also expressed in the human placenta in the first trimester and is involved in placental calcium transport.[16] Calcium-selective ion channels (TPRV5, TPRV6) located at the apical surface of trophoblast cells facilitate maternal-fetal transplacental transfer of calcium.[17] Fetal serum calcitriol concentrations are a bit lower than those of the mother. Experimentally, fetal serum calcium values and mineralization of the fetal skeleton are normal in the presence of maternal vitamin D deficiency or an inactive vitamin D receptor (VDR). In the VDR-null fetal mouse, if the mother ingests a diet enriched with calcium and phosphate, indicating that the fetus does not have an absolute requirement for calcitriol or the VDR for normal mineral metabolism.[1,18]

In man, the fetal cartilaginous skeleton is present by the eighth week of gestation. Primary ossification centers appear in the long bones and vertebrae by the twelfth week, and secondary centers at the femoral ends are noted by the thirty-fourth week.[1] Fetal PTHrP secreted by

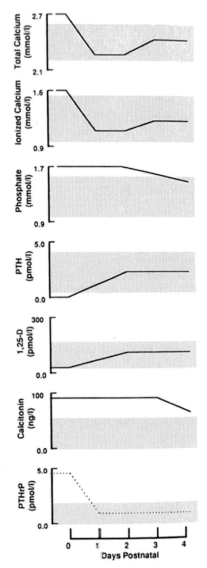

Figure 17-4 Schematic changes in mineral and calciotropic hormone values during the first 4 days of life in normal full-term neonates. The shaded areas represent normal adult ranges. The PTHrP values are depicted by a dashed line to indicate their speculative nature. To convert calcium in mmol/L to mg/dL, multiply by 4; to convert phosphate in mmol/L to mg/dL, multiply by 3.097; to convert PTH in pmol/L to pg/mL, multiply by 9.50; and to convert calcitriol in pmol/L to pg/mL, multiply by 0.4166. [Reproduced with permission from Kovacs CS, Kronenberg HM (1997). Maternal-fetal calcium and bone metabolism during pregnancy, puerperium, and lactation. Endocrine Reviews 18:832–872.]

50 IU/L. Thus, vitamin D supplementation (200–400 IU/day) is necessary during breast feeding.[6] Cow's milk formulas contain calcium at ~40 to 60 mg/dL, phosphate at ~30 to 40 mg/dL, and vitamin D at ~30 to 40 IU/dL. The bioavailability of calcium (that which is accessible for normal metabolic usage) varies dependent on its source and the formulaic content and source of protein, fat, and carbohydrates. For example, infants fed formulas that contain palm olein absorb less calcium than those receiving a formula fortified with another form of fat or human breast milk—and these infants have lower total body bone mineral content.[24]

Phytate (inositol hexaphosphate) present in soy formulas and infant cereals chelates calcium, and oxalate (a constituent of spinach) precipitates calcium—thereby reducing intestinal absorption of this mineral, a difficulty overcome by increasing dietary calcium content. Optimizing calcium, vitamin D intake, and bone mineralization during infancy (and childhood) may substantially contribute to achievement of an adult peak bone mass of sufficient density to avoid osteopenia and osteoporosis and their adverse consequences in later life.[6]

CHILD AND ADOLESCENT

During childhood and adolescence, serum concentrations of total calcium (8.8–10.8 mg/dL, depending on the analytical laboratory) and magnesium (1.7–2.2 mg/dL) remain relatively constant.[22] Serum phosphate levels are higher in children (4.5–6.2 mg/dL) than in adults (2.5–4.5 mg/dL), and attain maximum values several months before the peak height velocity of adolescence is achieved. The rise has been attributed to augmentation of the renal tubular reabsorption of phosphate due to the combined effects of the increased secretion of growth hormone (GH), IGF-I, and sex hormones—factors that contribute to the pubertal growth spurt.[25]

Total serum alkaline phosphatase activity is also higher in children than in adults, and increases transiently during the pubertal growth spurt. Levels of bone-specific alkaline phosphatase (the major isoform of this enzyme in normal adolescents) increase between 9 and 12 months before peak height velocity and reach maximum at Tanner male genital stage III. These levels are directly related to the secretion of testosterone in boys.[26] In females, serum bone-specific alkaline phosphatase activity peaks at Tanner stage III breast development and correlates with serum osteocalcin concentrations. Serum concentrations of PTH fluctuate very little during adolescence, whereas levels of calcitriol rise transiently.

Serum values of osteocalcin, a bone matrix γ-carboxyl-glutamic acid whose concentration reflects osteoblast activity, are higher during infancy than childhood and increase during adolescence—reaching peak values at 12 years of age in girls and at 14 years in boys.[27,28] Mean 24-hour levels of osteocalcin are not related to mean 24-hour GH concentrations or to growth rates in prepubertal children, but random and 24-hour mean osteocalcin concentrations are substantially lower in GH-deficient children than in children of normal stature. Serum levels of the carboxyl-terminal propeptide of procollagen type I (PICP) also reflect osteoblast activity. These levels are highest in infancy, fall during childhood, increase briefly during puberty, and then decline to adult values.

Serum levels of the amino-terminal extension of procollagen type III (PIIINP) reflect soft-tissue growth and to a limited extent bone formation. Values decline between infancy and childhood, increase during adolescence, and then fall to adult concentrations.[29,30] Mean 24-hour concentrations of PICP and PIIINP correlate with mean 24-hour GH values and growth rates. Their levels are significantly lower in GH-deficient children than in normal children.[31]

Serum concentrations of cross-linked carboxyl-terminal telopeptide of type I collagen (ICTP) and urinary excretion of the nonreducible pyridinium compounds and the carboxyl- (CTx) and amino-terminal (NTx) telopeptides of type I collagen are markers of bone resorption. Values of ICTP peak between 9 and 13 years in girls at Tanner stage III breast development and at 14 years and Tanner male genital stage IV in boys. In both cases, they then decline.[32] Pyr (hydroxylysyl-pyridinoline; present in bone and cartilage) and Dpd (lysyl-pyridinoline; found primarily in bone) are derivatives of the amino acids lysine and hydroxylysine, respectively—which cross-link adjacent telopeptide regions of collagen fibers in mature bone.[33]

The urinary excretion of both compounds is independent of diet and reflects collagen degradation. The urinary excretion of the pyridinium cross-links fluctuates diurnally with highest values in the morning. The 24-hour urinary excretion of both pyridinium compounds is greatest in the child 2 to 10 years of age, declines between 11 and 17 years, and still further thereafter as values approach adult levels.[28] Urinary levels of NTx, a reliable index of bone resorption, may be determined in spot or 24-hour urine specimens and are expressed as nmol of bovine cartilage equivalent (BCE) units/mmol of creatinine. Values are highest in infancy and decline steadily with age.[34]

The urinary excretion of hydroxyproline is a less specific marker of bone resorption because it is present in the collagen of connective tissue in many sites other than bone—particularly skin, as well as in dietary protein. Urinary excretion increases during puberty, and in girls peaks (150 mg/day) in the year before menarche coincident with maximal growth rate.[29] Tartrate-resistant acid phosphatase activity (TRAP), a marker of osteoclast activity, is released when bone collagen is degraded. In adolescents, markers of bone formation (bone-specific alkaline phosphatase, osteocalcin, and PICP) and of bone resorption (TRAP, ICTP, and urine excretion of NTx and the pyridinolines) increase to a similar extent and then decline in tandem—reflecting the tight link between bone formation and resorption. In females, these measurements correlate inversely with serum concentrations of estradiol—reflecting the maturational effect of estrogen on epiphyseal cartilage and its inhibitory effect on growth.[35]

The rate of bone accretion is steady throughout childhood, and increases substantially during adolescence—the physiologic interval in which up to 50% of adult bone mass is acquired. Indeed, in the 2 years that bracket the peak growth rate of puberty 25% of peak bone mineral mass is accumulated.[36] Approximately 90% of peak bone mass is accrued by 18 years of age in normal subjects, and peak BMC is achieved between 20 and 25 years of age. During puberty, trabecular bone volume and mineralization increase appreciably in response to GH, IGF-I, estrogens, and androgens and are maximal by the end of the second decade of life in females (and perhaps in the male).

However, the timing of peak bone mass of the axial skeleton is more variable—being attained between 17 and 35 years of age. Most often this occurs near the age when adult sexual maturity is achieved. At all ages, vertebral cross-sectional size is smaller in females than in males—even when controlling for height. However, femoral dimensions are similar in both genders when matched for height and weight. Trabecular bone mass becomes greater in black than in white subjects at adolescence, when trabecular bone mineral density increases 34% in black and 11% in white subjects. The difference persists thereafter. The cross-sectional area of the femur is also greater in black than in white adolescents and adults.

Disorders of Mineral Homeostasis in the Neonate and Infant

HYPOCALCEMIA

Clinical manifestations of hypocalcemia (total calcium <7.5 mg/dL; Ca^{2+}_e <1.20 mmol/L) in neonates include irritability, hyperacusis, jitteriness, tremulousness, facial spasms, neuromuscular excitability (tetany), laryngospasm, and focal or generalized seizures.[20] Nonspecific symptoms such as apnea, tachycardia, cyanosis, emesis, and feeding problems may also occur. Traditionally, neonatal hypocalcemia develops after 3 days of age in offspring born in the late winter to early spring of the year to multiparous women of lower socioeconomic status with inadequate intake of vitamin D or exposure to sunlight. Causes of neonatal hypocalcemia may be considered in relation to the age of onset (before or after 72 hours of life, Table 17-1).

Early Neonatal Hypocalcemia

In the absence of hypoproteinemia, hypocalcemia occurring within the first 72 hours after birth is considered "early neonatal hypocalcemia." It occurs most commonly in premature or small-for-gestational-age, low birth weight, or asphyxiated neonates—or in those born to women with gestational or permanent forms of diabetes mellitus. It occurs as a consequence of suppression of PTH secretion, prolonged secretion of calcitonin, and/or hypomagnesemia.[20] Total calcium and Ca^{2+}_e concentrations decline more rapidly and to lower nadir values in preterm than in term neonates. In premature infants, early neonatal hypocalcemia has been attributed to blunting of the physiologic postnatal rise in PTH secretion and to the relative resistance of the renal tubule to PTH-mediated phosphate excretion—leading to hyperphosphatemia.

Prolonged elevation of circulating levels of calcitonin also contributes to early neonatal hypocalcemia. In low birth weight (LBW) neonates, hypocalcemia may be further attributed to the rapid accretion of skeletal calcium in the presence of relative resistance to the calcium absorptive and reabsorptive effects of calcitriol on the intestinal tract and bone, respectively. Offspring of severely vitamin-D-deficient mothers may become hypocalcemic shortly after birth. Hypocalcemia develops in approximately 33% of asphyxiated newborns who are products of complicated and compromised deliveries. In these infants, increased phosphate load due to cellular injury, reduced calcium intake, and hypercalcitonemia

TABLE 17-1

Causes of Hypocalcemia

I. Neonatal

A. Maternal Disorders

1. Diabetes mellitus
2. Toxemia
3. Hyperparathyroidism
4. High intake of alkali or magnesium sulfate

B. Neonatal

1. Low birth weight, intrauterine growth retardation
2. Asphyxia, sepsis
3. Hyperbilirubinemia, phototherapy, exchange transfusion
4. Hypomagnesemia, hypermagnesemia
5. Acute/chronic renal insufficiency
6. Nutrients/medications: high dietary phosphate, fatty acids, phytates, bicarbonate, citrated blood, anticonvulsants, aminoglycosides
7. Hypoparathyroidism
8. Vitamin D deficiency or resistance
9. Osteopetrosis type II

II Hypoparathyroidism

A. Congenital

1. Transient neonatal
2. Dysgenesis/agenesis of the parathyroid glands
   a. Isolated hypoparathyroidism (*GCM2, PTH, SOX3*)
   b. Hypercalciuric hypocalcemia *(CASR)*
   c. DiGeorge syndrome (*TBX1*)
   d. Sanjad-Sakati syndrome (short stature, retardation, dysmorphism - HRD)
      Kenny-Caffey syndrome 1 (short stature, medullary stenosis) *(TCBE)*
   e. Barakat syndrome (sensorineural deafness, renal dysplasia - HDR) *(GATA3)*
   f. Lymphedema-hypoparathyroidism-nephropathy, nerve deafness
   g. Mitochondrial fatty acid disorders (Kearns-Sayre, Pearson, mitochondrial encephalopathy, lactic acidosis, stroke-like - MELAS)
3. Insensitivity to parathyroid hormone
   a. Blomstrand chondrodysplasia (*PTHR1*)
   b. Pseudohypoparathyroidism - type IA *(GNAS)*
   • Pseudohypoparathyroidism - type IB
   • Pseudohypoparathyroidism - type IC
   • Pseudohypoparathyroidism - type II
   • Pseudopseudohypoparathyroidism
   c. Hypomagnesemia

4. Dyshormonogenesis

B. Acquired

1. Autoimmune polyglandular syndrome - type I (*AIRE1*)
2. Activating antibodies to the calcium-sensing receptor
3. Post surgical, radiation destruction
4. Infiltrative [excessive iron (hemochromatosis, thalassemia) or copper (Wilson disease) deposition; granulomatous or neoplastic invasion; amyloidosis, sarcoidosis]
5. Maternal hyperparathyroidism
6. Hypomagnesemia

III. Vitamin D Deficiency

IV. Other Causes of Hypocalcemia

A. Calcium Deficiency

1. Nutritional deprivation
2. Hypercalciuria

B. Hypomagnesemia/Hypermagnesemia

1. Congenital
   a. Malabsorption
   b. Hypermagnesuria
   • Primary *(CLDN16)*
   • Bartter syndrome (3)
   • Renal tubular acidosis
2. Acquired
   a. Acute renal failure
   b. Chronic inflammatory bowel disease, intestinal resection
   c. Diuretics

C. Hyperphosphatemia

1. Renal failure
2. Phosphate administration (intravenous, oral, rectal)
3. Tumor cell lysis
4. Muscle injuries (crush, rhabdomyolysis)

D. Miscellaneous

1. Hypoproteinemia
2. Hyperventilation
3. Drugs - furosemide, bisphosphonates calcitonin, anticonvulsants, ketoconazole, anti-neoplastic agents (plicamycin, asparaginase, cisplatinum, cytosine arabinoside, doxorubicin), citrated blood products
4. Hungry bone syndrome
5. Acute and critical illness - sepsis, acute pancreatitis, toxic shock
   a. Organic acidemia - propionic, methylmalonic, isovaleric

Modified from Thakker RV (2006). Hypocalcemia: Pathogenesis, differential diagnosis, and management. In Favus MJ (ed.), *Primer on the metabolic bone diseases and disorders of mineral metabolism, Sixth edition*. Washington, D.C.: American Society for Bone and Mineral Research 213–215; from Goltzman D, Cole DEC (2006). Hypoparathyroidism. In Favus MJ (ed). *Primer on the metabolic bone diseases and disorders of mineral metabolism, Sixth edition*. Washington, D.C.: American Society for Bone and Mineral Research 216–219; from Levine MA (2006). Parathyroid hormone resistance syndromes. In Favus MJ (ed.), *Primer on the metabolic bone diseases and disorders of mineral metabolism, Sixth edition*. Washington, D.C.: American Society for Bone and Mineral Research 220–224; and from Carpenter TO (2006). Neonatal hypocalcemia. In Favus MJ (ed.), *Primer on the metabolic bone diseases and disorders of mineral metabolism, Sixth edition*. Washington, D.C.: American Society for Bone and Mineral Research 224–229.

are important pathogenetic factors in the development of hypocalcemia.

Fifty percent of infants of mothers with diabetes mellitus develop early neonatal hypocalcemia. The incidence may be reduced by strict maternal glycemic control.[2,20] Its causes are multifactorial and include reduced placental transfer of calcium due to substantial maternal urinary excretion of calcium and magnesium, decreased neonatal secretion of PTH, hypercalcitonemia, hypomagnesemia (occurring in 40% of offspring), and limited intake and impaired absorption of ingested calcium.[37]

Maternal hypercalcemia due to unsuspected hyperparathyroidism leads to increased transfer of calcium to the fetus, and still further increase in fetal calcium concentrations that suppress fetal PTH synthesis and release and stimulate calcitonin secretion—aberrations in homeostatic mechanisms that persist postpartum and may result in hypocalcemic tetany/seizures in the mother's offspring. Suppression of PTH secretion may persist for several months and be undetected until symptomatic hypocalcemia develops after weaning of the infant from breast milk to higher-phosphate-containing cow's milk formula. Maternal ingestion of large quantities of calcium carbonate in antacids has also led to neonatal hypocalcemia.[38]

Hypocalcemia has occurred in neonates with hyperbilirubinemia undergoing exchange transfusion and in those exposed to phototherapy.[39] Neonates with acute rotavirus infection and severe diarrhea may present with hypocalcemic seizures.[40] Aminoglycoside antibiotics (e.g., gentamycin) increase urinary excretion of calcium and magnesium and facilitate the development of neonatal hypocalcemia. Compounds that complex with and sequester calcium—such as citrate (present in transfused blood), phosphates (that alter the calcium X phosphate product), and fatty acids (given as caloric supplements)—lower Ca^{2+}_e levels. Bicarbonate administered to correct acidosis increases calcium binding to albumin and thus lowers Ca^{2+}_e values. Hypocalcemia may also occur in hyperventilated infants with severe respiratory alkalosis, as well as in those with other causes of metabolic alkalosis. Phytates in soy milk bind calcium and phosphate and interfere with their absorption. Neonates with osteopetrosis type II and impaired osteoclastogenesis may present with early or late neonatal manifestations of hypocalcemia.[41,42]

Late Neonatal Hypocalcemia

Hypocalcemia developing after 72 hours of postnatal age may be due to increased intake of phosphate, hypomagnesemia, hypoparathyroidism, or vitamin D deficiency (Table 17-1). One of the most frequent causes of late neonatal hypocalcemia is excessive phosphate intake in evaporated milk or modified cow's milk formulas. Phosphate forms poorly soluble calcium salts and limits the intestinal absorption of calcium while raising serum phosphate values. Premature introduction of fiber-containing cereals into the infant's diet also decreases calcium absorption. Affected infants may have an associated defect in renal phosphate excretion or a coexisting deficiency in vitamin D.

Hyperphosphatemia and hypocalcemia may initially suggest hypoparathyroidism, but serum PTH concentrations are high in infants with excessive phosphate loading in response to reciprocal reduction in serum calcium values. Newborns and infants with chronic renal insufficiency due to renal hypoplasia or obstructive nephropathies are often hypocalcemic and hyperphosphatemic, with elevated serum PTH levels as well. However, they are also azotemic. Hypomagnesemia leads to impaired secretion of PTH and decreased peripheral responsiveness to PTH, and may be transient or related to congenital abnormalities of intestinal absorption or renal tubular reabsorption of magnesium.[20] Hypermagnesemia may occasionally be associated with neonatal hypocalcemia.

Hypocalcemia due to fetal/neonatal deficiency of vitamin D occurs in offspring of mothers deprived of vitamin D (for cultural or socioeconomic reasons). Impaired renal 25-hydroxyvitamin D-1α hydroxylase activity and loss-of-function mutations of the vitamin D receptor also lead to hypocalcemia (and hypophosphatemia). Hypovitaminosis D may develop in the breast-fed infant of a vegetarian mother who shields herself from sunlight and ingests a diet low in vitamin D. However, marginal deficiency of vitamin D in neonates and infants is likely much more common than has been recognized heretofore.[8,9,11,43]

Late neonatal hypocalcemia occurs in premature infants with osteopenia at 3 to 4 months of age in whom the intake of calcium, phosphate, and vitamin D has been marginal. It is perhaps due to avid deposition of all available calcium into bone.[20] Hypocalcemia due to vitamin D deficiency may develop acutely, and in the absence of clinical or radiographic signs of rickets, in the older infant and young child ingesting an elimination diet low in vitamin D because of severe allergies and/or maintained indoors with limited exposure to sunlight.

Hypoparathyroidism

Hypoparathyroidism presenting in infancy is most often transient and related to delayed developmental maturation of PTG function. It frequently resolves within the first several weeks of life. When prolonged, hypoparathyroidism is often due to an error in the embryogenesis of the PTGs. Occasionally, it may be due to defects in the synthesis of PTH or to peripheral unresponsiveness to PTH. Hypercalciuric hypocalcemia is a form of autosomal-dominant hypoparathyroidism (OMIM 146200) due to gain-of-function mutations in CASR (Table 17-2) that result in enhanced sensitivity to Ca^{2+}_e. A lowered set-point enables PTH secretion to be suppressed, and renal tubular reabsorption of calcium to be depressed, by extremely low concentrations of Ca^{2+}_e. This disorder may present in the newborn period.[44,45] Mutations may be scattered throughout the gene, but occur predominantly in the extracellular domain of the CaSR.

Activating mutations (Cys141Trp) of the CaSR may also inhibit function of the renal outer medullary potassium channel (KCNJ1, OMIM 600359), leading to a Bartter-like syndrome with hypokalemic metabolic alkalosis, hyperreninemia, and hyperaldosteronism as well as hypercalciuric hypocalcemia. The paired metabolic defects are in part responsive to treatment with hydrochlorothiazide and low doses of calcitriol.[46]

Children with hypercalciuric hypocalcemia due to gain-of-function mutations in CASR are very sensitive to even low doses of calcitriol that can lead to even more marked hypercalciuria and to nephrocalcinosis. Thus, management of these patients has been quite difficult. Administration of recombinant human PTH^{1-34} (0.7 μg/kg/day) to a 14-month-old hypocalcemic male infant with a de novo nonsense mutation in CASR (Leu727Gln) for 17 months in part restored calcium homeostasis, with increased but still subnormal serum levels of calcium (whereas urinary excretion of calcium decreased into the normal range).[47] During treatment, the child was

TABLE 17-2

Genetic Origins of Disorders of Mineral, Cartilage, and Bone Metabolism

Gene	Chromosome	OMIM	Disease	OMIM
ACVR1	2q23-q24	102576	Fibrodysplasia ossificans progressiva	135100
AIRE1	21q22.3	607358	Autoimmune polyendocrine syndrome, type I	240300
ALPL	1p36.1-p34	171760	Hypophosphatasia, infantile	241500
			Hypophosphatasia, childhood	241510
			Hypophosphatasia, adult	146300
CA2	8q22	259730	Osteopetrosis - renal tubular acidosis	259730
CASR	3q13.3-q21	601199	Hereditary hypocalciuric hypercalcemia	145980
			Neonatal severe hyperparathyroidism	239200
			Hypercalcemic hypercalciuria	601199
			Hypoparathyroidism, familial isolated	146200
			Acquired hypocalciuric hypercalcemia	145980
CLCN5	Xp11.2	300008	X-linked recessive hypophosphatemic rickets	300554
			Dent disease	300009
			Nephrolithiasis, X-linked recessive	310468
CLCN7	16p13	602727	Osteopetrosis, autosomal recessive	259700
			Osteopetrosis, autosomal dominant	166600
CLDN16	3q27	603959	Primary hypomagnesemia	248250
CLDN19	1p34.2	610036	Hypomagnesemia, hypercalciuria, visual impairment	248190
COL1A1	17q21.31-q22	120150	Osteogenesis imperfecta type I	166200
			Osteogenesis imperfecta type IIA	166210
			Osteogenesis imperfecta type III	259420
			Osteogenesis imperfecta type IV	166220
COL1A2	7q22.1	120160	Osteogenesis imperfecta type IIA	166210
			Osteogenesis imperfecta type III	259420
			Osteogenesis imperfecta type IV	166220
CRTAP	3p22	605497	Osteogenesis imperfecta type IIB	610854
			Osteogenesis imperfecta type VII	610682
CTSK	1q21	601105	Pycnodysostosis	265800
CYP2R1	11p15.2	608713	25-Hydroxylase deficiency, selective	600081
CYP27B1	12q13.1-q13.3	609506	25α-Hydroxyvitamin D-1α-hydroxylase deficiency (Vitamin D-dependent rickets, type I)	264700
DMP1	4q21	600980	Hypophosphatemic rickets, autosomal recessive	241520
ELN	7q13.23	120160	Williams-Beuren syndrome	194050
FGF23	12p13.3	605380	Hypophosphatemic rickets, autosomal dominant	193100
			Familial tumoral calcinosis	211900
			Hyperostosis hyperphosphatemia syndrome	610233
GALNT3	2q24-q31	601756	Familial tumoral calcinosis	211900
			Hyperostosis hyperphosphatemia syndrome	610233
GATA3	10p13-14	131320	Hypoparathyroidism, sensorineural deafness, renal disease (HDR/Barakat syndrome)	146255
GCM2	6p24.2	603716	Hypoparathyroidism, familial isolated	146200
GNAS	20q13.2	139320	Pseudohypoparathyroidism, type 1A	103580
			Pseudohypoparathyroidism, type 1B	603233
			Osseous heteroplasia, progressive	166350
			Fibrous dysplasia/McCune-Albright	174800
GNPTAB	12q23.2	607840	Mucolipidosis type II	252500
HNRPA1	12q13.1	164017	Vitamin D-dependent rickets type II	600785
HRPT2	1q24-q31	607393	Familial hyperparathyroidism 2 jaw tumor syndrome	145001
IKBKG	Xq28	300248	Osteopetrosis, anhidrotic ectodermal dysplasia, lymphedema	300301
KCNJ1	11q24	600359	Antenatal Bartter syndrome type 2	600839
LEPRE1	1p34	610339	Osteogenesis imperfecta type VIII	610915
LRP5	11q13.4	603506	Osteoporosis-pseudoglioma syndrome	259770
			Idiopathic juvenile osteoporosis	259750
			High bone mass variation	601884
			Van Buchem disease, type 2	607636
MEN1	11q13	131100	Multiple endocrine neoplasia type I	131100

TABLE 17-2

Genetic Origins of Disorders of Mineral, Cartilage, and Bone Metabolism—Cont'd

Gene	Chromosome	OMIM	Disease	OMIM
NPR2	9p21-p12	108961	Acromesomelic dysplasia (Maroteaux)	602875
OSTM1	6q21	607649	Osteopetrosis, autosomal recessive	259700
PHEX	Xp22.2-p22.1	300550	Hypophosphatemic rickets, X-linked dominant	307800
PTH	11p15.3-p15.1	168450	Hypoparathyroidism, familial isolated	146200
PTHR1	3p22-p21.1	168468	Blomstrand osteochondrodysplasia	215045
			Murk-Jansen metaphyseal chondrodysplasia	156400
			Enchondromatosis (Ollier disease)	166000
RET	10q11.2	164761	Multiple endocrine neoplasia type IIA	171400
			Multiple endocrine neoplasia type IIB	162300
			Familial medullary carcinoma of thyroid	155240
SLC12A1	15q15-q21.1	600839	Antenatal Bartter syndrome type I	601678
SLC34A3	9q34	609826	Hypophosphatemic rickets with hypercalciuria, hereditary	241530
SLC7A7	14q11.2	603593	Lysinuric protein intolerance	222700
SOST	17q12-q21	605740	Sclerosteosis	269500
			Hyperostosis corticalis generalisata (Van Buchem disease type 1)	239100
SOX3	Xq26.3	313430	Hypoparathyroidism, X-linked	307700
STX16	20q13.32	603666	Pseudohypoparathyroidism, type 1B	603233
TBX1	22q11.12	602054	DiGeorge syndrome	188400
TBCE	1q42-q43	604934	Sanjad-Sakati (HRD) syndrome	241410
			Kenney-Caffey syndrome, type 1	244460
TGFB1	19q13.1	190180	Progressive diaphyseal dysplasia	131300
TCIRG1	11q13.4-q13.5	604592	Osteopetrosis, autosomal recessive	259700
TNFRSF11A	18q22.1	603499	Polyostotic osteolytic dysplasia, hereditary (familial) expansile	174810
TNFRSF11B	8q24	602643	Paget disease, juvenile	239000
TRPM6	9q22	607009	Familial hypomagnesemia with hypocalcemia	602014
VDR	12q12-q14	601769	Vitamin-D-dependent rickets, type II	277440

See Table 17-12 for genes associated with osteochondrodysplasias.

clinically asymptomatic, did not develop nephrocalcinosis, and tolerated the drug well.

The most common form of dysgenesis of the PTGs in neonates and infants is that associated with the DiGeorge syndrome (DGS, OMIM 188400), a disorder that occurs with a frequency of 1:4,000 to 1:8,000 births and is present in approximately 70% of children with isolated hypoparathyroidism.[48,49] The DGS is a neurocristopathy, the result of disturbed migration of cervical neural crest cells and consequent maldevelopment of tissues of neural crest origin derived from the third and fourth pharyngeal pouches and first to fifth branchial arches. It is usually associated with microdeletions of chromosome region 22qll.2 (del22q11.2, DGCR) and is thus a contiguous gene syndrome (a disorder caused by deletion of several adjacent genes that when individually mutated may result in a distinctive clinical feature and when collectively lost lead to a group of apparently unrelated clinical findings).

Although the clinical severity and phenotype of patients with this chromosomal anomaly are variable, characteristically subjects with DGS have the triad of hypocalcemia due to hypoplasia of the PTGs (often manifest in the neonatal period but which may not be detected until an older age), defective T-lymphocyte function and impaired cell-mediated immunity due to partial or complete absence of thymic differentiation (leading to increased frequency of viral and fungal infections), and conotruncal defects of the heart or aortic arch (Tetralogy of Fallot, truncus arteriosus, interrupted or right aortic arch, aberrant right subclavian artery).[20,48,50] Indeed, delq2211 has been associated with three overlapping disorders—DGS and the conotruncal anomaly face and velocardiofacial syndromes.

Collectively, these syndromes are associated with a quite typical face (ocular hypertelorism, lateral displacement of inner canthi, short palpebral fissures, swollen eyelids, dysmorphic segmented nose, small mouth, low-set ears with abnormally folded pinnae, short philtrum, micrognathia, malar hypoplasia, velopharyngeal insufficiency (with/without cleft palate), olfactory dysfunction, short stature, nonverbal learning disabilities, and various psychological maladies.[49,51,52] DGS may occur sporadically or be transmitted as an autosomal-dominant characteristic. Takao velocardiofacial syndrome (included in OMIM 188440) consists primarily of the typical cardiac defects described previously, which may also be associated with hypocalcemia.

Shprintzen velocardiofacial syndrome (OMIM 192430) is characterized by craniofacial and palatal defects and cardiac anomalies. Cayler cardiofacial syndrome (OMIM 125520) is associated with partial unilateral facial paresis (due to hypoplasia of the depressor angularis muscle) and with anomalies of the heart and aorta. These syndromes have been grouped as the CATCH-22 syndromes of Cardiac defects, Abnormal face, Thymic hypoplasia, Cleft palate, and Hypocalcemia. In addition to the anomalies and clinical findings listed, a litany of abnormalities may be seen in patients with del22q11.2.[53] Disparate manifestations of these syndromes may be observed in different members of the same family, indicating the variable clinical expressions that accompany del22q11.2.[54]

A two-megabase microdeletion at chromosome 22q11.2 leads to loss of several contiguous genes within this region, including *HIRA* (histone cell cycle regulation, OMIM 600237)—a transcription factor (expressed in developing heart and upper body neural crest elements) necessary to normal cardiac development.[55] Also within this region is *TBX1* encoding T-BOX-1, a transcription factor with a highly conserved DNA-binding sequence (the T-box) essential for organogenesis and pattern formation and expressed in the pharyngeal arches and pouches. Experimental disruption of *Tbx1* impairs development of the pharyngeal arch arterial vasculature, whereas introduction of null mutations in *Tbx1* results in anomalies of the cardiac outflow track and hypoplasia of the thymus and PTGs.[56]

Evaluation of patients with clinical characteristics of the CATCH-22 syndromes but intact 22q11.2 has revealed heterozygous loss-of-function mutations in *TBX1* in patients with the DGS (Phe148Tyr, Gly310Ser) and Shprintzen velocardiofacial syndrome.[49,57] Thus, haploinsufficiency of *TBX1* alone can account for the cardiac defects, abnormal face, thymic and parathyroid hypoplasia, and velopharyngeal insufficiency with cleft palate but not for the developmental delay characteristic of CATCH-22. Another candidate gene for the DGS sited at chromosome 22q11.2 is *UFD1L* (ubiquitin fusion degradation 1-like, OMIM 601754), whose product is important in the posttranslational processing of proteins and/or their degradation by interaction with the ubiquitin fusion protein.

Experimentally, the DGS and related disorders have also been linked to genes encoding endothelin-1, vascular endothelial growth factor, and fibroblast growth factor-8 (a target gene for TBX1)—as well as to genes within the DGCR at chromosome 22q11.2 [CRKL (*OMIM* 602007) and DGCR6 (OMIM 601279)]. In the mouse hypomorphic for *Fgf8,* there are cardiovascular, craniofacial, parathyroid, and thymic defects—an experimental phenocopy of the human del22q11.2 syndrome.[58] Fgf8 functions through stimulation of transcription of *Crkl.* Its product is an adaptor protein that transduces intracellular signals from several tyrosine kinase receptors, one of which is the receptor for Fgf8, Interestingly, Fgf8 interacts with Tbx1 as well. The DGS has also been associated with microdeletions of chromosomes 10p13, 18q21.33, and 4q21.2-q25—indicative of the cascade of genes likely involved in the generation of this phenotype.

There are several other syndromes with multisystem involvement and hypoparathyroidism. The Barakat or HDR syndrome (OMIM 146255) of hypoparathyroidism, sensorineural deafness, and renal disease (steroid-resistant nephrosis with progressive renal failure) has been attributed to haploinsufficiency of *GATA3*—a zinc-finger transcription factor important in the embryonic development of the PTGs, kidneys, and inner ear and in normal function of the immune system as an essential T-cell receptor enhancer.[59]

The PTGs of these children are dysgenetic (hypoplastic or absent). Hypocalcemia may be present in the newborn period or unrecognized until later childhood.[60] Heterozygous deletions, insertions, and missense and nonsense mutations in *GATA3* have been identified in patients and families with HDR.[61,62] Interestingly, subjects with isolated loss of *GATA3* function do not have other features common to patients with larger terminal deletions of 10p—such as growth and developmental retardation, dysmorphic facial features, and congenital heart disease.

Biallelic mutations in the gene encoding tubulin-specific chaperone E *(TBCE)* have been identified in the Sanjad-Sakati syndrome of hypoparathyroidism mental retardation dysmorphism (HRD, OMIM 241410) and the Kenny-Caffey syndrome type 1 of hypocalcemia, cortical thickening, and medullary stenosis (KCS1, OMIM 244460). Children with HRD are short, developmentally delayed, and seizure prone. They have medullary stenosis and other skeletal anomalies. They are microcephalic, with faces characterized by deeply recessed eyes or microphthalmia, depressed nasal bridge, beaked nose, long philtrum, thin upper vermillion border, micrognathia, and large earlobes. The HRD syndrome often presents in infancy with symptomatic hypocalcemia associated with low serum concentrations of PTH and normal phosphaturic response to exogenous PTH.

The cardiovascular system of these patients is intact, but as infants they are susceptible to life-threatening pneumococcal infections.[63] Neonates with KCS1 are severely hypocalcemic early in the neonatal period. As children they are short, with craniofacial anomalies (due to absence of diploic space in the skull), osteosclerosis, and thickening of the cortices of the long bones with narrowing of the medullary compartment and normal or mildly delayed development. They too are susceptible to recurrent bacterial infections. TBCE is essential for formation of microtubules—cytosolic structures composed of heterodimeric α- and β-tubulin subunits that form the cytoskeleton, mitotic apparatus, cilia, and other cellular components. This chaperonin assists in the correct folding of α- and β-tubulin subunits and the formation of α- β-tubulin heterodimers.

The α- and β-tubulin subunits and TCBE are necessary to normal embryogenesis of the PTGs. Mutations in *TCBE* result in lowered microtubule formation and consequently in decrease in subcellular components such as the golgi apparatus and endosomal compartments required for normal intracellular movement of proteins. Interestingly, the identical mutation in *TCBE* (a homozygous 12 bp deletion in exon 2) may result in the HRD or KCS1 phenotype in a specific family.[64] A child with autosomal-recessive HRD syndrome and intact *TCBE* has been identified, suggesting that this disorder is likely to be genetically heterogeneous.[65] In KCS type 2 (OMIM 127000), the phenotype is similar to that of KCS1 but transmission is as an autosomal-dominant trait for which no gene mutation has been identified to date.

Familial isolated congenital or later-onset hypoparathyroidism may be transmitted as an autosomal-recessive, autosomal-dominant, or X-linked recessive trait. It has been associated with loss-of-function mutations of GCM2, PTH, and possibly SOX3, and gain-of-function mutations in CaSR. GCM2 encodes a 506-aa DNA-binding protein whose expression is restricted to the PTGs. Knockout of Gcm2 in mice leads to agenesis of the PTGs and hypoparathyroidism. Biallelic intragenic deletion or homozygous missense mutations of GCM2 result in hypoparathyroidism in humans.[66-68]

Homozygous loss-of-function mutations in PTH have been detected in neonates with autosomal-recessive familial isolated hypoparathyroidism. In one family, substitution of proline for serine at the −3 position of the signal peptide of prepro-PTH likely prevented its normal post-translational processing and accelerated protein product degradation within the endoplasmic reticulum.[69] As previous described, hypoparathyroidism due to a heterozygous activating mutation in CASR have been found in a hypocalcemic neonate. One mutation (Phe806Ser) occurred in the sixth transmembrane domain of this G-protein–coupled receptor (GPCR) near its site of interaction with $G_s\alpha$.[44] X-linked hypoparathyroidism (OMIM 307700) is associated with agenesis of the PTGs. The disorder has been mapped to Xq27 and may involve a deletion-insertion mutation that adversely affects the position of SOX3.[70] Because Sox3 is expressed in embryonic mouse PTGs, it is likely an important transcription for normal embryologic development of the PTGs.

In the neonate with Blomstrand osteochondrodysplasia (OMIM 215045), hypocalcemia is secondary to loss-of-function mutations in PTHR1 and hence insensitivity to the calcemic effects of PTH.[71] Transmitted as an autosomal-recessive trait, its clinical characteristics include polyhydramnios, hydrops fetalis, short-limbed dwarfism, facial anomalies, aberrant tooth development, aplasia of the nipples and breasts, hypoplastic lungs, and preductal aortic coarctation. Serum concentrations of PTH are elevated. Skeletal maturation is advanced. Histologically, the proliferative zone of the cartilage growth plate is narrowed—with relatively few resting and proliferating chondrocytes—whereas the hypertrophic zone is composed of irregular columns of chondrocytes.

Although Blomstrand osteochondodysplasia has been lethal to date, skeletal malformations may be more (type I) or less severe (type II). Mutations in PTHR1 that result in complete absence of product (e.g., Arg104Ter) lead to type I, whereas mutations that permit some PTHR1 synthesis (Pro132Leu) result in type II.[72] Loss-of-function mutations in GNAS, the gene encoding the $G_\alpha s$ subunit of the activating G protein, lead to PTH insensitivity and pseudohypoparathyroidism (PHP)—a disorder that may be suspected in the neonate with hypocalcemia in whom hyperthyrotropinemia has been detected in the neonatal screening study for congenital hypothyroidism.[73] As a consequence of the loss-of-function mutation in GNAS in the thyroid gland, the $G_\alpha s$ subunit required by the thyrotropin GPCR is also impaired. In some neonates with elevated serum concentrations of PTH and phosphate and blunted phosphaturic response to PTH, neonatal pseudohypoparathyroidism is transient and resolves within the first few months of life.[74]

Abnormalities of the mitochondrial genome have also been associated with hypoparathyroidism. In addition, patients with the Kearns-Sayre syndrome (OMIM 530000) manifest ophthalmoplegia, retinal pigmentation, and cardiomyopathy. Point mutations, duplications, and deletions of various length of the mitochondrial genome (16,569 bp) have been found in these patients. Hypoparathyroidism has been observed in patients with the syndrome of mitochondrial encephalopathy, lactic acidosis, and stroke-like episodes (MELAS) and the mitochondrial trifunctional protein deficiency syndrome (MTPDS)—a disorder of fatty acid oxidation.[71,75]

Evaluation and Management

Evaluation of the neonate with hypocalcemia begins with review of the maternal, gestational, peripartum, postnatal, and family histories and physical examination (Figure 17-5). Historical data include those related to maternal parity and complications of pregnancy such as maternal diabetes mellitus (gestational, types I or II), toxemia of pregnancy or ingestion of excessive alkali, or abnormalities of delivery, low birth weight, neonatal sepsis, or other early postpartum illnesses. The family history is examined for members with abnormalities of mineral metabolism such as renal calculi, rickets, or hypocalcemia (e.g., seizure disorders).

The social history provides information about the socioeconomic status of the mother and her cultural beliefs that may have impacted on maternal diet and exposure to sunlight during gestation. The physical examination (abnormal face, cardiac murmur) may suggest a complex form of hypocalcemia. Determination of a complete blood count; serum concentrations of total calcium, Ca^{2+}_e, magnesium, phosphate, creatinine, intact PTH, calcidiol, and calcitriol; and urinary calcium and creatinine concentrations in a spot urine should precede initial therapy of the hypocalcemic newborn whenever possible.

Decreased serum concentrations of PTH are common in neonates with early-onset hypocalcemia, but persistently low PTH levels suggest impaired PTH secretion. High PTH concentrations are present in patients with vitamin D deficiency or insensitivity, PTH resistance due to loss-of-function mutations in PTHR1 or GNAS, or impaired renal function. Low levels of calcidiol signify decreased maternal (and hence fetal) vitamin D stores or rarely a defect in vitamin D-25 hydroxylase, whereas calcitriol concentrations are inappropriately low in subjects with severely compromised renal function, hypoparathyroidism, or deficiency of 25OHD-1α-hydroxylase. Elevated calcitriol values suggest vitamin D resistance due to an abnormality in VDR, a disorder that may be associated with alopecia. Skeletal radiographs may disclose osteopenia, whereas chest X-ray may not identify a thymic shadow (an unreliable sign in a severely ill or

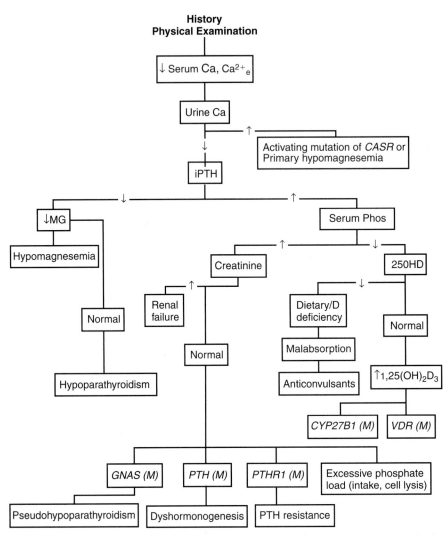

Figure 17-5 Evaluation of hypocalcemia. Abbreviations: Ca (serum total calcium), Ca²⁺ₑ (extracellular ionized calcium), Phos (serum phosphate), Mg (magnesium), PTH (parathyroid hormone), 25OHD [25-hydroxyvitamin D (calcidiol)], 1, 25 (OH)₂ D₃ [1, 25-dihydroxy vitamin D₃ (calcitriol)] PTHR1 (PTH receptor), VDR (vitamin D receptor), D (vitamin D), and M (mutation).

stressed neonate). Serum levels of calcium, Ca²⁺ₑ, phosphate, and intact PTH should be measured in the mothers of neonates with unexplained hypocalcemia.

In neonates with hypocalcemia not otherwise explained, evaluation for possible DGS should be undertaken—particularly when physical examination reveals an abnormal face and a congenital anomaly of the outflow tract of the heart. The white blood and T (CD4) lymphocyte counts are low in DGS, and the thymic shadow often absent. The diagnosis of the DGS is confirmed by the presence of a microdeletion of chromosome 22q11.2 as demonstrated by fluorescent in situ hybridization (FISH).

Occasionally, sequence analysis of *TBX1* may be needed to establish this diagnosis if the *FISH* study is normal. Because the DGS may be heritable, examination of the karyotype of the parents of a DGS infant is indicated (as well as those of the siblings if the parent also has delq22.11). It should be noted that the majority of neonates and infants with DGS are recognized primarily because of cardiac anomalies and that subjects without

these lesions may not be identified until mid or late childhood or adolescence.[76] Neonates with PHP type I usually do not have the characteristic skeletal phenotype (brachymetacarpals) of Albright hereditary osteodystrophy, but if this diagnosis is suspected analysis of GNAS is indicated.

Early neonatal hypocalcemia is often asymptomatic, but nevertheless treatment is indicated when the total serum calcium concentration is below 6 mg/dL in the preterm infant and less than 7 mg/dL in the term infant.[20] Asymptomatic neonates are most easily managed by increasing the oral intake of calcium and establishing an overall ratio of calcium:phosphate intake of 4:1 (including that in feedings with a low phosphate formula such as Similac PM 60/40ᴿ, calcium:phosphate ratio 1.6:1), with calcium glubionate or calcium carbonate administered in divided doses every 4 to 6 hours (Table 17-3).

Eucalcemia is almost always restored in these subjects within 3 weeks after birth, and often earlier. In the hypocalcemic infant with tetany or frank seizures, 10% calcium gluconate (elemental calcium 9.3 mg/mL) at a dose of

TABLE 17-3

Preparations of Calcitriol, Calcium, Magnesium, and Phosphate

Medication	Content	Elemental Mineral
Vitamin D		
Vitamin D	8,000 IU/mL	
	25,000 or 50,000 IU/tablet	
Calcidiol	20 or 50 μg/tablet	
Calcitriol	1 μg/mL	
	0.25 μg or 0.5 μg/casule	
Dihydrotachysterol	0.2 μg/5 mL	
	01.25, 0.2, 0.4 mg/tablet	
Calcium		
Calcium gluconate (iv)	93 mg/g	93 mg/10 mL
Calcium glubionate (solution)	64 mg/g	115 mg/5 mL
Calcium carbonate	400 mg/g	500 mg/tablet
Calcium carbonate (suspension)	1,250 mg/5 mL	500 mg/5 mL
Calcium citrate	210 mg/g	200 mg/tablet
Magnesium		
Magnesium sulfate (50% im soln)		49 mg/mL
Magnesium oxide	603 mg/g	241 mg/tablet
Mg gluconate	54 mg/g	27 mg/tablet
Magnesium chloride	120 mg/g	64 mg/tablet
Phosphorus		
Sodium phosphate (phospha-soda)		127 mg/mL
Sodium/potassium phosphate (Neutraphos)		250 mg/packet (powder)
Potassium phosphate (Neutraphos-K)		250 mg/packet (powder)
Potassium phosphate (K-Phos Original)		114 mg/tablet
Sodium/Potassium phosphate (K-Phos MF)		126 mg/coated tablet
Sodium/Potassium phosphate (K-Phos #2)		250 mg/coated tablet
Sodium/Potassium phosphate (K-Phos Neutral)		250 mg/tablet

Compiled from Alon US (2006). Hypophosphatemic vitamin D-resistant rickets. In Favus MJ (ed.), *Primer on the metabolic bone diseases and disorders of mineral metabolism, Sixth edition*. Washington, D.C.: American Society for Bone and Mineral Research 342–345; from Bringhurst FR, et al. (2003). Hormones and disorders of mineral metabolism. In Larsen PR, Kronenberg HM, Melmed S, Plonsky KS (eds.), *Williams textbook of endocrinology, Tenth edition*. Philadelphia: Saunders/Elsevier 1303–1371; from Favus MJ (ed.), *Primer on the metabolic bone diseases and disorders of mineral metabolism, Sixth edition*. Washington, D.C.: American Society for Bone and Mineral Research 496; and from Levine B-S, Carpenter TO (1999). Evaluation and treatment of heritable forms of rickets. The Endocrinologist 9:358–365.

1 to 3 mg/kg and rate of less than 1 mL/minute and a total dose not to exceed 20 mg of elemental calcium/kg may be administered by intravenous infusion. Often seizures will cease after 1 to 3 mL of 10% calcium gluconate has been administered.[20,22] Cardiac rate and rhythm must be carefully monitored to prevent bradycardia and asystole.

Further intravenous bolus doses of calcium (~10 mg/kg at 6-hour intervals) should be used sparingly because they result in wide excursions in serum calcium values. These infants too should receive supplemental oral calcium. Depending on the cause of the hypocalcemia, supplemental vitamin D or calcitriol may also be needed. Serum and urine calcium and creatinine levels should be determined frequently, and treatment modified to maintain eucalcemia and the urine calcium/creatinine ratio <0.2 in an effort to avoid iatrogenic hypercalcemia, hypercalciuria, nephrocalcinosis, and renal insufficiency.

After restoration of eucalcemia in the infant with DGS, the other components of this disorder must be addressed. Cardiac anomalies usually require surgical correction, as do palatal clefts. In DGS infants with immunocompromise and recurrent infections due to thymic aplasia, ap-

propriate anti-infectious therapy is mandatory. Transplantation of fetal or cultured postnatal thymic tissue, bone marrow, or peripheral blood mononuclear cells has restored immune function in infants with the DGS.[77,78] Supplemental calcitriol (20–60 ng/kg/day) and calcium are necessary for restoration and maintenance of eucalcemia in infants with hypoparathyroidism. Poor growth due to feeding difficulties and learning disabilities due to developmental delay must be managed on an individual basis and illustrate the need for a multidisciplinary approach to the care of DGS patients.[76] Hypocalcemia due to hypomagnesemia is managed acutely by the intravenous infusion or intramuscular injection of 50% magnesium sulfate at a dose of 0.1 to 0.2 mL/kg while monitoring cardiac status.

HYPERCALCEMIA

Although hypercalcemia in neonates and very young infants is defined as total blood calcium concentration >10.8 to 11.3 mg/dL (depending on the analytical laboratory), substantial symptoms (anorexia, gastroesophageal reflux and emesis, constipation, lethargy and hypotonia, or irritability and seizures) usually do not occur until the total calcium level exceeds 12 to 13 mg/dL.[22,79] These infants frequently have polyuria, and may become dehydrated due to renal resistance to antidiuretic hormone if oral fluid intake is restricted.

Due to the vasoconstrictive effect of calcium, the hypercalcemic infant may be hypertensive. Hypercalcemia also shortens the S-T segment and can lead to heart block and ultimately to asystole. In older infants and young children with chronic hypercalcemia, poor growth and failure to thrive are often presenting manifestations. Hypercalcemia also leads to hypercalciuria and the complications of nephrocalcinosis and nephrolithiasis.

Etiology

Neonatal/infantile hypercalcemia may be iatrogenic in origin (e.g., administration of excessive calcium or vitamin D) at times in the breast milk of mothers ingesting large amounts of cholecalciferol. It may also be due to maternal ingestion of thiazide diuretics that increase renal tubular absorption of calcium or purposeful restriction of phosphate that leads to hypophosphatemia and reciprocal increase in serum calcium concentrations as hypophosphatemia stimulate renal tubular 25OHD-1α-hydroxylase activity, calcitriol synthesis, and increased intestinal absorption of calcium (Table 17-4). Hypercalcemia, hypophosphatemia, hyperphosphatasemia, and radiographic evidence of rickets develop in premature infants receiving intravenous alimentation deficient in phosphate or in those fed only human breast milk—the phosphate content of which is low.

The problem may be prevented or treated by increasing the amount of parenteral phosphate administered to the extent possible or by the use of breast milk fortified with phosphate.[80] Adequate extrauterine mineralization of the preterm skeleton requires intakes of calcium and phosphate of approximately 200 mg/kg/day. Extracorporeal life support may also be associated with hypercalcemia in neonates.[81]

Hypervitaminosis D may be due to prolonged feeding of an improperly prepared formula or commercial dairy milk containing excessive vitamin D; iatrogenic prescription of vitamin D, calcidiol, or calcitriol; or increased endogenous production of calcitriol from inflammatory sites.[79] In infants with severe birth trauma or perinatal asphyxia, subcutaneous fat necrosis may develop in tissues that have sustained direct trauma and be manifested by indurated extremely firm violaceous nodules on the cheeks, trunk, buttocks, and legs.[22] Hypercalcemia may be present when the lesions first appear or develop as the nodules resolve several weeks later.

Histologically, the skin lesions are composed of adipocytes, an inflammatory lymphohistiocytic infiltrate, and multinucleated giant cells in a bed of calcium crystals. The hypercalcemia of subcutaneous fat necrosis is attributable not only to reabsorption of precipitated calcium but to extrarenal synthesis of calcitriol by local macrophages and resultant hyperabsorption of ingested calcium. The 25OHD-1α-hydroxylase activity of these inflammatory macrophages is not under the control of PTH, calcium, or phosphate levels but is suppressible by glucocorticoids.[22]

TABLE 17-4

Causes of Hypercalcemia

I. Neonate/Infant
A. Maternal Disorders
1. Excessive vitamin D ingestion, hypoparathyroidism, pseudohypoparathyroidism

B. Neonate/Infant
1. Excessive intake of calcium or vitamin D
2. Phosphate depletion
3. Subcutaneous fat necrosis
4. Williams-Beuren syndrome
5. Familial hypocalciuric hypercalcemia/neonatal severe hyperparathyroidism
6. Metaphyseal chondrodysplasia, Jansen type
7. Persistent parathyroid hormone related protein
8. Bartter syndrome with excessive production of prostaglandin E
9. Lactase/disaccharidase deficiency
10. Infantile hypophosphatasia
11. Mucolipidosis type II
12. Post bone marrow transplantation for osteopetrosis
13. Idiopathic
14. Endocrinopathies: primary adrenal insufficiency, severe congenital hypothyroidism, hyperthyroidism

II. Hyperparathyroidism
A. Sporadic
B. Familial
1. Neonatal severe hyperparathyroidism (*CASR*)
2. Multiple endocrine neoplasia, type I (*MEN1*)
3. Multiple endocrine neoplasia, type IIa (*RET*)
4. McCune-Albright syndrome (*GNAS*)
5. Familial hyperparathyroidism 2 -jaw tumor syndrome (*HRPT2*)
6. Jansen's metaphyseal dysplasia (*PTHR1*)

C. Secondary/Tertiary
1. Postrenal transplantation
2. Chronic hyperphosphatemia

D. Ectopic Production of PTHrP

III. Familial Hypocalciuric Hypercalcemia (CASR)
A. Loss-of-Function Mutations in *CASR*
B. Inhibitory Autoantibodies to the Calcium-Sensing Receptor

IV. Excessive Intake of Calcium or Vitamin D
1. Nutritional - milk-alkali syndrome
2. Exogenous ingestion (vitamin D) or topical application (calcitriol or analog)
3. Ectopic production of calcitriol associated with granulomatous diseases: sarcoidosis, inflammatory bowel disease; tuberculosis, histoplasmosis, coccidioidomycosis, leprosy; human immunodeficiency virus; neoplasia: lymphoma, dysgerminoma

V. Immobilization

VI. Other Causes
A. Neoplasia: Osseous metastases, production of PTHrP, cytokines/osteoclast activating factors
B. Hypophosphatasia
C. Drugs: thiazide diuretics, lithium, vitamin A and analogs, calcium, alkali, anti-estrogens, aminophylline
D. Total parenteral nutrition
E. Endocrinopathies: hyperthyroidism, hypoadrenocorticism, pheochromocytoma
F. Vasoactive intestinal polypeptide-secreting tumor
G. Acute or chronic renal failure/administration of aluminum
H. Juvenile rheumatoid arthritis, cytokine mediated

Excessive production of prostaglandin E and interleukins (IL) -1 and -6 further contributes to hypercalcemia in this disorder by increasing the rate of bone turnover.[82] Hypercalcemia attributable to subcutaneous fat necrosis is managed by the ingestion of a low-calcium formula, avoidance of vitamin D, and administration of fluids, furosemide, calcitonin, glucocorticoids, or bisphosphonate (etidronate, pamidronate) as needed.[83] Hypercalcemia due to subcutaneous fat necrosis has also been observed in older children with major trauma or disseminated varicella.[79] Congenital lactase deficiency has been associated with infantile hypercalcemia, perhaps due to increased intestinal absorption of calcium directly promoted by lactose.

Neonatal severe hyperparathyroidism (NSHPT) is a potentially lethal form of familial (hereditary) hypocalciuric hypercalcemia (HHC), with very high serum calcium concentrations. NSHPT is most commonly due to homozygous or compound heterozygous inactivating mutations of *CASR* that greatly increase the serum concentration of Ca^{2+}_e needed to suppress PTH synthesis and secretion. However, in several infants with NSHPT there have been heterozygous inactivating mutations of *CASR* (e.g., Arg185Gln, Arg227Leu)—suggesting that the products of these mutations possibly exert a dominant-negative effect on the normal allele, perhaps by interfering with migration of wt receptors to the cell surface or inactivation of wt receptor by linking to the mutated CaSR once embedded in the cell membrane, or by sequestration of G-proteins.[84]

In addition, the heterozygous fetus who has inherited only one inactivated CaSR allele from an affected father and is delivered by a normal mother may have been relatively hypocalcemic in utero, leading to hyperplasia of the fetal PTGs that persists after birth. Conversely, homozygous mutations near the amino terminal of *CASR* (e.g., Leu13Pro) may not become manifest until mid childhood or even adulthood.[85,86] The clinical spectrum of NSHPT ranges from mild—(constipation, polyuria) with calcium concentrations ranging from 12 to 13 mg/dL—to severe and life-threatening (dysrhythmia, respiratory distress due to hypotonia, demineralization and fractures of the ribs) when calcium levels exceed 15 mg/dL.[87]

NSHPT may present within the first few days of life to several months of age, depending on the degree of hypercalcemia. Search of the family history may identify members with autosomal-dominant HHC1. The serum calcium concentration is usually markedly elevated (>14–17 mg/dL), as is the PTH value. There are hypermagnesemia, normal to low serum phosphate levels, hyperphosphatasemia, elevated calcitriol values, low renal tubular reabsorption of phosphate, and relative hypocalciuria. Radiographically, osteopenia, metaphyseal widening and irregularity, subperiosteal resorption, and varus angulation of the hips may be seen in response to the bone resorptive effects of PTH.

Treatment of NSHPT includes induction of sodium diuresis (fluids, furosemide) in order to increase urinary calcium excretion and intravenous administration of a bisphosphonate (pamidronate, zoledronic acid) to acutely lower serum calcium values. Calcimimetic drugs that act directly on the CaSR have also been effective in lowering

serum calcium values in infants with NSHPT.[88,89] Parathyroidectomy may be a requisite life-saving measure at times. Children with NSHPT who remain hypercalcemic are anorectic, fail to thrive, and are at risk for developmental delay.[22]

Secondary hyperparathyroidism in the neonate may be the result of maternal hypocalcemia due to hypoparathyroidism or PHP.[22] Maternal hypocalcemia reduces placental transport and net delivery of calcium to the fetus, resulting in relative fetal hypocalcemia and leading to hyperplasia of the fetal PTGs and secondary hyperparathyroidism proportional to the maternal calcium deficit. Although 25% of infants of hypocalcemic mothers are hypercalcemic, most have skeletal changes that reflect PTH excess that vary from severe demineralization with fractures to osteopenia detectable only by absorptiometry. Secondary hyperparathyroidism usually resolves within a few weeks after birth as the infant ingests adequate calcium and phosphate.

Another cause of neonatal secondary hyperparathyroidism is mucolipidosis type II (OMIM 252500). This Hurler-like disorder is characterized by facial abnormalities (asymmetry, flat nasal bridge), hepatosplenomegaly, skeletal deformities (dysostosis multiplex), and developmental delay and is due to inactivating mutations in a gene (*GNPTAB*- N-acetyglucosamine-1-phosphotransferase, α/β subunits) encoding a phosphotransferase required for synthesis of mannose 6-phosphate.[90] In this disease, maternal calcium concentrations are normal but placental histology is abnormal—suggesting impaired placental transport of calcium and fetal hypocalcemia, leading to compensatory increase in in utero PTH generation. In turn, skeletal evidence of PTH excess (osteopenia, fractures) develops. Secondary hyperparathyroidism and its adverse effects remit within the first several weeks to months after birth.

Murk-Jansen metaphyseal chondrodysplasia (OMIM 156400) is an autosomal-dominant chondrodystrophy associated with marked hypercalcemia as a consequence of heterozygous mutations that lead to constitutive ligand-independent activation of PTHR1 expressed in the kidney, bone, and growth plate chondrocytes.[91] Phenotypically, there are marked short-limbed dwarfism; deformities of the long bones, digits, spine, and pelvis; choanal atresia; highly arched palate; micrognathia; widely open cranial sutures (in infancy); sclerosis of the basal cranial bones; disorganization of the metaphyses (delayed chondrocyte differentiation, irregularly calcified cartilage protruding into the diaphysis); and excessive loss of cortical bone but normal trabecular bone.

Interestingly, birth length and physical appearance are usually normal in these neonates—although radiographic evidence of the chondrodysplasia is present. In affected neonates and infants, there are hypercalcemia, hypophosphatemia, increased serum concentrations of calcitriol, and elevated urinary excretion of nephrogenous cyclic adenosine monophosphate but low or undetectable serum levels of PTH and PTHrP. Constitutively activating mutations of *PTHR1* in these subjects include His223Arg at the junction of the first intracellular loop and second transmembrane domain and Thr410Pro in the sixth transmembrane domain—sites specifically important in conferring ligand-independent activity upon PTHR1.[79,92] Excessive secretion of PTHrP and resultant hypercalcemia have been observed in infants with neonatal iron storage disease and embryonal renal tumors (Wilms', mesoblastic nephroma). In these infants, intravenous pamidronate (0.5 mg/kg in 30 mL of normal saline over 4 hours repeated once or twice) has restored eucalcemia.[93]

The Williams-Beuren syndrome (OMIM 194050) is characterized by intrauterine and postnatal growth retardation; hypercalcemia in infancy in 15% of patients that usually resolves by 1 year of age but may occasionally persist into adulthood; consistent hypercalciuria; supravalvular aortic stenosis in 30% of subjects; stenoses of the pulmonary, renal, mesenteric, and celiac arteries; microcephaly; elfin face (epicanthal folds, stellate iris pattern, esotropia, short nose with full nasal tip, arched upper and prominent lower lips, long philtrum, full cheeks with flattened malar eminences, dental malocclusion); hoarse voice; radioulnar synostosis; renal hypoplasia or unilateral agenesis; hypertension; and developmental delay (poor visual-motor integration, attention deficit disorder, IQ 20–106).[22]

Although most patients with the Williams-Beuren syndrome are developmentally challenged, they have unique and proficient verbal skills with a large vocabulary and enhanced auditory memory (particularly for names), adept social language skills, and exceptional musical aptitude—including the ability to memorize and sing many musical compositions and play many instruments.[79] The pathophysiology of hypercalcemia in this syndrome is unknown. No consistent abnormalities of vitamin D metabolism or of PTH or calcitonin secretion have been found in patients with the Williams-Beuren syndrome. Interestingly, many patients with this disorder have hypoplasia of the thyroid gland and elevated serum concentrations of thyrotropin. However, the significance of these findings to the pathophysiology of the syndrome itself is unclear.[94]

The Williams-Beuren syndrome may be transmitted as an autosomal-dominant trait. It has been localized to chromosome 7q11.23, where microdeletions of 0.9 to 2.5 Mb and hemizygous loss of perhaps as many as 17 contiguous genes combine to produce the syndromic phenotype. The microdeletions may arise in the maternal or paternal seventh chromosome. Hemizygous deletions of *ELN* have been found in more than 90% of patients with the Williams-Beuren syndrome and likely account for the abnormalities of vascular connective tissue present in these subjects, but not the other manifestations of this disorder. Singular deletion and intragenic loss-of-function mutations of *ELN* lead to isolated supravalvular aortic stenosis without other features of the Williams-Beuren syndrome.

Hemizygosity for *ELN* leads to compensatory increase in the number of rings of smooth muscle and elastic lamellae, resulting in arterial thickening and increased risk of obstruction.[95] Additional genes at chromosome 7q11.23 whose haploinsufficiency may be responsible for aspects of the Williams-Beuren phenotype include *RFC2* (OMIM 600404, encoding a subunit of a DNA replication factor whose loss might account for disturbed growth), *LIMK1*

(OMIM 601329, encoding LIM kinase-1, a protein expressed in the brain that may be important in visual-spatial constructive cognition), *GTF2I* (OMIM 601679, a constituent of a growth factor signal transduction pathway whose hemizygous loss may contribute to developmental delay), *GTF2IRD1* (OMIM 604318, a transcription factor whose heterozygous loss may lead to abnormalities of neurologic development and craniofacial and somatic growth).

CYLN2 (OMIM 603432) is a cytoplasmic protein that links membranous organelles and microtubules and whose haploinsufficiency results in mild growth retardation and neural defects.[96] Microdeletions of chromosome 7q11.23 arise by unequal crossing over of chromosomal segments between homologous seventh chromosomes during meiosis or by intrachromosomal recombination. The Williams-Beuren phenotype has also been associated with interstitial deletion of chromosome 6q22.2q23 as well as defects in chromosomes 4, 11, and 22, implying that the syndrome is quite genetically heterogeneous (involving a number of genetic cascade systems). The diagnosis of the Williams-Beuren syndrome is suspected on the basis of the characteristic clinical phenotype (with/without hypercalcemia) and confirmed by demonstration of the microdeletion at chromosome 7q11.23 or of *ELN* by FISH, although a normal chromosome analysis does not entirely eliminate this diagnosis. Hypercalcemia is managed by ingestion of a low-calcium, vitamin-D-free formula. Occasionally, short-term glucocorticoid therapy may be necessary to restore eucalcemia.

Idiopathic infantile hypercalcemia is clinically similar to the Williams-Beuren syndrome (hypertension, hyperacusis, strabismus, radioulnar synostosis), and the distinction between the two entities is sometimes difficult.[79] Prolonged hypercalcemia and elevated serum concentrations of the amino-terminal fragment of PTHrP have been recorded in some children with this disorder in the absence of a neoplasm, but in the majority of patients the pathophysiology of this disorder is not known. In most patients, hypercalcemia resolves within the first several years of life (but may persist to older ages). Avoidance of vitamin D, low dietary calcium intake, and glucocorticoids to reduce intestinal absorption of calcium are therapeutic modalities for this disorder.

Antenatal Bartter syndromes, type 1 (OMIM 601678) and type 2 (OMIM 600839), are quite similar clinically and biochemically and are due to loss-of-function mutations in genes controlling transepithelial transport of chloride and potassium (respectively) across the renal tubular thick ascending limb of the loop of Henle (TALH). Affected fetuses develop polyhydramnios, leading to premature delivery with postnatal salt wasting, hypokalemic metabolic alkalosis, hypercalciuria (and occasionally hypercalcemia), failure to thrive, and often death. The type 1 disorder is due to inactivating mutations of the gene encoding sodium/potassium/chloride cotransporter-2 (*SLC12A1*)—the mediator of active reabsorption of sodium chloride in the TALH. The type 2 syndrome is due to an inactivating mutation in the gene encoding an inwardly rectifying potassium channel (*KCNJ1*).[97]

Hypokalemia (occasionally transient hyperkalemia in the type 2 syndrome), reduced intravascular volume, and increased levels of angiotensin sum to increase renal and systemic production of prostaglandin E2 that further inhibits sodium and chloride reabsorption in the TALH and enhances juxtaglomerular renin release. Hypochloremic, hypokalemic alkalosis, hyperprostaglandin E, hypercalciuria leading to nephrocalcinosis and osteopenia, and hypercalcemia suggest neonatal Bartter syndrome. Replacement of fluid and electrolytes and administration of potassium-sparing diuretics and the cyclooxygenase inhibitors (indomethacin or a specific inhibitor of cyclooxygenase type 2) are usually effective in ameliorating the biochemical and clinical manifestations of the disease.

Perinatal hypophosphatasia is a lethal disorder manifested during gestation by marked skeletal hypomineralization. At times only the base of the skull may be calcified. Usually, the calvarium and vertebrae are partially mineralized, rachitic changes are present at the distal ends of the long bones, and fractures are common.[98] Infantile hypophosphatasia (OMIM 241500) is an often fatal autosomal-recessive disorder recognized clinically by 6 months of age and characterized by rickets, demineralization of the calvarium and peripheral skeleton, increased intracranial pressure, flail chest, hypercalcemia, and hypercalciuria. Radiographically, spurs of cartilage and bone extend from the sides of the knee and elbow joints. The disease is due to defective osteoblast synthesis of tissue non-specific alkaline phosphatase because of loss-of-function missense, nonsense, and donor splice site mutations of ALPL.

The lethal homozygous or compound heterozygous mutations of ALPL are located within or near the enzyme domain and/or the homodimer and tetramer interfaces.[99,100] Decreased alkaline phosphatase activity leads to a deficit in phosphate ions for combination with calcium at the site of hydroxyapatite formation, whereas continued intestinal calcium absorption results in hypercalcemia. Inappropriately low serum bone alkaline phosphatase activity differentiates this condition from other rachitic states in which alkaline phosphatase activity is usually elevated.

Increased urine phosphoethanolamine and serum inorganic pyrophosphate and pyridoxal-5'-phosphate values are consistent with the diagnosis of hypophosphatasia, whereas analysis of ALPL identifies the gene mutation(s) itself. Hypophosphatasia can be diagnosed prenatally by ALPL genotyping.[98] The hypercalcemia of infantile hypophosphatasia is managed by hydration, diuretics that act at the TALH (e.g., furosemide), and administration of bisphosphonates (pamidronate), calcitonin, or glucocorticoids as necessary. Dietary calcium intake should be restricted, and vitamin D and its metabolites avoided. Bone marrow transplantation and stem cell boosts of transfused donor osteoblasts have also been used to treat affected patients.

Evaluation and Management

After completing the historical review (during which the family history is explored for members with mineral disorders and the patient's intake of calcium, phosphate, and vitamin D are estimated) and physical examination (searching for the facial and cardiovascular signs of

Williams-Beuren syndrome, the subcutaneous nodules associated with subcutaneous fat necrosis, or the deformities of metaphyseal chondrodysplasia and infantile hypophosphatasia), evaluation of the hypercalcemic neonate and infant continues with total calcium and Ca^{2+}_e, phosphate, alkaline phosphatase, PTH, calcidiol, and calcitriol measurements as indicated and appropriate (Figure 17-6). In infants with suspected Williams-Beuren syndrome, FISH analysis of chromosome 7q11.23 or for ELN should be undertaken.

Treatment of hypercalcemia in neonates and infants must be directed to its cause and severity. Use of a formula low in calcium and avoidance of vitamin D (excessive intake or sunlight) are helpful in the majority of neonates with modest hypercalcemia.[22] Significantly elevated serum calcium levels that must be rapidly decreased may require infusion of 0.9% sodium chloride (10–20 mL/kg over 1 hour), followed by an intravenous bolus injection of furosemide (1–2 mg/kg) when adequate urine flow has been established. Hydrocortisone (1 mg/kg intravenously every 6 hours) reduces intestinal calcium absorption, and salmon calcitonin (10 units/kg subcutaneously) inhibits calcium mobilization from bone.

Currently, bisphosphonates (analogs of pyrophosphate that adsorb to the surface of hydroxyapatite crystals in bone and inhibit osteoclast function and bone resorption) are the agents of choice for the treatment of

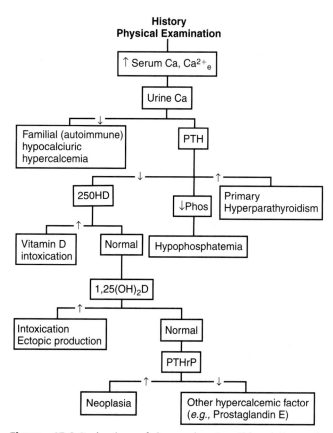

Figure 17-6 Evaluation of hypercalcemia. Abbreviations: Ca (serum total calcium), Ca^{2+}_e (extracellular ionized calcium), Phos (serum phosphate), PTH (parathyroid hormone), 25OHD [25-hydroxyvitamin D (calcidiol)], and 1,25(OH)₂ D-[1,2,5-RTHnP RTH related protein dihydroxyvitamin D (calcitriol)].

substantial hypercalcemia in infants. Etidronate (5 mg/kg twice daily orally) and pamidronate (0.5–2.0 mg/kg in 30 mL normal saline intravenously over 4 hours) have been successfully employed in infants with hypercalcemia due to vitamin D intoxication, subcutaneous fat necrosis, and other causes.[83,101-103] Parathyroidectomy may be urgently required in the newborn with NSHPT and life-threatening hypercalcemia.

DISORDERS OF BONE MINERALIZATION

Low Bone Mass and Rickets

Approximately 80% of total bone calcium in the full-term neonate is accrued in the last trimester of pregnancy as the in utero rate of calcium deposition increases more than twofold between 28 and 36 weeks of gestation. LBW (<1,500 g) and very low birth weight (VLBW <1,000 g) infants are particularly vulnerable to the development of bone disease of prematurity because they are unable to maintain the in utero rate of synthesis of organic bone matrix (osteoid) or the rate of calcium and phosphate deposition into osteoid from the minerals provided via the gastrointestinal tract or by parenteral nutrition.[104] Decreased calcification of bone matrix results in low bone mineral content (BMC), whereas depressed calcification of the cartilage growth plate leads to rickets and its characteristic deformities.

In general terms, osteopenia may be defined as too little bone tissue with decreased thickness of bone cortex and/or decreased thickness or number of bone trabeculae. Osteoporosis is present when bone mass is so low that fractures occur after minor trauma.[104] (Thus, in this population of LBW and VLBW neonates these terms are not necessarily defined by the same quantitative measurements of bone density as employed in adults.) Postpartum, hypocalcemia, and decrease in spontaneous movement against the force exerted by the muscular wall of the uterus depress the rate of bone mineral acquisition—whereas an increased rate of bone resorption further decreases skeletal mass in premature infants.[105,106]

Approximately 30% of preterm infants with birth weights <1,500 g develop bone disease.[107] Birth weight and rate of postnatal weight gain, as well as umbilical cord concentrations of IGF-I, are important determinants of bone mass in premature infants.[108,109] Necrotizing enterocolitis, a disorder that affects approximately 10% of LBW infants, increases the rate of bone resorption as assessed by measurement of serum (ICTP) and urinary (Dpd) markers of this process.[110] Interestingly, neonatal sepsis is not associated with increase in levels of bone resorption markers.[110,111] Malrotation of the intestinal tract or catastrophic necrotizing enterocolitis leading to intestinal infarction requiring extensive small bowel resection substantially increases the risk of malabsorption and subsequent low bone mass.

Parenteral alimentation of LBW or VLBW neonates restricts administration of fluid, calcium, and phosphate (in part, because of the incompatibility of the coinfusion of these ions in high concentrations). Excessive aluminum in parenteral fluids also adversely affects bone formation. Another factor that may contribute to the bone disease of

prematurity is decreased synthesis of glucagon-like peptide 2 (GLP2, OMIM 138030, chromosome 2q36-q37), a 33-aa post-translational derivative of proglucagon whose production is depressed by small intestinal resection or atrophy during prolonged parenteral alimentation. GLP-2 promotes intestinal calcium absorption and depresses osteoclastic activity.[110] Increased maternal parity, male gender, severe systemic disease (bronchopulmonary dysplasia), immobility, and pharmacologic agents (glucocorticoids, methylxanthines such as theophylline, diuretics such as furosemide) also adversely impact bone formation in these neonates.[106,112]

Theophylline and furosemide increase urinary excretion of calcium.[113] A polymorphic variant of estrogen receptor α with multiple TA repeats (>18) at 1174 bp upstream appears to protect LBW neonates from development of bone disease of prematurity, and a variant with a low number of TA repeats increases the risk of bone disease. The mechanism of this effect is not known at present.[107] Two prenatal factors that contribute to low bone mass in VLBW and LBW neonates include intrauterine growth retardation (possibly by reducing placental transport of calcium and decreasing the rate of bone formation) and prenatal exposure to large amounts of magnesium sulfate administered repeatedly to the mother in preterm labor that leads to hypocalcemia and osteopenia by suppressing PTH secretion through its interaction with the CaSR and by competing with calcium for deposition at bone surfaces, respectively.[114]

In preterm neonates, serum levels of total and bone-specific alkaline phosphatase, PICP, and osteocalcin (markers of osteoblast activity and bone formation) are elevated relative to full-term neonates and older infants and continue to rise over the first 10 weeks of life.[115] Urinary hydroxyproline and Pyr/Dpd values (markers of osteoclast activity and bone resorption) are also increased, although serum concentration of ICTP (another marker of bone resorption) decline during the first 10 weeks after premature delivery.

Overall, the data indicate that intrauterine and postnatal rates of bone turnover in preterm newborns are rapid and persistently elevated through 40 weeks postconceptual age—a conclusion confirmed by bone histomorphometry.[105,112,116] By photon absorptiometry and quantitative ultrasonography, bone mass of preterm infants appears to decline during the first several weeks after birth.[116a] Serum levels of alkaline phosphatase and osteocalcin and urinary excretion of Pyr and calcium may remain elevated in LBW infants with bone disease of prematurity relative to values in LBW infants without bone disease for the first year of life, even though radiographic improvement in skeletal mineralization is usually evident by 6 months of age.[107]

Because standard roentgenograms may not detect low bone mineralization before deficits of 20 to 30% or greater have occurred in the second month of life, estimation of BMC by dual-energy X-ray absorptiometry (DEXA) has become the preferred method of assessing bone mineralization in infants because of its accuracy, reproducibility, rapidity of performance, and low radiation exposure (2–3 mrems).[12,117] Mean total body BMC in the first 2 days of life ranges from 21.7 g in newborns with birth weights of 1,001 to 1,500 g to 78.8 g in neonates with birth weights of 3,501 to 4,000 g, whereas BMD varies from 0.146 mg/cm² (1,001–1,500 g) to 0.234 gm/cm² (3,501–4,000 g). In full-term healthy neonates, the mean whole-body BMC measured by newly introduced fan beam DEXA is 89.3 (SD ∀ 14.1) g.[118]

BMC and BMD increase through the first year of life and beyond as measured by DEXA (see Chapter 3, Table 8). No racial, gender, or seasonal factors affect bone mineralization at this age. Body weight is best correlated with bone mass.[119] There is increasing use of quantitative ultrasound (QUS) to assess bone integrity and strength in preterm and other LBW infants because the study may be performed at the crib side, there is no exposure to radiation, and it may be repeated as frequently as necessary.[120] QUS measures the speed of sound (SOS) through a bone (humerus, tibia, radius, patella, os calcis, metacarpal, phalanx), a measurement correlated with the strength of the bone. Mineral content is but one of several skeletal components (elasticity, cortical thickness, microstructure) that collectively contribute to bone strength.

QUS also permits calculation of bone transmission time, a measurement that determines the difference in the velocity of sound as it travels through bone and surrounding soft tissue. There is considerable overlap of SOS values at various ages and somatic sizes. However, bone transmission times may discriminate to a greater extent between these parameters. Humeral QUS measurements are lower in preterm than term infants and correlate positively with gestational age, length, and weight.[121] In neonates with intrauterine growth retardation, tibial SOS levels may be appropriate for gestational age or may even be elevated.[122,123]

With prolonged deprivation of calcium, phosphate, and vitamin D, not only does the LBW infant lag in accumulation of bone mass but clinical and radiographic evidence of rickets also develops—usually between the sixth and twelfth postnatal weeks—and fractures may occur in as many as 24% of VLBW infants.[116a] The LBW neonate at risk for low bone mass and/or rickets is best managed preventively by the daily enteral administration of as much of the needed amounts of calcium (140–160 mg/100 kcal), phosphate (95–108 mg/100 kcal of formula), and vitamin D (400 U)—as well as protein (for collagen synthesis) and energy (carbohydrates, lipids)—as possible.

When parenteral administration of nutrients is necessary in the LBW or VLBW neonate, an attempt should be made to administer the maximum amounts of calcium and phosphate safely attainable. The solubility of calcium and phosphate depends not only on their quantities but on the forms selected for infusion (i.e., calcium chloride, gluconate, glycerophosphate, monobasic phosphate, or dibasic phosphate). Utilizing monobasic phosphate and glycerophosphate, it is possible to infuse as much as 86 mg of calcium/kg/dL and 46 mg/kg/dL of phosphate.[12] Enteral feeding should begin as soon as possible in the LBW infant. Fortification of human breast milk with calcium glycerophosphate (calcium 170 mg/kg/day, phosphate 87 mg/kg/day) permits 57% absorption and 91% retention (88 mg/kg/day) of calcium and 94% absorption and 61% retention (50 mg/kg/day) of phosphate.[12]

Prepared formulas for feeding of LBW neonates can also provide up to 90 mg/kg/day of retained calcium and 40 mg/kg/day of retained phosphate. The type of prepared formula (sources of protein, fat, and carbohydrates) and its lipid and mineral additives determine the rate of intestinal calcium absorption and retention. Therefore, the choice of formula must be carefully considered before it is selected.[6] Nevertheless, parenteral nutrition, fortified human milk, and current preterm formulas are unable to provide the amounts of calcium and (in particular) phosphate that would normally accrue to the fetus in utero. Vitamin D 400 IU/day should also be provided to the preterm infant either enterally or parenterally.

Monitoring of serum levels of calcium, phosphate, creatinine, and alkaline phosphatase (and urinary excretion of calcium, phosphate, and creatinine) is essential in order to prevent hypercalcemia, hypercalciuria, and nephrocalcinosis. It is also important to avoid hypocalcemia because of the avidity of bone matrix for calcium once remineralization has commenced (hungry bone syndrome). Passive physical activity (daily range of motion with extension/flexion of all joints of each extremity in the supine infant for 4 weeks, beginning after the neonate has been stabilized between 2 and 6 weeks of postnatal age) with or without gentle massage of the prone infant from head to toe increases serum levels of markers of bone formation as well as bone mineralization by DEXA and QUS changes consistent with augmented bone strength.[116a,124]

Administration of estrogen and progesterone to VLBW female infants in sufficient amounts to maintain intrauterine levels of these hormones for 6 weeks postnatally does not increase the retention of calcium or phosphate during this interval or bone mineralization in later infancy.[125,126] The efficacy and safety of bisphosphonates or of PTH[1-34] in the management of osteopenia of prematurity remain to be examined. Although in the prematurely born infant bone mass may remain low through infancy and early childhood, bone mineralization eventually catches up to the norms.[127-130]

Osteogenesis imperfecta congenita (OIC) [type II (OMIM 166210)] is a perinatal lethal disorder most commonly associated with heterozygous newly developed loss-of-function mutations in the genes encoding collagen-α1(I) (COL1A) or collagen-α2(I) (COL1A2). The mutations may be partial gene deletions resulting in decreased synthesis of type I collagen or missense mutations that lead to amino acid substitutions (e.g., arginine, aspartic acid, cysteine) for the glycine residues essential to the normal three-dimensional conformation of collagen-α1(I) and synthesis of the triple helix and structural integrity of type I collagen in extracellular matrix of bone upon which hydroxyapatite is deposited. Osteogenesis imperfecta type II may rarely be transmitted as an autosomal-dominant trait by a parent mosaic for a heterozygous mutation in collagen-α1(I) or -α2(I).[131]

Clinical manifestations of OIC are variable and include fractures present at birth (which may also occur in newborns with osteogenesis imperfecta types I and III), deformities of the long bones, osteopenia of the skull with large fontanelles, intrauterine growth retardation, premature delivery, and death (usually in infancy) due to respiratory insufficiency. Radiologically, OIC has been categorized into three subgroups: A (short, broad, and crumpled long bones, angulation of the tibia, and continuous beading of the ribs), B (similar femoral and tibial configurations but incomplete beading of the ribs), and C (thin long bones with many fractures and thin beaded ribs). The diagnosis of OIC is most often made clinically by its differentiation from campomelic dysplasia, achondrogenesis type I, thanatophoric dysplasia, and perinatal hypophosphatasia and is confirmed by quantitation of subnormal amounts of collagen synthesis by fibroblasts in vitro and identification of the mutation in *COL1A1* or *COL1A2* by direct genotyping.

The lethal mutations in collagen-α1(I) are clustered at sites at which the collagen monomer binds integrins, matrix metalloproteinases, fibronectin, and cartilage oligomeric matrix protein. Those in collagen-α2(I) coincide with binding sites for proteoglycans. Administration of the bisphosphonate pamidronate has been helpful in infants with severe manifestations of osteogenesis imperfecta types III and IV but has been ineffective in the lethal form of osteogenesis imperfecta type II.[132,133]

Lysinuric protein intolerance (OMIM 222700) is an autosomal-recessive disorder of hepatic and renal tubular transport of dibasic amino acids (lysine, arginine, ornithine) that manifests itself in infancy and childhood by vomiting, diarrhea, failure to thrive, developmental delay, hepatomegaly, and cirrhosis. Affected infants and children have impaired urea synthesis due to decreased hepatic uptake of ornithine but are episodically hyperammonemic with increased urinary excretion of the dibasic amino acids. There is extremely low bone mass due to marked protein deprivation and perhaps due to increase in cytokine-induced bone resorption.[134] Administration of citrulline has been reported to increase growth and bone mass in some of these patients. Lysine protein intolerance is due to loss-of-function deletion, duplication, missense, nonsense, and splice-site mutations in *SLC7A7* encoding an amino acid transporter.[135]

INCREASED BONE MASS

Increased bone mass may be generalized or localized. Osteosclerosis refers to thickening of trabecular bone, and hyperostosis refers to increase in cortical bone mass.[136] The infantile malignant form of osteopetrosis (OMIM 259700) is an autosomal-recessive disorder due to abnormal osteoclast differentiation or function resulting in defective resorption of the mineral phase of bone. Affected infants manifest failure to thrive, delayed development, nasal obstruction, loss of sight, hearing and other cranial nerve functions, and intense bone overgrowth leading to pancytopenia and increased susceptibility to infection, hepatosplenomegaly as sites of extramedullary hematopoiesis, increased susceptibility to fracture because of decreased bone strength despite high bone mass, mandibular osteomyelitis, and death (often within the first several years of life) due to sepsis, anemia, or hemorrhage.

Physical examination reveals impaired linear growth, enlarged head circumference, nystagmus, and hepatosplenomegaly. The radiographic hallmark of infantile osteopetrosis is relatively uniform increase in bone density of the skull, vertebrae, and axial skeleton, Ehrlenmeyer flask deformity at the distal ends of the long bones

in older children, and alternating bands of sclerotic and lucent bone in the iliac wings. This usually lethal form of osteopetrosis may be due to homozygous or compound heterozygous loss-of-function mutations in one of three genes: *TCIRG1, CLCN7,* and *OSTM1. TCIRG1* encodes a subunit of the vacuolar proton pump within the osteoclast ruffled border through which hydrogen ions are transported from the cytosol into the subosteoclast resorption lacuna.

CLCN7 encodes a chloride channel required for movement of this cation into and acidification of the resorption lacuna. *OSTM1* encodes a subunit of CLCN7 necessary to its normal post-translational processing. In selected subjects, bone marrow transplantation effectively supplies sufficient osteoclast precursors to halt the progression of this disorder—albeit often with substantial residual deficits. Transient but substantial hypercalcemia may occur after this procedure. Osteopetrosis (OMIM 259730) due to deficiency of *CA2* encoding carbonic anhydrase II may present in infancy with failure to thrive or fracture with insignificant trauma. Disproportionate short stature is the cardinal manifestation of pycnodysostosis (OMIM 265800) and is manifest during infancy or early childhood.[136]

In subjects with pycnodysostosis, there is relative macrocranium with open fontanelles and cranial sutures, dysmorphic facial features (fronto-occipital prominence, proptosis, bluish sclerae, hypoplastic maxilla, micrognathia, highly arched palate, malocclusion, beaked nose), stubby and clubbed fingers with hypoplastic nails, narrow thorax, pectus excavatum, lumbar lordosis, kyphoscoliosis, and increased fracture risk. Radiographically, there is marked osteosclerosis that increases with age, open fontanelles and cranial sutures, thin clavicles with hypoplastic lateral ends, erosion and hypoplasia of the distal phalanges and ribs, and dense vertebrae yet normal transverse processes. Histologically, there are decreased numbers of osteoblastic and osteoclastic activity.

Pycnodysostosis is due to homozygous or compound heterozygous loss-of-function mutations (stop, missense, nonsense) in *CTSK*, the gene encoding cathepsin K—a lysosomal cysteine protease expressed in osteoclasts. Loss of cathepsin K activity impairs degradation of collagen and the resorption of organic matrix but not that of the mineral component of bone.[137] Isolated decreased stimulated secretion of GH has been recorded in some subjects. Administration of GH has improved the rate of linear growth of some patients with pycnodysostosis, but no effective treatment of the abnormal bone mineralization has been reported.[138]

Disorders of Magnesium Metabolism

In serum, magnesium is present complexed to proteins and ionized or free. Approximately 50% of body magnesium stores are deposited within bone adsorbed to the surface of hydroxyapatite. The CaSR binds magnesium as well as calcium. Magnesium regulates the secretion but not the synthesis of PTH and the generation of calcitriol.[20] In addition, experimental magnesium deficiency leads to decreased bone mineralization in mice, and magnesium oxide supplements increase BMC in healthy girls.[139,140]

HYPOMAGNESEMIA

Hypomagnesemia (serum total magnesium concentration <1.5 mg/dL) leads to hypocalcemia by inhibiting the release of PTH and by interfering with its peripheral action and may mimic congenital hypoparathyroidism, which is itself often associated with hypomagnesemia. In neonates and infants, hypomagnesemia may be clinically silent or present with neuromuscular irritability or seizures often in association with hypocalcemia. Hypomagnesemia occurs in infants born to mothers deficient in magnesium, those with preeclampsia or gestational or type 1 diabetes mellitus, and in neonates with low birth weight (prematurity or intrauterine growth retardation).[141]

Prolonged nasogastric suctioning, malabsorption disorders due to extensive intestinal resection (short gut syndrome), intestinal fistulas, or other diseases associated with chronic diarrhea and steatorrhea also lead to infantile hypomagnesemia. In renal tubular disorders such as Gitelman (OMIM 263800) and Bartter (OMIM 242200) syndromes, as well as in subjects exposed to diuretics and nephrotoxic (cisplatin, cyclosporin, mercury, gentamycin) agents, hypermagnesuria leads to hypomagnesemia.[97,142]

In children and adolescents, hypomagnesemia is manifested by heightened neuromuscular irritability (carpal pedal spasm, tetany, seizures)—and when prolonged and profound by muscle wasting, weakness, apathy, and tachycardia with prolonged PR and QT intervals by electrocardiography. In these age groups, hypomagnesemia may be primary and due to a specific defect in the intestinal absorption of magnesium or in the renal tubular resorption of filtered magnesium. It may also be secondary and due to gastrointestinal losses (chronic vomiting or diarrhea or malabsorptive states due to inflammatory bowel disease, bowel resection or fistulas, or pancreatitis); to associated renal tubulopathies (Gitelman and Bartter syndromes); to exposure to alcohol, diuretics, and chemotherapeutic agents; or to specific endocrinopathies (diabetes mellitus, primary hyperparathyroidism, hyperaldosteronism).[143]

Familial hypomagnesemia with hypocalcemia (OMIM 602014) is an autosomal-recessive disorder pathophysiologically due to a selective small intestinal defect in magnesium absorption. The disease presents with hypocalcemic tetany and/or seizures in the neonatal period and can lead to myocardial, renal, and arterial calcinosis. Renal excretion of magnesium is normal in subjects with this disease. Hypocalcemia is attributable to decreased secretion of and peripheral sensitivity to PTH. This disorder is due to biallelic loss-of-function mutations in *TRPM6* (transient receptor potential cation channel, subfamily M, member 6), encoding a 2,022-aa bifunctional protein with two domains: a calcium- and magnesium-permeable ion channel domain and a protein tyrosine kinase domain expressed in the kidney and colon.[144]

For full functional activity, TRMP6 must team with its homolog TRPM7 (OMIM 605692) and form a functional TRPM6/TRPM7 complex at the surface of the cell.[145] Although most mutations of *TRPM6* associated with this disease (nonsense, deletion) have resulted in extensive loss of product, the naturally occurring missense mutation Ser141Leu specifically disrupts formation of the complex. Oral ingestion of large quantities of magnesium is

effective therapy for this illness. Primary hypomagnesemia (OMIM 248250) is an autosomal-recessive disorder due to decreased renal tubular resorption of filtered magnesium linked to biallelic loss-of-function mutations in *CLDN16*.[146]

This disease often presents in infancy and is associated with tetany, hypermagnesuria, hypercalciuria, mild hypocalcemia, nephrocalcinosis, impaired renal function, and secondary hyperparathyroidism. Claudin 16 (also termed paracellin 1) is a 305-aa protein with four transmembrane domains and intracellular amino and carboxyl terminals that is expressed within the intercellular tight junctions of renal epithelial cells in the TALH and distal convoluted tubule, where it facilitates paracellular transport and reabsorption of magnesium and calcium from the renal tubule. The first extracellular loop of claudin 16 bridges the intercellular space and is the site of paracellular conductance of ions. A number of missense mutations in *CLDN16* have been identified in this gene, particularly at leucine 151 (Leu151Phe, Leu151Trp, Leu151Pro).[147]

Most of the mutations in *CLDN16* impair its normal movement to the renal epithelial cell's lateral surface. In other mutations (Ala62Val, His71Asp), products localize to the tight junctions but are functionally defective.[148] Oral administration of 20 times the normal daily requirement of magnesium has been successful therapy in these subjects.[149] Hypomagnesemia, hypercalciuria, and visual impairment (macular colobomata, myopia, nystagmus; OMIM 248190) have been associated with loss-of-function mutations in CLDN19—a second renal epithelial tight junction protein localized to the distal renal tubule and eye and necessary for paracellular transport of calcium and magnesium.[150] Calcium and magnesium are also reabsorbed from the renal tubule by transcellular passage from apical to basolateral surfaces of the renal epithelial cell.

The presence of hypomagnesemia is identified by measurement of serum magnesium concentrations, whereas its pathophysiologic etiology is determined by concurrent assay of calcium, phosphate, sodium, potassium, chloride, bicarbonate, creatinine, PTH, and vitamin D levels and assessment of its urinary loss and intestinal absorption.[141] Hypomagnesemic hypocalcemic seizures are only transiently responsive and sometimes resistant to parenteral administration of elemental calcium alone. Intravenous or intramuscular administration of a 50% solution of magnesium sulfate ($MgSO_4.7H_2O$ 0.05–0.1 mL/kg, or 2.5–5.0 mg/kg elemental magnesium with cardiac monitoring) is often necessary to control convulsions in the hypomagnesemic neonate.[20,141] Oral magnesium supplements may also be helpful (50% $MgSO_4.7H_2O$, 0.2 mL/kg/day). Chronic hypomagnesemic states are treated with oral magnesium supplements as tolerated because large doses may lead to diarrhea.

HYPERMAGNESEMIA

Hypermagnesemia (>2.5 mg/dL) is frequently recorded in the neonatal period because magnesium sulfate has been administered to pregnant women with hypertension, preeclampsia, or toxemia of pregnancy. Most neonates with hypermagnesemia are asymptomatic. However, when serum magnesium concentrations are exceptionally high hypotonia and depression of the central nervous system may be present—and when extended, metabolic bone disease may develop.[141] Thus, prolonged (9–10 weeks) administration of intravenous magnesium sulfate to women with multiple fetuses who have entered labor prematurely has been associated not only with hypermagnesemia but with marked hypocalcemia in the offspring (and with significant osteopenia).[114]

Hypermagnesemia may also result from its parenteral administration or oral ingestion of magnesium-containing antiacids or enemas. In large amounts, magnesium sulfate suppresses secretion of PTH and decreases renal tubular reabsorption of calcium—factors contributing to hypocalcemia. The hypermagnesemic neonate is most appropriately managed by adequate hydration to permit urinary excretion of the high magnesium load. If the newborn is also hypocalcemic and osteopenic, administration of calcium and calcitriol is indicated. Hypermagnesemia may also develop in patients with renal insufficiency receiving magnesium-containing antiacids. Magnesium concentrations are modestly increased in patients with familial hypocalciuric hypercalcemia.

Disorders of Mineral Homeostasis in the Child and Adolescent

HYPOCALCEMIA

Etiology

Causes of hypocalcemia in the child and adolescent are listed in Table 17-1. Hypocalcemia is defined by the norms of the analytical laboratory and is dependent on the age of the subject (total calcium concentrations: 1–5 years, 9.4–10.8; 6–12 years, 9.4–10.2; >20 years, 8.8–10.2 mg/dL).[22] Total calcium levels are low in the hypoalbuminemic patient. A correction for hypoalbuminemia may be calculated by adding 0.8 mg/dL to the recorded total calcium concentration for every decrease in albumin concentration of 1 g/dL.[151] For this and other reasons, it is appropriate to measure total and Ca^{2+}_e values when evaluating the hypocalcemic child. However, reliance on Ca^{2+}_e determinations alone is discouraged given the technical difficulties with this assay.

Hypocalcemia develops as a consequence of too little inflow of calcium from the gastrointestinal tract, bone, or kidney into the extracellular and vascular spaces or excessive loss of calcium from these spaces into urine, stool, and bone. Thus, hypocalcemia may be due to decreased intake or absorption or excessive loss of calcium, decreased production of bioactive PTH due to congenital abnormalities of PTG development or PTH synthesis or of the CaSR, destruction of PTGs by autoantibodies, metal overload (copper, iron), surgical or radiation insults, granulomatous infiltration, or impaired cellular responsiveness to PTH. Restricted exposure to sunlight or reduced intake, absorption, metabolism, or activity of vitamin D leads to hypocalcemia.

Hypomagnesemia impairs the secretion of (but not the synthesis of PTH), and blunts tissue responsiveness to,

PTH. Hypocalcemia occurs in the very ill child or after exposure to a number of drugs and medications. Hypocalcemic tetany may develop after the administration of phosphate-containing enemas by rectum or laxatives by mouth.[152] At times, the hypocalcemic child or adolescent may be asymptomatic and identified by chemical screening for an unrelated problem—or may present with intermittent muscular cramping at rest or during exercise (when the increase in systemic pH due to hyperventilation lowers still further the concentration of Ca^{2+}_e); paresthesias of fingers, toes, or circumoral regions; tetany (carpopedal spasm, laryngospasm, bronchospasm); or seizures (grand mal, focal, petit mal, adynamic, or syncopal). Physical examination often reveals a positive Chvostek and/or Trousseau sign (carpopedal spasm) and hyperreflexia. However, a Chvostek sign is commonly present in normal adolescents also.

Hypoparathyroidism may occur as a solitary disorder, as part of a multidimensional autoimmune polyendocrinopathy, or as one manifestation of a group of complex congenital anomalies (DiGeorge, HRD, Kenny-Caffey, Barakat, Blomstrand, and other syndromes). There are sporadic and familial forms of hypoparathyroidism. When familial, hypoparathyroidism may be transmitted as an autosomal-dominant, autosomal-recessive, or X-linked recessive trait (Tables 17-1 and 17-2). Abnormalities in the development of the PTGs, transcription of PTH, and processing of the translated product have been associated with inherited forms of hypoparathyroidism.

In a family with autosomal-dominant dyshormonogenic hypoparathyroidism, a $T\Psi C$ transition in codon 18 of the 25-aa signal peptide of prepro-PTH that altered cysteine to arginine (Cys18Arg) has been identified.[153] This heterozygous mutation within the hydrophobic region (aa 10 to 21) of the signal sequence (a domain necessary for efficient transport of protein from the ribosome and interaction of prepro-PTH with the signal recognition particle) impairs movement of the precursor peptide into and exit from the rough endoplasmic reticulum, its cleavage by a signal peptidase, and its incorporation into a secretory granule.[154] The autosomal-dominant transmission of hypoparathyroidism in this family suggests that the mutant pre-pro-PTH exerted a dominant-negative effect on the synthesis of normal PTH directed by the wild-type allele.

Autosomal-recessive dyshormonogenic hypoparathyroidism has been associated with a homozygous $G\Psi C$ transversion in nucleotide 1 of intron 2 of PTH within the signal sequence that prevented normal cleavage of prepro-PTH and decreased secretion of PTH.[155] However, inactivating mutations in PTH are uncommon in patients with sporadic idiopathic hypoparathyroidism.[156] Isolated hypoparathyroidism may be found in patients with del22q11.2 but no other signs or symptoms of the DGS or the velocardiofacial syndrome.[157]

Autosomal-dominant hypoparathyroidism (OMIM 146200) due to heterozygous gain-of-function mutations in the extracellular, transmembrane, and intracellular domains of *CASR* (OMIM 600199) that transcribe a CaSR that is not intrinsically constitutively active but is exceptionally sensitive to and easily activated by very low serum Ca^{2+}_e concentrations may be identified in infancy or in

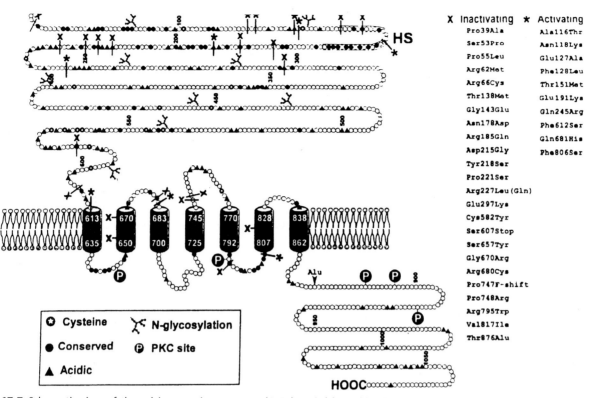

X Inactivating	★ Activating
Pro39Ala	Ala116Thr
Ser53Pro	Asn118Lys
Pro55Leu	Glu127Ala
Arg62Met	Phe128Leu
Arg66Cys	Thr151Met
Thr138Met	Glu191Lys
Gly143Glu	Gln245Arg
Asn178Asp	Phe612Ser
Arg185Gln	Gln681His
Asp215Gly	Phe806Ser
Tyr218Ser	
Pro221Ser	
Arg227Leu(Gln)	
Glu297Lys	
Cys582Tyr	
Ser607Stop	
Ser657Tyr	
Gly670Arg	
Arg680Cys	
Pro747F-shift	
Pro748Arg	
Arg795Trp	
Val817Ile	
Thr876Alu	

Figure 17-7 Schematic view of the calcium-sensing receptor (CaSR). Gain(*)- and loss(X)-of-function missense and nonsense mutations associated with autosomal-dominant hypoparathyroidism, familial hypocalciuric hypercalcemia, and neonatal severe hyperparathyroidism are depicted. Abbreviations: NCM (normal amino acid-codon-mutation), SP (signal peptide), and HS (hydrophobic segment). [Reproduced with permission from Brown EM, et al. (1997). Familial benign hypocalciuric hypercalcemia and other syndromes of altered responsiveness to extracellular calcium. In Krane SM, Avioli LV (eds.), *Metabolic bone diseases, Third edition.* San Diego: Academic Press 479–499.]

older subjects (Figure 17-7).[84] Even at hypocalcemic levels, Ca^{2+}_e binds avidly to the CaSR and activates phospholipase C-β1—increasing cytosolic levels of inositol phosphate and Ca^{2+}_i and stimulating the mitogen-activated protein kinase (MAPK) signal transduction pathway in parathyroid chief cells (suppressing PTH synthesis and secretion). In the kidney, it decreases renal tubular calcium and magnesium resorption—leading to urinary wasting of these cations (hypercalciuric hypocalcemia). Urinary concentrating ability is also depressed.

Serum levels of phosphate are increased and magnesium values decreased. PTH concentrations are low or inappropriately normal in these subjects. Affected patients frequently have symptomatic hypocalcemia such as tetany and seizures. They are very sensitive to vitamin D, and its administration can lead to hypercalciuria (even when serum calcium levels remain subnormal), nephrocalcinosis, and functional renal insufficiency. Administration of recombinant human (rh)PTH[1-34] restores calcium homeostasis in this disorder, although experience with treatment in childhood is limited at present.[47,158] There has been reluctance to administer rhPTH to children because there is an increased incidence of bone tumors in young rats receiving very large amounts of this agent. However, primates appear to be less susceptible to PTH-induced bone tumor formation than rodents.[159]

Development of stimulatory autoantibodies to the CaSR results in an acquired variant of spontaneous hypoparathyroidism that may be isolated or part of a complex autoimmune endocrinopathy.[160,161] Indeed, in perhaps as many as one-third of patients with acquired isolated idiopathic hypoparathyroidism antibodies directed against epitopes in the extracellular domain of the CaSR may be present. This form of acquired hypoparathyroidism may be reversible, as these antibodies do not destroy the PTGs. In patients with other forms of autoimmune hypoparathyroidism, the antibodies are likely cytotoxic and accompanied by lymphocytic infiltration, atrophy, and fatty replacement of parathyroid tissue.

In mid-childhood and adolescence, acquired hypoparathyroidism may be a late manifestation of a congenital abnormality (e.g., DGS). However, it is also likely to be the result of destruction of the PTGs by autoimmune disease or surgical removal or operative trauma to the vascular supply of these structures. Unusual causes of acquired hypoparathyroidism in this age group include infiltration by iron (hemochromatosis, thalassemia) or copper (Wilson's hepatolenticular degeneration), granulomatous diseases, or radiation (mantle radiation for Hodgkin/non-Hodgkin lymphoma or radioiodine therapy of hyperthyroidism).[162,163]

Autoimmune hypoparathyroidism may occur as an isolated disorder or as part of the complex of autoimmune polyendocrinopathy syndrome type I.[163,164] Development of an autoimmune endocrinopathy begins with presentation of a peptide specific for a target organ to a subgroup of T cells that recognize that peptide. When immunologic tolerance for that peptide is lost, clones of

CD4 T cells for the peptide expand. Type 1 helper T cells secrete inflammatory cytokines such as interferon-γ, whereas type 2 helper T cells stimulate B-cell function and lead to autoantibody-mediated inflammation. Loss of immune tolerance may be the consequence of the postinfectious inflammatory state due to activation of the innate immune system or due to a gene mutation that depresses immune tolerance and permits expansion of a CD4 T-cell clone after exposure to quantitatively small amounts of antigen.

Genetic variations within the major histocompatibility complex (HLA-DQ, HLA-DR) that determines peptide (antigen) presentation to CD4 T cells join with genetic abnormalities in immune regulation to induce autoimmune disease. As noted, in 30% of patients with isolated idiopathic hypoparathyroidism the disorder is due to antibodies to the extracellular domain of the CaSR and thus functionally inhibitory but potentially reversible. In approximately 33% of patients, serum antibodies to other components of the parathyroid chief cell may be present.[160,161]

Autoimmune polyendocrinopathy syndrome type I (OMIM 240300) is an autosomal-recessive disorder with the classic triad of autoimmune polyendocrinopathy, mucocutaneous candidiasis, and ectodermal dystrophy (APECED).[165] In a Finnish cohort of 91 patients with APECED, the cardinal manifestations were mucocutaneous candidiasis involving the nails and mouth occurring in 100% of patients (often in the first two years of life), hypoparathyroidism, and hypoadrenocorticism (both of the latter illnesses developed in 80% to 90% of affected subjects).[166] Hypoparathyroidism occurred most often between 2 and 10 years of age, and hypoadrenocorticism developed between 5 and 15 years of age.

Almost all females with APECED developed hypoparathyroidism, whereas 80% of affected males did so. Hypomagnesemia, often severe and recalcitrant to therapy, was common in patients with hypoparathyroidism due to APECED. The most frequent presenting manifestations of APECED were mucocutaneous candidasis (60%), hypoparathyroidism (32%), and hypoadrenocorticism (5%). The disease first became apparent between 2 months and 18 years of age. However, 10% of patients presented with another manifestation of APECED. In addition to hypoparathyroidism and hypoadrenocorticism, other endocrinopathies encountered in APECED included autoimmune oophoritis leading to ovarian failure (70%), orchitis resulting in testicular failure (30%), diabetes mellitus (30%), thyroiditis (30%), and hypophysitis (4%). Besides mucocutaneous candidiasis, dermatologic manifestations and complications of APECED in the Finnish cohort included alopecia (40%), vitiligo (30%), and rashes with fever (15%).

Keratoconjunctivitis developed in 20% of affected subjects, pernicious anemia in 30%, hepatitis in 20%, and chronic diarrhea in 20%. In a Norwegian population of 36 patients with APECED, 13 had clinical evidence of disease at or before 5 years of age—and an additional 15 subjects presented at or before 15 years of age.[167] Clinical manifestations of APECED and their age of onset vary between subjects and even between siblings. Later manifestations of APECED include esophageal and oral squamous cell carcinoma, asplenia, and interstitial nephritis. The diagnosis of APECED usually requires the presence of two of three of its primary manifestations (mucocutaneous candidiasis, hypoparathyroidism, hypoadrenocorticism), but occasionally hypoparathyroidism may be its only sign.

Autoimmune polyendocrinopathy syndrome type I is due to homozygous or compound heterozygous loss-of-function mutations in *AIRE* (autoimmune regulator), a 14-exon gene with 1,635 base pairs encoding a 545-aa with two zinc-finger motifs that is expressed in nuclei of thymic medullary epithelial cells and in lymph nodes, spleen, monocytes, and other tissues where it functions as a transcription factor.[168] AIRE also serves as an E3 ubiquitin ligase, an essential component of the ubiquitin-proteasomal system for protein modification and destruction involved in cellular division and differentiation, protein transport, and intracellular signaling.[169]

Structurally, AIRE contains two plant homeodomains in an amino acid sequence composed of an octet of cysteines and histidines that coordinate two zinc ions. The first plant homeodomain is essential to the E3 ubiquitin ligase activity of the protein, and the second plant homeodomain is required for its transcription-regulating action. Functionally, AIRE may assist in the elimination of forbidden clones of T cells from the thymus—or it might promote expression of peripheral antigens in the thymus, thereby increasing immune tolerance.[164] In the Finnish population with APECED, the most common loss-of-function mutation in *AIRE* was a homozygous truncating mutation at codon 257 (Arg257Ter). More than 55 pathogenic mutations in *AIRE* [missense, nonsense (Arg139Ter), insertion, and deletion (e.g., 13 base pair deletion; 964del13, NT 1094, exon 8)] that alter the subcellular distribution of AIRE and/or decrease its transcriptional activation capacity and/or its E3 ubiquitin ligase activity have been detected in patients with APECED.[168,169]

Pseudohypoparathyroidism (PHP) is a heterogeneous group of disorders associated with resistance to the action of PTH—classified as types IA, IB, IC, and II and pseudopseudohypoparathyroidism (PPHP). PHP is due to inactivating mutations in *GNAS* (guanine nucleotide-binding protein, α-stimulating activity polypeptide 1). PHP type IA (OMIM 103580) is the result of heterozygous inactivating mutations in *GNAS,* a gene with a complex structure of 13 exons that encodes the α subunit of stimulatory G protein ($G_s\alpha$).[170,171] After binding of PTH to the PTHR1, the receptor is linked through its carboxyl terminal to a stimulatory signal transduction protein whose $G_s\alpha$ subunit then binds guanosine triphosphate (GTP). GTP-binding proteins (G proteins) are heterotrimers with α, β, and γ subunits. Individual genes encode each of 16 α, 5 β, and 11 γ peptides—leading to multiple potential combinations and functions primarily defined by the Gα subunit.[172]

After binding of PTH (or PTHrP) to PTHR1, there is a change in the three-dimensional configuration of PTHR1 leading to replacement of guanosine diphosphate (GDP) on $G_s\alpha$ by GTP. $G_s\alpha$ then dissociates from its βγ companion subunit complex and stimulates membrane-bound adenylyl cyclase activity, generating in turn cyclic adenosine monophosphate (AMP) and activating protein kinase A and phosphorylating serine and tyrosine residues of specific proteins. Interaction of PTH with its receptor also leads to activation of $G_q\alpha$ and $G_{11}\alpha$, with stimulation of phospholipase C and breakdown of membrane phosphoinositides resulting in increase in intracellular $Ca^{2+}{}_i$ levels and stimulation of signal transduction pathways that lead to cellular action and the physiologic response(s) to PTH. $G_s\alpha$ has two distinct domains. One of these is a GTPase domain that degrades GTP to inactive GDP, thus terminating $G_s\alpha$ activity. Within this domain are binding sites for GTP/GDP, the GPCR, and the intracellular second messenger effector protein.

The second domain is a helical domain that may be necessary for maintenance of guanine nucleotide binding.[173] Upstream (5') of exon 2 of *GNAS* are four alternative first exons that can link to exons 2 through 13 of *GNAS*. The most upstream of these promoters is termed *NESP55*, which generates a transcript for a chromogranin-like protein with a coding region limited to the specific first exon. Exons 2 through 13 form its 3' untranslated region (Figure 17-8). NESP55 is expressed in neuroendocrine tissues and is parentally imprinted. Thus, it is only expressed by the maternally transmitted allele. (There is also a NESP antisense transcript in this region.)

The next promoter (XLαs) yields a $G_s\alpha$ isoform also specific for neuroendocrine tissues and identical to $G_s\alpha$ except that it has a very long amino terminal sequence of amino acids. XLαs is also imprinted. It is expressed only by the paternally acquired allele. Exon 1A contains a differentially methylated region (DMR) that is methylated on the maternal allele and unmethylated on the paternal allele and is expressed only by the paternal allele. Exon 1A generates an untranslated mRNA transcript. Exon 1 (and thus $G_s\alpha$) is generally expressed in most tissues by both parental alleles.

However, in the renal proximal tubules, thyroid, pituitary, and ovaries $G_s\alpha$ is expressed primarily by the maternal allele.[171] Tissue-specific parental imprinting of $G_s\alpha$ is not related to differential methylation within its CpG island but rather with differences in the extent of methylation of histone H3 lysine 4 in the region of exon 1 of *GNAS*. Thus, *GNAS* has several independent imprinting

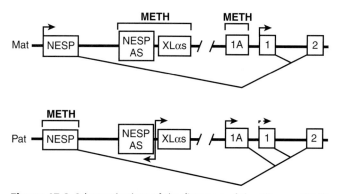

Figure 17-8 Schematic view of the first two of the 13-exon *GNAS* gene complex. Three alternate exons (NESP55, XLas, and 1A) are upstream of exon 1. The pattern of methylation, and hence the expression of the alternate exons, is dependent on the parent of origin of the allele and the specific tissue in which GNAS is expressed. [Reproduced with permission from Weinstein LS, Liu J, Sakamoto A, et al. (2004). GNAS: Normal and abnormal functions. Endocrinology 145:5459–5464.]

sites and mechanisms. Bioactive isoforms of $G_s\alpha$ are also formed by inclusion (long transcript variant of $G_s\alpha$ = $G_s\alpha$-L) or exclusion (short transcript variant of $G_s\alpha$ = $G_s\alpha$-S) of exon 3 in the mRNA transcript.[174]

Patients with PHP type IA have the distinct phenotype of Albright hereditary osteodystrophy (AHO), including short stature, husky to obese body habitus, shortening of the third through fifth metacarpal bones and distal phalanx of the first finger (brachydactyly), syndactyly between the second and third toes, round face, flat nasal bridge, short neck, subcutaneous calcifications (heterotopic ossification), and cataracts—and in some subjects developmental delay in association with hypocalcemia, hyperphosphatemia, hyperphosphaturia, and elevated serum concentrations of PTH. Administration of exogenous PTH ($rhPTH^{1-34}$) does not increase serum concentrations of calcium or urinary excretion of nephrogenous cyclic AMP or phosphate.

The phenotype of AHO but with normal serum calcium, phosphate, and PTH concentrations and response to exogenous PTH^{1-34} is termed PPHP. Normocalcemic PHP (eucalcemia with elevated serum concentration of PTH) has also been described.[174] Clinically, subnormal thyroid function with hyperthyrotropinemia is a common presenting manifestation of PHP type IA—particularly in infants less than 2 years of age.[175] Subcutaneous calcifications also appear early in life. Hypocalcemia is commonly identified in infancy but may not be recognized until mid-childhood or early adolescence.

Heterozygous loss-of-function mutations in *GNAS* (nonsense, missense, splice site, and base pair deletions) have been identified throughout the genomic structure of *GNAS* in subjects with PHP-IA and PPHP. These mutations lead to abnormal transcription and translation of *GNAS* and decreased expression of the mutated allele, resulting in approximately 50% of normal $G_s\alpha$ activity in most cells. Because $G_s\alpha$ is essential for normal chondrocyte differentiation by mediating the effects of PTH and PTHrP on this process, the skeletal manifestations of AHO reflect partial loss of $G_s\alpha$ activity in chondrocytes.[176]

If the mutated *GNAS* allele is of maternal origin, the kidney, thyroid, pituitary, and ovary have extremely low levels of $G_s\alpha$ activity and function in these tissues is almost nil—resulting in renal tubular resistance to PTH, thyroid insensitivity to thyroid-stimulating hormone, somatotroph resistance to GH-releasing hormone, and ovarian resistance to gonadotropins.[173,177,178] Thus, PHP type IA occurs in the offspring when mutated *GNAS* is transmitted from mother to child. In PPHP, the clinical phenotype is that of AHO but the patient is eucalcemic. Because the mutated *GNAS* has been transmitted from father to child and the proximal renal tubule, thyroid gland, pituitary somatotroph, and ovary express the intact maternal *GNAS* allele, near-normal $G_s\alpha$ activity is retained in these tissues. However, chondrocyte differentiation is impaired because in this tissue *GNAS* is expressed from both the maternal and paternal alleles and levels of $G_s\alpha$ activity are only one-half normal.

Mutations in $G_s\alpha$ can also result in progressive osseous heteroplasia (POH, OMIM 166350)—severe ectopic ossification of skin, skeletal muscle, and deep connective tissue—because $G_s\alpha$ and cyclic AMP play important inhibitory roles in the differentiation of osteoblasts.[171,173] The same mutation in *GNAS* can manifest itself clinically in the same family as POH or AHO. Localized dermal calcifications are frequently encountered in subjects with AHO/PHP type IA. Olfactory sense may also be decreased in patients with PHP type IA and IB. More than 80 heterozygous loss-of-function mutations in *GNAS* have been described to date. A four base pair deletion in exon 7 (codons 188 and 189) in *GNAS* that leads to a frame-shift and premature stop codon has been found in a number of families with PHP type IA and appears to be an amutational hotspot because it impairs DNA polymerization and replication.

Other mutations alter intracellular movement of GNAS protein (Leu99Pro, Ser250Arg), increase the rate of release of GDP (Arg258Trp, Ala366Ser), or impair coupling of G protein to PTHR1 (Arg385His). In the only mutation identified in exon 3 to date, insertion of adenosine in codon 85 led to a frame-shift and a stop sequence at codon 87 in exon 4—resulting in isolated deficiency of only the long transcript variant of $G_s\alpha$.[174] $G_s\alpha$ activity was 75% of normal in the tissues of this patient, who had the AHO phenotype, developmental delay, and hyperthyrotropinemia. Serum calcium levels were normal, but PTH values increased (normocalcemic PHP).

In patients with PHP type IB (OMIM 603233), the phenotype is normal but $G_s\alpha$ activity is deficient in the proximal renal tubule and thyroid. Thus, these patients are resistant to PTH (and in part to thyrotropin) and develop hypocalcemia and hyperphosphatemia.[171,173] This disorder is the result of an epigenetic defect: loss of the maternal pattern of *GNAS* expression due to an imprinting error and failure of methylation of the DMR of maternal exon 1A. Thus, in PHP type IB both *GNAS* alleles have a paternal imprinting pattern (nonmethylation of exon 1A on both alleles; i.e., a paternal epigenotype). Thus, there is a quantitatively normal amount of $G_s\alpha$ in most tissues (including the osteoblast and chondrocyte accounting for the normal skeletal phenotype).

When occurring sporadically, the primary abnormality in PHP type IB may lie within the DMRs of antisense NESP and/or exon 1A. When transmitted as a familial autosomal-dominant characteristic, PHP type IB develops only in the offspring of female obligate carriers and might at times be the result of partial deletion of *STX16* (Syntaxin 16)—a gene centromeric to NESP55 and exon 1A of *GNAS* that contains a cis-acting element(s) that regulates imprinting (methylation) of the DMR in maternal exon 1A of *GNAS*.[173,179] Loss of this element within the maternal *STX16* perhaps results in failure of methylation of the DMR in exon 1A of maternal *GNAS* and consequently a paternal pattern of *GNAS* expression with decreased synthesis of $G_s\alpha$ in the proximal renal tubule.

As anticipated, uniparental paternal disomy for chromosome 20 or familial mutations within *GNAS* itself may also result in the PHP type IB phenotype.[180] Epigenetic defects in methylation of structurally intact *GNAS* have also been described in patients with PHP type IA, variable $G_s\alpha$ activity in peripheral tissues, and mild skeletal abnormalities (designated PHP type IC).[171,181] In PHP type II, the phenotype is normal, serum calcium concentrations are low, phosphate and PTH levels elevated, and in response to exogenous PTH urinary cyclic AMP excretion increases but phosphate excretion does not.

The pathogenesis of this disorder is unknown but may be related to unsuspected deficiency of vitamin D.[171] In several unrelated boys with PHP type IA/AHO, Ala366Ser and Arg231His mutations in *GNAS* have been associated with gonadotropin-independent isosexual precocity. Their mutated $G_s\alpha$ products were quickly degraded at body temperature, leading to PHP type IA, but quite stable at scrotal temperature—resulting in increased Leydig cell function.[182,183]

Hypocalcemia occurs in patients with deficiency of vitamin D intake, metabolism, or bioactivity.[75] In the subject with skeletal demineralization due to marked vitamin D deficiency, serum calcium concentrations may fall precipitously after administration of even small amounts of vitamin D as renewed mineralization of bone matrix due to accelerated osteoblastic activity consumes calcium and phosphate (the "hungry bone" syndrome). After parathyroidectomy for primary hyperparathyroidism, calcium concentrations often decline rapidly by the same mechanism. Drugs that inhibit PTH secretion (excessive magnesium), osteoclast resorption of bone (bisphosphonates), or renal resorption of calcium (furosemide) may lead to hypocalcemia.

Intravenous infusion or rectal administration of phosphate (in enemas), acute cellular destruction by tumor cell lysis or rhabdomyolysis, and acute and chronic renal failure increase serum phosphate levels and lead to reciprocal decline in calcium values. Serum calcium concentrations decline in patients receiving multiple transfusions of citrated blood or during plasmapheresis. In subjects with acute pancreatitis, calcium complexed with free fatty acids generated by pancreatic lipase is deposited in necrotic tissue.[184] Acute severe illness of diverse pathogenesis is often associated with hypocalcemia. This has been attributed to hypoalbuminemia, functional hypoparathyroidism, hypercalcitonemia, hypomagnesemia, decreased calcitriol synthesis, alkalosis and increased serum concentrations of free fatty acids (the latter increase binding of Ca^{2+}_e to albumin), and increased cytokine activity.

Evaluation

Figure 17-5 outlines the evaluation of the child/adolescent with hypocalcemia. Hypocalcemia may be asymptomatic until detected by a multiassay chemical profile obtained for another purpose. It may be first identified during evaluation of a long QT interval noted by electrocardiography obtained for evaluation of a functional heart murmur or arrhythmia.[185] Clinical symptoms that suggest hypocalcemia include paresthesias, muscular cramping (particularly during vigorous exercise), tetany (uncontrollable muscular contractions, including laryngospasm), carpal-pedal spasm (flexion of the elbow and wrist, adduction of the thumb, flexion of the metacarpal/metatarsal-phalangeal joints, and extension of the interphalangeal joints), or seizure.[151]

Review of the past medical history may reveal symptoms consistent with or illnesses associated with hypocalcemia (recurrent infections, congenital cardiac anomalies, surgical procedures in the neck, cervical radiation, infiltrative diseases), or the family history may reveal members with hypoparathyroidism, dysmorphic physical characteristics, autoimmune endocrinopathies, or hypomagnesemia. Physical examination will disclose characteristic abnormalities in children with PHP type IA in whom the AHO phenotype is present (short stature, round face, subcutaneous hard nodules, brachymetacarpals), the DGS (typical face, recurrent infections, cardiac murmur), and familial autoimmune polyendocrinopathy syndrome type I (chronic mucocutaneous candidiasis and other ectodermal abnormalities such as vitiligo, alopecia, keratoconjunctivitis)—whereas rachitic deformities in the hypocalcemic child imply the presence of a form of hypovitaminosis D.

Most commonly, however, the physical examination reveals no striking abnormality in the hypocalcemic child other than those of increased neuromuscular irritability: hyperreflexia [e.g., positive Chvostek sign (twitching of the circumoral muscles when tapping lightly over the seventh cranial nerve)], Trousseau sign (carpal pedal spasm when maintaining the blood pressure cuff 20 mm Hg above the systolic blood pressure for three minutes), and occasionally cataracts, papilledema, or abnormal dentition. (Tetany also occurs in subjects with hypo- and hypernatremia, hypo- and hyperkalemia, and hypomagnesemia. A positive Chvostek sign may be found in many normal adolescents.)

After confirmation of the hypocalcemic state (by measuring serum total calcium and Ca^{2+}_e levels, the latter to exclude hypoalbuminemia as a cause of a low total calcium value), urine calcium excretion is determined. In most hypocalcemic patients, urine calcium excretion is low (Figure 17-5). If the urine calcium excretion is inappropriately normal or high, disorders such as autosomal-dominant hypoparathyroidism (gain-of-function mutation in *CASR*) may be considered. *CASR* may then be analyzed or antibodies to CaSR determined as clinically indicated. The frequency with which antibodies to the CaSR are detected in patients with autoimmune hypoparathyroidism depends on the method employed for their identification.

Thus, antibodies to CaSR have been found in 86% of subjects with APECED employing an immunoprecipitation assay with the full-length CaSR expressed in human embryonic kidney cells and in 50% of the same subjects utilizing a flow cytometry assay but in none of these patients applying a radiobinding assay.[186] The serum levels of intact PTH, magnesium, phosphate, creatinine, and alkaline phosphatase are to be measured. Determination of the serum concentration of intact PTH (by ultrasensitive assay) permits differentiation between low (or inappropriately anormal) and high PTH secretory states.

The child/adolescent with hypocalcemia, hypocalciuria, hyperphosphatemia, and low or undetectable serum PTH concentration (and normal or only slightly low serum magnesium level) likely has hypoparathyroidism due to a primary defect in PTH synthesis or secretion related to congenital malformation or acquired destruction of the PTGs. Patients with hypoparathyroidism often have low serum concentrations of calcitriol, normal levels of calcidiol, decreased excretion of urinary nephrogenous cyclic AMP, and increased renal tubular reabsorption of phosphate.[163] The DGS may be identified by abnormal FISH analysis of chromosome 22q11.2 or by *TBX1* genotyping. Analysis of *GCM2* or *SOX3* and genes associated with syndromic hypoparathyroidism (*TCBE, GATA3*) is indicated in the appropriate clinical context (Table 17-1).

The diagnosis of autoimmune polyendocrinopathy syndrome type I is based on clinical and laboratory findings and genotyping of *AIRE*. The presence of two of three of its major manifestations (candidasis and/or ectodermal dystrophy, hypoparathyroidism, hypoadrenocorticism) is accepted for its clinical diagnosis, but isolated hypoparathyroidism may occasionally be its only manifestation. Antibodies to the CaSR or other cellular components of the PTGs, the adrenal glands (side-chain cleavage, 21-hydroxylase, 17α-hydroxylase enzymes), neurotransmitters (aromatic L-amino acid decarboxylase, tryptophan hydroxylase), and interferons-α and -ω may be determined. Antibodies to interferon-ω are commonly present in patients with APECED.[167]

Genotyping of *AIRE* and identification of the mutations confirm the diagnosis of APECED. There is wide variability in the clinical expression of APECED between families and among siblings because the phenotype is not directly related to the genotype.[187] In patients with isolated idiopathic hypoparathyroidism, a search for antibodies to the CaSR and/or to parathyroid tissue is warranted. In hypomagnesemic subjects, magnesium and PTH levels are quite low—and PTH secretion increases rapidly after intravenous administration of magnesium. Primary hypomagnesemia should be considered when hypocalcemia and hypercalciuria coincide and serum PTH and magnesium values are low. Urinary magnesium excretion should then be quantitated and *CLDN16* genotyped. Because hypomagnesemia may also be due to a selective small intestinal defect in magnesium absorption, mutations in *TRPM6* should be examined as warranted. Primary hypomagnesemia must be differentiated from that due to the Gittleman and Bartter syndromes.

An elevated serum concentration of PTH in a hypocalcemic subject suggests that the patient is secreting an abnormal PTH molecule, is resistant to PTH, or is experiencing a compensatory (secondary) PTH secretory response to hypocalcemia (Figure 17-5). Physicochemical characterization of the PTH molecule and analysis of *PTH* enable one to define the abnormality in PTH synthesis, post-translational processing, secretion, or activity leading to the functionally hypoparathyroid state. Analysis of *GNAS* and its pattern of imprinting permit identification of the specific genetic defect in the majority of patients with clinical PHP type IA and PPHP.

Skeletal and renal responsiveness to PTH may be assessed if warranted by measurement of changes in serum calcium, phosphate, cyclic AMP, and calcitriol concentrations and measurement of urinary nephrogenous cyclic AMP and phosphate excretion following administration of biosynthetic PTH[1-34] (Elsworth-Howard test). In the normal subject and in the patient with primary hypoparathyroidism, urinary cyclic AMP excretion increases tenfold to twentyfold and that of phosphate several fold. In the patient with PHP types IA and IB, there is less than a threefold increase in the excretion of cyclic AMP.

The diagnosis of PHP type IB may be established by examining the imprinting pattern of GNAS (paternal pattern only) and analysis of STX16 as indicated. In the child with vitamin D deficiency, serum levels of calcidiol are subnormal. In patients with decreased renal $25OHD_3$-1α-hydroxylase activity, serum concentrations of calcidiol are normal and those of calcitriol are inappropriately low. Increased concentrations of calcitriol suggest the presence of a defect in its nuclear receptor. The patient with renal failure is recognized by an increased serum creatinine value. Other findings in hypocalcemic subjects include prolongation of the QT interval by electrocardiography and calcification of the basal ganglia by cranial computerized tomography.

Management

The primary goal in the care of the hypocalcemic child and adolescent is to increase serum calcium concentrations to levels at which the patient is asymptomatic and as close to the lower range of normal as possible. The secondary goal is to identify the cause of hypocalcemia as quickly as possible in order to provide disease-specific management.[75,163] Asymptomatic hypocalcemia (total calcium >7.5 mg/dL) may not require immediate intervention. With lower serum calcium levels or when hypocalcemia is symptomatic (tetany, seizures), acute management may require the intravenous administration of calcium gluconate (93 mg of elemental calcium/10 mL vial) at a slow rate (not greater than 2 mL/kg over 10 minutes) while closely monitoring pulse rate (and the QT interval).

Acutely, intravenous administration of calcium is intended to ameliorate the more serious consequences of hypocalcemia such as seizures—not to restore and maintain the eucalcemic state. Intravenously, calcium should not be administered with phosphate or bicarbonate because these salts may co-precipitate. Extravascular extravasation of calcium is to be avoided because it may precipitate and cause local tissue injury. After the acute symptoms have resolved, calcium gluconate (10 mL in 100 mL 5% dextrose/0.25 N saline) may be temporarily infused intravenously at a rate sufficient to maintain calcium levels in the asymptomatic low-normal range while the cause of the hypocalcemia is identified and more specific therapy for persistent hypocalcemia prescribed. The evaluation should proceed as rapidly as possible, and oral therapy begun reasonably quickly. In the child with marked hyperphosphatemia as a cause of hypocalcemia, in addition to parenteral calcium administration infusion of normal saline sufficient to maintain urine output at or above 2 mL/kg per hour is necessary.[152] Frequent measurement of serum calcium and phosphate concentrations permits rapid adjustment of fluid and electrolyte therapy.

After stabilization, patients with hypoparathyroidism or PHP may be treated with calcitriol (20–60 ng/kg/day) and supplemental calcium (calcium glubionate or calcium citrate 30–75 mg elemental calcium/kg/day in divided doses, Table 17-3) to restore eucalcemia. The serum calcium concentration should be maintained within the low-normal range. Each patient must be carefully monitored to avoid hypercalcemia, hypercalciuria, nephrocalcinosis, and nephrolithiasis. Basal and periodic measurements of serum concentrations of calcium, phosphate, and creatinine and urinary calcium and creatinine excretion and renal sonography are mandatory. Children with autosomal-dominant hypoparathyroidism due to gain-of-function mutations in CASR are extremely sensitive to vitamin D and its metabolites.

Even small doses of calcitriol may lead to hypercalciuria, with minimal increase in serum calcium levels. In this instance, addition of hydrochlorothiazide (0.5–2.0 mg/kg/day) may increase renal tubular reabsorption of calcium and lower the calcitriol requirement. In adults with primary hypoparathyroidism due to a variety of causes, the use of rhPTH[1-34] (0.5 µg/kg every 12 hours subcutaneously) together with calcium carbonate (1,000 mg/day of elemental calcium in four equally divided doses) has proven effective and safe for as long as 3 years—perhaps even safer than calcitriol because rhPTH[1-34] did not lead to hypercalciuria.[158] rhPTH[1-34] led to acceleration of bone turnover, as reflected by increases in serum alkaline phosphatase and osteocalcin and urinary Pyr and Dpd values without substantial changes in bone mass.

Because PHP type IA is associated with resistance to a number of peptide hormones that act through GPCRs, periodic assessment of pituitary-thyroid and pituitary-ovarian function and GH secretion is necessary—and hormone replacement therapy begun as indicated. In general, the short stature of PHP type IA reflects the AHO phenotype and not GH deficiency. Transient hypoparathyroidism of infancy may be the initial manifestation of later-onset hypoparathyroidism. Thus, it is important to assess calcium homeostasis in such subjects throughout childhood. Patients with apparently isolated hypoparathyroidism of unknown etiology should be reevaluated periodically to identify the development of autoimmune disorders in the patient or family. Assessment of thymic function is important in those subjects with findings suggestive of the DGS.

When hypomagnesemia is symptomatic, administration of magnesium sulfate parenterally may be necessary (50% solution, 0.1–0.2 mL/kg intramuscularly, repeated after 12–24 hours if needed). The patient with primary hypomagnesemia may require daily parenteral (intramuscular, intravenous) doses of magnesium sulfate in order to prevent tetany, seizures, and other neurological symptoms (slurred speech, choreo-athetoid movements, weakness) and to enable normal growth and development.[188] Calcitriol alone raises serum calcium levels in hypomagnesemic subjects but is ineffective in the prevention of tetany. Continuous overnight nasogastric infusion of magnesium may help alleviate the gastrointestinal side effects of multiple large doses of oral magnesium. More mild and transient forms of hypomagnesemia may be treated with oral magnesium gluconate or tribasic magnesium citrate (Table 17-3).

HYPERCALCEMIA

Etiology

Causes of hypercalcemia in children and adolescents are listed in Table 17-4. In the presence of a normal serum protein concentration, hypercalcemia occurs when the rate of entry of calcium into the extracellular and circulatory compartments exceeds its rate of loss and develops when the set-point for serum Ca^{2+}_e is increased due to a loss-of-function mutation in *CASR*, when the resorption rate of bone mineral (e.g., excessive secretion of PTH or PTHrP, constitutive activation of PTHR1, increased production of osteoclast-activating inflammatory cytokines, localized osteolytic processes such as metastatic neoplasms) or the absorption rate of intestinal calcium (hypervitaminosis D) exceeds the renal excretory capacity for calcium, or when there is augmented renal tubular absorption of calcium (e.g., administration of calcium-sparing diuretics such as thiazides).[151]

The total serum calcium concentration is increased in the presence of hyperalbuminemia, whereas the Ca^{2+}_e concentration is normal. Venous stasis (e.g., by tourniquet) results in spuriously altered local pH and Ca^{2+}_e values. Familial hypocalciuric hypercalcemia type 1 (HHC1, OMIM 145980) is an autosomal-dominant disorder with 100% penetrance at all ages characterized by PTH-dependent usually asymptomatic, total and ionized hypercalcemia with hypocalciuria, slight hypermagnesemia, hypomagnesuria, and hypophosphatemia due to heterozygous loss-of-function mutations in *CASR*.[189] Serum concentrations of PTH may be normal or slightly elevated, but inappropriately high for the Ca^{2+}_e level. Calcidiol and calcitriol values are normal.

In children, HHC1 is most commonly suspected initially by the presence of unexpected hypercalcemia (11–14 mg/dL) in a chemistry profile or through family screening of a parent or other relative with hypercalcemia. Older subjects with HHC1 may complain of fatigue, weakness, or polyuria. There is a slightly increased incidence of relapsing pancreatitis, cholelithiasis, chondrocalcinosis, and premature vascular calcification in HHC1. However, bone mass and fracture rate are normal. Because of decreased parathyroid chief cell membrane CaSR number and/or function, the set-point for Ca^{2+}_e suppression of PTH secretion is reset upward.[84,189] The PTGs are slightly hyperplastic.

In renal tubular cells, decreased CaSR number and activity lead to increased renal tubular reabsorption of calcium and relative hypocalciuria (ratio of calcium clearance to creatinine clearance <0.01). Renal tubular reabsorption of magnesium is also increased. Urinary concentrating ability and other measures of renal function are normal. In hypercalcemia of other pathogenesis, urinary calcium excretion is increased and renal concentrating ability depressed. Usually, HHC1 requires no therapy—but must be differentiated from mild primary hyperparathyroidism in which hypomagnesemia and hypercalciuria are present. Subtotal parathyroidectomy in HHC1 does not lower calcium levels as the residual PTGs hypertrophy. Total parathyroidectomy is unnecessary except in infants with NSHPT.

Approximately 70 nonsense, missense, insertion, and deletion mutations in *CASR* associated with HHC1 or NSHPT have been identified—mostly in the receptor's extracellular Ca^{2+} binding domain. These mutations decrease receptor affinity for Ca^{2+} or alter intracellular processing of the CaSR (glycosylation, dimerization; e.g., Arg66His, Asn583Stop) in the endoplasmic reticulum, preventing its translocation to the surface of the cell membrane[190] (Figure 17-7). Many of the mutations are located in the extracellular domain of CaSR between codons 39 and 300, a region rich in aspartate and glutamate residues in which Ca^{2+} may nestle.[71]

Glycosylation is necessary for dimerization and trafficking of the CaSR. Missense mutations involving arginine at codon 66 (Arg66His, Arg66Cys) result in a product that is able to be only partly glycosylated. It can form homodimers in the endoplasmic reticulum but cannot enter the golgi apparatus and be transported to the cell plasma membrane.[190] Mutations in *CASR* tend to be unique to the affected family. In approximately one-third of families with HHC, no mutations in the coding region of *CASR* have been identified. They may have a mutation in a noncoding region of *CASR* or an abnormality in genes associated with the HHC phenotype that have been identified on chromosomes 19p13.3 (HHC2, OMIM 145981) and 19q13 (HHC3, OMIM 600740).[189] Autoantibodies against the amino-terminal extracellular domain of the CaSR that reversibly inhibit receptor activity have been identified in a few patients with acquired HHC. This disorder may be responsive to glucocorticoid therapy.[191] In some patients with primary or uremic secondary hyperparathyroidism, there is reduced expression of *CASR* and an increased set-point for suppression of PTH secretion.[192]

Primary hyperparathyroidism is an unusual childhood disorder with an incidence of 2–5/100,000 compared to that in adults of approximately 100/100,000.[193,194] In adults with hyperparathyroidism, females outnumber males 3:1. In children, the female/male ratio is closer to one. In older children and adolescents, primary hyperparathyroidism is most often a sporadic disease and usually the result of a single parathyroid adenoma. It also occurs as an autosomal-dominant disorder in familial isolated primary hyperparathyroidism (OMIM 145000) due to germline mutations in the genes responsible for multiple endocrine neoplasia (MEN) type I *(MEN1)*, the hypoparathyroidism-jaw tumor syndrome *(HPRT2)*, or HCC1.[75,79,193,195]

Many children (80% to 90%) with hyperparathyroidism and hypercalcemia are symptomatic at the time of diagnosis [headache, fatigue, abdominal pain, nausea and vomiting, polydipsia, and behavioral changes (particularly depression)] or present with symptoms reflecting the consequences of this disorder, including flank pain due to renal calculi (hypercalciuria) and pathologic fractures (through areas of osteopenia or lesions of osteitis fibrosa cystica).[194] It is unusual to palpate a cervical mass in these patients.

Hypercalcemia, hypophosphatemia, and elevated serum concentrations of intact PTH are present in the majority of children with hyperparathyroidism. Ultrasonography, magnetic resonance imaging, computed tomography, and radionuclide scans (^{99m}Tc-SestaMIBI) have been employed to localize the abnormal PTG(s). Occasionally, the parathyroid tumor may be located ectopically in the thymus, thyroid gland, or mediastinum.

In subjects with primary hyperparathyroidism, hypercalcemia is the result of increased secretion of PTH due to loss of the normal relationship between the set-point of serum Ca^{2+}_e and PTH synthesis and release and to Ca^{2+}-independent (constitutive) PTH secretion related to the mass of parathyroid tissue.[193] Pathologically, hyperparathyroidism in children is most often due to a chief cell adenoma involving one PTG. Hyperplasia (particularly in MEN) and rarely carcinoma of the chief cells may occur. The majority of PTG neoplasms are monoclonal in origin. That is, a single mutant cell develops into a tumor.

In adolescents, parathyroid tumors may rarely develop after external radiation of the neck for treatment of lymphoma. In some parathyroid tumors, increased expression of cyclin D1 (encoded by *CCND1,* OMIM 168461, chromosome 11q13) has been demonstrated. Cyclins are intracellular proteins that regulate cyclin-dependent protein kinases that control the rate of transition of G1 to S in the cycle of cell division.[71] Overexpression of *CCND1* in parathyroid chief cells is at times the result of a somatic chromosome mutation-inversion (rotation) of regions 11p15 and 11q13 in which the promoter region of PTH is repositioned to serve as a promoter for CCND1, thereby increasing the rate of chief cell division whenever the (hypocalcemic) stimulus for PTH generation is received and leading ultimately to (benign) tumor formation.

However, in many parathyroid adenomas there is increased activity of cyclin D1 without this chromosomal rearrangement.[193] In patients with parathyroid adenomas and carcinomas, overexpression of the retinoblastoma and p53 tumor-suppressor genes (whose products inhibit the cell cycle at the G1/S step) has been demonstrated.[71] Chronic renal insufficiency leads to secondary hyperparathyroidism due to hyperplasia of the PTGs and to monoclonal parathyroid tumors (tertiary hyperparathyroidism) associated with somatic chromosomal deletions. In approximately 17% of sporadic parathyroid adenomas, a somatic loss-of-function mutation of the tumor suppressor factor menin (the germ-line aberration in patients with MEN type I) can be identified.[196] Germ-line loss-of-function mutations in *MEN1* and *CASR* have also been detected in patients with isolated hyperparathyroidism in association with multiglandular involvement. In this instance, patients with *CASR* mutations did not have the typical biochemical findings of HHC1.[195,197]

Autosomal-dominant familial primary hyperparathyroidism associated with multiple ossifying fibromas of the jaw (HRPT2, OMIM 145001) is due to loss-of-function heterozygous germ-line mutations in the tumor suppressor gene encoding parafibromin *(HRPT2).*[198] Hyperparathyroidism occurs in 80% of subjects with a mutation in *HRPT2* at a mean age of 32 years, but may also appear in children before 10 years of age.[199]

In these patients, the parathyroid lesion may be an atypical potentially premalignant cystic adenoma (65%), hyperplasia (20%), or even carcinoma (15%). The parathyroid tumor may be isolated or associated with maxillary and/or mandibular tumors composed of ossified fibrous tissue. Renal (Wilms' tumor, papillary renal cell carcinoma, hamartoma, polycystic kidney), pancreatic (carcinoma), and uterine (tumor) lesions may also develop in these patients.[71,195] Lesions within the PTGs may develop asynchronously. *HRPT2* is a 17-exon gene that encodes parafibromin, a 531-aa protein that is a component of a complex of accessory factors that modulate RNA polymerase II activity, gene transcription, and cell proliferation.

For a parathyroid tumor to develop, a second hit must occur that results in loss-of-heterozygosity (i.e., the germline inactivating mutation of *HRPT2* on one allele must be matched by a mutation in or deletion of *HRPT2* in the remaining normal allele).[200] When a germ-line mutation in *HRPT2* has been detected, screening of family members for this mutation and longitudinal evaluation of affected subjects is recommended because asymptomatic individuals with atypical adenoma or carcinoma of the PTGs may be so identified.[201] Somatic mutations in HPRT2 have also been identified in atypical parathyroid adenomas and carcinomas, but are distinctly unusual in the typical sporadic parathyroid adenoma.[202] Familial isolated hyperparathyroidism type 3 (HRPT3, OMIM 610071) has been linked to chromosome 2p14-p13.3, but a specific mutated gene in this region has not as yet been identified.

The syndromes of multiple endocrine neoplasia (MEN) are familial autosomal-dominant diseases of high penetrance associated with the development of tumors in two of three primary endocrine tissues (PTG, pituitary, pancreas) within the same person and multiple tumors in the same tissue (Table 17-5).[195,203-206] Within a single family, there is a high degree of uniformity in the clinical expression of MEN1. Hyperparathyroidism (due to a parathyroid adenoma or tumors within or hyperplasia of all four parathyroid glands) is the most common manifestation of MEN1, occurring in more than 90% of affected patients. It is the most frequent endocrinopathy in children with MEN1, at times appearing before 10 years of age. There are equal numbers of males and females with hyperparathyroidism in MEN1.

Pituitary tumors secreting prolactin and/or GH often (30% of MEN1 subjects) develop, as do gastrin- (Zollinger-Ellison syndrome), insulin-, and glucagon-secreting tumors of the pancreatic islets (40% of patients). These neoplasms also occur in children and adolescents with MEN1.[71,204] The Cushing syndrome that develops in patients with MEN1 may be due to excessive secretion of adrenocorticotropin by a pituitary adenoma or ectopically by a neoplasm or to a primary adrenal tumor. Benign and malignant thyroid tumors occur in 25% of patients with MEN1. Nonendocrine tumors such as facial angiofibroma (90%), collagenomas (72%), lipomas (34%), intestinal and bronchial carcinoids, and other intestinal neoplasms are reasonably common in subjects with MEN1.

Indeed, the dermatologic manifestations of MEN1 (more than three angiofibromas and any collagenomas) are extremely sensitive and specific indicators of this disease.[207] Patients with MEN1 may also develop a Schwannoma or a pheochromocytoma, the latter a tumor most often present in patients with MEN types IIA and IIB. Although most of the tumors that develop in MEN1 are benign but functionally hyperactive, those of pancreatic, intestinal, and foregut origin may be malignant. Germ-line mutations in *MEN1,* a 10-exon gene that encodes a 610-aa nuclear protein termed menin, have been demonstrated in the majority of patients with familial and sporadic forms of MEN1.[204] Menin localizes to the nucleus through two nuclear localization signals in its carboxyl terminus (aa 479-498, 589-608), where it is involved directly in the regulation of transcription, replication, and the cell cycle.

TABLE 17-5

Multiple Endocrine Neoplasia Syndromes

Subtype	Gene	Chromosome	Tumors	Sites of Frequent Mutations

MEN I	*MEN1*	11q13	Parathyroid (90%)
			Pancreatic (50%) - gastrinoma, insulinoma
			    pancreatic polypeptide, glucagonoma, VIPoma
			    somatostatinoma, nonfunctional
			Anterior pituitary (35%) - prolactinoma, GH,
			    ACTH, TSH, nonfunctional
			Adrenocortical (25%) - diffuse and nodular
			    hyperplasia, adenoma, carcinoma
			Intestinal - foregut carcinoid tumor, gastric
			    enterochromaffin-like
			Carcinoid - gastric, thymic, bronchial
			Other: facial angiofibroma, collagenoma, lipoma,
			    pheochromocytoma (rare)
				Intron 4 N:5168 G→A (10%)
				Codons 83-84 (4%)
				Codons 118-119 (3%)
				Codons 209-211 (9%)
				Codon 418 (4%)
				Codon 516 (7%)

MEN II Familial MCT MEN IIA	*RET*	10q11	 MCT (100%) MCT (95%) Pheochromocytoma (50%) Parathyroid hyperplasia (30%) Cutaneous lichen amyloidosis Megacolon	 Codon 618 (>50%) Codon 634 (Cys→Arg >80%)
MEN IIB			MCT (100%) Pheochromocytoma (50%), ganglioneuroma Associated: Marfanoid habitus (100%) Mucosal neuromas (90%) Medullated corneal nerves	Codon 918 (Met→Thr >95%)

MCT - Medullary
  carcinoma of
  thyroid				

Compiled from Marx SJ, et al. (1999). Multiple endocrine neoplasia type 1: Clinical and genetic features of the hereditary endocrine neoplasias. Rec Prog Horm Res 54:397–438; from Marx SJ, Simonds WF (2005). Hereditary hormone excess: Genes, molecular pathways, and syndromes. Endocrine Reviews 26:615–661; from Root AW (2000). Genetic disorders of calcium and phosphorus metabolism. Crit Rev Clin Lab Sci 37:217–260; and from Thakker RV (1998). Editorial: Multiple endocrine neoplasia, syndromes of the twentieth century. J Clin Endocrinol Metab 83:2617–2620.

Menin is a tumor suppressor factor. By binding directly to JunD, menin blocks JunD-mediated inhibition of transcription of activating protein-1 (and consequently cell division). Many of the mutations in *MEN1* in patients with MEN1 cluster in exon 4 and interrupt the binding of these two proteins (between menin aa 139-142 and 323-428). However, loss of inhibition of JunD is but one of several mechanisms that lead to unrestricted cell growth in targeted MEN1 tissues.[208] By interacting with SMAD3 (OMIM 603109, chromosome 15q21-q22), menin inhibits signaling by transforming growth factor (TGF) β and impairs TGFβ-mediated inhibitory control of cell replication.[209] Interaction of menin with the SMAD 1/5 complex inhibits signaling by bone morphogenetic protein (BMP) 2. Menin also inhibits the transcription-regulating protein nuclear factor κB (NFκB).[71,210]

In subjects with heterozygous germ-line loss-of-function mutations in *MEN1*, unregulated cell growth and tumor formation occur when a second insult leads to loss of *MEN1* on the normal allele within susceptible tissues. As with *HPRT2*, the two-hit hypothesis of tumorigenesis in MEN1 denotes that the patient receives germ-line suscepti-

bility to neoplasia superimposed on which is a second insult leading to loss of heterozygosity for chromosome segment 11q13 and biallelic loss of *MEN1*. The second hit may be deletion of a segment of chromosome 11 that includes 11q13 or a mutation (missense, frame-shift) within the wt *MEN1* allele itself, an observation that also extends to MEN type I tumors with somatic mutations in *MEN1*.[195,204,211]

Several hundred germ-line mutations in MEN1 have been identified in patients with MEN1, of which 25% have been nonsense mutations, 15% missense mutations, and 45% frame-shift insertions or deletions. More than 80% have led to the synthesis of an inactive product due to loss of the nuclear localization signal or the ability to bind to JunD or other downstream factor (Figure 17-9).[204,212] Especially susceptible germ-line mutational hot spots in *MEN1* are nucleotide 5168 G→A transition that results in a novel splice site in intron 4 (codons 83, 84, 118, 119, 209–211, 418, and 516), where collectively mutations have been identified in 37% of patients with MEN1.[213]

On either side of many of these sites are segments of repeat DNA sequences of single nucleic acids or of

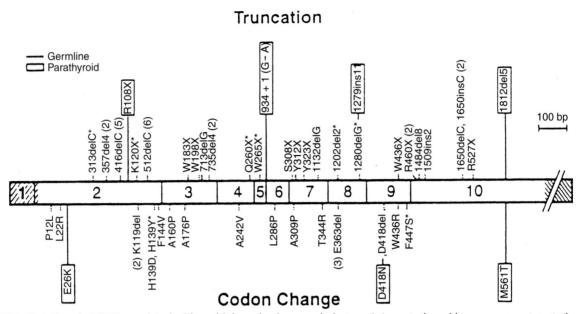

Figure 17-9 Mutations in MEN1 associated with multiple endocrine neoplasia type 1. Long tethered boxes represent mutations in isolated parathyroid tumors. Nonsense, frame-shift, and splice site mutations are depicted above, and missense and in-frame deletions below the outline of the codons of *MEN1*. [Reproduced with permission from Marx SJ, et al. (1998). Germline and somatic mutation of the gene for multiple endocrine neoplasia type 1 (MEN1). J Intern Med 243:447–453.]

dinucleotides to octanucleotides. This configuration may lead to increased susceptibility to replication-slippage because of misalignment of the nucleotide repeat segments during DNA replication, permitting deletion or insertion of nucleotides at inappropriate sites. To date, no significant correlation between genotype and phenotype has been recognized in MEN1. The tissue-specific susceptibility to tumor formation with a mutation in *MEN1* remains unexplained at present.[195]

Mutations in *MEN1* have been detected in approximately 75% to 95% of patients with familial MEN1. In only 7% of patients with a variant of MEN1 in which only tumors of the PTG and the adenohypophysis are present has a mutation in MEN1 been identified.[214] Familial autosomal-dominant isolated primary hyperparathyroidism has been variably associated with germline mutations (e.g., Val184Glu, Glu255Lys, Gln260Pro) in *MEN1* as well.[215] Somatic mutations in *MEN1* have also been identified in patients with sporadic isolated tumors of the PTGs, pancreatic islet cells, anterior pituitary, and adrenal cortex.[71]

Clinically apparent disease due to mutations in *MEN1* increases with advancing age. At 10 years of age, 7% of children with a mutation in *MEN1* have a detectable endocrinopathy. Fifty-two percent of affected 20-year-old subjects manifest one or more tumors. Penetrance increases to 87% by 30 years, to 98% by 40 years, and to 100% by 60 years.[216] New mutations of *MEN1* occur sporadically in 10% of patients with MEN1. In 5% to 20% of families with MEN1, no mutation in the coding region of *MEN1* has been identified—suggesting that there may be mutations in the untranslated regions of *MEN1* or that another unrecognized gene(s) may be involved in the pathogenesis of the MEN1 phenotype.

Medullary carcinoma of the thyroid (MCT) is the most common neoplasm encountered in MEN IIA, occurring in 95% of patients (OMIM 171400, Table 17-4). These subjects also develop pheochromocytomas, parathyroid hyperplasia or adenoma, localized cutaneous lichen amyloidosis (suprascapular pruritic deposits of subepidermal keratin), and partial or complete megacolon. In addition to MCT and pheochromocytoma, patients with MEN IIB (OMIM 162300) have a Marfanoid habitus, mucosal neuromas of the lips and tongue, and gastrointestinal ganglioneuromas.[195,206,217] Familial isolated MCT is a variant of these disorders. Germline gain-of-function mutations in the *RET* proto-oncogene underlie the pathogenesis of the type II hereditary endocrine neoplasias (Figure 17-10). *RET* is a 20-exon gene encoding three isoforms of a glycosylated cell membrane tyrosine kinase receptor with extracellular, transmembrane, and intracellular domains that is expressed in tissue of neural crest origin (sympathetic ganglia, adrenal medulla, thyroid parafollicular cells).

The natural ligand of this receptor is glial-cell-line-derived neurotrophic factor (GDNF, OMIM 600837, chromosome 5p13.1-p12).[218] Constitutively activating mutations among five cysteine residues in the extracellular domain of RET, particularly at codon 634 (Cys→Arg), are present in patients with MEN IIA. Loss of but one cysteine residue facilitates receptor homodimerization without ligand binding, activation of the RET intracellular tyrosine kinase domain, autophosphorylation of critical tyrosine residues (particularly at codons 1015 and 1062), and subsequent signal transduction.[195]

An activating mutation has been identified at codon 918 (Met→Thr) in more than 95% of patients with MEN IIB. This site lies within the tyrosine kinase domain and this mutation permits signal transduction and neural cell transformation and differentiation in the absence of ligand binding and receptor homodimerization. Missense mutations at codons 618 (Cys→Arg/Gly) or 620 (Cys→Arg/Ser) permitting receptor dimerization in the absence

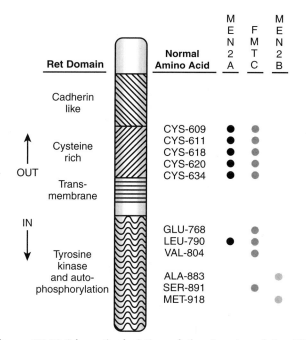

Figure 17-10 Schematic depiction of the domains of the *RET* proto-oncogene with sites of activating mutations in *RET* associated with multiple endocrine neoplasia types IIA and IIB and familial medullary carcinoma of the thyroid. [Reproduced with permission from Marx SJ, Simonds WF (2005). Hereditary hormone excess: Genes, molecular pathways, and syndromes. Endocrine Reviews 26:615–661.]

of GDNF have been found in more than 50% of patients with familial MCT. Mutations within the tyrosine kinase domain (Val804Leu) have also been identified in some of these families.

Two co-receptors, GFRA1 and GFRA2, interact with *Ret* protein—but the role of the co-receptors in the pathogenesis of MEN II, if any, has not been identified. In addition to the disorders designated multiple endocrine neoplasia, other familial syndromes associated with multiple tumors of the endocrine system include Von-Hipple Lindau (adrenal medulla, pancreas, neuroendocrine), Carney complex (adrenal cortex, testes, pituitary, thyroid), McCune-Albright (pituitary, adrenal cortex), and neurofibromatosis type I (adrenal medulla, thyroid).[195,217] In children, hyperparathyroidism is an unusual manifestation of the McCune-Albright syndrome due to a postzygotic activating mutation of *GNAS*.[219]

Ingestion of excessive amounts of vitamin D or calcitriol for therapeutic reasons (treatment of rickets, hypoparathyroidism, or other causes of hypocalcemia), megavitamin intake, and inappropriate fortification of milk are the major causes of hypervitaminosis D.[220-222] Topical application of creams containing vitamin D or an analogue (e.g., 22-oxacalcitriol) for treatment of psoriasis might also lead to hypercalcemia, particularly if the urinary excretion of calcium is compromised.[223,224]

Patients with granulomatous diseases (noninfectious sarcoidosis, berylliosis, eosinophilic granuloma, subcutaneous fat necrosis, and inflammatory bowel disease and infectious tuberculosis, histoplasmosis, coccidioidomycosis, candidiasis, and cat-scratch disease) and neoplastic disorders (B-cell lymphoma, Hodgkin disease, dysgermi-

noma) develop hypercalcemia due to associated monocytic (macrophage and other cells) expression of $25OHD_3$-1α-hydroxylase activity and production of calcitriol.[225] Unlike renal tubular cells (in which this enzyme is within mitochondria and the transcription of *CYP27B1* is closely regulated by PTH, calcitriol, calcium, and phosphate), in monocytes $25OHD_3$-1α-hydroxylase is microsomal in location and its gene is constitutively expressed and calcitriol synthesis regulated by the amount of substrate.

The monocytic expression of *CYP27B1* is very sensitive to stimulation by interferon-γ and its postreceptor signal transducer nitric oxide, as well as by leukotriene C_4. It is easily suppressed by glucocorticoids, ketoconazole, and chloroquine. Subjects with acquired immunodeficiency disease may become hypercalcemic because of being infected with granuloma-forming organisms or by osteoclast-activating cytokines elaborated during the course of this disorder. Elevated serum calcium concentrations have been recorded in children with congenital hypothyroidism, primary oxalosis, congenital lactase deficiency, and trisomy 21.[226]

Hypercalcemia has occurred in adolescents with juvenile rheumatoid arthritis due to increased synthesis of the osteoclast-activating cytokine interleukin-1β.[227] In some hypercalcemic children, excessive prostaglandin production may be of pathogenetic significance. Hypercalcemia develops frequently in the infantile form of hypophosphatasia, likely a consequence of the dissociation of the rates of low bone formation and normal bone resorption.[228] Hypercalcemia may follow successful bone marrow transplantation in infants with osteopetrosis because functional osteoclasts rapidly reabsorb excess bone mineral.

Oncogenic hypercalcemia may be the consequence of secretion of PTHrP, (rarely) PTH, or calcitriol—or of direct invasion and destruction of bone by the neoplasm.[229] Although hypercalcemia occurs in less than 1% of children with cancer, it may develop in patients with leukemia, Hodgkin and non-Hodgkin lymphoma, rhabdomyosarcoma, hepatoblastoma, neuroblastoma, and Ewing sarcoma.[230] Acute immobilization of the rapidly growing child with a femoral fracture or a spinal cord injury results in decreased bone mineral accretion and uncoupling of the interaction of osteoblasts and osteoclasts with increased rate of bone resorption, leading to hypercalciuria and "acute disuse osteoporosis."[231]

When the rate of bone resorption exceeds the renal tubular capacity for excretion of calcium, hypercalcemia ensues. Acute disuse osteoporosis and hypercalcemia can even occur in the immobilized hypoparathyroid or vitamin-D-depleted individual. Increased intake of calcium and absorbable alkali (milk or calcium-containing antacids such as calcium carbonate) for peptic ulcer disease or as dietary supplements leads to absorptive hypercalcemia, hypercalciuria, and nephrocalcinosis. Parenteral nutrition with excessive calcium or aluminum or too little phosphate also leads to hypercalcemia. Hypophosphatemia of various etiologies leads to hypercalcemia as the body attempts to maintain the calcium X phosphate product over 30.

Drugs causing hypercalcemia include thiazide diuretics (which increase renal tubular resorption of calcium and decrease plasma volume), vitamin D and analogs (which increase intestinal absorption of calcium), vitamin A and its retinoic acid analogs (which stimulate bone resorption), and lithium (which increases the set-point for PTH secretion, thereby increasing serum calcium concentrations while lowering urinary calcium excretion and thus mimicking HHC1). In the thyrotoxic subject, hypercalcemia is the result of thyroid-hormone-mediated stimulation of osteoclast function and subsequent increase in the rate of bone resorption. Pheochromocytomas and some islet cell tumors may be associated with hypercalcemia, in some instances because of co-secretion of PTHrP. Hypercalcemia in the hypoadrenal patient is of uncertain pathogenesis but is not related to increased serum concentrations of PTH, calcidiol, or calcitriol—or with augmented bone resorption.

During recovery from acute renal failure, serum calcium levels may increase due to mobilization of calcium from ectopic sites in which it had been deposited during the hyperphosphatemic phase of the illness. Hypercalcemia can develop in patients with chronic renal failure due to a combination of factors, including immobilization, aluminum toxicity, excessive ingestion of calcium antacids or vitamin D or its analogs, and hyperparathyroidism. After renal transplantation, hypercalcemia is the result of secondary hyperparathyroidism due to hypertrophy and hyperplasia of parathyroid chief cells that occurred in response to the PTH stimulatory effects of hyperphosphatemia, hypocalcemia, and decreased synthesis of and response to calcitriol during the period of chronic renal insufficiency.

In patients with compromised renal function, mild hypocalcemia and calcitriol deficiency develop when the glomerular filtration rate falls below 80 to 60 mL/min/1.73 m^2—whereas phosphate retention occurs after the glomerular filtration rate has fallen to 60 to 30 mL/min/1.73 m^2.[232] The secretion of PTH rises in these patients in an effort to increase the synthesis of calcitriol, raise calcium levels, and lower phosphate values. Prolonged uncontrolled secondary hyperparathyroidism can lead to relatively autonomous parathyroid hyperfunction ("tertiary hyperparathyroidism") and hypercalcemia, primarily in patients with chronic renal failure.

Hyperplasia of chief cells is followed by defects in function of the CaSR and loss of effective down-regulation of PTH secretion refractory to increased serum concentrations of Ca^{2+}_e. There is an expanded number of monoclonal chief cells in which the expression of *CASR* and the number of vitamin D nuclear receptors have declined. Secondary and tertiary hyperparathyroidism have occurred in patients with prolonged nutritional vitamin D deficiency rickets and in subjects with X-linked hypophosphatemic rickets receiving large amounts of phosphate.[232,233] Enhanced but transient secretion of PTH may accompany the administration of GH to adolescents with chronic renal failure, likely the result of superimposing upon a high basal rate of PTH secretion further increase in the rate of bone remodeling related to GH and sex hormones.[234] In acutely ill adults, GH administration has been associated with hypercalcemia as well.[231]

Isolated hypercalciuria in the eucalcemic child may be idiopathic or due to renal medullary or tubular dysfunction, mutations in the gene encoding the CLCN5 chloride chan-

nel, demineralizing disorders such as juvenile rheumatoid arthritis, hyperalimentation, metabolic acidosis, excessive protein ingestion, diabetes mellitus, hypomagnesemia, Bartter syndrome, and other disorders.[235] Secondary hyperparathyroidism (in which by definition serum calcium concentrations are normal) also develops in patients with inadequate dietary calcium, impaired intestinal absorption of calcium (lactose intolerance, ingestion of phytates, malabsorption syndromes due to pancreatic insufficiency or celiac disease), or excessive calcium loss in the urine or soft tissues.[232]

Evaluation

When hypercalcemia is mild (total calcium concentration <12 mg/dL), there may be few (if any) symptoms. Such children/adolescents are often identified by a multichannel screening study obtained for some other purpose. Hypercalcemia may also be detected during studies for renal calculi, abnormal bone mass, pathologic fractures, or during screening of families for associated problems. It should also be recognized that an elevated serum (total or ionized) calcium concentration in a single specimen may reflect assay variability and must be verified by repeated determinations in a reliable laboratory. Pseudohypercalcemia is the presence of persistently elevated total calcium concentrations while the Ca^{2+}_e is normal and is found in hyperalbuminemia and other dysproteinemic states.[226]

Symptoms attributable to hypercalcemia are independent of its cause and are related to the degree of hypercalcemia and include intestinal symptoms [anorexia, nausea, vomiting, abdominal pain (peptic ulceration, acute pancreatitis)] and constipation, urinary symptoms [polydipsia, nocturia, and polyuria (calcium acts as an osmotic diuretic while hypercalcemia impairs the concentrating function of the distal renal tubule)], skeletal symptoms (bone pain), and nervous system symptoms [headache, muscular weakness, impaired ability to concentrate, increased requirement for sleep, altered consciousness (ranging from lethargy and confusion to irritability, delirium stupor, and coma)]. On occasion, depression may be the major presenting concern in an adolescent with hypercalcemia.[151,236,237]

In the toddler and young child, hypercalcemia is manifested by anorexia, constipation, poor weight gain, and impaired linear growth (failure to thrive). In a series of 52 children and adolescents with hypercalcemia due to primary hyperparathyroidism, 80% were symptomatic. The most common symptoms were fatigue/lethargy (35%), headache (35%), nausea (29%), vomiting (23%), and polydipsia (21%).[194] Bone involvement (low bone mass, fractures) was present in 30%, and 14% of these subjects were depressed. All of the children (N = 17) with nephrolithiasis in this series were symptomatic.

Evaluation of the hypercalcemic child begins with the historical review (Figure 17-6), during which the family/patient is queried not only about symptoms related to hypercalcemia and its consequences (renal calculi) but about possibly excessive intake of vitamin D, vitamin A, and related compounds (such as retin A for treatment of acne); of calcium (perhaps to "prevent" osteoporosis), and of alkali or drugs that affect calcium metabolism (thiazide diuretics may "unmask" hyperparathyroidism by increasing renal tubular resorption of calcium and thereby raising borderline calcium concentrations into the hypercalcemic range). The family history is explored for members with known disorders of calcium metabolism (HHC1, hyperparathyroidism, renal calculi) or familial neoplasms (galactorrhea as a sign of a prolactinoma, and severe peptic ulcer disease as an indicator of a gastrinoma and the Zollinger-Ellison syndrome).

Except in extreme instances [when hypertension (if normally hydrated) or bradycardia, dehydration, decreased muscular strength, or altered consciousness may be present or in the subject with MEN IIB], physical examination of the hypercalcemic child and adolescent is usually normal. Rarely is a paratracheal (parathyroid) mass palpable in the hyperparathyroid patient. Subjects with hypercalcemia due to subcutaneous fat necrosis have firm to hard irregular movable masses scattered about the trunk and extremities. Those with the Williams-Beuren syndrome have a typical face, whereas those with Jansen metaphyseal chondrodysplasia have characteristic skeletal deformities.

After confirming the presence of total and ionized hypercalcemia, the urinary excretion of calcium is next measured (Figure 17-6). If calcium excretion is low, it is most probable that the patient has HHC1. This diagnosis can be substantiated by the finding of asymptomatic hypocalciuric hypercalcemia in one of the parents and further defined by identification of the inactivating mutation in *CASR*. If the patient is hypercalciuric, other causes of hypercalcemia should be sought. With highly sensitive and moderately specific immunoradiometric and immunochemiluminometric assays for intact PTH[1-84] (these assays may also measure larger carboxyl-terminal fragments of PTH; e.g., PTH[7-84]) in comparison to serum calcium values, separation of patients with hyperparathyroidism from those with other causes of hypercalcemia in whom PTH values are low or normal is usually possible.

In the absence of secondary hyperparathyroidism (chronic renal insufficiency, malabsorption syndromes, ingestion of thiazide diuretics or lithium), consistently elevated PTH concentrations in the hypercalcemic, hypophosphatemic, hypercalciuric child or adolescent are consistent with primary hyperparathyroidism. Although the diagnosis of primary hyperparathyroidism is usually quite apparent in children and adolescents, there is an occasional patient in whom serum calcium and/or PTH values may not be elevated in a single specimen and in whom repeated measurements of serum and urine calcium and PTH values are necessary before this diagnosis can be established. In the series of 52 children/adolescents with hyperparathyroidism previously described, serum calcium values were normal in 10% and PTH levels in 15%. However, in all subjects the PTH concentration was inappropriately increased relative to the calcium level.[194]

Phosphate values are usually low for age in this group. Osteitis fibrosa cystica, brown tumors (localized non-neoplastic areas of bone resorption composed of osteoclast-like multinuclear giant cells, fibroblast-like spindle-shaped cells, and hemorrhagic infiltrates), and subperiosteal and endosteal bone resorption can be detected radiographically in some children with hyperparathyroidism. Cortical (distal radial) bone mineral density is likely to be decreased in these subjects. Nonspecific findings in the hypercalcemic subject of diverse etiology include shortening of the QT interval by electrocardiography because the rate of cardiac repolarization is increased by increased calcium levels, bradycardia, and first-degree atrioventricular block—and nephrocalcinosis and renal calculi detected by abdominal ultrasonography. Serum concentrations of PTHrP should be measured when clinical and laboratory findings are consistent with primary hyperparathyroidism, but PTH values are low and humoral hypercalcemia of malignancy is suspected. When PTH concentrations are low in the hypercalcemic patient, metabolites of vitamin D (calcidiol, calcitriol) should be measured and other causes of hypercalcemia sought.

Preoperatively, a parathyroid adenoma may be localized by high-resolution ultrasonography, computed tomography, magnetic resonance imaging, or radionuclide scanning with ^{99m}Tc-sestamibi. The latter radionuclide is taken up by the thyroid and parathyroid glands but quickly washed out from the thyroid gland. Thus, two scans obtained 2 hours apart permit differentiation of parathyroid from thyroid tissue.[193] Alternatively, a simultaneously administered second radionuclide selectively accumulated by the thyroid (^{123}iodine) may be employed to visualize parathyroid tissue.

Scans may be obtained by conventional two-dimensional or computed tomographic techniques, the latter offering a three-dimensional image. Only occasionally is it necessary to undertake selective venous catheterization with sampling of local PTH levels and/or arteriography to identify the site of a parathyroid adenoma. Evaluation for associated endocrine tumors is necessary if the family history suggests the possibility of MEN I or MEN IIA or if there are clinical findings (galactorrhea, excessive growth, hypertension) to suggest the presence of a prolactinoma, somatotropinoma, or pheochromocytoma.

Patients at risk for MEN may be screened by determining basal and stimulated serum concentrations of prolactin, GH, IGF-I, gastrin, glucagon, pancreatic polypeptide, calcitonin, catecholamines, and other substances as warranted. Indeed, it is reasonable to consider screening children with hyperparathyroidism preoperatively for an associated pheochromocytoma or tumors of the maxilla and mandible and for mutations in *RET, MEN1,* and *HPRT2*.[195,204] Prior to surgery, survey of the pattern of bone mineralization for preferential loss of cortical rather than cancellous bone might also be considered.

In the patient with hypercalcemia due to ingestion of excessive amounts of vitamin D, serum concentrations of calcidiol are markedly elevated. In those receiving exogenous calcitriol or in hypercalcemic patients with granulomatous, chronic inflammatory and lymphomatous diseases serum levels of calcitriol are increased. Other disorders associated with hypercalcemia (Table 17-4) should be eliminated by appropriate historical findings and laboratory studies.

Management

Appropriate management of the patient with hypercalcemia depends on the severity and the cause of the high calcium levels. It is important to identify the patient with a pathologic cause of hypercalcemia so that effective medical and surgical therapy may be initiated promptly. It is equally important to recognize the child/adolescent with HHC1 so that aggressive therapy is avoided. When the calcium concentration is <12 mg/dL in the asymptomatic subject, treatment may be delayed until the cause of the hypercalcemia is understood. In the interim, it is reasonable to recommend that the patient increase fluid intake, avoid calcium and vitamin D supplements, and discontinue drugs associated with hypercalcemia if possible.

The child with HHC1 often has serum total calcium concentrations between 11 and 13 mg/dL but no clinical symptoms and requires no therapy under usual circumstances. In the absence of HHC1, if the total serum calcium concentration exceeds 12 mg/dL or if the child is symptomatic efforts to lower this level are necessary because of the adverse effects of hypercalcemia on cardiac, central nervous, renal, and gastrointestinal function. In these children, diagnostic studies as outlined previously and treatment should begin simultaneously.

The first tool of therapy of severe hypercalcemia is hydration [with 0.9% saline (twice maintenance volume over 24-48 hours), which restores intravascular volume, dilutes and decreases serum Ca^{2+}_e levels, increases glomerular filtration of Ca^{2+}, decreases reabsorption of Ca^{2+} in the proximal and distal renal tubules, and promotes calciuresis]. Hydration alone usually lowers the total serum calcium concentration 1 to 3 mg/dL. A second tool is calciuresis. Intravenous infusion of the loop diuretic furosemide (1 mg/kg slowly) initiated only after restoration of extracellular fluid volume with saline further lowers calcium levels by inhibiting resorption of calcium (and sodium) by the TALH. Thiazide diuretics are to be avoided because they increase renal tubular reabsorption of calcium and increase serum calcium concentrations and are clearly contraindicated in the management of hypercalcemia. A third tool is inhibition of bone resorption. If hypercalcemia does not respond to the above measures, specific inhibitors of osteoclast function may need to be employed.

Bisphosphonates (pamidronate, etidronate, zoledronic acid) are the agents of choice in the acute management of hypercalcemia in children and adolescents. Bisphosphonates are phosphatase-resistant analogs of pyrophosphate. In vivo, they inhibit osteoclast function by impeding osteoclast differentiation. By binding to and coating the hydroxyapatite crystal beneath the osteoclast, they interfere with its attachment and functional ability to dissolve bone.[236] Pamidronate (0.5–1.0 mg/kg/dose by intravenous infusion over 4–6 hours) has effectively lowered serum calcium concentrations in hypercalcemic infants and children.[102,103,230]

The hypocalcemic effect of bisphosphonates is variable in duration (days to weeks). Transient systemic side effects (fever, myalgia) may accompany the administration of pamidronate and other bisphosphonates. Salmon calcitonin also acts rapidly, but transiently, to lower serum calcium concentrations by inhibiting osteoclast activity and increasing urinary calcium excretion. It must be administered by multiple daily subcutaneous injections (2–4 U/kg/injection every 6–12 hours). Calcitonin may be paired with a bisphosphonate at the beginning of treatment of hypercalcemia in order to lower serum calcium levels more rapidly.[151]

Glucocorticoids do not lower calcium levels in patients with hyperparathyroidism or solid tumor malignancies but are quite effective in the management of hypercalcemia due to excess vitamin D ingestion or calcitriol production by activated monocytes or hematologic malignancies. Rarely, it may be necessary to dialyze (peritoneal or hemodialysis) with low- or zero-calcium dialysate the severely hypercalcemic patient resistant to conventional therapy. During acute treatment of hypercalcemia, Ca^{2+}_e concentrations may be assessed indirectly by monitoring the (shortened) QT interval by electrocardiography.

Although in older adults (>50 years) with asymptomatic primary hyperparathyroidism (without bone disease or renal stones) no immediate intervention may be advised at times, in younger adults, children, and adolescents with hyperparathyroidism surgical intervention is recommended when the diagnosis is established. Although hyperparathyroidism in youth is most often (>60%) due to an adenoma, hyperplasia of the parathyroid glands is also common (~30%).[194] In the pediatric population, efforts are undertaken to localize a parathyroid adenoma before its removal by a surgeon with experience and expertise in parathyroid surgery.[238]

In adults and older adolescents, minimally invasive procedures for removing a parathyroid adenoma(s) may be employed. ^{99m}Tc-sestamibi is administered 2 hours before surgery in conjunction with single-photon emission computed tomography. If the scan is consistent with an adenoma, skin and subcutaneous tissue are infiltrated with a local anesthetic, a horizontal 2.5-cm incision is made on the side of and slightly above the suspected parathyroid adenoma, and dissection directed by insertion of a handheld gamma probe until the adenoma is located and removed. Video assistance is an alternative method for localization of a parathyroid adenoma.

A complementary technique for assessing the completeness of the removal of the adenoma intraoperatively is to measure peripheral levels of PTH by rapid immunoassay before and 10 minutes after removal of the adenoma. A 50% decline in PTH levels indicates complete excision. If the PTH concentration does not decline following removal of suspected abnormal parathyroid tissue, further exploration is undertaken and additional tissue removed as guided by the serum PTH level. These procedures are reported to be cost effective because they decrease operative time and patient morbidity. Many patients return home within hours after leaving the operating suite. These techniques have been applied to the surgical management of the child and infant with a parathyroid adenoma or hyperplasia of multiple PTGs.

If there is parathyroid hyperplasia, subtotal (3.5 glands) or total parathyroidectomy is performed and autotransplantation of small fragments of one gland to a forearm pocket considered. Following removal of a parathyroid adenoma, many patients develop transient hypocalcemia that may be managed by the administration of supplemental oral calcium. When there is severe osteitis fibrosa cystica and marked demineralization, substantial hypocalcemia may occur as a result of the "hungry bone" syndrome. Other complications of surgery include (transient) vocal cord dysfunction and the need for further operations because of development of a second adenoma. If permanent hypoparathyroidism develops postoperatively, it is treated by the administration of calcitriol and supplemental calcium as needed.

Calcimimetic agents (phenylalkylamines) bind to and activate the membrane CaSR on the parathyroid chief cell and thereby increase cytosolic levels of $Ca^{2+}{}_i$ and depress secretion of PTH in adults with mild primary hyperparathyroidism.[193] The use of these agents in children and adolescents with this disorder remains to be assessed, but they offer a potential treatment pathway for subjects with diffuse parathyroid hyperplasia. The secondary hyperparathyroidism of chronic renal disease is best managed by lowering serum phosphate concentrations to the extent possible by limiting intake and by administration of oral phosphate binding agents and by maintaining serum $Ca^{2+}{}_e$ levels within the low-normal range by the administration of calcitriol or analogue. Calcimimetic agents (e.g., cinacalcet) may also be useful in this situation.[239] Parathyroidectomy may be necessary for effective management of refractory secondary and tertiary hyperparathyroidism as manifested by severe renal osteodystrophy, hypercalcemia, and systemic symptoms such as pruritus and bone pain.[232]

Hypercalcemia due to hypervitaminosis D or excessive production of calcitriol by granulomatous and chronic inflammatory tissues may be treated with glucocorticoids to suppress activity of $25OHD_3$-1α-hydroxylase. Ketoconazole (3–9 mg/kg/day in three divided doses) is an antifungal agent that also inhibits $25OHD_3$-1α-hydroxylase activity, and that promptly lowers calcitriol and calcium values in children and adults with similar disorders.[240] Side effects of therapy with ketoconazole include nausea, vomiting, abdominal pain, depressed secretion of gonadal steroids, and adrenal production of cortisol. Therefore, careful monitoring of patients receiving ketoconazole is essential.

Glucocorticoids ameliorate the hypercalcemia related to excessive interleukin-1β production in adolescents with juvenile rheumatoid arthritis.[227] An attempt should be made to prevent hypercalcemia in the immobilized child or adolescent by ingestion of a low-calcium diet, avoidance of vitamin D, copious fluid intake, and early mobilization. Serum and urine calcium levels should be monitored frequently, and fluids increased still further if hypercalciuria occurs.

Once present, hypercalcemia is best treated by mobilization. Saline diuresis and/or bisphosphonate administration may be necessary until eucalcemia is restored. Restriction of dietary calcium and limitation of exposure to sunlight may be appropriate in the long-term management of some patients with hypercalcemia not amenable to more specific treatment. Antiprostaglandin agents may be useful in the child with hypercalcemia associated with excessive production of these compounds. Specific treatment of diseases accompanied by hypercalcemia (thyrotoxicosis, hypoadrenocorticism) restores the eucalcemic state.

Disorders of Bone Mineralization and Formation

Bone formation may be impaired because of lack of minerals (calcium and/or phosphate) or because of deficient production of bone matrix. Bone mineralization may be excessive because of increase in the rate of mineral deposition or decrease in the rate of resorption of the mineral phase of bone. Ectopic calcification of extraskeletal tissues may occur when local calcium and phosphate levels are high, whereas extraskeletal ossification may ensue when the regulation of bone formation is deranged.

RICKETS

Rickets and osteomalacia are disorders that result from decreased mineralization of bone matrix due to deficiencies of calcium and/or phosphate[241-243] (Table 17-6). During endochondral bone formation in children, matrix is elaborated and subsequently mineralized. When endochondral osteoid is not fully mineralized, the ends of the long bones (particularly those that are weight bearing) deform and rickets ensues. During the processes of modeling and remodeling of trabecular bone and the periosteal and endosteal surfaces of cortical bone, osteoid is formed by osteoblasts. Failure to mineralize bone matrix in these regions results in osteomalacia.

During intervals of calcium and/or phosphate deprivation, the actively growing weight-bearing child with open cartilage growth plates develops rickets and osteomalacia—whereas adults develop only osteomalacia during remodeling as unmineralized bone matrix accumulates. Thus, rickets is the expression of defective endochondral mineralization at the growth plate and osteomalacia is the failure of mineralization of bone cortex and trabeculae. Clinically, rickets is manifested by skeletal deformities such as delayed closure of the fontanelles, craniotabes (reversible compression of the skull's outer table), frontal bossing (expansion of cranial bones), and occasional craniosynostosis in infants; delayed tooth eruption with poor enamel formation and propensity to caries; pectus carinatum, prominence of the costochondral junctions, and flaring of the lower rib cage; scoliosis and kyphosis; and genu varum and/or valgum, flaring of the metaphyses of the long bones, and tibial or femoral torsion.

Radiographically, rickets is characterized by cupping, splaying, and fraying of the metaphyses of long bones and demineralization. Osteomalacia is associated with increased fracture risk as well as limb deformities. Histologically, as a consequence of impaired calcification within the cartilage growth plate the pattern of chondrocyte differentiation and maturation is disrupted and disorganized—whereas osteoid seams widen at other sites of bone formation.[241] In subjects deprived of phosphate, it is the trabeculae that are primarily undermineralized. Impaired mineralization of osteoid may be due to dietary deficiencies or depressed intestinal absorption of calcium, phosphate, or vitamin D; inadequate amounts of these nutrients in fluids utilized in total parenteral nutrition; metabolic errors in the metabolism or action of

TABLE 17-6

Disorders of Bone Mineralization: Rickets

I. Vitamin D Deficiency

A. Decreased Intake, Endogenous Synthesis, Retention, or Sequestration

1. Maternal vitamin D deficiency - breast feeding
2. Reduced skin synthesis - sunlight deprivation, sunscreen use, increased skin pigmentation
3. Malabsorption - celiac disease, hepatobiliary dysfunction, short gut syndrome, cystic fibrosis, inflammatory bowel disease, gastric bypass surgery
4. Drugs - anticonvulsants, glucocorticoids, cholestyramine
5. Nephrotic syndrome
6. Obesity

B. Metabolic Errors

1. Deficiency of 25-hydroxylase
a. Loss-of-function mutation of *CYP2R1*
b. Hepatic dysfunction
2. Deficiency of 25OH-vitamin D_3-1-hydroxylase
a. Loss-of-function mutation of *CYP27B1*
b. Decreased renal mass - hypoplasia, chronic renal insufficiency
3. Loss-of-function mutation of vitamin D receptor (*VDR*)

II. Calcium Deficiency

A. Nutritional Deprivation

B. Hypercalciuria - Hyperprostaglandin E2 Syndromes

III. Phosphate Deficiency

A. Nutritional Deprivation

1. Low-birth-weight infant
2. Aluminum-containing antacids

B. Hyperphosphaturia

1. X-linked-dominant familial hypophosphatemic rickets (*PHEX*)
2. Autosomal-dominant hypophosphatemic rickets (*FGF23*)
3. Autosomal-recessive hypophosphatemic rickets with hypercalciuria (*SLC34A3*)
4. Autosomal-recessive hypophosphatemic rickets (*DMP1*)
5. X-linked-recessive hypophosphatemic rickets (*CLCN5*)
6. Oncogenic hypophosphatemic osteomalacia (*FGF23, sFRP4, MEPE, FGF7*)
7. Renal tubular acidosis
a. Renal tubular acidosis - Fanconi syndrome
  • Heritable - cystinosis, tyrosinemia, hereditary fructose intolerance, galactosemia, idiopathic (AD, AR, XLR)
  • Acquired - nephrotic syndrome, vitamin D deficiency, renal vein thrombosis, cadmium, lead, bismuth, outdated tetracycline, 6-mercaptopurine, valproic acid, ifosfamide, saccharated ferric oxide

IV. Hypophosphatasia

A. Perinatal, Infantile, Childhood, and Adult Forms (ALPL)

B. Odontohypophosphatasia

C. Pseudohypophosphatasia

V. Inhibitors of Mineralization

A. Aluminum - Parenteral

B. Bisphosphonates

C. Fluoride

---

rarely to a defect in its metabolism to the active metabolite calcitriol or in its cellular action), to decreased intake of calcium or its excessive loss in urine, or phosphopenic (related to renal phosphate wasting due to primary renal tubular defects in phosphate reabsorption or to generation of excessive amounts of phosphatonins, compounds that inhibit normal renal handling of phosphate). Thus, nutritional rickets may be due to decreased intake of vitamin D (or inadequate exposure to sunlight) or calcium or to marginal intakes of both nutrients. Dietary deficiency of phosphate is unusual, given its wide availability. However, this nutrient may be deficient in parenteral fluids. Bone mineralization may also be directly impaired by abnormalities of alkaline phosphatase generation or by agents such as aluminum or fluoride.[241]

Calciopenic Rickets

Neonates born to severely vitamin-D-deficient mothers may display signs of rickets at birth, including fractures and hypocalcemia. Clinical manifestations of rickets in preambulatory infants include bowing of the forearms, craniotabes, frontal bossing, and delayed closure of the cranial fontanelles.[243] In older infants and children, genu varum or valgum (bowed legs or knock knees) or a windswept deformity involving both legs, flaring (widening) of the metaphyses of the long bones with markedly enlarged wrists, prominence of the costochondral junctions (rachitic rosary), and indentation of the lower anterior thoracic wall (Harrison's groove) are noted. Tooth eruption may be delayed, and the enamel hypoplastic (predisposing to dental caries). Short stature and suboptimal weight are also frequently present.[244]

Because vitamin D has so many extraskeletal sites of action, there are a number of nonosseous systemic symptoms observed in children with vitamin-D-deficiency rickets. These include muscular weakness (manifested by hypotonia and delay in walking), anorexia, and increased susceptibility to infection—particularly pneumonia (due both to the lack of the stimulatory effect of vitamin D on the immune system and weakness of the thoracic wall).[245] Occasionally, reversible cardiomyopathy may develop.

Hypocalcemia, tetany, and seizures may occur in a severely vitamin-D-deficient infant without gross clinical or radiographic signs of rickets. Rarely, vitamin D deficiency in an adolescent may be associated with hypocalcemic seizures and fractures.[246] Radiographically, osteopenia with cortical thinning and thin stress fracture lines—as well as cupping, widening, and irregularity (fraying) of the distal metaphyses of the long bones—are observed in the rachitic subject.[12,242] Areas of osteitis fibrosa cystica associated with secondary hyperparathyroidism may sometimes develop. Bone pain is the most common symptom of osteomalacia in the adult.

After the introduction of cod liver oil as a dietary supplement in 1918 (and the later fortication of infant formulas and milk and other foods with irradiated ergosterol) and the discovery in 1919 that exposure to sunlight prevented development of rickets, nutritional deficiency of vitamin D became relatively unusual in North America—only to reemerge seven decades later.[247] Presently, deficiency of vitamin D occurs predominantly in darkly

---

vitamin D; defects in renal tubular conservation of phosphate or calcium; or abnormalities of alkaline phosphatase generation and function (Table 17-6).

Broadly, rickets may be considered calciopenic—usually related to nutritional deprivation of vitamin D (or

skinned black or brown infants and young children who ingest a diet low in vitamin D (breast milk from a vegetarian or poorly nourished mother or one with little or no dietary milk, meat, eggs, or fish) without supplemental vitamin D and who have limited exposure to sunlight because they are confined indoors due to illness, the climate, or parental choice or because they wear clothing that shields the entire body from sunlight.[244,245]

More than half of 30 infants with nutritional vitamin D deficiency cared for at two North Carolina medical schools between the years 1990 and 1999 were identified in 1998 and 1999, suggesting an increasing incidence of this problem. The median age at diagnosis was 15.5 months. Presenting complaints included failure to thrive, skeletal deformities, and hypocalcemic tetany/seizures.[244] During the same interval, 30 infants with vitamin-D-deficient rickets were identified in Maryland. All were black and had been breast fed for 6 or more months, and 90% had not received vitamin D supplements.[248] Vitamin D deficiency is more common in breast-fed black infants than in white infants due in large part to increased maternal skin pigmentation and decreased endogenous synthesis of cholecalciferol that coupled with socioeconomic circumstances leads to lower levels of 25OHD in maternal serum and of vitamin D in breast milk. These infants are also more likely to be weaned to diets low in calcium and vitamin D.[241]

Subtle forms of vitamin D deficiency or insufficiency are prevalent throughout the North American population, particularly in the winter months when there is little sunlight exposure and the ultraviolet light requisite for endogenous synthesis of vitamin D is limited.[12,43] In a group of 307 healthy urban male and female adolescents 11 to 18 years of age in the northeastern United States, 42% had serum concentrations of 25OHD less than 20 ng/mL.[249] The prevalence of very low 25OHD values (<15 ng/mL) was most common in black (36%) and Hispanic subjects (22%), whereas 6% of white students had such levels. There was an inverse relationship between serum levels of 25OHD and PTH, with secondary hyperparathyroidism present in many subjects and with low 25OHD concentrations implying the likelihood of incipient metabolic bone disease.

In addition to skin pigmentation and northern latitude, low 25OHD values were attributable to meager consumption of milk and multivitamins due to a large intake of phosphate-containing soft drinks and to increase in fat mass into which vitamin D had been deposited and thus not bioavailable. Similar findings have been recorded in otherwise healthy adolescent females in the United Kingdom.[250] Interestingly, women with low milk intake during childhood are at increased risk for low bone mass and increased fracture rate as adults.[251] Inasmuch as there is reasonable evidence that serum values of 25OHD below 30 to 32 ng/mL are suboptimal, the prevalence of vitamin D deficiency or insufficiency may be far greater than is currently acknowledged.[43,252]

Assuming a reliable assay such as those employing liquid chromatography-tandem mass spectrometry that measure both 25OHD$_2$ and 25OHD$_3$, 25OHD concentrations below 12 to 15 ng/mL in children clearly indicate vitamin D deficiency and values between 15 to 31 ng/mL are consistent with vitamin D insufficiency.[241,253] Serum levels of 25OHD that exceed 60 to 100 ng/mL are indicative of vitamin D excess. Subtle dietary deficiency of calcium may accentuate the adverse effects of borderline vitamin D stores.[254]

Vitamin D deficiency may also be the consequence of intestinal malabsorptive disorders (such as celiac disease, biliary obstruction, gastric resection or bypass, or pancreatic exocrine insufficiency), ingestion of calcium-binding agents such as cholestyramine, or the accelerated degradation by anticonvulsant drugs (such as phenytoin) of vitamin D to water-soluble forms that increase its urinary loss.[43] In the majority of infants and children with rickets due to vitamin D deficiency, serum concentrations of total calcium are borderline-normal or low, phosphate levels low, and alkaline phosphatase activity and PTH concentrations increased (Table 17-7). Secondary hyperparathyroidism develops as the intestinal absorption of calcium is reduced, resulting in lowered serum levels. PTH increases urinary phosphate loss and lowers serum phosphate concentrations while enhancing the rates of bone resorption and turnover.[242]

PTH also increases synthesis of calcitriol, which may increase the rate of calcidiol metabolism and further deplete the body's store of vitamin D.[241] Typically, in vitamin D deficiency serum concentrations of calcidiol are low—whereas calcitriol values may be normal, high, or low (depending on whether vitamin D deficiency is modest, moderate, or severe). Serum concentrations of osteocalcin are low. Serum levels of PICP (a marker of bone formation) and ICTP and urinary excretion of NTx (markers of bone resorption) are substantially increased in infants with vitamin D deficiency rickets, indicating increased collagen turnover in this disorder.[255] With treatment, these values increase transiently and then fall to age-appropriate norms before radiographic healing of the rachitic lesions is complete.

Prevention of vitamin D deficiency is its most effective management. Because the amount of vitamin D in human breast milk is approximately 20 IU/L and vitamin D supplementation of the breast-feeding mother may be inadequate to ensure normal calcidiol levels in her infant (unless she is receiving approximately 2000 IU per day), it is important that all breast-fed infants receive a supplement of vitamin D daily (200–400 IU/day). By extension, this recommendation is also appropriate for infants who are not receiving adequate amounts of vitamin D in their prepared formulas or diet or have suboptimal exposure to sunlight.[43,241,243,244,247,256] It is somewhat ironic that an increase in the incidence of vitamin D deficiency in infants and children coincides with well-intentioned recommendations that exposure to sunlight be limited by sunscreen and protective clothing.

Vitamin D supplementation (at least 400 IU/day and perhaps as high as 800 to 1,000 IU/day) is appropriate throughout life if sunlight exposure is limited.[43,252] In the active lightly dressed white child with skin that normally tans with exposure to sunlight and who plays outdoors 30 minutes thrice weekly, endogenous vitamin D synthesis is usually sufficient to obviate the need for supplementation.[241,243] A brown or black-skinned child requires several fold longer sunlight exposure for a comparable biologic effect. The latitude in which the child lives, season of the

TABLE 17-7

Laboratory Data in Rickets of Varying Pathogenesis

Type	Calcium	Phosphate	Alkaline Phosphatase	Calcidiol	Calcitriol	PT
Calcium deficiency	↓↓	↓	↑↑	N	↑	↑
Phosphate deficiency	N, ↑	↓↓	↑↑	N	↑	N,↓
Vitamin D deficiency						
Mild	N,↓	N,↓	↑	↓	N	N
Moderate	N,↓	↓	↑↑	↓	↓,N,↑	↑
Severe	↓	↓	↑↑	↓↓	↓	↑↑
Loss-of-function *CYP2R1* (25-hydroxylase)	↓	↓	↑	↓	↓	↑
Loss-of-function *CYP27B1* (25OHD-1α-hydroxylase)	↓↓	↓↓	↑↑↑	N	↓↓↓	↑↑↑
Loss-of-function *VDR* (Resistance to calcitriol)	↓↓	↓↓	↑↑↑	N	↑↑↑	↑↑↑
Loss-of-function *PHEX* (X-linked hypophosphatemic rickets)	N	↓	↑	N	N,↓	N

N = normal, ↓ = low, ↑ = high.

year, time of day, local environmental pollutants, amount of clothing, and use of sunscreen affect the time required for sunlight exposure to evoke adequate vitamin D synthesis in the individual child.[256] Between November and February, little or no vitamin D can be synthesized above 35 degrees latitude (Atlanta, GA)—but vitamin D insufficiency is also prevalent in lower latitudes.[43,257]

Once established, vitamin D deficiency in the child or adolescent may be treated by the oral ingestion of vitamin D$_3$ 2,000 to 10,000 IU daily for 4 to 6 weeks or 50,000 IU weekly for 8 weeks or by the administration of a single oral (or intramuscular) dose of 150,000 to 600,000 units of vitamin D$_3$—depending on patient age and other individual circumstances.[43,220,241] At the beginning of treatment, elemental calcium (40 mg/kg/day in divided doses) must also be administered to the vitamin-D-deficient child receiving vitamin D in order to avoid the hypocalcemia that accompanies rapid remineralization of bone matrix (the hungry bone syndrome). Serial measurement of total and/or bone-specific alkaline phosphatase values is an effective tool for monitoring the efficacy of treatment as levels decline progressively in tandem with the roentgenographic healing of the rachitic lesions.[255] Care should be exercised to avoid hypercalcemia, hypercalciuria, and nephrocalcinosis.

Rickets due primarily to low dietary intake of calcium has been observed in infants who ingest low-calcium-containing formulas and in children from developing countries receiving a diet with 200 mg (or less) of elemental calcium per day despite normal intake of phosphate and adequate endogenous stores of vitamin D as determined by serum calcidiol levels.[241] Calcium intake in these infants and children is well below that recommended (375 mg/day in infants, 500 mg/day in children below 4 years of age, 800–1300 mg/day in older children and adolescents). Histologically, bone biopsies from children with calcium-deficiency rickets reveal widened seams of unmineralized osteoid and low bone turnover rates—findings compatible with rickets.

In Nigerian infants, rickets due to vitamin D deficiency is most prevalent between 4 and 12 months of age. In 123 older Nigerian children (34–63 months of age) with rickets, low serum concentrations of calcium, normal phosphate levels, normal to low calcidiol, and elevated calcitriol concentrations, administration of calcium alone (1,000 mg daily in divided doses orally over 24 weeks) resulted in more rapid decline in serum levels of alkaline phosphatase and in radiographic healing of rickets than did administration of vitamin D (600,000 IU intramuscularly at inception of the study and at +12 weeks)—data supportive of the concept that calcium deficiency alone was the cause of the rickets in this population.[258]

Interestingly, calcidiol values rose and calcitriol levels declined with calcium supplementation alone—suggesting that a low-calcium diet and attendant calcium deficiency led to increased secretion of PTH and accelerated conversion of calcidiol to calcitriol. Calcium deficiency rickets also occurs in the United States when after completion of breast feeding infants and children are weaned to low-calcium-containing foods.[254] Calcium deficiency rickets may also develop as a consequence of impaired intestinal absorption of dietary calcium that has been bound by ingestion of high fiber- and phytate-containing cereals. Calcium deficiency is best addressed by its prevention, ensuring adequate intake of this element according to established guidelines for growing children and adolescents. When present, calcium deficiency rickets may be effectively treated by ensuring an intake of 1,000 mg of elemental calcium daily for 6 months—with provision of normal amounts of vitamin D by sunlight exposure or supplementation.[242]

Dietary phosphate deficiency is unusual because it is present in large amounts in most foods. Phosphate deficiency occurs in patients receiving parenteral nutrition with fluids low in this cation, in those ingesting large amounts of aluminum-containing antiacids as aluminum and phosphate co-precipitate in the intestinal tract, and in premature infants drinking human breast milk without supplemental phosphate.[242] In very premature infants receiving long-term parenteral nutrition, development of metabolic bone disease is frequent and related to deficiencies of calcium, phosphate, and vitamin D and to excess aluminum in the infusates.

Infants receiving large amounts of aluminum-containing antiacids over prolonged periods for treatment of gastroesophageal reflux may also have substantially low bone mass. Aluminum lowers the rate of bone formation by several mechanisms. Administered orally, aluminum binds intestinal phosphate—thereby impeding its absorption and leading to phosphate depletion. Administered intravenously during total parenteral nutrition or during hemodialysis, aluminum inhibits osteoblastic function and prevents mineralization of osteoid. It also impairs the secretion of PTH and decreases 25OHD-1α hydroxylase activity.[242] Patients requiring total parenteral nutrition should receive as much calcium and phosphate as can be administered safely—as well as supplemental vitamin D 400 IU/day.

Periodic measurements of serum levels of calcium, phosphate, alkaline phosphatase, PTH, and calcidiol (and serial skeletal radiographs and estimations of skeletal mineralization) are recommended in patients receiving total parenteral nutrition. If metabolic bone disease develops in spite of these efforts, serum aluminum levels should be measured. If they are elevated (>100 μg/L), a search for the source of the aluminum should be initiated and that product eliminated from the infusate if possible. Cadmium, fluoride, and saccharated ferric oxide are also able to impede normal bone mineralization.[242]

Metabolic and functional defects of vitamin D lead to rare forms of rickets. Rickets due to a defect in 25-hydroxylation has been described in two brothers of Nigerian origin in whom a homozygous loss-of-function mutation (Leu99Pro) in CYP2R1 eliminated hydroxylase activity of this 501aa protein.[259,260] Hypocalcemia, hypophosphatemia, skeletal abnormalities of rickets, and low plasma levels of 25OHD were present in these siblings. Vitamin-D-dependent rickets type 1 (OMIM 264700) or pseudovitamin D deficiency rickets (PDDR) type 1 is due to loss-of-function mutations in CYP27B1—the enzyme in the renal proximal tubule that catalyzes 1α-hydroxylation of 25OHD to 1,25(OH)$_2$D or calcitriol, the biologically active metabolite of vitamin D.[261,521] PDDR type 1 is an autosomal-recessive disease whose clinical manifestations [including bone deformities (bowing of the forearms), growth retardation, weakness, and/or seizures] appear in the first year of life. Biochemically, hypocalcemia, hypophosphatemia, hyperphosphatasemia, and markedly elevated serum levels of PTH are typical. Radiographs reveal rachitic deformities of the long bones.

The diagnosis of PDDR type 1 is established by finding normal serum concentrations of calcidiol but extremely low calcitriol values that do not increase after administration of vitamin D or calcidiol. The diagnosis is confirmed by identification of the mutation in CYP27B1 (Table 17-7). The clinical, biochemical, and radiographic manifestations of PDDR resolve completely and reason-

ably rapidly following treatment with physiologic amounts of calcitriol (10–20 ng/kg/day). Serum calcium concentrations often begin to rise within the first 24 hours of treatment. Life-long therapy is necessary, and calcitriol doses usually need to be increased during pregnancy. PDDR type 1 is found with high frequency in a Quebec French-Canadian population but occurs in all races and in diverse geographic regions.

CYP27B1 encodes a 508aa mitochondrial cytochrome P450 hydroxylase with conserved sites that bind ferrodoxin and heme. Many loss-of-function missense, nonsense, splicing, and duplication or deletion/frame-shift mutations in CYP27B1 lead to inactive or truncated protein products that are unable to bind substrate (calcidiol) or heme—the latter defect preventing electron transfer and inhibiting catalysis (Figure 17-11).[262] The most common mutation in CYP27B1 in the Quebec French-Canadian population at risk for PDDR type 1 is deletion of guanine at nucleotide 958 (codon 88, exon 2), which changes the reading frame and results in premature termination of translation and an inactive product (the Charlevoix mutation). A second common mutation in this population is triplication of a normally duplicated sequence in exon 8. However, this mutation is also found in patients of other ethnicities (Asian, Hispanic).

Homozygous or compound heterozygous inactivating mutations of VDR, the gene encoding the vitamin D receptor, lead to resistance to the biologic effects of calcitriol (autosomal-recessive vitamin-D-dependent rickets type II or vitamin-D-resistant rickets, OMIM 277440).[261,263] In addition to the radiographic findings of rickets, clinical and biochemical manifestations of resistance to calcitriol include severe infantile-onset bony deformities characteristic of rickets, growth retardation, varying degrees of alopecia, hypocalcemia, hypophosphatemia, and extraordinarily high serum concentrations of calcitriol (300–1,000 pg/mL) and PTH. Serum levels of 24,25-dihydroxyvitamin D are often low (Table 17-7).

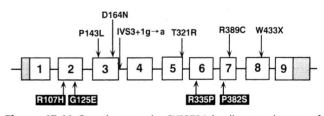

Figure 17-11 Genetic errors in CYP27B1 leading to absence of P450c1α activity, decreased synthesis of calcitriol, and pseudovitamin D deficiency rickets. IVS3 + 1g6a is guanine-to-adenosine transition in the first nucleotide of intron 3, resulting in retention of intron 3 in the transcribed product and introduction of a premature stop codon. Mutations have been identified in each of the nine exons of CYP27B1—including Q65H (exon 1), W241Ter (exon 4), S323Y (exon 6), R429 P (exon 8), P497R (exon 9)—and in introns 2, 3, 6, and 7. Abbreviations: C (cysteine), D (aspartic acid), E (glutamic acid), G (glycine), H (histidine), L (leucine), N (asparagine), P (proline), Q (glutamine), R (arginine), S (serine), T (threonine), W (tryptophan), Y (tyrosine), and X (termination). [Reproduced with permission from Kitanaka S, et al. (1999). No enzyme activity of 25-hydroxyvitamin D$_3$ 1α-hydroxylase gene product in pseudovitamin D deficiency rickets, including that with mild clinical manifestation. J Clin Endocrinol Metab 84:4111–4117.]

The high calcitriol values reflect the combined stimulatory effects of hypocalcemia, hypophosphatemia, and secondary hyperparathyroidism on the activity of 25OHD₃ 1α-hydroxylase together with decrease in its rate of catabolism due to depressed calcitriol-dependent 1,25α-dihydroxyvitamin D₃ 24-hydroxylase activity. Alopecia is the result of impaired vitamin D function in epithelial nuclei and those of the outer root-sheath cells of the hair follicle. Loss-of-function mutations (particularly in the DNA-binding region) of *VDR* result in a phenocopy of the generalized alopecia associated with loss of *HR* function (Hairless, OMIM 602302, chromosome 8p21.2). Interestingly, the role of the VDR in the maintenance of normal hair growth is not dependent on its binding to ligand.[261,264]

Although striking in infancy and early childhood, clinical manifestations of this disorder may vary and patients with milder defects in VDR may not be identified until adolescence or adulthood. The *VDR* consists of DNA-, ligand-, and retinoid-X-receptor-binding domains and a transactivation domain to which many co-modulators of VDR function are recruited. Loss-of-function mutations have been found in each of these domains. The mutated VDR may be unable to bind calcitriol because of decreased receptor number or affinity for ligand, incapable of forming heterodimers with the retinoid X receptor or translocating to the targeted gene in the nucleus, unable to bind to the vitamin D response element (VDRE) or to initiate gene transcription once bound to the VDRE (Figure 17-12).

Spontaneous remission of the rachitic process may occur rarely, most often between 7 and 15 years of age and when the patient enters puberty.[265] The diagnosis of vitamin-D-resistant rickets is suggested by the finding of elevated serum concentrations of calcitriol in the rachitic patient and confirmed by identification of the loss-of-function mutation in *VDR*. In general, patients with vitamin-D-resistant rickets without alopecia may be more responsive to treatment.[263] Administration of high doses of calcitriol (1 to 6 μg/kg/day) and supplemental calcium (1 to 3 g of elemental calcium

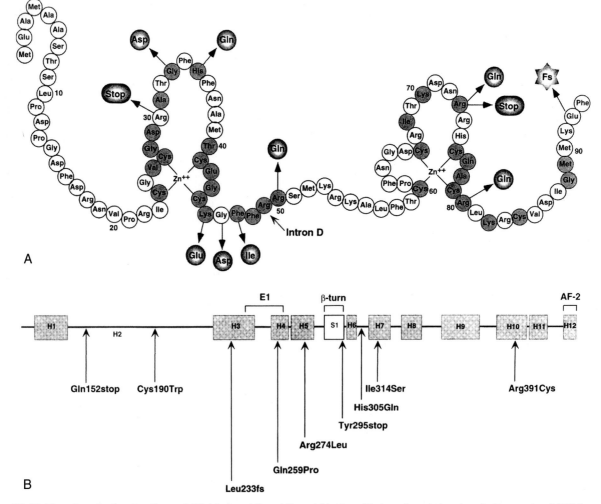

Figure 17-12 Mutations in the zinc-finger DNA-binding (*A*) and ligand-binding (*B*) domains of the vitamin D receptor (VDR) in patients with end-organ insensitivity to vitamin D. Shaded amino acids are conserved. Large circled amino acids denote missense mutations. Abbreviations: FS (frame-shift), H (α helixes), E1 (helixes within the ligand binding domain involved in transactivation), β-turn (change in spatial orientation of the VDR protein). [Reproduced with permission from Malloy PJ, et al. (1999). The vitamin D receptor and the syndrome of hereditary 1,25-dihydroxyvitamin D-resistant rickets. Endocrine Reviews 20:156–188.]

daily) has been effective in increasing serum calcium concentrations and healing rickets in patients with nonsense and missense mutations in *VDR* that lead to decreased affinity for ligand or alter nuclear targeting. It is appropriate to provide a trial of high-dose calcitriol/calcium therapy to each patient with vitamin-D-resistant rickets regardless of the *VDR* mutation.[261,263]

During treatment, serum values of calcium, phosphate, alkaline phosphatase, creatinine, and PTH; urinary calcium and creatinine excretion; skeletal radiographs; and renal ultrasounds for development of nephrocalcinosis are monitored serially. In patients refractory to oral therapy, continuous intravenous or intracaval administration of large amounts of calcium (0.4–1.4 g of elemental calcium/m^2/day) normalizes calcium, phosphate, alkaline phosphatase, and PTH values; heals rickets; and increases growth rate in selected children. If this mode of therapy is employed, careful monitoring for catheter sepsis and cardiac arrhythmia (as well as hypercalcemia, hypercalciuria, and nephrocalcinosis) is mandatory.

After healing of the rickets by parenteral calcium, maintenance therapy with large doses of oral calcium (3.5–9 grams of elemental calcium/m^2/day) is appropriate. In younger infants with vitamin-D-resistant rickets prior to development of florid rickets, high doses of oral calcium may ameliorate the rachitic process. These clinical observations indicate that the major defect in patients with vitamin-D-resistant rickets is lack of calcium. With treatment, growth may normalize in patients with vitamin D resistance. However, if alopecia is present the condition is unlikely to resolve.[265]

Genetically engineered mice in which the VDR has been inactivated by ablation of the second zinc finger in the DNA-binding domain *(Vdr^/-^)* are normal at birth, but develop an expanded zone of hypertrophic chondrocytes in the cartilage growth plate at 15 days, hypocalcemia at 21 days, alopecia at 28 days, and rickets by 35 days of age.[266] Except for alopecia, all of these abnormalities can be prevented (including the histomorphometric abnormalities characteristic of calciopenic rickets) by feeding these animals a diet known to prevent rickets in vitamin-D-deficient rats that is high in calcium (2% versus 1%), phosphorus (1.5% versus 0.67%), and lactose (20% versus none, lactose being a disaccharide that increases intestinal mucosal transport of calcium) beginning at 16 days of age.[266,267]

Clinical and experimental observations suggest that despite its known effects on osteoblast and osteoclast differentiation and function the primary role of the vitamin-D/VDR system in bone formation is to increase intestinal absorption of calcium in order to provide sufficient amounts of this cation for hydroxyapatite formation. Furthermore, in the mouse model of vitamin-D-resistant rickets maintenance of eucalcemia prevents secondary hyperparathyroidism—indicating that Ca^{2+} is a more potent regulator of PTH expression than is calcitriol and that secondary hyperparathyroidism is of fundamental pathophysiologic importance in the development of rickets of different etiologies.

A second form of vitamin D resistance (OMIM 600785) but with intact VDR and a phenotype similar to that of vitamin-D-dependent rickets type II (except for alopecia)

is due to inhibition of binding of the VDR-retinoid X receptor heterodimer to the VDRE by a member of a family of heterogeneous nuclear ribonucleoproteins.[268,269] *HNRPA1* encodes one of several ribonucleoproteins that are able to bind the VDRE and to inhibit its transactivation by the VDR-retinoid X receptor heterodimer. The mechanism by which overexpression of these otherwise normal ribonucleoproteins occurs is unknown at present.

Phosphopenic Rickets

Hypophosphatemia in childhood may be due to hereditary or acquired disorders (Table 17-8). Acute hypophosphatemia is accompanied by paresthesias, muscle weakness, and confusion. Chronic hypophosphatemia is often manifested by rickets. One of the most common (1:20,000

TABLE 17-8
Disorders of Phosphate Homeostasis in Children

I. Hypophosphatemia

A. Decreased Intestinal Absorption

1. Decreased intake/absorption - parenteral hyperalimentation, antacid abuse, starvation (anorexia nervosa)
2. Malabsorption - vitamin D deficiency, metabolism, function

B. Increased Urinary Excretion

1. Hypophosphatemic rickets - X-linked (*PHEX*), autosomal dominant (*FGF23*), autosomal recessive (*DMP1*), autosomal recessive with hypercalciuria (*SLC34A3*), X-linked recessive (*CLCN5*), tumor-induced osteomalacia, fibrous dysplasia (*GNAS*)
2. Renal tubular defects - Dent and Fanconi syndromes, postrenal transplantation, hypomagnesemia, fructose intolerance, macrophage activation syndrome
3. Hyperparathyroidism, acidosis, respiratory alkalosis
4. Drugs - diuretics, bicarbonate, glucocorticoids, calcitonin
5. Expansion of extracellular fluid volume

C. Shift from Extracellular to Intracellular Space

1. Recovery from diabetic ketoacidosis/insulin administration, sepsis, salicylate intoxication
2. Administration of glucose, nutritional repletion, hungry bone syndrome

II. Hyperphosphatemia

A. Increased Intake

1. Intravenous, oral, rectal

B. Decreased Urinary Excretion

1. Renal insufficiency
2. Hypoparathyroidism, acromegaly
3. Pseudohypoparathyroidism (*GNAS*)
4. Familial tumoral calcinosis (*FGF23*, *GALNT3*)
a. Hyperostosis hyperphosphatemia syndrome (*FGF23*, *GALNT3*)
5. Drugs - growth hormone, bisphosphonates

C. Excess Bone Resorption

1. Severe illness - acidosis (metabolic or respiratory), hemolytic anemia, diabetic ketoacidosis, hepatitis, catabolic states, rhabdomyolysis, hyperthermai
2. Drugs - cytotoxic therapy

Modified from Hruska KA (2006). Hyperphosphatemia and hypophosphatemia. In Favus MJ (ed.), *Primer on the metabolic bone diseases and disorders of mineral metabolism, Sixth edition.* Washington, D. C.: American Society for Bone and Mineral Research 233–242; and from Ward LM (2005). Renal phosphate-wasting disorders in childhood. Pediatr Endocrinol Rev 2:342–350.

births) forms of clinically evident rickets encountered in developed countries is X-linked hypophosphatemic rickets (XHR, OMIM 307800). XHR is an X-linked dominant disorder manifested in affected hemizygous males and heterozygous females, albeit with substantial inter- and intrafamilial variability in its clinical expression. Physical findings in children with XHR include short stature, genu varum or valgum that develops when the infant begins to walk, flaring of the metaphyses, rachitic rosary, frontal bossing, increased frequency of dental decay and/or periradicular abscesses in teeth free of caries, and bone, muscle, and joint aching and stiffness.

Craniotabes, tetany, and muscular weakness are not found in patients with XHR as they are in those with vitamin D deficiency. Adults with XHR have osteomalacia and increased fracture rate, dental abscesses, and bone pain. They may also develop stenosis of the spinal canal. Enesopathy (calcification of tendons, ligaments, and joint capsules) is common in adults and may be present in children with XHR. Whereas serum levels of total calcium and Ca^{2+}_e are normal, hypophosphatemia is marked due to urinary wastage because of substantially decreased renal tubular reabsorption of filtered phosphate and limited intestinal absorption of this anion. Serum concentrations of PTH and calcidiol are normal, but calcitriol values are inappropriately low for the degree of hypophosphatemia. Serum alkaline phosphatase activity is increased.[270]

Because the serum Ca^{2+}_e concentration is normal, secondary hyperparathyroidism does not occur unless the patient receives excessive amounts of supplemental phosphate. Phosphate induces differentiation and death of hypertrophic chondrocytes in the cartilage growth plate by activating the mitochondrial apoptotic pathway that is caspase 9 dependent.[261,271] Thus, hypophosphatemia leads to delayed loss and increased numbers of hypertrophic chondrocytes and expansion of the growth plate characteristic of rickets. Histomorphometrically in XHR, unmineralized osteoid accumulates along the trabeculae within cancellous bone.

Classic XHR is caused by loss-of-function mutations in *PHEX* (phosphate-regulating endopeptidase homolog, X-linked).[272] *PHEX* is a 22-exon gene that encodes a 749-aa integral membrane protein with very long extracellular (702 aa), transmembrane (27 aa), and short intracellular (20 aa) domains that structurally resembles several neutral endopeptidases (endothelin-converting enzyme-1, Kell antigen). The extracellular domain has 10 conserved cysteine residues and a pentapeptide motif (His-Glu-Phe-Thr-His) characteristic of zinc metallopeptidases that may either convert propeptides to active forms or degrade and inactivate their substrates. *PHEX* is expressed in bone (osteoblasts), muscle, lung, liver, testis, and ovary. Its expression by osteoblasts is down-regulated by calcitriol.[273]

In most patients with XHR, inactivating mutations of *PHEX* have been found primarily in the extracellular domain and include frame-shift deletions (16%), duplications, insertions (8%), deletional-insertional, splice site (15%), nonsense (27%), and missense (34%) mutations—many in exons 15 and 17. A mutation has also been identified in the 5'-untranslated region (A→G transver-

sion 429 bp upstream of the ATG initiation site, Figure 17-13).[272,274,275] Because PHEX is a glycosylated protein, failure of glycosylation leads to its sequestration within the endoplasmic reticulum—thus impeding its movement (trafficking) to the cell membrane. Other mutations interfere with the catalytic function of the protein or its three-dimensional conformation.[276] Mutations in *PHEX* arise spontaneously in more than 20% of patients with XHR. There is no correlation between the location or type of mutation in *PHEX* and the clinical manifestations or severity of the disease.[277,278]

Fibroblast growth factor (FGF)-23 (OMIM 605380, chromosome 12p13.3), is a phosphate-wasting element present in high concentrations in the serum of patients with XHR and serum concentrations of FGF23 correlate with the degree of hypophosphatemia.[279] FGF23 is a 251-aa that inhibits sodium-dependent phosphate uptake by renal proximal tubular cells and depresses 25OHD-1α hydroxylase activity and thus synthesis of calcitriol—characteristics that define a phosphatonin (a family of phosphaturic agents that includes in addition to FGF23, matrix extracellular phosphoglycoprotein and serum frizzled related protein-4).[280] FGF23 inhibits phosphate reabsorption by down-regulating expression of the genes encoding type II (a and c) sodium-phosphate co-transporters present in the apical membrane of the renal tubule. FGF23 is expressed and secreted primarily by osteoblasts and osteocytes.

FGF23 is coexpressed with PHEX in these cells. Normally, FGF23 is cleaved to biologically inactive products between amino acids Arg179 and Ser180 by metallic endopeptidases such as PHEX. Although the natural endogenous substrate for PHEX was thought likely to be FGF23, this peptide is not a substrate for PHEX action.[281,282] Rather, FGF23 is cleaved by subtilisin-like proprotein and furin-like convertases. In normal adults, the mean serum FGF23 concentration utilizing an immunometric assay that detects intact FGF23 is 29 pg/mL. FGF23 levels decline in response to phosphate deprivation and increase with phosphate loading, consistent with an important role for FGF23 in the normal regulation of serum phosphate concentrations and phosphate homeostasis.[283]

In the Hyp mouse model of XHR, there is increased expression of *Fgf23* in bone and in osteoblasts in vitro. Because normally *PHEX* is also expressed in bone, these observations suggest that decreased expression of *PHEX* in the Hyp mouse (and the patient with XLH) may up-regulate expression of *Fgf23*.[282] Although serum levels of matrix extracellular phosphoglycoprotein have been reported to be increased in some patients with XHR, it plays no role in the pathogenesis of XHR in the Hyp mouse (and its role in the human disorder is likely to be limited).[280,284]

When renal function is normal, rickets of diverse pathogenesis is commonly associated with hypophosphatemia. Secondary hyperparathyroidism as a cause of hypophosphatemia may be suspected by the presence of elevated serum concentrations of PTH (e.g., vitamin D deficiency). Serum PTH values are normal in subjects with primary hypophosphatemia due to an abnormality in renal tubular resorption of phosphate intrinsic to the renal cell or mediated by a circulating phosphatonin.[272]

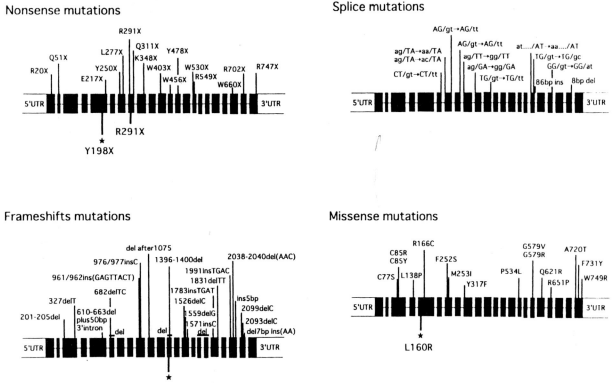

Figure 17-13 Nonsense, splice, frame-shift, and missense mutations in PHEX in patients with X-linked hypophosphatemic rickets. [Reproduced with permission from Sato K, et al. (2000). Three novel *PHEX* gene mutations in Japanese patients with X-linked hypophosphatemic rickets. Pediatr Res 48:536–540.]

The diagnosis of XHR is established when the typical family history (if the patient is not the initial mutant), clinical findings (deformities of the lower extremities, flaring of the metaphyses), and roentgenographic (rachitic changes) and laboratory data (hypophosphatemia, hyperphosphaturia, inappropriately low serum level of calcitriol, normal serum concentration of PTH, calcium, creatinine, and 25OHD) are present and when other causes of hypophosphatemia and hyperphosphaturia have been excluded (Tables 17-6 through 17-8).

The diagnosis of XHR may be confirmed by identification of the *PHEX* mutation, although occasionally no mutation is detected by current methods.[277] Rarely, somatic and germ-line mosaicism for a mutation in *PHEX* may mimic autosomal-dominant transmission of hypophosphatemic rickets.[285] The primary therapeutic agents employed in the treatment of XHR are calcitriol (25–70 ng/kg/day) administered in two doses (with the larger dose given at night when PTH secretion tends to increase) and elemental phosphorus 0.25 to 3 g daily (beginning at a dose of 30 mg/kg/day and increasing to 70 mg/kg/day) administered in four to six divided daily doses depending on age, size, compliance, and response to therapy.[272]

Table 17-3 lists the preparations of oral phosphate. Infants and young children may tolerate a phospha-soda solution more readily than other preparations. When able, most older children prefer a chewable phosphate tablet to the powder form that is dissolved in water or juice. Acidic potassium phosphate products are preferred because they do not increase intravascular volume and phosphate excretion and because they acidify the urine, thereby increasing the solubility of calcium phosphate. Calcitriol (Rocaltrol, Roche Pharmaceuticals) is available as an oral solution at a concentration of 1 μg/mL and as capsules with either 0.25 or 0.5 μg per capsule.

If hypercalcemia or hypercalciuria (urine calcium excretion more than 4 mg/kg/day) occurs during treatment, the dose of calcitriol should be lowered. If that leads to exacerbation of the rachitic process, an agent (e.g., amiloride) that increases renal tubular resorption of calcium may be added cautiously to the therapeutic program. Frequent (every 3 months) clinical evaluation and measurement of serum and urine calcium, phosphate, alkaline phosphatase, and creatinine levels and serum intact PTH values are essential to avoid hypercalcemia, hypercalciuria, nephrocalcinosis, and secondary hyperparathyroidism because high doses of phosphate may lead to counterproductive secondary (and sometimes tertiary) hyperparathyroidism.

Two goals of therapy of XHR are to maintain serum phosphate concentrations determined before a daytime dose of phosphate in the low normal range and alkaline phosphatase values within the high normal range. Renal sonograms prior to treatment and at 12-month intervals during therapy to identify early-stage nephrocalcinosis (and yearly skeletal radiographs to assess the degree of healing of the rickets) are recommended. Complete radiologic healing of XHR is often difficult to attain. Development of nephrocalcinosis (and compromise of renal function in some patients) is directly related to the amount of phosphate the patient receives. Hyperoxaluria has also been implicated in the pathogenesis of nephrocalcinosis.

Co-management with an experienced orthopedist is important because the orthopedist may prescribe braces, or in patients with extreme and progressive deformities perform corrective osteotomies. However, bracing is unpredictable and poorly tolerated—and osteotomies are often followed by complications. Femoral and tibial hemiepiphysiodeses may offer alternative surgical procedures for the correction of lower limb deformities in children with XHR younger than 10 years of age.[286]

The birth length of children with XHR is normal, but growth rate is slow during the first several years of life—leading to progressive shortening of height. Many children with XHR are significantly short by 5 years of age, although some patients (particularly girls) with minimal involvement may grow normally.[287] Treatment of the older child with XHR with calcitriol and phosphate may improve growth rate, in part due to correction of the deformities of the lower extremities.[288] During puberty, gain in height is normal in boys (+28.2 cm) and girls (+24.2 cm) with XHR. Thus, the compromised adult stature in XHR is related to impaired early childhood and preadolescent growth.

In a series of 19 closely monitored children with XHR, initiation of treatment with calcitriol and phosphate at a mean chronologic age of 4.2 months (range of 7 weeks to 6 months, N = 8) resulted in greater adult stature [−0.2 versus −1.2 standard deviations (SD)] than when treatment began at a mean age of 2.1 years (range of 1.3 to 8.0 years, N = 11)—with no difference in complication rate (secondary hyperparathyroidism, nephrocalcinosis, craniosynostosis) between the two groups.[289] The enhanced growth response to early treatment was likely related to the normal length and mild skeletal and biochemical signs of rickets in early infancy and the prevention of more clinically significant bone disease as the child aged.

Despite close adherence to treatment, many children with XLH retain mild to moderate radiographic signs of rickets and mildly elevated serum alkaline phosphatase activities—although the extent of lower limb deformities is often ameliorated by good compliance. GH increases glomerular filtration rate, renal tubular resorption, serum concentrations of phosphate, and rate of accrual of bone mineral. In the short term (6–12 months), GH accelerates the velocity of linear growth of children with XHR.[290-292] Approximately 90 children with XHR who have been treated with rhGH combined with conventional therapy have been reported. The majority have experienced improved linear growth, and some have achieved normal adult stature.[293] Whether GH therapy will increase adult stature in larger series of XHR subjects remains a matter of further clinical investigation. Future treatment of XHR may include development of agents that decrease production of FGF23, accelerate its degradation, or block its action in the renal tubule.

The majority of untreated adults with XHR are hypophosphatemic. Serum alkaline phosphatase activity is increased, and osteomalacia is present on bone biopsy.

Nevertheless, these patients are often clinically asymptomatic except for frequent dental abscesses, degenerative hip disease due to deformities of the lower limbs, and hearing impairment.[272] Occasionally, a female with XHR may be clinically well despite isolated hypophosphatemia. Roentgenographic manifestations of XHR in adults include thickening of the spinous processes and fusion of the vertebrae and stenosis of the spinal canal.

BMD determined by single and dual-photon absorptiometry tends to be normal in adults with XHR (despite the histomorphologic abnormalities), suggesting that most of these subjects are not at increased risk for osteoporotic fractures. However, in approximately 25% of adults with XHR there is clinical evidence of osteomalacia such as progressive lower limb deformities, bone pain, fractures, and pseudofractures.[294,295] Treatment of these patients with calcitriol and phosphate can be beneficial.[296]

Autosomal-dominant hypophosphatemic rickets (ADHR, OMIM 193100) is a partial phenocopy of XHR with hyperphosphaturia and inappropriately low serum levels of calcitriol that is due to mutations (Arg176Gln, Arg179Trp) in FGF23 that render the product less susceptible to cleavage between amino acid residues 179 and 180 by furin, a pro-protein convertase.[297] ADHR may be incompletely penetrant, variable in age of onset (childhood to adult), and rarely self-limiting.[298] The clinical, biochemical, and radiographic findings in ADHR are similar to those of XHR except that ADHR subjects manifest muscle weakness as a consequence of hypophosphatemia.[299]

ADHR may be identified by its pattern of transmission and detection of a mutation in FGF23. Treatment involves administration of calcitriol and phosphate, with close serial monitoring for safety and because hyperphosphaturia may occasionally resolve spontaneously. Excessive production of FGF23 with hypophosphatemia and inappropriately low calcitriol values has also been documented in patients with autosomal-recessive hypophosphatemic rickets, fibrous dysplasia due to a gain-of-function mutations in GNAS, the linear nevus sebaceous syndrome associated with hypophosphatemic rickets (OMIM 163200), osteoglophonic dysplasia (OMIM 166250; craniosynostosis, rhizomelic shortening of the limbs, noncalcifying bone lesions), and opsismodysplasia [OMIM 258480, a spondylo(epi)metaphyseal dysplasia with delayed ossification, micromelia, platyspondyly, and vertebral hypoplasia].[280,300]

Tumor-induced osteomalacia/rickets is an acquired disorder due to excessive production of one of several phosphatonins by a tumor of mesodermal origin. The majority of such tumors have secreted FGF23, but these neoplasms have also synthesized secreted frizzled related protein-4, matrix extracellular phosphoglycoprotein, and FGF7—all of which increase urinary phosphate excretion and suppress renal synthesis of calcitriol, albeit perhaps not to the same extent as FGF23.[280,301] The identification of an FGF23-secreting tumor is dependent on the sensitivity of the FGF23 assay employed.[302]

Although unusual in children, tumor-induced osteomalacia/rickets has been described in this age group. For example, an 11-year-old girl had significant bone pain and functional limitation associated with biopsy-proven hypophosphatemic osteomalacia/rickets and markedly elevated serum levels of FGF23.[303] Following removal of a benign fibro-osseous tumor from a small exostosis on a distal ulnar metaphysis, serum FGF23 concentrations normalized within 7 hours postoperatively and phosphate levels were normal 2 weeks later. Clinical symptoms abated, and radiographic and histomorphometric abnormalities resolved within 1 year after surgery.

In an 11-year-old boy with severe bone pain, weakness progressing to confinement to a wheelchair, hyperphosphaturia, and hypophosphatemia, elevated levels of FGF23 (1874 RU/mL) declined to normal values (43 RU/mL) within 48 hours after removal of a FGF23-containing hemangiopericytoma from his left iliac wing.[304] This lesion had not been identified by routine roentgenograms, computed tomographic or magnetic resonance imaging, or technetium bone scan. The tumor was demonstrated only by gradient recall echo magnetic resonance imaging (Figure 17-14). Within 2 weeks after surgery, the lad was walking without assistance—and several weeks thereafter he resumed normal activity.

Autosomal-recessive hypophosphatemic rickets (ARHR, OMIM 241520) is clinically, biochemically, and histomorphometrically similar to XHR and ADHR except for its mode of transmission and for the development of osteosclerosis at the base of the skull and in the calvarial bones. Serum concentrations of FGF23 are elevated in these subjects, and calcitriol values are inappropriately normal. Urinary calcium excretion is normal. Familial ARHR has been associated with homozygous loss-of-function mutations in the gene encoding dentin matrix acidic phosphoprotein 1 (DMP1).[305,306] DMP1 is a member of a class of tooth and bone noncollagenous matrix proteins termed SIBLING proteins (small integrin-binding ligand, N-linked glycoproteins) that include osteopontin and bone sialoprotein.

These substances regulate phosphorylation of proteins essential to initial nucleation of calcium and phosphate, as well as to early formation of hydroxyapatite crystals and hence to mineralization of osteoid.[307] DMP1 is ex-pressed in osteocytes. Rickets and osteopenia develop in mice in whom Dmp1 has been deleted.[305,308] In osteocytes without Dmp1, the expression of Fgf23 is increased and secondarily hyperphosphaturia develops—suggesting that Dmp1 regulates expression of Fgf23. This disorder has permitted identification of a bone-renal axis essential to normal bone mineralization, although the mechanism by which Dmp1 may regulate expression of Fgf23 has not yet been elucidated.

Autosomal-recessive hereditary hypophosphatemic rickets with hypercalciuria (OMIM 241530) is due to renal wastage of phosphate and is the consequence of a loss-of-function mutation in SLC34A3 encoding sodium-dependent phosphate co-transporter type IIC (NPT2c). This 599aa protein with eight transmembrane domains is located in the brush border of juxtamedullary proximal renal tubular cells. Because calcitriol synthesis is normal in these subjects, its production is substantially elevated in response to hypophosphatemia. Thus, intestinal absorption of calcium and its urinary excretion are increased.

Heterozygotic carriers of inactivating mutations in SLC34A3 also have moderately increased serum concentrations of calcitriol, hyperphosphaturia, and hypercalciuria but do not have identified metabolic bone disease. Loss-of-function missense and nonsense mutations have been found throughout the coding region of SLC34A3, as well as deletions in introns 9 and 10.[309,310] This disorder may be treated with phosphate salts in conjunction with hydration and avoidance of a high-sodium diet. Supplemental vitamin D is not needed, and may even be detrimental.

Increased urinary phosphate excretion due to acquired and heritable disorders of the proximal renal tubule is characteristic of the metabolic bone disease that accompanies various forms of the Fanconi syndrome of renal tubular acidosis, glucosuria, and amino aciduria (heritable:cystinosis, tyrosinemia, galactosemia, oculo-cerebral-renal syndrome, fructose intolerance, and Wilson disease, and acquired renal transplantation,

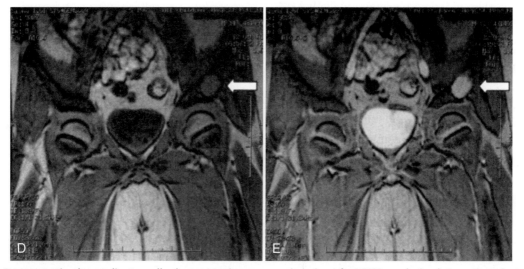

Figure 17-14 Demonstration by gradient recall echo magnetic resonance imaging of a FGF23 producing hemangiopericytoma in the left iliac wing of an 11-year-old boy with tumor-induced rickets. [Reproduced with permission from Shulman DI, et al. (2004). Tumor-induced rickets: Usefulness of MR gradient echo recall imaging for tumor localization. J Pediatr 144:381–385.]

nephrotic syndrome, renal vein thrombosis, mercury, lead and copper poisoning, and outdated tetracycline).[311,312] In addition to hypophosphatemia, acidosis contributes to the pathogenesis of bone disease in Fanconi syndrome by increasing the solubility of the mineral phase of bone, increasing urinary loss of calcium, and impairing conversion of calcidiol to calcitriol.

Inactivating mutations in *CLCN5* encoding a voltage-gated proximal renal tubular chloride channel lead to X-linked recessive hypophosphatemic rickets (XLRH, OMIM 300534); X-linked nephrocalcinosis, nephrolithiasis, and renal failure (OMIM 310468); and Dent disease (aminoaciduria, proteinuria, glycosuria, hypercalciuria, nephrocalcinosis, nephrolithiasis; OMIM 300009).[311,313] Mutations in different domains of this 12exon 746aa transmembrane chloride channel result in varying clinical and biochemical manifestations. The Ser244Leu mutation in *CLCN5* has ben particularly associated with X-linked recessive hypophosphatemic rickets.[314] Causes of hyperphosphatemia are also listed in Table 17-8.

Disorders of Alkaline Phosphatase

In its severe forms, hypophosphatasia is an autosomal-recessive disorder due to loss-of-function mutations in *ALPL*—the gene encoding the isoenzyme of tissue-nonspecific (bone/liver/kidney) alkaline phosphatase (TNSALP).[98] TNSALP is a homodimeric phosphomonoesterase anchored through its carboxyl terminal to the exterior of the cell membrane (i.e., an ectophosphatase) by a phosphatydylinositol-glycan moiety.[315] Pathophysiologically, decreased TNSALP activity leads to accumulation of its endogenous substrates pyrophosphate, pyridoxal 5'-phosphate, and phosphoethanolamine. Pyrophosphate is an inhibitor of osteoid mineralization. Calcification of bone matrix is impaired because pyrophosphate coats the surface of hydroxyapatite crystals, restricting crystal growth. In addition, inability to raise bone matrix phosphate levels to values sufficient to permit normal deposition of hydroxyapatite contributes to decreased bone mineralization.

Clinical manifestations of inactivating mutations of *ALPL* reflect the extent of loss of function of mutant ALPL. The younger the age of onset the more severe the disease is likely to be. The perinatal form is often a lethal disorder (at times in utero) due to marked osteopenia leading to cranial malformation; intracranial hemorrhage; pyridoxine-dependent seizures; short, bowed, and fractured extremities; and fractures of the ribs and deformities of the chest wall resulting in respiratory insufficiency and apnea. Survival is unusual. The infantile form (OMIM 241500) develops in the first 6 months of life and is characterized by anorexia, impaired linear growth and weight gain, deformities of the long bones and rib cage, widely open fontanelles and sutures (calvarial hypomineralization) with functional craniosynostosis with increased intracranial pressure manifested by prominence of the anterior fontanelle, proptosis, papilledema, pyridoxine-dependent seizures, hypotonia, constipation, hypercalcemia, hypercalciuria, and radiographic evidence of rickets with marked skeletal hypomineralization. Approximately 50% of these infants die of respiratory failure before their first birthday.

During childhood (OMIM 241510), clinical findings range from isolated premature shedding of deciduous teeth to physical and radiographic evidence of low bone mass and rickets. Spontaneous clinical improvement may occur during puberty and evolve into the adult form (OMIM 146300), which may be subclinical and identified when studying the family of an offspring with hypophosphatasia. The parent may have a history of premature loss of teeth, increased susceptibility to recurrent fractures predominantly of the metatarsal bones, pseudofractures of the proximal femur, chondrocalcinosis, or pseudogout due to articular deposition of calcium pyrophosphate dihydrate crystals.

Odontohypophosphatasia (OMIM 146300) is manifested only by premature shedding of primary teeth without radiologic abnormalities. Periodontitis may also develop. Pseudohypophosphatasia is phenotypically and biochemically similar to the classic disease, but serum alkaline phosphatase activity in vitro is normal—indicating that in this disorder enzyme activity toward fabricated substrates is preserved but alkaline phosphatase activity toward endogenous substrates is abnormal. The perinatal and infantile forms of hypophosphatasia are usually inherited as autosomal-recessive diseases, whereas childhood and adult forms may be transmitted as autosomal-recessive or autosomal-dominant traits.

In addition to the site(s) of mutation of *ALPL,* the clinical severity of hypophosphatasia is related inversely to the age at which skeletal disease is evident and to individual biologic factors that affect the expression of the disease. In the lethal perinatal form of hypophosphatasia, missense, nonsense, and frame-shift mutations in TNSALP cluster in crucial segments of the protein within (Ala94Thr, Arg-167Trp) or near (Gly103Arg, Gly317Asp) its enzyme active site or at the homodimer interface (Ala23Val, Arg374Cys).[315] These mutations interrupt binding to the phosphate ligand or destabilize attachment of necessary cofactors. On the other hand, *ALPL* mutations associated with infantile and childhood forms of hypophosphatasia (Arg119His, Asp361Val) tend to cluster on the three-dimensional surface of the enzyme molecule (at sites that relate to its tethering to the cell surface or its formation of tetramers) and retain substantial residual bioactivity.

In some patients with moderately severe hypophosphatasia, heterozygotic mutations in *ALPL* (Gly46Val, Arg167Trp, Asn461Ile) exert a dominant-negative effect on the intact TNSALP dimer. These mutations have been clustered at the enzyme active site or at the domain(s) involved with dimerization, tetramerization, or membrane anchoring.[316] Odontohypophosphatasia has been associated with heterozygotic mutations in *ALPL* (Pro-91Leu, Ala99Thr). In a mouse knockout model of hypophosphatasia with inactivating mutations of *Alpl,* the clinical, biochemical, radiographic, and histologic findings are similar to those in infants with this disease.[317]

These animals are small at birth, grow poorly, and succumb within the first several months of life. Bone roentgenograms and histology are normal at birth and through 8 days of age, even though no TNSALP activity can be demonstrated. They become increasingly abnormal thereafter. There is developmental arrest of chondrocyte differentiation, with failure of hypertrophic zone differentiation, formation of secondary ossification centers, and marked accumulation of unmineralized bone matrix—leading to skeletal deformities and fractures. In addition, these animals have seizures due to deficiency of pyridoxine—the product of TNSALP dephosphorylation of pyridoxal 5'-phosphate and the cofactor form of vitamin B_6 necessary for the synthesis of neural γ-aminobutyric acid.

Diagnostically, in addition to the clinical findings and radiographic features of rickets patients with hypophosphatasia have low serum levels of total and bone-specific alkaline phosphatase activity, increased serum concentrations of pyrophosphate and pyridoxal-5'-phosphate (~5,000 nM), and elevated urinary excretion of phosphoethanolamine (0.5–1.5 mmol/g of creatinine, control 0.15 mmol/g) and pyrophosphate (500–1,000 µmol/g of creatinine, control 200 µmol/g). In contrast to other forms of rickets, serum concentrations of calcium and phosphate are normal or even elevated—likely because intestinal absorption of calcium and renal tubular reabsorption of phosphate are normal, whereas the bone formation rate is depressed. In the perinatal and infantile forms of hypophosphatasia, hypercalcemia is frequent.[98,228]

There are normal serum levels of PTH and no evidence of secondary hyperparathyroidism. Although serum alkaline phosphatase activity in vitro is normal in patients with pseudohypophosphatasia, it is functionally inadequate in vivo—perhaps because the TNSALP protein is sequestered within the cell due to a defect in its transport to the cell surface or because the protein is active with artificial substrate but not with natural substrates at physiologic pH. There is no specific or effective therapy for hypophosphatasia currently available. Enzyme replacement by infusion of serum from patients with Paget disease and high alkaline phosphatase activity has been of only occasional and limited benefit. Administration of even small doses of vitamin D or its metabolites should be avoided because these patients easily develop hypercalcemia. Hypercalcemia in infants with hypophosphatasia responds to bisphosphonates and transiently to calcitonin.[318] Bone marrow transplantation may be effective therapy but requires further evaluation.[98] Seizures may be responsive to pyridoxine administration. Milder adult forms of hypophosphatasia may be responsive to teriparatide (rhPTH[1-34]).[318a]

Serum bone-specific alkaline phosphatase activity is normally increased during puberty and in response to skeletal injuries and reflects osteoblastic activity. Hyperphosphatasemia is encountered transiently in clinically well infants and children less than 5 years of age (median age 16 months). In this situation, serum activities of bone and liver alkaline phosphatases isoforms are increased, but there are no skeletal abnormalities. It is a self-limited process, with alkaline phosphatase values returning to normal within several months.[319] Rarely, hyperphosphatasemia may be familial and transmitted as a benign autosomal-dominant trait.[320] Occasionally, an adolescent with persistent nonfamilial benign hyperphosphatasemia may be encountered. In one family, familial hyperphosphatasemia has been associated with mental retardation (OMIM 239300).

Juvenile Paget disease (OMIM 239000), also termed *hyperostosis corticalis deformans juvenilis*, often begins in early childhood and is characterized clinically by expanded and bowed extremities, nontraumatic fractures of the long bones, kyphosis, macrocephaly, and muscular weakness. This disorder may progress to wheelchair dependence. Serum levels of alkaline phosphatase are markedly increased—a coupled response to increased osteoclastic action. Radiographic skeletal abnormalities include cortical thickening, osteosclerosis and osteopenia, coarse trabeculations, and progressive skeletal deformities. The disorder is due to biallelic loss-of-function mutations of *TNFRSF11B* encoding osteoprotegerin—a member of the tumor necrosis factor (TNF) receptor superfamily that functions as a decoy acceptor for receptor activator of nuclear factor κB-ligand (RANKL)—thereby modulating osteoclastogenesis. Hence, inactivating mutations of *TNFRSF11B* are associated with enhanced osteoclastic activity.

The severity of juvenile Paget disease depends on the site of mutation. Those that result in deletion of the entire gene or those in the ligand-binding domain that involved loss of cysteine residues result in marked clinical disease.[321-323] Treatment with recombinant osteoprotegerin has resulted in clinical and radiologic improvement.[324] Familial expansile osteolysis (OMIM 174810) is an autosomal-dominant disorder pathophysiologically similar to juvenile Paget disease but clinically and etiologically distinct.

Focal areas of increased bone turnover in the appendicular skeleton appear in the second decade of life, followed by medullary expansion, pathologic fractures, and skeletal deformities. Deafness and premature loss of dentition may occur. The disorder is due to monoallelic gain-of-function mutations (insertion duplications of 18 and 27 bases in the signal peptide region of exon 1) of the gene (*TNFRSF11A*) encoding RANK that result in an increase in NFκB signaling, as a consequence of which there is augmented osteoclastogenesis.[325]

RENAL OSTEODYSTROPHY

Renal osteodystrophy is the metabolic bone disease that accompanies chronic renal failure. It is most commonly associated with a high rate of bone remodeling (increased rates of bone resorption and formation) due to secondary hyperparathyroidism (high-turnover lesions of osteitis fibrosa). Dynamic (low-turnover) bone disease with relatively low PTH secretion and osteomalacia due to accumulation of aluminum may also occur. Generally, areas of low- and high-turnover skeletal abnormalities (termed mixed renal osteodystrophy) are detected by histomorphometry.[326,327] The pathogenesis of secondary hyperparathyroidism is multifactorial (Figure 17-15).

When the glomerular filtration rate declines to less than 30% of normal, urinary phosphate excretion is impaired—leading to its intracellular and extracellular accumulation, hyperphosphatemia, and very slight hypocalcemia (the latter two leading to secondary increase in PTH generation). In addition, down-regulation of the expression of *CASR* in uremic PTGs (raising of the set-point) contributes to chief cell hyperplasia and augmented PTH release—as do decline in calcitriol synthesis and relative skeletal insensitivity to PTH. Phosphate may also slow the rate of

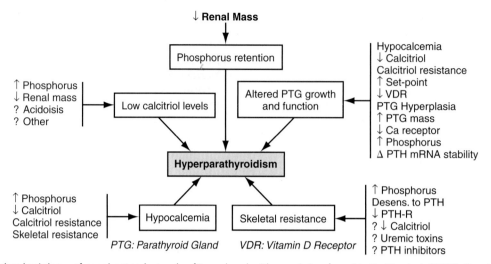

Figure 17-15 Pathophysiology of renal osteodystrophy. [Reproduced with permission from Martin KJ, et al. (2006). Renal osteodystrophy. In Favus MJ (ed.), *Primer on the metabolic bone diseases and disorders of mineral metabolism, Sixth edition.* Washington, D.C.: American Society for Bone and Mineral Research 359–366.]

degradation of PTH mRNA within the PTG and exert a direct enhancing effect on PTG growth.

Because calcitriol inhibits PTG growth and function, decrease in its synthesis also results in increased proliferation of parathyroid chief cells and synthesis of PTH. In the presence of elevated PTH secretion and various cytokines [IL-1, -6, and -11; TNF; and macrophage-colony stimulating factor (M-CSF)], osteoclastogenesis and the rates of bone resorption and formation are increased. Acidosis contributes to the dissolution of the mineral phase of bone directly and by impairing osteoprotegerin-mediated inhibition of osteoclast generation.

Chronic renal disease and osteodystrophy in children may be clinically silent except for failure of linear growth. As the disease progresses, deformities of the extremities, slipped epiphyses, fractures, bone and joint pain, and weakness and lassitude develop. In patients in whom the rate of bone formation is diminished and the volume of unmineralized bone (i.e., osteomalacia) increased, the process has been due to accumulation of aluminum at the mineralization front. However, with discontinuation of aluminum-containing phosphate binders osteomalacia in renal failure is now unusual.[326] In the absence of osteomalacia, adynamic bone disease in chronic renal failure is the result of decreased PTH generation due to improved control of serum phosphate levels, increased calcium stores, higher levels of PTH[7-84] and other carboxyl terminal fragments of PTH that inhibit bone resorption, and other factors that affect tissue response to PTH.

Biochemically, renal osteodystrophy is marked primarily by hyperphosphatemia and increase in serum PTH concentrations and alkaline phosphatase activity. Radiographic signs of rickets, low bone mass, and pseudofractures are often present in children with renal osteodystrophy. Therapeutically, the goals in treating a child with chronic renal failure in an effort to minimize renal osteodystrophy are to maintain (near) normal serum calcium, phosphate, and alkaline phosphatase values and to prevent the development or progression of secondary hyperparathyroidism. To do so, supplemental vitamin D

and calcium may be needed—and dietary phosphate restriction imposed.

Calcitriol is able to decrease the rate of bone formation in patients with chronic renal insufficiency by inhibiting osteoblast differentiation or function, decreasing PTH synthesis, altering intra-PTG degradation of PTH, and decreasing expression of *PTHR1*. Calcium-containing oral phosphate binders may also be useful. Dialysis fluids must be prepared with aluminum-free water. When indicated, suppression of PTH secretion may be further achieved with the use of calcitriol analogues such as paricalcitol or of a synthetic ligand of the CaSR (cinacalcet hydrochloride).[326]

After successful renal transplantation, secondary hyperparathyroidism may persist for months or years—its extent and intensity reflecting the severity and duration of chronic renal failure before renal transplantation, development of nodular or monoclonal hyperplasia of the PTGs, and the 20-year life span of the parathyroid chief cell.[328] In one study of 47 childhood kidney recipients, 3 years after renal transplantation iliac crest bone biopsies revealed normal bone formation in 65% but persistent mild hyperparathyroidism in 25% and adynamic bone disease in 10%.[329] In all children in whom prerenal transplantation iliac crest biopsy revealed normal bone formation rates, the post-transplantation biopsy was also normal.

In approximately 50% of those patients with an abnormal pretransplantation biopsy, normal bone formation rates were achieved in the post-transplantation period. However, in many subjects secondary hyperparathyroidism or adynamic bone disease persisted or evolved—and random measurements of serum PTH concentrations did not necessarily correlate with or predict the histologic picture. Five years after renal transplantation during childhood, serum concentrations of PICP, osteocalcin, and ICTP remain significantly increased—indicating accelerated bone turnover rate—whereas areal and volumetric bone mineral densities at the distal third of the nondominant radius are normal for height but subnormal for age.[330] Hypercalcemia and persistent secondary or tertiary hyperparathyroidism requiring parathyroidectomy may become apparent in children after renal transplantation.[331] The osteopenic effects of glucocorticoids and immune suppressive agents such as cyclosporin are observed in postrenal transplantation patients as well.

LOW BONE MASS

Osteopenia and osteoporosis (porous bone) designate states of reduced bone mass and abnormalities of bone microarchitecture that increase the risk for fracture (osteomalacia refers primarily to decrease in the mineral phase of bone).[332,333] Osteoporosis in adults is defined by the World Health Organization (WHO) as a BMD at a specific bone site that is −2.5 or more SD below the mean peak young adult value for gender (T score). In adults, osteopenia is present when the BMD lies between −1.1 and −2.4 SD below the mean peak young adult value for gender—and a normal BMD is one that is not more than 1 SD below or above the mean peak young adult value.

When the BMD is more than +2 SD above the mean for age and gender, bone mass is considered high. The WHO-designated categories of low bone mass do not necessarily apply to children and adolescents in whom variability in height, weight, and stage of sexual maturation affect bone mineralization. Use of the terms osteopenia and osteoporosis has been discouraged (although not eliminated) when describing mineralization in children. Presently, children may be identified as those with low bone density (Table 17-9) for chronologic age or height or stage of sexual maturation (reported as less than −2 SD or Z score for gender)—provided the method employed for determination of bone mineralization [DEXA, quantitative computed tomography (QCT), QUS] and the specific instrument, software version utilized for analysis, and ethnic mix of the reference population are stated.[334-337]

Despite its limitations (provision of areal rather than volumetric BMD data and failure to distinguish between trabecular and cortical bone), DEXA is the most widely employed bone densitometric method in children at this time—although peripheral (p) QCT may become the method of choice in the future. In infants, children, and adolescents, DEXA whole-body bone mineral measurement (BMC, BMD) rather than regional measurements is the currently preferred index of mineralization status. The inclusion or exclusion of head measurements in the determination of whole-body BMC and BMD by DEXA should also be stated.[338,339] Relative to bone strength determined by calculation of the stress-strain index of a long bone with data garnered by pQCT, the DEXA whole-body areal BMC (minus the skull) for height appears to afford the most reliable measurement for determining cortical bone strength and hence fracture risk.[338]

Although heritable factors account for 60 to 80% of optimal bone mineralization, modifiable factors that contribute to the development of osteopenia and osteoporosis in adulthood (weight-bearing exercise, nutrition, body mass, hormonal milieu) have their genesis in utero, infancy, childhood, and adolescence.[332,333] In children (as in adults), bone mass, composition, and size determine bone strength. Decreased bone strength is associated with

---

TABLE 17-9

Disorders of Bone Mineralization: Low Bone Mass

I. Primary
A. Osteogenesis Imperfecta (Types I–VIII)
B. Osteoporosis-Pseudoglioma Syndrome (*LRP5*)
C. Idiopathic Juvenile Osteoporosis
D. Marfan Syndrome (*FBN1*)
E. Ehlers-Danlos Syndrome (*COL1A1*)
F. Homocystinuria (*CBS*)
G. Idiopathic Hypercalciuria
H. Fibrous Dysplasia (*GNAS*)
I. Glycogen Storage Disease Type I (*G6PC*)
J. Menkes Kinky Hair Syndrome (*ATP7A*)
II. Secondary
A. Suboptimal Nutrition
1. Socioeconomic
2. Cultural
3. Excessive exercise
4. Anorexia nervosa
5. Malabsorption - cystic fibrosis, celiac disease, biliary atresia, short gut syndrome, gastric bypass

B. Endocrinopathies/Metabolic Diseases
1. Constitutional delay in growth and sexual development
2. Hypogonadism
   a. Hypergonadotropic - gonadal dysgenesis (Turner, Klinefelter syndromes), aromatase deficiency, estrogen receptor deficiency
   b. Hypogonadotropic - Kallmann syndrome, excessive physical activity, hyperprolactinemia
3. Diabetes mellitus
4. Hyperglucocorticoidism
5. Hyperthyroidism
6. Hyperparathyroidism
7. Growth hormone deficiency
8. Inborn errors - homocystinuria, lysinuric protein intolerance, propionic aciduria, methylmalonic aciduria

C. Disuse/Immobilization
1. Femoral fracture
2. Cerebral palsy
3. Muscular dystrophy
4. Quadriplegia/paraplegia
5. Spina bifida

D. Drugs
1. Glucocorticoids, immune suppressants, anticonvulsants, antiretroviral therapy, warfarin, lithium, methotrexate, cyclosporine A
2. Alcohol, tobacco

E. Chronic Illness
1. Rheumatologic disease
2. Inflammatory bowel disease
3. Hemoglobinopathies - thalassemia, sickle cell disease
4. Hemophilia
5. Cranial radiation
6. Renal failure, transplantation
7. Malignancy - leukemia, lymphoma
8. Human immunodeficiency virus infection

Adapted from Bachrach LK (2005). Osteoporosis and measurement of bone mass in children and adolescents. Endocrinol Metab NA 34:521–535; and from Rauch F, Bishop N (2006). Juvenile osteoporosis. In Favus MJ (ed.), *Primer on the metabolic bone diseases and disorders of mineral metabolism, Sixth edition.* Washington, D.C.: American Society for Bone and Mineral Research 293–296.

a greater risk of forearm fractures in children.[340] Because many youths consume excessive amounts of carbonated beverages and diluted fruit juices (thus limiting their intake of milk), most children and adolescents ingest only 55% to 70% of the recommended daily calcium allowance (1,300 mg/day)—although late pubertal males tend to consume more than do pubertal females.[341-343]

In adolescent and adult females, excessive intake of cola drinks with high phosphoric acid content lower body calcium content because of the sequestration of dietary calcium in the intestinal tract and the needed dissolution of bone mineral to neutralize acid—with consequent development of mild secondary hyperparathyroidism.[344,345] Sedentary non weight-bearing activities encouraged by television, video, and computer games also impair bone mineralization.[346] It had been suggested that fat may enhance bone mineralization through increased mechanical stress and estrogen production and through the stimulatory effects of leptin on osteoblast differentiation.

Although body weight and fat mass have correlated with bone mass in many studies, other data suggested that fat has a negative effect on the accrual of bone mass.[347,348] In a study of 300 male and female adolescents and young adults (13–21 years of age) employing DEXA assessment of body composition and QCT measurement of the axial and appendicular skeletons, a positive correlation between lean mass and all bone measurements was demonstrated in both genders—whereas fat mass had an inverse relationship or no relationship to bone mass. These observations strongly suggest that bone mass and strength are determined by dynamic muscular force and not by static load.[348] The mechanism(s) through which fat might exert an inhibitory effect on bone mass is unknown but may be related to the synthesis of cytokines that negatively affect bone accrual. An alternative postulated mechanism is through diversion of the mesenchymal stem cell (common to adipocytes and osteoblasts) into the adipogenic pathway.

The longer and more intense the weekly sporting activity (soccer, basketball, gymnastics, tennis) in children and adolescents the greater the vertebral and femoral BMDs independently of calcium intake.[343,346] In pre- and peripubertal children, simple school physical education programs utilizing jumping, hopping, and skipping exercises two to three times weekly significantly increase areal BMD at the femoral trochanter in as little as 8 months relative to children engaged in a standard physical education curriculum.[349-351] Thus, suboptimal nutrition and sedentary activities during childhood and adolescence (as well as consumption of colas and alcohol and smoking of cigarettes) prevent optimal bone mineralization and increase the likelihood of later development of osteoporosis and its complications.[342,352]

Because the risk of developing an osteoporotic fracture declines by 40% for every 5% increase in peak bone mineral mass, the foundation for the prevention of osteoporosis in the adult must be constructed in the child and adolescent by maintaining adequate calcium intake (1–3 years, 500 mg/day; 4–8 years, 800 mg/day; 9–18 years, 1,300 mg/day; >19 years, 1,000 mg/day), vitamin D stores (serum concentrations of 250 HD >30–32 ng/mL), and complementary weight-bearing activity during these formative years.[341,353] Discouragingly, combined quantitative analysis of multiple trials of calcium supplementation (usually of relatively short duration) in children revealed little effect on BMD or reduction of the risk of fracture.[354] However, the effects of sustained calcium supplementation over the many years of childhood and adolescence on future fracture risk has not been systematically examined.

Magnesium supplementation for 1 year increased BMC of the hip in healthy girls.[139] Sufficient protein, vitamins C and K, and copper must also be consumed for optimal bone matrix synthesis. It may be possible to identify the child or early pubertal subject at (genetic) risk for accrual of low peak bone mass and thus for later development of osteopenia/osteoporosis (e.g., offspring of a mother with osteopenia or osteoporosis). Axial and appendicular BMD and bone size determined by central or pQCT in the normal early pubertal boy and girl may accurately predict these measurements at sexual maturity.[355] If so, children at risk for low peak bone mass might benefit by a diet and exercise program during puberty that increases these values.

Nutritional deprivation depresses the rate of bone accrual, a process observed most dramatically in subjects with anorexia nervosa. The majority of postmenarchal late adolescent females with anorexia nervosa have significantly decreased total body, vertebral, and femoral neck areal BMDs—although volumetric BMDs may be normal for their small bone size.[356,357] In adolescent females with anorexia nervosa, decreased bone mineralization is associated with a slow rate of bone turnover—as demonstrated by lower serum concentrations of osteocalcin, estradiol, free testosterone, IGF-I, leptin, and bone-specific alkaline phosphatase and depressed urinary excretion of Dpd relative to normal-weight subjects.[356,358] In these patients, serum levels of osteoprotegerin correlate negatively with fat mass and leptin values and with lumbar spine areal and apparent BMDs. (by DEXA)

The decline in bone mass in adolescents with anorexia nervosa may be attributed to nutritional deprivation, chronic acidemia, and functional hypogonadism. Thus, the osteopenia encountered in patients with anorexia nervosa is the result of generalized nutritional deprivation with suboptimal intake of protein, calcium, and vitamin D; hypercortisolemia; and lowered IGF-I generation—leading to decreased osteoblast-mediated bone formation. Hypoestrogenism enhances to a limited extent osteoclast-stimulated bone resorption.[359] The bone loss of the patient with anorexia nervosa is not fully recovered even after return to normal weight, resulting in a several fold increase in fracture risk for these women.

In adolescents with anorexia nervosa, administration of estrogen/progestin does not increase bone mass or prevent its loss.[360] Bisphosphonates, IGF-I, and dehydroepiandrosterone have been reported to increase or maintain BMD in small series of patients with anorexia nervosa. However, their use should be limited presently to investigational studies.[359] Experimentally, in young adult female rats isocaloric restriction of protein alone lowers plasma concentrations of IGF-I—resulting in a decreased rate of periosteal cortical bone formation and impaired osteoblastic responsiveness to IGF-I.[361] The athletic triad of suboptimal body fat mass, amenorrhea in women, and osteoporosis is encountered in the highly trained female athlete and in male elite long-distance runners.

Acute immobilization of the healthy active child and adolescent leads to sudden reduction in weight bearing, and to consequent decrease in the mechanical load on bones and thus a lowered rate of bone formation. In the presence of continued bone resorption, hypercalciuria and later hypercalcemia and lowered bone mass develop.[362] In the chronically partially or fully immobilized child or adolescent (cerebral palsy, spastic quadriplegia, muscular dystrophy), the fracture rate (primarily of the femur) is high during such simple maneuvers as turning, dressing, or feeding. In this group of subjects, not only lack of weight bearing but the severity of the primary illness, body size and pubertal status, state of general nutrition, vitamin D and calcium intake, coexisting inflammatory states, medications (e.g., anticonvulsants, glucocorticoids), and indoor confinement adversely impact bone mass and fracture risk.[363-365]

In a study group of 117 patients (2 to 19 years of age) with moderate to severe cerebral palsy, distal femoral BMD Z scores were below −2.0 in 77%—and the incidence of low femoral and vertebral BMDs as well as fractures increased with advancing age.[363] Distal femoral and lumbar vertebral BMDs increase at slower than normal rates as the child with spastic cerebral palsy ages, resulting in diminution of BMD Z score in the older subject.[364] Intravenous administration of pamidronate in a small (N = 6) selected group of children with quadriplegic cerebral palsy increased distal femoral BMD by +88% over 18 months, with mean Z score increasing from −4.0 to −1.8 over the interval of treatment.[366] In 5 lads with spastic cerebral palsy, daily administration of recombinant human GH (0.35 mg/kg/week) increased vertebral BMD assessed by DEXA by +1.17 SD over 18 months of therapy without altering the quality of life of these subjects.[367] Assisted standing alone increases BMD in children with severe cerebral palsy.[368,369]

The fundamental importance of normal gonadal sex steroid secretion during age-appropriate sexual maturation is emphasized by the observation that in adult males with delayed sexual development radial, vertebral, and femoral areal BMDs are lower than in males with normal timing of pubertal maturation.[370] Volumetric BMD has been reported to be normal or subnormal in young adult men with a history of delayed adolescence.[371,372] In prepubertal children of both genders with constitutional delay in growth, areal vertebral (trabecular) and non-dominant radial (cortical) BMC and BMD are decreased relative to values in age and size-matched subjects with familial genetic short stature before and after correction for height, weight, bone age, and sex.[373,374] This finding suggests that factors other than sex hormones may also impair bone mineralization in short children with delayed skeletal maturation.

Osteoporosis with reduced bone mass and abnormal microarchitecture results in decreased skeletal strength and increased risk of fracture. Histomorphometrically, in sex-steroid-deprived osteoporotic bone there is

decrease in bone cortical width, trabecular number, osteoid, and mineralization activity.[375] As a consequence of estrogen (and androgen) deficiency, there is increase in the production but decline in the life span of osteoblasts and osteocytes—whereas osteoclastogenesis is stimulated and the life span of osteoclasts prolonged. These events reflect the sum of the activities of multiple pro-osteoclastogenic cytokines (including M-CSF, IL-1, IL-6, TNF, RANKL), whose synthesis is regulated by estrogen.[375,376]

Although osteopenia responsive to estrogen has been recorded in adult males with aromatase deficiency, mature women with complete androgen insensitivity are also osteopenic despite normal to increased estrogen production—clearly indicating that androgens are also important to normal bone mineralization.[377] In prepubertal children and in adolescents with Turner syndrome, there is osteopenia with decreased cortical and trabecular bone mass.[378] Although decreased relative to chronologic age, areal and volumetric BMDs may be normal relative to height or bone age in girls with Turner syndrome. Nevertheless, the frequency of wrist fractures is increased during childhood—as may be the general risk for fractures in adults with Turner syndrome.

Estrogens, GH, and particularly the administration of both agents increase bone calcium deposition and BMD in adolescents with Turner syndrome.[378-380] In adults with Turner syndrome, however, there appears to be intrinsic reduction in cortical bone that is independent of sex hormones and might possibly be related to elevated levels of follicle-stimulating hormone—which may have intrinsic proresorptive properties distinct from its effect on estrogen synthesis.[307,381]

Pubertal subjects with primary (Klinefelter syndrome, galactosemia, postradiation, or chemotherapy) or secondary hypogonadism (anorexia nervosa, excessive physical training, hypogonadotropism) also have decreased bone mineralization. By decreasing estrogen production, even short-term (6 months) use of the intramuscular contraceptive depot medroxyprogesterone acetate (MPA) results in significant loss in bone mass in adolescent females and young women (18–21 years of age) when BMD would ordinarily be increasing. However, bone mass increases over time after this agent is discontinued.[359]

The adverse impact of depot MPA on BMD may be prevented by concomitant administration of estrogen. Estrogen-/progestin-containing oral contraceptives do not decrease bone mass in adolescent females, although they do slow its rate of acquisition. After treatment of the child with central precocious puberty for 1 to 2 years with a gonadotropin-releasing hormone analogue that suppresses pituitary-gonadal function, there may be arrest or even decline in bone mineral accumulation in the peripheral and axial skeletons—a process that can be prevented or reversed by the co-provision of 1 g of calcium per day during analogue therapy.[382]

The low bone mass of glucocorticoid excess is the result of inhibition of osteoblastogenesis and increase in the rate of apoptosis of the osteoblast and osteocyte leading to decrease in the rate of bone matrix formation and microfracture repair, and of enhanced osteoclastogenesis and decrease in the rate of apoptosis of the osteoclast—permitting prolonged and excessive bone resorption.[383] Thus, during each remodeling cycle the amount of bone replaced is far less than the amount removed and skeletal microarchitecture is degraded—resulting in declining bone strength. At the molecular level, glucocorticoids suppress expression and synthesis of RUNX2 and BMP-2—factors essential to prenatal and postnatal osteoblast differentiation, respectively—and increase osteoblast expression of RANKL and decrease expression of osteoprotegerin, changes that favor osteoclastogenesis.[383-385]

Glucocorticoids inhibit synthesis of collagen type I and increase its rate of degradation. They impair IGF-I formation and function. To a limited extent, glucocorticoids inhibit normal vitamin D metabolism and thereby vitamin-D-dependent intestinal absorption of calcium. They also increase renal loss of calcium by a direct effect on the renal tubule, leading to secondary hyperparathyroidism.[383,384] Glucocorticoids also reduce production of sex hormones in the adolescent and adult. The muscle weakness of chronic glucocorticoid exposure reduces the impact of mechanical forces on bone formation. Finally, the disease for which glucocorticoids have been prescribed may contribute to decreased bone mass by impairing mobility and by elaboration of osteoclastogenic cytokines.

The risk of glucocorticoid-induced low bone mass is far greater with oral than with inhaled glucocorticoids in children with asthma.[386] However, in young adults with asthma there is an inverse relationship between vertebral and femoral BMDs and cumulative dose of inhaled glucocorticoid—with increasing fracture risk as the dose and duration of glucocorticoid administration increases. A cumulative dose of 5,000 mg leads to a 1 SD decline in vertebral BMD.[387] In adult women with 21-hydroxylase-deficient congenital adrenal hyperplasia treated with glucocorticoids, bone mineralization is modestly reduced—in part related to the extent of suppression of adrenal androgen production.[388]

In children experiencing adverse effects of glucocorticoids on growth and bone mineralization, it is important to lower their steroid dose to the greatest extent possible and to withdraw them if at all feasible. Increased weight-bearing exercise (walking) and supplemental calcium and active vitamin D metabolites may be helpful. In 7 of 10 children with juvenile rheumatoid arthritis and other rheumatic disorders and glucocorticoid/illness-mediated low bone mass, pamidronate at a dose to 2 to 4 mg/kg per infusion administered at 6-month intervals was followed by decline in bone pain, improved ambulation, and progressive increase in BMD of the lumbar spine.[389] PTH[1-34] increases bone mass in adults with glucocorticoid-induced osteoporosis, but its efficacy and safety in children with this problem have not yet been evaluated.[390]

Low bone mass is often encountered in GH-deficient children and in adults with GH deficiency of childhood or adult onset. In part, low bone mass may be attributed to the small bone size of the short child compared to age peers. It is also due to loss of direct and indirect actions of GH (particularly impaired local generation of IGF-I) on osteoblast differentiation, proliferation, and function.

GH enhances osteoblastic expression of IGF-I and IGF binding protein-3 and stimulates their synthesis of osteocalcin, bone-specific alkaline phosphatase, and procollagen type I—thus increasing bone matrix formation.[391] Secondarily, it increases osteoclastogenesis and bone resorption. Thus, administration of GH to GH-deficient children and adults increases the rates of bone formation and destruction—the latter predominating initially. Over long periods of treatment (12–18 months), GH increases BMD in these patients. To achieve peak bone mass, however, GH therapy must be continued into adulthood.

Nevertheless, in many untreated adults with congenital GH deficiency volumetric BMD is often normal—reflecting the smaller size of their bones.[392] In normal short children, GH administration also increases areal BMD.[393] Thyroid hormone, through direct action on the osteoblast, increases synthesis of osteocalcin, alkaline phosphatase, and IGF-I. It also enhances osteoclastogenesis, and thus the rate of bone resorption—the latter effect predominating.[394] With excess thyroid hormone there is increase in the rate of bone turnover but decrease in the length of the bone remodeling cycle (primarily due to shortening of the bone formation phase), resulting in a net loss of mineralized bone.

As in adults with thyrotoxicosis, whole-body, vertebral, and femoral BMDs are low in children and adolescents with hyperthyroidism—but substantially increase within the first 12 to 24 months after restoration of the euthyroid state.[395] Administration of physiologic replacement doses of thyroxine to children with acquired or congenital hypothyroidism does not adversely affect bone mineralization during childhood, although adults with congenital hypothyroidism have a 10% reduction in radial bone mass.[396] In adolescents with type 1 diabetes mellitus, whole-body, axial, and appendicular bone mass assessed by DEXA is decreased relative to control subjects and inversely related to hemoglobin A1c values—reflecting the adverse effects of chronic hyperglycemia and insulin deficiency on bone formation.[397,398] Utilizing pQCT in young prepubertal subjects with type 1 diabetes mellitus, cortical bone cross-sectional area and BMD were found to be decreased—implying an increased risk for fracture.[399]

Bone mass is decreased in 80% of children with acute lymphoblastic leukemia, and 40% sustain a fracture within the first 2 years of treatment.[400] Pathogenetic factors involved in the development of low bone mass in these subjects include adverse effects of the disease itself directly on bone; radiation injury of bone; inhibitory effects of glucocorticoid, chemotherapeutic, antibiotic, and immunosuppressive agents on bone formation; decreased caloric, protein, and vitamin D intake; sex hormone deficiency due to delayed or arrested adolescent development; and GH deficiency in children who have received cranial radiation. Cyclosporine A induces bone loss in organ transplant recipients by increasing osteoblast expression of RANKL and decreasing production of osteoprotegerin, thereby augmenting osteoclastogenesis.[401]

Leukemic patients should receive appropriate calcium and vitamin D supplements, and treatment with GH if they are GH deficient after the primary illness has been in prolonged remission. Adult survivors of childhood-onset acute lymphoblastic leukemia also have significant osteopenia of the lumbar spine, femur, and radius—primarily related to GH deficiency.[402] Decreased bone mineralization is common in the post-bone-marrow or post-solid-organ transplant subject. Its diverse pathogenesis includes the primary disease itself and the chronic illness that may accompany it, the use of high-dose glucocorticoids and antirejection medications, and altered intestinal and renal function.[403]

In addition to provision of adequate nutrition, calcium, and vitamin D, in adults the effects of transplantation may be partially ameliorated by administration of bisphosphonates. Their usefulness and safety in pediatric transplant patients has not yet been fully evaluated. In severely burned patients and in children with hemophilia, sickle cell disease, central diabetes insipidus, Marfan syndrome, homocystinuria, lysinuric protein intolerance, propionic, and methylmalonic aciduria, BMD is also decreased.[404,405]

Children with cystic fibrosis may have low vertebral and femoral neck BMD Z scores as a consequence of suboptimal nutrition, chronic inflammation, concomitant diabetes mellitus, pubertal delay, and drug therapy. However, approximately one-third of optimally managed cystic fibrosis patients with good clinical control may nevertheless have subnormal BMDs (Z score below −1 but seldom below −2.5)—although this is not necessarily translated into increased fracture risk.[406,407] Low bone mass and vertebral collapse may be early manifestations of chronic inflammatory bowel disease.[408]

Vitamin D deficiency and secondary hyperparathyroidism, as well as the chronic inflammatory state and therapeutic agents (such as glucocorticoids), likely contribute to decreased bone formation and increased bone resorption in this illness. That whole-body BMC in children, adolescents, and young adults with chronic inflammatory bowel disease is reportedly normal relative to lean body mass (although reduced relative to racial, age, and height norms) does not necessarily imply that bone strength in these patients is normal—as evidenced by the increased fracture risk of adults with this disorder.[409,410] Low bone mass is common in children and adults with celiac disease.[411]

In children and adolescents infected with the human immunodeficiency virus, whole-body BMD is decreased as a consequence of the infective agent itself, the chronic inflammatory state it induces, suboptimal nutrition, and the administration of highly active antiretroviral therapy that may have direct effects on osteoblast and osteoclast generation and function.[412,413] Despite clinical well-being and normal linear growth, the rate of accrual of bone mass is decreased in these subjects—whereas the rate of bone resorption is increased. Bone mass is reduced in children with a variety of rheumatic diseases (juvenile idiopathic arthritis, systemic lupus erythematosus, juvenile dermatomyositis) due to the chronic inflammatory state, production of pro-osteoclastic cytokines, and therapy with glucocorticoids.[414]

Idiopathic juvenile osteoporosis (OMIM 259750) is an unusual disorder of generalized low bone mass of unknown pathogenesis that appears in mid to late childhood and often resolves as sexual maturity is achieved.[415] In affected subjects, roentgenograms ob-

tained for evaluation of joint, muscle, and/or back pain; difficulty walking; foreshortening of the trunk; and/or the presence of kyphosis reveal biconcave vertebrae and/or vertebral compression and long bone radiolucent areas and fractures in the metaphyses. Chemical studies are normal. Histomorphometry reveals findings consistent with a low rate of bone turnover, with reduction in cancellous bone volume, trabecular thickness, and bone formation due primarily to decreased osteoblast activity on the endosteal but not the periosteal bone surface. There is no evidence of increased bone resorption.

Idiopathic juvenile osteoporosis is quite likely to be genetically heterogenous in origin. Mutation analyses of *COL1A1* and *COL1A2* have been normal in these subjects. In 15% of patients with juvenile osteoporosis, a familial heterozygous loss-of-function mutation in the gene encoding LDL receptor-related protein 5 (*LRP5*) has been detected.[416] Homozygous loss of *LRP5* results in the osteoporosis-pseudoglioma syndrome. The most difficult diagnostic problem is the clinical distinction between idiopathic juvenile osteoporosis and osteogenesis imperfecta type I (Table 17-10).

This form of osteogenesis imperfecta is characterized clinically by a positive family history, onset in early infancy, lifelong persistence, diaphyseal fractures, blue sclerae, abnormal dentition, wormian bones, and high bone turnover.[131,415] In children with idiopathic juvenile osteoporosis, symptomatic treatment is offered. In some patients, calcitriol or supplemental sodium fluoride has been of benefit. Although the disorder ameliorates and even disappears at puberty, treatment of the prepubertal patient with sex steroids does not seem to accelerate the healing process. Administration of the bisphosphonate pamidronate has been helpful in reducing bone pain and increasing vertebral BMD in a small group of children with idiopathic juvenile osteoporosis.[417]

The osteoporosis-pseudoglioma syndrome (OMIM 259770) is characterized clinically by congenital or early infantile onset of severe visual impairment due to hyperplasia of the vitreous (pseudoglioma that may be erroneously identified as retinoblastoma), leading to retinal detachment, glaucoma, and blindness; marked osseous fragility with craniotabes and fractures during late infancy, childhood, or adolescence; and variable cognitive impairment, ligamentous laxity, and hypotonia.[418] The disorder is transmitted as an autosomal-recessive trait and is due to biallelic (homozygous or compound heterozygous) inactivating [missense (Arg494Gln), nonsense (Arg428Ter), frame-shift, splice-site] mutations in *LRP5*—primarily located in the extracellular domain of this protein.[419]

Missense mutations likely prevent normal binding of LRP5 to the product of the mesoderm development gene (OMIM 607783, chromosome 15), a chaperone protein that directs LRP5 to the cell membrane. Although often asymptomatic, heterozygous carriers are usually osteopenic. However, vision is not impaired. Mutations in *LRP5* have also been associated with familial exudative vitreoretinopathy (OMIM 133780), a developmental disorder of retinal vasculature that may be transmitted as an autosomal-dominant (Leu145Phe) or autosomal-recessive (Arg570Gly, Arg752Gly) trait. These patients also have reduced

TABLE 17-10

Classification of Osteogenesis Imperfecta

Type - OMIM	Severity	Clinical features	Growth impairment	Blue sclera	Inheritance	Gene defect
I - 166200	Mild	Few fractures, little deformity, hearing loss in 50%; rarely dentinogenesis imperfecta	Minimal	Present	AD	Nonsense & frameshift mutations resulting in premature STOP codons in COL1A1
IIA - 166210	Perinatal lethal	Many rib & long bone fractures at birth, severe long bone deformities, unmineralized calvarium	—	Present	AD, parental mosaicism	A - Glycine substitutions in COL1A1 or COL1A2.
IIB - 610854					AR	B - Inactivating mutations of CRTAP
III - 259420	Severe, progressive deforming	Moderate to severe bowing, multiple fractures, dentinogenesis imperfecta, hearing loss	Severe	Present but lighten with age	AD	Glycine substitutions in COL1A1 or COL1A2
IV -166220	Moderately deforming	Mild to moderate bowing, fractures	Moderate, variable	Greyish or absent	AD	Glycine substitutions in COL1A1 or COL1A2
V - 610967	Moderately deforming, clinically similar to Type IV	Mild to moderate bone fragility, ossification of interosseous membranes of forearm, hypertrophic callus formation at fracture site	Mild to moderate	Absent	AD	Unknown
VI - 610968	Moderately to severely deforming, clinically similar to Type IV	Onset of fractures in infancy; increased osteoid, fish-scale@ pattern of lamellation	Moderate	Absent or faint	Unknown	Unknown
VII - 610682	Moderately deforming	Fractures present at birth with frequency declining with age, rhizomelia, limb deformities	Moderate	Absent or faint	AR	Inactivating mutation (duplication) of CRTAP
VIII - 610915	Severely deforming, overlaps type II & III	Phenotype overlaps those of types II and III	Severe	Absent	AR	Inactivating mutations of LEPRE1

Adapted and modified from Barnes AM, Chang W, Morello R, et al. (2006). Deficiency of cartilage-associated protein in lethal osteogenesis imperfecta. N Engl J Med 355:2757–2764; from Marini JC (2006). Osteogenesis imperfecta. In Favus MJ (ed.), *Primer on the metabolic bone diseases and disorders of mineral metabolism, Sixth edition.* Washington, D.C.: American Society for Bone and Mineral Research 418–421; from Rauch F, Glorieux FH (2004). Osteogenesis imperfecta. Lancet 363:1377–1385; and from Sillence DO, Senn A, Danks DM (1979). Genetic heterogeneity in osteogenesis imperfecta. J Med Genet 16:101–116.

AD, autosomal dominant; and AR, autosomal recessive.

bone mass. LRP5 is a membrane protein that transduces the signals of two extracellular ligands: Wnt10b (OMIM 601906, chromosome 12q13) and Norrin (OMIM 310600, chromosome Xp11.4).

Wnt signaling increases the accrual of bone by activating β-catenin, a transcription factor that enhances differentiation of pluripotential mesenchymal precursor cells into the pathway of chondrogenesis and osteogenesis and impedes their differentiation into the pathway of adipogenesis.[420] By stimulating Runx2, β-catenin further directs the osteochondroprogenitor cell into the osteoblastic track. In the mature osteoblast, β-catenin enhances expression of osteoprotegerin and hence depresses osteoclastogenesis.[421] Norrin signaling modulates vitreoretinal formation in the eye.

In addition to the primacy of genetic and hormonal factors, the most important considerations for the accrual and maintenance of bone mass are those that relate to diet (sufficient intake of calcium and protein), sustained normal vitamin D stores by exposure to sunlight or ingestion of supplements, and consistent weight-bearing exercise. Therapeutically, when trying to prevent bone loss or restore lost bone initial efforts are directed to the assurance that these basic approaches are being utilized to the fullest extent possible for the specific patient. Therapeutic agents that increase bone mass act by inhibiting resorption (antiresorptive or antiremodeling drugs) or by stimulating bone formation (anabolic medications).[390] The most widely employed antiresorptive medications are sex hormones, selective estrogen receptor modulators, calcitonin, and bisphosphonates.

Selective estrogen receptor modulators are triphenylethylene-, benzothiophene-, or naphthalene-related compounds (e.g., raloxifene) that bind with high affinity to estrogen receptor α (perhaps to estrogen receptor β as well) in specific tissues—where they alter the three-dimensional configuration of the receptor and recruit tissue-selective cohorts of various coactivating factors, thus inducing receptor function in targeted sites (e.g., bone).[422] These compounds decrease osteoclast formation primarily at trabecular bone sites.[307] Nasal salmon calcitonin inhibits osteoclast function directly and has modest bone restorative effects.

Bisphosphonates are analogues of pyrophosphate, with carbon substituted for the oxygen bridge between two phosphate groups. Also attached to the carbon atom are two side chains. R1 is usually a hydroxyl group that together with the phosphate residues binds tightly to and coats bone surface.[423,424] The bisphosphonates impede osteoclast function by hastening their death by one of two mechanisms. After entering the osteoclast by endocytosis, etidronate forms cytotoxic acyclic analogues of adenosine triphosphate (ATP) that interfere with cellular metabolic processes and lead to apoptosis. After endocytosis nitrogen-containing pamidronate and alendronate inhibit the mevalonate pathway and the activity of farnesyl diphosphate synthase, a property shared with statin drugs.[425]

The resulting failure of transfer of fatty acids (prenylation) to guanosine-triphosphate-binding proteins such as Ras renders them inactive, impairs cell metabolism, and in turn begins the apoptotic process. As osteoclast function declines, bone mass increases. In addition, bisphosphonates are incorporated into the surface of hydroxyapatite and thereby block its dissolution. The biologic activity of bisphosphonates on osteoclast function is observed immediately after its administration as serum calcium concentrations decline rapidly. Indeed, this rapid effect has been utilized in the treatment of hypercalcemic infants and children. In adults, the effects of bisphosphonates on bone mass last long after the agent has been discontinued (the residence time)—enabling some compounds (zolendronate) to be given as infrequently as once yearly.

Indeed, bisphosphonates remain in bone for extremely long intervals—and their long-term effects appear to be cumulative. Histomorphometric analysis has revealed that bisphosphonates increase bone mineralization by decreasing the number of resorption cavities (and thus the remodeling space), preserving cancellous (trabecular) bone architecture, and decreasing porosity of cortical bone.[390] Bisphosphonates have been useful in improving mineralization in children with osteogenesis imperfecta, as well as in those with glucocorticoid induced osteoporosis, osteoporosis-pseudoglioma syndrome, Menkes disease, and cerebral palsy. In most infants and children, intravenous pamidronate (1 mg/kg/day on 3 consecutive days every 3 to 6 months to 2–15 mg/kg/year administered once every 3 to 6 months) has been utilized—although a number of different regimens have been employed with reasonably similar increases in BMD, decline in fracture incidence, and improved well-being.[423]

Limited data indicate that oral bisphosphonates (pamidronate, alendronate, olpadronate) administered daily also increase BMD in children with osteogenesis imperfecta and connective tissue disease, but with lower efficacy than intravenous administration. Side effects of bisphosphonates have been acute (fever, myalgia, abdominal pain, vomiting, hypocalcemia) and chronic (inflammatory disorders of the eye, osteonecrosis of the jaw in the elderly, and induced osteopetrosis).[423,426] Experimentally and in adults receiving long-term therapy, bisphosphonates can suppress bone turnover and contribute to hypermineralization—the latter leading to reduced mechanical strength and increased fracture risk.[427] Therefore, when selecting a child for treatment with bisphosphonates one must carefully considered the primary diagnosis and whether the patient's low bone mass and fracture frequency merit therapy in view of the potential side effects of bisphosphonates.

In addition, there are many unanswered questions concerning which bisphosphonate to use, its route of administration, the dose of the drug, the duration of therapy, and the method of outcome analysis. At this time, the use of bisphosphonates should be confined to centers with experience in the care and management of children with bone disease.[423,424] Treatment with bisphosphonates several years prior to conception does not appear to have an adverse effect on fetal outcome, but treatment during pregnancy is contraindicated because of possible toxicity.[428]

Administered intermittently in small amounts, PTH and its analogue PTH[1-34] (teriparatide) preferentially accelerate the rates of bone remodeling and of bone formation relative to that of bone resorption by direct stimulatory effects on the osteoblast.[390] PTH also acts on the osteocyte to decrease the production of sclerostin, an inhibitor of bone synthesis that acts by repressing Wnt- and BMP-mediated bone formation.[429] The quantity of bone formed in each remodeling unit is increased, thus augmenting trabecular and cortical bone mass and strength. PTH[1-34] increases trabecular thickness and trabecular interconnectivity. By contrast, bisphosphonates preserve but do not alter trabecular architecture. PTH[1-34] increases periosteal new bone formation and cortical thickness and diameter (i.e., bone size)—thereby increasing bone strength and reducing fracture risk.[390]

Teriparatide is also capable of dissociating bone formation from resorption, doing so in part by decreasing the rate of osteoblast apoptosis. Side effects of PTH[1-34] administration include transient hypercalcemia, hypercalciuria, and development of antibodies to the peptide—all rather unusual events. Although osteosarcoma has been observed in mice receiving very high doses of PTH and PTH[1-34], no malignant disorders have been recorded in adults receiving either agent. To date, the pediatric use of PTH[1-34] has been limited to children with hypocalcemia due to a gain-of-function mutation in CASR and consequent hypercalciuric hypocalcemia—one form of familial isolated hypoparathyroidism. In development is an analogue of PTHrP (PTHrP[1-36]) that increases lumbar spine BMD in postmenopausal women with osteoporosis by stimulating bone formation selectively without inducing hypercalcemia.[430,431]

Denosumab is a human monoclonal antibody to RANKL that binds tightly to its ligand and prevents its interaction with RANK, thereby inhibiting osteoclastogenesis. Denosumab thus acts as a pseudo-osteoprotegerin. In postmenopausal women with decreased bone mineralization, denosumab decreases bone resorption and increases lumbar spine BMD.[432] Strontium renalate is another agent in development for treatment of low bone mass in adults. Strontium is incorporated into the structure of bone mineral.[433]

OSTEOGENESIS IMPERFECTA

Osteogenesis imperfecta (brittle bone disease) is a disorder of increased bone fragility due to low bone mass that varies in clinical severity from lethality in the perinatal period due to respiratory insufficiency to mildly increased susceptibility to fractures in later life.[132] The original Silence classification of four types of osteogenesis imperfecta based on clinical characteristics and disease course has been expanded to include four additional types of this disorder and identification of mutant genes to which the illnesses can be attributed (Table 17-10).[132,434] The hallmark of each type is increased bone fragility, but severity varies—with type II being a lethal form and type I being a relatively benign form. In decreasing order of severity, type II > type VIII ≥ type III > types IV, V, VI, and VII > type I.

In osteogenesis imperfecta types I through IV, heterozygous loss-of-function mutations have been identified in one of the two genes (COL1A1, COL1A2) encoding procollagen subunits α1(I) and α2(I), respectively—which intertwine to form collagen type I in bone, skin, ligaments, tendons, sclerae, and teeth.[131,132] [As previously described, the triple helical structure of type I collagen consists of two collagen α1(I) (COL1A1) peptides and one collagen α2(I) peptide—each of which consists of triple repeats of glycine and two additional amino acids (often proline, hydroxyproline, or lysine).] Transmitted as an autosomal-dominant trait, insertion, duplication, frame-shift, or point mutations within COL1A1 or COL1A2 reduce the amount of collagen synthesized or alter its structure and properties—interfering with the assumption of a normal three-dimensional configuration and leading to decreased bone formation, low bone mass, and increased fracture risk (Figure 17-16).[435]

To an extent, the site of the more than 800 mutations identified within COL1A1 or COL1A2 is related to the clinical phenotype of osteogenesis imperfecta types I through IV. Mutations that lead to a stop codon result in a truncated procollagen product that is rapidly degraded. Thus, only normal collagen type I is produced (but in reduced mounts). Lethal mutations in COL1A1 are those that alter an amino acid with a branched or charged side chain; those within the binding sites of the collagen monomer for integrins, matrix metalloproteins, fibronectin, and cartilage oligomeric matrix protein; and those that result in binding to and degradation of intact procollagen subunits.[131]

Lethal mutations in COL1A2 are those that interfere with its binding to proteoglycans. Mutations (Arg-134Cys) in COL1A1 may also be found in patients with classic Ehlers-Danlos syndrome (OMIM 130000) of hyperextensible skin and laxity of ligaments of the spine and large and small joints. Children with clinical features of osteogenesis imperfecta (osseous fragility) and Ehlers-Danlos syndrome have been described.[436] In these patients, the mutations have been concentrated within the first 90 aa of the helical region of collagen-α1(I) and prevent normal post-translational removal of the procollagen amino-propeptide. Although the mutant protein can be incorporated into collagen, the structural integrity of the product is impaired because its fibrils are thin and weak.[437]

Osteogenesis imperfecta type I (OMIM 166200) is an autosomal-dominant disorder (or new mutation in 33% of patients) due primarily to functionally null alleles—the result of splicing defects or point mutations that lead to insertion errors or truncation (COL1A1: Gly178Cys, Arg-963Ter, IVS26DS), which are mutations that result in decreased transport of procollagen-α1(I) into the cytoplasm or its release into matrix (thereby modestly decreasing production of intact procollagen type I). Its clinical manifestations are relatively benign: intensely blue sclerae present at birth that persist throughout adulthood, modestly low bone mass, infrequent fractures with little deformity (however, 15% of affected children develop deformities and 24% develop kyphoscoliosis before 10 years of age), low normal adult stature, hearing loss in 50%, mitral valve prolapse in 18%, and rarely dentinogenesis imperfecta (osteogenesis imperfecta type IB).

Mutations in COL1A2 less frequently lead to the phenotype of osteogenesis imperfecta type I. Subjects with mutations in COL1A1 more frequently have blue sclerae and taller stature than those with mutations in COL1A2. Osteogenesis imperfecta type II (OMIM 166210) is a disorder that is lethal in the perinatal period or in early infancy. It is

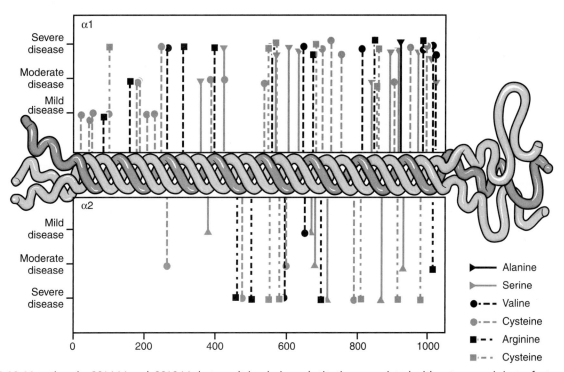

Figure 17-16 Mutations in *COL1A1* and *COL2A1* that result in glycine substitutions associated with osteogenesis imperfecta of variable clinical severity. [Reproduced with permission from Prockop DJ (2005). Type II collagen and avascular necrosis of the femoral head. N Engl J Med 352:2268–2270.]

usually the result of de novo heterozygous mutations in *COL1A1* or *COL1A2*, with alternative amino acid being substituted for glycine in the triple helical domains of the procollagen α1(I)/α2(I) chains (COL1A1: Gly94Cys, Gly391Arg, Gly1003Ser; COL1A2: Gly547Asp, Gly865Ser, Gly976Asp). These mutations lead to the synthesis of abnormal procollagen chains that bind to and thereby inactivate intact procollagen peptides in a dominant-negative manner, severely curtailing the synthesis of intact collagen type I.

Clinically, it is manifested by in utero fractures, long bone deformities, very little calvarial mineralization, and death due to respiratory insufficiency. A very similar phenotype (type IIB, OMIM 610854) is associated with homozygous loss-of-function mutations in the gene *(CRTAP)* encoding cartilage-associated protein. Osteogenesis imperfecta type III (OMIM 259420) is an autosomal-dominant trait due to point or frame-shift mutations in *COL1A1* (Gly154Arg, Gly844Ser) and *COL1A2* (Gly526Cys). It is characterized by recurrent fractures that lead to progressive bone deformities that are often apparent at birth, and by kyphoscoliosis, extreme short stature, blue sclerae that lighten with age, abnormal dentition (in 80% of children less than 10 years of age), and hearing loss.

Osteogenesis imperfecta type IV (OMIM 166220) is an autosomal-dominant disease usually associated with point mutations or small deletions in *COL1A2* (Gly586Val, Gly646Cys, Gly1012Arg) and occasionally in *COL1A1* (Gly175Cys, Gly832Ser). It is of variable severity, with prolonged survival, mild to moderate bone deformities, short stature, normal sclerae, dentinogenesis imperfecta, and hearing loss. One post-translational modification of type I procollagen is hydroxylation of proline and lysine residues by prolyl and lysyl hydroxylases, an essential step in nor-

mal collagen folding and stability. Prolyl 3-hydroxylase 1 [P3H1, also termed leprecan *(LEPRE1)*] specifically hydroxylates the proline residue at codon 986 in COL1A1, a reaction that requires interaction of P3H1 with CRTAP and cyclophilin B (chromosome 15, OMIM 123841).

CRTAP is expressed in the proliferative zone of developing cartilage and at the chondro-osseous junction. Cyclophilin B possesses peptidyl-prolyl cis-trans isomerase activity. *Crtap* knockout mice develop an osteochondrodysplasia (kyphoscoliosis, shortening of the proximal segment of the limbs consistent with rhizomelia) and severe osteopenia, the latter due to reduced production and alteration in the quality of osteoid and consequently decreased rate of mineral deposition.[438] Mice deficient in Crtap are unable to 3-hydroxylate the proline residue near the carboxyl terminus of bone COL1A1, leading to increased hydroxylation of lysine residues and resultant abnormal structure of the collagen fibril—changes that result in defective mineralization of bone collagen type I.

A recessive form of lethal osteogenesis imperfecta of unknown pathogenesis in which detailed analyses of *COL1A1* and *COL1A2* have been normal has been described. In 3 out of 11 patients with a recessive clinical form of lethal type II or severe osteogenesis imperfecta type III characterized by multiple fractures of the long bones (resulting in rhizomelic shortening of the limbs with externally rotated and abducted legs, poorly mineralized calvaria and ribs, proptotic eyes, and white or light blue sclerae), nonhydroxylated proline at codon 986 in bone COL1A1 has been demonstrated.[439]

This proved due to homozygous or compound heterozygous loss-of-function mutations in *CRTAP* [frame-shift (c.879delT), 16 bp duplication in exon 1, nonsense (Gly276Ter), missense (Met1Ile), splice donor site of exon 1 at the first intronic nucleotide (IVS1 + 1G→C)] that interfered with effective hydroxylation of the proline residue at codon 986 of bone procollagen α1(I). Loss-of-function mutations in *LEPRE1* lead to impaired P3H1 activity and a severe form of osteogenesis imperfecta designated type VIII.[434] It seems likely that a mutation in the gene encoding cyclophilin B as well as in others that post-translationally modify collagen subunits may be identified in different patients with similar clinical manifestations but intact *COL1A1* and *COL1A2*.

Currently, there are four forms of osteogenesis imperfecta (types V, VI, VII, VIII) in which extensive analyses of the structures of *COL1A1* and *COL1A2* have been normal.[131,132] Osteogenesis imperfecta type V (OMIM 610967) is phenotypically similar to type IV and is characterized by autosomal-dominant transmission, moderate to severe bone fragility, moderate to mild growth retardation, dislocation of the radial head, mineralization of interosseous membranes, exuberant callous formation at fracture sites, white sclerae, and intact dental development. Histologically, there is irregular arrangement of lamellae. Approximately 5% of patients with osteogenesis imperfecta appear to have type V, the molecular cause of which is as yet unidentified.

Osteogenesis imperfecta type VI (OMIM 610968) is also phenotypically similar to type IV. It is characterized by a fish-scale pattern of lamellation of bone on microscopic examination. Type VI is found in approximately 4% of patients with osteogenesis imperfecta. Its inheritance pattern is unknown. Osteogenesis imperfecta type VII (OMIM 610682) has been identified in northern Quebec in a Native American population. Clinically, it is an autosomal-recessive disorder in which fractures are present at birth but the frequency of fractures declines with advancing age—particularly after adolescence. The sclerae are slightly bluish, and there is progressive skeletal deformation that leads to rhizomelic shortening of the limbs and restricted ambulation.

In patients with type VII, a homozygous mutation in *CRTAP* has been identified: specifically, inclusion of 73 bp of intron 1 into the genome of *CRTAP* due to alteration of one nucleotide (c.472, 1021C→G) that generates a cryptic splice donor site that extends exon 2. However, this alteration results in a frame-shift that permits more rapid degradation of CRTAP and consequently leads to decreased 3-hydroxylation of proline 986 in bone COL1A1. Thus, inactivating mutations in *CRTAP* can result in at least two clinically distinct forms of osteogenesis imperfecta (types IIB and VII)—as do mutations in *COL1A1* and *COL1A2*. The phenotype of osteogenesis type VIII (OMIM 610915) overlaps with those of types II and III. In addition to osseous fragility, it is associated with substantial growth retardation, white sclerae, and bulbous metaphyses. It is due to loss-of-function mutations in *LEPRE1* encoding P3H1.[434]

In addition to diffusely low bone mass, thin cortices, metaphyseal flaring, and fractures and bone deformities resulting therefrom, radiographic findings in subjects with osteogenesis imperfecta include wormian skull bones (frequent but not pathognomonic of osteogenesis

imperfecta), platybasia that may compress overlying hindbrain, vertebral compression, and a triradiate pelvis.[131] Bone densitometry reveals decreased mineralization, the extent of which correlates to a degree with clinical manifestations. The diagnosis of osteogenesis imperfecta is established by clinical criteria and confirmed by genotyping of *COL1A1* and/or *COL1A2* or other pertinent gene(s)—although failure to detect a genetic mutation does not necessarily rule out this disorder. Occasionally, biopsy of the iliac crest and histologic examination of the bone may be necessary for subclassification of the disorder.

Determination of the rate of synthesis and forms of procollagen secreted by dermal fibroblasts in vitro permits identification of the forms and relative amounts of collagen subunits and intact proteins being synthesized (type I, type III, and so forth). Osteogenesis imperfecta type II can be identified prenatally by fetal ultrasonography. Types I, III, and IV can be determined prenatally by analysis of collagen synthesized by cells cultured from chorionic villus biopsies and by analysis of the procollagen genes.[440]

The basic management of patients with osteogenesis imperfecta is directed to prevention of fractures to the extent possible and to the treatment of fractures that occur by sound orthopedic procedures and by orthopedists familiar with this disorder. Rehabilitative services and physical therapy to improve muscle strength and mobility within the constraints of bone fragility are to be encouraged, as are protected ambulation and exercises such as swimming.[131] Introduction of bisphosphonates into the management of infants, children, and adolescents with osteogenesis imperfecta types I, III, and IV has been of substantial benefit. Patients with these disorders have responded to the intermittent intravenous administration of the bisphosphonate (pamidronate), with marked increase in bone mass and decline in fracture rate—as well as symptomatic improvement such as decreased pain and more facile mobility.[132,133,441]

Infants as young as 2 months of age have safely tolerated 4-hour intravenous infusions of pamidronate (0.5 mg/kg/day for 3 consecutive days every 6 to 8 weeks), realizing clinical improvement such as decline in bone pain (perhaps a placebo effect), increase in lumbar vertebral BMD of 86% to 227%, and decrease in fracture rate after 1 year of therapy.[131,442] In children (3–16 years of age), pamidronate administered as a 4-hour infusion (1.5–3.0 mg/kg/day) for 3 consecutive days every 4 months resulted in increases in lumbar spine BMD of 42% per year and increases in metacarpal cortical width of 27% per year. in decreased vertebral size, decline in vertebral fracture rate, and symptomatic improvement also occurred.

During 2 to 4 years of intravenous pamidronate administration, increase in vertebral (trabecular) bone mass and size are accompanied by decline in the extent of vertebral compression and fewer compressed vertebrae than in untreated patients.[443] In the iliac crest, bisphosphonates increase cortical bone thickness and trabecular number but not trabecular thickness. In metacarpals, bisphosphonates enhance cortical thickness. In treated subjects, the relative risk of long bone fracture may be a bit reduced—implying a beneficial effect of bisphosphonates on long bone cortical volume and hence on bone strength.[131,132,444] Oral alendronate (1 mg/kg/day) and intravenous pamidronate are reported to be equally effective in children with osteogenesis imperfecta, although data are limited and gastrointestinal side effects of oral bisphosphonate are of concern.[445]

Near-maximal benefits of bisphosphonates on lumbar vertebral BMD by DEXA (and on mean cortical width, cancellous bone volume, and trabecular bone formation rate by histomorphometric analysis of iliac crest bone biopsies) are achieved within the first 2 to 4 years of treatment, with little further change with more prolonged therapy.[446] Currently, because of the persistence of bisphosphonates in bone and their long-term effects it is suggested that these agents be administered to patients with osteogenesis imperfecta for approximately 2 to 4 years. Their positive effects on bone mass gain, reduced fracture rate, and functional well-being are often longer lasting.[447]

Care must be exercised when selecting a patient with osteogenesis imperfecta for treatment with bisphosphonates. It is currently recommended that these agents be employed only in patients with substantial disease, such as frequent fractures (more than two per year) and deformities of the long bones and vertebrae, irrespective of the specific mutation in the procollagen subunit, clinical type of osteogenesis imperfecta, or BMD.[133] Pamidronate has been the bisphosphonate most frequently administered to patients with osteogenesis imperfecta. Recent treatment recommendations utilizing this agent are: <2.0 years (0.5 mg/kg/day intravenously for 3 days every 2 months), 2.0 to 3.0 years (0.75 mg/kg/day for 3 days every 3 months), and >3.0 years (1 mg/kg/day to a maximum dose of 60 mg/day for 3 days every 4 months).[132]

Among the complications of bisphosphonate therapy are transient hypocalcemia and flu-like reaction of fever, vomiting, and rash after first exposure managed symptomatically. Although bisphosphonates decrease linear growth in experimental animals, experience in children indicates that over the span of several years these agents improve linear growth rate and height compared with untreated subjects with moderately severe forms of osteogenesis imperfecta.[441] Increase in the rate of linear growth has been reported during administration of recombinant human GH to children with osteogenesis imperfecta, but the effect has not been sustained—nor has treatment positively affected fracture risk.[132,441,448]

Bone marrow transplantation in five children with severe osteogenesis imperfecta has been reported to have been beneficial, but experience with this procedure has been variable.[449] As yet untested in osteogenesis imperfecta subjects is the use of PTH, PTH[1-34], or PTHrP[1-36]. Gene therapy of osteogenesis imperfecta remains a goal. Selective inactivation of wt or mutant COL1A1 in mesenchymal stem cells from two patients with severe forms of osteogenesis imperfecta (COL1A1: Gly773Ser, Gly1040Ser) has been accomplished. Cells in which survival and function of the wt gene and destruction of the mutant gene co-occur potentially permits their reintroduction into the affected host and normal collagen production.[450,451]

FIBROUS DYSPLASIA

Fibrous dysplasia involves the long bones and skull and may be monostotic, polyostotic, or panostotic. It primarily occurs in patients with the McCune-Albright syndrome (OMIM 174800) in association with large café-au-lait pigmentations and various endocrinopathies, including isosexual precocity, hypersomatotropism, thyrotoxicosis, and hyperadrenocorticism—as well as dysfunction in many other tissues (heart, liver, pancreas).[452] It is due to mosaicism for postzygotic somatic gain-of-function missense mutations (Arg201 to Cys, His, Ser, Gly) in GNAS, the gene encoding the α subunit of the Gs protein.[453]

The extent and severity of disease is determined by the point in development at which the mutation occurs and its tissue distribution. As a result of loss of intrinsic guanosine triphosphatase activity within the $G_s\alpha$ subunit, the stimulatory effect of $G_s\alpha$ on adenylyl cyclase is prolonged. The clones of mutated mesenchymal preosteoblasts proliferate, but their differentiation into mature osteoblasts is incomplete and their secreted matrix is abnormal. Continued expansion steadily erodes contiguous bone. These lesions can also synthesize FGF23 and lead to hyperphosphaturia, hypophosphatemia, and excess unmineralized osteoid and a rickets-like clinical state.[454]

Fibrodysplastic lesions are initially silent, whereas osteoclasts at the periphery of the lesions actively thin and compress bone cortices—ultimately resulting in bone pain and pathologic fractures of the long bones (particularly the proximal femoral metaphyses). Children between 6 and 10 years of age have the highest fracture rate (0.4 fractures per year). Within the skull base and facial bones, expansion of fibrous dysplastic lesions leads to disfiguration and compression of cranial nerves. Radiographically, the fibrodysplastic lesion is viewed as a cyst-like medullary structure with a ground-glass consistency. Histologically, there are abundant immature bone marrow stromal cells, incompletely differentiated osteoblasts, poorly formed bony trabeculae with excess undermineralized osteoid seams characteristic of osteomalacia, and islands of cartilage.

The clinical manifestations of fibrous dysplasia depend on the sites and extent of bone involvement and associated endocrinopathies, particularly GH excess.[455] Diagnosis of fibrous dysplasia is based on clinical characteristics and confirmation of the genetic mutation in GNAS. In addition to managing the multiple endocrinopathies and organ defects, attention must be paid to the osseous lesions. Fractures are repaired by standard techniques, including intramedullary nailing when indicated. Occasionally, it may be feasible to evacuate a fibrodysplastic lesion surgically and to fill the cavity with bone grafts. In children with fibrous dysplasia, the bisphosphonate pamidronate has proven useful in ameliorating bone pain (but not the skeletal lesions).[456,457]

HIGH BONE MASS

Abnormally increased bone mass is the consequence of disruption of the normal equilibrium between the velocities of bone formation and resorption. Thus, it may be due to decrease in the rate of bone resorption or to an increase in the rate of bone formation. Increase in cortical bone width is termed hyperostosis. Thickening of trabecular bone is termed osteosclerosis.[136] Table 17-11 lists selected dysplastic, metabolic, and other diseases associated with increased bone density in children and adolescents.

Failure of osteoclast-mediated bone resorption leads to osteopetrosis ("marble bone disease"), a group of heritable disorders with heterogeneous manifestations.[458] Histologically, osteopetrotic bone is characterized by quiescent osteoclasts with few ruffled borders and retained calcified cartilage formed during endochondral ossification (primary spongiosa) due to failure of reab-

---

TABLE 17-11
Disorders of Bone Mineralization: High Bone Mass

I. Decreased Bone Resorption
A. Osteopetrosis
1. Autosomal recessive (infantile) (*TCIRG1, CLCN7, OSTM1*)
a. Transient
2. Intermediate (*CLCN7*)
3. Autosomal dominant (adult) (*LRP5, CLCN7*)
4. Immunodeficiency, lymphedema, ectodermal dysplasia (*IKBKG*)
5. Carbonic anhydrase II deficiency (*CA2*)
6. Pycnodysostosis (*CTSK*)
7. Neuronal storage disease
8. Drug-induced - bisphosphonates

II. Increased Bone Formation
A. Activating Mutations of *LRP*
1. Autosomal-dominant high bone mass
2. Endosteal osteosclerosis (van Buchem disease type 2)

B. Inactivating Mutations of *SOST*
1. Sclerosteosis
2. Van Buchem disease type 1

III. Osteosclerosis
A. Dysplasias
1. Dysosteosclerosis
2. Infantile cortical hyperostosis (Caffey disease) (*COL1A1*)
3. Juvenile Paget disease (*TNFRSF11B*)
4. Metaphyseal dysplasia (Pyle disease)
5. Osteopoikilosis (*LEMD3*)
6. Progressive diaphyseal dysplasia (Camurati-Engelmann disease) (*TGFB1*)
7. Tubular stenosis, type 1 (Kenny-Caffey syndrome) (*TBCE*)

B. Metabolic Disorders
1. Fluorosis
2. Heavy metal poisoning
3. Hypervitaminosis A, D
4. Hypoparathyroidism, pseudohypoparathyroidism
5. Milk-alkali syndrome

C. Other
1. Hepatitis C-associated osteosclerosis
2. Ionizing radiation
3. Sarcoidosis
4. Sickle cell disease (*HBB*)
5. Tuberous sclerosis (*TSC1*)

Modified from Whyte MP (2006). Sclerosing bone disorders. In Favus MJ (ed.), *Primer on the metabolic bone diseases and disorders of mineral metabolism, Sixth edition.* Washington, D.C.: American Society for Bone and Mineral Research 398–414.

---

sorption of immature bone. Although densely packed with mineral, osteopetrotic bone is quite fragile because the abnormality in bone remodeling due to decreased osteoclastic bone resorption leads to incorporation of weak calcified growth plate cartilage into bone and to delay in repair of microfractures.

Radiographically, osteopetrosis is characterized by diffuse increase in bone mass, diaphyseal/metaphyseal widening with an Ehrlenmeyer flask appearance, alternating bands of sclerotic and lucent bone at the ends of the long bones, iliac crest and vertebrae, sclerotic changes at the base of the skull, narrow medullary cavities, and pathologic fractures.[136] Cranial computed tomography often reveals narrowing of the bony canals through which cranial nerves (II, III, IV, VII, VIII) pass. Classically, three clinical forms of osteopetrosis have been delineated. However, as knowledge of the genetic mutations responsible for this disease are being identified this classification is being replaced.

The infantile form of osteopetrosis (OMIM 259700) is an autosomal-recessive disorder (Albers-Schonberg disease) with attenuated growth (particularly of the limbs), delayed development, increased fracture rate, and failure of tooth eruption. Bony overgrowth leads to maldevelopment of the paranasal sinuses and to symptomatic nasal stuffness. Narrowing of cranial foramina compromises cranial nerve function (II, III, VII, VIII), with consequent blindness and deafness. Decrease in bone marrow volume leads to depressed intramedullary hematopoiesis, anemia, and leukopenia—partially compensated by extramedullary hematopoiesis and ensuing hepatosplenomegaly, with consequent increased susceptibility to infection and hemorrhage.

Retention of teeth within the sclerotic jaw leads to recurrent and persistent mandibular and maxillary osteomyelitis. Physical examination reveals short stature, macrocephaly, frontal bossing, and small facial features. Death usually occurs often within the first decade of life due to sepsis, anemia, or hemorrhage. Autosomal-recessive osteopetrosis may be due to biallelic mutations in a subunit of the osteoclast's vacuolar proton pump *(TCIRG1)*, its chloride channel *(CLCN7)*, or the osteopetrosis-associated transmembrane protein-1 *(OSTM1)*.

The intermediate form of osteopetrosis is transmitted as an autosomal-recessive trait and is associated with short stature, macrocephaly, recurrent fractures, variable compromise of cranial nerve function, abnormal dental development predisposing to osteomyelitis of the mandible or maxilla, and anemia. Pathogenetically, it likely represents the variable penetrance of one of the genetic mutations associated with the infantile form of osteopetrosis—predominantly of *CLCN7*. There are two clinical and radiographic forms of autosomal-dominant osteopetrosis previously thought to be manifested only in the adult.

Type I (OMIM 607634) is characterized by an enlarged and dense cranial vault and diffuse vertebral sclerosis, and is related to activating mutations of *LRP5*. It is not associated with an increase in fracture rate as bone strength is increased. Type II (OMIM 166600) is typified by thickening of the vertebral end plates, resembling "bone within bone" and resulting in a "rugger jersey spine" and sclerotic bands of bone in the pelvis and base of the skull.[459] It is a variant of Albers-Schonberg disease that results from heterozygotic mutations in *CLCN7*.[136,460] Affected subjects manifest cranial nerve compromise (16%), mandibular and nonmandibular osteomyelitis (19%), osteoarthritis of the hip (27%), and fractures (78%).[459]

Clinical evidence of the disease tends to worsen over time. However, the expression of the trait is variable. Thus, one-third of carriers of an inactivating mutation in *CLCN7* have no radiographic or clinical manifestations—although they do have significantly higher BMD than do subjects with the wt gene.[461] In one-quarter of clinically apparent patients with a heterozygous loss-of-function mutation in *CLCN7*, the expression of illness (fractures, osteomyelitis, compromised vision) is identifiable at birth or early in infancy or childhood. Patients with radiologic/clinical manifestations of this disorder have elevated serum concentrations of tartrate-resistant acid phosphatase and the BB isoform of creatine kinase elaborated by osteoclasts. These values are normal in unaffected carriers.[462]

Identification of many of the genes that regulate osteoclastogenesis and osteoclast function has greatly increased our understanding of the molecular mechanisms underlying experimental models of osteopetrosis. There are more than 17 murine models of osteopetrosis involving a litany of molecules that regulate osteoclastogenesis (Figure 17-17).[458,463] By mid 2007, five genetic mutations that impeded resorption of bone had been identified in patients with osteopetrosis. As anticipated, they related to abnormalities in osteoclastogenesis or function—particularly the efficiency of acidification of the resorption lacuna beneath the osteoclast's ruffled membrane and mineral dissolution or enzymatic degradation of organic bone matrix. The syndrome of osteopetrosis, lymphedema, anhidrotic ectodermal dysplasia, and immunodeficiency (OL-EDA-ID, OMIM 300301) has been linked to an inactivating mutation in a modulator of NFκB—an essential transcription factor for differentiation and function of osteoclasts.[464,465]

The inhibitor of the kinase of kappa light polypeptide gene enhancer in B cells gamma subunit (*IKBKG*) is also termed NFκB essential modulator (NEMO). IKBKG is a 412-aa component of the IκB kinase complex that activates NFκB. The substitution of guanine for adenine at N:1259 (A1259G) results in a change from a stop codon to tryptophan (Ter420Trp), permitting incorporation of an additional 27-aa component at the carboxyl terminus of the protein and resulting in decreased function of the product and 50% to 60% decline in activation of NFκB and hence in osteoclastogenesis.

Carbonic anhydrase II (one of several zinc metalloisoenzymes) is a protein expressed in osteoclasts, erythrocytes, brain, and kidney. It regulates the formation of carbonic acid from water and carbon dioxide (CO_2 + $H_2O \rightarrow H_2O_3$), which then dissociates to form proton/hydrogen (H^+) and bicarbonate (HCO_3^-) ions. Loss-of-function homozygous or compound heterozygous (Lys-17Glu, Tyr40Ter, His107Tyr) mutations in CA2 lead to an autosomal-recessive disease that presents in childhood with failure to thrive, short stature, visual impairment,

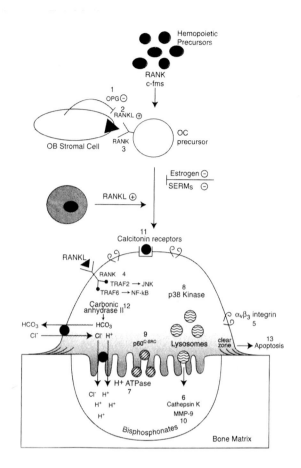

Figure 17-17 Sites at which pharmacologic agents may be targeted to affect osteoclast production and/or function: 1-4 (blockade of the RANK/RANK ligand/OPG signaling pathway of osteoclastogenesis), 5 (inhibition of $\alpha_v\beta_3$ integrin receptor binding to bone surface), 6 (antagonism of cathepsin K protease), 8 (inhibition of p38 kinase, an enzyme important in the inflammatory reaction), 9 (blocking of p60^{C-SRC} kinase, an enzyme important in osteoclast activation), 10 (inhibition of matrix metalloproteinase-9), 11 (agonist ligands of the calcitonin receptor with enhanced function), 12 (inhibition of carbonic anhydrase II), and 13 (enhancement of osteoclast death). [Reproduced with permission from Rodan GA, Martin TJ (2000). Therapeutic approaches to bone diseases. Science 289:1508–1514.)

and developmental delay in association with mild proximal and severe distal renal tubular acidosis, cerebral calcifications within the cortex and basal ganglia, and osteopetrosis with increased fracture risk.[136] Osteopetrosis is of modest severity and is usually nonprogressive. It may even improve at puberty.

After generation by carbonic anhydrase II, H^+ is extruded from the osteoclast into the subobsteoclastic resorption lacuna through transporters and proton pumps. *TCIRG1* (T-cell immune regulator 1) encodes an 822-aa 116-kDa protein that is a subunit of the osteoclast's vacuolar proton pump (H^+-ATPase). [By alternative splicing, this gene also encodes a 614-aa protein (TIRC7) essential to activation of T lymphocytes.] Biallelic-inactivating (missense, nonsense, deletion, splice site) mutations in *TCIRG1* whose loss impairs transport of H^+ and thus decreases bone mineral resorption have been found in 50% of subjects with the neonatal/infantile form of lethal osteopetrosis (OMIM 259700).[466,467]

Loss-of-function mutations in *CLCN7,* a chloride channel expressed in the ruffled membrane of the activated osteoclast, also impair acidification of the subosteoclastic resorption space and hence mineral dissolution. Heterozygotic-inactivating mutations (Arg767Trp) of *CLCN7* lead to the autosomal-dominant form of osteopetrosis (OMIM 166600)—whereas homozygous mutations (Leu766Pro) are found occasionally in infants with the lethal autosomal-recessive form of this disease (whose parents may even be clinically normal).[460,468] *CLCN7* is coexpressed with and complexed to osteopetrosis-associated transmembrane protein 1 *(OSTM1)* in endosomes and lysosomes and in the ruffled membrane of activated osteoclasts.[469] By decreasing post-translational stability of CLCN7, loss-of-function mutations in *OSTM1* have been pathogenetically related to autosomal-recessive lethal osteopetrosis in a subset of patients.[470,471]

The murine homolog of *OSTM1* is *Gl* (Grey-lethal), a mouse model of osteopetrosis. Related to the long-acting inhibitory effects of bisphosphonate on bone modeling and remodeling, administration of high doses of intravenous pamidronate (2800 mg) over a 3-year period resulted in an acquired osteopetrosis-like disorder in a 12-year-old boy with unexplained hyperalkaline phosphatasemia that persisted for at least several years after this agent was discontinued.[426] The metaphyses were extremely dense and club-shaped, the base of the skull sclerotic, and the vertebral endplates thickened. Histologically, iliac crest biopsy revealed bars of calcified cartilage and quiescent osteoclasts. Despite the severity of the radiographic and microscopic findings, the patient was clinically well—with normal growth and without evidence of bone marrow suppression or extramedullary hematopoiesis, although the risk for future fractures may have been increased.

A multidisciplinary team skilled in the management of patients with osteopetrosis is essential to the optimal care of infants and children with this disorder. In addition to appropriate orthopedic and neurosurgica input, medical therapy may at times be helpful. Nonspecific treatment with interferon-γ and high doses of calcitriol has led to arrest of disease progression and even its regression in some osteopetrotic children.[136,472] In this setting, calcitriol may act as an osteoclast-activating factor—whereas interferon γ indirectly stimulates osteoclast formation and increases generation of superoxide in osteoclasts, an important factor for osteoclast-mediated bone resorption.[473] Some children improve after bone marrow transplantation from human leukocyte antigen-identical donors with replacement of defective osteoclasts by normal osteoclast progenitor cells.[136]

Hypercalcemia may complicate the post-transplantation period as osteoclast function resumes. It can be managed with dietary restriction, calcitonin, and occasionally bisphosphonate administration. With improved treatment, there has been somewhat increased life span and improved developmental progress. Osteopetrosis due to deficiency of carbonic anhydrase II is not corrected by restoration of normal systemic acid-base balance, but bone marrow transplantation may be useful.[136] Identification and correction of the specific underlying gene defect may ultimately be feasible in patients with osteopetrosis.[467]

Pycnodysostosis (OMIM 265800) is clinically manifested by disproportionate short stature during infancy and childhood, with macrocranium and open cranial sutures, high forehead, small facial features, proptosis, bluish sclerae, beaked and pointed nose, micrognathia, highly arched palate, retained primary teeth, short fingers with hypoplastic nails, narrow thorax, pectus excavatum, and kyphoscoliosis with lumbar lordosis.[136] Radiologically, there is increased bone density that becomes progressively worse with age. Susceptibility to fractures is increased. The clavicles are slim and hypoplastic laterally. Ribs, distal phalanges, and hyoid bone may be partially or totally absent.

Laboratory data and bone histology are basically normal, although there is evidence of decreased osteoblastic and osteoclastic activity. An abundance of osteoclasts with ruffled borders surrounded by enlarged clear zones suggested that dissolution of bone mineral was normal but that degradation of matrix was abnormal in these patients. Indeed, pycnodysostosis is due to biallelic loss-of-function mutations in *CTSK.* This gene encodes cathepsin K, the osteoclast's lysosomal cysteine protease that degrades organic matrix after the mineral phase of bone has been reabsorbed.[137] Among the genetic abnormalities found in patients with pycnodysostosis have been unipaternal isodisomy for chromosome 1, with paternal *CTSK* harboring an inactivating Ala277Val mutation; Leu9Pro substitution in the signal peptide of the precursor form of the enzyme protein, preventing completion of its post-translational processing; and Ter330Trp substitution, permitting the addition of 19 amino acids to the carboxyl terminus of this enzyme.

In contrast with diseases that increase bone mass by decreasing bone resorption are those disorders that primarily increase bone formation. An example of the latter is the familial relatively benign form of autosomal-dominant high bone mass (OMIM 601884) that is associated with a heterozygous gain-of-function mutation (Gly171Val) in *LRP5.*[474] Loss-of-function mutations in the same gene are associated with idiopathic juvenile osteoporosis, the osteoporosis-pseudoglioma syndrome, and familial exudative vitreoretinopathy. LRP5 (and its homolog LRP6) is a co-receptor for Wnt proteins whose primary receptor is Frizzled.

After binding to LRP5 and Frizzled, the Wnt glycoprotein activates a canonical pathway that involves repression of glycogen synthase kinase 3 and leads to dephosphorylation of β-catenin—permitting its translocation to the nucleus, where it interacts with T-cell factor/lymphoid enhancing factor to control target genes that divert the mesenchymal stem cell into the track leading to osteoblastogenesis.[475] In the mature osteoblast, β-catenin stimulates expression of osteoprotegerin—thus impairing osteoclastogenesis. Dickkopf and sclerostin are proteins that bind to the extracellular domain of LRP5 and internalize the receptor complex, thereby blocking Wnt signaling.[476]

Mutations in *LRP5* associated with high bone mass are clustered near the amino terminal of its extracellular domain at the sites of binding to Dickkopf and sclerostin.[419] The Gly171Val mutation in *LRP5* interferes with the binding of LRP5 to Dickkopf and thus prolongs the interaction of LRP5 with Frizzled, thereby augmenting the Wnt signal and increasing bone formation.[477,478] Although generally benign, activating mutations of *LRP5* may also be associated with neurologic complications such as hearing loss, headaches, and pain in the extremities.[419]

In some families, heterozygous activating mutations (Ala242Thr) of *LRP5* and exuberant bone formation have been associated with autosomal-dominant generalized endosteal osteosclerosis (van Buchem disease type 2, OMIM 607636) or even osteopetrosis (Gly171Arg, Thr253Ile). However, the dense bones encountered in these subjects are not prone to fracture (as in classic forms of osteopetrosis). Sclerosteosis (OMIM 269500) is an autosomal-recessive disorder first manifested in childhood and characterized by very thick peripheral and cranial bones with calvarial overgrowth, leading to facial disfigurement, entrapment of cranial nerves VII and VIII, increased intracranial pressure, and brain stem compression.[136]

Affected patients also have variable asymmetric cutaneous or bony syndactyly of the index and middle fingers and excessive somatic growth. Sclerosteosis is due to biallelic loss-of-function mutations in *SOST,* the gene that encodes sclerostin—a 213-aa peptide secreted primarily by osteocytes embedded within bone. Normally, sclerostin inhibits Wnt-mediated bone formation by binding to and internalizing LRP5 (the co-receptor for Wnt).[475] When sclerostin activity is decreased, increased bone formation ensues. In heterozygous carriers of inactivating mutations in *SOST,* bone mass is increased (but not to pathologic levels).[479] van Buchem disease type 1 (OMIM 239100), an autosomal-recessive form of generalized osteosclerosis, is due to biallelic deletion of a 52-kb noncoding SOST-specific regulatory region approximately 35 kb downstream of the intact gene itself that results in loss-of-function of *SOST.*[480] Thus, van Buchem disease type 1 and sclerosteosis are allelic disorders.

Progressive diaphyseal dysplasia (Camurati-Englemann disease, OMIM 131300) is an autosomal-dominant cranial-peripheral hyperostotic disorder with variable expressivity that presents in children with problems such as limping, waddling gait, and/or leg pain, fatigue, and nonprogressive muscular weakness. Radiographically, there is symmetrical cortical thickening (hyperostosis) due to increased periosteal and endosteal bone formation in the diaphyses of the long bones, axial skeletons, and skull.[136,481] Pathogenetically, this disorder is primarily due to missense mutations within the latency-associated peptide domain of the precursor propeptide of TGFβ1 *(TGFB1).*

Normally, after post-translational processing two latency-associated peptides are noncovalently linked to two mature TGFβ1 peptides to form a latency complex. Mutations within the latency-associated peptide domain of *TGFB1* (particularly at codon 218, a mutational hot spot) impair this association, resulting in premature activation of TGFβ1 and consequent stimulation of bone formation and repression of bone resorption.[482] TGFβ1

also inhibits myogenesis and adipogenesis. Because of the inhibitory effects of glucocorticoids on bone formation and its stimulatory effects on bone resorption, short courses of these agents have been useful in alleviating many of the clinical symptoms and radiologic abnormalities in patients with progressive diaphyseal dysplasia.[481] However, long-term therapy with glucocorticoids is not advised.

ECTOPIC CALCIFICATION AND OSSIFICATION

Extraskeletal calcification may occur in a number of hypercalcemic, hyperphosphatemic, or dystrophic states (renal failure, hypo- and hyperparathyroidism, sarcoidosis, after cell lysis induced by cancer chemotherapy, subcutaneous fat necrosis, dermatomyositis, atherosclerosis)—as well as in specific diseases (e.g., PHP type IA, McCune-Albright syndrome).[483] Familial tumoral calcinosis (OMIM 211900) presents in childhood with recurrent bone pain, extensive cutaneous, periarticular and vascular calcifications, and periarticular hard and lobulated masses. In some patients, the ectopic calcifications may be confined to the eyelids. It is characterized radiographically by cortical hyperostosis, periosteal reaction, and mineral deposits around large joints (particularly hips and shoulders).[484-486]

Laboratory studies reveal marked hyperphosphatemia and relative hypophosphaturia due to increased renal tubular reabsorption of phosphate and inappropriately normal or elevated serum calcitriol levels, because despite hyperphosphatemia PTH secretion is not increased and synthesis of calcitriol and intestinal calcium absorption persist. The disorder is due to functional loss of FGF23 action and consequently unhindered renal tubular reabsorption of phosphate. The pathophysiology of this disorder is thus the mirror image of that associated with XHR, ADHR, and tumor-induced osteomalacia in which there is exaggerated FGF23 production and activity leading to hyperphosphaturia and consequent hypophosphatemia, rickets, and osteomalacia.

Familial tumoral calcinosis is genetically heterogeneous. Homozygous inactivating mutations (Met96Thr, Ser129Phe) in *FGF23* have been identified in a few patients with this disorder.[484,487] More commonly detected in patients with familial tumor calcinosis are biallelic loss-of-function microdeletions and splice site and missense mutations (Arg162Stop, Thr272Lys) in *GALNT3* (UDP-N-acetyl-alpha-D-galactosamine: polypeptide N-acetylgalactosaminyltransferase 3). The product of GALNT3 is a glycosyl transferase that initiates O-glycosylation in which N-acetylgalactosamine is the first sugar in the side chain, a step essential to secretion of intact and functional FGF23.[488] Failure to O-glycosylate FGF23 at Thr178 in the golgi apparatus permits its rapid intracellular cleavage between Arg179 and Ser180 to biologically inactive amino- and carboxyl-terminal fragments.[485,489]

Serum concentrations of intact FGF23 are low or nondetectable, whereas carboxyl-terminal FGF23 levels are elevated in patients with familial tumoral calcinosis due to either gene mutation. Therapy with an oral phosphate binder and the carbonic anhydrase inhibitor acetazolamide has resulted in hyperphosphaturia and reabsorption of ectopic calcifications without change in serum phosphate or calcium concentrations.[485,490] The hyperostosis hyperphosphatemia syndrome (OMIM 610233) is a clinical variant of familial tumoral calcinosis and is due to mutations in *FGF23* or *GALNT3*. Symptoms and signs may precede development of the more typical phenotype of familial tumoral calcinosis.[489,491]

Fibrodysplasia ossificans progressiva (FOP, OMIM 135100) is a disabling disorder of ectopic bone formation that may develop spontaneously or at sites of injury. It leads to ankylosis of all major joints, which severely limits mobility.[492] It is characterized by progressive ectopic ossification of muscle and connective tissue, leading to immobility of the mandible, neck, spine, hips, and other joints and to the development of a second skeleton that encases and imprisons the body. The disorder may be present at birth and is often manifest by 5 years of age. It is also associated with monophalangic big toes, deafness, scalp baldness, and mild developmental delay. Microscopically, there is normal endochondral osteogenesis occurring at an ectopic site.

Although primarily sporadic because affected subjects rarely reproduce, FOP can be transmitted as an autosomal-dominant trait. This disease is due to a highly specific (Arg206His) mutation in *ACVR1* (activin A receptor, type 1), to date the only mutation identified in these patients. Activins are members of the TGFβ superfamily that includes the BMPs as well as the inhibins and Mullerian-duct-inhibiting factor. The Arg206His mutation in *ACVR1* resides at the junction of the receptor's glycine-serine activation and tyrosine kinase domains and results in a constitutively active receptor product that directs the pluripotent mesenchymal stem cell into the chondrogenic pathway, leading to (ectopic) endochondral new bone formation. BMPs alone are able to stimulate complete endochondral osteogenesis in ectopic sites.[493]

BMP4 induces osteogenesis but is also required for commitment of the stem cell to the adipocyte pathway of development.[494] *BMP4* and the genes encoding its coreceptors (e.g., *BMPR1A*) are not mutated in patients with FOP. *BMP4* (but not *BMPR1A*) is overexpressed in cells from patients with FOP. However, there is an increased number of plasma membrane BMPR1A receptors in their cells due to a slow rate of ligand-mediated receptor internalization and consequently decreased rate of degradation—which might lead to prolonged BMP4-mediated intracellular signaling and function.[493] Overall, data suggest that BMP4-directed osteogenic activity is enhanced and the adipogenic pathway circumvented in patients with FOP. However, the role that the mutated ACVR1 plays in the pathogenesis of this disease is unclear at present. Management of these patients is primarily symptomatic to the extent possible, although immunosuppression may diminish the intensity of extraskeletal ossification.[495]

Progressive osseous heteroplasia (POH, OMIM 166350) is characterized by multiple foci of dermal membranous bone formation (osteoma cutis) beginning in infancy in the absence of any local injury or inflammatory insult. Lesions may develop on the trunk, extremities, or digits and may be asymptomatic or painful. Over time, ossification involving skeletal muscle and deep connective issue evolves. The disorder occurs in both genders. POH is transmitted as an autosomal-dominant trait and is due to inactivating mutations of the *GNAS* allele inherited from the father.[496,497] Identical mutations in *GNAS* may be clinically manifested as POH or PPHP in different members of the same family.

Osteochondrodysplasias

The osteochondrodysplasias form a heterogeneous group of malformations of cartilage and bone that have been grouped according to clinical and radiologic characteristics into those involving long bone growth alone (epiphyseal, metaphyseal, and/or diaphyseal dysplasias), long bones and vertebrae (spondyloepiphyseal and/or spondyloepimetaphyseal dysplasias), and variants thereof (Figure 17-18).[498] The genetic skeletal disorders have been classified into 37 groups based on the underlying genetic mutations and/or radiographic manifestations.[499] Mutations in one gene may give rise to several clinically defined disorders (Table 17-12).

These disorders are of interest not only because of the diagnostic and therapeutic clinical challenges they present but because they have identified many factors that normally regulate cartilage and bone development. Achondroplasia (OMIM 100800), the most common of the human chondrodystrophies (1/15,000–40,000 live births), is due to gain-of-function mutations in *FGFR3*—the gene

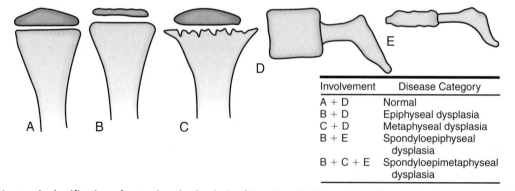

Involvement	Disease Category
A + D	Normal
B + D	Epiphyseal dysplasia
C + D	Metaphyseal dysplasia
B + E	Spondyloepiphyseal dysplasia
B + C + E	Spondyloepimetaphyseal dysplasia

Figure 17-18 Anatomic classification of osteochondrodysplasias. [Reproduced with permission from Shohat M, Rimoin DL (2007). The skeletal dysplasias. In Lifschitz F (ed.), *Pediatric endocrinology, Fifth edition.* New York: Informa Healthcare 145–162.]

TABLE 17-12

Human Osteochondrodysplasias: Selected Mutated Genes

Gene	Chromosome Locus	OMIM	Gene Product Function	Clinical Disorder (Syndrome)	Inheritance pattern	OMIM
Fibroblast Growth Factor Receptors						
FGFR1	8p11.2-p11.1	136350	Transmembrane tyrosine kinase receptor for FGFs	Pfeiffer	AD	101600
FGFR2	10q25.3-q26	176943		Apert	AD	101200
				Crouzon	AD	123500
				Jackson-Weiss	AD	123150
				Pfeiffer	AD	101600
				Antley-Bixler	AD	207410
				Beare-Stevenson cutis gyrata	AD	123790
FGFR3	4p16.3	134934		Achondroplasia	AD	100800
				Hypochondroplasia	AD	146100
				Thanatophoric dysplasia, Types I, II	AD	187600
				Severe with developmental delay and acanthosis nigricans	AD	134934
				Muenke nonsyndromic coronal craniosynostosis	AD	602849
Collagenopathies						
COL2A1	12q13.11- q13.2	120140	Extracellular matrix protein	Achondrogenesis type II	AD	200610
				Spondyloepiphyseal dysplasia congenita	AD	183900
				Spondylometaphyseal dysplasia	AD	184252
				Kneist dysplasia	AD	156550
				Spondyloepimetaphyseal dysplasia Strudwick type	AD	184250
				Stickler syndrome (1)	AD	108300
COL9A1	6q13	120210		Stickler syndrome	AR	
				Multiple epiphysea dysplasia	AD	
COL9A2	1p33-p32.2	120260		Multiple epiphyseal dysplasia (2)	AD	
COL9A3	20q13.3	120270		Multiple epiphyseal dysplasia (3)	AD	
COL10A1	6q21-q22.3	120110		Metaphyseal chondrodysplasia Schmid-type	AD	156500
COL11A1	1p21	120280		Stickler syndrome (2)	AD	604841
				Marshall syndrome	AD	154780
COL11A2	6p21.3	120290		Otospondylomega-epiphyseal dysplasia	AR	215150
				Stickler syndrome (3)	AD	184840
Sulfation Disorders						
SLC26A2	5q32-q33.1	606718	Transmembrane sulfate transporter	Diastrophic dysplasia	AR	222600
				Atelosteogenesis type II	AR	256050
				Achondrogenesis type IB	AR	600972
				Multiple epiphyseal dysplasia (4)	AR	226900
PAPSS2	10q22-q24	603005	3'-Phosphoadenosine 5'-phosphosulfate synthase 2	Spondyloepimetaphyseal dysplasia	AR	603005
ARSE	Xp22.3	300180	Arylsulfatase E	Chondrodysplasia punctata (1)	XLR	302950
CHST3	10q22.1	603799	Carbohydrate sulfotransferase 3	Spondyloepiphyseal dysplasia (Omani)	AR	608637

(Continued)

TABLE 17-12

Human Osteochondrodysplasias: Selected Mutated Genes—Cont'd

Gene	Chromosome Locus	OMIM	Gene Product Function	Clinical Disorder (Syndrome)	Inheritance pattern	OMIM
Perlecan Group						
HSPG2	1p36.1	142461	Heparan sulfate proteoglycan	Myotonic chondrodystrophy (Schwartz-Jampel, type 1)	AR	255800
Filamin Group						
FLNA	Xq28	300017	Actin-binding protein	Fronto-metaphyseal dysplasia	XLD	305620
				Otopalataldigital (1,2)	XLD	
FLNB	3p14.3	603381		Atelosteogenesis (1,3)	AD	108720, 108721
Pseudoachondroplasia Group						
COMP	19p12-13.1	600310	Cartilage oligomeric matrix protein	Pseudoachondroplasia	AD	177170
				Multiple epiphyseal dysplasia (Fairbank)	AD	132400
Metaphyseal Dysplasias						
RMRP	9p21-p12	157660	Mitochondrial RNA-processing endoribonuclease	Cartilage-hair hypoplasia	AR	250250
				Anauxetic dysplasia	AR	607095
PTHR1	3p22-p21.1	168468	Transmembrane G-protein receptor for PTH & PTHrP	Murk-Jansen metaphyseal chondrodysplasia	AD	156400
				Blomstrand chondrodysplasia	AR	215045
Mesomelic/Rhizo-mesomelic Dysplasias						
SHOX	Xpter-p22.32	312865	Homeobox gene Transcription factor	Leri-Weill dyschondrosteosis	XLD	127300
				Langer dysplasia (Idiopathic short stature) (Turner syndrome)	Biallelic	249700
Others						
RUNX2	6p21	600211	Osteoblast-specific transcription factor	Cleidocranial dysplasia	AD	119600
SOX9	17q24.1-q25.1	608160	Transcription factor	Campomelic dysplasia	AD	114290
Defects in Cholesterol Synthesis						
DHCR7	11q12-q13	602858	Δ^7-Dehydro cholesterol reductase	Smith-Lemli-Opitz syndrome	AR	270400
EBP	Xp11.22-p11.23	300205	3β-Hydroxysteroid Δ^8,Δ^7 isomerase	Chondrodysplasia punctata (2) (Conradi-Hunermann-Happle)	XLD	302960
DHCR24	1p33-p33.1	606418	3β-hydroxysterol-Δ^{24} reductase	Desmosterolosis	AR	602398
LRB	1q42.1	600024	3β-hydroxysterol-Δ^{14} reductase (Lamin B receptor)	Hydrops-ectopic calcification moth eaten dysplasia (Greenberg)	AR	215140
NSDHL	Xq28	300275	3β-hydroxysteroid C-4 sterol demethylase complex	Congenital hemidysplasia, icthyosiform erythroderma, limb defects	XLD	308050

AD, autosomal dominant; AR, autosomal recessive; CD, chondrodysplasia punctata; MED, multiple epiphyseal dysplasia; PTH, parathyroid hormone; PTHrP, PTH-related protein; SED, spondyloepiphyseal dysplasia; XLD, X-linked dominant; and XLR, X-linked recessive.

Adapted from Herman GE (2003). Disorders of cholesterol biosynthesis: Prototypic metabolic malformation syndromes. Hum Molec Genet 12:R75–R88; from Superti-Furga A, Unger S, and the Nosology Group of the International Skeletal Dysplasia Society (2007). International nosology and classification of genetic skeletal disorders: 2006 revision. Am J Med Genet 143A:1–18 (*www.isds.ch*).

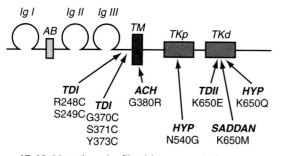

Figure 17-19 Mutations in fibroblast growth factor receptor-3 leading to achondroplasia (ACH), hypochondroplasia (HYP), thanatophoric dysplasia (TD) types I and II, and severe achondroplasia-developmental delay-acanthosis nigricans (SADDAN). [Reproduced with permission from Horton WA (2006). Molecular pathogenesis of achondroplasia. Growth Genet Horm 22:49–54.]

encoding fibroblast growth receptor 3. It is transmitted as an autosomal-dominant disorder but with a high rate of spontaneous mutations (primarily of the paternal allele). Clinically, it is manifested by short limbs but normal trunk length, large head, frontal bossing, and depressed nasal bridge. It is complicated by increased risk for cervical cord compression and spinal stenosis.[500,501]

FGFR3 is a transmembrane protein with three immunoglobulin domains in the extracellular region of the receptor and two tyrosine kinase domains in its intracellular portion (Figure 17-19). Three additional clinically distinct osteochondrodysplasias are associated with mutations in the same gene. Thanatophoric dysplasia is characterized by severe bony malformations, particularly of the skull, long bones, and ribs—the latter leading to respiratory insufficiency and early death. There are two radiographic forms of this disorder (I and II). Severe achondroplasia—developmental delay—acanthosis nigricans (SADDAN) is a clinical phenotype intermediate between those of thanatophoric dysplasia and achondroplasia. Hypochondroplasia is a clinically less severe manifestation of mild short-limbed (rhizomelic) short stature of variable severity that presents in mid-childhood.

Mutations in FGFR3 correlate with the clinical phenotype. Achondroplasia is most often (98%) associated with a missense mutation (Gly380Arg) in its transmembrane domain. Thanatophoric dysplasia type I is related to mutations (Arg248Cys, Gly370Cys) in the extracellular ligand-binding region next to the transmembrane region of the receptor. Type II is related to a mutation (Lys650Glu) in the distal tyrosine kinase domain. SADDAN is also the result of a Lys650Met mutation. Hypochondroplasia has been associated with mutations within the proximal (Asn540Gly in 60%) and distal (Lys650Gln) tyrosine kinase domains, respectively, as well in the immunoglobulin domains of the extracellular region (Ser84Leu, Arg200Cys) and transmembrane domain (Val381Glu) of FGF23.[501,502]

It is noteworthy that different mutations at Lys650 result in three distinct clinical phenotypes. Patients with Muenke nonsyndromic coronal craniosynostosis also have a mutation (Pro250Arg) in FGFR3. In chondrocytes, constitutively active FGFR3 initiates ligand-independent autophosphorylation of tyrosine residues within its

cytoplasmic domain that then propagate signal through the MAPK and signal transducer and activator of transcription pathways—resulting in inhibition of mitosis, matrix synthesis, and terminal (hypertrophic) differentiation. Thus, FGFR3 normally functions as a negative regulator of cartilage formation. As a single-gene disorder, it is possible to identify a mutation in FGFR3 in an affected fetus by analysis of fetal cell-free DNA in maternal plasma if the mother is unaffected.[503]

A loss-of-function mutation (Arg621His within the distal tyrosine kinase domain) in FGFR3 has been identified in a family whose members display the phenotype of tall stature, camptodactyly, and hearing loss.[504] Activating mutations in FGFR1 and FGFR2 have been associated with chondrodysplasias complicated by premature craniosynostosis (Pfeiffer, Apert, Crouzon, Jackson-White, and Beare-Stevenson cutis gyrata syndromes). Interestingly, mutations in FGFR1 have also been associated with hypogonadotropic hypogonadism (OMIM 147950), as FGFR1 is an essential neuronal migration factor.[505] Mutations in FGFR4 have not been associated with osteochondrodysplasias to date.

Defective formation of several types of collagen due to mutations in COL2A1, COL9A1, COL9A2, COL10A1, COL11A1, and COL11A2 result in a large number of skeletal malformations depending on the site and developmental timing of the synthetic error (Table 17-12). Abnormalities of sulfate transport, collagen matrix protein sulfation, and sulfatase activity have resulted in several chondrodysplasias. Spondyleptimetaphyseal dysplasia (OMIM 603005) is due to a biallelic loss-of-function mutation (Ser438Ter) in the gene (PAPSS2) encoding 3'-phosphoadenosine-5'-phosphosulfate synthase 2—an enzyme with dual activities. It catalyzes the synthesis of adenosine 5'-phosphosulfate and its phosphorylation to 3'-phospho-adenosine 5'-phosphosulfate, the universal sulfate donor necessary to sulfation of cartilage and bone matrix proteins.[506]

Clinical manifestations of this disorder include short limbs, kyphoscoliosis, brachydactyly, and enlarged knee joints. In the mouse model of this disease, there is decreased sulfation of matrix proteoglycans—resulting in short chondrocyte columns with irregularly aligned cells and decrease in the number and size of hypertrophic chondrocytes. Loss-of-function mutations (insertions, missense, nonsense) in SOX9, a transcription factor expressed in both developing chondrocytes (where it is coexpressed with COL2A1) and in the genital ridges during gonadal differentiation, cause campomelic dysplasia (OMIM 114290) and male-to-female sex reversal in 75% of affected 46XY subjects.

Clinically, this disorder is characterized by prenatal onset of bowing of tubular bones, hypoplastic scapulae, 11 ribs, cleft palate, and micrognathia—leading often to neonatal death. Heterozygous pseudoautosomal microdeletions and intragenic inactivating mutations (Leu 132Val, Arg195Ter) of the X (and Y) -linked pseudoautosomal gene SHOX (short stature homeobox-containing gene) resulting in haploinsufficiency are present in patients with Leri-Weill dyschondrosteosis (OMIM 127300)—typified by mesomelic limb shortening and growth retardation, Madelung deformity of the wrist, bowing of the radius, and ulnar dislocation.[507] Patients with idiopathic short stature and no identifying skeletal characteristics have also been observed to have heterozygous loss-of-function mutations in *SHOX*.

The Leri-Weill phenotype has been recorded in patients with intact *SHOX* but with microdeletions of downstream segments of the X chromosome pseudoautosomal region, implying the presence of modifying genes in this region.[508] Homozygous loss of *SHOX* leads to Langer mesomelic dysplasia (OMIM 249700). Endogenous *SHOX* is primarily expressed in hypertrophic and apoptotic chondrocytes within the cartilage growth plate. It is a transcriptional activator whose gene targets are as yet unidentified but whose expression in osteogenic cells results in arrest of the cell cycle and in apoptosis.[509]

Gain- and loss-of-function mutations of *PTHR1* lead to abnormalities of bone formation and growth.[510] Blomstrand chondrodysplasia (OMIM 215045) is an autosomal-recessive disorder that is lethal in utero and that may be identified in the fetus with short extremely dense long bones and markedly advanced skeletal maturation (as well as somatic anomalies such as aortic coarctation and facial anomalies). Pathologically, epiphyseal cartilage is reduced—and there are irregular columns and erratic distribution of chondrocytes within matrix. The abnormality is the result of inactivating mutations (deletions, missense mutations, Pro132Leu) of the gene encoding the PTH/PTHrP receptor.

Patients with Murk-Jansen metaphyseal chondrodysplasia (OMIM 156400) have short limbs and fingers, micrognathia, and deformities of the spine and pelvis but survive to adulthood. The average adult height is 125 cm, and child bearing is possible. Characteristically, these patients have hypercalcemia, hypophosphatemia, and low or undetectable serum levels of PTH or PTHrP. The disorder is due to activating mutations (His223Arg, Thr410Pro) of *PTHR1* and is associated with extraordinary delay in chondrocyte differentiation and decreased mineralization due to excessive bone resorption. Both disorders reflect the functional effect of PTHrP in developing cartilage, where it normally acts to slow differentiation and decrease the rate of chondrocyte apoptosis—thus prolonging chondrocyte proliferation and enhancing long bone growth.

Anauxetic dysplasia (OMIM 607095) is a spondylometaepiphyseal dysplasia transmitted as an autosomal-recessive disorder characterized by intrauterine growth retardation (birth length <40 cm), severely compromised adult height (<85 cm), hypodontia, and mild mental retardation. All bones are malformed, and there are few chondrocytes in the cartilage growth plates. It is due to loss-of-function mutations (insertions) in *RMRP* (RNA component of mitochondrial RNA-processing endoribonuclease), a gene that encodes the untranslated RNA subunit of the endoribonuclease RNase MRP.[511]

This enzyme is involved in the assembly of ribosomes (the structural units in which translation and protein synthesis takes place), the generation of RNA primers for replication of mitochondrial DNA, and the regulation of the cyclin-dependent cell cycle. The mutations that result in anauxetic dysplasia impair ribosome assembly and protein synthesis exclusively. Inactivating mutations

(duplications, insertions) in *RMRP* that modestly impair ribosomal assembly and regulation of the cell cycle have been found in patients with cartilage hair hypoplasia (OMIM 250250) and metaphyseal dysplasia without hypotrichosis (OMIM 250460).

Errors in the biosynthesis of cholesterol have been associated with several abnormalities of bone development (Table 17-12, Figure 17-20).[512] In patients with the Smith-Lemli-Opitz syndrome (OMIM 270400), inactivating mutations of the microsomal enzyme Δ^7-dehydrocholesterol reductase (DHCR7) impair synthesis of cholesterol and lead to intrauterine and postnatal growth retardation, short limbs, syndactyly and polydactyly, characteristic facial features (blepharoptosis, anteverted nares, broad alveolar ridges, cleft palate), congenital malformations of the heart and central nervous system, microcephaly, incomplete virilization of male external genitalia, hypoplastic thumbs, and developmental delay.[513] Stippled epiphyses are detected by radiologic examination. Hypocholesterolemia with elevated serum concentrations of 7-dehydrocholesterol are present.

Cholesterol covalently binds to the amino terminal and is essential to the function of Indian hedgehog, Sonic hedgehog, and Desert hedgehog—factors necessary to normal development of cartilage and bone, brain, and testes, respectively. However, substitution of 7-dehydrocholesterol for cholesterol does not impair the function of Sonic hedgehog. Therefore, it is likely that lack of cholesterol exerts its teratologic effect by impairing the intracellular signaling response(s) to these factors. Alternatively, the accumulation of precursors of cholesterol may exert toxic effects on the developing fetus. Cholesterol supplementation may improve the health, behavior, and growth of children with the Smith-Lemli-Opitz syndrome.

Chondrodysplasia punctata 2 (OMIM 302960) is an X-linked dominant disorder (Conradi-Hunermann-Happle syndrome) that is ordinarily lethal in the affected male and characterized clinically in the affected female by short stature with asymmetric short proximal limbs (rhizomelic dwarfism), frontal bossing, icthyosis in children and atrophic pigmentary lesions in adults, coarse hair with alopecia, and cataracts. Reflecting functional X-chromosomal mosaicism in females, the phenotype may vary from stillborn to mildly affected.[512] Radiographic examination reveals generalized osteosclerosis, irregular punctate calcification (stippling) of epiphyses in children, and hemivertebrae.

This disorder is due to loss-of-function mutations in *EBP* (emopamil-binding protein), the gene encoding 3β-hydroxysteroid-Δ^8,Δ^7isomerase—an enzyme important in sterol biosynthesis. In the serum of affected subjects, plasma concentrations of 8-dehydrocholesterol cholest-8(9)-en-3β-ol are elevated. This protein also binds many unrelated molecules. Its genetic designation derives from its ability to bind emopamil (i.e., EBP), a calcium ion antagonist. X-linked recessive and autosomal-recessive forms of the Conradi-Hunermann syndrome have also been reported, suggesting genetic heterogeneity for this phenotype. The X-linked recessive form of chondrodysplasia punctata (CDPX1, OMIM 302950) is due to inactivating mutations of the gene (*ARSE*) encoding aryl-sulfatase E. Affected males may

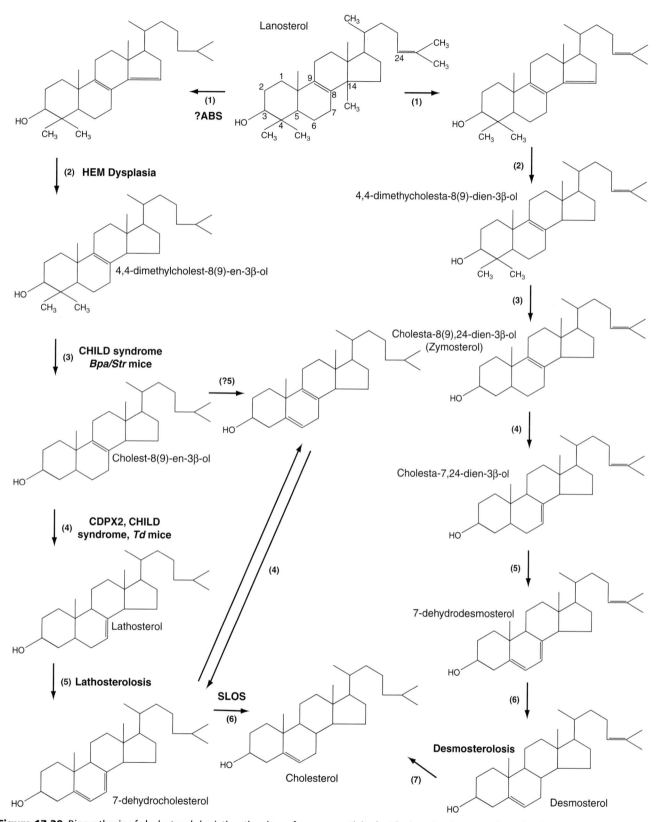

Figure 17-20 Biosynthesis of cholesterol depicting the sites of enzyme activity lost by inactivating mutations that lead to skeletal, genital, and other malformations. The numbers in parentheses denote specific enzymes: (1) lanosterol 14α-demethylase, (2) 3β-hydroxysteroid-Δ14-reductase, (3) 3β-hydroxysteroid C-4 sterol demethylase complex, (4) 3 β -hydroxysteroid-Δ8-Δ7-sterol isomerase, (5) 3β-hydroxysteroid-α5-desaturase, (6) 3β-hydroxysteroid-Δ7-reductase, and (7) 3β-hydroxysteroid-Δ24-reductase. [Reproduced with permission from Herman GE (2003). Disorders of cholesterol biosynthesis: Prototypic metabolic malformation syndromes. Hum Molec Genet 12:R75–R88.]

be stillborn or may survive, whereas female carriers may be asymptomatic or mildly affected.

Desmosterolosis (OMIM 602398) is an autosomal-recessive disorder whose skeletal manifestations include osteosclerosis, shortened limbs, macrocephaly, cleft palate, and thick alveolar ridges in addition to congenital heart disease and ambiguous genitalia in the affected female. It is due to inactivating mutations of the gene (DHCR24) encoding 3β-hydroxysterol-Δ^{24} reductase, the enzyme that converts desmosterol to cholesterol.[513,514] The rare lethal Greenberg dysplasia of hydrops ectopic calcification moth-eaten skeletal dysplasia (OMIM 215140) is transmitted as an autosomal-recessive trait associated with short-limbed dwarfism, polydactyly, and irregularly decreased calcification of the long bones together with calcification of the larynx and trachea. It is due to a loss-of-function mutation in the gene (LRB) encoding the lamin B receptor, a nuclear envelope inner membrane protein that not only binds lamin B but has 3β-hydroxysteroid-Δ^{14} reductase activity—an enzyme necessary to normal cholesterol biosynthesis.[515]

The CHILD syndrome (OMIM 308050) of congenital hemidysplasia with icthyosiform erythroderma (or nevus) and limb defects is remarkable for its unilateral distribution of anomalies that are confined to one-half of the body.[512] It is an X-linked disorder due to loss-of-function mutations in NSDHL (NADPH steroid dehydrogenase-like) encoding a sterol dehydrogenase or decarboxylase that is part of the 3β-hydroxysteroid C-4 sterol demethylase complex.

Concluding Remarks

In the past decade, our understanding of the complex mechanisms that underlie the pathophysiology of numerous illnesses that adversely affect the regulation of calcium, phosphate, and magnesium metabolism; chondrocyte differentiation and growth; and bone formation, mineralization, and strength has been transformed by the insights advances in genetics and proteomics have brought to these clinical problems. As further clarification of the very most basic mechanisms that underlie these disorders becomes available in the next decade, our ability to identify and specifically manage these problems will almost certainly experience another quantum leap forward.

REFERENCES

1. Kovacs CS (2006). Skeletal physiology: Fetus and neonate. In Favus MJ (ed.), *Primer on the metabolic bone diseases and disorders of mineral metabolism, Sixth edition.* Washington, D.C.: American Society for Bone and Mineral Research 50–55.
2. Kovacs CS, Kronenberg HM (1997). Maternal-fetal calcium and bone metabolism during pregnancy, puerperium, and lactation. Endocrine Reviews 18:832–872.
3. Kovacs CS, Kronenberg HM (2006). Skeletal physiology: Pregnancy and lactation. In Favus MJ (ed.), *Primer on the metabolic bone diseases and disorders of mineral metabolism, Sixth edition.* Washington, D.C.: American Society for Bone and Mineral Research 63–70.
4. Naylor KE, Iqbal P, Fledelius C, et al. (2000). The effect of pregnancy on bone density and bone turnover. J Bone Mineral Res 15:129–137.
5. Black AJ, Topping J, Durham B, et al. (2000). A detailed assessment of alterations in bone turnover, calcium homeostasis, and bone density in normal pregnancy. J Bone Miner Res 15:557–563.
6. Koo WWK, Warren L (2003). Calcium and bone health in infants. J Neonat Nurs 22:23–35.
7. Weisman Y (2003). Maternal, fetal, and neonatal vitamin D and calcium metabolism during pregnancy and lactation. Endocrine Devel 6:34–49.
8. Hollis BW, Wagner CL (2004). Vitamin D requirements during lactation: High dose maternal supplementation as therapy to prevent hypovitaminosis D for the mother and nursing infant. Am J Clin Nutr 80:1752S–1758S.
9. Hollis BW, Wagner CL (2006). Nutritional vitamin D status during pregnancy: Reasons for concern. CMAJ 174:1287–1290.
10. Ziegler EE, Hollis BW, Nelson SE, Jeter JM (2006). Vitamin D deficiency in breast fed infants in Iowa. Pediatrics 118:603–610.
11. Holick MF (2006). Resurrection of vitamin D deficiency and rickets. J Clin Invest 116:2062–2072.
12. Rigo J, De Curtis M, Pieltain C, et al. (2000). Bone mineral metabolism in the micropremie. Clin Perinatol 27:147–170.
13. Koo WWK, Hockman EM (2000). Physiologic predictors of lumbar spine bone mass in neonates. Pediatr Res 48:485–489.
14. Kovacs CS, Chafe LL, Fudge NJ, et al. (2001). PTH regulates fetal blood calcium and skeletal mineralization independently of PTHrP. Endocrinology 142:4983–4993.
15. Kovacs CS, Ho-Pao CL, Hunzelman JL, et al. (1998). Regulation of murine fetal-placental calcium metabolism by the calcium-sensing receptor. J Clin Invest 101:2812–2820.
16. Bradbury RA, Cropley J, Kifor O, et al. (2002). Localization of the extracellular Ca²⁺-sensing receptors in the human placenta. Placenta 23:192–200.
17. Moreau R, Daoud G, Bernatchez R, et al. (2002). Calcium uptake and calcium transporter expression by trophoblast cells from human term placenta. Biochim Biophys Acta 1564:325–332.
18. Rummens K, van Cromphaut SJ, Carmeliet G, et al. (2003). Pregnancy in mice lacking the vitamin D receptor: Normal maternal skeletal response, but fetal hypomineralization rescued by maternal calcium supplementation. Pediatr Res 54:466–473.
19. Hallak M, Cotton DB (1993). Transfer of maternally administered magnesium sulfate into the fetal compartment of the rat: assessment of amniotic fluid, blood and brain. Am J Obstet Gynecol 169:427–431.
20. Carpenter TO (2006). Neonatal hypocalcemia. In Favus MJ (ed.), *Primer on the metabolic bone diseases and disorders of mineral metabolism, Sixth edition.* Washington, D.C.: American Society for Bone and Mineral Research 224–227.
21. Bagnoli F, Bruchi S, Garosi G, et al. (1990). Relationship between mode of delivery and neonatal calcium homeostasis. Eur J Pediatr 149:800–803.
22. Hsu SC, Levine MA (2004). Perinatal calcium metabolism: Physiology and pathophysiology. Semin Neonatol 9:23–36.
23. Favus MJ (ed.) *Primer on the metabolic bone diseases and disorders of mineral metabolism, Sixth edition.* Washington, D.C.: American Society for Bone and Mineral Research 492, 496.
24. Koo WW, Hockman EM, Dow M (2006). Palm olein in the fat blend of infant formulas: Effect on the intestinal absorption of calcium and fat, and bone mineralization. J Am Coll Nutr 25:117–122.
25. Diamond FB Jr., Root AW (1992). Factors regulating the adolescent growth spurt in females. Adol Pediatr Gynec 5:48–49.
26. Krabbe S (1989). Calcium homeostasis and mineralization in puberty. Danish Med Bull 36:113–124.
27. McKay CP, Specker BL, Tsang RC, Chesney RW (1992). Mineral metabolism during childhood. In Coe FL, Favus MJ (eds.), *Disorders of bone and mineral metabolism.* New York: Raven Press 395–416.
28. Mora S, Pitukcheewanont P, Kaufman FR, et al. (1999). Biochemical markers of bone turnover and the volume and the density of bone in children at different stages of sexual development. J Bone Miner Res 14:1664–1671.
29. Root AW, Diamond FB Jr. (1993). Disorders of calcium and phosphorus metabolism in adolescents. Endocrinol Metab Clin NA 22:573–592.
30. Sorva R, Anttila R, Siimes MA, et al. (1997). Serum markers of collagen metabolism and serum osteocalcin in relation to pubertal development in 57 boys at 14 years of age. Pediatr Res 42:528–532.
31. Saggese G, Baroncelli GI, Bertelloni S, et al. (1994). Twenty-four-hour osteocalcin, carboxyterminal propeptide of type I procollagen, and aminoterminal propeptide of type III procollagen rhythms in normal and growth retarded children. Pediatr Res 35:409–415.
32. Crofton PM, Wade JC, Taylor MRH, Holland CV (1997). Serum concentrations of carboxyl-terminal propeptide of type I procollagen,

amino-terminal propeptide of type III procollagen, cross-linked carboxy-terminal telopeptide of type I collagen, and their interrelationships in school children. Clin Chem 43:1577–1581.

33. Miller PD, Baran DT, Bilezikian JP, et al. (1999). Practical clinical application of biochemical markers of bone turnover. J Clin Densitom 2:323–342.

34. Bollen A-M, Eyre DR (1994). Bone resorption rates in children monitored by the urinary assay of collagen type I cross-linked peptides. Bone 15:31–34.

35. Blumsohn A, Hannon RA, Wrate R, et al. (1994). Biochemical markers of bone turnover in girls during puberty. Clin Endocrinol 40:663–670.

36. Nelson DA, Norris SA, Gilsanz V (2006). Skeletal physiology: Childhood and adolescence. In Favus MJ (ed.), *Primer on the metabolic bone diseases and disorders of mineral metabolism, Sixth edition.* Washington, D.C.: American Society for Bone and Mineral Research 55–63.

37. Allgrove J (2001). Parathyroid disorders. Curr Paediatr 11:357–363.

38. Robertson WC (2002). Calcium carbonate consumption during pregnancy: An unusual cause of neonatal hypocalcemia. J Child Neurol 17:853–855.

39. Jain BK, Singh H, Singh D, Toor NS (1998). Phototherapy induced hypocalcemia. Indian Pediatr 35:566–567.

40. Foldenauer A, Vobeck S, Pohlandt F (1998). Neonatal hypocalcemia associated with rotavirus diarrhea. Eur J Pediatr 157:838–842.

41. Kurt A, Sen Y, Elkiran O, et al. (2006). Malignant infantile osteopetrosis: A rare cause of neonatal hypocalcemia. J Pediatr Endocrinol Metab 19:1459–1462.

42. Srinivasan M, Abinum M, Cant AJ (2000). Malignant infantile osteopetrosis presenting with neonatal hypocalcemia. Arch Dis Child Fetal Neonatal 83:F21–F23.

43. Holick MF (2007). Vitamin D deficiency. N Engl J Med 457:266–281.

44. Baron J, Winer KK, Yanovski JA, et al. (1996). Mutations in the Ca^{2+}-sensing receptor gene cause autosomal dominant and sporadic hypoparathyroidism. Human Molec Genet 5:601–606.

45. Shiohara M, Mori T, Mei B, et al. (2004). A novel gain-of-function mutation (F821L) in the transmembrane domain of calcium-sensing receptor is a cause of severe sporadic hypoparathyroidism. Eur J Pediatr 163:94–98.

46. Watanabe S, Fukumoto S, Chang H, et al. (2002). Association between activating mutations of calcium-sensing receptor and Bartter's syndrome. Lancet 360:692–694.

47. Mittleman SD, Hendy GN, Fefferman RA, et al. (2006). A hypocalcemic child with a novel activating mutation of the calcium-sensing receptor gene: Successful treatment with recombinant human parathyroid hormone. J Clin Endocrinol Metab 91:2474–2479.

48. Adachi M, Tachibana K, Masuno M, et al. (1998). Clinical characteristics of children with hypoparathyroidism due to 22q11.2 microdeletion. Eur J Pediatr 157:33–38.

49. Yagi H, Furutani Y, Hamada H, et al. (2003). Role of TBX1 in human del22q11.2 syndrome. Lancet 362:1366–1373.

50. Brauner R, Le Harivel de Gonneville A, Kindermans C, et al. (2003). Parathyroid function and growth in 22q11 deletion syndrome. J Pediatr 142:504–508.

51. Moss EM, Batshaw ML, Solot CB, et al. (1999). Psychoeducational profile of the 22q11.2 microdeletion: A complex pattern. J Pediatr 134:193–198.

52. Sobin C, Kiley-Brabeck K, Dale K, et al. (2006). Olfactory disorder in children with 22q11 deletion syndrome. Pediatrics 118:697–703.

53. Robin NH, Shprintzen RJ (2005). Defining the clinical spectrum of deletion 22q11.2. J Pediatr 147:90–96.

54. Shooner KA, Rope AF, Hopkin RJ, et al. (2005). Genetic analyses in two extended families with deletion 22q11 syndrome: Importance of extracardiac manifestations. J Pediatr 146:382–387.

55. Schinke M, Izumo S (1999). Getting to the heart of the DiGeorge syndrome. Nature Med 5:1120–1121.

56. Jerome LA, Papaioannou VE (2001). DiGeorge syndrome phenotype in mice mutant for the T-box gene, Tbx1. Nature Genet 27:286–291.

57. Paylor R, Glaser B, Mupo A, et al. (2006). Tbx1 haploinsufficiency is linked to behavioral disorders in mice and humans: implications for 22q11 deletion syndrome. Proc Natl Acad Sci USA 103:7729–7734.

58. Moon AM (2006). Mouse models for investigating the developmental basis of human birth defects. Pediatr Res 59:749–755.

59. Van Esch H, Groenen P, Nesbit MA, et al. (2000). GATA3 haploinsufficiency causes human HDR syndrome. Nature 406:419–422.

60. Watanabe T, Mochizuki H, Kohda N, et al. (1998). Autosomal dominant familial hypoparathyroidism and sensorineural deafness without renal dysplasia. Eur J Endocrinol 139:631–634.

61. Chiu W-Y, Chen H-W, Chao H-W, et al. (2006). Identification of three novel mutations in the GATA3 gene responsible for familial hypoparathyroidism and deafness in Chinese families. J Clin Endocrinol Metab 91:4587–4592.

62. Nesbit MA, Bowl MR, Harding B, et al. (2004). Characterization of GATA3 mutations in the hypoparathyroidism, deafness, and renal dysplasia (HDR) syndrome. J Biol Chem 279:22624–22634.

63. Hershkovitz E, Parvari R, Diaz GA, Gorodischer R (2004). Hypoparathyroidism-retardation-dysmorphism (HRD) syndrome: A review. J Pediatr Endocrinol Metab 17:1583–1590.

64. Parvari R, Hershkovitz E, Grossman N, et al. (2002). Mutation of TBCE causes hypoparathyroidism-retardation-dysmorphism and autosomal recessive Kenney-Caffey syndrome. Nature Genet 32:448–452.

65. Courtens W, Wuyts W, Poot M, et al. (2006). Hypoparathyroidism-retardation-dysmorphism syndrome in a girl: A new variant not caused by a TBCE mutation, clinical report and review. Am J Med Genet 140:611–617.

66. Baumber L, Tufarelli C, Patel S, et al. (2005). Identification of a novel mutation disrupting the DNA binding activity of GCM2 in autosomal recessive familial isolated hypoparathyroidism. J Med Genet 42:443–448.

67. Ding C, Buckingham B, Levine MA (2001). Familial isolated hypoparathyroidism caused by a mutation in the gene for the transcription factor GCMB. J Clin Invest 108:1215–1220.

68. Thomee C, Schubert SW, Parma J, et al. (2005). GCMB mutation in familial isolated hypoparathyroidism with residual secretion of parathyroid hormone. J Clin Endocrinol Metab 90:2487–2492.

69. Sunthornthepvarakul T, Churesigaew S, Ngowngarmratana S (1999). A novel mutation of the signal peptide of the preproparathyroid hormone gene associated with autosomal recessive familial isolated hypoparathyroidism. J Clin Endocrinol Metab 84:3792–3796.

70. Bowl MR, Nesbit MA, Harding B, et al. (2005). An interstitial deletion-insertion involving chromosomes 2p25.3 and Xq27.1, near SOX3, causes X-linked recessive hypoparathyroidism. J Clin Invest 115:2822–2831.

71. Thakker RV (2004). Genetics of endocrine and metabolic disorders: Parathyroid. Rev Endocrinol Metab Dis 5:37–51.

72. Hoogendam J, Farih-Sips H, Wynaendts CW, et al. (2007). Novel mutations in the parathyroid hormone (PTH)/PTH-related peptide receptor type 1 causing Blomstrand osteochondrodysplasia type I and II. J Clin Endocrinol Metab 92:1088–1095.

73. Pinsker JE, Rogers W, McLean S, et al. (2006). Pseudohypoparathyroidism type 1a with congenital hypothyroidism. J Pediatr Endocrinol Metab 19:1049–1052.

74. Fujisawa Y, Yamashita K, Hirai N, et al. (1997). Transient late neonatal hypocalcemia with high serum parathyroid hormone. J Pediatr Endocrinol Metab 10:433–436.

75. Thakker RV (2006). Hypocalcemia: Pathogenesis, differential diagnosis, and management. In Favus MJ (ed.), *Primer on the metabolic bone diseases and disorders of mineral metabolism, Sixth edition.* Washington, D.C.: American Society for Bone and Mineral Research 213–215.

76. Oskarsdottir S, Persson C, Eriksson BO, Fasth A (2005). Presenting phenotype in 100 children with the 22q11 deletion syndrome. Eur J Pediatr 164:146–153.

77. Bowen DC, Lederman HM, Sicherer SH, et al. (1998). Immune constitution of complete DiGeorge anomaly by transplantation of unmobilised blood mononuclear cells. Lancet 352:1983–1984.

78. Markert ML, Boeck A, Hale LP, et al. (1999). Transplantation of thymus tissue in complete DiGeorge syndrome. N Engl J Med 341:1180–1189.

79. Langman CB (2006). Hypercalcemic syndromes in infants and children. In Favus MJ (ed.), *Primer on the metabolic bone diseases and disorders of mineral metabolism, Sixth edition.* Washington, D.C.: American Society for Bone and Mineral Research 209–212.

80. Warner JT, Linton HR, Dunstan FDJ, Cartilidge PHT (1998). Growth and metabolic responses in preterm infants fed fortified human milk or a preterm formula. Intern J Clin Pract 52:236–240.

81. Fridriksson JH, Helmrath MA, Wessel JJ, Warner BW (2001). Hypercalcemia associated with extracorporeal life support in neonates. J Pediatr Surg 36:493–497.

82. Sharata H, Postellon DC, Hashimoto K (1995). Subcutaneous fat necrosis, hypercalcemia, and prostaglandin E. Pediatr Dermat 12:43–47.

83. Khan N, Licata A, Rogers D (2001). Intravenous bisphosphonate for hypercalcemia accompanying subcutaneous fat necrosis: A novel treatment approach. Clin Pediatr 40:217–219.

84. Yamaguchi T, Chattopadhay N, Brown EM (2000). G protein-coupled extracellular Ca^{2+} (Ca^{2+}$_o$)-sensing receptor (CaR): Roles in cell signaling and control of diverse cellular functions. In O'Malley B (ed.), *Hormones and signaling.* New York: Academic Press 209–253.

85. Chikatsu N, Fukumoto S, Suzawa M, et al. (1999). An adult patient with severe hypercalcaemia and hypocalciuria due to a novel homozygous inactivating mutation of calcium-sensing receptor. Clin Endocrinol 50:537–543.

86. Myashiro T, Kunii I, Manna TD, et al. (2004). Severe hypercalcemia in a 9-year-old Brazilian girl due to a novel inactivating mutation of the calcium-sensing receptor. J Clin Endocrinol Metab 89:5936–5941.

87. Brown EM (2005). Mutant extracellular calcium-sensing receptors and severity of disease. J Clin Endocrinol Metab 90:1246–1248.

88. Levine MA (2006). Spectrum of hyperparathyroidism in children. In *Endocrine Society 88th Annual Meeting.* [city]: Meet-The-Professor 390–396.

89. Steddon SJ, Cunningham J (2005). Calcimimetics and calcilytics: Fooling the calcium receptor. Lancet 365:2237–2239.

90. Sathasivam A, Garibaldi L, Murphy J (2006). Transient neonatal hyperparathyroidism: A presenting feature of mucolipidosis type II. J Pediatr Endocrinol Metab 19:859–862.

91. Nissenson RA (1998). Parathyroid hormone (PTH)/PTHrP receptor mutations in human chondrodysplasia. Endocrinology 139:4753–4755.

92. Schipani E, Langman CB, Parfitt AM, et al. (1996). Constitutively activated receptors for parathyroid hormone and parathyroid hormone-related peptide in Jansen's metaphyseal chondrodysplasia. N Engl J Med 335:708–714.

93. Buckmaster A, Rodda C, Cowell CT, et al. (1997). The use of pamidronate in PTHrP associated hypercalcemia in infancy. J Pediatr Endocrinol Metab 10:301–304.

94. Selicorni A, Fratoni A, Pavesi MA, et al. (2006). Thyroid anomalies in Williams syndrome: Investigation of 95 patients. Am J Med Genet 140A:1098–1101.

95. Li DY, Faury G, Taylor DG, et al. (1998). Novel arterial pathology in mice and humans hemizygous for elastin. J Clin Invest 102:1783–1787.

96. Morris CA, Mervis CB, Hobart HH, et al. (2003). GTF21 hemizygosity implicated in mental retardation in Williams syndrome: Genotype-phenotype analysis of five families with deletions in the Williams syndrome region. Am J Med Genet 123A:45–59.

97. Simon DB, Karet FE, Hamdan JM, et al. (1996). Bartter's syndrome, hypokalemic alkalosis with hypercalciuria, is caused by mutations in the Na-K-cotransporter NKCC2. Nature Genet 13:183–188.

98. Whyte MP (2006). Hypophosphatasia. In Favus MJ (ed.), *Primer on the metabolic bone diseases and disorders of mineral metabolism, Sixth edition.* Washington, D.C.: American Society for Bone and Mineral Research 351–353.

99. Mornet E (2000). Hypophosphatasia: The mutations in the tissue-nonspecific alkaline phosphatase gene. Hum Mutat 15:309–315.

100. Zurutuza L, Muller F, Ginrat JF, et al. (1999). Correlations of genotype and phenotype in hypophosphatasia. Hum Molec Genet 8:1039–1046.

101. Rice AM, Rivkees SA (19991). Etidronate therapy for hypercalcemia in subcutaneous fat necrosis of the newborn. J Pediatr 134:349–351.

102. Lteif AN, Zimmerman D (1998). Bisphosphonates for treatment of childhood hypercalcemia. Pediatrics 102:990–993.

103. Ezgu FS, Buyan N, Gunduz M, et al. (2004). Vitamin D intoxication and hypercalcaemia in an infant treated with pamidronate infusions. Eur J Pediatr 163:163–165.

104. Rauch F, Schoenau E (2002). Skeletal development in premature infants: A review of bone physiology beyond nutritional aspects. Arch Dis Child Fetal Neonatal Ed 86:F82–F85.

105. Beyers N, Alheit B, Taljaard JF, et al. (1994). High turnover osteopenia in preterm infants. Bone 15:5–13.

106. Miller ME (2003). The bone disease of preterm birth: A biomechanical perspective. Pediatr Res 53:10–15.

107. Funke S, Morava E, Czako M, et al. (2006). Influence of genetic polymorphisms on bone disease of preterm infants. Pediatr Res 60:607–612.

108. Atabek ME, Pirgon O, Yorulmaz A, Kurtoglu S (2006). The role of cord blood IGF-I levels in preterm osteopenia. J Pediatr Endocrinol Metab 19:253–257.

109. De Schepper J, Cools F, Vandenplas Y, et al. (2005). Whole body bone mineral content is similar at discharge in premature infants receiving fortified breast milk or preterm formula. J Pediatr Gastroenterol Nutr 41:230–234.

110. Cakir M, Mungan I, Karahan C, et al. (2006). Necrotizing enterocolitis increases the bone resorption in premature infants. Early Hum Devel 82:405–409.

111. Eliakim A, Shiff Y, Nemet D, Dolfin T (2003). The effect of neonatal sepsis on bone turnover in very-low birth weight preterm infants. J Pediatr Endocrinol Metab 16:413–418.

112. Aly H, Moustafa MF, Amer HA, et al. (2005). Gestational age, sex, and maternal parity correlate with bone turnover in premature infants. Pediatr Res 57:708–711.

113. Aladangady N, Coen PG, White MP, et al. (2004). Urinary excretion of calcium and phosphate in preterm infants. Pediatr Nephrol 19:1225–1231.

114. Kaplan W, Haymond MW, McKay S, Karaviti LP (2006). Osteopenic effects of MgSO$_4$ in multiple pregnancies. J Pediatr Endocrinol Metab 19:1225–1230.

115. Shiff Y, Eliakim A, Shainkin-Kestenbaum R, et al. (2001). Measurement of bone turnover markers in premature infants. J Pediatr Endocrinol Metab 14:389–395.

116. Tsukahara H, Miura M, Hori C, et al. (1996). Urinary excretion of pyridinium cross-links of collagen in infancy. Metabolism 45:510–514.

116a. Eliakim A, Nemet D (2005). Osteopenia of prematurity: The role of exercise in prevention and treatment. Pediatr Endocrinol Rev 2:675–682.

117. Nelson DA, Koo WWK (1999). Interpretation of absorptiometric bone mass measurements in the growing skeleton: Issues and limitations. Calcif Tissue Int 65:1–3.

118. Hammami H, Koo WWK, Hockman EM (2003). Body composition of neonates from fan beam duel energy X-ray absorptiometry measurements. J Parenteral Enteral Nutr 27:423–426.

119. Koo WWK, Walters J, Bush AJ, et al. (1996). Dual-energy x-ray absorptiometry studies of bone mineral status in newborn infants. J Bone Miner Res 11:997–1002.

120. Ritschl E, Wehmeijer K, de Terlizzi F, et al. (2005). Assessment of skeletal development in preterm and term infants by qualitative ultrasound. Pediatr Res 58:341–346.

121. Rubinacci A, Moro GE, Boehm G, et al. (2003). Quantitative ultrasound for the assessment of osteopenia in preterm infants. Europ J Endocrinol 149:307–315.

122. Littner Y, Mandel D, Mimouni FB, Dollberg S (2005). Bone ultrasound velocity of infants born small for gestational age. J Pediatr Endocrinol Metab 18:793–797.

123. McDevitt H, Tomlinson C, White MP, Ahmed SF (2005). Quantitative ultrasound assessment of bone in preterm and term neonates. Arch Dis Child Fetal Neonatal 90:F341–342.

124. Aly H, Moustafa MF, Hassanein SM, et al. (2004). Physical activity combined with massage improves bone mineralization in premature infants: A randomized trial. J Perinatol 24:305–309.

125. Trotter A, Bokelmann B, Sorgo W, et al. (2001). Follow-up examination at the age of 15 months of extremely preterm infants after postnatal estradiol and progesterone replacement. J Clin Endocrinol Metab 86:601–603.

126. Trotter A, Maier L, Pohlandt F (2002). Calcium and phosphate balance of extremely preterm infants with estradiol and progesterone replacement. Am J Perinatol 19:23–29.

127. Fewtrell MS, Prentice A, Jones SC, et al. (1999). Bone mineralization and turnover in preterm infants at 8-12 years of age: The effect of early diet. J Bone Miner Res 14:810–820.

128. Ichiba H, Shintaku H, Fujimaru M, et al. (2000). Bone mineral density of the lumbar spine in very-low-birth-weight infants; a longitudinal study. Eur J Pediatr 159:215–218.

129. Weiler HA, Yuen CK, Seshia MM (2002). Growth and bone mineralization of young adults weighing less than 1500 grams at birth. Early Hum Devel 67:101–102.

130. Yeste D, Almar J, Clemente M, et al. (2007). Areal bone mineral density of the lumbar spine in 80 premature newborns: A prospective and longitudinal study. J Pediatr Endocrinol Metab 17:959–966.

131. Marini JC (2006). Osteogenesis imperfecta. In Favus MJ (ed.), *Primer on the metabolic bone diseases and disorders of mineral metabolism, Sixth edition.* Washington, D.C.: American Society for Bone and Mineral Research 418–421.

132. Rauch F, Glorieux FH (2004). Osteogenesis imperfecta. Lancet 363:1377–1385.

133. Rauch F, Glorieux FH (2005). Bisphosphonate treatment in osteogenesis imperfecta: Which drug, for whom, for how long? Ann Med 37:925–302.

134. Duval M, Fenneteau O, Doireau V, et al. (1999). Intermittent he-mophagocytic lymphohistiocytois is a regular feature of lysinuric protein intolerance. J Pediatr 134:236–239.

135. Borsani G, Bassi MT, Sperandeo MP, et al. (1999). SLC7A7, encoding a putative permease-related protein, is mutated in patients with lysinuric protein intolerance. Nature Genet 21:297–301.

136. Whyte MP (2006b). Sclerosing bone disorders. In Favus MJ (ed.), *Primer on the metabolic bone diseases and disorders of mineral metabolism, Sixth edition*. Washington, D.C.: American Society for Bone and Mineral Research 398–414.

137. Fujita Y, Nakata K, Yasui N, et al. (2000). Novel mutations of the cathepsin K gene in patients with pycnodysostosis and their characterization. J Clin Endocrinol Metab 85:425–431.

138. Soliman AT, Rajab A, Al Salmi I, et al. (1996). Defective growth hormone secretion in children with pycnodysostosis and improved linear growth after growth hormone treatment. Arch Dis Child 75:242–244.

139. Carpenter TO, DeLucia MC, Zhang JH, et al. (2006). A randomized controlled study of the effects of dietary magnesium oxide supplementation on bone mineral content in healthy girls. J Clin Endocrinol Metab 91:4866–4872.

140. Rude RK, Gruber HE (2004). Magnesium deficiency and osteoporosis: Animal and human observations. J Nutr Biochem 15:710–716.

141. Koo WWK (2007). Neonatal calcium, magnesium, and phosphorus disorders. In Lifshitz F (ed.), *Pediatric endocrinology, Fifth edition*. New York: Informa Healthcare 497–529.

142. Simon DB, Nelson-Williams C, Bia MJ, et al. (1996). Gitelman's variant of Bartter's syndrome, inherited hypokalemic alkalosis, is caused by mutations in the thiazide-sensitive Na-Cl cotransporter. Nature Genet 12:24–30.

143. Rude RK (2006). Magnesium depletion and hypermagnesemia. In Favus MJ (ed.), *Primer on the metabolic bone diseases and disorders of mineral metabolism, Sixth edition*. Washington, D.C.: American Society for Bone and Mineral Research 230–233.

144. Walder RY, Landau D, Meyer P, et al. (2002). Mutation of TRPM6 causes familial hypomagnesemia with secondary hypocalcemia. Nature Genet 31:171–174.

145. Chubanov V, Waldegger S, Mederos y Schnitzler M, et al. (2004). Disruption of TRPM6/TRPM7 complex formation by a mutation in the TRPM6 gene causes hypomagnesemia with secondary hypocalcemia. Proc Nat Acad Sci USA 101:2894–2899.

146. Simon DB, Lu Y, Choate KA, et al. (1999). Paracellin-1, a renal tight junction protein required for paracellular Mg^{2+} resorption. Science 285:103–106.

147. Weber S, Schneider L, Peters M, et al. (2001). Novel paracellin-1 mutations in 25 families with familial hypomagnesaemia with hypercalciuria and nephrocalcinosis. J Am Soc Nephrol 12:1872–1881.

148. Kausalya PJ, Amasheh S, Gunzel D, et al. (2006). Disease-associated mutations affect intracellular traffic and paracellular Mg^{2+} transport function of claudin-16. J Clin Invest 116:878–891.

149. Shalev H, Phillip M, Galil A, et al. (1998). Clinical presentation and outcome in primary familial hypomagnesemia. Arch Dis Child 78:127–130.

150. Konrad M, Schaller A, Seelow D, et al. (2006). Mutations in the tight-junction gene claudin 19 (CLDN19) are associated with renal magnesium wasting, renal failure, and severe ocular involvement. Am J Hum Genet 79:949–957.

151. Shane E, Irani D (2006). Hypercalcemia: Pathogenesis, clinical manifestations, differential diagnosis, and management. In Favus MJ (ed.), *Primer on the metabolic bone diseases and disorders of mineral metabolism, Sixth edition*. Washington, D.C.: American Society for Bone and Mineral Research 176–180.

152. Domico MB, Huynh V, Anand SK, Mink R (2006). Severe hyperphosphatemia and hypocalcemic tetany after oral laxative administration in a 3-month-old infant. Pediatrics 118:1580–1583.

153. Arnold A, Horst SA, Gardella TJ, et al. (1990). Mutation of the signal peptide-encoding region of the preproparathyroid hormone gene in familial isolated hypoparathyroidism. J Clin Invest 86:1084–1087.

154. Karaplis AC, Lim SK, Baba H, et al. (1995). Inefficient membrane targeting, translocation, and proteolytic processing by signal peptidase of a mutant preproparathyroid hormone protein. J Biol Chem 270:1629–1635.

155. Parkinson DB, Thakker RV (1992). A donor splice site mutation in the parathyroid hormone gene is associated with autosomal recessive hypoparathyroidism. Nature Genet 1:149–152.

156. Goswami R, Mohapatra T, Gupta N, et al. (2004). Parathyroid hormone gene polymorphism and sporadic idiopathic hypoparathyroidism. J Clin Endocrinol Metab 89:4840–4845.

157. Makita Y, Masuno M, Imaizumi K, et al. (1995). Idiopathic hypoparathyroidism in 2 patients with 22q11 microdeletions. J Med Genet 32:669.

158. Winer KK, Ko CW, Reynolds JC, et al. (2003). Long-term treatment of hypoparathyroidism: A randomized controlled study comparing parathyroid hormone-(1-34) versus calcitriol and calcium. J Clin Endocrinol Metab 88:4214–4220.

159. Tashjian AH Jr, Chabner BA (2002). Commentary on clinical safety of recombinant human parathyroid hormone 1-34 in the treatment of osteoporosis in men and postmenopausal women. J Bone Miner Res 17:1151–1161.

160. Kifor O, McElduff A, Leboff MS, et al. (2004). Activating antibodies to the calcium-sensing receptor in two patients with autoimmune hypoparathyroidism. J Clin Endocrinol Metab 89:548–556.

161. Mayer A, Ploix C, Orgiazzi J, et al. (2004). Calcium-sensing receptor antibodies are relevant markers of acquired hypoparathyroidism. J Clin Endocrinol Metab 89:4484–4488.

162. Bringhurst FR, Demay MB, Kronenberg HM (2003). Hormones and disorders of mineral metabolism. In Larsen PR, Kronenberg HM, Melmed S, Plonsky KS (eds.), *Williams textbook of endocrinology, Tenth edition*. Philadelphia: Saunders/Elsevier 1303–1371.

163. Goltzman D, Cole DEC (2006). Hypoparathyroidism. In Favus MJ (ed.), *Primer on the metabolic bone diseases and disorders of mineral metabolism, Sixth edition*. Washington, D.C.: American Society for Bone and Mineral Research 216–219.

164. Eisenbarth GS, Gottlieb PA (2004). Autoimmune polyendocrine syndromes. N Engl J Med 350:2068–2079.

165. Betterle C, Greggio NA, Volpato M (1998). Autoimmune polyglandular syndrome type 1. J Clin Endocrinol Metab 83:1049–1055.

166. Perheentupa J (2006). Autoimmune polyendocrinopathy-candidasis-ectodermal dystrophy. J Clin Endocrinol Metab 91:2843–2850.

167. Wolff ASB, Erichsen MM, Meager A, et al. (2007). Autoimmune polyendocrine syndrome type 1 in Norway: Phenotypic variation, autoantibodies, and novel mutations in the autoimmune regulator gene. J Clin Endocrinol Metab 92:595–603.

168. Bjorses P, Halonen M, Palvimo JJ, et al. (2000). Mutations in the AIRE gene: Effects on subcellular location and transactivation function of the autoimmune polyendocrinopathy-candidiasis-ectodermal dystrophy protein. Am J Hum Genet 66:378–392.

169. Uchida D, Hatakeyama S, Matsushima A, et al. (2004). AIRE functions as an E3 ubiquitin ligase. J Exp Med 199:167–172.

170. Germain-Lee EL, Schwindinger W, Crane JL, et al. (2005). A mouse model of Albright hereditary osteodystrophy generated by targeted disruption of exon 1 of the *Gnas* gene. Endocrinology 146:4697–4709.

171. Levine MA (2006a). Parathyroid hormone resistance syndromes. In Favus MJ (ed.), *Primer on the metabolic bone diseases and disorders of mineral metabolism, Sixth edition*. Washington, D.C.: American Society for Bone and Mineral Research 220–224.

172. Farfel Z, Bourne HB, Iiri T (1999). The expanding spectrum of G protein diseases. N Engl J Med 340:1012–1020.

173. Weinstein LS, Liu J, Sakamoto A, et al. (2004). GNAS: Normal and abnormal functions. Endocrinology 145:5459–5464.

174. Thiele S, Werner R, Ahrens W, et al. (2007). A disruptive mutation in exon 3 of the *GNAS* gene with Albright hereditary osteodystrophy, normocalcemic pseudohypoparathyroidism, and selective long transcript variant G$_s\alpha$ deficiency. J Clin Endocrinol Metab 92:1764–1768.

175. Gelfand IM, Eugster EA, DiMeglio LA (2006). Presentation and clinical progression of pseudohypoparathyroidism with multihormonal resistance and Albright hereditary osteodystrophy: A case series. J Pediatr 149:877–880.

176. Sakamoto A, Chen M, Kobayashi T, et al. (2005). Chondrocyte-specific knockout of the G protein G$_s\alpha$ leads to epiphyseal and growth plate abnormalities and ectopic chondrocyte formation. J Bone Miner Res 20:663–671.

177. Aldred MA (2006). Genetics of pseudohypoparathyroidism types Ia and Ic. J Pediatr Endocrinol Metab 19:635–640.

178. Juppner H, Bastepe M (2006). Different mutations within or upstream of the *GNAS* locus cause distinct forms of pseudohypoparathyroidism. J Pediatr Endocrinol Metab 19:641–646.

179. Linglart A, Gensure RC, Olney RC, et al. (2005). A novel *STX16* deletion in autosomal dominant pseudohypoparathyroidism type IB

redefines the boundaries of the cis-acting imprinting control element of *GNAS*. Am J Hum Genet 76:804–814.

180. Wu W-I, Schwindinger WF, Aparicio LF, Levine MA (2001). Selective resistance to parathyroid hormone caused by a novel uncoupling mutation in the carboxyl terminus of G-alpha(s). J Biol Chem 276:165–171.

181. Perez de Nanclares G, Fernandez-Rebollo E, Santin I, et al. (2007). Epigenetic defects of *GNAS* in patients with pseudohypoparathyroidism and mild features of Albright's hereditary osteodystrophy. J Clin Endocrinol Metab 92:2370–2373.

182. Farfel Z, Iiri T, Shapira H, et al. (1996). Pseudohypoparathyroidism, a novel mutation in the beta/gamma-contact region of Gs-alpha impairs receptor stimulation. J Biol Chem 271:19653–19655.

183. Iiri T, Herzmark P, Nakamoto JM, et al. (1994). Rapid GDP release from Gs-alpha in patients with gain and loss of endocrine function. Nature 371:164–168.

184. Downs RW Jr. (2006). Miscellaneous causes of hypocalcemia. In Favus MJ (ed.), *Primer on the metabolic bone diseases and disorders of mineral metabolism, Sixth edition*. Washington, D.C.: American Society for Bone and Mineral Research 227–229.

185. Bradley TJ, Metzger DL, Sanatani S (2004). Long on QT and low on calcium. Cardiol Young 14:667–670.

186. Gavalas NG, Kemp EH, Krohn KJE, et al. (2007). The calcium-sensing receptor is a target of autoantibodies in patients with autoimmune polyendocrine syndrome type 1. J Clin Endocrinol Metab 92:2107–2114.

187. Ishii T, Suzuki Y, Ando N, et al. (2000). Novel mutations of the autoimmune regulator gene in two siblings with autoimmune polyendocrinopathy-candidiasis-ectodermal dystrophy. J Clin Endocrinol Metab 85:2922–2926.

188. Cole DEC, Kooh SW, Vieth R (2000). Primary infantile hypomagnesemia: Outcome after 21 years and treatment with continuous nocturnal nasogastric magnesium infusion. Eur J Pediatr 159:38–43.

189. Marx SJ (2006). Familial hypocalciuric hypercalcemia. In Favus MJ (ed.), *Primer on the metabolic bone diseases and disorders of mineral metabolism, Sixth edition*. Washington, D.C.: American Society for Bone and Mineral Research 188–190.

190. Pidasheva S, Grant M, Canaff L, et al. (2006). Calcium-sensing receptor dimerizes in the endoplasmic reticulum: Biochemical and biophysical characterization of the CASR mutants retained intracellularly. Hum Molec Genet 15:2200–2209.

191. Pallais JC, Kifor O, Chen Y-B, et al. (2004). Acquired hypocalciuric hypercalcemia due to autoantibodies against the calcium-sensing receptor. N Engl J Med 351:362–369.

192. Korfor O, Moore FD Jr., Wang P, et al. (1996). Reduced immunostaining for the extracellular Ca^{2+}-sensing receptor in primary and uremic secondary hyperparathyroidism. J Clin Endocrinol Metab 81:1598–1606.

193. Bilezikian JP, Silverberg SJ (2006). Primary hyperparathyroidism. In Favus MJ (ed.), *Primer on the metabolic bone diseases and disorders of mineral metabolism, Sixth edition*. Washington, D.C.: American Society for Bone and Mineral Research 181–185.

194. Kollars J, Zarroug AE, van Heerden J, et al. (2005). Primary hyperparathyroidism in pediatric patients. Pediatrics 115:974–980.

195. Marx SJ, Simonds WF (2005). Hereditary hormone excess: Genes, molecular pathways, and syndromes. Endocrine Reviews 26:615–661.

196. Heppner C, Kester MB, Agarwal SK, et al. (1997). Somatic mutation of the MEN I gene in parathyroid tumors. Nature Genet 16:375–378.

197. Warner J, Epstein M, Sweet A, et al. (2004). Genetic testing in familial isolated hyperparathyroidism: Unexpected results and their implications. J Med Genet 41:155–160.

198. Carpten JD, Robbins CM, Villablanca A, et al. (2002). HRPT2, encoding parafibromin, is mutated in hyperparathyroidism-jaw tumor syndrome. Nature Genet 32:676–680.

199. Simonds WF, James-Newton LA, Agarwal SK, et al. (2002). Familial isolated hyperparathyroidism: Clinical and genetic characteristics of 36 kindreds. Medicine 81:1–26.

200. Rubin MR, Silverberg SJ (2005). HRPT2 in parathyroid cancer: A piece of the puzzle. J Clin Endocrinol Metab 90:5505–5507.

201. Guarnieri V, Scillitani A, Muscarella LA, et al. (2006). Diagnosis of parathyroid tumors in familial isolated hyperparathyroidism with HRPT2 mutation: Implication for cancer surveillance. J Clin Endocrinol Metab 91:2827–2832.

202. Krebs LJ, Shattuck TM, Arnold A (2005). HRPT2 mutational analysis of typical sporadic parathyroid adenomas. J Clin Endocrinol Metab 90:5015–5017.

203. Brandt ML, Gagel RF, Angeli A, et al. (2001). Guidelines for diagnosis and therapy of MEN type 1 and type 2. J Clin Endocrinol Metab 86:5658–5671.

204. Marx SJ, Agarwal SK, Kester MB, et al. (1999). Multiple endocrine neoplasia type 1: Clinical and genetic features of the hereditary endocrine neoplasias. Rec Prog Horm Res 54:397–438.

205. Root AW (2000). Genetic disorders of calcium and phosphorus metabolism. Crit Rev Clin Lab Sci 37:217–260.

206. Thakker RV (1998). Multiple endocrine neoplasia: Syndromes of the twentieth century. J Clin Endocrinol Metab 83:2617–2620.

207. Asgharian B, Turner ML, Gibril F, et al. (2004). Cutaneous tumors in patients with muliple endocrine neoplasm type 1 (MEN1) and gastrinomas: Prospective study of frequency and development of criteria with high sensitivity and specificity. J Clin Endocrinol Metab 89:5328–5336.

208. Agarwal SK, Guru SC, Heppner C, et al. (1999). Menin interacts with the AP1 transcription factor JunD and represses JunD-activated transcription. Cell 96:143–152.

209. Kaji H, Canaff L, Lebrun J-J, et al. (2001). Inactivation of menin, a Smad3-interacting protein, blocks transforming growth factor beta signaling. Proc Natl Acad Sci 98:3837–3842.

210. Heppner C, Bilimoria KY, Agarwal SK, et al. (2001). The tumor suppressor protein menin interacts with NF-kappaB proteins and inhibits NF-kappaB-mediated transactivation. Oncogene 20:4917–4925.

211. Pannett AAJ, Thakker RV (2001). Somatic mutations in MEN type 1 tumors, consistent with the Knudson "two-hit" hypothesis. J Clin Endocrinol Metab 86:4371–4374.

212. Marx SJ, Agarwal SK, Kester MB, et al. (1998). Germline and somatic mutation of the gene for multiple endocrine neoplasia type 1 (MEN1). J Intern Med 243:447–453.

213. Turner JJO, Leotela PD, Pannett AAJ, et al. (2002). Frequent occurrence of an intron 4 mutation in multiple endocrine neoplasia type 1. J Clin Endocrinol Metab 87:2688–2693.

214. Ozawa A, Agarwal SK, Mateo CM, et al. (2007). The parathyroid/pituitary variant of multiple endocrine neoplasia type 1 usually has causes other than $p27^{Kip\,1}$ mutations. J Clin Endocrinol Metab 92:1948–1951.

215. Teh BT, Kytola S, Farnebo F, et al. (1998). Mutation analysis of the *MEN1* gene in multiple endocrine neoplasia type 1, familial acromegaly and familial isolated hyperparathyroidism. J Clin Endocrinol Metab 83:2621–2626.

216. Bassett JHD, Forbes SA, Pannett AAJ, et al. (1998). Characterization of mutations in patients with multiple endocrine neoplasia type I. Am J Hum Genet 62:232–244.

217. Stratakis CA, Ball DW (2000). A concise genetic and clinical guide to multiple endocrine neoplasias and related syndromes. J Pediatr Endocrinol Metab 13:457–465.

218. Santoro M, Melillo RM, Carlomagno F, et al. (1998). Molecular biology of the *MEN2* gene. J Intern Med 243:505–508.

219. Lumbroso S, Paris F, Sultan C (2004). Activating Gsα mutations: Analysis of 113 patients with signs of McCune-Albright syndrome, a European collaborative study. J Clin Endocrinol Metab 89:2107–2113.

220. Cesur Y, Caksen H, Fundem A, et al. (2003). Comparison of low and high dose of vitamin D treatment in nutritional vitamin D deficiency rickets. J Pediatr Endocrinol Metab 16:1105–1109.

221. Chan W, Sheehan S, Miller LC, Sadeghi-Najad A (2006). Hypercalcemia in a newly arrived international adoptee. J Pediatr Endocrinol Metab 19:1249–1250.

222. Holick MF, Shao Q, Liu WW, Chen TC (1992). The vitamin D content of fortified milk and infant formula. N Engl J Med 326:1178–1181.

223. Kawaguchi M, Mitsuhashi Y, Kondo S (2003). Iatrogenic hypercalcemia due to vitamin D3 ointment (1,24(OH)2D3) combined with thiazide diuretics in a case of psoriasis. J Dermatol 30:801–804.

224. Ohigashi S, Tatsuno I, Uchida D, et al. (2003). Topical treatment with 22-oxacalcitriol (OCT), a new vitamin D analogue, caused severe hypercalcemia with exacerbation of chronic renal failure in a psoriatic patient with diabetic nephropathy: A case report and analysis of the potential for hypercalcemia. Intern Med 42:1202–1205.

225. Adams JS, Hewison M (2006). Hypercalcemia caused by granuloma-forming disorders. In Favus MJ (ed.), *Primer on the metabolic bone diseases and disorders of mineral metabolism, Sixth edition*.

Washington, D.C.: American Society for Bone and Mineral Research 200–202.

226. Jacobs TP, Bilezikian JP (2005). Clinical review: Rare causes of hypercalcemia. J Clin Endocrinol Metab 90:6316–6322.

227. Schurman SJ, Bergstrom WH, Root AW, et al. (1998). Interleukin-1 beta mediated calciotropic activity in serum of children with juvenile rheumatoid arthritis. J Rheumatol 25:161–165.

228. Mochizuki H, Saito M, Michigami T, et al. (2000). Severe hypercalcemia and respiratory insufficiency associated with infantile hypophosphatasia caused by two novel mutations of the tissue-nonspecific alkaline phosphatase gene. Eur J Pediatr 159:375–379.

229. Horwitz MJ, Stewart AF (2006). Hypercalcemia associated with malignancy. In Favus MJ (ed.), *Primer on the metabolic bone diseases and disorders of mineral metabolism, Sixth edition*. Washington, D.C.: American Society for Bone and Mineral Research 195–199.

230. Kutluk MT, Hazar V, Akyuz C, et al. (1997). Childhood cancer and hypercalcemia: Report of a case treated with pamidronate. J Pediatr 130:828–831.

231. Wysolmerski JJ (2006). Miscellaneous causes of hypercalcemia. In Favus MJ (ed.), *Primer on the metabolic bone diseases and disorders of mineral metabolism, Sixth edition*. Washington, D.C.: American Society for Bone and Mineral Research 203–208.

232. Prince RL (2006). Secondary and tertiary hyperparathyroidism. In Favus MJ (ed.), *Primer on the metabolic bone diseases and disorders of mineral metabolism, Sixth edition*. Washington, D.C.: American Society for Bone and Mineral Research 190–195.

233. Bereket A, Casur P, Firat P, Yordam Y (2000). Brown tumour as a complication of secondary hyperparathyroidism in severe long-lasting vitamin D deficiency rickets. Eur J Pediatr 159:70–73.

234. Picca S, Cappa M, Rizzoni G (2000). Hyperparathyroidism during growth hormone treatment: A role for puberty? Pediatr Nephrol 14:56–58.

235. Thomas SE, Stapleton FB (2000). Leave no stone unturned: Understanding the genetic bases of calcium-containing stones in children. Adv Pediatr 47:199–221.

236. Guise TA, Mundy GR (1998). Cancer and bone. Endocrine Reviews 19:18–54.

237. Solomon BL, Schaaf M, Smallridge RC (1994). Psychologic symptoms before and after parathyroid surgery. Am J Med 96:101–106.

238. Bornemann M (1998). Management of primary hyperparathyroidism in children. South Med J 91:475–476.

239. Ix JH, Quarles LD, Chertow GM (2006). Guidelines for disorders of mineral metabolism and secondary hyperparathyroidism should not be modified. Nature Clin Pract Nephrol 2:337–339.

240. Saggese G, Bertelloni S, Baroncelli GI, Di Nero G (1993). Ketoconazole decreases the serum ionized calcium and 1,25-dihydroxyvitamin D levels in tuberculosis-associated hypercalcemia. Am J Dis Child 147:270–273.

241. Pettifor JM (2005). Rickets and vitamin D deficiency in children and adolescents. Endocrinol Metab Clin NA 34:537–553.

242. Pettifor JM (2006). Nutritional and drug-induced rickets and osteomalacia. In Favus MJ (ed.), *Primer on the metabolic bone diseases and disorders of mineral metabolism, Sixth edition*. Washington, D.C.: American Society for Bone and Mineral Research 330–338.

243. Wharton B, Bishop N (2003). Rickets. Lancet 362:1389–1400.

244. Kreiter SR, Schwartz RP, Kirkman HN Jr., et al. (2000). Nutritional rickets in African American breast-fed infants. J Pediatr 137:153–157.

245. Joiner TA, Foster C, Shope T (2000). The many faces of vitamin D deficiency rickets. Pediatr in Rev 21:296–302.

246. Schnadower D, Agarwal C, Oberfield SE, et al. (2006). Hypocalcemic seizures and secondary bilateral femoral fractures in an adolescent with primary vitamin D deficiency. Pediatrics 118:2226–2230.

247. Welch TR, Bergstrom WH, Tsang RC (2000). Vitamin D-deficient rickets: The reemergence of a once-conquered disease. J Pediatr 137:143–145.

248. Peng LF, Serwint JR (2003). A comparison of breastfed children with nutritional rickets who present during and after the first year of life. Clin Pediatr 42:711–717.

249. Gordon CM, DePeter KC, Feldman HA, et al. (2004). Prevalence of vitamin D deficiency among healthy adolescents. Arch Pediatr Adolesc Med 158:531–537.

250. Das G, Crocombe S, McGrath M, et al. (2006). Hypovitaminosis D among healthy adolescent girls attending an inner school. Arch Dis Child 91:569–572.

251. Kalkwarf HJ, Khoury JC, Lanphear BP (2003). Milk intake during childhood and adolescence, adult bone density, and osteoporotic fractures in U.S. women. Am J Clin Nutr 77:257–265.

252. Hollis BW (2005). Circulating 25-hydroxyvitamin D levels indicative of vitamin D insufficiency: Implications for establishing a new effective dietary intake recommendation for vitamin D. J Nutr 135:317–322.

253. Hollis B (2004). The determination of circulating 25-hydroxyvitamin D: No easy task. J Clin Endocrinol Metab 89:3149–3151.

254. DeLucia MC, Mitnick ME, Carpenter TO (2003). Nutritional rickets with normal circulating 25-hydroxyvitamin D: A call for reexamining the role of dietary calcium intake in North American infants. J Clin Endocrinol Metab 88:3539–3545.

255. Baroncelli GI, Bertelloni S, Ceccarelli C, et al. (2000). Bone turnover in children with vitamin D deficiency rickets before and during treatment. Acta Paediatr 89:513–518.

256. Misra M, Pacaud D, Petryk A, et al. (2007). Nutritional rickets and its management: Review of current knowledge and recommendations. Lawson Wilkins Pediatric Endocrine Society, personal communication to members.

257. Tangpricha V (2007). Vitamin D deficiency in the southern United States. South Med J 100:384–385.

258. Thacher TD, Ighogboja SI, Fischer PR (1997). Rickets without vitamin D deficiency in Nigerian children. Ambulatory Child Health 3:56–64.

259. Casella SJ, Reiner BJ, Chen TC, et al. (1994). A possible genetic defect in 25-hydroxylation as a cause of rickets. J Pediatr 124:929–932.

260. Cheng JB, Levine MA, Bell NH, et al. (2004). Genetic evidence that human CYPR1 enzyme is a key vitamin D 25-hydroxylase. Proc Natl Acad Sci USA 101:7711–7715.

261. Demay MB (2006). Rickets caused by impaired vitamin D activation and hormone resistance: Pseudovitamin D deficiency rickets and hereditary vitamin D-resistant rickets. In Favus MJ (ed.), *Primer on the metabolic bone diseases and disorders of mineral metabolism, Sixth edition*. Washington, D.C.: American Society for Bone and Mineral Research 338–341.

262. Miller WL, Portale AA (1999). Genetic disorders of vitamin D biosynthesis. Endocrinol Metab Clin NA 28:825–840.

263. Malloy PJ, Pike JW, Feldman D (1999). The vitamin D receptor and the syndrome of hereditary 1,25-dihydroxyvitamin D-resistant rickets. Endocrine Reviews 20:156–188.

264. Skorija K, Cox M, Sisk JM, et al. (2005). Ligand-independent actions of the vitamin D receptor maintain hair follicle homeostasis. Mol Endocrinol 19:855–862.

265. Nicolaidou P, Tsitsika A, Papadimitriou A, et al. (2007). Hereditary vitamin D-resistant rickets in Greek children: Genotype, phenotype, and long-term response to treatment. J Pediatr Endocrinol Metab 20:425–430.

266. Li YC, Pirro AE, Amling M, et al. (1997). Targeted ablation of the vitamin D receptor: An animal model of vitamin D-dependent rickets type II. Proc Natl Acad Sci USA 94:9831–9835.

267. Amling M, Priemel M, Holzmann T, et al. (1999). Rescue of the skeletal phenotype of vitamin D receptor-ablated mice in the setting of normal mineral ion homeostasis: Formal histomorphometric and biomechanical analyses. Endocrinology 140:4982–4987.

268. Hewison M, Rut AR, Kristjansson K, et al. (1993). Tissue resistance to 1,25-dihydroxyvitamin D without a mutation of the vitamin D receptor gene. Clin Endocrinol 39:663–670.

269. Chen H, Hewison M, Hu B, Adams JS (2003). Heterogeneous nuclear ribonucleoprotein (hnRNP) binding to hormone response elements: A cause of vitamin D resistance. Proc Natl Acad Sci USA 100:6109–6114.

270. Carpenter TO (1997). New perspectives on the biology and treatment of X-linked hypophosphatemic rickets. Pediatr Clin NA 44:443–446.

271. Sabbagh Y, Carpenter TO, Demay M (2005). Hypophosphatemia leads to rickets by impairing caspase-mediated apoptosis of hypertrophic chondrocytes. Proc Natl Acad Sci USA 102:9637–9642.

272. Alon US (2006). Hypophosphatemic vitamin D-resistant rickets. In Favus MJ (ed.), *Primer on the metabolic bone diseases and disorders of mineral metabolism, Sixth edition*. Washington, D.C.: American Society for Bone and Mineral Research 342–345.

273. Ecarot B, Desbarats M (1999). 1,25-$(OH)_2D_3$ down-regulates expression of *PHEX*, a marker of the mature osteoblast. Endocrinology 140:1192–1199.

274. Filisetti D, Ostermann G, von Bredow M, et al. (1999). Non-random distribution of mutations in the PHEX gene, and under-detected missense mutations at non-conserved residues. Eur J Hum Genet 7:615–619.

275. Sato K, Tajima T, Nakae J, et al. (2000). Three novel PHEX gene mutations in Japanese patients with X-linked hypophosphatemic rickets. Pediatr Res 48:536–540.

276. Sabbagh Y, Boileau G, Campos M, et al. (2003). Structure and function of disease-causing missense mutations in the PHEX gene. J Clin Endocrinol Metab 88:2213–2222.

277. Cho HY, Lee BH, Kang JH, et al. (2005). A clinical and molecular genetic study of hypophosphatemic rickets in children. Pediatr Res 58:329–333.

278. Holm IA, Nelson AE, Robinson BG, et al. (2001). Mutational analysis and genotype-phenotype correlation of the PHEX gene in X-linked hypophosphatemic rickets. J Clin Endocrinol Metab 86:3889–3899.

279. Yamazaki Y, Okazaki R, Shibata M, et al. (2002). Increased circulatory level of biologically active full-length FGF-23 in patients with hypophosphatemic rickets/osteomalacia. J Clin Endocrinol Metab 87:4957–4960.

280. White KE, Larsson TE, Econs MJ (2006). The roles of specific genes implicated as circulating factors in normal and disordered phosphate homeostasis: Frizzled related protein-4, matrix extracellular phosphoglycoprotein, and fibroblast growth factor 23. Endocrine Reviews 27:221–241.

281. Benet-Pages A, Lorenz-Depiereux B, Zischka H, et al. (2004). FGF23 is processed by proprotein convertases but not by PHEX. Bone 35:455–462.

282. Liu S, Guo R, Simpson LG, et al. (2003). Regulation of fibroblast growth factor-23 expression but not degradation by PHEX. J Biol Chem 278:37419–37426.

283. Burnett SAM, Gunawardene SC, Bringhurst FR, et al. (2006). Regulation of C-terminal and intact FGF-23 by dietary phosphate in men and women. J Bone Miner Res 21:1187–1196.

284. Liu S, Brown TA, Zhou A, et al. (2005). Role of matrix extracellular phosphoglycoprotein in the pathogenesis of X-linked hypophosphatemia. J Am Soc Nephrol 16:1645–1653.

285. Goji K, Ozaki K, Sadewa AH, et al. (2006). Somatic and germline mosaicism for a mutation of the *PHEX gene* can lead to genetic transmission of X-linked hypophosphatemic rickets that mimics an autosomal dominant trait. J Clin Endocrinol Metab 91:365–370.

286. Novais E, Stevens PM (2006). Hypophosphatemic rickets: The role of hemiepiphysiodesis. J Pediatr Orthop 26:238–244.

287. Steendijk R, Hauspie RC (1992). The pattern of growth and growth retardation of patients with hypophosphatemic vitamin D-resistant rickets: A longitudinal study. Eur J Pediatr 151:422–427.

288. Verge CF, Lam A, Simpson JM, et al. (1991). Effects of therapy in X-linked hypophosphatemic rickets. N Engl J Med 325:1843–1848.

289. Makitie O, Doria A, Kooh SW, et al. (2003). Early treatment improves growth and biochemical and radiographic outcome in X-linked hypophosphatemic rickets. J Clin Endocrinol Metab 88:3591–3597.

290. Wilson DM (2000). Growth hormone and hypophosphatemic rickets. J Pediatr Endocrinol Metab 13:993–998.

291. Baroncelli GI, Bertelloni S, Ceccarelli C, Saggese G (2001). Effect of growth hormone treatment on final height, phosphate metabolism, and bone mineral density in children with X-linked hypophosphatemic rickets. J Pediatr 138:236–243.

292. Haffner D, Nissel R, Wuhl E, Mehls O (2004). Effects of growth hormone treatment on body proportions and final height among small children with X-linked hypophosphatemic rickets. Pediatrics 113:e593–e596.

293. Baroncelli GI, Bertelloni S, Dati E, Cavallo L (2007). Linear growth during growth hormone treatment in X-linked hypophosphatemic rickets: Report of two patients. J Pediatr Endocrinol Metab 20:351–356.

294. Reid IR, Hardy DC, Murphy WA, et al. (1989). X-linked hypophosphatemia: A clinical, biochemical, and histopathologic assessment of morbidity in adults. Medicine 68:336–352.

295. Reid IR, Murphy WA, Hardy DC, et al. (1991). X-linked hypophosphatemia: Skeletal mass in adults assessed by histomorphometry, computed tomography, and absorptiometry. Am J Med 90:63–69.

296. Sullivan W, Carpenter T, Glorieux F, et al. (1992). A prospective trial of phosphate and 1,25-dihydroxyvitamin D3 therapy in symptomatic

adults with X-linked hypophosphatemic rickets. J Clin Endocrinol Metab 75:879–885.

297. Takeda E, Yamamoto H, Nashiki K, et al. (2004). Inorganic phosphate homeostasis and the role of dietary phosphorus. J Cell Mol Med 8:191–200.

298. Econs MJ, McEnery PT (1997). Autosomal dominant hypophosphatemic rickets/osteomalacia: Clinical characterization of a novel renal phosphate-wasting disorder. J Clin Endocrinol Metab 82:674–681.

299. Jan de Beur SM, Levine MA (2002). Molecular pathogenesis of hypophosphatemic rickets. J Clin Endocrinol Metab 87:2467–2473.

300. Zeger MD, Adkins D, Fordham LA, et al. (2007). Hypophosphatemic rickets in opsismodysplasia. J Pediatr Endocrinol Metab 20:79–86.

301. Carpenter TO, Ellis BK, Insogna KL, et al. (2005). Fibroblast growth factor 7: An inhibitor of phosphate transport derived from oncogenic osteomalacia-causing tumors. J Clin Endocrinol Metab 90:1012–1020.

302. Imel EA, Peacock M, Pitukcheewanont P, et al. (2006). Sensitivity of fibroblast growth factor 23 measurements in tumor-induced osteomalacia. J Clin Endocrinol Metab 91:2055–2061.

303. Ward LM, Rauch F, White KE, et al. (2004). Resolution of severe, adolescent-onset hypophosphatemic rickets following removal of an FGF-23-producing tumour of the distal ulna. Bone 34:905–911.

304. Shulman DI, Hahn G, Benator R, et al. (2004). Tumor-induced rickets: Usefulness of MR gradient echo recall imaging for tumor localization. J Pediatr 144:381–385.

305. Feng JQ, Ward LM, Liu S, et al. (2006). Loss of DMP1 causes rickets and osteomalacia and identifies a role for osteocytes in mineral metabolism. Nature Genet 38:1310–1315.

306. Lorenz-Depiereux B, Bastepe M, Benet-Pages A, et al. (2006). DMP1 mutations in autosomal recessive hypophosphatemia implicate a bone matrix protein in the regulation of phosphate homeostasis. Nature Genet 38:1248–1250.

307. Zaidi M (2007). Skeletal remodeling in health and disease. Nature Med 13:791–801.

308. Ling Y, Ross HF, Myers ER, et al. (2005). DMP1 depletion decreases bone mineralization in vivo: An FTIR imaging analysis. J Bone Miner Res 20:2169–2177.

309. Bergwitz C, Roslin NM, Tieder M, et al. (2006). SLC4A3 mutations in patients with hereditary hypophosphatemic rickets with hypercalciuria predict a key role for the sodium-phosphate cotransporter NaP(1)-IIc in maintaining phosphate homeostasis. Am J Hum Genet 78:179–192.

310. Ichikawa S, Sorenson AH, Imel EA, et al. (2006). Intronic deletions in the *SLC34A3* gene cause hereditary hypophosphatemic rickets with hypercalciuria. J Clin Endocrinol Metab 91:4022–4027.

311. Scheinman SJ, Guay-Woodford LM, Thakker RV, Warnock DG (1999). Genetic disorders of renal electrolyte transport. N Engl J Med 340:1177–1187.

312. Tebben PJ, Thomas LF, Kumar R (2006). Fanconi syndrome and renal tubular acidosis. In Favus MJ (ed.), *Primer on the metabolic bone diseases and disorders of mineral metabolism, Sixth edition.* Washington, D.C.: American Society for Bone and Mineral Research 354–358.

313. Ward LM (2005). Renal phosphate-wasting disorders in childhood. Pediatr Endocrinol Rev 2:342–350.

314. Oudet C, Martin-Coignard D, Pannetier S, et al. (1997). A second family with XLRH displays the mutation S244L in the CLCN5 gene. Hum Genet 99:781–784.

315. Zuruta L, Muller F, Gibrat JF, et al. (1999). Correlations of genotype and phenotype in hypophosphatasia. Hum Molec Genet 8:1039–1046.

316. Lia-Baldini AS, Muller F, Taillandier A, et al. (2001). A molecular approach to dominance in hypophosphatasia. Hum Genet 109:99–108.

317. Fedde KN, Blair L, Silverstein J, et al. (1999). Alkaline phosphatase knock-out mice recapitulate the metabolic and skeletal defects of infantile hypophosphatasia. J Bone Miner Res 14:2015–2026.

318. Barcia JP, Strife F, Langman CB (1997). Infantile hypophosphatasia: Treatment options to control hypercalcemia, hypercalciuria, and chronic bone demineralization. J Pediatr 130:825–828.

318a. Whyte MP, Mumm S, Deal C (2007). Adult hypophosphatasia treated with teriparatide. J Clin Endocrinol Metab 92:1203–1208.

319. Stein P, Rosalki SB, Foo AY, Hjelm M (1987). Transient hyperphosphatasemia of infancy and early childhood: Clinical and biochemical features of 21 cases and literature review. Clin Chem 33:313–318.

320. Rosalki SB, Foo AY, Dooley JS (1993). Benign familial hyperphosphatasemia as a cause of unexplained increase in plasma alkaline phosphatase activity. J Clin Pathol 46:738–741.

321. Chong B, Hegde M, Fawkner M, et al. (2003). Idiopathic hyperphosphatasia and TNFRSF11B mutations: Relationships between phenotype and genotype. J Bone Miner Res 18:2095–2104.

322. Middleton-Hardie C, Zhu Q, Cundy H, et al. (2006). Deletion of aspartate 182 in OPG causes juvenile Paget's disease by impairing both protein secretion and binding to RANKL. J Bone Miner Res 21:438–445.

323. Whyte MP, Obrecht SE, Finnegan PM, et al. (2002). Osteoprotegerin deficiency and juvenile Paget's disease. N Engl J Med 347:175–184.

324. Cundy T, Davidson J, Rutland M.D., et al. (2005). Recombinant osteoprotegerin for juvenile Paget's disease. N Engl J Med 353:918–923.

325. Hughes AE, Ralston SH, Marken J, et al. (2000). Mutations in TNFRSF11A, affecting the signal peptide of RANK, cause familial expansile osteolysis. Nature Genet 24:45–48.

326. Martin KJ, Al-Aly Z, Gonzalez EA (2006). Renal osteodystrophy. In Favus MJ (ed.), *Primer on the metabolic bone diseases and disorders of mineral metabolism, Sixth edition*. Washington, D.C.: American Society for Bone and Mineral Research 359–366.

327. Rauch F (2006). Watching bones at work: what we can see from bone biopsies. Pediatr Nephrol 21:457–462.

328. Koch Nogueira PC, David L, Cochat P (2000). Evolution of secondary hyperparathyroidism after renal transplantation. Pediatr Nephrol 14:342–346.

329. Sanchez CP, Salusky IB, Kuizon BD, et al. (1998). Bone disease in children undergoing successful renal transplantation. Kidney Int 53:1358–1364.

330. Reusz GS, Szabo AJ, Peter F, et al. (2000). Bone metabolism and mineral density following renal transplantation. Arch Dis Child 83:146–151.

331. Nieto J, Ruiz-Cuervas P, Escuder A, et al. (1997). Tertiary hyperparathyroidism after renal transplantation. Pediatr Nephrol 11:65–68.

332. Bachrach LK (2005). Osteoporosis and measurement of bone mass in children and adolescents. Endocrinol Metab NA 34:521–535.

333. Harvey N, Earl S, Cooper C (2006). Epidemiology of osteoporotic fractures. In Favus MJ (ed.), *Primer on the metabolic bone diseases and disorders of mineral metabolism, Sixth edition*. Washington, D.C.: American Society for Bone and Mineral Research 244–248.

334. Kalkwarf HJ, Zemel BS, Gilsanz V, et al. (2007). The bone mineral density in childhood study: Bone mineral content and density according to age, sex, and race. J Clin Endocrinol Metab 92:2087–2099.

335. Ward KM, Ashby RL, Roberts SA, et al. (2007). UK reference data for the Hologic QDR Discovery dual-energy X-ray absorptiometry scanner in healthy children and young adults aged 6-17 years. Arch Dis Child 92:53–59.

336. Writing Group for ISCD Position Development Conference (2004). Diagnosis of osteoporosis in men, premenopausal women, and children. J Clin Densitom 7:17–26.

337. Zemel BS, Leonard MB, Kalkwarf HJ, et al. (2004). Reference data for whole body, lumbar spine and proximal femur for American children relative to age, gender and body size. J Bone Miner Res 19:(1):S231.

338. Leonard MB, Shults J, Elliott DM, et al. (2004). Interpretation of whole body dual energy X-ray absorptiometry measures in children: Comparison with peripheral quantitative computed tomography. Bone 34:1044–1052.

339. Taylor A. Konrad PT, Norman ME, et al. (1997). Total body bone mineral measurements in young children: Influence of head bone mineral density. J Bone Miner Res 12:652–655.

340. Jones IE, Taylor RW, Williams SM, et al. (2002). Four-year gain in bone mineral in girls with and without past forearm fractures: A DEXA study. J Bone Miner Res 17:1065–1072.

341. Bachrach LK (2000). Making an impact on pediatric bone health. J Pediatr 136:137–139.

342. Golden NH (2000). Osteoporosis prevention: A pediatric challenge. Arch Pediatr Adolesc Med 154:542–543.

343. Ruiz JC, Mandel C, Garabedian M (1995). Influence of spontaneous calcium intake and physical exercise on the vertebral and femoral bone mineral density of children and adolescents. J Bone Miner Res 10:675–682.

344. Wyshak G (2000). Teenaged girls, carbonated beverage consumption, and bone fractures. Arch Pediatr Adolesc Med 154:610–613.

345. Tucker KL, Morita K, Qiao N, et al. (2006). Colas, but not other carbonated beverages, are associated with low bone mineral density in older women: The Framingham Osteoporosis Study. Am J Clin Nutr 84:936–942.

346. Janz KF, Burns TL, Torner JC, et al. (2001). Physical activity and bone measures in young children: The Iowa bone development study. Pediatrics 107:1387–1393.

347. Weiler HA, Janzen L, Green K, et al. (2000). Percent body fat and bone mass in healthy Canadian females 10 to 19 years of age. Bone 27:203–207.

348. Janicka A, Wren TAL, Sanchez MM, et al. (2007). Fat mass is not beneficial to bone in adolescents and young adults. J Clin Endocrinol Metab 92:143–147.

349. McKay HA, Petit MA, Schutz RW, et al. (2000). Augmented trochanteric bone mineral density after modified physical education classes: A randomized school-based exercise intervention study in prepubescent and early pubescent children. J Pediatr 136:156–162.

350. Petit MA, McKay HA, MacKelvie KJ, et al. (2002). A randomized school-based jumping intervention confers site and maturity-specific benefits on bone structural properties in girls: A hip structural analysis study. J Bone Miner Res 17:363–372.

351. Specker B, Binkley T (2003). Randomized trial of physical activity and calcium supplementation on bone mineral content in 3- to 5-year old children. J Bone Miner Res 18:885–892.

352. Lorentzon M, Mellstrom D, Haug E, Ohlsson C (2007). Smoking is associated with lower bone mineral density and reduced cortical thickness in young men. J Clin Endocrinol Metab 92:497–503.

353. Weaver CM, Peacock M, Johnston CC Jr. (1999). Adolescent nutrition in the prevention of postmenopausal osteoporosis. J Clin Endocrinol Metab 84:1839–1843.

354. Winzenberg TM, Shaw K, Fryer J, Jones G (2006). Calcium supplementation for improving bone mineral density in children. Cochrane Database of Systematic Reviews 2:CD005119.

355. Loro LM, Sayre J, Roe TF, et al. (2000). Early identification of children predisposed to low peak bone mass and osteoporosis later in life. J Clin Endocrinol Metab 85:3908–3918.

356. Soyka LA, Grinspoon S, Levitsky LL, et al. (1999). The effects of anorexia nervosa on bone metabolism in female adolescents. J Clin Endocrinol Metab 84:4489–4496.

357. Stone M, Briody J, Kohn MR, et al. (2006). Bone changes in adolescent girls with anorexia nervosa. J Adolesc Hlth 39:835–841.

358. Misra M, Soyka LA, Miller KK, et al. (2003). Serum osteoprotegerin in adolescent girls with anorexia nervosa. J Clin Endocrinol Metab 88:3816–3822.

359. DiVasta AD, Gordon CM (2006). Bone health in adolescents. Adolesc Med 17:639–652.

360. Gordon NH, Lanzkowsky L, Schebendach J, et al. (2002). The effect of estrogen-progestin treatment on bone mineral density in anorexia nervosa. J Pediatr Adolesc Gynecol 15:135–143.

361. Bourrin S, Ammann P, Bonjour JP, Rizzoli R (2000). Dietary protein restriction lowers plasma insulin-like growth factor I (IGF-I), impairs cortical bone formation, and induces osteoblastic resistance to IGF-I in adult female rats. Endocrinology 141:3149–3155.

362. Zacharin M (2004). Current advances in bone health of disabled children. Curr Opin Pediatr 16:545–551.

363. Henderson RC, Lark RK, Grka MJ, et al. (2002). Bone density and metabolism in children and adolescents with moderate to severe cerebral palsy. Pediatrics 110:e5.

364. Henderson JK, Kairalla JA, Barrington JW, et al. (2005). Longitudinal changes in bone density in children and adolescents with moderate to severe cerebral palsy. J Pediatr 146:769–775.

365. King W, Levin R, Schmidt R, et al. (2003). Prevalence of reduced bone mass in children and adults with spastic quadriplegia. Dev Med Child Neurol 45:12–16.

366. Henderson RC, Lark RK, Kecskemethy HH, et al. (2002). Bisphosphonates to treat osteopenia in children with quadriplegic cerebral palsy: A randomized, placebo-controlled clinical trial. J Pediatr 141:644–651.

367. Ali O, Shim M, Fowler E, et al. (2007). Growth hormone therapy improves bone mineral density in children with cerebral palsy: A preliminary pilot study. J Clin Endocrinol Metab 92:932–937.

368. Caulton JM, Ward KA, Alsop CW, et al. (2004). A randomised controlled trial of standing programme on bone mineral density in non-ambulant children with cerebral palsy. Arch Dis Child 89:131–135.

369. Chad KE, Bailey DA, McKay HA, et al. (1999). The effect of a weight-bearing physical activity program on bone mineral content and estimated volumetric density in children with spastic cerebral palsy. J Pediatr 135:115–117.

370. Finkelstein JS, Klibanski A, Neer RM (1996). A longitudinal evaluation of bone mineral density in adult men with histories of delayed adolescence. J Clin Endocrinol Metab 81:1152–1155.

371. Bertelloni S, Baroncelli GI, Ferdeghini M, et al. (1998). Normal volumetric bone mineral density and bone turnover in young men with histories of constitutional delay of puberty. J Clin Endocrinol Metab 83:4280–4283.

372. Finkelstein JS, Klibanski A, Neer RM (1999). Evaluation of lumbar spine bone mineral density (BMD) using dual energy X-ray absorptiometry (DEXA) in 21 young men with histories of constitutionally-delayed puberty. J Clin Endocrinol Metab 84:3403–3404.

373. Moreira-Andres MN, Canizo FJ, de la Cruz FJ, et al. (1998). Bone mineral status in prepubertal children with constitutional delay of growth and puberty. Eur J Endocrinol 139:271–275.

374. Moreira-Andres MN, Canizo FJ, de la Cruz FJ, et al. (2000). Evaluation of bone mineral content in prepubertal children with constitutional delay of growth. J Pediatr Endocrinol Metab 13:591–597.

375. Reid IR (2006). Menopause. In Favus MJ (ed.), *Primer on the metabolic bone diseases and disorders of mineral metabolism, Sixth edition.* Washington, D.C.: American Society for Bone and Mineral Research 68–70.

376. Manolagas SC (2000). Birth and death of bone cells: Basic regulatory mechanisms and implications for the pathogenesis and treatment of osteoporosis. Endocrine Reviews 21:115–137.

377. Couse JF, Korach KS (1999). Estrogen receptor null mice: What have we learned and where will they lead us? Endocrine Reviews 20:358–417.

378. Rubin K (1998). Turner syndrome and osteoporosis: Mechanisms and prognosis. Pediatrics 102:481–485.

379. Beckett PR, Copeland KC, Flannery TK, et al. (1999). Combination growth hormone and estrogen increase bone mineralization in girls with Turner syndrome. Pediatr Res 45:709–713.

380. Sas TC, De Muinck Keizer-Schrama SM, Stijnen T, et al. (2000). A longitudinal study on bone mineral density until adulthood in girls with Turner's syndrome participating in a growth hormone injection frequency-response trial. Clin Endocrinol 52:531–536.

381. Bakalov VK, Axelrod L, Baron J, et al. (2003). Selective reduction in cortical bone mineral density in Turner syndrome independent of ovarian hormone deficiency. J Clin Endocrinol Metab 88:5717–5722.

382. Antoniazzi F, Bertoldo F, Lauriola S, et al. (1999). Prevention of bone demineralization by calcium supplementation in precocious puberty during gonadotropin releasing hormone agonist treatment. J Clin Endocrinol Metab 84:1992–1996.

383. Van Staa TP (2006). The pathogenesis, epidemiology and management of glucocorticoid-induced osteoporosis. Calcif Tissue Int 79:129–137.

384. Sambrook PN (2006). Glucocorticoid-induced osteoporosis. In Favus MJ (ed.), *Primer on the metabolic bone diseases and disorders of mineral metabolism, Sixth edition.* Washington, D.C.: American Society for Bone and Mineral Research 296–302.

385. Tsuji K, Bandyopadhyay A, Harfe BD, et al. (2006). BMP2 activity, although dispensable for bone formation, is required for initiation of fracture healing. Nature Genet 38:1424–1428.

386. Allen DB (2006). Effects of inhaled steroids on growth, bone metabolism, and adrenal function. Adv Pediatr 53:101–110.

387. Wong CA, Walsh LJ, Smith CJP, et al. (2000). Inhaled corticosteroid use and bone mineral density in patients with asthma. Lancet 355:1399–1403.

388. King JA, Wisniewski AB, Bankowski BJ, et al. (2006). Long-term corticosteroid replacement and bone mineral density in adult women with classical congenital adrenal hyperplasia. J Clin Endocrinol Metab 91:865–869.

389. Noguera A, Ros JB, Pavia C, et al. (2003). Bisphosphonates, a new treatment for glucocorticoid-induced osteoporosis in children. J Pediatr Endocrinol Metab 16:529–536.

390. Hodsman AB, Bauer DC, Dempster DW, et al. (2005). Parathyroid hormone and teriparatide for the treatment of osteoporosis: A review of the evidence and suggested guidelines for its use. Endocrine Reviews 26:688–703.

391. Ohlsson C, Bengtsson B-A, Isaksson OG, et al. (1998). Growth hormone and bone. Endocrine Reviews 19:55–79.

392. Maheshwari HG, Bouillon R, Nijs J, et al. (2003). The impact of congenital, severe, untreated growth hormone (GH) deficiency on bone size and density in young adults: Insights from genetic GH-releasing hormone receptor deficiency. J Clin Endocrinol Metab 88:2614–2618.

393. Lanes R, Gunczler P, Weisinger JR (1999). Decreased trabecular bone mineral density in children with idiopathic short stature: Normalization of bone density and increased bone turnover after 1 year of growth hormone treatment. J Pediatr 135:177–181.

394. Robson H, Siebler T, Shalet SM, Williams GR (2003). Interactions between GH, IGF-I, glucocorticoids, and thyroid hormones during skeletal growth. Pediatr Res 52:137–147.

395. Lucidarme N, Ruiz JC, Czernichow P, Leger J (2000). Reduced bone mineral density at diagnosis and bone mineral recovery during treatment in children with Graves disease. J Pediatr 137:56–62.

396. Tumer L, Hasanoglu A, Cinaz P, Bideci A (1999). Bone mineral density and metabolism in children treated with L-thyroxine. J Pediatr Endocrinol Metab 12:519–523.

397. Heap J, Murray MA, Miller MC, et al. (2004). Alterations in bone characteristics associated with glycemic control in type 1 diabetes mellitus adolescents. J Pediatr 144:56–62.

398. Moyer Mileur LJ, Dixon SB, Quick JL, et al. (2004). Bone mineral acquisition in adolescents with type 1 diabetes. J Pediatr 145:662–669.

399. Bechtold S, Dirlenbach I, Raile K, et al. (2006). Early manifestation of type 1 diabetes in children is a risk factor for changed bone geometry: Data using peripheral quantitative computed tomography. Pediatrics 118:627–634.

400. Atkinson SA, Halton JM, Bradley C, et al. (1998). Bone and mineral abnormalities in childhood acute lymphoblastic leukemia: Influence of disease, drugs and nutrition. Int J Cancer Suppl 11:35–39.

401. Hofbauer LC, Heufelder AE (2000). The role of receptor activator of Nuclear Factor-κB ligand and osteoprotegerin in the pathogenesis and treatment of metabolic bone diseases. J Clin Endocrinol Metab 85:2355–2363.

402. Hoorweg-Nijman JJG, Kardos G, Roos JC, et al. (1999). Bone mineral density and markers of bone turnover in young adult survivors of childhood lymphoblastic leukaemia. Clin Endocrinol 50:237–244.

403. Cohen A, Ebling P, Sprague S, Shane E (2006). Transplantation osteoporosis. In Favus MJ (ed.), *Primer on the metabolic bone diseases and disorders of mineral metabolism, Sixth edition.* Washington, D.C.: American Society for Bone and Mineral Research 302–309.

404. Barnes C, Wong P Egan B, et al. (2004). Reduced bone density among children with severe hemophilia. Pediatrics 114:e177–e181.

405. Buison AM, Kawchak DA, Schall JI, et al. (2005). Bone area and bone mineral content deficits in children with sickle cell disease. Pediatrics 116:943–949.

406. Gronowitz E, Mellstrom D, Strandvik B (2004). Normal annual increase of bone mineral density during two years in patients with cystic fibrosis. Pediatrics 114:435–442.

407. Rovner A, Zemel BS, Leonard MB, et al. (2005). Mild to moderate cystic fibrosis is not associated with increased fracture risk in children and adolescents. J Pediatr 147:327–331.

408. Thearle M, Horlick M, Bilezikian JP, et al. (2000). Osteoporosis: An unusual presentation of childhood Crohn's disease. J Clin Endocrinol Metab 85:2122–2126.

409. Burnham JM, Shults J, Semeao E, et al. (2004). Whole body BMC in pediatric Crohn disease: Independent effects of altered growth, maturation, and body composition. J Bone Miner Res 19:1961–1968.

410. Van Staa TP, Cooper C, Brusse LS, et al. (2003). Inflammatory bowel disease and the risk of fracture. Gastroenterology 125:1591–1597.

411. Cellier C, Flobert C, Cormier C, et al. (2000). Severe osteopenia in symptom-free adults with a childhood diagnosis of coeliac disease. Lancet 355:806.

412. Arpradi S, Horlick M, Shane E (2004). Metabolic bone disease in human immunodeficiency virus-infected children. J Clin Endocrinol Metab 89:21–23.

413. Mora S, Zamproni I, Beccio S, et al. (2004). Longitudinal changes of bone mineral density and metabolism in antiretroviral-treated human immunodeficiency virus-infected children. J Clin Endocrinol Metab 89:24–28.

414. Rouster-Stevens KA, Klein-Gitelman MS (2005). Bone health in pediatric rheumatic disease. Curr Opin Pediatr 17:703–708.

415. Rauch F, Bishop N (2006). Juvenile osteoporosis. In Favus MJ (ed.), *Primer on the metabolic bone diseases and disorders of mineral metabolism, Sixth edition*. Washington, D.C.: American Society for Bone and Mineral Research 293–296.

416. Hartikka H, Makitie O, Mannikko M, et al. (2005). Heterozygous mutations in the LDL receptor-related protein 5 (LRP5) gene are associated with primary osteoporosis in children. J Bone Miner Res 20:783–789.

417. Shaw NJ, Boivin CM, Crabtree NJ (2000). Intravenous pamidronate in juvenile osteoporosis. Arch Dis Child 83:143–145.

418. Ai M, Heeger S, Barteks CF, et al. (2005). Clinical and molecular findings in osteoporosis-pseudoglioma syndrome. Am J Hum Genet 77:741–753.

419. Balesman W, Van Hul W (2007). The genetics of low density Lipoprotein Receptor-Related Protein 5 in bone: A story of extremes. Endocrinology 148:2622–2629.

420. Glass DA II, Karsenty G (2007). In vivo analysis of Wnt signaling in bone. Endocrinology 148:2630–2634.

421. Baron R, Rawadi G (2007). Targeting the Wnt/β-catenin pathway to regulate bone formation in the adult skeleton. Endocrinology 148:2635–2643.

422. McDonnell DP (1999). The molecular pharmacology of SERMs. Trends Endocrinol Metab 10:301–311.

423. Shaw NJ, Bishop NJ (2005). Bisphosphonate treatment of bone disease. Arch Dis Child 90:494–499.

424. Speiser PW, Clarkson CL, Eugster EA, et al. (2005). Bisphosphonate treatment of pediatric bone disease. Pediatr Endocrinol Rev 3:87–96.

425. Rogers MJ (2006). From molds and macrophages to mevalonate: A decade of progress in understanding the molecular mode of action of bisphosphonates. Calcif Tissue Int 75:451–461.

426. Whyte MP, Wenkert D, Clements KL, et al. (2003). Bisphosphonate-induced osteopetrosis. N Engl J Med 349:457–463.

427. Odvina CY, Zerwekh JE, Sudhaker R, et al. (2005). Severely suppressed bone turnover: A potential complication of alendronate therapy. J Clin Endocrinol Metab 90:1294–1301.

428. Chan B, Zacharin M (2006). Maternal and infant outcome after pamidronate treatment of polyostotic fibrous dysplasia and osteogenesis imperfecta before conception: A report of four cases. J Clin Endocrinol Metab 91:2107–2020.

429. Bellido T, Ali AA, Gubrij I, et al. (2005). Chronic elevation of parathyroid hormone in mice reduces expression of sclerostin by osteocytes: A novel mechanism for hormonal control of osteoblastogenesis. Endocrinology 146:4577–4583.

430. Horwitz MJ, Tedesco MB, Grundberg C, et al. (2003). Short-term, high-dose parathyroid hormone-related protein as a skeletal anabolic agent for treatment of postmenopausal osteoporosis. J Clin Endocrinol Metab 88:569–572.

431. Horwitz MJ, Tedesco MB, Sereika SM, et al. (2006). Safety and tolerability of subcutaneous PTHrP(1-36) in healthy human volunteers: A dose escalation study. Osteoporosis Int 17:225–230.

432. McClung MR, Lewiecki EM, Cohen SB, et al. (2006). Denosumab in postmenopausal women with low bone mineral density. N Engl J Med 354:821–831.

433. Sambrook P, Cooper C (2006). Osteoporosis. Lancet 367:2010–2018.

434. Cabral WA, Chang W, Barnes AM, et al. (2007). Prolyl 3-hydroxylase 1 deficiency causes a recessive metabolic bone disorder resembling lethal/severe osteogenesis imperfecta. Nature Genet 39:359–365.

435. Byers PH (1995). Disorders of collagen biosynthesis and structure. In Scriver CR, Beaudet AL, Sly WS, Vale D (eds.), *The metabolic and molecular bases of inherited disease, Seventh edition*. New York: McGraw-Hill 4029–4077.

436. Cabral WA, Makareeva E, Colige A, et al. (2005). Mutations near amino end of alpha-1(I) collagen cause combined osteogenesis imperfecta/Ehlers-Danlos syndrome by interfering with N-propeptide processing. J Biol Chem 280:19259–19269.

437. Marakeeva E, Cabral WA, Marini JC, Leikin S (2006). Molecular mechanism of alpha-1(I)-osteogenesis imperfecta/Ehlers-Danlos syndrome: Unfolding of an N-anchor domain at the N-terminal end of the type I collagen triple helix. J Biol Chem 281:6463–6470.

438. Morello R, Bertin TK, Chen Y, et al. (2006). CRTAP is required for prolyl 3-hydroxylation and mutations cause recessive osteogenesis imperfecta. Cell 127:291–304.

439. Barnes AM, Chang W, Morello R, et al. (2006). Deficiency of cartilage-associated protein in lethal osteogenesis imperfecta. N Engl J Med 355:2757–2764.

440. Pepin M, Atkinson M, Starman BJ, Byers PH (1997). Strategies and outcomes of prenatal diagnosis for osteogenesis imperfecta: A review of biochemical and molecular studies completed in 129 pregnancies. Prenatal Diag 17:559–570.

441. Plotkin H (2007). Growth in osteogenesis imperfecta. Growth Genet Horm 23:17–23.

442. DiMeglio LA, Ford L, McClintock C, Peacock M (2004). Intravenous pamidronate treatment of children under 36 months of age with osteogenesis imperfecta. Bone 35:1038–1045.

443. Land C, Rauch F, Munns CF, et al. (2006). Vertebral morphometry in children and adolescents with osteogenesis imperfecta: Effect of intravenous pamidronate treatment. Bone 39:901–906.

444. Letocha AD, Cintas HL, Troendle JF, et al. (2005). Controlled trial of pamidronate in children with types III and IV osteogenesis imperfecta confirms vertebral gains but not short-term functional improvement. J Bone Miner Res 20:977–986.

445. DiMeglio LA, Peacock M (2006). Two-year clinical trial of oral alendronate versus intravenous pamidronate in children with osteogenesis imperfecta. J Bone Miner Res 21:132–140.

446. Rauch F, Travers R, Glorieux FH (2006). Pamidronate in children with osteogenesis imperfecta: Histomorphometric effects of long-term therapy. J Clin Endocrinol Metab 91:511–516.

447. Rauch F, Munns C, Land C, Glorieux FH (2006b). Pamidronate in children and adolescents with osteogenesis imperfecta: Effect of treatment discontinuation. J Clin Endocrinol Metab 91: 1268–1274.

448. Marini JC, Hopkins E, Glorieux FH, et al. (2003). Positive linear growth and bone responses to growth hormone treatment in children with types III and IV osteogenesis imperfecta: High predictive value of the carboxyterminal propeptide of type I procollagen. J Bone Miner Res 18:237–243.

449. Horwitz EM, Prockop DJ, Gordon PL, et al. (2001). Clinical responses to bone marrow transplantation in children with severe osteogenesis imperfecta. Blood 97:1227–1231.

450. Chamberlain JR, Schwarze U, Wang P-R, et al. (2004). Gene targeting the stem cells from individuals with osteogenesis imperfecta. Science 303:1198–1201.

451. Prockop DJ (2004). Targeting gene therapy for osteogenesis imperfecta. N Engl J Med 350:2302–2304.

452. Collins MT, Bianco P (2006). Fibrous dysplasia. In Favus MJ (ed.), *Primer on the metabolic bone diseases and disorders of mineral metabolism, Sixth edition*. Washington, D.C.: American Society for Bone and Mineral Research 415–418.

453. Weinstein LS (2006). $G_s\alpha$ mutations in fibrous dysplasia and McCune-Albright syndrome. J Bone Miner Res 21(2):P120–P124.

454. Yamamoto T, Imanishi Y, Kinoshita E, et al. (2005). The role of fibroblast growth factor 23 for hypophosphatemia and abnormal regulation of vitamin D metabolism in patients with McCune-Albright syndrome. J Bone Miner Res 23:231–237.

455. Collins MT (2006). Spectrum and natural history of fibrous dysplasia of bone. J Bone Miner Res 21(2):P99–P104.

456. Glorieux FH, Rauch F Collins MT (2006). Medical therapy of children with fibrous dysplasia. J Bone Miner Res 21(2):P110–P113.

457. Plotkin H, Rauch F, Zeitlin L, et al. (2003). Effect of pamidronate treatment in children with polyostotic fibrous dysplasia of bone. J Clin Endocrinol Metab 88:4569–4575.

458. Tolar J, Teitelbaum SL, Orchard PJ (2004). Osteopetrosis. N Engl J Med 351:2839–2849.

459. Benichou OD, Laredo JD, De Vernejoul MC (2000). Type II autosomal dominant osteopetrosis (Albers-Schonberg disease): Clinical and radiological manifestations in 42 patients. Bone 26:87–93.

460. Cleiren E, Benichou O, Van Hul E, et al. (2001). Albers Schonberg disease (autosomal dominant osteopetrosis, type II) results from mutations in ClCN7 chloride channel gene. Hum Molec Genet 10:2861–2867.

461. Waguespack SG, Hui SL, DiMeglio LA, Econs MJ (2007). Autosomal dominant osteopetrosis: Clinical severity and natural history of 94 subjects with a chloride channel 7 gene mutation. J Clin Endocrinol Metab 92:771–778.

462. Waguespack SG, Hui SL, White KE, et al. (2002). Measurement of tartrate-resistant acid phosphatase and the brain isoenzyme of creatine kinase accurately diagnoses type II autosomal dominant osteopetrosis but does not identify gene carriers. J Clin Endocrinol Metab 87:2212–2217.

463. Rodan GA, Martin TJ (2000). Therapeutic approaches to bone diseases. Science 289:1508–1514.

464. Doffinger S, Smahi A, Bessia C, et al. (2001). X-linked anhidrotic ectodermal dysplasia with immunodeficiency is caused by impaired NF-κB signaling. Nature Genet 27:277–285.

465. Dupuis-Girod S, Corradinin N, Hadj-Rabia S, et al. (2002). Osteopetrosis, lymphedema, anhidrotic ectodermal dysplasia, and immunodeficiency in a boy and incontinentia pigmenti in his mother. Pediatrics 109:1–6.

466. Sobacchi C, Frattini A, Orchard P, et al. (2001). The mutational spectrum of human malignant autosomal recessive osteopetrosis. Hum Molec Genet 10:1767–1773.

467. Susani L, Pangrazio A, Sobachhi A, et al. (2004). TCIRG1-dependent recessive osteopetrosis: Mutation analysis, functional identification of the splicing defects, and in vitro rescue by U1 snRNA. Hum Mutat 24:225–235.

468. Kornak U, Kasper D, Bosl MR, et al. (2001). Loss of the ClC-7 chloride channel leads to osteopetrosis in mice and man. Cell 104:205–215.

469. Lange PF, Wartosch L, Jentsch TJ, Fuhrmann JC (2006). ClC-7 requires Ostm1 as a β-subunit to support bone resorption and lysosomal function. Nature 440:220–223.

470. Chalhoub N, Benachenhou N, Rajapurohitam V, et al. (2003). Grey-lethal mutation indices severe malignant autosomal recessive osteopetrosis in mouse and human. Nature Med 9:399–406.

471. Ramirez A, Faupel J, Goebel I, et al. (2004). Identification of a novel mutation in the coding region of the grey-lethal gene OSTM1 in human malignant infantile osteopetrosis. Hum Mutat 23:471–476.

472. Key LL Jr., Rodriguez RM, Willi SM, et al. (1995). Recombinant human interferon gamma therapy for osteopetrosis. N Engl J Med 332:1594–1599.

473. Gao Y, Grassi F, Ryan MR, et al. (2007). IFN-γ stimulates osteoclast formation and bone loss in vivo via antigen-driven T cell activation. J Clin Invest 117:122–132.

474. Boyden LM, Mao J, Belsky J, et al. (2002). High bone density due to a mutation in LDL-receptor-related protein 5. N Engl J Med 346:1513–1521.

475. Ott SM (2005). Sclerostin and Wnt signaling: The pathway to bone strength. J Clin Endocrinol Metab 90:6741–6743.

476. Shoback D (2007). Update in osteoporosis and metabolic bone disorders. J Clin Endocrinol Metab 92:747–753.

477. Patel MS, Karsenty G (2002). Regulation of bone formation and vision by LRP5. N Engl J Med 346:1572–1574.

478. Van Wesenbeeck L, Cleiren E, Gram J, et al. (2003). Six novel missense mutations in the LDL receptor-related protein 5 (LRP5) gene in different conditions with increased bone density. Am J Hum Genet 72:763–771.

479. Gardner JC, van Bezooijen RL, Mervis B, et al. (2005). Bone mineral density in sclerosteosis: Affected individuals and gene carriers. J Clin Endocrinol Metab 90:6392–6395.

480. Loots GB, Kneissel M, Keller H, et al. (2005). Genomic deletion of a long-range bone enhancer misregulates sclerostin in Van Buchem disease. Genome Res 15:928–935.

481. Janssens K, Vanhoenacker F, Bonduelle M, et al. (2007). Camurati-Engelmann disease: Review of the clinical, radiological, and molecular data of 24 families and implications for diagnosis and treatment. J Med Genet 43:1–11.

482. Janssens K, ten Dyke P, Janssens S, Van Hul W (2005). Transforming growth factor-beta 1 to the bone. Endocrine Reviews 26:743–774.

483. Whyte MP (2006). Extracellular (ectopic) calcification and ossification. In Favus MJ (ed.), *Primer on the metabolic bone diseases and disorders of mineral metabolism, Sixth edition*. Washington, D.C.: American Society for Bone and Mineral Research 436–437.

484. Benet-Pages A, Orlik P, Strom TM, Lorenz-Depiereux B (2005). An FGF23 missense mutation causes familial tumoral calcinosis with hyperphosphatemia. Hum Molec Genet 14:385–390.

485. Ichikawa S, Imel EA, Sorensen AH, et al. (2006). Tumoral calcinosis presenting with eyelid calcifications due to novel missense mutations in the glycosyltransferase domain of the *GALNT3* gene. J Clin Endocrinol Metab 91:4472–4475.

486. Whyte MP (2006). Tumoral calcinosis. In Favus MJ (ed.), *Primer on the metabolic bone diseases and disorders of mineral metabolism, Sixth edition*. Washington, D.C.: American Society for Bone and Mineral Research 437–439.

487. Araya K, Fukumoto S, Backenroth R, et al. (2005). A novel mutation in fibroblast growth factor 23 gene as a cause of tumoral calcinosis. J Clin Endocrinol Metab 90:5523–5527.

488. Kato K, Jeanneau C, Tarp MA, et al. (2006). Polypeptide GalNAc-transferase T3 and familial tumoral calcinosis: Secretion of fibroblast growth factor 23 requires O-glycosylation. J Biol Chem 281:18370–18377.

489. Frishberg Y, Ito N, Rinat C, et al. (2007). Hyperostosis-hyperphosphatemia syndrome: A congenital disorder of O-glycosylation associated with augmented processing of fibroblast growth factor 23. J Bone Miner Res 22:235–242.

490. Garringer HJ, Fisher C, Larsson TE, et al. (2006). The role of mutant UDP-N-acetyl-alpha-D-galactosamine-polypeptide N-acetylgalactos-aminyltransferase 3 in regulating serum intact fibroblast growth factor 23 and matrix extracellular phosphoglycoprotein in heritable tumoral calcinosis. J Clin Endocrinol Metab 91:4037–4042.

491. Narchi H (1997). Hyperostosis with hyperphosphatemia: Evidence of familial occurrence and association with tumoral calcinosis. Pediatrics 99:745–748.

492. Shore EM, Xu M, Feldman GJ, et al. (2006). A recurrent mutation in the BMP type I receptor ACVR1 causes inherited and sporadic fibrodysplasia ossificans progressiva. Nature Genet 38:525–527.

493. Kaplan FS, Fiori J, Serrano de la Pena L, et al. (2006). Dysregulation of the BMP-4 signaling pathway in fibrodysplasia ossificans progressiva. Ann NY Acad Sci 1068:54–65.

494. Bowers RR, Kim JW, Otto TC, Lane MD (2006). Stable stem cell commitment to the adipocyte lineage by inhibition of DNA methylation: Role of the BMP-4 gene. Proc Natl Acad Sci USA 103:13022–13027.

495. Kaplan FS, Glaser DL, Shore EM, et al. (2007). Hematopoietic stem-cell contribution to ectopic skeletogenesis. J Bone Joint Surg 89:347–357.

496. Chan I, Hamada T, Hardman C, et al. (2004). Progressive osseous heteroplasia resulting from a new mutation in the *GNAS1* gene. Clin Exper Dermatol 29:77–80.

497. Shore EM, Ahn J, Jan de Beur S, et al. (2002). Paternally inherited inactivating mutations of the *GNAS1* gene in progressive osseous heteroplasia. N Engl J Med 346:99–106.

498. Shohat M, Rimoin DL (2007). The skeletal dysplasias. In Lifschitz F (ed.), *Pediatric endocrinology, Fifth edition*. New York: Informa Health Care 145–162.

499. Superti-Furga A, Unger S, and the Nosology Group of the International Skeletal Dysplasia Society (2007). International nosology and classification of genetic skeletal disorders: 2006 revision. Am J Med Genet 143A:1–18 (*www.isds.ch*).

500. Brook CGD, de Vries BBA (1998). Skeletal dysplasias. Arch Dis Child 79:285–289.

501. Horton WA (2006). Molecular pathogenesis of achondroplasia. Growth Genet Horm 22:49–54.

502. Heuertz S, Le Merrer M, Zabel B, et al. (2006). Novel FGFR3 mutations creating cysteine residues in the extracellular domain of the receptor cause achondroplasia or severe forms of hypochondroplasia. Eur J Hum Genet 14:1240–1247.

503. Saito H, Sekizawa A, Morimoto T, et al. (2000). Prenatal DNA diagnosis of a single gene disorder from maternal plasma. Lancet 356:1170–1171.

504. Toydemir RM, Brassington AE, Bayrack-Toydemir P, et al. (2006). A novel mutation in FGFR3 causes camptodactyly, tall stature, and hearing loss (CATSHL) syndrome. Am J Hum Genet 79:935–941.

505. Pitteloud N, Acierno JS Jr., Meysing A, et al. (2006). Mutations in fibroblast growth factor receptor 1 cause both Kallmann syndrome and idiopathic hypogonadotropic hypogonadism. Proc Natl Acad Sci USA 103:6281–6286.

506. Haque MF, King LM, Krakow D, et al. (1998). Mutations in orthologous genes in human spondyloepimetaphyseal dysplasia and the brachymorphic mouse. Nature Genet 20:157–162.

507. Belin V, Cusin V, Viot G, et al. (1998). SHOX mutations in dyschondrosteosis (Leri-Weill syndrome). Nature Genet 19:67–69.

508. Benito-Sanz S, Thomas NS, Huber C, et al. (2005). A novel class of pseudoautosomal region 1 deletions downstream of SHOX is associated with Leri-Weill dyschondrosteosis. Am J Hum Genet 77:534–544.

509. Marchini A, Marttila T, Winter A, et al. (2004). The short stature homeodomain protein SHOX induces cellular growth arrest and apoptosis and is expressed in human growth plate chondrocytes. J Biol Chem 279:37103–37114.

510. Nissenson RA (1998). Parathyroid hormone (PTH)/PTHrP receptor mutations in human chondrodysplasia. Endocrinology 139:4753–4755.

511. Thiel CT, Horn D, Zabel B, et al. (2005). Severely incapacitating mutations in patients with extreme short stature identify RNA-processing endoribonuclease *RMRP* as an essential cell growth regulator. Am J Hum Genet 77:795–806.

512. Herman GE (2003). Disorders of cholesterol biosynthesis: prototypic metabolic malformation syndromes. Hum Molec Genet 12: R75–R88.

513. Opitz, JM (1999). RSH (so-called Smith-Lemli-Opitz) syndrome. Curr Opin Pediatr 11:353–362.

514. Waterham HR, Koster J, Romeijn GJ, et al. (2001). Mutations in the 3 beta-hydroxysterol delta 24-reductase gene cause desmosterolosis, an autosomal recessive disorder of cholesterol biosynthesis. Am J Hum Genet 69:685–694.

515. Waterham HR, Koster J, Mooyer P, et al. (2003). Autosomal recessive HEM/Greenberg skeletal dysplasia is caused by 3 β-hydroxysterol Δ^{14}-reductase deficiency due to mutations in the lamin B receptor gene. Am J Hum Genet 72:1013–1017.

516. Levine B-S, Carpenter TO (1999). Evaluation and treatment of heritable forms of rickets. The Endocrinologist 9:358–365.

517. Hruska KA (2006). Hyperphosphatemia and hypophosphatemia. In Favus MJ (ed.), *Primer on the metabolic bone diseases and disorders of mineral metabolism, Sixth edition.* Washington, D.C.: American Society for Bone and Mineral Research 233–242.

518. Sillence DO, Senn A, Danks DM (1979). Genetic heterogeneity in osteogenesis imperfecta. J Med Genet 16:101–116.

519. Brown EM, Bai M, Ollak M (1997). Familial benign hypocalciuric hypercalcemia and other syndromes of altered responsiveness to extracellular calcium. In Krane SM, Avioli LV(eds.), *Metabolic bone diseases, Third edition.* San Diego: Academic Press 479–499.

520. Kitanaka S, Murayama A, Sakai T, et al. (1999). No enzyme activity of 25-hydroxyvitamin D_3 1α-hydroxylase gene product in pseudo-vitamin D deficiency rickets, including that with mild clinical manifestation. J Clin Endocrinol Metab 84:4111–4117.

521. Kim CJ, Kaplan LE, Perwad F, et al. (2007). Vitamin D 1α-hydroxylase gene mutations in patients with 1α-hydroxylase deficiency. J Clin Endocrinol Metab 92:3177–3182.

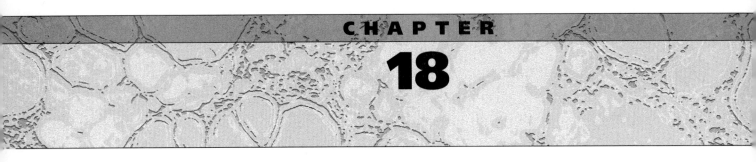

Autoimmune Polyglandular Syndromes

MICHAEL J. HALLER, MD • WILLIAM E. WINTER, MD
• DESMOND A. SCHATZ, MD

Introduction

The autoimmune polyglandular syndromes (APS) I and II are uncommon constellations of organ-specific autoimmune diseases characterized by the occurrence of more than one autoimmune disease in an affected individual. More commonly, autoimmune disease of endocrine glands occurs in only a single organ. However, multiorgan involvement of endocrine and nonendocrine organs and tissues may be present.

Tolerance is an active state in which the immune system does not mount a reaction against self-antigens.[1-3] If tolerance is not established or is lost, autoimmunity and subsequent autoimmune disease can result. Although the breakdown in self-tolerance remains unexplained in most human autoimmunities, our improved understanding of normal immunologic processes has identified a number of possible mechanisms. To comprehend these mechanisms, a brief overview of how tolerance is maintained is essential.

Mechanisms Underlying Generation of Autoimmunity

INTRODUCTION

In a normal immune response, the host organism must differentiate self from non-self, generate an immune response to non-self, and eliminate non-self to protect the host from injury, organ dysfunction, and even death.[1-3] Endogenous antigens represent self, whereas exogenous antigens represent non-self. The adaptive immune system assumes the all exogenous (foreign) antigens are potentially harmful and acts to eliminate non-self. Self/non-self discrimination is carried out by the adaptive (specific) immune system through the use of T- and B-cell surface receptors.[4]

These receptors recognize distinctive peptides or epitopes and are the keys to the specificity of the adaptive immune response. Whereas B cells and their receptors recognize soluble antigen or antigens on cell surfaces, T cells and their receptors only perceive short polypeptides presented by specialized cell-surface molecules encoded by the major histocompatibility complex (MHC).[5-7] The human MHC is termed the *human leukocyte antigen* (HLA) *complex*. Class I MHC (e.g., HLA-A, HLA-B, and HLA-C molecules) present peptides derived from the cell cytoplasm to CD8 T cells, whereas class II MHC (e.g., HLA-DP, HLA-DQ, and HLA-DR molecules) present peptides derived from the extracellular space and intravesicular space to CD4 T cells.

Regulation of self-tolerance occurs at two major levels. First, through a process of negative selection thymic medullary epithelial cells project an immunologic "self-shadow" and signal the removal or silencing of self-reactive thymocytes (central tolerance).[3,8] Negative selection occurs when double positive (CD4+, CD8+) alpha/beta T cells bind too tightly to dendritic cells and/or macrophages at the corticomedullary border in the thymus and are triggered to undergo apoptosis. Second, in lymphoid and non-lymphoid tissues mature self-reactive T cells are deleted or anergized (peripheral tolerance) when their receptors engage peptides plus MHC molecules in the absence of appropriate co-stimulatory molecules (Figures 18-1 and 18-2). Nevertheless, recent data have demonstrated that proteins

Development of Tolerance to Self-Antigens

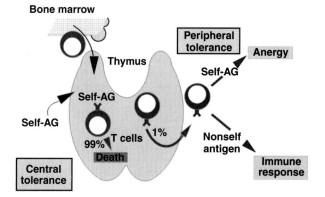

Figure 18-1 Normal tolerance pathways. T-cell precursors initially arise in the bone marrow. These progenitors enter the thymus and encounter self-antigen. Strong self-antigen stimulation of developing T cells induces apoptosis, with approximately 99% of all developing T cells dying. This is *central immunologic tolerance*, where strongly anti-self T cells are eliminated. Naive T cells that do leave the thymus can be subsequently tolerized to self-antigens if they encounter self-antigen without the normal co-stimulatory signals (B7-CD28; see Figure 18-3). Induction of tolerance outside the thymus is termed *peripheral tolerance* (top right), which is a complementary mechanism to central tolerance. Peripheral tolerance is functionally expressed as anergy: autoreactive cells are present but are inactive (top right). If non-self antigen is encountered, a normal immune response ensues (bottom right).

Autoimmunity: Failure of Tolerance to Self-Antigens

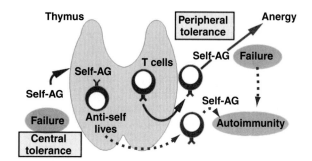

Figure 18-2 Autoimmunity: failure of tolerance to self-antigens. With a failure of central tolerance (bottom left), anti-self T cells survive that should not normally survive. When such anti-self T cells leave the thymus, autoimmunity may result (dashed arrows). Alternatively, with a failure of peripheral tolerance (top right) if anergy (solid arrow) does not occur after contact with self-antigen, an autoimmune response can occur (red arrow).

previously thought to be expressed only in peripheral tissues are expressed in the developing thymus and therefore play a critical role in establishing tolerance.[9]

Although many of the mechanisms involved in establishing tolerance remain poorly understood, recent characterization of the autoimmune regulatory gene (AIRE) has improved understanding of positive and negative T-cell selection. AIRE plays a critical role in the expression of peripheral antigens and provides for the negative selection of autoreactive T-effector cells.[10] Deletions in the mouse AIRE homologue result in multiorgan autoimmunity, and mutations in the human AIRE gene result in APS I.[11,12]

Tolerance is initially developed in utero. During gestation and early life, tolerance is most easily induced by exposure of the host to a specific antigen. Although the thymus atrophies during puberty, residual thymic tissue provides for T-cell development throughout life. T cells do not require exposure to large doses of antigen to achieve tolerance during their thymic development. However, larger doses of antigen are required to induce B-cell tolerance (which is often short lived). B cells are produced by the bone marrow continuously throughout life. Tolerance is immunologically specific, learned or acquired, most easily induced in immature or developing lymphocytes, and potentially induced in mature lymphocytes when co-stimulatory signals are absent at the time of peptide recognition by the T lymphocyte.

CENTRAL T-CELL TOLERANCE

T cells are educated to distinguish self and non-self in the thymus.[13-15] Central T-cell tolerance is the process by which anti-self T cells are eliminated in the thymus. As many as 99% of developing thymocytes die in the thymus and never reach the periphery. T-cell tolerance is a function of the selection of the T-cell receptor (TCR) repertoire that exits the thymus. In the thymic cortex CD4+, CD8+ (double positive) T cells bearing alpha/beta TCRs that bind to self-MHC initially survive (positive selection). In this way, the thymus initially chooses for survival T cells that bind to self-MHC—as opposed to TCRs that might bind to other self-molecules, leading to ineffective communication. This positive selection resulting from self-peptide-MHC presentation is carried out by thymic nurse epithelial cells in the cortex.

At the corticomedullary junction of the thymus, if such saved TCRs bind to self-MHC too tightly autoreactivity is possible and these T cells then undergo negative selection and suffer apoptotic death. The cells inducing negative selection are macrophages and dendritic cells. This process of positive selection for MHC binding in the thymic cortex and negative selection (at the thymic corticomedullary border) against tight binding to self-peptides accounts for central (thymic) immunologic tolerance.[3,8,10]

PERIPHERAL T-CELL TOLERANCE

Once in the circulation and in secondary lymphoid organs (e.g., lymph nodes and spleen), naive T cells still require multiple signals to become activated.[16] The initial signal is the presentation of antigen-specific peptides to TCRs by MHC molecules. CD4 and CD8 molecules on these T-cell subsets serve as antigen-nonspecific co-receptors binding to nonpolymorphic portions of the class II MHC molecules and class I MHC molecules, respectively. The second signal is antigen nonspecific and is provided by the B7 molecule of the antigen-presenting cell interacting with the CD28 molecule on the T-cell surface.

When both signals are perceived by the T cell, a cascade of intracellular signaling events occurs—leading to T-cell activation. Activated CD4 T cells express cytokines (including IL-2, IL-4, IL-5, and so on), cytokine receptors, and CTLA-4. Activated CD4 T cells then down-regulate TCR expression and acquire class II MHC expression. It is unknown why activated human T cells express class II MHC (activated T cells in mice do not express class II MHC). CTLA-4 expression by the activated T cell and its interaction with B7 provides an immunosuppressive signal to the T cell down-regulating the T-cell immune responses. Thus, CTLA-4 and CD28 act antithetically: B7-CD28 turns on T cells, whereas B7-CTLA-4 down-regulates them (Figure 18-3).

Functionally, helper CD4 T cells are predominantly subdivided into Th1 cells (which activate cell-mediated and some antibody responses) and Th2 cells, which predominantly activate antibody-mediated responses.[17] Th1 cells can activate macrophages, natural killer cells, and B cells—and they secrete predominantly IL-2, gamma interferon (IFN-γ), and IL-12. Th2 cells elaborate IL-4, IL-5, IL-6, and IL-10. Cross talk between Th1 and Th2 cells occurs: IFN-γ from Th1 cells suppresses Th2 cells and IL-10 from Th2 cells inhibits Th1 cells. Another subset of CD4 T cells has been described as regulatory T cells that secrete the immunomodulatory cytokines IL-10 and/or transforming growth factor-beta (TGF-beta).

Regulatory T cells include CD4+CD25+ T cells and Tr1 and Th3 cells. Tr1 and Th3 cells express CD4 but do not express CD25 (the IL-2 receptor alpha chain). Tr1 cells secrete IL-10 and TGF-beta, whereas Th3 cells secrete IL-4, IL-10, and TGF-beta. Although CD4+CD25+ T cells can

Role of B7, CD28, and CTLA-4 in T-Cell Activation

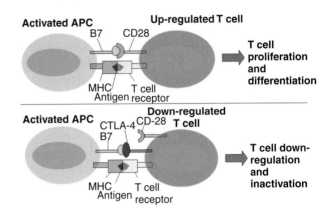

Figure 18-3 Role of B7, CD28, and CTLA-4 in T-cell activation. An activated antigen-presenting cell (APC) presents antigen on the multiple histocompatibility complex (MHC) and expresses B7 co-stimulators. When B7 is bound by CD28 and MHC is bound by a T-cell receptor, T-cell proliferation and differentiation of naive T cells ensues. Conversely, an activated T cell will now express CTLA-4 and bind to B7—thereby inducing down-regulation and inactivation of T cells.

secrete IL-10 and TGF-beta, their regulatory action on autoreactive T cells appears to occur through cell-to-cell contact. Upon activation, CD8 T cells (often with the help of Th1 cells supplying IFN-γ to up-regulate B7 expression on antigen-presenting cells) become functional cytotoxic T killer cells.

The requirement for two signals to activate naive T cells accounts for peripheral T-cell tolerance. When the naive T cell perceives antigen peptide presented by MHC molecules without the necessary co-stimulatory signal (e.g., B7-CD28), the T cell becomes unresponsive. This state of unresponsiveness is termed *anergy*. The T cell may also undergo apoptosis (programmed cell death) to be completely removed from the T-cell repertoire. Anergic T cells can generally not be restimulated with antigen peptide displayed by the antigen-presenting cell. Tolerance may also exist because the TCR does not come into contact with the relevant peptide. This has been termed *T-cell ignorance.*

Improvements in the characterization of regulatory T cells have recently allowed for further understanding of the peripheral tolerance pathway. Regulatory T cells play a critical role in suppressing the activity of effector T cells that escape negative selection to self-antigen in the thymus.[18] Functional regulatory T cells are able to anergize previously self-reactive T effector cells, resulting in improved tolerance to self. The expression of the forkhead transcription factor, FOXP3, is specific for identification of the CD4+CD25+ cell (T$_{reg}$) population.

First identified in the Scurfy mouse, a mouse model of immune dysfunction and polyendocrinopathy, abnormal FOXP3 expression is now known to be responsible for the failure in tolerance in humans affected with a similar polyendocrinopathy (discussed in material following).[19,20] The absence of normal FOXP3 expression in humans leads to an extremely rare recessively inherited (yet X-linked) and typically fatal autoimmune lymphoproliferative disease known as IPEX (immune dysregulation, polyendocrinopathy, enteropathy, and X-linked inheritance). Defects in the forkhead transcription factor responsible for IPEX map to Xp11.23-Xq13.3.

B-CELL TOLERANCE

B cells are partially educated in the bone marrow to be anergized or undergo apoptosis in response to self-antigen when they are at the stage of development of the naive immature B cell (central B-cell tolerance). In the bone marrow, naive immature B cells that see multivalent antigens become anergized (unresponsiveness to subsequent stimulation)—whereas exposure to highly polyvalent antigens can induce apoptosis.

Naive immature B cells express IgM on their surface but are not yet IgD positive, as observed in naive mature B cells. Anergized B cells do not instantly die, but will live no longer than unstimulated naive immature B cells. Naive mature B cells expressing IgD on their surface require T-cell help for realization of their full potential through affinity maturation and class switching. The absence of T-cell help leads to B-cell tolerance.

AUTOIMMUNE DISEASES

The organ-specific nature of many autoimmune diseases results from abnormal immune system recognition of tissue-specific self-antigens. In many autoimmune endocrinopathies, the target molecule is a tissue-specific or tissue-limited (i.e., the protein is not unique to one tissue but is clearly restricted in its distribution) enzyme or cell-surface receptor[21,22] (Table 18-1).

TABLE 18-1

Autoantigens in Autoimmune Endocrine and Associated Diseases

Disease	Confirmed Autoantigens	Putative Autoantigens
Addison disease	P450c21	P450c17, P450scc
Hashimoto thyroiditis	Thyroid peroxidase Thyroglobulin	
Graves' disease	Thyrotropin receptor	
Diabetes	Insulin	Proinsulin
	Glutamic acid decarboxylase-65	Carboxypeptidase H ICA69
	IA-2 (ICA 512)	Glima 38
	IA-2β	
Premature gonadal failure		P450c17 P450scc 3BHSD
Pernicious anemia	H+/K+ ATPase Intrinsic factor	
Myasthenia gravis	Acetylcholine receptor	
Vitiligo		Tyrosinase Tyrosinase-related protein-2
Celiac disease	Transglutaminase	Reticulin Gliadin Endomyseum

The criteria for classification of a disease as autoimmune are not universally agreed upon.[23] However, major criteria generally accepted as strong evidence that the disease is autoimmune include detection of autoantibodies or autoreactive T cells, including lymphocytic infiltration of the targeted tissue or organ; disease transfer with antibodies or lymphocytes; disease recurrence in transplanted tissue; and ability to abrogate the disease process with immunosuppression or immunomodulation. Few, if any, human autoimmune diseases meet all four of these criteria. Further information supportive of (but not diagnostic for) an autoimmune disease includes increased disease frequency in women compared to men, presence of other autoimmune diseases in affected individuals, and increased frequencies of particular HLA alleles in affected individuals compared to an unaffected control population.

DEFECTS IN TOLERANCE THAT CAUSE AUTOIMMUNE DISEASES

Several hypotheses explaining defects in tolerance have been proposed.[24] Theoretically, autoimmunity may develop because tolerance never developed to specific self-antigens or because established tolerance was lost. If self-antigen is not efficiently presented in the thymus, tolerance may not be established during T-cell education within the thymic cortex.[25] For example, variations in the insulin gene VNTR (variable number of tandem repeats; ~500 base pairs upstream of the insulin gene promoter) influence the extent of insulin gene expression in the thymic cortex. Risk of developing type 1 diabetes is enhanced when certain VNTR alleles are present, which leads to lower mRNA expression of insulin in the thymus.

Specifically, class III alleles (greater number of VNTR) are associated with increased thymic expression of insulin and a decreased risk of developing type 1 diabetes—whereas class I alleles (smaller number of VNTR) are associated with decreased thymic expression of insulin and an increased risk of developing diabetes.[26] If there is failure to delete an autoreactive clone of T cells, autoimmunity could develop. If autoimmunity does result from defects in thymic tolerance, the defects must be antigen specific because organ-specific autoimmune diseases are usually extremely selective. For example, in type 1 diabetes the beta cells are attacked and ultimately destroyed by a cell-mediated autoimmune process but the remaining islet cells (including alpha cells, delta cells, and pancreatic polypeptide-producing cells) are unscathed.

Defects in peripheral tolerance could result from concurrent T-cell stimulation by self-antigen/MHC plus T-cell co-stimulation (e.g., B7-CD28), leading to aberrant T-cell activation and an autoimmune response. If tolerance has not been developed because an antigen is sequestered intracellularly or is not expressed in the thymus during T-cell ontogeny, T-cell reactivity in the periphery would not be abrogated. However, several antigens initially thought to be sequestered intracellularly have now been shown to circulate in low concentrations in normal individuals. Thyroglobulin is such a self-antigen in autoimmune thyroid disease.

The development of thyroglobulin autoantibodies was believed to follow the release of thyroglobulin from the thyroid gland as part of viral attack, trauma, or some other form of environmental damage. Hypothetically, this immunization then leads to an antithyroglobulin humoral response and autoimmune thyroid disease. However, we now know that thyroglobulin does circulate in low but appreciable quantities in normal individuals who show no serologic evidence of thyroid autoimmunity. Furthermore, thyroid follicular cell destruction in Hashimoto thyroiditis is cell mediated (not humorally mediated).

If sequestered antigens do play a role in autoimmune disease, viral infections, trauma, ischemia, or irradiation are all mechanisms that could disturb cellular integrity and lead to release of intracellular antigens.[27] Some self-antigens may never normally come into contact with the immune system unless there is a breakdown of anatomic barriers within the body. An example is the occurrence of autoimmunity to the eye following orbital trauma. Although a rare consequence of orbital damage, initiation of an autoimmune response to eye proteins in adjacent lymph nodes can generate autoreactive T cells that can invade and damage the contralateral eye (sympathetic ophthalmia).[28] Removal of the inciting damaged tissues and immunosuppression may be required to sustain vision in the undamaged eye. Similarly, transient autoantibody reactivity to cardiac myosin following myocardial infarction has also been described.[29]

Hypothetically, tolerance may not develop if self-antigen expression is delayed during negative selection. When the self-antigen is ultimately expressed, if tolerance has not previously been established the autoantigen is perceived as foreign and autoreactivity develops. No spontaneous examples of this process have been described. However, in experimental systems in which transgenes are placed under control of promoters that can be turned on by exogenous agents such as metals, autoreactivity can be elicited when gene expression is stimulated after the neonatal period.

Alteration of self-antigens as a result of infection or neoplasia is believed to be a plausible theory explaining some types of autoimmunity. As environmental triggers, viral infections could lead to modification of self-proteins and neoantigen expression (e.g., a new antigen is present on self-cells). Alternatively, a self-antigen may be partially degraded—leading to a "new" antigenic target for the adaptive immune system. This new antigen is recognized as foreign by the immune system, and the immune response to these new antigens results in autoimmunity.

Some self-cells/tissues may suffer unintended autoimmune damage when substances bind to the cells and elicit an initial immune response. For example, certain drugs bind to red blood cells and result in an immune hemolytic anemia. If an antibody response to the red-cell-bound drug is elicited, the antigen-antibody complex present on the red blood cell can lead to red blood cell destruction. This can occur through red blood cell phagocytosis by the monocyte-macrophage system or via complement-mediated lysis of the red blood cell. Thus, the red blood cell is an innocent bystander to the antidrug humoral immune response. Theoretically, this could also occur with viruses that serendipitously attach to tissues.

Molecular mimicry is one of the most popular explanations for autoimmunity.[27] Due to exposure to a dietary, viral, or bacterial antigen (e.g., infection) and molecular mimicry (similarity) between the self-antigen and the foreign antigen, the immune response to the foreign antigen leads to cross reactivity with self-antigen, autoimmunity, and disease.[30-32] For this theory to work, tolerance must not previously exist to the self-antigen. This might be true if the self-antigen is truly sequestered and the immune system has never developed tolerance to the self-antigen. Alternatively, the self-antigen peptides may be present in too low a concentration to elicit an immune response and initial immune system tolerization has not occurred.

Only with infection or novel dietary exposure would there be a sufficient degree of self-immunization to develop immune autoreactivity. With immune autoreactivity, self is now recognized as foreign during the response to the cross-reactive pathogen. If the self-antigen is a cell surface antigen, the "pathogen-induced" autoantibodies could fix to self and produce disease via complement fixation—or the antibodies could act as opsonins for fixed or circulating phagocytes (antibody-dependent-cell cytotoxicity). In rheumatic fever, cross reactivity between *Streptococcus M* protein and cardiac myosin have been described. In ankylosing spondylitis, cross reactions between Klebsiella nitrogenase and HLA-B27 have been described. In rheumatoid arthritis there is cross reactivity between cartilage protein and a mycobacterial proteoglycan wall component.

Aberrant class II MHC expression was a theory in vogue in the mid 1980s. In this hypothesis, cells elicit autoimmune reactions by presenting their own self-peptides via self-expressed class II MHC molecules. Indeed, class II MHC expression has been identified on various cells that are targets of autoimmune-mediated cell destruction. Examples include pancreatic islet beta cells in type 1 diabetes, biliary tract cells in primary biliary cirrhosis, and thyroid follicular cells in Hashimoto thyroiditis.

However, there are strong counterarguments to this theory. First, class II MHC molecules do not present intracytoplasmic antigens (which are often targets of attack). Instead, class II MHC molecules present peptides derived from extracellular proteins. Second, accessory molecules are typically needed to activate naive T cells. If, for example, pancreatic beta cells present peptides via their class II MHC molecules without B7 the naïve T cells seeing these peptides in the absence of B7 will actually be tolerized. Indeed, aberrant (or ectopic) class II MHC expression may be a mechanism cells use to actually induce a state of tolerance to down-regulate an immune response. Aberrant class II MHC expression may therefore serve an anti-inflammatory role in modulating an immune response to a lower level of intensity. Costimulator expression (e.g., B7) is highly regulated even among professional antigen-presenting cells. For example, in the basal state neither macrophages nor B cells express B7. Upon phagocytosis of bacteria species, macrophages will express class II MHC and B7. Whereas B cells express class II MHC in their basal state, internalization of bacterial antigen bound to their cell surface receptor antibody molecules will induce B7 expression.

Some cases of autoimmunity may result from superantigens initiating an anti-self immune response as part of the polyclonal immune activation process. Superantigens are polycolonal T-cell stimulators that have the ability to cross-link TCR beta chains and MHC molecules. Superantigens have been reported to activate as many as a third of all T cells in the body. In such cases, systemic disease can develop from massive cytokine release. This is the case in toxic shock syndrome, wherein a staphylococcal exotoxin acts as a superantigen. Mycobacterial antigens have been promulgated as possible superantigens in Crohn disease.[33] This theory presupposes that T cells bearing anti-self TCRs have not been deleted or permanently anergized. T cells with anti-self receptors may be stimulated, and if they encounter self-antigen they may further proliferate to develop an autoimmune response.

Similar to polyclonal T-cell activation, polyclonal B-cell stimulation has also been implicated in humoral autoimmunity. Indeed, autoreactive B cells can be found in normal individuals. If an autoreactive clone of B cells encounters self-antigen and a co-stimulator (which might be nonspecific, such as Epstein Barr virus or a bacterial product such as lipopolysaccharide), autoantibodies could be produced—bypassing the need for T-cell help.

However, which of these speculative theories applies to the APS is unknown. Human disease most often results from an interaction of environmental and genetic factors.[34] Many environmental factors are implicated in various autoimmune diseases: wheat gliadin ingestion and celiac disease, penicillamine exposure and myasthenia gravis, methimazole and autoimmune hypoglycemia from insulin autoantibodies, and amiodarone and thyroiditis. Cytokine exposure is also associated with autoimmune disease in the case of alpha interferon use in hepatitis and the apparent development of thyroiditis. Even cancer can be associated with the development of autoimmunity: thymoma and myasthenia gravis are associated, as are ovarian carcinoma and cerebellar degeneration, and breast cancer and stiffman syndrome. How this interaction among genes, the environment, and the immune system actually leads to autoimmunity and disease clearly needs to be elucidated.

Classification of the Autoimmune Polyglandular Syndromes

APS I, also known as APECED (autoimmune polyendocrinopathy-candidiasis-ectodermal dystrophy), is an autosomal-recessive disorder mapped to a single gene (the autoimmune regulator or AIRE gene) on chromosome 21q22.3.[11,12] The presence of two of the following three conditions are prerequisites for diagnosis: adrenocortical failure (Addison disease) or serologic evidence of adrenalitis (e.g., adrenal autoantibodies), hypoparathyroidism, and mucocutaneous candidiasis.[35-37]

APS II is defined by the coexistence of autoimmune adrenocortical insufficiency or serologic evidence of adrenalitis with autoimmune thyroiditis (Schmidt syndrome) and/or type 1 diabetes mellitus (Carpenter syndrome, which is Schmidt syndrome plus type 1 diabetes) or serologic evidence of thyroid or islet autoim-

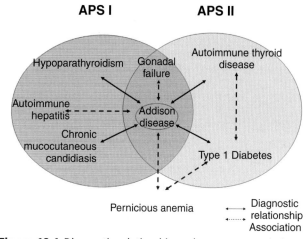

Figure 18-4 Diagnostic relationship and common associations of APS I and APS II. The solid lines indicate diagnostic relationships. The dashed lines indicate common associations. The diagnosis of APS I depends on the coexistence of Addison disease (or adrenal autoantibodies) and hypoparathyroidism or chronic mucocutaneous candidiasis, or both. The diagnosis of APS II depends on the coexistence of Addison disease (or adrenal autoantibodies) and autoimmune thyroid disease or type 1 diabetes, or both (or their associated autoantibodies).

munity[38-41] (Figure 18-4). The presence of thyroiditis without adrenal disease but associated with type 1 diabetes mellitus, pernicious anemia, vitiligo, or alopecia has been referred to as APS III. However, because APS II and III differ only by the presence or absence of adrenocortical disease and share similar susceptibility genes and immunologic features we do not recognize APS III as a unique syndrome and consider it an extension of the APS II constellation.

Clinical Aspects

APS I

The major disease components, frequencies, and differences between APS I and II are outlined in Table 18-2. APS I (APECED) may occur sporadically or in families. Although the disease is not common, cohorts of patients have been reported from Finland and the United States and among Iranian Jews. Males and females are equally affected in this autosomal-recessive disorder.[35,37,42] Persistent mucocutaneous candidiasis is usually the first sign, which commonly appears during the first year or two of life. However, it may also have its onset in adulthood. Candidal infections in the region of the diaper area often present early, with vulvovaginal candidiasis commonly developing at puberty in females.

Colonization of the gut can lead to intermittent abdominal pain and diarrhea. The nails may be affected with chronic candidiasis, leading to a darkened discoloration, thickening, or erosion. Retrosternal pain occurring in patients with confirmed oral candidiasis suggests esophageal candidiasis and can be confirmed by esophagoscopy. It is extremely important that the candidiasis be

TABLE 18-2

The Autoimmune Polyglandular Syndromes I and II

Disease Characteristic	APS I	APS II
Comparative frequency	Less common	More common
Onset	Infancy/early childhood	Late childhood, adulthood
Heredity	Autosomal recessive	Polygenic
Gender	Males = females	Female predominance
Genetics	AIRE gene; no HLA association	HLA associated; DR/DQ
Hypoparathyoidism	77-89%	None
Mucocutaneous candidiasis	73-100%	None
Ectodermal dysplasia	77%	None
Addison disease	60-86%	70-100%
Type 1 diabetes	4-18%	41-52%
Autoimmune thyroid disease	8-40%	70%
Pernicious anemia	12-15%	2-25%
Gonadal failure		
Females	30-60%	3.5-10%
Males	7-17%	5%
Vitiligo	4-13%	4-5%
Alopecia	27%	2%
Autoimmune hepatitis	10-15%	Rare
Malabsorption	10-18%	Rare

aggressively treated. Carcinoma of the oral mucosa with its high mortality is well described in APS I patients with chronic mucosal candidiasis.

Any patient with refractory mucocutaneous candidiasis should be thoroughly investigated not only for a T-lymphocyte abnormality (absolute lymphocyte count, enumeration of T-cell subpopulations, assessment of T-cell function) but for the presence of a polyendocrinopathy. The largest cohort of longitudinally followed APS I patients resides in Finland. In Perhentupa's recent review of these 91 APS I patients, 60% presented with candidaisis as the first sign of APS I, 96% developed candidiasis by 20 years of age, and 100% developed candidiasis by 40 years of age.[35]

Addison disease is found in more than 85% of APS I patients, yet the disease is often missed—with the diagnosis commonly made late or at the time of a life-threatening adrenal crisis. Autoimmune adrenocortical failure usually has its peak onset before adolescence, when it is associated with APS I. However, Addison disease may have its onset in adulthood. Deficiencies of cortisol, aldosterone, and adrenal andogens may present simultaneously or may evolve over months to several years. The initial clinical features of Addison disease are often nonspecific mimicking psychiatric or gastrointestinal disease. These include fatigue, weight loss, myalgias, arthralgias, behavioral changes, nausea and vomiting, abdominal pain, and diarrhea. Hyperpigmentation (due to elevated ACTH) in non sun-exposed areas and postural hypotension can usually be found on careful examination. Unexplained hypotonic dehydration should raise the suspicion of Addison disease. Adrenal crises with hyponatremia, hyperkalemia, and hypoglycemia may be fatal unless recognized early and treated appropriately.

Like other components of APS I, hypoparathyroidism usually presents before puberty. Severe hypocalcemia as evidenced by seizures, carpopedal spasms, muscle twitching, and laryngospasm may be presenting features. Hyperphosphatemia with a low intact parathyroid hormone (PTH) level is diagnostic. These symptoms may, however, be masked in the presence of adrenal insufficiency.

Ectodermal dystrophy unrelated to hypoparathyoidism or to mucocutaneous candidiasis has been well characterized in the Finnish patients with APS I. Dental enamel hypoplasia of permanent (but not deciduous) teeth, as well as nail dystrophy, is commonly found. There may be complete absence of the enamel or transverse hypoplastic bands alternating with zones of well-formed enamel. Dystrophy of nails is manifest by 0.5- to 1-mm pits. Nearly a third of the Finnish patients also had calcification of the tympanic membranes.[43]

Premature gonadal failure is more common in females and may present in puberty. Less than 30% of men with APS I develop testicular failure, whereas more than 50% of women with APS I develop ovarian failure by 20 years of age.[35] In younger female patients, gonadal failure often presents with primary amenorrhea—and in time menstrual irregularities, polycystic ovaries, or infertility may manifest.[35,44]

As shown in Table 18-2, in contrast to patients with APS II type 1 diabetes and autoimmune thyroiditis occur far less frequently in APS I. When present, thyroiditis is typically atrophic rather than goitrous. Atrophic gastritis occurs in 15% to 30% of APS I cases, with a mean age of onset of 16 years.[35,43] Gastric-parietal cell autoimmunity, which leads to atrophic gastritis with resultant achlorhydria and intrinsic factor deficiency, typically presents as iron deficiency anemia or vitamin B_{12}-deficient pernicious anemia.

Nonendocrine organ-specific diseases include alopecia, vitiligo, autoimmune hepatitis, and malabsorption. All types of alopecia may occur, but progression to alopecia totalis (total loss of scalp hair) or universalis (total loss of all body hair including eyelashes, eyebrows, and scalp hair)—which are most common—usually occurs before puberty. Vitiligo presents initially as small pale pigment-lacking skin patches. These may be missed unless specifically sought with ultraviolet light examination of the skin.

The appearance of clay-colored stools, dark urine, and jaundice confirms the diagnosis of chronic active hepatitis—which is not related to infectious hepatitis. Hepatitis occurs in 10% to 15% of APS I patients and is the leading cause of death in these patients. Consequently, all patients suspected of having APS I should have their liver function regularly monitored. Intermittent malabsorption (typically of fat) has been linked to hypoparathyroidism, bacterial and fungal overgrowth, gluten sensitivity, and IgA deficiency. There have also been rare reports of APS I and associated diabetes insipidus, growth hormone deficiency, ACTH deficiency, rheumatoid arthritis, Sjögren's disease, and myopathy.[45]

APS II

APS II is the most common of the polyendocrinopathies, and unlike APS I usually has its onset in adulthood—particularly during the third or fourth decades. APS II is at least three times more common in females than in males. In 1926, Schmidt first described the association of adrenocortical and thyroid gland failure—and Carpenter extended this in 1964 to include insulin-dependent diabetes mellitus.[38,39] In 1957, the autoimmune nature of these diseases was suggested by Doniach and Roitt's discovery of thyroglobulin autoantibodies in patients with Hashimoto thyroiditis.[46] APS II was originally defined by the occurrence of adrenocortical insufficiency (Addison disease) in conjunction with autoimmune thyroid disease and/or type 1 diabetes mellitus.

Adrenocortical failure is the presentation in approximately 50% of APS II cases. The disease usually has its onset between ages 20 and 50 years, although it is not unusual to find cases before or after these ages.[41,47,48] Several of the disease components may be present at diagnosis. Type 1 diabetes coexists in nearly 50% of patients with Addison disease, whereas autoimmune thyroid disease (AITD) coexists in about two-thirds of patients with Addison disease. Thus, type 1 diabetes and AITD should be vigorously sought in any patient presenting with Addison disease.

The most common component of the APS II to occur as an isolated condition is AITD. AITD affects nearly 4.5% of the U.S. population,[49] and because of a strong female predominance 80% to 90% of all cases occur in females. AITD has an increased incidence during the teen years, with a peak appearing in the fifth and sixth decades. Chronic lymphocytic thyroiditis (Hashimoto disease) is by far the most common form of AITD, although Graves disease or postpartum thyroiditis may also occur. Several studies have reported on the coexistence of anti-islet immunity (3%-8%) or even overt type 1 diabetes and AITD.[50,51] Just 1% of patients with otherwise isolated thyroiditis have serologic evidence of adrenal autoimmunity.

Although polyglandular involvement in patients with autoimmune thyroid disease is infrequent, thyroid autoimmunity or a family history of thyroiditis is common in patients with pernicious anemia, vitiligo, alopecia, myasthenia gravis, and Sjögren syndrome.[52-54] More patients with APS I than APS II have vitiligo, but because APS I is far less common most patients with vitiligo who have another autoimmune disease have APS II. Twenty to 40% of vitiligo patients have another component of APS II, with thyrogastric autoimmunity being the most common.[55,56]

Thyrogastric autoimmunity is a descriptive term for the high frequency of concurrent AITD and autoimmune lymphocytic gastritis. Many of these patients with vitiligo are asymptomatic, and evidence of their autoimmunity can only be ascertained by autoantibody screening. Segmental vitiligo with involvement of dermatomal regions is not associated with autoimmunity, however.[57] Up to 15% of patients with alopecia (areata, totalis, universalis) and 5% of their first-degree relatives have thyroid disease.

Nearly 30% of patients with myasthenia gravis (autoimmune disease characterized by muscle weakness worsening during muscular contraction and caused by anti-acetylcholine receptor autoantibodies) have AITD. Both Hashimoto thyroiditis and Graves disease may occur in patients affected with myasthenia gravis.[58,59] Interestingly, these subjects with AITD appear more likely to have a milder expression of their myasthenia gravis and a lower incidence of thymic disease or autoantibodies to the acetylcholine receptor α-chain than AITD-negative patients. The proportion of ocular myasthenia is higher in patients with Graves disease.

Type 1 diabetes mellitus is also a diagnostic component of APS II. The worldwide incidence of type 1 diabetes continues to rise, particularly in children less than 5 years of age. The disease has a peak incidence during the teen years, with a smaller but increasing incidence occurring in the preschool years.[60] Nevertheless, the disease may have its onset at any age. Approximately 10% to 15% of diabetes patients with disease onset after 40 years actually have slowly progressive autoimmune disease [latent autoimmune diabetes of adults (LADA)], rather than insulin-resistant forms of diabetes (classic type 2 diabetes).[61] A gender bias is not present in patients with isolated type 1 diabetes. However, a female predominance occurs in APS II patients whose disease constellation includes type 1 diabetes.

This female bias in APS II is almost certainly related to the coexistence of AITD. The presence of thyroid microsomal (thyroid peroxidase) and/or thyroglobulin autoantibodies documents thyroiditis (often asymptomatic) in 20% to 25% of females with type 1 diabetes.[47] A female bias is also found in APS II patients with type 1 diabetes and gastric parietal cell autoimmunity. Gastric parietal cell autoantibodies (PCA) are present in approximately 10% of females and 5% of males with type 1 diabetes.[62] Although pernicious anemia typically affects women after the fifth decade, children at increased risk for pernicious anemia should be closely monitored when PCA are detected.

Atrophic gastritis may lead to the development of a megaloblastic anemia due an inability to produce intrinsic factor, and consequently to an inability to absorb vitamin B_{12}. Iron deficiency anemia secondary to an inability to absorb iron consequent to decreased acid production (achlorhydria) has also been reported in adolescents and adults.[63] Adrenocortical autoimmunity is much less frequent among patients with type 1 diabetes, with serologic evidence reported in 1.5% of cases.[64,65] Antibodies suggestive of celiac disease are present in up to 10% patients with type 1 diabetes. Endomysial or transglutaminase autoantibodies can be used to screen for celiac disease.[66] Although celiac disease should be suspected in patients with unexplained diarrhea, weight loss, failure to gain weight, or failure to thrive, biopsy-proven celiac disease is seen in less than 6% of type 1 diabetes patients.[67,68]

Approximately 10% of women with APS II who are less than 40 years of age develop ovarian failure presenting as primary or secondary amenorrhea. A female sex bias also occurs in the relationship between adrenocortical and gonadal autoimmunities. Among females with biopsy-proven lymphocytic oophoritis, adrenocortical failure or subclinical adrenal autoimmunity is often present.[69] Progression to gonadal failure is very rare among males with Addison disease, even in the presence of the high-risk steroidal cell autoantibodies (SCA) that mark the disease in women. Pituitary involvement is occasionally seen in APS II.[70,71] Hypophysitis and empty sella syndrome have been described, usually leading to isolated failure of secretion of GH, ACTH, TSH, FSH, or LH. Several nonendocrinologic conditions have been reported in association with APS II. These include ulcerative colitis,[72] primary biliary cirrhosis,[73] sarcoidosis,[74,75] achalasia,[76] myositis,[77] and neuropathy.[78]

IPEX

In addition to the classic diagnoses of APS I and II, an improved understanding of abnormal FoxP3 expression and T-cell function has led to the characterization of yet another autoimmune polyendocrinopathy. As previously stated, the absence of normal FoxP3 expression leads to the extremely rare recessively inherited X-linked and typically fatal autoimmune lymphoproliferative disease known as IPEX.[79-82]

Neonatal onset type 1 diabetes can be observed in IPEX, as well as dermatitis, enteropathy, thyroiditis, hemolytic anemia, and thrombocytopenia. To date, long-term immunosuppression or bone marrow transplantation appears to be the only effective therapy for IPEX. Bone marrow transplantation may be effective due to the normalization of FOXP3 expression in T cells even in patients with only partial chimerism. Increased expression of FOXP3 has recently been shown to reprogram effector T cells to act as regulatory T cells.[83,84] Thus, enhancement of FOXP3 expression to augment the number and function of regulatory T cells has significant potential to treat human autoimmune diseases.

Diagnostic Approach and Follow-up

The approach to diagnosing polyglandular syndromes is threefold. First, autoantibody screening is used to verify the autoimmune nature of the suspected endocrinopathy and to test for the involvement of other organs and tissues. Second, a full assessment of endocrine function is required in patients with confirmed autoantibodies—as well as in those who may be autoantibody negative but in whom disease may be suspected clinically. Third, mutation analysis can now be used to confirm the diagnosis and to screen siblings and other relatives for their carrier status.

Recognition of multiorgan autoimmune diseases prior to their symptomatic phases is the best way to minimize their associated morbidity and mortality. A thorough history and physical examination should always be performed, and a high index of suspicion should be maintained. Another clue to the identification of asymptomatic polyglandular disease may come from the history of a relative who has a different component disease than the proband or has typical multiorgan disease.

Any patient with suspected APS should be screened with a panel of autoantibodies (Figure 18-5). These include adrenal cortex cytoplasmic autoantibodies or autoantibodies directed against 21 hydroxylase (markers for autoimmune Addison disease); GADA, IA-2A, IAA, and ICA (for type 1 diabetes); thyroid microsomal/thyroperoxidase and thyroglobulin autoantibodies (for autoimmune thyroid disease); steroidal cell autoantibodies (for ovarian failure); and endomysial or transglutaminase autoantibodies (for celiac disease). Other autoantibodies have been reported in autoimmune adrenal disease and/or gonaditis, such as those against 17-hydroxylase, the

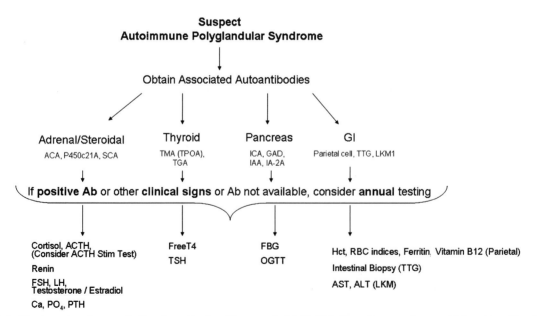

Figure 18-5 Antibody and end-organ testing in patients with suspected APS. This flow diagram shows which autoantibodies should be obtained when APS is suspected due to clinical signs and symptoms. Following autoantibody positivity, annual testing of end-organ function should be obtained as shown.

side-chain cleavage enzyme, and 3-hydroxysteroid dehy-drogenase. However, clinical testing is only available for the adrenal cytoplasmic autoantibodies (as detected by indirect immunofluorscence) and 21-hydroxylase autoan-tibodies. There is a clear link between the presence of organ-specific autoantibodies and the presence of preex-isting disease and subsequent progression to disease. However, in patients with APS the number of associated disorders that will develop and their age of appearance are clinically unpredictable. Thus, clinical long-term fol-low-up is necessary in both autoantibody positive and negative subjects.

All patients with a single autoimmune disease must be considered at risk for other autoimmune diseases. Whether and when to screen for other autoantibodies is based on the likelihood of finding another autoimmune disease, on cost effectiveness, and on the likelihood that screening will prevent morbidity and mortality from other diseases (e.g., diabetic ketoacidosis, Addisonian crisis, or hypocalcemia with seizures) in the future.

Because of the high incidence of AITD in patients with type 1 diabetes, we recommend that such patients have thyroid microsomal/thyroperoxidase and thyroglobulin autoantibodies measured biannually. This approach is preferred to assessing thyrotropin levels because autoan-tibody seroconversion is a much earlier event in the evolution of thyroid disease. In addition, measurement of thyroid microsomal/thyroperoxidase and thyroglobulin autoantibodies has close to 90% sensitivity. In those sub-jects who are positive, thyrotropin levels are measured annually. Most patients with isolated Hashimoto thyroid-itis will not develop additional endocrine disease, but when they do the thyroid disease has usually been pre-ceded by the overt failure of another gland.

Screening for APS is not recommended in patients with isolated autoimmune thyroid disease. However, several reports have demonstrated an increased incidence of pari-etal cell autoantibodies in patients with isolated autoim-mune thyroid disease.[63,85] Thus, screening for parietal cell autoantibodies in children with AITD can be considered. In hypothyroid patients with confirmed APS, evidence for adrenal autoimmunity must also be sought before starting thyroid hormone replacement therapy because thyroid hormone replacement can precipitate an adrenal crisis in patients with marginal adrenocortical function (by increas-ing metabolism and catabolism of steroid hormones).

Delayed diagnoses and even preventable deaths un-fortunately still occur in patients with undiagnosed adre-nocortical failure. As mentioned previously, the presenta-tion is often vague and nonspecific until an Addisonian crisis ensues. In patients with type 1 diabetes, unex-plained hypoglycemia or other unexplained improve-ment in blood glucose control might be a clue to the diagnosis of Addison disease. Improved glycemia may represent the loss of anti-insulin activity associated with glucocorticoid deficiency.

As mentioned previously, any patient with prolonged or unexplained chronic mucocutaneous candidiasis or hypoparathyoidism should be evaluated for APS I. Screen-ing for APS should also be performed in females with premature ovarian failure or young patients with vitiligo. Assessment of end-organ function in any patient with

autoantibodies is recommended annually (Figure 18-5). Fasting and/or 2-hour postprandial blood glucose testing and testing of calcium, phosphate, and PTH and TSH levels can effectively assess pancreatic islet, parathyroid, and thyroid function in asymptomatic individuals. Go-nadal failure can be diagnosed by the finding of elevated FSH and LH levels with concomitant low sex steroids.

Obtaining a hemoglobin and hematocrit together with indices can assess progression to atrophic gastritis in pa-tients with gastric autoimmunity. The findings of a megalo-blastic anemia with an elevated mean corpuscular volume (MCV) suggest vitamin B_{12} deficiency, whereas a microcytic hypochromic anemia confirms iron deficiency. However, vitamin B_{12} levels should be followed in all patients with parietal cell autoantibodies because neuropathy can de-velop without anemia. It is useful to obtain a vitamin B_{12} level and an iron profile prior to starting therapy. Methyl-malonic acid levels are not routinely needed in patients with gastric autoimmuinity but can be helpful if the vitamin B_{12} levels are borderline low.[86] Liver function tests and antimitochondrial autoantibodies should be obtained in patients with APS I. Patients testing positive for endomysial or transglutaminase autoantibodies should have an intesti-nal biopsy to confirm the diagnosis of celiac disease.

Low early morning cortisol levels, electrolyte abnor-malities (hyponatremia/hyperkalemia), and hypoglyce-mia represent late changes occurring at or just before the onset of adrenal insufficiency. Just as the natural history of pre type 1 diabetes has now been well de-scribed (see Chapter 10), there is now data to predict the subsequent development of adrenocortical insuffi-ciency once adrenal autoantibodies are first recognized (Figure 18-6). During the development of adrenocortical insufficiency in adrenocortical autoantibody positive subjects, a regular progression of sequential findings is exhibited. Stage 1 involves increased plasma renin ac-tivity, with normal to low aldosterone. Stage 2 involves

Natural History of Autoimmune Endocrinopathies

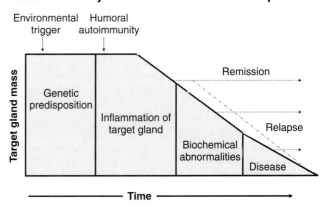

Figure 18-6 Proposed model of the natural history of an organ-specific autoimmune disease. In genetically susceptible individu-als, the onset of autoimmunity (identified by the presence of se-rum autoantibodies) is thought to be triggered by environmental agents. These organ-specific autoantibodies can be identified months to years before the disease becomes clinically manifest—thus allowing for the prediction and early diagnosis of the disease before the clinical manifestations or metabolic abnormalities can usually be detected.

TABLE 18-3

Stages in the Development of Autoimmune Addison Disease

Stage	Renin	Aldosterone	Basal Cortisol	Cortisol Post-ACTH	Basal ACTH
1	Elevated	N or Low	N	N	N
2	Elevated	N or Low	N	Low	N
3	Elevated	N or Low	N	Low	Elevated
4	Elevated	Low	Low*	Low	Elevated

*Clinical Addison disease.
ACTH, adrenocorticotropic hormone; and N, normal.

decreased cortisol response after parenteral ACTH administration. Stage 3 involves elevated basal ACTH. Stage 4 involves low basal cortisol (Table 18-3).[87,88] In those individuals with adrenocortical autoantibodies, screening with mid-afternoon or later ACTH levels together with a supine renin should be carried out. Complete assessment of adrenocortical function should be carried out in those with ACTH levels >55 pg/mL or in those with elevated renins.

Treatment

Hormone replacement or other therapies for the component diseases of APS I and APS II are similar whether the ailments occur in isolation or in association with other conditions. Specific therapies are described in the individual chapters.

Genetics of APS I

For some time it had been recognized that APS I could be inherited in an autosomal-recessive fashion.[89] Unlike APS II, specific HLA alleles are not associated with APS I.[90] APS I was initially mapped to chromosome 21q22.1 in Finnish families, and the AIRE gene was subsequently cloned.[11] Individuals with APS I were found to be homozygous (possess two mutated copies) for the AIRE gene, with their parents being heterozygous for the mutated gene. AIRE is expressed in the thymus, lymph nodes, fetal liver, pancreas, adrenal cortex, and testes. The gene spans 11.9 kb and contains 14 exons. The predicted protein contains 545 amino acids.[12]

Initially, five AIRE mutations were described: one nonsense mutation and four frame-shift mutations.[11,90] Multiple shared and unique mutations in the gene have now been defined in Sardinians, Britains, Italians, Finns, Japanese, and North Americans.[37] Sequence analysis of the AIRE protein demonstrates that the predicted AIRE protein displays features common to other proteins that function as transcription factors (proteins that bind to the regulatory elements in the DNA regulatory region of genes).[3,91] Transcription factors act to modulate the rate of gene transcription, whereas regulatory elements include the promoter region, enhancers, silencers, and metabolic response units. Further understanding of the AIRE protein

function may provide fundamental insights into the nature of polyglandular and uniglandular autoimmunity.

With recognition that APS I can be predicted in families with an index case, the focus of future therapy should be on the diagnosis of affected individuals using direct AIRE gene analysis, prediction of disease using autoantibody measurements, functional assessment (described previously), and the treatment of physiologic deficits prior to their clinical expression. More than 50 different mutations in the AIRE gene have now been reported, and mutations can be confirmed in more than 95% of patients with clinical diagnoses of APS I.[36,92-94] Thus, screening for mutations in the AIRE gene can be considered if the diagnosis is unclear. Mutational analysis should be offered to siblings of affected children in order to determine carrier status and possibly to allow for the diagnosis of endocrinopathies before the onset of symptoms. Despite the availability of mutational analysis, more studies are needed to determine the relative sensitivity and cost effectiveness of mutational analysis screening versus primary antibody screening.

Genetics of APS II

Whereas APS I displays an autosomal-recessive Mendelian pattern of inheritance, APS II is not inherited as a single gene mutation. APS II is much more typical of other autoimmune endocrinopathies wherein cases occur sporadically or within families. Overall, patients with APS II have HLA associations similar to those of patients with type 1 diabetes—especially having increased frequencies of HLA-DR3 (DQB1*0201) and DR4 (DQB1*0302).[95] This is not surprising because type 1 diabetes, a frequent component of APS II, is strongly HLA associated. However, when patients with type 1 diabetes are removed from the APS II subject group the association between HLA-DR alleles and APS II disappears.

Thus, in the absence of type 1 diabetes HLA-DR is not a major locus for the development of APS II. Previous studies have shown not only that Addison disease and type 1 diabetes share the major risk DR3/DR4 genotype but that Addison disease is particularly associated with DRB1*0404 and DRB1*0301 haplotypes.[96] It is estimated that 1 in 20 patients with type 1 diabetes with this haplotype will have adrenal autoantibodies.[97,98] Another high-risk allele for Addison disease is DRB5 (DQB1*0301). Graves disease is more often associated with HLA-DR3 as opposed to Hashimoto thyroiditis, which is associated with HLA-DR4 or DR5.[99,100] Autoimmune hypoparathyroidism and mucocutaneous candidiasis do not display associations with specific HLA alleles.

Because the association of APS II with specific HLA alleles is only modest, other genes must be important in providing susceptibility. To identify non-HLA genes that influence susceptibility to APS II genome-wide scan or linkage studies are necessary. The G allele of the CTLA-4 exon 1 A/G diallelic polymorphism has been associated with Addison disease in APS II, and less strongly associated with isolated Addison disease.[101]

Autoantibodies in Autoimmune Polyglandular Syndromes

Autoantibodies are antibodies (predominantly IgG) that bind to self-antigens (e.g., autoantigens). Autoantibodies may be pathogenic, as observed in Graves disease or myasthenia gravis. In Graves disease, agonistic autoantibodies directed against the thyroid follicular cell TSH receptor stimulate overproduction of thyroid hormone—producing hyperthyroidism.[102] In myasthenia gravis, autoantibodies directed against the motor end plate acetylcholine receptor located on myocytes stimulate internalization of the acetylcholine receptor—producing weakness. Alternatively, autoantibodies may serve solely as serologic markers of autoimmunity—as in type 1 diabetes, in which islet cell cytoplasmic autoantibodies (ICA) and glutamic acid decarboxylase autoantibodies (GADA) are indicators of ongoing autoimmunity.[103,104]

Detection of autoantibodies in relation to autoimmune polyglandular syndromes serves several important functions. First, detection of autoantibodies implicates an autoimmune etiology as the cause of disease and allows a specific diagnosis to be established.[105] Second, autoantibody detection in asymptomatic individuals indicates an increased risk for the later development of clinical disease.[64] Third, the diagnosis of one autoimmune disease in an individual (or detection of predilection to one autoimmune disease by the presence of autoantibodies) suggests that this individual is at risk for associated autoimmune diseases.

ADRENAL CYTOPLASMIC AUTOANTIBODIES

Adrenal cytoplasmic autoantibodies (ACA) were first detected using a complement-fixation technique with saline extracts of adrenal tissue, and soon afterward by indirect immunofluorescence.[106] Usually, all layers of the adrenal cortex fluoresce—whereas the medulla does not usually fluoresce.[87] The microsomal localization of autoantigens has been confirmed using ultracentrifuged cellular components.[107] Other assays for adrenal autoantibodies include solid-phase radioimmunoassays and nonradioactive enzyme-linked immunoabsorbent assays.[88,108]

Up to 75 to 80% of new-onset subjects with Addison disease exhibit ACA.[87] In up to approximately half of

asymptomatic ACA-positive individuals, Addison disease develops in less than 3 years. In a follow-up of 20 ACA-positive children followed for up to 11 years, the cumulative risk for developing Addison disease was 100%.[87] ACA are also predictive of the development of Addison disease in adults, although less frequently than in children. Higher titers of ACA and complement-fixing ACA might be associated with an increased risk of displaying clinical disease.[109]

Autoantibodies to the surface of adrenal cortical cells have been described but are not detected routinely because of the difficulty in obtaining fresh human or animal adrenal tissue that can be used for such assays. However, almost 90% of individuals with Addison disease were reported to exhibit such autoantibodies.[110] ACA are detected in all forms of autoimmune Addison disease, be it isolated Addison disease or as part of APS I or APS II. As stated previously, subjects with other forms of organ-specific autoimmune disease exhibit increased frequencies of ACA. In such circumstances, ACA predict an increased risk for developing biochemical and clinical evidence of adrenal insufficiency.

ADRENAL ENZYME AUTOANTIBODIES

Typical of many organ-specific autoimmune diseases, major autoantigens that serve as targets of autoantibodies in the autoimmune polyglandular syndromes are enzymes. Such enzymes are typically expressed in the tissues that are being targeted for humoral and/or cell-mediated autoimmune attack. Examples of various autoimmune diseases where enzymes are targeted are outlined in Table 18-1. (Adrenal hormone synthesis is discussed in Chapter 12.)

21-hydroxylase (P450c21) is a major autoantigen recognized by sera from patients with Addison disease.[111] There is a strong correlation between positivity for ACA and P450c21 autoantibodies.[112] Other enzymes have been identified as autoantigens in patients with isolated autoimmune Addison disease or in patients with an autoimmune polyglandular syndrome, including P450 cholesterol side-chain cleavage enzyme (P450scc), 17α-hydroxylase (P450c17), and 3β-hydroxysteroid dehydrogenase (not a P450 enzyme).[112]

ADRENAL ENZYME AUTOANTIBODIES IN APS I

Although autoantibodies to P450c21 (21-hydroxylase), P450ssc (side-chain cleavage enzyme), and P450c17 (17α-hydroxylase) have been reported, autoantibodies to P450c21 are most commonly identified in patients with adrenal autoimmunity. Nearly 75% of APS I and APS II patients reportedly have P450c21 autoantibodies present.[87] The autoantigenic epitopes of the P450c21 enzyme are located in the C-terminal end and in a central region of the enzyme.[113] Peterson et al. found that two of four epitopes recognized by P450c17 autoantibodies cross-reacted with P450c21, indicating that reactivity to one of these autoantigens could actually reflect molecular mimicry between such epitopes.[114] Except for the N-terminal amino acids 1-40 and the C-terminal amino acids 456 to 521, immunoreactive epitopes have been described throughout P450c21.[115]

Higher titers of ACA and higher concentrations of P450c21 autoantibodies appear to correlate with more severe impairment of adrenocortical function and the predicted development of Addison disease.[87] Autoantibody concentrations appear to rise until the development of clinical Addison disease, at which time autoantibody reactivity disappear. This is consistent with the concept that once an autoantigen is completely destroyed the immune system is no longer stimulated to produce autoantibodies—with autoantibody prevalence and concentration diminishing.

ADRENAL ENZYME AUTOANTIBODIES IN APS II

When clinical or preclinical Addison disease is present, there is no unique combination of adrenal or gonadal antibodies that separate APS I from APS II.[105,116,117] The differentiation of APS I from APS II is made on clinical grounds or by detecting an autoantibody characteristic of a nonadrenal APS II–associated autoimmune disease. Furthermore, there are no unique epitopes recognized by P450c21 autoantibodies that allow differentiation of Addison disease as to etiology (e.g., isolated autoimmune Addison disease versus APS I versus APS II) other than indicating that the disease is indeed autoimmune.[118]

Autoantibodies to P450c21, P450scc, and P450c17 are common in APS II. Most patients with APS I or II with Addison disease have autoantibodies to one or more of these enzymes, compared to less than 25% of APS patients without adrenal insufficiency.[119] In one study (using an immunoprecipitation assay with ^{125}I-labeled 21-hydroxylase) it was demonstrated that nearly all patients with Addison disease and APS II were positive for autoantibodies to P450c21—compared to 92% of patients with APS-I, 72% of patients with isolated Addison disease, and 80% of non-Addisonian patients who were ACA positive.[120] Technical differences in the performance of the various assays contribute to the differences in reported frequencies as well as the presence or absence of SCA.

ADRENAL ENZYME AUTOANTIBODIES IN ISOLATED ADDISON DISEASE

Autoantibodies to P450c21 are common in Addison disease patients, whether isolated or part of APS I or APS II, and are rare in the absence of Addison disease.[87,121] P450c21 appears to be the major adrenal autoantigen in cases of isolated Addison disease, being detected in nearly 75% of patients. Autoantibodies to P450scc and P450c17 have been reported but are less frequently found (<30%) than P450c21 antibodies.[112]

STEROIDAL CELL/GONADAL AUTOANTIBODIES

In some individuals with ACA, their sera has also been shown to react with reproductive-steroid-producing tissues such as the theca interna of the graffian follicle,

Leydig cells of the testis, and/or syncytiotrophoblastic layer of the placenta.[98,122] Sera that recognize antigens in adrenal and reproductive-steroid-producing tissues whose immunoreactivity cannot be absorbed with adrenal extracts are considered SCA. Sera may react to all tissues or to just one. The significance of whether a serum reacts with a single tissue or multiple tissues in defining SCA is unknown. Such variability may represent variations in the autoimmune epitopes recognized by the serum or differences in the tissue substrates relating to autoantigen densities or epitope availability.

SCA are associated with an increased risk of developing primary autoimmune gonadal failure that is expressed predominantly in women as either primary amenorrhea or premature menopause. Men are usually asymptomatic. When ACA are present in the absence of SCA, gonadal failure is unlikely to develop.[98] About a third of individuals with ACA upon initial screening using adrenal as the sole substrate have SCA using ovary, testis, or placenta as the antigen source. SCA can be observed in APS II patients, although gonaditis is more common in APS I than in APS II. It is estimated that 60% of subjects with APS I and Addison disease express SCA, versus 30% of subsets with APS II.

Primary hypogonadism can be observed in APS I or APS II manifesting as hypergonadotropic ovarian, or rarely as testicular failure. Premature ovarian failure independent of APS can also occur as a consequence of autoimmunity.[123] Nevertheless, Addison disease coexists in approximately 2% to 10% of women with ovarian failure.[124] Autoimmune ovarian failure is characterized histologically by ovarian infiltration with inflammatory cells.[125] Patients with isolated premature ovarian failure or premature ovarian failure associated with APS often express SCA. As early as 1968, SCA were described using indirect immunofluorescence.[126] Five of 5 women with SCA, all of whom also had ACA consistent with an autoimmune polyglandular syndrome, manifested ovarian failure. Autoantibodies reacting strongly to the pig zona pellucida as determined by indirect immunofluorescence were observed in 6 of 22 women with infertility.[127]

SCA, depending on the assay used, have been reported in 4% to 87% of women with premature ovarian failure.[122,128,129] SCA are also predictive of later gonadal failure in APS women with normal menses at the time of initial study. Ahonen et al. reported that 100% (11 of 11) of APS I patients who were positive for SCA developed primary ovarian failure during a follow-up period of up to 12 years.[130] The nature of the ovarian autoantigens in premature ovarian failure is controversial. Because the adrenal cortex and gonad share several synthetic pathways common to cells producing adrenocortical steroids and sex steroids, humoral autoimmunity to a shared autoantigen may be observed in adrenalitis and gonaditis.

The synthesis of sex and adrenal steroids requires P450scc, 3β-hydroxysteroid dehydrogenase, and P450c17. Therefore, it would be anticipated that these enzymes could also be autoantigens in some individuals with gonaditis. Data are however contradictory. In one study, SCA activity was removed by preabsorption with recombinant human 3β-hydroxysteroid dehydrogenase—suggesting that this enzyme was a major autoantigen detected by SCA-positive sera.[131] Another study suggested that SCA correlated best with reactivity to P450scc and a 51-kilodalton autoantigen that binds to the aromatic L-amino acid decarboxylase present in granulosa cells, placenta, liver, and pancreatic beta cells.[132]

In the absence of adrenal autoimmunity, autoantibodies to P450c21, P450c17, or P450scc are rarely found in women with premature ovarian failure.[122] This suggests that in the absence of APS few cases of idiopathic premature ovarian failure result from autoimmune damage to the ovary. In another study, no autoantibodies to P450c17 or P450scc in 48 women with isolated premature ovarian failure were identified—whereas only 2 of these women had SCA and only 1 had autoantibodies to 3β-hydroxysteroid dehydrogenase.[133] However, in another study autoantibodies to 3β-hydroxysteroid dehydrogenase were observed in women with premature ovarian failure who did not have coexistent autoimmune diseases.[134]

An alternative hypothesis attempting to explain premature ovarian failure is the potential existence of antagonist autoantibodies directed against the FSH or LH receptors. Support for this hypothesis is weak, however, because recent studies have not been able to confirm the presence of gonadotropin receptor autoantibodies in the sera of a large group of women with premature ovarian failure.[135]

AUTOANTIBODIES IN HYPOPARATHYROIDISM

Autoimmune hypoparathyroidism is a characteristic disorder essentially unique to APS I. Hypoparathyroidism is absent in subjects with APS II. In Blizzard's original report of parathyroid autoantibodies detected using indirect immunofluorescence, nearly 40% of patients with autoimmune hypoparathyroidism were found to have parathyroid cytoplasmic autoantibodies—versus 6% of controls.[136,137] However, other laboratories did not confirm the initial reports of such parathyroid cytoplasmic autoantibodies.[138,139] It was shown that autoantibodies detected by indirect immunofluoresence directed against the parathyroid gland could be preabsorbed with human mitochondria, indicating that such autoantibodies were not tissue specific.[139]

Autoantibodies have also been identified that are cytotoxic for cultured bovine parathyroid cells in patients with hypoparathyroidism.[140] These autoantibodies also bind to cultured bovine endothelial cells.[141] Unrelated to APS I or APS II, autoantibodies that bind to anti-PTH antibodies employed in a PTH immunoassay (e.g., anti-idiotypic PTH autoantibodies) have also been described in a patient with hypoparathyroidism.[142] More recently, autoantibodies to the extracellular domain of the calcium receptor have been described in patients with hypoparathyroidism.[143] Similarly, autoantibodies that block the calcium receptor have been described that cause hyperparathyroidism (e.g., autoimmune hypercalcemia).[144]

OTHER AUTOANTIBODIES IN APS I AND II

Autoantibodies to thyroid follicular cell organelles in autoimmune thyroid disease (e.g., thyroid microsomal autoantibodies), follicular cell enzymes (e.g., thyroperoxidase) and products (e.g., thyroglobulin), and autoantibodies to pancreatic beta cells in type 1 diabetes (e.g., islet cell cytoplasmic autoantibodies) and beta cell proteins (e.g., glutamic acid decarboxylase and insulinoma-associated antigen-2) and products (e.g., insulin and carboxypeptidase H) are well described in patients with autoimmune polyglandular syndromes. Their frequency is especially high in patients with APS II. However, the biology of these autoantibodies will not be reviewed here. (See the specific chapters that address autoimmune thyroid disease and type 1 diabetes.)

Celiac disease is accompanied by mucosal (especially) IgA autoantibodies to reticulin, endomysium, transglutaminase, and jejunum.[145] Retrospective studies show that tissue transglutaminase autoantibodies can provide 100% sensitivity and specificity for biopsy-proven celiac disease.[146] There is a high prevalence of various autoimmune disorders [including type 1 diabetes (6% of type 1 patients reportedly have antiendomyseal antibodies), autoimmune thyroiditis, dermatitis herpetiformis, autoimmune alopecia, autoimmune hepatitis, and collagen vascular diseases] in patients with celiac disease.[145] In one study, 3.6% of new-onset type 1 diabetes patients had celiac disease.[147]

Autoantibodies to tyrosine hydroxylase have been reported in ~40% of patients with APS I and correlate with alopecia areata.[148] Antibodies to liver/kidney microsome type 1 (LKM1) are found in nearly 100% of patients with type 2 autoimmune hepatitis.[149] Forty percent of such patients have associated autoimmune disease commonly seen in APS I. The hepatic autoantigens P450IA2 and P4502A6 have been reported as targets of these antibodies. Autoantibodies to aromatic L-amino acid decarboxylase have also been recognized in APS I and isolated cases of Addison disease.[132]

Autoantibodies to the adrenal medulla may also occur in various autoimmune conditions, but especially so in type 1 diabetes.[150,151] Adrenal-medullary autoimmunity has been linked to autonomic dysfunction in individuals with diabetes mellitus.[152] Pteridin-dependent hydroxylases have also been proposed as autoantigens in APS I.[153]

Summary

The autoimmune polyglandular syndromes result from a loss of tolerance to self-antigens. A thorough understanding of tolerance induction and defects in tolerance is required to fully understand the immunopathogenesis of APS. APS I, an autosomal-recessive disorder mapped to the AIRE gene, is defined by the presence of two of the following: adrenocortical autoimmunity, hypoparathyroidism, and mucocutaneous candidiasis. APS II is defined by the coexistence of autoimmune adrenocortical insufficiency or serologic evidence of adrenalitis with autoimmune thyroiditis and/or type 1 diabetes mellitus.

The occurrence of any component disease of an APS may be linked to the occurrence of others through shared autoimmunity background genes that lead to a loss of tolerance. As such, a high index of suspicion should be maintained whenever one autoimmune disorder is diagnosed. For example, in type 1 diabetes it is routine to screen for thyroid autoimmunity and celiac disease.

Treatment of APS should be aimed at optimal management of the specific underlying diseases. Screening for the presence of associated autoimmune disorders should be performed regularly. An improved understanding of the interaction among susceptibility genes, environmental triggers, and the development of impaired immune tolerance should prove to be the best path to improved diagnostic and therapeutic modalities in the care of patients with APS.

REFERENCES

1. Ballotti S, Chiarelli F, de Martino M (2006). Autoimmunity: Basic mechanisms and implications in endocrine diseases, Part II. Horm Res 66:142–152.
2. Ballotti S, Chiarelli F, de Martino M (2006). Autoimmunity: basic mechanisms and implications in endocrine diseases, Part I. Horm Res 66:132–141.
3. Anderson MS, Venanzi ES, Klein L, Chen Z, Berzins SP, Turley SJ (2002). Projection of an immunological self shadow within the thymus by the AIRE protein. Science 298:1395–1401.
4. Delves PJ, Roitt IM (2000). The immune system. N Engl J Med 343:37–49.
5. Unanue ER (2002). Perspective on antigen processing and presentation. Immunological Reviews 185:86–102.
6. Cresswell P, Ackerman AL, Giodini A, Peaper DR, Wearsch PA (2005). Mechanisms of MHC class I-restricted antigen processing and cross-presentation. Immunol Rev 207:145–157.
7. Holling TM, Schooten E, van Den Elsen PJ (2004). Function and regulation of MHC class II molecules in T-lymphocytes: Of mice and men. Human Immunology 65:282–290.
8. Mathis D, Benoist C (2004). Back to central tolerance. Immunity 20:509–516.
9. Kyewski B, Derbinski J, Gotter J, Klein L (2002). Promiscuous gene expression and central T-cell tolerance: More than meets the eye. Trends Immunol 23:364–371.
10. Anderson MS, Venanzi ES, Chen Z, Berzins SP, Benoist C, Mathis D (2005). The cellular mechanism of Aire control of T cell tolerance. Immunity 23:227–239.
11. Nagamine K, Peterson P, Scott HS, Kudoh J, Minoshima S, Heino M, et al. (1997). Positional cloning of the APECED gene. Nat Genet 17:393–398.
12. The Finnish-German APECED Consortium (1997). An autoimmune disease, APECED, caused by mutations in a novel gene featuring two PHD-type zinc-finger domains: Autoimmune Polyendocrinopathy-Candidiasis-Ectodermal Dystrophy. Nat Genet 17:399–403.
13. von Boehmer H, Aifantis I, Gounari F, Azogui O, Haughn L, Apostolou I, et al. (2003). Thymic selection revisited: How essential is it? Immunol Rev 191:62–78.
14. von Boehmer H, Kisielow P (1990). Self-nonself discrimination by T cells. Science 248:1369–1373.
15. Ramsdell F, Fowlkes BJ (1990). Clonal deletion versus clonal anergy: The role of the thymus in inducing self tolerance. Science 248:1342–1348.
16. Delves PJ, Roitt IM (2000). The immune system. N Engl J Med 343:108–117.
17. Abbas AK, Murphy KM, Sher A (1996). Functional diversity of helper T lymphocytes. Nature 383:787–793.
18. Lan RY, Ansari AA, Lian ZX, Gershwin ME (2005). Regulatory T cells: Development, function and role in autoimmunity. Autoimmun Rev 4:351–363.
19. Ziegler SF (2006). FOXP3: Of Mice and Men. Annu Rev Immunol 24:209–226.
20. Kyewski B, Klein L (2006). A central role for central tolerance. Annu Rev Immunol 24:571–606.
21. Kyewski B, Derbinski J (2004). Self-representation in the thymus: an extended view. Nat Rev Immunol 4:688–698.
22. Chiovato L, Latrofa F, Braverman LE, Pacini F, Capezzone M, Masserini L, et al. (2003). Disappearance of humoral thyroid autoimmunity after complete removal of thyroid antigens. Ann Intern Med 139:346–351.

23. Pisetsky DS (2006). Fulfilling Koch's postulates of autoimmunity: Anti-NR2 antibodies in mice and men. Arthritis & Rheumatism 54:2349–2352.
24. Goodnow CC, Sprent J, de St Groth BF, Vinuesa CG (2005). Cellular and genetic mechanisms of self tolerance and autoimmunity. 435:590–597.
25. Viret C, Sant'Angelo DB, He X, Ramaswamy H, Janeway CA Jr. (2001). A role for accessibility to self-peptide-self-MHC complexes in intrathymic negative selection. J Immunol 166:4429–4437.
26. Vafiadis P, Ounissi-Benkalha H, Palumbo M, Grabs R, Rousseau M, Goodyer CG, et al. (2001). Class III alleles of the variable number of tandem repeat insulin polymorphism associated with silencing of thymic insulin predispose to type 1 diabetes. J Clin Endocrinol Metab 86:3705–3710.
27. Cohen IR (2001). Antigenic mimicry, clonal selection and autoimmunity. Journal of Autoimmunity 16:337–340.
28. Damico FM, Kiss S, Young LH (2005). Sympathetic ophthalmia. Semin Ophthalmol 20:191–197.
29. Zhang M, Alicot EM, Chiu I, Li J, Verna N, Vorup-Jensen T, et al. (2006). Identification of the target self-antigens in reperfusion injury. J Exp Med 203:141–152.
30. Soulas P, Woods A, Jaulhac B, Knapp A-M, Pasquali J-L, Martin T, et al. (2005). Autoantigen, innate immunity, and T cells cooperate to break B cell tolerance during bacterial infection. J Clin Invest 115:2257–2267.
31. Olson JK, Croxford JL, Miller SD (2001). Virus-induced autoimmunity: Potential role of viruses in initiation, perpetuation, and progression of T-cell-mediated autoimmune disease. Viral Immunol 14:227–250.
32. Ziegler A-G, Schmid S, Huber D, Hummel M, Bonifacio E (2003). Early infant feeding and risk of developing type 1 diabetes-associated autoantibodies. JAMA 290:1721–1728.
33. McKay DM (2001). Bacterial superantigens: Provocateurs of gut dysfunction and inflammation? Trends in Immunology 22:497–501.
34. Tait KF, Gough SCL (2003). The genetics of autoimmune endocrine disease. Clinical Endocrinology 59:1–11.
35. Perheentupa J (2006). Autoimmune polyendocrinopathy-candidiasis-ectodermal dystrophy. J Clin Endocrinol Metab 91:2843–2850.
36. Buzi F, Badolato R, Mazza C, Giliani S, Notarangelo LD, Radetti G, et al. (2003). Autoimmune polyendocrinopathy-candidiasis-ectodermal dystrophysyndrome: Time to review diagnostic criteria? J Clin Endocrinol Metab 88:3146–3148.
37. Peterson P, Peltonen L (2005). Autoimmune polyendocrinopathy syndrome type 1 (APS1) and AIRE gene: New views on molecular basis of autoimmunity. Journal of Autoimmunity 25:49–55.
38. Schmidt M (1926). Eine biglandulare Erkrankung (Nebennieren und Schilddrusse) bei Morbus Addisonii. Verh Dtsch Ges Pathol Ges 21:212–221.
39. Carpenter CC, Solomon N, Silverberg SG, Bledsoe T, Northcutt RC, Klinenberg JR, et al. (1964). Schmidt's syndrome: Thyroid and adrenal insufficiency, A review of the literature and a report of fifteen new cases including ten instances of coexistent diabetes mellitus. Medicine (Baltimore) 43:153–180.
40. Eisenbarth GS, Gottlieb PA (2004). Autoimmune polyendocrine syndromes. N Engl J Med 350:2068–2079.
41. Betterle C, Dal Pra C, Mantero F, Zanchetta R (2002). Autoimmune adrenal insufficiency and autoimmune polyendocrine syndromes: Autoantibodies, autoantigens, and their applicability in diagnosis and disease prediction. Endocr Rev 23:327–364.
42. Kumar PG, Laloraya M, Wang CY, Ruan QG, Davoodi-Semiromi A, Kao KJ, et al. (2001). The autoimmune regulator (AIRE) is a DNA-binding protein. J Biol Chem 276:41357–41364.
43. Ahonen P, Myllarniemi S, Sipila I, Perheentupa J (1990). Clinical variation of autoimmune polyendocrinopathy-candidiasis-ectodermal dystrophy (APECED) in a series of 68 patients. N Engl J Med 322:1829–1836.
44. Maclaren N, Chen Q-Y, Kukreja A, Marker J, Zhang CH, Sun ZS (2001). Autoimmune hypogonadism as part of an autoimmune polyglandular syndrome. Journal of the Society for Gynecologic Investigation 8:S52–S54.
45. Gazulla Abio J, Benavente Aguilar I, Ricoy Campo JR, Madero Barrajon P (2005). Myopathy with trabecular fibers associated with familiar autoimmune polyglandular syndrome type 1. Neurologia 20:702–708.

46. Doniach D, Roitt IM (1957). Auto-immunity in Hashimoto's disease and its implications. J Clin Endocrinol Metab 17:1293–1304.

47. Betterle C, Lazzarotto F, Presotto F (2004). Autoimmune polyglandular syndrome Type 2: The tip of an iceberg? Clin Exp Immunol 137:225–233.

48. Hugle B, Dollmann R, Keller E, Kiess W (2004). Addison's crisis in adolescent patients with previously diagnosed diabetes mellitus as manifestation of polyglandular autoimmune syndrome type II: Report of two patients. J Pediatr Endocrinol Metab 17:93–97.

49. Hollowell JG, Staehling NW, Flanders WD, Hannon WH, Gunter EW, Spencer CA, et al. (2002). Serum TSH, T4, and Thyroid Antibodies in the United States Population (1988 to 1994): National Health and Nutrition Examination Survey (NHANES III). J Clin Endocrinol Metab 87:489–499.

50. Jaeger C, Hatziagelaki E, Petzoldt R, Bretzel RG (2001). Comparative analysis of organ-specific autoantibodies and celiac disease: Associated antibodies in type 1 diabetic patients, their first-degree relatives, and healthy control subjects. Diabetes 24:27–32.

51. Kordonouri O, Klinghammer A, Lang EB, Gruters-Kieslich A, Grabert M, Holl RW (2002). Thyroid autoimmunity in children and adolescents with type 1 diabetes: A multicenter survey. Diabetes Care 25:1346–1350.

52. Alkhateeb A, Fain PR, Thody A, Bennett DC, Spritz RA (2003). Epidemiology of vitiligo and associated autoimmune diseases in Caucasian probands and their families. Pigment Cell Research 16:208–214.

53. Ruggeri RM, Galletti M, Mandolfino MG, Aragona P, Bartolone S, Giorgianni G, et al. (2002). Thyroid hormone autoantibodies in primary Sjögren syndrome and rheumatoid arthritis are more prevalent than in autoimmune thyroid disease, becoming progressively more frequent in these diseases. J Endocrinol Invest 25:447–454.

54. Tsao CY, Mendell JR, Lo WD, Luquette M, Rennebohm R (2000). Myasthenia gravis and associated autoimmune diseases in children. J Child Neurol 15:767–769.

55. Zettinig G, Tanew A, Fischer G, Mayr W, Dudczak R, Weissel M (2003). Autoimmune diseases in vitiligo: Do anti-nuclear antibodies decrease thyroid volume? Clinical and Experimental Immunology 131:347–354.

56. Kakourou T, Kanaka-Gantenbein C, Papadopoulou A, Kaloumenou E, Chrousos GP (2005). Increased prevalence of chronic autoimmune (Hashimoto's) thyroiditis in children and adolescents with vitiligo. Journal of the American Academy of Dermatology 53:220–223.

57. Hann SK, Lee HJ (1996). Segmental vitiligo: Clinical findings in 208 patients. J Am Acad Dermatol 35:671–674.

58. Tanwani LK, Lohano V, Ewart R, Broadstone VL, Mokshagundam SP (2001). Myasthenia gravis in conjunction with Graves' disease: A diagnostic challenge. Endocr Pract 7:275–278.

59. Weetman AP (2005). Non-thyroid autoantibodies in autoimmune thyroid disease. Best practice and research. Clinical Endocrinology and Metabolism Autoimmune Endocrine Disorders 19:17–32.

60. Karvonen M, Viik-Kajander M, Moltchanova E, Libman I, LaPorte R, Tuomilehto J for the Diabetes Mondiale (DiaMond) Project Group (2000). Incidence of childhood type 1 diabetes worldwide. Diabetes Care 23:1516–1526.

61. Stenstrom G, Gottsater A, Bakhtadze E, Berger B, Sundkvist G (2005). Latent autoimmune diabetes in adults: Definition, prevalence, beta-cell function, and treatment. Diabetes 54:S68–S72.

62. Alonso N, Granada ML, Salinas I, Lucas AM, Reverter JL, Junca J, et al. (2005). Serum pepsinogen I: An early marker of pernicious anemia in patients with type 1 diabetes. J Clin Endocrinol Metab 90:5254–5258.

63. Segni M, Borrelli O, Pucarelli I, Delle Fave G, Pasquino AM, Annibale B (2004). Early manifestations of gastric autoimmunity in patients with juvenile autoimmune thyroid diseases. J Clin Endocrinol Metab 89:4944–4948.

64. Barker JM (2006). Type 1 diabetes-associated autoimmunity: Natural history, genetic associations, and screening. J Clin Endocrinol Metab 91:1210–1217.

65. Barker JM, Ide A, Hostetler C, Yu L, Miao D, Fain PR, et al. (2005). Endocrine and immunogenetic testing in individuals with type 1 diabetes and 21-hydroxylase autoantibodies: Addison's disease in a high-risk population. J Clin Endocrinol Metab 90:128–134.

66. Hansson T, Dahlbom I, Rogberg S, Dannaeus A, Hopfl P, Gut H, et al. (2002). Recombinant human tissue transglutaminase for diagnosis and follow-up of childhood coeliac disease. Pediatr Res 51:700–705.

67. Smith CM, Clarke CF, Porteous LE, Elsori H, Cameron DJ (2000). Prevalence of coeliac disease and longitudinal follow-up of anti-gliadin antibody status in children and adolescents with type 1 diabetes mellitus. Pediatric Diabetes 1:199–203.

68. Not T, Tommasini A, Tonini G, Buratti E, Pocecco M, Tortul C, et al. (2001). Undiagnosed coeliac disease and risk of autoimmune disorders in subjects with Type I diabetes mellitus. Diabetologia 44:151–155.

69. Welt CK, Falorni A, Taylor AE, Martin KA, Hall JE (2005). Selective theca cell dysfunction in autoimmune oophoritis results in multi-follicular development, decreased estradiol, and elevated inhibin B levels. J Clin Endocrinol Metab 90:3069–3076.

70. Cemeroglu AP, Bober E, Dundar B, Buyukgebiz A (2001). Autoimmune polyglandular endocrinopathy and anterior hypophysitis in a 14 year-old girl presenting with delayed puberty. J Pediatr Endocrinol Metab 14:909–914.

71. Zung A, Andrews-Murray G, Winqvist O, Chalew SA (1997). Growth hormone deficiency in autoimmune polyglandular syndrome. J Pediatr Endocrinol Metab 10:69–72.

72. Govindarajan R, Galpin OP (1992). Coexistence of Addison's disease, ulcerative colitis, hypothyroidism and pernicious anemia. J Clin Gastroenterol 15:82–83.

73. Ko GT, Szeto CC, Yeung VT, Chow CC, Chan H, Cockram CS (1996). Autoimmune polyglandular syndrome and primary biliary cirrhosis. Br J Clin Pract 50:344–346.

74. Papadopoulos KI, Hornblad Y, Liljebladh H, Hallengren B (1996). High frequency of endocrine autoimmunity in patients with sarcoidosis. Eur J Endocrinol 134:331–336.

75. Watson JP, Lewis RA (1996). Schmidt's syndrome associated with sarcoidosis. Postgrad Med J 72:435–436.

76. Fritzen R, Bornstein SR, Scherbaum WA (1996). Megaoesophagus in a patient with autoimmune polyglandular syndrome type II. Clin Endocrinol 45:493–498.

77. Heuss D, Engelhardt A, Gobel H, Neundorfer B (1995). Myopathological findings in interstitial myositis in type II polyendocrine autoimmune syndrome (Schmidt's syndrome). Neurol Res 17:233–237.

78. Watkins PJ, Gayle C, Alsanjari N, Scaravilli F, Zanone M, Thomas PK (1995). Severe sensory-autonomic neuropathy and endocrinopathy in insulin-dependent diabetes. QJM 88:795–804.

79. Wildin RS, Freitas A (2005). IPEX and FOXP3: Clinical and research perspectives. Journal of Autoimmunity 25:56–62.

80. Bennett CL, Christie J, Ramsdell F, Brunkow ME, Ferguson PJ, Whitesell L, et al. (2001). The immune dysregulation, polyendocrinopathy, enteropathy, X-linked syndrome (IPEX) is caused by mutations of FOXP3. Nat Genet 27:20–21.

81. Wildin RS, Ramsdell F, Peake J, Faravelli F, Casanova JL, Buist N, et al. (2001). X-linked neonatal diabetes mellitus, enteropathy and endocrinopathy syndrome is the human equivalent of mouse scurfy. Nat Genet 27:18–20.

82. Zavattari P, Deidda E, Pitzalis M, Zoa B, Moi L, Lampis R, et al. (2004). No association between variation of the FOXP3 gene and common type 1 diabetes in the Sardinian population. Diabetes 53:1911–1914.

83. Hori S, Nomura T, Sakaguchi S (2003). Control of regulatory T cell development by the transcription factor FoxP3. Science 299:1057–1061.

84. Hori S, Takahashi T, Sakaguchi S (2003). Control of autoimmunity by naturally arising regulatory CD4+ T cells. Adv Immunol 81:331–371.

85. Bright GM, Blizzard RM, Kaiser DL, Clarke WL (1982). Organ-specific autoantibodies in children with common endocrine diseases. J Pediatr 100:8–14.

86. Elin RJ, Winter WE (2001). Methylmalonic acid: A test whose time has come? Arch Pathol Lab Med 125:824–827.

87. Coco G, Dal Pra C, Presotto F, Albergoni MP, Canova C, Pedini B, et al. (2006). Estimated risk for developing autoimmune Addison's Disease in Patients with Adrenal Cortex Autoantibodies. J Clin Endocrinol Metab 91:1637–1645, 2006.

88. Betterle C, Coco G, Zanchetta R (2005). Adrenal cortex autoantibodies in subjects with normal adrenal function. Best Practice & Research Clinical Endocrinology & Metabolism Autoimmune Endocrine Disorders 19:85–99.

89. Ahonen P (1985). Autoimmune polyendocrinopathy-candidosis-ectodermal dystrophy (APECED): Autosomal recessive inheritance. Clin Genet 27:535–542.

90. Aaltonen J, Bjorses P, Sandkuijl L, Perheentupa J, Peltonen L (1994). An autosomal locus causing autoimmune disease: Autoimmune polyglandular disease type I assigned to chromosome 21. Nat Genet 8:83–87.

91. Zuklys S, Balciunaite G, Agarwal A, Fasler-Kan E, Palmer E, Hollander GA (2000). Normal thymic architecture and negative selection are associated with AIRE expression, the gene defective in the autoimmune-polyendocrinopathy-candidiasis-ectodermal dystrophy (APECED). J Immunol 165:1976–1983.

92. Trebusak Podkrajsek K, Bratanic N, Krzisnik C, Battelino T (2005). Autoimmune regulator-1 messenger ribonucleic acid analysis in a novel intronic mutation and two additional novel AIRE gene mutations in a cohort of autoimmune polyendocrinopathy-candidiasis-ectodermal dystrophy patients. J Clin Endocrinol Metab 90:4930–4935.

93. Meloni EF, Corda D, Perniola R, Cao A, Rosatelli MC (2005). Two novel mutations of the AIRE protein affecting its homodimerization properties. Human Mutation 25:319.

94. Ulinski T, Perrin L, Morris M, Houang M, Cabrol S, Grapin C, et al. (2006). Autoimmune polyendocrinopathy-candidiasis-ectodermal dystrophy syndrome with renal failure: Impact of posttransplant immunosuppression on disease activity. J Clin Endocrinol Metab 91:192–195.

95. Wallaschofski H, Meyer A, Tuschy U, Lohmann T (2003). HLA-DQA1*0301-associated susceptibility for autoimmune polyglandular syndrome type II and III. Horm Metab Res 35:120–124.

96. Robles DT, Fain PR, Gottlieb PA, Eisenbarth GS (2002). The genetics of autoimmune polyendocrine syndrome type II. Endocrinol Metab Clin North Am 31:353–368.

97. Brewer KW, Parziale VS, Eisenbarth GS (1997). Screening patients with insulin-dependent diabetes mellitus for adrenal insufficiency. N Engl J Med 337:202.

98. Myhre AG, Undlien DE, Lovas K, Uhlving S, Nedrebo BG, Fougner KJ, et al. (2002). Autoimmune adrenocortical failure in Norway autoantibodies and human leukocyte antigen class II associations related to clinical features. J Clin Endocrinol Metab 87:618–623.

99. Hunt PJ, Marshall SE, Weetman AP, Bunce M, Bell JI, Wass JAH, et al. (2001). Histocompatibility leucocyte antigens and closely linked immunomodulatory genes in autoimmune thyroid disease. Clinical Endocrinology 55:491–499.

100. Levin L, Ban Y, Concepcion E, Davies TF, Greenberg DA, Tomer Y (2004). Analysis of HLA genes in families with autoimmune diabetes and thyroiditis. Human Immunology 65:640–647.

101. Vaidya B, Imrie H, Geatch DR, Perros P, Ball SG, Baylis PH, et al. (2000). Association analysis of the cytotoxic T lymphocyte antigen-4 (CTLA-4) and autoimmune regulator-1 (AIRE-1) genes in sporadic autoimmune Addison's disease. J Clin Endocrinol Metab 85:688–691.

102. Schott M, Minich WB, Willenberg HS, Papewalis C, Seissler J, Feldkamp J, et al. (2005). Relevance of TSH receptor stimulating and blocking autoantibody measurement for the prediction of relapse in Graves' disease. Hormone and Metabolic Research 741–744.

103. Winter WE, Harris N, Schatz D (2002). Immunological markers in the diagnosis and prediction of autoimmune type 1a diabetes. Clin Diabetes 20:183–191.

104. Winter WE, Harris N, Schatz D (2002). Type 1 diabetes islet autoantibody markers. Diabetes Technol Ther 4:817–839.

105. Soderbergh A, Myhre AG, Ekwall O, Gebre-Medhin G, Hedstrand H, Landgren E, et al. (2004). Prevalence and clinical associations of 10 defined autoantibodies in autoimmune polyendocrine syndrome type I. J Clin Endocrinol Metab 89:557–562.

106. Blizzard RM, Kyle M (1963). Studies of the adrenal antigens and antibodies in Addison's disease. J Clin Invest 42:1653–1660.

107. Drexhage HA, Bottazzo GF, Bitensky L, Chayen J, Doniach D (1981). Thyroid growth-blocking antibodies in primary myxoedema. Nature 289:594–596.

108. Betterle C, Volpato M, Pedini B, Chen S, Rees Smith B, Furmaniak J (1999). Adrenal-cortex autoantibodies and steroid-producing cells autoantibodies in patients with Addison's disease: Comparison of immunofluorescence and immunoprecipitation assays. J Clin Endocrinol Metab 84:618–622.

109. Betterle C, Volpato M, Smith BR, Furmaniak J, Chen S, Greggio NA, et al. (1997). Adrenal cortex and steroid 21-hydroxylase autoantibodies in adult patients with organ-specific autoimmune diseases: Markers of low progression to clinical Addison's disease. J Clin Endocrinol Metab 82:932–938.

110. Khoury EL, Hammond L, Bottazzo GF, Doniach D (1981). Surface-reactive antibodies to human adrenal cells in Addison's disease. Clin Exp Immunol 45:48–55.

111. Husebye ES, Bratland E, Bredholt G, Fridkin M, Dayan M, Mozes E (2006). The substrate-binding domain of 21-hydroxylase, the main autoantigen in autoimmune Addison's disease, is an immunodominant T cell epitope. Endocrinology 147:2411–2416.

112. de Carmo Silva R, Kater C, Dib S, Laureti S, Forini F, Cosentino A, et al. (2000). Autoantibodies against recombinant human steroidogenic enzymes 21-hydroxylase, side-chain cleavage and 17alpha-hydroxylase in Addison's disease and autoimmune polyendocrine syndrome type III. Eur J Endocrinol 142:187–194.

113. Nikoshkov A, Falorni A, Lajic S, Laureti S, Wedell A, Lernmark K, et al. (1999). A conformation-dependent epitope in Addison's disease and other endocrinological autoimmune diseases maps to a carboxyl-terminal functional domain of human steroid 21-hydroxylase. J Immunol 162:2422–2426.

114. Peterson P, Krohn KJ (1994). Mapping of B cell epitopes on steroid 17 alpha-hydroxylase, an autoantigen in autoimmune polyglandular syndrome type I. Clin Exp Immunol 98:104–109.

115. Liiv I, Teesalu K, Peterson P, Clemente M, Perheentupa J, Uibo R (2002). Epitope mapping of cytochrome P450 cholesterol side-chain cleavage enzyme by sera from patients with autoimmune polyglandular syndrome type 1. Eur J Endocrinol 146:113–119.

116. Falorni A, Laureti S, Santeusanio F (2002). Autoantibodies in autoimmune polyendocrine syndrome type II. Endocrinol Metab Clin North Am 31:369–389.

117. Betterle C, Lazzarotto F, Presotto F (2004). Autoimmune polyglandular syndrome type 2: The tip of an iceberg? Clinical and Experimental Immunology 137:225–233.

118. Nikoshkov A, Falorni A, Lajic S, Laureti S, Wedell A, Lernmark A, et al. (1999). A conformation-dependent epitope in Addison;s disease and other endocrinological autoimmune diseases maps to a carboxyl-terminal functional domain of human steroid 21-hydroxylase. J Immunol 162:2422–2426.

119. Uibo R, Perheentupa J, Ovod V, Krohn KJ (1994). Characterization of adrenal autoantigens recognized by sera from patients with autoimmune polyglandular syndrome (APS) type I. J Autoimmun 7:399–411.

120. Tanaka H, Perez MS, Powell M, Sanders JF, Sawicka J, Chen S, et al. (1997). Steroid 21-hydroxylase autoantibodies: Measurements with a new immunoprecipitation assay. J Clin Endocrinol Metab 82:1440–1446.

121. Boe A, Bredholt G, Knappskog P, Hjelmervik T, Mellgren G, Winqvist O, et al. (2004). Autoantibodies against 21-hydroxylase and side-chain cleavage enzyme in autoimmune Addison's disease are mainly immunoglobulin G1. Eur J Endocrinol 150:49–56.

122. Dal Pra C, Chen S, Furmaniak J, Smith B, Pedini B, Moscon A, et al. (2003). Autoantibodies to steroidogenic enzymes in patients with premature ovarian failure with and without Addison's disease. Eur J Endocrinol 148:565–570.

123. Goswami D, Conway GS (2005). Premature ovarian failure. Hum Reprod Update 11:391–410.

124. Bakalov VK, Vanderhoof VH, Bondy CA, Nelson LM (2002). Adrenal antibodies detect asymptomatic auto-immune adrenal insufficiency in young women with spontaneous premature ovarian failure. Hum Reprod 17:2096–2100.

125. Santoro N (2001). Research on the mechanisms of premature ovarian failure. Journal of the Society for Gynecologic Investigation 8:S10–S12.

126. Irvine WJ, Chan MM, Scarth L, Kolb FO, Hartog M, Bayliss RI, et al. (1968). Immunological aspects of premature ovarian failure associated with idiopathic Addison's disease. Lancet 2:883–887.

127. Shivers CA, Dunbar BS (1977). Autoantibodies to zona pellucida: A possible cause for infertility in women. Science 197:1082–1084.

128. Falorni A, Laureti S, Candeloro P, Perrino S, Coronella C, Bizzarro A, et al. (2002). Steroid-cell autoantibodies are preferentially expressed in women with premature ovarian failure who have adrenal autoimmunity. Fertility and Sterility 78:270–279.

129. Reimand K, Peterson P, Hyoty H, Uibo R, Cooke I, Weetman AP, et al. (2000). 3β-hydroxysteroid dehydrogenase autoantibodies are rare in premature ovarian failure. J Clin Endocrinol Metab 85:2324–2326.

130. Ahonen P, Miettinen A, Perheentupa J (1987). Adrenal and steroidal cell antibodies in patients with autoimmune polyglandular disease type I and risk of adrenocortical and ovarian failure. J Clin Endocrinol Metab 64:494–500.

131. Uibo R, Aavik E, Peterson P, Perheentupa J, Aranko S, Pelkonen R, et al. (1994). Autoantibodies to cytochrome P450 enzymes P450scc, P450c17, and P450c21 in autoimmune polyglandular disease types I and II and in isolated Addison's disease. J Clin Endocrinol Metab 78:323–328.

132. Soderbergh A, Rorsman F, Halonen M, Ekwall O, Bjorses P, Kampe O, et al. (2000). Autoantibodies against aromatic L-amino acid decarboxylase identifies a subgroup of patients with Addison;s disease. J Clin Endocrinol Metab 85:460–463.

133. Reimand K, Peterson P, Hyoty H, Uibo R, Cooke I, Weetman AP, et al. (2000). 3beta-hydroxysteroid dehydrogenase autoantibodies are rare in premature ovarian failure. J Clin Endocrinol Metab 85:2324–2326.

134. Arif S, Vallian S, Farzaneh F, Zanone MM, James SL, Pietropaolo M, et al. (1996). Identification of 3 beta-hydroxysteroid dehydrogenase as a novel target of steroid cell autoantibodies: Association of autoantibodies with endocrine autoimmune disease. J Clin Endocrinol Metab 81:4439–4445.

135. Tonacchera M, Ferrarini E, Dimida A, Agretti P, De Marco G, De Servi M, et al. (2004). Gonadotrophin receptor blocking antibodies measured by the use of cell lines stably expressing human gonadotrophin receptors are not detectable in women with 46,XX premature ovarian failure. Clinical Endocrinology 61:376–381.

136. Blizzard RM, Chee D, Davis W (1966). The incidence of parathyroid and other antibodies in the sera of patients with idiopathic hypoparathyroidism. Clin Exp Immunol 1:119–128.

137. Irvine WJ, Scarth L (1969). Antibody to the oxyphil cells of the human parathyroid in idiopathic hypoparathyroidism. Clin Exp Immunol 4:505–510.

138. Chapman CK, Bradwell AR, Dykks PW (1986). Do parathyroid and adrenal autoantibodies coexist? J Clin Pathol 39:813–814.

139. Betterle C, Caretto A, Zeviani M, Pedini B, Salviati C (1985). Demonstration and characterization of anti-human mitochondria autoantibodies in idiopathic hypoparathyroidism and in other conditions. Clin Exp Immunol 62:353–360.

140. Brandi ML, Aurbach GD, Fattorossi A, Quarto R, Marx SJ, Fitzpatrick LA (1986). Antibodies cytotoxic to bovine parathyroid cells in autoimmune hypoparathyroidism. Proc Natl Acad Sci USA 83:8366–8369.

141. Fattorossi A, Aurbach GD, Sakaguchi K, Cama A, Marx SJ, Streeten EA, et al. (1988). Anti-endothelial cell antibodies: detection and characterization in sera from patients with autoimmune hypoparathyroidism. Proc Natl Acad Sci USA 85:4015–4019.

142. McElduff A, Lackmann M, Wilkinson M (1992). Antiidiotypic PTH antibodies as a cause of elevated immunoreactive parathyroid hormone in idiopathic hypoparathyroidism, a second case: Another manifestation of autoimmune endocrine disease? Calcif Tissue Int 51:121–126.

143. Kifor O, McElduff A, LeBoff MS, Moore FD Jr., Butters R, Gao P, et al. (2004). Activating antibodies to the calcium-sensing receptor in two patients with autoimmune hypoparathyroidism. J Clin Endocrinol Metab 89:548–556.

144. Kifor O, Moore FD Jr., Delaney M, Garber J, Hendy GN, Butters R, et al. (2003). A syndrome of hypocalciuric hypercalcemia caused by autoantibodies directed at the calcium-sensing receptor. J Clin Endocrinol Metab 88:60–72.

145. Schuppan D (2000). Current concepts of celiac disease pathogenesis. Gastroenterology 119:234–242.

146. Nemec G, Ventura A, Stefano M, Leo GD, Baldas V, Tommasini A, et al. (2006). Looking for celiac disease: Diagnostic accuracy of two rapid commercial assays. The American Journal of Gastroenterology 101:1597–1600.

147. Barera G, Bonfanti R, Viscardi M, Bazzigaluppi E, Calori G, Meschi F, et al. (2002). Occurrence of celiac disease after onset of type 1 diabetes: A 6-year prospective longitudinal study. Pediatrics 109:833–838.

148. Hedstrand H, Ekwall O, Haavik J, Landgren E, Betterle C, Perheentupa J, et al. (2000). Identification of tyrosine hydroxylase as an autoantigen in autoimmune polyendocrine syndrome type I. Biochem Biophys Res Commun 267:456–461.

149. Diamantis I, Boumpas DT (2004). Autoimmune hepatitis: Evolving concepts. Autoimmunity Reviews 3:207–214.

150. Ejskjaer N, Arif S, Dodds W, Zanone MM, Vergani D, Watkins PJ, et al. (1999). Prevalence of autoantibodies to autonomic nervous tissue structures in type 1 diabetes mellitus. Diabet Med 16:544–549.

151. Brown FM, Kamalesh M, Adri MN, Rabinowe SL (1988). Anti-adrenal medullary antibodies in IDDM subjects and subjects at high risk of developing IDDM. Diabetes Care 11:30–33.

152. Granberg V, Ejskjaer N, Peakman M, Sundkvist G (2005). Autoantibodies to autonomic nerves associated with cardiac and peripheral autonomic neuropathy. Diabetes Care 28:1959–1964.

153. Ekwall O, Hedstrand H, Haavik J, Perheentupa J, Betterle C, Gustafsson J, et al. (2000). Pteridin-dependent hydroxylases as autoantigens in autoimmune polyendocrine syndrome type I. J Clin Endocrinol Metab 85:2944–2950.

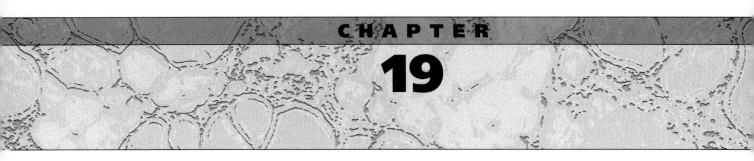

Disorders of Energy Balance

ROBERT H. LUSTIG, MD • RAM WEISS, MD

Introduction

Energy balance is the "final frontier" of endocrinology. Prior to 1994, with the discovery of leptin, the disorders of energy balance were not even considered endocrine diseases. Today, obesity can account for up to 25% of pediatric endocrine practice referrals—and type 2 diabetes accounts for up to 30% of the new referrals for diabetes, virtually all of whom are also obese. Since the discovery of leptin, the negative feedback pathway of energy balance has been elucidated—and endocrinologists have embraced disorders of energy balance as part of their portfolio.

Thus, the study of energy balance has become a matter of continuing education for pediatric endocrinologists. The entire field is a "work in progress," which is problematic because our knowledge, diagnostic armamentarium, and treatment options are still in their infancy. This chapter conveys a clear and up-to-date basic understanding of the energy balance pathway, and provides a clinical rationale and formulation for evaluating and treating patients with energy balance disorders.

Neuroendocrine Regulation of Energy Balance

The negative feedback axis of energy balance and its function during homeostasis has been largely delineated through studies in animal models. Human data are presented where available. The axis consists of three arms (Figure 19-1). The first is the afferent arm, which conveys in the form of hormonal and neural inputs peripheral information on hunger and peripheral metabolism to the hypothalamus. The second is a central processing unit, consisting of various areas within the hypothalamus. The ventromedial hypothalamus [VMH, consisting of the ventromedial (VMN) and arcuate (ARC) nuclei] integrates the afferent peripheral signals, along with other central stimuli. The paraventricular nuclei (PVN) and lateral hypothalamic area (LHA) serve as a gated neurotransmitter system to alter neural signals for changes in feeding and energy expenditure. The third component is the efferent arm, which consists of a complex network of autonomic effectors that regulate energy intake and monitor energy expenditure versus storage.[1,2] Anatomic disruptions or genetic or metabolic alterations of the afferent, central processing, or efferent arms can alter energy intake or expenditure in stereotyped ways—which can lead to obesity or cachexia.

THE AFFERENT SYSTEM

Alimentary Afferents

Hunger. *The afferent vagus:* The vagus nerve is the primary neural connection between the brain and the gut. The afferent vagus nerve conveys information regarding mechanical stretch of the stomach and duodenum and sensations of gastric fullness to the nucleus tractus solitarius (NTS).[3] Of note is that each of the alimentary neuropeptide effects on hunger and satiety discussed in the material following is obviated by concomitant vagotomy, implicating the afferent vagus as the primary mediator of alimentary energy balance signals.[4-6]

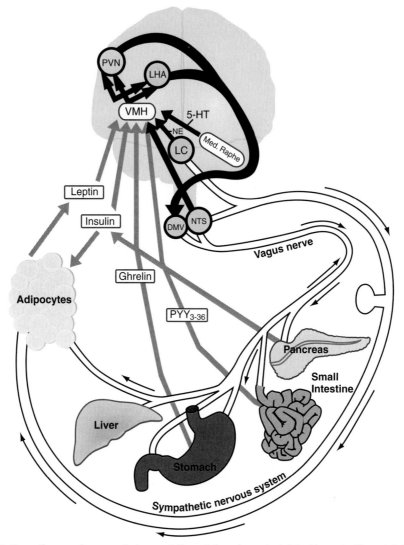

Figure 19-1 The homeostatic pathway of energy balance. Afferent (gray), central (black), and efferent (white) pathways are delineated. The hormones insulin, leptin, ghrelin, and peptide YY(3-36) (PYY3-36) provide afferent information to the ventromedial hypothalamus regarding short-term energy metabolism and energy sufficiency. From there, the ventromedial hypothalamus elicits anorexigenic (α-melanocyte-stimulating hormone, cocaine-amphetamine-regulated transcript) and orexigenic (neuropeptide Y, agouti-related protein) signals to the melanocortin-4 receptor in the paraventricular nucleus and lateral hypothalamic area. These lead to efferent output via the locus coeruleus, via the nucleus tractus solitarius, which activates the sympathetic nervous system—causing the adipocyte to undergo lipolysis. Alternatively, this is achieved via the dorsal motor nucleus of the vagus, which activates the vagus nerve to store energy by increasing pancreatic insulin secretion and (in rodents) by increasing adipose tissue sensitivity to insulin. 5-HT, serotonin (5-hydroxytryptamine); DMV, dorsal motor nucleus of the vagus; LC, locus coeruleus; LHA, lateral hypothalamic area; NE, norepinephrine; NTS, nucleus tractus solitarius; PVN, paraventricular nucleus; and VMH, ventromedial hypothalamus. [From Lustig RH (2006). Childhood obesity: Behavioral aberration or biochemical drive? Reinterpreting the first law of thermodynamics. Nature Clin Pract Endo Metab 2:447–458. Courtesy of Nature Publishing Group, with permission.]

Ghrelin: Ghrelin, an octanoylated 28-amino-acid peptide, was discovered serendipitiously while looking for the endogenous ligand of the growth hormone (GH) secretagogue receptor (GHS-R).[7] Ghrelin induces rat GH release through stimulation of the pituitary GHS-R. The endogenous secretion of ghrelin from the fasting stomach is high, but is decreased by nutrient administration. Volumetric stretching of the stomach wall has no effect. However, ghrelin also binds to the GHS-R in the VMH—which increases hunger, food intake, and fat deposition.[8,9]

Ghrelin also increases the respiratory quotient (RQ) in rats, suggesting a reduction of fat oxidation and promotion of fat storage. Ghrelin appears to tie the lipolytic effect of GH with the hunger signal, and is probably important in the acute response to fasting. In humans, ghrelin levels rise with increasing subjective hunger—and peak at the time of voluntary food consumption.[10] This suggests that ghrelin acts on the VMH to trigger meal initiation. Ghrelin infusion increases food intake in humans.[11] However, plasma ghrelin levels are low in obese individuals—and increase with fasting,[12] suggesting that ghrelin is a response to (rather than a cause of) obesity.

Satiety. *Peptide YY$_{3-36}$ (PYY$_{3-36}$):* A recently identified hormonal signal to control meal volume is PYY$_{3-36}$.[13] This peptide fragment is secreted by intestinal L cells in response to exposure to nutrient, crosses the blood-brain barrier, and binds to the Y_2 receptor in the VMH. Activation of this receptor causes a decrease in NPY mRNA in neurons of the orexigenic arm of the central processing system. In nonobese humans, infusion of PYY_{3-36} during a 12-hour period decreased the total amount of food ingested from 2,200 to 1,500 k/cal—but without effect on food ingested during the next 12-hour interval.[13] Although the pharmacology of this peptide is being elucidated, its specific role in obesity is not yet known.

Glucagon-like peptide-1 (GLP-1): Those same intestinal L cells produce GLP-1 through post-translational processing of pre-proglucagon. Two equipotent forms of GLP-1 are generated: a glycine-extended form called $GLP-1_{(7-37)}$ and the amidated peptide $GLP-1_{(7-36)}$ amide.[14] GLP-1 acts on the stomach to inhibit gastric emptying. This prolongs the time of absorption of a meal. GLP-1 also activates its receptor on pancreatic β-cells to stimulate cAMP production, protein kinase A activation, and insulin secretion (Figure 19-2)—thereby improving glucose tolerance (a mechanism of the "incretin" effect). GLP-1 also acts on β cells to stimulate neogenesis, thereby increasing β-cell mass.[15]

GLP-1 also exerts potent effects on reduction of appetite, through reduction in gastric emptying and through direct decreases of corticotropin-releasing hormone (CRH) signaling in the PVN and increasing leptin signaling in the VMH.[16]

Cholecystokinin (CCK): CCK is an 8-amino-acid gut peptide released in response to a caloric load. It circulates and binds to CCK_A receptors in the pylorus, vagus nerve, NTS, and area postrema to promote satiety.[3]

Metabolic Afferents

Leptin. Energy intake versus expenditure is normally regulated very tightly (within 0.15% per year) by the hormone leptin. Leptin is a 167-amino-acid hormone produced by adipocytes, which transmit the primary long-term signal of energy depletion/repletion to the VMH.[17,18] Leptin's primary neuroendocrine role is to mediate information about the size of peripheral adipocyte energy stores to the VMH. Leptin is a prerequisite signal to the VMH for the initiation of high-energy processes, such as puberty and pregnancy.[19,20] Leptin reduces food intake and increases the activity of the sympathetic nervous system (SNS).[21]

Conversely, low leptin circulating levels infer diminished energy stores (which signal via the VMH to reduce energy expenditure), inhibit metabolic processes and increase appetite. Serum leptin concentrations drop precipitously (in excess of body fat loss) during periods of short-term fasting,[22,23] and it seems likely that leptin functions primarily as a peripheral signal to the hypothalamus of inadequate caloric intake rather than specifically as a satiety signal.[24]

In the fed state, circulating levels of leptin correlate with percentage of body fat.[25,26] Leptin production by adipocytes is stimulated by insulin and glucocorticoids,[27,28] and is inhibited by β-adrenergic stimulation.[24] Programming of relative leptin concentrations by early caloric intake may be one mechanism that links early overnutrition with later obesity.[29]

Leptin binds to its receptor (a member of the cytokine receptor superfamily) on target VMH neurons. There are four receptor isoforms formed by differential mRNA splicing: ObRa (an isoform with a shortened intracellular domain, which may function as a transporter), ObRb (the intact full-length receptor), ObRc (also with a short intracellular domain), and ObRe (without an intracellular domain, but which may function as a soluble receptor).[30] As leptin binds to its VMH receptor, three neuronal signals are transduced.

The first is opening of an ATP-sensitive potassium channel, which hyperpolarizes the neuron and decreases its firing rate.[31] The second is the activation of a cytoplasmic Janus kinase 2 (JAK2), which phosphorylates a tyrosine moiety on proteins of a family called signal transducers and activators of transcription 3 (STAT-3).[32] The phosphorylated STAT-3 translocates to the nucleus, where it promotes leptin-dependent gene transcription.[33] However, leptin also activates the insulin receptor substrate 2/phosphatidyl inositol-3-kinase (IRS2/PI3K) second-messenger system in VMH neurons—which increases neurotransmission of the central anorexigenic signaling pathway.[34]

Insulin. Insulin plays an extremely important role in energy balance[35] because it is part of the afferent and efferent systems. On the afferent side, there is a significant insulin receptor density in a subpopulation of VMH neurons[36]—and there is coordinated transport of insulin across the blood-brain barrier.[37] This suggests a central role for this hormone. In animals, acute intracerebroventricular (ICV) infusions of insulin decrease feeding behavior and induce satiety.[38-40] The data on acute and chronic peripheral insulin infusions are less clear.

Studies of overinsulinized diabetic rats demonstrate increased caloric intake (to prevent subacute hypoglycemia) and the development of peripheral insulin resistance.[41,42] Chronic experimental peripheral insulin infusions decrease hepatic and skeletal muscle glucose uptake by decreasing Glut4 expression, but do not alter adipose tissue glucose uptake.[43,44] One study in humans showed that injecting short-term insulin peripherally during meals did not have an effect on satiety.[45]

Insulin normally activates the insulin receptor substrate 2/phosphatidyl inositol-3-kinase (IRS2/PI3K) second-messenger system in VMH neurons,[46] which increases neurotransmission of the central anorexigenic signaling pathway. The importance of CNS insulin action was underscored by the construction of a brain/neuron-specific insulin receptor knockout (NIRKO) mouse, which cannot transduce a CNS insulin signal.[47] Such mice become hyperphagic, obese, and infertile—with high peripheral insulin levels. These data suggest that peripheral insulin mediates a satiety signal in the VMH to help control energy balance.[48] Various knockouts of the insulin signal transduction pathway that reduce insulin signaling lead to an obese phenotype,[49,50] whereas those that increase insulin signaling lead to a lean phenotype.[51,52]

CENTRAL PROCESSING

The peripheral afferent signals outlined previously reach neurons in the VMH, where they are integrated by a gated neural circuit designed to promote or diminish energy intake and expenditure (Figure 19-2). This circuit consists

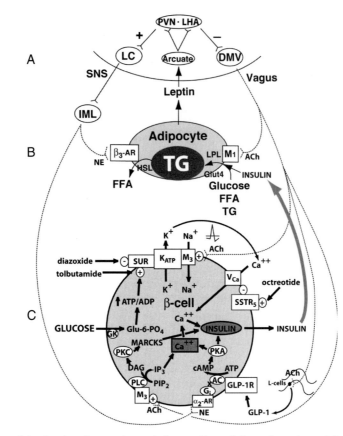

Figure 19-2 Central regulation of leptin signaling, autonomic innervation of the adipocyte and β cell, and the starvation response. *(A)* The arcuate nucleus transduces the peripheral leptin signal as one of sufficiency or deficiency. In leptin sufficiency, efferents from the hypothalamus synapse in the locus coeruleus—which stimulates the sympathetic nervous system. In leptin deficiency or resistance, efferents from the hypothalamus stimulate the dorsal motor nucleus of the vagus. *(B)* Autonomic innervation and hormonal stimulation of white adipose tissue. In leptin sufficiency, norepinephrine binds to the β₃-adrenergic receptor—which stimulates hormone-sensitive lipase, promoting lipolysis of stored triglyceride into free fatty acids. In leptin deficiency or resistance, vagal acetylcholine increases adipose tissue insulin sensitivity (documented only in rats to date), promotes uptake of glucose and free fatty acids for lipogenesis, and promotes triglyceride uptake through activation of lipoprotein lipase. *(C)* Autonomic innervation and hormonal stimulation of the β cell. Glucose entering the cell is converted to glucose-6-phosphate by the enzyme glucokinase, generating ATP—which closes an ATP-dependent potassium channel, resulting in cell depolarization. A voltage-gated calcium channel opens, allowing for intracellular calcium influx—which activates neurosecretory mechanisms, leading to insulin vesicular exocytosis. In leptin sufficiency, norepinephrine binds to α_2-adrenoceptors on the β-cell membrane to stimulate inhibitory G proteins and decrease adenyl cyclase and its product cAMP—and thereby reduce protein kinase A levels and insulin release. In leptin deficiency or resistance, the vagus stimulates insulin secretion through three mechanisms. First, acetylcholine binds to a M_3 muscarinic receptor, opening a sodium channel—which augments the ATP-dependent cell depolarization, increasing the calcium influx and insulin exocytosis. Second, acetylcholine activates a pathway that increases protein kinase C—which also promotes insulin secretion. Third, the vagus innervates L cells of the small intestine, which secrete glucagon-like peptide-1—which activates protein kinase A, contributing to insulin exocytosis. Octreotide binds to a somatostatin receptor on the β cell, which is coupled to the voltage-gated calcium channel—limiting calcium influx and the amount of insulin released in response to glucose. α_2-AR, α_2-adrenergic receptor; β₃-AR, β₃-adrenergic receptor; AC, adenyl cyclase; ACh, acetylcholine; DAG, diacylglycerol; DMV, dorsal motor nucleus of the vagus; FFA, free fatty acids; G_i, inhibitory G protein; GK, glucokinase; GLP-1, glucagon-like peptide-1; GLP-1R, GLP-1 receptor; Glu-6-PO₄, glucose-6-phosphate; Glut4, glucose transporter-4; HSL, hormone-sensitive lipase; IML, intermediolateral cell column; IP₃, inositol triphosphate; LC, locus coeruleus; LHA, lateral hypothalamic area; LPL, lipoprotein lipase; MARCKS, myristoylated alanine-rich protein kinase C substrate; NE, norepinephrine; PIP₂, phosphatidylinositol pyrophosphate; PKA, protein kinase A; PKC, protein kinase C; PLC, phospholipase C; PVN, paraventricular nucleus; SSTR₅, somatostatin-5 receptor; TG, triglyceride; V_{Ca}, voltage-gated calcium channel; VMH, ventromedial hypothalamus; and SUR, sufonylurea receptor. [From Lustig RH (2006). Childhood obesity: Behavioral aberration or biochemical drive? Reinterpreting the first law of thermodynamics. Nature Clin Pract Endo Metab 2:447–458. Courtesy of Nature Publishing Group, with permission, and also reprinted with permission of Springer Science and Business media.]

of two arms: the anorexigenic arm [which contains neurons expressing the colocalized peptides pro-opiomelanocortin (POMC) and cocaine/amphetamine-regulated transcript (CART)] and the orexigenic arm, which contains neurons with the colocalized peptides neuropeptide Y (NPY) and agouti-related protein (AgRP). Ghrelin receptor-immunoreactivity colocalizes with NPY and AgRP neurons, whereas insulin and leptin receptors are located on POMC/CART and NPY/AgRP neurons in the VMH[53]—suggesting divergent regulation of each arm. These two arms compete for occupancy of melanocortin receptors (MC₃R or MC₄R) in the PVN and LHA.

Anorexigenesis, POMC/α-MSH, and CART

POMC is differentially cleaved in different tissues and neurons. The ligand α-melanocyte-stimulating hormone (α-MSH) is the primary product involved in anorexigenesis. Overfeeding and peripheral leptin infusion induce the synthesis of POMC and α-MSH within the ARC.[54] α-MSH induces anorexia by binding to melanocortin receptors within the PVN or LHA. CART is a hypothalamic neuropeptide induced by leptin and reduced by fasting. Intrahypothalamic infusion blocks appetite, whereas antagonism of endogenous CART increases caloric intake.[55]

Orexigenesis, NPY, and AgRP

NPY and AgRP colocalize to a different set of neurons within the ARC, immediately adjacent to those expressing POMC/CART.[56] NPY has numerous functions within the hypothalamus, including initiation of feeding, initiation of puberty, regulation of gonadotropin secretion, and adrenal responsiveness.[57,58] NPY is the primary orexigenic peptide. ICV infusion of NPY in rats rapidly leads to hyperphagia, energy storage, and obesity[59,60] mediated through Y_1 and Y_5 receptors.

Fasting and weight loss increase NPY expression in the ARC, accounting for increased hunger—whereas PYY_{3-36} (through Y_2 receptors) and leptin decrease NPY mRNA.[13,61] AgRP is the human homolog of the protein agouti, which is present in abundance in the yellow (A^y-a) mouse.[62] This protein is an endogenous competitive antagonist of all MCRs, accounting for the yellow color in these mice. In the presence of large amounts of AgRP at the synaptic cleft in the PVN, α-MSH cannot bind to the MC_4R to induce satiety.[63]

Other Neuroendocrine Modulators of Energy Balance

Norepinephrine. Norepinephrine (NE) neurons in the locus coeruleus synapse on VMH neurons to regulate food intake.[64] The actions of NE on food intake seem paradoxical because intrahypothalamic NE infusions stimulate food intake through effects on central $α_2$- and β-adrenergic receptors,[65] whereas central infusion of $α_1$-agonists markedly reduces food intake.[66]

Serotonin. 5-HT has been implicated in the perception of satiety based on many lines of evidence: injection of 5-HT into the hypothalamus increases satiety, particularly with respect to carbohydrate;[67] central administration of $5-HT_{2c}$ receptor agonists increases satiety, whereas antagonists induce feeding;[68] administration of selective 5-HT reuptake inhibitors induces early satiety;[69] leptin increases 5-HT turnover;[70] and the $5-HT_{2c}R$-KO mouse exhibits increased food intake and body weight.[71] The role of 5-HT in the transduction of the satiety signal may have central and peripheral components because intestinal 5-HT is secreted into the bloodstream during a meal, where it may impact on gastrointestinal (GI) neuronal function and muscle tone and may bind to 5-HT receptors in the NTS to promote satiety.[72]

Melanin-concentrating Hormone. MCH is a 17-amino-acid peptide expressed in the zona incerta and LHA. MCH neurons synapse on neurons in the forebrain and locus coeruleus. MCH appears to be important in conditions such as anxiety and aggression around food.[73] Expression of this peptide is upregulated in *ob/ob* mice. MCH-knockout mice are hypophagic and lean,[74] whereas transgenic MCH-overexpressing mice develop obesity and insulin resistance.[75] ICV administration of MCH stimulates food intake, similar to that seen with NPY administration.[76]

Orexins A and B. These 33- and 28-amino acid peptides, respectively, have been implicated in energy balance and autonomic function in mice.[77] Orexin-knockout mice demonstrate narcolepsy, hypophagia, and obesity[78]—suggesting that orexins bridge the gap between the afferent and efferent energy balance systems.[79] Orexins in the LHA stimulate NPY release, which may account for their effects on orexigenesis. They also stimulate the corticotropin-releasing factor (CRF) and SNS output to increase wakefulness and energy expenditure, learning and memory, and the hedonic reward system.[80] Conversely, orexin neurons in the perifornical and dorsomedial hypothalamus regulate arousal and response to stress.

Endocannabinoids. It has long been known that tetrahydrocannibinol stimulates food intake. This observation led to the identification of endogenous ECs and their receptor, termed CB1.[81] The CB_1 receptor is expressed in corticotropin-releasing hormone (CRH) neurons in the PVN, in CART neurons in the VMN, and in MCH- and orexin-positive neurons in the LHA and perifornical region. Fasting and feeding are associated with high and low levels of ECs in the hypothalamus, respectively. For example, CB_1 receptor-knockout mice have increased CRH and reduced CART expression.

In the *ob/ob* mouse, hypothalamic EC levels are increased—whereas leptin infused intravenously reduces these levels, indicating that a direct negative control is exerted by leptin on the EC system. Glucocorticoids increase food intake by stimulating EC synthesis and secretion, whereas leptin blocks this effect.[82] Finally, the presence of CB_1 receptors on afferent vagal neurons suggests that endocannabinoids may be involved in mediating satiety signals originating in the gut.

Melanocortin Receptors and Central Neural Integration

The human MC_4R localizes to chromosome 2 and is a 7-transmembrane G-coupled receptor encoded by an intronless 1-kB gene. The binding of hypothalamic α-MSH to the MC_4R in the PVN and LHA results in a state of satiety, whereas ICV administration of MC_4R antagonists stimulate feeding—suggesting that MC_4R transduces satiety information on caloric sufficiency. In the MC_3R knockout mouse, a different phenotype is seen. These animals are obese, but they are instead hypophagic and have increased body fat for their lean mass. They gain weight on low- or high-fat chow, and do not change caloric oxidation in response to changes in dietary fat content—suggesting a defect in energy expenditure.[83] Thus, these two hypothalamic MCRs appear to modulate different aspects of energy metabolism. One hypothesis is that the MC_4R modulates energy intake and the MC_3R modulates energy expenditure.[84]

THE EFFERENT SYSTEM

The MCRs in the PVN and LHA transduce the anorexigenic and orexigenic information coming from the VMH in order to modulate activity of the SNS, (which promotes energy expenditure) and of the efferent vagus, which promotes energy storage (Figure 19-2). In this way, peripheral energy balance can be modulated acutely to provide requisite energy for metabolic needs and to store the rest.

The Sympathetic Nervous System and Energy Expenditure

Anorexigenic pressure increases energy expenditure through activation of the SNS.[85] For instance, leptin adminstration to *ob/ob* mice promotes increased brown adipose tissue lipolysis, thermogenesis, renovascular activity, and increased movement—all associated with increased energy expenditure, which assists in weight loss.[86] Similarly, insulin administration acutely increases SNS activity in normal rats and in humans.[87,88] The magnitude of energy expenditure also has a salutary effect on quality of life. Those factors that reduce resting energy expenditure (REE; e.g., hypothyroidism) reduce quality of life, whereas those factors that increase REE (e.g., caffeine) increase quality of life (at least acutely).

The SNS increases energy expenditure in four ways: by innervating the hypothalamus and appetite centers in the medulla to reduce appetite, by increasing TSH secretion to increase thyroid hormone release and energy expenditure, by innervating skeletal muscles to increase energy expenditure, and by innervating β_3-adrenergic receptors in white adipose tissue to promote lipolysis. Activation of the SNS increases energy expenditure at the skeletal muscle by activating β_2-adrenergic receptors,[89] which in turn increase the expression of numerous genes in skeletal muscle[90]—especially those involved in carbohydrate metabolism. SNS activation stimulates glycogenolysis, myocardial energy expenditure, glucose and fatty acid oxidation, and protein synthesis.[91]

Activation of the SNS in rodents stimulates the β_3-adrenergic receptor of brown adipose tissue to promote lipolysis.[92] In humans, activation of the β_3-adrenergic receptor increases cAMP—which activates protein kinase A (PKA). PKA acts in two separate molecular pathways to increase energy expenditure. First, PKA phosphorylates cyclic AMP response element binding protein (CREB)—which induces expression of PPARγ-coactivator-1α (PGC-1α). PGC-1α then binds to enhancer elements on the uncoupling protein-1 (UCP1) gene, which increases the expression and activity of uncoupling proteins (UCPs) 1 and 2.[93,94] UCPs reduce the proton gradient across the inner membranes of mitochondria, which thereby diverts protons from storage in the form of ATP to heat production. Originally, UCPs were discovered in brown adipose tissue and were found to be responsible for thermogenesis.

UCP1 is an inner membrane mitochondrial protein that uncouples proton entry from ATP synthesis.[95] Therefore, UCP1 expression dissipates energy as heat—thus reducing the energy efficiency of the adipose tissue. However, UCP2 has been found in most tissues and UCP3 in skeletal muscle. Second, PKA activation acti-

vates the enzyme hormone-sensitive lipase (HSL), which is responsible for lipolysis of intracellular triglyceride to its component free fatty acids (FFAs). The FFAs also induce UCP1, further increasing energy expenditure. The FFAs released from the adipocyte also travel to the liver, where they are utilized for energy by metabolizing into two-carbon fragments. Lipolysis reduces leptin expression. Thus, a negative feedback loop is achieved between leptin and the SNS (Figure 19-2).

The Efferent Vagus and Energy Storage

In response to declining levels of leptin and/or persistent orexigenic pressure, the LHA and PVN send efferent projections residing in the medial longitudinal fasciculus to the dorsal motor nucleus of the vagus nerve (DMV)—activating the efferent vagus.[96] The efferent vagus opposes the SNS by promoting energy storage in four ways: by slowing the heart rate, myocardial oxygen consumption is reduced; the vagus nerve promotes alimentary peristalsis, pyloric opening, and energy substrate absorption; through direct effects on the adipocyte, the vagus nerve promotes insulin sensitivity to increase the clearance of energy substrate into adipose tissue; and through effects on the β cells, the vagus increases postprandial insulin secretion—which promotes energy deposition into adipose tissue.[97-100]

Retrograde tracing of white adipose tissue reveals a wealth of efferents originating at the DMV.[100] These efferents synapse on the M_1 muscarinic receptor on the adipocyte, which increases insulin sensitivity of the adipocyte. Denervation of white adipose tissue results in reduction of glucose and FFA uptake and in induction of HSL, which promotes lipolysis—both of which reduce the efficiency of insulin-induced energy storage. Thus, vagal modulation of the adipocyte augments storage of glucose and FFAs by improving adipose insulin sensitivity[101] (Figure 19-2).

The DMV also sends efferent projections to the β cells of the pancreas.[102] This pathway is responsible for the "cephalic" (preabsorptive) phase of insulin secretion, which is glucose independent and can be blocked by atropine.[103] Overactive vagal neurotransmission increases insulin secretion from β cells in response to an oral glucose load through the following three distinct but overlapping mechanisms[104] (Figure 19-2).

- Vagal firing increases acetylcholine availability and binding to the M_3 muscarinic receptor on the β cell, which is coupled to a sodium channel within the pancreatic β-cell membrane.[105] As glucose enters the β cell after ingestion of a meal, the enzyme glucokinase phosphorylates glucose to form glucose-6-phosphate—increasing intracellular ATP, which induces closure of the ATP-dependent potassium channel. Upon channel closure, the β cell experiences an ATP concentration-dependent β-cell depolarization[106,107] and opening of a separate voltage-gated calcium channel within the membrane. Intracellular calcium influx increases acutely, which results in rapid insulin vesicular exocytosis. Concomitant opening of the sodium channel by vagally mediated acetylcholine augments β-cell depolarization, which in turn augments the intracellular calcium influx and results in insulin hypersecretion.[108-110]

- Vagally mediated acetylcholine increases phospholipases A$_2$, C, and D within the β cell—which hydrolyze intracellular phosphatidylinositol to diacylglycerol (DAG) and inositol triphosphate (IP$_3$).[104] DAG is a potent stimulator of protein kinase C (PKC),[111] which phosphorylates myristoylated alanine-rich PKC substrate (MARCKS)—which then binds actin and calcium-calmodulin and induces insulin vesicular exocytosis.[112] IP$_3$ potentiates release of calcium within β cells from intracellular stores, which also promotes insulin secretion.[113]
- The vagus also stimulates the release of GLP-1 from intestinal L cells, which circulates and binds to a GLP-1 receptor within the β-cell membrane. Activation of this receptor induces a calcium-calmodulin-sensitive adenyl cyclase, with conversion of intracellular ATP to cAMP—which then activates PKA. PKA causes the release of intracellular calcium stores and the phosphorylation of vesicular proteins, each contributing to an increase in insulin exocytosis.[14,114]

In the efferent pathway, insulin is responsible for shunting blood-borne nutrients into adipose for storage. Indeed, the primary hormonal signal for adipogenesis is insulin.[115] Within the adipocyte, insulin increases Glut4 expression, acetyl-CoA carboxylase, fatty acid synthase, and lipoprotein lipase.[116] Thus, the net effect of insulin on the adipocyte is the rapid clearance and storage of circulating glucose and lipid. Thus, insulin promotes energy storage.

NEGATIVE FEEDBACK MODULATION OF ENERGY BALANCE: THE STARVATION RESPONSE

The regulation of the components of the energy balance system is manifest during the starvation response. Everyone has a "personal leptin threshold" (probably genetically set) above which the brain interprets a state of energy sufficiency.[117] Thus, the leptin-replete state is characterized by increased physical activity, decreased appetite, and increased feelings of well-being. However, in response to caloric restriction leptin levels decline even before weight loss is manifest[22,23]—which is interpreted by the VMH as starvation. Gastric secretion of ghrelin is increased, which increases pituitary GH release in order to stimulate lipolysis to provide energy substrate for catabolism.

Ghrelin stimulates NPY/AgRP to antagonize α-MSH/CART. Decline of leptin reduces α-MSH/CART as well. This leads to decreased MC$_4$R occupancy. The resultant lack of anorexigenic pressure on the MC$_4$R results in increased feeding behavior and energy efficiency (with reduced fat oxidation) in order to store energy as fat. In response, the efferent pathway of energy balance coordinates efforts at improving energy efficiency and increasing energy storage. Total and resting energy expenditure decline in at attempt to conserve energy.[118] Specifically, UCP1 levels within adipose tissue decline[119] as a result of decreased SNS activity in response to starvation.[120]

However, in spite of decreased SNS tone at the adipocyte there is clearly an obligate lipolysis (due to insulin suppression and up-regulation of HSL)—which is necessary to maintain energy delivery to the musculature and brain in the form of liver-derived ketone bodies. In addition, in the starved state vagal tone is increased in order to slow the heart rate and myocardial oxygen consumption, increase β-cell insulin secretion in response to glucose, and increase adipose insulin sensitivity—all directed at increasing energy storage.[120] These revert back to baseline once caloric sufficiency is reestablished, and leptin levels rise.

THE HEDONIC PATHWAY OF FOOD REWARD

The negative feedback pathway delineated previously is not the only site of central regulation of food intake. Complementary to insulin and leptin's ability to alter energy balance, these hormones also modify the *hedonic pathway*—the pleasurable and motivating responses to food. This is the same pathway that responds to drugs of abuse, such as nicotine and morphine. The hedonic pathway comprises the ventral tegmental area (VTA) and the nucleus accumbens (NA), with input from various components of the limbic system—including the striatum, amygdala, hypothalamus, and hippocampus.

Food intake is a readout of the hedonic pathway. Administration of morphine to the NA increases food intake in a dose-dependent fashion.[121] When functional, the hedonic pathway helps curtail food intake in situations in which energy stores are replete. However, dysfunction of this pathway can increase food intake—leading to obesity. The VTA appears to mediate feeding on the basis of palatability rather than energy need. The dopaminergic projection from the VTA to the NA mediates the motivating, rewarding, and reinforcing properties of various stimuli (such as food and addictive drugs). Leptin and insulin receptors are expressed in the VTA, and both hormones have been implicated in modulating rewarding responses to food and other pleasurable stimuli.[122] For instance, fasting and food restriction (where insulin and leptin levels are low) increase the addictive properties of drugs of abuse—whereas ICV leptin can reverse these effects.[123]

In rodent models of addiction, increased addictive behavior and pleasurable response from a food reward (as measured by dopamine release and dopamine receptor signaling) are greater after food deprivation.[124] Acutely, insulin increases expression and activity of the dopamine transporter—which clears and removes dopamine from the synapse. Thus, acute insulin exposure blunts the reward of food.[125] Furthermore, insulin appears to inhibit the ability of VTA agonists (e.g., opioids) to increase intake of sucrose.[126] Finally, insulin blocks the ability of rats to form a conditioned place preference association to a palatable food.[127] However, insulin resistance of this pathway may lead to increased reward of food. The role of the hedonic pathway in human obesity is not yet elucidated, but may be surmised.

LEPTIN RESISTANCE

Most obese children have high leptin levels but do not have receptor mutations, manifesting what is commonly referred to as leptin resistance. Leptin resistance prevents exogenous leptin administration from promoting weight loss.[128] The response to most weight loss regimens plateaus rapidly due to the rapid fall of peripheral leptin levels below a personal "leptin threshold,"[129] which is likely genetically determined. Leptin decline causes the VMH to sense a reduction in peripheral energy stores, which modulates a decrease in REE to conserve energy—analogous to the starvation response[118] but occurring at elevated leptin levels.

The cause of leptin resistance is unknown, but may have several etiologies. Leptin crosses the blood-brain barrier via a saturable transporter, which limits the amount of leptin reaching its receptor in the VMH.[130,131] Activation of the leptin receptor induces intraneuronal expression of suppressor of cytokine signaling 3 (SOCS-3), which limits leptin signal transduction.[51] Dietary fat limits access of peripheral leptin to the VMH, and interferes with leptin signal transduction upstream of STAT-3 (its primary second messenger).[132]

Two clinical paradigms have been shown to improve leptin sensitivity. After weight loss through caloric restriction, exogenous administration of leptin can then increase REE back to baseline and permit further weight loss[133,134]—suggesting that the weight loss itself improves leptin sensitivity. Second, suppression of insulin correlates with improvement in leptin sensitivity and promotes weight loss[135]—suggesting that hyperinsulinemia promotes leptin resistance by interfering with leptin signal transduction in the VMH and VTA.[136] Indeed, insulin reduction strategies can be effective in promoting weight loss in children with hyperinsulinemia by improving leptin sensitivity.[137] This has led to the hypothesis that chronic hyperinsulinemia functions to block leptin signal transduction at the VMH and VTA, which turns a negative feedback cycle into a vicious feed-forward cycle[18] (Figure 19-3). However, this hypothesis remains to be proven.

Energy Excess: Obesity

The rise in the prevalence of obesity in children and adolescents is one of the most alarming public health issues facing the world today. Obesity is associated with significant health problems in children and is an early risk factor for much of adult morbidity and mortality.[138] It is also a major contributor to increasing health care expenditures. Importantly, childhood obesity tends to track to adulthood and thus represents an early beginning of a potentially lethal pathologic process.

DEFINITION

The theoretical definition of obesity is a degree of somatic overweight that causes detrimental health consequences.[139] Based on morbidity and mortality statistics, and with a desire to prevent future risk of morbidity, we practically define obesity as a statistical magnitude of overweight for a population—keeping in mind that morbidity and mortality vary with degree of overweight in different racial, ethnic, and socioeconomic groups[140] and indeed among individuals. The World Health Organization[141] categorizes adult overweight into four subgroups based on body mass index [BMI; weight (kg) ÷ height (m^2)]: BMI 25 to 30 (overweight); BMI 30 to 35, grade 1 (moderately obese); BMI 35 to 40, grade 2 (severely obese); and BMI >40, grade 3 (morbidly obese). Some make a further delineation at BMI >60, denoting this as "superobesity" because even surgical therapies are less effective in this range.

The majority of obesity in adulthood has its origins in childhood,[142,143] making obesity a pediatric concern—and the prevention and treatment of obesity a pediatric goal. BMI is also the accepted marker in children.[144] In childhood, comparison of BMI to normal curves for age[145] allows for categorization of BMI above the 85th percentile as overweight and above the 95th percentile as obese (Figure 19-4A and B).

PREVALENCE AND EPIDEMIOLOGY

The prevalence of childhood obesity in the United States has increased dramatically during the past 30 years,[146,147] although the comparison of longitudinal and cross-sectional data is difficult due to different definitions and measurement parameters among epidemiologic studies. The most recent estimates of obesity prevalence in the United States are based on data from the 1999-2000 National Health and Nutrition Examination Survey (NHANES IV).[147] NHANES demonstrates that the epidemic of childhood obesity is occurring at earlier ages. Based on the

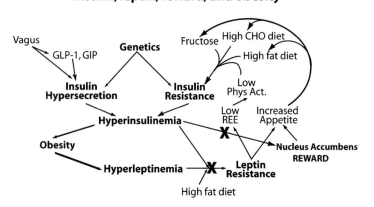

Insulin, leptin, reward, and obesity

Figure 19-3 Postulated algorithm describing the role of hyperinsulinemia in the dysfunction of the energy balance pathway by promoting energy storage into adipocytes; by interfering with leptin signal transduction in the hypothalamus, promoting the starvation response; and by interfering with dopamine clearance at the nucleus accumbens, thereby increasing the reward of food. Each of these alterations turns a negative feedback pathway into a "vicious cycle." [From Isganaitis E, Lustig RH (2005). Fast food, central nervous system insulin resistance, and obesity. Arterioscler Thromb Vasc Biol 25:2451-2462. Courtesy of the American Heart Association, with permission.]

1999-2000 NHANES, 20.6% of 2- to 5-year-old U.S. children were overweight, defined as BMI for age ≥85th percentile.

The prevalence of obesity in older children was even higher: 30.3% of 6- to 11-year-old children and 30.4% of adolescents (12-19 years old) have now become obese. The prevalence of obesity (defined as weight for length ≥95th percentile in 2-year-old children or younger, or BMI greater than 95th percentile in older children) among children aged 0 to 23 months, 2 to 5 years, 6 to 11 years, and adolescents were 11.4%, 10.4%, 15.3%, and 15.5%, respectively. The prevalence of obesity among both sexes was not significantly different. It was slightly higher in 2- to 5-year-old females (11.0% versus 9.9%), 6- to 11-year-old males (16.0% versus 14.5%), and similar (15.5%) in adolescents. In all age ranges, the prevalence has increased compared with the previous report by NHANES III (1988-1994)—with the greatest change (from approximately 11% to 15%) among 6- to 19-year-olds.

GLOBAL PREVALENCE

Obesity has overtaken AIDS and malnutrition as the number one public health problem in the world.[148] The global prevalence of childhood obesity has been increasing worldwide at an alarming rate during the past 20 years. Rates have increased 2.7-fold to 3.8-fold over 29 years in the United States,[147] 2.0-fold to 2.8-fold over 10 years in England, 3.4-fold to 4.6-fold over 10 years in Australia, and 3.4-fold to 3.6-fold over 23 years in Brazil. In Asia, the prevalence has increased 1.1-fold to 1.4-fold over 6 years in China and 2.3-fold to 2.5-fold over 26 years in Japan. In Africa, the prevalence has increased 3.9-fold over 18 years in Egypt,

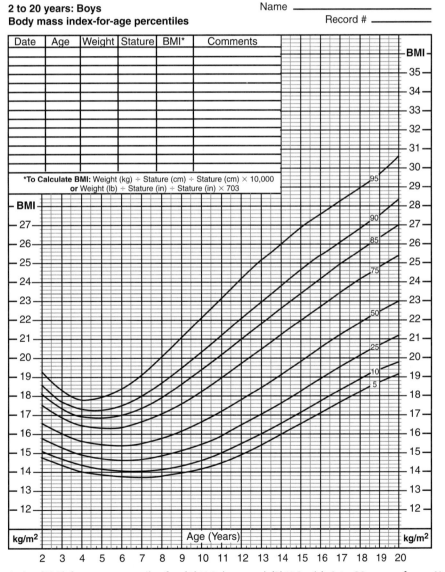

Figure 19-4 Body mass index (BMI)-for-age percentiles for *(A)* U.S. boys and *(B)* U.S. girls 2 to 20 years of age. Note that the 95th percentile signifies obesity. The adiposity rebound occurs at approximately 5 years of age in both sexes. The earlier the adiposity rebound occurs the more likely an organic etiology for the weight gain can be inferred. [From [Author] (2001). BMI curves. http://www.cdc.gov/growthcharts. National Center of Health Statistics, 2000.]

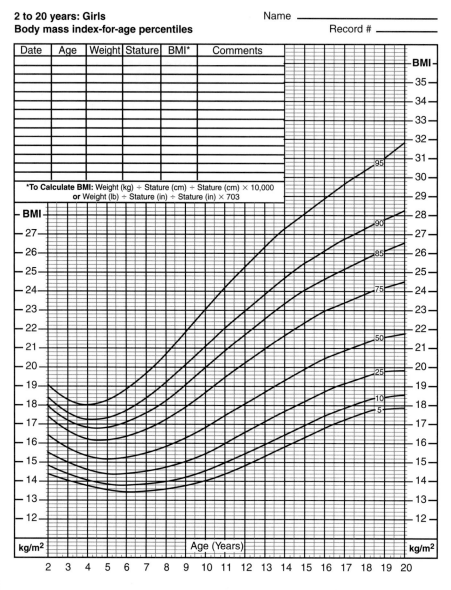

2 to 20 years: Girls
Body mass index-for-age percentiles

Name _____

Record # _____

*To Calculate BMI: Weight (kg) ÷ Stature (cm) ÷ Stature (cm) × 10,000
or Weight (lb) ÷ Stature (in) ÷ Stature (in) × 703

Figure 19-4 (cont'd)

3.8-fold over 6 years in Ghana, and 2.5-fold over 5 years in Morocco.[149] Even in Japan, the rate has doubled from 5% to 10% in the last 10 years.[150,151]

In developed countries, the urban poor are more susceptible to obesity, presumably due to poor dietary practices and limited opportunity for physical activity.[152,153] In contrast, obesity is more frequent in the upper socioeconomic class of developing countries—probably due to transition to a more Western lifestyle, with a more energy-dense diet consisting of higher fats and sugar (which tend to be more palatable at a lower cost).[154,155] This may be due to specific properties of processed food, which promote leptin resistance.[136]

RACIAL AND ETHNIC CONSIDERATIONS

The NHANES surveys only list prevalence among Caucasians, African Americans, and Hispanics despite the fact that Native Americans, Pacific Islanders, Asians, and other racial/ethnic groups are experiencing rapid in-

creases in prevalence as well. Across racial groups, there is a marked dichotomy in the prevalence and rate of increase in childhood obesity.[147,156] For instance, the prevalence among African-American (23.6%) and Hispanic (23.4%) adolescents is twice that than among white adolescents (12.7%)—and the rate of increase in the prevalence of obesity among African-American and Hispanic adolescents almost doubled between 1988 to 1994 and 1999 to 2000, from 13.4% to 23.6% in African Americans and from 13.8% to 23.4% in Hispanics.

Analyses based on the adult definition of obesity (BMI ≥30 kg/m²) indicated that 11.2% of adolescents in general (but approximately 20% of African-American female adolescents) fit into this category. Within these high-risk groups, female African-American adolescents and male 6- to 19-year-old Hispanics exhibit the highest prevalence of obesity (26.6%-27.5%). In the NHLBI Growth and Health Study,[157] the prevalence of obesity in 9-year-old African-American girls was 17.7% and in 9-year-old Caucasian girls 7.7%—and both of these prevalences doubled over the 10 years of study. These prevalences are true at younger ages as well.

The 1994 Pediatric Nutrition Surveillance System (PedNSS) indicated that 12% of 2- to 4-year-old Native American children were overweight, which is similar to Hispanic children at the same age (12%) but much higher than white children (6%). The prevalence of overweight at 5 to 6 years in Native Americans is twice that in U.S. youth in general, and the prevalence of obesity is three times higher.[158] Among infants and toddlers less than 2 years of age, the prevalence of obesity is highest in African Americans (18.5%)—compared to 10.1% in Caucasians and 13.7% in Hispanics. It is possible that different dietary practices may account for some of these differences. For instance, a study of 2-year-old Latino children in California correlated obesity with early consumption of sugar-sweetened beverages.[159]

Within racial populations, ethnic variability in the prevalence of childhood obesity has also been noted. The United States National Longitudinal Study of Adolescent Health (Add Health) indicated that the BMI ≥85th percentile in adolescent Hispanics was more common among Mexican Americans (32.1%) and Puerto Ricans (30.3%) compared with Cuban Americans (27.1%) and Central/South Americans (26.2%).[153] Only 25% of first-generation Hispanic adolescents were overweight based on BMI≥ 85th percentile compared with 32% of second- and third-generation Hispanics.

The prevalence of overweight in Asian-American adolescents in this study was 20.6%, with comparable prevalence among Filipinos (18.5%) and Chinese (15.3%). Again, only 12% of first-generation Asian Americans were overweight—compared with 27% and 28%, respectively, of second and third generations. In Native Americans, among the studies performed between 1990 and 2000 there is great variation in the prevalence of obesity (12%-77%) based on tribe, age group, measurement tool, and cutoff value.[158] These studies indicate that obesity in Native Americans begins very early in childhood.

PREDICTIVE FACTORS

The higher the BMI during childhood the more likely adult obesity will manifest. In general, children with a BMI ≥95th percentile have a very high risk for adult obesity.[160] Obesity in adolescence is a primary risk factor for obesity in adulthood, with an increased odds ratio from 1.3 for obesity at 1 to 2 years of age to 17.5 for obesity at 15 to 17 years of age.[161] The change of BMI during and after adolescence was the most important predictive variable for adult obesity.[162] Long-term studies suggest that between 50% and 75% of all obese adolescents will become obese adults, and more than one-third of 18-year-olds with BMI greater than the 60th percentile will also be overweight as adults. Children and adolescents with BMI ≥95th percentile have a 62% to 98% chance of being obese at 35 years of age, with a 50% chance in males aged ≥13 years and 66% chance in girls aged ≥13 years.[163]

The age of adiposity rebound, the point of the BMI nadir before the body fatness begins to rise (between 5 and 6 years of age; Figure 19-4A and B), is also an important predictor for adult obesity.[164] Girls tend to have slightly earlier adiposity rebound than do boys. Children with early adiposity rebound have a fivefold greater chance of becoming obese as adults, compared with those with late adiposity rebound. At the age of adiposity rebound, children already overweight have a sixfold greater risk for adult obesity compared to lean children. Therefore, the earlier the onset of childhood obesity the greater the risk for adult obesity.

Infant overnutrition plays an extremely important role in the future development of obesity. Numerous studies have implicated bottle feeding as a specific risk factor.[165] The prevalence of obesity in children who were never breast fed was 4.5%, compared with 2.8% in breast-fed children—and a clear time-response effect was identified for the duration of breast feeding on the decline in prevalence of obesity.[166] Early overnutrition has been correlated with elevated leptin concentrations in later life.[29] Differences in volume and composition of commercial formula versus breast milk have been proposed as etiologic factors.

Parental obesity is also an important predictor of childhood obesity. Children with at least one overweight parent at the age of adiposity rebound have a four- to fivefold greater chance of becoming obese adults. Lean children 5 years or younger have a thirteenfold risk of adult obesity if both parents are obese. Conversely, older children (10–14 years of age) who are obese have a 22.3-fold increased risk of adult obesity regardless of parental weight.[143] Parental obesity is related to early adiposity rebound, suggesting that genetic influences predominate in childhood weight gain.[167] Obesity and type 2 diabetes often run in families, particularly in minorities with lower socioeconomic backgrounds.[168]

Metabolic Impact of Childhood Obesity

Many of the metabolic and CV complications of obesity are already evident during childhood, and are closely related to the development of insulin resistance and hyperinsulinemia—the most common biochemical abnormality seen in obesity. The obesity-related co-morbidities that emerge early in childhood are alterations in glucose metabolism, dyslipidemia, and hypertension. Although an accelerated atherogenic process is present in obese children, thrombotic CV events do not usually appear until adulthood. The clustering of these manifestations is termed the *metabolic syndrome*. In addition, nonalcoholic fatty liver disease (NAFLD) and polycystic ovarian syndrome are often related—as are other nonendocrine morbidities.

LIPID PARTITIONING

The term *lipid partitioning* refers to the distribution of excess body fat in various organs and compartments. The majority of excess fat is stored in its conventional subcutaneous depot, yet other potential storage sites exist—such as the intra-abdominal (visceral) fat compartment and insulin-sensitive tissues such as muscle and liver. One hypothesis to explain the relation between obesity and insulin resistance is the "portal-visceral" paradigm.[169] Associations among visceral adiposity, insulin resistance, and co-morbidities have been demonstrated across most age groups and ethnicities.[170] This hypothesis claims that increased adiposity causes accumulation of fat in the visceral depot, leading to an increased portal and systemic free fatty acid (FFA) flux.[171] Increased circulating FFA inhibits insulin action in insulin-sensitive tissues by a "competitive" mechanism, proposed by Randle.[172] Of note, studies of *in vivo* FFA fluxes from the visceral and the subcutaneous truncal and abdominal depots have failed to demonstrate a substantial difference in net fluxes between these depots.

Recent studies demonstrate that subcutaneous fat, which does not drain into the portal system, is strongly related to insulin resistance in healthy obese and in diabetic men.[173] Similarly, truncal subcutaneous fat mass has been demonstrated to independently predict insulin resistance in obese women. Visceral and subcutaneous fat differ in their biologic responses,[174] with visceral fat more resistant to insulin and more sensitive to catecholamines. These observations emphasize that visceral and subcutaneous abdominal fat can contribute to insulin resistance, possibly by different mechanisms.[175]

An alternative theory to explain the relation between obesity and insulin resistance is the "ectopic lipid deposition" paradigm.[176] This theory is based on the observation that lipid content in muscle is increased in obesity and in type 2 diabetes mellitus (T2DM) and is a strong predictor of insulin resistance.[177] Moreover, in conditions such as lipodystrophies all fat is stored in liver and muscle due to lack of subcutaneous fat tissue—causing severe insulin resistance and diabetes.[178] In obese adults (BMI >30), muscle attenuation on CT (representing lipid content) is a stronger predictor of insulin resistance than is visceral fat.[179] Studies performed in vivo using ^{1}H-NMR spectroscopy demonstrated that increased intramyocellular lipid (IMCL) content is a strong determinant of insulin resistance in humans.[180]

Thus, obesity co-morbidity may begin when the subcutaneous fat reaches its capacity to store excess fat and begins to shunt lipid to ectopic tissues (such as liver and muscle)—leading to peripheral insulin resistance.[181] Another postulated cause of intramuscular lipid accumulation is a reduction of fat oxidation,[182] related to low aerobic capacity or reduced SNS tone. The effect of IMCL accumulation on peripheral sensitivity is postulated to be due to an alteration of the insulin signal transduction pathway in muscle caused by derivates of fat such as long-chain fatty acyl-CoA and diacylglycerol within the myocyte. These derivates activate the serine/threonine kinase cascade and cause serine phosphorylation of IRS-1, which inhibits insulin signaling.[183] A comparable mechanism has been demonstrated in the liver, where accumulation of lipids (in particular, diacylglycerol) activates the inflammatory cascade by inducing c-jun N-terminal kinase (JNK-1)—which causes serine rather than tyrosine phosphorylation of IRS-1, leading to inhibition of hepatic insulin signaling.[184,185]

Studies in obese children have shown a strong association between IMCL accumulation and peripheral insulin sensitivity.[186] In addition, IMCL is greater in those with impaired glucose tolerance in comparison to more insulin-sensitive adolescents with normal glucose tolerance.[184] Similarly, an inverse relation between the degree of visceral adiposity and insulin sensitivity has been shown in obese children.[187] These observations imply that IMCL and hepatic lipid accumulation may play a pivotal role in the development of peripheral insulin resistance.

ADIPOCYTOKINES

Leptin

The discovery of leptin in 1994 has dramatically changed the view of adipose tissue in the regulation of energy balance.[17] Adipocytes secrete several proteins that act as regulators of glucose and lipid homeostasis.[188] These proteins have been collectively referred to as adipocytokines because of their structural similarity with cytokines. Circulating leptin levels correlate with the degree of obesity. As stated previously, the primary role of leptin is to serve as an adiposity sensor to protect against starvation. Leptin probably has a permissive role in high-energy metabolic processes such as puberty, ovulation, and pregnancy. However, its role in states of energy excess is less known. In obesity, the development of leptin resistance may result in a breakdown of the normal partitioning of surplus lipids in the adipocyte compartment.[189]

Adiponectin

The cytokine adiponectin is peculiar in obesity because in contrast to the other adipocytokines its level is reduced in obesity.[190] The adiponectin gene is expressed exclusively in adipose tissue and codes a protein, a carboxyl-terminal globular head domain, and an amino-terminal collagen domain—which is structurally reminiscent of the complement factor 1q.[191] The gene is located on chromosome 3q27, a location previously linked to the development of type 2 diabetes and the metabolic syndrome. Several single-nucleotide polymorphisms (SNPs) in the adiponectin gene have been reported to be associated with the development of type 2 diabetes in populations around the world, suggesting that adiponectin plays a major role in glucose metabolism.[192]

Adiponectin circulates in plasma in three major forms: a low-molecular-weight trimer, a middle-molecular-weight hexamer, and a high-molecular-weight 12- to 18-mer.[193] Circulating plasma adiponectin concentrations demonstrate a sexual dimorphism (females have greater concentrations), suggesting a role for sex hormones in the regulation of adiponectin production or clearance. Dietary factors such as linoleic acid or fish oil versus a high carbohydrate diet or increased oxidative stress have been shown to increase or decrease adiponectin concentrations, respectively. These observations suggest that the circulating levels of adiponectin are regulated by complex interactions between genetic and environmental factors.[194]

The receptors for adiponectin have recently been characterized in rodent models and cloned. Two receptors (ADIPOR1 and ADIPOR2) have been characterized. ADIPOR1 is expressed in numerous tissues, including muscle—whereas ADIPOR2 is largely restricted to the liver. Both receptors are bound to the cell membrane, yet are unique in comparison to other G-protein–coupled receptors in the fact that the C terminal is external and the N terminal is intracellular.[195] ADIPOR1 and ADIPOR2 are receptors for the globular head of adiponectin and serve as initiators of signal transduction pathways that lead to increased PPARα and AMP kinase activities, which promote glucose uptake and increased fatty acid oxidation. Adiponectin has been shown to have potent antiatherogenic functions because it accumulates in the subendothelial space of injured vascular walls to reduce the expression of adhesion molecules and the recruitment of macrophages.[196]

Studies in obese children and adolescents have shown that adiponectin is inversely related to the degree of obesity, insulin sensitivity visceral adiposity, and IMCL—whereas weight loss increases adiponectin. A fall in adiponectin has been shown to coincide with the onset of insulin resistance[197] and the development of diabetes in monkeys.[198] All of these observations, along with human clinical data, support a pivotal role for adiponectin in the prevention of the co-morbidities of the metabolic syndrome.

Inflammatory Cytokines

Recent accumulating evidence indicates that obesity is associated with subclinical chronic inflammation.[199] The adipose tissue serves not merely as a simple reservoir of energy stored as triglycerides but as an active secretory organ releasing many peptides, including inflammatory cytokines, into the circulation. In obesity, the balance among these numerous peptides is altered such that larger adipocytes and macrophages embedded within them produce more inflammatory cytokines (e.g., TNF-α, IL-6) and fewer anti-inflammatory peptides such as adiponectin.[200]

One theory posits that as energy accumulates in adipocytes the perilipin border of the fat vacuole breaks down, causing the adipocyte to die.[201] Cell death recruits macrophages in the adipose tissue, especially the visceral compartment, which in the process of clearing debris also elaborate inflammatory cytokines—initiating a proinflammatory milieu that predates and possibly drives the development of systemic insulin resistance, diabetes, and endothelial dysfunction.[202,203]

Systemic concentrations of C-reactive protein (CRP) and IL-6, two major markers and participants of the inflammatory process, are increased in obese children and adolescents. CRP levels within the high-normal range have been shown to predict CV disease[204] and the development of T2DM[205] in adults. Elevated levels of CRP correlate with other components of the metabolic syndrome in obese children.[206,207] Thus, inflammation may be one of the links between obesity and insulin resistance—and may promote endothelial dysfunction and early atherogenesis.

Other Adipocytokines

Several other novel adipocytokines have been identified recently, but their clinical significance in humans is unclear. Among them is visfatin,[208] which is secreted exclusively from adipose tissue, is correlated with the amount of visceral fat, and has insulin mimetic effects on adipogenesis in vitro. Another novel adipocytokine is resistin, a 12.5-kDa polypeptide hormone produced by adipocytes in rodents and by immunocompetent cells in humans. In rodents, resistin appears to have an important role in the development of hepatic insulin resistance. However, its role in humans is less clear but may be related to involvement in the regulation of inflammatory processes rather than in tissue-specific insulin sensitivity.

INSULIN RESISTANCE

Insulin resistance presents in the obese child as altered glucose metabolism manifest as impaired glucose tolerance or overt T2DM, dyslipidemia, vascular changes culminating in hypertension, NAFLD, and/or polycystic ovarian syndrome (PCOS). The development of T2DM is covered in depth in Chapter 10. However, it is worth noting that impaired glucose tolerance (IGT)—known as pre-diabetes—is a relatively common condition in obese children and adolescents. The prevalence of IGT among obese children and adolescents is reported to be greater than 20%.[209] Higher prevalence rates of IGT have been reported in obese children from Thailand and the Philippines, in Latino children living in the United States,[210] and in Germany[211]—whereas a lower prevalence rate (15%) was found in obese children in France. IGT in obese youth is typically characterized by obesity with an unfavorable pattern of lipid partitioning, with increased deposition of fat in the visceral and IMCL compartments.[212]

VASCULAR CHANGES

Early stages of the atherosclerotic process may be detected in obese children. In recent years, it has become clear that endothelial dysfunction represents a key early step in the development of atherosclerosis.[213] The hallmark and cause of endothelial dysfunction is impairment in nitric oxide (NO)-mediated vasodilatation.[214] This is due to decreased NO production by endothelial nitric oxide synthase (eNOS), which has been postulated to result from high levels of FFAs and inflammatory cytokines (IL-6, TNF-α; in insulin-resistant obese individuals), from increased reactive oxygen species, or from increased uric acid (which inhibits eNOS activity).[215]

Decreased NO bioavailability leads to an imbalance between vasodilating and vasoconstricting factors (such as endothelin), which leads to impaired vascular smooth-muscle relaxation, increased adhesion of inflammatory cells to the endothelium, increased expression of plasminogen activator inhibitor-1 (PAI-1; a prothrombotic molecule), and increased vascular smooth-muscle cell proliferation. Thus, decreased NO bioavailability is thought to create a proinflammatory prothrombotic environment that promotes atherosclerosis.[216] Endothelial function represents an integrated index of the overall CV risk burden in any given individual.

During the last decade, noninvasive techniques for the assessment of endothelial function [including high-resolution external vascular ultrasound to measure flow-mediated endothelium-dependent dilatation (FMD) of the brachial artery during hyperemia] have been developed.[217,218] Impaired FMD correlates with arterial wall stiffness, coronary dilatation, and endothelial dysfunction in obese children.[219] Similarly, anatomic changes in peripheral arterial vessels [such as increased intimal medial thickness (IMT)] have also been demonstrated in obese children and adolescents.[220] These changes mimic early coronary pathology and predict adverse CV outcomes.

The landmark Bogalusa heart study demonstrated that CV risk factors present in childhood are predictive of coronary artery disease in adulthood.[221,222] Among these risk factors, LDL cholesterol and BMI measured in childhood were found to predict IMT in young adults.[223] There is now substantial evidence that the insulin resistance of childhood obesity creates the metabolic platform for adult CV disease.[224-226] Moreover, the constellation of peripheral insulin resistance, an unfavorable adipocytokine profile, subacute inflammation, and endothelial dysfunction work in parallel to promote the pathologic processes of aging.

THE METABOLIC SYNDROME

The association and clustering of T2DM, hypertension, dyslipidemia, and CV disease in adults has led to the hypothesis that they may arise from a common antecedent. The World Health Organization argues that this antecedent is insulin resistance and defines this association as the metabolic syndrome.[227-230] An alternative definition is provided by the National Cholesterol Education Program (NCEP) Adult Treatment Panel (ATP) III, which categorizes adults deemed to have the syndrome as meeting at least three of the following five criteria: elevated blood pressure, high triglyceride level, low HDL-cholesterol level, high fasting glucose, and central obesity. The metabolic syndrome affects approximately 25% of the U.S. adult population.[231] Because of its wide prevalence, the metabolic syndrome is of enormous clinical and public health importance even at its earliest stages.

Although still debated, one scheme of the pathophysiology of the metabolic syndrome is shown in Figure 19-5. According to this paradigm, the impact of obesity is determined by the pattern of lipid partitioning (i.e., the specific depots in which excess fat is stored). This pattern of lipid storage determines the adipocytokine secretion profile on circulating concentrations of inflammatory cytokines and on the flux of FFA. The combined effect of these factors determines the sensitivity of insulin target organs (such as muscle and liver) to insulin and impacts the vascular system by affecting endothelial function. Peripheral insulin resistance and endothelial dysfunction are the early promoters of overt pathology, culminating in T2DM and CVD. Of note is that formal criteria for the diagnosis of the metabolic syndrome in children have not yet been agreed upon.[232]

OTHER CO-MORBIDITIES RELATED TO INSULIN RESISTANCE

Nonalcoholic Fatty Liver Disease

NAFLD represents fatty infiltration of the liver in the absence of alcohol consumption.[233] The spectrum of NAFLD ranges from pure fatty infiltration (steatosis) to

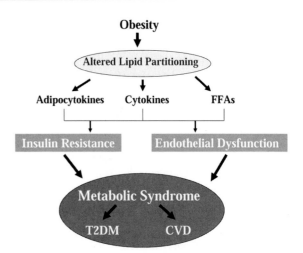

Figure 19-5 A hypothesis on the relation between obesity and the metabolic syndrome. The metabolic impact of obesity is determined by the pattern of lipid partitioning. Lipid storage in insulin-sensitive tissues such as liver or muscle and in the visceral compartment is associated with a typical metabolic profile characterized by elevated free fatty acids and inflammatory cytokines alongside reduced levels of adiponectin. This combination can independently lead to peripheral insulin resistance and to endothelial dysfunction. The combination of insulin resistance and early atherogenesis (manifested as endothelial dysfunction) drives the development of altered glucose metabolism and of cardiovascular disease.

inflammation (nonalcoholic steatohepatitis, or NASH) to fibrosis and even cirrhosis.[234] NAFLD was found in the NHANES III survey to be more prevalent in obese African-American and Hispanic males with T2DM, hypertension, and hyperlipidemia.[235] These associations have led to the hypothesis that NAFLD may precede the onset of T2DM in some individuals.

NAFLD is now the most common liver disease among children in North America.[236,237] NAFLD in children is associated with increased visceral fat deposition,[238] and may progress to cirrhosis and related complications.[239] The association between abdominal obesity and fatty liver may be partially explained by sustained exposure of the liver to an increased flux of FFA from the visceral depot.[175] NAFLD may represent an early manifestation of ectopic lipid deposition in the liver and represents a challenge to the clinician due to the contrast of its minimal early manifestations and its potential serious outcomes.

Recent data indicate that insulin plays a key role in regulating transcription factors, such as sterol response element binding protein-1c (SREBP-1c), which are abundantly expressed in the liver.[240] SREBP-1c is pivotal in the control of hepatic lipogenesis and is increased in proportion to circulating insulin levels.[241] These data raise the possibility that fasting hyperinsulinemia may contribute to hepatic steatosis, rather than vice versa. Alternatively, inflammatory cytokines released by visceral fat or by the hepatic immunoreactive cells may contribute to altered hepatic lipid metabolism.[233]

The majority of patients probably experience NAFLD without progressing to NASH. It is likely that subsequent inflammation or increased oxidative stress is necessary to promote progression to NASH (the "second hit" theory).[239] As hepatic imaging modalities improve, noninvasive quantification of hepatic lipid deposition may enable us to use it as a target for intervention. For the time being, NAFLD can be surmised by an elevated ALT or GGT—although the sensitivity and specificity of these enzymes are low.

Polycystic Ovary Syndrome

The association of hyperandrogenism and oligomenorrhea or amenorrhea (termed *PCOS*) in females is a frequent co-morbidity of obesity that can often be traced to childhood. This disorder is covered in detail in Chapter 14. A 2003 consensus statement[242] defined the diagnostic criteria for PCOS as two out of the following three (after exclusion of other hyperandrogenic disorders): oligo/anovulation, clinical or biochemical manifestations of hyperandrogenism, and polycystic ovaries by ultrasound. PCOS is the most common cause of infertility due to anovulation and a major risk factor for development of the metabolic syndrome and altered glucose metabolism in females. The antecedents of PCOS have been identified in prepubertal girls, suggesting a developmental lesion.[243]

About two-thirds of patients with classic PCOS have hirsutism, acne, or male-pattern alopecia—with a similar portion having manifestations of anovulation such as amenorrhea, dysfunctional uterine bleeding, or oligomenorrhea.[244] The biochemical manifestations of classic PCOS may include evidence of hyperandrogenism and an increased LH level (or an increased LH/FSH ratio) or the demonstration of polycystic ovaries by ultrasound. The nonclassic form of PCOS includes females with manifestations of hyperandrogenism and anovulation without evidence of alterations of gonadotropin levels or of polycystic ovaries on ultrasound.

Obesity characterizes about 50% of women with classic PCOS,[245] although it is even more common among adolescents. Increased peripheral insulin resistance occurs in approximately 50% of patients with PCOS, and almost certainly plays a role in the pathogenesis of this condition. On the other hand, almost all forms of severe insulin resistance (such as T2DM or rare lipodystrophy syndromes) are also associated with PCOS. Insulin resistance has not been included as a diagnostic criterion for PCOS mainly because it is difficult to measure or define.

Fasting hyperinsulinemia and an increased insulin secretory response to an oral glucose load have been demonstrated in girls with PCOS.[246] Indeed, obese adolescent girls with PCOS have been shown to be 50% more insulin resistant than weight-matched controls without PCOS.[247] The constellation of metabolic abnormalities typically seen in insulin-resistant individuals is commonly encountered in obese adolescents with PCOS, including NAFLD[248] and T2DM.[249] The increased prevalence of the metabolic syndrome may be related to the hyperandrogenism independent of obesity-related insulin resistance.[250] Early markers of accelerated atherogenesis are already present in young females with PCOS,[251] indicating that early intervention aimed at reducing CV risk may be beneficial.

Metabolic examination of patients with PCOS demonstrates hepatic and muscle resistance, but not ovarian insulin resistance—possibly accounting for insulin stimulation of theca cell androgen production.[252] The correlation between insulin resistance and hyperandrogenism begs a unifying hypothesis as to their pathogenesis, which is proffered by the "serine phosphorylation hypothesis"—which suggests that P450c17 and the insulin receptor are aberrantly serine phosphorylated. In the case of P450c17, this leads to excess activity and increased androgen production.[253] In the case of the insulin receptor, this leads to tissue-specific insulin resistance.[254] However, this hypothesis remains to be proven.

OTHER ENDOCRINE CO-MORBIDITIES

Obesity causes changes in other hormonal systems, some of which confer specific morbidities. The age at which pubertal initiation occurs continues to decrease, particularly in African Americans. This phenomenon is explained in part by the increasing overnutrition and BMI seen in this population.[255] Infertility in older adolescents and adult women may occur as a manifestation of PCOS due to excessive ovarian androgen production in females or to excessive aromatization of androgen to estrogen by peripheral adipose tissue (with suppression of the hypothalamic-pituitary gonadal axis in both sexes).[256] The hyperestrogenemia may also promote gynecomastia in males.[257] In addition, the hypercapnia associated with obstructive sleep apnea can suppress hypothalamic GnRH function—leading to a syndrome of delayed puberty.[258]

Obesity is associated with decreased GH secretion, and indeed most obese subjects (despite normal or excessive statural growth) fail GH stimulation testing. However, caloric restriction for 24 hours can restore normal GH responsivity.[259] Despite the functional GH inadequacy, statural growth is accelerated, bone age is advanced, and peripheral total and free IGF-1 levels are normal or elevated in obesity—suggesting normal or accentuated GH sensitivity[260] or the suppression of IGFBP-1 and the effects of hyperinsulinemia on activation of the growth plate IGF-1 receptor.[261] Free thyroxine levels tend to be lower and TSH higher in obese children, although still within the normal range. The mechanism is unknown. Last, obesity can be associated with increased cortisol exposure—possibly due to conversion of circulating cortisone to cortisol by the enzyme 11β-hydroxysteroid dehydrogenase-1 (11β-HSD1) located within visceral adipocytes.[262]

OTHER CO-MORBIDITIES

Childhood obesity is associated with numerous other co-morbidities. Pseudotumor cerebri[263] is a rare and poorly understood condition leading to incracranial hypertension, whose manifestations include papilledema and headache. Treatment includes serial lumbar puncture, acetazolamide to reduce CSF production, and occasionally optic nerve sheath fenestration to save eyesight. Obstructive sleep apnea occurs frequently in morbidly obese children, presumably due to the large amount of retropharyngeal fat (which compresses the upper airway during sleep).[264] Affected patients snore, often stop breathing for more than 20 seconds during sleep, and wake up during the night with headache. Treatment includes nocturnal positive airway pressure, and when appropriate tonsilloadenoidectomy. However, symptoms often recur.

Obese children manifest numerous orthopedic difficulties, including fractures, knee pain, anatomic lower limb malalignment, and impairment in mobility.[265] Cholelithiasis occurs in approximately 2.5% of obese adolescents, especially in females, but is not usually seen in prepubertal obese children.[266] Last, psychological distress (including clinical depression) is clearly manifested in obese children.[267] These various co-morbidities all appear to be associated with BMI Z score in a curvilinear fashion.[268] Thus, the more obese the more likely patients will manifest co-morbidity.

Factors Associated with the Current Epidemic of Obesity

GENETICS

The association between obesity and genetics owes to two separate lines of investigation: the discoveries of monogenic disorders of the energy balance pathway, and studies of specific racial and ethnic groups in which obesity seems prevalent (such as the Pimas and other Hispanics in the Southwest United States).[269,270] These observations are combined with an attractive theory (termed the *thrifty gene hypothesis*[271]) on the natural selection of individuals in response to drastic environmental/ecologic pressure (e.g., famine) to yield a very strong driving force for the elucidation of specific genetic loci in the pathogenesis of obesity.[272]

However, the rapid timescale of increased prevalence of childhood obesity cannot possibly reflect a population genetic change. Therefore, the current model is that obesity is a result of gene-environment interactions—an ancient genetic selection to deposit fat efficiently that is maladaptive with our current food overabundance. In the common forms of obesity, relating single-nucleotide polymorphisms with associated risks for obesity is difficult because the effects are uncertain and the results not always confirmed. Despite feverish searches for specific candidate genes, none has thus far been discovered.[273]

EPIGENETICS AND FETAL AND NEONATAL PROGRAMMING

Follow-up studies of newborns born small for gestational age (SGA), large for gestational age (LGA), and premature have noted markedly increased risks for obesity and the metabolic syndrome. The "fetal origins hypothesis"[274] states that some aspect of the in utero environment contributes to the development of obesity and chronic disease in later life. The specific developmental aberration that promotes obesity remains unknown. However, each of these three antenatal conditions is associated with insulin resistance.

Documentation of the relationship of SGA with adult obesity and CV disease started with studies of the Dutch famine during World War II and its aftermath.[275] Several studies of newborns born SGA demonstrate that they are hyperinsulinemic and insulin resistant at birth, exhibit rapid catch-up growth in the early postnatal period, and develop obesity in childhood—which remains and promotes persistent insulin resistance and the metabolic syndrome.

An analysis of Indian newborns born in India versus in the United Kingdom[276] demonstrates that despite those born in India weighing 700 g less at birth, their glucose and insulin levels are markedly elevated. After adjustment for birth weight, the India-born babies demonstrate increased adiposity and four times higher insulin and two times higher leptin levels than the U.K.-born babies. Thus, these babies are insulin resistant even at birth—which translates into increased adiposity. Following such babies into childhood, there are numerous studies documenting insulin resistance during early childhood.[277-279]

Babies born LGA are hyperinsulinemic at birth.[280] Although LGA in most babies is due to gestational diabetes mellitus (GDM) and exposure to hyperglycemia throughout the pregnancy, this is not always the cause. Follow-up of LGA babies without GDM demonstrates a doubling of prevalence of insulin resistance and metabolic syndrome, whereas LGA babies resulting from GDM manifest a threefold increase.[281,282] Indeed, the "vertical" transmission of maternal diabetes to the offspring in the form of later obesity and diabetes has been documented in studies of Pima Indians.[283,284] Last, weight gain during pregnancy increases the risk for LGA and poor outcomes.[285]

Although there are no studies documenting hyperinsulinemia at birth in premature infants due to technical reasons, follow-up of these babies into early childhood also demonstrates increased weight gain—as well as insulin resistance and compensatory insulin secretion that are inappropriately high for the degree of weight gain.[286] The protective effect of breast feeding against development of future obesity has long been known,[166] and there appears to be a dose response (i.e., the longer the breast feeding the more protective).[287] However, this may be complicated by confounding factors such as socioeconomic status, maternal smoking in pregnancy, and maternal BMI.[288] The mechanism of breast feeding's antiobesity effect is also unclear. Some think infant feeding self-regulation is most relevant, whereas a recent study suggests that leptin in breast milk may contribute to this protection.[289] Concern regarding fructose/sucrose content in infant formula has also received attention.

ENVIRONMENT

Numerous environmental factors have also been associated with the obesity epidemic, particularly in children. However, most of these associations are cross-sectional rather than longitudinal—and in many cases a mechanism remains lacking.[290]

Stress and Cortisol

In humans, elevated cortisol or markers of HPA axis dysregulation correlate with abdominal fat distribution and the metabolic syndrome.[291] Although circulating cortisol is clearly important in determining visceral adiposity, the recent identification of reduction of circulating cortisone to cortisol within visceral fat tissue by the enzyme 11β-hydroxysteroid dehydrogenase-1 (11βHSD1) has also been linked to the metabolic syndrome.[262,292] These data suggest that cortisol is important in increasing visceral adiposity and promoting the metabolic syndrome.

In adults, job stress and depression stress cause increased cortisol secretion[293]—which leads to insulin resistance and the metabolic syndrome. Psychosocial stresses correlate with risk of myocardial infarction in adults.[294] It is assumed that such patients exhibit increased HPA axis activation.[295] Even exogenous glucocorticoid administration is a risk factor for CV events.[296] Evidence of associations between elevated cortisol and psychological distress with abdominal fat distribution in adults is compelling. For instance, urinary glucocorticoid excretion is linked to aspects of the metabolic syndrome—including blood pressure, fasting glucose, insulin, and waist circumference.[291]

Although circulating cortisol is clearly important in determining visceral adiposity, the recent identification of reduction of circulating cortisone to cortisol within visceral fat tissue by 11βHSD1 has also been linked to the MetS. The role of cortisol in mediating visceral fat accumulation, insulin resistance, and T2DM has been elegantly demonstrated by the transgenic knockout and overexpression of 11βHSD1.[262,292] These data suggest that cortisol is important in increasing visceral adiposity and promoting the MetS—equivalent to Cushing syndrome of the abdomen.[297] However, the role of stress and cortisol in childhood obesity is currently speculative.

Sleep Deprivation

Americans get significantly less sleep than they did three decades ago. Adults in the United States currently average less than 7 hours of sleep per night, which is almost 2 hours less than in 1980 (and about one-third of them get less than 6 hours per night).[298] Analyses of data from the first NHANES revealed that adults (ages 32 to 49) who got less than 7 hours of sleep were more likely to be obese 5 to 8 years later than those who got 7 or more hours of sleep.[299] Similarly, a 13-year prospective cohort study in which participants were interviewed at ages 27, 29, 34, and 40 years of age found that sleep duration correlated negatively with obesity.[300]

The link between short sleep duration and obesity has also been observed among children.[301] Like adults, increasing numbers of children are chronically sleep deprived. This is especially true of obese children, who have been found to get less sleep than those of normal weight. In addition to its other effects, sleep is one of the most powerful cross-sectional[302] and longitudinal[303] predictors of childhood obesity in prepubertal children. Although relatively little is known about the mechanism for the sleep-obesity relationship, especially among children, there are reasons to assume increased stress and altered activity of various hormones (such as leptin, ghrelin, and cortisol).

Television Viewing and "Screen Time"

Television watching is considered one of the most modifiable causes of childhood obesity.[304] There are four possible mechanisms linking television watching and obesity. First, television watching may increase stress levels and cortisol—causing increased food intake and promotion of obesity.[305] Second, television watching displaces physical activity and reduces voluntary energy expenditure (VEE). Most studies find inverse correlations between television watching and physical activity and fitness.[306,307] Third, television watching increases calorie consumption from eating during viewing or from the effects of food advertising. Television viewing is also associated with increased high-fat food intake, decreased fruit and vegetable consumption, and increased soft drink intake.[308]

Junk food is the most frequently advertised product category on children's television. Last, REE and nonexercise associated thermogenesis (NEAT) appears to be decreased during television watching.[309] According to NHANES III (1988-1994), the prevalence of childhood obesity is lowest among children watching television ≤ 1 hour/day and highest among those watching 4 hours/day.[310] The relationship between television watching and obesity has been examined in large number of cross-sectional epidemiologic studies but in few longitudinal studies.[304]

Several experimental studies of reducing television watching have been conducted, and their results support the suggestion that reduced television watching may help to reduce the obesity risk or help promote weight loss in obese children.[311] These studies represent the strongest direct evidence that altering television watching alone is a promising strategy for prevention of childhood obesity. Other forms of "screen time," such as video games, computers, and cell phones, are also implicated in obesity pathogenesis.

Dietary Fat Versus Carbohydrate

Fat is generally considered more obesigenic than other macronutrients, given its more energy-dense, highly palatable, and effective conversion to body fat.[312] A high-fat meal induces decreased thermogenesis and a higher positive fat balance than an isocaloric and isoproteic low-fat meal.[313] Excessive fat intake is believed to cause weight gain,[314] but the relationship between dietary fat intake and childhood adiposity remains controversial.[315]

The prevalence of overweight in the United States has increased despite a decreased percentage of dietary energy derived from fat. A meta-analysis of 12 studies in overweight or obese adults who were given dietary advice on low-fat diet and followed for 6 to 18 months suggested that low-fat diets are no better than calorie-restricted diets in long-term weight loss.[316] Similarly, in children total fat consumption expressed as a percentage of energy intake has decreased.[317] This decrease in fat consumption is largely due to increased total energy intake in the form of carbohydrates. Much of this imbalance is attributed to changing beverage consumption patterns characterized by declining milk intake and substantial increases in soft drink consumption,[318] which may have its own etiopathogenesis. Most interventions with a low-fat heart-healthy diet have not been successful in childhood overweight prevention.[319]

Reduction in carbohydrate intake is taken to the extreme in the Atkins diet, which restricts adult subjects to less than 25 g/d of ingested carbohydrate. Adult evaluations of the diet for weight control have been disappointing long-term,[320,321] and the popular diet has been abandoned recently. There are currently no data in children or adolescents. However, it should be noted that the ketogenic diet used for seizure control is similar in composition to the Atkins diet. A 2-year study of the ketogenic diet demonstrated persistent decreases in weight Z scores in children who were above average upon diet initiation, without significant compromise in general nutrition or in height.[322]

Glycemic Index and Fiber

Not all sugars exert the same insulinogenic response. Complex carbohydrates can take two forms: a combination of α1-4 linkages and α1-6 linkages that gives the starch a globular stucture called amylopectin (as seen in bread, rice, pasta, potatoes, and glycogen) or a linear polymer of α1-4 linkages called amylose (as seen in beans, lentils, and other legumes). Digestion and absorption of the former in the intestine is rapid due to the simultaneous actions of α1-4 and α1-6 glucosidases, whereas that of the latter is much slower because the α1-4 glucosidase can only cleave single glucose moieties on either side of the polymer. This phenomenon constitutes the basis of the glycemic index (GI),[323] which refers to the glucose area under the curve after consumption.

High-GI foods lead to an accentuated insulin response, which can shunt energy substrate to adipose tissue.[324] In children, controlled studies with a high-GI diet demonstrate that energy intake is 53% higher than on low-GI diet.[325] One adolescent study demonstrated that an ad libitum low-GI diet was more effective in promoting weight loss than an energy-restricted low-fat diet.[326] Therefore, the GI may be a simple concept to institute—although the "toxic environment" of American foodstuffs may make it difficult to maintain.

Dietary fiber consists of the nonstarch polysaccharide portion of plant foods, including cellulose, hemicellulose, pectins, β-glucans, fructans, gums, mucilages, and algal polysaccharides. Major sources of dietary fiber include whole grains, fruits, vegetables, legumes, and nuts. Fiber content accounts for 50% of the variability in glycemic load (GL; GI × volume) among foods. Cohort studies of adults demonstrate that fiber intake is inversely associated with weight gain, fasting insulin levels, and risk of T2DM.[327,328] Fiber may influence body weight regulation by several mechanisms involving intrinsic, hormonal, and colonic effects—which eventually decrease food intake by promoting satiation (lower meal energy content) or satiety (longer duration between meals) or by increasing fat oxidation and decreasing fat storage.[329] A fiber-rich meal is processed more slowly and has less caloric density, fat, and added sugars.

Fiber-containing foods engender slower glucose absorption, which lessens the postprandial insulin surge and decreases lipogenesis.[330] In addition, high-fiber meals allow for delivery of undigested triglyceride to the colon—where fermentation to short-chain fatty acids and their absorption improve lipids and insulin sensitivity.[331] Archeologists surmise that our ancestors used to consume 100 to 300 g of fiber a day.[332] However, the dietary fiber intake throughout childhood and adolescence currently averages approximately 12 g/day and has not changed during the past 30 years.[333] Therefore, parents and school foodservice personnel should strive to offer fiber-rich foods to children so that their acceptance and consumption of them will be increased.[334]

Fructose

The most commonly used sweetener in the U.S. diet is the disaccharide sucrose (i.e., table sugar), which contains 50% fructose and 50% glucose. However, in North America and many other countries non-diet soft drinks are sweetened with high-fructose corn syrup (HFCS)—which contains up to 55% of the monosaccharide fructose. Because of its abundance, sweetness, and low price, HFCS has become the most common sweetener used in processed foods. It is not that HFCS is biologically more ominous than sucrose. It is that its low cost has made it available to everyone, especially low socioeconomic groups.

HFCS is found in processed foods ranging from soft drinks and candy bars to crackers to hot dog buns to ketchup. Average daily fructose consumption has increased by more than 25% over the past 30 years. The growing dependence on fructose in the Western diet may be fueling the obesity and T2DM epidemics.[335] Animal models demonstrate that high-fructose diets lead to increased energy intake, decreased resting energy expenditure, excess fat deposition, and insulin resistance[336]—which suggest that fructose consumption is playing a role in the epidemics of insulin resistance and obesity and T2DM in humans.[337] The metabolism of fructose differs significantly from that of glucose (Figure 19-6). Fructose is absorbed in the intestine and enters the liver without insulin regulation. There, fructose is converted to fructose-1-phosphate and enters the glycolytic pathway without regulation. This leads to an excess accumulation of citrate outside the mitochondria, which then undergoes de novo lipogenesis and is reassembled into free fatty acids (which promote insulin resistance), very low-density lipoproteins (which promote atherogenesis and serve as a substrate for obesity),[338] and triglycerides (some of which precipitate in the liver, activate the inflammatory pathway, and cause nonalcoholic steatohepatitis).[339] Fructose also does not suppress secretion of the "hunger hormone" ghrelin, levels of which correlate with perceived hunger.

In sum, fructose consumption has metabolic and hormonal consequences that facilitate development of obesity and the metabolic syndrome.[340] The highest fructose loads are soda (1.7 g/oz) and juice (1.8 g/oz). Although soda has received most of the attention,[159,341] high fruit juice intake is also associated with childhood obesity—especially in lower income families.[342] Nonetheless, the American Academy of Pediatrics recommends that fruit juice consumption be allowed to 4 to 5 oz/day for 1- to 6-year-old children and 8 to 12 oz/day for 7- to 18-year-old children.[343]

Calcium and Dairy

There have been several reports of an inverse relationship between dietary calcium and obesity indices.[344,345] Dietary calcium plays an important role in energy metabolism

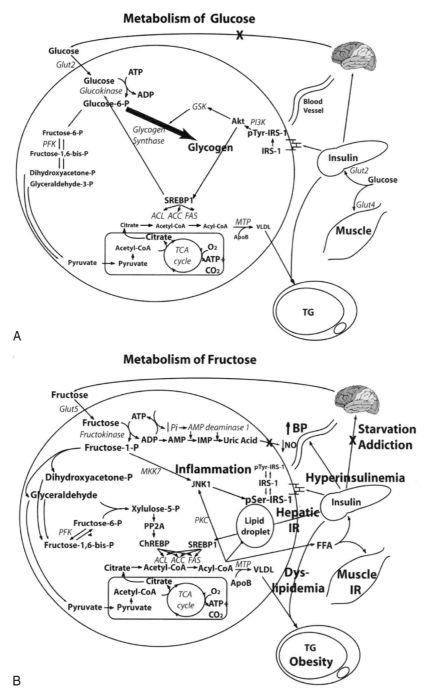

Figure 19-6 Hepatic (*A*) glucose and (*B*) fructose metabolism. Only 20% of an ingested glucose load is metabolized by the liver, whereas 100% of a fructose load is hepatically metabolized. Thus, in a 120-calorie glucose load (two slices of white bread) 24 calories are hepatically metabolized—whereas in a 120-calorie sucrose load (an 8-oz. glass of orange juice) a bolus of 72 calories reach the liver. In contrast to glucose, fructose induces substrate-dependent hepatocellular phosphate depletion, which increases uric acid and contributes to hypertension through inhibition of endothelial nitric oxide synthase and reduction of nitric oxide (NO); stimulation of de novo lipogenesis and excess production of VLDL and serum triglyceride, promoting dyslipidemia; accumulation of intrahepatic lipid droplets, promoting hepatic steatosis; production of FFA, which promotes muscle insulin resistance; c-jun N-terminal kinase (JNK-1) activation, which serine phosphorylates and the hepatic insulin receptor—rendering it inactive and contributing to hepatic insulin resistance, which promotes hyperinsulinemia and influences substrate deposition into fat; and CNS hyperinsulinemia, which antagonizes leptin signaling (see Figure 19-3) and promotes continued energy intake.

regulation. Increased calcitriol (1,25-dihydroxyvitamin D) in response to low-calcium diets stimulates Ca^{2+} influx in human adipocytes may lead to stimulation of lipogenic gene expression and lipogenesis, as well as inhibition of lipolysis.[345] This may result in an expansion of adipocyte triglyceride stores, which can promote adiposity.

Increased dietary calcium reduces calcitriol levels and leads to reduction of fat mass without caloric restriction in mice,[346] and this antiobesity effect of dietary calcium is supported by human clinical and epidemiologic studies.[347] Vitamin D deficiency correlates with increasing BMI, especially in African Americans.[348] However, it is not known if this is due to substitution of soft drinks for dairy, to lactose intolerance, or to other factors. One adult study[349] revealed a consistent effect of higher calcium intake on lower body weight and body fat. However, pediatric studies are lacking.

Trace Minerals

Chromium and vanadium appear to be involved in the insulin signaling process. In diabetic animals, chromium or vanadium supplementation results in improvement in insulin sensitivity and glycemic control[350,351]—and there is a suggestion of decreased weight. It is not yet known whether the pathogenesis of insulin resistance in humans involves a deficiency of a trace mineral. However, inadequate dietary intakes of vitamins and minerals are widespread—most likely due to excessive consumption of energy-rich micronutrient-poor refined food. Inadequate intake of micronutrients may result in chronic metabolic disruption, mitochondrial decay, DNA damage, oxidant leakage, and cellular aging associated with late-onset diseases such as obesity and cancer.[352]

Infectious Causes

The pattern of increase in prevalence during the current obesity epidemic is reminiscent of an infectious transmission. Studies in animals implicate adenovirus-36 in the conversion from lean to obese.[353] Studies in adults thus far demonstrate correlation between BMI and antibodies to this virus,[354] but mechanism is lacking. Alternatively, the predominance of certain human intestinal flora species (firmicutes versus bacteroides) may predispose animals and humans to obesity[355]—possibly by increasing efficiency of energy absorption. However, factors that determine their predominance are unknown.

Medications

Numerous medications promote excessive weight gain in children. The most commonly prescribed are pharmacologic doses of glucocorticoids (e.g., prednisone, methylprednisolone, dexamethasone), used for their antiinflammatory and antineoplastic activities. Patients so treated frequently become obese,[356,357] and develop many of the features of Cushing syndrome (e.g., visceral adiposity, hyperlipidemia, hypertension, glucose intolerance)—which typify the metabolic syndrome.[296]

Sex hormone administration also promotes excessive weight gain, presumably by inducing insulin resistance.[358]

In an effort to improve type 1 diabetes glycemic control, many physicians will overinsulinize the patient—but at the expense of excessive weight gain.[359] Last, more and more children are being placed on the atypical antipsychotics risperidone, olanzapine, quetiapine, clozepine, aripriprazole, and ziprasidone to affect mood and behavior.[360] These medications induce insulin resistance, which foments persistent hyperphagia and weight gain and increases risk for the metabolic syndrome.[361]

Disorders of Obesity

The concept that obesity is a phenotype of numerous pathologies is evident from the examination of specific endocrine disorders leading to obesity in early childhood (Table 19-1). Some involve neural mechanisms, others classical hormonal mechanisms, and still others dysregulation of increased energy intake, decreased energy expenditure, and/or increased energy storage at the adipocyte.

CLASSIC ENDOCRINE DISORDERS WITH AN OBESITY PHENOTYPE

In children, linear or statural growth accounts for up to 20% of ingested calories. Endocrine states that allow for normal energy intake for age but inhibit linear growth will of necessity lead to excessive energy storage. This is the case for the four "classic" endocrine disorders associated with obesity. These can be distinguished from other causes of pediatric obesity on the basis of their suboptimal growth rate—as opposed to overnutrition, which tends to increase the rate of growth and skeletal maturation (probably due to excess insulin cross-reacting with the IGF-1 receptor).[261]

Hypothyroidism (see Chapter 1) results in a lower REE due to insufficient circulating T_3, along with decreased VEE due to fatigue. The decrease in total energy expenditure, despite a relatively low caloric intake, promotes persistent energy storage and increases adiposity. Thyroid hormone replacement is sufficient to increase growth, REE, and VEE to resolve the obesity over time.

Cushing syndrome (see Chapter 12) results in growth arrest and cortisol-induced hyperphagia,[362] with a decrease in REE and VEE due to muscle wasting. Reduction of circulating glucocorticoid through medical or surgical means usually reverses the obesity to some degree. Exogenous glucocorticoid therapy can result in the same obesity phenotype. Hypercortisolism may be more related to obesity than previously realized, due to the transgenic model of 11βHSD1 overexpression in visceral adipose tissue—which converts inactive circulating cortisone to cortisol.[262] However, its role in human obesity is not clear because correlations between 11βHSD1 polymorphisms and BMI or waist:hip ratio were weak at best[363]—and enzyme activity was not elevated in one human study.[364]

GH deficiency (see Chapter 8) prevents lipolysis and promotes visceral adiposity, although obesity is usually not severe. GH deficiency is also associated with fatigue and decreased VEE. GH deficiency is often accompanied by other pituitary hormone deficiencies (e.g., central hypothyroidism), which can also decrease REE. GH therapy

TABLE 19-1

Classification of Childhood Obesity Disorders

Mongenetic Disorders of the Energy Balance Pathway
- Leptin deficiency
- Leptin receptor deficiency
- POMC mutation ("red" hair, adrenal insufficiency)
- Prohormone convertase-1 deficiency
- MC_3R mutation
- MC_4R mutation
- SIM-1 mutation

Syndromic Disorders (Mental Retardation Prominent)
- Prader-Willi syndrome
  - Short stature
  - Hypogonadism
  - Hypotonia
  - Ghrelin overproduction
- Bardet-Biedl syndrome
  - Retinitis pigmentosa
  - Polydactyly
  - Hypogonadism
- TrkB mutation
  - Hypotonia
  - Impaired short-term memory
  - Decreased nociception
- Börjeson-Forssman-Lehmann syndrome
  - Microcephaly
  - Large ears
  - Hypogonadism
- Carpenter syndrome
  - Variable craniosynostosis
  - Brachdactyly, polydactyly, syndactyly
  - Congenital heart disease
  - Hypogonadism
- Cohen syndrome
  - Persistent hypotonia
  - Microcephaly
  - Maxillary hypoplasia
  - Prominent incisors
- Alström syndrome
  - Hypogonadism
  - Short stature
  - Neurosensory deficits

Classic Endocrine Disorders (Short Stature and Growth Failure Prominent)
- Hypothyroidism
  - Primary
  - Central
- Cushing syndrome (adrenal hypercorticism)
  - Adrenal adenoma/carcinoma
  - Adrenal micronodular hyperplasia
  - Pituitary ACTH-secreting tumor
  - Ectopic ACTH-secreting tumor
  - Exogenous glucocorticoid administration
- Growth hormone deficiency
- Pseudohypoparathyroidism 1a
  - Maternal transmission (AHO + multihormone resistance)
  - Paternal transmission (pseudopseudohypoparathyroidism, AHO only)

Insulin Dynamic Disorders
- Hypothalamic obesity (insulin hypersecretion)
- Insulin resistance
- Leptin resistance

is able to reverse these defects, increase muscle mass, and promote weight loss.

Pseudohypoparathyroidism type 1a (PHP1a) (see Chapters 2 and 17) is an autosomal-dominant mutation of GNAS1, which codes for the $G_{s\alpha}$ subunit necessary to peptide hormone signal transduction. Maternal transmission leads to PHP1a (multihormone resistance), along with Albright's heriditary osteodystrophy (AHO)—of which a cardinal feature is obesity, probably due to the inability to stimulate cAMP in response to β-adrenergic stimulation within adipocytes (due to defective G-protein signal transduction).[365] Paternal transmission leads to AHO without multihormone resistance, also known as pseudopseudohypoparathyroidism. Unfortunately, this form of obesity is not responsive to current medications.

MONOGENETIC DISORDERS OF THE NEGATIVE FEEDBACK PATHWAY

The elucidation of the regulation of the energy balance pathway is exemplified by the discovery of specific defects within that pathway leading to early-onset obesity. Numerous obesity syndromes within the pathway have been described over the past 10 years, and are reviewed in detail elsewhere.[366,367]

Leptin Deficiency

Mutations of the leptin gene in humans recapitulate the phenotype of the *ob/ob* leptin-deficient mouse.[368] Approximately 11 such patients have been described, primarily of Pakistani and Turkish descent expressing the products of consanguinity. These patients manifest hyperphagia from birth, with obesity documentable as early as 6 months of age. The lack of leptin induces the starvation response in the form of reduced thyroid hormone levels, lack of sympathetic tone, lack of pubertal progression, and defective immunity.[369]

Despite the modest hypothyroidism, the concomitant hyperinsulinemia allows excess insulin to cross-react with the IGF-1 receptor in order to maintain growth rate and bone age until the usual time of puberty. However, because of the important role of leptin in initiating and maintaining puberty, untreated patients with leptin deficiency are short due to the lack of a pubertal growth spurt. The diagnosis is made by demonstrating extremely low or unmeasurable serum leptin levels. However, treatment with recombinant leptin is effective in restoring leptin signaling—resulting in reduction of hyperphagia, resolution of obesity, induction of puberty, and restoration of immune regulation.[369] Heterozygotes for leptin deficiency assume an intermediate phenotype.[370]

Leptin Receptor Deficiency

Three family members in France of Algerian extraction were found to have a mutation truncating the leptin receptor prior to its insertion in the membrane.[371] This family had symptoms and signs similar to those with leptin deficiency, although they had growth retardation, low thyroid levels, and low IGF-1 and IGFBP-3 levels. The reason for this dichotomy is not known. Diagnosis hinges on documenting extremely high leptin levels even for the degree of obesity. No other families have been described. Unfortunately, no treatment currently exists.

POMC Splicing Mutation

Inability to synthesize POMC due to missense or truncation mutations results in the inability to splice out α-MSH in the brain, leading to defective anorexigenesis at the MC₄R and early-onset obesity. In the periphery, this defect leads to "red" hair to due lack of α-MSH action at the skin MC₁R. In the pituitary, the defect results in inability to splice out ACTH—leading to secondary adrenal insufficiency.[372] Recently, a Turkish patient with this mutation was reported to have dark hair—indicating that pigmentation of the hair is not entirely explained by the mutation's effect on MC₁R.[373] Approximately six patients have thus far been reported, but are easily diagnosed due to their unusual phenotype, ACTH levels, and hypocortisolemia. There is currently no treatment for the obesity.

Prohormone Convertase-1 Deficiency

Defects in this enzyme lead to the inability to process various preprohormones to their active ligands, such as POMC to ACTH and α-MSH, proinsulin to insulin, and various gut propeptides to active hormones.[374] Only two unrelated patients have thus far been reported. They manifest severe early-onset obesity, ACTH deficiency, hypogonadism, hyperproinsulinemia, and small intestinal dysfunction—presumably on the basis of inability to cleave intestinal propeptides to their mature form. The diagnosis can be made by finding extremely high levels of proinsulin. No treatment currently exists for the obesity.

Melanocortin-3 Receptor Mutation

Two family members in Singapore with mutations of the MC₃R manifested with early-onset obesity.[375] This receptor appears to have a slightly different function from the MC₄R, as it seems to be involved in regulation of energy expenditure as opposed to energy intake.[84] Diagnosis can only be made by gene sequencing. No treatment currently exists.

Melanocortin-4 Receptor Mutation

Mutations in the MC₄R appear to account for up to 5% of morbid obesity, especially those beginning in childhood.[376,377] This mutation is transmitted as a co-dominant inheritance because homozygotes are more severely affected than heterozygotes, and not all carriers exhibit obesity. Patients exhibit early-onset hyperphagia and obesity, although not as severe as those with leptin deficiency. These patients grow rapidly, due to the hyperinsulinemia. Notably, their lean mass and their bone mineral density are increased commensurate with the adiposity.[377] The diagnosis is made by gene sequencing. There is currently no treatment for this disorder.

SIM-1 Mutation

SIM1 stands for "single-minded," a drosophila gene involved in neurogenesis—particularly the PVN, which expresses the MC₄R. SIM1 appears to act as a signal transduction mechanism integrating information downstream from MC₄R activation.[378] Heterozygous null mice for SIM1 are obese. The human homolog is on chromosome 6q. A girl with hyperphagia, obesity, and developmental delay with a balanced translocation between 1p22.1 and 6q16.2 was found to have a mutation of SIM1.[379] Only a few polymorphisms of SIM1 in obesity have been reported, and their significance is not yet established.[380]

PLEIOTROPIC OBESITY AND MENTAL RETARDATION DISORDERS

Approximately 30 different obesity syndromes have been described, and most (if not all) are associated with mental retardation.[381] Each has some other distinguishing phenotype, which makes the diagnosis obvious on clinical grounds. Various genetic linkages have been noted, but the etiologies for the obesity in these disorders remain obscure.

Prader-Willi Syndrome

Prader-Willi syndrome (PWS) is a defect in the paternal allele of chromosome 15q11-13[382] from deletion, mutation, defective imprinting, or uniparental disomy of chromosome 15. Subjects affected with PWS present with hypotonia and failure to thrive in the neonatal period, and as they get older they develop the classic findings of hypogonadism, short stature, mental retardation, and severe obesity.

PWS patients are classically described as voracious eaters, although they can be easily dissuaded from food if they are removed from behavioral signals for food intake. REE is approximately 60% of normal in PWS, promoting adiposity.[383] In addition, ghrelin levels are massively elevated in PWS[384]—which may be one etiology for their persistent hyperphagia. Others have suggested that the obesity in PWS is a function of GH deficiency, with defective lipolysis.[385]

Bardet-Biedl Syndrome

This syndrome is characterized by obesity, mild mental retardation, dysmorphic extremities (including polydactyly), retinitis pigmentosa, hypogonadism, and renal malformations. Its inheritance is complex, but is usually described as autosomal recessive. Eight different genetic loci have been implicated,[386] although their functions continue to remain elusive. The cause of the obesity remains unknown, but it is postulated to be due to failure of development of ciliated hypothalamic neurons.[387,388] Diagnosis usually rests on clinical grounds. Although there is no specific treatment available, anecdotal instances of efficacy of metformin exist.

TrkB Mutation

The NTRK2 gene codes for the ligand-specific subunit for the receptor TrkB, which has brain-derived growth factor (BDNF) as its ligand. TrkB is important for neural development. An 8-year-old boy with early hypotonia, developmental delay, impaired short-term memory, decreased responsiveness to nociception, and severe hyperphagia starting at 6 months culminating in morbid obesity was reported recently.[389] Examination of the NTRK2 gene demonstrated a A to G transition in codon 722, substituting cysteine for tyrosine, which inhibited phosphorylation of TrkB. A second patient with obesity, impaired cognitive function, and hyperactivity was found to have an isocentric inversion at the BDNF locus.[390] The etiology of the hyperphagia and obesity remain unclear.

Carpenter Syndrome

This syndrome consists of obesity plus variable craniosynostosis, brachdactyly, polydactyly, syndactyly, congenital heart disease, and hypogonadism. Its etiology remains obscure.

Cohen Syndrome

This disorder presents with persistent hypotonia, microcephaly, maxillary hypoplasia, and prominent incisors. The gene for Cohen syndrome has been mapped to chromosome 8q,[391] and it codes for a transmembrane protein of unknown function.

Alström Syndrome

This syndrome presents with neurosensory deficits, such as deafness, with various other endocrinopathies that cause an early-onset type 2 diabetes. The ALMS1 gene has been discovered.[392] It appears to be important in cilia function,[388] and may account for abnormal neuronal migration.

Börjeson-Forssman-Lehmann Syndrome

This syndrome is characterized by microcephaly, seizures, large ears, and hypogonadism. The defective gene is a zinc-finger protein of unknown function.[393]

INSULIN DYNAMIC DISORDERS

Hypothalamic Obesity and Insulin Hypersecretion

It is well known that bilateral electrolytic lesions or deafferentation of the VMH in rats leads to intractable weight gain,[109,110,394-396] even upon food restriction.[397] Originally, the obesity was felt to be due to damage to a satiety center—which promoted hyperphagia and increased energy storage.[398] However, we now understand that dysfunction of leptin signal transduction in the VMH due to hypothalamic damage secondary to CNS tumor, surgery, radiation, or trauma can alter the afferent and efferent pathways of energy balance and lead to severe and intractable weight gain.[399,400]

In this syndrome of "hypothalamic obesity," hypothalamic insult prevents integration of peripheral afferent signals. The VMH cannot transduce these signals into a sense of energy sufficiency and a subjective state of satiety.[54,395] Children with hypothalamic obesity exhibit weight gain even in response to forced caloric restriction.[401] This seems paradoxical, as one would expect that if hyperphagia were the reason for the obesity caloric restriction would be effective. The reason for this paradox is that similar to the *db/db* mouse these subjects exhibit "organic leptin resistance" (that is, the inability to respond to their own leptin due to the VMH damage).

Numerous assessments of weight gain following cancer therapy in children have been performed. Most of these evaluations have been retrospective, and performed in the acute lymphoblastic leukemia (ALL) survivor population.[402] An extremely high frequency of hypothalamic obesity of 30% to 77% has been documented after craniopharyngioma treatment.[403] In each of these cancer types, hypothalamic damage is the primary risk factor for development of this syndrome.[404] However, the syndrome has also been reported in cases of pseudotumor cerebri, trauma, and infiltrative or inflammatory diseases of the hypothalamus.[399] Aside from the symptoms of tumor-induced increased intracranial pressure, patients with hypothalamic obesity classically exhibit signs of limbic system involvement such as hypogonadism, somnolence, rage, and hyperphagia.[405] However, such classic presentations are actually rare.[396]

Hypothalamic obesity is the result of "organic" leptin resistance due to death of VMH neurons. This leads to defective autonomic neurotransmission.[99] This is akin to the starvation response in that it manifests defective activation of the SNS (which retards lipolysis and energy expenditure)[406,407] and overactivation of the vagus,[408] which promotes an obligate insulin hypersecretion and energy storage.[409] In animals and in humans, vagal hyperreactivity can be prevented by pancreatic vagotomy.[110,410-412]

Primary Insulin Resistance

Insulin resistance is a primary entity in some pediatric populations. It is associated with the development of the metabolic syndrome, especially in certain racial and ethnic groups.[413] For example, the Pima Indians of Arizona exhibit a 50% incidence of obesity and type 2 diabetes.[414] Insulin resistance correlates with abdominal adiposity and CV morbidity.[415,416] The presence of acanthosis nigricans, a hyperpigmented and hypertrophic patch of skin at extensor surfaces such as the nape of the neck, is a clinical marker of hyperinsulinemia[417] due to cross reactivity between insulin and the epidermal growth factor receptor of the skin.[418] Fasting hyperinsulinemia, an indicator of inherent insulin resistance in children, is an important predictor of adult obesity.[419,420]

This is further exacerbated by sex hormones (especially estrogen), contributing to the increased incidence of insulin resistance and obesity in teenage girls. The cause is unknown, but primary insulin resistance may be a manifestation of all three inciting factors (genetic, epigenetic, and environmental). There may be specific genetic predispositions[269] that have been enriched by natural selection. In addition, the high incidence of gestational DM in Pima mothers promotes obesity and T2DM in the offspring.[284]

Last, the consumption of low-quality processed food[136] made available by government subsidies promote continued obesity. It should be noted that in primary insulin resistance dietary and exercise interventions have been notoriously ineffective at reducing the obesity.[421,422] The locus of the resistance to insulin is not defined. Reduced numbers and function of insulin receptors may in part be secondary to the hyperinsulinemia itself, rather than due to a primary defect.

Evaluation and Treatment of the Obese Child

WORKUP

The key to successful obesity therapy is accurate diagnosis. Our diagnostic armamentarium is not yet fully developed, and thus matching treatment to diagnosis is still uncertain. Specific points in the evaluation and their rationale are listed in Table 19-2. In eliciting the history, birth weight, parents' BMIs, gestational diabetes, prematurity, history of breast feeding, and neonatal complications (especially CNS injury) are all relevant. The earlier the patient's obesity is noted (i.e., early adiposity rebound) the more likely an organic reason will be discerned. Neurodevelopmental abnormalities may signify the need for a genetics referral.

The medication list must be reviewed, especially for atypical antipsychotics. Orthopedic pain, headache, and snoring must be assessed. Dietary history must include skipping breakfast, daily ingestion of sodas and juices, and frequency and type of snacking. The degree of perceived stress by the patient is also likely a major contributor to visceral adiposity. A corollary is the number of caretakers of the child because this increases stress, family chaos, and lack of child supervision.

On physical examination, linear growth is key because classical endocrine evaluation [e.g., hypothyroidism, Cushing syndrome, GH deficiency, pseudohypoparathyroidism (PHP)] is not necessary if linear growth is not attenuated. However, hyperinsulinemia and insulin resistance usually cause accelerated growth due to cross reactivity of insulin with the IGF-1 receptor.[261] Important physical features to assess include acanthosis nigricans and waist circumference (both of which are associated with insulin resistance and the metabolic syndrome), fundoscopic examination to rule out pseudotumor cerebri, liver enlargement to suggest hepatic steatosis, hirsutism to suggest PCOS, and muscle tone to evaluate hypotonia and myopathy (which reduce energy expenditure).

TABLE 19-2

Diagnostic Workup of Childhood Obesity and Its Co-morbidities

Etiology/Co-Morbidity	Evaluation
Histroy	
• Genetic etiology	• Parent BMI, race, mental retardation
• Epigenetic etiology	• Birth weight, gestational difficulties, prematurity
• CNS etiology	• CNS insult, mental retardation or developmental delay
• Endocrine etiology	• Slowdown in linear growth, red hair
• Medication etiology	• Medication history, especially atypical antipsychotics
• Dietary etiology	• Calorie recall, especially sugar-containing liquids, breast-feeding Hx
• Physical activity etiology	• Exercise history, television, computer, and cell phone recall
• Stress etiology	• Socioeconomic status, number of caregivers, television recall, sleep status, atypical depression
• Sleep apnea	• History of snoring, headache, waking up with headache
• PCOS	• Hirsutism, oligomenorhea, amenorrhea
• Type 2 diabetes	• Polyuria, polydipsia, nocturia, recent weight loss
• Orthopedic morbidity	• Knee or hip pain, limitation of motion
• Depression	• Affect, activity level, school performance
Physical	
• Insulin resistance	• Acanthosis nigricans, skin tags, waist circumference
• Hypertension	• SBP or DBP >90th percentile for age
• Pseudotumor cerebri	• Papilledema
• Hepatic steatosis	• Hepatomegaly
• PCOS	• Hirsutism
• Precocious/delayed puberty	• Gonadal and pubic hair status
• Sleep apnea	• Tonsillar hypertrophy
• Myopathy	• Decreased muscle tone, hyporeflexia
• Syndromic obesity	• Specific neurocutaneous stigmata (see Table 19-1), retardation
Laboratory	
• Hepatic steatosis	• ALT, hepatic ultrasound
• Glucose intolerance	• Fasting glucose >100 or 2-hr glucose >140
• Type 2 diabetes mellitus	• Fasting glucose >125 or 2-hr glucose >200; HbA1c >6.5%
• Dyslipidemia	• Lipid profile with increased VLDL, TG:HDL >2.5
• Insulin resistance	• Fasting insulin, glucose
• Insulin hypersecretion	• 3-hour OGTT with insulin levels
• CNS lesion	• MRI, especially with hypothalamic coned-down views

Laboratory evaluation includes tests of obesity-related morbidity (e.g., AST, ALT, lipids, fasting glucose and HbA1c, knee and hip x-rays, and sleep studies as necessary). Specific diagnostic studies must be tailored to the individual patient. For instance, growth attenuation requires endocrine evaluation—including thyroid function tests, IGF-1 and IGFBP-3, 24-hour urinary cortisol or midnight serum cortisol, and possibly magnetic resonance imaging (MRI) of the hypothalamus and pituitary. Patients with developmental delay will require karyotype and MRI.

Severe obesity in a toddler may require a leptin level and genetic testing for a MC_4R mutation. Fasting insulin and glucose allow for the computation of indices of insulin resistance, such as the homeostatic model of insulin resistance (HOMA-IR).[423] However, an OGTT may become necessary to evaluate for type 2 diabetes and for insulin hypersecretion.[409] Luteinizing hormone (LH), follicle stimulating hormone (FSH), and testosterone levels may be appropriate when evaluating for delayed puberty in males or PCOS in females.

LIFESTYLE MODIFICATION

Lifestyle modification is and remains the cornerstone of obesity therapy, especially in children. This approach is common sense, and based on a handful of early studies demonstrating efficacy of lifestyle in a select handpicked group of children with intensive follow-up.[424] Indeed, the Diabetes Prevention Trial for T2DM demonstrated efficacy of lifestyle on weight loss in adults. However, the cost per patient of administering such an intervention was astronomical.[425] Data supporting the efficacy of lifestyle modification in the "real world" is not particularly persuasive.

Indeed, one analysis of numerous methodologies concluded that lifestyle modification was effective in modulating reported behaviors but had little effect on BMI or prevalence of pediatric obesity.[319] In addition, follow-up studies often find a rapidly diminishing effect once the study is completed. Another meta-analysis concluded that the results of well-controlled studies were too weak to be definitive.[426] Finally, a meta-analysis of 39 published intervention studies designed to prevent childhood obesity showed that 40% of the 33,852 participating children had reduction in BMI and that the remaining 60% exhibited no effect.[427]

Although weight loss is the conventional goal for intervention among adults, weight maintenance is recommended for the majority of children. The prevention of weight gain is easier, less expensive, and more effective than treating obesity itself[428]—and the prevention of overweight among children prior to the presence of risk-related behaviors is crucial to stem the obesity epidemic. The primary goal of obesity prevention should be to promote physical activity and healthy diet, with emphasis on improving overall health rather than weight loss.[429]

There are at least four reasons to promote interventions to improve nutrition and physical activity in children.[430] First, the child may receive immediate benefits such as better fitness or energy or micronutrient intake. Second, intervention at critical periods may improve adult health. Third, modifying chronic disease risks in childhood may lead to lower rates and risk factors in adults. Last, modification of children's behaviors may lead to improved behaviors in adulthood that would protect against chronic diseases.

Behavioral-cognitive therapy is designed to deal with both parent and patient, with behavior restructuring and reinforcement. Behavior changes include counseling sessions, teaching parenting skills, praise and contracts, self-monitoring tools, stimulus control within the home, role-modeling of behaviors by parents, and vigorous and long-term exercise programs. These programs have been successful in small studies with handpicked subjects by specific investigators[431,432] but have not yet been successful when attempted in clinic populations.

One new clinical approach involves motivational interviewing,[433] a method for helping patients work through their ambivalence about behavior change. This method has been shown to be effective for substance abuse and in adult diabetes. Whether it will be successful in pediatric obesity remains to be seen.[434]

Dietary Intervention

Dietary intervention is essential to the reduction of caloric intake and to reduction of the insulin response that promotes excessive energy deposition into adipose tissue. A myriad of studies demonstrate an association between consumption of high-calorie high-fat high-carbohydrate low-fiber foods and the development of pediatric obesity.[319] Specific maneuvers that have been successful in reducing obesity in children include elimination of sugar-containing beverages (including soda and juice)[435,436] and a shift to a low-glycemic-load diet.[326]

Other common sense approaches in adults (although pediatric efficacy data are lacking) include eating breakfast, reducing portion sizes, increasing fruit and vegetable consumption, reducing between-meal snacking, and reducing fast-food consumption.[437,438] However, dietary intervention alone is not a successful strategy for reducing pediatric overweight unless the treatment is very intensive[439]—in which case, the majority drop out. Furthermore, studies of nonsupervised dieting have demonstrated the opposite effect. That is, increased attempts in female adolescents predict a greater increase in weight and risk for obesity.[440]

Physical Activity Intervention

In adults, exercise is not an effective means of inducing weight loss unless combined with reduction of caloric intake. The role of exercise may have a greater impact on weight maintenance, rather than weight loss.[441] Similarly, there is question as to whether physical activity regimens for children can stabilize or reduce BMI.[442,443] Short-term studies show that vigorous exercise can result in short-term reductions in adiposity[444] and improved insulin resistance.[445] This amounts to a minimum of 30 minutes of vigorous exercise 5 days per week.

This is still under the recently proposed activity guidelines from the Institute of Medicine.[446] However, such interventions eventually plateau in their effectiveness—and even short-term cessation rapidly reverses any accrued benefit.[447] To succeed, physical activity interventions must be long-term, sustained, and incorporated into behavioral modifications aimed at the individual, at the family, at the school, and within the community in general.[444,447] In other words, to make physical activity work it must become a priority.

Appropriate interventions include making school-based physical education mandatory for every child and school, increasing access to after-school recreation, increasing culturally appropriate activities, reducing the competitive nature of sports so that more children will participate, increasing the incorporation of physical activity into daily life (e.g., stairs, walking to school as appropriate), and increasing participation of parents in physical recreation for their own weight management and as role models for their children.

Last, the effects of reducing sedentary behavior by restricting television viewing has been efficacious in small and large studies and in diverse ethnic groups[304]—although fitness is not improved. Restriction of television also has a secondary effect of reducing caloric intake while watching television. Results using dietary or exercise intervention alone are not encouraging. Those studies that use behavioral, dietary, and exercise components together appear to be more successful[319,448]—although long-term efficacy is lacking.

School Intervention

Numerous school-based interventions have focused on reducing obesity rates, most of which have not been successful—in part because school cafeteria fare in most districts remains problematic. However, interventions that increased time spent in vigorous physical activity (20 minutes in elementary schools and 30 minutes in middle schools) were more successful.[449] One approach is to improve self-esteem and self-efficacy of students, as opposed to simply educating them about eating disorders,[450] because this increases physical activity.[451] Schools can model health-promoting environments, provide appropriate health education, and engender increased self-efficacy in coping with stress—which can empower children to make healthy lifestyle choices.

Family Intervention

Invariably, the patient is not the only obese member of the family. There is frequently family chaos, which promotes obesity in other family members. Various caretakers (e.g., grandmothers, babysitters) will feed children and allow unrestricted television as a method of confining their activities indoors, particularly in dangerous neighborhoods. Some parents will not alter their shopping for junk food because they believe other sibs should not be deprived. Usually it is those same parents who do not want to be deprived.

Divorced parents will often use food as a reward for a child's love and loyalty. Thus, the family itself must be the target of lifestyle intervention. Parental involvement is critical, and the concept of "food is not love" must be emphasized. Families need training to modify behavior to make healthy dietary choices, increase activity, and reduce perceived stress. A recent meta-analysis of randomized trials of combined lifestyle interventions for treating pediatric obesity yielded a significant although underwhelming decrease in BMI of 1.5 kg/m², with targeted family intervention and a nonsignificant decrease in BMI of 0.4 kg/m² in those that targeted the patient alone.[452]

PHARMACOTHERAPY

Indications for Pharmacotherapy

Pharmacologic therapies in children must currently be considered adjuncts to standard lifestyle modification. At present, several limitations preclude physicians from early implementation of drug therapies for the treatment of childhood obesity, including: the youngest child for whom any obesity pharmacotherapy is currently Food and Drug Administration (FDA) approved is 10 years; the long-term use of pharmacologic intervention has not always proven to be more efficacious than behavior modification; there exists a limited number of well-controlled studies of safe and effective pharmacologic intervention in obese children; the relative risk for the development of adverse events in children must be weighed against the long-term potential for improvement of morbidity and mortality, which is difficult to estimate in children; and targeting the pathology is still in its infancy.

In addition, we cannot forget that many drugs used for treatment of adult obesity resulted in unforeseen complications—which resulted in their restriction (thyroid hormone, amphetamine) or recall (e.g., dinitrophenol, fenfluramine, dexfenfluramine, phenylpropanolamine, ephedra).[453-458] Despite these concerns, the negative health impact of childhood obesity may justify long-term medication to control its progression.

In the current pharmacopoeia of childhood obesity, nonspecific and specific strategies based on mechanisms of action within the energy balance negative feedback system are employed (Table 19-3). Currently, the approaches are suppression of caloric intake, limitation of the availability or absorption of nutrients, and insulin sensitization or suppression.

Reduction of Energy Intake: Sibutramine

Numerous anorexiant drugs have been used to treat obesity in adults. These drugs alter neurotransmission within the VMH in order to reduce caloric intake. Only sibutramine (a nonselective reuptake inhibitor of serotonin and norepinephrine) and dopamine are approved for children as young as 16 years.[459,460] Sibutramine effectively inhibits caloric intake[461] and stimulates thermogenesis in rats, although data on humans are contradictory.[462,463]

In adolescents, three randomized controlled trials (RCTs) document the safety and efficacy of sibutramine.[464-466] Tolerability and side effects of sibutramine are similar to adults.[466] Sibutramine can cause vasoconstriction and increase heart rate and blood pressure that persists even after significant weight loss.[454] Other adverse reactions include dry mouth, headache, insomnia, anxiety, nervousness, depression, somnolence or drowsiness, edema, palpitations,

TABLE 19-3

Medications for the Treatment of Pediatric Obesity

Drug	Dosage	Efficacy	Side Effects	Monitoring and Contraindications
Sibutramine Not FDA approved for <16 years of age.	5-15 mg PO qd	RCT: Wt 4.6 kg, BMI 4.5%, WC 5.4 cm over placebo at 6 months RCT: Wt 8.1 kg, BMI 2.5 kg/m² over placebo at 6 months	Tachycardia, hypertension, palpitations, insomnia, anxiety, nervousness, depression, diaphoresis.	Monitor HR, BP. Do not use with other drugs or MAO inhibitors.
Orlistat Not FDA approved for <12 years of age.	120 mg PO tid	Open-label: Wt 5.4 kg, BMI 2.0 kg/m² at 6 months; RCT: Wt 2.6 kg, BMI 0.85, WC 2.7 cm over placebo at 12 months	Borborygmi, flatus, abdominal cramps, fecal incontinence, oily spotting, vitamin malabsorption.	Monitor 25OHD₃ levels. MVI supplementation is strongly recommended. A lower dose preparation has been approved for over-the-counter sale.
Metformin Not FDA approved for treatment of obesity. Approved for 10 years of age for type 2 diabetes mellitus.	250-1,000 mg PO bid	RCT: BMI Z score 0.35 SD vs. placebo at 6 months RCT: Wt 2.7% vs. placebo at 6 months; Post hoc analysis: efficacy dependent on degree of insulin resistance; BMI Z score 0.23 SD in first 4 months, 0.12 SD in next year	Nausea, flatulence, bloating, diarrhea; usually resolves. Lactic acidosis not yet reported in children.	Do not use in renal failure or with intravenous contrast. MVI supplementation is strongly recommended.
Octreotide Not FDA approved for treatment of obesity; otherwise 18 years of age.	5-15 mcg/kg/d SQ ÷ tid	Open-label: Wt 4.8 kg, BMI 2.0 kg/m² in 6 months; RCT: 7.6 kg, BMI 2.5 kg/m² over placebo at 6 months Post hoc analysis: BMI Z score 0.70 SD in 6 months, dependent on insulin secretion and sensitivity	Gallstones, diarrhea, edema, abdominal cramps, nausea, bloating, reduction in thyroxine concentrations.	Monitor fasting glucose, FT₄, HbA₁c. Useful only for hypothalamic obesity. Ursodiol co-administration strongly recommended.
Leptin Not approved by FDA.	Titration of dose to serum levels, SQ	Anecdotal: BMI 19.0 kg/m² over 4 years	Local reactions.	Useful *only* in leptin deficiency.
Topiramate Not FDA approved for treatment of obesity.	96-256 mg PO qd	RCT: Wt 8.0% over placebo at 6 months	Paresthesias, difficulty with concentration/attention, depression, difficulty with memory, language problems, nervousness, psychomotor slowing.	No pediatric data.
Growth hormone Not FDA approved for treatment of obesity.	1-3 mg/m² SQ qd	Decreases in percentage body fat, with increases in absolute lean body mass	Edema, carpal tunnel syndrome, death in patients with preexisting obstructive sleep apnea.	Recommended only in Prader-Willi syndrome primarily to increase height velocity. It also decreases fat mass but should only be used in those have been after screening to rule out obstructive sleep apnea. Must closely monitor pulmonary function, glucose, HbA₁c.
Rimonabant Not FDA approved in the US. No pediatric data.	20 mg PO qd	RCT: Wt 4.8 kg over placebo at 12 months	Depressed mood, nausea, vomiting, diarrhea, dizziness, headache, anxiety.	40% dropout rate. No pediatric data.

Should be considered only after an unsuccessful 6-month trial of lifestyle intervention.
All drugs effective only when combined with appropriate lifestyle intervention.
RCT = randomized controlled trial, MVI = multivitamins.

diaphoresis, xerostomia, constipation, dizziness, paresthesias, mydriasis, and nausea. Sibutramine cannot be administered in conjunction with monoamine oxidase inhibitors or selective serotonin reuptake inhibitors.[453,467] Sibutramine is currently licensed in the United States for use in subjects 16 years of age and older. The FDA has extended the interval of treatment to 2 years.[466]

Reduction of Energy Absorption: Orlistat

This drug is a modified bacterial product that specifically inhibits intestinal lipase and can reduce fat and cholesterol absorption by approximately 30% in subjects eating a 30% fat diet.[468] Orlistat irreversibly binds to the active site of the lipase, preventing intraluminal deacylation of triglycerides—resulting in a 16 g/day increase in fecal fat excretion.[469] Orlistat does not inhibit other intestinal enzymes. It has minimal absorption and exerts no effect on systemic lipases.[470,471]

Although there have been several open-label trials of orlistat in adolescents, only two RCTs have been published.[472,473] The side effects with orlistat are predictable from its mechanism of action on intestinal lipase.[453] Orlistat appears to be well tolerated in adults, with the principal complaints being borborygmi, flatus, and abdominal cramps. The most troubling side effects are fecal incontinence, oily spotting, and flatus with discharge—which are highly aversive in the pediatric population. Orlistat does not affect the pharmacokinetic properties of most other pharmaceutical agents. Absorption of vitamins A and E and β-carotene may be slightly reduced, and this may require vitamin therapy in a small number of patients.

In one study,[474] vitamin D supplementation was required in 18% subjects despite the prescription of a daily multivitamin containing vitamin D—although in the company-sponsored study effects on vitamin levels were minor.[472] Orlistat must be taken with each meal, which reduces its attractiveness in children—who are in school during lunchtime. Orlistat is currently approved for treatment of children as young as 12 years. An over-the-counter lower-dose preparation recently obtained FDA approval.

Improvement of Insulin Resistance: Metformin

Metformin is a bisubstituted short-chain hydrophilic guanidine derivative used for the treatment of children and adults with T2DM.[475-478] Metformin also decreases fasting hyperinsulinemia, prevents T2DM,[479] and promotes weight loss in some obese individuals[480,481] by improving hepatic and muscle insulin sensitivity. Metformin has little effect on energy expenditure.[476] Although some believe that metformin promotes weight loss through a primary anorectic effect (as initial side effects of nausea and GI distress limit caloric intake acutely),[482] most believe that the decline in caloric intake observed with metformin is related to its enhancement of glucose clearance through reduction of hepatic glucose output and reduction in fasting hyperinsulinemia.[483,484]

Metformin improves hepatic insulin resistance by inducing hepatic AMP kinase,[485] which reduces hepatic gluconeogenesis. Therefore, pancreatic insulin secretion and peripheral insulin levels fall. Metformin also restores PI3-kinase and MAP kinase activity in muscle cells, improving muscle insulin sensitivity.[486] Another possible mechanism of metformin action is through stimulation of glucagon-like peptide-1 (GLP-1),[14,487] which may inhibit food intake through central actions on the VMH.[15]

Thus far, two RCTs and an observational prediction study in children and adolescents have been conducted.[488,489] Examination of the open-label responses to metformin in a multivariate analysis demonstrated two predictors for efficacy: race (Caucasian > African American) and the degree of insulin resistance prior to therapy.[137] Metformin has also been used "off-label" for treatment of polycystic ovarian syndrome and nonalcoholic steatohepatitis, with varying degrees of success.[490-495] One particular use for metformin may be to combat the weight gain associated with atypical antipsychotics.[496] However, cessation of metformin therapy leads to a rebound hypersinulinemia and rapid weight gain, which may negate any beneficial effects seen during the medication window.

Side effects with metformin include nausea, flatulence, bloating, and diarrhea at initiation of therapy—which appears to be self-limited and resolves within 3 to 4 weeks of initiation of the drug. Approximately 5% of pediatric patients discontinue metformin therapy because of severity of side effects. The most feared complication of metformin in adults is lactic acidosis, which is estimated to occur at a rate of 3 per 100,000 patient-exposure years—primarily in patients with contraindications to the use of metformin. However, no documented cases in children have been reported. Metformin increases the urinary excretion of vitamins B_1 and B_6, which are important in the tricarboxylic acid cycle and which may hasten lactic acidosis.[497]

Vitamin B_{12} deficiency has also been reported in as many as 9% of adult subjects using metformin. Therefore, prophylactic multivitamin supplementation is recommended with metformin use. Contraindications to metformin use include renal insufficiency, congestive heart failure or pulmonary insufficiency, acute liver disease, and alcohol use sufficient to cause acute hepatic toxicity. Metformin should also be withheld when patients are hospitalized with any condition that may cause decreased systemic perfusion, or when use of contrast agents is anticipated.[483] It should be noted that metformin is FDA approved for treatment of T2DM in children but is unlikely to be approved for childhood obesity or insulin resistance due to the short exclusivity interval afforded the makers of metformin by the FDA upon its introduction to the United States in 1996.

Suppression of Insulin Hypersecretion: Octreotide

It is well known that bilateral electrolytic lesions or deafferentation of the VMH in rats leads to intractable weight gain,[109,110,394-396] even upon food restriction.[397] In humans, hypothalamic damage due to CNS tumor, surgery, radiation, or trauma can alter the afferent and efferent pathway of energy balance and lead to severe and intractable weight gain.[399,400] In this syndrome of hypothalamic obesity, hypothalamic insult confers an "organic leptin resistance" as the

VMH senses starvation.[54,395] Therefore, energy intake is high and expenditure is low.[403] Children with hypothalamic obesity exhibit weight gain (even in response to forced caloric restriction[401]) secondary to overactivation of the vagus (which promotes an obligate insulin hypersecretion and energy storage) and to defective activation of the SNS, which retards lipolysis and energy expenditure.[99,402]

Insulin hypersecretion with normal insulin sensitivity is noted on oral glucose tolerance testing in these children.[409] This same phenomenon of insulin hypersecretion has also been documented in a subset of obese adults without CNS damage.[498] The voltage-gated calcium channel of the β cell is coupled to a somatostatin (SSTR$_5$) receptor.[499,500] Octreotide binds to this receptor, which limits the opening of this calcium channel, reduces influx of calcium into the β cells, and in turn reduces calmodulin activation and vesicle exocytosis—thereby acutely decreasing the magnitude of insulin response to glucose[501] (Figure 19-2), which results in weight loss or stabilization. Two RCTs and an observational prediction study using octreotide for obesity have been performed.[502,503] An examination of BMI responses to octreotide in pediatric hypothalamic obesity in a multivariate analysis demonstrated that insulin hypersecretion with concomitant retention of insulin sensitivity prior to therapy augured success.[137]

Octreotide is usually well tolerated. The most common side effects include diarrhea, abdominal cramps, nausea, and bloating—which are self-limited and usually resolve in 3 to 4 weeks.[504,505] Other adverse events include gallstones (which are preventable by coadministration of ursodiol), edema, development of sterile abscess at the injection sites, B$_{12}$ deficiency, suppression of GH and TSH secretion, and mild hyperglycemia—especially in those with severe insulin resistance.[506] At present, octreotide offers a promising approach to the treatment of insulin hypersecretion as seen in hypothalamic obesity but is not FDA approved for this use. The use of octreotide in obese children with acute glucose-stimulated insulin hypersecretion without cranial pathology has not yet been evaluated.

Other Targeted Therapies

Leptin. Mutations of the leptin gene in humans recapitulate the phenotype of the *ob/ob* leptin-deficient mouse.[368] Approximately 11 such patients have been described. They manifest hyperphagia from birth, with obesity documentable as early as 6 months of age. Leptin deficiency induces the starvation response,[369] with increased energy intake and decreased REE. The diagnosis is made by extremely low or unmeasurable serum leptin levels. In children with leptin deficiency, leptin therapy results in extraordinary loss of weight and fat mass[507,508]—along with reduction in hyperphagia, resolution of obesity, induction of puberty, and improvement in immunity.[369] Although leptin administration in adults did not prove effective by itself due to leptin resistance,[128] leptin may serve as an adjunct in combination with other medications after leptin sensitivity is ameliorated through weight loss.[133,509]

Growth Hormone. GH fosters anabolism and lipolysis. GH therapy has been shown to increase REE, promote linear growth, increase muscle mass, and decrease body fat percentage in Prader-Willi syndrome.[385,510] It has also been shown to decrease body fat percentage in children with GH deficiency[511] due to its effect on lipoprotein lipase.[512] However, it is not clear whether these reductions in body fat percentage are primary effects on the adipose tissue compartment or are due to the increase in lean body mass. Obesity results in a state of functional GH insufficiency, which can be ameliorated through weight loss.[513] GH therapy also improves the lipid profile in GH-deficient adults.[514] Currently, the role of GH therapy in the treatment of nonsyndromic childhood obesity is unclear and not approved.

The Future of Pediatric Obesity Pharmacotherapy

In response to the relative lack of efficacy of lifestyle interventions, the ever-expanding knowledge of the physiology of energy balance, and particularly as a business decision of potential financial reward, many pharmaceutical companies have launched obesity research programs. The agents discussed in the following are currently in human study. However, use of any of these new agents in children will depend on proof of safety and efficacy based on experience in adults. Oxyntomodulin is an analog of PYY(3-36), which has been shown in a 4-week RCT to reduce energy intake and weight in adults.[515]

Topiramate is a novel anticonvulsant that blocks voltage-dependent sodium channels, enhances the activity of the GABA$_A$ receptor, and antagonizes a glutamate receptor other than the N-methyl-D-aspartate (NMDA) receptor.[516] Topiramate promotes weight loss in a dose-dependent fashion.[517] A recent RCT in adults demonstrated a 9.1% weight loss in subjects taking topiramate 192 mg/day—along with significant improvements in blood pressure, waist circumference, and fasting glucose and insulin.[518] However, almost 33% of the subjects dropped out due to adverse events—which included paresthesias, somnolence, anorexia, fatigue, nervousness, decreased concentration, difficulty with memory, and aggression. There are currently no studies of topiramate in childhood obesity.

Rimonabant is an endocannabinoid receptor (CB$_1$) antagonist that reduces the reinforcement and reward properties of drugs of dependence at the level of the nucleus accumbens.[519] It also extinguishes the reward properties of food. A 1-year RCT in adults demonstrated a 6.6 ± 7.2 kg weight loss (p < 0.001), 6.5 ± 7.4 cm reduction in waist circumference (p < 0.001), and improvement in lipid profile.[520] Side effects included depressed mood, nausea, vomiting, diarrhea, dizziness, headache, and anxiety in 20% of subjects. Rimonabant was not FDA approved in the US and is under consideration for withdrawal in Europe due to these side effects.

BARIATRIC SURGERY
Indications for Bariatric Surgery

Conventional treatment of childhood obesity has proven to be time consuming, difficult, frustrating, and expensive. Although numerous short-term successes have been noted, long-term weight reductions are modest—and recidivism is the rule. In adolescents with extreme and morbid obesity that may be life-threatening, surgical therapy may be indicated in extreme and defined circumstances.[521,522] However, in comparison to adults stricter and more conservative criteria must be applied to adolescents due to the following factors.

- Not all obese adolescents will become obese adults.[523]
- Modestly improved rate of lifestyle and pharmacotherapeutic efficacy.
- Longer time interval before co-morbidities become life-threatening.
- The inability of adolescents to give legal consent.

Therefore, it is virtually impossible to perform RCT surgical studies in children. Efficacy of any given approach will continue to be suspect, and different procedures cannot be compared. For all of these reasons, an expert panel with representation from the American Pediatric Surgical Association and the American Academy of Pediatrics[522] suggested that bariatric surgery in adolescence could be justified in situations in which obesity-related co-morbid conditions threaten the child's health. They provided stringent recommendations that bariatric surgery be limited to those adolescents with BMI >40 kg/m² with presence of severe co-morbidity, or BMI >50 kg/m² with a less severe co-morbidity. However, these stringent criteria are undergoing careful scrutiny in an attempt to liberalize them.[524]

Particular care should be taken to avoid bariatric surgery at very late stages of obesity, when the presence of obesity-related co-morbidities and the inaccessibility of imaging (most MRI scanners have a weight limit of 450 lbs.) may affect surgical outcome. Indeed, a review of eight retrospective studies in adolescents found that bariatric surgery in adolescents can promote durable weight loss in most patients. However, there appears to be a significant complication and mortality rate.[525] Therefore, guidance is needed to determine the ideal circumstances in which the balance of risk versus benefit favors health preservation and reversal of complications with the lowest risk of morbidity and mortality from the procedure.

Bariatric procedures for weight loss can be divided into malabsorptive, restrictive, and combination procedures. Purely malabsorptive procedures aim to decrease the functional length or efficiency of the intestinal mucosa through anatomic rearrangement of the intestine. These procedures include the jejunoileal bypass and the biliopancreatic diversion with duodenal switch. Due to the high morbidity and mortality of these procedures, they cannot be recommended in children and will not be discussed further. The restrictive procedures reduce stomach volume to decrease the volume of food ingested. They include the bariatric intragastric balloon (no data in children) and laparoscopic adjustable gastric band (LAGB). The Roux-en-Y gastric bypass (RYGB) is a combination procedure.[526] Other bariatric procedures, such as gastric pacing, are still research modalities.

Restrictive: Laparoscopic Adjustable Gastric Banding

LAGB utilizes a prosthetic band to encircle and compartmentalize the proximal stomach into a small pouch and a large remnant.[526] The theoretical advantage of this technique is decreased risk of staple line dehiscence. The more recent introduction of a new laparoscopic approach and the use of an adjustable band (allowing the stomach size to change) make this procedure more attractive. Finally, this procedure is reversible (at least theoretically, but there are some surgeons who scoff at this notion)—or can be modified into the RYGB at a later date. Results vary widely in adults. However, several small studies support the safety and efficacy of LAGB in morbidly obese adolescents.

In one study of 11 morbidly obese adolescents (11-17 years old), LABG resulted in decreased mean BMI from 46.6 to 32.1 kg/m² at a mean follow-up of 23 months—with improved co-morbidities. No patient experienced operative or late complications.[527] In another study following LAGB, BMI in 7 adolescents (12-19 years old) fell from a preoperative median of 44.7 kg/m² to 30.2 kg/m² at 24 months—which corresponded to a 59.3% loss of excess weight.[528] In a 3-year follow-up study of 41 adolescents, BMI was reduced from 42 ± 8 to 29 ± 6—with an excess weight loss of 70%.[529] Again, complications were minor—although erosion of the band through the stomach serosa is documented. Although this procedure is considered safer than RYGB, it has not yet been approved by the FDA for use in adolescents—despite several studies that now support such use.

Combination: Roux-en-Y Gastric Bypass

RYGB involves dividing the stomach to create a small (15-30 mL) stomach pouch into which a segment of jejunum approximately 15 to 60 cm inferior to the ligament of Treitz is inserted—with the proximal portion of the jejunum that drains the bypassed lower stomach and duodenum reanastomosed 75 to 150 cm inferior to the gastrojejunostomy.[526] This procedure combines the restrictive nature of gastrectomy with the consequences of dumping physiology as a negative conditioning response when high-calorie liquid meals are ingested. In addition, RYGB is associated with decline in the circulating level of ghrelin—which may be in part responsible for the decrease in hunger associated with this procedure.[12]

RYGB appears to result in significant early weight reduction in adults.[526,530] However, long-term studies demonstrate weight regain in many patients.[531,532] Limited data are available regarding the efficacy of these surgical procedures to induce weight loss in severely obese children and adolescents, and most of these are case series from individual surgeons or institutions.[467] In a case review, 10 severely obese adolescents (BMI 52.5 ± 10.0 kg/m²) who underwent RYGB were followed for a mean of 69 months (range of 8-144 months).[533] In this series, weight loss was significant in 9 of 10 adolescents—and was maintained as long as 10 years. The average weight loss was 53.6 ± 25.6 kg, which represents approximately 59% excess weight lost. Weight loss was also associated with improvement of associated co-morbidities, including sleep apnea and hypertension.

Finally, a large retrospective series of 33 obese adolescents[534] age 16 ± 1 year with BMI 52 ± 11 (range of 38-91) and obesity co-morbidities followed these subjects up to

14 years after bariatric surgery (mostly RYGB). There were surgical complications in 13, which were treated. There were 2 sudden deaths, and 5 of the subjects regained their weight. However, the majority experienced significant weight loss—with resolution of their co-morbidities and improvement in quality of life. Adolescents participating in a multicenter study reported by the Pediatric Bariatric Study Group experienced excellent weight loss after laparoscopic RYGB, with mean BMI change from 58 kg/m^2 to 35.8 kg/m^2 at 1 year.[535] Gastrojejunostomy stenosis (21 patients) requiring endoscopic balloon dilation and internal hernia (14 patients) requiring laparoscopic or open reduction were the most common complications. This procedure appears to be safe and effective when candidates are carefully selected and the bariatric surgeon has advanced laparoscopic skills.

The most common reported complications of RYGB include iron-deficiency anemia (50%), transient folate deficiency (30%), and events requiring surgical intervention (40%: cholecystectomy in 20%, small bowel obstruction in 10%, and incisional hernia in 10%).[526] Because most of the stomach and duodenum is bypassed in this procedure, there is an increased risk for deficiencies in vitamin B$_{12}$, iron, calcium, and thiamine. Although beriberi has been reported in teenagers after RYGB,[536] compliance with daily supplementation and regular monitoring of patients can prevent such nutritional deficiencies.

Who Should Perform Bariatric Surgery in Children

Surgical outcomes in adults vary widely among surgeons and institutions.[537-539] Furthermore, there is a very clear learning curve because the morbidity of bariatric surgery varies inversely with the number of procedures performed.[540] In addition, because RCTs in adolescents are unlikely the only method to validate and refine the use of these procedures will come from following patients carefully and long-term. Last, the increased risk of readmission after bariatric surgery in adults[541] argues for close and careful follow-up and monitoring in adolescents. Therefore, it is essential that bariatric surgery in adolescents be performed in regional pediatric academic centers with programs equipped to handle the data acquisition and long-term follow-up involved in (and the multidisciplinary nature of) the treatment of these difficult patients.[522]

A multidisciplinary team with medical, surgical, nutritional, and psychological expertise should carefully select adolescents who are well informed and motivated to become potential candidates for LAGB or RYGB. Attention to the principles of growth, development, and compliance is essential to avoid adverse physical, cognitive, and psychosocial outcomes following bariatric surgery.[522] It must be clear to the subject and the parent that bariatric surgery is in fact an adjunct to a sincere commitment to lifestyle, rather than a "magic bullet." Indeed, evidence of recidivism in adults after RYGB is now commonplace.

Subjects and families must be well informed as to the risks and complications of such surgery. The medical team will require endocrine, GI, cardiology, pulmonary,

and otolaryngologic support. Prophylactic tracheostomy is rarely required to maintain airway patency and to allow for resolution of the hypercapnia prior to surgery.[542] Adolescents undergoing bariatric surgery require lifelong medical and nutritional surveillance postoperatively.[521] Extensive counseling, education, and support are required before and after bariatric surgery. Patients left to their own devices tend to regain weight over time. Indeed, studies in adults document an increased risk of hospitalization after RYGB due to difficulties from the procedure.[541] Monitoring of long-term weight maintenance, improvements in CV morbidity, and longevity are all necessary to determine the cost effectiveness of bariatric surgery in the pediatric population.

Energy Inadequacy

STARVATION VERSUS CACHEXIA

Although both are weight loss syndromes, understanding the neuroendocrine mechanisms that distinguish starvation from cachexia is integral to understanding and treating these disorders properly. In starvation, the negative feedback energy balance pathway is intact. The signal of leptin inadequacy from the weight loss is transduced by the VMH neuron into reduced sympathetic activity (to conserve energy) and increased vagal activity (to store energy). However, in cachexia this pathway is short-circuited by cytokine action on the hypothalamus. The VMH POMC neuron expresses receptors for various cytokines, including IL-1 and TNF-α[543]

In response to cytokine exposure, POMC neurons are activated—resulting in anorexigenesis, increased sympathetic activity, decreased vagal activity, and energy wastage.[544,545] Proinflammatory cytokines increase epinephrine, GH, and cortisol, and reduce insulin. These long-term hormonal changes accelerate muscle proteolysis (cortisol), increase resting energy expenditure (SNS), contribute to insulin resistance (glucagon and cortisol), increase catabolism (cortisol), and suppress appetite and intestinal transit (vagus). This is clearly adaptive in the short term during times of infection (to generate body heat to eradicate the organism) but maladaptive in the long term, when chronic cytokine signaling can lead to cachexia. Thus, even in the situations of leptin decline or inadequacy cytokine activation of POMC neurons will promote continued cachexia and weight loss through persistent SNS activation.

FAILURE TO THRIVE

Failure to thrive (FTT) is not a disease per se but rather a sign of multiple organic and nonorganic conditions and the interactions between them that lead to compromised growth at a young age. FTT still represents a common pediatric medical problem largely managed in the outpatient setting. Although FTT can rarely be a manifestation of critical illness, the majority of cases are the result of undernutrition due to the combination of biologic, environmental, and psychological factors. The diagnosis of FTT requires a thorough, prudent, and oriented history taking by the caregiver and is not always simple to establish. Moreover, this diagnosis may carry several legal implications (which are not within the scope of this text).

Definition

There is no consensus on a single definition of FTT. The condition reflects inadequate physical growth recorded over time using standard growth charts. The commonly used definitions in clinical practice include length and/or weight below the 5th percentile for age and gender, a downward cross of two major percentile lines of the growth chart over time, or a weight per height below the 10th percentile of expected. The practicality of usually using weight and not length curves evolves from the fact that undernutrition and chronic disease tend to primarily affect weight gain while preserving linear growth.

Ultimately, linear growth is also affected if these conditions persist. It is important to emphasize that single measurements without longitudinal follow-up growth points are inadequate to make the diagnosis of FTT, and a wrongful diagnosis may be established in infants who were born SGA or prematurely—and in some healthy infants growing along the lower percentiles.

Classification and Etiology

The traditional classification of FTT is to segregate organic and nonorganic causes. The nonorganic causes refer to environmental and psychological factors such as sensory deprivation, parental and emotional deprivation, and feeding difficulties of no organic source that occur in infancy. This traditional classification seems to lack the insight that the majority of cases suffer from a combination of the two, reflecting a mixed etiology.[546] A different approach is to classify the disorder based on the pathophysiology of the disorder (i.e., inadequate caloric intake, inadequate absorption, excess metabolic requirements, defective utilization of intake, and reduced growth potential).[547] Common causes of FTT based on this classification scheme are outlined in Table 19-4.

Of note, normal growth variation can confound the diagnosis of FTT because some infants may be born large for gestational age due to intrauterine causes (such as gestational diabetes) and later experience a "catch-down" pattern of growth during infancy toward the actual growth potential curves. Another cause of such negative crossing of percentiles can be constitutional growth delay. It is estimated that up to 25% of children can cross curves by more than 25 percentile lines (representing a cross of two major growth percentile lines) due to the previously cited reasons.[548] These infants reach a new point from which they display a normal growth rate and weight gain pattern, yet they do not have FTT.

Endocrine causes of FTT are uncommon, as typical hormonal deficiencies such as GH deficiency or hypothyroidism present as growth failure but with preserved or increased weight gain. Hyperthyroidism (representing a state of increased metabolic demands and characteristically manifested by increased linear growth) and disorders of salt metabolism (such as hypoaldosteronism and pseudohypoaldosteronism)

TABLE 19-4

Differential Diagnosis of Failure to Thrive

Inadequate Caloric Intake
- Poverty and low food resources
- Mechanical feeding difficulties (altered swallowing ability, congenital anomalies, central nervous system damage, severe gastroesophageal reflux)
- Wrongful preparation of infant formula (too diluted, too concentrated)
- Unsuitable feeding habits by parent
- Behavioral problems affecting eating
- Child neglect
- Poor parent-child interaction

Inadequate Absorption of Caloric Intake
- Reduced absorption surface area (short bowel syndrome, s/p necrotizing enterocolitis)
- Chronic liver disease, biliary atresia
- Celiac disease
- Cystic fibrosis
- Cow's milk allergy
- Chronic diarrhea
- Vitamin or mineral deficiencies (acrodermatitis enteropathica)
- Vomiting due to CNS abnormalities (tumor, raised ICP)

Increased Metabolism
- Hyperthyroidism
- Chronic infection (due to immune deficiency)
- Occult malignancy
- Congenital heart defects or acquired heart disease (mainly right to left shunts and heart failure)
- Chronic lung disease with hypoxemia (broncho-pulmonary dysplasia)
- Burns

Defective Utilization of Calories
- Renal failure, renal tubular acidosis
- Inborn errors of metabolism (storage diseases, amino acid disorders)

Reduced Growth Potential
- Genetic disorders (trisomies, skeletal dysplasias, Russel-Silver syndrome)
- Specific genetic syndromes
- Primordial dwarfism

---

may have FTT as part of their clinical manifestations.[549] Hypophosphatemic rickets may also present as FTT.

Diagnosis and Evaluation

The key to making the diagnosis of FTT is in plotting anthropometric data (weight and length) during a reasonable follow-up period. Although a prudent and focused history and physical examination are the keys to diagnosis, often the correct diagnosis is made in retrospect. The lack of an organic etiology to explain the findings is not enough to establish a diagnosis of nonorganic FTT. A response to an active intervention, manifested at least as a limited period of adequate growth while altering a behavioral element by the caregiver or child, can help establish a diagnosis of nonorganic FTT.

History should focus on the dietary and feeding history, past and present medical history, social environment, and family history. The dietary history is aimed at assessing as accurately as possible the actual caloric intake of the patient. An important tool for this assessment can be the use of food logs of several days. The important details are actual amounts of food, the way the food is prepared (specifically, relevant to the dilution technique of infant formulas and to cereals added to the formula), and beverages consumed (with specific emphasis on sweetened juices and formula). These details should allow the practitioner to estimate the caloric intake.

The important details regarding feeding begin with the location of the meals and their timing throughout the day. Who feeds the patient or supervises the feeding process is of major importance. The feeding technique should be appropriate to the developmental stage of the child. The timing is relevant in regard to frequent snacking between meals that may cause early satiety during mealtimes.

A standard pediatric medical history should be taken from all patients, yet it should be focused on details that may be relevant to the diagnosis of FTT. The pregnancy and birth history are important for differentiation of infants who were born SGA versus those who suffer from FTT. The timing at which poor weight gain began, especially in relation to changes in feeding, is critically important to the diagnosis. Chronic medical conditions such as congenital heart disease, asthma, multiple recurrent infections, and anemia can all be causes of organic FTT. Multiple hospitalizations and a history of injuries can raise the suspicion of parental neglect. GI manifestations of relevant medical conditions such as frequent vomiting (in cases of milk allergy or gastroesophageal reflux) and stool frequency and consistency (to rule out malabsorption, celiac, inflammatory bowel disease, or cystic fibrosis) should be elicited in detail.

The social history should focus on identifying the actual caregivers of the patient during the majority of the time and whether there are economic issues that may affect the ability to raise the patient adequately. Potential external and intrafamilial stressors that may affect the supply of food to the child should be sought (any stressor or life event that can affect the functioning of the caregiver in a way that could compromise the well-being of the child). The family history should focus on the body habitus of parents and siblings to obtain clues regarding genetic potential for height and weight. Medical conditions in siblings and relatives can suggest a predisposition to genetic disorders. The caregivers should be asked about mental illnesses (such as depression) that may hamper their ability to provide adequate care for the child. A family history of previous children who suffered from FTT should be investigated as well. A call to the local Department of Family Services may be warranted.

The physical examination begins with plotting the child's length, weight, and head circumference on standard growth charts—along with previous measurements (if available). The severity of the FTT can be estimated by assessing the present weight in comparison to the expected weight for age. If the weight is less than 60% of expected by the 50th percentile for age and length, the condition is severe—whereas a weight between the 60th and 75th percentile of expected is considered moderate FTT. Microcephaly accompanied by neurologic signs may suggest a CNS lesion. It should be remembered that head

circumference is the last parameter to change in FTT, and only in the severest cases.

Detection of dysmorphism may suggest a genetic cause of impaired growth and development. Measures of nutritional status (such as thickness of skin folds and body fat distribution) can be examined. It is important to carefully observe the interaction of the caregiver and the child during feeding. Impaired parent-child interactions can have a major impact on feeding habits, and their identification is critical to the design of effective behavioral interventions tailored to the patient and family.

The majority of children with FTT have no laboratory abnormalities, and no hormonal alterations. There is minimal literature available about comprehensive laboratory workups in children with FTT, although a classic manuscript about the workup of more than 180 infants in an in-patient setting found laboratory abnormalities in less than 1.4% of tests taken.[550] The choice of tests that may be beneficial should be based on the history and physical examination, and usually should be focused on the assessment of malnutrition in severe cases. A minimal workup (although not cost effective) may include a blood count, chemistry panel (including liver and renal function tests, electrolytes, serum protein and albumin concentrations, and blood acid-base status), and urinalysis with pH.

Additional tests should be oriented toward specific findings from the history and physical examination. No hormonal tests are warranted initially unless a clinical suspicion of a specific disorder arises. In children older than 6 months, screening for iron deficiency and lead poisoning is warranted. Hospitalization and in-patient workup does not add any yield to the workup[551] unless the degree of FTT is severe or if there are concerns of child safety and neglect.

Management

The management of FTT is based on the identification of the underlying cause and its correction. The vast majority of cases are handled by a combination of nutritional and behavioral intervention. Importantly, the intervention should begin before the workup is complete (i.e., from the first evaluation). All medical problems are treated independently of nutritional and behavioral interventions and should not delay or hamper them. The mainstay of treatment of all infants with FTT is a calorie-rich diet accompanied by frequent and close monitoring of weight response. An effective intervention will document a catch-up weight and height gain that is maintained over time.

Feeding and eating behaviors should be addressed, walking the fine line between encouragement and pressure to promote eating. Timing meals and snacks and eating as a family in a pleasant environment of low stress may be important to the acquisition of improved eating and feeding practices. The feeding intervention is dependent on the infant's age at presentation. For breast-feeding infants, it is beneficial to attempt to increase breast milk supply[552] by pumping milk, treatment with metoclopramide to induce oxytocin secretion,[553] improving maternal nutrition and fluid intake, and making adaptations at the home and workplace that can promote and simplify the breast-feeding process. Suckling problems in neurologically impaired infants can be solved by providing expressed human milk via bottle feeding. Bottle-fed and older infants allow more interventions to promote increased caloric content of the diet.

Infants with FTT should receive ~150% of the recommended daily caloric intake based on their expected weight (rather than based on their actual weight).[554] The enrichment of formula may be achieved by adding cereals, and toddlers may benefit from the addition of palatable high-energy-density foods (such as cheese and peanut butter) to their diet. High-calorie milk-based drinks (such as PediaSure, which provides 30 calories/oz.; in comparison to whole milk, which provides 19 calories/oz.) can be added alongside vitamin supplementation. Zinc supplementation has been shown to increase IGF-1 levels without affecting IGFBP-3 in infants with nonorganic FTT, yet this effect did not actually promote growth.[555]

Prognosis

The vast majority of infants and children with FTT show improvement with intervention. Others may even show progress when they achieve a more independent stage of development at which they can attain their own food. Those who require gastrostomy feeding due to neurologic dysfunction may require assisted enteral nutrition for life. The cognitive and intellectual function outcomes of those who suffered from FTT seem worse than their peers, although this association has only been well established in cases of iron deficiency anemia.[556]

It seems conceivable that deficiencies of other elements critical to brain development during infancy may have a similar adverse impact on intellectual properties at later ages, although this has not been studied systematically. The effects of nonorganic factors (such as emotional deprivation) on intellectual development, often coexisting with organic factors, may also contribute to decreased cognitive ability at later ages.

CANCER CACHEXIA

Cancer activates a complex set of CNS metabolic pathways, which result in cachexia[557] (Table 19-5). Peripheral cytokines gain access to the CNS through the central circumventricular organs that bypass the blood-brain barrier or through stimulation and amplification of CNS microglial cytokine or eicosanoid production. For instance, TNF-α stimulates VMH POMC neurons—which stimulates the SNS, which increases resting energy expenditure, increases cortisol and glucagon levels, and contributes to insulin resistance. IL-1 decreases neuropeptide Y within the VMH and thus decreases appetite. IL-1 also increases CRF, which indirectly inhibits appetite. IL-6 bears striking similarity to ciliary neurotrophic factor (CNTF), which has been shown to reduce weight by activating VMH POMC neurons through a leptin-independent mechanism.[558] Conversely, due to reduction in vagal activity, GI motility is impaired in cancer cachexia and is clinically manifest by early and inappropriate satiety—which occurs in 40% to 60% of cancer patients.

TABLE 19-5

Metabolic Changes in Cachexia

Expression of Cytokines
- Increased production of acute phase proteins (APP)
- Up-regulation of transcription factor NF Kappa B and AP-1
- Increased interleukin-1, IL-6, and tumor necrosis factor-α and interferon-γ
- Increased expression of tumor-specific cachexins (proteolysis-inducing factor, lipid-mobilizing factor, and anemia-inducing substance)
- Increased expression of ubiquitin, E_1, E_2, E_3, and proteasome components (cell death and removal)

Increased SNS Tone
- Increased expression of hormone-sensitive lipase in adipose tissue
- Up-regulation of uncoupling proteins (UCP2 and UCP3) in muscle and adipose tissue
- Increased hepatic gluconeogenesis

Reduced Vagal Tone
- Reduced lipoprotein lipase expression in adipose tissue
- Reduced intestinal transit
- Reduced hunger

In addition, cytokines have adverse peripheral effects. Uncoupling proteins are up-regulated by cytokines and contribute to increased energy expenditure. Cancer cachexia leads to overexpression of UCP1 in brown adipose tissue, UCP2 in brain, skeletal muscle and liver, and UCP3 in skeletal muscle. Levels of UCP2 and UCP3 in the liver and muscle are regulated by prostaglandins, and UCP3 is also regulated by triglycerides—all of which are increased in cancer.[559]

Cytokines cause insulin resistance in skeletal muscle, liver, and adipose tissue. TNF-α decreases insulin receptor and PPAR activity. In addition, there is an inverse correlation between interleukin-6 levels and insulin sensitivity.[560] Adipose tissue insulin resistance increases fat oxidation and decreases lipoprotein lipase activity, resulting in continued lipolysis.[561] The insulin resistance of cancer is not related to defective insulin clearance, and is therefore different than other forms of primary insulin resistance.[562]

Cancers are uniformly anaerobic and depend on glucose for survival. Thus, the glucose manufactured from gluconeogenesis secondary to hepatic insulin resistance is essential to tumor growth. Cancers release large amounts of lactate, which is converted in the liver back to glucose. Such gluconeogenesis consumes ATP, which also increases energy expenditure.[563] Additional raw materials for gluconeogenesis are alanine (derived from skeletal muscle proteolysis) and glycerol (from lipolysis).

Treatment is difficult. Many methods have been tried (SNS antagonists, prostaglandin inhibitors, omega-3 fatty acids, melatonin, thalidomide, interleukins, anticytokine monoclonal antibodies, IL-1 receptor antagonists, chemotherapy), but all are lacking. One promising new avenue is that of melanocortin antagonists,[543] but this is still in preclinical evaluation.

THE DIENCEPHALIC SYNDROME

Originally described by Russell in 1951,[564] this rare disorder presents in infants less than age 1 year and is an indication of a hypothalamic lesion—usually an anterior hypothalamic glioma or other neoplasm affecting hypothalamic function. Although the clinical spectrum is variable, emaciation with paucity of subcutaneous fat (but with normal linear growth and head circumference) is inviolate. Other frequent features include hyperalterness, hyperkinesis, nystagmus, and vomiting.[565,566]

Although numerous patients have been anecdotally reported and characterized, the cause of the emaciation remains unclear. Subjects with diencephalic syndrome have extremely elevated baseline GH levels, but with normal IGF-1 levels, suggesting a modicum of GH resistance.[565] It has been suggested that the high GH leads to lipolysis and accounts for the emaciation, but this finding is not consistent in all patients. Only one evaluation of energy balance has been performed, which demonstrated 30% to 50% greater REE in comparison to normal babies and 13% greater energy expenditure compared to intake.[567]

Treatment recommended is surgical extirpation of the lesion whenever feasible. Radiation is usually reserved for the very young patient. Frequently, these patients postoperatively manifest hypopituitarism—and ultimately develop hypothalamic obesity.[566]

ANOREXIA NERVOSA

Definition

Anorexia nervosa (AN) is an eating disorder that typically begins during adolescence and consists of persistent dieting and intense physical activity, usually accompanied by compulsive behavioral traits and sometimes with purging behavior and binge eating. Most subjects manifest a disturbed body image and a persistent fear of fatness, both of which promote further weight loss. The result of this behavior is a pathologic weight loss, with pathophysiologic consequences.

The risk of developing AN among females in Western societies is estimated to be between 0.5% and 1%.[568] There are two subtypes of anorexia: the food-restrictive type (characterized by very low caloric intake plus excessive exercise) and the purging type (characterized by varying levels of food purging, usually by way of self-induced vomiting and laxative abuse). Alongside the obvious mental elements, the definition in the *Diagnostic and Statistical Manual of Mental Disorders* (DSM-IV) includes anthropometric as well as metabolic components: a significantly low weight (defined as a sustained weight below the 85th percentile of the expected weight per height due to weight loss or failure to gain weight during growth and development) and secondary amenorrhea in pubertal girls and women (defined as no menses in 3 months).

Medical complications driven by the chronically reduced caloric intake, purging behavior, and excessive exercise may affect several organ systems. Typically, patients develop a marked loss of subcutaneous fat tissue, impaired menstrual function, bradycardia and orthostatic hypotension, hypothermia, and increased hair loss. Importantly, anorexia nervosa that develops during adolescence may create adverse clinical effects that persist into adulthood[569]—including osteopenia and osteoporosis,[570] higher rates of miscarriage, and reduced offspring birth weight.[571] Anorexia may also alter cognitive abilities (as during extreme weight loss), and a reduction of gray and white matter occurs. Conversely, during weight restoration white matter returns to premorbid levels but gray matter does not.[572]

Anorexia carries an increased mortality risk—specifically for suicide, yet also from medical causes such as starvation per se and purging-induced arrhythmias. Full recovery of body habitus and of growth and development occurs in 50% to 70% of treated adolescents, yet achieving a full physiologic and psychological recovery may take a comprehensive treatment intervention that may last as long as 5 to 7 years.[573] Greater weight loss, lower sustained weight, and the coexistence of other psychiatric disorders adversely affect the probability of recovery. The outcomes for adults with AN are poorer than those who are diagnosed and treated in adolescence.

Endocrine Associations

Obesity and malnutrition usually result in opposing effects on normal physiology and are both associated with changes in the hormonal profile. The majority of these changes represents an adaptive response yet should be considered part of the differential diagnosis of specific hormonal excess or deficiency disorders. Figure 19-7 shows the typical hormonal profile of patients with AN, aimed at energy preservation and the cessation of energetically costly and nonvital processes.

Hypothalamic-Pituitary-Thyroid Axis. The starvation status of AN may resemble the sick euthyroid syndrome. In patients with AN, serum total and free T_4, total and free T_3, TSH, and TBG are significantly lower than normal—whereas rT_3 levels are significantly greater than healthy controls.[574] Most AN patients have a hyporesponsive or delayed responsiveness of TSH to TRH stimulation. Of note, weight regain reverses the effects of AN on the hypothalamic-pituitary-thyroid axis back to normal. Thus, the reduction in thyroxinemia may actually be a normal adaptive physiologic response to starvation.

The differential diagnosis of hypothyroidism should be considered in patients with AN because both disorders are characterized by low T_4 and T_3 levels. In primary hypothyroidism, TSH levels will be greater than those seen in patients with AN—although in mild secondary hypothyroidism this distinction may be difficult. Obtaining a serum reverse T_3 (rT_3) level may be helpful in distinguishing a true thyroid disorder from the euthyroid sick syndrome associated with systemic illness.

Growth Hormone-IGF-1 Axis. Patients with AN typically have GH hypersecretion accompanied by low IGF-1 levels. Whether this profile is due to a primary hypothalamic dysfunction, peripheral target organ resistance to GH, or an impaired negative IGF-1 central feedback mechanism is unclear. An increased GH response to GHRH has been demonstrated in AN, possibly reflecting an impairment of beta-adrenergic suppression of GH

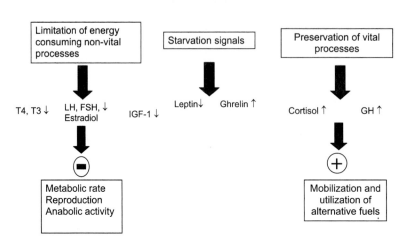

Figure 19-7 Hormonal changes in anorexia nervosa. The hormonal profile of the patient with anorexia nervosa represents an adaptive response aimed at conserving energy. Processes that require significant energy such as reproduction and growth are limited by a complete suppression of the gonadotropic axis and by reduced IGF-1 levels respectively. A seemingly chronic stress response characterized by increased growth hormone and cortisol is aimed at efficient utilization of the limited energetic sources present. Reduced leptin serves as a signal for down-regulating the hypothalamic-pituitary-gonadal axis. Reduced leptin also serves as a starvation signal, although this signal appears to be circumvented in this disorder.

secretion.[575] The clinical presentation of weight loss, cessation of menses, and cold intolerance alongside low levels of pituitary derived hormones may resemble panhypopituitarism—yet patients with AN present with GH hypersecretion.

Hypothalamic-Pituitary-Adrenal Axis. Patients with AN typically present with elevated cortisol levels in the presence of normal ACTH levels.[576] The elevated cortisol levels are apparently due to increased cortisol secretion alongside a reduction in cortisol clearance. Elevated CRH levels found in cerebrospinal fluid of patients with AN suggest that AN represents an overall state of activation of the hypothalamic stress response, manifested peripherally by hypercortisolemia. An abnormal response in the dexamethasone suppression test, mainly of reduced suppression, suggests that an element of decreased feedback sensitivity occurs in this disorder.

Bone Metabolism. Adolescence represents a critical period for the accumulation of bone mineral, thus building bone strength and density for later years. The achievement of peak bone mass is dependent on several hormonal effects characteristic of puberty (such as estradiol and IGF-1), as well as on being dependent on adequate nutrition—all of which are compromised in patients with AN. Adolescents and adults with AN have a low bone mineral density. Whereas in adults this is due to increased bone resorption and reduced bone formation, adolescents are characterized by an overall reduced bone turnover.[577]

The reduced bone density is caused by the typical hormonal profile of AN (i.e., reduced estrogens and androgens, low IGF-1, and relative hypercortisolemia). Moreover, the reduced lean body mass and lower mechanical forces acting on long bones may also contribute to the overall reduced BMD. Recent publications also suggest that elevated levels of gut-derived hormones

PYY(3-36) and ghrelin may also contribute to impaired bone metabolism in AN.[578] Importantly, resolution of AN with weight gain often does not bring full recovery of the bone mineral density status. Osteopenia resulting from undernutrition and the typical hormonal dynamics of AN is one of severe long-term complications of AN during adolescence, and thus is a major treatment target.

Hypothalamic-Pituitary-Gonadal Axis. Amenorrhea is one of the hallmarks of AN, yet it is not always explained by the severe weight loss. Thus, hypothalamic amenorrhea in AN often precedes weight loss and may persist after re-feeding and achievement of normal weight. Gonadotropin levels are reduced in patients with AN, and GnRH stimulation testing in patients with AN demonstrates a blunted LH response with a preserved FSH response and very low levels of estradiol. LH pulsatility may revert to prepubertal patterns in adolescents who have previously achieved pubertal status. The amenorrhea of AN is also marked by strikingly reduced leptin levels.

Leptin serves as a metabolic signal of energy status and nutritional reserve and thus may have a permissive role in the initiation of the complex hormonal dynamics necessary to normal reproductive function.[579] Teleologically, conservation of energy for immediate and necessary metabolic demands while suppressing energetically expensive processes such as reproduction serves as a protective measure in severely malnourished individuals (as seen in AN). The rise in leptin upon weight gain is associated with increases in gonadotropin secretion, suggesting that leptin serves a permissive role in the activation of the hypothalamic-pituitary-gonadal axis.

Fat-derived Hormones. Adipocytes secrete a wide array of adipocytokines, the normal profile of which is altered in AN. Patients with AN typically have very low plasma leptin concentrations alongside a marked disturbance of the leptin diurnal secretion profile.[580] The concentration of leptin-binding protein (the soluble isoform of leptin receptor) has been reported to be increased in patients with AN, contributing to a further reduction in concentration of free leptin.[581] Leptin has a major role in the neuroendocrine adaptations to the chronic starvation and undernutrition typical of AN, such as reduction in gonadotropins, reduction in thyroid hormone in order to conserve energy, a modified stress response manifested by hypercortisolemia, and elevated GH aimed at mobilizing and utilizing alternative energy sources.[582]

Weight gain in AN patients can induce relative hyperleptinemia in comparison to controls matched for BMI. Circulating leptin concentrations in AN patients thus traverse from subnormal to supranormal levels within a few weeks. Adiponectin is the only adipocytokine whose plasma concentrations are inversely related to fat mass. Conflicting results regarding adiponectin concentration in AN, ranging from hyperadiponectinemia[583] to hypoadiponectinemia,[584] have been reported. Interestingly, weight gain in AN is not necessarily associated with reciprocal changes in adiponectin concentration.[585]

Treatment

Indications for hospitalization and in-patient treatment of AN include dehydration, electrolyte disturbances (mainly hypokalemia), arrhythmias, CV instability (significant bradycardia, hypotension, and orthostatic changes), hypothermia, acute food refusal, acute complications of malnutrition (seizures, pancreatitis, cardiac failure), and psychiatric emergencies. Along with psychological interventions that may consist of psychotherapy and/or pharmacotherapy (based on the spectrum of psychiatric pathology), an increase in caloric intake must be part of the treatment protocol. Starting with 1,200 to 1,500 kcal per day and increasing by 500 kcal is aimed at a gain of 0.5 to 1 kg per week.[586] There is no superior feeding regimen as long as adequate caloric intake is supplied. Extreme cases may be handled through hospitalization in dedicated in-patient units, and caloric intake in this setting may initially be provided by nasogastric feeding—and in extreme cases by parenteral feeding.

One major treatment decision facing the caregiver of patients with AN is whether to utilize estrogen replacement therapy in order to treat amenorrhea and protect the skeleton from osteopenia. There is a lack of a proven efficacious beneficial effect of estrogen replacement therapy in regard to improved bone mass in AN in comparison to placebo,[587] although this treatment modality is still commonly used.[588] This treatment approach may have several adverse effects on the treatment of adolescents because it masks the beneficial effect of weight gain on the resumption of menses and may provide an erroneous sense of security in patients still at critically low weight status. Increased calcium intake alongside 400 IU of vitamin D to accelerate absorption should be encouraged in all patients with AN as another potential protective measure of bone status.

Conclusions

In childhood obesity, the overwhelming majority of cases are not due to a documentable genetic or neuroanatomic lesion. Indeed, although classic endocrinopathies account for less than 2% of childhood obesity in fact every obese patient does manifest an endocrine disturbance (e.g., insulin resistance and/or leptin resistance). We must acknowledge the obvious: that the child eats too much and exercises too little. The question physicians must internally pose when evaluating an obese patient is, "Where in the negative feedback energy balance pathway is this patient's dysfunction?" Only then can appropriate treatment be proffered. Similarly, in cachexia one must go beyond the lack of appetite to understand the reasons for the wasting and illness. These are endocrine paradigms that may permit modulation, especially with endocrine therapies. Understanding the energy balance pathway, and where these various disorders impair its regulation, is the key to further research and to successful prevention and treatment.

REFERENCES

1. .Morton GJ, Cummings DE, Baskin DG, Barsh GS, Schwartz MW (2006). Central nervous system control of food intake and body weight. Nature 443:289–295.
2. Coll AP, Farooqi IS, O'Rahilly S (2007). The hormonal control of food intake. Cell 129:251–262.
3. Hellstrom PM, Geliebter A, Naslund E, Schmidt PT, Yahav EK, Hashim SA, et al. (2004). Peripheral and central signals in the control of eating in normal, obese and binge-eating human subjects. Br J Nutr 92:S47–S57.
4. Date Y, Murakami N, Toshina IK, Matsukura S, Niijima A, Matsuo H, et al. (2002). The role of the gastric afferent vagal nerve in ghrelin-induced feeding and growth hormone secretion in rats. Gastroenterology 123:1120–1128.
5. Bi SM (2002). Actions of CCK in the control of food intake and body weight: Lessons from the CCK-A receptor deficient OLETF rat. Neuropeptides 36:171–181.
6. Abbott CR, Monteiro M, Small CJ, Sajedi A, Smith KL, Parkinson JRC, et al. (2005). The inhibitory effects of peripheral administration of peptide YY3-36 and glucagon-like peptide-1 on food intake are attenuated by ablation of the vagal-brainstem-hypothalamic pathway. Brain Res 1044:127–131.
7. Kojima M, Hosoda H, Date Y, Nakazato M, Matsuo H, Kangawa K (1999). Ghrelin is a growth-hormone-releasing acylated peptide from stomach. Nature 402:656–660.
8. Kamegai J, Tamura H, Shimizu T, Ishii S, Sugihara H, Wakabayashi I (2000). Central effect of ghrelin, an endogenous growth hormone secretagogue, on hypothalamic peptide gene expression. Endocrinology 141:4797–4800.
9. Tschöp M, Smiley DL, Heiman ML (2000). Ghrelin induces adiposity in rodents. Nature 407:908–913.
10. Cummings DE, Purnell JQ, Frayo RS, Schmidova K, Wisse BF, Weigle DS (2001). A prandial rise in plasma ghrelin levels suggests a role in meal initiation in humans. Diabetes 50:1714–1719.
11. Druce MR, Neary NM, Small CJ, Milton J, Monteiro M, Patterson M, et al. (2006). Subcutaneous administration of ghrelin stimulates energy intake in healthy lean human volunteers. Int J Obes 30:293–296.
12. Cummings DE, Weigle DS, Frayo RS, Breen PA, Ma MK, Dellinger EP, et al. (2002). Plasma ghrelin levels after diet-induced weight loss or gastric bypass surgery. N Engl J Med 346:1623–1630.
13. Batterham RL, Cowley MA, Small CJ, Herzog H, Cohen MA, Dakin CL, et al. (2002). Gut hormone PYY$_{3-36}$ physiologically inhibits food intake. Nature 418:650–654.

14. Kiefer TJ, Habener JF (1999). The glucagon-like peptides. Endocrine Reviews 20:876–913.

15. Drucker DJ (2005). Biologic actions and therapeutic potential of the proglucagon-derived peptides. Nature Clin Pract Endo Metab 1:22–31.

16. Gotoh K, Fukagawa K, Fukagawa T, Noguchi H, Kakuma T, Sakata T, et al. (2005). Glucagon-like peptide-1, corticotropin-releasing hormone, and hypothalamic neuronal histamine interact in the leptin-signaling pathway to regulate feeding behavior. FASEB J 19:1131–1133.

17. Zhang Y, Proenca R, Maffei M, Barone M, Leopold L, Friedman JM (1994). Positional cloning of the mouse obese gene and its human homologue. Nature 393:372–425.

18. Lustig RH (2006). Childhood obesity: Behavioral aberration or biochemical drive? Reinterpreting the first law of thermodynamics. Nature Clin Pract Endo Metab 2:447–458.

19. Chehab FF, Mounzih K, Lu R, Lim ME (1997). Early onset of reproductive function in normal female mice treated with leptin. Science 275:88–90.

20. Mantzoros CS, Flier JS, Rogol AD (1997). A longitudinal assessment of hormonal and physical alterations during normal puberty in boys: Rising leptin levels may signal the onset of puberty. J Clin Endocrinol Metab 82:1066–1070.

21. Mark AL, Rahmouni K, Correia M, Haynes WG (2003). A leptin-sympathetic-leptin feedback loop: Potential implications for regulation of arterial pressure and body fat. Acta Physiol Scand 177:345–349.

22. Boden G, Chen X, Mozzoli M, Ryan I (1996). Effect of fasting on serum leptin in normal human subjects. J Clin Endocrinol Metab 81:454–458.

23. Keim NL, Stern JS, Havel PJ (1998). Relation between circulating leptin concentrations and appetite during a prolonged, moderate energy deficit in women. Am J Clin Nutr 68:794–801.

24. Flier JS (1998). What's in a name? In search of leptin's physiologic role. J Clin Endocrinol Metab 83:1407–1413.

25. Hassink SG, Sheslow DV, de Lancy E, Opentanova I, Considine RV, Caro JF (1996). Serum leptin in children with obesity: relationship to gender and development. Pediatrics 98:201–203.

26. Guven S, El-Bershawi A, Sonnenberg GE, Wilson CR, Hoffman RG, Krakower GR, et al. (1999). Plasma leptin and insulin levels in weight-reduced obese women with normal body mass index: Relationships with body composition and insulin. Diabetes 48:347–352.

27. Barr VA, Malide D, Zarnowski MJ, Taylor SI, Cushman SW (1997). Insulin stimulates both leptin secretion and production by white adipose tissue. Endocrinology 138:4463–4472.

28. Kolaczynski JW, Nyce MR, Considine RV, Boden G, Nolan JJ, Henry R, et al. (1996). Acute and chronic effects of insulin on leptin production in humans: Studies in vivo and in vitro. Diabetes 45:699–701.

29. Singhal A, Farooqi IS, O'Rahilly S, Cole TJ, Fewtrell M, Lucas A (2002). Early nutrition and leptin concentrations later in life. Am J Clin Nutr 75:993–999.

30. Lee GH, Proenca R, Montez JM, Carroll KM, Darvishzadeh JG, Lee JI, et al. (1996). Abnormal splicing of the leptin receptor in diabetic mice. Nature 379:632–635.

31. Spanswick D, Smith MA, Groppi VE, Logan SD, Ashford ML (1997). Leptin inhibits hypothalamic neurons by activation of ATP-sensitive potassium channels. Nature 390:521–525.

32. Kishimoto T, Taga T, Akira S (1994). Cytokine signal transduction. Cell 76:252–262.

33. Banks AS, Davis SM, Bates SJ, Myers MG (2000). Activation of downstream signals by the long form of the leptin receptor. J Biol Chem 275:14563–14572.

34. Niswender KD, Schwartz MW (2003). Insulin and leptin revisited: Adiposity signals with overlapping physiological and intracellular signaling capabilities. Front Neuroendocrinol 24:1–10.

35. Porte D, Baskin DG, Schwartz MW (2005). Insulin signaling in the central nervous system: A critical role in metabolic homeostasis and disease from C. elegans to humans. Diabetes 54:1264–1276.

36. Baskin DG, Wilcox BJ, Figlewicz DP, Dorsa DM (1988). Insulin and insulin-like growth factors in the CNS. Trends Neurosci 11:107–111.

37. Baura GD, Foster DM, Porte D, Kahn SE, Bergman RN, Cobelli C, et al. (1993). Saturable transport of insulin from plasma into the central nervous system of dogs in vivo: A mechanism for regulated insulin delivery to the brain. J Clin Invest 92:1824–1830.

38. VanderWeele DA (1994). Insulin is a prandial satiety hormone. Physiology of Behavior 56:619–622.

39. McGowan MK, Andrews KM, Grossman SP (1992). Role of intra-hypothalamic insulin in circadian patterns of food intake, activity, and body temperature. Behav Neurosci 106:380–385.

40. Woods SC, Lotter EC, McKay LD, Porte D (1979). Chronic intra-cerebroventricular infusion of insulin reduces food intake and body weight of baboons. Nature 282:503–505.

41. Abusrewil SS, Savage DL (1989). Obesity and diabetic control. Arch Dis Child 64:1313–1315.

42. VanderWeele DA (1993). Insulin and satiety from feeding in pancreatic-normal and diabetic rats. Physiol Behav 54:477–485.

43. Assimacopoulos-Jeannet F, Brichard S, Rencurel F, Cusin I, Jeanrenaud B (1995). In vivo effects of hyperinsulinemia on lipogenic enzymes and glucose transporter expression in rat liver and adipose tissues. Metabolism 44(2):228–233.

44. Cusin I, Terrettaz J, Rohner-Jeanrenaud F, Zarjevski N, Assimacopoulos-Jeannet F, Jeanrenaud B (1990). Hyperinsulinemia increases the amount of GLUT4 mRNA in white adipose tissue and decreases that of muscles: A clue for increased fat depot and insulin resistance. Endocrinology 127:3246–3248.

45. Woo R, Kissileff HR, Pi-Sunyer FX (1984). Elevated post-prandial insulin levels do not induce satiety in normal-weight humans. Am J Physiol Regul Integ Comp Physiol 247:R776–R787.

46. Niswender KD, Morton GJ, Stearns WH, Rhodes CJ, Myers MG, Schwartz MW (2001). Intracellular signalling: Key enzyme in leptin-induced anorexia. Nature 413:794–795.

47. Brüning JC, Gautam D, Burks DJ, Gillette J, Schubert M, Orban PC, et al. (2000). Role of brain insulin receptor in control of body weight and reproduction. Science 289:2122–2125.

48. Schwartz MW, Figlewicz DP, Baskin DG, Woods SC, Porte D (1994). Insulin and the central regulation of energy balance: Update 1994. Endocrinol Rev 2:109–113.

49. Lin X, Taguchi A, Park S, Kushner JA, Li F, Li Y, White MF (2004). Dysregulation of insulin receptor substrate 2 in β-cells and brain causes obesity and diabetes. J Clin Invest 114:908–916.

50. Plum L, Ma X, Hampel B, Balthasar N, Coppari R, Munzberg H, et al. (2006). Enhanced PIP(3) signaling in POMC neurons causes K(ATP) channel activation and leads to diet-sensitive obesity. J Clin Invest 116:1886–1901.

51. Bjorkbaek C, Elmquist JK, Frantz JD, Shoelson SE, Flier JS (1998). Identification of SOCS-3 as a potential mediator of central leptin resistance. Molecular Cell 1:619–625.

52. Bence KK, Delibegovic M, Xue B, Gorgun CZ, Hotamisligil GS, Neel BG, Kahn BB (2006). Neuronal PTP1B regulates body weight, adiposity, and leptin action. Nat Med 12:917–924.

53. Elmquist JK, Ahima RS, Elias CF, Flier JS, Saper CB (1998). Leptin activates distinct projections from the dorsomedial and ventromedial hypothalamic nuclei. Proc Natl Acad Sci USA 95:741–746.

54. Thornton JE, Cheung CC, Clifton DK, Steiner RA (1997). Regulation of hypothalamic proopiomelanocortin mRNA by leptin in ob/ob mice. Endocrinology 138:5063–5066.

55. Kristensen P, Judge ME, Thim L, Ribel U, Christjansen KN, Wulff BS, et al. (1998). Hypothalamic CART is a new anorectic peptide regulated by leptin. Nature 393:72–76.

56. Broberger C, Johansen J, Johasson C, Schalling M, Hokfelt T (1998). The neuropeptide Y/agouti gene related protein (AGRP) brain circuitry in normal, anorectic, and monosodium glutamate-treated mice. Proc Natl Acad Sci USA 95:15043–15048.

57. Liebowitz SF (1995). Brain peptides and obesity: Pharmacologic treatment. Obes Res 3:573S–589S.

58. Kalra SP, Kalra PS (1996). Nutritional infertility: the role of the interconnected hypothalamic neuropeptide Y-galanin-opioid network. Front Neuroendocrinol 17:371–401.

59. Beck B, Stricker-Krongard A, Nicolas JP, Burlet C (1992). Chronic and continuous intracerebroventricular infusion of neuropeptide Y in Long-Evans rats mimics the feeding behavior of obese Zucker rats. Int J Obesity 16:295–302.

60. Stephens TW, Basinski M, Bristow PK, Bue-Valleskey JM, Burgett SG, Craft L, et al. (1995). The role of neuropeptide Y in the antiobesity action of the obese gene product. Nature 377:530–534.

61. Broberger C, Landry M, Wong H, Walsh JN, Hokfelt T (1997). Subtypes of the Y_1 and Y_2 of the neuropeptide Y receptor are respectively expressed in pro-opiomelanocortin and neuropeptide Y-containing neurons of the rat hypothalamic arcuate nucleus. Neuroendocrinology 66:393–408.

62. Shutter JR, Graham M, Kinsey AC, Scully S, Luthy R, Stark KL (1997). Hypothalamic expression of ART, a novel gene related to agouti, is up-regulated in obese and diabetic mutant mice. Genes and Development 7:454–467.

63. Graham M, Shutter JR, Sarmiento U, Sarosi I, Stark KL (1997). Overexpression of Agrt leads to obesity in transgenic mice. Nature Genet 17:273–274.

64. Wellman PJ (2005). Modulation of eating by central catecholamine systems. Curr Drug Targets 6:191–199.

65. Leibowitz S, Roosin P, Rosenn M (1984). Chronic norepinephrine injection into the hypothalamic paraventricular nucleus produces hyperphagia and increased body weight in the rat. Pharmacol Biochem Behav 21:801–808.

66. Wellman PJ, Davies BT (1992). Reversal of cirazoline-induced and phenylpropanolamine-induced anorexia by the alpha-1-receptor antagonist prazosin. Pharmacol Biochem Behav 42:97–100.

67. Liebowitz SF, Alexander JT, Cheung WK, Weiss GF (1993). Effects of serotonin and the serotonin blocker metergoline on meal patterns and macronutrient selection. Pharmacol Biochem Behav 45:185–194.

68. Wong DT, Reid LR, Threlkeld PG (1988). Suppression of food intake in rats by fluoxetine: Comparison of enantiomers and effects of serotonin antagonists. Pharmacol Biochem Behav 31:475–479.

69. Garattini S, Bizzi A, Caccia S, Mennini T (1992). Progress report on the anorectic effects of dexfenfluramine, fluoxetine, and sertraline. Int J Obesity 16:S43–S50.

70. Calapai G, Corica F, Corsonello A, Saubetin L, DiRosa M, Campo GM, et al. (1999). Leptin increases serotonin turnover by inhibition of nitric oxide synthesis. J Clin Invest 104:975–982.

71. Nonogaki K, Strack AM, Dallman MF, Tecott LH (1998). Leptin-independent hyperphagia and type 2 diabetes in mice with a mutated serotonin 5-HT$_{2c}$ receptor gene. Nature Med 4:1152–1156.

72. Simansky KJ (1996). Serotonergic control of the organization of feeding and satiety. Behavioral Brain Research 73:37–42.

73. Pissios P, Bradley RL, Maratos-Flier E (2006). Expanding the scales: the multiple roles of MCH in regulating energy balance and other biological functions. Endocr Rev 27:606–620.

74. Shimada M, Tritos NA, Lowell BB, Flier JS, Maratos-Flier E (1998). Mice lacking melanin-concentrating hormone receptor are hypophagic and lean. Nature 396:670–674.

75. Ludwig DS, Tritos NA, Mastaitis JW, Kulkarni R, Kokkotou E, Elmquist J, et al. (2001). Melanin-concentrating hormone overexpression in transgenic mice leads to obesity and insulin resistance. J Clin Invest 107:379–386.

76. Gomori A, Ishihara A, Ito M, Mashiko S, Matsushita H, Yumoto M, et al. (2003). Chronic intracerebroventricular infusion of MCH causes obesity in mice. Am J Physiol 284:E583–E588.

77. Taylor MM, Samson WK (2003). The other side of the orexins: Endocrine and metabolic actions. Am J Physiol 284:E13–E17.

78. Hara J, Beuckmann CT, Nambu T, Willie JT, Chemelli RM, Sinton CM, et al. (2001). Genetic ablation of orexin neurons in mice results in narcolepsy, hypophagia, and obesity. Neuron 30:345–354.

79. Harris GC, Aston-Jones G (2006). Arousal and reward: a dichotomy in orexin function. Trends Neurosci. 29:571–577.

80. Mieda M, Yanigasawa M (2002). Sleep, feeding, and neuropeptides: Roles of orexins and orexin receptors. Curr Opin in Neurobiol 12:339–346.

81. Pagotto U, Marsicano G, Cota D, Lutz B, Pasquali R (2006). The emerging role of the endocannabinoid system in endocrine regulation and energy balance. Endocr Rev 27:73–100.

82. Malcher-Lopes R, Di S, Marcheselli VS, Weng FJ, Stuart CT, Bazan NG, Tasker JG (2006). Opposing crosstalk between leptin and glucocorticoids rapidly modulates synaptic excitation via endocannabinoid release. J Neurosci 26:6643–6650.

83. Chen AS, Marsh DJ, Trumbauer ME, Frazier EG, Guan XM, Yu H, et al. (2000). Inactivation of the mouse melanocortin-3 receptor results in increased fat mass and reduced lean body mass. Nature Genet 26:97–102.

84. Butler AA, Cone RD (2002). The melanocortin receptors: Lessons from knockout models. Neuropeptides 36:77–84.

85. Rahmouni K, Haynes WG, Morgan DA, Mark AL (2003). Role of melanocortin-4 receptors in mediating renal sympathoactivation to leptin and insulin. J Neurosci 23:5998–6004.

86. Collins S, Kuhn CM, Petro AE, Swick AG, Chrunyk BA, Surwit RS (1996). Role of leptin in fat regulation. Nature 380:677.

87. Muntzel M, Morgan DA, Mark AL, Johnson AK (1994). Intracerebroventricular insulin produces non-uniform regional increases in sympathetic nerve activity. Am J Physiol 267:R1350–R1355.

88. Vollenweider L, Tappy L, Owlya R, Jequier E, Nicod P, Scherrer U (1995). Insulin-induced sympathetic activation and vasodilation in skeletal muscle: Effects of insulin resistance in lean subjects. Diabetes 44:641–645.

89. Blaak EE, Saris WH, van Baak MA (1993). Adrenoceptor subtypes mediating catecholamine-induced thermogenesis in man. Int J Obesity 17:S78–S81.

90. Viguerie N, Clement K, Barbe P, Courtine M, Benis A, Larrouy D, et al. (2004). In vivo epinephrine-mediated regulation of gene express in human skeletal muscle. J Clin Endocrinol Metab 89:2000–2014.

91. Navegantes LC, Migliorini RH, do Carmo Kettelhut I (2002). Adrenergic control of protein metabolism in skeletal muscle. Curr Opin Clin Nutr Metab Care 5:281–286.

92. Susulic VS, Frederich RC, Lawitts J, Tozzo E, Kahn BB, Harper ME, et al. (1995). Targeted disruption of the beta 3-adrenergic receptor gene. J Biol Chem 270:29483–29492.

93. Boss O, Bachman E, Vidal-Puig A, Zhang CY, Peroni O, Lowell BB (1999). Role of the b$_3$-adrenergic receptor and/or a putative b$_3$-adrenergic receptor on the expression of uncoupling proteins and peroxisome proliferator-activated receptor-$_g$ coactivator-1. Biochem Biophys Res Comm 261:870–876.

94. Lowell BB, Spiegelman BM (2000). Towards a molecular understanding of adaptive thermogenesis. Nature 404:652–660.

95. Klingenberg M, Huang SG (1999). Structure and function of the uncoupling protein from brown adipose tissue. Biochem Biophys Acta 1415:271–296.

96. Powley TL, Laughton W (1981). Neural pathways involved in the hypothalamic integration of autonomic responses. Diabetologia 20:378–387.

97. Peles E, Goldstein DS, Akselrod S, Nitzan H, Azaria M, Almog S, et al. (1995). Interrelationships among measures of autonomic activity and cardiovascular risk factors during orthostasis and the oral glucose tolerance test. Clin Autonom Res 5:271–278.

98. Rohner-Jeanrenaud F, Jeanrenaud B (1985). Involvement of the cholinergic system in insulin and glucagon oversecretion of genetic preobesity. Endocrinology 116:830–834.

99. Lustig RH (2003). Autonomic dysfunction of the β-cell and the pathogenesis of obesity. Rev Endocr Metab Dis 4:23–32.

100. Kreier F, Fliers E, Voshol PJ, Van Eden CG, Havekes LM, Kalsbeek A, et al. (2002). Selective parasympathetic innervation of subcutaneous and intra-abdominal fat-functional implications. J Clin Invest 110:1243–1250.

101. Boden G, Hoeldtke RD (2003). Nerves, fat, and insulin resistance. N Engl J Med 349:1966–1967.

102. D'Alessio DA, Kieffer TJ, Taborsky GJ, Havel PJ (2001). Activation of the parasympathetic nervous system is necessary for normal meal induced-insulin secretion in rhesus macaques. J Clin Endocrinol Metab 86:1253–1259.

103. Ahren B, Holst JJ (2001). The cephalic insulin response to meal ingestion in humans is dependent on both cholinergic and non-cholinergic mechanisms and is important for postprandial glycemia. Diabetes 50:1030–1038.

104. Gilon P, Henquin JC (2001). Mechanisms and physiological significance of the cholinergic control of pancreatic β-cell function. Endocr Rev 22:565–604.

105. Miura Y, Gilon P, Henquin JC (1996). Muscarinic stimulation increases Na$^+$ entry in pancreatic β-cells by a mechanism other than the emptying of intracellular Ca^{2+} pools. Biochem Biophys Res Comm 224:67–73.

106. Zawalich WS, Zawalich KC, Rasmussen H (1989). Cholinergic agonists prime the β-cell to glucose stimulation. Endocrinology 125:2400–2406.

107. Nishi S, Seino Y, Ishida H, Seno M, Taminato T, Sakurai H, et al. (1987). Vagal regulation of insulin, glucagon, and somatostatin secretion in vitro in the rat. J Clin Invest 79:1191–1196.

108. Komeda K, Yokote M, Oki Y (1980). Diabetic syndrome in the Chinese hamster induced with monosodium glutamate. Experientia 36:232–234.

109. Rohner-Jeanrenaud F, Jeanrenaud B (1980). Consequences of ventromedial hypothalamic lesions upon insulin and glucagon secretion by subsequently isolated perfused pancreases in the rat. J Clin Invest 65:902–910.

110. Berthoud HR, Jeanrenaud B (1979). Acute hyperinsulinemia and its reversal by vagotomy following lesions of the ventromedial hypothalamus in anesthetized rats. Endocrinology 105:146–151.

111. Tian YM, Urquidi V, Ashcroft SJH (1996). Protein kinase C in β-cells: Expression of multiple isoforms and involvement in cholinergic stimulation of insulin secretion. Mol Cell Endocrinol 119:185–193.

112. Arbuzova A, Murray D, McLaughlin S (1998). MARCKS, membranes, and calmodulin: Kinetics of their interaction. Biochimica et Biophysica Acta 1376:369–379.

113. Blondel O, Bell GI, Moody M, Miller RJ, Gibbons SJ (1994). Creation of an inositol 1,4,5-triphosphate-sensitive Ca^{2+} store in secretory granules of insulin-producing cells. J Biol Chem 269:27167–27170.

114. Rocca AS, Brubaker PL (1999). Role of the vagus nerve in mediating proximal nutrient-induced glucagon-like peptide-1 secretion. Endocrinology 140:1687–1694.

115. Marin P, Russeffé-Scrive A, Smith J, Bjorntorp P (1988). Glucose uptake in human adipose tissue. Metabolism 36:1154–1164.

116. Ramsay TG (1996). Fat cells. Endocrinol Metab Clin NA 25:847–870.

117. Leibel RL (2002). The role of leptin in the control of body weight. Nutr Rev 60:S15–S19.

118. Leibel RL, Rosenbaum M, Hirsch J (1995). Changes in energy expenditure resulting from alered body weight. N Engl J Med 332:621–628.

119. Champigny O, Ricquier D (1990). Effects of fasting and refeeding on the level of uncoupling protein mRNA in rat brown adipose tissue: Evidence for diet -induced and cold-induced responses. J Nutr 120:1730–1736.

120. Aronne LJ, Mackintosh R, Rosenbaum M, Leibel RL, Hirsch J (1995). Autonomic nervous system activity in weight gain and weight loss. Am J Physiol 269:R222–R225.

121. Kelley AE, Bakshi VP, Haber SN, Steininger TL, Will MJ, Zhang M (2002). Opioid modulation of taste hedonics within the ventral striatum. Physiol Behav 76:365–377.

122. Hommel JD, Trinko R, Sears RM, Georgescu D, Liu ZW, Gao XB, et al. (2006). Leptin receptor signaling in midbrain dopamine neurons regulates feeding. Neuron 51:801–810.

123. Shalev U, Yap J, Shaham Y (2001). Leptin attenuates food deprivation-induced relapse to heroin seeking. J Neurosci 21:RC129: 121–125.

124. Carr KD, Tsimberg Y, Berman Y, Yamamoto N (2003). Evidence of increased dopamine receptor signaling in food-restricted rats. Neuroscience 119:1157–1167.

125. Figlewicz DP, Szot P, Chavez M, Woods SC, Veith RC (1994). Intraventricular insulin increases dopaminergic transporter mRNA in rat VTA/substantia nigra. Brain Res 644:331–334.

126. Sipols AJ, Bayer J, Bennett R, Figlewicz DP (2002). Intraventricular insulin decreases kappa opioid-mediated sucrose intake in rats. Peptides 23:2181–2187.

127. Figlewicz DP (2003). Adiposity signals and food reward: expanding the CNS roles of insulin and leptin. Am J Phyisol Regul Integ Comp Physiol 284:R882–R892.

128. Heymsfield SB, Greenberg AS, Fujioka K, Dixon RM, Kushner R, Hunt T, et al. (1999). Recombinant leptin for weight loss in obese and lean adults: A randomized, controlled, dose-escalation trial. JAMA 282:1568–1575.

129. Rosenbaum M, Nicolson M, Hirsch J, Murphy E, Chu F, Leibel RL (1997). Effects of weight change on plasma leptin concentrations and energy expenditure. J Clin Endocrinol Metab 82:3647–3564.

130. Caro JF, Kolaczynski JW, Nyce MR, Ohannesian JP, Opentanova I, Goldman WH, et al. (1996). Decreased cerebrospinal fluid/serum leptin ratio in obesity: A possible mechanism for leptin resistance. The Lancet 348:159–161.

131. Banks WA, Kastin AJ, Huang W, Jaspan JB, Maness LM (1996). Leptin enters the brain by a saturable system independent of insulin. Peptides 17:305–311.

132. El-Haschimi K, Pierroz DD, Hileman SM, Bjorbaek C, Flier JS (2000). Two defects contribute to hypothalamic leptin resistance in mice with diet-induced obesity. J Clin Invest 105:1827–1832.

133. Rosenbaum M, Murphy EM, Heymsfield SB, Matthews DE, Leibel RL (2002). Low dose leptin administration reverses effects of sustained weight reduction on energy expenditure and circulating concentrations of thyroid hormones. J Clin Endocrinol Metab 87:2391–2394.

134. Rosenbaum M, Goldsmith R, Bloomfield D, Magnano A, Weimer L, Heymsfield S, et al. (2005). Low-dose leptin reverses skeletal muscle, autonomic, and neuroendocrine adaptations to maintenance of reduced weight. J Clin Invest 115:3579–3586.

135. Lustig RH, Sen S, Soberman JE, Velasquez-Mieyer PA (2004). Obesity, leptin resistance, and the effects of insulin suppression. Int J Obesity 28:1344–1348.

136. Isganaitis E, Lustig RH (2005). Fast food, central nervous system insulin resistance, and obesity. Arterioscler Thromb Vasc Biol 25:2451–2462.

137. Lustig RH, Mietus-Snyder ML, Bacchetti P, Lazar AA, Velasquez-Mieyer PA, Christensen ML (2006). Insulin dynamics predict predict BMI and z-score response to insulin suppression or sensitization pharmacotherapy in obese children. J Pediatr 148:23–29.

138. Dietz WH (1998). Health consequences of obesity in youth: childhood predictors of adulthood disease. Pediatrics 101:518–525.

139. Hubbard VS (2000). Defining overweight and obesity: What are the issues. Am J Clin Nutr 72:1067–1068.

140. Calle EE, Thun MJ, Petrelli JM, Rodriguez C, Heath CW (1999). Body-mass index and mortality in a prospective cohort of U.S. adults. N Engl J Med 341:1097–1105.

141. World Health Organization (1998). Report of a WHO consultation on obesity. Obesity: Preventing and managing the global epidemic. World Health Organization, Geneva.

142. Troiano RP, Flegal KM, Kuczmarski RJ, Campbell SM, Johnson CL (1995). Overweight prevalance and trends for children and adolescents. Arch Ped Adol Med 149:1085–1091.

143. Whitaker RC, Wright JA, Pepe MS, Seidel KD, Dietz WH (1997). Predicting obesity in young adulthood from childhood and parental obesity. N Engl J Med 337:869–873.

144. Dietz WH, Robinson TN (1998). Use of the body mass index (BMI) as a measure of overweight in children and adolescents. J Pediatr 132:191–193.

145. [Author] (2001). BMI curves. http://www.cdc.gov/growthcharts.

146. Gortmaker SL, Dietz WH, Sobol AM, Wehler CA (1987). Increasing pediatric obesity in the United States. Am J Dis Child 141:535–540.

147. Ogden CL, Flegal KM, Carroll MD, Johnson CL (2002). Prevalence and trends in overweight among US children and adolescents, 1999–2000. JAMA 288:1728–1732.

148. Brown LR (2000). Obesity epidemic threatens health in exercise-deprived societies. Worldwatch Institute internet release, www.worldwatch.org/chairman/issue/001219.html.

149. Ebbeling CB, Pawlak DB, Ludwig DS (2002). Childhood obesity: Public-health crisis, common sense cure. Lancet 360:473–482.

150. Matsushita Y, Yoshiike N, Kaneda F, Yoshita K, Takimoto H (2004). Trends in childhood obesity in Japan over the last 25 years from the national nutrition survey. Obes Res 12:205–214.

151. Yoshinaga M, Shimago A, Koriyama C, Nomura Y, Miyata K, Hashiguchi J, et al. (2004). Rapid increase in the prevalence of obesity in elementary school children. Int J Obes 28:494–499.

152. Gordon-Larsen P, Adair LS, Popkin BM (2002). Ethnic differences in physical activity and inactivity patterns and overweight status. Obes Res 10:141–149.

153. James WPT, Nelson M, Ralph A, Leather S (1997). Socioeconomic determinants of health: The contribution of nutrition to inequalities in health. BMJ 314:1545–1549.

154. Drewnowski A (1998). Energy density, palatability, and satiety: Implications for weight control. Nutrition Reviews 56:347–353.

155. Martorell R, Khan LK, Hughes ML, Grummer-Strawn LM (1998). Obesity in Latin-American women and children. Journal of Nutrition 128:1464–1473.

156. Strauss RS, Pollack HA (2001). Epidemic increase in childhood overweight, 1986–1998. JAMA 286:2845–2848.

157. Kimm SY, Barton BA, Obarzanek E, McMahon RP, Kronsberg SS, Waclawiw MA, et al. (2002). Obesity development during adolescence in a biracial cohort: The NHLBI Growth and Health Study. Pediatrics 110:e54.

158. Crawford PB, Story M, Wang MC, Ritchie LD, Sabry ZI (2001). Ethnic issues in the epidemiology of childhood obesity. Ped Clin NA 48:855–878.

159. Warner ML, Harley K, Bradman A, Vargas G, Eskenazi B (2006). Soda consumption and overweight status of 2-year-old Mexican-American children in California. Obesity 14:1966–1974.

160. Dietz WH (1998). Health consequences of obesity in youth: Childhood predictors of adult disease. Pediatrics 101:518–525.

161. Styne DM (2001). Childhood and adolescent obesity: Prevalence and significance. Ped Clin NA 48:823–854.

162. Guo SS, Huang C, Maynard LM, Demerath E, Towne B, Chumlea WC, et al. (2000). Body mass index during childhood, adolescence and young adulthood in relation to adult overweight and adiposity: The Fels Longitudinal Study. Int J Obesity 24:1628–1635.

163. Guo SS, Wu W, Chumlea WC, Roche AF (2002). Predicting overweight and obesity in adulthood from body mass index values in childhood and adolescence. Am J Clin Nutr 76:653–658.

164. Whitaker RC, Pepe MS, Wright JA, Seidel KD, Dietz WH (1998). Early adiposity rebound and the risk of adult obesity. Pediatrics 101:1–6.

165. Toschke AM, Vignerova J, Lhotska L, Oscanova K, Kolestzko B, von Kries R (2002). Overweight and obesity in 6- to 14-year-old Czech children in 1991. Protective effect of breast feeding. J Pediatr 141:764–769.

166. von Kries R, Koletzko B, Sauerwald T, von Mutius E, Barnert D, Grunert V, et al. (1999). Breast feeding and obesity: Cross sectional study. BMJ 319:147–150.

167. Dorosty AR, Emmett PM, Cowin S, Reilly JJ (2000). Factors associated with early adiposity rebound: ALSPAC study team. Pediatrics 105:1115–1118.

168. Glaser NS (1997). Non-insulin-dependent diabetes mellitus in childhood and adolescence. Ped Clin NA 44:307–337.

169. Bjorntorp P (1990). Portal adipose tissue as a generator of risk factors for cardiovascular disease and diabetes. Arteriosclerosis 10:493–496.

170. Bonora E (2000). Relationship between regional fat distribution and insulin resistance. Int J Obes 24:S32–S35.

171. Arner P (2002). Insulin resistance in type 2 diabetes: Role of fatty acids. Diab Metab Res Rev 18:S5–S9.

172. Randle PJ, Garland PB, Hales CN (1963). The glucose fatty acid cycle: Its role in insulin sensitivity and metabolic disturbances in diabetes mellitus. Lancet 1:7285–7289.

173. Abate N, Garg A, Peshock RM, Stray-Gundersen J, Adams-Huet B, Grundy SM (1996). Relationship of generalized and regional adiposity to insulin sensitivity in men with NIDDM. Diabetes 45:1684–1693.

174. Wajchenberg BL (2000). Subcutaneous and visceral adipose tissue: their relation to the metabolic syndrome. Endocr Rev 21:697–738.

175. Montague CT, O'Rahilly S (2000). The perils of portliness: Causes and consequences of visceral adiposity. Diabetes 49:883–888.

176. Ravussin E, Smith SR (2002). Increased fat intake, impaired fat oxidation, and failure of fat cell proliferation result in ectopic fat storage, insulin resistance, and type 2 diabetes mellitus. Ann NY Acad Sci 967:363–378.

177. Krssak M, Falk Petersen K, Dresner A, DiPietro L, Vogel SM, Rothman DL, et al. (1999). Intramyocellular lipid concentrations are correlated with insulin sensitivity in humans: A ^{1}H NMR spectroscopy study. Diabetologia 42:113–116.

178. Garg A (2004). Acquired and inherited lipodystrophies. N Engl J Med 350:1220–1234.

179. Goodpaster BH, Thaete FL, Simoneau JA, Kelley DE (1997). Subcutaneous abdominal fat and thigh muscle composition predict insulin sensitivity independently of visceral fat. Diabetes 46:1579–1585.

180. Perseghin G, Scifo P, De Cobelli F, Pagliato E, Battezzati A, Arcelloni C, et al. (1999). Intramyocellular triglyceride content is a determinant of in vivo insulin resistance in humans: A 1H-13C nuclear magnetic resonance spectroscopy assessment in offspring of type 2 diabetic parents. Diabetes 48:1600–1606.

181. Unger RH (2003). Weapons of lean body mass destruction: The role of ectopic lipids in the metabolic syndrome. Endocrinology 144:5159–5165.

182. Dobbins RL, Szczepaniak LS, Bentley B, Esser V, Myhill J, McGarry JD (2001). Prolonged inhibition of muscle carnitine palmitoyltransferase-1 promotes intramyocellular lipid accumulation and insulin resistance in rats. Diabetes 50:123–130.

183. Morino K, Petersen KF, Shulman GI (2006). Molecular mechanisms of insulin resistance in humans and their potential links with mitochondrial dysfunction. Diabetes 55:S9–S15.

184. Samuel VT, Liu ZX, Qu X, Elder BD, Bilz S, Befroy D, et al. (2004). Mechanism of hepatic insulin resistance in non-alcoholic fatty liver disease. J Biol Chem 279:32345–32353.

185. Hirosumi J, Tuncman G, Chang L, Görgün CZ, Uysal KT, Maeda K, et al. (2002). A central role for JNK in obesity and insulin resistance. Nature 420:333–336.

186. Sinha R, Dufour S, Petersen KF, LeBon V, Enoksson S, Ma YZ, et al. (2002). Assessment of skeletal muscle triglyceride content by (1)H nuclear magnetic resonance spectroscopy in lean and obese adolescents: Relationships to insulin sensitivity, total body fat, and central adiposity. Diabetes 51:1022–1027.

187. Bacha F, Saad R, Gungor N, Janosky J, Arslanian SA (2003). Obesity, regional fat distribution, and Syndrome X in obese black versus white adolescents: race differential in diabetogenic and atherogenic risk factors. J Clin Endocrinol Metab 88:2534–2540.

188. Saltiel AR (2001). You are what you secrete. Nature Med 7:887–880.

189. Unger RH (2004). The hyperleptinemia of obesity-regulator of caloric surpluses. Cell 117:145–146.

190. Arita Y, Kihara S, Ouchi N, Takahashi Y, Maeda K, Miyagawa JI, et al. (1999). Paradoxical decrease of an adipose-specific protein, adiponectin, in obesity. Biochem Biophys Res Comm 257:79–83.

191. Shapiro L, Scherer PE (1998). The crystal structure of a complement-1q family protein suggests an evolutionary link to tumor necrosis factor. Curr Biol 8:335–338.

192. Kondo H, Shimomura I, Matsukawa Y, Kumada M, Takahashi M, Matsuda M, et al. (2002). Association of adiponectin mutation with type 2 diabetes: A candidate gene for the insulin resistance syndrome. Diabetes 51:2325–2328.

193. Pajvani UB, Du X, Combs TP, Berg AH, Rajala MW, Schulthess T, et al. (2003). Structure-function studies of the adipocyte-secreted hormone Acrp30/adiponectin: Implications fpr metabolic regulation and bioactivity. J Biol Chem 278:9073–9085.

194. Kadowaki T, Yamauchi T (2005). Adiponectin and adiponectin receptors. Endocr Rev 26:439–451.

195. Yamauchi T, Kamon J, Ito Y, Tsuchida A, Yokomizo T, Kita S, et al. (2003). Cloning of adiponectin receptors that mediate antidiabetic metabolic effects. Nature 423:762–769.

196. Ouchi N, Kihara S, Arita Y, Okamoto Y, Maeda K, Kuriyama H, et al. (2000). Adiponectin, an adipocyte-derived plasma protein, inhibits endothelial NF-kappaB signaling through a cAMP-dependent pathway. Circulation 102:1296–1301.

197. Yatagai T, Nagasaka S, Taniguchi A, Fukushima M, Nakamura T, Kuroe A, et al. (2003). Hypoadiponectinemia is associated with visceral fat accumulation and insulin resistance in Japanese men with type 2 diabetes mellitus. Metabolism 52:1274–1278.

198. Hotta K, Funahashi T, Bodkin NL, Ortmeyer HK, Arita Y, Hansen BC, et al. (2001). Circulating concentrations of the adipocyte protein adiponectin: A decrease in parallel with reduced insulin sensitivity during the progression of type 2 diabetes in Rhesus monkeys. Diabetes 50:1126–1133.

199. Weisberg SP, McCann D, Desai M, Rosenbaum M, Leibel RL, Ferrante AW (2003). Obesity is associated with macrophage accumulation in adipose tissue. J Clin Invest 112:1673–1808.

200. Matsuzawa Y, Funahashi T, Nakamura T (1999). Molecular mechanism of metabolic syndrome X: Contribution of adipocytokines adipocyte-derived bioactive substances. Ann NY Acad Sci 892:146–154.

201. Cinti S, Mitchell G, Barbatelli G, Murano I, Ceresi E, Faloia E, et al. (2005). Adipocyte death defines macrophage localization and function in adipose tissue of obese mice and humans. J Lipid Res 46:2347–2355.

202. Yudkin JS, Kumari M, Humphries SE, Mohamed-Ali V (2000). Inflammation, obesity, stress and coronary heart disease: Is interleukin-6 the link? Atherosclerosis 148:209–214.

203. Pickup JC, Crook MA (1998). Is type 2 diabetes mellitus a disease of the innate immune system? Diabetologia 41:1241–1248.

204. Ridker PM, Hennekens CH, Buring JE, Rifai N (2000). C-reactive protein and other markers of inflammation in the prediction of cardiovascular disease in women. N Engl J Med 342:836–843.

205. Pradhan AD, Manson JE, Rifai N, Buring JE, Ridker PM (2001). C-reactive protein, interleukin 6, and risk of developing type 2 diabetes mellitus. JAMA 286:327–334.

206. Cook DG, Mendall MA, Whincup PH, Carey IM, Ballam L, Morris JE, et al. (2000). C-reactive protein concentration in children:

Relationship to adiposity and other cardiovascular risk factors. Atherosclerosis 149:139–150.

207. Ford ES, Galuska DA, Gillespie C, Will JC, Giles WH, Dietz WH (2001). C-reactive protein and body mass index in children: Findings from the Third National Health and Nutrition Examination Survey, 1988–1994. J Pediatr 138:486–492.

208. Fukuhara A, Matsuda M, Nishizawa M, Segawa K, Tanaka M, Kishimoto K, et al. (2005). Visfatin: A protein secreted by visceral fat that mimics the effects of insulin. Science 307:426–430.

209. Sinha R, Fisch G, Teague B, Tamborlane WV, Banyas B, Allen K, et al. (2002). Prevalence of impaired glucose tolerance among children and adolescents with marked obesity. N Engl J Med 346:802–810.

210. Goran MI, Bergman RN, Avila Q, Watkins M, Ball GD, Shaibi GQ, et al. (2004). Impaired glucose tolerance and reduced beta-cell function in overweight Latino children with a positive family history for type 2 diabetes. J Clin Endocrinol Metab 89:207–212.

211. Wiegand S, Maikowski U, Blankenstein O, Biebermann H, Tarnow P, Gruters A (2004). Type 2 diabetes and impaired glucose tolerance in European children and adolescents with obesity: A problem that is no longer restricted to minority groups. Eur J Endocrinol 151:199–206.

212. Weiss R, Dufour S, Taksali SE, Tamborlane WV, Petersen KF, Bonadonna RC, et al. (2003). Prediabetes in obese youth: A syndrome of impaired glucose tolerance, severe insulin resistance, and altered myocellular and abdominal fat partitioning. Lancet 362:951–957.

213. Calles-Escandon J, Cipolla M (2001). Diabetes and endothelial dysfunction: A clinical perspective. Endocr Rev 22:36–52.

214. Moncada S, Palmer RMJ, Higgs EA (1991). Nitric oxide: Physiology, pathophysiology, and pharmacology. Pharmacol Rev 43:109–142.

215. Nakagawa T, Tuttle KR, Short R, Johnson RJ (2006). Hypothesis: Fructose-induced hyperuricemia as a causal mechanism for the epidemic of the metabolic syndrome. Nat Clin Pract Nephrology 1:80–86.

216. Bonetti PO, Lerman LO, Lerman A (2003). Endothelial dysfunction: A marker of atherosclerotic risk. Arterio Thromb Vasc Biol 23:168–175.

217. Anderson TJ, Uehata A, Gerhard MD, Meredith IT, Knab S, DeLaGrange D, et al. (1995). Close relation of endothelial function in the human coronary and peripheral circulations. J Am Coll Cardiol 26:1235–1241.

218. Corretti MC, Anderson TJ, Benjamin EJ, Celermajer D, Charbonneau F, Creager MA, et al. (2002). Guidelines for the ultrasound assessment of endothelial-dependent flow-mediated vasodilation of the brachial artery: A report of the International Brachial Artery Reactivity Task Force. J Am Coll Cardiol 39.

219. Tounian P, Aggoun Y, Dubern BP, Varille V, Guy-Grand B, Sidi D, et al. (2001). Presence of increased stiffness of the common carotid artery and endothelial dysfunction in severely obese children: A prospective study. Lancet 358:1400–1404.

220. Meyer AA, Kundt G, Steiner M, Schuff-Werner P, Kienast W (2006). Impaired flow-mediated vasodilation, carotid artery intima-media thickening, and elevated endothelial plasma markers in obese children: The impact of cardiovascular risk factors. Pediatrics 117:1560–1567.

221. Li S, Chen W, Srinivasan SR, Bond Gene M, Tang R, Urbina EM, et al. (2003). Childhood cardiovascular risk factors and carotid vascular changes in adulthood. JAMA 290:2271–2276.

222. Berenson GS, Srinivasan SR, Bao W, Newman WP, Tracy RE, Wattigney WA (1998). Association between multiple cardiovascular risk factors and atherosclerosis in children and young adults: The Bogalusa Heart Study. N Engl J Med 338:1650–1656.

223. Raitakari TO, Juonala M, Kahonen M, Taittonen L, Laitinen T, Maki-Torkko N, et al. (2003). Cardiovascular risk factors in childhood and carotid artery intima-media thikness in adulthood. JAMA 290:2277–2283.

224. Pathobiological Determinants of Artherosclerosis in Youth (PDAY) Research Group (1990). Relationships in young men to serum lipoprptein cholesterol concentrations and smoking. JAMA 264:3018–3024.

225. Davis PH, Dawson JD, Riley WA, Lauer RM (2001). Carotid intimal media thickness is related to cardiovascular risk factors measured from childhood through middle age. Circulation 104:2815–2819.

226. Mahoney LT, Burns TL, Stanford W, Thompson BH, Witt JD, Rost CA, et al. (1996). Coronary risk factors measured in childhood and young adult life are associated with coronary artery calcification in young adults: The Muscatine Study. J Am Coll Cardiol 27:277–284.

227. Reaven GM (1988). Banting lecture 1988. Role of insulin resistance in human disease. Diabetes 37:1595–1607.

228. Haffner SM (1999). Epidemiology of insulin resistance and its relation to coronary artery disease. Am J Cardiol 84:11J–14J.

229. Hu FB, Stampfer JM, Haffner SM, Solomon CG, Willett WC, Manson JE (2002). Elevated risk of cardiovascular disease prior to clinical diagnosis of type 2 diabetes. Diab Care 25:1129–1134.

230. Alberti KG, Zimmet PZ (1998). Definition, diagnosis and classification of diabetes mellitus and its complications. Part 1: Diagnosis and classification of diabetes mellitus provisional report of a WHO consultation. Diabet Med 15:539–553.

231. Ford ES, Giles WH, Dietz WH (2002). Prevalence of the metabolic syndrome among U.S. adults: Findings from the Third National Health and Nutrition Examination survey. JAMA 287:356–359.

232. Speiser PW, Rudolf MCJ, Anhalt H, Camacho-Hubner C, Chiarelli F, Eliakim A, et al. (2005). Consensus statement: childhood obesity. J Clin Endocrinol Metab 90:1871–1887.

233. Angulo P (2002). Nonalcoholic fatty liver disease. N Engl J Med 346:1221–1231.

234. Ludwig J, Viggiano TR, McGill DB, Ott BJ (1980). Nonalcoholic steatohepatitis: Mayo clinic experience with a hitherto unnamed disease. Mayo Clin Proc 55:434–438.

235. Meltzer AA, Everhart JE (1997). Association between diabetes and elevated serum alanine aminotransferase activity among Mexican Americans. Am J Epidemiol 146:565–571.

236. Lavine JE, Schwimmer JB (2004). Nonalcoholic fatty liver disease in the pediatric population. Clin Liver Dis 8:549–558.

237. Roberts E (2003). Nonalcoholic steatohepatitis in children. Curr Gastroenterol Rep 5:253–259.

238. Burgert TS, Taksali SE, Dziura J, Goodman TR, Yeckel CW, Papademetris X, et al. (2006). Alanine aminotransferase levels and fatty liver in childhood obesity: Associations with insulin resistance, adiponectin, and visceral fat. J Clin Endocrinol Metab 91:4287–4294.

239. Day CP, James OF (1998). Steatohepatitis: A tale of two "hits"? Gastroenterology 114:842–845.

240. Shimomura I, Shimano H, Horton JD, Goldstein JL, Brown MS (1997). Differential expression of exons 1a an 1c in mRNAs for sterol regulatory element binding protein 1 in human and mouse organs and cultured cells. J Clin Invest 99:838–845.

241. Shimomura I, Matsuda M, Hammer RE, Bashmakov Y, Brown MS, Goldstein JL (2000). Decreased IRS2 and increased SREBP-1c lead to mixed insulin resistance and sensitivity in liver dystrophic and ob/ob mice. Mol Cell 6:77–86.

242. Rotterdam ESHRE/ASRM-Sponsored PCOS Consensus Workshop Group (2004). Revised 2003 consensus on diagnostic criteria and long-term health risks related to polycystic ovary syndrome (PCOS). Hum Reprod 19:41–47.

243. Ibanez L, Potau N, Francois I, de Zegher F (1999). Precocious pubarche, hyperinsulinism, and ovarian hyperandrogenism in girls: Relation to reduced fetal growth. J Clin Endocrinol Metab 84:2691–2695.

244. Buggs C, Rosenfield RL (2005). Polycystic ovary syndrome in adolescence. Endocrinol Metab Clin NA 34:677–705.

245. Azziz R, Woods KS, Reyna R, Key TJ, Knochenhauer ES, Yildiz BO (2004). The prevalence and features of the polycystic ovary syndrome in an unselected population. J Clin Endocrinol Metab 89:2745–2749.

246. Apter D, Butzow T, Laughlin GA, Yen SS (1995). Metabolic features of polycystic ovary syndrome are found in adolescent girls with hyperandrogenism. J Clin Endocrinol Metab 80:2966–2973.

247. Lewy VD, Danadian K, Witchel SF, Arslanian S (2001). Early metabolic abnormalities in adolescent girls with polycystic ovarian syndrome. J Pediatr 138:38–44.

248. Setji TL, Holland ND, Sanders LL, Pereira KC, Diehl AM, Brown AJ (2006). Nonalcoholic steatohepatitis and nonalcoholic fatty liver disease in young women with polycystic ovary syndrome. J Clin Endocrinol Metab 91:1741–1747.

249. Gambineri A, Pelusi C, Manicardi E, Vicennati V, Cacciari M, Morselli-Labate AM, et al. (2004). Glucose intolerance in a large

cohort of Mediterranean women with polycystic ovary syndrome: Phenotype and associated factors. Diabetes 53:2353–2358.

250. Coviello AD, Legro RS, Dunaif A (2006). Adolescent girls with polycystic ovary syndrome have an increased risk of the metabolic syndrome associated with increasing androgen levels independent of obesity and insulin resistance. J Clin Endocrinol Metab 91:492–497.

251. Vryonidou A, Papatheodorou A, Tavridou A, Terzi T, Loi V, Vatalas IA, et al. (2005). Association of hyperandrogenemic and metabolic phenotype with carotid intima-media thickness in young women with polycystic ovary syndrome. J Clin Endocrinol Metab 90:2740–2746.

252. Venkatsen AM, Dunaif A, Corbould A (2001). Insulin resistance in polycystic ovary syndrome: Progress and paradoxes. Recent Prog Horm Res 56:295–308.

253. Zhang LH, Rodriguez H, Ohno S, Miller WL (1995). Serine phosphorylation of human P450c17 increases 17,20-lyase activity: implications for adrenarche and the polycystic ovary syndrome. Proc Natl Acad Sci USA 92:10619–10623.

254. Dunaif A, Xia J, Book CB, Schenker E, Tang Z (1995). Excessive insulin receptor serine phosphorylation in cultured fibroblasts and in skeletal muscle: A potential mechanism for insulin resistance in the polycystic ovary syndrome. J Clin Invest 96:801–810.

255. Kaplowitz PB, Slora EJ, Wasserman RC, Pedlow SE, Herman-Giddens ME (2001). Earlier onset of puberty in girls: Relation to increased body mass index and race. Pediatrics 108:347–353.

256. Lustig RH, Hershcopf RJ, Bradlow HL (1990). The effects of body weight and diet on estrogen metabolism and estrogen-dependent disease. In Frisch RE (ed.), *Adipose tissue and reproduction*. Basel: Karger 107–124.

257. Braunstein GD (1999). Aromatase and gynecomastia. Endocrine-Related Cancer 6:315–324.

258. Kaplowitz P (1998). Delayed puberty in obese boys: Comparison with constitutional delayed puberty and response to testosterone therapy. J Pediatr 133:745–749.

259. Rose SR, Burstein S, Burghen GA, Pitukcheewanont P, Shope S, Hodnicak V (1999). Caloric restriction for 24 hours increases mean night growth hormone. J Ped Endocrinol Metab12:175–183.

260. Coutant R, Boux de Casson F, Rouleau S, Douay O, Mathieu E, Audran M, et al. (2001). Body composition, fasting leptin, and sex steroid administration determine GH sensitivity in peripubertal short children. J Clin Endocrinol Metab 86:5805–5812.

261. Olney RC, Mougey EB (1999). Expression of the components of the insulin-like growth factor axis across the growth plate. Mol Cell Endocrinol 156:63–71.

262. Masuzaki H, Paterson J, Shinyama H, Morton NM, Mullins JJ, Seckl JR, et al. (2001). A transgenic model of visceral obesity and the metabolic syndrome. Science 294:2166–2170.

263. Kesler A, Fattal-Valevski A (2002). Idiopathic intracranial hypertension in the pediatric population. J Child Neurol 17:745–748.

264. de la Eva R, Baur LA, Donaghue KC, Waters KA (2002). Metabolic correlates with obstructive sleep apnea in obese subjects. J Pediatr 140:654–659.

265. Taylor ED, Theim KR, Mirch MC, Ghorbani S, Tanofsky-Kraff M, Adler-Wailes DC, et al. (2006). Orthopedic complications of overweight children and adolescents. Pediatrics 117:2167–2174.

266. Kaechele V, Wabitsch M, Thiere D, Kessler AL, Haenle MM, Mayer H, et al. (2006). Prevalence of gallbladder stone disease in obese children and adolescents: Influence of the degree of obesity, sex, and pubertal development. J Pediatr Gastroenterol Nutr 42:66–70.

267. Young-Hyman D, Tanofsky-Kraff M, Yanovski SZ, Keil M, Cohen ML, Peyrot M, et al. (2006). Psychological status and weight-related distress in overweight or at-risk-for-overweight children. Obesity 14:2249–2258.

268. Bell LM, Byrne S, Thompson A, Ratnam N, Blair E, Bulsara M, et al. (2007). Increasing body mass index z-score is continuously associated with complications of overweight in children, even in the healthy weight range. J Clin Endocrinol Metab 92:517–522.

269. Baier LJ, Hanson RL (2004). Genetic studies of the etiology of type 2 diabetes in Pima Indians. Diabetes 53:1181–1186.

270. Butte NF, Cai G, Cole SA, Comuzzie AG (2006). Viva la Familia Study: Genetic and environmental contributions to childhood obesity and its comorbidities in the Hispanic population. Am J Clin Nutr 84:646–654.

271. Neel JV (1962). Diabetes mellitus: A thrifty genotype rendered detrimental by "progress." Am J Hum Genet 14:353–362.

272. Mutch DM, Clement K (2006). Genetics of human obesity. Best Pract Res Clin Endocrinol Metab 20:647–664.

273. Speakman JR (2006). Thrifty genes for obesity and the metabolic syndrome-time to call off the search? Diab Vasc Dis Res 3:5–6.

274. Barker DJ (2004). The developmental origins of chronic adult disease. Acta Paediatr Supp 93:26–33.

275. Roseboom TJ, van der Meulen JH, Ravelli AC, Osmond C, Barker DJ, Bleker OP (2001). Effects of prenatal exposure to the Dutch famine on adult disease in later life: An overview. Mol Cell Endocrinol 185:93–98.

276. Yajnik CS, Lubree HG, Rege SS, Naik SS, Deshpande JA, Joglekar CV, et al. (2002). Adiposity and hyperinsulnemia in Indians are present at birth. J Clin Endocrinol Metab 87:5575–5580.

277. Arends NJ, Boonstra VH, Duivenvoorden HJ, Hofman PL, Hokken-Koelega AC (2005). Reduced insulin sensitivity and the presence of cardiovascular risk factors in short prepubertal children born small for gestational age (SGA). Clin Endocrinol 62:44–50.

278. Potau N, Gussinye M, Sanchez Ufarte C, Rique S, Vicens-Calvet E, Carrascosa A (2001). Hyperinsulinemia in pre- and post-pubertal children born small for gestational age. Horm Res 56:146–150.

279. Yajnik CS, Fall CH, Vaidya U, Pandit AN, Bavdekar A, Bhat DS, et al. (1995). Fetal growth and glucose and insulin metabolism in four-year-old Indian children. Diabet Med 12:330–336.

280. Silverman BL, Landsberg L, Metzger BE (1993). Fetal hyperinsulinism in offspring of diabetic mothers: Association with the subsequent development of childhood obesity. Ann NY Acad Sci 699:36–45.

281. Silverman BL, Rizzo TA, Cho NH, Metzger BE (1998). Long-term effects of the intrauterine environment: The Nortwestern University Diabetes in Pregnancy Center. Diabetes Care 21(2):B142–B149.

282. Boney CM, Verma A, Tucker R, Vohr BR (2005). Metabolic syndrome in childhood: Association with birth weight, maternal obesity, and gestational diabetes. Pediatrics 115:e290–e296.

283. Knowler WC, Pettitt DJ, Savage PJ, Bennett PH (1981). Diabetes incidence in Pima Indians: Contributions of obesity and parental diabetes. Am J Epidemiol 113:144–156.

284. Dabelea D, Hanson RL, Lindsay RS, Pettit DJ, Imperatore G, Gabir MM, et al. (2000). Intrauterine exposure to diabetes coveys risk for type 2 diabetes and obesity: A study of discordant sibships. Diabetes 42:2208–2211.

285. Caughey AB (2006). Obesity, weight loss, and pregnancy outcomes. Lancet 368:1136–1138.

286. Hofman PL, Regan F, Jackson WE, Jefferies C, Knight DB, Robinson EM, et al. (2004). Premature birth and later insulin resistance. N Engl J Med 351:2179–2186.

287. Harder T, Bergmann R, Kallischnigg G, Plagemann A (2005). Duration of breastfeeding and risk of overweight: A meta-analysis. Am J Epidemiol 162:397–403.

288. Owen CG, Martin RM, Whincup PH, Davey-Smith G, Gillman MW, Cook DG (2005). The effect of breastfeeding on mean body mass index throughout life: A quantitative review of published and unpublished observational evidence. Am J Clin Nutr 82:1298–1307.

289. Miralles O, Sanchez J, Palou A, Pico C (2006). A physiological role of breast milk leptin in body weight control in developing infants. Obesity 14:1371–1377.

290. Keith SW, Redden DT, Katzmaryk PT, Boggiano MM, Hanlon EC, Benca RM, et al. (2006). Putative contributors to the secular increase in obesity: Exploring the roads less traveled. Int J Obes 30:1585–1594.

291. Andrew R, Gale CR, Walker BR, Seckl JR, Martyn CN (2002). Glucocorticoid metabolism and the Metabolic Syndrome: Associations in an elderly cohort. Exp Clin Endocrinol Diab 110:284–290.

292. Kotelevtsev YV, Holmes MC, Burchell A, Houston PM, Scholl D, Jamieson PM, et al. (1997). 11β-hydroxysteroid dehydrogenase type 1 knockout mice show attenuated glucocorticoid inducible responses and resist hyperglycaemia on obesity and stress. Proc Natl Acad Sci USA 94:14924–14929.

293. Chandola T, Brunner E, Marmot M (2006). Chronic stress at work and the metabolic syndrome: Prospective study. BMJ 332:521–525.

294. Rosengren A, Hawken S, Ounpuu S, Sliwa K, Zubaid M, Almahmeed WA, et al. (2004). Association of psychosocial risk factors with risk of acute myocardial infarction in 11,119 cases

and 13,648 controls from 52 countries (the INTERHEART study): Case-control study. Lancet 364:953–962.

295. Brunner EJ, Hemingway H, Walker BR, Page M, Clarke P, Juneja M, et al. (2002). Adrenocortical, autonomic, and inflammatory causes of the metabolic syndrome: Nested case-control study. Circulation 106:2659–2665.

296. Souverein PC, Berard A, Van Staa TP, Cooper C, Egberts AC, Leufkens HG, et al. (2004). Use of oral glucocorticoids and risk of cardiovascular and cerebrovascular disease in a population based case-control study. Heart 90:859–865.

297. Bujalska IJ, Kumar S, Stewart PM (1997). Does central obesity reflect "Cushing's disease of the omentum"? Lancet 349:1210–1213.

298. Spiegel K, Sheridan JF, Van Cauter E (2002). Effect of sleep deprivation on response to immunization. JAMA 288:1471–1472.

299. Gangwisch JE, Malaspina D, Boden-Albala B, Heymsfield SB (2005). Inadequate sleep as a risk factor for obesity: Analyses of the NHANES I. Sleep 28:1217–1220.

300. Hasler G, Buysse DJ, Klaghofer R, Gamma A, Ajdacic V, Eich D, et al. (2004). The association between short sleep duration and obesity in young adults: A 13-year prospective study. Sleep 27:602–603.

301. Taheri S (2006). The link between short sleep duration and obesity: We should recommend more sleep to prevent obesity. Arch Dis Child 91:881–884.

302. Sekine M, Yamagami T, Hamanishi S, Handa K, Saito T, Nanri S, et al. (2002). Parental obesity, lifestyle factors and obesity in preschool children: results of the Toyama birth cohort study. J Epidemiol 12:33–39.

303. Reilly JJ, Armstrong J, Dorosty AR, Emmett PM, Ness A, Rogers I, et al. (2005). Early life risk factors for obesity in childhood: Cohort study. BMJ 330:1357.

304. Robinson TN (2001). Television viewing and childhood obesity. Ped Clin NA 48:1017–1025.

305. Sgoifo A, Braglia F, Costoli T, Musso E, Meerlo P, Ceresini G, et al. (2003). Cardiac autonomic reactivity and salivary cortisol in men and women exposed to social stressors: Relationship with individual ethological profile. Neurosci Biobehav Rev 27:179–188.

306. Taras HL, Sallis JF, Patterson TL, Nader PR, Nelson JA (1989). Television's influence on children's diet and physical activity. J Devel Behav Pediatr 10:176–180.

307. DuRant RH, Baranowski T, Johnson M, Thompson WO (1994). The relationship among television watching, physical activity, and body composition of young children. Pediatrics 94:449–455.

308. Coon KA, Goldberg J, Rogers BL, Tucker KL (2001). Relationships between use of television during meals and children's food consumption patterns. Pediatrics 107:e7.

309. Dietz WH, Bandini LG, Morelli JA, Peers KF, Ching PL (1994). Effect of sedentary activities on resting metabolic rate. Am J Clin Nutr 556–559.

310. Crespo CJ, Smit E, Troiano RP, Bartlett SJ, Macera CA, Andersen RE (2001). Television watching, energy intake, and obesity in U.S. children: Results from the third National Health and Nutrition Examination Survey, 1988–1994. Arch Ped Adol Med 155:360–365.

311. Robinson TN (1999). Reducing children's television viewing to prevent obesity: A randomized controlled trial. JAMA 282:1561–1567.

312. Parsons TJ, Power C, Logan S, Summerbell CD (1999). Childhood predictors of adult obesity: A systematic review. Int J Obesity 23(8):S1–S107.

313. Maffeis C, Schutz Y, Grezzani A, Provera S, Piacentini G, Tato L (2001). Meal-induced thermogenesis and obesity: is a fat meal a risk factor for fat gain in children? J Clin Endocrinol Metab 86:214–219.

314. Jequier E (2001). Is fat intake a risk factor for fat gain in children? J Clin Endocrinol Metab 86:980–983.

315. Tucker LA, Seljaas GT, Hager RL (1997). Body fat percentage of children varies according to their diet composition. J Am Diet Assoc 97:981–986.

316. Pirozzo S, Summerbell C, Cameron C, Glasziou P (2002). Advice on low-fat diets for obesity. Cochrane Database Systems Review CD003640.

317. Kennedy E, Powell R (1997). Changing eating patterns of American children: A view from 1996. J Am Coll Nutr 16:524–529.

318. Harnack L, Stang J, Story M (1999). Soft drink consumption among U.S. children and adolescents: Nutritional consequences. J Am Diet Assoc 99:436–441.

319. Center for Weight and Health (2001). Pediatric overweight: A review of the literature. June, *http://www.cnr.berkeley.edu/cwh/news/announcements.shtml#lit_review.*

320. Foster GD, Wyatt HR, Hill JO, McGuckin BG, Brill C, Mohammed BS, et al. (2003). A randomized trial of a low-carbohydrate diet for obesity. N Engl J Med 348:2082–2090.

321. Stern L, Iqbal N, Seshadri P, Chicano KL, Daily DA, McGrory J, et al. (2004). The effects of low-carbohydrate versus conventional weight loss diets in severely obese adults: One-year follow-up of a randomized trial. Ann Int Med 140:778–785.

322. Vining EP, Pyzik P, McGrogan J, Hladky H, Anand A, Kriegler S, et al. (2002). Growth of children on the ketogenic diet. Dev Med Child Neurol 44:796–802.

323. Ludwig DS (2002). The glycemic index: physiological mechanisms relating to obesity, diabetes, and cardiovascular disease. JAMA 287:2414–2423.

324. Pawlak DB, Bryson JM, Denyer JS, Brand-Miller JC (2001). High glycemic index starch promotes hypersecretion of insulin and higher body fat in rats without affecting insulin sensitivity. J Nutr 131:99–104.

325. Ludwig DS, Majzoub JA, Al-Zahrani A, Dallal GE, Blanco I, Roberts SB (1999). High glycemic index foods, overeating, and obesity. Pediatrics 103:e261–e266.

326. Ebbeling CB, Leidig MM, Sinclair KB, Hangen JP, Ludwig DS (2003). A reduced-glycemic load diet in the treatment of adolescent obesity. Arch Ped Adolesc Med 157:773–779.

327. Ludwig DS, Pereira MA, Kroenke CH, Hilner JE, Van Horn L, Slattery ML, et al. (1999). Dietary fiber, weight gain, and cardiovascular disease risk factors in young adults. JAMA 282:1539–1546.

328. Liese AD, Schulz M, Fang F, Wolever TM, D'Agostino RB, Sparks KC, et al. (2005). Dietary glycemic index and glycemic load, carbohydrate and fiber intake, and measures of insulin sensitivity, secretion, and adiposity in the Insulin Resistance Atherosclerosis Study. Diab Care 28:2832–2838.

329. Pereira MA, Ludwig DS (2001). Dietary fiber and body weight regulation: Observations and mechanisms. Ped Clin NA 48:969–980.

330. Rigaud D, Paycha F, Meulemans A, Merrouche M, Mignon M (1998). Effect of psyllium on gastric emptying, hunger feeling and food intake in normal volunteers: A double blind study. Eur J Clin Nutr 52:239–245.

331. Slavin J (2003). Why whole grains are protective: Biological mechanisms. Proc Nutr Soc 62:129–134.

332. Leach JD (2007). Evolutionary perspective on dietary intake of fibre and colorectal cancer. Eur J Clin Nutr 61:140–142.

333. Martlett JA, McBurney MI, Slavin JL (2002). Position of the American Dietetic Association: Health implications of dietary fiber. J Am Diet Assoc 102:993–1000.

334. Ludwig DS, Pereira MA, Kroenke CJ, Hilner JE, van Horn L, Slattery ML, et al. (1999). Dietary fiber, weight gain, and cardiovascular disease risk factors in young adults. JAMA 282:1539–1546.

335. Gross LS, Li S, Ford ES, Liu S (2004). Increased consumption of refined carbohydrates and the epidemic of type 2 diabetes in the United States: An ecologic assessment. Am J Clin Nutr 79:774–779.

336. Jurgens H, Haass W, Castaneda TR, Schurmann A, Koebnick C, Dombrowski F, et al. (2005). Consuming fructose-sweetened beverages increases body adiposity in mice. Obes Res 13:1146–1156.

337. Havel PJ (2005). Dietary fructose: Implications for dysregulation of energy homeostasis and lipid/carbohydrate metabolism. Nutr Rev 63:133–157.

338. Fried SK, Rao SP (2003). Sugars, hypetriglyceridemia, and cardiovascular disease. Am J Clin Nutr 78:873S–880S.

339. Roden M (2006). Mechanisms of disease: Hepatic steatosis in type 2 diabetes-pathogenesis and clinical relevance. Nat Clin Pract Endo Metab 2:335–348.

340. Le KA, Tappy L (2006). Metabolic effects of fructose. Curr Opin Nutr Metab Care 9:469–475.

341. Ludwig DS, Peterson KE, Gortmaker SL (2001). Relation between consumption of sugar-sweetened drinks and childhood obesity: A prospective, observational analysis. Lancet 357:505–508.

342. Faith MS, Dennison BA, Edmunds LS, Stratton HH (2006). Fruit juice intake predicts increased adiposity gain in children from low-income families: Weight status-by-environment interaction. Pediatrics 118:2066–2075.

343. American Academy of Pediatrics Committee on Nutrition (2001). The use and misuse of fruit juice in pediatrics. Pediatrics 107:1210–1213.

344. Pereira MA, Jacobs DR, van Horn L, Slattery ML, Kartashov AI, Ludwig DS (2002). Dairy consumption, obesity, and the insulin resistance syndrome in young adults. JAMA 287:2081–2089.

345. Zemel MB, Shi H, Greer B, Dirienzo D, Zemel PC (2000). Regulation of adiposity by dietary calcium. FASEB J 14:1132–1138.

346. Shi H, Dirienzo D, Zemel MB (2001). Effects of dietary calcium on adipocyte lipid metabolism and body weight regulation in energy-restricted aP2-agouti transgenic mice. FASEB J 15:291–293.

347. Lin YC, Lyle RM, McCabe LD, McCabe GP, Weaver CM, Teegarden D (2000). Dietary calcium is related to changes in body composition during a two year exercise intervention in young women. J Am Coll Nutr 19:754–760.

348. Yanoff LB, Parikh SJ, Spitalnik A, Denkinger B, Sebring NG, Slaughter P, et al. (2006). The prevalence of hypovitaminosis D and secondary hyperparathyroidism in obese Black Americans. Clin Endocrinol 64:523–529.

349. Heaney RP, Davies KM, Barger-Lux MJ (2002). Calcium and weight: Clinical studies. J Am Coll Nutr 21:152S–155S.

350. Anderson RA (2000). Chromium in the prevention and control of diabetes. Diabetes Metabolism 26:22–27.

351. Fantus IG, Tsiani E (1998). Multifunctional actions of vanadium compounds on insulin signaling pathways: Evidence for preferential enhancement of metabolic versus mitogenic effects. Mol Cell Biochem 182:109–119.

352. Ames BN (2006). Low micronutrient intake may accelerate the degenerative diseases of aging through allocation of scarce micronutrients by triage. Proc Natl Acad Sci USA 103:17589–17594.

353. Pasarica M, Shin AC, Yu M, Ou Yang HM, Rathod M, Jen KL, et al. (2006). Human adenovirus 36 induces adiposity, increases insulin sensitivity, and alters hypothalamic monoamines in rats. Obesity 14:1905–1913.

354. Atkinson RL, Dhurandhar NV, Allison DB, Bowen RL, Israel BA, Albu JB, et al. (2005). Human adenovirus-36 is associated with increased body weight and paradoxical reduction of serum lipids. Int J Obes 29:281–286.

355. Turnbaugh PJ, Ley RE, Mahowald MA, Magrini V, Mardis ER, Gordon JI (2006). An obesity-associated gut microbiome with increased capacity for energy harvest. Nature 444:1027–1031.

356. Rogers PC, Meacham LR, Oeffinger KC, Henry DW, Lange BJ (2005). Obesity in pediatric oncology. Pediatr Blood Cancer 45:881–891.

357. Foster BJ, Shults J, Zemel BS, Leonard MB (2006). Risk factors for glucocorticoid-induced obesity in children with steroid-sensitive nephrotic syndrome. Pediatr Nephrol 21:973–980.

358. Bonny AE, Ziegler J, Harvey R, Debanne SM, Secic M, Cromer BA (2006). Weight gain in obese and nonobese adolescent girls initiating depot medroxyprogesterone, oral contraceptive pills, or no hormonal contraceptive method. Arch Pediatr Adol Med 160:40–45.

359. Quinn M, Ficociello LH, Rosner B (2003). Change in glycemic control predicts change in weight in adolescent boys with type 1 diabetes. Pediatr Diabetes 4:162–167.

360. Vieweg WV, Sood AB, Pandurangi A, Silverman JJ (2005). Newer antipsychotic drugs and obesity in children and adolescents: How should we assess drug-associated weight gain? Acta Psychiatr Scand 111:177–184.

361. Amamoto T, Kumai T, Nakaya S, Matsumoto N, Tsuzuki Y, Kobayashi S (2006). The elucidation of the mechanism of weight gain and glucose tolerance abnormalities induced by chlorpromazine. J Pharmacol Sci 102:213–219.

362. Tataranni PA, Larson DE, Snitker S, Young JB, Flatt JP, Ravussin E (1996). Effects of glucocorticoids on energy metabolism and food intake in humans. Am J Physiol 271:E317–E325.

363. Draper N, Echwald SM, Lavery GG, Walker EA, Fraser R, Davies E, et al. (2002). Association studies between microsatellite markers with the gene encoding human 11β-hydroxysteroid dehydrogenase Type 1 and body mass index, waist to hip ratio, and glucocorticoid metabolism. J Clin Endocrinol Metab 87:4984–4990.

364. Tomlinson JW, Sinha N, Bujalska I, Hewison M, Stewart PM (2002). Expression of 11beta-hydroxysteroid dehydrogenase type 1 in adipose tissue is not increased in human obesity. J Clin Endocrinol Metab 87:5630–5635.

365. Kaartinen JM, Kaar ML, Ohisalo JJ (1994). Defective stimulation of adipocyte adenylate cyclase, blunted lipolysis, and obesity in pseudohypoparathyroidism 1a. Pediatric Research 35:594–597.

366. Farooqi IS, O'Rahilly S (2004). Monogenic human obesity syndromes. Recent Prog Horm Res 59:409–424.

367. Farooqi IS, O'Rahilly S (2006). Genetics of obesity in humans. Endocr Rev 27:710–718.

368. Montague CT, Farooqi IS, Whitehead JP, Soos MA, Rau H, Wareham NJ, et al. (1997). Congenital leptin deficiency is associated with severe early-onset obesity in humans. Nature 387:903–908.

369. Farooqi IS, Matarese G, Lord GM, Keogh JM, Lawrence E, Agwu C, et al. (2002). Beneficial effects of leptin on obesity, T-cell hyporesponsiveness, and neuroendocrine/metabolic dysfunction of human congenital leptin deficiency. J Clin Invest 110:1093–1103.

370. Farooqi IS, Keogh JM, Kamath S, Jones S, Gibson WT, Trussell R, et al. (2001). Partial leptin deficiency and human adiposity. Nature 414:34–35.

371. Clement K, Vaisse C, Lahlou N, Cabrol S, Pelloux V, Cassuto D, et al. (1998). A mutation in the human leptin receptor gene causes obesity and pituitary dysfunction. Nature 392:398–401.

372. Krude H, Biebermann H, Luck W, Horn R, Brabant G, Grüters A (1998). Severe early-onset obesity, adrenal insufficiency, and red hair pigmentation caused by POMC mutations in humans. Nature Genet 19:155–157.

373. Farooqi IS, Drop S, Clements A, Keogh JM, Biernacka J, Lowenbein S, et al. (2006). Heterozygosity for a POMC-null mutation and increased obesity risk in humans. Diabetes 55:2549–2553.

374. Jackson RS, Creemers JW, Ohagi S, Raffin-Sanson ML, Sanders L, Montague CT, et al. (1997). Obesity and impaired prohormone processing associated with mutations in the prohormone convertase 1 gene. Nature Genet 16:303–306.

375. Lee YS, Poh LKS, Loke KY (2002). A novel melanocortin-3 receptor gene (MC3R) mutation associated with severe obesity. J Clin Endocrinol Metab 87:1423–1426.

376. Vaisse C, Clement K, Durand E, Hercberg S, Guy-Grand B, Frougel P (2000). Melanocortin-4 receptor mutations are a frequent and heterogeneous cause of morbid obesity. J Clin Invest 106:253–262.

377. Farooqi IS, Keogh JM, Yeo GS, Lank EJ, Cheetham T, O'Rahilly S (2003). Clinical spectrum of obesity and mutations in the melanocortin 4 receptor gene. N Engl J Med 348:1085–1095.

378. Kublaoui BM, Holder JL, Gemelli T, Zinn AR (2006). Sim1 haploinsufficiency impairs melanocortin-mediated anorexia and activation of paraventricular nucleus neurons. Mol Endocrinol 20.

379. Holder JL, Butte NF, Zinn AR (2000). Profound obesity associated with a balanced translocation that disrupts the SIM1 gene. Hum Mol Genet 9:101–108.

380. Hung CC, Luan J, Sims M, Keogh JM, Hall C, Wareham NJ, et al. (2007). Studies of the SIM1 gene in relation to human obesity and obesity-related traits. Int J Obes 31:429–434.

381. Gunay-Aygun M, Cassidy SB, Nicholls RD (1997). Prader-Willi and other syndromes associated with obesity and mental retardation. Behavioral Genetics 27:307–324.

382. Cassidy SB (1997). Prader-Willi syndrome. J Med Genet 34:917–923.

383. Bekx MT, Carrel AL, Shriver TC, Li Z, Allen DB (2003). Decreased energy expenditure is caused by abnormal body composition in infants with Prader-Willi Syndrome. J Pediatr 143:372–376.

384. Cummings DE, Clement K, Purnell JQ, Vaisse C, Foster KE, Frayo RS, et al. (2002). Elevated plasma ghrelin levels in Prader-Willi syndrome. Nature Med 8:643–644.

385. Carrel AL, Myers SE, Whitman BY, Allen DB (2002). Benefits of long-term GH therapy in Prader-Willi syndrome: A 4-year study. J Clin Endocrinol Metab 87:1581–1585.

386. Mykytyn K, Nishimura DY, Searby CC, Shastri M, Yen HJ, Beck JS, et al. (2002). Identification of the gene (BBS1) most commonly involved in Bardet-Biedl, syndrome, a complex human obesity syndrome. Nat Genet 31:435–438.

387. Mykytyn K, Mullins RF, Andrews M, Chiang AP, Swiderski RE, Yang B, et al. (2004). Bardet-Biedl syndrome type 4 (BBS4)-null mice implicate Bbs4 in flagella formation but not global cilia assembly. Proc Natl Acad Sci USA 101:8664–8669.

388. Badano JL, Mitsuma N, Beales PL, Katsanis N (2006). The ciliopathies: An emerging class of human genetic disorders. Ann Rev Genomics Hum Genet 22:125–148.

389. Yeo GSH, Hung CCC, Rochford J, Keogh J, Gray J, Sivaramakrishnan S, et al. (2004). A de novo mutation affecting human TrkB associated with severe obesity and developmental delay. Nature Neurosci 7:1187–1189.

390. Gray J, Yeo GS, Cox JJ, Morton J, Adlam AL, Keogh JM, et al. (2006). Hyperphagia, severe obesity, impaired cognitive function, and hyperactivity associated with functional loss of one copy of the brain-derived neurotrophic factor (BDNF) gene. Diabetes 55:3366–3371.

391. Chandler KE, Kidd A, Al-Gazali L, Kolehmainen J, Lehesjoki AE, Black GC, et al. (2003). Diagnostic criteria, clinical characteristics, and natural history of Cohen syndrome. J Med Genet 40:233–241.

392. Collin GB, Marshall JD, Ikeda A, So WV, Russell-Eggitt I, Maffei P, et al. (2002). Mutations in ALMS1 cause obesity, type 2 diabetes, and neurosensory degeneration in Alstrom syndrome. Nat Genet 31:74–78.

393. Lower KM, Turner G, Kerr BA, Mathews KD, Shaw MA, Gedeon AK, et al. (2002). Mutations in PHF6 are associated with Borjeson-Forssman-Lehmann syndrome. Nat Genet 32:661–665.

394. Jeanrenaud B (1985). An hypothesis on the aetiology of obesity: Dysfunction of the central nervous system as a primary cause. Diabetologia 28:502–513.

395. Satoh N, Ogawa Y, Katsura G, Tsuji T, Masuzaki H, Hiraoka J, et al. (1997). Pathophysiological significance of the obese gene product, leptin in ventromedial hypothalamus (VMH)-lesioned rats: evidence for loss of its satiety effect in VMH-lesioned rats. Endocrinology 138:947–954.

396. Bray GA, Inoue S, Nishizawa Y (1981). Hypothalamic obesity. Diabetologia 20:366–377.

397. Bray GA, Nishizawa Y (1978). Ventromedial hypothalamus modulates fat mobilization during fasting. Nature 274:900–902.

398. Sklar CA (1994). Craniopharyngioma: Endocrine sequalae of treatment. Ped Neurosurg 21:120–123.

399. Bray GA (1984). Syndromes of hypothalamic obesity in man. Ped Annals 13:525–536.

400. Daousi C, Dunn AJ, Foy PM, MacFarlane IA, Pinkney JH (2005). Endocrine and neuroanatomic predictors of weight gain and obesity in adult patients with hypothalamic damage. Am J Med 118:45–50.

401. Bray GA, Gallagher TF (1975). Manifestations of hypothalamic obesity in man: A comprehensive investigation of eight patients and a review of the literature. Medicine 54:301–333.

402. Lustig RH (2002). Hypothalamic obesity: The sixth cranial endocrinopathy. The Endocrinologist 12:210–217.

403. Harz KJ, Muller HL, Waldeck E, Pudel V, Roth C (2003). Obesity in patients with craniopharyngioma: Assessment of food intake and movement counts indicating physical activity. J Clin Endocrinol Metab 88:5227–5231.

404. Lustig RH, Post SM, Srivannaboon K, Rose SR, Danish RK, Burghen GA, et al. (2003). Risk factors for the development of obesity in children surviving brain tumors. J Clin Endocrinol Metab 88:611–616.

405. Reeves AG, Plum F (1972). Hyperphagia, rage, and dementia accompanying a ventromedial hypothalamic neoplasm. Archives of Neurology 20:616–624.

406. Schofl C, Schleth A, Berger D, Terkamp C, Von Zur Muhlen A, Brabant G (2002). Sympathoadrenal counterregulation in patients with hypothalamic craniopharyngioma. J Clin Endocrinol Metab 87:624–629.

407. Coutant R, Maurey H, Rouleau S, Mathieu E, Mercier P, Limal JM, et al. (2003). Defect in epinephrine production in children with craniopharyngioma: Functional or organic origin? J Clin Endocrinol Metab 88:5969–5975.

408. Lee HC, Curry DL, Stern JS (1989). Direct effect of CNS on insulin hypersecretion in obese Zucker rats: Involvement of vagus nerve. Am J Physiol 256:E439–E444.

409. Preeyasombat C, Bacchetti P, Lazar AA, Lustig RH (2005). Racial and etiopathologic dichotomies in insulin secretion and resistance in obese children. J Pediatr 146:474–481.

410. Tokunaga K, Fukushima M, Kemnitz JW, Bray GA (1986). Effect of vagotomy on serum insulin in rats with paraventricular or ventromedial hypothalamic lesions. Endocrinology 119:1708–1711.

411. Inoue S, Bray GA (1977). The effect of subdiaphragmatic vagotomy in rats with ventromedial hypothalamic lesions. Endocrinology 100:108–114.

412. Smith DK, Sarfeh J, Howard L (1983). Truncal vagotomy in hypothalmic obesity. Lancet 1:1330–1331.

413. Weiss R, Dziura J, Burgert TS, Tamborlane WV, Taksali SE, Yeckel CW, et al. (2004). Obesity and the metabolic syndrome in children and adolescents. N Engl J Med 350:2362–2374.

414. Sakul H, Pratley R, Cardon L, Ravussin E, Mott D, Bogardus C (1997). Familiality of physical and metabolic characteristics that predict the development of non-insulin-dependent diabetes mellitus in Pima indians. Am J Hum Genet 60:651–656.

415. Kissebah A, Krakower R (1994). Regional adiposity and mortality. Physiol Rev 74:791–811.

416. Bodkin NL, Hannah JS, Ortmeyer HK, Hansen BC (1993). Central obesity in rhesus monkeys: association with hyperinsulinemia, insulin resistance, and hypertriglyceridemia? Int J Obesity 17:53–61.

417. Mukhtar Q, Cleverly G, Voorhees RE, McGrath JW (2001). Prevalence of acanthosis nigrans and its association with hyperinsulinemia in New Mexico adolescents. J Adol Health 28:372–376.

418. Cruz P, Hud J (1992). Excess insulin binding to insulin-like gowth factor receptors: Proposed mechanism for acanthosis nigricans. J Invest Dermatol 98(6):82S–85S.

419. Odeleye OE, de Courten M, Pettitt DJ, Ravussin E (1997). Fasting hyperinsulinemia is a predictor of increased body weight gain and obesity in Pima Indian children. Diabetes 46:1341–1345.

420. Maffeis C, Moghetti P, Grezzani A, Clementi M, Gaudino R, Tato L (2002). Insulin resistance and the persistence of obesity from childhood into adulthood. J Clin Endocrinol Metab 87:71–76.

421. Luepker RV, Perry CL, McKinlay SM, Nader PR, Parcel GS, Stone EJ, et al. (1996). Outcomes of a field trial to improve children's dietary patterns and physical activity: The Child and Adolescent Trial for Cardiovascular Health. CATCH collaborative group. JAMA 275:768–776.

422. Davis SM, Going SB, Helitzer DL, Teufel NI, Snyder P, Gittelsohn J, et al. (1999). Pathways: A culturally appropriate obesity-prevention program for American Indian schoolchildren. Am J Clin Nutr 64:796S–802S.

423. Gungor N, Saad R, Janosky JE, Arslanian S (2004). Validation of surrogate estimates of insulin sensitivity and insulin secretion in children and adolescents. J Pediatr 144:47–55.

424. Epstein LH, Valoski S, Wing R, McCurley J (1990). Ten-year follow-up of behavioral, family-based treatment for obese children. JAMA 264:2519–2523.

425. Knowler WC, Barrett-Connor E, Fowler SE, Hamman RF, Lachin JM, Walker EA, et al. (2002). Reduction in the incidence of type 2 diabetes with lifestyle intervention or metformin. N Engl J Med 346:393–403.

426. Summerbell CD, Ashton V, Campbell KJ, Edmunds L, Kelly S, Waters E (2003). Interventions for treating obesity in children. Cochrane Database Syst Rev CD001872.

427. Flodmark CE, Marcus C, Britton M (2006). Interventions to prevent obesity in children and adolescents: A systematic literature review. Int J Obes 30:579–589.

428. International Obesity Task Force (1999). Assessment of childhood and adolescent obesity: Results from an international obesity task force workshop, Dublin, June 16, 1997. Am J Clin Nutr 70:117S–175S.

429. Barlow SE, Dietz WH (1998). Obesity evaluation and treatment: Expert committee recommendations. The Maternal and Child Health Bureau, Health Resources and Services Administration and the Department of Health and Human Services. Pediatrics 102:e29.

430. Baranowski T, Mendelein J, Resnicow K, Frank E, Cullen K, Baranowski J (2000). Physical activity and nutrition in youth: An overview of obesity prevention. Preventive Medicine 31:S1–S10.

431. Sothern MS, Schumacher H, von Almen TK, Carlisle LK, Udall JN (2002). Committed to kids: An integrated, 4-level team approach to weight management in adolescents. J Am Diet Assoc 102:S81–S85.

432. Epstein LH, Roemmich JN, Raynor HA (2001). Behavioral therapy in the treatment of pediatric obesity. Ped Clin NA 48:981–993.

433. Resnicow K, Davis R, Rollnick S (2006). Motivational interviewing for pediatric obesity: Conceptual issues and evdience review. J Am Diet Assoc 106:2024–2033.

434. Schwartz RP, Resnicow KA, Hamre R, Dietz WH, Slora E, Myers EF, et al. (2006). The healthy lifestyles pilot study. San Francisco, PAS meeting, abstr. 5430–5438.

435. James J, Thomas P, Cavan D, Kerr D (2004). Preventing childhood obesity by reducing consumption of carbonated drinks: Cluster randomised controlled trial. BMJ 328:doi:10.1136/bmj.38077.458438.EE.

436. Ebbeling CB, Feldman HA, Osganian SK, Chomitz VR, Ellenbogen SJ, Ludwig DS (2006). Effects of decreasing sugar-sweetened beverage consumption on body weight in adolescents: A randomized, controlled pilot study. Pediatrics 117:673–680.

437. Campbell K, Waters E, O'Meara S, Summerbell C (2001). Interventions for preventing obesity in childhood: A systematic review. Obesity Rev 2:149–157.

438. Dietz WH, Robinson TN (2005). Overweight children and adolescents. N Engl J Med 352:2100–2109.

439. Nuutinen O (1991). Long-term effects of dietary counseling on nutrient intake and weight loss in obese children. Eur J Clin Nutr 45:287–297.

440. Stice E, Cameron R, Killen J, Hayward C, Taylor CB (1999). Naturalistic weight reduction efforts prospectively predict growth in relative weight and onset of obesity among female adolescents. J Consult Clin Psychol 67:967–974.

441. Klem ML, Wing RR, McGuire MT, Seagle HM, Hill JO (1997). A descriptive study of individuals successful at long-term maintenance of substantial weight loss. Am J Clin Nutr 66:239–246.

442. Ravussin E, Danforth E (1999). Beyond sloth-physical activity and weight gain. Science 283:184–185.

443. Sothern M (2001). Exercise as a modality in the treatment of childhood obesity. Ped Clin NA 48:931–945.

444. Gutin B, Barbeau P, Owens S, Lemmon CR, Bauman M, Allison J, et al. (2002). Effects of exercise intensity on cardiovascular fitness, total body composition, and visceral adiposity of obese adolescents. Am J Clin Nutr 75:818–826.

445. McMurray RG, Bauman MJ, Harrell JS, Brown S, Gangdiwala SI (2000). Effects of improvement in aerobic power on resting insulin and glucose concentrations in children. Eur J Appl Physiol 81:132–139.

446. McKechnie R, Mosca L (2003). Physical activity and coronary heart disease: Prevention and effect on risk factors. Cardiology in Review 11:21–25.

447. Ferguson MA, Gutin B, Le NA, Karp W, Litaker M, Humphries M, et al. (1999). Effects of exercise training and its cessation on components of the insulin resistance syndrome in obese children. Int J Obesity 22:889–895.

448. Nemet D, Barkan S, Epstein Y, Friedland O, Kowen G, Eliakim A (2005). Short- and long-term beneficial effects of a combined dietary-behavioral-physical activity intervention for the treatment of childhood obesity. Pediatrics 115:e443–e449.

449. McMurray RG, Harrell JS, Bangdiwala SI, Bradley CB, Deng S, Levine A (2002). A school-based intervention can reduce body fat and blood pressure in young adolescents. J Adolesc Health 31:125–132.

450. O'Dea JA, Abraham S (2000). Improving the body image, eating attitudes, and behaviors of young male and female adolescents: A new educational approach that focuses on self-esteem. Int J Eating Dis 28:43–57.

451. Trost SG, Pate RR, Ward DS, Saunders R, Riner W (1999). Correlates of objectively measured physical activity in preadolescent youth. Am J Prev Med 17:120–126.

452. McGovern L, Kamath C, Johnson JN, Hettinger A, Singhal V, Paulo R, et al. (2007). Systematic review of randomized trials of obesity treatments. J Clin Endocrinol Metab (in press).

453. Yanovski SZ, Yanovski JA (2002). Drug therapy: Obesity. N Engl J Med 346:591–602.

454. Bray GA, Greenway FL (1999). Current and potential drugs for treatment of obesity. Endocr Rev 20:805–875.

455. Abenhaim L, Moride Y, Brenot F, Rich S, Benichou J, Kurz X, et al. (1996). Appetite-suppressant drugs and risk of primary pulmonary hypertension: International pulmonary hypertension study group. N Engl J Med 335:609–616.

456. Jick H, Vasilakis C, Weinrauch LA, Meier CR, Jick SS, Derby LE (1998). A population-based study of appetite-suppressant drugs and the risk of cardiac valve regurgitation. N Engl J Med 339:719–724.

457. Weintraub M (1985). Phenylpropanolamine as an anorexiant agent in weight control: A review of published and unpublished studies. In Morgan JP, Kagan DV, Bordy JS (eds.), *Phenylpropanolamine: Risks, benefits, and controversies*. New York: Praeger 53–79.

458. Morgan JP, Funderburk FR (1992). Phenylpropanolamine and blood pressure: A review of prospective studies. Am J Clin Nutr 55:206S–210S.

459. Ryan DH, Kaiser P, Bray GA (1995). Sibutramine: A novel new agent for obesity treatment. Obesity Res 3:S553–S559.

460. Bray GA, Blackburn GL, Ferguson JM, Greenway FL, Jain AK, Mendels CM, et al. (1999). Sibutramine produces dose-related weight loss. Obesity Res 7:189–198.

461. Heal DJ, Frankland AT, Gosden J, Hutchins LJ, Prow MR, Luscombe GP, et al. (1992). A comparison of the effects of sibutramine hydrochloride, bupropion and methamphetamine on dopaminergic function: Evidence that dopamine is not a pharmacological target for sibutramine. Psychopharmacology 107:303–309.

462. Seagle HM, Bessesen DH, Hill JO (1998). Effects of sibutramine on resting metabolic rate and weight loss in overweight women. Obesity Res 6:115–121.

463. Hansen DL, Toubro S, Stock MJ, MacDonald IA, Astrup A (1998). Thermogenic effects of sibutramine in humans. Am J Clin Nutr 68:1180–1186.

464. Berkowitz RI, Wadden TA, Tershakovec AM, Cronquist JL (2003). Behavior therapy and sibutramine for the treatment of adolescent obesity: A randomized controlled trial. JAMA 289:1805–1812.

465. Berkowitz RI, Fujioka K, Daniels SR, Hoppin A, Owen S, Perry AC, et al. (2006). Effects of sibutramine treatment in obese adolescents: A randomized trial. Ann Int Med 145:81–90.

466. James WPT, Astrup A, Finer N, Hilsted J, Kopelman P, Rössner S, et al. (2000). Effect of sibutramine on weight maintenance after weight loss: A randomized trial. Lancet 356:2119–2125.

467. Yanovski JA (2001). Intensive therapies for pediatric obesity. Ped Clin NA 48:1041–1053.

468. Mittendorfer B, Ostlund RJ, Patterson B, Klein SZ (2001). Orlistat inhibits dietary cholesterol absorption. Obesity Res 9:599–604.

469. Guerciolini R, Radu-Radulescu L, Boldrin M, Dallas J, Moore R (2001). Comparative evaluation of fecal fat excretion induced by orlistat and chitosan. Obesity Res 9:364–367.

470. Zhi J, Melia AT, Guercioloni R, Chung J, Kinberg J, Hauptman JB, et al. (1994). Retrospective population-based analysis of the dose-response (fecal fat excretion) relationship of orlistat in normal and obese volunteers. Clin Pharmcol Therap 56:82–85.

471. Reitman JB, Castro-Cabezas M, de Bruin TW, Erkelens DW (1994). Relationship between improved postprandial lipemia and low-density lipoprotein metabolism during treatment with tetrahydro-lipstatin, a pancreatic lipase inhibitor. Metabolism 43:293–298.

472. Chanoine JP, Hampl S, Jensen C, Boldrin M, Hauptman J (2005). Effects of orlistat on weight and body composition in obese adolescents: A randomized controlled trial. JAMA 293:2873–2883.

473. Maahs D, de Serna DG, Kolotkin RL, Ralston S, Sandate J, Qualls C, et al. (2006). Randomized, double-blind, placebo-controlled trial of orlistat for weight loss in adolescents. Endocr Pract 12:18–28.

474. McDuffie JR, Calis KA, Booth SL, Uwaifo GI, Yanovski JA (2002). Effects of orlistat on fat-soluble vitamins in obese adolescents. Pharmacotherapy 22:814–822.

475. Davidson MB, Peters AL (1997). An overview of metformin in the treatment of type 2 diabetes mellitus. Am J Med 102:99–110.

476. Stumvoll M, Nurjhan N, Perriello G, Dailey G, Gerich JE (1995). Metabolic effects of metformin in non-insulin-dependent diabetes mellitus. N Engl J Med 333:550–554.

477. DeFronzo RA, Goodman AM (1995). Efficacy of metformin in patients with non-insulin-dependent diabetes mellitus. N Engl J Med 333:541–549.

478. Jones KL, Arslanian S, Peterokova VA, Park JS, Tomlinson MJ (2002). Effect of metformin in pediatric patients with type 2 diabetes. Diab Care 25:89–94.

479. Diabetes Prevention Program Research Group (2002). Reduction in the incidence of type 2 diabetes with lifestyle intervention or metformin. N Engl J Med 346:393–403.

480. Mogul HR, Peterson SJ, Weinstein BI, Zhang S, Southren AL (2001). Metformin and carbohydrate-modified diet: A novel obesity treatment protocol: preliminary findings from a case series of nondiabetic women with midlife weight gain and hyperinsulinemia. Heart Disease 3:285–292.

481. Lee A, Morley JE (1998). Metformin decreases food-consumption and induces weight-loss in subjects with obesity with type-II non-insulin-dependent diabetes. Obesity Res 6:47–53.

482. Paolisso G, Amato L, Eccellente R, Gambardella A, Tagliamonte MR, Varricchio G, et al. (1998). Effect of metformin on food intake in obese subjects. European J Clin Invest 28:441–446.

483. Bailey CJ, Turner RC (1996). Metformin. N Engl J Med 334:574–579.

484. Lenhard JM, Kliewer SA, Paulik MA, Plunket KD, Lehmann JM, Weiel JE (1997). Effects of troglitazone and metformin on glucose and lipid metabolism: Alterations of two distinct molecular pathways. Biochem Pharmacol 54:801–808.

485. Zhou G, Myers R, Li Y, Chen Y, Shen X, Fenyk-Melody J, et al. (2001). Role of AMP-activated protein kinase in mechanism of metformin action. J Clin Invest 108:1167–1174.

486. Kumar N, Dey CS (2002). Metformin enhances insulin signalling in insulin-dependent and -independent pathways in insulin resistant muscle cells. Br J Pharmacol 137:329–336.

487. Mannucci E, Ognibene A, Cemasco F, Bardini G, Mencucci A, Pierazzuoli E, et al. (2001). Effect of metformin on glucagon-like peptide-1 (GLP-1) and leptin levels in obese nondiabetic subjects. Diab Care 24:489–494.

488. Freemark M, Bursey D (2001). The effects of metformin on body mass index and glucose tolerance in obese adolescents with fasting hyperinsulinemia and a family history of type 2 diabetes. Pediatrics 107:e55.

489. Kay JP, Alemzadeh R, Langley G, D'Angelo L, Smith P, Holshouser S (2001). Beneficial effects of metformin in normoglycemic morbidly obese adolescents. Metabolism 50:1457–1461.

490. Velasquez EM, Mendoza S, Hamer T, Sosa F, Glueck CJ (1994). Metformin therapy in polycystic ovarian syndrome reduces hyperinsulinemia, insulin resistance, hyperandrogenemia, and systolic blood pressure, while facilitating normal menses and pregnancy. Metabolism 43:647–654.

491. Pasquali R, Gambineri A, Biscotti D, Vicennatti V, Gagliardi L, Colitta D, et al. (2000). Effect of long-term treatment with metformin added to hypocaloric diet on body composition, fat distribution, and androgen and insulin levels in abdominally obese women with and without the polycystic ovary syndrome. J Clin Endocrinol Metab 85:2767–2774.

492. Jamieson MA (2002). The use of metformin in adolescents with polycystic ovary syndrome: for and against. J Ped Adol Gynecol 15:109–114.

493. Ibanez L, Valls C, Potau N, Marcos MV, de Zegher F (2000). Sensitization to insulin in adolescent girls to normalize hirsutism, hyperandrogenism, oligomenorrhea, dyslipidemia, and hyperinsulinism after precocious adrenarche. J Clin Endocrinol Metab 85:3526–3530.

494. Marchesini G, Brizi M, Bianchi G, Tomassetti S, Zoli M, Melchionda N (2001). Metformin in non-alcoholic steatohepatitis. Lancet 358:893–894.

495. Schwimmer JB, Middleton MS, Deutsch R, Lavine JE (2005). A phase 2 trial of metformin as a treatment for non-diabetic paediatric non-alcoholic steatohepatitis. Aliment Pharmacol Ther 21:871–879.

496. Morrison JA, Cottingham EM, Barton BA (2002). Metformin for weight loss in pediatric patients taking psychotropic drugs. Am J Psychiatr 159:655–657.

497. Silverman B, Franklin GM, Bolin R (1997). Lactic acidosis traced to thiamine deficiency related to nationwide shortage of multivitamins for total parenteral nutrition. MMWR 46(23):523–528.

498. Velasquez-Mieyer PA, Cowan PA, Buffington CK, Arheart KL, Cowan GSM, Connelly BE, et al. (2003). Suppression of insulin secretion promotes weight loss and alters macronutrient preference in a subset of obese adults. Int J Obesity 27:219–226.

499. Hsu WH, Xiang HD, Rajan AS, Kunze DL, Boyd AE (1991). Somatostatin inhibits insulin secretion by a G-protein-mediated decrease in Ca^{2+} entry through voltage-dependent Ca^{2+} channels in the beta-cell. J Biol Chem 266:837–843.

500. Mitra SW, Mezey E, Hunyady B, Chamberlain L, Hayes E, Foor F, et al. (1999). Colocalization of somatostatin receptor sst5 and insulin in rat pancreatic β-cells. Endocrinology 140:3790–3796.

501. Bertoli A, Magnaterra R, Borboni P, Marini MA, Barini A, Fusco A, et al. (1998). Dose-dependent effect of octreotide on insulin secretion after OGTT in obesity. Hormone Research 49:17–21.

502. Lustig RH, Hinds PS, Ringwald-Smith K, Christensen RK, Kaste SC, Schreiber RE, et al. (2003). Octreotide therapy of pediatric hypothalamic obesity: A double-blind, placebo-controlled trial. J Clin Endocrinol Metab 88:2586–2592.

503. Lustig RH, Greenway F, Velasquez-Mieyer P, Heimburger D, Schumacher D, Smith D, et al. (2006). A multicenter, randomized, double-blind, placebo-controlled, dose-finding trial of a long-acting formulation of octreotide in promoting weight loss in obese adults with insulin hypersecretion. Int J Obesity 30:331–341.

504. Krentz AJ, MacDonald LM, Schade DS (1994). Octreotide: A long-acting inhibitor of endogenous hormone secretion for human metabolic investigations. Metabolism 43:24–31.

505. Lamberts SWJ, Van Der Lely AJ, De Herder WW, Hofland LJ (1996). Drug therapy: Octreotide. N Engl J Med 334:246–254.

506. Tauber MT, Harris AG, Rochiccioli P (1994). Clinical use of the long-acting somatostatin analog octreotide in pediatrics. European J Pediatr 153:304–310.

507. Farooqi IS, Jebb SA, Langmack G, Lawrence E, Cheetham CH, Prentice AM, et al. (1999). Effects of recombinant leptin therapy in a child with congenital leptin deficiency. N Engl J Med 341:913–915.

508. Gibson WT, Farooqi IS, Moreau M, DePaoli AM, Lawrence E, O'Rahilly S, et al. (2004). Congenital leptin deficiency due to homozygosity for the d1333G mutation: report of another case and evaluation of response to four years of leptin therapy. J Clin Endocrinol Metab 89:4821–4826.

509. Shi ZQ, Chinookoswong N, Wang JL, Korach E, Lebel C, DePaoli A, et al. (2002). Additive effects of leptin and oral antiobesity drugs in treating diet-induced obesity in rats. Diabetes 51(2):1707.

510. Carrel AL, Moerchen V, Myers SE, Bekx MT, Whitman BY, Allen DB (2004). Growth hormone improves mobility and body composition in infants and toddlers with Prader-Willi syndrome. J Pediatr 145:744–749.

511. Kaplowitz PB, Rundle AC, Blethen SL (1998). Weight relative to height before and during growth hormone therapy in prepubertal children. Horm Metab Res 30:565–569.

512. Simsolo RB, Ezzat S, Ong JM, Saghizadeh M, Kern PA (1995). Effects of acromegaly treatment and growth hormone on adipose tissue lipoprotein lipase. J Clin Endocrinol Metab 80:3233–3238.

513. Williams T, Berelowitz M, Joffe SN, Thorner MO, Rivier J, Vale W, et al. (1984). Impaired growth hormone responses to growth hormone-releasing factor in obesity: A pituitary defect reversed with weight reduction. N Engl J Med 311:1403–1407.

514. Jorgensen JO, Pedersen SB, Borglum J, Moller N, Schmitz O, Christiansen JS, et al. (1994). Fuel metabolism, energy expenditure, and thyroid function in growth hormone-treated obese women: A double-blind, placebo-controlled study. Metabolism 43:872–877.

515. Wynne K, Park AJ, Small CJ, Patterson M, Ellis SM, Murphy KG, et al. (2005). Subcutaneous oxyntomodulin reduces body weight in overweight and obese subjects: A double-blind, randomized, controlled trial. Diabetes 54:2390–2395.

516. Teter CJ, Early JJ, Gibbs CM (2000). Treatment of affective disorder and obesity with topiramate. Ann Pharmacotherapy 34:1262–1265.

517. Wilkes JJ, Nelson E, Osborne M, Demarest KT, Olefsky JM (2005). Topiramate is an insulin-sensitizing compound in vivo with direct effects on adipocytes in female ZDF rats. Am J Physiol Endocrinol Metab 288:E617–E624.

518. Wilding J, Van Gaal L, Rissanen A, Vercruysse F, Fitchet M (2004). A randomized double-blind placebo-controlled study of the long-term efficacy and safety of topiramate in the treatment of obese subjects. Int J Obesity 28:1399–1410.

519. LeFoll B, Goldberg SR (2005). Cannabinoid CB_1 receptor antagonists as promising new medications for drug dependence. J Pharmacol Exp Ther 312:875–883.

520. Van Gaal LF, Rissanen AM, Scheen AJ, Ziegler O, Rossner S (2005). Effects of the cannabinoid-1 receptor blocker rimonabant on weight reduction and cardiovascular risk factors in overweight patients: 1-year experience from the RIO-Europe study. Lancet 365:1389–1397.

521. Strauss R (2002). Perspectives on childhood obesity. Curr Gastroenterol Rep 4:244–250.

522. Inge TH, Krebs NF, Garcia VF, Skelton JA, Guice KS, Strauss RS, et al. (2004). Bariatric surgery for overweight adolescents: Concerns and recommendations. Pediatrics 114:217–223.

523. Whitaker RC, Wright JA, Pepe MS, Seidel KD, Dietz WH (1997). Predicting obesity in young adulthood from childhood and parental obesity. N Engl J Med 337:869–873.

524. Inge TH, Xanthakos SA, Zeller MH (2007). Bariatric surgery for pediatric extreme obesity: Now or later? Int J Obes 31:1–14.

525. Apovian CM, Baker C, Ludwig DS, Hoppin AG, Hsu G, Lenders C, et al. (2005). Best practice guidelines in pediatric/adolescent weight loss surgery. Obes Res 13:274–282.

526. Mun EC, Blackburn GL, Matthews JB (2001). Current status of medical and surgical therapy for obesity. Gastroenterology 120:669–681.

527. Abu-Abeid S, Gavert N, Klausner JM, Szold A (2003). Bariatric surgery in adolescence. J Pediatr Surg 38:1379–1382.

528. Dolan K, Creighton L, Hopkins G, Fielding G (2003). Laparoscopic gastric banding in morbidly obese adolescents. Obes Surg 13:101–104.

529. Fielding GA, Duncombe JE (2005). Laparoscopic adjustable gastric banding in severely obese adolescents. Surg Obes Relat Dis 1:399–405.

530. Rubino F, Gagner M, Gentileschi P, Kini S, Fukuyama S, Feng J, et al. (2004). The early effect of the Roux-en-Y gastric bypass on hormones involved in body weight regulation and glucose metabolism. Ann Surg 240:236–242.

531. Sjostrom L, Lindroos AK, Peltonen M, Torgerson J, Bouchard C, Carlsson B, et al. for the Swedish Obese Subjects Study Scientific Group (2004). Lifestyle, diabetes, and cardiovascular risk factors 10 years after bariatric surgery. N Engl J Med 351:2683–2693.

532. Shah M, Simha V, Garg A (2006). Review: Long-term impact of bariatric surgery on body weight, co-morbidities, and nutritional status. J Clin Endocrinol Metab 91:4223–4231.

533. Strauss RS, Bradley LJ, Brolin RE (2001). Gastric bypass surgery in adolescents with morbid obesity. J Pediatr 138:499–504.

534. Sugerman HJ, Sugerman EL, DeMaria EJ, Kellum JM, Kennedy C, Mowery Y, et al. (2003). Bariatric surgery for severely obese adolescents. J Gastrointest Surg 7:102–107.

535. Lawson ML, Kirk S, Mitchell T, Chen MK, Loux TJ, Daniels SR, et al. (2006). One-year outcomes of Roux-en-Y gastric bypass for morbidly obese adolescents: A multicenter study from the Pediatric Bariatric Study Group. Ped Surg 41:137–143.

536. Towbin S, Inge TH, Garcia VF, Roehrig HR, Clements RH, Harmon CM, et al. (2004). Beriberi after gastric bypass surgery in adolescence. J Pediatr 145:263–267.

537. Mason EE, Scott DH, Doherty C, Cullen JJ, Rodriguez EM, Maher JW, et al. (1995). Vertical banded gastroplasty in the severely obese under age twenty-one. Obes Surg 5:23–33.

538. Greenstein RJ, Rabner JG (1995). Is adolescent gastric-restrictive anti-obesity surgery warranted? Obes Surg 5:138–144.

539. Breaux CW (1995). Obesity surgery in children. Obes Surg 5:279–284.

540. Nguyen NT, Paya M, Stevens M, Mavandadi S, Zainabadi K, Wilson SE (2004). The relationship between hospital volume and outcome in bariatric surgery at academic medical centers. Ann Surg 240:586–594.

541. Zingmond DS, McGory ML, Ko CY (2005). Hospitalization before and after gastric bypass surgery. JAMA 294:1918–1924.

542. Ray RM, Senders CW (2001). Airway management in the obese child. Ped Clin NA 48:1055–1063.

543. DeBoer MD, Marks DL (2006). Therapy insight: Use of melanocortin antagonists in the treatment of cachexia in chronic disease. Nat Clin Pract Endo Metab 2:459–466.

544. Walsh D, Nelson KA (2002). Autonomic nervous system dysfunction in advanced cancer. Support Care Cancer 10:523–528.

545. Barber MD, Ross JA, Fearon KC (2000). Disordered metabolic response with cancer and its management. World J Surg 24:681–689.

546. Gahagan S, Holmes R (1998). A stepwise approach to evaluation of undernutrition and failure to thrive. Ped Clin North Am 45:169–187.

547. Krugman SD, Dubowitz H (2003). Failure to thrive. Am Fam Phys 68:879–884.

548. Schmitt BD, Mauro RD (1989). Non-organic failure to thrive: an outpatient approach. Child Abuse Negl 13:235–248.

549. Kuhnle U, Lewicka S, Fuller PJ (2004). Endocrine disorders of sodium regulation: Role of adrenal steroids in genetic defects causing sodium loss or sodium retention. Horm Res 61:68–83.

550. Sills RH (1978). Failure to thrive: The role of clinical and laboratory evaluation. Am J Dis Child 132:967–969.

551. Berwick DM, Levy JC, Kleinerman R (1982). Failure to thrive: Diagnostic yield of hospitalization. Arch Dis Child 57:347–351.

552. Gahagan S (2006). Failure to thrive: A consequence of undernutrition. Pediatr Rev 27:e1–e11.

553. Gabay MP (2002). Galactogogues: Medications that induce lactation. J Hum Lact 18:274–279.

554. Maggioni A, Lifshitz F (1995). Nutritional management of failure to thrive. Ped Clin North Am 42:791–810.

555. Hershkovitz E, Printzman L, Segev Y, Levy J, Phillip M (1999). Zinc supplementation increases the level of serum insulin-like growth factor-I but does not promote growth in infants with nonorganic failure to thrive. Horm Res 52:200–204.

556. Lozoff B, Jimenez E, Wolf AW (1991). Long-term developmental outcome of infants with iron deficiency. N Engl J Med 325:687–694.

557. Davis MP (2007). Anorexia and cachexia in cancer. In Yeung S, Escalante C, Gagel RF (eds.), Internal medicine care of cancer patients. New York: Decker (in press).

558. Kelly JF, Elias CF, Lee CE, Ahima RS, Seeley RJ, Bjorbaek C, et al. (2004). Ciliary neurotrophic factor and leptin induce distinct patterns of immediate early gene expression in the brain. Diabetes 53:911–920.

559. Argiles JM, Busquets S, Lopez-Soriano FJ (2002). The role of uncoupling proteins in pathophysiological states. Biochem Biophys Res Comm 293:1145–1152.

560. Makino T, Noguchi Y, Yoshikawa T, Doi C, Nomura K (1998). Circulating interleukin 6 concentrations and insulin resistance in patients with cancer. Br J Surg 85:1658–1662.

561. Yoshikawa T, Noguchi Y, Doi C, Makino T, Okamoto T, Matsumoto A (1999). Insulin resistance is connected with the alterations of substrate utilization in patients with cancer. Cancer Lett 141:93–98.

562. Yoshikawa T, Noguchi Y, Doi C, Makino T, Nomura K (2001). Insulin resistance in patients with cancer: Relationships with tumor site, tumor stage, body-weight loss, acute-phase response, and energy expenditure. Nutrition 17:590–593.

563. Tayek JA, Katz J (1997). Glucose production, recycling, Cori cycle, and gluconeogenesis in humans: Relationship to serum cortisol. Am J Physiol 272:E476–E484.

564. Russell A (1951). A diencephalic syndrome of emaciation in infancy and childhood. Arch Dis Child 26:274.

565. Fleischman A, Brue C, Poussaint TY, Kieran M, Pomeroy SL, Goumnerova L, et al. (2005). Diencephalic syndrome: A cause of failure to thrive and a model of partial growth hormone resistance. Pediatrics 115:e742–e748.

566. Brauner R, Trivin C, Zerah M, Souberbielle JC, Doz F, Kalifa C, et al. (2006). Diencephalic syndrome due to hypothalamic tumor: A model of the relationship between weight and puberty onset. J Clin Endocrinol Metab 91:2467–2473.

567. Vlachopapadopoulou E, Tracey KJ, Capella M, Gilker C, Matthews DE (1993). Increased energy expenditure in a patient with diencephalic syndrome. J Pediatr 122:922–924.

568. Hoek HW, van Hoeken D (2003). Review of the prevalence and incidence of eating disorders. Int J Eating Dis 34:383–396.

569. Johnson JG, Cohen P, Kasen S, Brook JS (2002). Eating disorders during adolescence and the risk for physical and mental disorders during early adulthood. Arch Gen Psychiatry 59:545–552.

570. Rigotti NA, Neer RM, Skates SJ, Herzog DB, Nussbaum SR (1991). The clinical course of osteoporosis in anorexia nervosa: A longitudinal study of cortical bone mass. JAMA 265:1133–1138.

571. Bulik CM, Sullivan PF, Fear JL, Pickering A, Dawn A, McCullin M (1999). Fertility and reproduction in women with anorexia nervosa: A controlled study. J Clin Psychiatry 60:130–135.

572. Lambe EK, Katzman DK, Mikulis DJ, Kennedy SH, Zipursky RB (1997). Cerebral gray matter volume deficits after weight recovery from anorexia nervosa. Arch Gen Psychiatry 54:537–542.

573. Strober M, Freeman R, Morrell W (1997). The long-term course of severe anorexia nervosa in adolescents: Survival analysis of recovery, relapse, and outcome predictors over 10-15 years in a prospective study. Int J Eating Dis 22:339–360.

574. Tamai H, Mori K, Matsubayashi S, Kiyohara K, Nakagawa T, Okimura MC, et al. (1986). Hypothalamic-pituitary-thyroidal dysfunctions in anorexia nervosa. Psychother Psychosom 46:127–131.

575. Gianotti L, Arvat E, Valetto MR, Ramunni J, Di Vito L, Maccagno B, et al. (1998). Effects of beta-adrenergic agonists and antagonists on the growth hormone response to growth hormone-releasing hormone in anorexia nervosa. Biol Psychiatry 43:181–187.

576. Licinio J, Wong ML, Gold PW (1996). The hypothalamic pituitary adrenal axis in anorexia nervosa. Horm Res 62:75–83.

577. Misra M, Klibanski A (2006). Anorexia nervosa and osteoporosis. Rev Endo Metab Dis 7:91–99.

578. Misra M, Miller KK, Tsai P, Gallagher K, Lin A, Lee N, et al. (2006). Elevated peptide YY levels in adolescent girls with anorexia nervosa. J Clin Endocrinol Metab 91:1027–1033.

579. Welt CK, Chan JL, Bullen J, Murphy R, Smith P, DePaoli AM, et al. (2004). Recombinant human leptin in women with hypothalamic amenorrhea. N Engl J Med 351:987–997.

580. Balligand JL, Brichard SM, Brichard V, Desager JP, Lambert M (1998). Hypoleptinemia in patients with anorexia nervosa: Loss of circadian rhythm and unresponsiveness to short-term refeeding. Eur J Endocrinol 138:415–420.

581. Monteleone P, Fabrazzo M, Tortorella A, Fuschino A, Maj M (2002). Opposite modifications in circulating leptin and soluble leptin receptor across the eating disorder spectrum. Mol Psychiatry 7:641–646.

582. Chan JL, Mantzoros CS (2005). Role of leptin in energy-deprivation states: Normal human physiology and clinical implications for hypothalamic amenorrhoea and anorexia nervosa. Lancet 366:74–85.

583. Brichard SM, Delporte ML, Lambert M (2003). Adipocytokines in anorexia nervosa: A review focusing on leptin and adiponectin. Horm Metab Res 35:337–342.

584. Tagami T, Satoh N, Usui T, Yamada K, Shimatsu A, Kuzuya H (2004). Adiponectin in anorexia nervosa and bulimia nervosa. J Clin Endocrinol Metab 89:1833–1837.

585. Bosy-Westphal A, Brabant G, Haas V, Onur S, Paul T, Nutzinger D, et al. (2005). Determinants of plasma adiponectin levels in patients with anorexia nervosa examined before and after weight gain. Eur J Nutr 44:355–359.

586. American Psychiatric Association (2006). Treatment of patients with eating disorders, third edition. Am J Psychiatr 163:4–54.

587. Klibanski A, Biller BM, Schoenfeld DA, Herzog DB, Saxe VC (1995). The effects of estrogen administration on trabecular bone loss in young women with anorexia nervosa. J Clin Endocrinol Metab 80:898–904.

588. Robinson E, Bachrach LK, Katzman DK (2000). Use of hormone replacement therapy to reduce the risk of osteopenia in adolescent girls with anorexia nervosa. J Adolesc Health 26:343–348.

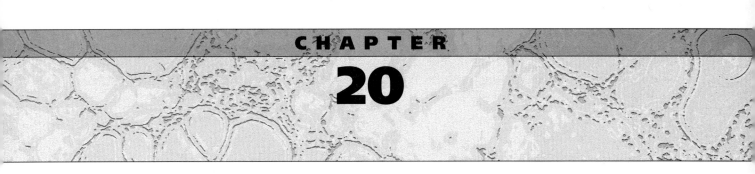

Lipid Disorders in Children and Adolescents

SARAH C. COUCH, PhD, RD • STEPHEN R. DANIELS, MD, PhD

Introduction

Cardiovascular disease (CVD) is a major cause of morbidity and mortality among adults in industrialized countries. Dyslipidemia (specifically elevated LDL cholesterol, low HDL cholesterol, and high triglycerides) has been identified as an independent risk factor in the development of CVD. There is strong evidence that lipoprotein levels track from childhood into adulthood and that abnormal levels of LDL cholesterol and perhaps other lipoproteins are associated with atherosclerosis and therefore with related adverse outcomes.

This chapter reviews the evidence for the role of cholesterol abnormalities in the early natural history of atherosclerosis. In addition, a general overview of lipoprotein metabolism is provided—followed by a review of genetic disorders in the metabolism of lipoproteins. Sec-ondary causes of high cholesterol are explained, including the increasing prevalence of obesity and metabolic syndrome as a cause of cholesterol abnormalities in the pediatric population. Standards and approaches to screening for hyperlipidemia in childhood are reviewed, as well as current approaches to the dietary and pharmacologic management of pediatric lipid disorders.

Metabolism

Lipid disorders in children and adolescents can result from defects in the production, transport, and/or degradation of lipoproteins. To understand the diverse causes of lipoprotein abnormalities, a brief review of lipoprotein structure, function, and metabolism is provided. Table 20-1 summarizes the lipoprotein subclasses, the source of

TABLE 20-1

Lipoprotein Subclasses and Associated Apolipoproteins and Lipid Constituents

Lipoprotein	Apolipoprotein	Source	Lipid Constituents
Chylomicrons	apoB-48, apoC-II*, apoC-III, apoE*	Intestine	Dietary triglycerides
VLDL	apoB-100, C-II*, C-III, apoE*	Liver	Endogenous cholesterol and triglyceride
IDL	apoB-100, apoE	VLDL metabolism	Cholesterol and triglyceride
LDL	apoB-100	VLDL metabolism	Cholesterol
HDL	apoA-I, apoA-II, apoC-II, apoE	Liver and intestine	Cholesterol and phospholipid

* Transferred from HDL.

each, and the constituent lipids and apolipoproteins associated with each particle.

Triglycerides, cholesterol esters, phospholipids, and plant sterols within food postingestion are digested to fatty acids, 2-monoglycerides, unesterified cholesterol, lysophospholipids, and unesterified plant sterols. These lipid-soluble products diffuse through the apical surface of the enteric membrane and are reaggregated into lipoproteins through the action of a microsomal triglyceride transfer protein (MTP). MTP (and perhaps an additional transfer protein) conjugate triglycerides with cholesterol ester (a phospholipid monolayer) and apolipoprotein B-48 (apoB-48) to create a mature chylomicron.[1]

Most of the plant sterol ingested and about half of the absorbed cholesterol are excreted from the intestinal cell back into the lumen by two ATP-binding cassette (ABC) half-transporters, thus limiting the amount of these sterols that are absorbed.[2,3] Once formed, chylomicrons are too large to penetrate the capillary membrane. Consequently, they are secreted into the lymphatic system and enter the venous plasma compartment through the thoracic lymph duct. As the nascent particles are released into the plasma, several apolipoproteins (including apoC-II and apoE) are preferentially transferred to the chylomicrons from other lipoproteins (e.g., high-density lipoproteins, HDL).[4] Figure 20-1 depicts chylomicron metabolism.

Chylomicrons transport dietary triglyceride and cholesterol to sites of storage or metabolism.[5] They are rapidly cleared from the circulation through the action of lipoprotein lipase (LPL). LPL is a triglyceride hydrolase found on the capillary endothelium of various tissues, with highest concentration in muscle and adipose tissues.[6] LPL is activated by apo-CII on the chylomicron. As the triglyceride contained within the chylomicron is hydrolyzed, the particle decreases in size. When approximately 80% of the initial triglyceride has been removed, apoC-II dissociates from its surface.[4] The triglyceride-depleted chylomicrons, now considered chylomicron remnants, are taken up by the liver through a receptor that recognizes apoE on the particle surface. A smaller fraction of remnants may also be internalized via a low-density lipoprotein (LDL) receptor-like protein (LRP)-mediated endocytosis.[7,8]

Very-low-density lipoproteins (VLDLs) originate from the liver, and like chylomicrons are triglyceride-rich particles (Figure 20-2). In contrast to the intestinally derived chylomicrons, however, the fatty acids contained within the VLDL triglyceride come from de novo synthesis from dietary carbohydrate, lipoprotein remnants, or circulating fatty acids internalized by the liver from plasma.[4] Within the hepatocyte, triglyceride and cholesterol ester are assembled by an MTP and surrounded with a phospholipid membrane associated with apoB-100.[1] The mature VLDL particles are released into the lymph and ultimately into the vascular space, where other apolipoproteins (including apoC-II and apoE) adsorb to the VLDL surface.

The metabolism of the VLDL particle follows a route similar to that of the chylomicron: apo C-II on its surface activates LPL, LPL hydrolyzes the VLDL triglyceride, the particle decreases in size (80% loss of triglyceride), and ultimately apoC-II dissociates—resulting in the formation

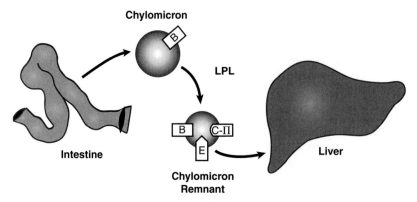

Figure 20-1 Exogenous lipoprotein metabolism. [Courtesy of Emilie Graham, University of Cincinnati.]

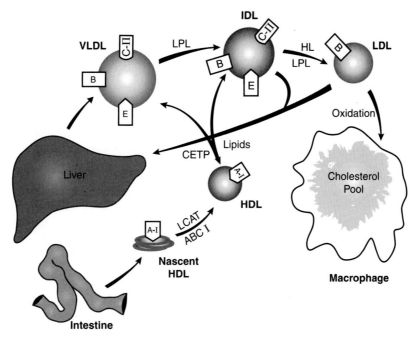

Figure 20-2 Endogenous lipoprotein metabolism. [Courtesy of Emilie Graham, University of Cincinnati.]

of VLDL remnants [also known as intermediate-density lipoproteins (IDLs)]. Approximately half of the IDL is then removed from plasma through the interaction of apoB with the apoB-100/apoE receptor on the surface of liver cells.[9] The rest of the IDL is converted to LDL through further hydrolysis of core triglycerides by hepatic triglyceride lipase (HL). ApoE is transferred from IDL to HDL during the transition of the remnant to LDL.[10]

LDL, the major carrier of cholesterol in plasma, is taken up into peripheral tissues and liver cells by the apoB-100/apoE receptor—which recognizes apoB-100 on the particle surface. Upon receptor binding, the LDL-receptor complex is rapidly internalized into clathrin-coated pits by endocytosis. Within the cell, the newly formed endosome becomes acidified through the action of an ATP-dependent proton pump.[11] Acidification causes degradation of the clathrin coat, dissociation of the receptor from LDL, and subdivision of the endosomal membranes. The endosome containing the LDL receptor recirculates back to the cell membrane for additional LDL uptake. It then fuses with lysosomes, where the lipoprotein is digested into its component parts: unesterified cholesterol, fatty acids, and free amino acids.[11]

The amount of cholesterol released from endosomal uptake regulates hepatic synthesis of LDL receptor and cholesterol. When cellular concentration of cholesterol is low, sterol receptor binding protein (SREBP) is released. SREBP is a nuclear factor that enhances the transcription of LDL receptor and hydroxy-methylglutaryl (HM6) CoA reductase, the rate-limiting enzyme of cholesterol biosynthesis.[12] In this way, intracellular hepatic cholesterol concentration regulates the amount of cholesterol internalized and synthesized by the cell.

When excess LDL is present in the plasma, the capacity of the LDL receptor to remove it is exceeded and LDL is more susceptible to oxidation. Oxidized LDL can be taken up by scavenger receptors on macrophages in the subendothelium of arteries and may contribute to the formation of atherosclerotic lesions.[13]

HDL transfers cholesterol and other lipids from peripheral tissues (including arterial atheroma) back to the liver. The particles are synthesized predominantly in the liver (and to a lesser extent in the intestine) as lipid-poor precursor particles (pre beta HDL) containing apoA-I. Nascent HDL interacts with the plasma membrane of cells, collecting lipid through an ATP-binding cassette transporter-A1 (ABCI) mechanism.[2,3] The cholesterol and phospholipids transferred through this process adsorb to the HDL, forming a disc-shaped particle referred to as HDL3. Within the plasma, HDL3 interacts with the enzyme lecithin cholesterol acyl transferase (LCAT)—which catalyzes the esterification of particle-associated cholesterol. ApoA-I on the HDL surface activates LCAT. Once formed, the cholesterol ester is more hydrophobic and moves to the interior of the particle—creating a sphere-shaped HDL particle known as HDL2.[14]

As HDL2 increases in size, the particle becomes substrate for cholesterol ester transfer protein (CETP). This enzyme promotes the exchange of esterified cholesterol within HDL2 for triglyceride contained within apoB-100-associated lipoproteins.[15] This lipid exchange is one mechanism whereby HDL indirectly participates in reverse cholesterol transport from tissues back to the liver. Two direct pathways in which HDL2 can transport cholesterol back to the liver involve holoparticle uptake via the apoB-100/apoE receptor and cholesterol ester transfer from HDL2 to the liver and other steroid-hormone-producing tissues through a scavenger receptor B1 (SRB1). This latter process may require the action of HL.[16]

Primary Dyslipidemias

Lipoprotein synthesis, transport, and metabolism occur in many steps and involve many specialized proteins. A number of genetic defects have been identified in these processes and are referred to as primary dyslipidemias. Most of these genetic defects present in childhood. Table 20-2 provides a summary of pediatric lipoprotein disorders with reference to the characteristic lipoprotein profile of each. The genetic and metabolic etiologies of these disorders are detailed in the material following.

DISORDERS OF CHOLESTEROL METABOLISM

Familial Hypercholesterolemia

Familial hypercholesterolemia (FH) is the most common single gene disorder of lipoprotein metabolism. FH is inherited as an autosomal-dominant trait with relatively low prevalence in western countries. The heterozygous form is found in 1 in 500 persons and the homozygous form is found in 1 in 1,000,000 persons. The disorder is caused by a mutation in the apoB-100/apoE receptor or LDL receptor (LDLR) gene.[17,18] More than 900 mutations in this gene have been identified, including those that affect receptor synthesis, intracellular transport, ligand binding, internalization, and recycling.[19] In the heterozygous form, inheritance of one defective LDLR gene results in plasma LDL cholesterol levels two to three times higher than normal.[17]

Individuals with heterozygous FH are at an increased risk of developing early-onset coronary artery disease (CAD), usually between the ages of 30 and 60 years.[17,18] In the homozygous form, individuals inherit a mutant allele for FH from both parents—resulting in plasma LDL cholesterol concentrations that are five to six times higher than normal. Due to the excessively high plasma cholesterol levels in these individuals, cholesterol deposits are common in the tendons (xanthomas) and eyelids (xanthelasmas)—generally by the age of 5 years.[20] In the heterozygous form, xanthomas occur only rarely and generally not until older adulthood. Children with homozygous FH have early-onset atherosclerosis, and often have myocardial infarction in the first decade of life and death from CAD in the second decade.[20]

Autosomal-Recessive Hypercholesterolemia

Autosomal-recessive hypercholesterolemia (ARH) is another inherited disorder resulting in marked elevations in LDL cholesterol levels. This disorder is caused by a defect in the ARH protein.[21] ARH protein binds to the LDLR and clathrin, suggesting a role for ARH in the recruitment and retention of LDLR in clathrin coated pits.[22] Several different mutations in this protein have been identified, all leading to a lack of (or suboptimal internalization of) the LDLR.[22,23] Cholesterol levels in individuals with ARH are five to six times higher than normal. Children with this disorder are clinically similar to those with homozygous FH. However, their parents usually have normal lipoprotein profiles.[23]

Familial Ligand-Defective apoB-100

Familial ligand-defective apoB-100 (FDB) is a monogenic disorder resulting in moderate to markedly high plasma LDL cholesterol levels. The disorder is caused by poor binding of the LDL particle to the LDLR due to a mutation in apoB-100.[24] Such deficient binding results in decreased clearance of LDL from plasma. The disorder is most common in individuals of European descent (1 per 1,000).[9] Patients with FDB are at moderate risk of developing CAD.

Phytosterolemia

Phytosterolemia is a rare autosomal-recessive disease caused by a mutation in two genes (ABCG5 and ABCG8) encoding the ABC half-transporters.[9,25,26] These proteins limit the absorption of cholesterol and plant sterols (and possibly shellfish sterols) in the gut. They also promote biliary and fecal excretion of cholesterol and phytosterols.[26] Defective proteins result in an abnormally high absorption of plant sterols (and to a lesser extent, cholesterol) into the enterocyte and decreased excretion of these sterols from the liver into the bile. Plasma cholesterol can be mildly, moderately, or markedly elevated—whereas plant sterol concentrations in the plasma are markedly increased.[25,26] Patients with phytosterolemia

TABLE 20-2

Pediatric Lipoprotein Disorders*

Lipoprotein Disorder	Lipoprotein Analysis	Blood Lipids
Familial hypercholesterolemia	↑↑ LDL	↑↑ Cholesterol
Autosomal recessive hypercholesterolemia	↑↑ LDL	↑↑ Cholesterol
Familial ligand-defective apoB-100	↑↑ LDL	↑↑ Cholesterol
Phytosterolemia	↑ LDL	↑ Cholesterol
Familial combined hyperlipidemia	↑ VLDL, ↑ LDL, ↓ HDL	↑ Cholesterol, ↑ triglycerides
Familial hypertriglyceridemia	↑↑ VLDL, ↓ HDL	↑ Triglycerides
Familial lipoprotein lipase deficiency	↑↑ Chylomicrons	↑↑ Triglycerides
Hypoalphalipoproteinemia	↓ HDL	Normal
Dysbetalipoproteinemia	↑↑ Chylomicron remnants, ↑↑ IDL	↑↑ Cholesterol, ↑↑ triglycerides

* ↑↑ very high; ↑ moderately elevated; and ↓ decreased.

develop premature CAD, xanthomas in childhood, and may develop aortic stenosis.[25,27]

DISORDERS OF OVERPRODUCTION OF VLDL

Familial combined hyperlipidemia (FCHL) is an autosomal-dominant disorder with variable phenotypic expression, even within members of the same family.[28] In most cases of FCHL, the disorder is caused by an overproduction of VLDL in the liver, a reduction in fatty acid uptake and retention by adipose tissue, and a decreased clearance of chylomicron remnants. The most common lipoprotein pattern is high LDL cholesterol, high triglycerides, and low HDL cholesterol.[29] LDL particles tend to be small and dense. The prevalence of this disorder is estimated to be 0.5% to 1% of the adult population.[21]

Several studies identify FCHL as three times as common in clinical practice as FH.[30,31] FCHL is diagnosed based on a primary hyperlipidemia, including hypercholesterolemia and/or hypertriglyceridemia; multiple lipoprotein phenotypes within a family; and a positive family history of premature CHD.[21] Tendon xanthomas are usually not present in patients with FCHL. Patients with FCHL often have concurrent problems with insulin resistance, central obesity, and hypertension—and are at an increased risk of premature cardiovascular disease.[28]

Syndromes with a similar phenotype are hyperapobetalipoproteinemia, LDL subclass pattern B, and the metabolic syndrome.[29,32-34] Of the three, the latter syndrome is much more prevalent in children. Rates of metabolic syndrome are continuing to rise with the prevalence of obesity in the pediatric population.[34] There appears to be a mechanistic link between central obesity, insulin resistance, and dyslipidemia—with central obesity generally preceding both glucose and lipid abnormalities.

DISORDERS OF MARKED HYPERTRIGLYCERIDEMIA

Familial Hypertriglyceridemia

Familial hypertriglyceridemia (FHTG) follows an autosomal-dominant inheritance pattern expressed predominantly in adulthood. However, the prevalence in children is increasing.[9] Obesity is an important factor that can expedite the expression of FHTG, and patients often have concurrent glucose intolerance. The phenotype for FHTG is moderate to markedly high serum triglycerides and low to normal LDL and HDL cholesterol levels. The metabolic cause of the disorder is hepatic secretion of large triglyceride-rich VLDL particles that are catabolized slowly.[28] The fundamental genetic defect for FHTG has not been identified.

Familial Lipoprotein Lipase Deficiency

Familial lipoprotein lipase (FLPL) deficiency is rare. The disorder is expressed as elevated serum chylomicron levels due to diminished or absent hydrolysis of chylomicron associated triglycerides by lipoprotein lipase.[28] In the heterozygous state, patients have low to moderate

levels of chylomicron catabolism and levels of serum triglycerides that range from 200 to 750 mg/dL.[9]

In patients in the homozygous state, serum triglycerides can reach 10,000 mg/dL or higher.[35] Blood from patients with homozygous FLPL has a viscous, creamy appearance due to the presence of large numbers of chylomicron particles. Risk for pancreatitis is increased in the homozygous state due to the markedly elevated serum triglycerides. In addition, eruptive xanthomas and neurologic symptoms may be apparent. The gene for LPL has been located on chromosome 8p22, and more than 50 different mutations have been identified in patients with FLPL.[36]

HYPOLIPIDEMIAS

Low HDL Cholesterol

In clinical practice, patients with low HDL cholesterol levels commonly have concurrent high triglycerides, with or without elevations in small dense LDL cholesterol.[37-39] These patients are usually obese, and the mechanistic explanation for this dyslipidemic triad is VLDL overproduction. Less common are familial disorders of HDL, including familial hypoalphalipoproteinemia, mutations of the apoA-1 protein, and Tangier disease. These disorders are characterized by low HDL level with no other lipid abnormality. Familial hypoalphalipoproteinemia follows an autosomal-dominant inheritance pattern.[9] ApoA-1 levels are also often low due to decreased production of HDL.

A number of mutations have been described in the apoA-1 gene and are associated with low HDL cholesterol and low apoA-1.[40,41] Tangier disease is due to mutations in the ABCI gene.[42,43] Patients affected by this disease are not able to actively withdraw cholesterol from cells onto nascent HDL particles, causing rapid degradation of the nascent HDL. ApoA-1 is rapidly cleared before it is able to acquire cholesterol.[43] In Tangier disease, HDL cholesterol levels are close to zero and the apoA-1 levels are less than 5 mg/dL. The risk of premature CAD in these patients is mild to moderate.[9]

Abetalipoproteinemia

Abetalipoproteinemia is associated with low serum cholesterol (<50 mg/dL) and triglycerides (2-45 mg/dL). Patients with this disorder present with steatorrhea and fatty liver. Without treatment, ataxia follows (with acanthocytosis and retinitis pigmentosis). Abetalipoproteinemia is caused by a defect in MTP.[28] Without MTP, no chylomicrons, VLDL, or LDL appear in the plasma. In these patients, HDL takes over as the primary cholesterol carrier. Thus, the defect is not fatal. Because of significant fat malabsorption, fat-soluble vitamin status is impaired.

In particular, because vitamin E absorption and cellular uptake require chylomicron and LDL transport, high doses of vitamin E are required to prevent retinal and sensory neuron degeneration. Additional dietary considerations include restricting long-chain dietary triglycerides to less than 15 g/day to alleviate the steatorrhea. Medium-chain triglycerides (MCT oils) can be used as an alternative source of energy.[44]

Hypobetalipoproteinemia

Hypobetalipoproteinemia is an autosomal-dominant disorder resulting from a defect in the apoB gene that produces a truncated apolipoprotein B.[28] Cholesterol levels in patients with heterozygous hypobetalipoproteinemia are usually 50% of those of an unaffected family member. The heterozygous form of this condition is benign. However, homozygous hypobetalipoproteinemia is associated with severe hypocholesterolemia, significant steatorrhea, fatty liver, acanthocytosis retinopathy, and peripheral neuropathy. Dietary considerations are the same as for patients with abetalipoproteinemia.[44]

DISORDERS WITH LIPOPROTEIN CLEARANCE VIA apoE PATHWAYS

Dysbetalipoproteinemia is characterized by elevated cholesterol and triglyceride levels.[28] The disorder results from the presence of a polymorphism of the apoE allele (apoE2, rather than the more common apoE3) along with the gene for FCHL.[44] Metabolically, this defect results in poor uptake of remnant particles and abnormal remnant catabolism because of the abnormal apoE. Increased remnants, VLDL, chylomicrons, and apoE are all present. Xanthomas may occur, and premature CAD has been reported. This lipoprotein disorder is rare in children and often presents in young adulthood.[28]

Secondary Causes

Secondary dyslipidemias can result from a variety of diseases and conditions (see Table 20-3 for a list). In the United States, the most prevalent cause of secondary dyslipidemia is overweight and obesity.[45] The dyslipidemic triad (namely, elevated triglycerides and small

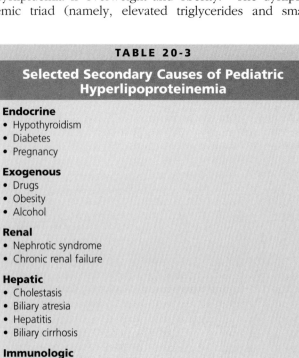

TABLE 20-3

Selected Secondary Causes of Pediatric Hyperlipoproteinemia

Endocrine
- Hypothyroidism
- Diabetes
- Pregnancy

Exogenous
- Drugs
- Obesity
- Alcohol

Renal
- Nephrotic syndrome
- Chronic renal failure

Hepatic
- Cholestasis
- Biliary atresia
- Hepatitis
- Biliary cirrhosis

Immunologic
- HIV infection/AIDS

dense LDL and low HDL cholesterol) is commonly associated with overweight (in particular, with central adiposity).[45,46] In addition to dyslipidemia, insulin resistance and elevated blood pressure may be present. This cluster of abnormalities characterizes the metabolic syndrome and is associated with increased cardiovascular disease risk.[47,48] The prevalence of metabolic syndrome appears to be increasing in children and adolescents, along with the prevalence of obesity.[47] The primary approach to treating this disorder is weight management.

Metabolic lipid perturbations in adult patients with type 1 and 2 diabetes mellitus are similar to those found in patients with the metabolic syndrome, but often are more severe.[49] Generally in adults with diabetes, triglycerides are elevated and HDL-cholesterol is low—and LDL cholesterol can be normal or mildly or moderately elevated. Diabetes in adults is considered a CHD risk equivalent according to the National Cholesterol Education Program (NCEP). This means that the risk for developing CAD in patients with poorly controlled diabetes is equivalent to those with established CHD.[50] For this reason, the NCEP recommends aggressive treatment of dyslipidemia in adult patients with diabetes.

Although type 1 diabetes is currently the main form of diabetes seen in children, in the United States a growing number of patients with type 2 diabetes are under the age of 18 years.[51] Change in the prevalence of type 2 diabetes in youth is likely related to the growing obesity epidemic occurring in the pediatric population.[51,52] Data on lipid concentrations in children and adolescents with diabetes are few, particularly in those with type 2 diabetes. The Search for Diabetes in Youth Study assessed the prevalence of serum lipid abnormalities among a representative sample of U.S. children and adolescents with type 1 and type 2 diabetes.[53]

Findings from this study showed a substantial number of diabetic children over the age of 10 years with abnormal serum lipids: nearly 50% had an LDL cholesterol level above the optimal level of 100 mg/dL. For children with type 2 diabetes, 37% had elevated triglyceride levels and 44% had low HDL cholesterol. These data highlight the importance of serum lipid screening in children with diabetes. Recommended approaches to managing dyslipidemia in children and adolescents with diabetes are discussed later in the chapter.

Other causes of secondary dyslipidemia include hypothyroidism, nephrotic syndrome, other renal diseases, liver diseases, and infection.[54] Dylipidemias can also result from the ingestion of a variety of medications. These medications include progestins, estrogens, androgens, anabolic steroids, corticosteroids, cyclosporine, and retinoids. Secondary causes of dyslipidemias should be identified by patient historical data and a careful physical examination. Laboratory tests (including thyroid, renal, and liver function panels) would confirm the diagnosis.

The risk of development of atherosclerosis with these conditions is unknown but is likely proportionate to the length of exposure and extent of elevation in serum LDL cholesterol levels. Cardiovascular disease is common in patients with chronic renal insufficiency.[55] The treatment of dyslipidemia in patients with secondary causes is focused on managing the underlying disease. Diet and physical activity changes may also be recommended to reduce elevated LDL cholesterol and triglyceride levels.

Vascular Changes and Dyslipidemia

It is well established that elevated concentrations of total cholesterol and LDL cholesterol in adult life are strong and reversible risk factors for CAD.[50] Whether dyslipidemia in childhood contributes to atherosclerotic lesions in coronary and other arteries has been a subject of debate, but accumulating evidence from pathologic and in vivo imaging studies favors a relationship. Atherosclerotic lesions result from deposits of lipid and cholesterol in the intima of the arterial wall.[56] Early lesions, called fatty streaks, are formed from the accumulation of macrophages filled with lipid droplets (foam cells).

Fatty streaks do not disorganize the normal structure of the intima and do not deform or obstruct the artery, and are in themselves not considered harmful.[57] However, some continue to accumulate macrophage foam cells and extracellular lipid and smooth muscle cells—forming raised plaques. From these, more advanced lesions may develop—with further deposition of extracellular lipid, cholesterol crystals, collagen, and potentially calcium.[58] It is these raised lesions that result in a myocardial infarction because of their increasing size and obstruction of the arterial lumen or because of rupture of the fibrous plaque, which results in the release of thrombogenic substances from the necrotic core.[56]

Pathobiologic studies of the coronary arteries of young individuals who died from causes unrelated to heart disease have been useful in documenting the progression of atherosclerosis by age and risk factor determinants. Stary et al. studied more than 500 postmortem samples of coronary arteries from persons younger than 30 years of age and found presence of fatty streaks in the majority of children less than 9 years of age, raised lesions in about half of adolescents, and more advanced lesions in about a third of the young adults studied.[59] In 93 autopsies of young adults for whom childhood risk factor data were available, Berenson and colleagues found that the extent of the surface of arteries covered with fatty streaks and fibrous plaques was positively associated with LDL cholesterol, triglycerides, blood pressure, and body mass index and negatively associated with HDL cholesterol levels in childhood.[60]

The Pathobiological Determinants of Atherosclerosis in Youth (PDAY) study reached similar conclusions from examination of more than 3,000 postmortem samples of coronary arteries of young adults who died from noncardiovascular events and who likewise had a variety of antimortem risk factor measures available.[61] In general, pathology studies have made important contributions to the identification of risk factors for early aspects of the atherosclerotic process. In conjunction with findings from longitudinal studies such as the Framingham Heart Study (in which risk factor assessments of participants preceded the development of cardiovascular disease)[62] a group of risk factors, often referred to as the traditional risk factors

for CAD, has been established. A complete list of pediatric risk factors for CAD is found in Table 20-4.

Recent advances in vascular imaging technology have provided a means of measuring early pathologic changes and functional abnormalities against coronary and other arteries in response to adverse changes in cardiovascular disease risk factors. The advantage in using this technology is that walls of superficial arteries can be imaged noninvasively in real time at high resolution, and changes to the arterial wall can be measured as a continuous variable from childhood to adulthood in patients with and without presence of risk factors for CVD.[63] Computed tomography (CT) scanning is considered one of the most sensitive noninvasive tools for imaging the extent and location of coronary artery calcium present in atheroma.[64]

The presence of coronary artery calcium has been associated with adverse cardiovascular disease outcomes in adults.[65] In adolescents, small studies have shown associations among hypercholesterolemia, BMI, and significant coronary artery calcium. In the Muscatine Study (in which participants were assessed for CVD risk factors during their school-age years and later assessed for cardiovascular changes by CT scan), 31% of men and 10% of women aged 29 to 37 years had significant coronary artery calcification.[66] Childhood risk factors associated with calcification were obesity, increased blood pressure, and low HDL cholesterol.

Vascular ultrasound imaging has been utilized to assess alterations in brachial artery flow-mediated dilation, which is a measure of endothelial function, and carotid intima-media thickness (IMT).[64] In adults, both measures have been associated with adverse changes in traditional cardiovascular disease risk factors,[67] respond to normalization of risk factors,[68] and are considered important early markers for the progression of atherosclerotic disease.[67-70] Although few studies have used ultrasound technology to evaluate coronary arteries in the young, children with hypercholesterolemia have been assessed using these measures and have been found to have abnormalities of carotid IMT and brachial artery vasodilation.[71-73]

Further, in young adults aged 33 to 42 years who had comprehensive risk factor assessments performed some 25 years prior Davis et al.[74] found an association between mean carotid IMT and elevations in total cholesterol and triglyceride concentrations during childhood. Lavrencic et al.[75] found that the mean carotid IMT was significantly

TABLE 20-4

Pediatric Risk Factors for Coronary Artery Disease

- Elevated LDL cholesterol (>130 mg/dL)
- Family history of premature (aged <55 years) coronary heart disease, CVD, or peripheral vascular disease
- Smoking
- Hypertension
- Low HDL cholesterol (<35 mg/dL)
- Obesity [>95th percentile weight for height on National Center for Health Statistics (NCH) growth chart]
- Physical inactivity
- Diabetes

greater in youth with FH compared with those in a control group—as well as being significantly greater in all subjects in regard to total cholesterol, LDL cholesterol, and systolic blood pressure. Similar risk factors have been associated with impaired vasodilation, indicating endothelial dysfunction.[76-78]

In summary, these studies confirm the utility of vascular imaging for detecting early pathologic and functional changes to coronary vessels and associations with modifiable CVD risk factors in the young. Clinically, vascular imaging by ultrasound may be a valuable means of estimating the benefit of treating multiple CVD risk factors in children and adolescents. CT scans may be less useful in younger patients because calcium depositions are uncommon before young adulthood.

Screening for Lipid Disorders

ROUTINE SCREENING

Data from pathologic and, more recently, in vivo imaging studies (as discussed previously) support the screening and treatment of children and adolescents with elevated LDL cholesterol levels and other risk factors. For more than a decade, pediatric guidelines established by the NCEP have provided the standard of care with respect to lipid screening and treatment of dyslipidemia in childhood.[79] An algorithm summarizing these diagnostic and therapeutic guidelines is presented in Figure 20-3. In brief, the guidelines recommend targeted blood choles-

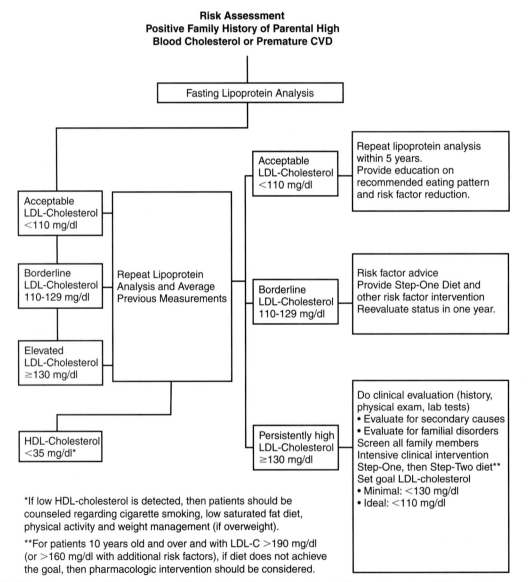

*If low HDL-cholesterol is detected, then patients should be counseled regarding cigarette smoking, low saturated fat diet, physical activity and weight management (if overweight).

**For patients 10 years old and over and with LDL-C >190 mg/dl (or >160 mg/dl with additional risk factors), if diet does not achieve the goal, then pharmacologic intervention should be considered.

Figure 20-3 Child treatment algorithm based on LDL cholesterol levels. [Reprinted with permission from Williams CL, Hayman LL, Daniles SR, Robinson TN, Steinberger J, Paridon S, et al. (2002). Cardiovascular health in childhood: A statement for health professionals from the Committee on Atherosclerosis, Hypertension, and Obesity in the Young (AHOY) of the Council on Cardiovascular Disease in the Young, American Heart Association. Circulation 106:143-160.]

terol screening if a child or adolescent has a parent with hypercholesterolemia (total cholesterol >240 mg/dL) or if a child has a parent or grandparent <55 years of age who has documented CVD.

CVD is defined as angina pectoris, myocardial infarction, established coronary atherosclerosis, peripheral vascular disease, cerebrovascular disease, or sudden cardiac death. Lipid screening of children with multiple risk factors for future CVD (e.g., smoking, hypertension, obesity, diabetes, poor diet quality, and sedentary lifestyle) is recommended by the NCEP. Screening children whose family histories are unknown is discretionary.

A fasting (12-hour) lipoprotein analysis is recommended for screening a child. A fasting lipoprotein analysis allows quantification of total cholesterol, HDL cholesterol, triglycerides, and calculation of LDL cholesterol. The Friedewald equation [LDL cholesterol = (total cholesterol − HDL cholesterol) − triglycerides/5] can be used to calculate LDL cholesterol as long as the serum triglyceride level is <400 mg/dL.[80] Direct measurement of LDL cholesterol concentration is available through some commercial laboratories and is indicated for individuals whose fasting triglyceride level is >400 mg/dL.

The NCEP defines cut-points for total cholesterol and LDL cholesterol in children based on data from the National Health and Nutrition Examination Survey (NHANES), performed from 1988 to 1994. The 75th and 95th percentiles for lipid values from this survey were used to define "borderline" and "high" risk categories, respectively. Acceptable, borderline, and high risk values for total and LDL cholesterol are outlined in Table 20-5. If a lipoprotein analysis reveals LDL cholesterol to be borderline or high, a repeat test should be performed and the average value of the two tests considered for clinical decision making.[46]

Clinical evaluation of children and adolescents at high risk for CVD based on LDL cholesterol levels should include careful review of the patient's medical and family history and physical examination to identify additional risk factors and secondary causes of dyslipidemia. Assessment should include the following: review of past medical or family history for hypertension, diabetes mellitus, medica-

tion use, obesity, poor dietary habits (including excessive intake of saturated fat), sedentary behavior, and tobacco use; measurement of height, weight, and calculation of BMI; Tanner staging to assess pubertal growth; blood pressure measurement; physical inspection of skin, eyes, and tendons for lipid deposition and palpitation of the thyroid gland and liver for signs of enlargement; and laboratory tests (including thyroid, renal, and liver function panels). Glucose and insulin levels should be measured to assess for the presence of metabolic syndrome or diabetes.

Several limitations have been identified regarding the NCEP guidelines for the identification of children and adolescents at high risk for CVD. First, several studies have noted that selectively screening children and adolescents for elevated cholesterol based on parental history may be inadequate to identify a substantial proportion of the population with elevated LDL levels.[81-83] In general, studies have shown that approximately 30% to 60% of pediatric patients with elevated cholesterol would be missed using the NCEP screening approach based on family history.[82,83] A second limitation is that current guidelines give no significant consideration to variation in LDL cholesterol level according to race, gender, age, and level of sexual maturation.

There is considerable variation in LDL cholesterol with age during growth and development. This is especially true during the period of puberty.[84,85] Total and LDL cholesterol levels tend to decline during puberty, meaning that some adolescents will appear normal when in fact they will have elevated levels after puberty. A third limitation is that guidelines were published at a time when the epidemic of overweight and obesity was not yet obvious, and the guidelines do not address screening for low HDL cholesterol and high triglycerides. Recent data from pathobiologic and vascular imaging studies show adverse changes in vascular structure and function in adulthood related to low HDL cholesterol and high triglyceride levels in childhood. These data support pediatric assessment of triglyceride and HDL cholesterol levels. The American Heart Association[86] has recommended that triglyceride levels >130 mg/dL and HDL cholesterol levels <35 mg/dL be considered abnormal for children and adolescents (Table 20-5).

GENETIC TESTING

Increasingly, DNA-based tests are being used to confirm the diagnosis of FH in patients with a family member who has a mutation or in a young patient with high LDL cholesterol with tendon xanthomas or atherosclerotic disease.[87] Currently, three genes (LDLR, APOB, PCSK9) have been identified in association with mutations that cause this disorder.[88] In addition to LDLR, most laboratories test for the apolipoprotein B gene r500Q mutation. Rapid and relatively inexpensive methods have been developed to test a selected subset of the LDLR mutations. However, more expensive "complete gene scans" are needed for mutation-negative samples.[88] Once a mutation is identified, testing of relatives can be performed rapidly and cheaply.

At present, it is unclear whether knowledge of specific mutations will lead to improved treatment. Several studies have shown that the degree of cholesterol lowering

TABLE 20-5			
Normal Plasma Lipid and Lipoprotein Concentrations for Children and Adolescents*			
Category	Acceptable	Borderline	High
Total cholesterol	<170	170-199	≥200
LDL cholesterol	<110	110-129	≥130
Triglycerides			
0-9 years	<75	75-99	≥100
10-19 years	<90	90-129	≥130
Category	Acceptable	Borderline	Low
HDL cholesterol	>45	35-45	<35

LDL, low-density lipoprotein; and HDL, high-density lipoprotein.

* Values for plasma lipids and lipoproteins are from the National Cholesterol Education Program Expert Panel on Cholesterol Levels in Children.

achieved by statins is influenced by the type of mutation (e.g., individuals with the APOB r3500Q mutation showed a strong positive response to statin therapy).[89,90] In addition, the diagnosis of FH based on genetic testing improved uptake and adherence to treatment in several studies.[91,92] Concerns about long-term benefits and side effects from life-long treatment for identified children remain. As progress in this area continues, current treatment algorithms may need modification to describe the role of genetic testing in clinical practice.

Diet Therapy in Managing Dyslipidemia

The NCEP guidelines outline a two-pronged approach to managing pediatric hypercholesterolemia: one geared to the population in general and the second to individualized treatment of elevated LDL cholesterol levels in high-risk patients. The population-based approach stipulates that all children older than 2 years of age should consume a low-fat diet, referred to as the Step 1 diet.[79] This recommendation is viewed as a primary preventive measure to reduce serum lipids, thereby reducing risk of CAD in the pediatric population at large. The individual patient approach recommends that all children and adolescents with elevated LDL cholesterol first be treated with the Step 1 diet.

If after 3 to 6 months of dietary compliance LDL cholesterol levels remain abnormal further restriction of dietary saturated fat and cholesterol, referred to as the Step 2 diet, is recommended. Repeated studies have shown that this stepwise dietary approach to lowering LDL cholesterol levels is safe and efficacious in children with hypercholesterolemia.[93-95] The nutrient composition of the Step 1 diet is 30% or less of calories from total fat, less than 10% of calories from saturated fat, and less than 300 mg/day of cholesterol—with adequate energy to support growth and development.[79] The dietary restriction on total fat is not intended to be a daily recommendation but rather averaged over several days.[96]

Further, these recommendations are not intended for children younger than 2 years of age because infants and young children are thought to require a higher level of dietary saturated fat and cholesterol to support development of the central nervous system. To prevent overzealous implementation of a very-low-fat diet for children with high cholesterol, which could lead to failure to thrive,[97] the American Academy of Pediatrics (AAP) recently set a lower limit for percentage of energy from fat at 20% of calories.[98] In most cases, with dietary compliance the Step 1 diet should normalize borderline-high LDL cholesterol levels. The reported response to the diet in children with LDL cholesterol levels <130 mg/dL has ranged from 3% to 10%.[46,99]

For children with persistently high LDL cholesterol levels, further reduction of dietary saturated fatty acids and cholesterol is recommended. Specifically, the Step 2 diet calls for restricting saturated fat intake to <7% of calories and cholesterol to <200 mg/day.[79] Based on clinical evidence, these dietary restrictions should achieve an additional LDL cholesterol reduction of 4% to 14%.[100,101]

However, the extent to which LDL cholesterol is lowered may depend on previous dietary intake and baseline LDL cholesterol levels.

To achieve the NCEP dietary goals for saturated fat and cholesterol, key sources of these nutrients must be the focus of intervention. Foods high in saturated fat and cholesterol include red meats, poultry with skin, whole-milk dairy products, and egg yolks. The NCEP recommends that red meats be limited to modest amounts of lean cuts (e.g., 5-6 oz per day) and that dairy products be limited to skim or low-fat varieties (24-32 oz/day).[79] Skin should be removed from chicken and turkey, and intake limited to white meat. Processed meats should contain no more than 3 g of fat per serving, and egg yolks should be limited to 4 per week, on the Step 1 diet (2 egg yolks per week on the Step 2 diet). Oils used in cooking should be unsaturated, and soft margarines used in place of butter. Table 20-6 highlights some additional practical dietary strategies for lowering saturated fat and cholesterol in the diets of the young.

To ensure children prescribed low-fat diets consume adequate calories and nutrients to support growth and development, high-fat foods omitted from the diet should be replaced with lower-fat versions of the same. For example, whole-milk dairy products contribute calcium, phosphorus, and protein to the diet—along with substantial amounts of saturated fat and cholesterol. Children should be encouraged to replace whole-milk dairy foods with low-fat or nonfat milk, yogurt, cottage cheese, and frozen desserts to ensure overall nutrient adequacy. Breads, cereals, grains, fruits, and vegetables should comprise the largest proportion of energy in children's diets. Most choices within these food groups are low in fat, cholesterol free, and high in fiber—and will help displace energy sources containing saturated fat. Children should be encouraged to choose 6 to 10 servings of whole-grain cereals, breads, and pasta and to consume at least five servings of fruits and vegetables per day.

TABLE 20-6

Practical Dietary Strategies for Lowering Saturated Fat and Cholesterol

- Eat 5 to 9 servings of fresh, frozen, or canned fruits and vegetables daily.
- Use vegetable oils and soft margarines low in saturated fat and trans fatty acids instead of butter or most other animal fats in the diet.
- Eat whole-grain breads and cereals rather than processed grain products.
- Use nonfat (skim) or low-fat milk and dairy products daily.
- Eat more fish, especially oily fish (broiled or baked).
- Eat lean cuts of meat, and trim any obvious fat from red meat before cooking.
- Take the skin off chicken or turkey and eat only the white meat.
- Avoid processed meats such as hotdogs, sausage, and bologna.
- Avoid creams or sauces made with butter or whole-milk dairy products.
- Choose low-fat snacks such as ginger snaps, graham crackers, pretzels, plain popcorn, animal crackers, and vanilla wafers.
- Use recommended portion sizes on food labels when preparing and serving food.

Although pediatric dietary recommendations do not include specific guidelines for lowering serum triglycerides or raising HDL cholesterol, diets containing high levels of sucrose and excess calories have been associated with adverse changes in these lipids/lipoproteins.[102] For this reason, children should be counseled to reduce intake of simple sugars from processed foods such as cookies and desserts, and limit intake of sugared beverages. Weight management should be a goal of diet therapy for children with a BMI >85th percentile.

Weight reduction approaches should focus on decreasing the child's weight-for-height percentile while maintaining linear growth.[101] Although weight loss may temporarily lower HDL cholesterol, weight stabilization at a new lower level will lead to a gradual increase in HDL cholesterol over time.[103] Moderate caloric restriction can be achieved by following the Step 1 diet. Increased physical activity should be encouraged, and sedentary activities (such as television viewing and playing computer and video games) should be limited to no more than 2 hours per day.

Pharmacologic Management

For many children with moderately or severely elevated LDL cholesterol, diet alone will not lower their cholesterol levels to the acceptable or even borderline range. Long-term drug therapy is associated with decreased incidence of heart disease and overall mortality in adults.[50] However, no studies directly demonstrate the efficacy of administering lipid-lowering drug therapy in children to prevent CAD. In addition, long-term safety studies for some of the newer medications have not been performed.

The pediatric panel of the NCEP recommends using medication only in patients who are at least 10 years of age and whose post-dietary LDL cholesterol level is >190 mg/dL or whose LDL cholesterol level is >160 mg/dL with a family history of early CVD, with two or more risk factors for CVD, or with the metabolic syndrome present (Figure 20-3). A follow-up LDL cholesterol assessment is recommended 6 weeks after starting drug therapy, and every 3 months thereafter until LDL cholesterol goals are met. Thereafter, follow-up can be less frequent.

For children in general, the goal for LDL cholesterol is <130 mg/dL. For children with diabetes, the goal for LDL cholesterol is <100 mg/dL.[104,105] The lower LDL cholesterol goal for children with diabetes reflects a synthesis of pediatric guidelines and treatment recommendations for adults with diabetes that now consider the presence of diabetes a coronary heart disease risk equivalent.[50] Table 20-7 summarizes the recommendations of the American Diabetes Association for lipid screening and management of children and youth with diabetes. Medications used in the treatment of specific lipid abnormalities are summarized in Table 20-8 and are reviewed in the material following.

BILE ACID BINDING AGENTS

Bile acid binding agents lower serum cholesterol indirectly by binding with bile acids in the gastrointestinal tract. This action prevents their reabsorption into the enterohepatic circulation, resulting in their loss from the body and removal from the cholesterol pool.[106] To compensate for this loss, the liver increases endogenous cholesterol synthesis and up-regulates LDL-receptor synthesis—thereby lowering LDL cholesterol levels in the blood. In bile-acid resin trials in children, a dose of 8 g/day while on a cholesterol-lowering diet resulted in a decrease in LDL cholesterol ranging from 10% to 20%.[107,108]

TABLE 20-7

American Diabetes Recommendations for Management of Children and Adolescents with Diabetes*

	Type 1 Diabetes	Type 2 Diabetes
Screening	After glycemic control	
	>2 years at diagnosis if other CVD risk factors; otherwise at 12 years; if normal, rescreen every 5 years	At diagnosis regardless of age; if normal, rescreen every 2 years
Lipid goals	LDL <100 mg/dL	
	HDL >35 mg/dL	
	Triglycerides <150 mg/dL	
Treatment strategies	Glycemic control	
	Diet	
	Physical activity	
	Weight reduction if appropriate	
	Medication indications if initial management fails:	
	• Age >10 years	
	• If LDL >160 mg/dL	
	• If LDL 130–159 mg/dL consider based on CVD risk profile	
	• Statins with or without resins	
	• Fibrates if TG >1,000 mg/dL	
	• Manage other CVD risk factors (Table 20-4) if appropriate	

* Recommendations are from the American Diabetes Association. American Diabetes Association (2005). Standards of medical care in diabetes. Diabetes Care 28(1):S4–S36.

TABLE 20-8

Drugs Used in the Treatment of Pediatric Lipid Disorders

Class of Medication	Common Name	Starting Daily Dose	Change in Lipid Profile	Adverse Effects
Bile acid binding agents	Cholestyramine	80 mg/kg	↓ LDL	Constipation
	Colestipol	5 g	↑ TG	Abdominal cramping
HMG Co-A reductase inhibitors*	Atorvastatin	10 mg	↓ LDL	Dyspepsia
	Simvastatin	5 mg	↓ TG	↑ Liver transaminases
	Pravastatin	10 mg	↑ HDL	↑ CK
	Rosuvastatin	5 mg		Myositis
	Lovastatin	10 mg		
	Fluvastatin	20 mg		
Fibrates*	Bezafibrate	200 mg TID	↓ TG	Constipation
	Clofibrate	500 mg BID	↑ HDL	Myositis
	Fenofibrate	48 mg		Anemia
	Gemfibrozil	600 mg BID		
Niacin*	Niaspan	500 mg @ HS	↓ LDL	Flushing
			↓ TG	Headache
			↑ HDL	↑ Liver transaminases
Cholesterol absorption blocker*	Ezetimibe	10 mg	↓ LDL	Not reported in children or adolescents

* Long-term safety and efficacy has not been established in children and adolescents.
CK = creatine kinase; LDL = low density lipoprotein; TG = triglycerides; and HDL = high-density lipoproteins.

Bile-acid resins come in powder and tablet form. The powder is usually taken twice daily (4-g scoop) mixed with water or juice. Resins in this form tend to be gritty in texture and children complain that they are unpleasant to drink. Tablets are more palatable, but are large and difficult for some children to swallow. Overall, studies report poor to fair compliance with the medication.[106,109] Side effects are few and are mainly gastrointestinal in nature, including constipation and gas. These can be minimized with increased intake of water and fiber. Resins may increase triglyceride levels and may interfere with the absorption of certain medications and fat-soluble vitamins.[110] Supplementation with a multivitamin and folate (1 mg daily) is usually recommended.[106]

HMG-CoA REDUCTASE INHIBITORS

HMG-CoA reductase inhibitors (also known as statins) lower LDL cholesterol in the blood by blocking hepatic HMG Co-A reductase, the rate-limiting enzyme in cholesterol biosynthesis.[111] This action depletes the intracellular cholesterol pool, leading to an up-regulation of LDL receptors and a decrease in serum cholesterol. Doses ranging from 5 to 40 mg/day have resulted in a 20% to 40% lowering of LDL cholesterol, and slight increases in HDL cholesterol levels have been reported in children.[112-114]

In vivo imaging studies have demonstrated improvements in surrogate markers for atherosclerosis with statin therapy. Reversal of endothelial dysfunction and regression of carotid IMT have been reported in children treated with statins over a 2-year period.[115,116] This latter finding suggests that initiation of lipid-lowering statins in childhood may inhibit progression or might even lead to regression of atherosclerosis.

Adverse effects of the medication are few but have included GI complaints, elevated liver transaminase and creatine kinase (CK) levels, and myositits.[106,110,115] For this reason, statins would not be recommended for patients with liver disease. Follow-up of patients treated with statins should include laboratory assessment of liver transaminase and CK levels and identification of adverse physical symptoms such as muscle cramps.

Because statins are potentially teratogenic, it is essential that physicians determine that adolescent girls are not pregnant or likely to become pregnant before initiating therapy.[106] The longest statin trials have been 2 years in length. Thus, whether statins adversely affect long-term growth and development and are safe for lifelong use has not been ascertained. Longer-term safety and efficacy studies are needed, particularly with follow-up of vascular endpoints.

INHIBITORS OF CHOLESTEROL ABSORPTION

Ezetimibe is a new cholesterol-lowering agent that prevents the absorption of cholesterol and plant sterols by inhibiting the passage of sterols across the intestinal wall.[117] The reduction in cholesterol absorption leads to a decrease in hepatic cholesterol uptake and availability. As a result, there is a compensatory increase in hepatic cholesterol biosynthesis, an up-regulation of LDL receptor expression, and an overall decrease in blood LDL cholesterol levels.

In adult trials, a daily intake of 10 mg/day reduced LDL cholesterol by approximately 18%.[117-120] Although Ezetimibe has already been approved for children older than 10 years who have FH, it has not been adequately studied in this group of patients. Such studies are needed to confirm adult findings and to assess the safety and efficacy of this medication for use in children and adolescents.

FIBRIC ACID DERIVATIVES

Fibric acid derivatives (also known as fibrates) lower blood triglyceride levels by reducing the hepatic production of VLDL.[106,117] The drug also increases the production of apoA-I, resulting in higher HDL cholesterol levels. Side effects are similar to those for statins and include GI complaints, elevated liver transaminase activity, and myopathy.[106] For this reason, fibrates are not recommended for used with statins. No cut-points for initiating fibrate therapy in children and adolescents have been established. Because the major risk of elevated triglyceride (pancreatitis) does not increase until triglycerides levels reach 750 to 1,000 mg/dL, many experts recommend withholding fibrate use in children until the triglycerides are persistently >350 mg/dL or a random level is >700 mg/dL.[106]

NIACIN

Niacin decreases hepatic VLDL production, leading to decreased production of LDL cholesterol.[106,117] Children with heterozygous FH treated with 1,000 to 2,250 mg of niacin daily over an average of 8 months showed a 23% to 30% reduction in LDL cholesterol.[120] However, 76% of the children had adverse effects from therapy (e.g., flushing, headache, nausea, glucose intolerance, myopathy, abnormal liver function) and 38% discontinued the drug. Niacin is generally not used to treat children with FH unless LDL cholesterol is persistently elevated or unusual hypertriglyceridemia and low HDL cholesterol are present.[106] Niacin given in combination with statins has been used to treat homozygous FH. Niacin is available in immediate and slow-release forms (Niaspan, Slo-Niacin).

DIETARY ADDITIVES AND SUPPLEMENTS

Plant sterols and stanols consumed at levels of 2 g per day have been shown to reduce LDL cholesterol levels by 9% to 20% in adults.[50] Foods containing these additives (e.g., margarines and salad dressings) lower serum cholesterol by preventing dietary cholesterol absorption in the gastrointestinal tract.[121] In children with familial hypercholesterolemia, use of 2 g/day of plant sterols decreased LDL cholesterol by 14% but did not improve endothelial function.[122] This suggests that LDL cholesterol must be reduced to a certain threshold level before improvement of endothelial function can occur.

More studies examining the long-term effects of plant sterols on the vascular endothelium are warranted. Concern has been raised about the potential for the malabsorption of fat and fat-soluble vitamins in children consuming plant sterols chronically. The AHA recommends reserving the use of foods supplemented with plant sterols/stanols to children with moderate to severe elevation in cholesterol, and monitoring fat-soluble vitamin status.[123]

Dietary supplements containing soluble fiber, garlic, and omega-3 fatty acids have been used to treat pediatric hyperlipidemia with unremarkable findings. In a randomized controlled trial, Dennison et al.[124] studied the effect of psyllium fiber versus placebo on change in blood cholesterol levels of 5- to 17-year-old children. Psyllium fiber (6 g/d) and the placebo were added to a ready-to-eat cereal. Although compliance was excellent, there were no significant effects of the added psyllium on total, LDL, or HDL cholesterol levels over a 5-week period. Garlic extract therapy (300 mg × 3 doses per day) was studied in a randomized controlled trial for effects on serum lipoproteins in 8- to 18-year-old children with FH.[125]

Garlic extract was given in 3 daily doses of 300 mg versus a placebo for 8 weeks. No significant effects of garlic treatment versus placebo were noted on total, LDL, or HDL cholesterol. Omega-3 fatty acids, as found in fish oils, are known to reduce serum triglyceride levels in adults.[50] In a randomized crossover study, children with FH and FCH were supplemented with either 1.2 g/day of docosahexaenoic acid (DHA) or a placebo for 6 weeks.[126] All children were given counseling on the NCEP Step 2 diet. Outcomes studied included triglycerides, LDL and HDL-cholesterol, and endothelial function as measured by flow-mediated dilation (FMD) of the brachial artery.

Findings showed that DHA supplementation was associated with increased levels of total, LDL, and HDL cholesterol but no change in triglycerides compared to the placebo group. FMD improved significantly after DHA supplementation compared to baseline in both groups, and the change was greater in the DHA-treated group versus the controls. This finding suggests that in children DHA may not be effective for positively modifying serum lipids. However, the endothelium may be a therapeutic target for DHA in hyperlipidemic children.

Conclusions and Future Directions

Increasing evidence indicates that extreme elevation in LDL cholesterol is associated with vascular pathology in youth. Fortunately, appropriate therapy can reverse these changes. Pediatric clinical trials of lifestyle and drug therapy to treat lipid abnormalities suggest similar effectiveness and safety to that observed in adults. The majority of studies, however, have been short term in design. Longer-term safety and efficacy studies are needed, particularly with follow-up of vascular endpoints.

Few clinical data are available to document at what age drug therapy should be appropriately and safely started. More work is needed in this regard to support clinical judgments on what age and dosage should be used in children at high risk for CHD. Importantly, current diagnostic and treatment algorithms should be updated to reflect recent advances in the field—including the role of genetic testing in the confirmation and management of genetic hyperlipidemias.

REFERENCES

1. Shoulders CC, Shelness GS (2005). Current biology of MTP: Implications for selective inhibition. Curr Top Med Chem 5(3):283–300.
2. Choudhuri S, Klaassen CD (2006). Structure, function, expression, genomic organization, and single nucleotide polymorphisms of human ABCB1 (MDR1), ABCC (MRP), and ABCG2 (BCRP) efflux transporters. Int J Toxicol 25:231–259.
3. Cavelier C, Lorenzi I, Rohrer L, von Eckardstein A (2006). Lipid efflux by the ATP-binding cassette transporters ABCA1 and ABCG1. Biochim Biophys Acta 1761:655–666.

4. Sook Sul H, Storch J (2006). Cholesterol and lipoproteins: Synthesis, transport and metabolism. In Stipanuk MH (ed.), *Biochemical, physiological, and molecular aspects of human metabolism, Second edition*. Saint Louis: Saunders/Elsevier 492–516.

5. Daniels, SR (2003). Lipid metabolism and secondary forms of dyslipoproteinemia in children. Prog Ped Card 17:135–140.

6. Otarod JK, Goldberg IJ (2004). Lipoprotein lipase and its role in regulation of plasma lipoproteins and cardiac risk. Curr Atheroscler Rep 6:335–342.

7. Twinckler TB, Dallinga-Thie GM, Cohn JS, Chapman MJ (2004). Elevated remnant-like particle cholesterol concentration: A characteristic feature of the atherogenic lipoprotein phenotype. Circulation 109:1918–1925.

8. Yu KC-W, Chen W, Cooper AD (2001). LDL receptor-related protein mediates cell-surface clustering and hepatic sequestration of chylomicron remnants in LDLR-deficient mice. J Clin Invest 107:1387–1394.

9. Clauss SB, Kwiterovich PO (2003). Genetic disorders of lipoprotein transport in children. Prog Ed Card 17:123–133.

10. Zambon A, Bertocco S, Vitturi N, Polentarutti V, Vianello D, Crepaldi G (2003). Relevance of hepatic lipase to the metabolism of triacylglycerol-rich lipoproteins. Biochem Soc Trans 31(5):1070–1074.

11. Beglova N, Blacklow SC (2005). The LDL receptor: How acid pulls the trigger. Trends Biochem Sci 30(6):309–317.

12. Ory DS (2004). Nuclear receptor signaling in the control of cholesterol homeostasis: Have the orphans found a home? Circ Res 95:660–670.

13. Riggoti A (2000). Scavenger receptors and atherosclerosis. Biol Res 33:97–103.

14. Krimbou L, Marcil M, Genest J (2006). New insights into the biogenesis of human high-density lipoproteins. Curr Opin Lipidol 17:258–267.

15. Schaefer EJ, Azstalos BF (2006). Cholesteryl ester transfer protein inhibition, high-density lipoprotein metabolism and heart disease risk reduction. Curr Opin Lipidol 17:394–398.

16. Ohashi R, Mu H, Wang X, Yao Q, Chen C (2005). Reverse cholesterol transport and cholesterol efflux in atherosclerosis. QJM 98:845–856.

17. Ose L (2002). Familial hypercholesterolemia from children to adults. Card Drugs Ther 16:289–293.

18. Goldstein JL, Hobbs HH, Brown MS (2001). Familial hypercholesterolemia. In Scriver C, Beaudet A, Sly W, Valle D (eds.), *The metabolic and molecular bases of inherited disease, Eighth edition*. New York: McGraw-Hill 2863–2913.

19. Rader DJ, Cohen J, Hobbs HH (2003). Monogenic hypercholesterolemia: New insights in pathogenesis and treatment. J Clin Invest 111:1795–1803.

20. Naoumova RP, Thompson GR, Soutar AK (2004). Current management of severe homozygous hypercholesterolemia. Curr Opin Lipidol 15:413–422.

21. Wood Holmes K, Kwiterovich PO (2005). Treatment of dyslipidemia in children and adolescents. Curr Card Rep 7:445–456.

22. Arca M (2002). Autosomal recessive hypercholesterolemia in Sardinia, Italy, and mutations in ARH: A clinical and molecular genetic analysis. Lancet 359:841–847.

23. Lind S, Olsson AG, Erickson M (2004). Autosomal recessive hypercholesterolemia: Normalization of plasma LDL cholesterol by ezetimibe in combination with statin treatment. J Inter Med 256:406–412.

24. Innerarity TL, Mahley RW, Weisgraber KH, et al. (1990). Familial defective apolipoprotein B-100: A mutation of apolipoprotein B that causes hypercholesterolemia. J Lipid Res 31:1337–1349.

25. Patel MD, Thompson PD (2006). Phytosterols and vascular disease. Atherosclerosis 186:12–19.

26. von Bergmann K, Sudhop MD, Lütjohann D (2005). Cholesterol and plant sterol absorption: Recent insights. Am J Cardiol 96(1A):10D–14D.

27. Lutjohann D, Bjorkham I, Beil VF, von Bergmann K (1995). Sterol absorption and sterol balance in phytosterolemia evaluated by deuterium-labeled sterols: Effect of sitostanol treatment. J Lipid Res 36:1763.

28. Durrington P (2003). Dyslipidemia. Lancet 362:717–731.

29. Kwiterovich PO Jr. (2000). The metabolic pathways of HDL, LDL and triglycerides: A current review. Am J Cardiol 86(1):5–10.

30. Cortner JA, Coates PM, Gallagher PR (1990). Prevalence and expression of familial combined hyperlipidemia in childhood. J Pediatr 116:514–524.

31. Aguilar CA, Zamora M, Gomez-Diaz RA, Mehta R, Perez FJG, Rull JA (2004). Familial combined hyperlipidemia: Controversial aspects of its diagnosis and pathogenesis. Semin Vasc Med 4:203–209.

32. Kwiterovich PO (2002). Clinical relevance of the biochemical, metabolic and genetic factors that influence low density lipoprotein heterogeneity. Am J Cardiol 90(8A):30i–48i.

33. Sniderman AD, Scantlebury T, Cianflione K (2001). Hypertriglyceridemic hyperapob: The unappreciated atherogenic dyslipoproteinemia in type 2 diabetes mellitus. Ann Intern Med 135:447–459.

34. Eckel RH, Grundy SM, Zimmet PZ (2005). The metabolic syndrome. Lancet 365:1415–1428.

35. Gilbert T, Rouis M, Griglio S (2001). Lipoprotein lipase (LPL) deficiency: A new patient homozygous for the preponderant mutation Gly 188 Glu in the human LPL gene and review of the reported mutations; 75% are clustered in exons 5 and 6. Ann Genet 44:25–32.

36. Deeb SS, Peng R (1989). Structure of the human lipoprotein lipase gene. Biochemistry 28:4131–4135.

37. Wright CM, Parker L, Lamont D, Craft AW (2001). Implications of childhood obesity for adult health: Findings from thousand families cohort study. BMJ 323:1280–1284.

38. Sierovogel RM, Wisemandle W, Maynard LM, Guo SS, Roche AF, Chumlea WC, et al. (1998). Serial changes in body composition throughout adulthood and their relationships to changes in lipid and lipoprotein levels: The Fels Longitudinal Study. Arteriosclerosis Thromb Vasc Biol 18:1759–1764.

39. Cortner, JA, Coates PM, Liacouras CA, Jarvik GP (1994). Familial combined hyperlipidemia in children: Clinical expression, metabolic defects, and management. Curr Probl Pediatr 24:295–305.

40. Remaley AT, Rust S, Rosier M, et al. (1999). Human ATP-binding cassette transporter a (ABC1): Genomic organization and identification of the genetic defect in the original Tangier disease kindred. PNAS 96:12685–12690.

41. Bodzioch M, Orso E, Klucken E, et al. (1999). The gene encoding ATP-binding cassette transporter 1 is mutated in Tangiers Disease. Nat Genet 22:347–351.

42. Assmann, G, Von Ekardstein A, Brewer HB Jr. (2001). Familial analphalipoproteinemia: Tangier disease. In Scriver C, Beaudet A, Sly W, Valle D (eds.), *The metabolic and molecular bases of inherited disease, Eighth edition*. New York: McGraw-Hill 2937–2960.

43. Brewer HB, Remaley AT, Neufeld EB, et al. (2004). Regulation of plasma high density lipoprotein levels by the ABCA1 transporter and emerging role of high density lipoprotein in the treatment of cardiovascular disease. Arterioscler Thromb Vasc Biol 24:1755–1760.

44. Smelt AH, de Beer F (2004). Apolipoprotein E and familial dysbetalipoproteinemia: Clinical, biochemical and genetic aspects. Semin Vasc Med 4:249–257.

45. Deckelbaum RJ, Williams CL (2001). Childhood obesity: the health issue. Obes Res 9:239S–243S.

46. Williams CL, Hayman LL, Daniels SR, Robinson TN, Steinberger J, Paridon S, et al. (2002). Cardiovascular health in childhood: A statement of health professionals from the Committee on Atherosclerosis, Hypertension, and Obesity in the Young (AHOY) of the Council on Cardiovascular Disease in the Young, American Heart Association. Circulation 106:143–160.

47. Steinberger J (2003). Diagnosis of the metabolic syndrome in children. Curr Opin Lipidol 14:555–559.

48. Steinberger J, Daniels SR (2003). Obesity, insulin resistance, diabetes, and cardiovascular risk in children: An American Heart Association scientific statement from the Atherosclerosis, Hypertension and Obesity in the Young Committee (Council on Cardiovascular Disease in the Young) and the Diabetes Committee (Council on Nutrition, Physical Activity and Metabolism). Circulation 107:1448–1453.

49. Chahil TJ, Ginsberg HN (2006). Diabetic dyslipidemia. Endocrinol Metab Clin North Am 35:491–510.

50. Expert Panel on Detection, Evaluation, and Treatment of High Cholesterol in Adults (2001). Executive Summary of the Third Report of the National Cholesterol Education Program (NCEP) Expert Panel on Detection, Evaluation, and Treatment of High Blood Cholesterol in Adults (Adult Treatment Panel III). JAMA 285:2486–2497.

51. Kaufman FR (2002). Type 2 diabetes mellitus in children and youth: A new epidemic. J Pediatr Endocrinol Metab 15:737–744.

52. American Diabetes Association (2003). Management of dyslipidemia in children and adolescents with diabetes. Diabetes Care 26:2194–2197.

53. Kershnar AK, Daniels ST, Imperatore G, Palla SL, Pettitt DB, Pettitt DJ, et al. (2006). Lipid abnormalities are prevalent in youth with type 1 and type 2 diabetes: The Search for Diabetes in Youth Study. J Pediatr 149:314–319.

54. Daniels SR (2003). Lipid metabolism and secondary forms of dyslipoproteinemia in children. Progr Pediatr Cardiol 17:135–140.

55. Galley R (2006). Improving outcomes in renal disease. JAAPA 19:20–25.

56. Badimon L, Martinez-Gonzalez J, Llorente-Cortes V, Rodriguez C, Padro T (2006). Cell biology and lipoproteins in atherosclerosis. Curr Mol Med 6:439–456.

57. Moore MJ, Freeman MW (2006). Scavenger receptors in atherosclerosis: Beyond lipid uptake. Arterioscler Thromb Vasc Biol 26:1702–1711.

58. Kher N, Marsh JD (2004). Pathobiology of atherosclerosis: A brief review. Sem Throm Hemostasis 30:665–672.

59. Stary HC, Stoll JD, Yin J, Fallon KB, Yu Z (1996). The natural history of atherosclerosis in the aorta in the first forty years of life. In [editor] (ed.), *Syndromes of atherosclerosis: Correlations of clinical imaging and pathology.* Armonk, NY: Futura Publishing 225–238.

60. Berenson GS, Srinivasan SR, Bao W, Newman WP III, Tracy RE, Wattigney WA (1998). Association between multiple cardiovascular risk factors and atherosclerosis in children and young adults: The Bogalusa Heart Study. N Eng J Med 338:1650–1656.

61. McGill HC, McMahan CA, Herderick EE, Zieske AW, Malcom GT, Tracy RE, et al. (2002). Pathobiological Determinants of Atherosclerosis in Youth (PDAY) Research Group. Circulation 105:2712–2718.

62. Lloyd-Jones DM, Wilson PW, Larson MG, Beiser A, Leip EP, D'Agostino RB, et al. (2004). Framingham risk score and prediction of lifetime risk of coronary heart disease. Am J Cardiol 94:20–24.

63. de Groot, E, Hovingh K, Wiegman A, Duriez P, Smit AJ, Fruchart JC, et al. (2004). Measurement of arterial wall thickness as a surrogate marker for atherosclerosis. 109:III33–III38.

64. Sankatsing RR, de Groot E, Jukema JW, de Feyter PJ, Pennell DJ, Schoenhagen P, et al. (2005). Surrogate markers for atherosclerosis disease. Curr Opin Lipidol 16:434–441.

65. Keelan PC, Bielak LF, Ashai K, JamJoum AE, Denktas JA, Rumberger PF, et al. (2001). Long term prognostic value of coronary calcification detected by electron-beam computed tomography in patients undergoing coronary angiography. Circulation 104:412–417.

66. Mahoney LT, Burns TL, Staford W, et al. (1996). Coronary risk factors measure in childhood and young adults are associated with coronary artery calcification in young adults: The Muscatine Study. J Am Coll Cardiol 27:277–284.

67. Kobayashi K, Akishita M, Yu W, Hashimoto M, Ohni M, Toba K (2004). Interrelationship between non-invasive measurements of atherosclerosis: Flow mediated dilation of brachial artery, carotid intima-media thickness and pulse wave velocity. Atherosclerosis 173:13–18.

68. Watanabe K, Sugiyama S, Kugiyama K, Honda O, Fukushima H, Koga H, et al. (2005). Stabilization of carotid atheroma assessed by quantitative ultrasound analysis in nonhypercholesterolemic patients with coronary artery disease. J Am Coll Cardiol 46:2022–2030.

69. Teregawa H, Kato M, Kurokawa J, Yamagata T, Matsuura H, Chayama K (2001). Usefulness of flow-mediated dilation of the brachial artery and/or the intima-media thickness of the carotid artery in predicting coronary narrowing in patients suspected of having coronary artery disease. Am J Cardiol 88:1147–1151.

70 Furomoto T, Fujii S, Saito N, Mikami T, Kitabatake A (2002). Relationships between brachial artery flow mediated dilation and carotid artery intima-media thickness in patients with suspected coronary artery disease. Jpn Heart J 43:117–125.

71. Raitakari OT, Juonala M, Kahonen M, Taittonen L, Laitinen N, Maki-Torkko MJ, et al. (2003). Cardiovascular risk factors in childhood and carotid artery intima-media thickness in adulthood: The Cardiovascular Risk in Young Finns Study. JAMA 290:2277–2283.

72. Sanchez A, Barth JD, Zhang L (2000). The carotid artery wall thickness in teenagers is related to their diet and the typical risk factors of heart disease among adults. Atherosclerosis 152:265–266.

73. Tonstad S, Jokimsen O, Stensland-Bugge E, Leren TP, Ose L, Russell D, et al. (1996). Risk factors related to carotid intima-media thickness and plaque in children with familial hypercholesterolemia and control subjects. Ateriosclero Thromb Vasc Biol 16:984–991.

74. Davis PH, Dawson JD, Riley WA, Lauer RM (2001). Carotid intima-media thickness is related to cardiovascular risk factors measured from childhood through middle age. Circulation 104:2815–2819.

75. Lavrencic A, Kosmina B, Keber I, Videcnik V, Keber D (1996). Carotid intima-media thickness in young patients with familial hypercholesterolemia. Heart 76:321–325.

76. Leeson CP, Kattenhorn M, Morley R, Lucas A, Deanfield JE (2001). Impact of low birth weight and cardiovascular risk factors on endothelial function in early adult life. Circulation 103:1264–1268.

77. Meyer AA, Kundt G, Lenschow U, Schuff-Werner P, Kienast W (2006). Improvement of early vascular changes and cardiovascular risk factors in obese children after a six-month exercise program. J Am Coll Cardiol 48:1865–1870.

78. Meyer AA, Kundt G, Steiner M, Schuff-Werner P, Kienast W (2006). Impaired flow-mediated vasodilation, carotid-arter intim-media thickening, and elevated endothelial plasma markers in obese children: The impact of cardiovascular risk factors. Pediatrics 117:1560–1567.

79. National Cholesterol Education Program (NCEP) (1992). Highlights of the Report of the Expert Panel on Blood Cholesterol Levels in Children and Adolescents. Pediatrics 89:495–501.

80. Warnick GR, Knopp RH, Fitzpatrick V, Branson L (1990). Estimating low-density lipoprotein cholesterol by the Friedewald equation is adequate for classifying patients on the basis of nationally recommended cutpoints. Clin Chem 36:15–19.

81. Starc TJ, Belamarich PF, Shea S, Dobrin-Seckler BE, Dell RB, Gersony WM, et al. (1991). Family history fails to identify many children with severe hypercholesterolemia. Am J Dis Child 145:61–64.

82. Kelishadi R, Ardalan G, Gheiratmand R, Ramezani A (2006). Is family history of premature cardiovascular diseases appropriate for detection of dyslipidemic children in population-based preventive medicine programs? CASPIAN Study. Prediatr Cardiol 27:729–736.

83. Resnicow K, Cross D, Lacosse J (1993). Evaluation of a school-site cardiovascular risk factor screening intervention. Prev Med 22:838–856.

84. Morrison JA (2003). A longitudinal evaluation of the NCEP-Peds guidelines for evaluated total and LDL cholesterol in adolescent girls and boys. Prog Pediatr ardiol 17:159–168.

85. Labarthe DR, Dai S, Fulton JE (2003). Cholesterol screening in children: Insights from Project HeartBeat! And NHANES III. Prog Pediatr Cardiol 17:169–178.

86. Kavey RE, Daniels SR, Lauer RM, Atkins DL, Hayman LL, Taubert K (2003). American Heart Association guidelines for primary prevention of atherosclerotic cardiovascular disease beginning in childhood. Circulation 107:1562–1566.

87. Vergopoulos A, Knoblauch H, Schuster H (2002). DNA testing for familial hypercholesterolemia: Improving disease recognition and patient care. Am J Pharmacogenetics 2:253–262.

88. Hadfield SG, Humphries SE (2005). Implementaion of cascade testing for the detection of familial hypercholesterolemia. Curr Opin Lipidol 16:428–433.

89. Miltiadous G, Xenophontas S, Bairaktarik K, Ganatakis M, Cariolou M, Elisaf M (2005). Genetic and environmental factors affecting the response to statin therapy in patients with molecularly defined familial hypercholesterolemia. Pharmacog Genomics 15:219–225.

90. Humphries SE, Whittall RA, Hubbart CS, Maplebeck S, Cooper JA, Soutar AK, et al. for the Simon Broome Familial Hyperlipidemia Register Group and Scientific Steering Committee (2006). Genetic cause of familial hypercholesterolemia in patients in the UK: Relation to plasma lipids and coronary heart disease risk. J Med Genetics 43:943–949.

91. Umans-Eckenhausen MA, Defesche JC, Sijbrands EJ (2001). Review of the first 5 years of screening for familial hypercholesterolemia in the Netherlands. Lancet 357:165–168.

92. Leren TP, Manshaus T, Skovholt U, et al. (2004). Application of molecular genetics for diagnosing familial hypercholesterolemia in Norway: Results from a family based screening program. Semin Vasc Med 4:75–85.

93. Lauer RM, Obarzanek E, Hunsberger S, A et al. (2000). Efficacy and safety of lowering dietary intake of total fat, saturated fat and cholesterol in children with elevated LDL-cholesterol: The Dietary Intervention Study in Children. Am J Clin Nutr 72:1332S–1342S.

94. Obarzanek E, Kimm SY, Barton BA, et al. (2001). Long-term safety and efficacy of a cholesterol lowering diet in children with elevated low-density lipoprotein cholesterol: Seven year results of the Dietary Intervention Study in Children. Pediatrics 107:256–264.

95. Jacobson MS, Tomopoulus S, Williams CL, et al. (1998). Normal growth in high risk hyperlipidemic children and adolescents with dietary intervention. Prev Med 27:775–780.

96. Couch SC, Daniels SR (year). Current concepts of diet therapy for children with hypercholesterolemia. Prog Pediatr Cardiol 17:179–186.

97. Lifshitz F, Moses N (1989). A complication of dietary treatment of hypercholesterolemia. Am J Dis Child 143:537–542.

98. American Academy of Pediatrics Committee on Nutrition (1998). Cholesterol in childhood. Pediatrics 101:141–147.

99. Tershakovec AW, Shannon BM, Achterberg CL, et al. (1998). One-year follow-up of nutrition education for hypercholesterolemic children. Am J Public Health 88:258–261.

100. Kuehl KS, Cockerham JT, Hitchings M, Slater D, Nixon G, Rifai N (1993). Effective control of hypercholesterolemia in children with dietary intervention based in pediatric practice. Prev Med 22:154–166.

101. Gidding SS, Dennison BA, Birch LL, Daniels SR, Gilman MW, Lichtenstein AH, et al. for the American Heart Association (2006). Dietary recommendations for children and adolescents: A guide for practitioners. Pediatrics 117:544–559.

102. Starc TJ, Shea S, Cohn LC, Mosca L, Gersony WM, Deckelbaum RJ (1998). Greater dietary intake of simple carbohydrate is associated with lower concentrations of high-density lipoprotein cholesterol in hypercholesterolemic children. Am J Clin Nutr 67:1147–1154.

103. Reinehr R, de Sousa G, Toschke AM, Andler W (2006). Long-term follow-up of cardiovascular disease risk factors in children after an obesity intervention. Am J Clin Nutr 84:490–496.

104. American Diabetes Association (2005). Standards of medical care in diabetes. Diabetes Care 28(1):S4–S36.

105. American Diabetes Association (2003). Management of dyslipidemia in children and adolescents with diabetes. Diabetes Care 26:2194–2197.

106. McCrindle BW (2003). Drug therapy of hyperlipidemia. Prog Pediatr Cardiol 17:141–150.

107. McCrindle BW, O'Neill MB, Cullen-Dean G, Helden E (1997). Acceptability and compliance with two forms of cholestyramine in the treatment of hypercholesterolemia in children: A randomized, crossover trial. J Pediatr 130:266–273.

108. Tonstad S, Knudtzon J, Sivertsen M, et al. (1996). Efficacy and safety of cholestyramine therapy in peripubertal and prepubertal children with familial hypercholesterolemia. J Pediatr 129:42–49.

109. McCrindle BW (2006). Hyperlipidemia in children. Thromb Res 118:49–58.

110. McCrindle BW, Helden E, Cullen-Dean G, Conner WT (2002). A randomized crossover trial of combination pharmacologic therapy in children with familial hyperlipidemia. Pediatr Res 51:715–721.

111. Rodenburg J, Vissers MN, Trip MS, Wiegman A, Bakker HD, Kastelein JJP (2004). The spectrum of statin therapy in hyperlipidemic children. Sem Vasc Med 4:313–320.

112. Knipscheer HC, Boelen CC, Kastelein JJ, van Diermen DE, Groenemeijer BE, van den EA, et al. (1996). Short-term efficacy and safety of pravastatin in 72 children with familial hypercholesterolemia. Pediatr Res 39:867–871.

113. Lambert M, Lupien PJ, Gagne C, Levy E, Blaichman S, Langlois S, et al. (1996). Treatment of familial hypercholesterolemia in children and adolescents: Effects of lovastatin. Canadian lovastatin in children study group. Pediatrics 97:619–628.

114. Stein EA, Illingworth DR, Kwiterovich PO Jr., Liacouras CA, Siimes MA, Jacobson MS, et al. (1999). Efficacy and safety of lovastatin in adolescent males with heterozygous familial hypercholesterolemia: A randomized controlled trial. JAMA 281:137–144.

115. Arambepola C, Farmer AJ, Perera R, Neil HA (2006). Statin treatment for children and adolescents with heterozygous familial hypercholesterolemia: A systematic review and meta-analysis. Atherosclerosis 2006 (in press).

116. Weigman A, Hutten BA, de Groot, et al. (2004). Efficacy and safety of statin therapy in children with familial hypercholesterolemia: A randomized controlled trial. JAMA 292:331–337.

117. Rodenburg J, Vissers MN, Daniels SR, Wiegman A, Kastelein JJ (2004). Lipid-lowering medications. Pediatr Endocrinol Rev 2(1):171–180.

118. Pearson GJ, Francis GA, Romney JS, Gilchrist DM, Opgenorth A, Gyenes GT (2006). The clinical effect and tolerability of ezetimibe in high risk patients managed in a speciality cardiovascular risk reduction clinic. Can J Cardiol 22:939–945.

119. Wierzbicki AS, Doherty E, Lumb PJ, Chik G, Crook MA (2005). Efficacy of ezetimibe in patients with statin-resistant and statin-intolerant familial hyperlipidemia. Curr Med Res Opin 21:333–338.

120. Colletti RB, Neufeld EJ, Roff NK, McAuliffe TL, Baker AL, Newburger JW (1993). Niacin treatment of hypercholesterolemia in children. Pediatrics 92:78–82.

121. Ostlund RE Jr. (2004). Phytosterols and cholesterol metabolism. Curr Opin Lipidol 15:37–41.

122. Jakulj L, Vissers MN, Rodenburg J, Wiegman A, Trip MD, Kastelein JJP (2006). Plant sterols do not restore endothelial function in prepubertal children with familial hypercholesterolemia despite reduction in low-density lipoprotein cholesterol levels. J Pediatrics 148:495–500.

123. Lichtenstein AH, Deckelbaum RJ (2001). Stanol/sterol ester-containing food and blood cholesterol levels: A statement for healthcare professionals from the nutrition committee of the council on nutrition, physical activity and metabolism of the American Heart Association. Circulation 103:1177–1179.

124. Dennison BA, Levine DM (1993). Randomized double-blind, placebo-controlled, two period crossover clinical trial of psyllium fiber in children with hypercholesterolemia. J Pediatr 123:24–29.

125. McCrindle BW, Helden E, Conner WT (1998). Garlic extract therapy in children with hypercholesterolemia. Arch Pediatr Adolesc Med 152:1089–1094.

126. Engler MM, Engler MB, Malloy M, Chiu E, Besio D, Paul S, et al. (2004). Docosahexaenoic acid restores endothelial function in children with hyperlipidemia: Results from the EARLY study. Int J Clin Pharmacol Ther 42:672–679.

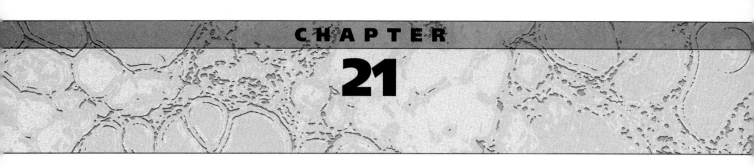

Laboratory Methods in Pediatric Endocrinology

ROBERT RAPAPORT, MD • RUSSELL GRANT, PhD
• SHARON J. HYMAN, MD • MARK STENE, PhD

Introduction

Pediatric endocrinology is a specialty that relies greatly on laboratory testing for evaluating and monitoring children with suspected or known endocrine conditions. It is therefore essential that those involved in the care of children understand all variables involved in proper prescribing, sample collecting, performance, and interpretation of laboratory tests. Appropriate use and application of hormonal assays can improve the health care of children by helping to avoid unnecessary detailed and invasive examinations. We hope this chapter will lend sufficient guidance to help clinicians appropriately select and evaluate endocrine hormone tests. The principles of molecular endocrinology testing are discussed elsewhere in this textbook.

Endocrine hormone assays have evolved from radio-immunoassay (RIA) technology by using monoclonal antibodies, sensitive detection techniques, extensive automation, and most recently tandem mass spectrometry (MS/MS). With extensive automation, the sudden availability of platforms with a menu of commonly demanded hormone tests rapidly broadened access of endocrine testing to more than 1,600 laboratories today.[1]

The distribution of endocrine testing now likely resembles the overall medical testing industry, in which hospitals perform 55% of testing, commercial laboratories perform 24%, physician office laboratories perform 11%, and others (such as nursing homes) perform 10%. As of 2003, laboratory testing at $40 billion accounted for 2.9% of all American health care expenditures. Specialized testing, including endocrinology, consisted of about $3.7 billion.[2] Despite the vast number of testing laboratories, most endocrine testing is concentrated on only a handful of automated analyzers manufactured by a small number of companies.

Recent advances in information technology are also changing the physician, hospital, and laboratory interaction. Similar to computer-computer interfaces, laboratory web-based information systems for ordering testing and receiving results are now increasingly available. These systems may reduce certain types of errors while potentially creating others.[3] How these systems will reliably populate hospital systems, handheld devices, and electronic medical records or practice management systems is an emerging variable.

Changes in the reimbursement environment have influenced the structure of hospital, commercial, and physician-office laboratories. Today, these laboratories employ only laboratory generalists and depend largely on these simple-to-operate platforms. Although practical, such systems have limited accuracy in certain applications. Their ease of installation and tacit interchangeability are also potential limitations. In most laboratories, appropriate technical knowledge of endocrinology and analytic systems is diminished and is often outsourced to device manufacturers whose continued focus is further integration and consolidation. Although these comments apply primarily to the current situation in the United States, they are likely to reflect trends in all developed countries.

Hormonal Assay Methods

PREANALYTIC VARIABLES

Normal endocrine physiology, nonendocrine illness,[4] sample collection, and handling influence measured hormone levels (Table 21-1). Under normal circumstances in the basal state, many hormones are secreted in an episodic manner. Chronologic age, pubertal stage, emotional and physical stress, nutritional status, and postural effects contribute to the variation. Consequently, some hormones, growth factors, or surrogate markers may have very wide normal basal ranges and large intrasubject variability. Intrasubject variability can be remarkable for 24-hour integrated concentrations[5,6] and for dynamic responses.[7]

Proper collection, documentation, and storage are needed to ensure accurate hormonal determinations.[8,9] Most steroid, thyroid, peptide, and protein hormones (and nearly all measured antibodies) are relatively resistant to collection and handling factors—including freezing and thawing. Generally, a serum sample drawn under normal conditions should be allowed to clot at room temperature for an hour, separated, and frozen until analysis is adequate. See Table 21-2 for patient preparation, sample collection, handling requirements, and relevant information regarding certain hormone assays. For best results, always consult with the specific laboratory to understand its collection and handling requirements.

STANDARDIZATION

Unlike routine chemistries, most quantitative hormone assays can vary widely in absolute terms. To simplify research and clinical findings, standardization of hormone methods has been a long sought after and continuing goal.[10] Standardization of steroid and other small-molecule hormone assays is relatively simple because these hormones are of low molecular weight and are synthesized and highly purified using physical and chemical methods. Such standards are typically available as preparations that can be reliably prepared and stably stored.[11]

By contrast, peptide hormones, protein hormones, and antihormone antibody standards are of high molecular weight and higher complexity (with many circulating isoforms)—making an absolute assignment more difficult. Recombinant technology and the availability of pharmaceutical-grade hormone are enabling improvement.[12] Despite better standards, similarly designed assays often yield different absolute results.[13] Some differences happen for proprietary reasons, but others are reflecting the complexity of the circulating and standard hormone preparations and variances in recognition of these hormones by capture and detection antibody systems. Testing proficiency data from automated systems show that identical systems have not reduced variability substantially for all hormones.

REFERENCE RANGES

For the clinician, basal and dynamic testing reference data appropriate to the method result is more important than the absolute standardization. As outlined in Tables 21-3 through 21-5, ideally reference data should be available for all patient groups commonly making use of the test.[14] These data must be established comprehensively, especially for new analytes, and must account for all factors that partition circulating hormone levels. For existing analytes, a reference method with an extensive normal data set allows for a less costly and more accessible way of establishing reference ranges.

A subset of normal samples can be used to confirm the reference database if the newly implemented method is similar in design and the reference population is the same.[14] Laboratories increasingly rely on device manufacturers to provide this base data set against which the smaller internally derived normal data are statistically evaluated for transference.[15] Current practice may fall short of these requirements because method differences and bias between methods are sometimes unrelated to the differences in reference intervals.[16]

TABLE 21-1

Preanalytic Variables Affecting Hormonal Measurements

Variable	Hormone
Episodic secretion	Pituitary hormones, cortisol
Exercise (acute)	Adrenocorticotropic hormone (ACTH), anti-diuretic hormone (ADH), aldosterone, cortisol, epinephrine, glucagon, growth hormone (GH), prolactin, norepinephrine, testosterone
Circadian rhythm, diurnal variation	ACTH, cortisol, dehydroepiandrosterone sulfate (DHEAS), epinephrine, estradiol, follicle-stimulating hormone (FSH), GH, luteinizing hormone (LH), norepinephrine, prolactin, testosterone
Seasonal variation	Estradiol, prolactin, testosterone
Postural change	Aldosterone, epinephrine, norepinephrine, renin
Nutrition	C peptide, estradiol, glucagon, insulin-like growth factor-I (IGF-I), insulin-like growth factor binding protein-1 (IGFBP-1), insulin, proinsulin, thyroxine-binding globulin (TBG)

TABLE 21-2

Hormone Assays: Preanalytic and Other Considerations

Hormone	Patient Preparation, Sample Collection, and Hormone Stability	Assay Notes
ACTH	• EDTA • 6-hr RT, 4° C • Ship frozen • Avoid FT	• 1-24 ACTH, used for stimulation studies, and pro-opiomelanocortin (POMC) fragments can lower ACTH levels as measured by two-site methods.
ADH	• EDTA • Avoid FT • Ship frozen	• Solid-phase purification.
Aldosterone	• Patient: posture and sodium • Stability: 1 day at RT, 2 days at 4° C	• Spironolactone and tetrahydroaldosterone 3-glucuronide may cross-react in some assays.
Calcitonin	• 1 day at RT • 1 day at 4° C	• Large calcitonin and others cross-react in some RIA methods. • High dose suppression of values possible with two-site methods. • Heterophile antibodies and human anti-animal antibodies may give falsely elevated results in two-site methods.
Cortisol, urine-free cortisol	• With boric acid 5 days at RT and 14 days at 4° C	• Prednisolone and 6-beta-hydroxycortisol may cross-react.
C peptide	• EDTA: 1 day at RT • RT: 1 day at 4° C • Ship frozen	• C peptide immunoreactivity may be unstable. • Some immunoassays may be affected by anti-insulin antibodies.
Dopamine, epinephrine, norepinephrine	• Patient preparation: posture and activity • Stability: 0 days at 4° C • Must freeze sample ASAP	• Very unstable analytes present in low concentrations.
Estradiol	• 2 days at RT • 6 days at 4° C	• RU-486, Efavirez, and steroid-binding proteins may interfere with some assays.
Free IGF-I	• Avoid FT • Ship frozen	• Direct methods controversial.
GH	• 2 days at RT • 2 days at 4° C	• 20-kD GH react in certain RIA methods. • Human placental lactogen (hPL) may augment or suppress hGH levels. • 44-191 GH in RIA methods. • High hGH concentrations may require sample dilution if accurate results are needed. • After treatment, anti-GH antibodies may suppress GH levels in sandwich assays.
Glucagon	• EDTA • Avoid FT • Ship frozen	• Unstable; keep frozen.
IGF-I	• 2 days at RT • 2 days at 4° C	• IGF binding proteins react in methods that do not exclude or block. • Variable reactivity with therapeutic IGFI and IGFI/IGFBP3 complex with some assays.
Insulin	• 6 hours at RT • 1 day at 4° C • Ship frozen	• Variable reactivity with various recombinant insulins. • On treatment, hook effect possible for two-site assays. • Human anti-insulin antibodies may interfere (use free and total measurements to avoid this issue). • Assays typically most reactive with human insulin, less reactive with porcine insulin, and least reactive with bovine insulin.
IPTH, intact parathyroid hormone	• EDTA • 4 hours at RT • 1 day at 4° C	• Assay terminology: second-generation N-terminal anti-1-24, third-generation N-terminal anti-1-6. • Second and third generations typically use C-terminal anti-39-84. • Midrange PTH RIAs (MPTH) recognize PTH molecules containing amino acid sequences 44-68. • C-terminal (CPTH) assays recognize molecules containing amino acids 39-84. • Circulating PTH fragments are not biologically active unless they have key N-terminal residues (1-24) and can lower or raise results from two-site methods. • Third-generation assays do not detect PTH 7-84 that is not biologically reactive. • Fragments are especially high with renal failure. • Human anti-PTH antibodies may interfere with assays.

Continued

TABLE 21-2
Hormone Assays: Preanalytic and Other Considerations—cont'd

Hormone	Patient Preparation, Sample Collection, and Hormone Stability	Assay Notes
LH and FSH	• 2 days at RT • 2 days at 4° C	• HCG for stimulation or due to tumor may augment RIA values and suppress two-site methods. • Some RIAs more sensitive to degradation.
Osteocalcin	• EDTA • Avoid FT	
Proinsulin	• 1 day at RT • 1 day at 4° C	• High insulin levels associated with treatment may suppress proinsulin levels in two-site assays. • Human antibodies specific to insulin or proinsulin.
Prolactin	• 2 days at RT • 2 days at 4° C	• Macroprolactin or big prolactin a complex of prolactin and IgG lacks biologic activity because not freely available to tissues. • Two-site assays may demonstrate suppression (high-dose hook) at extremely high prolactin levels associated with macroprolactinomas.
PTH-rP, parathyroid-hormone-related protein	• Plasma with protease inhibitor • Avoid FT • Ship frozen	• Unstable; collect with inhibitor and keep frozen. • PTHrp N terminal contains key PTH sequences and is biologically active. • Also known as the humoral hypercalcemina of malignancy factor.
Renin	• EDTA • Process at RTsSnap Freeze • Ship frozen • Do not leave cold	• Process ambient and freeze rapidly to avoid plasma renin activity (PRA) increases due to cold-activated proteases. • Activity assays known as PRA. • Also direct renin assays.
Testosterone	• 2 days at RT • 6 days at 4° C	• RU-486, testolactone, and steroid binding proteins may interfere in some assays.
Thyroglobulin	• 2 days at RT • 2 days at 4° C	• Circulating anti-TG antibodies significantly suppress two-site methods. • RIA methods are less likely to be impacted.
TSH, thyroid-stimulating hormone	• 2 days at RT • 2 days at 4° C	• βHCG or alpha subunit with some methods causing falsely lower results. • Heterophile antibodies have been reported as causing falsely high values. • Controversy about TSH reference ranges.
Vitamin D 25 OH	• Avoid FT • Ship frozen	• Assays may or may not efficiently measure D2 form and C-3 epimer.

Notes: Stability: RT = room temperature. FT = freeze/thaw cycle. Stability studies using normal sera have shown that all hormone levels except ACTH, ADH, dopamine, epinephrine, glucagon, insulin, norepinephrine, osteocalcin, IPTH, and renin are relatively stable when kept at ambient temperature (20-25° C) for 1 day. Stability may be worse for patient samples and for samples kept at elevated temperatures, and may vary with the method. For most reliable hormone data, patient samples generally should be separated as soon as possible and kept frozen until measurement. Consult your laboratory for proper handling. Circulating antihormone antibodies will usually suppress two-site assay data. Hormone assay precision, the 95% confidence interval for a hormone level, ranges from ±10-20% to ±15-30%— depending on the absolute hormone concentration and the method used.

TABLE 21-3
IGF-I (ng/mL) Pediatric Normal Data for an Acid Ethanol Extracted Blocking Method

Children and Young Adults	Male Range	Male Average	Female Range	Female Average
1-2	30-122	76	56-144	100
3-4	54-178	116	74-202	138
5-6	60-228	144	82-262	172
7-8	113-261	187	112-276	194
9-10	123-275	199	140-308	224
11-12	139-395	267	132-376	254
13-14	152-540	346	192-640	416
15-16	257-601	429	217-589	403
17-18	236-524	380	176-452	314
19-20	281-510	371	217-475	323

Source: Esoterix/LabCorp.

Like method-specific normals for basal testing, many dynamic tests can only be interpreted correctly if the method has been validated and normal ranges developed in response to various stimuli.[17,18] If these data are not available, a clinician must rely on information from the literature, from similar assay methods, or from their own clinical experience with the assay method and the provocative stimuli.

METHOD VALIDATION

Underlying our belief in hormone testing is the assumption that the results correlate to biologic action and clinical findings. Such faith is only possible with analytic and clinical validation. Key elements of analytic validation are:

• *Sensitivity:* What is the lowest concentration of hormone detected by the method with less than 20% variation between assay runs?

TABLE 21-4

Baseline Steroid Levels and Steroid Responses to a 0.25-mg Bolus of ACTH in Normal Females

Steroid	Group 1 (<1 Year)	Group 2 (1-5 Years)	Group 3 (6-12 Years)	Group 4 (T II- III)	Group 5 (T IV-V)
17 OH preg. (ng/dL) 0 minutes	298 ± 272 61.9-829	23.6 ± 12.0 10-47	58.6 ± 43.3 11-141	137.9 ± 111 58-452	221 ± 154 52-543
17 OH preg. (ng/dL) 60 minutes	1612 ± 801 898-3178	282 ± 233 45-733	355 ± 187 70-657	559 ± 171 251-802	953 ± 306 503-1604
17 OH prog. (ng/dL) 0 minutes	32.4 ± 28.8 12.9-106	21.5 ± 26.5 5-90	27.1 ± 14.9 7.0-55.9	56.6 ± 54.6 18.2-220	98.3 ± 62.6 36.1-197.3
17 OH prog. (ng/dL) 60 minutes	142 ± 49.7 85-207	186 ± 98 50-354	134 ± 52.6 75-218	200 ± 103 88-424	166 ± 45 80-226
Cortisol (ug/dL) 0 minutes	12.8 ± 7.1 4.2-23	10.2 ± 4.1 7.3-19	8.3 ± 3.4 3.0-12	8.8 ± 3.7 4.3-16	10 ± 2.8 6.0-15
Cortisol (ug/dL) 60 minutes	40 ± 8.1 32.1-60.1	31.8 ± 5.3 24-40	22.4 ± 3.4 17-28	22 ± 4.2 16-32	26 ± 5.1 18-35
DOC (ng/dL) 0 minutes	20.8 ± 13.6 7-52	8.3 ± 3.6 4.3-15.9	6.94 ± 3.31 1.99-12.9	6.62 ± 3.64 1.99-11.9	7.28 ± 1.66 4.97-9.93
DOC (ng/dL) 60 minutes	64.9 ± 39.1 19.9-158	67.9 ± 33. 8 26.1-143.3	38.7 ± 14.9 19.2-61.2	37.4 ± 14.6 12.9-63.2	28.5 ± 5.96 23.2-40.0

Note: Selected hormones shown.

TABLE 21-5

Baseline Steroid Levels and Steroid Responses to a 0.25-mg Bolus of ACTH in Normal Males

Steroid	Group 1 (<1 Year)	Group 2 (1-5 Years)	Group 3 (6-12 Years)	Group 4 (T II- III)	Group 5 (T IV-V)
17 OH preg. (ng/dL) 0 minutes	283 ± 284 13.9-767	38.3 ± 28.6 12-103	84.6 ± 59 31-186	102 ± 115 19.9-364	120 ± 91.6 32-297
17 OH preg. (ng/dL) 60 minutes	1243 ± 755 394-3291	207 ± 171 55-738	261 ± 132 114-498	399 ± 202 88.3-676	517 ± 190 220-860
17 OH prog. (ng/dL) 0 minutes	59.6 ± 49 10.9-173	40.4 ± 33.8 3.97-114	34.4 ± 18.9 13.9-69.2	47 ± 40.4 11.9-131	101 ± 38.4 51-190
17 OH prog. (ng/dL) 60 minutes	197 ± 85 108-468	146 ± 56.9 65.2-269	144 ± 32.1 115-197	160 ± 70.8 69.2-313	157 ± 41.4 105-230
Cortisol (ug/dL) 0 minutes	12.6 ± 5.3 3.0-21	12 ± 5.8 5.7-25	9.2 ± 3.1 5.7-15	8.1 ± 2.7 4-13	9.5 ± 2.9 5.0-15
Cortisol (ug/dL) 60 minutes	38 ± 4.4 32-40	28 ± 3.9 22-37	24 ± 1.6 22-27	21 ± 8.2 15-45	22 ± 3.2 18-27
DOC (ng/dL) 0 minutes	24.5 ± 14.9 6.95-57.3	14.6 ± 13.9 3.97-49	15.9 ± 8.94 8.94-34.1	9.93 ± 8.28 3.97-30.1	8.94 ± 2.98 4.97-13.9
DOC (ng/dL) 60 minutes	78.1 ± 25.8 38.1-110	79.1 ± 30.1 34.1-139	89.4 ± 42.4 33.1-139	38.1 ± 14.9 11.9-74.1	31.45 ± 9.93 19.2-46

Note: Selected hormones shown.

- *Specificity:* Does the method measure the intended hormone specifically without interference from other related molecules?
- *Precision:* How variable are data from repeated testing of the same sample?
- *Accuracy:* Does the method yield an absolute value as expected based on adding defined standard to matrix, and does the method render proportional data when the sample is diluted progressively?
- *Carryover:* Is each analysis free from influence by previously measured samples?

- *Reportable range:* Over what range are sensitivity and precision sufficient to allow for validated results?[19,20]

Clinical validation often proves more difficult, and for existing tests is often replaced by testing sets of patient samples having a range of values (for excellent correlation and small, uniform bias).[21] Newly developed analytes especially require careful and detailed assessment of each proposed clinical use prior to widespread acceptance, ideally including calculation of clinical sensitivity, clinical specificity, positive predictive value, negative predictive value, and full receiver-operating characteristic (ROC) analysis.[18,22]

Immunoassay Techniques

Competitive protein binding methods are the basis of some platform methods (Figure 21-1, Table 21-6), but manual RIAs are infrequently used today (yet still have an important role in certain esoteric applications). RIAs use reagents, antibodies, or hormone receptors/binding proteins that bind the analyte in a specific way—commonly called an analyte-specific reagent (ASR).[23] The ASR is added in limited quantity and the endogenous hormone competes with radiolabeled hormone for binding with the ASR. The principle advantage of RIAs in a clinical setting is resistance to autoantibody interference and their relatively broad reactivity with the hormone in its various forms.

The primary limitation of competitive methods is their broader reactivity, often with related molecules that are not biologically relevant. Despite this limitation, for some applications (such as monitoring for residual tumor) broader reactivity may actually be desired. RIAs, but not methods using newer sensitive detection techniques, are also relatively insensitive. RIA technology is still commonly used in select situations, depending on the laboratory. Examples are growth hormone (GH), insulin-like growth factor-I (IGFI), insulin-like growth factor binding protein-3 (IGFBP3), leptin, thyroglobulin, urinary gonadotropins, and numerous steroid hormone methods.

Noncompetitive protein binding methods are widely used as manual and automated platform methods (Figure 21-2, Table 21-6). The methods are commonly known as sandwich methods and are named in part based on the detection method used: IRMA for immunoradiometric (radioisotope detection) assay, ELISA for enzyme-linked immunosorbent assay (enzyme transformation of a colorless substrate to a colored product-spectrophotometric detection), ICMA for immunochemiluminometric assay (chemiluminescent detection), and IFMA for immunofluorimetric assays (time-resolved fluorescent detection). These methods use complementary antibody pairs to capture and detect the analyte of interest.[23]

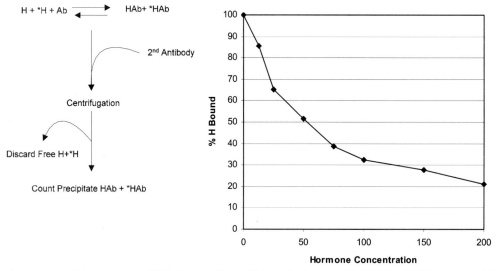

Figure 21-1 Basic hormone radioimmunoassay (RIA). For traditional RIA methods, reagent antibody (Ab) is harvested from the serum of animals. Rabbits or goats are immunized following a prescribed immunization protocol and schedule. Small nonimmunogenic molecules (haptens) such as steroid hormones are first conjugated to irrelevant proteins prior to immunization. Larger human peptide and protein hormones are typically immunogenic in these animals without conjugation. Animals are bled during the schedule, and each lot is evaluated for concentration (titer), affinity, and specificity. The "bleed" with the highest titer, optimal affinity, and specificity is selected for RIA without or with further purification. Hybridoma technology is frequently used to develop monoclonal antibodies (MAbs) from immunized mice. These MAbs are typically used in noncompetitive immunoassay configurations. As shown for RIA (top left), hormone (H) in patient, control, or standard is incubated with purified radiolabeled hormone (*H in this case is [125]H) and the reagent antibody (Ab)—shown here in an equilibrium-type reaction. Two key elements for RIA, a competitive immunoassay, is that H and *H are as similar as possible and that they compete for a limiting amount of antihormone antibody (Ab). The antihormone-specific antibody is referred to as the first antibody. For this example, a second antibody (reactive with the animal immunoglobulin of the first antibody) is used along with centrifugation to separate free hormone (H and *H) from hormone bound to the first antibody (HAB and *HAB). The bound fractions (HAB-2nd Ab and *HAB-2nd Ab) precipitate and are then "counted" (counts/min or CPM) in a gamma counter. The bound CPM are converted to % H bound and plotted versus the standard hormone concentration. "Unknown" % H bound from patient samples or controls are converted into hormone concentration. A number of algorithms are used to automatically deduce the most statistically valid standard curve from which unknown responses (% H bound) for patient and control samples are converted into hormone concentration. All hormone assays, including mass spectrometry methods, create some type of dose-response relationship (with standard hormone as a basis for determining hormone levels in patient samples and controls). Most curves are displayed to the operator as a simple linear plot. Shown (top right) is a simple point-to-point plot rarely used today. These data create a linear dose-response curve when plotted as the Logit function versus log of hormone concentration. Based on simple equilibria of binding, the affinity and binding sites (concentration) of an antisera, binding protein, or receptor can also be estimated using Scatchard analysis of data from a set of properly designed experiments.

TABLE 21-6

Immunoassay Techniques

Method and Principle	ASR	Separation of Unbound Label (Effectiveness)	Sensitivity	Specificity	Precision Interassay (% CV)
RIA analyte and tracer competition for ASR	Polyclonal antisera limited	Second antibody (good)	>0.5 ng/mL	Varies. More likely to measure multiple forms related to hormone. Some not biologically reactive.	8-12
ELISA or IRMA two-site capture and detection, noncompetitive	Paired monoclonal or affinity-purified polyclonal antisera	Physical removal of solid phase is manual, gel filtration or magnetic (excellent)	>0.1 ng/mL	Can be excellent. More likely to measure intact biologically active hormone.	7-10
ICMA or IFMA	Paired monoclonal or affinity-purified polyclonal antisera	Physical removal of solid phase is manual, gel filtration or magnetic (excellent)	>1 pg/mL	Can be excellent. More likely to measure intact biologically active hormone.	3-9

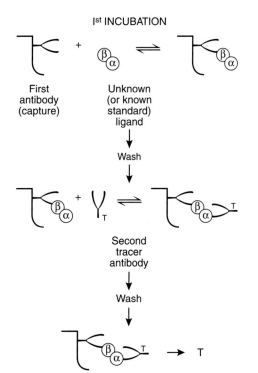

Figure 22-2 Depiction of an assay system with two antibodies in a sandwich system. The first antibody is solid phase (attached to the wall of the vessel) and binds a specific portion of the ligand. After all of the ligand is bound, the reaction vessel is washed. The second antibody is added, which binds to a specific epitope on the other end of the ligand. This antibody contains the tracer, and thus after washing out the excess second antibody the amount of ligand within the sandwich can be quantified as indicated (T, lower right). The tracer can be radioactive, enzymatic, fluorescent, chemiluminescent, or other. Most direct immunoassays add capture and label antibody at the same time, thus eliminating the requirement for an intermediate wash. The format often depends on the characteristics of the antibody pair and the technical requirements of the assay method. Showing the α and β subunits also allows one to see how high levels of the free subunits could actually suppress the apparent hormone levels. Generally, the capture antibody to label antibody stoichiometry is such that the capture is present at a 10:1 ratio or more than the label. High-level cross reactants that bind the label phase can therefore suppress binding.

The antibodies are selected against two noninteracting epitopes, hopefully unique within the hormone of interest. Ideally, both epitopes are essential to the biologic activity of the hormone—giving the assay excellent correlation with hormone bioactivity. The two-site design improves the assay specificity by eliminating smaller partially cross-reactive molecules from detection. Variations of these methods are used on many automated platforms. The primary limitations of these methods are greater interference from nonspecific binding of hormone, autoantibodies, heterophile antibodies (human anti-rabbit or anti-goat antibodies), and reactivity or suppression of reactivity by smaller molecules containing a selected epitope.[24]

Most hormones today are measured by noncompetitive protein binding methods. Examples are adrenocorticotropic hormone (ACTH), follicle-stimulating hormone (FSH), GH, luteinizing hormone (LH), thyroid-stimulating hormone (TSH), and many others. Depending on the analyte, the methods described previously are suitable for direct analyses or may require significant pretreatment (such as solvent extraction and chromatography) prior to immunoassay to remove interfering analytes. Unlike steroid hormones, which are very similar chemically and immunologically, most protein hormones or factors can be measured accurately in relatively direct methods.

CONSOLIDATED ANALYZERS

Today, 10 manufacturers are supporting more than 25 immunoassay analyzers—of which 5 are used widely for performing hormone immunoassays (Table 21-7). Nearly all of the devices perform typical thyroid testing. Many add reproductive hormones, but few offer less frequently ordered hormone tests. All of these methods consolidate more than 20 or 30 hormone or other assays on a single platform that can operate in batch or random access mode with unattended capability, timely turnaround, and cost-effective throughput.

These methods are calibrated automatically and ideally are designed to maintain calibration for long periods and to have procedures that call for as little as one quality control event every 24 hours. The methods are essentially free from user-related bias and require minimal training to operate. Competitive immunoassays and noncompetitive immunoassays combined with sensitive detection techniques are used to maximize analytic sensitivity and specificity to the extent possible with such simple techniques. Limitations vary, depending on the hormone being measured and the sample population being tested. In general, the methods are subject to the same type of interferences associated with other competitive or noncompetitive manual or semiautomated immunoassays.[25]

MASS SPECTROMETRY

Mass spectrometry is a technique that selects and measures the presence and quantity of molecules within a sample. Steroid hormones, for example, are charged in an interface and then accelerated as gas-phase ions into a mass spectrometer operated under vacuum. In tandem mass spectrometry (MS/MS), molecules (gas-phase ions) of interest are selected and fragmented—and products specific to the analyte are again selected for detection. Filter paper bloodspot testing for 17-hydroxyprogesterone (17-OHP) is a new application for LC-MS/MS methods.[26,27] 17-OHP is the marker for 21-hydroxylase deficiency, the most common form of congenital adrenal hyperplasia (CAH).

TABLE 21-7

Commonly Used Analyzers

Analyzer	No. Units	Method(s)	Protein Hormone	Steroid Hormone	Thyroid Hormone
Abbott AxSym Plus	2,400 USA, 10,000 worldwide	Competitive FPIA, noncompetitive MEIA	FSH, hCG, LH, prolactin, TSH, anti-TPO, anti-TG	Cortisol, estradiol, progesterone, testosterone	T3, T4, free T3, free T4, T3 uptake
Bayer Advia Centaur	>1,300 USA, >3,100 worldwide	Competitive chemiluminescent with magnetic particle separation	FSH, hCG, LH, prolactin, TSH, anti-TPO, anti-TG, IPTH, C peptide, insulin	Cortisol, estradiol, progesterone, testosterone	T3, T4, free T3, free T4, T3 uptake
Beckman Coulter Access 2	>1,300 USA	Noncompetitive chemiluminescent assay with magnetic particle separation	FSH, hCG, LH, prolactin, TSH, anti-TG, GH, ostase, TG, insulin	DHEAS, estradiol, unconjugated estriol, cortisol, progesterone, testosterone	T3, T4, T3 uptake
Diagnostic Products Corp. Immunlite 2000	>3,600 worldwide	Noncompetitive chemiluminescent assay with bead separation	Thyroglobulin, TBG, anti-TG, anti-TPO, ACTH, IPTH, hCG, FSH, LH, prolactin, GH, IGFI, IGFBP3, calcitonin, IPTH, gastrin, SHBG	Cortisol, estradiol, unconjugated estriol, progesterone, testosterone, androstenedione	T3, T4, FT3, FT4

Notes: This is a partial listing of platforms and available methods. Check with manufacturer for current configurations. FPIA = fluorescence polarization immunoassay and MEIA = microparticle enzyme immunoassay.

MS sensitivity gains made possible serum testing for CAH follow-up, and for measuring other serum steroids.[28-34] New-generation LC-MS/MS steroid assays have shown improved accuracy, precision, sensitivity, and selectivity (specificity) over simple direct and complex reference immunoassays.[31-34] LC-MS/MS methods using isotope dilution typically use more than five degrees of selectivity to provide quantitative results. Selectivity requirements are greatest when analyzing steroid hormones in pediatric and hormone-deficient samples.

Numerous steroids circulate physiologically that cannot be separated by tandem MS/MS alone—such as cortisol/cortisone,[28] estradiol/estrone,[33] and 17-hydroxyprogesterone/11-deoxycorticosterone.[34] Selectivity in steroid analysis using LC-MS/MS technologies represents the greatest challenge during analysis. For example, estradiol measurement using MS/MS requires resolution of 24 interfering steroids/medications.[35] In Figure 21-3, an isotope dilution LC-MS/MS assay that uses additional preparative steps to remove interfering steroids is compared with an automated direct competitive

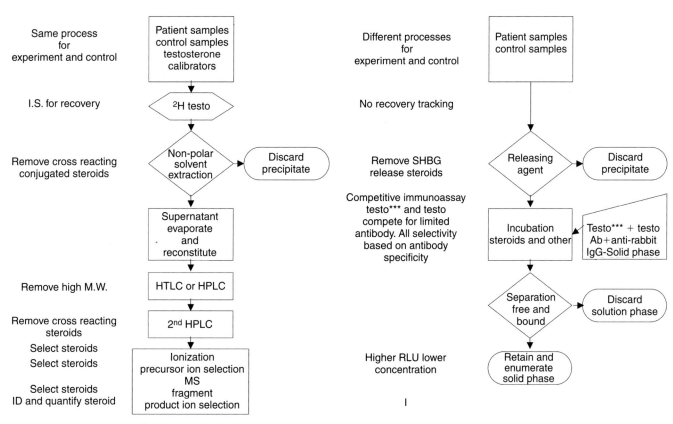

Figure 21-3 Comparison of a direct method of testosterone measurement and an isotope dilution HTC-LC-MS/MS method. *LC/MS/MS:* The isotope dilution protocols follow the general outline shown (top left). First, a stable isotopically labeled mimic [also known as an internal standard (IS)] of the hormone is added to calibrators, quality control samples, and patient samples. Following sample mixing, extraction of the hormone and internal standard are performed off-line using liquid/liquid extraction, solid-phase extraction, or sample dilution/precipitation or on-line using turbulent flow chromatography. This type of sample preparation reduces sample complexity prior to LC-MS/MS detection by removing unwanted sample constituents such as albumin, lipids, salts, and so on. It also enables concentration of analyte. The IS corrects for potential losses of hormone during these processing steps and during MS/MS. Fractionation of the sample is then usually accomplished by liquid chromatography (LC) separation based on hydrophobic differences between potential cross-reacting hormones. This LC fractionation step is critical to the removal of cross-reacting steroids that would otherwise impact the accuracy of steroid measurements by MS/MS. Following LC separation, the effluent flows into an interface—where the hormone solution and IS are converted to gas-phase ions and solvents are removed. The hormone and IS are then detected using MS/MS. MS/MS is depicted in Figure 21-4. See the American Society of Mass Spectrometry (ASMS.org) for more detail and references on this complex technology. Calibration curves based on standards performed in each assay batch are plotted as concentration (X axis) and hormone/IS ratio (Y axis). The concentration of samples is back-calculated against the calibration curve based on the hormone/IS response ratio observed. In comparison with existing immunoassays, calibration curves are linear over 3 to 4 orders (i.e., 3–4 logs$_{10}$). When all components of the isotope dilution LC-MS/MS experiment are considered, it is apparent that in excess of 5 degrees of selectivity are generally used to provide quantitative results. *Direct platform method:* This automated competitive immunoassay follows the outline shown (top right). Samples are treated to release testosterone and other steroids from specific binding proteins, such as SHBG (sex-hormone-binding globulin). Then chemiluminescent-tagged testosterone is added to compete with a limit amount of first antibody directed against testosterone and a solid-phase antibody reactive against the antibody species of the first antibody. After incubation, the solid phase is separated and enumerated. The response information is compared to a stored calibration curve. The instrument requires a two-point calibration every 7 days. Two quality controls are evaluated each day.

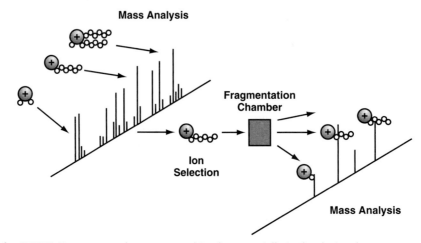

Figure 21-4 Schematic for MS/MS. Two mass analyzers are combined sequentially in the devices known as a tandem mass spectrometry or MS/MS. This method is helpful in identifying and measuring specific hormones within complex mixtures. As shown (top), the first mass analyzer selects ions of a desired mass (more correctly stated, the desired mass/charge ratio) for steroid hormones. Then the selected ions are fragmented into hormone-characteristic ions that are analyzed in the second mass analyzer and enumerated. In this way, the tandem MS device adds analytic specificity to the hormone assay.

immunoassay method for testosterone. A graphical description of MS/MS is provided in Figure 21-4.

Note that development, validation, and operation of MS-based hormone methods require expertise that is in short supply. Facilities suitable for MS and ancillary core competencies are not currently available in many commercial testing laboratories in the private or academic setting. At present, only a handful of laboratories have reported using MS for steroid hormone proficiency testing.[36] To date, LC-MS/MS steroid tests include androstenedione, dehydroepiandrosterone (DHEA), estradiol, estrone, estrone sulfate, progesterone, testosterone, 17-hydroxypregenolone (17-OPN), 17-OHP, pregnenolone, 25-hydroxy-vitamin D_3, and others. Reference methods have been reported for some peptide hormones, such as thyroxine, c peptide, insulin, renin, and others.

Quality Assurance and Quality Control

Laboratory quality assurance (QA) programs include internal and external mechanisms to ensure laboratory quality. The overriding goal of QA and quality control systems is to ensure that results meet or exceed expected operating parameters. Key components of an internal program at the method level are method validation, instrument qualification, assay batch or daily quality control, and data review before reporting. Proficiency testing, laboratory certification, and on-site quality audits are important external systems for laboratory quality. Clinicians are most likely to encounter assay inaccuracy, assay imprecision, or sample errors.

Repeated measurement data typically have a normal distribution, with the difference from the average value being distributed about both sides of the mean without cumulative bias. As such, these data should be reported with a 95% confidence interval [±2 SD or ±2 * (% CV), % CV = Stdev/Average * 100] representing the likely range of true values for a particular sample. For example, the value 10 ng/mL should be reported as 10 ng/mL ± 2 ng/mL if the assay has a variation of 10% in that analytic range. Because data are not reported with an associated variance, it is important to consider such potential variance—especially when reviewing clinically borderline results. Variance for nearly all assay systems is greatest at low levels of detection.

Inaccuracy of a particular assay should always be considered when results are unusual for the clinical presentation, especially when evaluations are being performed on certain patient populations (such as infants and patients with renal impairment) for whom cross reactants are unusually elevated. Although most assay data are reliable, it is estimated that significant medical errors are as frequent as 5%—whereas estimates of laboratory errors, exclusive of blood banking, range from 0.05% to 0.61% (with preanalytic errors accounting for 31%-75%, analytic errors for 13%-32%, and postanalytic errors for 9%-31%).[37] Table 21-8 lists common errors associated with laboratory results.

Case Studies, Common Diagnoses, and Testing

17-OHP

In the United States, most state governments now have mandatory screening for 21-hydroxylase deficiency—by measuring 17 hydroxyprogesterone on filter paper blood spots taken from newborns. By design, these tests have high clinical sensitivity but low clinical specificity. Most positive screens tests will test negative when properly evaluated by a reference method. Reference methods should be completely free of interference from cross-reacting steroids present during the newborn period. A male patient positive on state screening 17-OHP was

TABLE 21-8

Common Errors

Frequency	Type of Error	Error	Example(s)
Very common	Preanalytic	Biological variance	Testosterone, DHEA, prolactin and other pituitary hormones. More consistent results are achieved by pooling multiple draws.
Common	Preanalytic	Wrong patient's samples	Improperly labeled sample, or sample mix-up during draw or in laboratory.
Common	Preanalytic	Incorrect date of birth (DOB) information	With the wrong DOB pediatric samples may not get extraction or other necessary steps and may have incorrect normal data provided with the report.
Common	Preanalytic	Wrong sample type	Serum required for most total calcium determinations, sodium fluoride tubes for glucose and EDTA for ACTH. Most assays are not validated for samples other than serum or plasma.
Common	Preanalytic	Improper patient preparation	Examples; A) Fasting for glucose, cpeptide, insulin, B) Posture for aldosterone, catecholamines and renin.
Common	Preanalytic	Improper sample handling	Examples ACTH, plasma catecholamines, IPTH, renin and PTHrp often problematic. Ambient stability can decline at elevated summer temperatures.
Common	Preanalytic	Systemic illness	Hormone levels may be impacted by systemic illness. Most well recognized is the impact of illness on thyroid hormone levels.
Infrequent	Preanalytic	Drug interference	Many pharmaceuticals directly or indirectly influence hormone levels. Pay attention to time since last dose. Most assays not validated to deal with this type of interference.
Very common	Analytic	Typical assay variance	Tests have inherent variability. Contact the laboratory to discuss borderline results. 95% confidence interval for most hormone immunoassays is at least ±10%-20%.
Common	Analytic	Test used not sufficiently specific for patient in question	Direct measurement of steroids, 17-OHP, and testosterone not appropriate especially for infants, children, and women.
Common	Analytic	Test used not sufficiently sensitive for patient in question	ACTH, calcitonin, GH (acromegaly), estradiol, IGFI, testosterone, and other methods require better analytic sensitivity for certain applications.
Common	Analytic	Patient sample contains cross-reacting substances that raise or lower results for improperly designed or improperly used methods	Stimulation doses of 1-24 ACTH, cortisone, dexamethasone, HCG, antihormone antibodies and others may affect otherwise valid methods. Conjugated steroids and others steroids such as cortisol that circulate at high levels.
Infrequent	Analytic	Assay out of calibration	Method improperly calibrated initially or loses calibration.
Infrequent	Analytic	Assay reporting reference data that are inappropriate for the method	Reference data used not sufficient or insufficiently validated and inappropriate.
Infrequent	Postanalytic	Wrong data	Manual or automated data entry error especially a problem for referred testing.

Notes: Errors that can lead to erroneous hormone reports are included. The errors can be preanalytic, analytic, or postanalytic. Other errors (such as improper test or test method selection) are more difficult to track. An assay designed for use in adults may not be suitable for use with samples from infants and children. Review the laboratory directory of service for proper assay selection, patient preparation, sample collection, and handling.

examined and lacked any hallmarks of CAH. A follow-up serum sample was obtained and referred to a commercial laboratory for 17-OHP measurement.

The laboratory reported a result more than 10 times the upper limit for the reported age. As the data were not congruent with the clinical picture, another serum sample was obtained and referred to an endocrine reference laboratory that reported the value just at the upper limit of normal. Upon further investigation, the first confirmation sample was discovered as being submitted with a transcription or data entry error—changing the patient

age from newborn to early childhood. The initial referral laboratory, being aware of cross-reacting steroids present in the newborn, performs extractions prior to 17-OHP determinations on samples from newborns and infants but not from older children.[38]

TESTOSTERONE

An infant with prenatal chromosomes 46XY was born with normal female genitalia. Testosterone by an automated direct immunoassay method was unexpectedly measured as being four times the upper limit of normal for newborn females in a reference method. Based on the case presentation and laboratory data, a diagnosis of androgen insensitivity was considered. Later, extracted samples were evaluated in an "in-house" RIA and found to be close to what would be an upper limit of normal for female infants. The diagnosis was reconsidered, and at 10 months of age baseline and human chorionic gonadotropin (HCG) stimulation samples had undetectable testosterone levels. Gonadotropins were markedly elevated after luteinizing-hormone-releasing hormone (LHRH) and a repeat ultrasound revealed an infantile uterus. Based on these data, the diagnosis was changed to 46XY complete gonadal dysgenesis.[39]

Summary

Preanalytic patient and sample-related variables must be considered before hormonal sampling is underway. Co-existent illness (including extreme body mass index, emotional well-being, posture, activity level, and recent or current exposure to therapeutic or nutritional products) may affect hormonal concentrations. Studies on normal subjects have also shown that many endocrine hormones exhibit large intrasubject variation, as reflected in broad cross-sectional normal reference ranges. Sample collection errors are important as well but are largely avoidable by following proper collection and handling procedures and by carefully labeling samples and creating accurate and legible requests.

All laboratories must have active and thorough QA programs that include assay validation reports and continuous quality control data. Standard hormone preparations and consolidation of many tests on a few predominant platforms have led to greater comparison of some hormone assays among laboratories. Comparable normal reference data must be confirmed by each laboratory each time they significantly modify or change methods. Pediatric reference data, especially for steroid hormones and insulin-like growth factors, by design must be different for simple methods when compared to complex reference methods.

For these reasons, longitudinal test data are most reliable when all testing is done with a single method—preferably at one laboratory location. When testing is controlled in this way, variation is limited but still typically ranges from 10% to 30%—depending on the method and the hormone concentration being evaluated The other common systematic error relates directly to using simple methodology for complex samples, such as those from infants and children and from patients with kidney disease. Newer automated methods, such as LC-MS/MS coupled with other purification techniques, are beginning to correct a decline in the quality of these complex analyses. However, widespread application of such methods awaits improvements in usability, training, and instrument cost.

The physician and other health care providers as the final line of quality control can influence testing decisions and can intervene when individual patient data seem inappropriate. Ongoing interaction between laboratories and clinicians also contributes to clinical investigation that is integral to the provision of quality care to children with endocrine disorders.

REFERENCES

1. College of American Pathologists (2006). Surveys 2006 K/KN-C. Ligand [volume]:1–33.
2. Klipp J (2005). Lab Industry Strategic Outlook 2005. Market Trends and Analysis. 1–222.
3. Kilpatrick ES, Holding S (2001). Use of computer terminals on wards to access emergency test results: A retrospective audit. BMJ 322:1101–1103.
4. Kempers MJE, Lanting CI, van Heijst AFJ, van Trotsenburg ASP, Wiedijk BM, de Vijlder JJM et al. (2006). Neonatal screening for congenital hypothyroidisms based on thyroxine, thyrotropin and thyroxine binding globulin measurements: Potentials and pitfalls. J Clin Endocrinol Metab 91:3370–3376.
5. Albertsson-Wikland K, Rosberg S, Lannering B, Dunkel L, Stelstam G, E Norjavaara (1997). Twenty-four-hour profiles of luteinizing hormone, follicle-stimulating hormone, testosterone, and estradiol levels: A semilongitudinal study throughout puberty in healthy boys. J Clin Endocrinol Metab 82:541–549.
6. Albertsson-Wikland K, Rosberg S (1992). Reproducibility of 24-hour growth hormone profiles in children. Acta Endocrinol (Copenh) 125:109–112.
7. Cacciari E, Tassoni P, Parisi G, Pirazzoli P, Zucchini S, Mandini M, et al. (1992). Pitfalls in diagnosing impaired growth hormone (GH) secretion: Retesting after replacement therapy of 63 patients defined as GH deficient. J Clin Endocrinol Metab 74:1284–1289.
8. Flower L, Ahuja RH, Mohamed-Ali V (2000). Effects of sample handling on the stability of interleukin 6, tumour necrosis factor-α and leptin. Cytokine 12(11):1712–1716.
9. Wenk RE (1998). Mechanism of interference by hemolysis in immunoassays and requirements for sample quality. Clinical Chemistry 44(12):2554.
10. Binkley N, Krueger D, Cowgill CS, Plum L, Lake E, Hansen KE, et al. (2004). Assay variation confounds the diagnosis of hypovitaminosis D: A call for standardization. J Clin Endocrinol 89:3152–3157.
11. Bangham DR (1983). Reference materials and standardization. In Odell WD, Franchimont P (eds.), *The principles of competitive protein binding assays, Second edition.* New York: John Wiley and Sons 85–106.
12. Rafferty B, Das RG (1999). Comparison of pituitary and recombinant human thyroid stimulating hormone (rhTSH) in a multi-center collaborative study: Establishment of the first world health organization reference reagent for rhTSH. Clinical Chemistry 45:2207–2215.
13. Spencer CA, Bergoglio M, Kazarosyan M, Fatemi S, LoPresti JS (2005). Clinical impact of thyroglobulin (Tg) and Tg autoantibody method differences on the management of patients with thyroid carcinomas. J Clin Endocrinol Metab 90:5566–5575.
14. Sasse EA, Doumas BT, Miller WG, D'Orazio PD, Eckfeldt JH, Evans SA, et al. (2000). How to define and determine reference intervals in the clinical laboratory. NCCLS 20(13):1–37.
15. Linnet K (2000). Nonparametric estimation of reference intervals by simple and bootstrap-based procedures. Clinical Chemistry 46(6):867–869.
16. Sacks SS (2005). Analytical commentary: Are routine testosterone assays good enough? Clin Biochem Rev 26:43–45.
17. Lashansky G, Saenger P, Fishman K, Gautier T, Mayes D, Berg G, et al. (1991). Normative data for adrenal steroidogenesis in a healthy pediatric population: Age- and sex-related changes after adrenocorticotropin stimulation. J Clin Endocrinol Metab 73:674–686.
18. Biller BMK, Samuels MH, Zagar A, Cook DM, Arafah BM, Bonert V, et al. (2002). Sensitivity and specificity of six test for the diagnosis of adult GH deficiency. J Clin Endocrinol Metab 87:2067–2079.
19. Shah VP, Midha KK, Dighe S, McGilveray IJ, Skelly JP, Yacobi A, et al. (1992). Analytical methods validation: Bioavailability, bioequivalence and pharmacokinetic studies. Pharmaceutical Research 9(4):588–592.
20. Grant RP, Curtin W, Morr M, Chandler W (2007). Validation strategy for TFC-LC-MS/MS assays used in endogenous analyte quantification for clinical diagnostics. Clinical Chemistry (in press).

21. Bland JM, Altman DG (1986). Statistic methods for assessing agreement between two methods of clinical measurement. The Lancet [volume]:307–311.

22. Zweig MH, Campbell G (1993). Receiver-operating characteristic (ROC) plots: A fundamental evaluation tool in clinical medicine. Clinical Chemistry 39:561–577.

23. Wide L (1983). Non competitive versus competitive binding assays. pp 243-254 In O'Dell WD, Franchimont P (eds.), *The principles of competititve protein-binding assays, Second edition.* New York: John Wiley & Sons.

24. Kricka LJ (1999). Human anti-animal antibody interferences in immunological assays. Clinical Chemistry 45(7):942–956.

25. Ford A (2006). Move to integrated analyzers well underway. CAP Today [volume]:14–48.

26. Minutti CZ, Lacey JM, Magera MJ, et al. (2004). Steroid profiling by tandem mass spectrometry improves the positive predictive value of newborn screening for congenital adrenal hyperplasia. J Clin Endocrinol Metab 89(8):3687–3693.

27. Lacey JM, Magera MJ, Di Bussolo JM, Tortorelli S, Hahn S, Rinaldo P, et al. (2006). Rapid determination of steroids for newborn screening for congenital adrenal hyperplasia (CAH) by turbulent flow liquid chromatography tandem mass spectrometry. ASMS [volume:pages].

28. Taylor RL, Machacek D, Singh RJ (2002). Validation of a high-throughput liquid chromatography-tandem mass spectrometry method for urinary cortisol and cortisone. Clinical Chemistry 48(9):1511–1519.

29. Kushnir MM, Rockwood AL, Nelson GJ, Terry AH, Meikle AW (2003). Liquid chromatography-tandem mass spectrometry analysis of urinary free cortisol. Clinical Chemistry 49(6/1):965–967.

30. Nelson RE, Grebe SK, OKane DJ, Singh RJ (2004). Liquid chromatography-tandem mass spectrometry assay for simultaneous measurement of estradiol and estrone. Clinical Chemistry 50(2):373–384.

31. Wagner A, Kallal T, Curtin B, Chandler DW, Grant RP (2004). LC-MS/MS analysis of steroids for clinical evaluation of endocrine disorders. ASMS [volume:pages].

32. Clarke NJ, Goldman M (2005). Clinical applications of HTLC-MS/MS in the very high-throughput diagnostic environment. ASMS [volume:pages].

33. Morr M, Wagner A, Patel M, Grant RP (2006). Quantitative LC-MS/MS analysis of endogenous biomarkers for clinical diagnosis in endocrinology. ASMS [volume:pages].

34. Grant RP, Morr M, Wagner A (2006). Evaluation of a multiplexed enhanced pressure pumping system for clinical diagnosis. ASMS [volume:pages].

35. Wagner A, Morr M, Grant RP (2006). Ultra low level quantitation of endogenous biomarkers. Bioanalytical Land of Lakes [volume:pages].

36. College of American Pathologists (2006). Surveys 2006 Y-C. Ligand [volume]:1–18.

37. Bonini P, Plebani M, Ceriotti F, Rubboli F (2002). Errors in laboratory medicine. Clinical Chemistry 48:691–698.

38. Lynch J (2006). personal communication, Jane Lynch, M.D.

39. Tomlinson C, Wallace AM, Ahmed SF (2004). Erroneous testosterone assay causing diagnostic confusion in a newborn infant with intersex anomalies. Acta Paediatr 93:1004–1006.

40. Stene M, Panagiotis N, Tuck ML, Sowers JR, Mayes D, Berg G (1980). Plasma norepinephrine levels are influenced by sodium intake, glucocorticoid administration and circadian changes in normal man. J Clin Endocrinol Metab 51:1340–1345.

41. Mitamura R, Yano K, Suzuki N, Ito Y, Makita Y, Okuno A (2000). Diurnal rhythms of luteinizing hormone, follicle-stimulating hormone, testosterone and estradiol secretion before the onset of female puberty in short children. J Clin Endocrinol Metab 85:1074–1080.

42. Bjornerem A, Straume B, Oian P, Berntsen GKR (2006). Seasonal variation of estradiol, follicle stimulating hormone and dehydroepi-androsterone sulfate in women and men. J Clin Endocrinol Metab 91:3798–3802.

43. Dorgan JF, Hunsberger SA, McMahon RP, Kwiterovich PO Jr., Lauer RM, Van Horn L, et al. (2003). Diet and sex hormones in girls:findings from a randomized controlled clinical trial. J Natl Cancer Inst 95:132–141.

44. Jones JC, Carter GD, MacGregor GA (1981). Interference by polar metabolites in a direct radioimmunoassay for plasma aldosterone. Ann Clin Biochem 18(1):54–59.

45. Sadee W, Finn AM, Schmiedek P, Baethmann A (1975). Aldosterone plasma radioimmunoassay interference by a spirolactone metabolite steroids. 25(3):301–311.

46. Uwaifo GI, Remaley AT, Stene M, Reynolds JC, Yen PM, Snider RH, et al. (2002). A case of spurious hypercalcitoninemia: A cautionary tale on the use of plasma calcitonin assays in the screening of patients with thyroid nodules for neoplasia. J Endocrinol Invest 25:197.

47. Leboeuf R, Langlois M, Martin M, Ahnadi C, Fink GD (2006). Clinical case seminar "hook effect" in calcitonin immunoradiometric assay in patients with metastatic medullary thyroid carcinoma: Case report and review of the literature. J Clin Endocrinol Metab 91:361–364.

48. Sinicco A, Raiteri R, Rossati A, Savarino A, Di Perri GE (2000). Favirenz interference in estradiol ELISA assay. Clin Chem 46(5):734–735.

49. Tejada F, Cremades A, Monserrat F, Penafiel R (1998). Interference of the antihormone RU486 in the determination of testosterone and estradiol by enzyme-immunoassay. Clin Chim Acta 275(1):63–69.

50. Markkanen H, Pekkarinen T, Valimaki MJ, Alfthan H, Kauppinen-Makelin R, Sane T, et al. (year). Effect of sex and assay method on serum concentrations of growth hormone in patients with acromegaly and healthy controls. Clinical Chemistry 52:468–473.

51. Jansson C, Boguszewski C, Rosberg S, Carlsson L, Albertsson-Wikland K (1997). Growth hormone (GH) assays: Influence of standard preparations, GH isoforms, assay characteristics, and GH-binding protein. Clinical Chemistry 43(6):950–956.

52. Blum WF, Brier BH (1994). Radioimmunoassays for IGFs and IGFBPs. Growth Regulation 4(1):11–19.

53. Owen WE, Roberts WL (2004). Cross-reactivity of three recombinant insulin analogs with five commercial insulin assays. Clinical Chemistry 50:257–259.

54. Boudou P, Ibrahim F, Cormier C, Chabas A, Sarfati E, Souberbielle J (2005). Third- or second-generation parathyroid hormone assays: A remaining debate in the diagnosis of primary hyperparathyroidism. J Clin Endocrinol Metab 90:6370–6372.

55. Cantor T, Yang Z, Caraiani N, Ilamathi E (year). Lack of comparability of intact parathyroid hormone measurements among commercial assays for end-stage renal disease patients: Implications for treatment decisions. Clinical Chemistry 52:1771–1776.

56. Gibney J, Smith TP, McKenna TJ (2005). The impact on clinical practice of routine screening for macroprolactin. J Clin Endorinol 90:3927–3932.

57. Key TJ, Moore JW (1988). Interference of sex-hormone binding globulin in a no-extraction double-antibody radioimmunoassay for estradiol. Clin Chem 34(6):1357–1358.

58. Sapin R, d'Herbomez M, Schlienger JL, Wemeau JL (1998). Anti-thyrotropin antibody interference in thyrotropin assays. Clinical Chemistry 44(12):2557–2559.

59. Wartofsky L, Dicker RA (2005). Controversy in clinical endocrinology: The evidence for a narrower thyrotropin reference range is compelling. J Clin Endocrinol Metab 90:5483–5488.

60. Surks ML, Goswami G, Daniels GH (2005). Controversy in clinical endocrinology: The thyrotropin reference range should remain unchanged. J Clin Endocrinol Metab 90:5489–5496.

61. Lensmeyer GL, Wiebe DA, Binkley N, Drezner MK (2006). HPLC method for 25-hydroxyvitamin D measurement: Comparison with contemporary assays. Clinical Chemistry 52:1120–1126.

62. Singh RJ, Taylor RL, Satyanarayana GS, Grebe SKG (2006). C-3 epimers can account for a significant proportion of total circulating 25-hydroxyvitamin D in infants, complicating accurate measurement and interpretation of vitamin D status. J Clin Endocrinol 91:3055–3061.

63. Advia Centaur 111751 Rev. J, 2004-03.

64. American Society for Mass Spectrometry (1998). *What is mass spectrometry, Third edition.* [city: publisher] 22.

65. Fuqua JS, Sher ES, Migeon CJ, Berkovitz GD (1995). Assay of plasma testosterone during the first sex months of life: Importance of chromatographic purification of steroids. Clinical Chemistry 41:1146–1149.

Index